FUNDAMENTALS OF NURSING
A Framework for Practice

FUNDAMENTALS OF NURSING
A Framework for Practice

Brenda Bigelow-Kemp, R.N., M.S.N.
Associate Professor, Division of Nursing
D'Youville College, Buffalo, New York

Adele Pillitteri, R.N., M.S.N.
Professor, College of Nursing
Niagara University, Niagara Falls, New York

LITTLE, BROWN AND COMPANY
BOSTON / TORONTO

10 9 8 7 6 5 4 3 2

Library of Congress Catalog Card No. 83-81694

ISBN 0-316-48818-6

Printed in the United States of America

DON

To my sons, **Erich, Steven, and Jonathan,**
with love and pride,
and to my parents, **Carol and Walker Bigelow,**
with love and appreciation
B. B-K.

To **Joe,** *with love*
R. A. P.

CONTENTS

VII. NURSING PROCESS IN ACTION: SELF-ESTEEM NEEDS

VIII. NURSING PROCESS IN ACTION: SAFETY NEEDS

IX. NURSING PROCESS IN ACTION: BODY MAINTENANCE NEEDS

X. HEALTH CARE IN ACTION

APPENDIXES

LIST OF PROCEDURES

CONTRIBUTORS AND REVIEWERS

Susan G. Asmus, R.P.T.
Assistant Director, Department of Physical Therapy, Millard Fillmore Hospital, Buffalo, New York

Patricia Brown, R.N., B.S., M.S.
Assistant Professor, School of Nursing, Adelphi University, Garden City, New York
Contributor, Quick Reference Stops: Research

Michele Farrell, M.L.S.
Assistant Professor, Librarian, D'Youville College Library Resources Center, D'Youville College, Buffalo, New York

Ann L. Garrigues, R.N., M.S.N.
Instructor, School of Nursing, Associate Degree Nursing Program, University of Arkansas, Fayetteville, Fayetteville, Arkansas

Mary Bigelow Huntoon, R.N., M.S.N.
Former Clinical Instructor, School of Nursing, Boston University, Boston

Harry Peery, B.S., M.S.
Assistant Professor, Division of Allied Health and Nursing, Tompkins Cortland Community College, Dryden, New York

Patricia Pierson, R.N., B.S.N., M.S.N.
Director of Nursing, Mary Sherman Hospital, Sullivan, Indiana; former Assistant Professor, Philip Hahn School of Nursing, University of San Diego, San Diego, California

William Andrew Regan, J.D.
William Andrew Regan and Associates, Attorneys-at-Law, Providence, Rhode Island

Kenneth J. Trzecki, R.P.T.
Director, Department of Physical Therapy, Millard Fillmore Hospital, Buffalo, New York

PREFACE

Fundamentals of Nursing: A Framework for Practice has been written for students in basic nursing courses. The content stresses application of biopsychosocial principles through the nursing process, an intrinsic component of basic nursing practice. As such, this text is also appropriate as a reference for nurses returning to practice who need to update their knowledge of nursing fundamentals or for practicing nurses who simply wish to review these concepts.

Throughout the text we emphasize several themes that we consider vital in the study of nursing fundamentals. Our approach includes:

Emphasis on the importance of learning scientific principles rather than memorizing facts so that the student can adapt care to individual circumstances or settings.

Emphasis on the nursing process as the basis for nursing care. Throughout, the nursing process is applied to the management of patient problems. To help review, examples of complete nursing care plans or records with evaluations are provided at the ends of chapters.

Emphasis on the ability to form a nursing diagnosis from assessment data. Nursing diagnoses from the Fourth Annual Conference on Nursing Diagnosis are included as examples within chapters and are listed in Appendix C. Care plans at the ends of chapters are based on these diagnoses.

Emphasis on viewing patients throughout the life cycle. We feel that, among the concepts and skills learned in nursing fundamentals, the ability to assess developmental stage and plan care accordingly is one of the more important. Age is a factor not only in physical response to illness and treatment, but in psychological response to hospitalization, readiness for learning, and ability to maintain a healthy lifestyle. We have applied life span concepts to the topics in each chapter; we have also added modifications for children and older patients to the procedures, where appropriate.

Discussion of the role of the nurse in both ambulatory and in-patient settings.

Integration of concepts of health maintenance and disease prevention as well as health restoration and acceptance of death.

Emphasis on the holistic approach to patient care so that beginning students will view their patients as total beings whose health is influenced by their environment.

Emphasis on the role of the nurse as a patient advocate and on the active participation of the consumer. A nurse is viewed as a person capable of independent thought and as an important contributor to the health care delivery system.

Emphasis on the importance of nursing research as a contributing factor in the continuous delivery of high quality nursing care. To underscore this often neglected component of nursing, we have included 14 research presentations (each entitled Quick Reference Stop: Research), which highlight some recent investigations that relate directly to aspects of patient care discussed in the text.

Each chapter has been organized to provide a complete learning experience. Important elements include:

Learning Objectives. Included at the beginning of each chapter, Learning Objectives point out the most important concepts to be covered and help the student understand what behavioral outcomes are expected after mastering the material in that chapter.

Terms. Each chapter also opens with a list of terms essential to an understanding of that chapter's content; these terms are defined in the Glossary at the end of the book.

Procedures. Techniques of common procedures with accompanying rationales are boxed and presented in outline format for easy reference. Illustrations often accompany the procedures to clarify technique. A list of these procedures appears on page xi.

Quick Reference Stops. Interspersed throughout the book and boxed for quick reference, these points of information fall into eight categories: nutrition, pharmacology, advocacy, safety, research, health teaching, community considerations, and psychological considerations. Quick Reference Stops provide important and interesting information in an accessible format.

Suggested Readings. Near the end of each chapter appears an extensive list of up-to-date readings relevant to the topics discussed in that chapter. References have been chosen that will be readily available in most nursing school libraries.

Questions for Review. Each chapter concludes with a list of questions designed to help the student review the material covered in that chapter. The answers to these questions, which appear in a variety of formats, are provided in Appendix I.

The chapters in this text were designed to be independent of each other: they may be used in the order presented or assigned in a differing sequence, depending on the requirements of your program. The current order of chapters reflects our view that a student, before she can begin to understand her role as a nurse, must become acquainted with the dimensions of nursing as a profession, the health care system as the environment within which nursing care is provided, and the concepts of health and health adaptation that affect all people. Only then can the nursing process be presented as the means by which patient problems are assessed and nursing care is given.

In Part I the student is introduced to nursing as a profession through topics such as the evolution of modern nursing, standards and theories of nursing, ethical and legal considerations of nursing, organization of nursing practice, and the role of the nurse as a researcher. The contribution of the nurse to quality care and the role of the consumer as an active participant in his care are stressed in Part II, in which the health care delivery system and the interrelationship of system, health care provider, and consumer are discussed.

Part III introduces the student to the concept that health is a relative state influenced by life span, individuality, and ethnicity, as well as an individual's level of stress. The total role of the nurse as protector and promoter of health is emphasized.

In Part IV, the nursing process and the role of the nurse as a patient advocate and change agent are discussed. The nursing process is presented according to the format chosen by the ANA Council of State Boards of Nursing: assessment, analysis (including nursing diagnosis), planning, implementation, and evaluation. Throughout the text, the nursing process is applied to specific patient problems with explanations on how to establish and prioritize nursing diagnoses, establish a locus of decision-making, set patient goals, and establish evaluation criteria.

Parts V and VI present those activities necessary to implement the nursing process: effective communication, including teaching-learning theories and documentation of care; and assessment by interviewing, physical examination, and laboratory testing. Parts VII through IX apply the nursing process to patient needs, specifically, self-esteem needs, safety needs, and body maintenance needs. Throughout these chapters all the necessary skills and tools for quality patient care are presented as appropriate to specific problems.

In the final part, the nursing process is used to help the student incorporate fundamentals of practice into two common nursing situations: admission and discharge, and preoperative, intraoperative, and postoperative nursing care.

For consistency, the term "patient" was chosen to describe a person for whom a nurse provides care. It is used in its present broad definition to indicate a person during health and illness. We recognize that the term "client" is used in many schools of nursing to emphasize the self-care potential of all persons. Here, the choice of term is one of semantics: we believe that persons cared for should have input into their care, no matter which term is used to describe them.

To avoid the use of confusing pronouns, the feminine pronoun "she" is used to refer to all health care personnel and the masculine pronoun "he" is used to refer to all persons for whom care is provided. This is done for the sake of readability; we do not mean to imply that health care personnel cannot be male any more than that persons cared for cannot be female. Also for readability, those people significant to a patient are referred to as "support people" or "family" rather than the redundant "significant others."

To help instructors get the most out of this text, an *Instructors' Manual* has been prepared by Patricia Brown, R.N., B.S., M.S. This manual provides objectives, summaries, teaching strategies, and test questions for every text chapter as well as an overview discussion of objective, teaching, and evaluation strategies.

It is hoped that *Fundamentals of Nursing: A Framework for Practice* will provide students with the basic knowledge—fundamental and introductory in nature, but broad enough in scope—needed to meet the challenges offered by modern nursing practice.

Brenda Bigelow-Kemp
Adele Pillitteri

ACKNOWLEDGMENTS

The number of people who make contributions to a textbook of this size is obviously large. We would like to express our sincere appreciation to:

Brian S. Smistek and Timothy R. Palaszewski, Department of Medical Photography, Children's Hospital, Buffalo, New York, for their personal concern as well as their photographic skill.

Robert E. Pope, Director, and the staff of the Department of Public Relations and Development, Millard Fillmore Hospital, Buffalo, New York, for their interest and photographic skill.

Eileen Walsh, Graphic Designer, Niagara University, Niagara Falls, New York, for her excellent illustrations.

Ceia Barbara, typist, without whose skill and willingness we could not have completed the manuscript.

Friends and colleagues who offered suggestions and support, especially Ellen Pedersen, R.N., Ed.M., Lucy Krull, R.N., M.S.N., Rosemary Saccomando, R.N., M.S.N., Janice Feigenbaum, R.N., M.S.N., Patricia Mulvey, R.N., M.S.N., and Janet Rittenhouse, B.A.

Families and friends, for their love and steadfast encouragement.

Staff and administration of Children's Hospital, Buffalo, New York, and Millard Fillmore Hospital, Buffalo, New York, for their interest and cooperation in the project.

Nursing students for their encouragement and their willingness to be photographed.

Julie Stillman, former Editor, Ann West, Nursing Editor, and Elizabeth Welch, Book Editor, of Little, Brown and Company, for their editorial assistance and guidance throughout the project.

B. B-K.
R. A. P.

NOTICE

The indications and dosages of all drugs in this book have been recommended in the medical literature and conform to the practices of the general medical community. The medications described do not necessarily have specific approval by the Food and Drug Administration for use in the diseases and dosages for which they are recommended. The package insert for each drug should be consulted for use and dosage as approved by the FDA. Because standards for usage change, it is advisable to keep abreast of revised recommendations, particularly those concerning new drugs.

I. THE NURSE

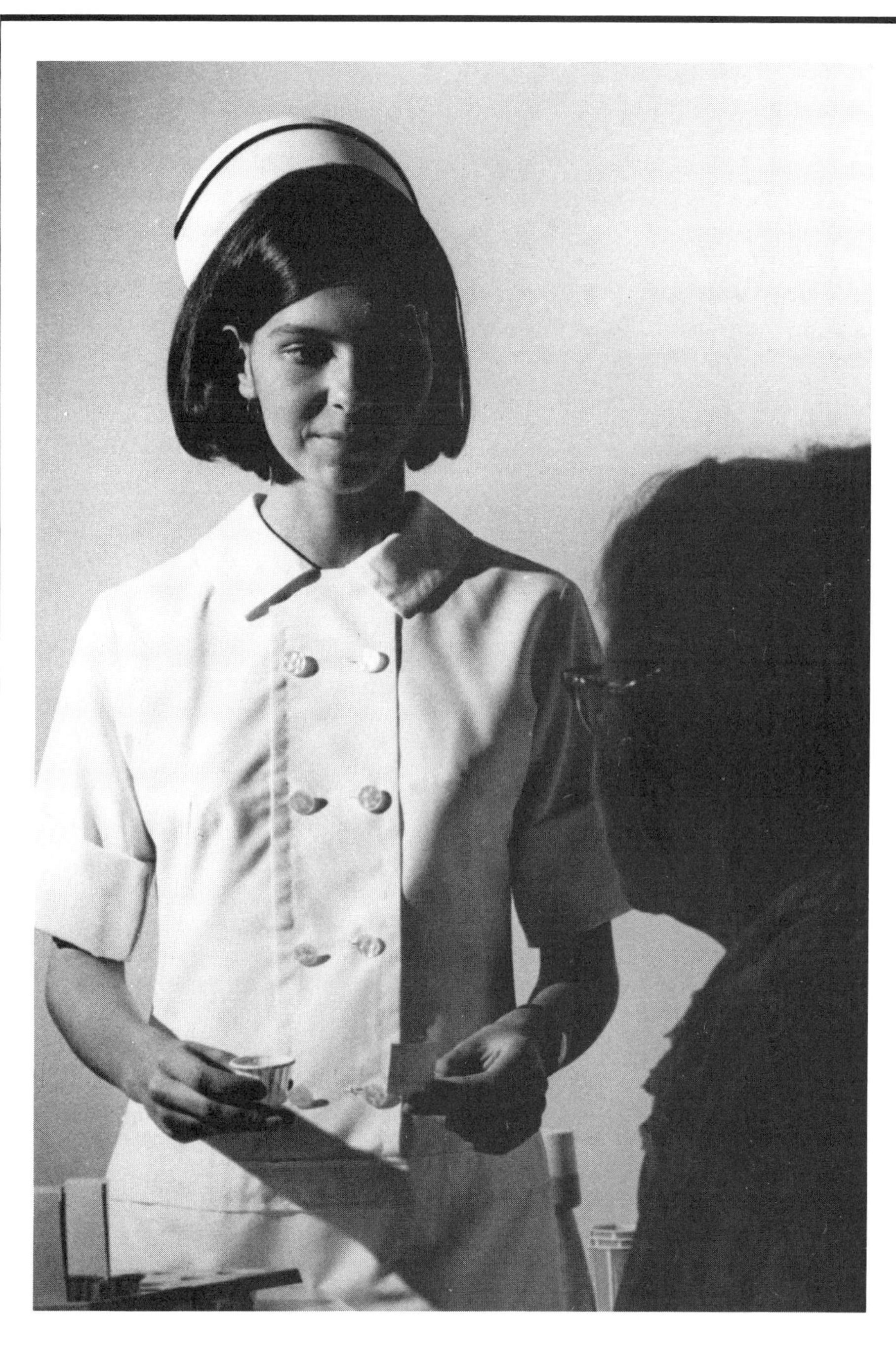

1. THE PROFESSION OF NURSING PRACTICE

OBJECTIVES

Upon mastery of the material in this chapter, you should be able to:

1. Describe ways that nursing has changed throughout its history.
2. Compare three definitions of nursing.
3. Describe the criteria for a profession and decide whether nursing meets those criteria.
4. Describe differing types of programs for nursing education.
5. Describe the role of professional organizations.
6. Describe settings in which nurses frequently practice today.

TERMS

The terms important for an understanding of this chapter are shown below and defined in the glossary:

nurse
nursing
profession

A newborn baby cries; hands reach out to comfort and warm him. A 4-year-old steps on a rusty nail; hands reach out to administer a tetanus immunization inoculation to her. A 12-year-old worries that growing up will not be much fun; hands reach out to comfort and offer reassurance that coming of age is a solvable crisis. A 20-year-old worries how she can spend the rest of her life living with diabetes; hands reach out to help her learn how to administer her daily insulin. A 40-year-old feels pain from surgery; hands reach out to change his position to take away the pain. An 80-year-old knows that she is dying; hands reach out to reassure her that she will not die alone.

These hands are the hands of nurses.

Nursing is a profession that touches people at almost all the critical phases of their lives. It is a profession that makes an important difference in people's lives at the times that it touches them. To understand what nursing is today, it is important to understand the history and development of nursing practice.

THE HISTORY OF NURSING

Nursing care has always existed, even in very primitive times. Signs of many common illnesses that we know today such as pneumonia, arteriosclerosis, appendicitis, tuberculosis, and kidney stones have been found in mummies of ancient Egypt; bones of our earliest ancestors contain evidence of arthritis, sinusitis, and bone tumor. Ancient skeletons also reveal that even in the beginning of civilization forms of therapy must have been undertaken for disease, as ancient skeletons show trepanned skulls (skulls with holes carved in them) as if a letting-out of evil spirits must have been practiced as a type of cure.

If disease was always present and there was always therapy for disease, it follows that even in very early times there must have been people who were adept at caring for ill persons and that a nursing role existed. In early civilizations these people were probably close relatives; in Egypt priests in temples apparently served in these roles. Early papyrus records from Egypt describe special diets for the ill, how to make linen and wood splints for broken bones, and how to aid in childbirth, all nursing responsibilities.

Nursing in Greek and Roman Civilizations

Hippocrates (460—379 B.C.), often called the Father of Medicine, wrote extensively of observations he made of patients with illnesses and rituals for treatment. Although he did not call the people who helped him to make his required observations nurses, he stated that such people must be "well educated and informed," qualities even more appreciated today as nursing becomes more complex every year. These observers of Hippocrates tended to be priests; nursing at this stage was largely a profession of men.

Medieval Nursing

Jewish and Christian traditions of charity influenced the growth of medicine and nursing during the Middle Ages. Taking care of the ill or the handicapped was not only a duty; through these influences it became an honor or a virtue. Early churches had forms of outpatient clinics supervised by church deacons and deaconesses where people came for consultation or care. As early as the third century each church diocese was urged to construct a *nosokomeion* (house of the sick) to improve care. By the twelfth century the word *nosokomeion* was replaced by the word *hospital* which means "house of God." The term nosocomial infections, which is now used to describe infections that arise in hospitals, is derived from the early word for hospital.

There was no formal schooling for nurses during the Middle Ages; both males and females were apprenticed to practicing nurses for about a year's period. At the end of this time they were given permission to serve as nurses in monastery- or convent-affiliated hospitals.

Nursing and the Reformation

As Protestantism swept across Europe, convent and monastery hospitals were closed, and the nursing orders affiliated with them were dissolved. A major effect of this change was that when nursing orders were reinstituted in association with government-sponsored hospitals, they were organized primarily for women; from 1500 until about 1940 men were almost totally excluded from the profession of nursing.

With few formal nursing schools existing, many women began nursing during this time not to improve people's state of health but for what they could gain from the experience. Charles Dickens' famous character Sairey Gamp, with doubtful morals and a tendency to drink more than was wise, is representative of the quality of nurses and nursing care during this period.

The Age of Florence Nightingale

Florence Nightingale, named for the city of Florence, Italy, where she was born, was the daughter of well-to-do English parents. In the 1800s in England, at the time she grew to adulthood, it was unusual for a woman of her social class to be interested in nursing, since nursing was practiced only by women who could not better themselves in any other way. She attended the School of Sisters of Charity in Paris over the opposition of her parents for a short time but did not complete her nursing courses there as she was called back to England to care for her ill grandmother.

In 1854, when Florence Nightingale was 30, England found itself involved in the Crimean War. The secretary of war, concerned about the large number of injured soldiers who were dying not on the battlefield but at the army's hospital, asked Florence Nightingale if she would take a group of nurses to Scutari in Turkey to provide some sort of nursing care to the hundreds of wounded soldiers there. She agreed and in four days assembled supplies, transportation, and 38 women to accompany her as nurses. Some of the women chosen were religiously affiliated and wore their designated apparel; for the others she designed a uniform that included a hat, which to her was a sign of an English lady and marked her companions as women finer and better educated than the average nurses of the day.

Nightingale improved sanitary conditions at the army hospital in Scutari to such an extent that the hospital became a place where many could recover. Almost singlehandedly she changed the concept of nurse in England from that of Sairey Gamp to that of someone loyal, courageous, and caring.

In order that her system of nursing would not be lost, Nightingale put her theory of nursing into writing (Nightingale, 1859) and the following year opened her own school of nursing at St. Thomas Hospital in London. The period of education for her nurses was one year; her first class had 15 students. Students wore brown uniforms and the Nightingale mark of a well-bred woman: a cap on their heads. Quickly, graduates of the school spread to hospitals around the world.

When Florence Nightingale died, she left behind the legacy that in order to perform quality nursing people must be well educated. Her graduates were so loyal to her that at her death they fixed a black mourning band to their caps in memory of her. Today, the cap of a registered nurse (RN) is differentiated from that of the licensed practical nurse (LPN) by the black mourning band on the cap.

Modern Nursing

Nursing changed during the Nightingale era from a profession of ill respect to one of great respect, from one of intuition to one of scientific reasoning. A great many more changes occurred during World War II. During this time, when nurses had to make many independent judgments because physicians were serving in the armed forces, it was realized that nurses were able to make these types of decisions safely and effectively. Taking a blood pressure is an example of a technical skill that was a physician's responsibility at the beginning of the war and a nurse's by the end of it.

In recent years the theoretical body of knowledge of nursing has grown so much that its base has moved from the hospital to the university. Many university programs of nursing have substituted a navy blue or other colored band on their caps to demonstrate that they are no longer mourning nursing's founder but looking forward to the future of nursing.

Nursing has evolved from a profession that was largely dependent and based solely on a medical model to one that has a strong independent component and operates on its own theoretical base; from a profession whose members were "trained" to one whose members are educated in institutions of higher learning. It is a profession still in the process of change, one that offers a challenge to students to both learn and care about people, and one that is both a science and an art.

COMMON DEFINITIONS OF NURSING

As nursing has changed and expanded over the years, so have definitions of nursing. Both nursing theorists and professional organizations of nursing have established definitions of what they believe nursing should be, or what beliefs and attitudes should be incorporated into nursing practice. In the United States nursing practice is also *legally* defined by state laws; each state has its own nurse practice act which sets forth the extent and limitations of nursing practice allowed in that state.

Definitions of Nursing Theorists

A nursing theorist is a person who has tried to systematically define the basis and principles of nursing practice. It is interesting to compare how nursing theorists view nursing.

FLORENCE NIGHTINGALE

Florence Nightingale can be viewed as the first nursing theorist in that she advanced a new concept of nursing by viewing it as based on a separate body of knowledge from that of medicine. Although her definition of nursing was written over a century ago, it continues to be applicable today. Florence Nightingale described nursing as the art of utilizing the environment of the patient to assist him in his recovery. In this way the nurse by her actions is able "to put the patient in the best condition for nature to act on him" (Nightingale, 1969).

Many nursing actions today are based on the fact that a person's environment is important to him and are directed toward helping him to change those things in his world that are changeable and to accept those things that are not.

VIRGINIA HENDERSON

Virginia Henderson was one of the first modern nurses to attempt to define nursing. According to Henderson (1966),

> The unique function of the nurse is to assist the individual sick or well, in the performance of those activities contributing to health or its recovery (or to a peaceful death) that he would perform unaided if he had the necessary strength, will or knowledge. And to do this in such a way as to help him gain independence as rapidly as possible. This aspect of her work, this part of her function, she initiates and controls; of this she is master.

Henderson identified 14 needs (such as "to breathe normally") that are basic to human function. She sees the nurse as assisting the patient to meet these needs until such time as he is able to meet them on his own, thereby helping the patient move from a dependent to an independent state as he is able. Many nursing actions are based on the concept of doing for people what they cannot do for themselves, and teaching them to do those things when they are again able.

DOROTHEA OREM

As the focus of nursing expands, definitions of nursing begin to reflect greater individual patient and community responsibility. For example, Dorothea Orem is a nursing theorist who affirms some general concepts of Henderson's theory and yet focuses on the individual's need for self-care action, which she calls *universal self-care.* Her theory is particularly compatible with care being rendered by nurses in the community or home setting as she sees the nurse acting chiefly to assist the individual to care for himself. Orem defines nursing as "the ability to assist others in the design, provision, and management of systems of self-care to improve or to maintain human function at some level of effectiveness" (Orem, 1971). This definition is based not on the medical model of *cure* but on the concept of *care* and on facilitating patient independence as much as possible.

Definitions of Professional Organizations of Nursing

THE INTERNATIONAL COUNCIL OF NURSES

The International Council of Nurses (ICN) is a federation of national nurses' associations from 93 countries. It was founded in 1899 and has as its purpose the sharing of nursing knowledge so that nursing practice throughout the world can be strengthened and improved. The organization serves as a spokesman for nurses at an international level.

In 1975 the ICN defined the nurse as follows (*Int. Nurs. Rev.* 1975):

> A nurse is a person who has completed a programme of basic nursing education and is qualified and authorized in her/his country to practice nursing. Basic nursing education is a formally recognized programme of study which provides a broad and sound foundation for the practice of nursing and for post-basic education which develops specific competency. At the first level, the educational programme prepares the nurse, through study of behavioural, life and nursing sciences and clinical experience, for effective practice and direction of nursing care, and for the leadership role. The first level nurse is responsible for planning, providing and evaluating nursing care in all settings for the promotion of health, prevention of illness, care of the sick and rehabilitation; and functions as a member of the health team. In countries with more than one level of nursing personnel, the second level programme prepares the nurse, through study of nursing theory and clinical practice, to give nursing care in co-operation with and under the supervision of a first level nurse.

THE AMERICAN NURSES' ASSOCIATION

The American Nurses' Association (ANA) is nursing's professional organization in the United States. Registered nurses from all states and territories are members. The ANA was founded in 1896 to work for the improvement of health standards and the availability of health care services for all people, to foster high standards of nursing, and to stimulate and promote the professional development of nurses and advance their economic and general welfare.

The definition of nursing formulated by the ANA in 1973 and published in *Standards of Nursing Practice* states, "Nursing practice is a direct service, goal oriented, and adaptable to the needs of the individual, the family and community during health and illness" (ANA, 1973). Note that this definition of nursing stresses a broad scope for practice (caring for people both sick and well; consideration for both individuals and the community), responsibility for care to be planned (goal oriented), and the need for care to be based on individual needs. Because nursing has enlarged its focus to this extent, the knowledge needed to function as a nurse has expanded over a hundred times what it was even ten years ago.

Common Themes of Definitions

Major themes of these and other definitions of nursing are shown in the box below. As mentioned, later definitions of nursing reflect a greater degree of patient responsibility for self-recovery than earlier definitions did. Also, the focus of decision making has changed from that of the nurse to that of a nurse-patient one. As an example of this, 30 years ago the nurse cared for a patient with poliomyelitis; today she teaches the importance of poliomyelitis immunization to prevent the disease. Fifteen years ago the nurse made a home visit to exercise a patient's arm; today the nurse would make the same home visit but teach the patient or his family how to do the exercises themselves so the patient can be independent. Her time spent in nursing activities has not changed; her goal of care and the level of concern have changed to reflect an increasingly sophisticated and broader body of nursing knowledge.

COMMON COMPONENTS OF DEFINITIONS OF NURSING

- Nurses offer care and concern for persons as individuals.
- Nurses plan care of the person as a whole or consider that man is more than the sum of his body parts.
- Implementation of nursing care includes direct contact between the patient and the nurse, by either a "laying on of hands" or communication between patient and nurse.
- Care of the individual, family, and community are all stressed; these systems are interrelated.
- Nurses play an important role in health as well as in illness; the preventive aspects of nursing care are as important as the therapeutic aspects.
- It is important to recognize and encourage the role the patient plays in his own recovery; the nurse assists the patient until he is able to care for himself.
- If a person cannot fully recover from an illness, he should be helped to maintain as high a level of functioning as possible or to die with dignity.
- Health education is an important nursing role.
- Nurses are effective leaders; they improve care by the use of research and further education.
- A nurse acts on behalf of the patient or serves as the patient's advocate.

IS NURSING A PROFESSION?

In its beginning, nursing was closer to a technical trade than a profession. In the 1940s, as the body of knowledge of nursing began to expand, people started to ask: When will nursing be a true profession, the same as medicine and pharmacy? There is still some debate as to whether nursing is truly a profession or not. In order to evaluate this debate, it is useful to review common criteria or characteristics of a profession. These are:

- Practice is based on a theoretical, well-defined body of knowledge that is used in practice and continues to be enlarged upon.
- It is altruistic in nature or provides necessary human services.
- It is autonomous or sets its own policies or standards in matters of practice.
- Its members practice under a code of ethics particular to that profession.

Theoretical Base of Knowledge

In the early years, nurses learned about diseases from physicians; and about nursing care from nurses. The nurse was viewed primarily as the physicians's handmaiden or assistant. Today nursing theorists have developed a knowledge base that is specific to nursing. This change in focus from a strictly disease-oriented model to a nursing model that incorporates the study of disease into nursing theory about health promotion is what makes today's nursing care total patient care.

Altruism as a Base of Practice

Nursing has strong concepts of human service. A nurse is at various times a teacher, a nurturer, a comforter, a planner, a healer, a coordinator, an advocate, and a protector. All these roles are altruistic—that is, they are characterized by a selfless concern for others.

Autonomy

A profession is autonomous if it regulates itself and sets its own standards. It is a current issue among nurses today as to how much autonomy nurses have in regulating their own practice because of their close alliance with other health care providers and the need for all health care disciplines to act in unison in many instances in order to administer quality health care. As a step toward nursing autonomy the American Nurses' Association has defined Standards of Nursing Practice; these are discussed in Chap. 2.

An Ethical Code for Nursing

Nursing practice is guided by both ethical and legal considerations. Both the International Council of Nursing and the American Nurses' Association have published ethical standards for nursing, as discussed in Chap. 3. Such standards guide both the quality and kinds of nursing practice.

THE GROWTH OF PROFESSIONALISM IN NURSING

As the body of nursing knowledge and the responsibility involved in nursing care increase yearly, the education for nursing changes in requirements and depth.

Educational Requirements

Today more than ever before nurses are educated in colleges and universities. The majority of nurses, regardless of the type of nursing program, complete some designated college and university courses in preparation for the study of their major, nursing.

The American Nurses' Association Position Paper on Education for Nurses states that, "Education for those who work in nursing should take place within the general education system" (ANA, 1965). In 1978 the ANA passed a resolution to support this position further. This states that by 1985 entry into professional practice be at the baccalaureate level (ANA, 1979). The National League for Nursing at its 1983 convention voted to retain its position calling for the baccalaureate degree as the academic preparation for professional nurse practice (NLN), 1983). The rationale for education at the baccalaureate level is to ensure that nurses are liberally educated people as well as practitioners of nursing.

Educational Opportunities

Basic education for nursing is possible in three kinds of undergraduate programs: baccalaureate, associate degree, and diploma. All programs require some liberal arts and biological and social sciences as the foundation upon which the nursing major is built. The knowledge, skills, and behavior necessary for practice evolve from a combination of the knowledge provided in this framework.

These three programs do differ, however, in philosophy, scope of knowledge and practice, and expected outcomes of the graduate. Successful completion of study in an approved school in any one of these types of programs allows the graduate to take the National Council Licensure Examination (State Board Examination) for Registered Nurse licensure.

Baccalaureate degree programs, located in universities and colleges, are generally four-year courses of study. The degree conferred is a Bachelor of Science in Nursing (BSN).

Associate degree programs, located in community and junior colleges, are two years in length. The degree conferred is an Associate Degree (AD) or an Associate of Applied Science (AAS).

Diploma programs are hospital-based programs that are two or three years in length. The student earns college credit for those courses completed at an institution of higher learning. Upon graduation the student receives a diploma in nursing issued by the hospital program.

External degree programs present a newer nontraditional format for nursing education. These are college-based programs that give credit for previous learning experiences. In addition, the student individually arranges to meet the requirements of her professional course of study. This nontraditional approach to nursing education does not focus on classroom attendance but on content to be mastered, and the length of time necessary to complete this type of program varies. A highly motivated and independent learner can be awarded an associate or baccalaureate degree in nursing through this type of contractual learning.

The career ladder approach to basic nursing education is based on the premise that a nurse may choose initially to enter a diploma or associate degree nursing program and then choose to continue her education on a college level in order to enhance her preparation for professional practice. In this type of program, as one step builds on the next, the student receives credit for all courses completed at an earlier level. She may enter the college program with advanced standing or she may be enrolled in a separate "track" for RN nursing students, depending on the college or university philosophy and curriculum design.

Educational opportunities vary, and the decision regarding what type of nursing education to pursue is usually made after much investigation; however, in light of the complex nature of modern nursing, it is little disputed today that a baccalaureate program in nursing is best able to provide the liberal arts and scientific background of the educated person who is also a registered professional nurse. The decision whether to achieve this goal in an initial program or to build up to it in steps is an individual one.

Status of Practice

As previously stated, currently there is no difference among graduates of diploma, associate degree, and baccalaureate programs in terms of legal licensure. Many nursing leaders, however, believe that education at a professional level requires baccalaureate preparation. The American Nurses' Association supported this view in a position paper in 1965 and a resolution in 1978. In both, the nursing association also differentiated between professional and associate nursing: a *professional* nurse was defined as one who is educated in a senior college or a university; *associate* nurse as one who is educated in an associate degree or diploma program (ANA, 1965, 1979).

As each state is autonomous in its determination of nursing practice, there have been widely differing responses to these proposals. For example, in 1974 the New York State Nurses' Association (NYSNA) approved what has come to be called the 1985 resolution. This resolution proposes that beginning in 1985 the level of education for beginning professional nurse practice will be the baccalaureate level. According to this resolution, "the *professional* nurse is one who diagnoses and treats human responses to actual and potential health problems through such services as case-finding, health teaching, health counseling, and provision of care supportive to or restorative of life and well-being" (NYSNA, 1974).

An *associate* nurse is one who "executes functions in the treatment of human responses to actual or potential health problems, within the framework of case-finding, health teaching, health counseling and provision of supportive and restorative care, in keeping with a nursing regimen established by a licensed or otherwise legally authorized nurse" (NYSNA, 1974).

By this definition a baccalaureate-prepared nurse would be responsible, for example, for planning a patient's program of care and carrying out all phases of that care, and for changing the plan or modifying it as necessary as the patient's condition changed. The associate nurse would be responsible for completing care but would have to refer the initial plan for care or changes in care back to the professional nurse before she could proceed.

Each year NYSNA proposes the 1985 resolution in an Entry into Practice bill, which is introduced into the New York State Legislature. However, in 1983 the legislative proposal did not state a specific year for enactment but rather that a change in licensure would occur four years after passage of the law. If approved by the New York State Legislature, this Entry into Practice bill will mandate separate licensure for nurses from different programs. Henceforth, only the graduate of a baccalaureate program in nursing would be eligible for professional licensure in New York State. The graduate of an associate degree program in a two-year college would take a separate examination and would be eligible for associate nurse licensure. This legislation provides for what is commonly known as a "grandfather clause." This provides for all previously licensed graduates of diploma and associate degree programs to retain their title of professional nurse.

The proposed resolution would apply only to New York State nurses and only to those educated after the four years from passage time frame. Many people have reservations about the resolution and its implications for nursing practice. It is a beginning step in addressing consistent entry to professional practice, however.

Overall, it seems necessary to resolve the problem of multiple preparation for professional practice and make educational preparation for nursing equal in order that both nurses and consumers of health care can understand better what nursing is today and to make the educational level comparable to that of related professions and appropriate for current practice.

Continuing Education

It is generally acknowledged that in a rapidly changing area such as nursing one's education should be updated at least every five years in order for a person's knowledge to remain current.

If there is controversy over this issue, it lies with the question of whose responsibility it is to provide continuing education: If it is a personal responsibility, will everyone comply and in what depth? If it is mandated by states, can it be enforced in an impartial manner?

At the present time many nurses, as responsible professionals, willingly and eagerly expand their knowledge and improve their skills through educational programs offered by colleges, universities, professional organizations, staff development programs sponsored by hospitals and community agencies such as the American Heart Association, and community-sponsored programs for professional and interested lay persons such as programs on women's health issues. Continuing education programs can take many forms: formal classes, lectures by professional leaders, demonstrations, one- or several-day seminars or workshops, either multidisciplinary in scope or concentrated on a single topic.

Individual states can set their own continuing education requirements, as the legal scope of the practice of nursing in the United States is determined at the state level and therefore varies from state to state. Certain states have already mandated a specific number of hours of continuing education credit necessary for nursing relicensure. Any program that meets certain educational requirements and is approved by the regional accrediting committee of the American Nurses' Association may grant continuing education credit.

Master's Degree Programs in Nursing

A student graduating from a baccalaureate program in nursing is a generalist in nursing theory and equipped to practice in any nursing setting (hospital, home, community, nursing home, extended health facility, etc.) at a beginning level of practice. In order to gain expertise in a specialized area, she completes a master's degree program in nursing. Master's programs are commonly offered in education, administration, clinical specialist, nurse practitioner, community health, and mental health. Part of the requirement for such programs is generally a research study—the graduate must be able to complete research to expand or further some aspect of nursing care.

Doctorate Programs in Nursing

The nurse who wishes to specialize further in nursing can complete a doctorate program (a D.N.Sc., Ph.D., or Ed.D. degree). Doctorate programs have a strong research component; the graduate must initiate independent nursing research and further advance the body of knowledge of nursing in order to qualify.

Certification in Nursing

Certification is a credentialing program whereby a nurse completes an American Nurses' Association or specialty organization examination and perhaps submits further written documentation describing her level of practice in order to demonstrate that she understands the theory of and practices with a high quality of care. Certification is a mark of pride and a way that nurses can experience satisfaction by knowing that their level of practice is the best in their field. Recognized by an employing agency, it has implications for advancement or promotion.

PROFESSIONAL ORGANIZATIONS

Nursing, as well as other professions, is represented by professional organizations. The role of professional organizations is the maintenance of standards of professional practice and education. Overall, professional nursing organizations seek to represent and safeguard the interests of the consumer of health care as well as the provider of such care, the nurse. Membership and participation in professional nursing organizations may be at the local, state, national, or international level. Although membership is voluntary, you, as a student nurse, and later as a practicing registered nurse, have a professional responsibility to be a participant member of a professional organization. Appendix A lists the addresses of professional nursing organizations if you wish additional information on them.

International Council of Nurses

The ICN, as previously mentioned, maintains a global look at nursing and its impact on world health standards. Every nurse who is a member of a national professional nursing organization is also a member of the ICN; the presidents of member organizations serve as its governing body. The ICN has published an international ethical code for nurses. The organization publishes *The International Nursing Review.*

American Nurses' Association

The ANA is composed of 50 state nursing associations plus those of the District of Columbia and U.S. territories. A nurse may belong at the state level only but preferably holds national as well as state membership. Functions of the ANA include setting standards of nursing practice; establishing a code of ethics; setting requirements for certification; providing legislative lobbying; publishing professional literature such as *The American Journal of Nursing (AJN)*—the official publication of the ANA; sponsoring conferences and workshops; determining continuing education policies; funding nursing research; and in some instances serving as a labor relations representative.

National League for Nursing

The National League for Nursing (NLN) is open to all RNs, health-related agencies, and interested lay individuals. The overall goal of this organization is the improvement of both nursing practice and health care for the consumer. Major tasks are the promotion of quality education programs to prepare nurses for practice, accreditation of educational programs in nursing, provision of a testing service to evaluate nursing level competency, and provision of information on nursing to the public. The NLN publishes the journal *Nursing and Health Care.*

National Student Nurses' Association

Established in 1953, the National Student Nurses' Association (NSNA) is a national organization whose membership is open to all undergraduate nursing students. It is the largest independent preprofessional student organization in the United States and the only national organization for student nurses. NSNA assists the student nurse in the development of a professional role. This is accomplished through such functions as contributing to nursing education and standards of practice in the form of programs of professional concerns, providing and encouraging student involvement in areas of professional interest, promoting interdisciplinary communication and action, and publishing *Imprint*, the NSNA journal. The NSNA is an advocate of student nurse rights and has been active in student recruitment, in particular among minority groups.

Additional Professional Groups

There are also professional organizations concerned with specialty nursing practice such as the Association of Operating Room Nurses, political groups (Nurses' Coalition for Action in Politics—NCAP), and honorary societies such as the National Honor Society of Nursing (Sigma Theta Tau). In certain instances an invitation, special interest, or preparation is necessary in order to qualify for membership in these organizations.

AREAS OF NURSING PRACTICE

At one time the only area of nursing practice available was in a hospital. Today nursing opportunities are found

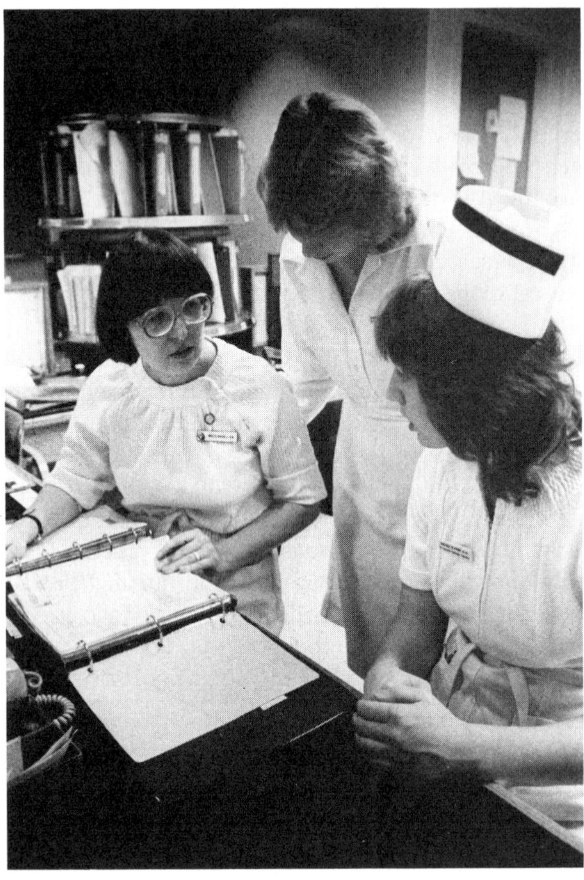

FIGURE 1-1. Most nurses today are employed in hospital settings.

in the home, in community settings such as industry, in schools, and in ambulatory services such as clinics or health maintenance organizations, nursing homes, and nursing care centers. In all these settings the nurse not only offers direct care but serves as an advocate, educator, and change agent, and also helps to determine public policy.

Hospital Settings

The greatest number of nurses still practice in hospital settings. Hospitals employ such a great number of nurses because most patients go to hospitals for care; hospitals never close and nursing care is necessary around the clock. A hospital staff nurse usually works an eight-hour shift and a five-day, 40-hour week. In many localities nurses may work 12-hour shifts or a three-day, 36-hour week (Fig. 1-1).

Hospitals are acute-care facilities where ill persons receiving specific treatment are cared for. Patients are assigned to hospital units based on their problem area (mental health or physical health), body system affected (such as heart or kidney), seriousness of their medical or surgical condition (general care unit or intensive care unit), or by age group (child or adult). Child health units may be further divided by age and developmental status. A hospital stay is generally of short or limited duration. A patient in need of professional long-term care is transferred to an extended or convalescent care center in his home community.

A staff nurse (beginning level nurse) collaborates with other members of the nursing team such as the nursing care coordinator or head nurse, and specialty nurse clinicians. The physician diagnoses medical illness and prescribes treatment, directing the patient's medical care while he is in a hospital; nurses are coordinators of patient care, implementing the nursing process, reporting and recording information, delegating certain patient care activities or task-oriented functions to other members of the nursing service, and coordinating the services of other health care personnel such as the nutritionist, pharmacist, psychologist, respiratory therapist, and physical and occupational therapists.

Many years ago people thought that being admitted to a hospital meant that they were "sick enough to die." Today the hospital is generally considered to be a "place to go to get better." The hospital is still principally a disease cure and control institution, however, although its community role in health promotion is of ever-increasing importance. Most hospitals provide ambulatory or outpatient care and in some instances offer satellite services in suburban and rural areas. These ambulatory services include health screening, health teaching, and developmental assessment as well as continuation and follow-up of medical treatment. Ambulatory services in the area of mental health such as counseling and rehabilitation can be of long duration.

Community Settings

The nurse most commonly identified in a community setting is the community health nurse (public health nurse). She may be employed by a state, county, or city health department or by a voluntary community agency such as the Visiting Nurses' Association of America. She functions in clinics, schools, industry, community centers, and homes. Her role encompasses assessment of physical and developmental abilities, control of communicable disease (through immunization clinics and sexually transmitted disease clinics), and assistance to the family in learning to care for one of its members in the home setting such as a low-birth-weight infant or a person recently discharged from the hospital. Overall, her role is that of health teacher to the community. State health departments may employ nurses to function in community settings in health promotion, disease control, consultant, and evaluative roles (Fig. 1-2).

The primary role of such a nurse in the school is preventive in nature. She performs or assists with health appraisals (physical examinations), conducts state-mandated screening programs such as the detection of scoliosis (curvature of the spine), and maintains a health record for each child. In the school health office she administers first-aid and supervises student self-care (a child who must take prescribed medication during

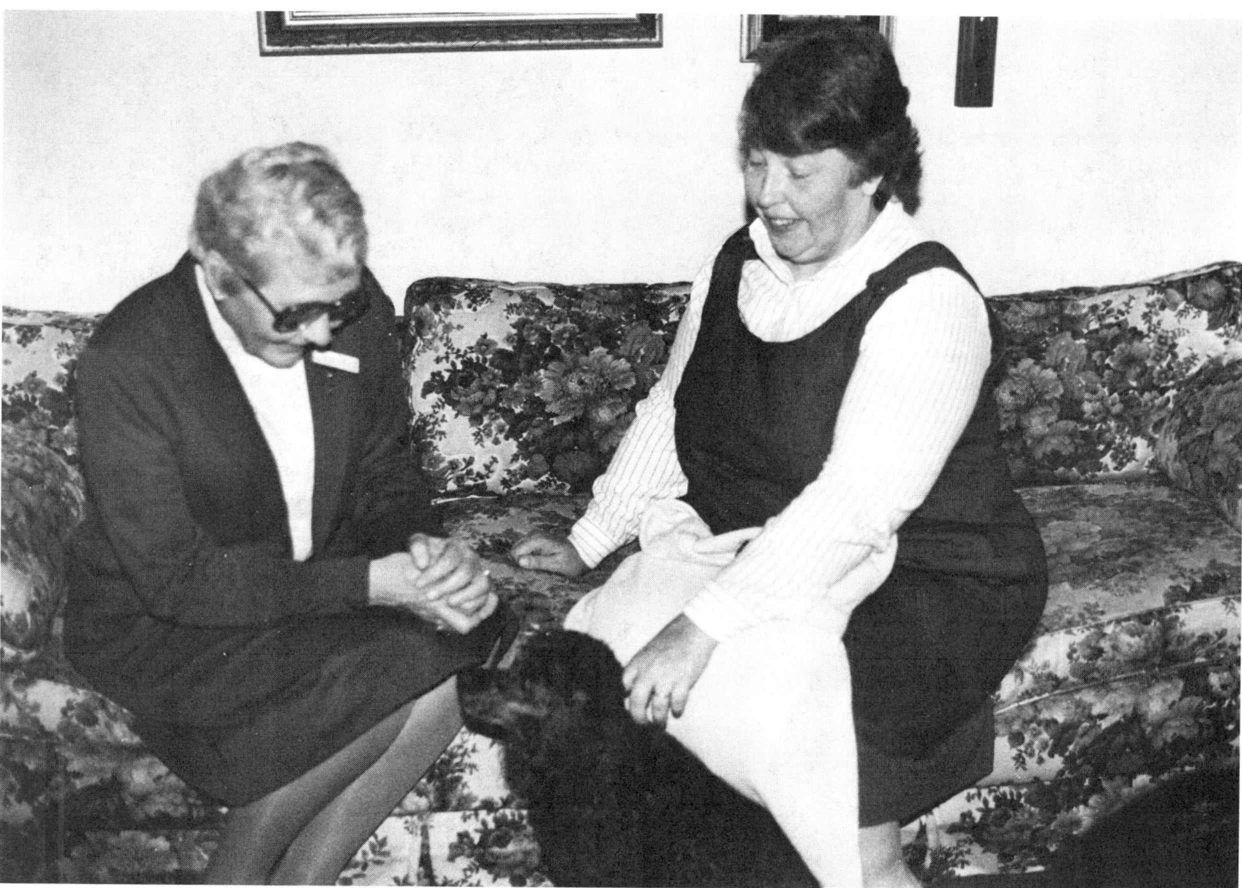

FIGURE 1-2. A community health nurse counsels a patient regarding home care. Note that the nurse greets the family dog, an important step in establishing rapport.

school hours); she refers ill students to home and/or medical follow-up care.

In certain states such as New York a nurse with advanced academic preparation and certification may be employed as a school nurse-teacher. Her status in the school system is comparable to that of a classroom teacher. In addition to responsibilities in the school health office, the nurse-teacher may present age-related preventive health content (hygiene, health, family life, sex education) in the classroom. The nurse-teacher may counsel the student and, at times, his family in matters such as preparation for hospitalization.

Still other nurses in the community are employed as industrial or occupational health nurses. A nurse in an industrial setting generally has assessment skills and in some instances trauma nursing experience. Health teaching is an important part of the role of the industrial nurse as well as supervising safe manufacturing practices so that occupational illnesses such as lung cancer from exposure to asbestos products do not occur.

Expanding Roles in Hospital and Community Settings

The previously described roles of both the hospital- and community-based nurse are traditional in nature. The term *expanded role* is used to denote a nurse who by virtue of advanced education and/or experience functions in a specialty role. The nurse who practices in such a role gains increased professional recognition, may increase her sense of personal accomplishment, and can receive increased monetary return from practicing in such a capacity.

NURSE PRACTITIONER

A nurse practitioner is a nurse who has educational preparation (usually at a master's degree level) and clinical experience beyond her basic nursing education. She is skilled at obtaining health histories, performing physical assessments, offering guidance and counseling, and treating minor illness with the consultation of a physician. Nurse practitioners generally work in ambulatory or out-of-hospital settings. They can have a large impact in improving the quality of health care by offering comprehensive care and health education to people whom they serve (Fig. 1-3).

Nurse practitioners may practice in schools as school nurse practitioners. This role encompasses certain designated responsibilities of the school nurse and the school nurse-teacher. Additionally, the role includes school-home liaison: A school nurse practitioner may meet with a child's classroom teacher as well as with his family in order to assist the child in coping with a

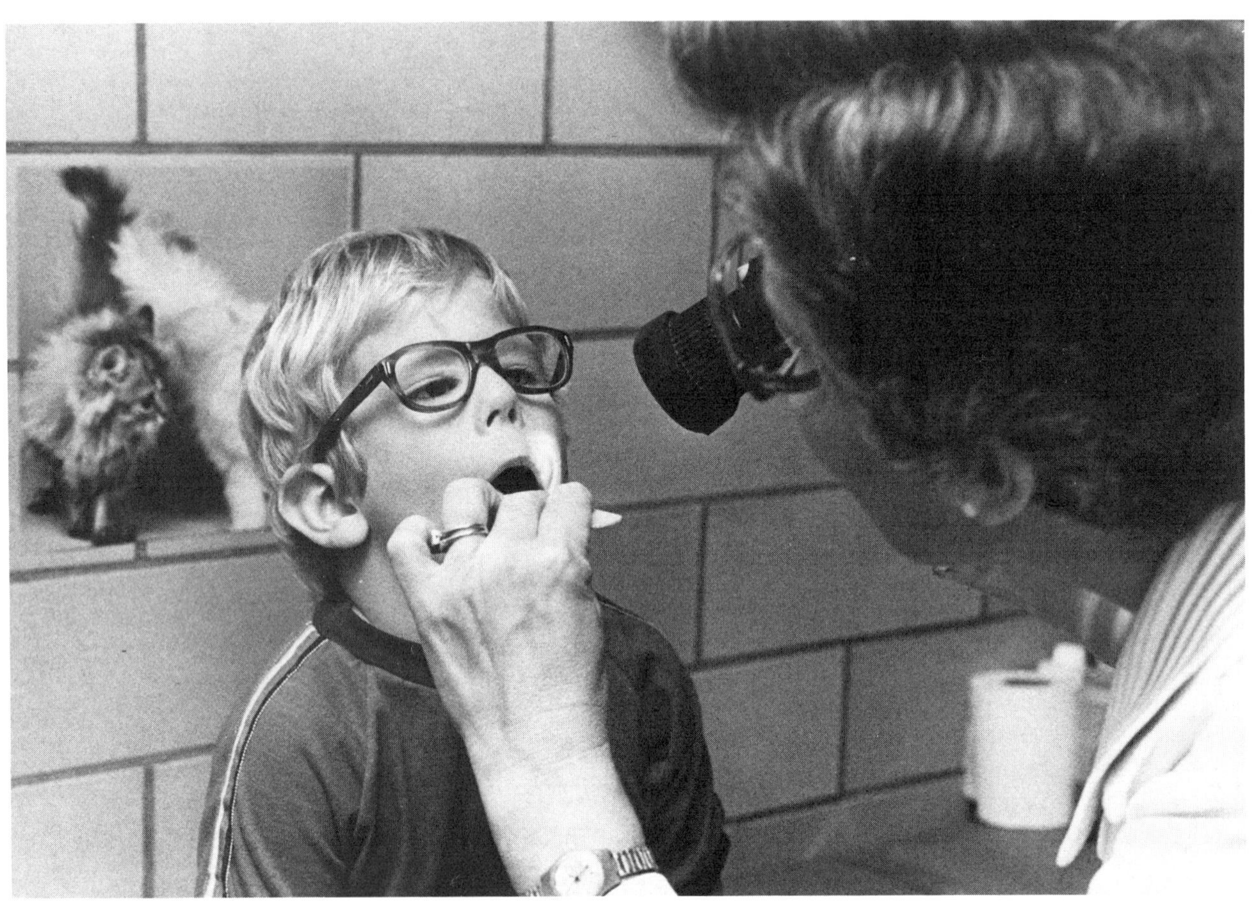

FIGURE 1-3. Nurse practitioners are nurses with extended skills. They generally practice in ambulatory settings.

stressful situation. In this way the child may be assisted in securing and maintaining his position both as a member of his class and as a member of his family.

INDEPENDENT NURSE PRACTITIONER

The legal scope of the independent nurse practitioner practice varies from state to state and is determined by the nurse practice act of that state. Such a nurse may be in private practice or be in joint practice. Joint practice involves collaboration with other health care professionals. These frequently include physicians, social workers, and other nurses. The area of practice may be the family or may be specialized such as mental health, child health, or the care of women. For example, the role of an independent nurse practitioner engaged in the care of women would include assessing, counseling, and teaching women to monitor their own health.

CLINICAL NURSE SPECIALIST

A clinical nurse specialist possesses expertise in a particular area of nursing practice. Preparation for this role is most usually obtained at the master's degree level. A clinical nurse specialist practices her speciality in either a hospital or community setting. She may provide direct patient care as well as supervise and coordinate care given by others, in particular other nurses. The clinical nurse specialist is expected to possess and maintain current knowledge in her area of nursing practice; thus, as she gives direct care, teaches, and guides, she presents herself as a role model of excellence in nursing practice.

PATIENT ADVOCATE

An advocate is a person who speaks for another. A nurse is always a patient advocate in that she helps the person to explain his needs and seek help as necessary for himself. As part of this role, she is a change agent and leader. A nurse may serve in a formal position as patient advocate in a health care setting, representing all patients admitted to that health care facility.

NURSE CONSULTANT

Nurses often serve as consultants to community, industrial, and governmental agencies in order to improve the health care of citizens or to plan new health care systems for that agency. Nurse consultants can safeguard the health of many individuals in this way and can be instrumental in initiating new programs for care.

NURSE RESEARCHER

Few nurses are full-time researchers, although their numbers are increasing, and many nurses have the potential to be. Every nurse who reads a research study reported in a professional nursing journal is a consumer of research. Every student nurse enrolled in a basic undergraduate program in nursing has the capacity to be an active research participant, now and in the future.

Methodologies for research are included in the curriculum of baccalaureate, master's, and doctoral programs. Nurses with this preparation are encouraged to initiate research in whatever setting they practice. It is through nursing research that the unique functions of the profession are explained, documented, and recorded. *Nursing Research* and *Nursing Educator* are two journals in which many nursing studies are reported.

NURSE AUTHOR

Knowledge gained and not recorded will probably be lost. Nurses are encouraged to submit material for publication to professional journals; both nurse educators in college and university settings and nurses in practice publish articles in professional journals and textbooks. Nurse researchers are professionally obligated to publish the results of their studies. Two examples of nursing journals where articles on nursing care are published are *The American Journal of Nursing* and *Nursing Forum.*

NURSING TOMORROW

It would have been difficult 20 years ago to predict the level of responsibility or number of skills that nurses would be expected to be able to accomplish today. As an example, 20 years ago nurses in intensive care units were told that reading an electronic monitor printout of a patient's heartbeat pattern was a physician's responsibility; 10 years ago nurses were expected to read this type of printout and notify the physician of changes in the pattern so that he could begin treatment; today nurses read such monitor printouts and administer potent medication based on their independent assessment and judgment of the pattern.

In order to reach this level of expertise, a nurse needs a solid foundation in the fundamentals of nursing practice and a thorough framework for nursing practice. Twenty years ago nursing was both a science and an art. Today, looking forward to tomorrow, it is not only a science and an art but also a challenge. Nursing is a profession that requires better preparation for practice than ever before.

SUGGESTED READINGS

American Nurses' Association. ANA's first position paper on education for nurses. *Am. J. Nurs.* 65:106, 1965.

American Nurses' Association. *Standards of Nursing Practice.* Kansas City, Mo.: The Association, 1973.

American Nurses' Association. *A Case for Baccalaureate Preparation in Nursing.* Kansas City, Mo.: The Association, 1979.

American Nurses' Association. *Nursing: A Social Policy Statement.* Kansas City, Mo.: The Association, 1980.

Barnard, K. Social policy statement can move nursing ahead. *Am. Nurse* 15(1):4, 1983.

Bullough, B., and Bullough, V. (Eds.) *Expanding Horizons for Nurses.* New York: Springer, 1977.

Byrnes, M. A. The nurses state their case: Non-nursing functions. *Am. J. Nurs.* 82:1089, 1982.

Dohevy, M. O., Cook, C. B., and Stopper, M. C. *The Discipline of Nursing.* Bowie, Md.: Brody, 1982.

Donaldson, S., and Crawley, D. The discipline of nursing. *Nurs. Outlook* 26:113, 1978.

Douglass, L., and Bevis, E. *Nursing Management and Leadership in Action* (3rd ed.). St. Louis: Mosby, 1979.

Field, L., et al. Five nurse leaders discuss social policy statement. *Am. Nurse* 15(2):4, 1983.

Gramer, M. The ideology of professionalism. *Nurs. Outlook* 27:108, 1979.

Grandbouche, A. It's time to put a proper price on nursing. *R.N.* 45:24, 1982.

Gray, J., et al. Do graduates of technical and professional nursing programs differ in practice? *Nurs. Res.* 26:365, 1977.

Henderson, V. *The Nature of Nursing.* New York: McGraw-Hill, 1966.

Hillsmith, K. From RN to BSN: Student perceptions. *Nurs. Outlook* 26:98, 1978.

Hirsch, G. A. Nursing: Art or science? *Can. Nurse* 79(1):4, 1983.

ICN adopts definition of "nurse." *Int. Nurs. Rev.* 22:163, 1975.

Kalisch, P., and Kalisch, B. *The Advance of American Nursing.* Boston: Little, Brown, 1978.

Kalisch, B. J., et al. Improving the image of nursing. *Am. J. Nurs.* 83(1):48, 1983.

Kelly, L. Y. *Dimensions of Professional Nursing* (3rd ed.). New York: Macmillan, 1981.

McGriff, E., and Simms, L. New York nurses debate the 1985 proposal. *Am. J. Nurs.* 76:930, 1976.

National Student Nurses' Association. *Getting the Pieces to Fit: How to be an NSNA Constituent.* New York: National Student Nurses' Association, 1980.

Nightingale, F. *Notes on Nursing.* New York: Dover Publications, 1969.

NLN votes to retain position on basic education. *Am. Nurse,* July—August, 1983.

NYSNA. *A Blueprint for the Education of Nurses in New York State.* Guilderland, N.Y.: NYSNA, 1967.

NYSNA. Adoption of "1985 Resolution" (voting body action). NYSNA convention, Rochester, N.Y., Oct. 1974.

Orem, D. *Nursing: Concepts of Practice.* New York: McGraw-Hill, 1971.

Riehl, J., and Roy, C., Sr. *Conceptual Models for Nursing Practice* (2nd ed.). New York: Appleton-Century-Crofts, 1980.

Simms, E. Preparation for independent practice. *Nurs. Outlook* 25:114, 1977.

QUESTIONS FOR REVIEW*

1. Florence Nightingale is best known for:
   a. Introducing men to nursing.
   b. Founding the American Nurses' Association.
   c. Founding the first baccalaureate program of nursing.
   d. Changing the image of the nurse to one of respect.

2. As definitions of nursing become more modern, they mention:
   a. Greater similarities to medical care.
   b. A more limited scope of practice.
   c. Increased patient responsibility for own care.
   d. Decreased responsibility for nurses.

3. Which of the following is *not* a criterion for a profession?
   a. Members are educated in institutions of higher learning.
   b. Members are well paid.
   c. Members set their own standards.
   d. Members work within a theoretical base of knowledge.

4. A graduate of which of the following nursing programs is eligible to take a National Council Licensure Examination?
   a. Baccalaureate program.
   b. Associate program.
   c. Diploma program.
   d. All of the above.

5. A continuing education program is one that:
   a. Is taught in the senior year of a nursing program.
   b. Is required before a student can graduate.
   c. Is required as part of a state board examination.
   d. Expands knowledge after graduation.

6. The National Council Licensure Examination is an examination:
   a. To qualify a graduate for beginning nursing practice.
   b. To determine who is eligible for graduate study.
   c. Written by the federal regulatory board for nurses.
   d. To help nurses learn more about nursing.

7. The American Nurses' Association is an organization:
   a. All nurses must belong to in order to practice.
   b. Professional nurses should feel an obligation to join.
   c. That is a nursing honor society.
   d. That only hospital-employed nurses can join.

8. A community health nurse is one who:
   a. Knows several languages.
   b. Cares for people in their homes.
   c. Designs new hospital units.
   d. Maintains an independent practice.

*Answers to the Questions for Review, which appear at the end of each chapter, are shown in Appendix I.

9. The following is a BINGO card. To begin, cover the right hand column. Locate the answer to each question in the left hand column on the BINGO card and cross it off. As soon as you have BINGO—five squares in a row or all four corners—look in the right hand column to see if you are correct.

1. Degree granted by a 2-year community college nursing program.
2. A hospital-based program of nursing.
3. The setting where most nurses work today.
4. The legislative level at which nursing practice is controlled in the United States.
5. The basic concept of Florence Nightingale's theory of nursing.
6. The journal published by the American Nurses' Association.
7. The degree granted by a four-year university program of nursing.
8. A nurse with expanded skills and knowledge.
9. The people who performed most nursing care in ancient Greece.
10. A criterion for a profession.

No, you shouldn't have a BINGO yet. Recheck your answers.

No, not yet. Recheck your answers.

No, not yet. Recheck your answers.

No, not yet. Recheck your answers.

No, not yet. Recheck your answers.

RIGHT. All squares under the I should be marked.

You're right that this makes a 4-corner BINGO. Recheck your answers, however; you should have scored before this.

B	I	N	G	O
ASSOCIATE DEGREE	HOSPITALS	*AMERICAN JOURNAL OF NURSING*	FEDERAL LEVEL	ENVIRONMENTAL CONTROL
DEPENDENT FUNCTION	DIPLOMA PROGRAM	WOMEN	CLINICS	LICENSED PRACTICAL NURSE PROGRAM
ADAPTATION	NURSE PRACTITIONER	FREE SPACE	COMMUNITY HEALTH NURSE	PHYSICIAN FUNCTION
INTERPERSONAL BASIS	STATE LEVEL	PEOPLE'S HOMES	NURSING FUNCTION	NATIONAL LEAGUE OF NURSING
BACCALAUREATE DEGREE	MEN	SELF-CARE THEORY	INDUSTRY	SETS OWN STANDARDS

2. STANDARDS AND THEORIES OF NURSING PRACTICE

OBJECTIVES

Upon mastery of the material in this chapter, you should be able to:

1. Describe the reasons that standards of nursing practice were devised.
2. Describe the basic tenets of the American Nurses' Association Standards of Nursing Practice.
3. Compare several nursing theories.
4. Describe the role of nursing theorists in establishing a basis of nursing knowledge.
5. Describe the similarities and differences between case, functional, team, and primary nursing systems of care.
6. Describe the advantages and disadvantages of functional, team, and primary nursing staffing patterns.

TERMS

The terms important for an understanding of this chapter are shown below and defined in the glossary:

standard
theory

STANDARDS OF NURSING PRACTICE

Because nurses practice in so many settings and provide such a wide range of types of care, it is difficult at first to picture how nursing fits into the overall scene of health care delivery or even to identify the factors that unify nurses and allow them to practice with consistency of care in so many settings. A major unifying force of nursing is consistent standards of nursing practice. A common theoretical basis of knowledge and the organization of care are other factors.

ANA Standards

In order to measure one level of nursing care against others and to maintain nursing care at a quality level, the American Nurses' Association has developed Standards of Nursing Practice (1973) for general care and for each specific area in nursing such as maternal-child health, community health, and psychiatric nursing. The standards for general practice are listed below, each standard followed by its rationale and a discussion of the ways that nurses meet the standard and problems that may arise in meeting it. These standards are stated according to a systematic approach based on the five steps of the nursing process: assessment, analysis, planning for care, implementation of care, and, finally, evaluation of care. The term *client/patient,* rather than *patient,* is used. The nursing process is defined and described in detail in Chap. 13.

STANDARD 1

The collection of data about the health status of the client/patient is systematic and continuous. The data are accessible, communicated, and recorded.

Rationale: Comprehensive care requires the complete and ongoing collection of data about the client/patient to determine the nursing care needs of the client/patient. All health status data about the client/patient must be available for all members of the health care team.

In order to fulfill this standard, a nurse must collect patient data in many different areas. One must elicit information on growth and development; emotional, physical, cultural, religious, and socioeconomic status; important support people; environmental factors; and health goals. Such information is obtained from interview, physical assessment, and axillary sources such as laboratory reports or previous medical records. It is important that assessment data be collected systematically to avoid gaps in information. Important findings gained by assessment must be recorded and communicated. Assessment must be thought of as an ongoing process so that new information is not missed. The nursing knowledge necessary to obtain a complete health history by interview, perform physical assessment, and interpret the meaning of laboratory data grows yearly.

For example, Mrs. Engles, a 24-year-old woman admitted to a hospital because she fell on ice and fractured her tibia, underwent surgery to have the bone stabilized. Assessing that she is in severe pain, is anxious about the care of her two children (two years and two months of age) at home, and is angry at her inability to carry out self-care activities such as using the bathroom because of her bulky cast are examples of ways that you would fulfill this standard. They are important assessments because they are the factors that make Mrs. Engles different from other patients on the nursing unit and serve as the foundation for planning care for her that will be specific to her needs.

STANDARD 2
Nursing diagnoses are derived from health status data.

Rationale: The health status of the client/patient is the basis for determining the nursing care needs. The data are analyzed and compared with norms when possible.

Once the data collection is complete, the person's limitations and capabilities are identified, and the present and potential health problems that a nurse can supply solutions to are defined. Although these problems are compatible with the problems that the person's physician establishes as the basis for care, they are uniquely those that a nurse can best solve. The physician, for example, would list Mrs. Engles' chief problem as a fractured tibia (this is the medical diagnosis which serves as the basis of her medical care). Separating out problems that are specific to nursing establishes the basis for nursing care. You would probably identify Mrs. Engles' nursing problems as anxiety related to child care; pain related to recent surgery; and interference with self-care related to a large cast. These problems are constructed from assessment data; they make her care complete (the healing of a bone will be little gain if her two-year-old burns himself playing with matches while she is hospitalized due to inadequate supervision at home).

STANDARD 3
The plan of nursing care includes goals derived from the nursing diagnoses.

Rationale: The determination of the results to be achieved is an essential part of planning care.

In planning patient care, you must be careful that all goals set are congruent with other planned therapies; goals are stated in realistic and measurable terms, and sensible time limits are set for goals to be reached. In order for goals to be realistic, the patient must be included in planning and goal setting. Three goals for Mrs. Engles, for example, could be: (1) Patient will do own self-care within limitations of the cast by 24 hours post surgery; (2) patient will develop a plan of child care in 4 hours; and (3) patient will have pain reduced to tolerable level in 20 minutes.

Helping people to develop goals not only aids them in recovering from a present illness but also enables them to gain skill in planning ways to stay well and avoid illness in the future by organizing better what it is they hope to accomplish. For example, it is unrealistic to think that Mrs. Engles would be able to do all her own care or that of her children by 24 hours post surgery. Helping her to see that the sensible goal is to make child care arrangements, not to plan on being able to give this care herself, keeps her from putting herself under unnecessary pressure or stress trying to do the impossible. In the matter of the pain, setting a goal of reduction rather than absence of pain assures her that healing is taking place as expected; if she thought that you expected her to be completely painfree in 24 hours, she would become worried at that time when she found that her leg was not yet at that stage of healing.

Some people are better planners than others, and goal setting is a step that those who find planning difficult may tend to bypass. Performing nursing care without a picture of what the outcome of the care should be, however, is the same as traveling without a road map. Goal setting is included as a standard of practice to ensure that nursing care is a productive and meaningful activity.

STANDARD 4
The plan of nursing care includes priorities and the prescribed nursing approaches or measures to achieve the goals derived from the nursing diagnoses.

Rationale: Nursing actions are planned to promote, maintain, and restore the client's/patient's well-being.

It is important that care be individualized for each patient. Both physiological and psychosocial concerns should be considered in planning. Teaching points, changes in environment, and changes in the individual should be included.

Plans must be tailored to individual circumstances. It would be easy to advise Mrs. Engles, for instance, that to solve her child care concern she suggest that her husband stay home from work for a few days, that her mother watch the children for her, or that she hire a baby sitter for the length of her hospital stay. Only Mrs. Engles can say, however, whether these are good suggestions or not. Suppose her husband is stationed overseas with the army; her mother has a serious heart condition and cannot care for an active 2-year-old; and she barely has enough money for food and rent each month, certainly none for a full-time baby sitter for a week. If so, none of the above suggestions are workable. A nurse who practices by standards of nursing care does not expect always to have easy answers to problems, since she realizes that individual circumstances change solutions.

Priority setting allows you to develop plans for the most important aspects of care first so that you meet critical needs immediately. Initiating a plan or means of care to reduce Mrs. Engles' pain, for example, would seem to be a priority problem, because as long as pain is present she may be so distracted by her discomfort that she is unable to deal with her other concerns. Child care is certainly also a priority problem because the safety of the children is at stake.

STANDARD 5
Nursing actions provide for client/patient participation in health promotion, maintenance, and restoration.

Rationale: The client/patient and family are continually involved in nursing care.

Participation in his own care offers a person a sense of independence and of being well again. Patients can participate in their care by planning alternative methods for carrying out procedures, by learning about their illness, and by doing as much of their own care as possible. Participating in actions to make oneself well again builds confidence and skills useful for keeping well and avoiding illness in the future.

An important way that Mrs. Engles could participate is by learning methods of self-care. If she participates in decision making (Will it be better for her to transfer from the right side of her bed or the left side to reach a chair? When she goes home should she sleep downstairs on the couch to avoid having to negotiate stairs on crutches? How will she carry her 2-month-old baby and walk on crutches? Can she manage at home without help with a large cast, crutches, and a 2-month-old baby?) she can solve many problems in advance of their actually becoming problems. Only by actively participating in learning skills such as crutch-walking will she be able to care for herself until the cast is removed.

STANDARD 6
Nursing actions assist the client/patient to maximize his health capabilities.

Rationale: Nursing actions are designed to promote, maintain, and restore health.

When nursing actions are consistent with the plan of care, are based on scientific principles, are individualized to the specific situation, and include the use of appropriate resources, they are instrumental factors in helping a patient to avoid becoming ill and in aiding him to become well again. Helping Mrs. Engles learn what foods are high in calcium and protein to promote bone and tissue healing and assisting her to learn crutch-walking (more difficult than usual perhaps because she may decide to carry her baby by a "back pack") are examples of nursing actions that would allow Mrs. Engles to return to health and usual functioning at the earliest possible date.

STANDARD 7
The client's/patient's progress or lack of progress toward goal achievement is determined by the client/patient and the nurse.

Rationale: The quality of nursing care depends upon a comprehensive and intelligent determination of nursing's impact upon the health status of the client/patient. The client/patient is an essential part of this determination.

It is easy to think once nursing care planning has been accomplished and activities of care finished that the job is done. This is not necessarily the case, however. In most instances, the person himself is in the best position to judge whether his progress is satisfactory, so it is important to evaluate his feelings. Even if you feel that the person's progress has been good, if he feels that it has been less than that, he will not feel comfortable about his state of health.

Suppose by the fifth day following surgery Mrs. Engles has still not been able to go to the physical therapy department to learn crutch-walking because her requisition for therapy was lost in transit. You and she both anticipated that she would be ready for discharge on this day but now she is a good two days away because of this confusion in communication; your goal has not been reached. The expected level of health has not been achieved. Only if outcomes are compared to goals in this way can it be recognized that a goal has not been achieved. Evaluation of Mrs. Engles' care also reveals deficiencies in a system; in order to ensure that care is better coordinated for future patients, whatever caused the lack of communication needs to be corrected.

STANDARD 8
The client's/patient's progress or lack of progress toward goal achievement directs reassessment, reordering of priorities, new goal setting, and revision of the plan of nursing care.

Rationale: The nursing process remains the same, but the input of new information may dictate new or revised approaches.

Patient care is never static but changes as patient conditions change. With new assessment following the change, new problems, new goals, and new actions are established. If Mrs. Engles is not able to be discharged on the day planned, she will have to make continued child care arrangements, for example. The problem of poor communication among hospital departments will have to be solved.

Standards of nursing care are important not only as a source of guidelines for a level of practice; because they serve as a level of practice, they have ethical and legal implications as well. The ethical and legal aspects of nursing practice are discussed in Chaps. 3 and 4. Specific ways that standards of nursing practice serve as a basis for care are further discussed in Chap. 13, The Nursing Process.

THEORETICAL BASIS OF NURSING

Nursing leaders are making an effort to define a theoretical basis for nursing practice so that nurses can understand more fully not only what it is they are doing but why and how they are doing it. Most current theories of nursing address three separate issues: How is the person who is to be nursed to be viewed; what are the goals of nursing care; and what are the activities of nursing care. The first facet, that of characterizing the person to be nursed, seems at first to be an unnecessary question. People who are to be cared for are certainly people who are ill. However, in addition to caring for the ill, today's nurse cares for people who are well in order to help them learn methods to use to stay well and also helps detect those people who are sick. Nursing theorists help to determine the most helpful ways to view people so that nursing activities can best meet their needs—seeing the patient, for example, not simply as a physical form but as a dynamic force with important psychosocial needs as well.

The overall goal of nursing care has changed along with the current scope of nursing. At one time the goal of nursing could have been stated as to care and comfort the injured and ill; today this goal would be thought of by most nurses as very limited, as they are equipped to do much more. Nursing theorists help to identify the present goal of nursing to be certain that nursing is striving to be all that it can be in today's world. A current all-encompassing goal for nursing might be to promote the health of individuals and communities.

As nursing's goals become broader so do nursing's activities. For example, when the goal of nursing was considered to be care of the ill, nursing actions were mainly bathing, feeding, and providing comfort. Today, with promotion of health as a goal, teaching, counseling, supporting, and advocacy are also common nursing roles.

It is important that nurses continue to examine the basis of nursing practice so that it can best meet the health needs of people and continue to change in the future as people's health needs change.

Table 2-1 summarizes the major components of several theorists' concepts of nursing. It also indicates how these theories may be applied in a specific situation, that of Mrs. Brown, a 40-year old woman recently hurt in an automobile accident who has suffered damage to her right side and probably will not regain full use of her right arm or leg.

Nursing schools may base their curricula on one theorist's concepts or integrate a number of theorists' concepts throughout a program. At first glance it may appear to be a confusing situation if nurses practice differently because of differing theories of nursing. By examining the third column of Table 2-1, however, you can see that although the theoretical basis of how nursing care is organized may be different, the end result of every theory is to provide a high level of nursing care. Differing views of nursing theory are in the end not contradictory; you will experience no difficulty in working with nurses who base their care on an alternate theory of nursing.

At the present time, no one theory of nursing appears to be unanimously superior to any other. Until one theory does prove to be superior, it is likely that schools of nursing and individual nurses will continue to use diverse theories for care. Knowing that individual theories exist increases your basic knowledge of nursing; using any theorist's basic assumptions as a framework for organization offers increased opportunity for depth and thoroughness in assessment, planning, and implementation of nursing practice.

SYSTEMS FOR ORGANIZATION OF CARE

Different nursing units use different methods of organizing care based on the specific needs of the patients cared for on that unit and on the number and type of personnel available to give care. As a beginning student it is helpful to be familiar with the usual methods of organizing staff and care in health care agencies so that you can appreciate the relationship of nurses both to each other and to other health care personnel with whom you coordinate procedures or information.

Staffing in Health Care Agencies

Health care agencies are, as a rule, large organizations employing thousands of health care providers. Whether the health care agency is a hospital, an extended-care facility, an ambulatory clinic, or a community health department, the overall structure is generally divided into departments. One of these departments is the department of nursing. The person responsible for the functioning of all nurses in the department is a director of nurses (sometimes titled an associate hospital administrator). The director is responsible for formulating agency policy in relation to nursing; she plans, organizes, directs, coordinates, and evaluates the activities of the nursing staff. She interviews and hires new staff nurses.

Nursing supervisors (sometimes called nursing care coordinators) work under the director of nurses. Nursing supervisors are responsible for the quality of nursing care administered in a number of selected nursing units (or division offices if in community health).

Directly in charge of each nursing unit (a section of the health agency containing a limited number of beds or a section of the community) is a head nurse (sometimes called a patient care coordinator). She is responsible for the quality of nursing care on that particular nursing unit for 24 hours every day. She has assistants (called charge nurses) who supervise care in the hours she is not actually there. The head nurse serves as teacher, role model, and coordinator for all the nursing personnel who work under her and actually perform patient care.

TABLE 2-1. SUMMARY OF NURSING THEORIES

Nursing Theorist	Major Concept of Theory	Emphasis of Care
Faye Abdellah	The role of the nurse is to identify and correct needs according to 21 identified areas. Needs may be overt (apparent) or covert (hidden or unknown to the patient).	Assess Mrs. Brown as to her health care needs according to the 21 areas of concern. Care is not complete until all needs are met.
Lydia Hall	Nursing care consists of 3 interlocking circles: care, cure, and core. Care is nurturing; cure is assisting with medical needs; core is the therapeutic use of self or helping the patient to grow in self-identity.	As rehabilitation progresses, cure functions grow less; care and core functions increase. Meet Mrs. Brown's basic needs and help to accept limitations and reach the best level of functioning possible.
Virginia Henderson	Basic nursing care is provided to the patient in order to meet 14 identified human needs. The role of the nurse is to assist the patient until such time as he can care for himself, or gain independence within a framework of supportive care.	To provide hygiene, assess Mrs. Brown's ability to wash her hands and face. Allow her to do as much as she can and then continue with the bath. Reassess her ability for responsibility for bathing every day.
Dorothy Johnson	A person is composed of 8 subsystems which must remain in balance for optimal functioning. Any actual or potential threat to this balance is a nursing concern.	Assess the effect of lack of limb function on person as a whole. Establish stability to increase functioning.
Imogene King	The central focus of nursing is man. Nursing is a process of action, reaction, interaction, and transaction. Needs are identified based on patient's social system, perceptions, interpersonal relationships, and health.	Discuss with Mrs. Brown the way she views herself and illness. She sees herself as being able to return to previous role of mother and part-time worker. Structure care to help her meet these perceptions.
Myra Levine	Nursing is human interaction. Nursing interventions are to conserve energy, and structural, personal and social integrity.	Give as much care as Mrs. Brown needs to conserve strength; allow choices in care as much as possible to preserve identity; maintain family contact to preserve social integrity.
Florence Nightingale	The role of the nurse is viewed as changing or structuring elements of the environment such as ventilation, temperature, odors, noise, and light to assist the patient in his recovery.	Turn Mrs. Brown's bed into the sunlight; provide adequate covers for warmth; leave her comfortable and with reading material to occupy her time.
Dorothea Orem	The focus of nursing is on the individual; patients are assessed in terms of ability to complete self-care. Care given may be wholly compensatory (patient has no role); partly compensatory (patient participates in care); or supportive-educational (patient performs own care).	To provide hygiene, prepare a raised seat to allow Mrs. Brown to sit at the bathroom sink to wash self.
Ida Jean Orlando	The focus of the nurse is interaction with the patient. Effectiveness of care depends on patient behavior, nurse's reaction to behavior, and the nursing action appropriate to patient needs. Patient should define his own needs.	Ask Mrs. Brown what she feels is her main need. She says worry over children at home is her main problem. Stress solution to this problem as you meet health and hygiene needs.
Hildegard Peplau	The promotion of health is viewed as the forward movement of the personality. This is accomplished through interpersonal process including orientation, identification, exploitation, and resolution.	Plan care together with Mrs. Brown. As she is unable to assume full responsibility for bathing, encourage her to speak of children and job accomplishments to retain self-esteem.
Martha Rogers	The purpose of nursing is to move man toward optimal health. The nurse should view man as a whole, constantly changing, and help him to interact in the best way possible with the environment.	Help Mrs. Brown to make use of her left side as much as possible so that she returns to optimal health and functioning as soon as possible.
Sister Callistra Roy	The role of the nurse is to aid man to adapt to the change caused by illness. Levels of adaptation depend on the degree of environmental change and state of coping ability. Full adaptation includes physiological factors, self-concept, role function, and interdependence.	Assess Mrs. Brown's ability to use her left hand to replace her right hand functions which are now lost. Direct nursing care toward replacing deficit with other skills.

Students in a nursing program may either work under the guidance of the head nurse or that of a school-employed instructor, depending on school philosophy.

The registered nurse on a hospital unit or employed by a community agency carries out the most difficult types of patient care on the unit, since she is the person (along with the head nurse) with the most education and knowledge of care procedures. She is also the best informed person on the unit for patient teaching.

A licensed practical nurse (also called a vocational nurse) is a graduate of a nursing program of about one year in length that emphasizes technical skills and a much simpler background of physical and social sciences than that of the registered nurse. She works under the direction of registered nurses; typical care activities she might do are bed baths, hot and cold applications, and dressing changes. With an additional course from a health care agency, she may be allowed to administer medicine.

Nurse's aides and orderlies have completed a 6- to 12-week course in basic care procedures such as bed making, bathing, positioning, and the taking of temperatures, pulses, and respirations. They keep the unit well stocked with supplies and help transport patients and specimens to other hospital departments.

Additional unit personnel that may or may not be present depending on the personnel structure of the agency are a ward clerk (concerned with filling out requisitions for supplies, answering the telephone, and keeping patient charts in order), dietary aides (concerned with preparing food trays for patients and helping to distribute and collect them), and transport aides (concerned with safely transporting patients to other hospital departments such as x-ray).

Support Department Personnel

Many diagnostic studies and some treatments for patients are carried out not on the nursing unit at the patient's bedside but in other hospital departments such as x-ray, physical therapy, occupational therapy, and radionuclear medicine. These departments are structured like that of nursing with a department director and levels of personnel under the director actually per-

FIGURE 2-1. Relationship of health care agency departments.

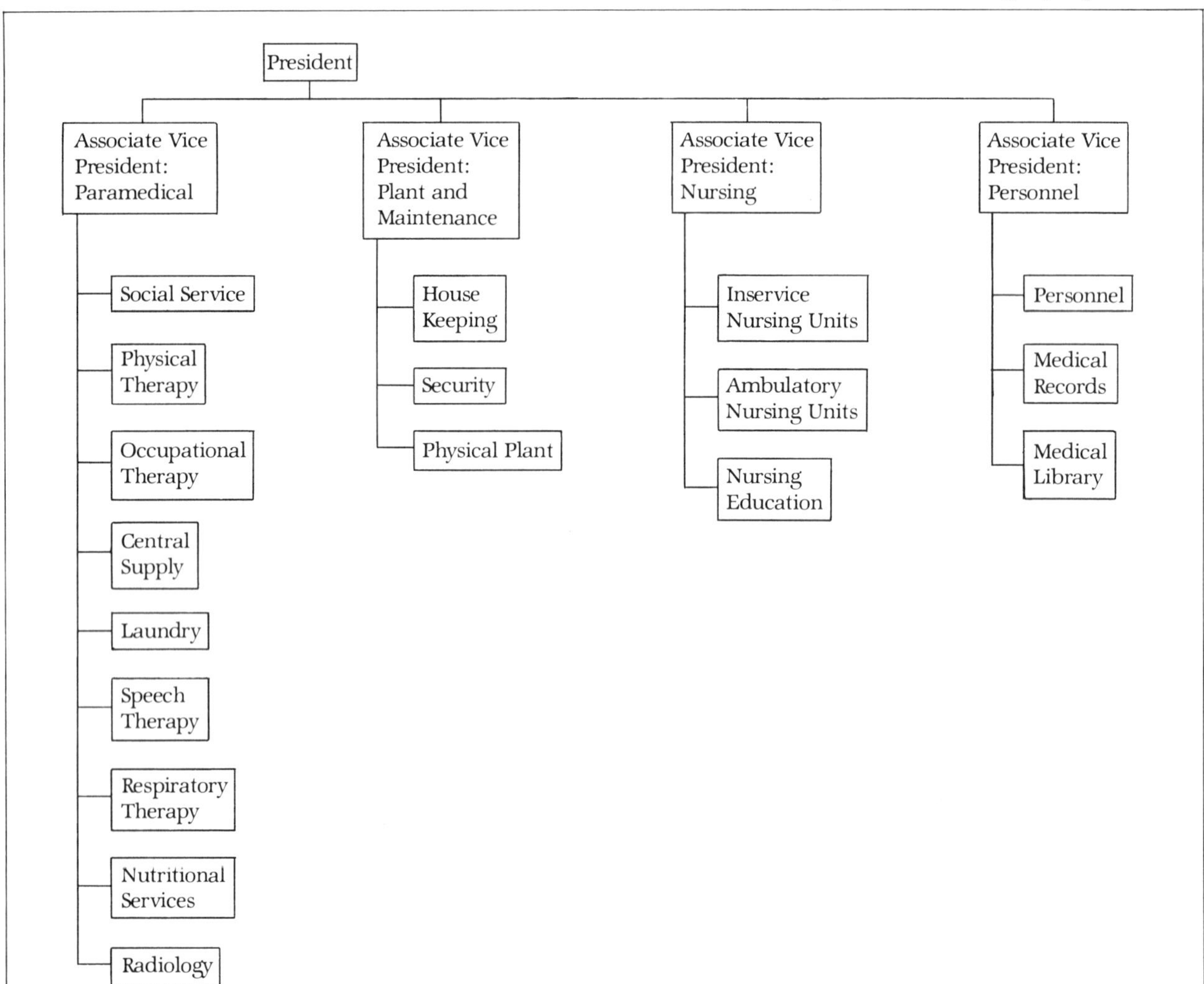

forming care. Figure 2-1 shows a typical diagram of a total hospital structure. Notice that other departments such as dietary, medical records, and so forth are on an equal level with nursing. In the course of a day's time representatives of any of these departments may contact you or your patient to consult on care or how their aspects of care coordinate with yours (or you may want to make the contact yourself to find out those same things) (Fig. 2-2). Remember that in a typical agency structure these people are your equals. This means that when a patient is scheduled for physical therapy, for example, it must be not only when it is convenient for you but at a time that is convenient for the other department as well. Sometimes lack of information as to the relationship of other agency departments causes misunderstandings that could have been avoided with more information.

METHODS OF ORGANIZING NURSING CARE

Because a nursing unit has different levels of health care providers, it must have an organizational plan so that all personnel can administer their level of care without duplication or gaps of care that no one takes as their responsibility. Methods of organizing nursing care have changed over the years and still continue to change in order that the most effective yet cost-efficient method can be devised. Types of systems of care that are helpful to be familiar with are the case method, functional nursing, team nursing, and primary nursing.

FIGURE 2-2. Collaboration between the nurse and other health care professionals enhances comprehensive patient care.

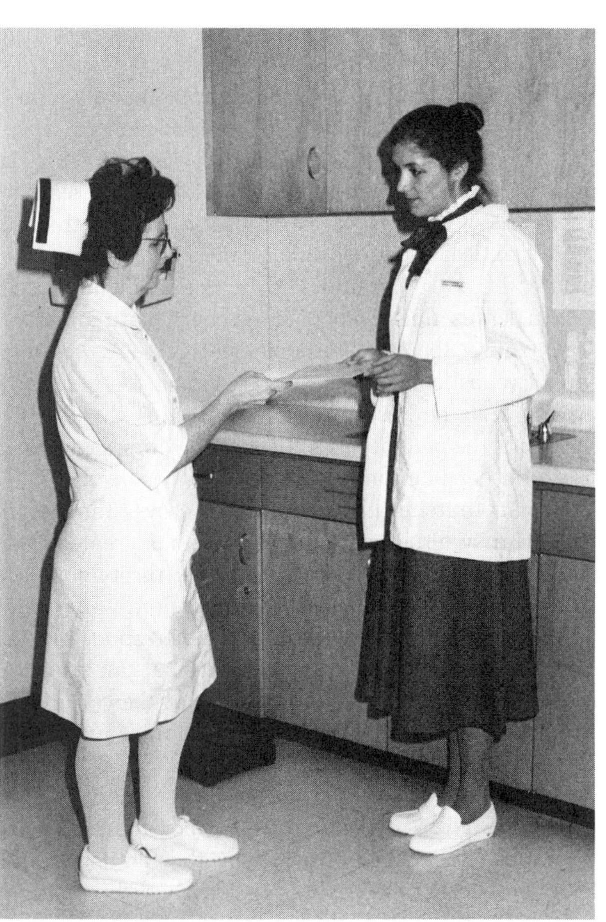

Individual Care (Case Method)

Prior to the 1940s nurses were assigned the full care of everyone assigned to them. In other words, all the time they were on duty they performed all those activities that a patient needed for care (temperature taken, bath given, abdominal dressing changed, diet supervised, for examples). This type of assignment of nursing care was necessary because much nursing was done in the home, and a patient truly had his own nurse for the length of time nursing care was needed.

Functional Nursing

In the 1940s during World War II so many nurses left community hospitals to staff armed forces hospitals that more time-effective methods of organizing care had to be devised. The most efficient way to be certain that all patient care is done is to organize it on a functional basis or divide the nursing staff on the unit so that each member of the staff carries out a small portion of care for all patients (a nurse's aide takes temperatures for all patients on the unit; a licensed practical nurse makes all the beds; a registered nurse changes all postsurgical dressings). This "assembly line" type of organization (shown in Fig. 2-3A) is efficient because a person does a small portion of care over and over and thereby grows very proficient at doing it. However, the quality of care may suffer under such a system because the patient's care is fragmented (no one takes care of the total person). Parts of the person's care may not be done (everyone assumes someone else did it). Care may not be individualized because a person responsible for a single task may tend to do it as a matter of a routine and neglect to take into account individual preferences. When care is not individualized, it becomes inconsistent (the person changing dressings today does it differently from the person who did it yesterday).

Although functional nursing fulfilled its purpose as a method of organizing care when health care agencies were very short of nursing staff, it is little used today because it must look like Fig. 2-3B to the patient. It falls short in accountability, individuality of care, consistency, and generally in job satisfaction for nurses (it grows boring, and the nurse misses the satisfaction of seeing a person grow well again because she never sees the total picture). The administration of medicine or the taking of temperatures may still be done by this system because these are two nursing functions that are easily separated out from other aspects of care.

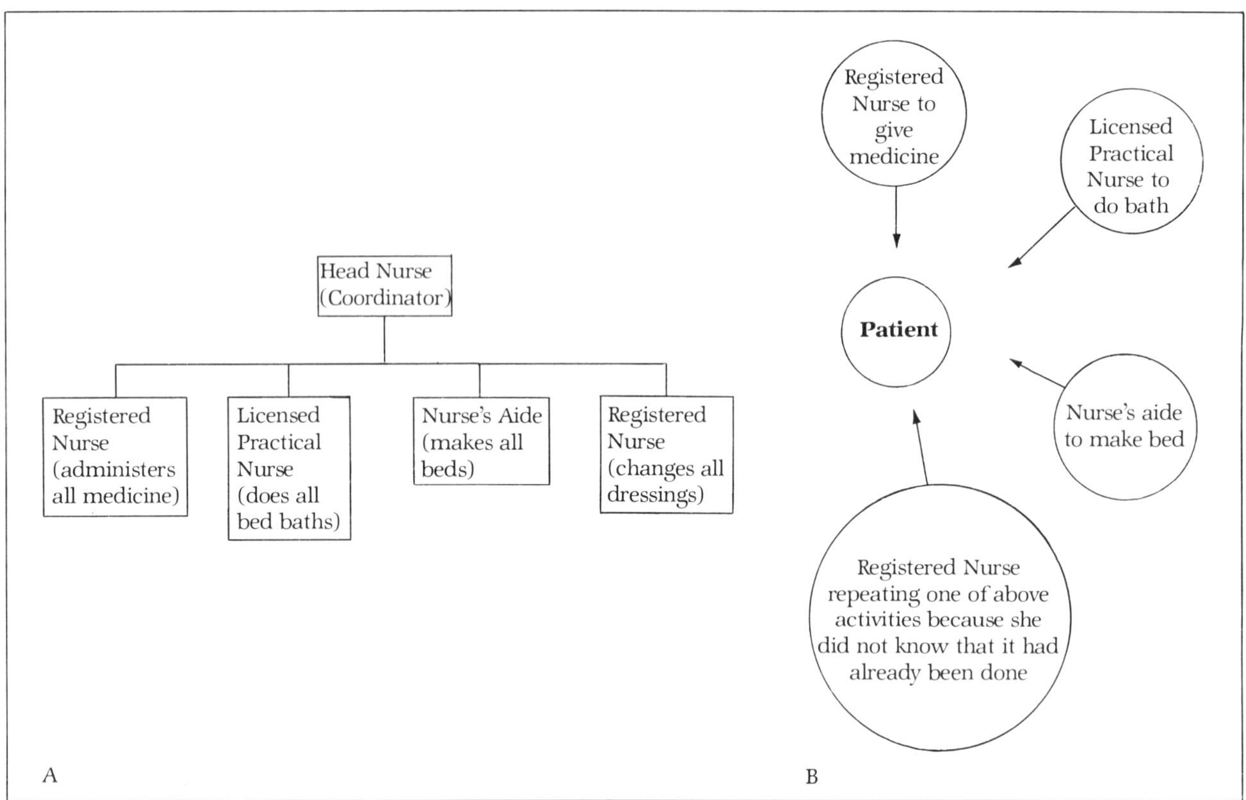

FIGURE 2-3. A. Functional nursing. B. Functional nursing from a patient standpoint.

Team Nursing

In the 1950s team nursing was introduced as a solution to improving the quality of nursing care. By this system a number of team leaders (skilled registered nurses) work under the head nurse. The remainder of the nursing staff is divided to work under the team leaders. Each team on the unit is responsible for the total care of the number of patients assigned to it. Each member of a team does that level of care which is consistent with education and experience (the nurse's aide on the team changes beds, the licensed practical nurse gives bed baths, the registered nurse changes sterile dressings and administers medication) (Fig. 2-4). A team conference, held daily, alerts all members of the team to each patient's care and progress. Team method is shown diagrammatically in Fig. 2-5A.

Team nursing is a forward step in reducing the number of persons giving care in any one day, but fragmented care can still result, especially if members of a team are too busy to meet for a daily conference. Team nursing from a patient standpoint must look like Fig. 2-5B. Although team nursing is still used in many settings and as a student you may be assigned a position on a team, the system falls short in terms of accountability, individuality of care, consistency, and, if team members are changed frequently or communication breaks down, job satisfaction for nurses.

Primary Nursing

Primary nursing is yet another manner of organizing nursing care. By this method a patient is assigned a nurse (his primary nurse) when he is admitted to a health care agency. This nurse completes the patient's health history and isolates patient problems; she establishes goals and organizes and implements care measures to meet the goals established (Fig. 2-6). She is responsible for the patient's welfare for 24 hours a day for as many days as the patient is in the health care agency, and she is responsible for discharge planning to ensure that care continues to be consistent after the person leaves that particular agency. This method of organization for care is shown in Fig. 2-7A. A nurse cannot realistically be with a patient for the length of time he may be hospitalized; when she is not directly caring for the patient himself, associate nurses give care based on her plan and goals.

Primary nursing has the advantage over functional and team systems in that it provides for greater continuity of care (one person gives care throughout an illness; care is better coordinated shift to shift) and maintains accountability (one person is responsible for care, not several people). It is a system that can lead to a high level of job satisfaction because of the continuity and a sense of progression and accomplishment for nurses.

Primary nursing as it must appear to a patient is shown in Fig. 2-7B. Nurses must be thorough and conscientious to practice in this way as they do not have a team or backup system to provide care should they forget. Some nurses may feel isolated by this system; they

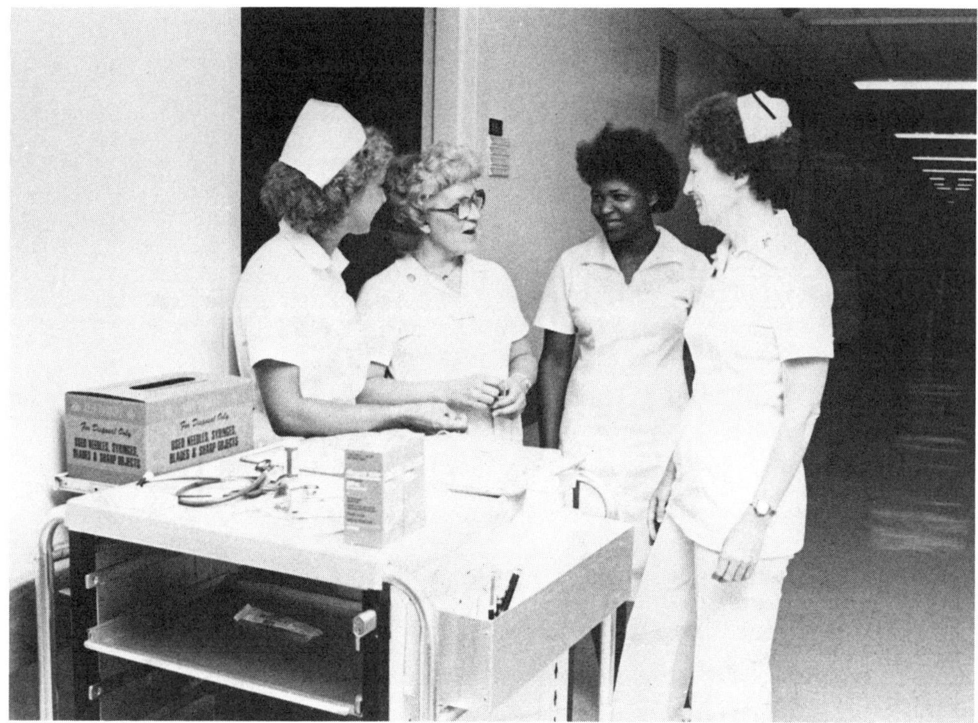

FIGURE 2-4. Nursing team members (LPN, student nurse, and nurse's aide) informally confer with the team leader, a registered nurse.

FIGURE 2-5. A. Team nursing. B. Team nursing from a patient standpoint.

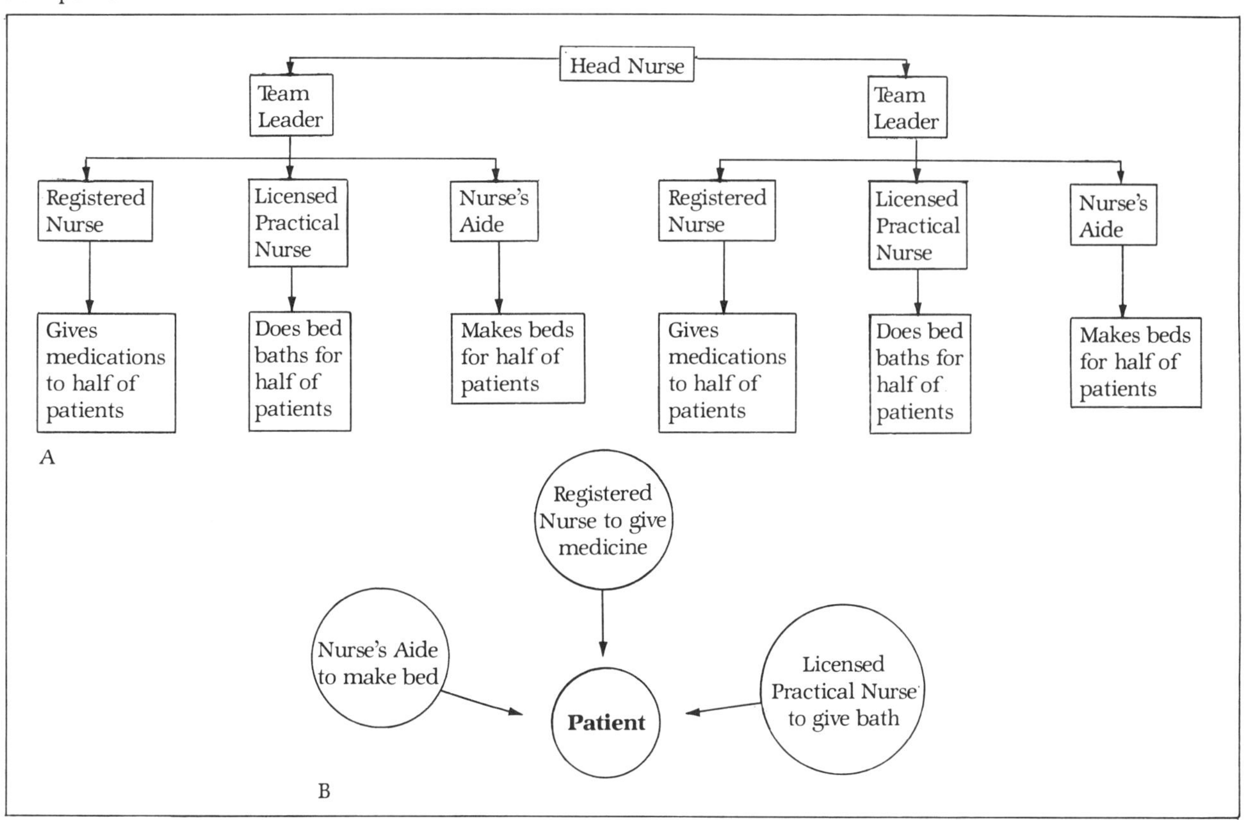

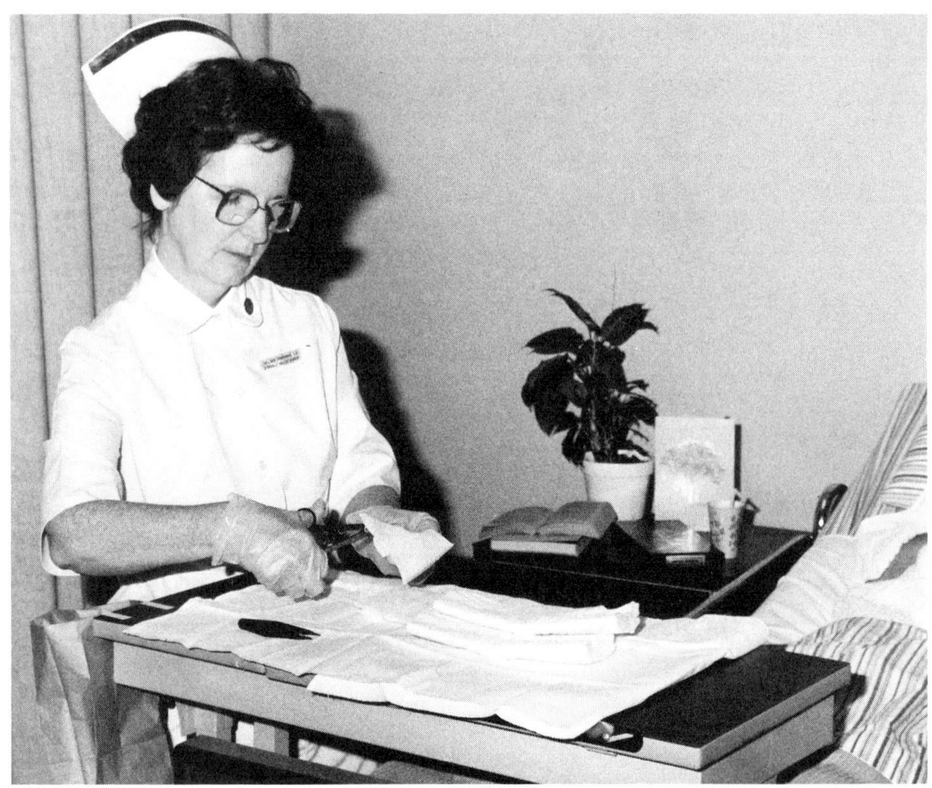

FIGURE 2-6. The primary nurse prepares to change the patient's surgical dressing; the same plan and procedure would be implemented on subsequent shifts by the associate nurse.

FIGURE 2-7. A. Primary nursing. B. Primary nursing from a patient standpoint.

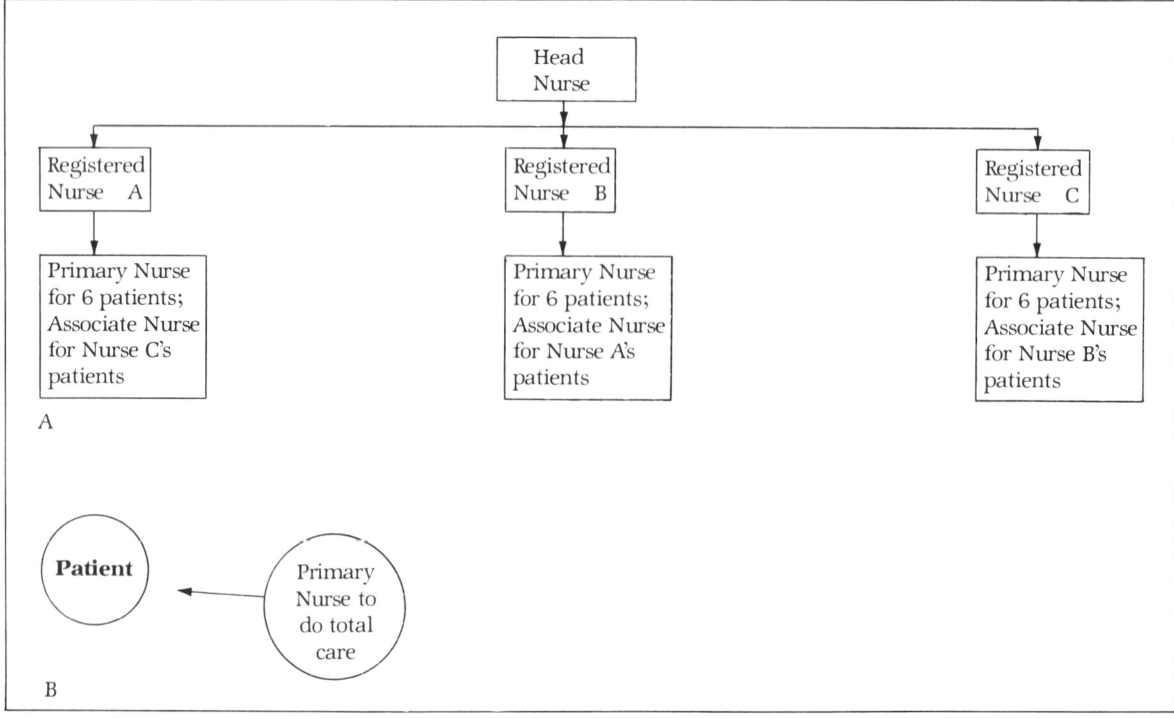

☐ **QUICK REFERENCE STOP 2-1: RESEARCH**
Primary Nursing

Primary nursing has been applauded as the most efficient and most effective method for delivery of nursing care to patients. Numerous researchers have tested this belief in many studies. A sample of the research in this area is reported below.

DOES PRIMARY NURSING RESULT IN ACTUAL DIFFERENCES IN NURSING CARE DELIVERY?

A small sample of 12 patients was utilized by researchers (Hamera and O'Connell, 1981) to assess whether there were differences in number of patient contacts, nurturance of patients, and patient involvement with care under the primary nursing vs. the team nursing approach. Although the findings failed to demonstrate an increase in the amount of patient contact with primary nursing, there are indications that the quality of care improved.

HOW DO PATIENTS LIKE PRIMARY NURSING?

An experimental study was conducted to evaluate the effectiveness of implemented primary nursing care. Specifically, patient satisfaction was examined. Two nursing units contributed subjects to the study—one unit implemented primary nursing while the other unit utilized a team/functional approach in the delivery of nursing care. No difference in patient satisfaction was found between the subjects on the two units. The researchers suggest, however, that the effects of primary nursing may not effectively be assessed through the use of patient satisfaction as an evaluation measure and that further research in the area is necessary (Ventura et al., 1982).

HOW DO NURSES LIKE PRIMARY NURSING?

Another study analyzed the job satisfaction, by questionnaire, of 180 staff-level registered nurses from 27 nursing units. It compared the job satisfaction of nurses working the primary system vs. that of nurses working the team system. Overall, the results showed greater job satisfaction among primary system nurses than team system nurses. Primary system nurses felt that they had more opportunity for accountability. The data suggested, however, that both systems are perceived as limiting in self-fulfillment, decision making, independent judgment, and prestige (Carlsen and Malley, 1981).

SUGGESTED READINGS

Carlsen, R. H., and Malley, J. D. Job satisfaction of staff registered nurses in primary and team nursing delivery systems. *Res. Nurs. Health* 4:251, 1981.

Hamera, E., and O'Connell, K. A. Patient-centered variables in primary and team nursing. *Res. Nurs. Health* 4:183, 1981.

Ventura, M. R., Fox, R. N., Corley, M. C., and Mercurio, S. M. A patient satisfaction measure as a criterion to evaluate primary nursing. *Nurs. Res.* 31:4, 226, 1982.

may prefer to be part of a team rather than work independently (see QRS 2-1).

Primary nursing is becoming the organizational method most used today. It is the system of care most consistent with the teaching method used most in schools of nursing (you give total care to a patient during the time you are with him).

Integration of Organizational Structures

On many nursing units two or three methods of organizing nursing care are used: Medicine is administered by a functional system; patients who are hospitalized for long-term care are assigned a primary nurse; patients who are admitted for only short-term diagnostic procedures or stays are cared for by team members.

It is important for you as a student in nursing to be aware of the method used for the organization of care on a nursing unit where you receive experience so that you can recognize the people you will be responsible to (a head nurse, a team leader, or a primary nurse) besides your instructor. Knowing these relationships as well as the importance of standards of nursing and the role of nursing theorists helps you to add to continuity of care during the hours when you are not actively administering patient care.

SUGGESTED READINGS

American Nurses' Association. *Standards of Nursing Practice.* Kansas City: American Nurses' Association, 1973.

Aspinall, M. J., and Tanner, C. A. *Decision Making for Patient Care.* New York: Appleton-Century-Crofts, 1981.

Beck, J. The standards as a guide for nursing care plans. *Oncol. Nurs. Forum* 7:28, 1980.

Betz, M., et al. Cost and quality: Primary and team nursing compared. *Nurs. Health Care* 1:150, 1980.

Beyer, M., and Phillips, C. *Nursing Management for Patient Care.* Boston: Little, Brown, 1979.

Clark, J. Development of models and theories on the concept of nursing. *J. Adv. Nurs.* 7:129, 1982.

Cox, C. L. An interaction model of client health behavior: Theoretical prescription for nursing. *ANS* 5(1):41, 1982.

Evans, R. W., et al. A model for evaluating primary nursing. *Nurs. Admin. Q.* 5:93, 1981.

Ferrin, T. One hospital's successful implementation of primary nursing. *Nurs. Admin. Q.* 5:1, 1981.

Floyd, J. A. Research using Rogers' conceptual system: Development of a testable theorem . . . regarding the sleep-wakefulness rhythm. *ANS* 5(2):37, 1983.

Hall, M. B. How do students learn on a primary nursing care unit. *Nurs. Outlook* 25:370, 1977.

Henderson, V. *The Nature of Nursing.* New York: Macmillan, 1966.

Hymovich, D. P. How children, mothers and nurses view primary and team nursing. *Am. J. Nurs.* 80:2041, 1980.

Iveson-Iveson, J. A two-way process . . . Theories in nursing practice . . . Peplau's nursing model. *Nurs. Mirror* 155(18):52, 1982.

Iveson-Iveson, J. Standards of behavior . . . Theories of nursing practice . . . The Johnson model. *Nurs. Mirror* 155(20):38, 1982.

Joiner, C., et al. Is primary nursing the answer? *Nurs. Admin. Q.* 5:69, 1981.

Kimbro, C. D. The nursing staff organization: A needed development. *Nurs. Outlook* 28:610, 1980.

McClure, M. The long road to accountability. *Nurs. Outlook* 26:47, 1978.

McMurrey, P. H. Toward a unique knowledge base in nursing. *Image* 14:12, 1982.

Milne, M. A. Training for team care. *J. Adv. Nurs.* 5:579, 1980.

Nightingale, F. *Notes on Nursing.* New York: Dover Publications, Inc., 1969.

Nursing Theories Conference Group. *Nursing Theories.* Englewood Cliffs, N.J.: Prentice-Hall, 1980.

Orem, D. *Nursing: Concepts of Practice.* New York: McGraw-Hill, 1971.

Perkel, L. The role of concepts and theories in research. *Fla. Nurse* 30(8):12, 1982.

Roberts, L. E. primary nursing: Do patients like it—are nurses satisfied—does it cost more? *Canad. Nurse* 76:20, 1980.

Rogers, M. *An Introduction to the Theoretical Basis of Nursing.* Philadelphia: F. A. Davis, 1970.

Roy, S. C. *Introduction to Nursing: An Adaptation Model.* Englewood Cliffs, N.J.: Prentice-Hall, 1976.

Simons, B. J. Decentralizing nursing services—six months later. *Superv. Nurse* 11:59, 1980.

Wandelt, M. A., et al. Why nurses leave nursing and what can be done about it. *Am. J. Nurs.* 81:72, 1981.

Winstead-Fry, P. The need to differentiate a nursing self. *Am. J. Nurs.* 77:1452, 1977.

QUESTIONS FOR REVIEW

1. Commonly accepted standards of nursing practice have been written by:
   a. Association of nursing practice.
   b. American Nurses' Association.
   c. American Hospital Association.
   d. Association for graduate nurses.

2. The purpose of standards of nursing is to:
   a. Make each nurse's care identical.
   b. List tasks that a nurse cannot do.
   c. Separate nurse from physician tasks.
   d. Provide guidelines for quality practice.

3. Which of the following statements reflects a standard of nursing practice?
   a. Nurses do not evaluate their own care.
   b. Patients should participate in their own care.
   c. Prioritizing problems is done after planning is complete.
   d. Collection of data about a patient is done only once.

4. The goal of modern nursing might be *best* stated:
   a. To restore people to complete wellness.
   b. To make people feel better.
   c. To help everyone who wants to get well to do so.
   d. To promote health of individuals and communities.

5. Nursing theorists add to the basic knowledge of nursing by:
   a. Defining better how the person nursed is to be viewed.
   b. Writing specific procedures such as how to count a pulse rate.
   c. Limiting the role of nurses to improving sanitary conditions.
   d. Writing standards to improve the appearance of nurses.

6. In a functional organization of nursing care, the registered nurse would:
   a. Act as an outside consultant.
   b. Do all nursing care activities for one patient.
   c. Do all nursing care activities for six or more patients.
   d. Repeat one procedure over and over for all patients.

7. In a team nursing organizational structure, the registered nurse would:
   a. Not be required to meet standards of nursing practice.
   b. Carry out a task such as administration of medicine.
   c. Work independently to give patient care.
   d. Work directly under the head nurse.

8. Primary nursing organizational structure is becoming more popular because it promotes:
   a. An assembly-line technique.
   b. Job satisfaction.
   c. Increased nursing dependence.
   d. The increased use of nurse's aides.

3. ETHICAL CONSIDERATIONS OF NURSING PRACTICE

OBJECTIVES

Upon mastery of the material in this chapter, you should be able to:

1. Describe the concepts of personal and professional ethics.
2. Describe the application of the American Nurses' Association Code of Ethics to nursing practice.
3. Describe the use of values clarification to determine personal values.
4. Describe ways that ethical considerations arise in nursing practice today.

TERMS

The terms important for an understanding of this chapter are shown below and defined in the glossary:

value
values clarification

Laws are a society's formal rules of conduct or action, recognized as enforceable by a controlling authority. Ethics are a set of moral principles or values that informally govern individuals in a society.

The word *ethics* comes from the Greek *ethos* meaning "guided belief" or "custom." Everyone has personal values or a personal set of ethics. All professions establish ethical codes of conduct for their members. Members not only agree to subscribe to these rules to govern their own conduct but to monitor other members of the profession to see that they subscribe to them as well.

PERSONAL ETHICS

Every person develops, as he matures, a code of behavior which he adheres to (not stealing, not consciously causing harm to another, or spending time in worthwhile activities). Such personal ethical codes vary greatly from person to person depending on religious, cultural, and individual family influences. The more you learn about people the more you will come to appreciate how varied are people's ethical standards and how almost no one has standards exactly like yours. It is important when working with people that you appreciate these differences so that you do not expect others to adjust to your standards and you do not feel obligated to adjust to theirs.

If you believe that everyone should work at a productive job if he is able, you may have difficulty discussing a patient goal that reflects less effort (a person who, following hospital discharge, plans to extend his illness as long as possible in order to receive all sickness benefits) or a goal that will lead to an occupation that you find distasteful (such as prostitution) unless you accept differences in people and different value choices in a nonjudgmental way. It is difficult to be truly unbiased because you are first a person and people tend to be judgmental.

Life Span Concepts and Personal Ethics

Values are taught not so much by words as by actions. The mother who neglects to tell the grocery store clerk that she was handed too much change and the father who wheels a shopping cart home with him from the grocery store are both saying by their actions louder than any words they speak that honesty and respect for property are not highly valued by them. Children who do not have a strong commitment to honesty may ask you to "cheat" for them: Don't give me the medicine—I'll tell everyone that you did; let me have something to eat—I won't tell anyone. When a child is ill, it is often not a good time to teach ethical judgment (and you should not impose your standards on others), but it is an effective time for role-modeling behavior because what you do speaks more strongly than what you say in these same instances.

THE INFANT

Children under three years of age have few ethical values and little understanding of right and wrong. They initiate actions not out of conscience but out of a desire to please the person who is their primary caretaker.

THE TODDLER AND PRESCHOOLER

A toddler learns that it is wrong for him to touch articles on the coffee table or to hit his younger brother, but he learns this mostly from conditioning not reasoning (every time he touches an article on the table or approaches his brother, his mother frowns and says "No").

At preschool age the child begins to develop a conscience. This is the reason that a preschooler can share and wait his turn in line. Preschoolers operate at an elemental level of ethics development, however. If you ask a preschool child why it would be wrong to enter his neighbor's house and steal money from him, the child usually answers "because mother would punish me." The possible consequences of his acts, not really the right or wrong of the situation, control his actions.

THE SCHOOLAGER AND ADOLESCENT

Schoolagers gain deeper convictions but still do not operate at an adult level of conscience. If you ask a school-age child why it would be wrong to enter his neighbor's house and steal money, he will probably answer, "The police would put me in jail" (his world has widened but his sense of control is derived from external not internal controls).

A school-age child tends to do unkind things such as forming a club and excluding a third child from the club because, with only external controls operating, at any point that he does not receive enough guidance he may not manage to be fair. School-age children are old enough that, when asked to put themselves in the other child's place, they can see that their activity was not a kind one.

Part of adolescent identity is deciding what kind of person one is going to become not only in terms of being a plumber, an accountant, or a salesman but also in terms of what ethical standards one is going to adopt (be an honest person or not, one who can be trusted or not).

An adolescent begins to use adult reasoning in connection with ethical decision making. Asked the same question about stealing, an adolescent will usually respond, "It is wrong to steal because taking something from my neighbor would deprive or hurt him." This change in conceptual thinking—rejecting an action because it is harmful to another—represents an internal control basis for decision making and is a big step toward being able to function as an adult. However, many adolescents do not readily view that stealing from a large corporation or department store can hurt (this is the reason for the high rate of shoplifting in the adolescent population).

THE ADULT

Young adults try out the patterns of values they choose to think of as theirs when they are identity building. Young adults who enter professions that have codes of ethics may find that their personal codes conflict with those of the professional organization. In the helping professions problems may arise with situations of abortion, euthanasia (mercy-killing), artificial insemination, or termination of life.

Ethical values as a rule do not change drastically through life, although values may be modified. As people grow into middle and older age, they have been living with an ethical framework for such an extended period of time that they may have difficulty adapting it to changing times. They may not be able to accept a person as a roommate in a health care agency whose illness was the result of an action that they do not approve of (a man injured while robbing a bank; a woman who has an infection following an abortion). Remember that as you grow away from young adulthood, your ethical standards may tend to become more fixed. If you find yourself saying, "Isn't that terrible?" about a patient's actions, learn to stop and ask yourself, "Weighed by whose standards?" If the answer is "mine," you may need to reevaluate your tendency to judge people according to your standards; such judging can interfere with unbiased nursing care.

Many parents grow disappointed during middle age as they realize that their children are not planning to enter the occupations they had always anticipated for them (a son announces he does not want to enter the family business; a daughter expresses a wish to become a space engineer rather than a gradeschool teacher). One thing that most parents are not even aware of is that what they hoped for their children's ethical values has come true. Since these standards are learned subtly, early in life, they often tend to mimic very closely those of one's parents (for better or worse, depending on the code of ethics of the parents).

Selection of Values

What you value and what you do not comes from the interplay of many influences: family, friends, sex, religion, community, country. Something may be prized because it was hard to come by (a rare mineral); is expensive (a figurine); has unusual artistic quality (a painting); causes good (peace) or has high personal attachment (honesty). Sometimes a value is important to you because it is something you have always had and would miss greatly if you should lose it; other values are important because they reflect something that you collected, categorized, and cared for over the years (Fig. 3-1). You might also value something that you have never had and so would like to have. Money is a material

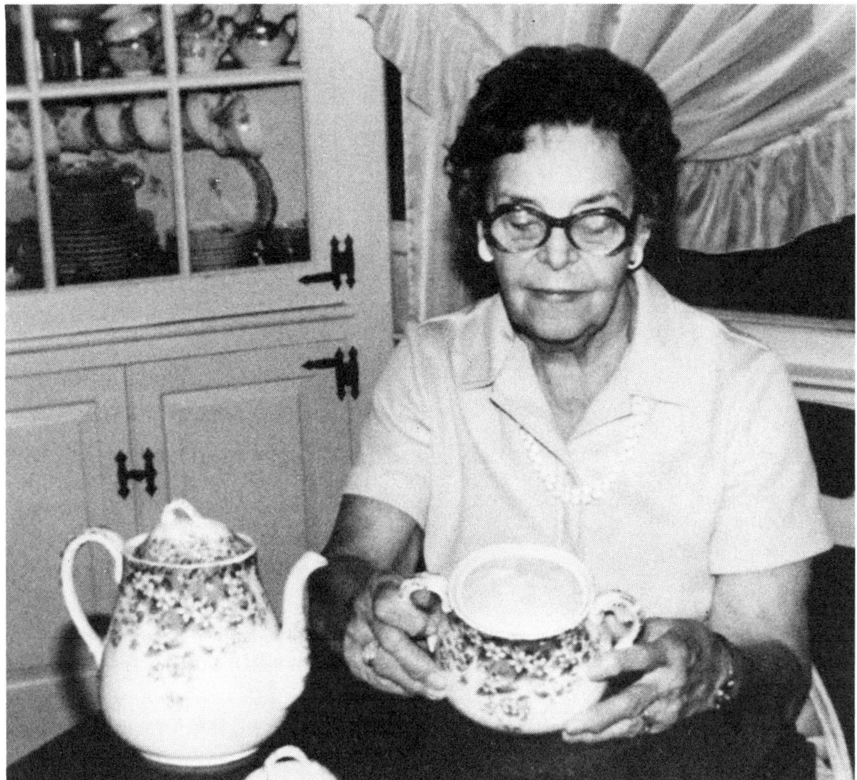

A

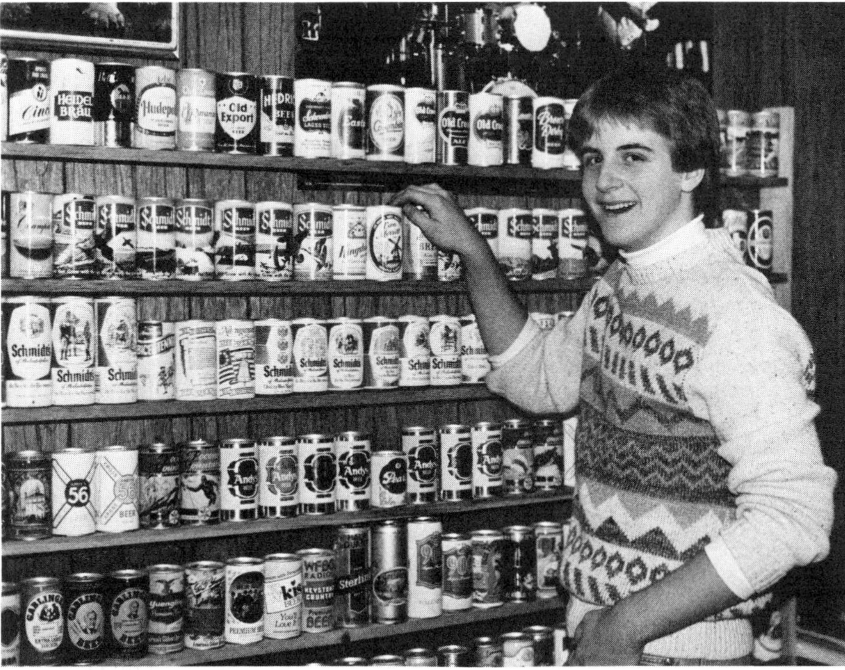

B

FIGURE 3-1. A. To this woman, her mother's china is a value. B. A collection of 500 different empty beer cans is a value to this boy who started the collection in grade school and continued to add to and refine his collection through his teen years.

value that most people rate highly; peace is a conceptual value that people in countries both free of war and at war generally list as a priority.

Because values may not be constant throughout life but change depending on age, environmental influences, and life situations, everyone needs to periodically review his values. Otherwise, a person may spend a great deal of effort trying to accomplish or obtain something, and then, after he has it in his hands, realize little enjoyment from it. His values may change to the extent that, by the time he achieves the goal, it no longer is important to him.

Age as a Determinant of Values

A preschool child generally names as values things that he knows that his mother also values. An adolescent may name values that are exactly opposite those of his parents (if they value religion, he states religion is not important; if they value neatness, he leaves his room in a constant mess). A person is inseparable from his values, so in many cases the easiest way for an adolescent to show that he is rejecting his parents is to reject their values. With greater maturity the young adult realizes that he can make a statement for independence without rejecting his parent's values and again affirms similar ethical concerns.

As a person moves from young adulthood to middle age, his values may change again. If a couple's values do not change similarly (a wife values material things, her husband values free time), they may find their relationship strained as they try to adapt to the other's value system.

Environmental Influences

Before the Great Depression in the 1930s people may or may not have listed financial security as a priority value; most people who lived through the Depression find financial security very important (hold it as a priority value). Because financial security in the 1940s and 1950s was very important to a large segment of the population in the United States, many federally funded programs were originated to prevent people from ever suffering such financial loss again. Today, as the average citizen no longer remembers what that degree of financial disaster was like, cuts in federal programs are apparent.

Environmental influences such as a high crime rate in a neighborhood may make people place a higher value on safe housing or law enforcement than people in other neighborhoods. During a period of exceptionally cold weather, people may list warmth as a high value; in the summer the same people may list a day of cool weather as something they want very much.

Situational Influences

People often find their values changing as their situation in life changes. A young married couple, for example, may both value their freedom to travel; this makes them compatible as a couple. Following the birth of their first child, they may find that their values are turning more toward purchasing a permanent home and establishing security. Marriages often suffer considerable stress when one partner's values change and the other partner's do not.

State of health influences people's values greatly. The average person rarely notes the ability to see as a high value; the person with failing eyesight probably gives this very high priority. The average person rarely lists the ability to stand as a value while a person confined to a wheelchair may value such a simple act very highly. Because illness changes values in these ways, helping people with values clarification is often an intrinsic part of patient care.

VALUES CLARIFICATION

Values clarification is a process for examining and determining the things you value (believe in or desire) most. It is important to remember that when you are helping others with value clarification, it is your role to help them determine *what* they value; it is never your role to tell them what *to* value—that is a personal choice.

Determining or clarifying values should be done by a step-by-step process, the same as any other controlled investigation. These seven steps are as follows:

Listing Values

The first step in values clarification is to list those things that you think you value (health, comfort, a sense of humor, love). Be honest in listing values, not censoring. If money is a value, for example (and it is for most people), list it despite the fact that someone else thinks money is the root of all evil (a statement that reflects that person's value system). When working with patients, urge them to be honest about values. If a person values the sensation he feels after the injection of a drug, being honest with himself about this feeling is important, not only for himself but for you; although it may not make his behavior what you would like it to be, it explains his constant drug-seeking behavior and the reason he sets health care goals as he does.

Examining the Possible Consequences of Value Choices

When listing values that are important to you, it helps to examine the consequences if that value were sought and also the consequences if it were not (termed risk-benefit). Suppose you list "becoming a registered nurse" as a value. The consequences of seeking out that value are at least two years of education, many hours of study, many hours of feeling vulnerable and under constant scrutiny from instructors, considerable expense, and so forth. Assuming you are a student in a program of nursing, you must have weighed those consequences at some point and decided that you were willing to accept them in order to achieve what you value. Others in your high school class may have weighed those same consequences and decided that, although they would like to achieve that goal, they did not feel strongly enough about it to accept the consequences (the risk outweighed the benefit).

The following box describes the steps in values clarification that could result in the decision to choose or not

Steps in Values Clarification

Problem: What is important to me as a life's vocation?

Step	*Example*
List alternatives	Helping people, teaching, and making people feel good about themselves are values for me. I could do these things as either a teacher, nurse, social worker, or parent.
Examine possible consequences	Being a teacher will offer more free time. Being a nurse is more science oriented; I do well in science courses. I think that I like more "hands on" contact than social work offers. "Parent" will not support me financially.
Choose freely	All school programs involve equal expense and are available in my area.
Feel good about choice	I feel satisfaction at the end of a day's clinical experience with patients.
Affirm the choice	I am pleased to tell people that I am a student in nursing.
Act on choice	I am conscientiously completing a program in nursing.
Act with a pattern	I find myself incorporating nursing process or a system of planning in activities outside nursing studies.

Conclusion: Becoming a nurse is a value for me.

Problem: What is important to me as a life's vocation?

Step	*Example*
List alternatives	Helping people, teaching, and making people feel good about themselves are values for me. I could do these things as either a teacher, nurse, social worker, or parent.
Examine possible consequences	Being a teacher will offer me more free time. I am not sure that I will like touching people in order to provide intimate care. I enjoy counseling, so social work appeals to me. "Parent" will not support me financially.
Choose freely	All school programs involve equal expense and are available in my area.
Feel good about choice	I feel that I have not accomplished much at the end of a day's nursing care.
Affirm the choice	I generally tell people that I am in college, not that I am a nursing major.
Act on choice	I am just "getting by" in my nursing program.
Act with a pattern	I rarely think of nursing actions when away from a clinical area.

Conclusion: I think that I do not value becoming a nurse as much as I originally thought.

choose to pursue nursing as a professional career. In order to help others in clarifying their own values, it is important to recognize the process and place of values clarification in your own life. Why *did* you decide to become a student nurse?

A person may say that improving his cardiovascular functioning is a value but not feel powerfully enough about it that he is willing to follow a weight reduction diet; or he may say that improved lung function is a value but he does not want to stop smoking cigarettes or do daily breathing exercises to achieve it. In these instances, the improved cardiovascular and lung function are not important values or the person would be ready to accept the consequences that accompany achieving the value.

Choosing Freely

Values must be chosen freely in order to be meaningful. Some people work at the job they do, not because it is what they wanted to do in life, but because there was no money available for them to go to college or they had family or home commitments that forced them to begin earning a salary immediately out of high school. If this type of worker is told that for some health reason he cannot perform this work any longer, he may feel little remorse. On the other hand, some people choose the same positions freely; for them loss of such a position might be devastating.

Realizing that values are only true values when they are chosen freely, not by coercion from family, teachers, or friends or pressure from a sensation such as fear, often explains people's reactions to medical diagnoses and helps you to establish health care goals with them.

Feelings About the Choice

When a person states that honesty is a value yet does not feel happy about the fact that he does not cheat on his income tax, it is questionable whether honesty is really of value to him (perhaps gaining money is a higher value). A person who says that he values walking should feel happy about going to physical therapy to learn how to do it, or the fact that the value is really important to him is in doubt.

Some people derive satisfaction from being ill (ordinarily the people around them pay little attention to them; when they are ill, every day two physicians, a medical student, a student nurse, three registered nurses, three nurse's aides, a dietician, a physical therapist, and some friend from work stops to give them special attention). If illness is valued in this way, the person may derive little satisfaction from participating in treatments that will make him well again; instead he feels good about the state of being ill.

Affirming the Choice

If a person truly believes in something, he is willing to defend it verbally, should the occasion arise. Very often proposed social reforms (preventing a neighborhood playground from being converted into an apartment building, protesting air pollution from a local industry, for example) are lost causes because although people in the neighborhood seem interested in these issues they are not committed enough to the value (adequate play space, clean air) to make their views known at a city government meeting. Sometimes people who say that good lung function is important to them not only are unwilling to commit themselves to stop smoking (unable to accept the consequences that accompany believing in a value) but also are unwilling to state to their friends that clean air is important to them and therefore will not ask family members or friends to stop smoking in the same room.

Acting on the Choice

Values are deep commitments; the commitment is so deep that some action that shows the value to be intrinsic to a person naturally follows. A person with honesty as a value immediately tells an instructor that she has accidentally been handed an examination key with the answers marked rather than a blank examination paper; a person who values honesty less spends a few minutes glancing over answers before she returns it.

Actions are closely associated with verbal confirmation and often are even more revealing. "Actions speak louder than words" is an old proverb that implies that, no matter what people say, the way they act reveals what they really believe.

Acting with a Pattern

Values are so intrinsically woven into the fabric of a person's being that once a value is established as important, it pervades not only one aspect of a person's life but all aspects. The person's behavior always reflects that value. A person who truly values kindness, for example, does not spend her working hours as a nurse being very kind and then spend the next 16 hours at home being less than that; she does not have good days and bad days in relation to kindness. People who value fame and money structure their entire life patterns to achieve these things. If illness forces them to change in some way, remember that it is not a one-time act they have to change; it is a total life style or behavior pattern that has to change, and that is a very difficult thing to do.

Sources of Values

Certainly a large number of a person's values are derived from family, customs, and religion. Others are acquired as a result of motivating forces such as needs or interests.

NEEDS

Maslow's (1970) theory is that a hierarchy of needs is a strong determinant of people's actions and values. True to this theory, people seek food, shelter, and space to breathe above everything else. Basic food, shelter, and breathing space, however, do not usually reflect values but simply unmet needs because free choice is not involved in seeking these (a person must eat, keep warm, and breathe to live). The *type* of food a person selects, the *kind* of shelter he builds for himself, and the type of breathing (supposing a disease condition presents a choice) can represent values.

People recovering from suicide attempts may discover that life itself is a value (or attempt suicide again when they clarify that it is not a value for them). In these instances even eating basic food, seeking shelter, and breathing may represent actions toward achieving a newly recognized value.

INTERESTS AND FEELINGS

Interests may represent values (the person is interested in preserving the neighborhood playground because he values free-form play) or they may merely reflect a passing fancy (the property had momentary appeal or the person enjoyed the attention of seeing his photograph in the newspaper as a community picket). Feelings, as a rule, are at a more shallow level than values. Feelings may also only reflect a temporary situation (one person feels angry because money was taken from his paycheck for union dues; his work partner feels angry because he values active not passive participation in organizations). On a particular issue one person will talk but do nothing, while another will take action; this represents the difference between feelings and values.

BELIEFS

Beliefs is a word often interchanged with value but often reflects, rather than a free choice, a pattern that a person has subtly gained from his parents or an organized religious system. Prejudice against certain people, for example, makes people react in certain ways. If you examine these feelings in yourself, however, you will probably discover that you did not freely choose these beliefs, that they have been with you as long as you can remember. Beliefs are confusing if followed as if they were values because following a belief does not offer the satisfaction that following a value does; if not based on fact but inaccurate knowledge, they can lead a person to less than ideal behavior.

Using Values Clarification

Without clear values a person often acts with uncertainty or inconsistency. He may flounder, not knowing where to put his best efforts or his actions, and find little satisfaction in what he achieves, no matter how strong is his effort to achieve it.

In order to help people clarify their values, you need to help them think about what is important or not important to them. This is done best by asking them how they feel about their actions or decisions (Fig. 3-2).

Values are determined from a range of alternatives. A major role of a nurse in any situation is to be certain that a person is aware of all his alternatives and that he has spent time thinking about them, by asking such questions as “Are there any other things you are considering?” or “What do you think you'll gain by doing that?” Helping a person to explore whether he chose freely can be initiated by a question such as “Did that just happen or did you have a choice?” or “Did you have any say in that decision?”

Sometimes people are reluctant to think about whether they feel good about a choice or not (if they realize they don't feel good, it means they have made a bad choice and that is a demeaning feeling). Helping people to examine their feelings can be done sensitively by a question such as “How do you feel about that now?” or “Some people feel good when they make a decision, some feel bad; how do you feel?”

To determine if a person is ready to verbally or physically act on his decision, a question such as “Will it be difficult to tell your family about this?” or “Have you done anything to show that you really feel this way?” would probably be effective. To help a person determine if he consistently acts in a pattern, a question such as “Would you do that again? or “How many times have you done that?” would be helpful.

Notice that in all these examples the question asked of the person is one that assists him in thinking through his thoughts on a subject or is a clarifying question. The response is never your opinion (“I don't think that is the right thing to do”), a disapproving remark (“That's not right”), or a teaching point (“It would be better if you did it this way”). Although all these responses may have merit at other times (when the person asks you for your personal opinion or when you must prevent the person

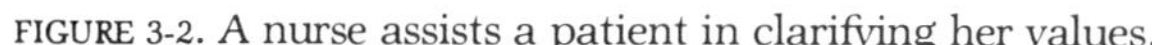

FIGURE 3-2. A nurse assists a patient in clarifying her values.

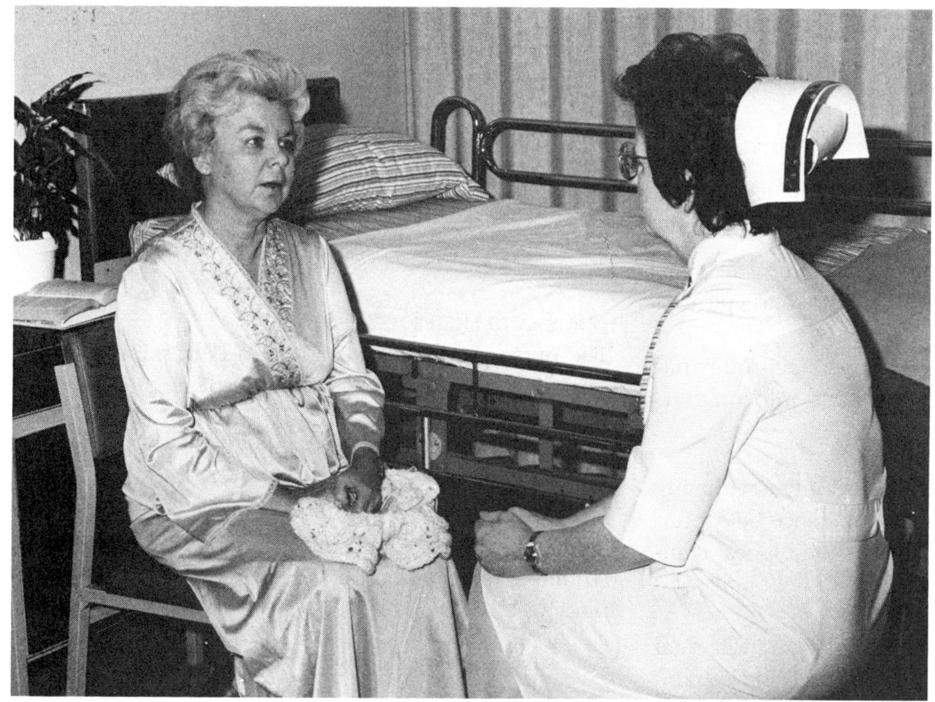

from harming himself or others), they are not effective in clarifying values and are actually confusing because they impose your values on another.

The Effect of Personal Values

What a person values affects and guides how he acts. Any time you are puzzled by a course of action, take the time to ask yourself, "What are my values in this situation? What do I really want to gain from this situation?" Any time you see a person acting in a way that seems incongruent with the way you assumed he would act, ask, "Did I read his values wrongly? Is there another value he must want more than I thought he did that is influencing him to act this way?" Help people to clarify their values so that they can better understand what motivates them to action. Know your own values so that you can act decisively in situations where value judgments must be made and to ensure that your personal ethical system does not conflict with your professional ethical system.

PROFESSIONAL ETHICS

All true professions have codes of ethics. These set guidelines to demonstrate levels of optimal practice and to maintain standards of conduct within the profession. They also allow people outside the profession to be assured that a member of that profession will consistently act in a certain way. It is important for you to know the Code of Ethics for nursing because as a nurse you are expected to adjust your conduct to these statutes.

International Council of Nurses Code of Ethics

In 1973 the International Council of Nurses adopted and published a code of ethics for nurses around the world (see box). By this code of ethics the nurse is expected not only to provide nursing care but to promote a suitable environment for care, maintain effective relationships with other health care providers, advance nursing knowledge, and initiate and support action to improve general health.

American Nurses' Association Code of Ethics

In 1950 the American Nurses' Association adopted and published a code of ethics. This code, as revised in 1968 and again in 1976 (ANA, 1976). It is important to be familiar with the sections of this code, because although an ethical code is not a law, not following such standards could be reason for a state board of nursing to suspend a

International Council of Nurses Code for Nurses: Ethical Concepts Applied to Nursing

The fundamental responsibility of the nurse is fourfold: to promote health, to prevent illness, to restore health, and to alleviate suffering.

The need for nursing is universal. Inherent in nursing is respect for life, dignity, and rights of man. It is unrestricted by considerations of nationality, race, creed, color, age, sex, politics, or social status.

Nurses render health services to the individual, the family, and the community and coordinate their services with those of related groups.

NURSES AND PEOPLE

The nurse's primary responsibility is to those who require nursing care.

The nurse, in providing care, promotes an environment in which the values, customs, and spiritual beliefs of the individual are respected.

The nurse holds in confidence personal information and uses judgment in sharing this information.

NURSES AND PRACTICE

The nurse carries personal responsibility for nursing practice and for maintaining competence by continual learning. The nurse maintains the highest standards of nursing care possible within the reality of a specific situation.

The nurse uses judgment in relation to individual competence when accepting and delegating responsibilities.

The nurse when acting in a professional capacity should at all times maintain standards of personal conduct which reflect credit upon the profession.

NURSES AND SOCIETY

The nurse shares with other citizens the responsibility for initiating and supporting action to meet the health and social needs of the public.

NURSES AND CO-WORKERS

The nurse sustains a cooperative relationship with co-workers in nursing and other fields. The nurse takes appropriate action to safeguard the individual when his care is endangered by a co-worker or any other person.

NURSES AND THE PROFESSION

The nurse plays the major role in determining and implementing desirable standards of nursing practice and nursing education.

The nurse is active in developing a core of professional knowledge.

The nurse, acting through a professional organization, participates in establishing and maintaining equitable social and economic working conditions in nursing.

Source: International Council of Nurses, *Code for Nurses: Ethical concepts applied to nursing.* Geneva: Imprimeries Populaires, 1973. Reprinted with permission.

nurse's license or an employing agency to terminate employment.

STANDARD 1
The nurse provides services with respect for human dignity and the uniqueness of the client unrestricted by considerations of social or economic status, personal attributes, or the nature of health problems.

Standard 1 of this code of ethics is important because if everyone follows it, all those seeking health care can be assured that they will receive the same quality of care as others. If such a standard were not followed, people of minority groups or those with less than perfect personalities or with an illness that altered their physical appearance might worry that they will not (and in fact might not) receive quality nursing care. Because everyone relates more easily to some people than to others, and one may enjoy caring for people with one illness rather than another (or caring for ill people rather than helping well people to remain well), this standard is not always easy to follow. Understanding the importance of it—that following it is the patient's guarantee of quality care—marks the difference between a good nurse and a less than good one.

Another action that this standard implies is that a nurse does not accept tips or other gifts for services rendered. This extends to accepting a piece of candy from a box on a bedside stand or uneaten food from a patient's tray. These practices are also *unsafe:* The number of bacteria that may have settled onto a box of candy on a bedside stand in just an hour could be very high; a patient who coughed while eating could have seriously contaminated the food on his tray. It also implies that a nurse does not take for herself unused supplies such as medicine or sterile dressings that were charged to a patient (which would be indirectly taking a tip because the patient is paying for these items). You can decline a tip gracefully by saying that accepting one is against school or agency policy or by explaining that the service which was so appreciated was a part of your normal care. Only in rare instances will such a statement be misinterpreted as a rejection on your part.

STANDARD 2
The nurse safeguards the client's right to privacy by judiciously protecting information of a confidential nature.

Because this standard exists, people can feel free to relate their concerns and history of past illnesses to their health care providers. If privacy of personal information were not guaranteed, eliciting a history from people on admission to a health care facility would be very difficult. Illnesses could then be diagnosed incorrectly, medicine could be prescribed wrongly, and the chances of people returning to good health as quickly as possible would be greatly reduced. This standard is not always easy to follow because sometimes the information you read on a patient's chart or is told to you is of considerable interest (a prominent politician in your city has been admitted to the hospital for treatment of a thromboembolus—a blood clot—in his leg; the blood clot occurred because he injects heroin into the veins of that leg). Be careful that lunchtime conversations do not involve confidential information of this type, and guard the patient's identity on written or oral reports that you submit for class assignments by using only the person's initials. People have a legal right not to have this type of information spread about indiscriminately, since such information could interfere with obtaining employment or insurance or with personal relationships. When confidentiality is, in addition, stated as an ethical standard, the patient is twice assured that it will be maintained.

STANDARD 3
The nurse acts to safeguard the client and the public when health care and safety are affected by the incompetent, unethical, or illegal practice of any person.

This standard puts responsibility on you not only to maintain a high standard of care for yourself but to monitor the standards of care of those people around you as well. If everyone did this conscientiously, overall care would be improved. Like other ethical standards, such a rule is not always easy to follow (if you found a friend not performing a nursing procedure correctly, it might be difficult to decide where to place your loyalty—with the patient or with your friend). This standard makes it clear that your duty would be to correct her (or report to a nursing supervisor the inadequacy of her care if she did not change her technique); safe care from everyone who is in contact with him is the minimum that a patient has a right to expect.

STANDARD 4
The nurse assumes responsibility and accountability for individual nursing judgments and actions.

This standard puts responsibility on you not to undertake actions that are beyond your ability and not to proceed to perform care with inadequate knowledge as to individual circumstances and requirements. Accountability is also a legal responsibility. You have a strong obligation always to be aware of not only those things you know how to do safely but also those procedures you are not able to do, and to seek help or consultation with the latter. If everyone follows this standard, patients are assured safe care.

STANDARD 5
The nurse maintains competence in nursing.

The fifth standard assures patients that the nurse caring for them has kept her knowledge in her area of care current. Nursing knowledge is not static; it changes so swiftly that a nurse who graduated from a nursing school as little as ten years ago would have difficulty functioning safely on a nursing unit today without an update in knowledge of some kind. This can be achieved by reading journal articles and by attending workshops or continuing educational programs.

This standard also implies that nurses remain competent in appearance (not so overweight that they present a poor role model; not gum chewing or with hair so unmanageable that they look more adolescent than adult; not smoking cigarettes in patient care areas so that their advice on keeping well becomes "do as I say, not as I do"). For many people these are personal standards of conduct; when written in a code of ethics, they become a professional standard as well.

STANDARD 6
The nurse exercises informed judgment and uses individual competence and qualifications as criteria in seeking consultation, accepting responsibilities, and delegating nursing activities to others.

This standard reinforces your responsibility for personal accountability. it places responsibility on you to be certain that when you assign a task to a nurse's aide, for example, you are certain the aide knows how to do the task well and will do it at the same level of care that you would have used. Delegating authority in this way has legal implications as well (you are legally accountable to oversee the aide's actions if you assigned her part of your patient's care). This is stipulated so that people can be assured that they will receive quality care no matter which member of a health care team approaches their bedside or arrives at their home to actually carry out the care.

STANDARD 7
The nurse participates in activities that contribute to the ongoing development of the profession's body of knowledge.

Standard 7 places responsibility on you to participate in the nursing research projects of others (provided you are assured that patients' rights have been protected) and to initiate nursing research of your own. It places responsibility on you to share your areas of expertise with others through writing journal articles or by participating in in-service programs. Learning to do research begins with being a critical consumer of it. Chapter 5 discusses ways to evaluate research projects at this beginning level.

STANDARD 8
The nurse participates in the profession's efforts to implement and improve standards of nursing.

This standard urges you to participate in nursing education by serving as a preceptor or instructor to students, serving as a role model, and, as prescribed by the previous standard, putting in writing your suggestions for improvements in nursing care. It also places responsibility on you to join a nursing professional organization whose interests are improving standards of nursing care.

STANDARD 9
The nurse participates in the profession's efforts to establish and maintain conditions of employment conducive to high quality nursing care.

This standard was written to ensure people that not only will the health care they receive be of a high quality but also the environment around them will be safe for their care. It would be unethical for you to ignore conditions that you felt were unsafe from a fire safety, mental health, or sanitary standpoint. Some nurses interpret this standard as making it obligatory for them to strike, if necessary, in order to secure working conditions optimal for quality care. Other nurses have difficulty viewing an action such as a strike as compatible with nursing's first obligation for patient safety.

STANDARD 10
The nurse participates in the profession's effort to protect the public from misinformation and misrepresentation and to maintain the integrity of nursing.

This standard prevents a nurse from advertising or endorsing products. To do so might be misleading, since some people might assume that a nurse would have special knowledge about the product and that it was therefore better than competing brands. It also places responsibility on you to help patients interpret advertising claims. You should also monitor newspaper articles or television programs as to the image they project of nurses or nursing.

STANDARD 11
The nurse collaborates with members of the health professions and other citizens in promoting community and national efforts to meet the health needs of the public.

This last statement makes it necessary for a nurse to look beyond her immediate work situation to the community around her to see if there are unmet needs that she could help meet (recognizing there are no classes for prepared childbirth available and beginning to teach some). If every nurse did this conscientiously, the comprehensiveness of care and concern that would result would improve total health care.

ETHICAL PROBLEMS IN NURSING

Ethical problems in nursing arise from conflict in three main categories: between what an individual nurse believes and the way in which the code of nursing ethics determines that she should act; between an individual nurse's beliefs or the code of nursing ethics and those of the agency where she works; between the code of nursing ethics and a patient's beliefs.

Conflicts between Nurses' Values and the Code of Ethics

Various situations arise in nursing that may bring personal and professional ethics into conflict. Suppose, for example, that you do not believe that having an abortion is a woman's individual choice and right. If you are assigned to care for a woman who is scheduled for a therapeutic abortion, what should you do? Refuse the assignment? Take the assignment but give poor care? Take the assignment but tell the young woman that you do not approve of her action? Take the assignment and proceed to give the same level of care as if she were undergoing a type of surgery that you do approve of? Look for yet another option?

This is not an easy question to answer, because each option compromises you in some way. The first three suggested solutions compromise the first professional ethical standard (providing service with respect for human dignity and the uniqueness of the patient unrestricted by considerations of social or economic status, personal attributes, or the nature of the health problem). The fourth option compromises your personal values. Is there a fifth option?

Fortunately, as nurses are concerned with respect for human dignity, so is the average health care agency that supplies nursing care. Before you accept a nursing position, you should discuss with the employing agency areas where your values may conflict with professional ethics. Ask not to be assigned such patients; this is a more responsible action than refusing an assignment later. It allows the health care agency the opportunity to schedule other nurses to do this care or even to choose at that early stage whether they want to hire you based on your criteria for employment. If after accepting you on these conditions the health care agency insists that you care for this type of patient, you should consider finding another place to work. An agency that does not respect your personal ethics probably has little concern for patients' values either. You would be happier in an agency with more responsible standards of care.

Ethical and legal aspects of care are often interconnected. Legally, once you begin care for a patient (establish a nurse-patient relationship), you are committed to continue care for that patient unless appropriately relieved. This is the reason that you should make clear in advance that you do not choose to care for a patient. Once you begin care, you are legally committed and your personal values may have to be compromised to avoid legal entanglements.

For the same reason it is important as a student that you make this type of personal value clear to an instructor who will be choosing your patient assignment *before* assignments are made. If, after you have made it clear that because of personal values you do not want to accept a particular type of patient assignment, an instructor insists that you do so, you need to discuss the problem with your instructor's immediate superior. As a last resort, you might consider transfer to another school of nursing, unless the instructor has a valid argument that you can meet a required objective only by taking care of this type of patient. This is the same problem that arises when a nurse is working in a health care agency that shows little respect for personal values. Check your student manual or college bulletin for statements in regard to this situation. A school of nursing is legally bound by the language in these publications.

This type of values conflict might also arise with a teaching assignment. If you are asked to teach a group of women about birth control and have moral reservations about birth control, what should you do? Teach the class and compromise your values? Refuse to teach and therefore receive a failing grade? Teach but state that you do not believe in what you are saying? Search for a fourth alternative?

Again, on most issues where your personal values conflict with professional role expectations the problem can be solved in a way that maintains and respects your values and yet allows you to function professionally. The objective of such an assignment is probably not to teach birth control as such but to demonstrate that you are knowledgeable about methods of birth control and that you can teach effectively. Make your values known and suggest alternatives such as writing a paper to demonstrate that you know the required material and teaching another subject (bathing a baby, breast-feeding techniques, stimulation techniques for young infants). If the problem arises as part of a work assignment (someone on the nursing staff must teach this information), it is part of your contract obligation and a matter you should have discussed before being hired for the position. However, you can usually solve such problems by trading off an equal-time task with someone who has no objection to the assignment. This is what the agency wants: the task done well, not any one person to do it.

Whenever personal values and professional ethics conflict, be firm so that your personal values are not compromised and also that patients never receive less than quality care. Ensure that the person who will be giving the care in your place is as capable at giving it as you would have been if the conflict of values had not arisen.

Conflicts Between Personal Beliefs and Agency Policy

Suppose you believe that people who are dying should be told the truth if they ask; agency policy is that only a physician should answer questions about this subject. Unfortunately, this administrative directive is difficult to carry out when a person asks "Am I dying?" and you are the only person standing at the side of the bed.

In most instances this type of situation can be solved

without compromising beliefs on either side if you examine closely what it is you truly believe—that a person should know he is dying, not that *you* give him this information. You can answer his question by saying, "The rules here don't allow me to answer that question for you; only Dr. Jones can. When she makes rounds this morning, I'll tell her you asked me that so she can talk to you about it." Follow through by telling Dr. Jones of the direct request. Most physicians do not enjoy talking about death; Dr. Jones cannot help but feel that in some way she has failed when one of her patients is dying and so avoids the subject until a need to discuss it is drawn to her attention. Most physicians appreciate your accompanying them when they discuss painful subjects such as a poor surgery outcome or death.

A policy such as the one in question probably should be reviewed by an agency policy committee. It is most likely a remnant of a former time and should be replaced by one that recognizes a modern nurse's expertise to discuss this type of information with patients.

Another example of this nature might be your discovery that a physician visiting a patient preoperatively is obviously inebriated. You know that she is going from the patient's unit to surgery to begin operating. Your personal values tell you that it's not nice to be a "tattletale"; your common sense tells you that the patient's life may be at stake; your professional ethics tells you that you have an obligation to safeguard the patient against incompetent practice. You are also aware that the physician is the sister of the personnel manager who can block any chance you have for promotion or even retention at this agency. What should you do?

In this instance, because a person's life is at stake, your common sense and your professional ethics make it imperative that you report to a supervisor what you have seen. This is also a legal responsibility. It is not always easy to stand up and be counted when a personal value is at stake; it is not always easy to be counted when a professional issue is at stake either.

Guidelines Helpful for Ethical Decision Making

1. *Know your values.* Take some time and use values clarification to determine those things that you value highly enough that you are willing to defend them. This is important to ensure that you do not compromise an important value, not realizing at the time that it was that important to you, or that you do not spend time fighting for a value that in the end is not important to you (winning battles but losing wars).
2. *Do not allow your values to be compromised.* Giving in to a situation may temporarily solve a problem, but in the end it can breed disrespect for yourself and the agency or person asking you to compromise. You can not continue to function well if you do not feel good about yourself or the people around you. This type of compromise is often very destructive and negatively affects the nursing care you give.
3. *Know professional nursing ethics.* Knowing what is expected of you ethically as a nurse is as important as knowing what is expected of you in any other area. Acting within ethical guidelines is what makes you a professional nurse; it makes your actions dependable and helps to ensure quality care.
4. *Do not allow your nursing ethics to be compromised.* In the same way that allowing your personal ethics to be violated leads to disrespect, so does violation of professional ethical standards.
5. *Do not be disappointed that not everyone meets your standards.* Values differ among people. Feeling angry with someone because he does not value something as highly as you do is destructive to your relationship. Such a person may have a higher value in another area, and in the end you may wish that you were not so quick to feel superior to him and resist working with him.
6. *Do not force your personal values on others.* Personal values are just that: personal. What works for you may not work at all for another; trying to remake others in your image is not often workable.

Conflicts with Patient Beliefs

Patients' beliefs may at times conflict with nurses' ethical beliefs. Parents of children born with birth defects, for example, must make decisions at birth about the child's care and future. In some instances, the decisions to be made are harsh ones; the ones that parents arrive at may not be those you would have liked to see them make. Infants born with Down's syndrome, a mental retardation syndrome, are often also frequently born with heart defects and atresias (complete blockage) of the duodenum. At one time parents were told by their physicians at the child's birth that the best therapy for the infant would be surgery for the duodenal obstruction immediately and for the heart at a later date; parents signed the necessary permissions for surgery without any real consideration as to what they wanted—they merely followed the doctor's orders. Such a course of action was recommended because while the child might die in early infancy because of the heart defect, he would die in a week's time from starvation from the complete intestinal obstruction. Today, it is a recognized constitutional right of parents to participate in making this type of decision, and they may decide that they do not want the surgery performed.

If this decision is in opposition to your personal values—if you believe that mentally retarded persons have the right to live and become all that they can become—it is difficult to stand by and let the decision go unchallenged, a course that will surely kill the child from starvation. Such a decision is in opposition to your professional ethics, since it does not respect human dignity or uniqueness.

Fortunately, as in most instances where patients or parents make decisions not in a person's best interests, the decision was based on inadequate information as to alternatives available. People who make this type of decision are really making the decision not to raise the child; they invariably do not realize that there are other alternatives such as signing the responsibility for the child's rearing over to the state. The state will authorize the surgery to correct the physical defects and arrange for the infant to be initially cared for in an institutional setting or foster home. In many instances an informed, caring adoptive family can be found and formal adoption proceedings can be accomplished.

Informing such patients of all their alternatives protects the child and solves the ethical problem of a conflict of beliefs.

PRINCIPLES OF ETHICAL DECISION MAKING

Ethical decision making is a difficult form of decision making because there are no black and white solutions as to what is the right or wrong answer. In actual practice situations are very complex because of many more interrelated factors than those in the examples given.

Because they involve feelings more than facts, it is easy for people not to reason as much as argue when ethical issues are involved. The preceding box contains a number of guidelines that are helpful in making this type of decision. It is most important to be aware of the interplay of your own personal value system and the standards of the nursing code of ethics so that you have firm guidelines for ethical decision making and action.

SUGGESTED READINGS

American Nurses' Association. *Code for Nurses.* Kansas City: American Nurses' Association, 1976.

Aroskar, M. A. Anatomy of an ethical dilemma: The theory . . . the practice. *Am. J. Nurs.* 80:658, 1980.

Bayles, M. D. The value of life—By what standard? *Am. J. Nurs.* 80:2226, 1980.

Beyrer, M. K., et al. Ethics for the eighties. *Health Educ.* 11:9, 1980.

Carper, B. A. The ethics of caring. *Adv. Nurs. Sci.* 1:11, 1979.

Creighton, H. Withdrawal of life support systems. *Superv. Nurse* 11:52, 1980.

Crisham, P. Measuring moral judgment in nursing dilemmas. *Nurs. Res.* 30:104, 1981.

Curtin, L., and Flaherty, M. J. *Nursing Ethics.* Bowie, Md.: Robert J. Brady, 1982.

Davis, A. J. When parents disagree on treatment. *Am. J. Nurs.* 80:2080, 1980.

Davis, A. J. Ethical considerations in gerontological nursing research. *Geriatr. Nurs.* 2:269, 1981.

Eldridge, T. M. Adolescent health care: The legal and ethical implications. *Pediatr. Nurs.* 5:51, 1979.

Fromer, M. J. Solving ethical dilemmas in nursing. *Top. Clin. Nurs.* 4:15, 1982.

Harris, E., et al. Nothing but the truth? . . . How much information to give a patient. *Am. J. Nurs.* 83(1):121, 1983.

Levine, M. Nursing ethics and the ethical nurse. *Am. J. Nurs.* 77:845, 1977.

Maslow, A. *Motivation and Personality.* New York: Harper and Row, 1970.

Maurice, S., et al. Ethics in professional nursing practice. *JOGN Nurs.* 8:327, 1979.

McNally, J. M. Values. *Superv. Nurse* 11:27, 1980.

Prato, S. A. Ethical decisions in daily practice. *Superv. Nurse* 12:18, 1981.

Robbins, D. Developing your ethical perspective. *JEN* 8:100, 1982.

Ryden, M. B. An approach to ethical decision making. *Nurs. Outlook* 26:705, 1978.

Scott, D. W. Ethical issues in nursing research: Access to human subjects. *Top. Clin. Nurs.* 4:74, 1982.

Simon, S., and Kirschenbaum, H. *Values Clarification.* New York: Hart, 1972.

Smith, S. J., et al. Ethical dilemmas: Conflicts among rights, duties and obligations. *Am. J. Nurs.* 80:1462, 1980.

Steele, S. M., and Harmon, V. M. *Values Clarification in Nursing.* New York: Appleton-Century-Crofts, 1979.

Thompson, H. O., et al. Ethical decision-making in nursing. *MCN* 6:21, 1980.

Uustal, D. Values clarification: Application to practice. *Am. J. Nurs.* 78:2058, 1978.

QUESTIONS FOR REVIEW

1. Which of the following is a true statement regarding the nursing code of ethics?
   a. Such a code determines your legal responsibility.
   b. The American Nurses' Association code of ethics lists salary standards.
   c. A code of ethics offers a guideline of "right" actions.
   d. Such a code must reflect your personal values or you cannot practice nursing.

2. Which of the following statements is true of personal values?
   a. Personal values are instinctive and not learned.
   b. The terms *personal value* and *goal* are synonymous.
   c. A person's personal values guide his actions.
   d. Personal values remain constant throughout life.

3. An indication that someone believes strongly in a value is:
   a. He defends it verbally.
   b. He learned it from his parents.
   c. He didn't have to choose it.
   d. He learned it after age 21.

4. Which of the following is *not* a statement of the American Nurses' Association code of ethics?
   a. The nurse maintains competence in nursing.
   b. The nurse acts to safeguard the patient.
   c. The nurse provides service with respect for human dignity.
   d. The nurse requires patient participation in care.

5. The manufacturer of a new brand of aspirin asks you to appear in uniform in a commercial. Your ethical response to this should be:
   a. It is all right as long as he does not pay you.
   b. Nurses cannot ethically advertise products.
   c. You must have conclusive proof that it is a good product first.
   d. It is illegal for nurses to advertise medicine.

6. You are assigned to care for Mrs. Smith, a patient who is ill because she swallowed 100 aspirin in an apparent suicide gesture. When you begin to care for her, you realize that she is a neighbor. At dinnertime, your mother asks you what person you cared for at the hospital. Which of the following answers is best ethically?
   a. A patient named Mary Smith who swallowed aspirin.
   b. Mary Smith, a patient who attempted suicide.
   c. A person from the neighborhood who attempted suicide.
   d. A patient who swallowed aspirin.

7. On the second day you care for Mrs. Smith, she offers you a dollar for going to the news stand for her to buy cigarettes. Which act would be best for you ethically?
   a. Take the money but tell her she needn't have offered it.
   b. Take it because it is under $5.
   c. Take it and offer to buy coffee for the nursing staff with it.
   d. Refuse the money; you consider the errand part of her care.

8. You are working as a staff nurse and the agency you work for has bought a new type of intravenous infusion pump. You have difficulty getting it to work correctly, and your nursing supervisor chides you because you did not read the article in a current nursing journal on such a pump. She says your action is unethical. On what statement from the American Nurses' Association code of ethics does she base this?
   a. Nurses should subscribe to nursing journals.
   b. Nurses have particular responsibility in regard to intravenous fluid.
   c. Nurses have an obligation to maintain competence in nursing.
   d. Nurses have a particular responsibility in regard to electrical equipment.

9. On a busy day in a clinical area you do not have time for lunch. A patient offers you the dessert from her lunch tray. Your ethical responsibility in regard to this is:
   a. Refuse it (the dessert is part of her care).
   b. Refuse the dessert and state that you do not eat people's food because it is so germ laden.
   c. Accept it and thank her for her consideration.
   d. Accept it (it does not involve a financial matter).

10. Mr. Burrows is a difficult patient to care for because he makes sexual advances while you give care. Which decision reflects the most ethical course of action?
    a. Refuse to care for Mr. Burrows and ask to have him moved to another unit.
    b. Give less than quality care so Mr. Burrows asks to be transferred.
    c. Maintain quality care despite the difficulty.
    d. Agree to give quality care if Mr. Burrows changes his behavior.

4. LEGAL CONSIDERATIONS OF NURSING PRACTICE

OBJECTIVES

Upon mastery of the material in this chapter, you should be able to:

1. Describe the sources and types of United States law.
2. Describe the special characteristics of the patient-nurse relationship.
3. Define the terms *negligence*, *malpractice*, *libel*, *slander*, *false imprisonment*, *assault*, *battery*, and *invasion of privacy*.
4. Describe the reason for Good Samaritan Acts.
5. Describe the nurse's role in filling out incident reports.
6. Describe the nurse's role in obtaining informed consent.
7. Describe the characteristics of a suit-prone nurse and patient.

TERMS

The terms important for an understanding of this chapter are shown below and defined in the glossary:

assault
battery
civil law
common law
criminal law
defendant
libel
plaintiff
slander
tort

Nursing care should always be directed toward the optimal well-being of the patient. It should always be carried out thoroughly and with deliberate thought (quality care). A philosophy of care that always directs you toward that end is to think of every patient you care for as your *first* patient, your *only* patient, and your *last* patient. Legally, nurses are required to offer a level of care that is reasonable under the circumstances.

SOURCES OF LAW

Legislative Law

Legislative law is legislated or originated by a government body. Since the supervision and licensing of nursing is delegated to the state level, the state legislative body is an influential and controlling body on nursing. State legislatures, for example, originate nursing practice acts (the written statement of what a nurse is allowed and forbidden to do in that state). Speed limits, zoning ordinances, and building codes are other examples of legislative law.

Common Law

Common law is a second source of law, derived from English tradition. It is sometimes referred to as the law of *precedent* or judge-made (judicial) law. This second source of law is necessary because state, federal, and local legislatures cannot anticipate every crime that people will commit or every civil law violation that will require a judicial remedy.

For example, speed limits (legislative laws) originally only referred to automobiles. There was no clear state statute to say whether a motorcyclist was as responsible as an automobile driver to abide by speed limits. The first time a person on a motorcycle broke a speed limit a judge had to review the situation and make a decision as to the motorcyclist's liability. Common law decisions of this nature are just as binding as legislative law. After one common law decision in a given state on a particular subject has been rendered (a motorcyclist must obey speed limits), all other decisions involving the same circumstances will be rendered in the same manner and will follow the precedent set by the first case (all motorcyclists must obey speed limits). Common law decisions often serve as an interim measure until new legislation on the subject can be established. As many legal questions of nursing involve new procedures or new roles where the legislature has not established statutes, common law decisions in every state have important relevancy to nursing.

TYPES OF LAW

Criminal Law

Criminal law is designed to protect the physical safety and property of people at large. It is divided into *felonies* and *misdemeanors*. The most commonly recognized felonies are murder, arson, manslaughter, robbery, and rape. Misdemeanors include assault, motor vehicle violations, and many so-called white-collar crimes. If a person is found guilty of a criminal law, he pays a penalty to the governing body that originated the law (imprisonment or a fine or both).

Civil Law

Civil law is law controlling most offenses against individuals. If a person is found legally liable for a civil law violation, he pays a sum of money to the offended individual. Most legal controversies in which nurses are involved are civil actions. Violations of civil law causing injury or serious inconvenience to individuals are sometimes described as *torts*.

THE NURSE'S RESPONSIBILITY OR LEGAL ACCOUNTABILITY FOR CARE

A nurse's responsibility or relationship to her patient's need is recognized, legally speaking, to be on a higher level than an everyday person-to-person relationship. A nurse must take her responsibility for patient care seriously and conscientiously. A patient-nurse relationship may be established by the simple introduction, "Hello, I'm Miss Jones (or Mary Jones); I'm going to be caring for you today," or by beginning care. The fact that it may be begun by giving care and not only by an oral or written commitment means that your relationship with an unconscious patient or a child under the age of reason is just as binding as your relationship with a patient where oral contract is made. Once a nurse-patient relationship is established, you are required to render quality care to that individual until such time as you are relieved by another health care provider (Fig. 4-1).

Abandonment

Part of the nursing-patient relationship implies that you will provide or supervise the care of a patient until properly relieved. If you should leave a person without care and harm should come to him during that time, your departure and absence might be labelled as *abandonment*. This legal pitfall is why it is important to notify someone before you leave a patient unit to run an errand, to eat lunch, or to leave for the day. Someone should be observing your patients while you are absent and should be made aware of any special problems or concerns of yours concerning your patients.

Remember that a nurse-patient relationship is established by the act of beginning care. If you should agree to assist a physician with a procedure in an operating room, for example, and after arriving in the room and beginning care discover that the procedure is a distasteful one to you (or, in the instance of abortion, one immoral to you), you cannot merely announce at that time that you will not assist and leave. If harm should result from your absence, this could be interpreted as abandonment or irresponsibility. Abandonment could result in (1) a lawsuit, and (2) suspension or loss of one's nursing license. The time to announce that you do not wish to assist with the procedure because of personal religious or ethical beliefs is at the time of employment or as soon as you become aware that you may be called upon to so assist. By putting your hospital on early notice, you ensure that they have sufficient time to contact persons who will be able to competently assist and

FIGURE 4-1. A nurse renders special care to a patient.

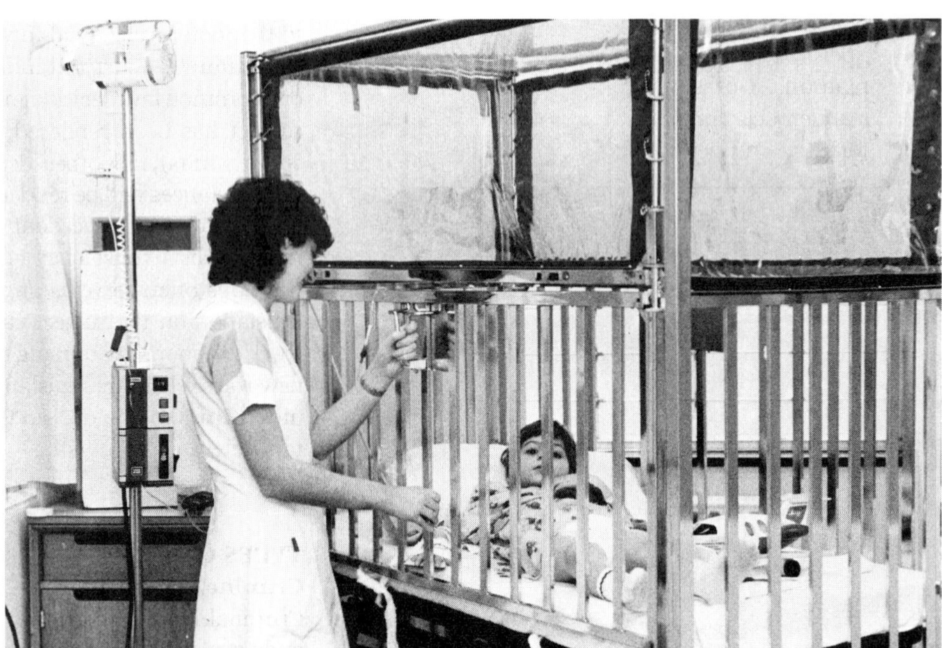

follow through with the care of such patients. The nurse-patient relationship is a special bond respected by law and must not be initiated lightly or irresponsibly.

Respondeat Superior

Respondeat superior is a Latin phrase that means "Let the master answer." It implies that an employer is responsible for the work of his employees. If you take your watch to a jewelry shop, for example, and speak with the owner of the shop about having it repaired, you expect that the repair will be of the quality that you agreed upon, no matter who actually does the repair—the shop owner or someone to whom he delegates the repair of that particular brand. People being seen for health care have the same right to know that no matter who gives them care—a nurse, an aide, a student nurse—the employer involved will be legally liable for any negligence involved in the rendering of such care. A nurse as the representative of the employer is responsible for the actions of auxiliary clinical personnel who work with her. If, for example, a nurse asks an aide to take some medicine to Mr. Smith in Room 312 (a duty far beyond an aide's job description for that agency) and the aide administers it to Mr. Smith's roommate instead and harm results from the wrong administration, the nurse would be just as responsible for the error as if she had given the wrong medicine. This means that when you ask an auxiliary worker to help you with patient care, you must be certain that it is a type of care that the aide is qualified to do and is authorized to do by law and by the aide's job description.

Student nurses are legally accountable for their own actions. A nursing instructor might also be found liable if the action of a student nurse resulted in injury to a patient and if it could be shown that the student was not properly instructed or supervised. Many times your instructor is asking you about your patient, your actions, or the principle behind what you are doing to evaluate your progress. At other times she is asking you these questions to be certain that you are proceeding safely. Her reputation and perhaps her nursing license are intrinsically tied to yours by legal as well as caring reasons.

This doctrine of *respondeat superior* extends upward as well as downward in lines of authority. A hospital is responsible for the actions of its nurses. If you, as a nurse employee, should negligently cause harm to a patient, the hospital and you can be sued. If you were acting within the scope of your employment and following hospital policy, the entire out-of-court settlement or court judgment for money damages would probably be paid by the hospital because of the *respondeat superior* doctrine.

Each nurse graduate or student is ultimately responsible for her own actions, however. If you were not following hospital policy and if a patient was injured as a result of this and sued your hospital, after the law suit was settled and the hospital paid a money settlement, the hospital might choose to sue you to recover damages. Nurses working as private-duty nurses are always regarded as independent contractors and so do not have the insurance protection usually provided by the hospital or health agency for its employees.

THE NURSE'S RESPONSIBILITY FOR HER ACTIONS

As mentioned, most nursing legal controversies involve areas of civil law (torts) or are a violation of a duty owed to the patient by the provider of care. Such instances center around the areas of negligence and malpractice.

Negligence

Negligence laws apply to all citizens. Negligence is the omission (not doing) or the commission (doing) of an act that the average prudent (sensible) person would or would not do. The average reasonable person, for example, stops at stop signs when driving his automobile and proceeds across the intersection when it is safe to do so. Running a stop sign and, by so doing, causing injury to a person or property is negligence by commission.

If you were sitting in a hospital lobby with your umbrella in the center of a busy aisle and someone tripped over it and was injured, you might be held negligent. Carelessness in some paperwork duties of nurses such as preparing laboratory forms which led to improper treatment might fall under the category of negligence doctrine because these duties are outside direct patient care.

Malpractice

Malpractice is negligence at a nursing level. It consists in the omission (not doing) or commission (doing) of an act that the average prudent (reasonable) nurse would or would not do. Negligent actions of nurses (aside from some paperwork as mentioned above or actions outside nursing time) are described as acts of malpractice rather than common negligence.

ELEMENTS OF MALPRACTICE

In order for malpractice to be established, three criteria must be present: a patient injury, a nursing error, and an association between the two (proximate cause).

For example, suppose you thoughtlessly break a rule of medicine administration (always check the patient's identification band before administration) and unintentionally administer some oral penicillin meant for Mr. Smith to his roommate Mr. Clyde. Fortunately no harm results from the ingestion. It would be difficult for Mr. Clyde to establish malpractice even though you have committed an error (you gave him medicine not ordered for him) because no harm resulted from your action. On the other hand, if Mr. Clyde had a penicillin allergy, and if after you gave him the penicillin by error, he became short of breath and before adequate help could arrive, he died, all the ingredients of malpractice would be present: injury (death), error (wrong patient), proximate cause (your error caused the injury).

For another example, suppose before you administer the penicillin you check Mr. Smith's chart for any indication that he is allergic to penicillin. Again, just before you hand it to him, you ask him if he has ever had a penicillin allergy (common sense measures before administering a drug that has known allergy reactions). Mr. Smith replies that he has no allergies and you find no notation to that effect on his chart, so you administer the penicillin. He swallows it and within minutes becomes short of breath; before adequate help can arrive, he dies. Although there is injury (death) and proximate cause (your administration of penicillin caused the reaction), it would be difficult to establish malpractice because the third component (nurse error) is not present (you did everything that a reasonable thoughtful nurse would do, even though death resulted).

In yet another example, suppose that you erroneously administer the medicine to Mr. Clyde and no harm results. Mr. Clyde returns home for a month and is then readmitted to the hospital with a blood clot (thrombus) in his leg. He says he is going to bring suit because the clot was caused by his worrying about the wrong medicine he was administered. Injury is present (thrombus); error is present (your medication error); proximate cause is not (there is no documented finding that worry leads to blood coagulation).

It is important to remember the three components that are essential for malpractice to be proven (and it is the patient's responsibility to prove it exists) in charting nursing actions. Always chart the precautions that you took to make a procedure safe as well as the procedure and the procedure outcome.

Practice Standards

Various means are used by the lawyer for the plaintiff (person bringing legal action) to prove that the nurse being accused did not act according to the way that a reasonable and prudent nurse would act.

NURSE PRACTICE ACT

Every nurse is responsible for practicing nursing within the limitations and the full scope of the Nurse Practice Act in the state where the nurse is employed. These acts vary from state to state but have many common features. The following box shows the Nurse Practice Act of New York state as signed into law in 1972.

Contrary to what many people assume, nurse practice acts are not detailed lists of actions that nurses may and may not do. Such a listing would have to be updated at least every six months as new equipment is designed or new procedures are originated. State legislatures would spend an inordinate amount of time regulating professions (and still always be behind current practice) if that were true. Instead, practice acts specify broad categories of duties (case finding, health teaching, executing medical regimes) that are within the scope of practice and equally broad categories that are excluded. For example, the nurse may not vary a medical regime; such an action by a nurse would be interpreted as practicing medicine. A nurse is allowed to evaluate patient response to illness

Excerpts from the New York State Nurse Practice Act: Legal Definition of Nursing Practice

SECTION 6901

Definitions. As used in Section 6902:

1. "Diagnosing" in the context of nursing practice means the identification of and discrimination between physical and psychosocial signs and symptoms essential to effective execution and management of the nursing regimen. Such diagnostic privilege is distinct from a medical diagnosis.
2. "Treating" means selection and performance of those therapeutic measures essential to the effective execution and management of the nursing regimen, and execution of any prescribed medical regimen.
3. "Human Responses" means those signs, symptoms and processes which denote the individual's interaction with an actual or potential health problem.

SECTION 6902

Definition of the practice of nursing.

1. The practice of the profession of nursing as a registered professional nurse is defined as diagnosing and treating human responses to acute or potential health problems through such services as casefinding, health teaching, health counseling, and provision of care supportive or restorative of life and well-being, and executing medical regimens prescribed by a licensed or otherwise legally authorized physician or dentist. A nursing regimen shall be consistent with and shall not vary any existing medical regimen.
2. The practice of nursing as a licensed practical nurse is defined as performing tasks and responsibilities within the framework of casefinding, health teaching, health counseling, and provision of supportive and restorative care under the direction of a registered professional nurse or licensed or otherwise legally authorized physician or dentist.

SECTION 6906

2. Nothing in this article shall be construed to confer the authority to practice medicine or dentistry.

but not diagnose disease, because then the nurse would be practicing medicine, not nursing.

Every nurse always works under the provisions of the Nurse Practice Act for the state where the nurse is licensed. A nurse not meeting the standard of practice would be legally liable for not doing what the average nurse does.

Standards of Nursing Care

The American Nurses' Association has published Standards of Nursing Care for the profession. These standards are published for nursing in general and for individual areas of nursing such as maternal-child health and community nursing. These Standards of Care are discussed in detail in Chap. 2. A nurse practicing outside the stipulations of these standards could be found liable for not practicing as does the average nurse.

Health Agency Policies and Procedures

All health care agencies have written policies and procedures that specify how actions should be carried out. The average nurse works in accordance with the policy and procedures of the health agency by which the nurse is employed. Not following these guidelines leaves any nurse potentially open for liability for not doing as the average nurse does.

If a policy is written in a way that is not practical (the amount of intravenous fluid that has infused must be recorded on the patient's chart every 15 minutes, for example), you should make every effort with the nursing policy committee to have the directive changed rather than just ignore it. In this instance, checking the amount of fluid absorbed in a short period of time is theoretically a good policy, but having to return to the desk area every 15 minutes to record it would seriously interfere with accomplishing nursing care and therefore is not practical; a recording interval of an hour is a more practical time frame.

Job Descriptions

The average nurse works within the bounds of her job description. When you apply for a nursing position, ask for a copy of the job description for the position for which you are applying and study the description thoroughly. If the description does not coincide with your interests and experience, you may be legally wise to refuse the position rather than to take it and work outside the description. If you desire the position but have reservations about your ability to perform some of the duties, express your concern to your employer and ask for as much in-service education as is necessary to bring you up to date and allow you to safely meet the requirements of the position.

Periodicals and Textbooks

Nursing periodicals and textbooks set out commonly accepted standards of care. If most textbooks state, for example, that the patient's vital signs (temperature, pulse, respirations, and blood pressure) are always recorded on hospital admission, and you fail to take such vital signs, you are not practicing nursing as does the average nurse. It is a nurse's responsibility to keep current in her field and know the latest developments as they apply to her care. At one time, for example, all patients with shock (low blood pressure, rapid pulse) from blood loss were placed in a Trendelenburg (head down) position to encourage blood perfusion to the brain and support brain cells; a nurse would have been remiss not to do so. Today it is becoming common practice *not* to use a Trendelenburg position, as it has been found that this may increase cerebral pressure to such a degree that it actually causes harm; a nurse would therefore be remiss today if she were to place a person in a Trendelenburg position without a specific order. Begin the habit of reading current nursing literature to keep updated on current exemplary nursing practices.

Expert Witness

Nurses with a broad range of professional expertise are occasionally called upon to serve as expert witnesses. A nurse expert witness may be asked to testify in court as to whether she considers the action of the nurse defendant to be consistent with what the average nurse, under those same circumstances, with the same background, education, and experience, would have done. Although nurse expert witnesses are generally nursing instructors or care coordinators, many nurses are considered experts at general nursing care by reason of years of experience and so might be asked to be an expert witness in court.

Patient Rights

Almost all health care agencies have printed patient rights (see The Patient's Bill of Rights, Chap. 17, for a typical example). The average nurse protects patients' rights and arranges her care in accordance with them. Violating patients' rights is outside the framework of exemplary nursing practice.

THE NURSE'S RESPONSIBILITY FOR PATIENT SAFETY

A nurse has a high degree of responsibility for keeping patients safe both physically and psychologically while in her care. A number of legal concerns center directly on patient safety.

Assault and Battery

Assault is the *threat* of harm to someone; battery is the *actual* intentional touching of another person's body without his consent. Shouting "Take this medicine or I'll give you an injection" is assault; giving an injection without the alert, oriented person's consent is battery. Both are tort offenses. Make a habit of speaking to people before you touch them; explain procedures before you initiate any action, not only to guard the person's right to know what you are going to do, but also because this action prevents you from unwittingly being responsible for battery. When faced with patient opposition, use better interaction techniques than threatening (such as re-explaining; asking for the basis for a person's lack of cooperation; reconsidering whether your action is the best) to avoid the risk of assault.

False Imprisonment

Freedom is a basic constitutional right. Keeping an alert, conscious person in a health care facility against his will is therefore illegal. Threatening a person to make him stay ("You can't leave until you pay your bill") carries the same weight as if you actually imprisoned him behind a door.

RIGHT TO REFUSE CARE

An alert, conscious person has the right to refuse health care if he so desires. Every health care facility has a refusal of medical care form which people choosing to leave the agency against their physician's advice are asked to sign. A court order may be obtained to restrain a patient from leaving a health care facility in certain instances such as a pregnant woman, a minor, or a person without adequate intellectual ability to make responsible decisions. In other instances, such as advanced pathology which has affected intellectual functioning, when the person has a communicable disease, or when the person is under heavy sedation, court intervention may be possible.

USE OF RESTRAINTS

Using restraints to hold a body part secure or to confine a person to a bed are a form of imprisonment and therefore cannot usually be instituted without a physician's order. A nurse can always apply as much restraint as necessary, however, to prevent a patient from hurting himself or hurting another person, even in the absence of a medical order.

When a physician's order for patient restraints is obtained, responsibilities concurrent with restraints must be thoughtfully followed (assess the patient or patient's extremity at least hourly for symptoms of constriction or interference of circulation). Judgment must be utilized as to whether a manual restraint is the best safety precaution or whether quietly sitting with the patient, repeating instructions and explanations, or asking the physician for a sedative medication order might be the preferred safety measure.

Invasion of Privacy

A person has a right to have his medical condition or other personal information about himself kept confidential. This means that communicating information about a patient to people outside his immediate health care team may be an invasion of privacy. Suppose, for example, the wife of Mr. Smith (hospitalized for abdominal surgery) asks you about the diagnosis of Mr. Clyde (hospitalized for a urinary problem) in the bed next to her husband. It sounds like a simple conversational question; however, to answer it would be an invasion of Mr. Clyde's privacy. These laws were established because this type of information might be detrimental to Mr. Clyde's welfare: If Mrs. Smith were to mention his illness to his insurance company representative or a potential employer, the information might result in loss of money or job. Student nurses should be careful, when preparing school assignments concerned with patients they have cared for, not to identify patients by name (use Mr. B., Joseph C., whatever). Do not irresponsibly leave notes taken from a chart in a library or other public area; if you do so, you might violate a patient's privacy. Informing another nurse in your hospital unit or clinic of a person's diagnosis is good communication; telling a school friend or someone in the hospital cafeteria is gossip (and a blatantly unprofessional action).

Defamation of Character

Defamation of character is making a derogatory statement about someone. Interestingly, whether the statement is true or not is not relevant in court. If the derogatory statement is written, it is *libel.* If it is spoken, it is *slander.*

Nurses are rarely involved in issues of libel. Being certain when charting that you quote what people tell you rather than drawing conclusions about what they are saying ("Patient says, 'I am always sick'" not "I think patient is a hypochondriac") prevents this. To avoid slander, choose carefully not only what you say but to whom you say it. For example, if Mr. Clyde's doctor is having difficulty establishing his diagnosis, he would appreciate your informing him that Mr. Clyde was hospitalized two months before for protracted gonorrhea (an illness that can lead to urinary tract obstruction). On the other hand, if you mention Mr. Clyde's previous diagnosis to his fiancee, that is potentially derogatory and slanderous.

THE NURSE'S RESPONSIBILITY FOR EMERGENCY CARE

The circumstances of health care vary as to whether the setting is an emergency one or not, but, providing for the presence of the emergency situation, a high standard of care must still be provided.

Good Samaritan Laws

No nurse is legally required to stop at the scene of an accident to give care, although one may feel morally obligated to do so. At one time, because of the laws in existence, it was almost detrimental for a nurse to give care at an accident scene. For example, suppose you stopped at the site of an automobile accident where you found a woman bleeding profusely from her arm. You took a clean handkerchief and applied pressure (the first aid measure of choice for bleeding). An ambulance arrived and transported the woman to the hospital where she had sutures placed to halt bleeding. Unfortunately, the woman developed an infection in the arm and was left with a permanent deformity. In the past, the woman could have sued you for placing a clean, not sterile, compress on an open cut and causing the infection (even though you saved her life), because as a nurse you should know never to place anything less than a sterile compress on an open wound. Consequently, nurses and physicians were reluctant to stop at accident scenes.

Good Samaritan Laws were passed to ensure that as long as a health care provider followed the best procedure *under the circumstances*, he could not be held responsible that the circumstances were less than perfect. Using a clean handkerchief for a compression bandage in the above example was a sensible solution under roadside conditions; using a greasy rag from the car trunk, on the other hand, would not be a sensible alternate for care.

Emergency Room Care

In many states all hospitals must provide emergency room care (Rhode Island, Vermont, and Maine are exceptions). A hospital does not have to admit a patient into the hospital after emergency care, however; it could transfer him to another facility at that point. This service for meeting emergency trauma and crisis needs must be independent of the patient's ability to pay.

FIGURE 4-2. A nurse witnesses the signing of a consent form.

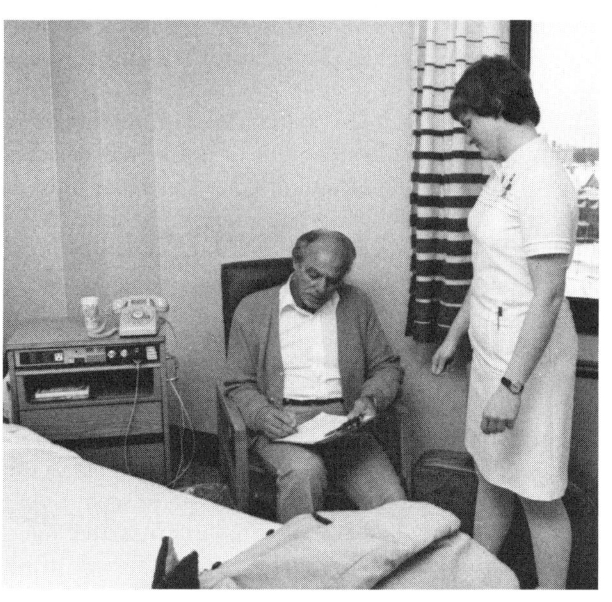

THE NURSE'S RESPONSIBILITY FOR INFORMED CONSENT

People have a right to choose whether they desire medical care or not. Before any health care is begun, the person is asked to sign a consent form detailing what care he desires. This consent, to be legal, must be *informed.* Before he signs, the patient must be told what the treatment consists of, what the relevant risks are, and what alternatives to the therapy could be considered. Nurses are frequently asked to witness a patient's signature (Fig. 4-2). Before you serve as a witness, you must listen to the physician's explanation of the procedure so that you are certain that what you are witnessing is *informed* consent. Consent is not informed if the explanation of the procedure was given when the person was too sleepy or otherwise too distraught to process the information; if a sedative or preoperative medication had been given; if the explanation was so technical that it could not be comprehended by the person; or if it was incomplete (no risks were mentioned). People on admission to a health care facility sign a general health care consent form; for a specific procedure that carries risk (surgery, biopsy, lumbar puncture, research, for example), additional consent must be obtained. Consent is not necessary for lifesaving procedures such as tracheotomy, intubation, or cardiopulmonary resuscitation when the time involved in giving the explanation would interfere with the emergency measure. It is assumed that the average person would consent to lifesaving measures such as these.

Do not witness a consent that you recognize as not an informed one. Ask the physician to repeat the explanation if you did not hear it or explain why in your opinion it is not an informed situation.

Emancipated minors are adolescents who provide the bulk of their own financial support or are the mother or father of a child. Even though such adolescents are not of legal age, they may sign for their own medical care or the care of their children.

HIGH-RISK AREAS OF PRACTICE

A number of nursing duties are more apt to involve legal controversies than others.

Medicine Administration

Medicine administration is always a high risk-area because it is an area of nursing where error may readily occur. Make a firm habit from the beginning of always following seven basic rules of medicine administration: right person, right time, right dose, right route, right medication, right information, and right precautions. Be certain you are aware of the action and purpose and usual dose of every drug you administer (Fig. 4-3).

You have the responsibility not only to carry out a medication order as it is written but also to recognize an order that is written incorrectly. You have the right to

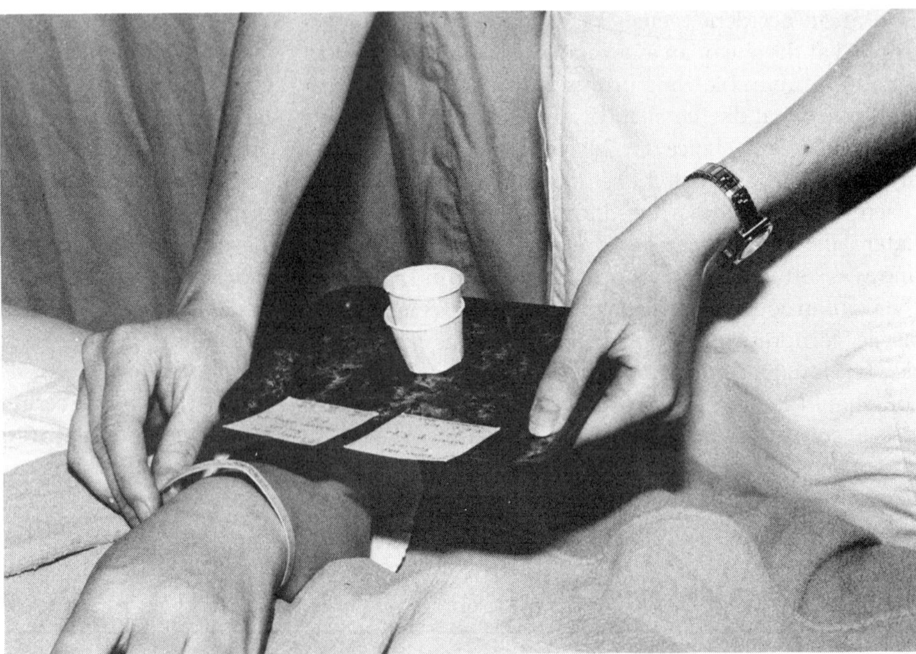

FIGURE 4-3. A nurse checks a patient's identification band before medicine administration.

delay administering a medication if, in your judgment, it is the wrong medication for the situation (you discover a physician has written an anticoagulation drug order for a person with heavy bleeding), the wrong dosage of a drug, or the wrong method of administration. In these instances, contact the physician and let her know your concern or otherwise follow your health care facility policy in this matter. You are entitled to such information as is necessary to resolve your concern about the appropriateness of the medication order.

Application of Heat

Application of heat is always a high-risk area because it invariably involves the potential for a burn to occur and, if an electrical apparatus is involved, the potential for electrical injury. Never use electrical equipment that is not well grounded (has a three-prong plug) or that has a frayed or damaged cord. Do not use electrical equipment around water. Be certain that heat lamps are placed a minimum of 12 inches from the patient. Time heat applications carefully so that a burn does not occur from overexposure to a heat source. If people are receiving sedatives or analgesics or have conditions that interfere with their perception of heat, your responsibility for keeping them safe increases in proportion to the degree of their loss of sensation.

New Equipment

Always be certain that you understand thoroughly how a new piece of equipment operates before you begin to work with it. Stating that you were unfamiliar with the equipment is no defense if patient injury should occur.

Transfers and Ambulation

Helping patients ambulate or transfer to a wheelchair or stretcher is always a high-risk area because of the possibility that the person may fall. Not using adequate siderails and leaving beds in high positions are also situations that invite patient injury.

Teaching

In order for a person to make decisions regarding his health care, he needs to be well informed of medications or treatments that he is receiving. You must be certain that the information you are supplying to patients is accurate. If you do not know the answer to a patient's question, simply answer, "I don't know—but I'll find out," rather than trying to guess what the answer would be.

If you neglect to tell a patient that drowsiness is a common side effect of an antihistamine he will begin to take after leaving the hospital, he might injure himself driving a car or working with a piece of machinery. Teaching is not a nicety of nursing; like almost all aspects of nursing it has legal implications.

Poor Communication

Some instances of legal liability occur not because of an action a nurse took but because she neglected to communicate her action or her assessment findings to the patient's physician or the care coordinator so that that party was aware of the necessity to initiate further measures of care. Be certain that you know precisely what

SUBJECT IDENTIFICATION-SECTION 1

1. I.R. # 755193 | 2. HOSPITAL NAME | 3. HOSP. CODE | 4. INCIDENT DATE | 5. TIME (CIRCLE) A P | 6. SHIFT (CIRCLE) D. E. N.

7. SUBJECT NAME | 8. CLASS USE TABLE 1 | 9. DATE OF BIRTH | 10. SEX (CIRCLE) M F | 11. MARITAL STATUS (CIRCLE) SING. WID. DIV. MARRIED LEG. SEP. | 12. SOC. SECURITY NO.

13. MEDICAL RECORD NO. | 14. STREET ADDRESS | 15. CITY & STATE | 16. ZIP CODE

17. HOME PHONE NO. | 18. BUSINESS PHONE NO. | 19. ATTENDING PHYSICIAN

20. (CIRCLE) PVT. SRV. | 21. STATION | 22. ROOM | 23. BED | 24. PRE-INCIDENT DIAGNOSIS

25. NAME OF CHARGE PERSON | 26. NAME OF PRIVATE DUTY NURSE

27. NAME OF PATIENT'S ROOMMATE | 28. NAME OF PATIENT'S ROOMMATE

CONDITIONS PRIOR TO INCIDENT-SECTION 2

29. AMBULATORY PRIVILEGES USE TABLE 2 | 30. INFORMED CONSENT (CIRCLE) YES NO | 31. MEDICATION PRIOR (CIRCLE) A) NONE B) 0-3 HRS. C) 3-6 HRS. | 32. COMMUN. STATUS USE TABLE 3 | 33. PHYSICAL STATUS USE TABLE 4 | 34. MENTAL STATUS USE TABLE 5 | 35. PHYSICAL ACTIVITY USE TABLE 6

CONDITIONS DURING INCIDENT-SECTION 3

36A. GENERAL LOCATION OF INCID. USE TABLE 7A | 36B. SPECIFIC LOCATION OF INCID. USE TABLE 7B | 37. LOC. VISIBILITY USE TABLE 8 | 38. LOC. PHYS. CONDITION USE TABLE 9 | 39. CALL SYSTEM USE TABLE 10 | 40. EQUIP. CONDITION USE TABLE 11 | 41. SEVERITY OF INCID. USE TABLE 12 | 42. NATURE OF INCID. USE TABLE 13

43. DESCRIBE BRIEFLY ANY INCIDENT NOT COVERED BY TABLE 13 INCIDENT CODES OR USE THIS SPACE TO ELABORATE-BE FACTUAL.

44. NAME OF OTHER PERSON(S) INVOLVED | 45. CLASS USE TABLE 1 | 46. NAME OF OTHER PERSON(S) INVOLVED | 47. CLASS USE TABLE 1

48. DESCRIPTION OF PERSONAL PROPERTY INVOLVED | 49. VALUE CLAIMED | 50. DESCRIPTION OF PERSONAL PROPERTY INVOLVED | 51. VALUE CLAIMED

CONDITIONS FOLLOWING INCIDENT-SECTION 4

52. EXAM (CIRCLE) Y N R | 53. EXAMINED BY: | 54. CLASS USE TABLE 1 | 55. TREATED? (CIRCLE) Y N R | 56. TREATED BY: | 57. CLASS USE TABLE 1

58. X-RAY (CIRCLE) Y N | 59. INCIDENT RELATED DIAGNOSIS/OBSERVATION | 60. PHYSICAL STATUS USE TABLE 4 | 61. MENTAL STATUS USE TABLE 5 | 62. PHYS. ACTIVITY USE TABLE 6

63. IF EQUIPMENT INVOLVED IN INCIDENT, DESCRIBE | 64. EQUIPMENT CONTROL NO. | 65. WAS REPAIR ORDERED? (CIRCLE) YES NO | 66. WAS EQUIP. REPAIRED OR TAKEN OUT OF SERVICE? (CIRCLE) YES NO

67-73 DID YOU NOTIFY? (CIRCLE)
CHARGE NURSE Y N SECURITY Y N
RESPONSIBLE PHYSICIAN Y N POLICE DEPT. Y N
RISK MANAGER Y N MED. EXAMINER Y N
SUPERVISOR Y N

74-75 WAS THE CHART DOCUMENTED- (CIRCLE)
BY THE NURSE? YES NO
BY THE PHYSICIAN? YES NO

76. WITNESS NAME-
ADDRESS-
PHONE-
| 77. CLASS USE TABLE 1 | 78. EMPLOYEE DISCOVERING INCIDENT | 79. CLASS USE TABLE 1

82. NAME OF REPORTER (PRINT) | 83. EMPLOYEE NO. | 84. CLASS USE TABLE 1

80. WITNESS NAME-
ADDRESS-
PHONE-
| 81. CLASS USE TABLE 1 | 85. SIGNATURE OF REPORTER | 86. DATE | 87. RISK MANAGER'S INITIALS | 88. CHECK IF S.N.F. INVOLVED ☐

H.U.M. COPY

FIGURE 4-4. An example of a hospital incident report form.

assessments you are expected to make on patients (not "Watch him" but "Take his pulse every 15 minutes and report if it rises above 100 beats per minute") or what procedures you are expected to do (not "Give him a lot of fluid" but "Give him a minimum of 100 ml every hour for the next 4 hours"). This type of instruction not only clarifies your actions but alerts you to an expected point of communication.

THE NURSE'S RESPONSIBILITY FOR INCIDENT REPORTS

An incident report (Fig. 4-4) is a report made to document any occurrence of patient injury or potential injury. In many states incident reports are admissible as evidence in court, so that when filling one out, remember that such a report should be factual but not self-incriminating. Remember that in every situation your actions are evaluated by determining whether they were proper under the circumstances that existed at the time. An incident report is your opportunity to explain the circumstances as they existed and the safeguards you took to make the procedure safe. You use an incident report to demonstrate that it was not your fault that, unfortunately, despite all your precautions, an injury did occur.

Incident reports should not include angry statements such as "This is a good example of why we need more in-service education programs" or "I think this brand of equipment is cheap and hard to use." Such statements are self-incriminating (you are saying that you knew that you needed more instruction on the use of the equipment) and immature (you want to convey a feeling of competency, not one of irresponsibility). Seek recourse and remedies for these problems through other sources.

A physician must be notified that an injury or potential injury has occurred. Record on the form that she was notified, the time of notification, and her action.

THE LAWSUIT-PRONE NURSE

Some nurses practice as if to attract lawsuits. People in general bring lawsuits against health care personnel because they are unhappy with the quality or outcome of care. Their happiness with care has a great deal to do with the concern or attitude of those who give that care. A nurse who practices impersonally—not extending people the courtesy of calling them by name or remembering their names, not explaining procedures before they are done, not explaining what medications are being given and how they will work, not explaining what can be expected from a treatment or laboratory test—is asking for people to be unhappy with her. Obviously, a nurse who practices on the edge of safety—knowing a little but not very much about the danger signs of illness, the drugs she administers, or the equipment she works with—is suit-prone and is not practicing as a good nurse.

THE SUIT-PRONE PATIENT

Illness is always a time of stress. People under stress need support people around them to serve as buffers. If they do not have this type of support, they turn to health care personnel. If they do not receive support from health care people, they may turn to lawyers.

A major role of a nurse is to serve as a supportive, concerned person for people who need this kind of interaction during particularly stressful times in their lives (Fig. 4-5). People who have a poor outcome from illness become angry and may manifest this anger in the form of lawsuits against their health care providers. People who do not understand what has happened to them are angry at being surprised and may initiate a lawsuit as a consequence of this form of anger.

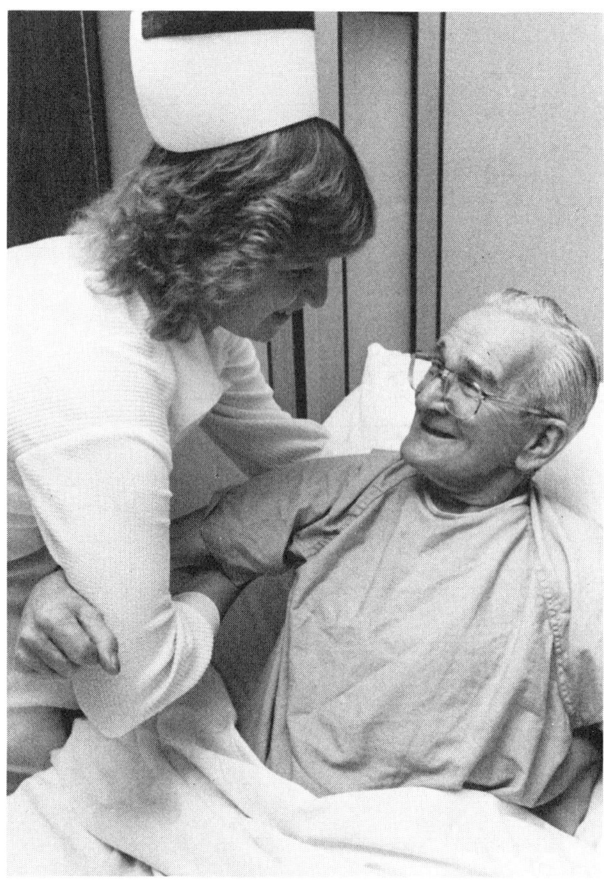

FIGURE 4-5. The nurse serves in a supportive, concerned role.

Patients who are at high risk for initiating lawsuits, therefore, are those who are surprised, angry, disappointed, depressed, stressed, or lonesome. People who are less apt to initiate lawsuits are those who have a constructive, open relationship with their health care personnel and have been fully informed about their care.

STATUTE OF LIMITATIONS

If you commit an error in nursing practice today, you would not be completely free of the possibility of being sued until enough time has passed so that a malpractice suit could no longer be brought against you. All states have statutes of limitations or time spans within which people can bring suit. After that period of time has passed, the threat of lawsuit is over. In most states the time span is three to five years. The exception to that is the maternal-child health area of nursing. There are instances in which, although the parents chose not to bring a lawsuit against health care personnel concerning a child's injury, when the child reached legal age, he was allowed to bring the suit himself. This privilege has implications for charting. No one can remember what he or she did or was thinking three or five years previously, much less twenty years. Always write nursing notes as if a long span of time will intervene before you

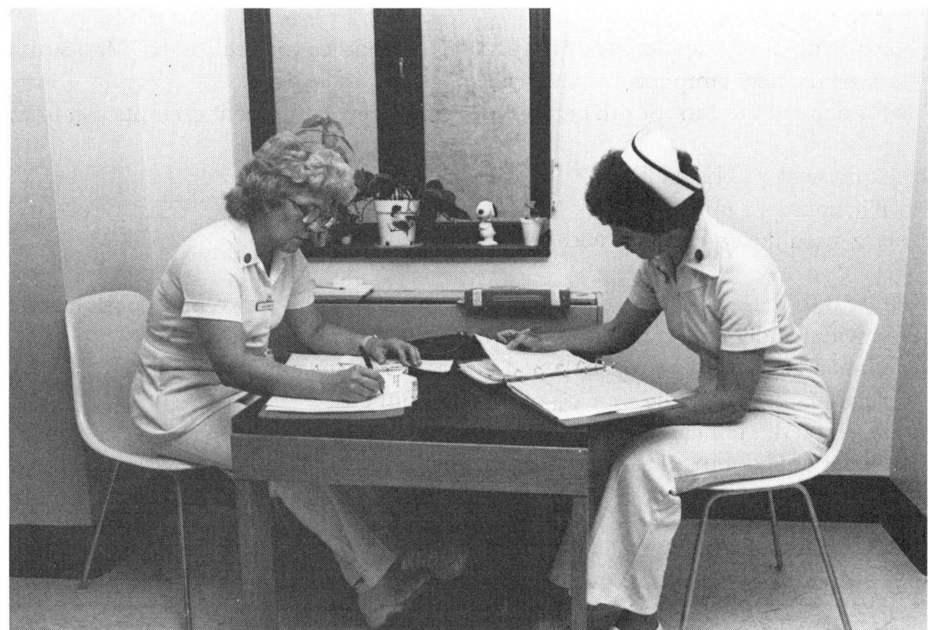

FIGURE 4-6. Nurses prepare their nursing notes, which are a legal record of care.

read them again. Be certain that they are clear and concise so that they can be interpreted clearly after a long period of time (Fig. 4-6).

LEGAL RESPONSIBILITY AND NURSES

Nursing grows more complex daily. The responsibilities undertaken by modern nurses were not imagined by nurses even ten years ago. As nursing grows more complex, it must continue to remain safe or technical advances will in the end not be therapeutic. Functioning at a safe level of practice with patients who are well informed as to the actions and procedures you are taking with them is your best assurance that you are working within the legal dimensions of quality patient care.

SUGGESTED READINGS

Annas, G. J. Invasion of privacy in the hospital. *Nurs. Law Ethics* 2:3, 1981.

Creighton, H. *Law Every Nurse Should Know* (3rd ed.). Philadelphia: Saunders, 1975.

Creighton, H. Legal concerns of nursing research. *Nurs. Res.* 26:337, 1977.

Creighton, H. Law for the nurse manager. Should nurses report negligence in medical treatment? *Nurs. Manage.* 14(1):47, 1983.

Cushing, M. A judgment on standards . . . circumstances under which a patient should be placed in seclusion. *Am. J. Nurs.* 81:797, 1981.

Cushing, M. "No code" orders: Current developments and the nursing director's role. *J. Nurs. Adm.* 11:22, 1981.

Doll, A. What to do after an incident. *Nursing 80* 10:73, 1980.

Doudera, A. E. Legal responsibility for nursing negligence. *Today's OR Nurse* 2:12, 1980.

Eldridge, T. M. Adolescent health care: The legal and ethical implications. *Pediatr. Nurse* 5:51, 1979.

Greenlaw, J. When leaving siderails down can bring you up on charges. *RN* 45(12):75, 1982.

Hollowell, E. E. What every nurse should know about tort liability. *Hospitals* 51:97, 1977.

Horsley, J. E. Think twice before you give advice. *RN* 43:95, 1980.

Horsley, J. E. Short staffing means increased liability for you. *RN* 44:73, 1981.

Horsley, J. E. You can't escape the Good Samaritan role—or its risks. *RN* 44:87, 1981.

Kreitzer, M. Legal aspects of child abuse: Guidelines for the nurse. *Nurs. Clin. North Am.* 16:149, 1981.

Mancini, M. Nursing, minors and the law. *Am. J. Nurs.* 78:124, 1978.

Nardecchia, M. A., et al. The policy manual: A basis for legal protection. *Nurs. Admin. Q.* 5:57, 1980.

Newton, M., et al. Guidelines for handling drug errors. *Nursing 77* 7:62, 1977.

Northrup, C. E. Responding to the malpractice crisis. *Am. J. Nurs.* 80:2245, 1980.

O'Sullivan, A. L. Privileged communication. *Am. J. Nurs.* 80:947, 1980.

Regan, W. A. You don't have to tolerate substandard hospital practices. *RN* 44:99, 1981.

Regan, W. A. The nurse as expert witness: Are you ready? *RN* 45:75, 1982.

Rozovsky, L. E. Answers to the 15 legal questions nurses usually ask. *Nursing 78* 8:73, 1978.

Shindul, J. A. legal restraints on restraint . . . civil commitment. *Am. J. Nurs.* 81:393, 1981.

Wiemerslage, D. Informed consents. *Crit. Care Update* 9:39, 1982.

QUESTIONS FOR REVIEW

1. You are using a new type of heat lamp as ordered for Mrs. Smith. After 10 minutes you realize that Mrs. Smith has been burned because you used the new lamp incorrectly. Legally,
   a. You cannot be held liable for damages to Mrs. Smith because the use of new equipment exempts you from blame.
   b. The manufacturer of the equipment will be liable.
   c. You are liable for your own actions as a nurse.
   d. You are liable only if you have used the equipment twice before.

2. You begin care for Mrs. Smith at 3:00 P.M.; at 3:30 P.M. your nursing shift is over but no evening nurse has yet arrived. If you leave without providing adequate supervision for Mrs. Smith's care:
   a. You might be held guilty of abandonment if injury happened to Mrs. Smith in your absence.
   b. You owe Mrs. Smith no obligation after the time your usual nursing shift ends.
   c. You owe no legal obligation as you did not care for her one full hour.
   d. You would not be held liable for abandonment as long as you stated in your notes that you were leaving.

3. Mr. Jones is sleeping when you go to administer an injection to him. If you give it without waking him, you might be guilty of:
   a. Negligence.
   b. Assault.
   c. Battery.
   d. Libel.

4. If you write something that is derogatory to Mr. Jones' reputation, you could be guilty of:
   a. Slander.
   b. Negligence.
   c. Libel.
   d. Assault.

5. If you make an error in medication administration, you might be legally guilty of:
   a. Malpractice.
   b. *Respondeat Superior.*
   c. Negligence.
   d. Carelessness.

6. In the United States the legal control of nursing is at which level?
   a. Federal.
   b. State.
   c. County.
   d. City.

7. A patient-nurse relationship is established when you:
   a. Chart your first nursing note.
   b. Begin care.
   c. Have given care for 1 hour.
   d. Have given care for 8 hours.

8. If you suspect the dosage of a medication order is too high, your *best* action in regard to this would be:
   a. Delay giving it until an adequate explanation is given you for the dosage.
   b. Give it one time; do not repeat the medication until the dosage is confirmed.
   c. Give it if it is an oral medication; delay it if it is an injection.
   d. Give the dose you know is appropriate.

9. Three criteria necessary to prove malpractice are:
   a. Injury, error, assault.
   b. Error, proximal cause, lack of consent.
   c. Proximal cause, negligence, nurse error.
   d. Error, injury, proximal cause.

10. To review the definitions of legal terms, match the definitions in column 2 with the statements in column 1.

a. A spoken statement of a derogatory nature.
b. The omission or commission of an act that another sensible person would do or not do.
c. A report detailing a patient injury.
d. A written statement of a derogatory nature.
e. Touching someone without their permission.
f. A type of law concerned with offenses against the individual.
g. The omission or commission of an act that another sensible nurse would or would not do.
h. A threat to commit bodily harm.
i. Leaving a patient without adequate supervision of care.
j. Consent is only legal if it is this.

1. Malpractice
2. Libel
3. Battery
4. Negligence
5. Assault
6. Informed
7. Abandonment
8. Incident
9. Civil
10. Slander

5. RESEARCH CONSIDERATIONS OF NURSING PRACTICE

OBJECTIVES

Upon mastery of the material in this chapter, you should be able to:

1. Define nursing research.
2. Describe common types of research studies.
3. List reasons for conducting nursing research.
4. Define common terms used in research articles.
5. Describe steps to use in evaluating a research study.
6. Describe the importance of nursing research.

TERMS

The terms important for an understanding of this chapter are shown below and defined in the glossary:

assumptions
control group
correlation
data
deductive reasoning
dependent variable
frequency distribution
Hawthorne effect
hypothesis
independent variable
inductive reasoning
mean
median
mode
population
sample
statistical significance
variable

IMPORTANCE OF RESEARCH

Research is the controlled investigation of a problem using the scientific method. Bodies of professional knowledge grow and expand to the extent that people in that profession plan and carry out research. Nursing research is the controlled investigation of a problem that has implications for nursing practice. It is the method by which the foundation for nursing grows and expands and improves.

Even as a beginning student in nursing it is time to begin to think of yourself as a possible researcher for not only what you can learn from nursing but what you can contribute to nursing's body of knowledge some day. In your everyday care of patients you may be asked to make assessments or observations as part of another person's research project. You might wonder whether a practice could be accomplished another way; for example, would it be possible for patients who feel well to take their own temperatures? Many reading assignments are based on conducted research. Presentations made at workshops or conferences are often based on the speaker's research results. It is helpful to have an elemental understanding of the research process and a beginning ability to evaluate a research study in order to read journal articles and listen to research presentations meaningfully.

PURPOSE OF RESEARCH

A number of reasons exist for conducting nursing research. One reason is to improve the quality of nursing care (by proving that one way of doing something is better than other ways); to document the benefit of nursing care (patients who had a nurse with them in the first hour after surgery had better outcomes than those patients who had a nursing assistant with them); and to develop a scientific basis for nursing practice. One of the definitions of a profession is that it carries on research; nursing cannot be said to fill the requirements of a profession unless its members initiate and carry on original research.

One of the earliest nursing researchers was Florence Nightingale who recorded detailed observations about her nursing care during the Crimean War. Today, in order to obtain a master's or doctoral degree in nursing, persons must complete some form of research utilizing sound research procedure. All nurses need to develop a problem-solving attitude, read, and share research findings.

LOCATING RESEARCH PROBLEMS

Research is basically problem solving or learning more about people or their behavior in some way. A potential for research exists whenever a problem interferes with people's well-being or behavior. As nursing is a practice profession, nursing research problems typically arise from practice settings. A nurse looks around her and

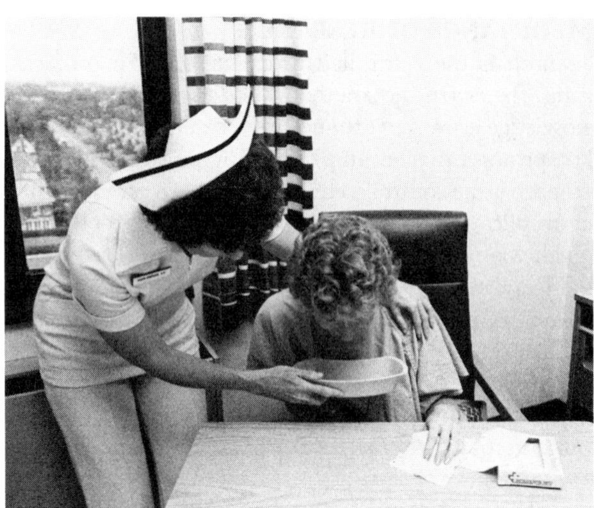

FIGURE 5-1. Nursing research problems arise from practice settings.

asks, "Why does this always happen?" or "What would happen if . . .?", and an idea for research is born (Fig. 5-1).

Some people never become researchers because they are willing to accept an answer such as "That's just the way things are" or "I don't think anyone can change that." Others recognize that if the real reason for the problem can be isolated, a solution to the problem may be found. These people are researchers.

Other studies in nursing research are conducted to enlarge the overall knowledge of nursing or to improve the process by which nurses plan and implement care. A person's experience, the areas in which she practices, and suggestions from others' research articles are sources for research studies.

PATIENT RIGHTS IN RELATION TO RESEARCH

The rights of people in research studies today are based on guidelines established after World War II known as the Nuremberg Articles. Such guidelines were established after it was discovered that people had been forced to participate in research studies by German physicians without informed consent or knowledge of the research being conducted. Justification for these research studies was that the research was so worthwhile that consent was not necessary. Today, the rights of people participating in research studies must be carefully considered and respected, and a person's informed consent to participate in a study must be obtained.

The Bill of Rights for Hospitalized Patients of the American Hospital Association that is issued to all patients in hospitals approved by the Joint Accreditation Committee of Hospitals includes the following statement concerning the rights of patients and research: "The patient has the right to be advised if the hospital proposes to engage in or perform human experimentation affecting his care or treatment. The patient has the right to refuse to participate in such research projects" (AHA, 1973).

Federal regulations require that a person involved in research receive a fair explanation of the procedures and of the risks and benefits involved, an assurance of confidentiality, a description of alternatives available to him, and the option to withdraw from the research at any time. Never participate in a research project unless you have assurance that these guidelines have been followed.

Nursing Ethics and Research

Any activity that a nurse performs must be consistent with the Nursing Code of Ethics. Research participated in or conducted by nurses must also meet these standards. One of the statements of the Code of Ethics—"The nurse participates in the profession's efforts to implement and improve standards of nursing" (ANA, 1976)—suggests that research is not only ethical (providing you have assurances that patient rights will be respected and the research will add to nursing's body of knowledge) but that not participating in it would be viewed as unethical.

Both the American and Canadian Nurses' Associations have printed guidelines for ethical considerations specific to nursing research. The following box lists the statements of the CNA.

TYPES OF RESEARCH

Research is a creative endeavor and it therefore can be conducted according to a number of different patterns.

Historical

Historical research is the study and interpretation of past events in order to explain present-day phenomena. An example of historical research is a description of the treatment of the many people who died in the 1917 flu epidemic. The strength of historical research is that patterns of behavior over a long time frame may be studied; a weakness is that a solution to a problem that worked in the past may no longer be applicable due to changing circumstances.

Case Study or Longitudinal

In case study research a researcher examines one person or one situation in detail, such as describing a patient condition every day following the onset of an illness. The strength of such research is its exactness and extensive detail; a disadvantage is that it may be faulty to generalize conclusions derived from the study of one individual or happening to others.

Survey

In survey research people are polled by the use of questionnaires or interviews in order to obtain information about some aspect of their lives or knowledge. Polling to learn people's opinions on candidates before elections is an example of this. A strength of such a technique is that

Canadian Nurses' Association Ethics of Nursing Research

THE SUBJECT

Respect for the value of human life, for the worth and dignity of human beings, and their rights to knowledge, privacy, and self-determination must underlie research practices in nursing as in other health disciplines. The legitimacy of involving human subjects in nursing research must be assessed within the context of these values. The right of the subject to informed consent, confidentiality, positive risk value, and competence of the investigator must be assured.

FREE AND INFORMED CONSENT

When individuals are involved as subjects of research, the researcher must obtain free and informed consent. Informed consent implies that every effort be made to have the subject understand the purpose and nature of the research and the use or uses to which the findings will be put, in such a way that he can appreciate the implications of participation or non-participation. He must also be informed that if any significant change in purpose, nature, or use of findings is contemplated, he will also be informed and have the right to consent or refuse to participate further.

Free consent means that the relationship between the researcher and the subject, and persons or institutions involved in his care will not place him under any obligation to agree to take part in the project against his own personal inclinations. It also means that his refusal to take part, or his withdrawal after having once consented, should not lead to any repercussions or recriminations. Free consent implies informing the subject that he has the right to withdraw at any point during the research.

If the nature of the research is such that fully informing subjects before the study would invalidate results, then this fact must be stated to the subject, together with whatever explanations can be given. There must be provision for appropriate explanation to the subject on completion of the study.

If the subject for any reason is unable to appreciate the implications of participation, informed consent must be obtained from the legal guardian or an impartial committee acting on behalf of the subject. If the research should impinge on the privacy or other rights of any third party, such as the spouse of the subject, this person's consent must also be obtained.

CONFIDENTIALITY

Subjects must be assured that confidentiality will be respected. Where anonymity is promised, it must be provided. Hidden coding to enable the researcher to identify individuals must not be resorted to. Every effort must be made to ensure that individuals and institutions cannot be identified.

INJURY, RISK, AND PRIORITIES

Research subjects must be assured protection against physical, mental or emotional injury. Should the research involve risk of injury, such risks must be weighed against the good to be achieved. Should the risk outweigh the positive value of the research, the project must not be pursued.

Where there is conflict between the rights of the subject and the needs of the researcher for freedom of inquiry, the conflict must be resolved with priority given to the concerns and rights of the subject.

THE RESEARCHER

In order to maintain high ethical standards, the nurse researcher must possess knowledge and skills compatible with the demands of the investigation to be undertaken. The researcher has responsibility to acknowledge personal limitations and to correct misrepresentations made by others. The researcher is obligated to develop the design and procedures appropriate to the study.

The researcher is accountable in varying ways to those participating in the investigation. The purpose of the research must be honestly represented, and any uses to which the findings may be put, made known to persons or institutions involved. In order to justify the investigation, the researcher must ensure that the purposes and anticipated outcomes are compatible with the financial investment and the people and resources used.

In order to ensure the integrity of the investigation, the researcher must present the project for review to a group of professional peers. With certain studies, ongoing reviews by a peer group may be mandatory.

THE SETTING

The milieu in which an investigation is to be conducted must be assessed in terms of the potential for a nurse researcher to conduct a study that is consistent with these guidelines. While the board and/or administrators of an institution or agency may require approval by its research committee of a nursing study as well as of any other proposal, any such approval body should include nursing representation. There should be ongoing provisions for coping with setting-related ethical problems during the course of the investigation.

Nurse researchers ought to be the principal investigators in the study of nursing problems and must be collaborators with other researchers in the study of interprofessional problems of health care. This interprofessional involvement indicates that a common code of ethics for health research should be developed to facilitate research in nursing and its related professions.

Source: Canadian Nurses' Association, Ethics of nursing research. *Canadian Nurse*, 68:23, 1972. Reprinted with permission.

a large number of people can be included in the sample; a weakness is that the cause of happenings or beliefs of the people surveyed—why such happenings occur or beliefs are held—may not be investigated.

Explanatory

Explanatory research investigates in detail a population the same as a survey technique but also examines what factors affect or cause the behavior that was determined to exist, such as the age, sex, or life experiences of people in the survey. A strength of such research is that it suggests ways that behavior is caused (so suggests ways that it could be modified); a disadvantage is that unless the surveyed population is large, conclusions as to causal relations may be as faulty as they would be with a single case study.

Empirical

Empirical investigation uses experimental designs and measures differences between two groups of individuals or settings. Comparing the illness rate of people who have periodic health checkups with that of those who do not would be an example of this type. A strength of such research is that, if properly conducted, results can be duplicated again and again; a disadvantage is that results can be interpreted wrongly if the research design allowed uncontrolled phenomena to interfere with the investigation.

EVALUATING RESEARCH STUDIES

Nursing research is reported most frequently in *Nursing Research*, a journal published six times annually since 1952, although many professional nursing journals publish articles based on a research study. Research studies are generally reported according to a commonly accepted format, which allows the researcher to describe how she conducted the research and the results and interpretations of the research. Understanding what each section includes allows you to evaluate as you read whether you can truly have confidence in the results and whether they will be applicable to your practice. In evaluating a research study, begin with an examination of the research sponsor and author.

Research Sponsor

A research article should describe or at least footnote any source of funding used for the study. Always read this to alert yourself to possible conflicting interests that could be present. A study to evaluate which brand of surgical instruments wears longest that was funded by the company that makes Brand A may be a legitimate study but it could also be heavily biased in preference of Brand A. One can have greater confidence in such a study if it is funded by an impartial source.

Qualifications of Researcher

Any nurse knowledgeable about the research process is capable of research, so a list of credentials or titles following a researcher's name does not ensure or distract from the quality of the research. Such credentials or titles are listed, however, because as with funding a researcher's title might reveal a conflict of interest (a person with the title of coordinator is probably very interested in showing that activities are well coordinated in his department). Some research is done as part of the requirements of a master's or doctoral degree; if this is so, this fact will be included in the description of the researcher's credentials. Such a statement usually implies that the research is valid and well done, but such time limits are imposed by this type of study that very often the number of people included in a sample population is very small. The smaller the sample of people studied, the more difficult it is to make generalizations from the study to the population at large.

Title

Research articles are titled to describe the research problem being considered, not for their ability to arrest attention. The title of a research article, therefore, often seems ponderous in relation to other articles: "A study of the reliability of self-temperature-taking in adult females" rather than "Self-care: Does it really work?" or "Good news: Patients can take their own temperatures." Do not let the titles of research articles intimidate you.

Statement of the Problem

Research studies begin with a statement of the problem that the researcher was interested in investigating. An example would be a description of how it is well documented that infection following childbirth is a grave and even fatal complication of childbirth. Infection is often first revealed by the presence of an elevated temperature. Nurses have always taken patients' temperatures because they must have a reliable assessment in such critical points in life. On the other hand, women following childbirth feel well; they have a need to "take hold" or function independently in order to prove to themselves that they are ready to take on the care of helpless newborns. Could women reliably take and record their own oral temperatures for the three days following childbirth? Would this be an acceptable area in which to encourage self-care?

As a rule, the statement of the problem is brief. If it is lengthy, it may indicate that the exact problem was not clearly delineated in the researcher's mind before the study was begun. A report introduced by a lengthy discussion of the importance of the problem suggests that the researcher was nervous that it would not stand on its own merits without some embroidery.

Ask yourself about a problem statement: Is it a problem that you agree is important? Is it one that will provide information relevant to your daily practice?

Review of the Literature

A review of the literature is a review of the same type of research that has been done in the past, in order to demonstrate that this new research study was done in order to duplicate (and therefore verify) earlier research or was originated as an extension of previous research because of a suggestion of a previous researcher. A published research article only contains a representative number of all the articles that were read by the researcher before preparing her research design, but it should include at least a number of references pertaining to similar research studies. If there are conflicting opinions concerning the research area, both sides should be represented. Accompanying the problem statement on the example of temperature-taking should be citations of previous studies on both temperature-taking and the reliability of adults at performing self-care. Review of the literature helps you to view the role of the current research in the perspective of other research and, again, is an aid in helping you to perceive how you will be able to use the research results in practice.

Ask yourself about the literature review: Is the scope of the articles cited comprehensive? Are recent research studies included? Are primary not secondary sources cited (to refer to Selye's concepts of stress, for example, the conscientious researcher quotes Selye's articles—a primary source, not Smith's article on Selye—a secondary source)?

Conceptual Framework

The conceptual framework, sometimes termed the study background, defines terms that are important for understanding the study, basic assumptions, and any other material that helps to place the study in a perspective for easy reading and comprehension. Although this type of information may not always strike you as interesting, always take a few minutes to investigate this section. Without this background knowledge, some of the conclusions of the study or the interpretation of the data may not be clear to you.

DEFINITIONS

A researcher should define any term she uses in the study, so that if you choose to duplicate the study at a later time or use the findings of the study, you can be certain that you understand exactly what procedure she used. Suppose, for example, a researcher chose a hospital for her study where there was an "adequate nurse-patient relationship." This term needs to be defined or qualified for specific settings so that you can be certain that your concept of adequate is the same as the researcher's (you may think one nurse to six patients is adequate; she may use the term to mean one to ten). In a study of independent temperature-taking, the terms *adult* and *temperature* would probably be defined.

ASSUMPTIONS

Assumptions listed in a research study are statements that everyone recognizes as facts (the sun always sets in the west and rises in the east). In a study of adult females taking their own temperatures, the meaning of *female* would probably be an assumption. If the study dealt with a phase of homosexuality or sexual deviation, the term would need to be defined as it might be necessary for interpretation of the study that the definition of female be precise.

VARIABLES

A research variable is a condition that may affect the outcome of the study or must be considered in evaluation of the information gained from the study. In a study of adult females taking their own temperatures, the thermometer used would be a variable. If one-third of the women used glass thermometers, one-third a new disposable type, and the other third an electronic thermometer, it would be difficult to group all the data obtained because three different types of data have been collected. An *independent* variable is one that can be controlled (if all women use glass, small-bulb thermometers, this variable becomes controlled); a *dependent* variable is the effect or response being measured, so is not controlled (in the above-mentioned study, the women's temperatures). In this section of a report the researcher explains how variables were controlled (temperature of the room was regulated, eyesight of the women was evaluated as normal, and so forth).

Ask yourself about this section of the report: Were all terms well defined? Are the author's assumptions true assumptions (everyone really believes these things)? Were all variables controlled except for the dependent one to be measured (would climate, family composition, physical setting, religion, intelligence, or other factors cause a difference in results)?

Hypothesis

A hypothesis is a statement of cause and effect or a statement of the expected relationship between the phenomena being studied. A good hypothesis is clear and understandable; it is stated so that it is testable. It is a refinement of the problem statement, a move from asking "What will happen if . . ." to "This will happen if. . . ."

In its best form it should imply not only that which is being studied but that which is not: The hypothesis "Adult female patients can take and record their 8:00 A.M. temperatures accurately during the first three days following childbirth" indicates that the women being studied are hospitalized (those not hospitalized are not studied); the 8:00 A.M. temperature recording is the measurement being studied (the 12:00 noon and 4:00 P.M. measurements are not); adult patients are being studied (adolescent girls hospitalized on the same unit were excluded from the study).

Ask yourself about a hypothesis statement: Is it well defined? Is it testable? (It does not matter whether it is worded in a negative or positive way—women can take their own temperatures or women cannot take their temperatures.)

Methodology

The methodology section of a research report describes the setting of the study, the population of people used, any measurement tools used, and how the collected data have been analyzed. In order to evaluate this category of information, you need to ask a few common sense questions about each division.

SETTING

The setting of a study is the geographic or environmental location in which the research was carried out. The setting chosen depends on the research question to be answered. If, for example, the researcher wanted to know what people being admitted to a hospital thought was important information to be told on admission, obviously the best place to investigate this question would be in a hospital or in the homes of people recently discharged from the hospital. If the question concerned disease incidence in a nursing home, the only possible setting for the investigation would be a nursing home. In some instances setting is not important, and the research can be conducted in college or specially designed research laboratories. Ask yourself: Was the setting chosen the best place to gather the information?

POPULATION SAMPLE

In most instances, if a researcher tried to investigate all the people or situations that could help answer her research question, the number of people involved would be so great that the research could never be practically conducted. Instead of attempting to do this, therefore, a researcher uses a sample or a representative group of people or instances rather than the entire population.

In order for the conclusions of the study to be valid, the sample population selected must represent the characteristics of the whole population. If a person mailed out 100 questionnaires, for example, and only five were returned, she does not have a sufficient sample group to predict any information. Such a small sample may not accurately represent the whole group; more likely it is composed of people with a special point to make. If a researcher states that her research findings will apply to people of all ages, the sample must include not just adults but children and infants of both sexes as well. For the temperature-taking study mentioned previously, obviously all people included in the sample must be adult females who have just given birth.

TABLE 5-2. TABLE OF RANDOM NUMBERS

10	8	26	11	55
5	96	2	64	69
23	65	44	73	60
14	72	81	34	17
38	12	72	47	93

Don't be misled into thinking that a random sample group was chosen by a researcher saying casually, "I think I'll use this person; I won't use that person." Most sample groups are chosen by the use of published random sample tables such as that shown in Table 5-2. To use the table, the researcher would use the tenth, then the next fifth, then the next twenty-third person admitted to the unit, and so forth. If the census of the patient unit was very small, the researcher might use the total admission number. There is no set size a sample must be. Questionnaire return rate should be over 50 percent in order to be acceptable. Otherwise, the size of samples is influenced by the individual study.

In any instance, the researcher should state how she arrived at her sample. Ask yourself about the population used: Were these the best people to use for this study? Was the sample size adequate so that I can trust the results?

INSTRUMENTS OR MEASUREMENT TOOLS

The researcher should explain and perhaps show an illustration of the actual measurement tool used to collect the data or information. This might be a tool such as a questionnaire, an interview format, an observational guide, an intelligence test, or measures of physical responses such as a sweat test, blood pressure determination, or pulse rate. In the temperature-taking study the only way that a researcher could know that the research subject did take her temperature accurately would be for the researcher to take the woman's temperature within a time frame close to when the woman took it (5 or 10 minutes). To analyze the information, the two recordings would be compared (Fig. 5-2).

Ask yourself: Was the measurement tool sensible to measure what was needed? If people under some form of stress were asked to fill out a questionnaire involving over 100 items, for example, you might question whether they answered the last 75 questions seriously or merely filled in numbers to finish the questionnaire quickly. If a researcher used a sophisticated psychological measurement tool such as a Rorschach (ink blot) test, was she qualified to interpret it (or did she seek qualified help)?

The more truly measurable phenomena a researcher

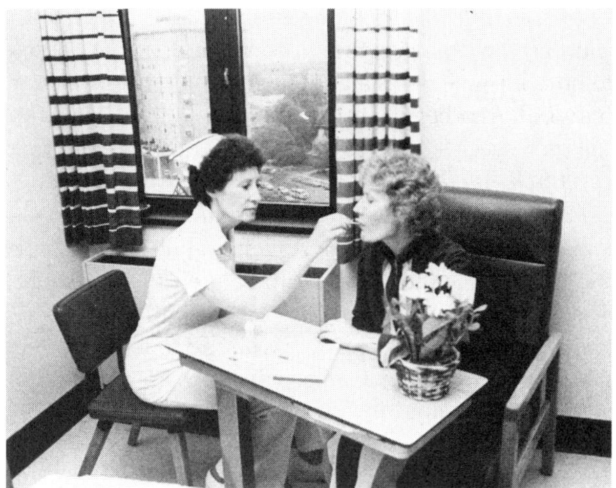

FIGURE 5-2. Both the woman and the nurse take and record a temperature reading.

uses, the more apt is the research to be reliable (measuring a pulse rate increased as a result of stress is more reliable than trying to assess whether the person appeared anxious). Subjective impressions tend to be biased depending on what the researcher expected to observe.

ANALYSIS

A research report should state how the data obtained were analyzed. It is often tempting to skip over this description as it can be technical. A major point to look for is whether the procedure seems logical. If a million questionnaires were returned, computer analysis should have been employed. Otherwise, the mental demands of evaluation of such a large number of questionnaire returns will almost surely have led to analytical error.

In examining this section, knowledge of a few statistical terms is helpful.

Frequency Distribution. Many researchers show the frequency distribution or align the numerical values obtained from the study in an order from the highest value to the lowest (or vice versa) to show the scope of the data obtained. Table 5-3 shows the frequency distribution of the 8:00 A.M. temperature recordings that were obtained by 14 patients on themselves. Three measures of central tendency (measures to determine the midpoint of the distribution) are frequently discussed. The *mean* of a distribution is the average number (all the numbers are totaled and divided by the number of values present); in this frequency distribution the mean is 99.3° (1390.2° divided by 14). The *median* is the middle value when the values are arranged in ascending or descending order; in this study the median is 98.8°. The *mode* of a frequency distribution is the most frequently occurring number; in this distribution it is 98.8°.

Various measures of variability—how far values vary from the central tendency—are also usually discussed. The *range* is the span between the highest and lowest

TABLE 5-3. FREQUENCY DISTRIBUTION OF 8:00 A.M. TEMPERATURES

101.2
100.6
100.2
100.2
99.8
99.8
98.8
98.8
98.6
98.6
98.6
98.4
98.4
98.2

values in a set of measurements—101.2° to 98.2° in this frequency distribution. The *standard deviation* is a description of the average deviation or distance of scores from the mean. Reporting the standard deviation of a group of figures alerts you to how spread apart was the range of scores (the greater the standard deviation, the greater distance between scores or the greater the spread of scores). One standard deviation from the mean includes 68 percent of all the values; two standard deviations include 95 percent; three standard deviations include 100 percent.

Common measurement tools that use median and standard deviation material are standardized height and weight growth charts (see App. D). The midline on such a chart is the median of the frequency distribution (the 50th percentile). The top and bottom percentiles (90th and 10th percentiles) represent 95 percent of the population studied or correspond to two standard deviations from the midpoint. These concepts should therefore not be completely unfamiliar; they are the basis for measures that you had your height and weight plotted against every time you had a health checkup until you reached age 18.

TEST OF STATISTICAL SIGNIFICANCE

One of the dangers of research is that differences in material obtained from two research groups may seem to be genuine but actually appear different only because of chance. Suppose that in the temperature-taking study the mean of the temperature recordings made by the researcher was 99.2°, while the mean of the temperature recordings made by the patients themselves was 98.8°. These figures suggest that the study hypothesis is not true, that patients cannot take their temperatures reliably, since the average of their recordings is different from the average of those obtained by the researcher. Is this really a difference, however? Suppose the researcher had 100,000 temperature recordings to analyze rather than 14? With this number of figures, would there still be a difference?

In order to determine this, researchers apply a test of statistical significance to their data. Frequently used tests are chi square and t tests. If the results of one of these tests reveal a figure less than .05 (abbreviated <.05), it is unlikely that the differences observed occurred by chance (the chances of the two figures being alike are only 5 in 100); if the results reveal a figure less than .01 (abbreviated <.01), it is *highly* unlikely that the differences observed occurred by chance (1 chance in 100).

Ask yourself: Was the data obtained adequately described? Were tests of statistical significance applied? If not, the researcher has little more to tell you than what she told you originally, that she thought there was a correlation or no correlation between two things; only if she applied a test of statistical significance can she say that there is truly a difference.

Interpretation

Following analysis of the data, a discussion of the findings and interpretation of their importance follows. Results are always discussed in the past tense and consist of the simple stating of facts, not generalizations to all situations: not "Adult women are capable of taking their own temperatures accurately" but "Adult women took their temperatures accurately." Researchers rarely state that they "proved" their hypothesis but that the hypothesis was supported and accepted or not supported and rejected. This is more than a matter of semantics; it reflects the researcher's willingness to admit that no conclusion is truly definite but open to further investigation.

Evaluate whether the stated conclusions really follow from the collected data. In the temperature-taking study, for example, a correlation between the temperatures recorded by both patients and nurses at 8:00 A.M. does not automatically lead to the conclusion that women can reliably take their temperatures at other times of the day. That would call for further investigation; it might turn out that some women are too tired by midafternoon to take their own temperatures and record them accurately.

THE HAWTHORNE EFFECT

The Hawthorne effect is an interesting phenomenon first noticed in 1920 during a research study at the Hawthorne Western Electric Plant in Chicago: When people know that they are being studied, they become more conscientious, take fewer work breaks, and speed up their productivity. If the study continues for a length of time, this effect wears off. If the study you are reviewing was of limited duration, see if the researcher mentioned that the Hawthorne effect could have been operating.

INDUCTIVE AND DEDUCTIVE REASONING

Researchers reach conclusions by using two types of reasoning. *Deductive* reasoning is reasoning that begins with general information and spreads to the specific. Detectives use this type of reasoning (a man has been murdered with a gun by someone who had easy access to him; his wife owns a gun; he may have been killed by his wife). Another example would be: Human beings are the only species capable of abstract thinking; Mr. Jones can think abstractly; Mr. Jones must be a human being.

Inductive reasoning is reasoning that starts with facts and spreads to the general: A woman kills her husband with a gun; therefore, guns can be used to kill people.

Ask yourself: Which form of reasoning is the researcher using? Either process will lead to faulty conclusions if generalizations or specifications are made without all the required information.

Discussion

The last section of a research report is a discussion of the implications of the results and suggestions for areas where further investigation is needed. The researcher points out limitations of the study such as a small sample size or a short time frame. In the example of temperature-taking, a topic for a follow-up study might be: Could adolescents also be depended on to take their temperatures while hospitalized? If that were true, it would be good practice to let them do so because adolescents like independent behavior.

Ask yourself about the discussion section: Can the implications truly be drawn from the results? Suppose the researcher stated that an implication of the temperature-taking study was that all hospitalized women could be depended on to take their morning temperatures accurately. That is a faulty generalization because an additional variable (feeling ill) is present in the average hospitalized woman. Women following childbirth are often exhausted, but because childbirth is a natural process are not usually ill.

PARTICIPATION IN RESEARCH

You may participate in research in three different ways.

Participation in Others' Research

At any stage in a nursing career you may be asked to participate in a research study such as the evaluation of new equipment. A health care agency, for example, might be experimenting to see which brand of syringe is most convenient for nurses to use. After using Brand A or Brand B you might be asked to record some information, such as whether the barrel of the syringe allowed any medicine to leak from it, whether you had any difficulty attaching the needle hub to the syringe, or whether breaking the syringe to dispose of it was difficult. At the end of a set period of time, an agency administrator would tabulate the information obtained and, based on nurse comments, decide whether to purchase Brand A or Brand B.

Be certain that, when you participate in this type of research, you do it with an open mind and not a biased one based on familiarity or what you think the answer will be. Otherwise, you tend to see qualities (either good or bad) that are not there but that you imagine are there.

Participating as a Research Subject

As a student in nursing or as a graduate nurse (or at the supermarket as a consumer) you may be asked to volunteer as a research subject. Before serving as a research subject, be certain you understand the scope and purposes of the study and exactly what will be expected of you. Nothing is more disappointing to a researcher than to have a subject withdraw from a study while it is in progress. If you don't feel you have the time or interest to participate as a research subject, it is usually better to decline in the beginning and allow the researcher to obtain a more willing subject.

Independent Research

Following a course in nursing research and statistical analysis, nurses may conduct independent research studies. Such a study might be to investigate what technique of nursing is superior to others; it might be a study that adds to the theoretical basis of nursing. Nurses conducting independent research may ask you to help them record observations or to be a research subject for them. Necessary elements in any research study are accuracy and an unbiased mind. Be certain that any contributions you make contain these two ingredients.

Preparing to be an independent researcher is as much a responsibility of nurses as preparing to administer physical care, serve as a patient advocate, or act as a counselor. Beginning to read research studies in a meaningful way is the start of preparation.

INTEGRATING RESEARCH INTO NURSING PRACTICE

Nursing research can certainly be a contributing factor in the delivery of high quality nursing care and its constant improvement. Yet many nurses do not integrate nursing research findings into their nursing care. A number of factors are probably responsible for this problem. Lack of research knowledge may result in the inability to understand research reports. Nurses often claim a lack of time to spend on reading that often appears "too elite." Finally, many nurses have simply not been exposed to nursing research that is very practical and applicable to their practice.

In order to assist you, the student, to view nursing research as appropriate and practical to your future nursing practice, Quick Reference Stops on research have been included in various chapters throughout the text. The intent of these presentations is to expose you to some aspects of nursing care currently being questioned and/or investigated. It is hoped that these will assist you in developing a questioning attitude regarding current nursing practice.

Nursing care can *always* be improved. The way nurses do things may not really be the best way. Research helps to determine why and how we need to improve our care.

SUGGESTED READINGS

American Hospital Association. *A Patient's Bill of Rights.* New York: American Hospital Association, 1973.

American Nurses' Association. *Code For Nurses.* Kansas City: The Association, 1976.

Arminger, B., Sr. Ethics of nursing research: Profile, principles, perspective. *Nurs. Res.* 26:330, 1977.

Barnard, K. Research designs: Descriptive method. *MCN* 6:243, 1981.

Barnard, K. The case study method: A research tool. *MCN* 8(1):36, 1983.

Batra, C. Motivating nurses to do nursing research. *Nurs. Health Care* 4(1):18, 1983.

Brossard-Bryant, P. Problem-solving via research. *Superv. Nurse* 12:36, 1981.

Creighton, H. Legal concerns of nursing research. *Nurs. Res.* 26:337, 1977.

Cruise, R. J., et al. Research for practicing nurses . . . an introduction for all nurses who can and should be doing nursing research. *Superv. Nurse* 10:52, 1979.

Davis, A. Ethical considerations in gerontological nursing research. *Geriatr. Nurs.* 2:269, 1981.

Dean, P. G. Facilitating research. *Nurs. Manage.* 13:23, 1982.

Diers, D. *Research in Nursing Practice.* Philadelphia: Lippincott, 1979.

Downs, F. S., and Newman, M. A. *A Source Book of Nursing Research* (2nd ed.). Philadelphia: Davis, 1977.

Fawsett, J. On research and the professionalization of nursing. *Nurs. Forum* 19:310, 1980.

Gordon, M. Determining study topics. *Nurs. Res.* 29:83, 1980.

Gortner, S. R. Nursing Research: Out of the past and into the future. *Nurs. Res.* 29:204, 1980.

Gortner, S. R. The history and philosophy of nursing science and research. *ANS* 5(2):1, 1983.

Hunt, J. Indicators of nursing practice: The use of research findings. *J. Adv. Nurs.* 6:189, 1981.

Jacox, A. Strategies to promote nursing research. *Nurs. Res.* 29:213, 1980.

King, K. Disseminating the results of nursing research. *Nurs. Outlook* 29:164, 1981.

Miller, J., and Messenger, S. Obstacles to applying research findings. *Am. J. Nurs.* 78:632, 1978.

Moore, F. Research in a clinical setting: Promises and potential. *Superv. Nurse* 11:36, 1980.

Nerone, B. J. Profile of a nurse researcher. *Imprint* 29:41, 1982.

Polit, D., and Hungler, B. *Nursing Research: Principles and Methods.* Philadelphia: Lippincott, 1983.

Sweeney, M. A. *An Introduction to Nursing Research.* Philadelphia: Lippincott, 1981.

Tinkle, M. B., et al. Toward a new view of science: Implications for nursing research. *ANS* 5(2):27, 1983.

Treece, E. W., and Treece, J. W., Jr. *Elements of Research in Nursing* (2nd ed.). St. Louis: Mosby, 1977.

Trussell, P., Brandt, A., and Knapp, S. *Using Nursing Research: Discovery, Analysis, and Interpretation.* Wakefield, Mass.: Nursing Resources, 1981.

QUESTIONS FOR REVIEW

To check your understanding of commonly used research and statistical terms, unscramble the word in the right-hand column to match the definition in the left. Write in the unscrambled word; copy the circled letters over at the bottom and unscramble one more time to spell out a role of a professional nurse.

1. Reasoning that proceeds from the general to the specific.

E	D	C	U	T	I	E	V	D

2. The most frequently occurring value in a distribution of values.

O	E	D	M
			○

3. A representative number of subjects.

M	A	E	P	L	S
○					

4. An isolated characteristic to be studied.

A	A	R	B	L	V	I	E

5. Reasoning that proceeds from the specific to the general.

I	V	E	I	T	U	N	C	D
				○				

6. A statement recognized as a fact.

P	I	O	M	U	S	S	A	T	N

7. The sum of values divided by the number of values.

A	N	E	M
		○	

8. The degree of relationship between two factors.

T	E	L	C	O	R	I	R	O	N	A
		○								

9. A characteristic of people to be carefully respected in a research study.

T	I	R	H	G	S
○					

10. The middle value when values are arranged in order of magnitude.

D	E	M	N	I	A
	○				

11. The span between the highest and lowest values in a set of measurements.

E	G	N	A	R
○				

12. Pieces of information gained by a study.

D	A	A	T

13. Statement of the expected relationship between phenomena being studied.

S	Y	H	P	I	S	E	T	O	H
○									

14. The subjects being studied.

T	U	P	O	O	P	I	A	L	N

15. A frequently used test of statistical significance.

T	T	T	E	S
		○		

A role of a professional nurse:

○	○	○	○	○	○	○	○	○	○

II. HEALTH CARE DELIVERY SYSTEM AND THE CONSUMER

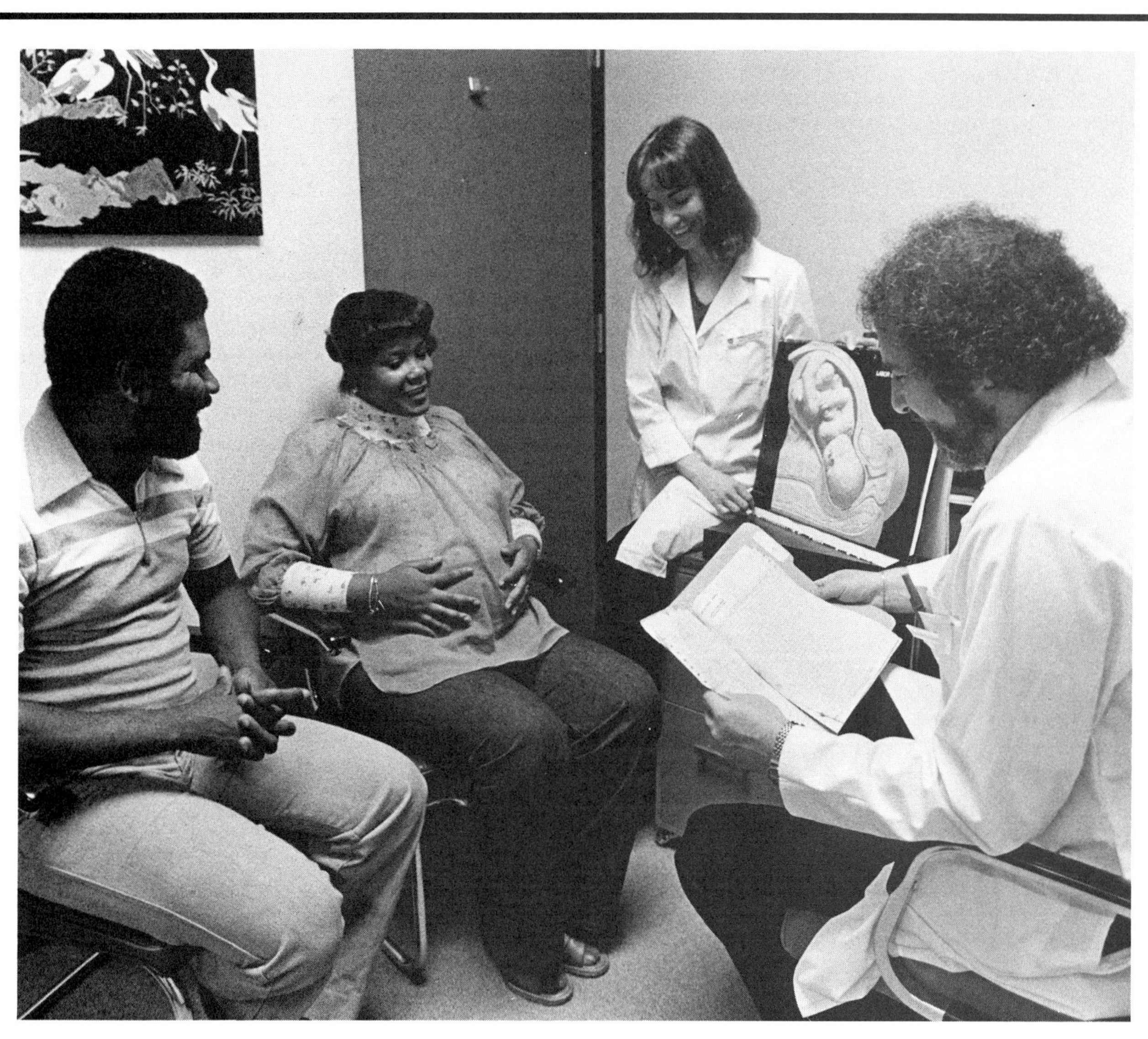

6. THE HEALTH CARE DELIVERY SYSTEM

OBJECTIVES

Upon mastery of the material in this chapter, you should be able to:

1. Define a system.
2. Describe the requirements of open and closed systems.
3. Describe the current health care delivery system in the United States.
4. List the functions of a Health Systems Agency.
5. Describe five methods of financing health care.
6. Describe the differences between official and voluntary health care agencies.
7. List examples of health care settings that offer comprehensive or episodic care and primary, secondary, and tertiary prevention.
8. List the major problems with health care delivery in the United States today.
9. Describe the major role of nurses in the health care delivery system.

TERMS

The terms important for an understanding of this chapter are shown below and defined in the glossary:

health care delivery system
system

The United States Declaration of Independence states that all men have the right to life, liberty, and the pursuit of happiness. Happiness is generally considered to include a feeling of being in good health. For this reason it has long been accepted by United States' citizens that every citizen has the right to a form of quality health care that promotes wellness, prevents disease, treats disease, and restores an ill person to his previous well state (rehabilitation).

The World Health Organization (1966) has stated that health care is a *universal* human right. The American Nurses' Association (1971) strongly supported this view. The system that provides health care for people in a country is termed its health care delivery system. Before examining the health care delivery system of the United States, it is helpful to look at the function of systems in general.

GENERAL SYSTEMS THEORY

General systems theory was first described in the early 1950s (Gray and Rizzo, 1969). By this theory a system, no matter how extensive or limited, can be examined in terms of its functions and components.

A system can be defined as a set of interrelated parts linked together to produce a meaningful whole that is greater than the sum of the parts. The test of whether something is a system is whether the parts are truly interrelated and whether they do form a meaningful whole. A clock, for example, is a system in that its parts (wheels, numbers, a cuckoo bird) form a meaningful whole (a time keeper). Many of these same parts (numbers, wheels, a plastic bird) could be found in a child's toy box, but in this situation they do not relate to each other to form a meaningful whole and are not a system (unless they are the component parts of a child's entertainment system).

Requirements of a System

In order for something to be a true system, it must fulfill the requirements of having (1) purpose (a reason for being), (2) content (parts), and (3) process (functions of the parts). The roles or function of the parts are generally fairly fixed and not interchangeable. All parts do not have to be of equal importance but must function together if the system is to operate effectively.

In addition to the above, a system has four activities: (1) It receives information, (2) it processes the information, (3) it initiates an action, and (4) it receives feedback. Receiving information is often called a system's *input;* processing it is termed *thruput;* the response or action is termed *output* (Fig. 6-1).

The toy shown in Fig. 6-2 works by a hand-wound key at the back: Winding the key tightens a spring inside; immediately after tightening, the spring unwinds and the legs of the soldier move up and down, which causes him to walk a distance of about 2 feet. Is the toy a system?

It has interrelated parts (the key, the spring, the legs),

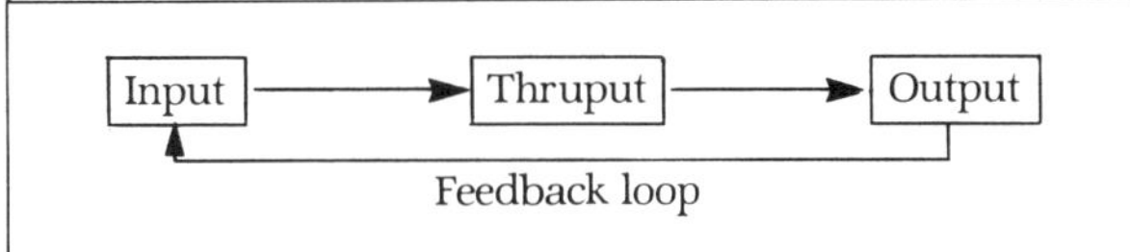

FIGURE 6-1. Requirements of a system.

Common Terms Used in Health Care Delivery

promotion of health educating consumers to be aware of good health practices through teaching and role modeling to encourage optimal health.

prevention of illness interventions to maintain health when risk of illness is present but symptomatic signs or symptoms are not yet apparent through techniques such as immunization and case finding.

health maintenance providing wellness care to assist a person to function at his optimal level of health; includes both promotion of health and prevention of illness aspects.

restoration of health the prompt diagnosis of illness and interventions to return the person to wellness most promptly.

acute care provision of health care to meet the immediate needs of the patient during the first phase of an illness.

long-term care provision of health care to meet the needs of the patient whose illness extends past a period of acute care.

primary prevention prevention to keep people well; health promotion and prevention of disease aspects of care.

secondary prevention prompt diagnosis of illness and interventions to prevent an illness from becoming severe.

tertiary prevention prevention of further complications from an illness, bringing an ill person back to the best state of wellness possible, or helping him to accept inevitable death.

which produce a meaningful whole (a toy that walks). Separate, these parts are nonfunctional; together they form a toy that is greater than the sum of the parts. It has purpose (it amuses); content (the spring, the legs), and process (the spring unwinding). It receives information (the key winds it); it processes the information (the winding tightens the spring); it initiates an action (the soldier's legs move up and down and he appears to walk). It receives feedback in that if he walks under a 2-foot distance, a tap on his head will make him walk the rest of his usual distance.

It is a system.

Subsystems

The parts of a system can usually be grouped together and examined as subsystems of the whole. The more subsystems that can be identified within a system, the more complex is the system. Because subsystems work together to form the whole, the effect of a nonfunctional subsystem will be felt and cause dysfunction in the whole. This can be demonstrated by the example of the wind-up toy: If the spring or one of the legs were to break, it would no longer be able to function as an amusing toy.

As nursing deals with people, it is helpful to consider whether people are systems. If they are, then any time a subsystem is not functioning (a person has a cold and therefore his respiratory subsystem is not filtering air as it should), this will affect the whole body.

A person *is* a system. He has purpose (to maintain life), content (lungs, heart, kidneys), and process (e.g., ability to concentrate or dilute urine, constrict or dilate blood vessels). He has subsystems such as a respiratory and a gastrointestinal system. When caring for ill people, it is important to remember that loss of function in a subsystem affects the whole. A great deal of nursing care consists of not only helping one body system to maintain its function in the face of illness, but also offering care aimed at helping other subsystems function temporarily without the help of the involved subsystem (holistic or comprehensive nursing care). People react to input, evidence thruput and output, and respond to feedback (Fig. 6-3A).

Because people are never isolated but are a part of families and communities, examining whether communities and families are systems helps to understand if illness or hospitalization (removal of a subsystem from a system) will have a major impact on a family or community.

A family *is* a system. It has purpose (the well-being and growth of its members), components (mother, father, and children), and process (the activities of mother, father, and children). It has educational, industrial, maintenance, and sanitation subsystems. When one subsystem is no longer functioning (the father—the

FIGURE 6-2. An amusing child's toy. Is it a system?

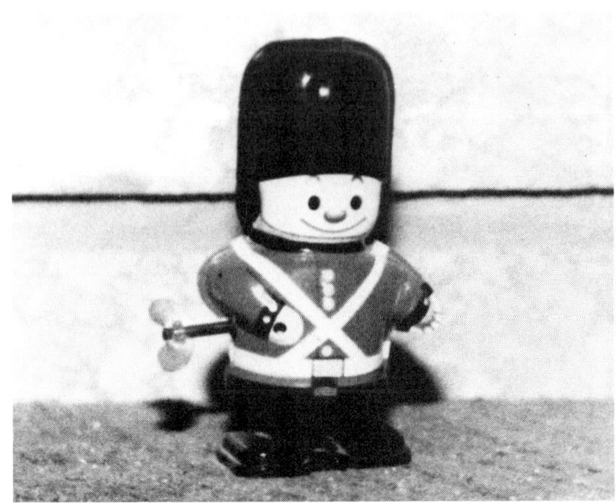

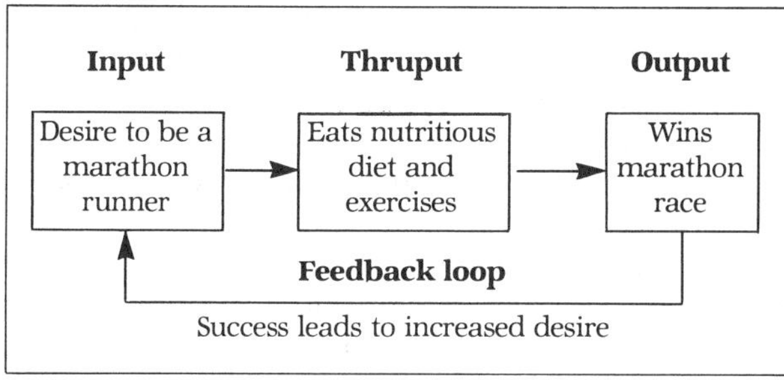

A

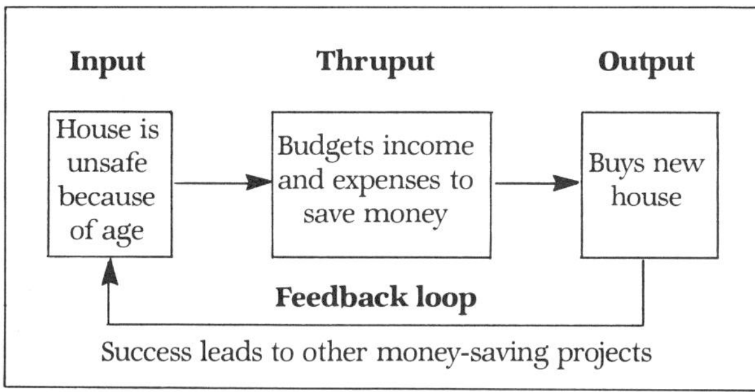

B

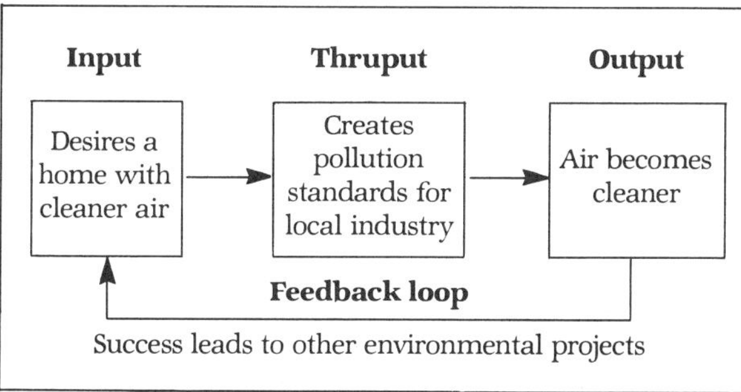

C

FIGURE 6-3. A. A person as a system. B. A family as a system. C. A community as a system.

industrial subsystem—is hospitalized, for example), the entire system feels the effect. It reacts to input, evidences thruput and output, and responds to feedback (Fig. 6-3B).

A community is a system in that it is a set of interrelated parts that are bound together to form a meaningful whole. Separately, people in a community have little power; united, they are capable of electing that official who will benefit them the most or be effective at bringing better services to their community. A community has purpose (the well-being and growth of the people who live there), components (people), and process (the activities the different people perform). It has subsystems of protection (fire and police departments), education, health maintenance, industry, and so forth. That it is a system can be demonstrated by the effect on the whole when one subsystem breaks down: A strike of sanitation workers which leaves garbage piled on the sidewalks causes a threat to transportation and to the health of the entire community. A community, therefore, is as much a system as is a single person (Fig. 6-3C).

In thinking of ways to keep people well and in caring for ill persons, it is important to remember that both families and communities are systems. Illness, therefore, will not only cause disruption in the person who is ill, but because he is a subsystem of a family and that family is a subsystem of a community, both the family and the community will be affected by his illness.

Environmental Effects on Systems

Systems have two types of environments: an internal and an external one. *Internal environment* refers to those surroundings or emotional tone that influence the workings of the system from within (genetic structure, temperament, intelligence in a person system). *External environment* refers to the surroundings in which the system exists (hot or cold temperature, accepting or rejecting surroundings of a person system).

Closed and Open Systems

A system is *closed* if it does not interact with its external environment. A terrarium, sealed with a glass cover, is an example of a closed system; it operates independently without any input from the outside (i.e., water). A system is *open* if it does interact with its surroundings (exchanges energy, matter, or information). A community, a family, a person, and the wind-up toy in Fig. 6-2 are all open systems.

Disruption of a System

If the feedback that a system receives alerts it to the fact that it is no longer fulfilling its purpose, an open system will change or adapt to the feedback information to move into a steady or productive state. Until successful adaptation can be completed, however, the system experiences tension or stress. The condition that is causing it to dysfunction is termed the *stressor.* A little stress and tension generally is productive to a system (a little stage fright may sharpen an actress's portrayal of a role). Stress greater than the system can adapt to, however, leads to chaos and loss of function (with too much stage fright, the actress cannot even walk out on stage). Similarly, a little tension can cause a heart to beat rapidly to enable a person to respond promptly to threat; too much stress cannot be adjusted to, and the heart will race until it fails. The health care delivery system is an example of a system that is continually under stress because of the numbers of people who need to be served and increasing technology, which makes health care complex and, unfortunately, expensive.

THE HEALTH CARE DELIVERY SYSTEM

The health care delivery system in the United States is the second largest industry in the country (the retail trade industry is the only one larger). More than four million people are employed in health-related roles. Over $100 billion are spent yearly for health care purposes.

The health care delivery system is a true system in that it has purpose (to guard the well-being of individuals), content (consumers and providers), and process (services such as immunization programs for children, administration of treatments to restore health, and rehabilitation exercises to restore optimal health).

Purposes of Health Care Delivery

The purposes of modern health care delivery are many-faceted but basically can be grouped in three categories: health maintenance; restoration of health; and assistance in accepting inevitable death with dignity.

Health maintenance is further subdivided into the areas of promotion of health and prevention of illness. Restoration of health includes both acute care (therapy immediately following the diagnosis of an illness or injury to bring the person quickly back to wellness) and long-term care (care of the individual with a condition that may not be curable but which he can learn to accept and with which he can function within limitations at the optimal level possible.) Refer to page 72 for complete definitions of these terms. Table 6-1 shows nursing activities that are typically carried out in each of these phases of health care delivery in relation to different age groups.

Factors Affecting Health Care Delivery

Health care and its method of delivery varies in different countries depending on the value placed on health care, the resources allotted to such care, and the technical knowledge and personnel available in that country.

VALUES AND HEALTH CARE

As mentioned, it is generally accepted in the United States that health is a right as basic as the right to pursue happiness. Health care delivery is usually, therefore, also considered a right. This belief has implications for the provision of health care in that it can cause a discrepancy between how you and the people you are caring for feel about the service: You may feel that you are expending a great deal of effort and thought in someone's care; he may view your service as nothing more than what he has a right to expect.

A closely associated current value is the emphasis on comprehensive health care—that health care needs should be met at one health care visit rather than dealing with each aspect in several different settings (at an agency a man can have his cold treated at the same time as his toothache; his injured foot cared for as well as his emotional reaction to injury). This value is a positive one for nursing, as nurses have always approached health care from a total viewpoint and organized care in a comprehensive way.

FINANCING

Health care is an entity that needs federal or private funding over and above that which individual consumers can supply in order to function because of the extremely high costs of equipment and personnel. Government funding programs vary with the degree of commitment of the present administration in Washington to issues of health care. As a nurse, you should become aware of which of your local, state, and federal legislators are most sympathetic to health-related causes. If all other qualifications are equal, you might want to think of them as the legislators to support.

TECHNOLOGY

Space exploration and computer technology in recent years have brought many improvements in the monitoring of patients' health. In some small community settings the major problem of health care delivery is how to afford this expensive equipment and the salaries of the personnel required to operate it effectively.

TABLE 6-1. PHASES OF HEALTH CARE DELIVERY: REPRESENTATIVE NURSING ACTIVITY BY AGE SPAN

Type of Care	Infant and Preschooler	Schoolager and Adolescent	Adult	Older Adult
Health maintenance				
Promotion of health (primary prevention)	Teaching tooth brushing	Teaching traffic safety	Teaching stress reduction	Teaching nutrition
Prevention of illness (primary prevention)	Administering immunizations	Screening for scoliosis	Administering yearly physical exam	Screening for hypertension
Restoration of health				
Acute care (secondary prevention)	Care of the child with a birth defect	Care of the child with tonsillitis	Care of a man following a heart attack	Care of a woman following surgery for cancer
Long-term care (tertiary prevention)	Care of the child who wears leg braces	Care of the child with asthma	Care of a woman with hypertension	Care of a man following a cerebral vascular accident (stroke)
Acceptance of death with dignity (tertiary prevention)	Helping parents accept the death of a premature infant	Helping parents and child accept a diagnosis of leukemia	Helping the person accept his impending death from cancer	Helping the person adjust to death from congestive heart disease

CONSUMER INPUT

Yet another factor that affects health care delivery is the amount of consumer input that occurs. The women's movement, for example, has been instrumental in changing care practices: Its efforts have led to the acceptance of the view that childbirth be conducted in more relaxed settings and to the provision of overnight facilities for parents in hospital units for children. Consumer input is expected to continue and to have an even greater effect on health care delivery in the future.

THE CONSUMERS OF HEALTH CARE

Everyone in a given population is a potential consumer (receiver) of health care. At some time in life every person will have sufficient illness or concern about the possibility of being ill to contact a provider for some form of health care. How much and what kinds of health care are needed in a community vary in accordance with the characteristics of the population such as age (old and young people typically need more care); sex (more childbearing health care will be needed in a primarily female population than in a typical male-dominated army base); education (people knowledgeable about health needs are better able to make health care decisions themselves and so need less care); occupation (some industries such as the coal-mining industry have a high risk of disease); life style (a community where camping is prevalent may need rattlesnake antivenom stocked at all clinic locations, while clinics in the heart of New York City do not need this as a routine item); culture and attitudes toward health care (whether people view health care as a positive service or not); and geographic location (dense population centers need more health care sites than areas with a sparse population). Many health care programs are not successful because the characteristics of the community were not examined before the service was initiated.

Health Statistics

A number of statistical measures are commonly used to compare the health of people in one community or country with that of people in another or the health of people from year to year. *Morbidity* refers to the number of people ill each year. *Mortality* is the number of deaths per 1,000 population each year; this rate for 1960 to 1982 is shown in Table 6-2. As expected, the age groups 55 years of age and older have the highest mortality. The next age group with a high mortality is that of infants less than one year of age. This type of information is used to determine what health care services a community needs (if it includes many infants less than one year, health care is required more than if it has many children of school age, since mortality is higher in the former age group).

Infant mortality is a common measure used to compare the effectiveness of health care from one country to another. Table 6-3 indicates that in 1980 the United States had a higher infant mortality than 12 other countries. This information suggests that the health care delivery systems of these countries are superior to that of the United States at least in supplying care to women during pregnancy and to children during their first year of life.

TABLE 6-2. MORTALITY RATES BY AGE: 1960—1982

Age	1960	1970	1980	1982
Under 1 yr	27.0	21.4	14.2	11.6
1—4	1.1	0.8	0.7	0.4
5—14	0.5	0.4	0.3	0.4
15—24	1.1	1.3	1.2	1.0
25—34	1.5	1.6	1.4	1.3
35—44	3.0	3.1	2.4	2.1
45—54	7.6	7.3	6.1	5.5
55—64	17.4	16.6	14.1	12.9
65—74	38.2	35.8	30.2	29.0
75—84	87.5	80.0	71.6	63.5
85 and over	198.6	163.4	146.8	149.7

Source: Monthly Vital Statistics Report, Vol. 32, No. 1. Hyattsville, Md.: U.S. Department of Health and Human Resources, Public Health Service, National Center for Health Statistics, 1983.

TABLE 6-3. INFANT MORTALITY (PER 1,000 LIVE BIRTHS) FOR SELECTED COUNTRIES, 1980

Country	Rate
Sweden	8.3
Japan	9.3
Denmark	10.3
Netherlands	10.6
Switzerland	10.7
Finland	11.0
Norway	11.1
England and Wales	14.2
France	14.7
Scotland	14.8
Hong Kong	14.9
Canada	15.0
United States	15.2

Source: Health in the United States. Hyattsville, Md.: U.S. Department of Health and Human Resources, Public Health Service, National Center for Health Statistics, 1980.

Table 6-4 shows the proportion of people in differing age groups. Notice the large number of people in the 5- to 17-year age group compared to that in any other age group. Health Systems Agencies must ask themselves if there are adequate health care facilities for this age group in their health systems area.

Table 6-5 shows the most frequent causes of deaths in each age group. Health care services must be primarily directed toward preventing and treating disease condi-

TABLE 6-4. PERCENTAGE OF THE TOTAL POPULATION BY AGE GROUP, July 1982

Age Group (years)	Percentage
Under 5	7.5
5—17	19.5
18—24	13.1
25—34	17.0
35—44	12.1
45—54	9.6
55—64	9.5
65 and over	11.6

Source: U.S. Bureau of the Census, Estimates of the population of the United States, by age, race and sex: 1980—1982. *Current Population Reports,* Series p. 25, No. 929. Washington, D.C.: U.S. Government Printing Office, 1983.

TABLE 6-5. COMMON CAUSES OF DEATH IN THE UNITED STATES BY AGE GROUP

Age Group	Cause of Death
Preschooler	Accidents, congenital anomalies, influenza and pneumonia
Schoolager	Accidents, malignant neoplasms, congenital anomalies
Adolescent	Accidents, homicide, suicide
Young adult	Accidents, diseases of the heart, malignant neoplasms
Middle-aged adult	Diseases of the heart, malignant neoplasms, cerebrovascular disease
Older adult	Diseases of the heart, malignant neoplasms, cerebrovascular disease

tions that occur frequently rather than those that are rarely seen.

THE PROVIDERS OF HEALTH CARE

The number of different types of providers of health care increases every year. Figure 6-4 shows diagrammatically health care providers as subsystems of the larger system of health care delivery. Effective health care delivery depends on cooperation between subsystems of providers, as no subsystem can achieve total health care by itself (a physician does not offer dental care; a nurse can not prescribe medicine), but together, since subsystems work together to produce a whole greater than the sum of all the parts, effective and comprehensive health care is possible.

Health Systems Agencies

In 1975 the National Health Planning and Resource Development Act divided the United States into a network of health service areas. Health care in each service area is supervised by a Health Systems Agency (HSA). The major purposes of HSAs are to prevent unnecessary duplication of health services, restrain increases in the cost of health services, reduce deficiencies of health services, and, by so doing, improve the overall health of residents of the area.

Each HSA is governed by a board that is responsible for developing a health care service plan that is responsive to the needs of all the people in that area. In order to assure that a HSA meets the needs of all the people in the community, 51 to 60 percent of the board's membership must be composed of consumers (health care receivers). These consumers must represent the varied special interests (industrial, racial, social divisions) of that community. The board must also have members representing providers of health care. A nurse, therefore, might serve on a Health Systems Agency board as either a provider or a consumer of health care.

Health Systems Agencies are currently being asked to make very difficult decisions as to how many obstetrical beds an area should maintain in the light of the present decrease in the birth rate or how many expensive CT (computerized tomography) scanners are needed. Health Systems Agency recommendations are often reported in local newspapers. A recommendation such as suggesting that a local hospital's obstetrical service be closed may not be popular with all the citizens in the area.

SETTINGS OF HEALTH CARE DELIVERY

Two major types of health care settings are those that are tax-supported (official agencies) and those supported by private funds (voluntary agencies).

Official Agencies

Federal, state, or local tax money may be the source of an official agency's revenue. Tax-supported agencies, as a category, are established to meet broad health needs or

FIGURE 6-4. Relationship of nursing to the health care delivery system. Nursing is a subsystem, as are medicine, pharmacy, and nutrition.

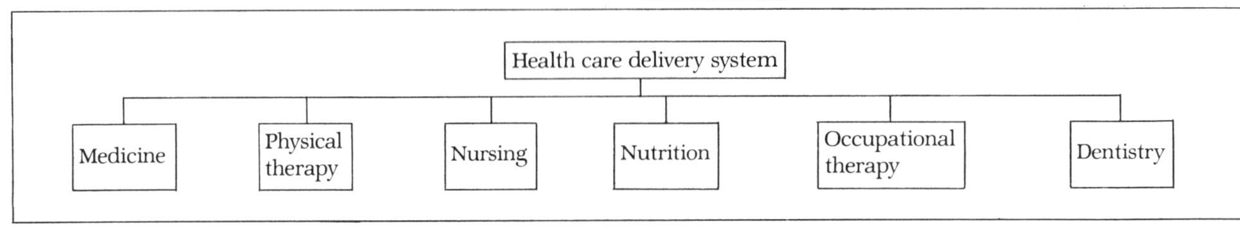

those of a wide variety of individuals. Although an agency receives its funding from a tax source, this does not mean that health care is supplied free to all people who utilize the service. People who have the means to pay are generally expected to contribute at least a portion of the cost of the service.

WORLD LEVEL HEALTH AGENCIES

An interest in health as a worldwide concern began about 1831 when programs to control the spread of plague in Europe were established. In 1948 the concept of world health became a reality with the establishment of the World Health Organization, a specialized agency of the United Nations.

The main purposes of the World Health Organization are (WHO, 1966):

1. To assist governments, upon request, in strengthening health services.
2. To promote improved standards of teaching and training in health, medical, and related professions.
3. To provide information, counsel, and assistance in the field of health.
4. To promote maternal and child health and improvement of nutrition, housing, sanitation, recreation, economic or working conditions, and other aspects of environmental hygiene.
5. To promote and conduct research in the field of health.

The World Health Organization employs nurses in both consultative and direct-care roles in order to fulfill these purposes.

FEDERAL LEVEL HEALTH AGENCIES

A diagram of the official health agency structure of the United States is shown in Fig. 6-5. The Department of Health and Human Services (formerly the Department of Health, Education and Welfare) is a major department of the federal government at the same level as the Department of the Interior. The Public Health Service is one of the divisions of this department. In 1798 John Adams, the second U.S. president, signed a bill that established care for sick and disabled seamen. From this simple beginning the Public Health Service today comprises the following six operating subdivisions.

Food and Drug Administration. The Food and Drug Administration (FDA) is responsible for enforcing a number of laws governing the safety and labeling of drugs, food, and cosmetics. The federal Food, Drug and Cosmetic Act requires not only that food, drugs, medical devices, and cosmetics be safe for ingestion or use but also that they be truthfully labeled. The FDA tests drugs to be certain that their performance is as expected before they can be released to the public. The Fair Packaging and Labeling Act requires that foods be properly labeled so that consumers can compare the values of competing brands. The Radiation Control for Health and Safety Act protects consumers from unnecessary exposure to radiation from sources such as x-ray machines, microwave ovens, and color television sets.

The Public Health Services Act gives the FDA authority to regulate vaccine and blood products and to establish safe food-handling practices in restaurants and interstate travel carriers such as airplanes.

Centers for Disease Control. The Centers for Disease Control (CDC) began in 1946 as an agency interested only in communicable disease. Today it tabulates the incidence of many health problems and offers assistance and recommendations to state and local organizations on ways to protect against outbreaks of illness. The National Institute of Occupational Safety and Health, a subdivision of the CDC, is responsible for safeguarding the health of people from occupational hazards such as chemicals and insecticides and, by regulating entry to

FIGURE 6-5. Structure of the United States federal official health agencies.

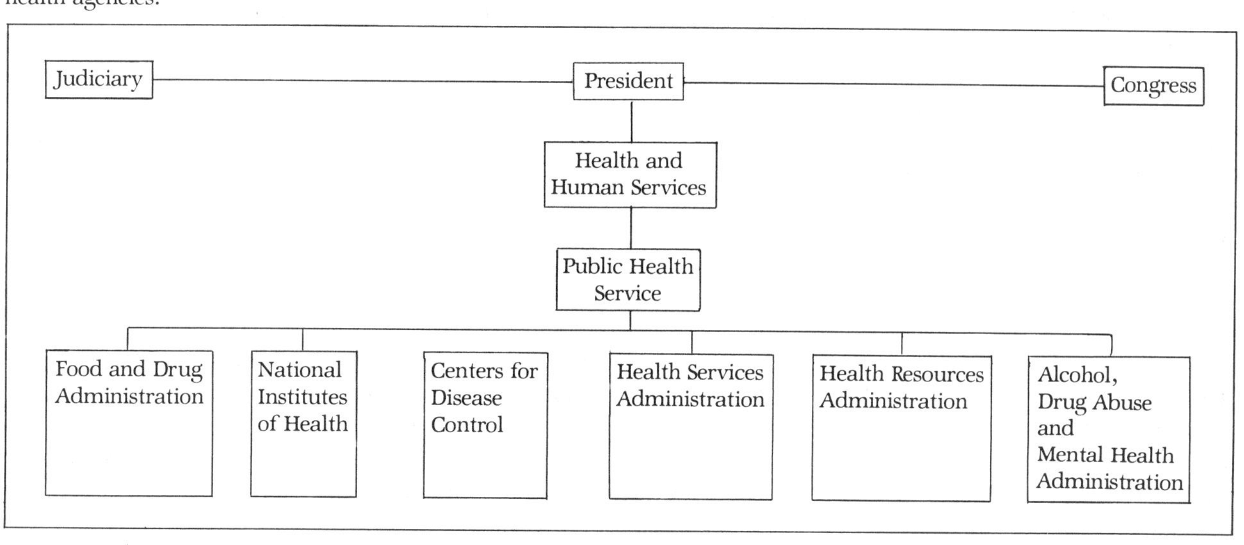

the United States, for preventing the spread of disease from other countries.

Health Services Administration. The Health Services Administration (HSA) has three bureaus. The Bureau of Community Health Services sponsors programs to improve the health care of migrant workers, mothers and infants, and children with mental retardation and handicapping conditions. The Bureau of Medical Services supervises emergency medical services and operates health care facilities for the Coast Guard, federal employees, and people in prison. The Indian Health Service is responsible for providing a system of health care delivery for native Americans and native Alaskans.

Health Resources Administration. The Bureau of Health Manpower of the Health Resources Administration (HRA) is responsible for supplying funding for health education programs and for construction of buildings and purchase of equipment to maintain health education programs. Nursing is a health care area that has benefited greatly from HRA improvement fundings.

Alcohol, Drug Abuse and Mental Health Administration. The National Institute of Mental Health conducts and supports research into the cause, treatment, and prevention of mental disorders. It promotes community mental health centers. The National Institutes of Alcohol and Drug Abuse support programs to make treatment available and promote the preventive and rehabilitation aspects of alcohol and drug use.

National Institutes of Health. The National Institutes of Health (NIH) has divisions on aging, cancer, allergy and infection, child health, general medicine, environmental health, and heart and lung, eye, dental, neurological, metabolic, and digestive diseases. Each division promotes programs dealing with the prevention, treatment, research, rehabilitation, and recovery from the diseases or conditions represented. Nurses are employed by national level health care organizations as consultants and coordinators of programs for direct care.

STATE LEVEL HEALTH AGENCIES

State health departments are official organizations at the state level. They are concerned with such factors as environmental health, communicable disease control, laboratory services, health education, mental health services, vital and health statistics, and adult and child services. State level agencies serve as consultants for local health agencies.

LOCAL LEVEL HEALTH AGENCIES

Local health services (county or city) are responsible for the above services on the local level plus direct services to consumers such as nursing care. Nurses working for a health department as community health nurses play a vital role in helping people to improve their health and to care for themselves during illness while remaining in their own homes.

Voluntary Organizations

The concept that people should have input into their health care organizations has led to the establishment of voluntary organizations. The first of these was the antituberculosis society formed in Philadelphia in 1892. They now comprise as large a network as that of official agencies.

PRIVATE, NONPROFIT SETTINGS

A private, nonprofit setting is one that is financed without tax revenue. Charges to people who use the service are limited to the costs of operating the service. A local hospital, for example, is usually established as a private, nonprofit organization.

PRIVATE, PROFIT-MAKING SETTINGS

Most physicians, dentists, and nursing homes operate on a private, hopefully profit-making basis. One of the criticisms of a system of health care delivery that is dependent on many profit-making persons is the possibility that these persons will be more concerned with making a profit than serving the best interests of the population. It is difficult to promote preventive care with many profit-making settings in a system. While people will usually pay an agency to cure them of an illness, they are less apt to pay for counseling or nutrition education programs to keep themselves well.

SPECIAL INTEREST AGENCIES

Some agencies depend on endowments or contributions of individual people to supply them with funds. The focus is often on one particular health problem. The National Foundation (formerly called the March of Dimes) and the American Heart Association are examples of this type of agency. They are generally governed by a board of directors, and although they may provide direct service (the Cancer Society, for example, provides supplies free to people with that disease), they primarily focus on educational services (pamphlets and television announcements on the danger of high blood pressure and steps to take to reduce it, for example). They also assess community needs, perform research, support health legislation, and serve as advisors to official agencies.

INDIVIDUAL ENTRY INTO THE HEALTH CARE DELIVERY SYSTEM

Table 6-1 shows examples of health care delivery according to the classification of health maintenance, restoration of health, and acceptance of inevitable death. If a health care delivery system is to be effective in safeguarding the health of consumers in the system, it must put its concentration not only on helping ill people become well again, but on promoting health and preventing illness. Another way to categorize services, therefore, is to list them according to the different levels of preventive strategies they employ. There are three levels of prevention: a *primary* preventive stage, which includes active preventive measures such as teaching and immunizations (the health maintenance section of Table 6-1); a *secondary* prevention stage, which includes early diagnosis of illness so that treatment can be offered (the acute care division of Table 6-1); and a *tertiary* prevention stage, which prevents an individual with an illness from becoming more ill (the long-term illness and acceptance of inevitable death phase of Table 6-1).

Primary Prevention Agencies

Voluntary agencies such as the American Heart Association tend to be involved at the primary prevention level. They educate the public about the danger of a specific illness (such as heart disease, one of the leading causes of death) and the steps a person can take to avoid the danger (such as avoiding being overweight and taking measures to keep blood pressure and cholesterol levels as near normal as possible). The Department of Health and Human Services and state and local health departments play large roles in primary prevention by means of education and immunization and screening programs (holding a screening clinic for diabetes at a shopping mall, for example).

Secondary Prevention Agencies

Ambulatory care facilities (people visit the setting but do not remain overnight) and hospital inpatient areas are the usual sites where secondary prevention is carried out. At this stage a person already has an illness. Emphasis is on treatment and preventing complications so that the person can recover fully.

Tertiary Prevention Agencies

At the third stage a person has had an illness that has left some impairment (a man has had his leg amputated due to poor blood circulation perhaps). Tertiary prevention measures are designed to prevent him from thinking of himself as ill and to restore him to a level of health where he can feel competent despite his limitations. Nursing homes (generally privately owned), extended care facilities of hospitals (private, nonprofit agencies), and voluntary agencies such as the Association for Cerebral Palsy are agencies that help handicapped persons to avoid becoming more ill and to achieve as high a level of health as the residual effects of their illness will allow. A hospice is a health care setting that concentrates on helping persons whose death is imminent to die without pain and with dignity.

EPISODIC VERSUS COMPREHENSIVE CARE

Department stores and shopping malls are popular places for people in the United States to shop because the average person can be assured that he can find all the different items he is seeking in one setting or by making one stop. For similar reasons the average consumer would probably like to have all his health care needs met in one setting rather than having to consult one physician because his back is painful, another if he is concerned about being overweight, and yet a third to have a cut on his child's leg sutured. Health care agencies can be divided into those that provide episodic care and those that offer comprehensive or total (holistic) care.

Episodic Care Settings

Many people use the health care delivery system only for episodic care. They do not benefit as much from services as they could if they went to more comprehensive settings.

DELIVERY ROOMS

Almost all children enter the health care delivery system at birth as they receive their first physical examination and have a record made concerning their health at this time. Delivery rooms offer only temporary health supervision, however. Following this introduction to the system, they are seen and followed in ambulatory settings for primary preventive care.

Some children are immediately placed in a secondary preventive level of care at birth because they are born with a congenital defect or develop an illness within hours after birth. It is important that all children continue to be seen by health care providers during their growing-up years to ensure that they remain in good health. It is very important that children who are born ill receive supervised continuing care so that they can become all that they are capable of becoming despite the handicapping condition. Nurses are important members of the health care team in a delivery room; nurses in the extended role of midwife supervise home births or those in hospital birthing rooms.

WELL CHILD CONFERENCES

Well child conferences (popularly called baby clinics) are clinics operated by local health departments to supply immunizations, nutrition and behavior counseling, and a physical examination to all children up to five years of age. These conferences are free and are generally situated in low socioeconomic areas. The difficulty with this type of health maintenance setting is that a child cannot be seen there if he is ill, which makes his wellness-illness care fragmented. Nurses may work in well child conferences in conjunction with a physician or, in the extended role of a pediatric nurse practitioner, independently manage such clinics.

EMERGENCY ROOMS

Some people use the emergency rooms of local hospitals as their primary health care setting. Because these services are staffed by rotating hospital personnel, a person treated at such a facility rarely sees the same staff members on subsequent visits. This type of service also leads to fragmented care as there is no provision for advice and counseling to keep people well. Follow-up care is allocated to another hospital division or another care person, increasing the episodic aspects of care. Nurses are important members of emergency room staffs and often are the people in such settings who offer any degree of continuity to follow-up care.

HEALTH OFFICES AT SCHOOL OR WORK

A child with a health problem or one whose parents have difficulty evaluating a potential illness in him often relies on a school health office for evaluation and advice on his health problem. The same applies to the health offices in industrial settings. Because schools and industries have limited means of follow-up care, this type of contact, while an essential means of entry into the system, leads to fragmented and, by itself, inadequate care. Nurses are the primary health care providers in both settings capable of providing adequate referral service to ensure that the care offered in such settings is coordinated with that required from other sources.

AMBULATORY OR SPECIALTY SERVICES

An adult who has a kidney disease may attend a specialized clinic for people with this disease; a child born with a heart defect is treated at a clinic that specializes in the care of children with heart disease; a person with dental cavities attends a dental clinic. These specialty areas of hospitals are important in providing quality care, but they can lead to a fragmented type of health care.

It is not unusual to discover that a child who regularly attends a specialty clinic has not received basic immunizations, because immunizations represent more comprehensive care than the setting offers. Nurses employed in such settings can be instrumental in being certain that the patient receives a comprehensive type of health care.

MOBILE UNITS

Mobile units are vans equipped with supplies for screening tests and examining equipment. They travel from place to place in a given area, providing ambulatory services to communities that otherwise would have no health services of this kind. Mobile units tend to offer fragmented care because their follow-up ability is limited. Nurses are employed by such services for both health education and direct care.

HOSPITALIZATION

If someone is very ill at the time of his first contact with health care providers, he may be admitted to a hospital as his first important health care delivery system interaction. Although a person may spend a considerable amount of time in a hospital, the care he receives there is not necessarily comprehensive. He may have prolonged treatment for the injury or illness that required hospitalization, such as injuries from an automobile accident, but a secondary problem of poor eyesight may be ignored, because hospital personnel tend to be specialized. A nurse is the person best prepared to ensure that not only a first concern, but a second, third, or fourth one is also assessed and solved during the hospitalization, converting this type of care from episodic to comprehensive care (Fig. 6-6).

Settings That Offer Comprehensive Care

Comprehensive health care facilities are growing in number as both consumers and health care providers become more aware of the advantages of total care.

HEALTH MAINTENANCE ORGANIZATIONS

Members of Health Maintenance Organizations (HMOs) sign a contract to pay a specified amount to the health care agency, similar to subscribing to an insurance policy. For this base price, the person can attend the agency as many times as is necessary to keep him well and is hospitalized as necessary for acute illness care or surgery. This type of plan concentrates on maintaining wellness rather than restoration of illness; it encourages

FIGURE 6-6. Nurses play an important role in ensuring that hospitalized patients receive comprehensive care.

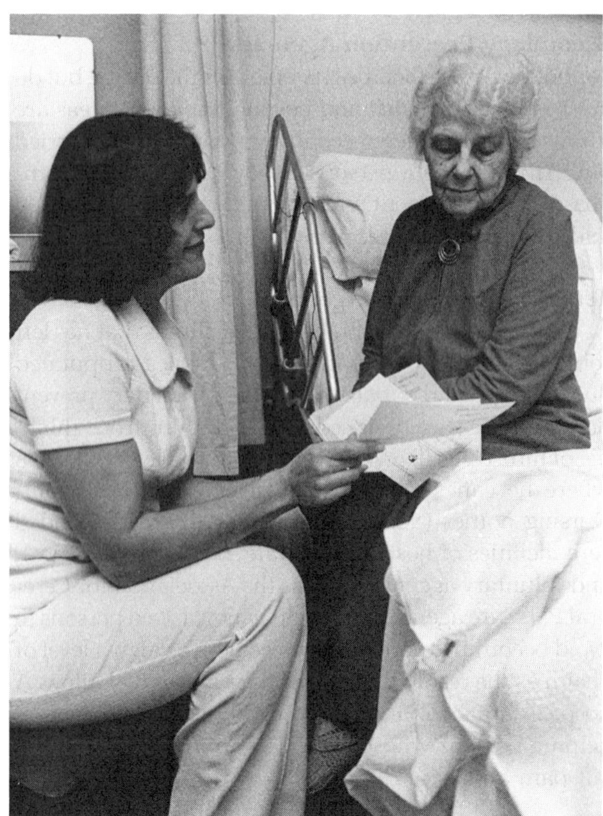

a person to visit the agency for immunizations or discussion of his health, because the more visits he makes, the more he gets for his money. Health Maintenance Organizations are not yet available in all communities; they are increasing rapidly, however, because they are a workable solution to providing comprehensive care. Nurses are primary members of HMO health care teams.

COMMUNITY HEALTH CENTERS

Community health centers are facilities set up in heavily populated areas to meet the needs of a particular population. People visit such centers for ambulatory care, and physicians follow and supervise patients during hospitalization. As with health maintenance organizations, the emphasis is on preventing illness. Such centers have consumer input as to policies; fees for services are usually scaled so that all members of the community can receive quality health care. Nurses work in community health centers in both consultation and direct care roles.

PRIVATE DOCTORS' OFFICES

A general practitioner provides comprehensive care to his patients by either supplying the care they need himself or referring them to specialists to provide intense short-term care. He sees them during both health and illness and so provides comprehensive care. The average physician in private practice employs a nurse to assist with health education and provide direct nursing care in the office setting.

EXTENDED CARE FACILITIES OR NURSING HOMES

Many elderly people who have illnesses so serious that they cannot be cared for at home live in skilled nursing facilities (extensions of hospital units) or freestanding nursing homes. Many of these facilities provide for all of the patient's health needs and so are comprehensive in the nature of their care. Nurses are employed to supervise and offer direct nursing care in such settings.

NURSES IN PRIVATE PRACTICE

A new concept in health care delivery is that of the nurse in private practice. Such a nurse has education in addition to that provided by a basic nursing program; she is called a nurse practitioner. She provides some patient services herself (advice, counseling, health teaching) and refers patients to other health care providers for intense short-term care as does a private physician. By doing so, she can provide comprehensive care.

HOSPICES

Hospices are settings where a person who is aware that he is dying and wants no heroic measures carried out for him (is prepared for his death) comes for care. Such a setting is comprehensive in scope; it provides for all his needs and offers support and comfort to his family as well. Caring for people who are dying is a sensitive role and requires skilled professional capability.

FINANCING HEALTH CARE

Many people do not receive adequate health care because they cannot afford to pay for services or are not aware of the financing arrangements that are available to them. Basically, there are five different ways that a person can pay for health services: (1) personal payment, (2) voluntary insurance, (3) social insurance, (4) industry insurance, and (5) charitable sources.

Personal Payment

A person may pay the full cost of his health care in cash or by writing a personal check. With the cost of current health care (a stay in an intensive care unit may cost as much as $500—$1,000 a day), payment by this means is becoming less and less common.

Voluntary Insurance

As many as 85 percent of people under 65 years of age in the United States subscribe to voluntary (private) insurance plans. The person pays a periodic premium; the policy may cover either an individual or his entire family. In many instances a portion or all the cost is paid for by an employer as a work benefit. In a region where there is high unemployment, many people may no longer have health insurance coverage as they are unable to continue the insurance payments on their own. Blue Cross/Blue Shield is presently the most common insurance of this type. Health Maintenance Organizations are voluntary insurance plans that not only pay for illness care but include health prevention visits as well.

Social Insurance

Insurance is provided by the government for particular segments of the population who, without this help, may not be able to afford coverage and therefore health care. *Medicare*, which provides for a portion of health care services for elderly people, and *Medicaid*, which provides coverage for people on public assistance or with special needs, are examples of social insurance.

A national health insurance program to provide federally funded protection to all United States citizens has been discussed in Congress for the past 10 years. If this type of insurance is approved, it will be a form of social insurance.

SOCIAL SECURITY BENEFITS

Under the Social Security plan during working years a proportion of one's earnings is deducted from each paycheck; these funds are held in special trust funds, and payments are made upon retirement or earlier if the person should become disabled. If the person should die, monthly payments are made to a surviving wife or husband. Nine out of every 10 working people in the

United States are covered by this program. Many elderly people depend on Social Security funds to pay their living expenses.

SUPPLEMENTAL SECURITY INCOME

People who are blind, disabled, or 65 or older may be eligible for monthly cash payments from special United States treasury funds called Supplemental Security Income (SSI) benefits. This may be in addition to Social Security payments; it is also available to those people who are not eligible for Social Security. This money is not specifically restricted to health care but is often used to purchase medicine or cover other expenses of long-term care.

MEDICARE

People receiving Social Security payments are eligible for Medicare health care insurance. Thus, Medicare is available not only to elderly people (people over 65 routinely receive Social Security income) but also to some handicapped persons eligible for Social Security payments. People needing dialysis or kidney transplant for chronic kidney disease are also eligible for Medicare. Medicare has two separate portions: hospital insurance or coverage of care when the person is confined in a hospital, extended care facility, or even in some instances in his own home; and medical insurance to pay physicians' expenses. The patient is required to pay the first part of his health care expense (the first $60 each year, for example); then the program will pay up to 80 percent of the remainder of the cost.

MEDICAID

Medicaid is a federal (but state administered) program that provides health care funds for low-income families. The funding is very comprehensive: People covered by Medicaid have all their health costs including prescriptions for medicine paid for fully. Without this funding program many low-income families would be completely without health care.

WORKMEN'S COMPENSATION INSURANCE

Since 1910, if a worker is injured in his work setting, he may collect Workmen's Compensation Insurance payments to sustain him during the time of his illness. Depending on the seriousness of the injury and his disability, hospital, physician, and other health care costs will be partially or totally paid by this method. Employers routinely pay into the Workmen's Compensation Fund so that funding is available when accidents happen.

Industrial Insurance

Industrial insurance is a policy furnished by a particular industry for its employees. In some instances the policy begins to cover health care expenses when a person's voluntary insurance payments are exhausted. A person loses his eligibility for this type of insurance upon termination of employment.

Charitable Resources

Charitable resources are provided mainly by religious organizations and special interest groups (people in a neighborhood solicit money to pay the cost of buying a dialysis machine for a community member). The type and amount of resources available vary widely from community to community.

PROBLEMS WITH THE CURRENT HEALTH CARE DELIVERY SYSTEM

The present system of health care delivery in the United States has problems that arise mainly because of its size. It is difficult for a large agency to respond to feedback because changing one aspect affects so many people and places. Some problems arise because agencies were formulated first as stop-gap measures; planning and coordination efforts came later. Health Systems Agencies are designed to reverse this process: Planning is now done before a new agency is originated.

Another problem is that the system emphasizes illness care, not prevention. In many instances the cost of preventive health care is prohibitive. In some areas there is a poor distribution of services (many pediatricians may have offices on the north side of a city, while there are no pediatricians on the south side). As a whole, lack of consumer participation prevents health facilities from truly meeting the health needs of people. Increased consumer participation is needed so that facilities can truly offer the type and extent of service desired.

Goals for the future should include: Reduce the financial burden of services to a workable level; provide personal, individualized care; provide comprehensive, not episodic care; and increase participation by people in decision making about their health care.

DETERMINING STANDARDS OF HEALTH CARE

Two programs have been designed to set standards for health care delivery and improve the level of health care available.

Professional Standards Review Organization

The Professional Standards Review Organization (PSRO) was organized in 1972 to mandate professional review of health care delivery supported by Medicare and Medicaid and maternal-child health programs to ensure that federal money allocated to these programs was well spent.

The program seeks to determine that care given is

Ways that Nurses can Respond to Problems with the Health Care Delivery System

Problem	*Response*
It is difficult for large agencies to respond to consumer feedback.	Be alert to consumer needs. Question bureaucratic solutions such as "That's against the rules" or "That doesn't work." Initiate new programs or methods of care.
Many agencies are Stop-gap in nature.	Be active in health care planning. Attend local government meetings such as city council meetings. Serve on a Health Systems Agency.
Stress is present in health as well as in illness.	Always include health teaching for promotion of health in your care. Support legislators who are advocating money for wellness or prevention care.
Consumer input is lacking.	Encourage people to voice their opinions of health care. Seek help for patients who are "lost in the system." Encourage patients to participate in setting their own health goals.
Health care is costly.	Always evaluate care in terms of not only effectiveness but efficient use of time and money. Suggest cost-saving ideas to your superiors.
Health care is routine, not individualized.	Always individualize care according to age, sex, growth and development of a patient, and circumstances present. Suggest ways that a hospital unit or ambulatory setting could be more personalized.
Health care is episodic, not comprehensive.	Always structure your care to be holistic. Keep lines of communication open between health care agencies so exchange of information is possible. Coordinate care between departments of an agency or different agencies to achieve comprehensive care.

necessary, safe, and according to professional standards, and is provided economically and with regard to the proper care setting. PSRO committees in health care agencies examine the admission records of patients at hospitals and nursing homes to be certain that the admissions were necessary and review progress charts periodically during an institutional stay to be certain that hospitalization is still required. Nursing notes are considered in this committee's review as documentation of patient status.

Quality Assurance Programs

The Joint Accreditation of Hospitals (JACH) is a voluntary, not-for-profit organization founded in 1951 to assure a high standard of health care in institutions such as hospitals. Many insurance companies reimburse facilities only if they are JACH-accredited, so agencies have high motivation to seek such accreditation. Hospitals maintain audit committees to review patient care in order to offer assurance that they are meeting JACH standards. The quality of nursing care is audited by the general hospital audit committee and by a second nursing audit committee. Various institutions may ask you to record your nursing notes in specified ways in order to meet the criteria of their audit committee.

FIGURE 6-7. Immunization administration is an example of primary prevention.

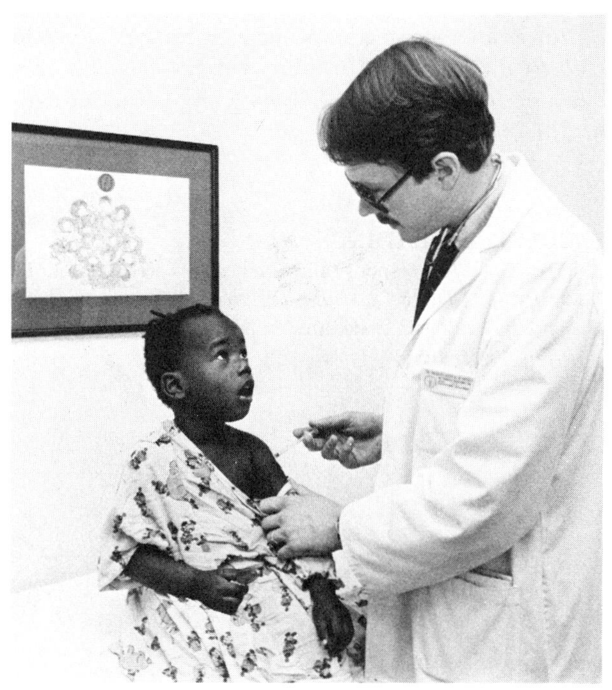

THE NURSE'S ROLE IN HEALTH CARE DELIVERY

Nursing is a subsystem of the major health care delivery system and works in cooperation with other subsystems such as medicine, physical therapy, and occupational therapy. Nurses function in almost every setting of health care possible. The box lists ways in which nurses can help to improve health care based on the problems of the current health care delivery system.

When a person has discomfort or in some other way realizes that he is ill, he readily visits a health care facility for care. People do not return for follow-up or reassessment care or seek primary preventive advice to keep well as readily, however. They come for these kinds of care only if they feel welcome at health care facilities and the care they receive seems adequate and meets their individual needs.

Nurses can help to structure care toward individualized preferences or needs. They can also help people to participate in their own care. They set the feeling tone for an agency (whether it is one of acceptance or rejection), and they can be instrumental in seeing that care is comprehensive and not sporadic in nature so that the greatest number of people receive the best care possible in health care settings.

Nurses work with other health care providers to promote health by teaching good health practices; they prevent illness by being the organizers of immunization or screening programs (Fig. 6-7); they restore health by hospital-based nursing care and help people return to a former level of functioning through long-term care in extended nursing care facilities. They are instrumental in helping people to accept an impending death in any setting.

Nurses are the integrators and coordinators of health care as they function in every setting of health care delivery; the health care delivery system of today cannot function without nurses.

SUGGESTED READINGS

Alderman, K. Self-responsibility in health care promotion: Motivational factors. *J. School Health* 50:22, 1980.

Alexander, A. Adolescent health: Challenge of the 80s. *J. School Health* 50:47, 1980.

American Nurses' Association. *Statement on the Essential Elements of a Health Care System.* Kansas City, Mo.: The Association, 1971.

Blum, R. W., et al. A school-based comprehensive health clinic for adolescents. *J. Sch. Health* 52(8):486, 1982.

Colt, A., et al. Home health care is good economics. *Nurs. Outlook* 25:632, 1977.

Crawford, C. C. The health of rural children. *Child. Contemp. Soc.* 13:58, 1980.

Curtin, L. L. Is there a right to health care? *Am. J. Nurs.* 80:462, 1980.

Defriese, G. H., et al. Child health and the problem of access to care. *Fam. Community Health* 4:71, 1982.

Enthovan, A. C. Consumer-centered vs. job-centered health insurance. *J. Nurs. Adm.* 10:19, 1980.

Fasano, N. F., et al. Futurism scenario: Commencement address to the Class of 2010. *JNE* 21(3):20, 1982.

Forthofer, R. N., et al. Utilization of services of an HMO by new enrollees. *Am. J. Public Health* 69:1127, 1979.

Gray, W., and Rizzo, N. History and Development of General Systems Theory. In W. Gray, F. Duke, and N. Rizzo (Eds.), *General System Theory and Psychiatry.* Boston: Little, Brown, 1969.

Griffith, H. M. Strategies for direct third-party reimbursement for nurses. *Am. J. Nurs.* 82:408, 1982.

Hain, M., Sr., and Chen, S. Health needs of the elderly. *Nurs. Res.* 25:433, 1976.

Isaacs, M. Toward a national health policy: A realist's view. *Am. J. Nurs.* 78:848, 1978.

Johnston, M. Ambulatory health care in the 80s: Decade of dilemmas. *Am. J. Nurs.* 80:76, 1980.

Lairson, P. D. Why informed consumers are choosing HMOs. *Patient Care* 16(18):67, 1982.

Lewis, C. E., et al. Child-initiated health care. *J. School Health* 50:144, 1980.

Mauksch, I. G. On national health insurance. *Am. J. Nurs.* 78:1323, 1978.

Moscovice, I. S., et al. Rural health care delivery amidst federal retrenchment: Lessons from the Robert Wood Johnson Foundation's Rural Practice Project. *Am. J. Public Health* 72(12):1380, 1982.

Ostrow, P. C. The historical precedents for quality assurance in health care. *AJOT* 37(1):23, 1983.

Raffel, M. W. *The United States Health System: Origins and Functions.* New York: Wiley, 1980.

Wingert, W. A., et al. Migrant health question . . . United States. *Pediatr. Nurse* 5:19, 1979.

World Health Organization. *The Album.* Geneva: World Health Organization, 1966.

QUESTIONS FOR REVIEW

1. Which of the following are components of all systems?
   a. Initiation, action, closed communication.
   b. Environmental interaction, progress.
   c. Purpose, content, process.
   d. Stimulation, feedback, openness.

2. An "open" system interacts with:
   a. Its component parts.
   b. The environment.
   c. System processers.
   d. Evaluators.

3. You are asked to join the board of a Health Systems Agency. You would qualify for such a position:
   a. Only if you do not have health insurance.
   b. Because you are a health care consumer.
   c. Only if you spend over $1,000 a year on health care.
   d. Only if you live in a large city.

4. A purpose of a Health Systems Agency is to:
   a. Prevent duplication of health care services.
   b. Carry out immunizations against common diseases.
   c. License health care providers.
   d. Sponsor educational programs on keeping well.

5. A state health department is an example of which type of agency?
   a. Voluntary.
   b. Profit-making.
   c. Private, nonprofit.
   d. Official.

6. The office of Dr. Smith, a pediatrician, represents which type of agency?
   a. Involuntary.
   b. Private, profit-making.
   c. Official.
   d. Federal.

7. A local community hospital generally represents which type of agency:
   a. Voluntary.
   b. Private, profit-making.
   c. Governmental additive.
   d. Official.

8. Mortality is a statistical term that refers to:
   a. The amount of illness in a community.
   b. The number of deaths of infants each year.
   c. The number of deaths per 1,000 population per year.
   d. The number of deaths of people over 65 each year.

9. Which of the following health care agencies offer comprehensive care?
   a. School health offices.
   b. Well child conferences.
   c. Emergency rooms.
   d. Health Maintenance Organizations.

10. Which of the following is true of the health care delivery system in the United States today?
    a. Health care is easily affordable by everyone.
    b. Health care facilities are evenly distributed among people.
    c. The focus of health care is on illness care.
    d. Health care delivery is always comprehensive.

7. COMMUNITY CONSIDERATIONS FOR HEALTH PROMOTION

OBJECTIVES

Upon mastery of the material in this chapter, you should be able to:

1. Describe the focus of community health nursing.
2. Describe the importance of identifying support people in the community.
3. Describe the areas of care of community health nursing.
4. Describe different family structures and family stages.
5. Describe important facets to assess about a community.

TERMS

The terms important for an understanding of this chapter are shown below and defined in the glossary:

community
community assessment
community health nurse
family
preventive focus

For many people the word *nurse* denotes someone who gives care in a hospital setting. Although most nurses are employed in hospitals, a hospital-based role is only one area of nursing practice. Other roles take the nurse into the community and settings such as schools, industry, ambulatory clinics, and homes. A nurse working in these settings is fulfilling a role in community health.

THE FOCUS OF COMMUNITY HEALTH NURSING

Community health nursing has a strong *preventive* focus. It is concerned mainly with keeping people well rather than beginning care after they are already ill and helping to restore health again. Community health nurses participate in all three levels of prevention: primary, secondary, and tertiary. For a review of representative activities at these levels see Table 6-1.

AREAS OF CARE OF THE COMMUNITY HEALTH NURSE

All care of patients must be family oriented in order to be successful because people are never totally separate from their families, even when they are physically separated from them due to hospitalization or illness. This concept is especially true in community health nursing when the patient is visited and cared for in his own home with his family present.

Direct Patient Care

Many people are discharged from health care agencies following an illness or surgery before they are completely ready to care for themselves. They receive follow-up care by returning to ambulatory settings such as clinics or a physician's office or by having a community health nurse care for them in their homes.

Local public health departments employ nurses for these services; many communities have privately funded organizations that employ nurses in community health roles as well. In contrast to a hospital-based nurse, the community health nurse typically wears a blue uniform and street stockings and shoes or average street clothing. She carries with her to the person's home the supplies she will need for care such as syringes to administer medicine (Fig. 7-1). Direct services of this nature often include not only physical care but also psychological support to give the person confidence to carry out his own care, to learn to live with a degree of handicap, or to educate him to a new way of self-care. The nurse's role may be as an advocate for him in the community.

Family Care

If a person has difficulty carrying out his own care or accepting a health problem, it is very likely that his family is also experiencing difficulty with the adjust-

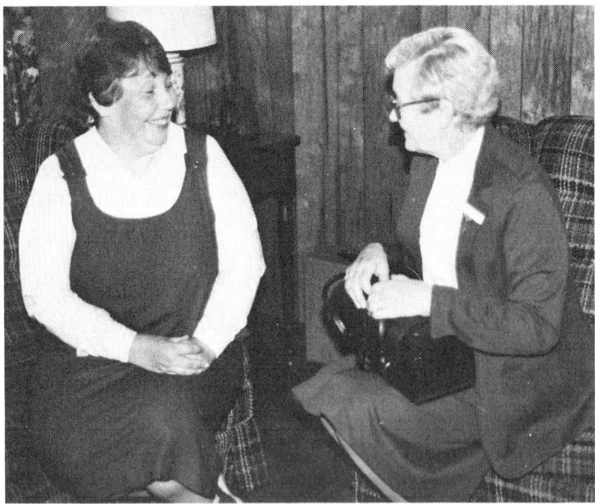

FIGURE 7-1. The community health nurse carries with her to the person's home the supplies she will need for care. Supplies are carried in a specially equipped bag such as the one this nurse holds on her lap.

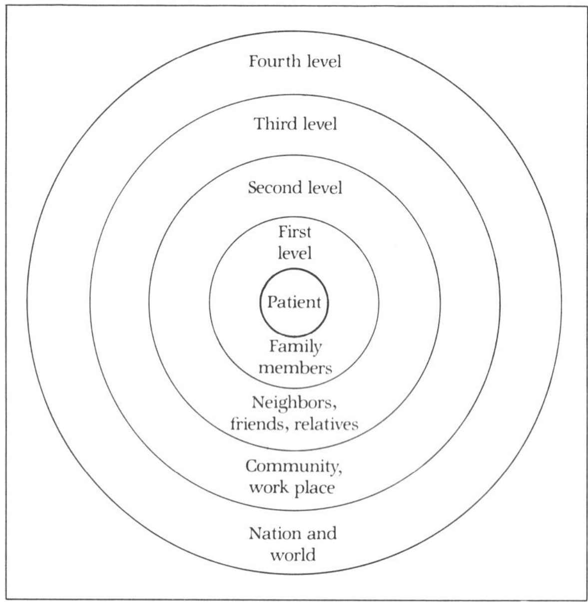

FIGURE 7-2. Levels of support people.

ment. To change a person's nutritional state, for example, you often have to talk not just to the person who is going to eat a new diet, but to the person who is going to prepare it as well. In order to ensure an infant's health, you have to consider the health of his caregivers and often the physical condition of his home: Are there screens on the windows to keep out flies? Are there rodents that can kill a newborn baby? Is there refrigeration if he is going to be formula fed?

Community Care

Just as the state of health of a member of a family depends on the family's health, the state of a family's health depends on that of the community. Community health nurses are concerned with problems of pollution or a low immunity level in the community, as these problems will eventually be reflected as ill health in individuals in the community.

In this role nurses are active as consultants or participants on planning and advisory boards concerning health problems and as health educators to inform people of potential dangers. The nurse may serve as an organizer of services needed in the community (recognizing the need for a hospice or a facility for the support of persons who are dying and helping to organize one) or as a liaison or coordinator of health care between home, hospital, workplace, or school.

IDENTIFYING SUPPORT PEOPLE

A person's support people are those people to whom he turns when he is in need of advice or physically dependent for care. Such people are termed *significant others* by sociologists. The average person has four circles or levels of support people he can call on as needed (Fig. 7-2).

First Level

First level support people are those individuals who live in close proximity to the person or have strong emotional attachments to him. In most instances these people are the person's family members. People who have no family (an older adult who has outlived other family members or a young adult living independently perhaps) may have no first level support people and must identify (often with your help) what would ordinarily be second level support people to use in this capacity. Being able to assess a patient's family is helpful in identifying which people are a patient's strongest support people.

Second Level

Second level support people are those people to whom a person would turn if his first level people are absent or if no first level people exist. These are typically friends, neighbors, and relatives outside the immediate family. The ability of second level support people to be effective is influenced by distance, transportation, and their feelings of responsibility to fill the role.

Third Level

The third level of support people is composed of individuals in the person's community, workplace, or school, or members of organizations to which the person belongs. Religious affiliation as a source of social contact is generally considered a third level support system, although an individual with a strong religious faith may well feel that his religious strength is a first level support system. In times of illness this ring of support people becomes very important because those at the first and second level may be so overwhelmed by the occurrence of illness in a loved one that they are no longer effective. A mother who has been told her child has diabetes, for example, may receive more support from an association of parents of children with diabetes for the first six months of her child's illness than her own family can supply to her. Careful assessment of a community to familiarize yourself with its services and facilities enables you to locate this ring of support people.

Fourth Level

The fourth level of support people is one that is almost unnoticed by the average person. It is the national or world population. People whose homes are devastated by an earthquake or flood become aware of this ring of support, as funds from this level become available to them for reestablishing their lives. For a person involved in a severe disaster, fourth ring support may be his most important support system.

TYPES OF FAMILIES

The support that a person receives from his family depends a good deal on the status of the family. People come from different types of families and families change in structure as they mature or are affected by such happenings as divorce or death of a marriage partner.

The Nuclear Family

A nuclear family is composed of husband, wife, and children. As a rule, a person receives his strongest support and is most strongly influenced by the values of his nuclear family. As most young people move away from their parents when they marry or establish housekeeping, more and more families today are nuclear in structure (no grandparents, aunts, or uncles live in the home). Although a person receives strong support from such a family structure, in time of illness or other crisis the nuclear family may offer limited support (the family members are as worried or frightened as the ill person and so cannot be effective in offering support).

The Extended Family

An extended family is one that includes not only the nuclear family but also other family members such as grandmothers, grandfathers, aunts, uncles, cousins, and grandchildren. Extended families offer more people to serve as resources in times of crisis and more role models for behavior and learning values. In an extended family a person's strongest support person or a child's primary caregiver may not be the person you first assume it to be; the grandmother may give the largest amount of child care, even though the child's mother is present every day as well.

The Single-Parent Family

In as many as 50 percent of families with school-age children today, only one parent lives in the home, due both to the high divorce rate and to the increasingly common practice of women raising children outside marriage. A health problem in a single-parent family is almost always compounded, because if the parent is ill, there is no backup person for child care. If a child is ill, there is no close support person to give reassurance or a second opinion on whether the child is becoming better again.

Low income is often an additional problem encountered by single-parent families, as the parent is most often a woman (nationally, women's incomes are lower than men's). Single parents often have difficulty with role modeling or identifying their own role in the family (they want to "mother" but they also must be father and breadwinner). Trying to fulfill two parental roles is not only time consuming but mentally and physically fatiguing and, in many instances, not satisfying. Such a woman may feel low self-esteem (if her husband left her or if the father of her child refused to marry her); low self-esteem interferes with decision making and thereby impedes effective daily functioning.

The Single-Adult Family

Many people live by themselves in apartments or rooming houses separate from family members; there is also a growing trend for people to live singly in private homes. Such people may lack support people in a crisis situation but generally have at least a neighbor or a family member close by on whom they know they can call at such times. The community health nurse's role might include helping a person to appreciate the importance of asking for help, as once a person declares his independence from a family, he may consider it face-losing to have to ask them for help. Many people living alone have a close attachment to a pet. Worrying about the welfare of a well-loved pet during a period of illness can be as devastating to some people as worrying over another person would be.

The Communal Family

Communes are composed of groups of people who have chosen to live together as an extended family group; their relationship to each other is social-value or interest motivated rather than kinship based. The values of commune members are often more freedom and free-choice oriented than those of a traditional family structure, and members may have fewer set roles. People with this philosophy may have difficulty conforming with health care regimes (health care itself may be seen as an established system which they are rejecting). On the other hand, people who reject traditional values may be the most creative people in a community and most interested in participating in their own care and so may have the best outcomes from therapy.

Cohabitation Families

Cohabitation families are couples who are raising children but remain unmarried by choice. Such people can offer as much support to each other as those formally married to each other. Although the relationship may be temporary in some cases, in others it is as long-lasting and as meaningful as more traditional alliances.

Homosexual Unions

Homosexual unions are persons of the same sex living together as married partners for both companionship and sexual fulfillment. Although such marriages are currently contradictory to the majority of people's value system, they offer firm support in times of crisis comparable to that offered by a traditional nuclear family. Children reared in his type of household need some exposure to traditional male-female roles so that they have the opportunity to make a more traditional life-style decision for themselves if they choose.

FAMILY LIFE CYCLES

Families, like individuals, pass through predictable developmental stages. Recognizing the stage of a family is as important as knowing an individual's developmental stage. Currently accepted developmental stages of families as identified by Duvall (1977) are shown in Table 7-1.

Stage I: Marriage

During the first stage of family development, members work to achieve three separate identifiable tasks: establishing a mutually satisfying marriage, relating well to their families, and reproductive life planning. Establishing a mutually satisfying marriage includes not only adjusting to each other in terms of routines (sleeping, eating, housecleaning) but also sexual and economic aspects. The first stage of family development is a tenuous one, as evidenced by the high divorce rate today at this stage. Illness of a member at this stage may be enough to destroy the still lightly formed bonds of partners, if the partners do not receive support from their former family members or from alert health care providers.

TABLE 7-1. FAMILY LIFE CYCLES

Stage	Characteristics
Stage I: Marriage	Two partners learning to manage finances, leisure time, decision making, and life style.
Stage II: Early childbearing	Two partners with one or more infant children accepting the responsibility for child care.
Stage III: Families with preschool children	Parents are maturing; childrearing has become a way of life.
Stage IV: Families with schoolage children	Parents reach middle age; begin to reach peak of earning power.
Stage V: Families with teenagers	Family changes goal to loosen, not strengthen, family ties so children can be independent.
Stage VI: Launching center families	Partners become a two-member family again as children leave home. Must readjust to new life style.
Stage VII: Families of middle years	Return to two-member family is complete.
Stage VIII: Families in retirement or old age	Family may become a single-member family if one partner dies. A final "rounding out" phase of life.

Source: E. M. Duvall, *Marriage and Family Development* (5th ed.). Philadelphia: Lippincott, 1977.

Stage II: Early Childbearing

The birth of a first baby is a stress to a family because of the economic and social role changes that are required. An important nursing role during this period is health education concerning well child care. It is a developmental step to change from being able to care for a well baby to caring for an ill baby. One way of determining whether a parent has made this change is to ask what the new parent has tried to do to solve a child-rearing or health problem. Even if what the person answers is not therapeutic or the best solution to the problem, as long as it is sensible (not "I don't do anything when the baby's sick; I just take him right to my mother" but "I've been trying to give him a little water and keep him warm"), it probably means the parent has mastered this developmental step. Parents who have difficulty with this step need a great deal of support and counseling from health care providers to be able to care for ill children at home or to give care to the child during a hospitalization.

Stage III: Families with Preschool Children

A family with preschool children is a busy family because children of this age demand a great deal of time due to the number of questions they ask daily and the amount of safety precautions which must be provided for them. Accidents are a major health concern during this family stage. If a child is hospitalized, parents may have difficulty facing the fact of his injury due to their guilt over the cause of his accident. It may be difficult for parents to visit due to the care requirements of other young children at home. Because it is such a busy time in the family life cycle, a family in this stage often needs continued support and help from a community health nurse in order to provide necessary health care for an ill member.

Stage IV: Families with Schoolage Children

Parents of schoolage children have the important responsibility of preparing their children to be able to function in a complex world while at the same time maintaining their own satisfying marriage relationship. For many families this is a trying time. Illness imposed at this stage adds to the burdens already present and may be enough to dissolve the marriage. Support systems within a family may be deceptive in that while family members are obviously physically present, if internal tension exists, they may not provide emotional support. Many families during this period will need to turn to the tertiary support level (friends, church organizations, health organizations) for adequate support.

Accidents—mainly motor vehicle ones—account for about half of the deaths of children of this age group. Many children are beginning to develop risk factors for heart disease, obesity, hypertension, and high blood cholesterol level.

Important concerns of a community health nurse during this family stage are monitoring the children's health in terms of immunization, dental care, and health care assessments; monitoring child safety related to electrical or automobile accidents; and encouraging a meaningful school experience that will make learning a lifetime occurrence, not merely a 12-year one.

Stage V: The Family with Teenagers

A family with teenagers has a different goal than in its previous stages. Prior to this time, one of its major objectives was strengthening family ties and maintaining family unity. Now the family must loosen family ties to allow adolescents more freedom and prepare them for life on their own. As technology advances at a rapid rate, the gap between generations increases; life when the parents were young was very different from what it is for their teenagers, making this a trying family stage for both children and adults.

Violence—accidents, homicide, and suicide—is the major cause of death in children in this age group. The nurse working with families at this stage, therefore, spends time counseling members on safety (driving defensively and not under the influence of alcohol), proper care and respect for firearms, and drug abuse. If a generation gap exists between parents and children, children are unable to talk to parents about these problems, particularly those of controversial nature such as sexual responsibility. A community health nurse is a neutral person who can assist families at this stage when communication difficulties exist.

Stage VI: Launching Center Families

For many families the stage at which children leave to establish their own households is the hardest stage, because it appears to represent the breaking up of the family. Parental roles change from those of mother or father to once-removed support persons or guideposts. The stage may represent a loss of self-esteem for parents who feel themselves being replaced by other people in their children's lives. They may feel old for the first time and less able to cope with their responsibilities. In an extended family older members may no longer be fully able to care for themselves, and decisions as to whether they should remain at home or go to an extended care facility may have to be made. Illness imposed on a family at this stage may be very detrimental to the family structure, acting as the "straw" that breaks up an already disorganized and uncohesive group.

A community health nurse, again, serves as counselor to such a family. She should help the parents to gain a better perspective of what is happening, to understand that their children are doing what they taught them to do, and that it is a positive not a negative situation. Major health concerns that arise in this stage are alcohol abuse (an estimated 10 million Americans are problem drinkers); continued routine supervision of health (even if parents have symptoms of disease such as a sign of cancer they may neglect going for health evaluation, trying to deny that anything so serious could happen to them); good nutrition; and adequate techniques for coping with stress.

Stage VII: Families of Middle Years

When a family returns to a two-partner nuclear unit, the same as it was prior to childbearing, the partners may view this stage either as the prime time of their lives (with opportunity to travel, economic independence, time to spend with hobbies) or as a period of gradual decline (lacking the constant activity and stimulation of children in the home; finding life boring without them; experiencing an "empty nest" syndrome). Diseases such as heart and kidney disorders occur with increased frequency at this stage. Because the family has returned to a two-partner union, support people may not be as plentiful as they were before. They may therefore need increased support from their health care providers.

Stage VIII: Family in Retirement or Old Age

The number of families of retirement age approximate 15 percent of the population. As a group Stage VIII members are more apt to suffer from chronic and disabling conditions than members in younger age groups. A community health nurse working with a family at this stage monitors health (taking medications that cause counteractive effects is an important problem at this age), encourages such individuals to stay active, not only physically but mentally, and promotes good nutrition (sometimes difficult if finances or transportation to shopping facilities are problems).

FAMILY ASSESSMENT

It is necessary to assess families for various characteristics, since the amount of support a person can expect from his family depends a great deal on these factors. If a patient you are caring for will need continued care after he returns home, you may want to identify and contact the nurturing member of the family as it will probably be this person who will supervise or give the needed care at home. Be aware that although nurturing has typically been thought of as a female characteristic, many men are just as nurturing as women and in some families it is the man who fulfills this role.

If a patient's illness will cause a major change in life style for the family, you may want to identify and contact the person in the family who is the decision maker or the person who is the problem solver (not necessarily the same). If the patient's illness will involve increased expense, you may want to identify and contact the wage earner for the family.

Knowledge of a family's safety and health consciousness is also important in helping you to plan care for a person. Identifying the family's support people helps you to evaluate the family's ability to cope with stress such as an ill family member. The following box lists areas of family assessment to consider and questions to ask to elicit this information.

Family Assessemnt

Area of Assessment	*Questions to Ask*
Type of family	Is the family nuclear, extended, communal, etc.?
Family characteristics	What is the socioeconomic level? What is their ethnic background? What is their religious affiliation?
Dominant family figure	Who makes decisions, particularly in the areas of finances and leisure time?
Nurturing figure	Who is the primary caregiver to children or any handicapped member?
Finances	Who is the family provider? Are finances adequate? If more than one person earns money, is it fairly divided?
Safety	Is the home safe from fire or accidents? Does a family member know the technique of CPR?
Health	Does the family eat a nutritious diet? Do they receive adequate sleep? Are immunizations current? Is there a balance between work and recreation? Can they cope with problems adequately?
Problem solver	Who does everyone turn to if they have a problem?
Support within family	Do they eat together or spend an equal amount of time with each other daily? Do they band together to defend each other from outsiders?
Outside support	Is the family active in community organizations or activities? Do they visit (or are visited by) friends and relatives? Can the family name one person they can always rely on for help in a time of crisis?

COMMUNITY ASSESSMENT

Community is a term that can be defined in many ways but it is generally accepted to refer to a limited geographic area in which the residents relate to and interact among themselves. When asked what community they are from, therefore, people may mention the entire city, a school district, a geographic district ("the east side"), a street name ("Pine Street area"), or a natural marking ("the lower creek area").

Because the health of individuals is influenced by the health of their community, it is important to become acquainted with the communities where you practice. If you are caring for a patient from a community unknown to you, it is important to assess his community to see if there are aspects about it that contributed to his illness (and that therefore need to be corrected) and to determine whether he will be able to return to such a community without extra help and counseling from you or some other health care provider.

Community assessment consists of examining the various systems that are present in almost all communities to see if they are functioning adequately.

Housing System

The condition of homes in a community is influenced by the financial structure and age of the community. Learn whether the average house in a community is a single- or multiple-family one; whether there is adequate heat and the means of heat (oil heat is expensive but also even and consistent); whether there is indoor plumbing and an adequate hot water supply.

The average age of houses in the community may tell you something about the average age of the persons living there. Homes 20 years old were probably purchased by couples then in their early twenties; the average couple in the community is probably now middle-aged. If the houses are 40 to 50 years old, the average person living there is likely 60 to 70 years old. Alternatively, older homes may have been divided into apartments which are occupied by a transient young population. If the neighborhood is composed primarily of apartment complexes, the population is also probably primarily young adults.

Knowing the condition of homes alerts you to many problems associated with health care services: If the home is old and in need of repairs, available funds may have to be spent on home repair rather than medicine; if there is no hot water, heating a sufficient amount to soak an infected arm will require more of an effort than if hot water were readily available; if the house is a second- or third-floor apartment with no elevator, exercise and activity following an illness may be a problem. Houses built before 1940 were painted with paint very high in lead content, which if eaten by preschool children, causes lead poisoning (plumbism), with permanent neurological damage and mental retardation. Children of this age should not be living in houses with lead-based paint if it can possibly be avoided.

Knowing the closeness of houses or buildings alerts you to potential health problems: If houses are well spaced with long driveways and large lawns, the people living in them may have less daily exposure to other people and may grow lonely if confined to their home because of illness; the physical activity involved in maintaining the lawns or shoveling snow from long driveways may cause an increased risk of cardiovascular disease in men (Fig. 7-3). If the population is transitory, a person may be discharged after a long hospitalization and no longer know the people living near him. Be aware that communities with resident schools, universities, or colleges and resort communities have different populations, depending on whether school, the ski season, or the beach season is bringing people into the area. In such communities people may need to locate two separate support systems, one for the busy time of the year, another for when the community seems deserted. Be familiar with the housing provided at resident schools; dormitory rooms located at a distance from a bathroom or a supervising adult may cause problems for a person returning to them after a hospitalization.

FIGURE 7-3. Ensuring that someone is there to shovel the walk in winter may make the difference for an older person who otherwise may be afraid to go outside.

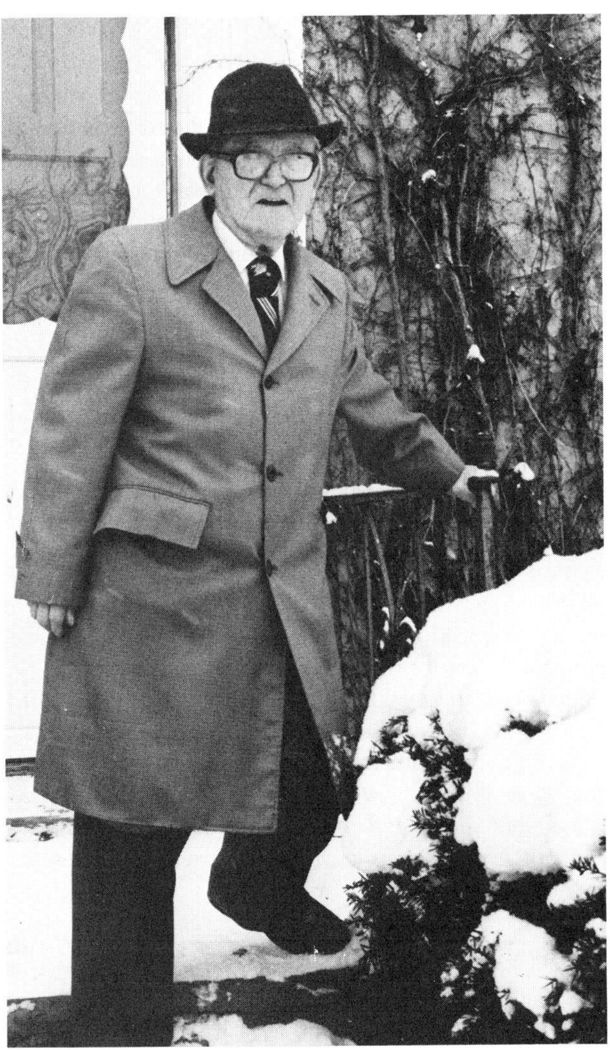

Too many people in a household can cause an increase in communicable disease and psychological stress (lack of privacy, increased noise level). In children five to fourteen years of age, the number of people per household appears to be an important factor. One study shows that a high mortality in children one to five years of age is associated with a high number of individuals per household, lack of hot water and inside lavatory space, and decreased owner occupancy (Brennan, 1978).

Transportation System

Knowing a community's transportation system alerts you to the ease or difficulty a person may have returning to a health care facility for follow-up care or visiting one for diagnosis at the first symptoms of illness. Poor transportation facilities may also prevent someone from obtaining medicine or attending an educational program on how to keep well.

In communities where bus service is frequent and convenient, many people do not own cars; if some condition prevents them from using a bus (a large bulky cast, inability to wait in the cold), or if public transportation should be on strike, they are virtually trapped in a small, walkable area. In other communities there is no public transportation and a person must depend on automobile transportation. If he cannot drive, visits to a health care facility will present a problem. The cost of using taxicabs for transportation may be prohibitive if frequent visits are required. In still other communities freeways are built across communities, cutting them in two and making it physically impossible to get from one section to another without major expense.

A large number of automobiles in a community increases the amount of environmental pollution (a problem for people with lung disease and possibly a cause of high lead contamination). Heavy use of automobiles also leads to an increased auto accident rate.

The transportation present in a community may alert you to health teaching needs (children need special auto safety seats and to be taught good street safety). In the vicinity of a railroad station your health education plans specific for that community should include measures to prevent children playing near tracks or with boxcars.

Educational System

The educational system of a community reflects the overall interest of the people to learn new skills or new knowledge. If a community is educationally oriented (the school is open not just during the day but in the evening for adult classes as well), learning about disease, self-care, and ways to stay well will be accepted as another educational process. If the community is not education focused, becoming a student again may be a painful transition for a person, even when something as serious as his own health is concerned.

Be aware of what kinds of health education programs are stressed in different communities. If a school district has a strong antidrug abuse program in all grades, for example, that may be an area in which you will need to do little teaching and which you may even want to avoid to prevent overkill. Know the frequency with which classes in cardiopulmonary resuscitation (CPR) are taught in order to estimate the proportion of people in the community who have at least a working acquaintance with this skill.

Age-Span System

The age-span system of a community influences the illnesses seen and the necessary health care facilities. A community formed of mostly older adults, for example, will have few resources either in direct health care facilities or in support people for the young woman expecting her first child. A community with a high incidence of children must provide health care services for the frequent lacerations and minor illnesses of childhood; such health care services might have difficulty fully meeting the needs of older adults with long-term illnesses. Assess what an individual outside the normal age span of the community could do to improve health care for himself at the point he needs it.

Sociocultural System

The sociocultural system of a community refers to the values or beliefs and life styles of the people in the community. A person's values and life style influence when and how much health care and health education he seeks; they also influence the level of health that people accept as wellness.

Many people from one ethnic group have a mistrust of or at least a suspicious attitude toward members of another ethnic group. This attitude may make it more difficult for a person of an ethnic group different from yours to accept health information from you until you prove yourself trustworthy and he sees you as "different" but helpful. A combination of different ethnic groups in a community may require specific programs to help groups accept each other to establish a sense of community.

The diet that people ingest is strongly influenced by their culture. Black Americans, for example, tend to eat a diet high in salt; people of Italian heritage use a great deal of pasta daily. Stores in the community stock those foods that are asked for most often; a person without these preferences may have to leave the immediate area to find the particular foods he enjoys. Dietary patterns contribute to the amount of obesity, iron-deficiency anemia, and cardiovascular disease in a community.

Culture also influences the standards of the community for work and recreation. If the members of a community believe that all citizens should be striving for a five-day work week or that men should be the total breadwinners of the family, the person who can no longer meet this standard because of illness may have a more difficult time adjusting than one in a community where work ethics are not so regulated. What activities are appropriate for women varies a great deal from community to community and is based largely on sociocultural influences.

Financial-Occupational System

The work that people do influences their health. A fishing population may be ingesting a high level of environmental contaminants such as mercury; workers producing asbestos may be inhaling lung irritants; workers with chemical substances may be handling potential cancer-causing agents. In communities where most men work in coal mines, the incidence of "black lung disease" (chronic occupational lung disease) is higher than in other communities. In areas where the average man works in an office of a corporation where he deals with a high level of stress, peptic ulcer (a stress-related erosion of the stomach lining) may be more common than normal. Men who work at desk jobs tend to have lower sperm counts than those who do not (increased scrotal heat decreases sperm motility), so fertility rates in such communities may be affected.

Occupations also determine financial levels, which influence the community's housing, education, and recreation systems. They can also influence dietary patterns. If the average person in the community packs a lunch, you need to include in your diet advice ways to adapt a diet to a brown bag. In dairyland areas people typically eat the products of their work (butter, milk, and cream), and blood cholesterol levels may be higher than in those communities where dairy products are not so easily obtained (dairy products contain saturated fat which increases blood cholesterol levels). Dairy families may also drink unpasteurized milk, which carries the risk of tuberculosis and brucellosis.

Political System

The political system of a community influences the way that public money is spent. The amount of money spent on health education programs or health care facilities is often influenced strongly by the ease or difficulty by which federal, state, or county money can be obtained. Whether a community is active in a political sense (the majority of people vote in elections) reflects the overall intent of the citizens in the community to regulate their lives. A person who views active participation as a necessary activity in his life is probably more interested in learning self-care following an illness than a person who does not.

Recreational System

Communities differ a great deal in the number and kinds of recreational opportunities available to their members. Recreational activities can both improve and present risks to health. Jogging, for example, is healthful in terms of aerating lung tissue, but it may lead to knee cartilage disorders or injury from auto accidents. Football leagues for young boys may result in a high incidence of knee and other injuries. If lakes where people swim in unsupervised settings are located in the community, a high incidence of drowning or near drowning may result; near-by mountains may lead to a high incidence of sprained ankles and poison ivy.

The number of recreational activities also usually reflects the view of the people in the community about the value of recreation. In a community where everyone plays in a local baseball league, the person who can no longer participate in this sport due to illness may feel this to be more of a handicap than would the person whose community does not place a high value on this activity.

Safety-Protection System

Protection systems include fire, law enforcement, and sanitation (garbage and water purification) systems. If law enforcement is inadequate, people may be unable to follow a simple instruction such as "Walk around the block daily": They worry that they will be "mugged" on the street or that their apartment will be ransacked while they are gone. In communities where people mainly use well water rather than a chlorinated-fluoridated water supply, there is a greater potential for spread of infectious diseases such as salmonella (diarrhea), and there is generally a high incidence of dental disease from the lack of fluoride protection.

Religious System

The religious system of a community and the values of its members influence the activities and facilities. If there is a strong Roman Catholic population, there are probably few local reproductive life planning facilities; if there is a strong Jewish influence, nursing homes for the elderly are probably well regulated and maintain high standards, as a Jewish community tends to place high value on the care of its older members.

Churches and synagogues also sponsor many of the recreational and social activities in the community. If there are few synagogues or churches in the area, such opportunities may be limited.

A person's religious system can serve as a strong support system for him particularly at a time of crisis. For those without a strong religious system, health care providers may need to fulfill this support function.

Environmental System

Some communities have much greater environmental problems or hazards than others. Any community near industry has the potential for having its air filled with pollutants noxious to good respiratory function; if the industry contaminates a stream or river nearby, irritants may be present in the water supply. Farming communities may have high contact levels of insecticides. A person with a chronic respiratory illness may be almost free of symptoms in an air-conditioned hospital but begin to develop acute symptoms within 24 hours after his return to his home downwind from a chemical plant.

Environment also includes the "milieu" or the psychological tone of the community. If the community is one of mainly young "on-the-way-up" executives, the psychological tension within the community may not be conducive to mental health. If the community is near a nuclear reactor or known contaminated chemical dumpsite, the anxiety level of the community may be higher than in a community where concern about the safety of such facilities does not exist.

Health Care System

Health care is not consistent from community to community. Learn what facilities are available in different areas of the community where you practice. In an area where there is an adequate number of physicians for the population, people typically visit a physician at the first sign of an illness. If the nearest physician is 50 miles away, however, a person may delay some time before he makes that long a trip.

In some communities there are actually too many hospitals, and health care providers are stretched too thin to offer the highest level of care they could if services were consolidated. Other communities have gaps in care (no service for women's health, neurological diagnosis, health teaching).

Not only the number of such services but the accessibility to them is important. Services at a distance from public transportation may be very difficult for some members of a community to reach and will not be used effectively.

USING COMMUNITY ASSESSMENT

Knowing the components of a community allows you to understand why people admitted for hospitalization reach the condition they do before they come for help (a woman living alone in a city has no transportation avail-

Community Assessment for Discharge Planning

Area of Assessment	*Questions to Ask*
Age span	Is the person within the usual age span of the community and thereby assured of third-ring support people?
Education	If the person is school age, is there provision for his schooling? Is there a library for self-education? Is there easy access to such places if the person is handicapped? If a special program such as diet counseling is needed, does it exist?
Environment	Are there environmental risks present such as air pollution? Busy highways? Train yards? Pools or water where frequent drownings occur? Will hypothermia be a problem from cold weather?
Finances, occupation	Is there a high rate of unemployment in the community? What is the average occupation? Will this person have adequate finances to manage comfortably? Are there supplemental aid programs available?
Health care delivery	Is there a health care agency the person can attend for comprehensive care? Is it convenient in terms of finances and transportation?
Housing	Are houses mainly privately owned or apartments? Are homes close enough together to afford easy contact? Are they in good repair? Is upkeep such as constant repair or extensive lawn mowing a problem?
Political	Is the community active politically? Can the person reach a local polling place to vote or does he know how to apply for absentee ballots?
Recreational	Are there recreational activities available of interest to the person? Are they economically feasible for him?
Religion	Is there a facility where the person can worship as he chooses? Is there easy transportation to it?
Safety, protection	Is there adequate protection so that the person can feel safe to leave his home or remain home alone? Does he know about "hot lines" available to him? Local and fire department numbers? Is his home safe from fire?
Sociocultural	What is the dominant culture in the community? Does the person fit into this environment? Are foods that are culturally significant to him available?
Transportation	Is there public transportation? Will the person have access to it if he is handicapped?

able to her until her son comes home from work; a man tried to ignore his chronic cough because other men were being laid off and he was worried that too much sick time would look bad on his record; a five-year-old child develops measles because there were no free immunization services in the community). You can better prepare people for return to their community after hospitalization if, for example, you know whether the Pine Street area has well or city water before you give discharge instructions; how many flights of stairs someone from the Stevens Plaza area will have to walk to reach his apartment; the availability of public transportation before you tell a mother to bring her child back every day for a dressing change. The preceding box summarizes areas of community assessment to use in discharge planning and questions to ask to elicit this information.

UTILIZING NURSING PROCESS

Mrs. Carmen Zarratini is a 65-year-old woman who is going to be discharged in four days following a persistent urinary tract infection. She is to continue taking an oral antibiotic for 10 more days and is to return to Urology Clinic for a follow-up visit in two weeks. The following example of a discharge summary note shows what kind of information should be included on her record.

NURSING DIAGNOSIS

Adult female with potential for independent community functioning related to supportive environment.

ASSESSMENT

Discharge status: Ability to function in community.

Physical Status: Patient is able to care for own needs including self-medication. Has a reminder chart prepared to take home with her to tape to refrigerator door so she remembers medication. Urged to return to normal level of activity by one week post discharge and to continue to drink at least one quart of fluid daily. Advised about necessity of good perineal hygiene. Not sexually active following death of husband three years ago.

Housing: Patient lives upstairs in apartment over delicatessen. Has adequate heat, hot water, and furnishings; indoor plumbing.

Support People: Patient has telephone in working order and states that her daughter-in-law phones her daily to check on her. Visits son and his family once a week, usually for Sunday dinner. Had difficulty accepting her daughter-in-law at one time because of cultural differences (daughter-in-law is English-Irish) but states now, "If I ever really need anything, I know Briar (daughter-in-law) would do it for me." Called daughter-in-law to bring her to hospital when symptoms of infection were first noticed. Has friends in neighborhood; these and delicatessen employees visit her frequently.

Occupation: Patient receives Social Security benefits plus a small monthly pension check from husband's former place of employment. Works three afternoons a week as housekeeper for parish priest. States "I'm comfortable," although was unable to buy the winter coat she wanted until it went on sale this spring.

Transportation: Patient does not drive but uses public transportation without difficulty; calls on daughter-in-law to drive her to any location not accessible by bus lines.

Recreation: Plays Bingo once a week at church. Knits. Chats in delicatessen downstairs.

Self-esteem: Thinks of herself as an active, busy person who has functioned well following husband's death three years ago. Has one son in medical school here in city; another son in California she speaks of proudly.

Safety: States she feels safe in apartment and on streets near apartment. Uses electric stove, has good vision and mobility, so falls should not be a problem.

Religious: Attends church once a week. Can talk any time with parish priest who is her employer.

Health Care: Does not have private physician. Uses the ambulatory services of hospital as primary health care provider. Has telephone number of hospital if she should need assurance or consultation before follow-up appointment.

RECOMMENDATIONS

Should do well with self-medication regime at home due to active and responsible life-style and presence of available support people.

SUGGESTED READINGS

Allor, M. T. The "community profile" . . . To better understand the community, its strengths and areas of potential or actual need. *JNE* 22(1):12, 1983.

Balik, B., et al. Developing a community-based parent education support group. *JOGN Nurs.* 10:197, 1981.

Brennan, M. W., and Lancashire, R. Association of childhood mortality with housing status and unemployment. *J. Epidemiol. Community Health* 32:28, 1978.

Community program serves released psychiatric patients. *Hospitals* 64(2):28, 1983.

Duvall, E. M. *Marriage and Family Development* (5th ed.). Philadelphia: Lippincott, 1977.

Friedman, M. *Family Nursing.* New York: Appleton-Century-Crofts, 1981.

Getty, C., and Humphreys, W. *Understanding the Family.* New York: Appleton-Century-Crofts, 1981.

Kline, M. M., et al. Quality assurance in public health. *Nurs. Health Care* 1:192, 1980.

Leininger, M. *Transcultural Nursing 1979.* St. Paul, Minn.: Masson, 1980.

McPhee, A. T. Sharing: Let the family in. *Nursing* 13(1):120, 1983.

Nass, G. *Marriage and the Family.* Menlo Park: Cal.: Addison-Wesley, 1978.

Pinckney, C. A., et al. Public health nurse: Generalist or specialist? *Am. J. Nurs.* 83(1):86, 1983.

Ray, D. W., et al. Competition vs. cooperation in community health nursing. *Nurs. Outlook* 28:626, 1980.

Robbins, M., et al. Family hierarchies. *Am. J. Nurs.* 82:284, 1982.

Robischon, P., and Smith, J. A. Family Assessment. In A. M. Reinhardt and M. D. Quinn (Eds.), *Current Practice in Family-Centered Community Nursing.* St. Louis: Mosby, 1977.

Shamansky, S. L., et al. A community is . . . . *Nurs. Outlook* 29:182, 1981.

Weissbourd, B., et al. Family focus: Supporting families in the community. *Child. Today* 10:6, 1981.

QUESTIONS FOR REVIEW

1. Match the problem in the right column that is most apt to occur in the family stage shown in the left column.

a. Stage I—Marriage	1. Many things to do every day
b. Stage II—Early Childbearing	2. Adjusting to two partner relationship again
c. Stage III—Preschool Children	3. Feeling useless due to an "empty nest" syndrome
d. Stage IV—Schoolage Children	4. Marriage partners adjusting to each other's life styles
e. Stage V—Adolescent Children	5. Difficulty meeting good nutrition
f. Stage VI—Launching Center	6. Teaching children to be independent
g. Stage VII—Middle Years	7. Teaching children responsibility
h. Stage VIII—Retirement or Old Age	8. Realizing the responsibility involved in creating a new life.

2. Various different types of family structures are shown in column I. Select the characteristic from column II that matches each situation in column I.

a. Homosexual union	1. Many traditional values rejected
b. Communal family	2. Limited financial resources
c. Single-parent family	3. Limited support persons available
d. Nuclear family	4. Limited sexual role modeling present
e. Extended family	5. Many child caregivers available

8. CONSUMER RIGHTS AND HEALTH CARE

OBJECTIVES
Upon mastery of the material in this chapter, you should be able to:

1. Describe the concept of health care delivery as a product and patients as consumers of that product.
2. Describe the circumstances that led to the development of Bills of Rights.
3. Describe common entities of various patient bills of rights.
4. Describe commonly accepted nurses' rights.
5. Describe the association between nursing ethics and patient rights.

TERMS
The terms important for an understanding of this chapter are shown below and defined in the glossary:

Bill of Rights
consumer

A *consumer* is someone who uses a product. Almost everyone is a consumer of products such as breakfast cereal, toothpaste, and city water. For most of history health care was not thought of as a product and so the people who benefited from it (patients) were not thought of as consumers. Today health care *is* viewed as a product; like breakfast cereal, it is a commodity that is purchased. Once you begin to think of health care this way, you begin to ask yourself, as a consumer, what kind of guarantees do I have of consistency in health care the same as I expect from breakfast cereal? Obviously, health care is not the same as breakfast cereal so some variability can be expected, but consumers should have some guarantee of consistency and safeguards from one setting of health care delivery to another.

As part of the increased consumer awareness movements of the 1960s and 1970s, the concept of health care has changed: Instead of thinking of health care as a *privilege*, we now regard it as a *right*. The preamble of the constitution of the World Health Organization (1966) states that this organization views good health as a right of all people. This statement implies that health *care* then is also a right, as health care is necessary to maintain health or return people to a state of wellness. The Declaration of Independence of the United States guarantees to every citizen the right to the pursuit of happiness. Many people interpret this to mean the right to health as it is difficult to be happy unless you have physical and mental well-being.

BILLS OF RIGHTS

Like the Bill of Rights of the nation's Constitution, which guarantees basic rights such as the right to assembly and freedom of speech, patient bills of rights are written to safeguard the rights of people when they come for health care and to provide guidelines as to how they can expect to be treated by health care providers.

The American Hospital Association Bill of Rights

In 1972 the American Hospital Association published a list of rights for hospitalized patients. These patient rights were devised to inform patients about what they could expect from their physician-patient relationship or the hospital-patient relationship. Indirectly, they apply to the rights of the patient with regard to all health care providers who contact him. It is suggested that a copy of such rights be distributed to people on admission to all Joint Accreditation (JACH) hospitals.

Patient rights are shown on page 100. As nurses are the people who put many of the physician's wishes into action, they have strong implications for nurses. They are discussed below in relation to nursing care.

A Patient's Bill of Rights

1. The patient has the right to considerate and respectful care.
2. The patient has the right to obtain from his physician complete current information concerning his diagnosis, treatment, and prognosis, in terms that the patient can be reasonably expected to understand. When it is not medically advisable to give such information to the patient, the information should be made available to an appropriate person in his behalf. He has the right to know by name the physician responsible for coordinating his care.
3. The patient has the right to receive from his physician information necessary to give informed consent prior to the start of any procedure and/or treatment. Except in emergencies, such information for informed consent should include but not necessarily be limited to the specific procedure and/or treatment, the medically significant risks involved, and the probable duration of incapacitation. Where medically significant alternatives for care or treatment exist, or when the patient requests information concerning medical alternatives, the patient has the right to such information. The patient also has the right to know the name of the person responsible for the procedures and/or treatment.
4. The patient has the right to refuse treatment to the extent permitted by law and to be informed of the medical consequences of his action.
5. The patient has the right to every consideration of his privacy concerning his own medical care program. Case discussion, consultation, examination, and treatment are confidential and should be conducted discreetly. Those not directly involved in his care must have the permission of the patient to be present.
6. The patient has the right to expect that all communications and records pertaining to his care should be treated as confidential.
7. The patient has the right to expect that within its capacity a hospital must make reasonable response to the request of a patient for services. The hospital must provide evaluation, service, and/or referral as indicated by the urgency of the case. When medically permissible, a patient may be transferred to another facility only after he has received complete information and explanation concerning the needs for and alternatives to such a transfer. The institution to which the patient is transferred must first have accepted the patient for transfer.
8. The patient has the right to obtain information as to any relationship of his hospital to other health care and educational institutions insofar as his care is concerned. The patient has the right to obtain information as to the existence of any professional relationships among individuals by name, who are treating him.
9. The patient has the right to be advised if the hospital proposes to engage in or perform human experimentation affecting his care or treatment. The patient has the right to refuse to participate in such research projects.
10. The patient has the right to expect reasonable continuity of care. He has the right to know in advance what appointment times and physicians are available and where. The patient has the right to expect that the hospital will provide a mechanism whereby he is informed by his physician or a delegate of the physician of the patient's continuing health.
11. The patient has the right to examine and receive an explanation of his bill regardless of source of payment.
12. The patient has the right to know what hospital rules and regulations apply to his conduct as a patient.

Source: A Patient's Bill of Rights, published by the American Hospital Association, copyright 1975.

STANDARD 1
The patient has the right to considerate and respectful care.

The right of respectful care has direct meaning for nursing as nurses have the most contact with patients in a hospital setting. Respectful care implies that such factors as individual preferences, developmental needs, cultural and religious practices, and age differences are considered and incorporated into care.

You must be certain not only that you yourself give respectful care but that those you supervise such as nurse's aides offer this same level of care. If a conflict arises in this area, it may result from an individual's interpretation of "respectful care."

STANDARD 2
The patient has the right to obtain from his physician complete current information concerning his diagnosis, treatment, and prognosis, in terms that the patient can be reasonably expected to understand.

In many instances people under stress do not "hear" well (or hear only what they expect or want to hear). Even though a physician offers a person a thorough explanation of his illness or planned treatment, after the

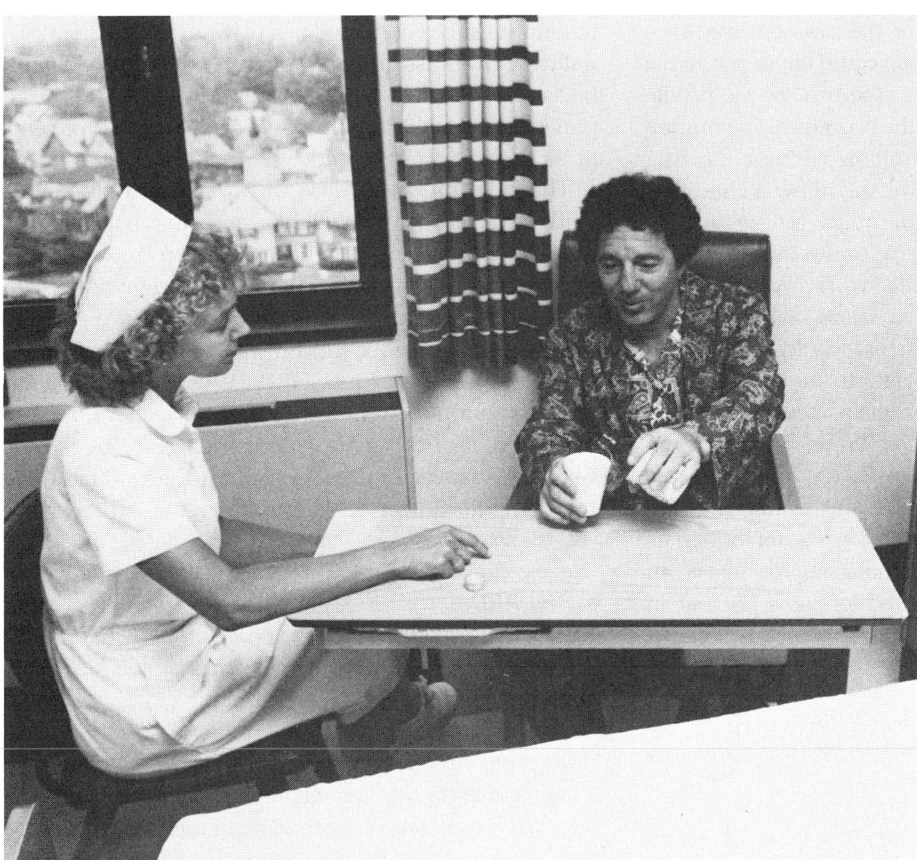

FIGURE 8-1. Nurses are often asked by patients to explain what the doctor said.

physician leaves, the person may turn to you and say, "What did she say? What kind of medicine did she mean?" Answering this type of question helps to ensure compliance as well as to fulfill a basic right of a hospitalized patient (Fig. 8-1).

In some instances a physician has used such technical language ("You have pneumonia and I'm going to start you on ampicillin") that you need to interpret the explanation in layman's terms ("You have an infection in your lungs; Dr. Jones is going to order a drug for you that cures infections"). Be careful when offering this type of information that you give factual explanations. Don't guess; if you don't know what the physician said, an honest "I wasn't listening to what she said, I'm sorry," or until your ability to interpret medical jargon increases, "To be honest, I didn't understand what she meant either," is your best approach. Then follow up by getting the information or alerting the physician that her explanation was not well understood. It is not disgraceful to lack knowledge of medical terminology as a beginner in nursing. It is disgraceful to try to fake an explanation based on inadequate knowledge, as this may result in the patient's receiving two different explanations of what is to happen to him. Almost nothing is so confusing and confidence-threatening as being given contradictory explanations.

Prognosis refers to an estimation of the ultimate outcome of the person's disease or condition. Early in the course of an illness it may be difficult for a physician to predict the outcome. She may speak of "guarded results" or say "Wait and see." These are not instances of trying to avoid offering a full explanation but rather of avoiding offering premature predictions. Many times you can help the patient to understand why an explanation seems vague by explaining that it is difficult to predict anything concrete at that point ("I'm sure Dr. Jones is waiting to see what your blood test shows before she says anything more to you"). As with any explanation, be certain that your words are based on facts, not hunches, to avoid confusion. Be certain that your explanations are clear and in terminology that the average person would understand.

STANDARD 3
The patient has the right to receive from his physician the information necessary to give informed consent.

Ten years ago, if a person was to have a procedure such as a lumbar puncture (where a needle is inserted into the spinal canal under sterile conditions and cerebral spinal fluid is withdrawn for analysis), the physician merely announced to the patient what she was going to do and added little more than "Don't worry, it's a simple procedure." Today in these same circumstances the physician must legally name the risks involved (the needle could strike a nerve which could cause paralysis; infection could be introduced at the time of the needle insertion), and alternatives to the procedure (beginning treatment for a supposed condition without the best information might be ineffective and allow a condition to grow worse). Although this approach is necessary for the patient's informed consent (a legal requirement), it also invariably adds a great deal of worry. A person may turn to you after a physician leaves and say, "I wish she hadn't told me all the things that could go wrong." Explaining that it is a person's right to know the risks as well as the benefits of treatment helps people to understand why the physician's explanation was in such detail. The average person appreciates the honesty of the explanation because he recognizes this as treating him as an adult with decision-making power, even though he may have found it easier in the days when a physician acted more as a father figure and less as a partner in care.

STANDARD 4
The patient has the right to refuse treatment to the extent permitted by law and to be informed of the medical consequences of his action.

The right to refuse treatment is easy to ignore, because when it is obvious to you that a course of treatment will make a person feel better, it seems bizarre for a patient to object to it. Usually the reason a person refuses treatment is that he does not fully understand its importance or effect (the benefits of treatments such as heat application or range of motion exercises are not obvious at first). Often explaining the purpose, therefore, is the answer to the problem. In other instances, a procedure will be acceptable if it is modified. In all instances you should learn why the person is refusing the treatment. In some cases it may not be the treatment he is refusing but the thought of having to stay in bed or remain in the hospital. In other instances a cultural or religious factor is interfering with acceptance; Jehovah's Witnesses, for example, generally refuse to have blood transfusions. Parents may refuse treatments such as intravenous therapy for their children because they do not want to see them hurt by the insertion of a needle.

If after an explanation of the procedure and its necessity the person still refuses it, remember that such action is his right. Health care is a right, not a requirement; a hospital stay is a purchased commodity, not a sentence. Good planning of care, including goal setting that includes the patient in planning, tends to reduce the problem of people refusing therapy.

STANDARD 5
The patient has the right to every consideration of his privacy.

Privacy is an easy right to forget in a busy hospital unit. It means that a discussion between you and the patient must be conducted in a private area, not a public hallway. Class assignments must not identify a patient by name or position. You must be careful not to discuss a patient or his condition in the hearing of other patients or as gossip among friends.

The right to privacy also means that people not directly involved in the patient's care must have his permission to be present when care is given. You also have the responsibility to ask people if it is all right with them if you look at some disease sign they have if you are interested in seeing the sign only to enlarge your scope of knowledge and not to give care. When your instructor comes into a patient's room, it is your responsibility to introduce her with a statement such as "This is Mrs. Clark, my instructor. Do you mind if she watches what I'm doing for a minute?" (And it might be difficult for you if the patient says, "Yes, I do mind").

STANDARD 6
The patient has the right to expect that all communications and records pertaining to his care should be treated as confidential.

To protect the right of confidentiality, be careful that you do not leave a patient chart in a place where it could be read by someone other than the patient or authorized personnel. Laboratory slips should contain no information other than that needed by the laboratory to process a sample or specimen. You may have to remind health care personnel such as volunteers, candy-stripers or dietary aides that a person's records are confidential and not to be discussed at home or with friends.

STANDARD 7
The patient has the right to expect that within its capacity a hospital must make reasonable response to the request of a patient for services.

Many times, as a nurse, you are the person who will be coordinating services for patients such as occupational therapy appointments, x-rays, and diagnostic studies. It is a patient's right not only that ordinary services such as these be provided, but also that they be provided in an order that is most convenient and shortens a hospital stay as much as possible. As a coordinator of care, you may need to justify to one hospital department why their service must follow the service of another in order for service to be most convenient for the patient.

STANDARD 8
The patient has the right to obtain information as to any relationship of his hospital to other health care and educational institutions or hospital personnel to each other.

Patients have the right to know whether a hospital is affiliated religiously or with a university or an extended care facility because these relationships may affect care.

A university-affiliated hospital, for example, is certain to have students giving care as part of their learning experiences; a hospital affiliated with an extended care facility may ask a patient to transfer to the adjoining setting sooner than if there were no associated facility. Such associations may be advantageous rather than detrimental for a person (a university-associated hospital usually uses the latest knowledge available; being transferred early to an extended care facility may save considerable expense). That a person should know professional relationships is included as a right so that a person could know that the specialist his physician asked to consult is the physician's sister. Although a relationship does not imply that such a consult was made to help out a relative rather than to provide the best care, being informed of the fact that such a relationship exists is a patient right. By this same standard patients have the right to know the title and status of the nurse caring for them and to refuse to have a student care for them.

STANDARD 9
The patient has the right to be advised if the hospital proposes to engage in or perform human experimentation affecting his care or treatment. He has the right to refuse to participate in such research projects.

The patient must be asked to sign a separate consent in addition to his consent for care if an experimental therapy or drug is proposed for him. He has the additional right of withdrawing from any research project at any point that he changes his mind. This right reflects the view that a person's basic responsibility is to himself, not to the advancement of medicine or science, and he has a right to refuse permission to anyone to touch his body.

STANDARD 10
The patient has the right to expect reasonable continuity of care.

The patient's right to continuity of physician care indirectly refers to nursing care as well. As a student, if you care for a person only one or two days a week, you have an obligation not to break continuity of care but to continue it in the same pattern that would have been followed if you were not there (providing that level of care is optimal for both the patient and his family). You have an obligation to familiarize yourself with a person's routines and preferences so that care does not become fragmented from differing caregivers. A patient who likes to take a shower in the evening, for example, should not have to bathe in the morning just because he has a student nurse assigned to him for the day.

STANDARD 11
The patient has the right to examine and receive an explanation of his bill regardless of source of payment.

There is a general tendency to think that because the cost of a hospital experience is covered by health insurance, the patient should be so grateful for such payment that he should not question any of the costs credited to him. Health care is a service, however; in the same way that a person has the right to expect his car mechanic to list in detail the parts and services included in a bill, so he has the right to expect a hospital to do the same. In using supplies you must be careful to use the minimum necessary to ensure safe care in order to limit the cost of hospitalization. Health insurance is not free. If the person is paying for it, he is doing so at the cost of money he could be spending in other ways each month; if an employer is paying for health insurance, the cost of the monthly payments is undoubtedly reflected in the cost of the product produced by the employer or the wages paid to his employees.

STANDARD 12
The patient has the right to know what hospital rules and regulations apply to his conduct as a patient.

Most health care agencies give patients an information booklet on admission that details such policies as smoking, visiting hours, and dietary services. A person under stress often has difficulty remembering oral instructions; this type of booklet allows him to review rules at his leisure. Reviewing or reminding patients of rules and regulations so that a patient can know what is expected of him is not a nicety; this information is a right of patients.

Quick Reference Stop 8-1 presents some interesting questions about patient's rights.

The Rights of People in Community Health Care

People who are cared for at home through a visiting health service have the same rights as people in a hospital. When working in a community setting, think of the American Hospital Association Bill of Rights as applying except for minor alterations in phrasing.

The Rights of Children

It has long been considered that because of children's immaturity they have a right to special safeguards of care over and above those offered to adults. In 1959 the 14th General Assembly of the United Nations approved a *Declaration of the Rights of the Child.* This document, shown on page 105, declares that the child "shall be entitled to grow and develop in health . . . shall have the right to medical services, and if handicapped, have special treatment, education and care required by his particular condition" (United Nations, 1959). This United Nations declaration serves as a guideline for care in all nations represented in the organization.

In 1970 the delegates to the White House Conference

☐QUICK REFERENCE STOP 8-1: RESEARCH: Patients' Rights

The patients' rights issue has brought the consumer into the forefront of health care decision making and has generated a number of professional concerns. Research in the area of patient rights has just begun to surface. This research needs to answer many questions: What do people and professionals know about patient rights? Do consumers act on their rights? Do professionals ensure that patient rights are met? The research presented here is just the beginning of much needed research in this area.

CAN PATIENTS COMPREHEND A PATIENT'S BILL OF RIGHTS?

A patient bill of rights is often made available to patients in an effort to inform them of their rights in the health care system. In essence, it is meant to be an educational tool. Iepson (1974) identified a potential problem in the efficacy of this tool in fostering patient comprehension of their rights: In a readability assessment of the document, she found it to be above high school level, a level of comprehension beyond that of 83 percent of the sample she utilized. Nurses need to examine carefully whether they are truly making patients aware of their rights.

WHAT DO HEALTH CARE WORKERS KNOW ABOUT PATIENT RIGHTS?

In a study that specifically looked at Maryland nursing homes, Ruth, et al. (1980) questioned caretakers' levels of knowledge and their compliance with specific aspects of care associated with patient rights. Findings demonstrated that nursing directors and other caretakers lacked knowledge and often did not comply with patient rights. Reported violations of patient rights existed. Professional education in this area seems necessary.

PATIENT AND PROFESSIONAL PERCEPTIONS OF INFORMED CONSENT

The ethical and legal implications of informed consent were studied by a Presidential Commission (1982). Various large studies confirmed the results of previous smaller studies done over the years. Many consumers did not know what informed consent meant, and there was a discrepancy between patients' desire for information and doctors' willingness to provide such information. Patients preferred shared decision making while physicians preferred unilateral decision making. Both groups felt that patient rights to information should be protected by law. The Commission leaned in favor of the consumer and recognized the positive role of professional nurses in educating patients and involving them in their own health care. It stated that "Nurses, as a practical matter, typically have a central role in the process of providing patients with information" (p. 147).

SUGGESTED READINGS

Iepson, L. *A Study of the Comparison of the Education Level of Patients to the Readability of the Patients' Bill of Rights.* Plan B Paper, University of Minnesota School of Nursing, July 1974.

President's Commission for the Study of Ethical Problems in Medicine and Biomedical and Behavioral Research. *Making Health Care Decisions.* A report on the ethical and legal implications of informed consent in the patient-practitioner relationship. Washington, D.C.: U.S. Government Printing Office, 1982. As cited in The patients' right to know—A reprisal. *Nurs. Outlook* 31:6, 1983.

Ruth, M. V., et al. *A Descriptive Study of Caretakers' Level of Knowledge in Relation to Five Aspects of Care Derived from the Patients' Bill of Rights and the Aging Process—Final Report.* University of Maryland School of Nursing, July 1980.

for Children and Youth (an organization that meets every 10 years to discuss and plan for the health of the nation's children and youth) set goals for the health care of United States' children. This document (White House Conference on Children, 1971) reads:

> Let us ask what we want for *our* children. Then let us ask not less for all children. We want for our children a home of love and understanding and encouragement. We want for our children a full opportunity for learning in an environment in which they can reach and grow and take pride in themselves. We want for our children the right to be healthy, to be free of sickness, but if sickness comes, to have the best care humanly possible.

The statements from the United Nations and the 1970 White House Conference are important guidelines to keep in mind to respect patient rights and administer safe and high quality care when you are working with children.

The Rights of Older Adults

The proportion of older adults in the population in the United States is growing yearly, so much so that by the year 2000 about 20 percent of the population will be over 65 years of age. There is growing concern for the rights of this segment of the population as, if illnesses such as loss of hearing or eyesight begin to become apparent, a person is more vulnerable to having his rights violated than when he was younger and healthier. A Bill of Rights for the elderly is shown on page 105. Protecting the rights of older adults is a major role of nurses. Rights of this age group must be recognized by everyone, if not

United Nations Declaration of the Rights of the Child

1. The right to affection, love, and understanding.
2. The right to adequate nutrition and medical care.
3. The right to free education.
4. The right to full opportunity for play and recreation.
5. The right to a name and nationality.
6. The right to special care if handicapped.
7. The right to be among the first to receive relief in times of disaster.
8. The right to learn to be a useful member of society and to develop individual abilities.
9. The right to be brought up in a spirit of peace and universal brotherhood.
10. The right to enjoy these rights, regardless of race, color, sex, religion, or national or social origin.

Source: Modified from United Nations, *Declaration of the Rights of the Child.* Geneva: United Nations, 1959.

Rights of Older Adults

1. The right to be useful.
2. The right to obtain employment, based on merit.
3. The right to freedom from want in old age.
4. The right to a fair share of the community's recreational, educational, and medical resources.
5. The right to obtain decent housing suited to needs of later years.
6. The right to the moral and financial support of one's family so far as is consistent with the best interests of the family.
7. The right to live independently, as one chooses.
8. The right to live with dignity.
9. The right of access to all knowledge available on how to improve the later years of life.

Source: United States Department of Health and Human Resources, *The Nation and Its Older People: Report of the White House Conference on Aging.* Washington, D.C.: U.S. Department of Health and Human Resources, 1961.

from a professional standpoint, then from a personal one: You may never be hospitalized in your lifetime and so may never have a personal experience with the rights of hospitalized patients. You *will* grow old and should be directly concerned that the rights of people in this age group are safeguarded well.

The Rights of People in Nursing Homes

People in nursing homes deserve to have the same rights as hospitalized people with additional rights to compensate for the long time span often involved in care. Appendix B shows the rights of people in nursing homes as defined by the Department of Health and Human Resources in 1974.

The Rights of Dying Patients

Although dying is an experience that everyone must eventually experience, it is rarely an easy one. It is therefore understandable that health care providers may draw back from a person who is dying in an attempt to unconsciously disassociate themselves from dying.

In order to protect the rights of persons who are dying, a separate Bill of Rights for the dying patient has been written (App. B). Notice that the majority of these rights are covered by the first statement of the American Hospital Association Bill of Rights, "A patient has the right to considerate and respectful care."

The Rights of Handicapped Persons

People who are handicapped (have less than average motor, sensory, or mental function) are more vulnerable to having their rights violated than are fully functional people. Appendix B lists Rights of Handicapped Individuals determined by the United Nations.

The United States has legal mandates that handicapped people must not be discriminated against in access to public buildings, schooling, employment, or health care. Any health care agency that employs more than 15 people must not refuse to administer care to an individual when a secondary handicap would complicate care. A hospital, for example, could not refuse to admit a person who is blind or hard of hearing for surgery when they realized that the extent of the person's handicap would complicate postoperative care because of the increased difficulty in giving care instructions. A health care agency must provide interpreters for people with language problems if the communication problem would interfere with safe care.

The Rights of Mentally Retarded Persons

Mentally retarded persons are yet another group of individuals who need special care and consideration in order that their rights be protected. Appendix B lists rights of mentally retarded persons as stated by the United Nations in 1971. You must be certain when working with persons with mental retardation to protect their rights, particularly in the area of consent forms. In order for a signed consent to be legal, it must be *informed;* you must be certain that the person fully understands the procedure and risks of the procedure to which he is agreeing, and that his mental not his chronological age has been considered.

The Rights of the Mentally Ill

Mental illness is a form of handicapping. Because a person with mental illness may be unable to make judgments or give consent for health care, specific rights for persons with mental illness have been written. Those stated by a patient group, the Mental Patients' Liberation Project, are shown in Appendix B. Of particular importance in this rights statement is the right to maintain communication with people outside the hospital or institution and the right to refuse drugs or treatments.

When a person is mentally ill, he maintains the same rights as a person who is physically ill.

The Rights of the Pregnant Woman

Pregnant women are a unique minority group in that they are vulnerable to having not only their own rights violated (because they may be more dependent than normally) but those of their unborn children as well. Caring for pregnant women is a double responsibility because of these circumstances. Rights of pregnant women are listed in Appendix B.

The Rights of Support People

Although as a nurse you give one-to-one care and establish a one-to-one relationship with a patient, you also always relate at least to some extent to the patient's family or friends or those people he relies on to help him through such an illness (his support people). Such people are sometimes referred to by sociologists as "significant others," a term that seems too paradoxic to be meaningful (if a person is an "other," he is not significant; if significant, he is more than an "other").

The rights of support people (App. B) reinforce the importance of support people and should help you to remember that a support person such as a parent sleeping overnight with a child in a health care agency, for example, needs a pillow and blanket provided in order to be comfortable; or that a spouse who has been sitting by a bedside for hours may need to be assured that you will stay with the patient for a space of time so that he can feel free to leave for lunch. Care for a patient is not "respectful" if it does not respect his support people as well.

CONSUMER RIGHTS AND NURSING ETHICS

In order to give quality care nurses must, in addition to following patient bills of rights, also be guided by the even stricter guidelines of the American Nurses Association Code of Ethics for Nurses. If you practice by the provisions of this code (discussed in detail in Chap. 3), you also will be following the tenets of patient bills of rights. The first statement of the Code of Ethics for Nurses, for example—the nurse provides services with respect for the dignity of man, unrestricted by considerations of nationality, race, creed, color, or status—is repeated over and over in patient bills of rights. Patient bills of rights are necessary because many of the people whom you supervise as a nurse (nurse's aides, orderlies, dietary aides, recreation leaders, volunteers) do not have a separate code of ethics.

LEGAL CONSIDERATIONS AND PATIENTS' RIGHTS

Many of the stipulations in patient bills of rights have legal implications for care. It is illegal, for example, to threaten a patient (that is technically assault); the patients' bill of rights makes this a violation of "respectful care."

It is illegal to violate a patient's privacy; doing so is also contradictory to the patient's bill of rights. Legally, a person has a right to "informed consent"; this is also a provision in most patient bills of rights.

Nurses' Bill of Rights

1. The right to find dignity in self-expression and self-enhancement through the use of our special abilities and educational background.
2. The right to recognition for our contribution through the provision of an environment for its practice and proper, professional economic rewards.
3. The right to a work environment that will minimize physical and emotional stress and health risks.
4. The right to control what is professional practice within the limits of the law.
5. The right to set standards for excellence in nursing.
6. The right to participate in policy making affecting nursing.
7. The right to social and political action in behalf of nursing and health care.

Source: C. M. Fagin, Nurses' rights. *Am. J. Nurs.* 75:82, 1975.

ADVOCACY AND PATIENT BILLS OF RIGHTS

Many health care agencies employ a person titled a patient advocate whose position is to ensure that patient rights are protected or, in instances where they are violated, to represent the patient in efforts to have his rights restored. Following such an occurrence, the patient advocate plans ways to prevent the violation from happening again, perhaps through better education of health care personnel about the extent of patient rights.

In many instances during a period of caring for a patient, a patient may ask you to act as an advocate for him. Chapter 18 discusses the role of advocacy and change and techniques of advocacy. Basically, the most important rule to remember is to follow lines of authority or seek a solution to the problem from the person next in line. A physician, for example, who carelessly uses Mr. Jones as a teaching example without Mr. Jones' permission will probably not mind having it pointed out to her that Mr. Jones resents medical students' listening to his chest unless he specifically gives permission; however, she might find your information offensive if it was communicated to her by the administrator of the health care agency because you "went over her head" to that person.

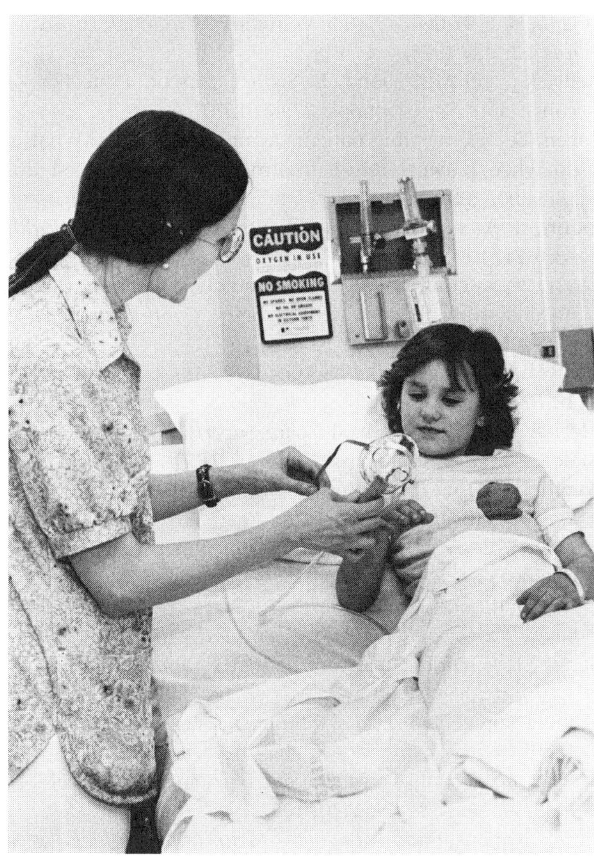

FIGURE 8-2. In order to protect a patient's rights, the nurse must explain what she is going to do before beginning a procedure. In the care of a child, an explanation to the family must also be included.

NURSES' BILL OF RIGHTS

Just as patients have rights, so do nurses. Fagin (1975), who outlined these rights in a seven-part statement, believes that nurses must set the highest possible standards for care. One way that nurses can protect their rights is by participation in the American Nurses' Association Nurses Coalition for Action in Politics (N-CAP) and by keeping informed about local, state, and federal legislation that will affect nursing practice or working conditions. The box on p. 106 lists the Nurses' Bill of Rights by Fagin. The address of N-CAP is noted in Appendix A.

ENCOURAGING RESPECT FOR PATIENT RIGHTS

The emergence of patient rights has put new responsibility on everyone concerned with health care to be certain that people understand as much about their illness as they wish to know; the reason for and steps of procedures; and the action and dosage of any medicine they will be taking. Whenever you begin to carry out a procedure with a patient, include an explanation of what you are going to do as a basic procedural step to be certain that your patient is adequately informed (Fig. 8-2).

The following is an imaginary conversation between Mrs. Rodrigues, a 24-year-old woman admitted to a hospital to have surgery to repair a fractured tibia, and her nurse. Following surgery, the patient had a long leg cast applied and was scheduled to learn crutch-walking on the third day postoperatively so that she could return home to care for her two young children by the fifth day following surgery. Due to an improperly completed requisition, however, the physical therapy department never scheduled Mrs. Rodrigues for crutch-walking lessons. Instead of being discharged five days following surgery, Mrs. Rodrigues must remain in the hospital two additional days to learn crutch-walking. Read the conversation and count how many of Mrs. Rodrigues's rights as a hospitalized patient were violated.

MRS. RODRIGUES: I really wanted to go home today.

NURSE: I heard Dr. Jones tell you before surgery that your tibia was communuted. You can't expect to heal quickly after that.

MRS. RODRIGUES: How much more will it cost me to stay two extra days?

NURSE: It won't matter. Your insurance will cover the cost.

MRS. RODRIGUES: Whose fault was it that I wasn't scheduled to go to physical therapy?

NURSE: Actually, you shouldn't expect the hospital to provide crutch-walking lessons for you. It's sort of a luxury.

MRS. RODRIGUES: The nurse yesterday said maybe I could try walking on my cast without crutches.

NURSE: That's not true. The kind of cast you have isn't strong enough for weight bearing.

MRS. RODRIGUES: Will someone explain to me exactly how much weight I can put on my leg?

NURSE: I imagine your doctor will do that.

MRS. RODRIGUES: What about which things I can do when I go home?

NURSE: I'll send a note to your employer explaining your limitations.

MRS. RODRIGUES: I wish I could have gone home today.

NURSE: All I know is that this isn't my fault. I just work here.

The preceding conversation would take less than five minutes, yet during it at least seven patient rights were violated. Telling a patient that she has a communuted tibia is not an explanation that a patient could be expected to understand; she does have a right to know her hospital costs, even if she won't be directly paying them; a hospital is expected to furnish common services such as crutch-walking instruction for people immobilized by casts; continuity of care between nurses was not provided or two nurses would not be offering Mrs. Rodrigues conflicting information; Mrs. Rodrigues has a right to know what rules apply to her, not be told that someone else will give her the necessary information; in order to protect patient privacy, the nurse has no right to send a note to an employer unless Mrs. Rodrigues gives her permission; the last comment of the nurse hardly reflects "considerate and respectful care."

Although statements made in a patient's bill of rights have legal implications, bills of rights for patients are not legal statements in themselves. They are guidelines for actions, however. If a health care agency accepts a patient's bill of rights as a guideline, they could have reason to terminate your employment if you did not follow them. Not following them also is questionable behavior from an ethical standpoint. If you were a consumer of health care, it would be important for you to have the people caring for you following such guidelines.

It is important for you as a nurse to know that your employer approves of and accepts the Nurses' Bill of Rights. An agency that does not do so may not be a preferred employer for you.

SUGGESTED READINGS

Annas, G. *The Rights of Hospital Patients.* New York: Avon, 1975.

Bandman, E. L. The Rights of Nurses and Patients: A Case for Advocacy. In E. L. Bandman and B. Bandman (Eds.), *Bioethics and Human Rights.* Boston: Little, Brown, 1978.

Bandman, E. L., and Bandman, B. There is nothing automatic about rights. *Am. J. Nurs.* 77:867, 1977.

Besch, L. B. Informed consent: A patient's right. *Nurs. Outlook* 27:33, 1979.

Chapman, C. M. The rights and responsibilities of nurses and patients. *J. Adv. Nurs.* 5:127, 1980.

Creighton, H. Recent developments in consent to treatment. *Superv. Nurse* 12:12, 1981.

Creighton, H. Rights of mental patients. *Superv. Nurse* 12:16, 1981.

Curtin, L. L. Informed consent: Rights, responsibilities and roles (editorial). *Nurs. Manage.* 13(10):7, 1982.

Curtin, L. L. Is there a right to health care? *Am. J. Nurs.* 80:462, 1980.

Dickman, R. L. The ethics of informed consent. *Nurse Pract.* 5:25, 1980.

Fagin, C. M. Nurses' rights. *Am. J. Nurs.* 75:82, 1975.

Halloran, M. C. S. Rational ethical judgments utilizing a decision-making tool. *Heart Lung* 11(6):566, 1982.

Hogan, N. S. Patient's rights: Voluntary or mandatory, *Hospitals* 52:111, 1978.

Kelly, K., and McClelland, E. Signed consent: Protection or constraint? *Nurs. Outlook* 27:43, 1979.

Laken, D. D. Protecting patients against themselves: What to do when patients refuse treatment. *Nursing* (Horsham) 13(1):90, 1983.

Lamb, G. A., et al. The age of consent. *Am. J. Public Health* 68:1071, 1978.

Laszlo, S. S., et al. The use of a simulation game in training hospital staff about patient rights. *J. Contin. Educ. Nurs.* 10:30, 1979.

Mancini, M. Rights of the handicapped. *Am. J. Nurs.* 79:2187, 1979.

McNally, J. M. A right to health care. *Superv. Nurse* 11:17, 1980.

Miller, P. A guide to informed consent. *DCCN* 1(5):304, 1982.

Newton, L. H. In defense of the traditional nurse. *Nurs. Outlook* 29:348, 1981.

Oberle, J. C. A mother's need, a hospital policy, a nurse's dilemma . . . Every mother needs the opportunity to breastfeed and bond if she chooses. *RN* 45(12):69, 1982.

Sklar, C. Was the patient informed? *Canad. Nurse* 76:18, 1980.

Starch, J. L. Patient teaching/patient rights. *Nurs. Adm. Q.* 4:107, 1980.

Trandel-Korenchuk, D., et al. Minor consent. *Nurse Pract.* 5:48, 1980.

Trandel-Korenchuk, D. M. Patient participation in decision-making. *Nurse Pract.* 7:46, 1982.

United Nations. *Declaration of the Rights of the Child.* Geneva: United Nations, 1959.

Vachon, M. L. Women as health care consumers. *Canad. Nurse* 77:46, 1981.

White House Conference on Children, 1970. *Report to the President.* Washington: U.S. Government Printing Office, 1971.

Wiemerslag, D. Informed consent. *Crit. Care Update* 9:39, 1982.

World Health Organization. *The Album.* Geneva: World Health Organization, 1966.

QUESTIONS FOR REVIEW

Mark whether the following statements are contained in the American Hospital Association Patient's Bill of Rights (true or false).

_____ 1. A patient has the right to know if his doctor is related to his physical therapist.
_____ 2. A patient has the right to refuse to participate in a research study.
_____ 3. A patient has the right to refuse surgery but not medication.
_____ 4. You should ask a patient not assigned to you for care if you can look at his cast because you have never seen that type before.
_____ 5. A patient has the right to know if a hospital is religiously affiliated.
_____ 6. A nurse has the right to enjoyable working conditions.
_____ 7. Telling a patient that he is going to have a laminectomy fulfills his right.
_____ 8. You do not have to give a patient an explanation of his bill on discharge if compensation insurance is going to pay the total cost.
_____ 9. It is a patient right to be told visiting hours.
_____10. A patient has the right to expect a hospital to supply him a vegetarian diet.

Mark the following statements true or false regarding consumer rights and health care.

_____11. A hospital is a consumer of health care.
_____12. The right to health care is guaranteed by the United States Constitution.
_____13. Volunteers in hospitals are excluded from following guidelines of patient bills of rights.
_____14. A hospital that refuses to admit a person who is blind because his handicap would complicate his care can still meet the Patient's Bill of Rights.
_____15. Health care is a product.

III. HEALTH AS A DYNAMIC FORCE

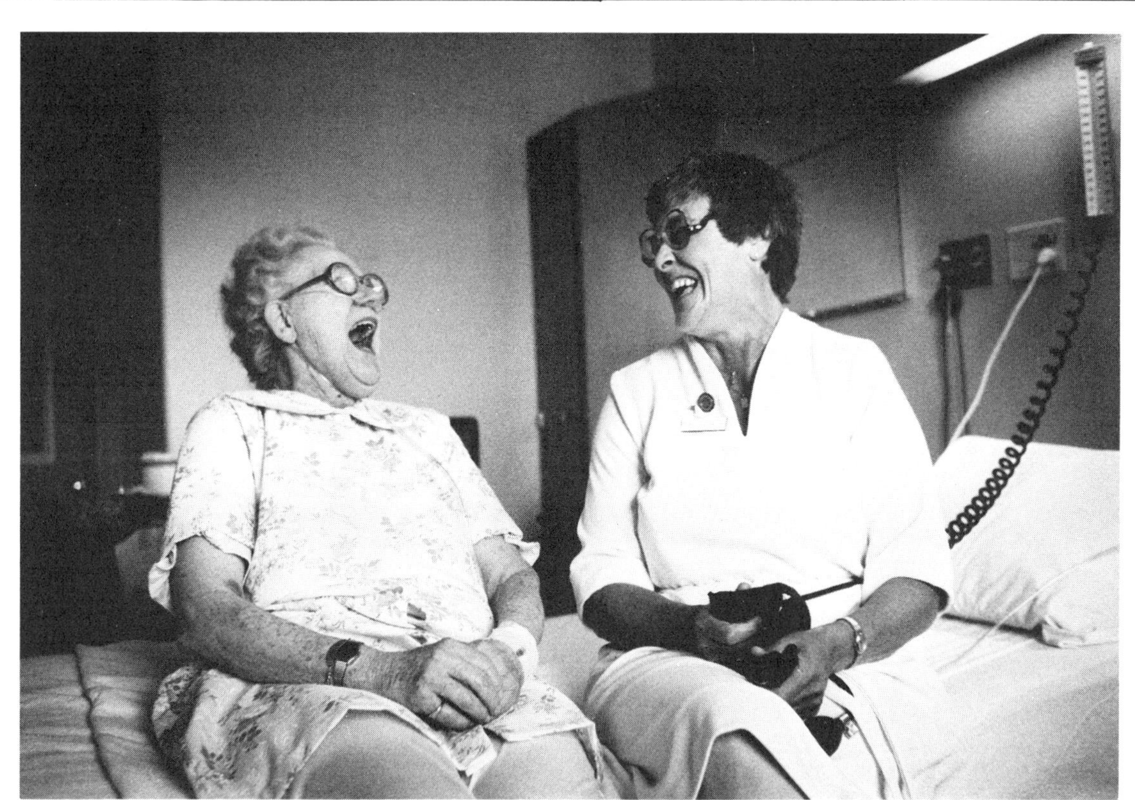

9. LIFE SPAN CONCEPTS

OBJECTIVES

Upon mastery of the material in this chapter, you should be able to:

1. List the eight stages of man as described by Erikson.
2. Describe the developmental task of each age group.
3. List common principles of growth and development.
4. Describe ways that growth and development are measured.
5. Describe common growth and developmental characteristics for each age group.
6. Describe the special considerations of care and the effect of illness on each age group.
7. Describe the difficulties a person with a handicap may have in achieving developmental tasks.

TERMS

The terms important for an understanding of this chapter are shown below and defined in the glossary:

accommodation
Apgar score
atrophy
Brazelton Neonatal Behavioral Assessment Scale
cephalocaudal
climacteric
cognitive development
conservation
Denver Developmental Screening Test (DDST)
development
developmental crisis
embryo
fetus
geriatrics
gerontology
growth
karyotype
meconium
menarche
menopause
neonate
placenta
puberty
Tanner Scale

A person changes greatly—not only in size but also in ability to reason, manipulate objects, speak, perform motor skills, and carry out social interaction—from the time he is a newborn until he becomes an older adult. Nursing care, therefore, must change as a person changes and adjust not only to a person's size but to his functional ability as well. In order to adjust nursing care in this manner it is necessary to have basic knowledge of the characteristics and abilities of all age groups.

GROWTH AND DEVELOPMENT

The terms *growth* and *development* are often used interchangeably but in fact they have different meanings. Growth is an increase in size (a quantitative change); it is measured in inches or centimeters, pounds or kilograms. Development is an increase in function (a qualitative change); it is measured by functional tests and observations of task accomplishment.

Principles of Growth and Development

All people grow and develop at slightly different rates but normal growth and development follow consistent principles. These are:

1. Development is *cephalocaudal* (proceeds from head to tail): A baby first begins to lift his head, then his chest, then straightens his back for sitting, then utilizes his legs for walking.
2. Development proceeds from the gross to the specific, from the proximal to the distal. A baby can handle a large ball before he can handle a small one and has use of large muscle groups before small ones.
3. Growth and development are continuous processes. Both occur very rapidly at some points in life (during intrauterine life and the first year after birth, for example) and more slowly at others (older age), but they are always active phenomena.
4. Growth and development are orderly. All people pass through the same predictable life stages and life crises.
5. People's passages through predictable stages occur at different rates. The age range for any life stage is wide and variable. Some people are ready to accept adult responsibility readily at age 18; others are well past 30 before they are ready to accept responsibility for their or other people's lives (and some are never truly ready).
6. All body tissue does not develop at the same rate. Neurological tissue matures rapidly in the first year of life. Reproductive tissue does not begin to develop to any extent until puberty. Lymphatic tissue develops rapidly to reach a peak at six years and then declines in growth (atrophies). Fig. 9-1 shows the sequence of the development of body tissue.
7. There is an optimal time for initiation of experiences or learning. A child cannot walk, for example, until

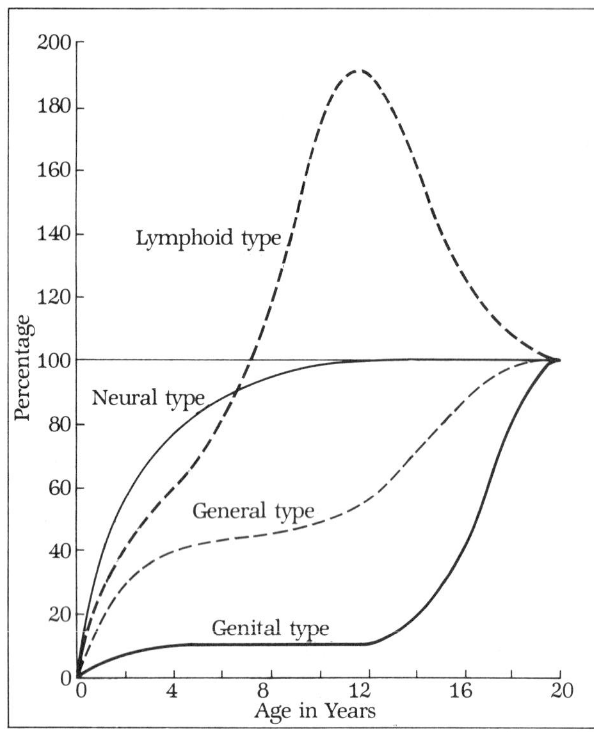

FIGURE 9-1. Main types of growth of various body systems.

his body has matured to a certain point. A person cannot tolerate adult levels of responsibility until his reasoning and coping abilities have progressed to a particular point of maturity. "Catching" a person at this point in time when he is ripe for learning a new skill makes teaching rewarding; attempting to teach that skill at any other time involves extensive work and even then may not be successful. Learning a skill at the point of maturity is interesting; learning it before that point is reached is frustrating; after that point it may be boring.

Factors Influencing Growth and Development

Genetic and environmental factors interact to influence growth and development outcomes.

GENETIC FACTORS

Genetic factors include intelligence level, race, health (free or not of a genetic or inherited disease), and sex; they set the upper limits a person can achieve in growth and development. A person cannot grow any taller or be any more intelligent or metabolize foods any more quickly than his genetic makeup dictates, no matter how much he wishes to do so or how much he spends on medications or special programs.

ENVIRONMENTAL FACTORS

Environmental factors influence whether the person's genetic potential will be reached. Nutrition, socioeconomic factors, parent-child relationship, ordinal position in the family, and health (free of diseases spread by environmental influences such as bacteria) all may influence final growth and development outcomes. The child who consistently eats a low protein diet, for example, is not apt to reach his genetic potential in height.

TABLE 9-1. LIFE SPAN STAGES

Stage	Age Span
Intrauterine	The 40 weeks before birth
Neonate	First 28 days of life
Infant	29 days to 1 yr
Toddler	1 to 3 yr
Preschooler	3 to 6 yr
Schoolager	6 to 12 yr
Adolescent	12 to 18 yr
Young adult	18 to 45 yr
Middle-aged adult	45 to 65 yr
Older adult	Over 65
Death and dying	No specific age

LIFE STAGES

In order that some generalities can be made about nursing care at different points in life, the span of life is usually divided into stages covering various time spans as shown in Table 9-1. Notice that death and dying are included in this table as the final stage of life; this period has developmental steps the same as other life stages.

Developmental Crises and Life Stages

A number of people have studied life stages in order to isolate those tasks best suited for that life stage and those consequences that generally occur during that particular time.

The Austrian psychoanalyst Sigmund Freud was one of the first theorists to relate happenings that occurred in childhood to later mental problems (Freud, 1946). Freudian stages of development for each age group are summarized in Table 9-2.

Erik Erikson, also a psychoanalyst, modified Freud's theories to center on the good rather than the bad happenings of life (those elements that lead to mental health rather than those that cause mental illness) (Erikson, 1963). He identified a developmental step for each life stage which, if accomplished, leads to individual fulfillment. These tasks are also summarized in Table 9-2.

Jean Piaget, a Swiss zoologist, studied cognitive or intellectual development and traced stages of development for reasoning or concept formation the same as earlier scientists traced motor development (Piaget, 1950). These stages of cognitive development are summarized in Table 9-3.

The concerns of these three theorists will be discussed as they apply to different age groups.

MEASURING GROWTH

Growth is measured by height and weight determinations. Taking and recording these measurements is part of basic nursing assessment. It is easy to think of measur-

TABLE 9-2. DEVELOPMENTAL THEORIES

Age Group	Freud	Erikson	Developmental Task
Infant	Oral stage	Sense of trust vs. sense of mistrust	Infant learns to love and be loved.
Toddler	Anal stage	Sense of autonomy vs. shame or doubt	Toddler learns independence.
Preschooler	Phallic stage	Sense of initiative vs. guilt	Child learns how to do things (basic problem solving).
Schoolager	Latent stage	Sense of industry vs. inferiority	Child learns how to do things well.
Adolescent	Genital stage	Sense of identity vs. role confusion	Child learns who he is and what kind of person he will be.
Young adult		Sense of intimacy vs. isolation	Individual learns to establish deep and lasting relationships.
Middle-aged adult		Sense of generativity vs. stagnation	Individual learns commitment to community and world.
Older adult		Sense of integrity vs. despair	Individual appreciates role and status in life; accepts inevitability of death.

TABLE 9-3. PIAGET'S THEORY OF COGNITIVE DEVELOPMENT

Age	Phase of Development	Learning Accomplishment
0 to 2 yr	Sensorimotor	Preverbal behavior: Able to coordinate simple motor activities; reacts and learns basically through five senses; learns permanence (that objects and people exist even when out of sight).
3 to 7 yr	Preoperational	Child is egocentric; employs "magical thinking" (what he wants to be he imagines as being); uses language as symbols of objects.
7 to 11 yr	Concrete operations	Able to understand relationships as to size and time and space; solves basic problems; appreciates other people's viewpoints; recognizes that there may be more than one way to do a task.
11 to 15 yr	Formal operations	Can use formal logic to scientifically reason; can do adult problem solving.

ing weight and height as a routine assessment rather than an important one; however, whether people are gaining or losing in weight and height is an excellent determination of their overall state of health. Techniques of height and weight measurement are discussed in Chap. 19 with other physical assessment techniques.

MEASURING DEVELOPMENT

Development is measured by means of standardized tests and observations of ability to function and to perform certain tasks.

TABLE 9-4. BEHAVIORS ASSESSED BY THE BRAZELTON NEONATAL BEHAVIORAL ASSESSMENT SCALE

Behavior	Description
Habituation	A newborn is capable of diminishing his response to stimuli such as light, sound, and a pinprick to his heel. When first stimulated, he startles easily; gradually he shuts out the stimulus and does not respond to it (habituation).
Orientation	When a newborn is given an auditory or visual stimulus, he turns toward or at least "attunes" to it.
Motor maturity	The organization of the newborn's motor coordination is assessed by his ability to respond to the examiner's interventions.
Variation	Infants have variable degrees of excitement and general activity and periods of alertness and sleep.
Self-quieting ability	When disturbed, a newborn uses interventions to console himself such as sucking on his fist.
Social behavior	A newborn naturally responds to being held closely by cuddling.

Source: T. B. Brazelton, Neonatal Behavioral Assessment Scale. In *Clinics in Developmental Medicine*, Vol. 50. Philadelphia: Lippincott, 1973.

The Brazelton Neonatal Behavioral Assessment Scale

A scale developed by T. Barry Brazelton (1973) is used to evaluate a newborn's capacity or ability to respond to set stimuli. Six major categories of behavior—habituation, orientation, motor maturity, variation, self-quieting ability, and social behavior—are assessed. These terms as used in the scale are defined in Table 9-4. A total evaluation takes 20 to 30 minutes. Since many infants have uncoordinated behavior for the first 48 hours after delivery, it is suggested that the infant be evaluated on the third day of life.

A major discovery that has arisen from use of this scale is the documented evidence that newborns are not

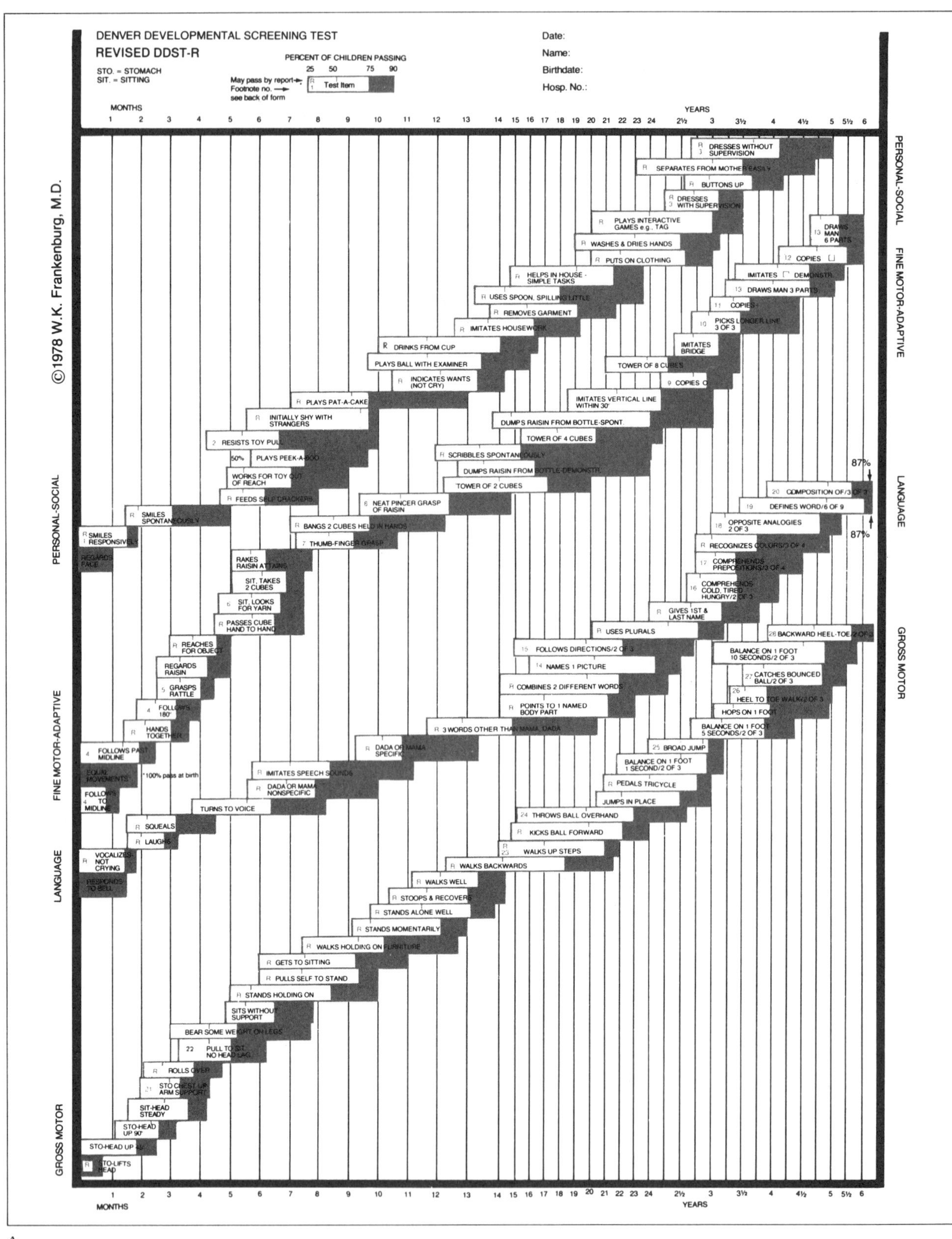

A

passive, nonhearing, unseeing, and unresponsive at birth and certainly are not alike. Many of the items tested by the scale, such as how the infant alerts (eyes widen, head is held as if listening) or orients himself to sound (turns toward the direction of his mother's voice), are excellent newborn behaviors to point out to parents. The more they know about their new baby, the easier it is for them to view him as an individual and begin to meet his needs.

Experience with newborns and specific instruction in assessment techniques are necessary before you can rate newborns by the Brazelton Behavioral Scale. It is men-

DIRECTIONS

DATE
NAME
BIRTHDATE
HOSP. NO.

1. Try to get child to smile by smiling, talking or waving to him. Do not touch him.
2. When child is playing with toy, pull it away from him. Pass if he resists.
3. Child does not have to be able to tie shoes or button in the back.
4. Move yarn slowly in an arc from one side to the other, about 6" above child's face. Pass if eyes follow 90° to midline. (Past midline; 180°)
5. Pass if child grasps rattle when it is touched to the backs or tips of fingers.
6. Pass if child continues to look where yarn disappeared or tries to see where it went. Yarn should be dropped quickly from sight from tester's hand without arm movement.
7. Pass if child picks up raisin with any part of thumb and a finger.
8. Pass if child picks up raisin with the ends of thumb and index finger using an over hand approach.

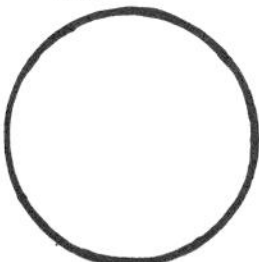
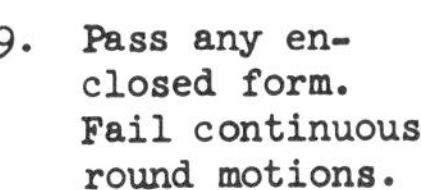
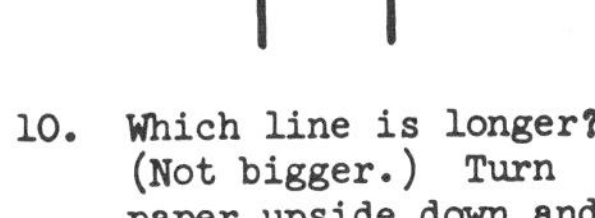
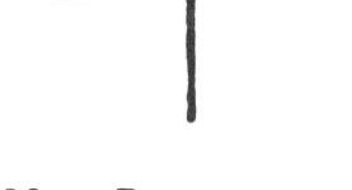
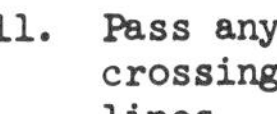

9. Pass any enclosed form. Fail continuous round motions.
10. Which line is longer? (Not bigger.) Turn paper upside down and repeat. (3/3 or 5/6)
11. Pass any crossing lines.
12. Have child copy first. If failed, demonstrate

When giving items 9, 11 and 12, do not name the forms. Do not demonstrate 9 and 11.

13. When scoring, each pair (2 arms, 2 legs, etc.) counts as one part.
14. Point to picture and have child name it. (No credit is given for sounds only.)

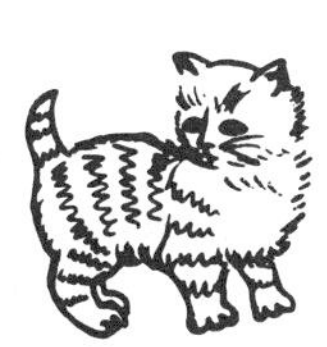
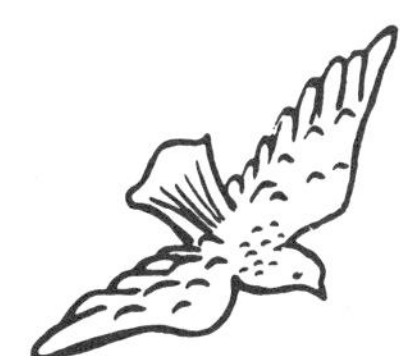
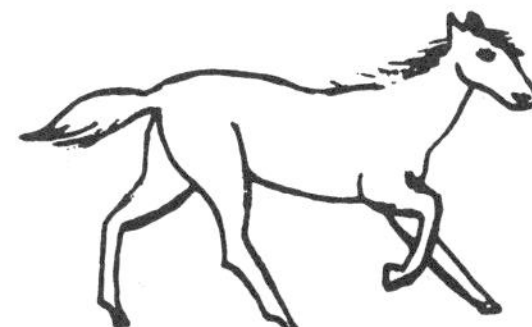
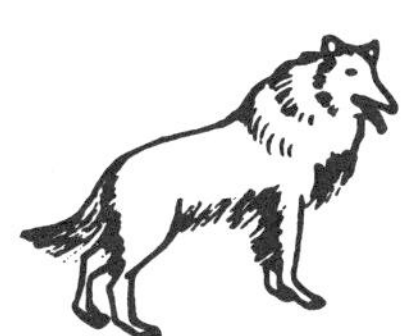
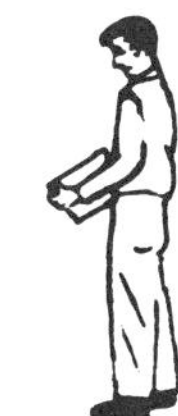

15. Tell child to: Give block to Mommie; put block on table; put block on floor. Pass 2 of 3. (Do not help child by pointing, moving head or eyes.)
16. Ask child: What do you do when you are cold? ..hungry? ..tired? Pass 2 of 3.
17. Tell child to: Put block <u>on</u> table; <u>under</u> table; <u>in front</u> of chair, <u>behind</u> chair. Pass 3 of 4. (Do not help child by pointing, moving head or eyes.)
18. Ask child: If fire is hot, ice is ?; Mother is a woman, Dad is a ?; a horse is big, a mouse is ?. Pass 2 of 3.
19. Ask child: What is a ball? ..lake? ..desk? ..house? ..banana? ..curtain? ..ceiling? ..hedge? ..pavement? Pass if defined in terms of use, shape, what it is made of or general category (such as banana is fruit, not just yellow). Pass 6 of 9.
20. Ask child: What is a spoon made of? ..a shoe made of? ..a door made of? (No other objects may be substituted.) Pass 3 of 3.
21. When placed on stomach, child lifts chest off table with support of forearms and/or hands.
22. When child is on back, grasp his hands and pull him to sitting. Pass if head does not hang back.
23. Child may use wall or rail only, not person. May not crawl.
24. Child must throw ball overhand 3 feet to within arm's reach of tester.
25. Child must perform standing broad jump over width of test sheet. (8-1/2 inches)
26. Tell child to walk forward, heel within 1 inch of toe. Tester may demonstrate. Child must walk 4 consecutive steps, 2 out of 3 trials.
27. Bounce ball to child who should stand 3 feet away from tester. Child must catch ball with hands, not arms, 2 out of 3 trials.
28. Tell child to walk backward, toe within 1 inch of heel. Tester may demonstrate. Child must walk 4 consecutive steps, 2 out of 3 trials.

<u>DATE AND BEHAVIORAL OBSERVATIONS</u> (how child feels at time of test, relation to tester, attention span, verbal behavior, self-confidence, etc,):

B

FIGURE 9-2. A. Revised Denver Developmental Screening Form (DDST-R). B. Instructions for administering specified items.

tioned here because, as its use grows in popularity, it is referred to more and more often; reports on children may include a summary of the results of the scale as it was administered early in life.

The Denver Developmental Screening Test

The Denver Developmental Screening Test (standardized on a large cross-section of children in Denver, Colorado) was designed to detect developmental delays during infancy and the preschool years. Four main categories of development are rated: personal-social development, fine motor adaptive development, language development, and gross motor development.

The materials needed for administering the test must be purchased as a kit. They are a skein of red wool, a box of raisins, a small bottle with a narrow neck opening, a bell, a rattle, a tennis ball, eight 1-inch brightly colored blocks, a test form, and a pencil.

Although administration of the DDST is not difficult, it should not be attempted except by nurses or other personnel educated specifically in its procedures and interpretation. This precaution is necessary to ensure the validity of the test. The parent is told prior to administration that it is a test not of intelligence but of development.

DDST test form is available in both the original and a revised DDST-R format (Fig. 9-2). Use of the DDST-R provides for the recording of test items in a step fashion that resembles a growth curve. The DDST-R format does not replace the DDST but is an optional form.

On the test form each of the test items is represented by a bar showing the ages by which 25 percent, 50 percent, 75 percent, and 90 percent of the children normally have mastered that developmental trait. The left end of the bar indicates the age for 25 percent, the tick mark at the top of the bar, 50 percent; the left end of the gray area, 75 percent; and the right end of the bar, 90 percent. For example, in the area of personal-social development, the item "imitates housework" is passed by 25 percent of children between 12 and 13 months, 50 percent between 13 and 14 months, 75 percent between 16 and 17 months, and 90 percent by 19 to 20 months.

The DDST is usually administered to infants at about 3 or 4 months of age, again at 10 months, and again at 3 or 4 years. Interpretation of test performance is detailed in the test manual. Developmental tests administered while a child is ill are unreliable and must be interpreted with extreme caution.

Achievement Tests

The development of schoolage and adolescent children is measured by standardized achievement tests administered at various points throughout their school years or in preparation for college. Nurses are not instrumental in administering these tests, but results can be secured from school administrators (with child or parent permission) if necessary for inclusion in a health appraisal. A Scholastic Achievement Test (SAT) is an example.

Assessment of Activities of Daily Living

The development level of adults can best be assessed by observation of the person's ability to complete activities of daily living such as feeding and dressing himself and managing his life style and finances; his degree of responsibility for others; and his capacity for good decision making. A mature adult, for example, is capable of living independently because he can meet his own needs in a healthful life style, can provide adequate finances for himself, and is capable of making judgments that reflect thoughtful consideration.

MEASURING INTELLIGENCE

Intelligence can be defined as the ability to think abstractly, to adjust to new situations, and to profit from experience. This type of learning—gaining concepts—is termed *cognitive* learning. It is measured by intelligence tests.

Almost everyone has had his intelligence quotient (IQ) rated at some point in his school career. Although nurses do not administer these tests, results can be obtained (with child or parent permission) from school administrators if necessary for inclusion in a health appraisal.

An intelligence quotient is the ratio of mental age as measured by an intelligence test to chronological age. The formula for this is

$$\frac{\text{mental age}}{\text{chronological age}} \times 100 = \text{IQ}$$

It is difficult to test the very young child with any degree of accuracy because he lacks the ability to complete tasks in the areas used for scoring intelligence tests: comprehension, imagination, reasoning, memory problems, and vocabulary. Labeling any age child as to IQ is often unfair, especially if the test was administered in a group setting in which he could be easily distracted. Table 9-5 shows the usual classification of intelligence quotients and predicted functional levels of these groups. IQ results vary according to a person's culture

TABLE 9-5. CLASSIFICATION OF INTELLIGENCE QUOTIENTS

Intelligence Quotient	Interpretation	Nursing Implications
0—20	Severely retarded	Dependent on others for care
21—50	Moderately retarded but trainable	Able to learn tasks of daily living
51—75	Mildly retarded but educable	Can function at the level of an 8—12 year old
76—89	Slightly retarded	Needs special attention to improve level of functioning
90—109	Average	Functions at an average level
110—139	Above average	Excels at learning
Over 140	Gifted	Needs a special education program to allow achievement of potential

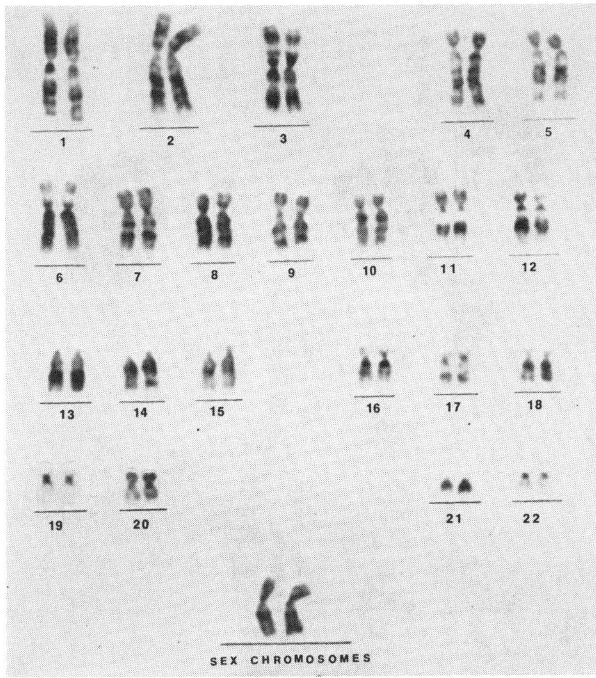

A

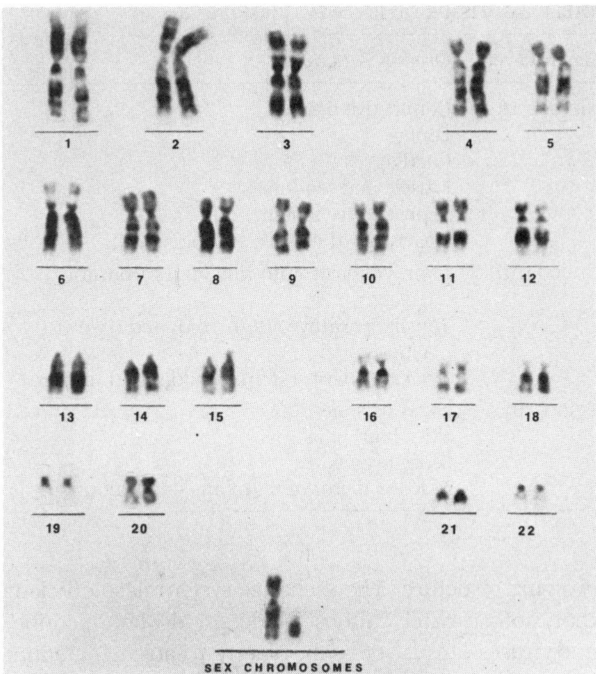

B

FIGURE 9-3. Photomicrographs of human chromosomes (karyotypes). A blood sample is taken, and the white cells are examined at the mitotic division phase of reproduction, transferred to slides, and photographed under high-power magnification. Individual chromosomes can then be cut from the photograph and arranged according to size and shape. A. Normal female karyotype. B. Normal male karyotype.

and experience. They are, at best, only an estimation, not a certainty, of a person's potential. Intelligence tests administered when a child is ill are unreliable and must be interpreted with extreme caution.

INTRAUTERINE GROWTH AND DEVELOPMENT

Life begins when an ovum (an egg cell from the woman) and a spermatozoon (a germ cell from the man) meet in a fallopian tube and fuse. This fused structure is termed a *zygote.*

The growing zygote contains 46 chromosomes (23 supplied by the ovum, 23 from the spermatozoon). The sex of the new individual as well as traits such as eye color, presence or absence of genetic disease, and blood type are determined by the chromosomes of the spermatozoon and ovum. Fig. 9-3 shows karyotypes or photographic studies of female and male chromosome patterns. The twenty-third pair of chromosomes determines sex. The ovum supplies the large X-shaped chromosome in both instances. The spermatozoon supplies either a second large X-shaped chromosome (Fig. 9-3A) or a smaller Y-shaped one (Fig. 9-3B). The child's sex will be female if two X-shaped chromosomes are present, male if one X-shaped and one Y-shaped chromosome are present. It is the spermatozoon's contribution that determines the child's sex.

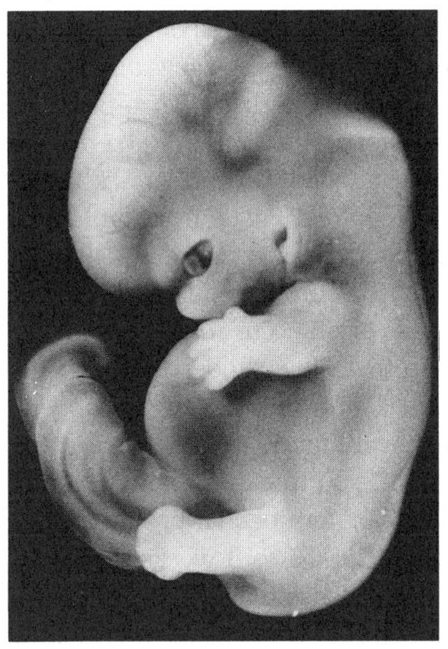

FIGURE 9-4. Human embryo at 48 days.

A zygote floats free in the uterine cavity for about 3 days, then touches against the soft endometrial bed prepared for it and implants or attaches to the inner uterine wall; it is then termed an *embryo* (Fig. 9-4). Over the next weeks the structure differentiates into three distinct types of tissue that will not only form the growing child but also provide an efficient nutrient supply system separate from but dependent on the mother's blood system and a protective insulating layer of fluid (amniotic fluid). The *placenta* is the support system that allows oxygen and nutrients to osmose across a thin membrane system to supply needed nourishment to the

TABLE 9-6. TISSUE DIVISION BY GERM LAYER

Germ Layer	Organs Generated
Mesoderm	Connective tissue
	Bones
	Cartilage
	Muscle and tendons
	Reproductive system
	Heart, blood vessels, and blood cells
Endoderm	Lining of gastrointestinal and respiratory tracts
	Tonsils, parathyroid, thyroid, and thymus glands
	Lower urinary system (bladder and urethra)
Ectoderm	Nervous system
	Skin, hair, nails
	Sense organs
	Mucous membranes of anus and mouth

growing structure. The exchange system is so efficient that, unfortunately, almost all drugs, alcohol, nicotine, and viruses can also cross the placenta, causing potential harmful effects in the growing child.

The three layers of tissue in the growing embryo are called the mesoderm, endoderm, and ectoderm. Different body structures arise from each germ or tissue layer (Table 9-6). The fact that different body parts arise from different tissue layers explains why birth defects occur as they do. Teratogens (substances detrimental to embryo growth) generally affect only one tissue layer and birth defects involve body structures of only that layer. Esophageal-tracheal defects are common, for example, because both structures arise from the endoderm; spinal cord and rectal anomalies often occur together because both body parts develop from the ectoderm layer. German measles (rubella) is one of the few teratogens known that affect all germ layers. When caring for women who are pregnant, you must double check any medicine you administer for teratogenic properties.

The embryo period, the first 5 to 8 weeks after implantation, is a time when the growing structure is very susceptible to injury from teratogens. After the fifth to eighth week, the structure is known as a *fetus* (meaning *offspring* in Latin). Milestones of embryo and fetal growth are summarized in Table 9-7 for easy reference.

Psychosocial Aspects of Pregnancy

The time span required for physical maturation of the fetus is also needed by the parents for adjustment to the psychological implications of pregnancy and the new responsibilities that will be asked of them (Fig. 9-5). The first pregnancy is a major life happening for both mother and father because at the end of the pregnancy they will assume completely different roles from the ones they played previously. A woman changes from being a daughter or wife at the beginning, to "being pregnant" by the fourth month, to being a mother at the end. The man changes in the same way from a son to a father.

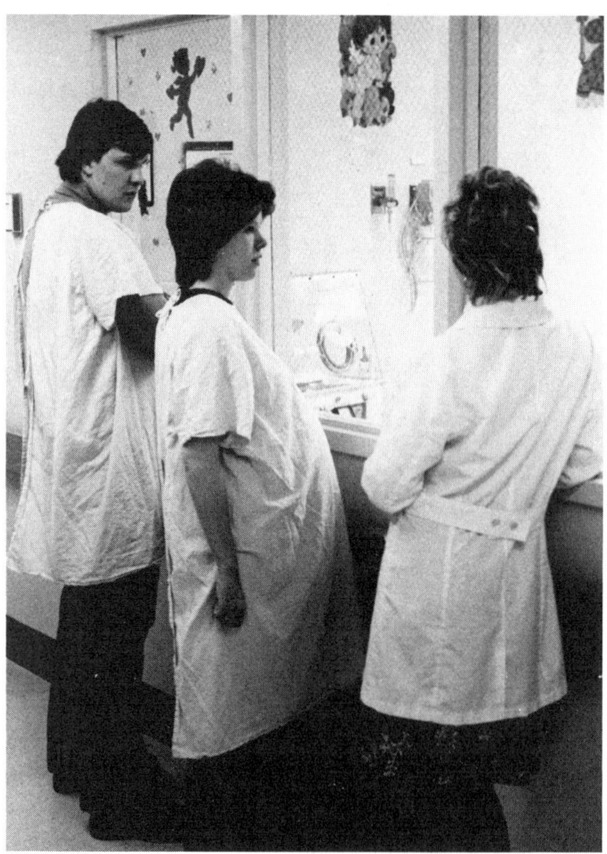

FIGURE 9-5. These soon-to-be parents are touring the hospital maternity unit as part of their preparation for a childbirth experience. Notice the rapt attention given the nurse as she describes the nursery and newborn care.

Important times when prospective parents are most apt to spend time thinking about their new roles occur when the pregnancy is confirmed (2 to 3 months of pregnancy), when the mother feels the fetus move (termed *quickening*, this occurs at 4 1/2 to 5 months of pregnancy), and when they begin to prepare a room and clothing and choose a name for the child (7 to 9 months of pregnancy). Pregnancy is a family event as illustrated in Fig. 9-6. It is important that parents work through their feelings about becoming parents during every pregnancy; otherwise at the time of the birth they may have difficulty accepting responsibility for the baby's care, a condition that may interfere with *bonding* or close attachment to the child.

Certain situations such as illness or loss of a support person during pregnancy are labeled high risk because they interfere with parents' psychological working through of their changing roles. In addition, happenings at birth such as the child being born with a health problem of some type or being separated from the mother due to illness of the child or mother may inhibit bonding.

Although as many as 80 percent of pregnancies may be unplanned and at the moment of conception and diagnosis unwanted, the majority of women change their minds about the pregnancy at the time of quicken-

TABLE 9-7. INTRAUTERINE GROWTH BY MONTH

Body System	4 Weeks	8 Weeks	12 Weeks	16 Weeks	20 Weeks	24 Weeks	28 Weeks	32 Weeks	36 Weeks	40 Weeks
General appearance	Arm and leg buds present; tightly curled body; tail present; placenta beginning to form	Fingers present; tail disappearing; eye, ears, and mouth present; head larger than body	Toe and fingernails present; skin pink and delicate; sex apparent; rapid growth in length	Rapid growth in length continuing; lanugo forming	Vernix caseosa present; mother feels movement	Vernix caseosa abundant; eyebrows and eyelashes present; eyelids open	Skin wrinkled; hair lengthening	Lanugo disappears from face; nails reach end of fingers; subcutaneous fat forming	General growth continues	Subcutaneous fat well formed; nails protrude beyond fingers
Cardiovascular system	Heart appears as a hollow tube; major vessels present; heart beat present	Immature red blood cells form; heart development complete	Blood forms in spleen and liver	Blood forms in bone marrow	Fetal heartbeat can be heard with stethoscope					Fetal hemoglobin begins to convert to adult structure
Respiratory system	Lung buds appear	Nostrils present but closed	Vocal cords present; lungs assume final shape	Bronchi complete	Nostrils open	Alveoli formed				Alveoli still incomplete; thinning to 1 cell thickness
Musculoskeletal system		Ossification of bones beginning	Tooth buds present	Joint cavities present	Movement is felt by mother	Movements stronger			Movements still stronger	Bones of skull are firm
Gastrointestinal system		Small intestine herniates into umbilical cord	Palate formed; intestine returns to abdomen	Meconium formed; fetus swallows amniotic fluid	Meconium in rectum					Digestive enzymes still immature but operable
Neurological system	Midbrain present; posterior neural groove closed	Cerebrospinal fluid forms	Brain configuration complete	Cerebellum prominent	Spinal cord myelination begins	Brain myelination begins				Spinal cord ends at L_3
Genitourinary system	Nephrons form in kidney; genital ridge that will define reproductive organs forming	Testes or ovaries present; renal tubules formed	Kidney excretes urine; sex observable	Testes high in abdomen; kidneys well placed			Testes in inguinal canal			Testes in scrotum; kidneys in final position

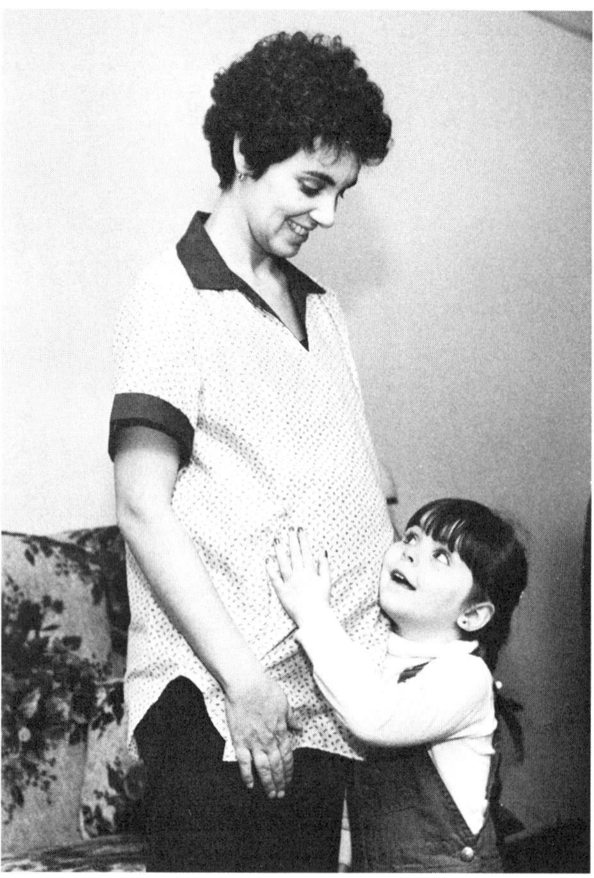

FIGURE 9-6. A preschooler "feels the baby move." The mother first feels fetal movement, termed *quickening*, at 4-1/2 to 5 months of pregnancy.

ing. Quickening is such a remarkable feeling that the average woman remembers for the rest of her life exactly where she was when she felt her first child move inside her. Mothers who do not welcome the pregnancy following quickening need continued assessment during the pregnancy and the child's birth to be certain that bonding or attachment does occur. Ineffective bonding places a child at high risk for neglect or abuse. Since abuse is highly associated with stress situations, it is discussed in Chap. 12 as a possible consequence of poor coping strategies.

Considerations for Care of the Pregnant Family

Embryos and fetuses are at high risk for interference in growth and development. Everyone who cares for a pregnant family must take responsibility to be certain that the woman understands that she must not take any medication that is not approved by her primary health care provider and must limit alcohol and nicotine intake. Some women may not be aware that this rule applies to over-the-counter medicine such as laxatives, cough syrups, and aspirin as well as to prescription drugs. The use of habit-forming drugs during pregnancy is exceptionally dangerous.

Pregnancy is a stress situation due to the increased responsibility not only for care of the fetus but for future care. As a result of this level of stress many women have decreased problem-solving ability during pregnancy. Some women need extra help in making decisions about health care or planning for the new family member. You need to establish which decisions the woman needs assistance with and which she can and wants to make herself. Increased nurturing during this period appears to have an overall positive effect on the mother's ability to give warm loving care to her newborn (she copies the kind, nurturing care given her in caring for her infant).

When planning care for the pregnant woman, observe as an overriding principle of care that you are always caring for at least two people: the woman and her unborn child. Any procedure that you undertake with the woman must be safe for both her and her child. In many instances you are caring for an entire family of mother, father, siblings, and unborn child. Ultimately all procedures must be safe for the entire family.

THE NEONATE

The neonatal period is the first 28 days (4 weeks) of life. A child during this period of his life is termed a *neonate.*

Birth

Almost as soon as a neonate is born, the placenta (his oxygen support system during pregnancy) begins to loosen, compromising his oxygen supply. When the child's body begins to register the effects of a lessening oxygen level, a buildup of carbon dioxide, and the stimulation of cooler room air, the respiratory center is stimulated to initiate the first breath.

A neonate generally cries (proof that he is breathing, as the sound is made by air being pulled past vocal cords) within 20 seconds after birth; this occurs whether the umbilical cord is cut or not.

Apgar Scoring

All newborns born under planned circumstances are assessed at one minute after birth and again at five minutes after birth by an *Apgar score,* a numerical indication of general heart and respiratory functioning, muscle tone, reflex activity, and color. A perfect score is 10; a score between 7 and 10 is normal (most newborns score a 9, not a 10); a score between 4 and 7 indicates that the baby needs some therapy such as oxygen administration; a score below 4 denotes an infant who is having extreme difficulty initiating respiration or heart function and needs intensive therapy such as ventilation or respiratory assistance.

Apgar scoring is apparently done most accurately by nurses (obstetricians tend to rate too high; pediatricians tend to underrate), so in most hospitals assigning this score is a nursing responsibility. As shown in Table 9-8, five signs are assessed and then scored 0, 1, or 2.

TABLE 9-8. APGAR SCORING CHART

	Score		
Sign	0	1	2
Heart rate	Absent	Slow (below 100)	Over 100
Respiratory effort	Absent	Slow, irregular; weak cry	Good; strong cry
Muscle tone	Flaccid	Some flexion of extremities	Well flexed
Reflex irritability (response to catheter in nostril or slap to sole of foot)	No response	Grimace	Cough or sneeze struggling against catheter; cry and withdrawal of foot
Color	Blue, pale	Body pink, extremities blue	Completely pink

Source: From V. Apgar, et al. Evaluation of the newborn infant—second report. *J.A.M.A.* 168:1985, 1958. Copyright © 1958 American Medical Association.

Newborn Appearance

A newborn is covered with a thick white cream-cheese-like substance termed *vernix caseosa*. This serves as a lubricant during the stay in utero and also prevents the newborn's skin from drying excessively on contact with air and linen. It should not be washed away unless it is obviously blood stained and the mother is concerned about the infant's appearance. Fine downy hair termed *lanugo* is present across the shoulders and upper arms. This hair serves to insulate the child from cold. It wears away from friction against bedclothes in 2 or 3 weeks.

The head of a newborn may seem large as body proportion is different in newborns than in adults: In adults the head is one-eighth of total body length; in the newborn the head is one-fourth of total body length. The head is 1 to 2 centimeters larger than the chest in diameter at birth. The chin may appear small, the neck short and thick (Fig. 9-7). The abdomen is round and protuberant. The legs appear short and slightly bowed.

FIGURE 9-7. The head of a newborn is one-fourth the total body length; the neck is short and thick. The eyes can follow an object as far as the midline.

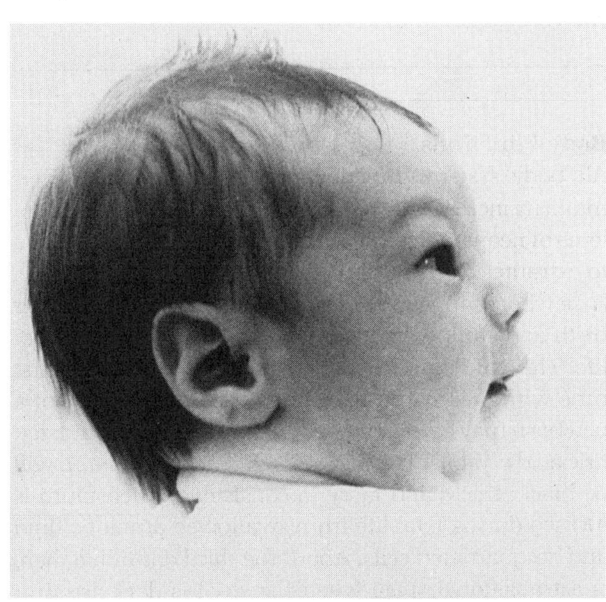

A newborn often has a few white pinpoint elevated lesions on his nose or across his cheeks termed *milia*. These are unopened sebaceous glands; they open spontaneously at about 2 weeks of age and disappear.

Black or oriental newborns may have a flat slate-gray surface patch most often on the sacral area. Termed a *mongolian spot*, this is an area of excessive pigmentation and fades in 3 or 4 years.

At the third day of life many newborns may appear yellowed. This condition is termed *physiological jaundice* and results from the presence of indirect bilirubin being released from red blood cells that were necessary during fetal life but are now no longer needed. Although the majority of jaundice that occurs in newborns is physiological and innocent, all newborns need careful evaluation of the actual indirect bilirubin blood level, because at an extreme point (20 mg indirect bilirubin per 100 ml blood) bilirubin begins to invade brain cells, causing mental retardation and reducing the newborn's ability to function.

Vital Statistics

The average temperature, pulse, respiration, and blood pressure of neonates are shown in Table 9-9. A newborn loses a small amount of weight (5 to 10 ounces) in the first few days following birth due to loss of the extra fluid he carried in fetal life that is no longer necessary. Most newborns are weighed daily to check that loss of weight amounts to no more than 5 to 10 percent of body weight.

Head Characteristics

In order for the fetus to pass safely through the birth canal, his head must be much more malleable than it will be later on in life when a hard unmoldable skull is needed for brain protection. A newborn's skull is malleable because of two fontanelles (unossified areas) that allow the head to adjust to the contour of the birth canal.

Senses

The senses of the newborn are active from birth. His eyes, slate blue, can fixate briefly and follow an object as far as the midline. That he can hear is documented by

TABLE 9-9. VITAL SIGNS BY AGE GROUP

Sign	Newborn	Infant	Toddler	Preschooler	Schoolager	Adolescent	Young Adult	Middle-Aged Adult	Older Adult
Temperature	98.6°F (37.0°C)	98.6°F (37.0°C)	98.6°F (37.0°C)	98.6°F (37.0°C)	98.6°F (37.0°C)	98.6°F (37.0°C)	98.6°F (37.0°C)	98.6°F (37.0°C)	98.6°F (37.0°C)
Pulse	120—140	120	110	100	90—100	75—85	70—80	70—80	70—80
Respiratory rate	30—50	20—40	20—30	20—30	17—22	15—20	16—20	16—20	16—20
Blood pressure	84/60	96/66	99/64	100/65	111/58	118/60	120/90	120/70	130/60

Source: From V. C. Vaughan, III and R. J. McKay, Jr. (Eds.), *Textbook of Pediatrics* (10th ed.). Philadelphia: Saunders, 1975; and R. B. Murray and J. P. Zenterner, *Nursing Assessment and Health Promotion Through The Life Span* (2nd ed.). Englewood Cliffs, N.J.: Prentice Hall, 1979.

TABLE 9-10. NEWBORN REFLEXES

Reflex	Description	Duration
Blink	Eyelid closes in response to bright light (to protect the eye)	Never fades
Rooting	Head turns if cheek is stroked by a corner of the mouth (to locate source of food)	About 6 weeks (fades when infant can see food source clearly)
Sucking	Child sucks on object touched to lips	6—9 months
Swallowing	Child swallows substances that touch posterior part of tongue	Never fades
Gag	Child expels substance entering airway	Never fades
Cough, sneeze	Child expels substances from airway	Never fades
Extrusion	Child extrudes tongue when substance is placed on the anterior portion (to protect against aspiration)	About 4 months
Palmar grasp	Child grasps any object placed against palm	3—4 months
Plantar grasp	Child grasps with toes any object placed against sole of foot	3—4 months
Step (walk-in-place)	Child takes quick prancing steps if sole of foot or anterior surface of lower leg is touched against hard surface	3—4 months
Tonic neck	When lying on back and head is turned to the side, child extends arm and leg on that side, flexes other arm and leg	3—4 months
Moro	When lying on back and head is lifted slightly, then dropped backward, infant flails out arms and legs, then flexes them back (to ward off attack); also elicited by a sudden noise or a jar to side of bassinet	5 months
Babinski	When sole of foot is stroked in a J-like arc, toes fan outward	3 months
Crossed extension	If one leg of a newborn is extended and the sole of that foot irritated, child will extend other foot to brush irritating object away (a test of spinal cord integrity)	3—4 months

the way he quiets to a soft soothing voice and startles at loud sounds. He also quiets to a gentle hand, demonstrating that his sense of touch is intact.

A newborn will draw away from sour or bitter tastes, showing that the sense of taste is intact. It is difficult to demonstrate an intact sense of smell, but the newborn probably locates breast milk by smell as well as vision.

Reflexes

Reflexes are involuntary responses to stimulation. Basically, these are survival or protective reactions that add to the infant's safety until he is more mature and can protect himself by more coordinated motor movements or strategic planning. Newborn reflexes are summarized in Table 9-10.

Body Functions

All body systems function at birth although greater maturity increases a system's efficiency. The major problems of neonates are adjusting their respiratory function to extrauterine life and maintaining body temperature. A newborn appears to be hungry only minutes after birth and can be breast-fed in the first few minutes of life. The child passes his first stool and voids for the first time within 24 hours after birth. The first voiding of a newborn may be slightly pink-tinged from accumulated uric acid crystals. The first stool, termed *meconium*, will be black, thick, and tarry in consistency. Meconium is formed during fetal life from swallowed amniotic fluid and desquamated cells. About the third day of life there is a transitional stage when the stool is dark green; it then becomes light yellow if the infant is breast-fed, bright yellow if formula-fed.

Patterns of Behavior Important for Care

Although all newborns may appear to look alike, all are different. Helping a mother to understand her infant's daily patterns enables her to care for him better and to feel more skilled and competent about herself as a mother.

SLEEP

Newborns sleep as many as 16 out of every 24 hours. Newborn sleep consists of a high proportion of rapid-eye-movement (REM) sleep, however, which is restless, stirring sleep. Mothers should have opportunities to watch their children sleep and should be informed that this seemingly disturbed sleep pattern is normal for newborns.

NUTRITION

The milk of choice for newborns is breast milk. Infants can be breast-fed immediately following birth; if they are going to be formula fed, they can be given glucose water one to four hours after birth.

ACTIVITY

Newborns are ready for toys that appeal to their senses: a mobile that they can watch move, a rattle or music box that they can easily hear. They quiet quickly to the sound of music and startle uncomfortably at noises that are loud or irritating. Newborns tend to spend more time focusing on their mothers' faces than on any other object.

SAFETY

The leading cause of death in very young infants is aspiration. Mothers may need to be reminded to hold infants with their heads elevated when feeding them so that aspiration does not occur. Be certain that no small objects are placed near an infant, as his natural grasp reflex will cause him to grasp the object and bring it to his mouth.

Concerns of Parents During the Newborn Period

The concerns of parents during the newborn period concentrate on the fact that parents are usually inexperienced. Even if a newborn is not their first child, they are as yet unfamiliar with the particular requirements of this new baby.

BONDING

Bonding or attachment to a baby is easiest if the mother is allowed to spend as much time as she wants with the infant at birth and during the newborn period. *Rooming-in* is the term for a hospital policy that allows the infant to be cared for by his mother in her own room rather than in a central nursery. Both mothers and fathers should be encouraged to become quickly involved in the care of their infant whenever circumstances permit to allow bonding to occur.

ASSESSMENT OF HEALTH

Becoming a parent is a developmental step for the neonate's mother and father. Assessing whether their infant is well or ill will be difficult until they grow more experienced with children. Taking care of the child should he become ill is a second developmental step.

All mothers need to learn how to take an infant's temperature (see Chap. 33) before they leave the hospital after his birth (or during the first days of life if he is born at home). The best way to determine whether a child is doing well is not frequent temperature taking, however, but by noting whether he is gaining in height and weight, maintaining his usual level of activity, and meeting motor, language, and social milestones. Plotting weight and height on a growth chart and performing a Brazelton Behavioral Assessment or a Denver Developmental Screening Test are other means of assuring a parent that a child is developing normally.

NUTRITIONAL REQUIREMENTS

Parents worry that their newborn may not be eating enough, particularly if he is breast-fed. At one time parents were taught to weigh their infant daily (or even before and after each feeding) as a means of gauging whether his intake was adequate. This approach tended to concentrate parents' attention on daily weight and actually increased their worry. Parents need to learn to judge intake adequacy on factors such as monthly weight gain, contentment between feeding times, and general overall sleeping and elimination patterns. As soon as the infant differentiates his cry (at about 2 months of age), it is easier for parents to determine the reason for the cry, and worry over whether he is hungry or not begins to decrease.

Considerations for Care of Newborns

When working with newborns you should keep in mind that a new mother is watching you for suggestions or role modeling of infant care. Your examples of safe care and active communication with the child will help her to imitate these behaviors and give care that is both stimulating and safe for her newborn.

Effect of Illness

Illness in a newborn may necessitate separation from the mother and interfere with mother-child bonding. If hospitalization should be necessary, make every effort to include the parent in the newborn's care. Unrestricted visiting hours should be allowed, so that the mother can spend time holding and rocking the neonate.

THE INFANT (1 to 12 months)

Both growth and development continue to proceed at a rapid rate during the infant year.

Physical Growth and Development
The child grows so rapidly during the first year of life that he doubles his birth weight in 4 or 5 months and triples it in a year. He gains 8 to 10 inches (20 to 25 cm) in height. He moves from reflex behavior to the complexities of standing, walking, feeding himself, and speaking. Milestones of motor, language, and social development of the infant year are shown in Table 9-11.

Developmental Task
Freud termed the infant period the oral stage, as a child's main interest during this period is sucking or oral pleasure. The developmental task of the infant year according to Erikson is that of achieving a sense of trust (versus mistrust). It might also be described as learning about love: The infant learns to love and be loved. A sense of trust develops because when the baby is hungry, his mother feeds him; when he is wet, she changes and dries him; when he is lonely, she comes and holds and comforts him. At the end of the first year of life, the child is able to expand this concept of loving one person to loving other family members and ultimately as he grows older, to loving people at a distance from him. He comes to think of the world as a friendly, responsive place to live.

Patterns of Behavior Important for Care
Parents have to be adjustable caregivers during the first year of life, as the infant's behavior changes continually throughout the year.

SLEEP
The amount of sleep needed daily by infants is reduced from 16 hours to about 12 (ten hours at night and two naps during the day). Infants may have difficulty falling asleep if they are overtired or overstimulated; providing a quiet time for them just before bed or nap time is often useful.

NUTRITION
Infants remain on breast milk or a balanced formula with iron for the first 5 to 6 months of life. At the midpoint in the infant year they are introduced to cereal (infant cereal), fruits, vegetables, and ground or strained meat. It is generally recommended that infants remain on breast milk or formula for the entire first year, as these forms of milk are much easier to digest than cows' milk, and the possibility of developing allergies to milk products is reduced.

After 6 months of age the infant's sucking reflex begins to fade; he is then "ripe" for gradual weaning from a bottle or breast to a small glass or cup for the majority of his fluid intake.

ACTIVITY
During the first year the child is most interested in developing motor skills—looking at his hands at 3 months, crawling at 9 months, cruising or walking from 10 to 12 months. Young infants are attracted to toys that appeal to their senses: brightly colored mobiles, blocks that are musical or rattle, stuffed toys of smooth or shaggy textures. At the end of the first year the infant enjoys toys that he can put into things and take out of things (small empty boxes that stack inside each other; concentric colored rings that stack on a center post).

SAFETY
The leading cause of death in infants is accidents. Parents may need to be cautioned not to leave an infant unsupervised on a couch or in his crib with the siderails down. Infants in automobiles should be contained in infant car seats (the best types place the infant's back toward the front of the car until the child is six months old).

Concerns of Parents During the Infant Year
Parents of infants often need help in assessing the seriousness of various health problems. Advise them about common conditions that they can deal with themselves, as well as those for which they need to contact a health care provider for assistance. Helping them to understand when they need additional aid is a nursing responsibility.

NIGHT BOTTLE SYNDROME
Infants who are put to bed at night with a propped bottle of formula have their teeth bathed in sweetened milk all night long. Bacteria grow freely in such an attractive medium and cause extensive tooth decay (see Chap. 34).

DIAPER RASH
To prevent diaper rash, infants need to be changed frequently so that wet diapers do not remain in contact with their skin for long periods of time (as urine stands, its ammonia content increases; it is the ammonia that inflames skin). At the time of a diaper change, the infant's skin should be washed with clear water, dried, and coated with an ointment such as A&D ointment. Occasionally diaper rash occurs because infants are sensitive to disposable diapers or laundry detergent. Some infants have such sensitive skin that despite extensive precautions rashes still occur.

Exposing the diaper area to air is often helpful for curing a diaper rash. If a rash is persistent, the mother should consult her primary health care provider.

SEBORRHEIC DERMATITIS (CRADLE CAP)
Cradle cap is a common condition of early infancy characterized by dirty-looking, adherent, yellow, crusting patches on the scalp or forehead. It can be prevented by frequent shampooing. Once such patches occur, lubricating them with mineral oil softens them and allows them to be removed with the next shampoo. Such crusting often occurs over the fontanelles, as mothers are afraid to wash over these "soft spots." They can be

TABLE 9-11. SUMMARY OF INFANT GROWTH AND DEVELOPMENT

Month	Nutrition	Activities	Play	Safety
0—1	Breast or iron-fortified commercial formula—117 cal/kg	Largely reflex behavior; able to follow object to midline; keeps hands fisted. Cognitive stage: sensorimotor	Enjoys watching face of primary caregiver, listening to soothing sounds	Aspiration is chief danger (from propped bottle or small object brought to mouth by grasp reflex)
2	Advise not to prop bottles to prevent aspiration and "night bottle syndrome" (cavities)	Makes cooing sounds, differentiates his cry, has social smile, focuses on objects well, head up when prone	Enjoys bright colored moving mobiles	Aspiration continues to be chief danger
3		Follows object past midline; head and chest up when prone; laughs out loud. Reflexes: grasp, stepping, tonic-neck fading	Spends time looking at hands or uses them as his toy during the month (hand regard)	Caution mothers that soon he will turn over; do not leave unattended on couch or bed
4		Turns front to back; no longer has head lag when pulled upright; bears partial weight on feet when held upright	Needs space in which to turn	Falls are major concerns
5		Turns both ways; Moro reflex fading	Handles rattles well	Be sure toys are big enough that when handled they can't be swallowed
6	Strained or mashed table foods introduced one at a time; continue iron-fortified commercial formula or breast-feeding	Reaches out in anticipation of being picked up; first tooth (central lower incisor) erupts; may say vowel sounds (oh-oh); sits unsteadily (still needs support)	Enjoys bathtub toys; rubber ring for teething	Can turn rapidly side to side; childproof large area
7	Calorie requirement decreases to 108 cal/kg	Transfers objects hand to hand; beginning fear of strangers	Likes objects that rattle and are good size for transfering	Check toy safety; beginning toys are 7 months old
8	Change to mashed table food if not aready using	Sits securely without support; fear of strangers (ability to tell known from unknown people) reaches peak	Enjoys manipulation, rattles and toys of different textures.	Caution mothers that he will creep in another month; childproof larger area of house
9		Creeps or crawls (abdomen off floor); says first word (da-da)	Needs space for creeping	Will soon pull to standing position; check higher areas for unsafe objects; poisoning becomes a problem from now until school age
10		Pulls himself to standing position; plays peek-a-boo and patty-cake. Cognitive: has concept of permanence	Plays games like patty-cake; uses pincer grasp (thumb and finger) to pick up objects	Can pick up very small objects; check table surfaces as he can reach them easily
11		"Cruises" (walks with support)	"Cruises"	Childproof larger area
12	Change to milk from formula or breast. Definitely change to table food if not already done	Says 2 words plus ma-ma and da-da; stands alone; some children take first step; holds cup and spoon well; helps to dress (pushes arm into sleeve)	Likes toys that fit inside each other (pots and pans); nursery rhymes; will like pull-toys as soon as he walks.	Childproof larger area of house

assured that the connective tissue covering these areas is strong, and washing the area will do no harm.

COLIC
Colic is abdominal pain that may occur in infants at about 2 weeks of age and reoccur intermittently until about 3 months of age. The pain is sharp; the infant pulls up his legs and cries loudly. The cause of colic is unknown but it is related to rapid swallowing of food and consequent accumulation of gas in intestines. It is a frightening illness for parents, as the infant appears to be extremely ill. It is baffling because the symptoms return over and over again, often at night when the parents are tired and have the most difficulty coping with the problem.

No nausea or vomiting occurs with colic; bowel movements and weight gain remain normal. The symptoms of colic are relieved best if the infant is fed slowly and bubbled frequently; placing him on his abdomen to put pressure on his abdomen after feedings may be helpful.

CONSTIPATION
Infants' faces often turn red and they make small grunting noises with bowel movements. It is easy for inexperienced parents to interpret these signs as those of constipation. As long as the infant's stool is soft, however, this is merely a normal infant response. Parents may need to be advised that there is no uniform "normal" pattern for bowel movements, that not having daily bowel movements may be normal for their infant.

TEETHING
Most infants acquire their first tooth at 5 to 6 months of age. The first tooth to appear is generally a front lower incisor. By the end of the infant period they have approximately six teeth. With teething, infants may be irritable and decrease their intake slightly as their gumline is tender.

THUMBSUCKING
Many infants suck their thumbs while still in utero. Sucking is a need of infants and many continue the practice through the first year of life. The best advice for parents in regard to thumbsucking is to recognize it as a normal need, be sure that the infant receives enough sucking pleasure in association with feeding, and then to ignore it. Making a point of thumbsucking may intensify the behavior, as it can also serve as a comforting, stress-relieving behavior. Use of a pacifier may be suggested to offer opportunity for sucking.

Considerations for Care of the Infant

Special care must always be taken with infants to be certain that parent-child relationships are developing (Fig. 9-8). This type of relationship grows best if the parents know what to expect next. Thus, they should be given anticipatory guidance of happenings that occur in the first year of life.

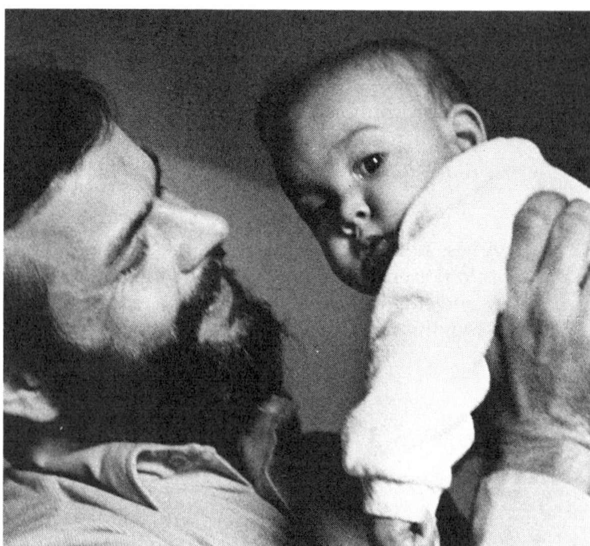

FIGURE 9-8. Father-infant bonding. Bonding occurs most readily if a father spends time with his child. (The baby's attention is momentarily diverted in the direction of the photographer.)

Because infant development is so rapid and dramatic during the first year, one of the major roles of the nurse during this time is to anticipate development of the infant and communicate this information to the parents so that they can provide safeguards to prevent injuries and not expect too much or too little of the child. This type of guidance includes such information as the child will turn shortly and will no longer be able to sleep in a bassinet; he will stand shortly so parents need to "child-proof" table levels.

Effect of Illness

To encourage a sense of trust try to limit the number of painful procedures done to infants: Draw no more blood than is absolutely necessary; regulate intravenous fluid carefully so that it does not have to be restarted. If painful procedures must be done, include holding and comforting the infant afterward as a basic procedural step, not a nicety to add "if there is time."

Try to present learning opportunities for the child at the time that particular developmental steps would normally occur. At nine months, for example, an infant generally begins crawling. Even an ill infant may need crawling space at this time so that he can practice the skill. Infants learn through play. Be certain that the hospitalized infant has enough toys and experiences around him to encourage continued learning.

THE TODDLER (1 to 3 years)

The child changes dramatically during the toddler period as he gains the ability to be responsible for a part of his own care.

TABLE 9-12. SUMMARY OF TODDLER GROWTH AND DEVELOPMENT

Age	Nutrition	Activities	Play	Safety
15 mo	Intake decreases due to lowered BMR (mothers may interpret this as feeding problem)	Walks alone well; can creep upstairs	Can stack 2 blocks; enjoys being read to; drops toys for adult to recover (exploring sense of permanence)	Will walk a city block if unsupervised outside; caution parents about pools, other unsafe areas; poisoning is big concern during toddler period
18 mo	Enjoys "finger foods"; provide some from each food group	Can run; walk up and down stairs; says about 20 words	Imitates household chores, dusting, etc.; begins parallel play (playing *beside* not *with* another child)	Can climb onto chairs, stools, etc.; anything not locked is accessible to him
24 mo	Wants to join family for meals	Walks up stairs, both feet on same step at same time; speaks in 2 word sentences ("daddy go," "me come") Cognitive: state of preoperational thought	Parallel play very evident	Can unscrew jar lids, turn doorknobs, so can go places he could not go before
30 mo		Makes simple strokes with pencil; jumps	Spends time "playing house;" imitating housework	Motor skills are ahead of judgment

Physical Growth and Development

Growth in the toddler period is slow compared with that of the infant period. During the entire period the child may grow only 7 inches (17 cm) and gain only 5 pounds (2.3 kg). This decrease in growth may cause his appetite to be small in contrast to his requirements as an infant.

Toddlers usually appear faintly chubby. They have a protuberant abdomen and a definite inward curving (lordosis) of their lower spine. They walk with a wide-based gait like a sailor on a rolling ship (hence the designation *toddler*).

By two years of age most children have all 20 of their temporary (deciduous) teeth. Table 9-12 summarizes normal toddler growth and development.

VITAL SIGNS

Usual vital signs for toddlers are shown in Table 9-9. Although blood pressure is shown in the table, it is not taken routinely on children until they reach 3 years of age because there are few instances when blood pressure is abnormal in younger children.

MOTOR DEVELOPMENT

The toddler can walk upstairs but does so by putting both feet at a time on each step. He runs, jumps, and climbs, spending the major part of his day in this type of active movement. Most toddlers have at least one bruise on their legs or knees from bumping into objects that are in their way of progress.

LANGUAGE

A major milestone of the 2-year-old is the ability to put together two-word sentences. Such sentences are composed of a noun and a verb ("me go," "Bobby see"). This is a major step in the child's ability to decipher not just how to pronounce words but how to use them.

Developmental Task

Freud termed the toddler period the anal stage because the child becomes concerned with toilet training and excretion or retention of stool during this time. Excessively strict toilet training may, according to Freud, result in adults who are overly concerned with neatness and rigidity or who are overly generous, giving away or placing little value on property.

According to Erikson, the developmental task of the toddler period is the achievement of a sense of autonomy versus shame and doubt. Another word for autonomy is independence. In order to learn how to do things for himself and feel independent, the child needs experience in self-feeding, self-dressing, and, when he shows signs of readiness, self-toileting. At the same time that he enjoys experimenting with independence, he also needs and wants "ground rules" to protect him. Most toddlers enjoy hearing the same nursery rhyme or the same story over and over again as an element of stability in their lives when almost everything else is changing.

Cognitive Development

Toddlers are still in the sensorimotor stage of cognitive thought. During this stage they are capable of simple concept formation: They can appreciate a concept such as chair; no matter how many different types of chair they see they can understand that they all fit into the same category.

Patterns of Behavior Important for Care

SLEEP

Toddlers need about 12 hours of sleep a day at the beginning of the period, closer to 10 hours by the end. They usually have one nap a day and have a great deal of difficulty falling asleep if overtired or overstimulated from their busy day.

NUTRITION

Since the toddler's appetite may not be as great as it was when he was an infant, his intake may actually be less than it was previously. Mothers need to be cautioned about this change or they can turn mealtime into an unhappy, nagging time. Toddlers like to use their fingers to eat and should be given finger foods: pieces of fruit, chunks of cucumber, crackers, and cheese.

ACTIVITY

Toddlers enjoy toys that they can manipulate in some way (pull toys, blocks that stack, tops that spin). When playing with other children, they engage in *parallel* play: They play beside, but not actually with, the other child. They have not yet learned sharing and argue frequently over whose toy is whose (Fig. 9-9).

SAFETY

Accidents are the major cause of death in toddlers. Toddlers have many falls because they underestimate the distance to be jumped; they do not appreciate the speed of moving automobiles and run in front of them to rescue balls. Another major cause of death is poisoning; in their efforts to explore the world around them, toddlers may swallow the contents of medicine or cleaning fluid bottles (Fig. 9-10). At health maintenance visits

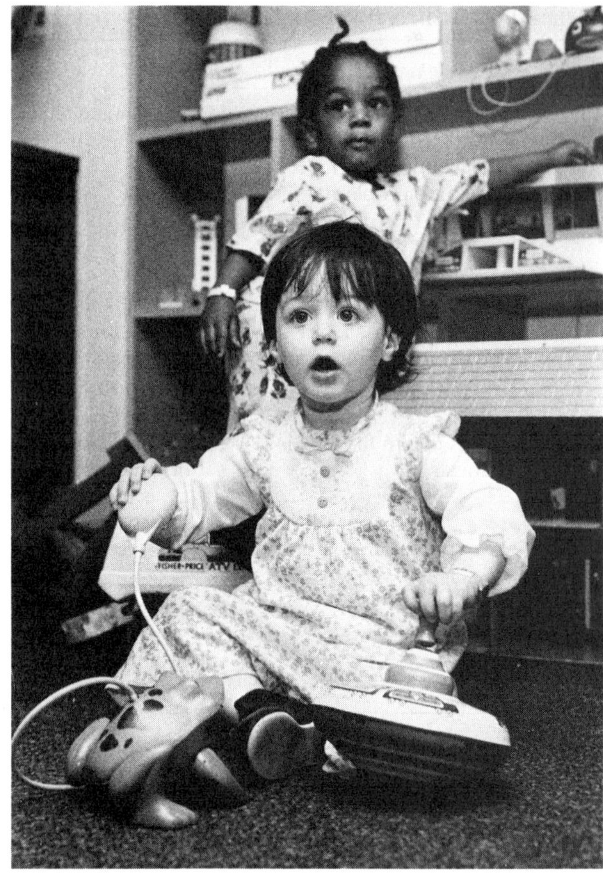

FIGURE 9-9. In the playroom these toddler girls choose toys they can manipulate. They play beside, not with, each other.

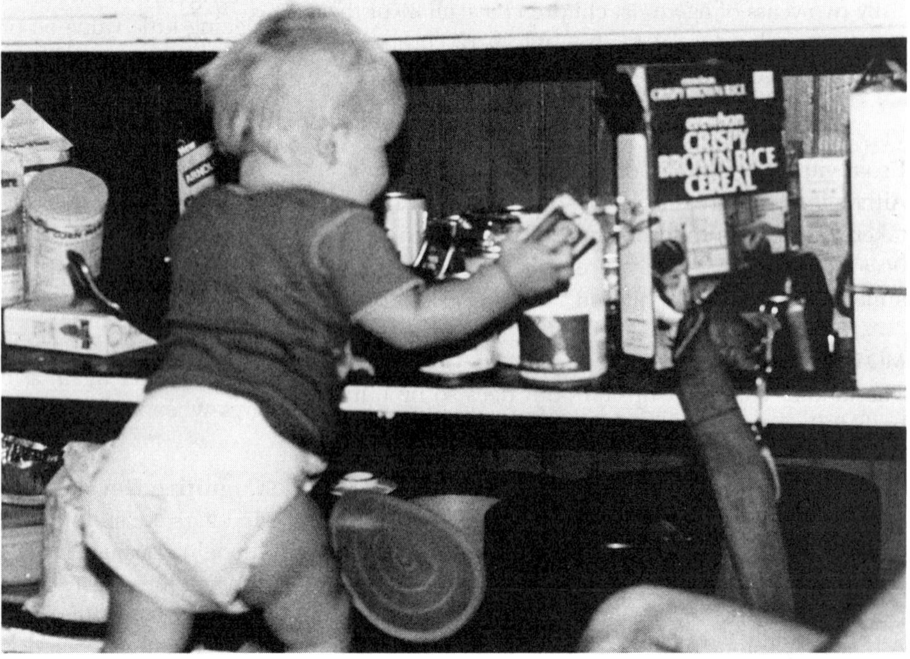

FIGURE 9-10. This young toddler explores the contents of a low cupboard. He needs constant supervision as poisoning is a major cause of accidents in infants and toddlers.

during the toddler period mothers should be instructed about the use of ipecac, an antiemetic which induces vomiting. Parents should contact the local poison control center before administering ipecac, however, because some materials such as lye cause less harm if not vomited after ingestion.

Common Concerns of the Toddler Period

Concerns of the toddler period center on conflicts that arise from the child's insistence on being independent in self-care, even though his knowledge is often inadequate for many tasks.

NEGATIVISM

In an effort to show how independent they are, toddlers typically answer "no" to every question asked them (whether they mean it or not). This makes planning care for a toddler or implementing it difficult, because the child appears to dislike everything you suggest.

The easiest way to discourage this type of behavior is to limit the number of questions you ask. For example, do not ask, "Would you like to take your bath now?" but say, "It's bathtime now." Not "Would you like to take your medicine now?" but "It's time to take your medicine."

On the other hand, eliminating decision making totally does not help the child to achieve a sense of autonomy or to move toward maturity. After announcing the primary task, therefore, offer a secondary choice the child can make a response to: "It's bathtime now. Do you want to play with your yellow duck or your frog?" "It's time to take your medicine. Do you want a drink of orange juice or water to go with it?" This technique both deals with the negativism and fosters the autonomy that you are striving to achieve.

TEMPER TANTRUMS

Temper tantrums occur in the toddler period because the child has definite ideas about what he wants to do or not do but has too little vocabulary to express his wants. A typical tantrum occurs when the child asks for a cookie just before mealtime and his mother answers no, he's going to eat in five minutes. Instead of saying, "I don't think I can wait even five minutes," the child lays down on the floor, kicks his heels, bangs his head, and cries. Some children hold their breath until they faint.

Temper tantrums are difficult to deal with because they are so explosive and violent that a parent is caught offguard. The principle for handling tantrums is to respect the child's right to protest (some assertiveness is a productive, desirable quality) but guide him into a more socially acceptable way of expressing anger. If using tantrums becomes a successful way of getting what he wants, the child will continue to use the method well past the toddler period. Almost everyone knows an adult who still uses temper tantrums—to the frustration of everyone around him.

When dealing with tantrums, evaluate first that your request of the child was reasonable—that you were not asking him something beyond his developmental level; that you have provided him with the proper material or equipment needed for the task; that he is not overtired (the incidence of temper tantrums rises near nap and bed time and on long shopping trips when the child is tired). If your request was reasonable, ignore the behavior for best results.

RITUALISM

At the same time that toddlers insist on being independent, they also demand rituals—some actions done the same way every day (the same bedtime story read every day; the same spoon used every day for breakfast). This type of consistency offers the child the same reassurance that strong guard posts on a steep mountain road offer adults. It aids them to move ahead in certain areas by being assured that other areas are always consistent and do not change.

TOILET TRAINING

Children are physiologically ready for toilet training by the time they walk, as this means that cephalocaudal development has proceeded along the spinal cord to the level of the anal and urethral sphincters. Cognitively, however, some children are not ready for toilet training until about 3 years of age.

The age that toilet training is achieved or introduced is culturally related. South Asian families do not typically use diapers on infants, and with more awareness of body functions such infants become trained much earlier. Some parents put undue stress on toilet training because they are anxious to be done with diapers; they may need to be reminded that they cannot rush development in this area any more than with any other.

Considerations in Care of the Toddler

Care of a toddler always involves a balance between allowing the child experiences that foster independence and experiences that promote security. It is not always easy to be a caregiver to a toddler because he seems to resist so many actions; on the other hand, it must not always be easy to be a toddler (your mind shows you many attractive possibilities that cannot yet be achieved because your motor ability has not kept pace).

Another important consideration is prevention of accidents, especially poisoning. Be certain that you do not allow the child's confident, I-can-do-it attitude about everything cause you to neglect necessary safeguards.

Effect of Illness

Illness during the toddler period can be devastating in terms of the child's achievement of a sense of autonomy, since he may be unable to do things for himself due to fatigue or specific symptoms. Remember when caring for ill toddlers to allow them secondary choices whenever possible so that they have some sense of control over the situation.

THE PRESCHOOLER (3 to 6 years)

Preschool age is a transition period from an age where the child can accomplish a few self-care skills to one where he is ready to leave home and care for himself for a large part of every day. It is the time in life when imagination is at its peak, which allows the child to learn new skills very rapidly but also brings problems as he may imagine situations as being more serious or more dangerous than they truly are.

Physical Growth and Development

The preschool period is another slow growth period: The child gains only about five pounds a year (2.25 kg); he grows about 2 inches a year (5 cm). His overall appearance changes from a paunchy, wide-stanced toddler to a thinner-appearing, better coordinated child. Table 9-13 is a summary of preschoolage growth and development.

Developmental Task

Freud viewed the preschool period as one in which the child became interested in his genital area (the phallic stage). It is a period certainly when children become involved in exploration of their bodies and of their sex roles. Freud describes an *Electra* complex in which the girl begins to compete with her mother for love of the father and an *Oedipus* complex where the boy competes with the father for the mother's love. If parents are good role models of their sex, at the end of the period the child identifies with his own sex and the Electra and Oedipus emphases fade. If something should happen to the parent with which the child is competing (a parent dies or leaves the home), the child may feel that he is so powerful that he can make his wishes come true. He also may have difficulty establishing his sex role at the end of the period as the role model is no longer present.

A single parent needs to be aware of his or her responsibility for modeling a sex role. He needs to try to provide the opposite role model for the child from a respected outside source (an aunt or uncle, a grandmother or grandfather, a nursery school teacher).

Erikson sees the developmental crisis of the preschool period as achieving a sense of initiative versus guilt. Achieving initiative is learning how to do things. The child watches carefully the people around him and pretends to be these people.

He enjoys material that he can use to create objects (play dough, mud pies, clay, finger paint). The child who is allowed to experiment in these ways will be better able to use creative expression as an adult in dancing,

TABLE 9-13. SUMMARY OF PRESCHOOLAGE GROWTH AND DEVELOPMENT

Age	Nutrition	Activity	Play	Safety
3 yr	Amount of food eaten is small because this is not a rapid growth time.	Can walk upstairs one step at a time; ride a tricycle; cognitive task: preoperational thought; vocabulary of 300—900 words; able to share for first time. Some mothers wait to begin toilet training until 3 years.	Markedly imaginative; enjoys molding clay, water play.	Motor skills proceed ahead of judgment; poisoning is still a threat; motor vehicle accidents increase.
4 yr	Continues to eat small amounts of food; may enjoy bright colors over more bland foods.	Constantly in motion as he practices motor skills of jumping, skipping; asks 300—400 questions (how, why, what) daily; can hop as new motor skill.	Imaginative play requires few "toys"; pretending is major activity.	Needs to be taught street safety as he will be outside home to nursery school or other experiences.
5 yr		New motor skill: throws overhand; may develop non-fluency (say "I want, want, want") as he tries to form sentences faster than tongue allows; ready for nursery school experience as long as he is assured that he will return home again.	Imaginative play continues.	Caution about outside safety.

writing, or problem solving. It is a crucial period for developing the ability to examine problems critically and move toward solving them.

Cognitive Development

The preschool child enters the preoperational period of thought. He is capable of elemental problem solving but has little experience on which to base sound decision making. He also is unable to view anyone else's side of a problem. In addition, he does not understand the concept of conservation: He cannot understand that there is the same amount of water in a large glass half filled as in a small glass fully filled. This distortion in judgment may make him argue over half-truths; because he only sees one side of the issue, however, he argues with the conviction of someone who is certain that he is correct.

Patterns of Behavior Important for Care

Although preschoolers are typically easy to relate to because they are so interested in learning new skills and interacting with people around them, conflicts can arise from everyday care measures relating to sleep and eating.

SLEEP

Preschoolers sleep 8 to 10 hours at night; most children continue to take an afternoon nap until they begin full-time school. Sleep during this period is often disturbed by nightmares, as the child's overactive imagination works even during sleep. Waking the child to be certain that the dream is interrupted and staying with him until he feels comfortable returning to sleep again is often necessary.

NUTRITION

Preschoolers do not have large appetites as this is a slow-growing period. They may be more interested in food that they helped prepare than a meal to which they made no contribution. Introducing a fork for eating if this skill has not yet been achieved may promote an interest in eating. As the child learns colors, the colors of foods may interest him. As a general rule, however, preschoolers are eating adequate amounts for their small weight gain; it just appears to adults to be insufficient.

ACTIVITY

Preschoolers spend most of their time with play materials that can be manipulated, such as a basin of water with soap bubbles, clay, or finger paint. When working with such media, they may not actually create anything but spend their time getting a feel for the medium and enjoying the creative effort rather than the finished product.

Preschoolers are capable of sharing, and they interact with the children around them much more than they did as toddlers when they played beside but not actively with others.

SAFETY

Many preschoolers begin a school experience. Before such experiences they need preparation in terms of bus and street safety. If there are specific hazards in a neighborhood such as electrical wires, swimming pools, or an unfriendly dog, they must be told to stay away from these dangers. Their natural curiosity and imagination take them into situations that interest them but are not necessarily safe.

Common Concerns of the Preschool Period

Most concerns about preschool children relate to the situations that result from the child's active imagination.

FEARS

Because the preschooler's imagination is so high, he typically experiences a number of fears: fear of the dark, of separation, of intrusive procedures. A teddy bear on the bedroom shelf may be viewed as a staring, open-eyed monster. When his mother goes to the coffee shop for 15 minutes, he may imagine that she has deserted him. When the needle of a syringe pierces only a half-inch under his skin, he may imagine it piercing his entire body.

These fears are very real and extremely frightening. Many children this age need to sleep with a night light and need frequent reassurance that their parents or you are close by. Try to limit the number of intrusive procedures used with preschoolers (no more blood drawn, temperatures taken, etc. than absolutely necessary) in order to reduce the level of stress.

TALL TALES

The child's active imagination often leads him into tall-tale telling. You may ask a child how many brothers he has; he has none, but your tone of voice implies that you expect him to have some, so he answers, "Twenty." If you ask him if his name is Bobby Jones and sound as if that is who you expect him to be, he will say yes. Tall-tale telling is not lying in that it is not meant to be a deceptive act but rather an effort to please.

Always keep this phenomenon in mind when caring for preschoolers. If you ask the child if he has pain, he may invent pain symptoms for you; if you ask if he already took his medicine, he may describe medicine taking that did not actually exist. Try to ascertain the truth without suppressing the active imagination. An effective way to do this might be to say, "That sounds like a lot of brothers to me. Is that a story you made up for me?" or "That's a good pretend answer. How many brothers do you really have?"

Do not encourage tall-tale telling by replying "You're lucky to have so many brothers," as if you believe the made-up story is true. Such a response leads the child to believe that his wish or thought may have magically come true, which is extremely frightening because the monster he thinks he sees in his bedroom or his worry that his mother will desert him may also become real in the same way.

LANGUAGE DEVELOPMENT

Preschoolers greatly expand their vocabulary from 300 to 900 words. They use these new words to ask questions almost constantly (as many as 300 to 400 daily). Many preschoolers are so eager to use their enlarged vocabulary that their language pattern sounds like stuttering (saying "I want want want to go"). This is not true stuttering but a common developmental phenomenon of the period termed *non-fluency.* It occurs most frequently when the child must hurry to say something (such as when he has to compete for time at the dinner table with siblings' stories of their activities).

Non-fluency passes most quickly if it is ignored and if the child is provided time to talk. Advice such as "Stop, slow down, start over" calls unnecessary attention to the problem and may make the child so self-conscious about his speech that he develops true stuttering.

DENTAL SUPERVISION

Preschoolers need to learn good toothbrushing habits. For many children brushing teeth well once a day is more effective than half-hearted attempts three or four times a day. At about 3 years of age the child should receive his first checkup with a dentist. At this early age the child usually needs little repair work; this introduction is mainly an informative, health promotion visit (Fig. 9-11).

FIGURE 9-11. A dental checkup need not be a frightening experience.

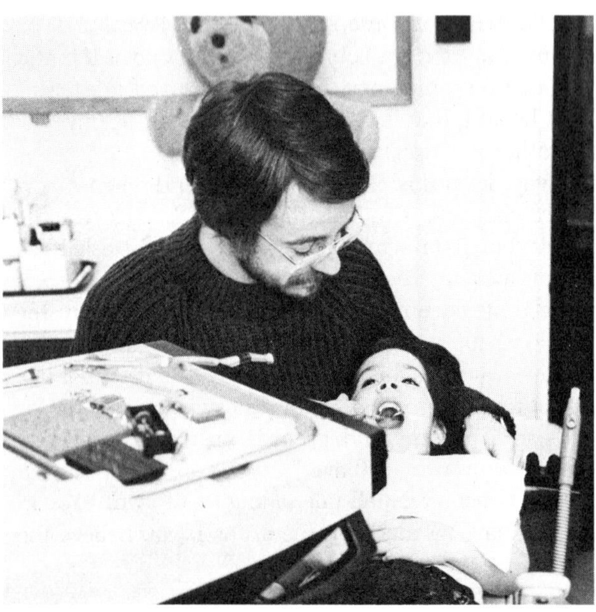

Considerations in Care of the Preschooler

Care of the preschooler should always include activities or experiences that promote creative or imaginative happenings. For parents who enjoy this type of activity themselves (an unscheduled trip to the zoo, an unplanned picnic), caring for a preschooler is fun. Parents who like a more structured schedule may be anxious for their child to pass through this question-asking phase.

Effect of Illness

Preschoolers have many upper respiratory infections, as this is the first time they have been exposed to so many other children. Some mothers need to be reminded that if the child has a severe sore throat or ear pain with a cold, the illness is no longer a simple one and she should consult her pediatrician for further care. (Some children are left with impaired hearing from the effect of scarring in the middle ear from improperly treated ear infections during the preschool period because an earache was disregarded.) All children need both hearing and vision screening performed before they begin grade school to be certain that they will be able to participate fully in school. Since the preschool child's eyes are not fully mature, he usually tests only 20/50 on a vision examination, rather than the 20/20 of the adult.

The preschool period is a time for the child to learn a great deal of information about his world. Evaluate whether children who are chronically ill are participating in activities like trips to the zoo or a shopping center so that their knowledge of common experiences remains on a par with that of children who are not ill. Such information is used in school as a base for further learning.

THE SCHOOLAGER (6 to 12 years)

Children change a great deal from the time they enter the schoolage period at six years until they leave it at 12. Their knowledge of the world and their sense of responsibility multiply many times during this time.

Physical Growth and Development

Growth at the beginning of the period is fairly slow; at the end of the period (10 years in girls; 12 years in boys) the child begins a preadolescent growth spurt of 6 to 12 inches. Because girls typically begin to grow first, all preadolescent girls tend to be taller than boys the same age. Boys tend to be slightly heavier than girls during the period despite the difference in height because of developing muscle mass. Table 9-14 summarizes normal schoolage growth and development.

VITAL SIGNS

Vital signs for the schoolage period are shown in Table 9-9. Toward the end of the period blood pressure begins to increase in boys over girls because of the former's larger muscle mass.

TABLE 9-14. SUMMARY OF EARLY SCHOOLAGE DEVELOPMENT

Age (years)	Physical Development	Psychosocial Development
6	A year of constant motion; skipping is a new skill; first molars erupt	First-grade teacher becomes authority figure; adjustment to all-day school may be difficult and lead to nervous manifestations of fingernail biting, etc.; he defines words by their use: a key is to unlock a door, not a metal object
7	Central incisors erupt; difference between sexes becomes apparent in play (bats like a girl, etc.); spends time in quiet play	A quiet year; striving for perfection leads to seventh year being called an *eraser* year. Conservation (water poured from tall container to a wide, flat one is the same amount of water) is learned; can tell time; can make simple change
8	Coordination makes definite improvement; playing with gang becomes important; eyes become fully developed	"Best friends" develop; whispering and giggling begin; can write as well as print; understands past, present, and future
9	All activities done with gang	"Gang age"; a 9-year-old club is formed to spite someone, has secret codes, is all boy or all girl; gangs disband and reform quickly
10	Coordination improves	Ready for a camp experience away from home; "collecting age"; likes rules; ready for competitive games

TEETH

Beginning at 6 or 7 years of age the child begins to lose his deciduous teeth and acquire his permanent ones. The first permanent teeth to develop are generally the first molars; these four teeth appear just posterior to the last deciduous teeth. Many children may not realize that these teeth are permanent because they do not replace deciduous teeth, and therefore they may not brush them as thoroughly as they should. This results in unfortunate decay of permanent teeth. By 12 years of age most children have all their permanent teeth with the exception of their third molars (wisdom teeth), which do not appear until 16 to 18 years of age.

TABLE 9-15. CHRONOLOGICAL DEVELOPMENT OF SECONDARY SEX CHARACTERISTICS

Age (years)	Boys	Girls
9—11	Prepubertal gain in weight	Breast: elevation of papilla with breast bed formation; areolar diameter enlarging; transverse diameter of hips enlarging
11—12	Sparse growth of straight, downy hair at base of penis; sebaceous gland secretion and perspiration increasing; testes and penis growth beginning	Straight hair along labia; pH of vagina becoming acid; slight mucous vaginal discharge present; dramatic growth spurt perspiration and sebaceous gland secretion increasing
12—13	Pubic hair present; penis lengthening; dramatic growth spurt beginning; breast growth beginning	Pubic hair growing darker; breasts enlarging, axillary hair present; menarche usually occurs
13—14	Growth spurt continuing; pubic hair abundant and curly; axillary and facial hair present; voice changes beginning	Pubic hair thick and curly; triangular in distribution; breast areola and papilla form a secondary mound; menstruation is ovulatory
15—16	Genitalia adult; scrotum dark and rugated; sperm production mature	Breast tissue adult; facial acne at peak incidence
16—18	Breast enlargement fades; facial acne at peak incidence; testes and penis reach final size	End of skeletal growth
18—21	End of skeletal growth	

SECONDARY SEXUAL CHARACTERISTICS

Puberty is the time of life when secondary sexual characteristics appear. *Menarche* is the term used to describe the beginning of menstruation in girls. At about 10 years in girls and 12 years in boys, the anterior pituitary gland, under stimulation by the hypothalamus, begins to secrete gonadotropin hormones that stimulate testes and ovaries to mature function. This is accompanied by a growth spurt, the secretion of 17-ketosteroids in urine (the breakdown product of androgen), pubic and axillary growth of hair, breast changes, and finally, menarche and sperm formation.

Secondary sexual characteristics appear in a specified order as shown in Table 9-15. It is helpful to recognize this natural progression to maturity in order to be able to assure children that they are changing normally and to detect abnormalities of growth. Notice that breast development occurs in both sexes. Termed *gynecomastia*, this change may be disturbing to boys. It occurs most predominantly in obese boys; it fades as androgen production becomes the dominant influence on their bodies. Some girls have their first menstrual period as late as 17 years and are still considered to be within normal limits. Girls who are concerned about their delayed development should be assessed but reassured by their primary health care provider on this point.

VISION

A child's eyes mature at 8 to 9 years of age. Following this time a child should test 20/20 on a standard eye examination. Children who do not meet these criteria need referral for further examination and probably corrective lenses so that they can continue to compete in school where good vision is a necessity.

Developmental Task

Freud described the schoolage period as a latent one; he did not consider schoolage activities to be important to mental health.

Erikson defines the developmental task of this period as achieving a sense of industry versus inferiority. During the preschool period the child learned how to do things; during this period he learns how to do them well. A sense of industry is important for operating as a responsible adult; without it an adult has difficulty holding a satisfactory job, completing school, voting or participating in community organizations, and even parenting.

Cognitive Development

The schoolage child is at the concrete operational level of thought. This means that he understands the concept of *conservation* (he can tell that a low level of water in a large glass is the same amount as a high level in a small glass) and develops the capacity for *accommodation* (he can visualize other people's points of view of a situation). A positive school experience enhances cognitive development and promotes a child's sense of industry and self-esteem.

The child learns the value of most coins by the second grade. He can determine change and make simple purchases the next year. He also learns how to tell time by second grade. During the next year he becomes interested in present, past, and future, as he applies the concept of time to the world around him.

Patterns of Behavior Important for Care

Schoolage children develop a great deal of common sense about how much sleep they need or what foods they need to eat if they were given experience in basic problem solving as preschoolers and are allowed to continue making judgments for themselves.

SLEEP

At the beginning of the schoolage period, some children may still need 10 hours of sleep a night; by the end of the period almost all need only about eight hours. Although schoolage children no longer nap, they may need a quiet time provided for them after school so that they do not become so tired that they cannot enjoy their evening activities.

NUTRITION

The appetite and food intake of the schoolage child differ a great deal depending on the child's activities for that day. Likes and dislikes for food are very apparent and are influenced by the attitude of peers (if a child's friend does not like green beans, then he may not either).

Schoolage children are responsible enough to learn simple food preparation such as salad making and defrosting frozen packages. Helping with food preparation often promotes increased interest in eating. If the child is learning about foods in nutrition classes at school, he may become very interested in what foods are high in common minerals and vitamins.

Late in the schoolage period when the growth spurt begins, children's appetites become ravenous. It is important that adequate protein, calcium, and vitamin D be provided at this time for optimal tissue and bone growth. As schoolagers eat at least one meal away from home almost every day, they need to be taught the importance of a balanced diet so that they will not trade their packed lunch or make unwise selections from a cafeteria menu.

ACTIVITY

Schoolage children play active, running, jumping, and climbing games. They are not old enough for competition in games before the age of 10 because they cannot tolerate the loss of self-esteem that comes with losing until that age. Parents should carefully evaluate structured competitive programs before the child enters such a program. If the program promotes winning above all other values, it may teach a philosophy that parents do not want their child exposed to (and that can be detrimental to the self-esteem of a child who causes a team to lose by a dropped pass or an infield out).

Most schoolage children have a best friend that they play with and share secrets with. It is a basic rule of the age group that while an even number of children of any size can play together, an odd number will usually quarrel, as the odd number leaves one child as "odd man out."

SAFETY

Schoolage children often injure themselves in sports activities by trying to perform beyond their limits or by playing without adequate training, preparation, or protective equipment. They are apt to swim too far on dares. School bus and street safety is vital.

Common Concerns of the Schoolage Period

The schoolage child is away from his parents for most of each day. This leaves him responsible for decision making for long stretches of time. Most concerns of the schoolage period arise from the child's making unwise or immature judgments in some aspect of self-care or conduct.

STEALING

Many children pass through a developmental phase of childhood stealing at about 7 years of age. This is the age when they are learning the value of money. They take money from parents' pockets, purses, or dresser tops. This type of stealing occurs because the child's concept of the value of money is stronger than his concept of property rights. He needs to have reviewed with him the concept of property rights: Some things are *his* property (his clothing), some things are his parent's (money in mother's purse), and some things are family property (food in the refrigerator). Children in large families where clothing and toys are passed freely from child to child may have the most difficulty recognizing property rights as everything appears to be family property.

GANGS

Nine-year-old children typically group into transitory but very intense gangs. A typical one is formed when two girls in a neighborhood make up a club and then exclude a third child from joining them. Nine-year-old groups typically have three common characteristics: They are a form of spite club (excluding someone); they have a secret password or code; and they are single sex groups.

The inclination to form gangs is part of the developmental step of identification; the child is trying to decide who he is (he is like the members of his group; he is not like the children he is excluding). Fortunately, such gangs last only short periods of time and then regroup (the girl who was excluded from the original club forms a club and excludes one of the first two). The excluded child is often one who is in some way different from the others: His parents are richer or poorer than others in the neighborhood, he is of a different religion; or he has a physical handicap. Of all the schoolage years the ninth is often the hardest for any child who is ill.

COLLECTING

Schoolage children enjoy collecting as a part of learning the cognitive step of conversation. Some of these collections do not seem important at first glance (a child may save all the salt and pepper packages from his hospital trays). These collections are a mark of worth, however, and need to be carefully protected as if they had monetary value. Many children appreciate a box with a lock as a present during the schoolage period because the box gives them assurance that their collection can be protected from tampering by young family members.

DRUG ABUSE

Drug abuse is a potential problem even for grade-school children. Sniffing airplane glue from a paper bag until it causes a giddy, floating feeling is one form of drug abuse that occurs at this age. This is a potentially harmful practice as the fumes can cause extensive liver damage.

In some communities hard drugs (amphetamines, barbiturates, PCP) and certainly alcohol, marijuana, and tobacco are available to schoolage children. Children need exposure to information on the danger of drug abuse. They need good role models (parents and health care personnel) who do not themselves abuse cigarettes and alcohol.

MENSTRUATION

Most parents are aware that if a girl is introduced to the function of menstruation before it occurs, her acceptance of becoming a woman will be greatly improved. Unfortunately, many parents are not prepared to explain menstruation; they rely heavily on health care personnel to do this for them. It is now well accepted than menstrual cramps resúlt mainly from prostaglandin release and only slightly from psychological influences. Girls need exposure to role models who demonstrate that being a woman is a worthy role; that menstruation is a signal of a potential for life not a "curse" or negative happening.

SCHOOL PHOBIA

School phobia is the appearance of physical illness symptoms in order to avoid attending school. Common symptoms are headache, nausea, dizziness, and abdominal pain. The child notices the symptoms early in the morning; by the time the school bus leaves or school begins, the symptoms disappear.

Such symptoms occur most frequently in single or youngest children; in many instances the parent may be as reluctant to allow the child to leave for school as the child is to leave. Children with school phobia should be urged to attend school despite the physical symptoms (after it has been firmly established that there is not a true physiological reason for them), as the more school the child misses, the more stressful the school situation becomes for him as he falls farther and farther behind his peer group. Some parents need counseling in order to appreciate that allowing a child increased freedom is necessary for his development.

Considerations in Care of the Schoolage Child

Schoolage children learn basic habits of self-care and responsibility that continue for the remainder of their lives. When caring for a schoolage child, you can help him achieve a sense of industry best by allowing him to complete frequent small projects rather than encouraging long complicated ones. As a small project is completed, the child sees immediately what he can achieve; he experiences the satisfaction and reward of accomplishment and is motivated to try another project. Long-term projects are not as satisfying because rewards are delayed. The Girl Scouts and Boy Scouts are organizations that have lasted for generations because they fulfill a sense of industry so well—they allow the child to complete frequent small merit-badge projects, feel good about himself, and then go on to yet another.

Effect of Illness

A big concern of illness in the schoolage child is that it may take the child out of school for an extended period of time and cause him to fall behind the level of his peer group. This is devastating to a sense of industry as it prevents the child from feeling good about his accomplishments. When caring for schoolage children, make a point of checking on homework and the effect of the illness on school progress. Asking an ill child to do homework may at first seem unfair but most children welcome being told that they must be responsible for homework as assurance that they are going to get well and return to school again. Figure 9-12 demonstrates how hospital "assignments" can foster a sense of accomplishment in schoolage children.

Two health problems that are age related are sinus headaches (frontal sinuses develop at about 6 years of age, and congestion and infection in this area can lead to pain) and scoliosis (sideways curvature of the spine) beginning at age 10. Scoliosis, especially, should be screened for at every health care encounter until the child reaches young adulthood.

THE ADOLESCENT (12 to 18 years)

Adolescence is a time when a person grows to both physical and psychological maturity. As this is not an easy adjustment—changing from a person who has little responsibility even for himself to someone who will be responsible not only for himself but young children as well—it is a difficult period of time. Many parents of adolescent children state that it is not easy for them to parent an adolescent. Helping parents to appreciate that likewise it is not easy to be an adolescent is a major nursing role for keeping the problem in perspective.

FIGURE 9-12. Her daily task of assisting the unit secretary is an important part of this schoolage girl's hospital experience. She is ready and waiting at the nurses' station to "do her job."

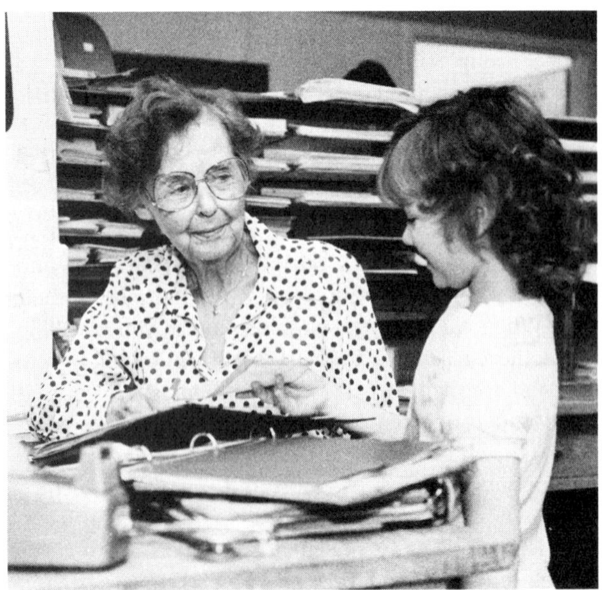

Physical Growth and Development

Physical growth and development continue to proceed at a rapid rate following the growth spurt just prior to adolescence.

HEIGHT AND WEIGHT

Girls have a gain in height of 2 to 8 inches (5 to 20 cm), boys an increase of 4 to 12 inches (10 to 30 cm) during the period. Accompanying this is a gradual increase in weight of 15 to 55 pounds (7 to 25 kg) for girls and 15 to 65 pounds (7 to 30 kg) for boys.

Growth of extremities is very noticeable, causing the adolescent to make clumsy movements at times (he reaches past objects, spills glasses of milk or bottles of ketchup at the table, bumps his elbows or knees on doorways or footstools). As the skeletal system temporarily outgrows the cardiovascular system, the adolescent notices extreme fatigue. He wants to stay up later than ever before, yet falls asleep earlier than he did the previous year. Toward the end of the adolescent period as the cardiovascular system grows and expands to meet his new needs, this constant fatigue ends.

SECONDARY SEXUAL CHARACTERISTICS

Changes in secondary sexual characteristics that began just prior to adolescence continue until maturity is reached. A commonly used scale for grading sexual maturity is the Tanner Stages of Maturity Scale. Illustrations of each stage are shown in Fig. 9-13. A child with the characteristics shown in the upper left corner of Fig. 9-13A would be listed on a physical examination report as being at a Tanner 2 stage of breast development.

VITAL SIGNS

Pulse and respiratory rates slow slightly during adolescence to reach adult levels at the end of the period, while blood pressure increases slightly to reach an adult level. As all of these determinations are affected by activity, there is apt to be inconsistency in readings from time to time when they are obtained on active adolescents. Normal averages, however, are shown in Table 9-9.

Developmental Task

Freud described the adolescent period as the genital period. It is the time when the child becomes aware of sexual response and takes an interest in lasting relationships. His activities are governed or induced by a *libido* force or sexual influences.

Erikson describes the developmental task of the adolescent as gaining a sense of identity versus role confusion. A person with a sense of identity has a strong feeling for who he is and expects to take responsibility for his actions. There are five main areas which adolescents typically work through in order to achieve a sense of identity.

ESTABLISHING A VALUE SYSTEM

Before an adolescent can know who he is, he has to arrive at a sense of what he believes in or values (is he a kind person or not, an honest one or not, does he want to be a rich one or not?). These are not always easy decisions, as many values are not as definite or well defined as they were in previous years (a father says he believes in obeying the law but always breaks the speed limit; a mother says she believes in honesty but never corrects a salesperson's error of wrong change). For the adolescent whose role models seem to have vague value systems you could be the first person that the child meets who knows firmly what she believes in. Adolescents sometimes test people by offhand comments about values to ascertain and evaluate their value systems.

ADJUSTING TO A NEW BODY IMAGE

An adolescent looks so different from his schoolage image that it is necessary for him to get reacquainted with the new person he sees in the mirror. Adolescents typically spend an inordinate amount of time studying their faces or hair, trying to get to know their new bodies and what they can expect from them.

Adolescents may be very disappointed with their new appearance (they were promised that they would become swans; instead they still look surprisingly like short brown ducks). It is not easy to cope with this disappointment until they gain greater maturity, which allows them to appreciate that physical appearance is only a small part of what influences relationships with others.

FIGURE 9-13. A. Female breast development; Tanner staging. Sex maturity rating 1 (not shown): prepubertal; elevation of papilla only. Sex maturity rating 2: breast buds appear; areola is slightly widened and projects as a small mound. Sex maturity rating 3: enlargement of the entire breast with no protrusion of the papilla or nipple. Sex maturity rating 4: enlargement of the breast and projection of areola and papilla as a secondary mound. Sex maturity rating 5: adult configuration of the breast with protrusion of the nipple; areola no longer projects separately from remainder of breast.

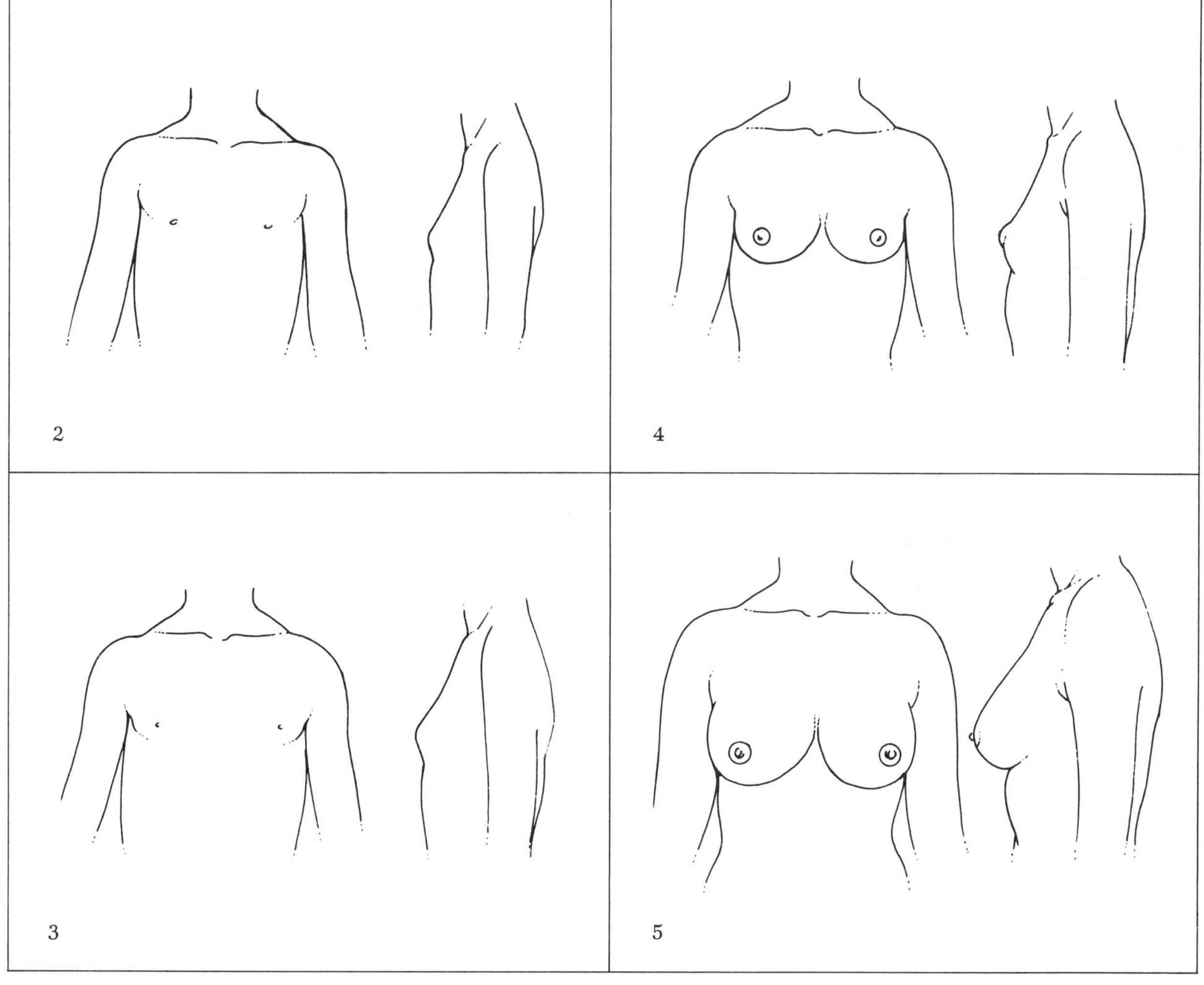

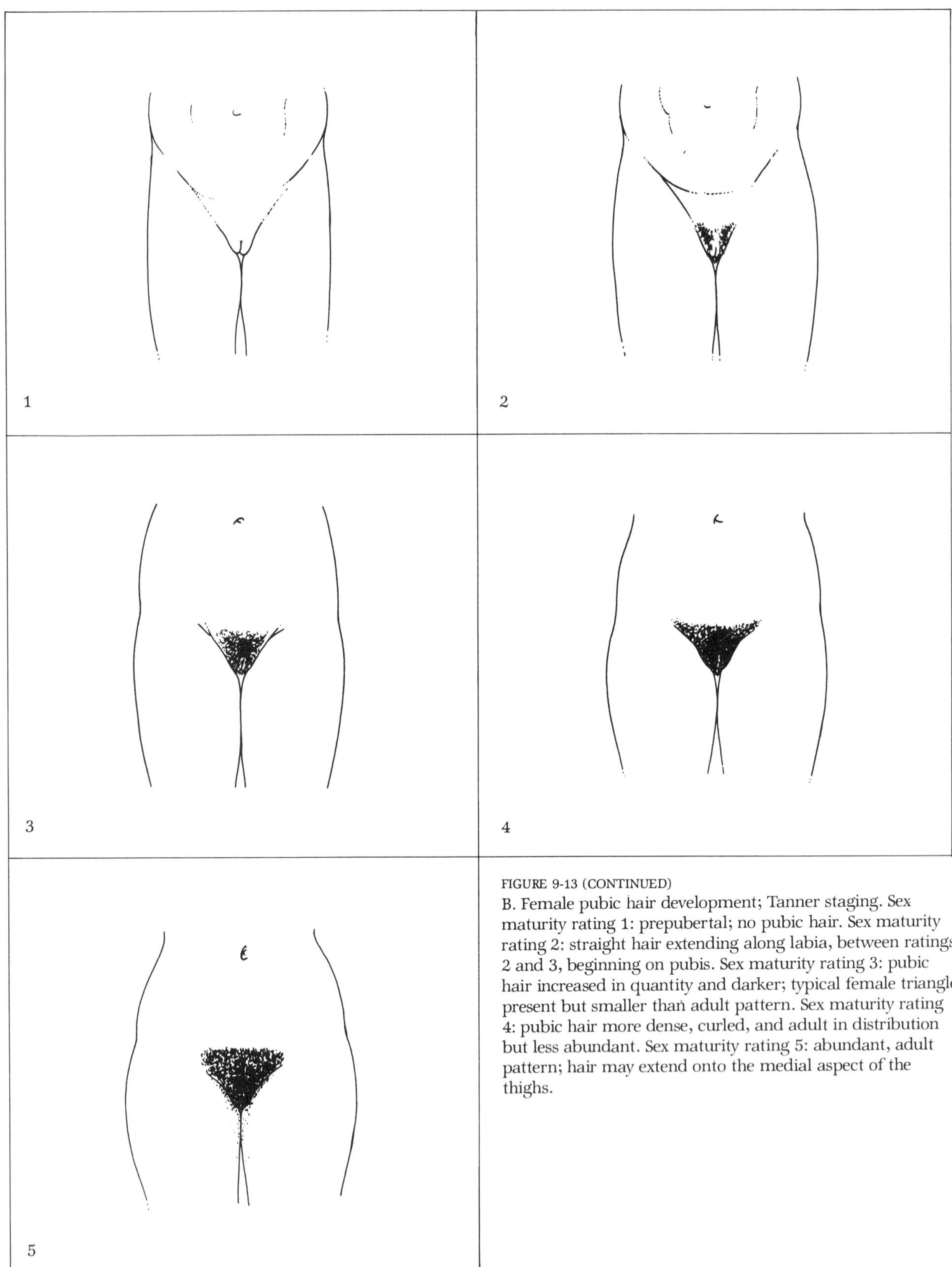

FIGURE 9-13 (CONTINUED)
B. Female pubic hair development; Tanner staging. Sex maturity rating 1: prepubertal; no pubic hair. Sex maturity rating 2: straight hair extending along labia, between ratings 2 and 3, beginning on pubis. Sex maturity rating 3: pubic hair increased in quantity and darker; typical female triangle present but smaller than adult pattern. Sex maturity rating 4: pubic hair more dense, curled, and adult in distribution but less abundant. Sex maturity rating 5: abundant, adult pattern; hair may extend onto the medial aspect of the thighs.

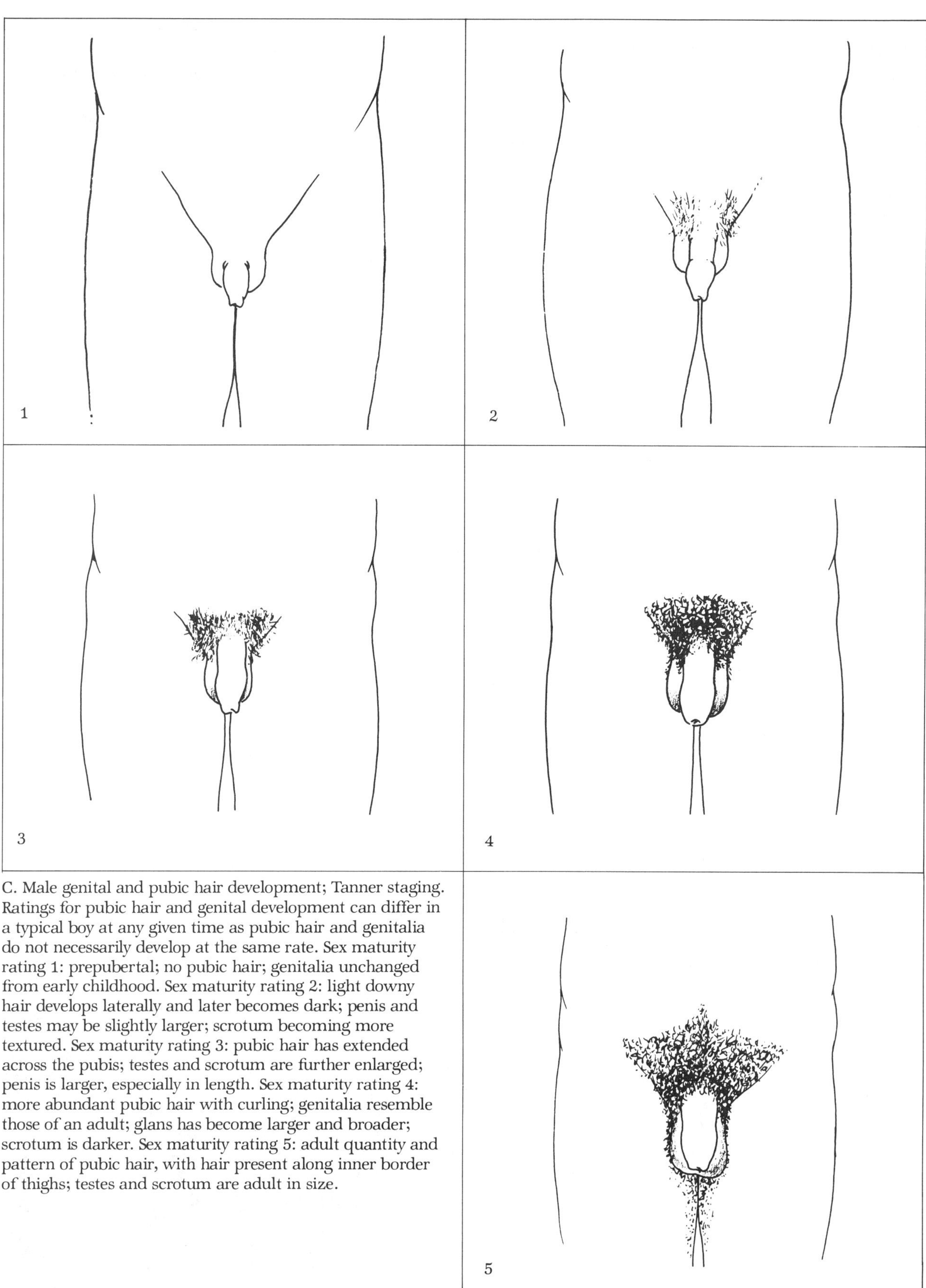

C. Male genital and pubic hair development; Tanner staging. Ratings for pubic hair and genital development can differ in a typical boy at any given time as pubic hair and genitalia do not necessarily develop at the same rate. Sex maturity rating 1: prepubertal; no pubic hair; genitalia unchanged from early childhood. Sex maturity rating 2: light downy hair develops laterally and later becomes dark; penis and testes may be slightly larger; scrotum becoming more textured. Sex maturity rating 3: pubic hair has extended across the pubis; testes and scrotum are further enlarged; penis is larger, especially in length. Sex maturity rating 4: more abundant pubic hair with curling; genitalia resemble those of an adult; glans has become larger and broader; scrotum is darker. Sex maturity rating 5: adult quantity and pattern of pubic hair, with hair present along inner border of thighs; testes and scrotum are adult in size.

EMANCIPATION FROM PARENTS

A person cannot be independent as long as he depends on his parents to make decisions or judgments for him. It is necessary for the adolescent, then, to reject his parents' decision making and do his own. Unfortunately, adolescents generally do not do this tactfully but forcefully, which often leads to hurt feelings and conflict between the child and his parents. It is important when caring for adolescents that you remember that to be independent is of great importance to adolescents. They reject health care providers' suggestions and advice at this time just as surely as they do their parents' if the advice takes the form of telling them what to do rather than an exploration of alternatives. Care should be planned with them so that the final decision is really theirs, not yours. The locus of decision making should always be the patient when dealing with adolescents, unless illness is so severe that it interferes to change this focus.

ESTABLISHING HETEROSEXUAL RELATIONSHIPS

Adolescents deal with their peers for the first time not as other children but as *male* and *female* people (Fig. 9-14). Learning how to deal with members of the opposite sex comes fairly easily for the child who has had good sexual role models around him (brothers, sisters, both parents). It may be more difficult for the child who has had little contact with people of the opposite sex (a 15-year-old girl living with her divorced mother, for example), particularly if members of the opposite sex not only are not present but have been portrayed as hateful and untrustworthy. For many children raised by a single female parent, male nurses may be the first role model of male caring ability that the child encounters.

Early in adolescence children tend to relate to members of their own sex; this is a way for them to grow comfortable with their own identity before they move on to heterosexual relationships. Such behavior leads to the formation of small groups of "best friends" as were established in middle school age. This is a normal consequence of early adolescence, however, and not a step backward. It is a part of learning more about oneself.

MAKING A VOCATIONAL CHOICE

In order to make future school plans, adolescents are asked to make vocational choices earlier and earlier in their school years. As the range of job opportunities for both sexes increases, the decision grows harder and harder to make. Hours may be spent pondering such decisions as whether to take physics or a foreign language. This may be another area that causes parent-child conflict if the parent's expectations for the child (he'll go to college and take over the family business) are different from what the adolescent wants (to be an auto mechanic). Successful completion of self-initiated projects and pride of accomplishment foster identity and can influence vocational choice (Fig. 9-15).

Cognitive Development

Adolescents are capable of formal operational thought—they have the ability to reason through situations at an adult level. Because an adolescent is capable of such reasoning, however, does not mean that he always uses it. A mark of an individual under stress is that problem-solving ability is decreased. Since the entire adolescent period is a high-stress period, adolescents typically have difficulty with problem solving.

Patterns of Behavior Important for Care

Adolescents want to make independent judgments about their self-care needs. However, their inexperience

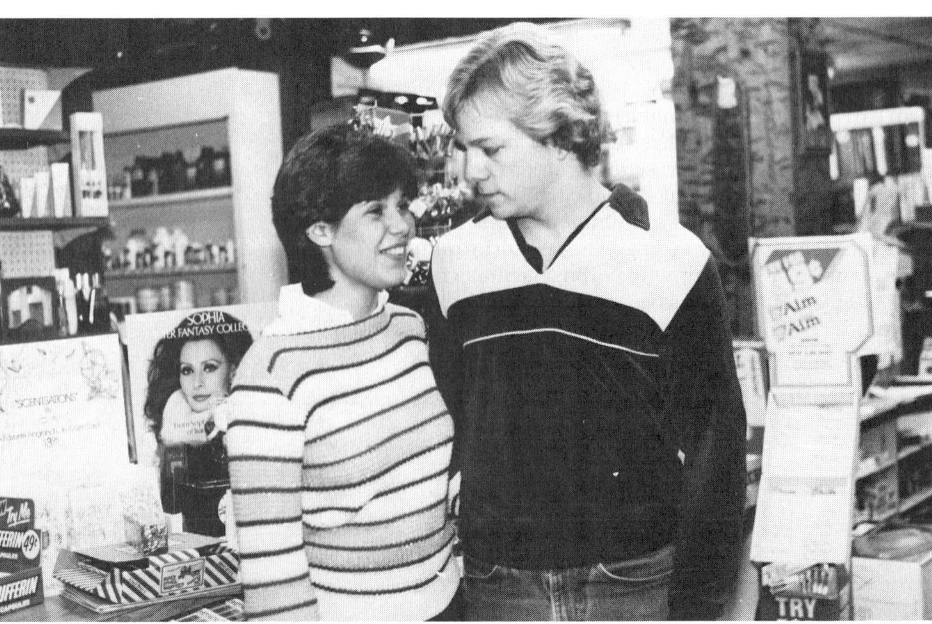

FIGURE 9-14. Relating to the opposite sex is an important task of adolescence, crucial to self-identity.

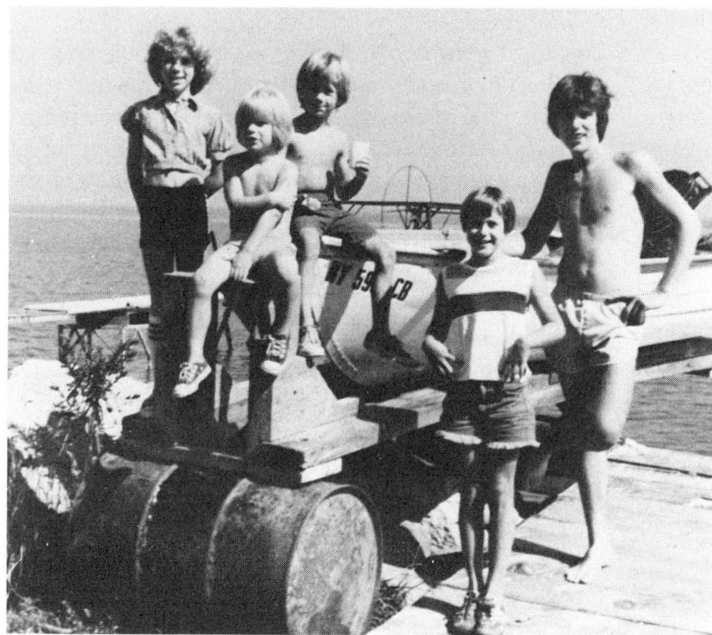

FIGURE 9-15. The 15-year-old boy on the right solely designed and constructed this boat ramp, which "works perfectly." Note his posture and how his young friends share his pride of accomplishment.

in many instances results in their not reaching the desired level of performance in such decision making.

SLEEP
Adolescents require more sleep than they did as younger children (about a total of 10 hours a night) because their skeletal growth is slightly ahead of their cardiovascular system growth and so extra rest is needed for thorough oxygenation of body cells. Some adolescents, not aware of this developmental need for sleep, try to stay up later than ever before. The consequent chronic fatigue they experience makes it difficult for them to function at their best level at home or school.

NUTRITION
Because the adolescent years are rapid growth years, the adolescent's need for calories increases by about 200 kcal daily over the requirement for childhood. As adolescents are always hungry, they need to be certain that they are not eating only empty calorie foods (doughnuts, cookies, pretzels) rather than foods that will not only alleviate hunger but supply nutrients as well. To sustain such rapid growth, the adolescent should have a diet high in protein, calcium, and vitamin D. Once menstruation begins, girls may need an iron supplement to counteract the iron loss with menstrual blood.

ACTIVITY
Despite the almost constant feeling of fatigue that many adolescents experience, they are almost continually active. Some adolescents may need to be cautioned to avoid unwise dieting regimes in order to qualify for athletic events such as wrestling matches. Adolescents who do not wish to compete in organized athletic events should be urged to establish a daily exercise or activity program.

SAFETY
The major cause of death in adolescents is from accidents, particularly motor vehicle accidents. Adolescents need to learn to keep their cars in safe working order and to recognize that alcohol and driving are not compatible (and to refuse to ride with a friend who does not appreciate the potential danger). When riding motorcycles they need to understand the importance of following traffic rules and using a safety helmet. Adolescents are so present- and self-oriented that they have a great deal of difficulty believing that traffic accidents could happen to them, even after episodes of close misses.

Common Concerns of the Adolescent Period

OBESITY
Children who became overweight as preadolescents generally have so much difficulty losing weight that their obesity continues in adolescence, and it will likely continue into adulthood if they do not change their intake and exercise habits. Hypertension is associated with obesity and begins to become apparent in obese adolescents. Obesity may also interfere with the child's ability to make friends and with his self-esteem if it prevents him from participating in athletic or other competitive activities.

PEPTIC ULCERS
Peptic ulcers are painful erosions of the lining of the stomach and the proximal duodenum. Excessive stomach acid levels occur whenever an individual is under tension or stress. As adolescence is a long-term

period of stress, the continual high level of hydrochloric acid present during the period can lead to excessive irritation and actual destruction of the mucus lining. Such ulcers are difficult to heal once they form. Therapy is aimed at helping the adolescent develop effective ways of coping with stress along with administration of anti-acid medication.

SEXUALLY TRANSMITTED DISEASE

A venereal disease (currently termed a *sexually transmitted disease* [STD]) is one transmitted through sexual intercourse. Although most illnesses are declining in incidence in the United States today, the incidence of venereal disease is increasing. In some communities it has reached epidemic proportions. The three most common sexually transmitted diseases are gonorrhea, syphilis, and herpes simplex type II infections. Adolescents and health care personnel caring for adolescents should be familiar with the symptoms of these illnesses. Many adolescents are not willing to admit that they might have these illnesses because they worry that their sexual activity or their partners will be revealed or because they have heard about painful treatments they are unwilling to submit themselves to. They can be assured that at health care visits their confidentiality will be respected; the treatment of both gonorrhea and syphilis consists of only one injection of penicillin or a suitable substitute if the child is allergic to penicillin. Treatment for herpes infections is limited to relieving the accompanying pain of the lesions.

SEXUAL ACTIVITY

Premarital sexual relations are accepted as expected behavior by many teenagers due to peer pressure. Children in this age group need education about the responsibility involved in such relationships and contraceptive information if they desire it. Contraceptive counseling for adolescents differs slightly from that for adults; it is discussed with adult methods in Chap. 21.

PREGNANCY

Although the birth rate is declining nationally, it is increasing among adolescent girls. An adolescent pregnancy is always a high risk pregnancy because psychologically the mother may not yet be able to adjust to mothering and physically she may find it difficult to provide enough nutrients for both the growing fetus and her own growing body. If the mother's pelvis is not fully mature, a normal delivery may not be possible.

Although not as well documented, adolescent fatherhood may be as traumatic psychologically as adolescent motherhood. If the girl chooses to have an abortion or place the child for adoption following birth, the father's grief at the loss may be great; his self-esteem may be severely damaged at finding himself legally helpless to halt the girl's actions.

ACNE

The most common health problem of adolescents is facial acne or *acne vulgaris*. Acne occurs due to oversecretion of the sebaceous glands stimulated by increased levels of androgen. With acne, there is plugging of sebaceous gland ducts with resulting stretching of the ducts (whiteheads) and an inflammatory reaction at the skin surface upon contact with surface bacteria (blackheads or comedones).

Medications effective for acne are vitamin A, antibiotics, and skin cleansers. The previous belief that the intake of chocolate aggravates the condition is now discounted. Acne will run a natural course until late in adolescence; when body hormones adjust more efficiently and androgen is no longer so prominent, the symptoms fade. Adolescents need a great deal of support while the condition is present. It is difficult to form a sense of optimal identity when your mirror image reflects a face that is acne inflamed or acne scarred.

DRUG ABUSE

Another problem that is increasing in incidence in adolescents is drug abuse. The drug most frequently abused is alcohol, a factor that causes the automobile accident rate in the age group to be so high. Other abused drugs are marijuana, amphetamines, hallucinogens, and barbiturates. The use of such substances is strongly associated with poor coping behavior and is discussed in detail in Chap. 12.

SUICIDE

Suicide is the leading cause of death in the late adolescent population. Like drug abuse, this is the result of poor coping ability and is discussed in Chap. 12.

Considerations of Care of the Adolescent

Care of the adolescent must be geared to protecting the child's right to participate in decision making while at the same time offering adequate guidance so that he is not so independent that he flounders. Adolescents are present oriented; it is difficult for them to carry out health care measures if they think the measure will benefit them only in the future, so their attention should be called to more immediate benefits.

Effect of Illness

Adolescents worry that an illness will separate them from their friends or in some way mark them as different from peers (Fig. 9-16). They may be poor at keeping appointments for health care as the appointment will almost invariably be considered secondary to another activity scheduled at the same time. They may follow health prescriptions poorly if the action in any way makes them different or causes them to stand out in a crowd.

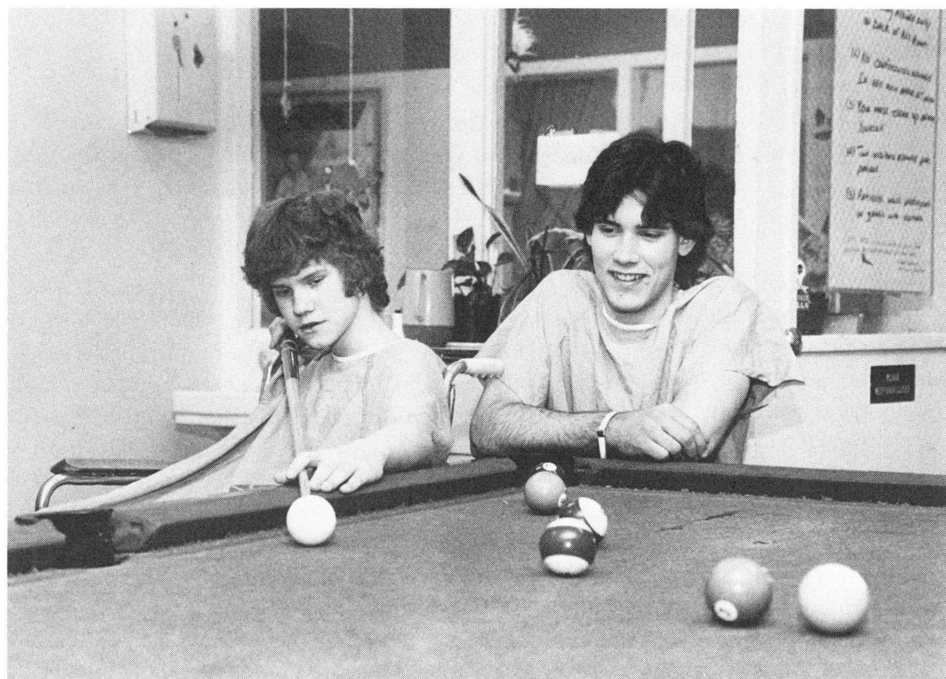

FIGURE 9-16. A "rec room" for hospitalized adolescents is as important as a playroom is for younger children: both are places for peer interaction. Note the self-made rules of behavior hand-lettered on the door.

As they are so extremely body conscious (this is the same phenomenon that makes everyone aware of flowers in the spring, as spring flowers are such a contrast to winter), they often worry about small problems that they would have ignored as a schoolage child. They appreciate being told at health maintenance visits that they are well. They may try to deny for a long time the fact that they are ill.

THE YOUNG ADULT (18 to 45 years)

Young adulthood is a period of life when people make final career and life style decisions; for many people it is a time of childbearing and child rearing, higher education, and beginning home management. It is the period during which people reach their physical peak. Emotionally, because of the responsibility involved in education, career decisions, and child rearing, it can be a period of stress as high as that experienced in adolescence.

The designation of 45 as the end of the young adult period may surprise you, if you think of people over 40 as old. When you consider that the life span of the average individual is 70 to 80 years, however, 45 *is* young. Some people past the age of 45 still think and operate as young adults in terms of life style.

Physical Growth and Development

In the early adult period a person has the fastest reflexes of any age group, and his physical endurance is better than at any other time. It is an ideal time for childbearing, as a woman's body is more than competent not only to sustain her own body systems but to nourish a growing fetus as well.

Most individuals reach their full height by the end of the adolescent period, although a few do continue to grow for an inch or two up to about 25 years of age.

Sexual maturity in males is reached at the end of adolescence and sexual interest also reaches a peak at this time. Although women's bodies are physically mature, the peak interest in sexual activity for many women does not occur until almost age 30. This discrepancy in interest may cause conflict between a couple if they do not openly discuss their differences.

Developmental Task

The developmental crisis of the young adult according to Erikson is achieving a sense of intimacy versus isolation. Intimacy is the ability to relate deeply with other persons. It is not only the ability to relate with members of the opposite sex (heterosexual relationships) but with one's own sex as well to form long-lasting friendships. This means that a person does not have to marry to achieve a sense of intimacy. The person who chooses a single life style or even a homosexual life style can be as fulfilled as the person who chooses a more conventional pattern.

A person needs a strong sense of identity before he is able to reach out fully to other people and offer deep friendship or love. Since you always run the risk of being rejected or being hurt when you offer love or friendship, you cannot offer it if you do not have confidence that you can cope with rejection.

Cognitive Development

Although capable of formal operational thought, adolescents do not always reason well. Young adulthood, then, becomes the time for application of mature reasoning or thought processes. If the person has not utilized his ability to problem-solve, he needs practice during this period in order to learn to do it well. He may need support and encouragement that he can problem-solve as he is so inexperienced in the process.

Patterns of Behavior Important for Care

Young adults are responsible for their own self-care and as a rule use common-sense guidelines.

SLEEP

The average young adult needs about 8 hours of sleep a night. Many people during this period do not get this much sleep as they crowd a busy school schedule and social life together or as parents of young children find themselves caring for children during the night. If problem-solving ability in a young adult seems to be at a low edge, ask about his recent sleep patterns. Spending some time first in sleep may be a step in the direction toward good problem solving.

NUTRITION

The young adult needs a well-balanced diet in order to supply enough calories and nutrients for a busy lifestyle. Many people in this age group tend to rely on fast food outlets for a major part of their food intake. It is possible to obtain adequate dietary intake from such sources but protein and vitamin C (meat and fresh fruits) may be hard to obtain in sufficient quantities.

ACTIVITY

Many young adults participate in active organized athletic programs or belong to exercise clubs. Young mothers, despite their busy days of child rearing, may be deficient in adequate exercise as many of their activities (standing in one place to cook dinner; sitting, rocking an infant; sitting, reading a story to a toddler) do not involve muscle-strengthening measures. Young adult men sitting long hours at desk jobs may have this same problem.

SAFETY

The high incidence of motor vehicle accidents continues from adolescence into early adulthood. Young adults think of their bodies as impregnable, so they fail to take usual, sensible precautions in traffic as they believe that no harm can come to them.

Common Concerns of Young Adulthood

Concerns of young adulthood center around the new responsibilities that arise as individuals try to fit into the adult world.

EDUCATION

Choosing whether to go to college, what college to attend, how many years of college to attend, whether to go to a vocational school, and whether to pursue education beyond college are all problems that the young adult must consider. In many instances the people he has relied on for advice in the past—parents, neighbors, teachers—are little help in this area. The world has changed so much since these people were his age that their advice may be 20 years out of date and no longer applicable.

Women's roles in society have changed so much that while once a college education for a woman was considered unique, today it is expected. Vocational training as a plumber's apprentice, jockey, or electrician is not considered unusual for women. For both sexes the range of occupations has increased so markedly with modern technology that decisions concerning the choice of education becomes more and more difficult to make.

OCCUPATION

Many people begin earning money during high school or college by short-term positions such as summer jobs or part-time after-school positions. A person's commitment to such a position may not be total (it is only for the summer), and his dedication to doing a good job may be less than optimal. It may be a shock to a young adult to realize that a full-time job employer expects total commitment.

LIFE STYLE

Most young adults choose to live away from home. For the person attending college or one who is earning little money due to an apprenticeship program, remaining at home may be necessary until he is more financially independent.

A person who is living away from home has to quickly assume responsibility for his total care. Food selection and preparation and good division of his time may be areas that are particularly difficult for him to master. If he becomes ill, locating support people for him who will help with meals, transportation, or hygiene may be a major problem.

For the young adult who remains at home, different value systems based on the differences in age of the people in the house may be a major area of stress. It is difficult for many persons to feel independent if they live at home; having to return home because of illness may make their struggle for independence even more difficult.

FORMING PERMANENT RELATIONSHIPS

More and more young people choose not to enter a traditional marriage arrangement today, at least not until they are more certain that the partner they have chosen is the right one for them. It is important when assessing relationships to appreciate that support people from these informal relationships may be as accountable and deeply supportive as those from formal marriage alliances.

Young adults struggle with defining whether their relationship is based on love or infatuation. As general rules, people choose mates who are compatible with them. Their needs and desires may be supplementary (similar) or complementary (needs are different and partners meet each other's needs). Many marriages end at the close of young adulthood (40 to 45 years of age) because as people mature they change. The people who had supplementary or complementary needs in early life may change so drastically as they mature that they no longer supplement or complement each other (or they may have underestimated in the first place how truly compatible they were).

BEGINNING A FAMILY

Formerly many married couples had their first child within the first year of marriage, but now more and more couples are delaying childbearing until they have been married a number of years. In many instances this secures a more solid financial status which is a positive factor; it also may make changing a life style from one without children to one with children a bigger adjustment. Another change in life styles is the trend for many single women to plan childbearing without a marriage partner.

The biggest change that a child brings to a relationship is the increased responsibility for care that becomes necessary. Parents are no longer free to engage in spontaneous activities; they may find time for travel or hobbies curtailed. Most parents accept these limitations willingly as an accepted part of parenthood. The parent who is not yet at this developmental step may have a difficult time adjusting to the birth of a child.

Fathers are accepting more and more responsibility for care of children, and household tasks of all kinds are increasingly shared between marriage partners. This is necessary as more and more women of childbearing age attend school or work part-time. Remember this when caring for a young adult male. Hospitalization may be very difficult for him because he is his children's primary caregiver.

People who never formed a sound sense of trust have difficulty developing a sense of intimacy with or transferring a sense of trust to their children. Role modeling can be an effective means of demonstrating good parenting skills. Providing anticipatory guidance as to what to expect of a growing child and relieving areas of stress when possible provide an atmosphere where bonding and the formation of a sense of trust can grow and deepen.

Considerations for Care of the Young Adult

In planning care for young adults, be certain that it provides for independence and use of problem-solving ability. In the same way that infants cannot be considered in planning apart from their parents, parents of young children cannot be considered apart from their children. Parents may transfer money and time and energy that should be spent on their own care to their children if they are forced to choose between their own and their child's needs.

Effect of Illness

Young adulthood is a well age; expecting to be well, some young adults ignore symptoms of illness, insisting that the symptoms really mean nothing. Many times hospitalization occurs as the result of motor vehicle accidents. Hospitalization can be devastating to this age group as they probably have few employment benefits due to short duration of employment (little sick leave, possibly reduced health insurance plans) and to beginning marriage relationships, which may be strong enough to support two well adults but not strong enough to survive when extra care and concern is needed because one member is ill.

Illness may disrupt an educational goal so much (the person is forced to fall behind a semester in school) that he drops out of school rather than try to catch up with work or continue in a program behind his classmates.

THE MIDDLE-AGED ADULT (45 to 65 years)

Middle age is a time of life when the person reaches the peak of his career success and often becomes actively involved in community and civic affairs. Young adulthood is the age that makes *families* grow and develop; middle age is the time of life that makes *communities* and the world function effectively.

Physical Growth and Development

Although most adults during early middle age function as well as they did during young adulthood, some changes do occur. Primarily, there is a slight decrease in metabolism rate. This almost automatically leads to a decrease in activity and stamina and a gain in weight. The gain in weight is most prominantly noticed as an increase in abdominal girth.

SEXUAL CHANGES

Menopause is the end of ovulation in women. At about 45 to 50 years of age, there is a decline in the ability of the ovary to respond to gonadotropic hormone from the pituitary; this leads to cessation of ovulation and therefore cessation of the menstrual cycle.

As the pituitary gland produces additional gonadotropic hormones in order to try to effect ovulation, many women experience vasomotor changes (termed hot flashes), heart palpitations, headaches, and dizziness. Because androgen levels remain normal while estrogen levels decrease, facial hair may become evident. Skin and mucus membrane gradually become drier. Vaginal secretions may decrease, in which case use of a lubricant may help to enhance sexual enjoyment. An active, fulfilling life style and positive attitude toward menopause as a normal life event do much to minimize the impact of the above described physical changes.

The mark of normal menopause is that menstrual periods decrease in amount of flow either gradually or suddenly. This might occur as normally spaced periods with lessened menstrual flow each time or the time between periods may continue to increase until they disappear. The annoying symptoms of menopause may be relieved by the administration of artificial estrogen. Long-term use of estrogen, however, is associated with breast and uterine cancer and is not recommended as a routine measure; it should be used only by those women whose systems are apparently estrogen dependent and who notice extreme depression following menopause.

Lessening sexual activity in the male at this time of life is termed the *climacteric* or *andropause*. This period occurs later in the male than the female menopause (50 to 60 years of age). Men rarely have dramatic symptoms associated with the climacteric as sex hormones gradually decrease. Although the male remains fertile, he may notice that he takes a longer period of time to achieve erection and ejaculation than formerly. This may increase the length of sexual foreplay and thus enhance sexual gratification for both partners. However, he may feel psychologically that he is not as competent as before, particularly, if other areas of his life are unsatisfactory.

MUSCULOSKELETAL SYSTEM

Some decalcification of bones (osteoporosis) occurs with middle age, although the process reaches its peak in older age. Some women develop a tightening or shrinking of intravertebral disks in the cervical and upper thoracic area known as a "dowager's hump." Overall, muscle bulk decreases late in middle age. The person notices that it takes him longer to restore energy after muscle work than it did previously.

SENSES

Presbyopia or decreasing power of accommodation occurs with middle age. People find that to read small print they must remove their glasses or hold the print at arm's length. Such a change in eyesight can be corrected by reading glasses or bifocals. Some decrease in hearing, specifically for high-pitched sounds, occurs.

CARDIOVASCULAR SYSTEM

As middle age persons gain weight, the cardiovascular system may become strained. Hardening changes in the system (arteriosclerosis) may result in mild hypertension as vessels become less elastic; atherosclerosis or fatty deposits on the blood vessels may lead to occlusion of the coronary blood vessels resulting in decreased blood supply to the heart and symptoms of angina or heart anoxic spasms.

Persons who smoke run a higher risk for cardiovascular disease than those who do not due to decreased blood perfusion through the lungs as a result of lung changes from smoking.

INTEGUMENT

One change that both men and women associate with growing old is the development of gray hair or baldness. Both gray hair and baldness are familial tendencies. The time and extent of their development vary widely. Most people develop some crease lines at the lateral aspect of their eyes (crows' feet) and under their eyes from loss of subcutaneous fat and a decrease in elasticity of skin. With decreasing estrogen levels women begin to notice the growth of facial hair.

Developmental Task

The developmental task of middle age is establishing a sense of generativity by which the person extends his concern from just himself and his family to the community and the world. He can handle stress better than he could previously because he has had so much more experience with it. He accepts challenges more readily for the same reason.

The middle-aged adult is interested in activities that change situations in the world around him. He may become politically active, participate in procedure-changing actions, or make far reaching community or world-based changes.

A person with a sense of generativity has a confident feeling in himself as a person. He is able to juggle his various lives (father, salesman, Little League coach, church member; mother, teacher, Republican chairperson, gourmet cook) without being overwhelmed.

People without a sense of generativity develop stagnation or self-absorption. Women who have devoted themselves to only one role (mother) or men who have involved themselves in only one role (businessman) are particularly apt to find themselves at the end of middle age with a narrow perspective and lack of ability to cope with changing situations. When these very limited roles change (children leave home and she is no longer a mother; the man retires and is no longer a businessman), they may become very depressed at realizing how little they have achieved in life.

Patterns of Behavior Important for Care

Middle-aged adults have well-established patterns of self-care; many are so busy with their children or work practices, however, that they often neglect health care.

SLEEP

The average middle-aged person needs 6 to 8 hours of sleep a night. Some people constantly manage on less, especially if they are holding two jobs or have returned to school for further education. Some people of this age have difficulty falling asleep at night because they are so tense from the day's activities that they cannot relax.

NUTRITION

With a decrease in metabolic rate, a middle-aged adult does not need the calories he needed as a young adult to maintain the same weight. Both men and women should reduce their daily caloric intake by about 200 kcal. If there is a high incidence of cholesterolemia in the family (high blood cholesterol levels), people are advised to sharply curtail their intake of saturated fats. However, it is still controversial whether diet is a major influence as hereditary factors are also involved in the formation of high blood cholesterol levels.

RECREATION

In order to prevent excess weight gain, a person must not only reduce his caloric intake but maintain an adequate exercise program as well. Regular exercise also seems to delay the aging process. Assess a person's exercise profile to determine whether it is appropriate for his physical condition and whether it is done regularly. Infrequent, vigorous exercise (playing volleyball all afternoon on a holiday and then not again until the next holiday) is a strain on the cardiovascular system.

SAFETY

As mentioned above, middle-aged adults need to plan their recreation sensibly or they will overdo activities. This also applies to work such as snow shoveling or heavy lifting. Many middle-aged adults need to be cautioned about the extent of their alcohol consumption or they will become as involved in automobile accidents as people in the younger age group as well as experience serious liver damage.

Common Concerns of the Middle-Aged Adult

Concerns of middle age center around roles with children, family, and community.

RELATIONSHIPS WITH CHILDREN

By the time a person reaches middle age, his children are typically adolescent or young adult. Because the world has changed so much since he was that age, he may have a great deal of difficulty relating to the concerns of his children. This situation is frequently termed a "generation gap." Parents react with emotion when a child chooses a life style that is in contrast to their own. The same as an adolescent has difficulty breaking away from parents if he loves them, so do parents have difficulty letting go of children whom they love strongly. Both parents and children need to concentrate on improving their ability to communicate therapeutically (helpfully) in order to close generation gaps. Techniques of therapeutic communication are discussed in Chap. 20.

RELATIONSHIP WITH FAMILY

As marriage partners reach middle age, they generally have more time to spend with each other than when small children were making demands on their time. For some couples this is time of reacquaintance because they both have changed a good deal from the way they were when they were first married. Some marriages end at this time because both partners realize that they no longer are compatible with each other because they have changed in such different ways.

COMMUNITY RESPONSIBILITY

Communities that have many young adults or many older adults are often not well coordinated because neither young families nor older adults have a strong sense of generativity. In a community of middle-aged adults many people are interested in seeing that their police department, fire department, and other community interests are run well. As women's roles change, this responsibility is as much a woman's as a man's role today. As children move out of the home or single adults grow secure in their jobs, greater attention can be devoted to community affairs and engaging in activities that had to be postponed when children's needs came first.

SELF-ESTEEM

Most people are able to accept the changes in appearance that come with middle age even if they do not like them. People who are not secure or have impaired self-esteem worry over signs of aging such as gray hair or increased weight and may attempt to change their image to one years younger than their actual age. Some may attempt to interact at a young adult level in order to feel better (younger) about themselves.

STRESS

As people reach the peak of their career or deal with family problems involving their spouse, their children, or their parents, they invariably find themselves under a degree of stress. Diseases that are highly stress related such as peptic ulcer occur with increasing frequency during this age period. Some people begin to use alcohol excessively as a means of reducing stress or improving their self-esteem. It is difficult for most people to believe that they have passed over the fine line between "social drinker" and "alcoholic" because they cannot see the devastation that their alcohol consumption is causing to family, job, health, and often automobile safety. Helping them to find help through an organization such as Alcoholics Anonymous is an important nursing responsibility.

AGING PARENTS

As people reach middle age, their parents and older relatives reach older age. If an older adult is ill, arrangements may be made to have him join the middle-aged family. This may cause problems relating to space, expenses, or life style. Concern over parents in all instances increases as the older adult begins to need more help with tasks of daily living or is left alone by the death of his spouse.

Considerations for Care of the Middle-Aged Adult

Most middle-aged adults have many people depending on them. It is often difficult, therefore, for them to assume a dependent role or be ill. They may be as worried about how the people who depend on them will manage as they are about their own condition. They may neglect their own health (return to work too soon after surgery, for example) in order to meet the needs of people who count on them.

Consistent exercise and activity appear to delay the effects of aging. Good nutrition to prevent excess weight gain may be important in preventing cardiovascular disease, the leading killer of middle-aged people.

Effect of Illness

Many middle-aged adults never visit a health care facility for health maintenance care, even though they know that a physical examination at least every 5 years is recommended for satisfactory health supervision. Because middle-aged adults do not come regularly for health care, they must be taught responsibility for monitoring their own health, particularly in regard to symptoms of malignancy (cancer) and cardiovascular diseases, as these are the leading causes of death in this age group.

Women should do self breast examination every month (see Chap. 19 for this technique), and men need to do testicular self-examination every month (see Chap. 19). Women should have a Pap test (a Papanicolaou smear) every 3 years to rule out uterine cancer. Men should be certain that a test for blood in stool (a guaiac test) is included as part of the physical examination; this is a test for the presence of colon cancer, which occurs frequently at this age (see Chap. 20).

Some people undergoing menopause or climacteric experience depression. Signs of depression are varied but generally are manifested as loss of appetite, inability to meet deadlines or appointments, neglect of personal hygiene or surroundings, fatigue, and expressing sadness or lack of self-esteem. People with such symptoms need a health care checkup so that the extent of the problem can be determined and help supplied as needed to assist them to accept this change in their life.

THE OLDER ADULT (65 years and over)

Gerontology is the science of aging and its process and problems. *Geriatrics* is the science of health care and treatment of older persons. As nurses give holistic care and are interested in more than a person's state of physical health, nurses deal more with gerontology concepts than geriatric ones.

Life expectancy has increased to the point that the average man can expect to live to be 72 years old; the average woman, 77 years. About 1 out of every 15 people in society today is over age 65; by the year 2000, 1 out of every 6 will be in this age group. Many people divide older age into young older age (65 to 75) and mature older age (past 76 years).

Physical Growth and Development

Although aging involves both physical and psychosocial processes and has been widely studied, why it occurs is poorly understood. Aging may be due to individual biologic time clocks, which are different for everyone and are why some people seem to be so much younger than others at any given age. Endrocrine changes which trigger other body events such as menopause may also be responsible for a general slowing down of all function. Breakdown or changes in cell RNA or DNA synthesis may account for lessened functioning of cells.

It is important that each older adult be evaluated carefully at each health care visit for his potential and any changes of aging that have occurred. The same as a 6-year-old is little like a 12-year-old yet both are school age, so a 65-year-old may be very different from an 80-year-old.

GASTROINTESTINAL CHANGES

Major gastrointestinal changes that occur with aging are decreases in taste sensation, peristaltic enzyme secretion, peristaltic action, and food absorption. These changes may lead to difficulty with digesting and absorbing some foods and cause constipation.

Assess dental health carefully. If the person has decayed teeth that need repair or dentures that are less than optimal, eating may be painful or at least difficult. Assess elimination. In addition to a diet rich in roughage, measures such as regularity of elimination, increased activity, and using natural laxatives such as prune juice should be instituted. If the person is immobilized due to illness, he may need a stool softener or artificial laxative in order to counteract constipation.

CARDIOVASCULAR CHANGES

The most serious effects of aging are changes in the cardiovascular system. Some degree of *atherosclerosis* or invasion of fatty deposits along the lumina of blood vessels tends to occur. This tendency appears to be inherited and affects some families more than others. If atherosclerosis becomes marked, the heart must work harder to push adequate blood through the narrowed vessels; pulse rate and blood pressure may not be increased in a resting state but rise very rapidly with even minimal activity. If the heart valves or walls of the heart as well as vessel walls become stiffened, cardiac output will fall. The overall effect will be loss of oxygen to vital organs and ultimately heart failure from the sustained work of the heart. Effects of inadequate oxygen to vital organs may result in kidney disease and memory loss (recent memory loss occurs before long-term loss).

When caring for older adults, be conscious that blood pressure may rapidly elevate with activity. Plan nursing care to allow for rest periods.

Be certain when helping an older adult to a sitting or standing position that you do it gradually to prevent *orthostatic hypotension.* Adjustment to a new position may leave the brain so devoid of blood flow that dizziness and fainting occur.

RESPIRATORY CHANGES

An older adult may develop some rigidity of the chest wall which reduces his vital capacity (maximum exhalation after a maximum inhalation). This combined with decreased blood flow through the lungs due to vessel hardening or stricture causes a decrease in oxygen diffusion across lung alveoli with a possibility of a decreased PO_2 (oxygen in blood) level.

Decreased vital capacity may also lead to an increase in respiratory infection as there is less turnover of air. This is particularly important to remember when caring for the older adult undergoing surgery. Deep breathing and coughing following surgery are very important to prevent respiratory infection due to stasis of lung secretions during anesthesia. Make sure also that position (arms should not be across chest) or restrictive clothing are not interfering with respiratory function.

NEUROLOGICAL CHANGES

Neurological changes in the older adult begin subtly. The person may notice a slower reaction time for both physical and mental responses. Both visual and auditory function may decrease. The person first has difficulty hearing high-pitched sound. This means that if you are a young female, your voice is in the range in which older persons first experience hearing loss. Loss of a sensation for pain may keep a person from seeking medical help as quickly as a younger person would; it means that you must be particularly careful with hot or cold applications because the person can be burned easily.

GENITOURINARY CHANGES

Kidney function decreases as blood flow decreases; also a certain percentage of nephrons decrease in function from direct age changes. This means that the kidney takes longer to clear the system of waste products than normally; the kidneys are not so efficient in clearing drugs from the bloodstream, so drug intoxication may occur.

Many women during this period have stress incontinence (involuntary voiding of urine on laughing, coughing, or quick movement) due to loss of muscle support from childbirth. Attempting to void frequently helps to reduce this problem.

Older adults need a good fluid intake to maintain circulating blood volume. If an older adult is taking a diuretic (a medication to stimulate kidney function), he often needs an oral potassium supplement to prevent him from becoming potassium deficient as this is eliminated from his body with the increased urine output.

Be aware that while prostatic hypertrophy is generally benign (harmless) overgrowth, it may also signal the development of carcinoma (cancer). All males with difficulty initiating or maintaining a urine stream need a physical examination to be certain that any hypertrophy causing the disorder is an aging change and not serious illness. Be aware also that postmenopausal bleeding may be innocent but can also be a prime sign of uterine malignancy. Such an occurrence always requires a physician's assessment for diagnosis.

INTEGUMENT CHANGES

Skin elasticity is decreased with aging; there is loss of subcutaneous tissue and skin tends to be dry. These conditions can lead quickly to skin breakdown or decubitus ulcer in an older adult. Using soap sparingly helps to prevent excessive dryness. Facial hair tends to increase in amount following menopause in women. Brittleness of finger and toe nails may cause them to break easily causing cuticle tears. Good fitting shoes are important to prevent skin irritation and damage to the skin on the feet (healing may be poor in feet due to impaired circulation).

MUSCULOSKELETAL CHANGES

The typical gait of an older adult is a stiff, small stepping one because of fibrotic changes in tendons which along with arthritic changes make joints stiff and less mobile. Bone becomes more porous as fewer cells are formed, making bone brittle and easily broken. This is termed *osteoporosis.* It is important that the older adult maintain a diet high in calcium, vitamin D, and fluoride in order for bone mineralization to continue at as near normal a rate as possible.

Arthritic changes cause swelling and pain in joints; many older people have such pain from arthritis that walking or doing fine motor tasks is difficult. Arthritis tends to be more painful on rainy or cold days. It is often worse early in the morning than later in the day.

SEXUAL FUNCTION

Although cessation of ovulation occurs in the middle-aged adult, women are capable of achieving orgasm and enjoying sexual relations throughout life. Erection and ejaculation may be slower in older males than when they were younger, but sperm formation is not noticeably decreased and males remain fertile throughout life.

Developmental Task

The developmental task of the older adult is to achieve a sense of integrity versus a sense of despair. A person with a sense of integrity feels fulfilled and worthwhile. He can look back on his life and although he identifies some things that he would do differently if he could live his life again, overall he is satisfied with the route he has taken and the goals he has reached. Without a sense of integrity he feels that his life has been a failure and that his achievements are less than those of people around him.

Most older individuals enjoy talking about their past life experiences. Describing events in their lives is part of developing a sense of integrity; it strengthens for them the feeling that their lives were filled with stimulating fulfilling experiences. Because memory may decrease as a person becomes older, a person may recount a particularly rewarding or amusing experience over and over, not aware that he has told it before. Remember that such repetition, sometimes called *life review*, aids in accomplishing the developmental task for the age group. This recognition will enable you to be patient in listening to the experience, the same as knowing that practicing stacking blocks independently leads to a sense of autonomy in a toddler allows you to patiently watch a child practice without interfering.

Changes in social and psychological functioning were described by Cumming and Henry (1961) as *disengagement* or society drawing away from older persons and older persons drawing away from society. Havighurst (1975) and Maddox (1974) have advanced a more modern *activity theory* that says aging does not have to include a lessening of social interaction. Those people who believe in a disengagement theory see social programs for the aging as not necessary (and not effective). Believing that activity is healthful for older adults makes optimal health care and social interaction imperative activities for the age group.

Patterns of Behavior Important for Care

It is important to respect the ways that the older adult prefers to do things, as he has deeply ingrained habits that may not be changed readily. They probably are right for him since they have worked well for such a long period.

SLEEP

The older adult needs less sleep than other age groups. Six hours a night is adequate for most people over age 65. Many older adults cat-nap in the daytime if their day is uninteresting and then find themselves unable to sleep at night. Being certain that an older adult is getting enough daily exercise and mental stimulation is a method of assuring that he will be able to sleep at night.

NUTRITION

Because of a decreased metabolic rate and more sedentary activity, the caloric total does not need to be as great for the older adult as it was formerly (see Chap. 34).

If the person notices decreased taste sensation, he may not find many foods that are appealing. Having to eat alone further decreases appetite and therefore food intake.

ACTIVITY

Older adults may continue to participate in sports activities such as bowling, golf, and bicycling. A person can judge if an activity is too strenuous for him by observing how quickly he recovers his breath and normal pulse rate following the activity. If recovery is not delayed, the activity is probably good not only for his physical well-being but for his psychological attitude toward himself and life as well.

SAFETY

If people have decreased hearing or vision, they need to consider carefully what effects these impairments will have on their everyday activities. Many older adults have decreased ability to accommodate to night vision, and driving a car with impaired vision is a dangerous practice. Persons with decreased vision must be careful when working at gas stoves that they judge carefully how close they put articles such as potholders to the open flame. Throw rugs or small pieces of furniture that if not seen easily could cause an accident should be removed from the homes of such persons.

With decreased sensation to pain, older adults also need to be careful to regulate bath water and heating pad temperature so that they do not burn themselves.

Concerns of the Older Adult

Concerns of the older adult tend to center on adjustment to a changed life pattern if they have recently retired or on offering assistance to a marriage partner who is in poor health.

RETIREMENT

At age 65 almost all people retire from the occupation they have enjoyed, either because of an employer's policy or because it is the "accepted" age for retirement. Although retirement brings increased time for hobbies or favorite projects, it may also bring a loss in social contacts, structured use of time, and social status (Fig. 9-17).

People should spend some time before retirement thinking through not only how retirement will change their financial status but how they will use their time and energy after retirement. People who will experience an extensive change of life style upon retirement (moving from a position of authority to one of non-authority, from 12-hour work days to no set responsibilities, from one part of the country to another) are particularly well advised to spend active time planning. Making plans to move to a warmer climate for retirement is a good plan in terms of avoiding snow shoveling, but it removes the person from his usual support systems, which, accompanied by loss of contact with work associates, may add greatly to a sense of loneliness.

The woman who was used to functioning independently in her home while her husband worked may be pleased that her husband will now be home with her following his retirement; however, she may find that she

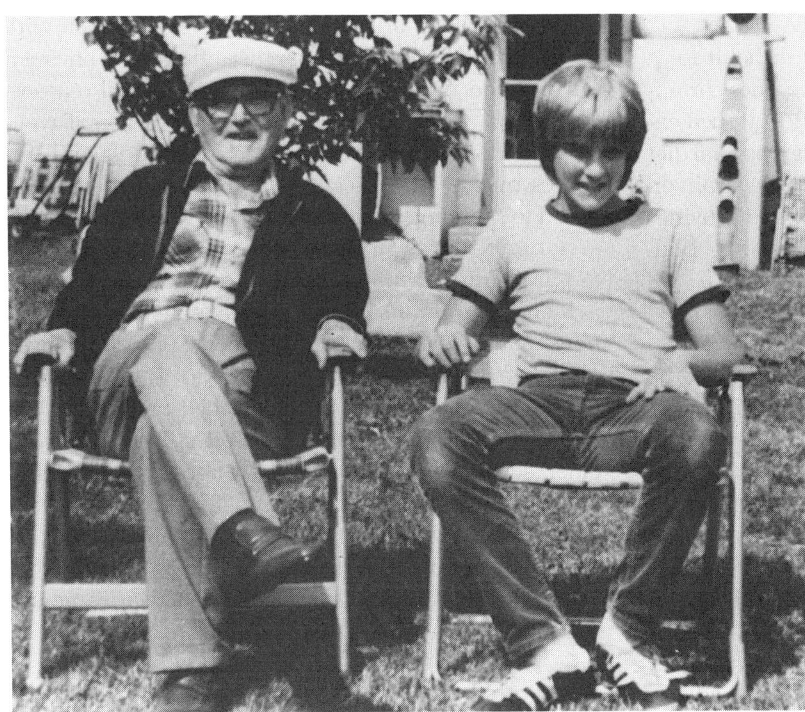

FIGURE 9-17. Grandfather and grandson (note imitating posture). Being retired, this man has more time to spend in leisure and family events.

misses her sense of independence, her ability to do things at her own pace and in her own way. She needs to plan for retirement as much as her husband, planning for activities that allow her freedom of choice and privacy. It is sometimes assumed that a woman who has held a full-time job will be anxious to retire so that she will have time to learn to sew or knit or spend time in her house. Actually, she likely will have the same difficulties at retirement as the man who is leaving a full-time job; if learning to knit was really important to her, she would have done so years before.

FINANCIAL RESOURCES

With retirement comes an almost automatic decrease in income. Although people receive Social Security and perhaps additional pension checks each month and their medical care is at least partially taken care of by a Medicare insurance plan, there are few people who continue to have as much income following retirement as they had before. Because pension and Social Security incomes are fixed, a year of high inflation affects this age group's income very markedly. Lack of funds may lead to poor nutritional patterns or inability to buy enough clothing or new furnishings. They worry that an illness or hospitalization will be so costly that it will take all their savings. Such a situation is destructive of self-esteem.

HOUSING

Older adults need to be close to shopping, religious, and health care facilities as they may no longer be able to drive as their reaction time and eyesight decrease. It may be difficult to use public transportation if it is expensive or requires rapid judgment or motion. If they have lived in the same home for years, it may need repairs that they cannot afford. If the neighborhood has deteriorated over the years, they may feel that their security is threatened. If going up or downstairs is a problem due to cardiac or arthritic changes, a two-story home may no longer be appropriate for them. The best home for an older adult is usually a one-story plan with floors that are not slippery, with well-lit rooms filled with familiar furnishings, and within easy walking distance of community services.

LOSS OF SOCIAL CONTACTS

For many people the most difficult aspect of retirement is being shut off from friends at work. Women who have worked until 65 or 70 discover that they have little in common with neighbors or women who are still working every day or who have never worked outside the home and find housework very time consuming. The recently retired woman finds hours of time on her hands as she had previously juggled both job and house. The retired man longs for "male talk" that he shared so freely with men at work.

Joining senior citizen groups, volunteer groups, or church clubs, or visiting in a park where other older adults congregate may be helpful in meeting this need for companionship. Older people need visits from their family members as well. Many older adults say they are particularly lonesome for the sound of children's laughter as in their "retirement village" this sound is absent. Social contacts of this nature help to keep an older adult active and his mental capabilities at full function.

LIVING WITH AN ILL SPOUSE OR COMPANION

Being independent becomes increasingly difficult for a couple if one member of the household becomes chronically ill. Illness may place a strain on finances if medication or hospitalization is involved. Cooking a special diet or providing exercises or other care may put a strain on an older person's energy. Inability to complete activities together may increase loneliness and depression for both partners.

ADJUSTING TO DEATH OF A SPOUSE

Statistically, men die at an earlier age than women; the average woman can, therefore, expect to live longer than her husband and have to adjust to being a widow or living without the person with whom she has shared the majority of her life. Grief is a well-studied process which involves specific stages. It takes about six weeks to complete the initial adjustment to such an acute loss; final resolution may not occur for 2 years (and maybe never). With resolution of grief will come a new awareness of life, an adjustment to living alone, and the formation of new relationships. Men may have more difficulty adjusting to the death of a spouse than women because they must adjust not only to the loss of someone close to them but to acquiring a new life style for themselves (cooking, cleaning, shopping—activities they may never have participated in before). Following the death of a lifetime partner, people are advised not to make any major changes in their lives such as selling the family home, moving to a new locale, or selling a business until at least six months. This delay prevents people from making decisions that will have a long-term effect before they have recovered sufficiently from the shock of death to be able to reason objectively.

Considerations of Care for the Older Adult

Be certain to maintain an older person's dignity when caring for him. An older adult may have loss of recent memory and may have difficulty remembering recent instructions for a procedure or an event such as what he ate for breakfast that morning. If this is a problem, give instructions again as necessary; do not put the responsibility for remembering fluid intake on a person who has difficulty with memory. Post reminders on the door to alert the person and those caring for him of what you want. If you use reminders, be certain that they are tasteful: intake and output, not "save urine"; older adults have grown up in a time when body functions were considered more private than they are today. On the other hand, do not assume that all older adults have loss of memory problems; the effects of aging are very individualized.

Respect older persons' names. Early in life you learned never to call people older than yourself by their first names; this rule should apply to people older than yourself until they give you permission to address them otherwise. Nicknames such as "pops" or "grandma" are always inappropriate and disrespectful.

Because older adults may have less contact with people than younger persons, they often enjoy having a nurse spend time with them for purely social reasons. Such social interaction helps to build a sense of well-being and companionship in the older adult and improves mental processes. Such an action can be compared to spending time playing with a child: Both on the surface appear as "niceties" of care; in reality they are required components of care for the two age groups.

Many older adults hunger for the more intimate relationship they enjoyed when their spouse or children lived with them (being hugged or kissed as a means of sharing happiness). They enjoy being touched or having their hand held during a painful procedure. Use touch with older adults as a general rule in liberal quantities (a hand on a person's shoulder while you talk to him, touching his face to convey reassurance) unless the person is the exception to the rule and does not enjoy this. Touch is also culturally influenced and varies greatly depending on a person's background.

Effect of Illness

Many older adults do not seek health care immediately when they realize something is wrong because they are unwilling to be involved in the expense of health care or they worry that hospitalization may be necessary. An expensive hospitalization could take them away from their home and with no close neighbors they worry that their property may be destroyed. The expense of the hospitalization could completely deplete their resources.

Ask at health visits if the person notices any difficulty with vision or hearing loss; many older people try to "make do" with broken hearing aids or glasses rather than have them repaired. Ask about ability to afford food, cook it, and eat it. Such problems as lack of money, poor vision, failing memory, or poorly fitted dentures all interfere with good nutrition.

Ask about living facilities (is there adequate heat, water, plumbing?). Can the person get safely to a shopping center or to church?

Ask about depression. Depression may be manifested as lessened physical hygiene, reduced exposure to people, and sedentary activities. It is often assumed that poor memory or disorientation in an older adult is the result of an organic illness. It may also be from depression over the loss of a life style or friends.

DEVELOPMENT IN THE HANDICAPPED PERSON

A handicap is any condition that interferes with normal psychologic or physical functioning. Such a condition may occur at birth (a child is born with a deformed arm, for example) or may occur at any point in life (a person is injured in an accident and is left with a permanently injured arm). Effects of long-term illnesses may affect the person's ability to achieve developmental tasks and therefore the person's ability to reach true maturity.

Sense of Trust

Many of the developmental events of the infant year (social smile, laughing aloud, reaching for an object, sitting, talking) are activities that encourage mother-child interaction, that make an infant fun to be with and naturally make a mother want to spend a great deal of time with her child. If the child is mentally retarded, he may not reach milestones such as social smile or first word. If he has physical limitations, he may not reach up and pat his mother's face as most infants do or reach to be picked up. If he cannot interact with her, she may be unable to interact with him.

Mother-child bonding does not happen readily if the child is separated from his mother at birth. This often happens when a child is born with a handicap and the child is immediately hospitalized for diagnosis and treatment. If the child leaves the hospital with a cast or other equipment necessary for care, the mother may be so concerned with the equipment that she is unable to do the everyday, relaxed, sitting, singing, playing activities with her child that she would have done if this illness had not happened.

Without a sense of trust a child has difficulty reaching out to others; he does not believe that he is lovable or that people will want to interact with him. People with a handicap need people around them to give them help at whatever point they are unable to fully meet their own needs. It is unfortunate that a handicapped child may be the one who is least able to reach out for help because he has not developed a sense of trust.

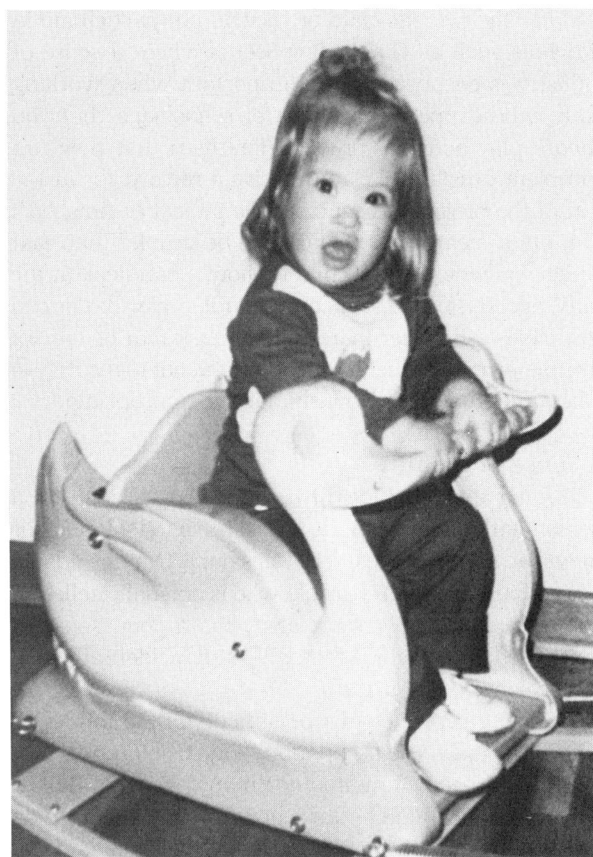

FIGURE 9-18. The parents of this handicapped toddler play an important role in promoting autonomy. Here she independently "rocks the duck," a toy appropriate for most toddlers.

Sense of Autonomy

It may be equally difficult for a child with a handicap to achieve a sense of autonomy or independence because, due to his limitations, he cannot be as independent as the average child. If he is on a special diet, for example, he may not be allowed foods that make good finger foods; if he is tube fed, he has no experience with finger foods at all. If he has physical limitations, he may be unable to explore freely; he may not have the physical ability to pound and manipulate toys as the average toddler does.

It is important for a person with a handicap to have a strong sense of autonomy so that he sees himself as able to do things by himself (see Fig. 9-18). It takes courage to move a wheelchair through a busy airport or rock concert crowd. It is unfortunate when a handicapped individual does not achieve a strong sense of autonomy that allows him to explore alternatives that open the world for him and give him intellectual stimulation and fulfillment.

Sense of Initiative

Learning how to do things when you have physical limitations is frustrating; not being able to understand how to do things when you have psychological or mental limitations is equally frustrating. Developing a sense of initiative, however, is learning problem solving. A person with a handicap needs problem-solving ability probably more than the average person, because even simple procedures (getting to work, fixing a meal, transferring to his bed) may be problems for him.

Many of the activities that preschoolers enjoy such as playing with mud, clay, or soap bubbles are messy activities. If the child is in bed, his mother may not offer him this type of experience, trying to keep the bedroom neat. A large tray of dry oatmeal or other dry breakfast cereal is a good substitute activity for a child on bedrest. Although not necessarily neater, such material is readily available even in a hospital setting and can be swept away easily at the finish of play.

A Sense of Industry

Gaining a sense of industry is learning how to do things well. A person with a handicap needs a sense of industry so that he will persevere with whatever measures he needs to accomplish to be as independent as possible. It is a sense of industry that allows him to practice muscle-strengthening exercises over and over again or to practice learning to write his name again after a cerebral vascular accident until his signature is readable.

People with a handicap may not develop a sense of industry if they are not given as many household chores to do as the average child or they do not participate in activities such as Girl or Boy Scouts where a sense of industry is encouraged. It is important when working with handicapped individuals of school age that you choose play activities or work for them that they can complete satisfactorily and receive a reward for at the end of the project (recognizing the project as finished). This often means that the task will be simpler than that which you would give a child without a handicap at the same age. It is better to choose a simpler task that he can complete well rather than a harder task that he cannot complete; on the other hand, be careful not to insult him with tasks that are obviously not age appropriate.

A Sense of Identity

Achieving a sense of identity is often very difficult for a person with a handicap. He has to learn to look past his handicap and at his real self: He is not a 16-year-old in a wheelchair; he is a 16-year-old who is normal intellectually, is a good conversationalist, has a good sense of humor, enjoys watching football—and incidentally, is in a wheelchair (Fig. 9-19).

Choosing a vocation may be difficult for the child with a handicap as some occupations may be closed to him because of specific limitations. Emancipation from parents may be difficult because he is forced to depend on them for some things. Establishing heterosexual relationships may be difficult if he has limited contacts with other children his own age. Many young people of this age have as much difficulty looking past a wheelchair or a physical limitation as does the person himself and do not offer friendship as freely as he would like.

An adolescent with a handicap needs opportunities to make decisions for himself. Many times he cannot make health care decisions for himself as he must do such things as remain on bedrest or wear a cast on his leg; find areas where he can make decisions and allow him experience in these areas.

A Sense of Intimacy

Gaining a sense of intimacy means establishing lasting relationships. An individual with a handicap may choose not to marry—or may not have the opportunity to—but this does not mean that he should be limited in his ability to form deep lasting relationships with people at his work or in his community. It is important for persons with handicaps to have a strong support network around them so that on a day they need help such as transportation to a special function they do not feel abandoned but are able to call and ask for help as needed. Your interest in such a person at a health care visit may be the reassurance he needs to feel good enough about himself to reach out to others to make friendships.

A Sense of Generativity

A sense of generativity or an interest in community and world concerns may be difficult to achieve for a person with a handicap because he may be limited in physical or psychological ways from actually participating in such activities. However, organizations such as political action groups, health care causes, and religious groups need the kind of help that often requires little physical movement such as telephone answering, typing, or mailing questionnaires. Participating in such groups adds to a sense of self-esteem and also enlarges the person's

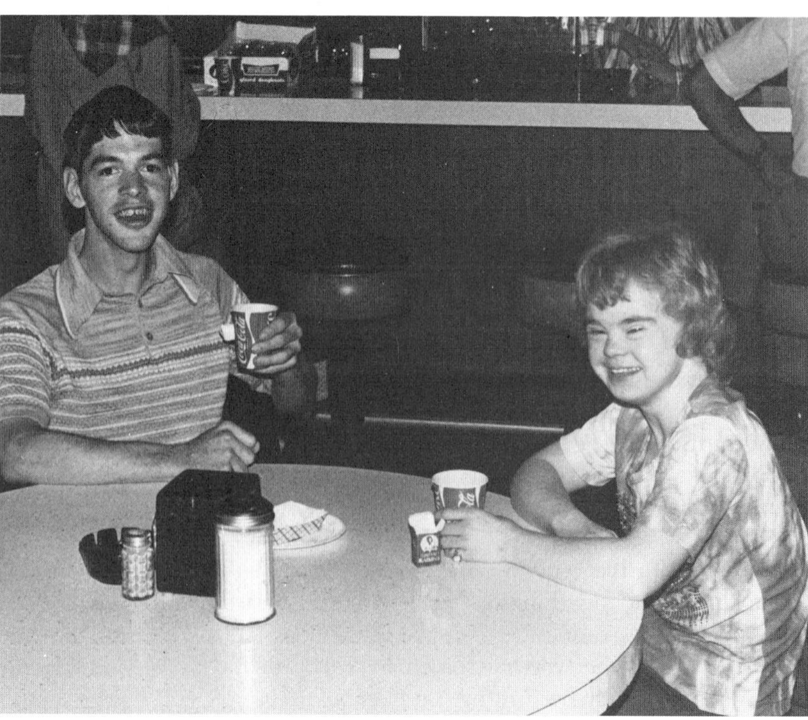

FIGURE 9-19. Living normally for retarded young adults means being able to enjoy social pastimes typical of their peers.

social contacts so that if at some point he needs additional help, he has a larger social network on which to rely.

A Sense of Integrity

A sense of integrity is a feeling of satisfaction in what you have become. Although a person with a handicap may feel that in some ways he has been cheated in life, all in all he should arrive at older age feeling that he has spent a good life. An older adult with a handicap may have outlived his family doctor; many old friends and support people may have died or moved away. Determine whether an older adult with a handicap still has support people around him; help him to locate new support people as necessary. Isolation due to lack of support people will defeat a sense of integrity.

HEALTH MAINTENANCE

Health maintenance is care aimed at helping individuals to remain well and prevent illness. Usual health maintenance measures suggested are shown in Table 9-16.

Notice how procedures vary according to the incidence or likelihood of a particular illness occurring at a certain age. Developmental assessment, for example, is concentrated in the young child; tests for cervical or colon cancer are concentrated in the adult (the age at which the illness tends to occur). Scoliosis (lateral curvature of the spine) occurs almost exclusively in late school age through early young adult ages, so special attention to the detection of this disorder is concentrated in these age groups. A health history and physical examination are done at every health care contact.

It is helpful to be familiar with the health promotion

TABLE 9-16. RECOMMENDED HEALTH MAINTENANCE MEASURES BY AGE GROUP

Measure	Infant	Toddler	Preschooler	Schoolager	Adolescent	Young Adult	Middle Age	Older Adult
Immunizations								
DPT[a]	2, 4, 6 mo	18 mo	3—4 yr					
TOPV[b]	2, 4, 6 mo	18 mo	3—4 yr					
MMR[c]		15 mo						
Td[d]					14—16 yr			
Tetanus[e]						Every 10 yr →	→	→
Health history	Every visit →	→	→	→	→	→	→	→
Physical exam	Every 1—3 mo	Every yr →	→	→	→	→	→	→
Dental exam			First visit at 3 yr	Yearly thereafter →	→	→	→	→
Height	At every visit →	→	→	→	→			
Weight	At every visit →	→	→	→	→	→	→	→
Screening procedures								
DDST[f]	3, 10 mo		3—4 yr					
Vision			3—4 yr	7—8 yr 10—12 yr	Every 2—3 yr thereafter →	→	→	→
Hearing			3—4 yr	Yearly	As indicated →	→	→	Yearly
Blood pressure			At each visit →	→	→	→	→	→
Bacteriuria[g]			3—4 yr (girls)	6—7 yr 10—12 yr	14—16 yr	19—20 yr		
Tuberculosis test	12 mo	As needed by incidence of tuberculosis in community →	→	→	→	→	→	→
Scoliosis[h]				10—12 yr	At each visit →	→	→	
Cervical cancer					Every 3 years →	→	→	→
Colon cancer							With every visit (males)	

[a]Diphtheria, pertussis (whooping cough), and tetanus vaccine.
[b]Trivalent oral poliomyelitis vaccine.
[c]Measles (rubeola), mumps (infectious parotitis), and rubella (German measles).
[d]Tetanus and diphtheria, adult type.
[e]Adult type tetanus immunization.
[f]Denver Developmental Screening Test.
[g]Bacteria in urine.
[h]Lateral curvature of the spine.

or health maintenance measures usually recommended for each age group so that you can monitor patterns of care of the people you interact with. These practices vary depending on different community needs and practices; they are suggested, not mandated procedures.

SUGGESTED READINGS

Growth and Development Across the Age Span

Blair, C., and Salerino, E. *The Expanding Family: Childbearing.* Boston: Little, Brown, 1976.

Duvall, E. *Family Development* (5th ed.). Philadelphia: Lippincott, 1977.

Erikson, E. *Childhood and Society* (2nd ed.). New York: Norton, 1963.

Freud, A. *The Ego and the Mechanisms of Defense.* New York: International Universities Press, 1946.

Gruber, H., and Voneche, J. *The Essential Piaget.* New York: Basic Books, 1977.

MacCarthy, D. Psychological influences affecting growth. *Health Visit.* 53:461, 1980.

Mullen, P.D. Promoting child health: Channels of socialization. *Fam. Commun. Health* 5:52, 1983.

Murray, R., and Zentner, J. *Nursing Assessment and Health Promotion Through the Life Span* (2nd ed.). Englewood Cliffs, N.J.: Prentice Hall, 1979.

Piaget, J. *The Psychology of Intelligence.* London: Routledge and Kegan Paul Ltd., 1950.

Weissbourd, B., et al. Family focus: Supporting families in the community. *Child. Today* 10:6, 1980.

Williams, L. Childhood immunizations. *Pediatr. Nurse* 8:18, 1982.

Yoos, L. A developmental approach to physical assessment. *MCN* 6:168, 1981.

The Newborn and Infant

Blackburn, S. Fostering behavioral development of high-risk infants. *J.O.G.N. Nurs.* 12(3):760, 1983.

Blosser, C. Avoiding potential behavior problems in children. *Pediatr. Nurse* 5:11, 1979.

Bradshaw, T. W. Teething. *Pediatr. Nurse* 7:15, 1981.

Brazelton, T. B. Neonatal Behavioral Assessment Scale. *Clinics in Developmental Medicine* No. 50. Spastics International Medical Pub. London: Heinemann Medical Books, 1973.

Brown, J. Infant temperament: A clue to childbearing for parents and nurses. *MCN* 2:228, 1977.

Davidson, S., et al. Appearance, behavior and capabilities: Teaching new parents infant ABC's. *Canad. Nurse* 77:37, 1981.

Frankenberg, K., et al. The revised Denver Developmental Screening Test: Its accuracy as a screening instrument. *J. Pediatr.* 79:988, 1971.

Jarrett, G. E. Childrearing patterns of young mothers. *MCN* 7:119, 1982.

Kraus, M. H., and Kennell, J. H. *Maternal-Infant Bonding.* St. Louis: Mosby, 1981.

Malnory, M. E. A prenatal assessment tool for mothers and fathers. *J. Nurse Midwife* 27(6):26, 1982.

Nelms, B. C. Attachment versus spoiling. *Pediatr. Nurs.* 9(1):49, 1983.

Reinhard, S. Nursing responsibility in infant car safety. *MCN* 5:26, 1980.

Riordan, J., et al. Basics of breast feeding. *JOGN Nurs.* 9:277, 1980.

Ventura, J. N. Parent coping behaviors, parent functioning, and infant temperament characteristics. *Nurs. Res.* 31(5):269, 1982.

The Toddler and Preschooler

Box, M. The developing child: Development assessment. *Health Visit.* 53:461, 1980.

Brown, M. S., et al. Effects of prior preparation on the preschooler's vision and hearing screening. *MCN* 7(5):323, 1982.

Cline, T. The second year of life. *Nurse Pract.* 6:45, 1981.

Ferullo, R. Objectivity in the assessment of preschool hearing-impaired bilingual Hispanic children. *J. Sch. Health* 53(2):131, 1983.

Fleming, R. Developing a child's self-esteem. *Pediatric Nurs.* 5:58, 1979.

Horner, M., et al. Toilet training: Ready or not? *Pediatr. Nurs.* 7:15, 1981.

Johnson, M. Teaching dental health to children. *Pediatr. Nurs.* 4:20, 1978.

Mitchell, S. H. Imaginary companions: Friend or foe? *Pediatr. Nurs.* 6:29, 1980.

Parcel, G. S. Health education for kindergarten children. *J. Sch. Health* 49:129, 1979.

Pipes, P. *Nutrition in infancy and childhood.* St. Louis: Mosby, 1977.

Seefeldt, C., et al. How older people view children. *Child. Today* 11:16, 1982.

Tush, B. A. Bruising in healthy 3-year-old children. *Matern. Child Nurs. J.* 11(3):165, 1982.

Vipperman, J., and Rager, P. Childhood coping: How nurses can help. *Pediatr. Nurs.* 6:11, 1980.

Weiss, R. S. Growing up a little faster: Children in single parent households. *Child. Today* 10:22, 1981.

The Schoolager and Adolescent

Adams, B. N. Adolescent health care: Needs, priorities, and services. *Nurs. Clin. North Am.* 18(2):237, 1983.

Amonker, R. G. What do teens know about the facts of life? *J. Sch. Health* 50:527, 1980.

Engel, N. S., et al. Nursing care for the adolescent urban nomad. *MCN* 8(1):74, 1983.

Erickson, C. J., et al. Understanding and evaluating adolescent behavior problems. *J. Sch. Health* 48:293, 1978.

Hagenbuch, V. Obesity and the school-age child. *Nurs. Clin. North. Am.* 17:207, 1982.

Howe, J. *Nursing Care of Adolescents.* New York: McGraw-Hill, 1979.

Langford, R. W. When your client has a weight problem: Teenagers and obesity. *Am. J. Nurs.* 81:556, 1981.

Leppirk, M. A. Adolescent sexuality. *Matern. Child Nurs. J.* 8:153, 1979.

Mercer, R. *Perspectives in Adolescent Health Care.* Philadephia: Lippincott, 1979.

Mowery, B. Family oriented approach to childhood obesity. *Pediatr. Nurs.* 6:40, 1980.

Peach, E. Counseling sexually active very young adolescent girls. *MCN* 5:191, 1980.

Perry, C. Enhancing the transition years: The challenge of adolescent health promotion. *J. Sch. Health* 52:307, 1982.

Rice, M., et al. Review: Identifying the adolescent substance abuser. *MCN* 8(2):139, 1983.

Russo, J. R. Adolescent menstrual disorders. *Female Patient* 5:19, 1980.

Segal, J., et al. The "problem" child—six ways to bring out the best in any child. *Fam. Health* 13:40, 1981.

Thackaberry, J. M. Nursing management of the school-age child with bowel incontinence: Utilizing Erikson's theory of psychosocial development. *J. Sch. Health* 53(3):189, 1983.

Wood, S. P. School aged children's perceptions of the causes of illness. *Pediatr. Nurs.* 9(2):101, 1983.

The Young and Middle-Aged Adult

Carroll, J. S. Middle age does not mean menopause. *Top. Clin. Nurs.* 4:38, 1983.

Dominian, J. Marital stress in the early years. *Health Visit.* 55:146, 1982.

Gaston, S. Death and mid-life crisis. *J. Psychiatr. Nurs.* 18:31, 1980.

Huber, H., et al. Teaching behavioral skills to parents: A preventative role for mental health. *Child. Today* 7:8, 1978.

Johnson-Saylor, M. T. Seize the moment: Health education for the young adult. *Top. Clin. Nurs.* 2:9, 1980.

Kiernan, B., and Scoloveno, M. Fathering. *Nurs. Clin. North Am.* 12:481, 1977.

Olson, J. K., et al. Helping families cope with elderly parents. *J. Gerontol. Nurs.* 6:151, 1980.

Peplau, H. Mid-life crises. *Am. J. Nurs.* 75:1791, 1975.

Perdue, B., et al. Mothering. *Nurs. Clin. North Am.* 12:491, 1977.

Roznoy, M. The young adult: Taking a sexual history. *Am. J. Nurs.* 76:1279, 1976.

Stanford, D. All about sex . . . after middle age. *Am. J. Nurs.* 77:608, 1977.

The Older Adult

Bozian, M. W., and Clark, H. M. Counteracting sensory changes in the aging. *Am. J. Nurs.* 80:473, 1980.

Butler, R. N., et al. Self-care, self-help and the elderly. *Int. J. Aging Hum. Dev.* 10:95, 1979—1980.

Cooper, S. Accidents and older adults. *Geriatr. Nurs.* 2:287, 1981.

Cozens, R. E. Obesity in the aged. *Nurs. Clin. North Am.* 17:227, 1982.

Cumming, E., and Henry, W. E. *Growing Old: The Process of Disengagement.* New York: Basic Books, 1961.

Dolan, M. B. Being old is not the same as being ill. *Nursing 80* 10:41, 1980.

Falk, G., and Falk, U. A. Sexuality and the aged. *Nurs. Outlook* 28:51, 1980.

Glassman-Feibuch, B. The socially isolated elderly. *Geriatr. Nurs.* 2:28, 1981.

Green, C. P. Fostering positive attitudes toward the elderly—a teaching strategy for attitude change. *J. Gerontol. Nurs.* 7:169, 1981.

Gioiella, E. C. Give the older person space. *Am. J. Nurs.* 80:898, 1980.

Havighurst, R. The future aged: The use of time and money. *Gerontologist* 15:10, 1975.

Kopac, C. Sensory loss in the aged: The role of the nurse and the family. *Nurs. Clin. North Am.* 18(2):373, 1983.

Maddox, G. L. Disengagement theory: a critical evaluation. *The Gerontologist* 4:80, 1974.

Megerle, J. Surviving. *Am. J. Nurs.* 83(6):892, 1983.

Stokes, S. A., et al. Health assessment—considerations for the older individual. *J. Gerontol. Nurs.* 6:328, 1980.

Talmadge, H., et al. Innovative home care program offers appropriate alternative for the elderly. *Hospitals* 64(2):50, 1983.

Wahl, P. R. Therapeutic relationships with the elderly. *J. Gerontol. Nurs.* 6:6260, 1980.

The Handicapped Individual

Baranowski, E. Childbirth education classes for expectant deaf parents. *MCN* 8(2):143, 1983.

Berg, W. E. Working with physically handicapped patients: Advocacy in a nursing home. *Health Soc. Work* 6:26, 1981.

Curry, M. F. Where are we with the education of the handicapped: New approaches to screening. *J. Sch. Health* 51:441, 1981.

Davis, A. J. Disability, home care and the care taking role in family life. *J. Adv. Nurs.* 5:475, 1980.

Foulk, D., et al. Emergency medical services and the handicapped patient. *EMT J.* 5:27, 1981.

Molla, P. M. Self concept in children with and without physical disabilities. *J. Psychiatr. Nurs.* 19:22, 1981.

Mori, A. A. Mildly handicapped children in the mainstream—implications for the health educator. *J. Sch. Health* 51:119, 1981.

Page, R. C., et al. Assertiveness training groups with the disabled. *J. Rehabil.* 47:52, 1981.

Rice, B. L. Nutritional problems of developmentally disabled children. *Pediatr. Nurs.* 7:15, 1981.

Rodgers, B. M., et al. Depression in the chronically ill or handicapped school age child. *MCN* 6:266, 1981.

Smigielski, P. A., et al. Teaching sex education to multiply handicapped adolescents. *J. Sch. Health* 51:238, 1981.

Stearns, S. E. Understanding the psychological adjustment of physically handicapped children in the classroom. *Child. Today* 10:12, 1981.

Stiles, K. et al. Training community health nurses in care of handicapped children. *J. Contin. Educ. Nurs.* 13:26, 1982.

Tabeek, E. S., et al. Teaching sexual awareness to the significantly disabled school-age child. *Pediatr. Nurs.* 7:21, 1981.

Zamerowski, S. T. Helping families to cope with handicapped children *Top. Clin. Nurs.* 4:41, 1982.

QUESTIONS FOR REVIEW

1. Match the statement in the first column with the corresponding developmental task.

a. ____ I don't think I would have done many things differently in life.
b. ____ I'm better at doing things than teaching others how to do them.
c. ____ I can do it myself.
d. ____ After 20 years my husband and I still love each other.
e. ____ I like to experiment and learn new things.
f. ____ I'm concerned that our highways are not well maintained.
g. ____ I don't like to leave projects half done.
h. ____ I always felt well loved as a child.

1. Sense of trust
2. Sense of autonomy
3. Sense of initiative
4. Sense of industry
5. Sense of identity
6. Sense of intimacy
7. Sense of generativity
8. Sense of integrity

2. Match the descriptions of common sleep patterns in the first column with the appropriate age group.

a. ____ Needs less sleep than any age group.
b. ____ May have difficulty sleeping from occupational stress.
c. ____ Sleeps 16 out of every 24 hours.
d. ____ Needs up to 10 hours of sleep a night to prevent fatigue.
e. ____ Often has nightmares during sleep.
f. ____ Begins to resist naps because he is so independent.

1. Newborn
2. Toddler
3. Preschooler
4. Adolescent
5. Middle-aged adult
6. Older adult

3. Match the descriptions of common safety precautions in the first column with the appropriate age group.

a. ____ Safety with firearms needs to be stressed.
b. ____ Auto accidents cause a high incidence of deaths.
c. ____ Alcoholism may become a problem resulting in accidents.
d. ____ Needs good lighting provided to prevent falls.
e. ____ Aspiration is a real danger.
f. ____ It is time to teach how to cross streets safely.

1. Infant
2. Schoolager
3. Preschooler
4. Young adult
5. Middle-aged adult
6. Older adult

4. Match the descriptions of common recreation patterns in the first column with the appropriate age group.

a. _____ Reflexes are at their peak.
b. _____ A main activity is watching his mother's face.
c. _____ May use unwise diets to qualify for sports teams.
d. _____ May need encouragement not to pursue all sedentary activities.
e. _____ Learns to crawl.
f. _____ Jumps, climbs, and runs constantly.
g. _____ Should plan regularly spaced activities, not sudden spurts of activity.
h. _____ First age that is old enough for competition.
i. _____ Enjoys parallel play.

1. Newborn
2. Infant
3. Toddler
4. Preschooler
5. Schoolager
6. Adolescent
7. Young adult
8. Middle-aged adult
9. Older adult

5. Match the special considerations for care in the first column with the appropriate age group.

a. _____ May neglect own care in place of occupational commitments.
b. _____ May be starved for touch.
c. _____ Important that he not be separated from mother.
d. _____ Needs a one-to-one relationship if at all possible.
e. _____ May be reluctant to be separated from gang.
f. _____ Try to limit intrusive procedures.
g. _____ May neglect own care because of needs of young children.
h. _____ May be particularly concerned about body image.

1. Newborn
2. Infant
3. Preschooler
4. Schoolager
5. Adolescent
6. Young adult
7. Middle-aged adult
8. Older adult

10. INDIVIDUALITY AND ETHNICITY

OBJECTIVES

Upon mastery of the material in this chapter, you should be able to:

1. Define culture and individuality.
2. Describe characteristics or influences that make individuals unique.
3. List basic rules to use to ensure that you respect individual differences in people.
4. Describe ways that cultural variations can affect behavior.
5. Describe common characteristics of differing culturally influenced groups with regard to their effects on health care.
6. Identify cultural values in yourself that might affect your nursing care.
7. Describe the importance of transcultural nursing.
8. Describe ways of improving health care for major cultural groups.

TERMS

The terms important for an understanding of this chapter are shown below and defined in the glossary:

culture
ethnic
ethnicity
individuality
maturity
temperament

Both innate characteristics and cultural influences are very strong determinants of human behavior. However, these factors operate in such a subtle way that a person is usually unaware that they are serving as bases for his actions.

It is important for nurses to be aware of individual and cultural differences regarding health care since these aspects influence the manner in which people accept or reject treatment. A nurse's individual and cultural perceptions may affect how she expects people to act in health care situations. If you are a member of a culture where the male is the authority figure, for example, you may expect a husband to always answer questions about his wife's health at an annual health visit; if you are from a culture where males are less dominant, you might find it annoying to hear a husband responding in this way. A nurse who has been culturally influenced to believe that stoic behavior is the "proper" response to pain may be agitated with a patient who has been influenced to believe that expressing his distress is "proper."

The United States is a country of many varied cultural groups, and under any circumstances you will see a wide range of behaviors exhibited. Because of the individual meaning of circumstances to people and the wide range of cultural mixing, any behavior can be considered "proper" for some individual at some time and place.

INDIVIDUALITY

A person's individuality refers to those characteristics that make him unique or not exactly like any other person. Some characteristics that differentiate people are maturity, intelligence, ordinal position in the family, temperament, state of health, sex, past experience, environment, education level, and life style.

Maturity

Maturity refers to a person's development in terms of judgment and reasoning ability. Maturity is associated with age level but is not synonymous; some people reach old age but never maturity, while some children are very mature even before legal adulthood.

A mature person is one who is able to delay immediate satisfaction for better or larger rewards at a later date, to view both sides of an argument, and to use progressive steps of problem solving to reach answers to questions. Maturity is not achieved at any specific point in life; it is usually a slow-growth process of about 20 years.

It is easy to recognize immature behaviors in children (a two-year-old crying because he wants a cookie just before dinner, unable to delay for even a short time; an adolescent slamming a bedroom door, unable to think of anyone's welfare but his own) and to accept these behaviors because at that point in time they are age appropriate. When older people display immature behaviors (a man shouting because he received no coffee on his lunch tray; a woman insisting on turning on her television set, even though other people in the room with her want to sleep), it is easy to become angry with them or to misinterpret their behavior as spiteful or threatening toward you. Maturity does not occur automatically with age, however, and a person's ability to display mature behavior is reduced when he is ill and under stress. Assess each person individually to determine his specific maturity level.

Intelligence

The higher a person's intelligence, the more easily is he apt to grasp principles for his care, and he will probably learn self-care techniques faster and more thoroughly than the less intelligent person.

People under stress may lose their problem-solving ability, however. As a result of stress a very intelligent person may become very frustrated because he cannot learn and change as easily as he expected.

People with less than average intelligence need special care and consideration from a safety standpoint. They may not realize that intravenous fluid, for example, must infuse at a certain rate and so increase the rate, causing an overload of fluid to the circulatory system. They often need additional instruction in health care so that they can return home or remain at home taking care of themselves to the point that they are able.

Educational Level

A person's education level often correlates with his intelligence level but not necessarily, as some people leave school early due to family or financial influences. Theoretically the more education a person has, the more broad-minded and tolerant he will be, and the better is his problem-solving ability. In actual practice, this is not always so because these abilities are influenced by factors other than education. If a person spent a high portion of his school time not actively learning, the number of years that he has spent in school is not necessarily the same as the number of years of his education.

Ordinal Position in the Family

No two children in a family are exactly alike; one factor responsible for individual differences is the birth order of children. First children are generally asked to assume responsibility for care of young children while the youngest child in the family has no opportunity to assume responsibility in this area. Consequently, first children may strive for more responsible positions as adults than do subsequent children. First-born children also usually have more restrictions on their behavior, such as having to go to bed earlier or not being able to date until later, than middle or younger children, because as parents become more skilled at caring for their children, they are able to relax their controlling measures. This situation increases the older child's ability to follow rules and promotes the younger child's problem-solving ability. Middle children may grow up feeling insecure because they feel that they are not "special" (neither the oldest nor the youngest); they may also be the most diplomatic people as they are used to being the "middleman" or the peacemaker in children's arguments.

Of equal importance in creating differences in children is the period in the family life cycle at which a child is born. If a child is born at a time when his parents are ripe for child rearing, the child is viewed by the parents as a "good" child; when he brushes an expensive vase off the coffee table the first time he pulls himself up to stand, the parent sees his action as "all boy" or "creative, exploring behavior." If a child arrives at a less than perfect time in a family's life (for example, when the father has no work, the marriage is failing, or the mother was planning to return to school and now feels that she cannot do so), knocking over a vase in the same way may be viewed as "trouble-making" or "bad" behavior. These emotions are subconscious; parents are not usually aware that they treat different children in different ways. A child who is told that he is bad and always starting trouble may as an adolescent view himself as only being capable of this role and enter adulthood as a person set to oppose rather than follow most of society's rules. Thus, a person's ordinal position in his family may affect his ability to accept or follow health care regimens insofar as it has influenced his sense of responsibility and attitude toward authority.

"Vulnerable" Children

A phenomenon that may distort a parent's perception of a child and thus the child's perception of himself may occur when a parent is told that a child is going to die but then the child lives. When parents believe that their child is dying, they begin anticipatory grieving for him or begin to think of him as already dead to protect themselves from the full shock when his death actually occurs. When the child does not die as predicted, parents may find that their grief reaction for the child was so complete that they are unable to reverse it; they cannot view the child as they did before, and they may treat him in a cold and unfeeling way as if he were not really there, as if the child that was theirs did die. Such children are termed *vulnerable* (Green, 1964). They may develop behavior problems as they grow older (acting-out behavior such as temper tantrums, stealing in school, shoplifting as adolescents), as if to say, "Notice me; I am not dead." If such behavior continues into adulthood, they may have serious difficulty relating to others and fitting into usual community settings. Such behavior may interfere with health care if the person uses rebellion against a health regimen as a means of demonstrating that he exists. He needs skilled counseling so that he will feel secure and consequently be willing to assume responsibility for his care.

Temperament

A person's *temperament* denotes his characteristic reaction pattern to situations. It is not a pattern that develops during childhood or in adult life but a trait that a person is born with. Manifestations of temperament become apparent when the child is about three months of age. A person's temperament determines whether he is passive or intense, quick or slow to react or adapt to situations, persistent or easily distracted. Thomas and Chess (1977) have identified nine different reactivity patterns by which temperament is manifested.

ACTIVITY LEVEL

Some people have a high level of motor activity and are rarely quiet. As infants they wiggle and squirm in their cribs as early as two weeks of age. They refuse to be controlled by a playpen. As children and adults they are constantly "on the go." A person with such a high activity level may have a difficult time if, for health reasons, he is placed on bedrest or in some other way has to limit his physical motion.

RHYTHMICITY

Some people from the beginning of life manifest a regular rhythm in their physiological functions. They wake at the same time each morning, feel hungry at similarly spaced intervals, have a bowel movement daily. As infants they are easy to care for as mothers learn early what to expect from them. A child without this innate sense of rhythm is much more difficult to care for, as the mother cannot easily plan a schedule for him. People with irregular rhythmicity may not follow a health regimen that requires them to carry out some daily procedure such as exercises or timed medicine-taking because each day is so different for them that they are unaccustomed to a regular pattern of activity.

APPROACH

Approach refers to the person's response on initial contact with a new situation. Some people do this in an unruffled manner; they explore new toys as children, new jobs as adults with little apprehension. Other people demonstrate withdrawal rather than approach. As children they cry at the sight of strangers, new foods, or new experiences such as starting school. As adults they may avoid new situations in order to avoid the sense of apprehension they feel at such times. Such a person may come for health care later than others; he may need extra preparation for procedures new to him such as surgery.

ADAPTABILITY

Adaptability is a person's ability to change his reaction to stimuli over a period of time. A person who cannot adapt will continue to withdraw from a situation even though he encounters it time and again. A person who can adapt quickly can "roll with the punch"; he may react inappropriately to a situation the first time he meets it but will handle it well subsequently. The greater adaptability a person has, the better he can be expected to accept health care, because as his health changes he can adapt to changes in his health care.

INTENSITY OF REACTION

Some people react to situations with their whole being, while others barely appear to respond. It is important to assess this characteristic in people so that you do not overestimate their anger at a situation (they are not extremely angry; it is their actions that are extreme) or underestimate their feelings (they are extremely angry but do not show it in their facial expressions). As a rule it is easier to care for people who react more intensely, because although their reactions may be startling, they are clearly revealed.

DISTRACTABILITY

Distractability is the ability to shift focus to a new activity. People who do not distract easily follow through on tasks; those who do distract easily may not complete one task before they move to another. Parents find the easy-to-distract child the easiest to care for, as they can easily direct him away from a hot stove or some other attractive but harmful object or activity. They describe the difficult-to-distract child as "bullheaded" or "stubborn." As an adult, however, some degree of persistence is necessary to achieve a goal and act as a responsible person. In terms of following health care instructions, it may be difficult for some people to move from a harmful routine to a more healthful one; it may be difficult for others to follow a schedule because they are so easily distracted into other behavior.

ATTENTION SPAN AND PERSISTENCE

The attention span of individuals varies widely from a few minutes to hours or days. Degree of persistence is also variable: Some people will keep trying to perform an activity even when they fail time after time, while others stop trying after one unsuccessful attempt. People need an adequate attention span and degree of persistence in order to perform health care activities such as taking a new medication or carrying out a breathing exercise; otherwise they will neglect to follow through with the activity.

THRESHOLD OF RESPONSIVENESS

Threshold of responsiveness is the intensity or level of stimulation necessary to evoke a response. People with a low threshold of responsiveness need very little stimulation to evoke a reaction; people with a high threshold level do not react or change their behavior until the stimuli become intense. As a rule, people with a low threshold of responsiveness come for health care sooner than those with a high threshold of responsiveness; they will be more aware of pain following surgery, more aggravated by having to wait to be seen by a health care provider, and more quickly upset by such things as dietary or motion restrictions. It is important to remember that although a person may reach his threshold of responsiveness slowly, at the point that he reaches it, his distress is as acute as that of the person who reached that point of agitation much sooner.

MOOD QUALITY

Mood is an overall feeling tone which people project to others. Some people may be always happy and cooperative, while others are always complaining and at least slightly unhappy. People with a negative mood quality may be difficult to care for because you cannot make them totally happy; on the other hand, it is easy to misinterpret the true concern of those with an overall positive mood quality, because even in the face of a bad medical prognosis, they do not project sadness or worry. Assess each person's individuality so that you can better understand his reactions to stress situations and how his type of temperament will probably cause him to react to a given situation.

State of Health

A person's state of health can influence his ability to adapt or respond to situations because if he is fatigued, nauseated, or in pain he does not have the adaptive resources or tolerance level that otherwise he might have had. The behavior of people on admission to a hospital, for example, when they are very ill, is very different from that seen on discharge when they feel well again. Be certain when assessing people for individual characteristics that you assess their level of health so that you neither over- nor underestimate their ability to cope with new situations when their state of health changes.

Sex

Men and women used to react to different situations presented to them in markedly different ways when male and female roles in life were more clearly delineated. Men were always assertive, women always restrained, for example. Sex roles in occupations and behavior now overlap; many men are involved in child rearing, many women contribute to the financial resources of the family, and the ways that men and women react to stimuli are no longer predictable by sex. Perception of sex role behavior can influence reactions, however, and must be a factor in assessment.

Past Experiences

What people are is closely related to what they have been. It is often important to ask people what past experiences they have had with health care providers as this may influence the way they will interact with you. If they had a poor outcome from a previous illness, they may not be anxious to participate in measures to restore themselves to health as you would expect them to be (they foresee that the outcome will be poor, no matter what they do).

Environment

People's reactions to situations may differ according to the situation. If you were working as a nurse in an industrial setting, for example, you might find the president of the company rarely demonstrating any qualities but stern control; if you visited him in his home as a community health nurse, however, you might find that he would be very willing—even anxious—to discuss how overwhelmed and out of control he feels at times. If you cared for him in a hospital setting close to the time of a frightening event such as surgery, you might find him sitting by his bed crying. If an employee visited, he would quickly regain his composure. His behavior differs when his environment and his perception of appropriate behavior change.

People in a hospital setting may feel that there is a certain way they should act—be patient, not expect special favors, follow a routine—and so do not make preferences known. In an ambulatory setting such as an emergency room where they do not feel that so many rules apply, you might be surprised to hear that they have strongly voiced opinions. The person does not change but his willingness to express his opinions or emotions may change, depending on the environment in which you care for him.

Life Style

Life style is the manner in which a person conducts his daily activities and responses. It is influenced by his other behavioral characteristics. Some people have a very rigid life style so that each day is more or less like the one before it; others operate with a free-flowing life style that invites constant change and stimulation. Some people choose a life style where they are constantly surrounded by people; others prefer one where they are more or less alone. Some include daily listening to music, working at a hobby, reading for enjoyment; others shun these activities and participate in physical sports. Life style also includes such factors as smoking or not smoking; using alcohol not at all, socially, or heavily; whether a person chooses marriage and children, a nontraditional cohabitation pattern, remaining single, or communal living.

Illness may cause a person to change his life style—to discontinue traveling or participation in sports, for example. If a life style has to be changed, the illness is apt to be perceived by the person as more serious than it would be if no life style modifications were necessary.

Individuality and Nursing Care

Because no two people ever react exactly alike to situations or live exactly identical lives, appropriate nursing care for two people with the same illness, the same physician's orders, and the same prognosis may be vastly different. The most beneficial measures to help people remain well or not become ill may differ widely.

There is a current tendency for some health care agencies to write standard nursing care plans for the

Assessment of Patient Needs Based on Characteristics of Individuality

1. What are the person's special needs based on his level of maturity or development?
2. What are his special needs based on his intelligence or level of education?
3. What are his special needs based on his state of health?
4. What are his special needs based on his environment?
5. What are his special needs based on his temperament?
6. What are his special needs based on his life style?
7. What are his special needs based on his sex?
8. What are his special needs based on the fact that he is unlike any other individual you have ever cared for before?

care of persons with common illnesses such as appendicitis, hernia, or pneumonia. In actuality, there is no such thing as a standard care plan; such plans may actually impede good nursing practice, as they do not focus on individualizing care. For example, Bob Fisher is a 15-year-old patient you must teach about daily insulin injections. You also plan to teach his father so that he can give the injections on any day that Bob does not feel well. Bob approaches new situations reluctantly; he finds the thought of daily injections difficult to adapt to. His father prides himself on quickly taking command of new situations and immediately initiating action. Your teaching plan for Bob, therefore, would probably include a day or two of quiet nonthreatening exploration of his knowledge of his illness and how a daily insulin regimen could be fit into his school schedule; you would not even produce a syringe and needle until the third or fourth day. For his father, on the other hand, you would probably demonstrate the use of syringe and needle on the first day after only a preliminary introduction. Temperament dictates learning styles, and different learning styles require different teaching strategies.

The above box lists different individual characteristics that are important to assess whenever planning care. Quick Reference Stop 10-1 lists basic rules for caring for people with individual characteristics different from your own.

☐ QUICK REFERENCE STOP 10-1: PSYCHOLOGICAL CONSIDERATIONS
Common Rules for Respecting Individual Differences

1. No behavior is right or wrong; any behavior in any situation may be "right" for that individual or moment in time.
2. Don't expect people to react to situations as you do; if their temperament or basic life style is different from yours, their reactions will be different.
3. Assume that people are doing the best they can for that particular circumstance; if their behavior is less than what you would like it to be, it is probably due to the intensity of the circumstances.
4. It is difficult to change basic individual characteristics; it is exceedingly difficult to change when under stress such as an illness.
5. The more people you become acquainted with, the easier it is to accept and appreciate individual differences. Make a point of meeting as many people as possible and discussing their life styles and values with them in order to better prepare yourself to individualize your nursing care based on specific characteristics.

☐ QUICK REFERENCE STOP 10-2: COMMUNITY CONSIDERATIONS
Commonly Accepted Facts Concerning Culture

1. Culture is an organized structure that guides behavior into "acceptable" ways for that group.
2. Each culture differs to some degree from every other; people are proud of cultural traits.
3. Culture is transmitted by formal and informal ways from generation to generation.
4. Although cultural ideas adapt from time to time, they tend to remain constant.
5. Cultural practices arise from environmental conditions (in a country where water is scarce, daily bathing is not practiced, in a country where meat is scarce, ethnic food recipes use little meat).
6. There is a wide variation within a culture as to values and actions because individuals make up the group and individually express their cultural heritage.

CULTURE

Culture may be defined as a view of the world and a set of traditions that a specific social group uses and transmits to the next generation. A person's culture influences his view of himself and his expectations and certainly his approach or lack of approach to health care. Quick Reference Stop 10-2 lists a number of commonly accepted facts concerning culture. Basic rules for respecting cultural differences are listed in Quick Reference Stop 10-3.

A person's *ethnicity* is the cultural group into which he was born. Ethnicity is sometimes used in a narrower context to mean only race. The term *minority* is used to refer to those people who belong to ethnic or cultural groups other than white ethnic groups such as English, Irish, or Swedish. Ethnic people of color (blacks and those of oriental heritage) comprise about 20 percent of the American population. Minority people tend to have a higher incidence of poverty than dominant ethnic groups; along with the problems that people of domi-

> ☐ **QUICK REFERENCE STOP 10-3: PSYCHOLOGICAL CONSIDERATIONS**
> **Basic Rules for Respecting Cultural Differences**
>
> 1. Learn as much about cultures different from your own as you can by reading about them or talking to people from different groups.
> 2. Look at yourself to see what cultural beliefs you hold that you may unconsciously believe are better than other people's beliefs.
> 3. Do not force your cultural values on others; they only work for you, not for everyone you meet.
> 4. Appreciate that cultural values are ingrained or very difficult to change (in yourself or in others).
> 5. Do not stereotype. Cultural behavior is learned; a person who looks Japanese may have more non-Japanese cultural values than the person next to him.
> 6. Remember that poverty is a problem of many minority culture groups. Many characteristics that are ascribed as being cultural are actually the consequence of poverty (seeking medical care late, for example). Solving these problems may have more to do with locating adequate financial sources than overcoming cultural limitations.

nant ethnic groups face, minorities often have the additional disadvantage of discrimination.

Most cultural groups have subcultures as well—smaller divisions of differences within the main group. In America, for example, a subculture (which has its own communication patterns, art forms, and values) is that of adolescents.

All people who move into a new community trade some of their traditions for those of the dominant culture as they become assimilated or *acculturized.* The more different or the more closely knit are the two cultures involved, the less likely will there be a high degree of assimilation or acculturation. *Mutual* culture assimilation may occur, as when Italians moved into American communities: The average Italian family coming to the United States learned to speak English; the average American family learned to cook spaghetti with Italian sauce.

Ethnocentrism is a belief that your own culture is superior to all others. A great deal of ethnocentrism stems from the 1800s when it was considered that the American way (which actually was the northern European way) was the "best" way. Some of this feeling of a "best" culture has been carried through to the present day. You cannot begin to understand how other people feel about situations or appreciate why they think the way they do unless you accept a philosophy that the world is large enough to accommodate a diversity of ideas and behaviors. "Best" for you may not be "best" for the person beside you; his "best" may be far too complicated an action for you to accept as "you." Being able to care for people from all cultures is termed *transcultural nursing* (Leininger, 1979).

Stereotyping

Stereotyping consists of expecting people to act in characteristic manners without regard to individual characteristics; it is generally derogatory in nature. Statements such as "Men never diaper babies well" or "Japanese women are never assertive" are examples of stereotyping. Stereotyping occurs because of lack of exposure to enough people in a particular group and consequently a lack of understanding of the wide range of differences among people. In the above examples, the first speaker, having seen three men change diapers poorly, assumed that these three represented the entire male population. The second example demonstrates lack of knowledge of a changing culture. If the person who believes that all Japanese females are nonassertive was exposed to more Japanese women, she certainly would find that her statement is not true. Using such stereotypes, you could plan health care that would be both inappropriate and resisted.

To avoid stereotyping, meet as many different people from cultures different from your own as you can. Assess each person you meet as an individual, not merely as one of a group. On the other hand, be aware that most people are proud of their cultural characteristics. Making a statement such as, "Hispanic women tend to be caring mothers," does not stereotype but supports a characteristic of which the members of the culture are proud.

Cultural Differences and Their Health Care Implications

When assessing whether cultural influences are present that will make special considerations of care necessary, you need to assess at least eight categories of information.

MALE-FEMALE ROLES

In most cultures the male is the dominant figure; if approval for hospitalization or therapy must be gained, it is usually the man who gives the approval. In a culture where the man is very dominant, the woman is extremely passive, perhaps so passive that she is unable to offer an opinion of her own health and is embarrassed to submit to a physical examination.

In contrast, in native American cultures the woman is often the dominant person in the family. The oldest woman in the home or tribe is the counselor; she would be the person who would have to give consent for hospitalization. It is important to evaluate male-female roles because knowing the dominant person in the household helps you to understand the meaning of the illness and the loss to the family. If a family's dominant person is sick and can no longer make his or her usual decisions, for example, the entire family is likely to be thrown into confusion; if a nondominant member is the ill person, you may have to act as advocate for his rights with the dominant person.

COMMUNICATION ABILITY

People who ordinarily associate only with members of their own culture may have great difficulty detailing a health history in English to a health care provider if English is not their native language. This is a problem not only because of the language barrier, but if the health history is given at a time when they are ill, their coping ability and ability to translate may be at a low point. The person may be able to converse well at work or in stores but not be able to recall the English words for symptoms such as nausea or dizziness; if so, he may omit mentioning the symptom rather than try to pantomime it or describe it in a different way.

Language problems arise not only with foreign languages but from dialects within a country. Something as simple as a New Englander adding an *r* sound to the end of words ending in *a* (idear, not idea) may make an explanation difficult to follow; the slow cadence of a person from the Deep South may seem strange to someone used to the rapid speech pattern of residents of New York City. People who feel that their speech patterns will not be understood may omit speaking, and therefore their needs may go unmet.

TIME ORIENTATION

The United States culture is geared toward punctuality regarding appointments; "time is money" is an often quoted axiom. Other cultures do not have this concern for time. They have a concept that time is to be enjoyed; for such a person there is no such thing as wasted time. In some South Asian cultures being late for appointments is not only a proper but a necessary sign of respect (giving the person you are meeting time to organize and be well prepared for your coming). People who are not accustomed to adhering to schedules may have difficulty following a strict medical regime. If they are told, for example, to take medication at 8 A.M., 12 noon, and 6 P.M. daily and to return for another appointment at 2 P.M. in a week's time, you may have to stress that the important aspect is that the medication be taken three times a day, not the specific times, and that returning for a checkup at a set time is important because the physician who will see them is only in the health care facility at that time.

WORK ORIENTATION

Anglo-American culture stresses that everyone should be employed productively (called the Protestant work ethic) and that work should be a pleasure and valued in itself (as important as the product of the work). Other cultures do not value work in itself but see it as a means to an end (you work to get money). A person with this orientation may be more distressed to learn that an illness will interfere with his ability to continue a hobby (going to baseball games) than with his occupation (teaching). Do not interpret this behavior as "lazy" or unproductive; it is merely a cultural variation.

Possession of material goods is highly valued in the United States, while other cultures revere people who are thinkers or philosophers rather than those who own the biggest cars or grandest homes. Having to take a job that will pay less but offer more free time may be perceived by the person who does not have a drive to possess material goods as a benefit of illness rather than a negative aspect.

PAST, PRESENT, AND FUTURE ORIENTATION

The dominant United States culture is present-future oriented; a person is expected not only to take care of himself at the present moment but at the same time to make plans for his future. Other cultures are past oriented—they carefully preserve past traditions and allow only the slightest change or variations in practices—and still others are present oriented; saving money for college or for retirement is not seen as a desirable action in these cultures. If a person's orientation is to the present or the past, he may have difficulty accepting a long-term rehabilitation plan (by six months he will be crutch walking; by one year he will be back at work and driving his car again); he may need to be motivated by present indications of progress (this afternoon he will be allowed to sit up for the first time; this evening he can begin to have periods of time without oxygen).

FAMILY ORIENTATION

The family structure most common in middle-class communities in America is that of the nuclear family (mother, father, and children). Some other cultures typically form extended families (nuclear family plus aunts, uncles, grandparents, and cousins); such extended families offer many more potential support people in crisis situations and so have many positive attributes. When caring for children from extended families, be certain to identify the child's primary caregiver before you give health care instructions, as the child's natural mother may not be fulfilling this role. Family traditions are well protected when there are many people to maintain them and so are difficult to change; information about the family may be carefully guarded and not given freely at health care visits as a way of keeping the family intact and unique. A family member may feel that he has to sacrifice a personal gain in order to maintain the family's welfare; in some instances such a choice could interfere with a person's regaining good health following an illness, as he might decide not to follow through with care in order to save the family money or might postpone needed surgery until after a child has left home.

PERCEPTION OF ILLNESS

It is generally assumed in the United States that illness is caused by documented factors such as bacteria, viruses, or trauma. In other cultures illness may be viewed primarily as a punishment from God or as caused by an evil spirit or by another person who wishes to harm the person. A person who believes that his own action (being sinful) caused an illness may not be highly motivated to take medication or other measures to get well again (he does not believe that a spoonful of penicillin will cure him). People from some cultures may receive more comfort from a spiritualist or witch doctor than from their physician; they may feel that it is necessary to suffer pain in order to be rid of the illness and are therefore reluctant to ask for medication to make the illness easier for themselves. Understanding this orientation allows you to respect their wishes and to work with them, even though their views are not the same as you would choose for yourself or a member of your family.

NUTRITION PRACTICES

Foods and their methods of preparation are strongly culturally related. In many instances hospital patients cannot find on the menu any foods that appeal to them. Advising a person to have a service such as Meals on Wheels supply him with food daily may be unsatisfactory if the food service is not geared to supplying foods that meet his cultural preferences. A Japanese diet, for example, includes many vegetables like bean sprouts, broccoli, mushrooms, water chestnuts, and alfalfa. Persons with this preference would probably tire very quickly of the corn and peas common to a middle-class American diet.

When a hospitalized person is not eating well, it is easy to conclude that it is due to the person's inactivity or his level of stress-related illness; try to remember that cultural implications may also be present. In most instances a person's family can provide food that appeals to him culturally and is still within his dietary limitations.

Cultural Groups

The United States has a large intermix of cultures because of the constant influx of people into the country. The cultural groups dominant in number or effect are discussed below. Remember that no individual fits all characteristics described since individuality also influences beliefs and actions.

MIDDLE-CLASS AMERICAN CULTURE

Middle-class Americans are the descendants of immigrants who have been in the country for at least two generations. The group is predominantly northern European influenced, white, Anglo-Saxon Protestant (WASPs).

Cultural Orientations. In the middle-class American household the father is the dominant authority figure; the mother, the home maker and child-rearer (although in many instances these roles are played more in public than they actually exist at home). As many as 50 percent of women of child-rearing age now hold at least part-time jobs outside their homes. The women's movement has encouraged women to be assertive and to insist on equal decision-making authority. Remember this when giving instructions to couples about health care. A course of action agreed to by a husband may be modified as soon as his wife is allowed time for her input. Most middle-class Americans have a high school education. The majority are conservative in terms of accepting new programs or actions, taking a middle-of-the-road approach to everything from car buying to food preferences to health care. They are very family oriented; they have a strong motivation to provide a better life for their children than they were provided by their parents and place a strong accent on higher education and increased financial security for their children. If illness interferes with a child's ability to achieve in these areas, it may be felt very strongly.

The Protestant work ethic is a strong influence: Men "ought" to work to support their families, and a man who does not is a failure. On the other hand, work should be accomplished within well accepted roles: For a male being a plumber is all right, while a male ballet dancer is suspect; a woman working as a secretary is respected, while her competing to be a surgeon is suspect. Young adults may need advocacy to help them meet goals that are different from those that their parents want for them. They may need exposure to a larger range of options than their middle-class culture presented to them.

Middle-class Americans tend to be very materialistic. A man measures his neighbor's success more by the make of car parked in his driveway than by the number of books he has read. Remember this when health teaching. If you are advising that an infant drink an iron-rich formula rather than a plain unenriched one, the family who might assume that the fortified milk would cost more may not comply with your advice unless you show them that, although both types cost the same, only the fortified milk has iron.

Middle-class Americans are future oriented. You will learn when you go for job interviews upon graduation from a school of nursing that a not infrequent question that you will be asked is what is your five-year plan or what is your long-term goal? This orientation also means that many people you care for may be more concerned with what an illness will mean to them in the future than its effect today.

The average American professes a personal faith in God but may or may not actively attend church. He may appreciate having a clergyman visit him when he is ill to support and renew a faith he has not practiced regularly.

Health Problems. The average American tends to think of himself as impervious to serious illness and, therefore, does not participate well in programs for promotion of health or prevention of illness unless he sees some concrete benefit from the program. Mothers are more likely to bring their infants to health care centers for well child examinations when they know that the visit will include an immunization rather than just a health history and physical examination.

Due to this avoidance of prevention programs, underimmunization of children is a major health problem. It is gradually being arrested by state laws that require a child to have at least a basic immunization series before attending public school. Cardiovascular illness in men occurs at a high rate due to the stress of being expected to provide financial support for the family and ingesting a diet high in saturated fats, which leads to atherosclerosis or narrowing of blood vessels. Cancer, particularly breast and uterine cancer in women and colon cancer in men, is common. The cause of cancer is unknown but a factor in colon cancer may be lack of roughage in the diet, which leaves pollutants or irritants in contact with the intestinal lining for long periods of time. Respiratory illnesses (lung cancer and emphysema) also occur at high rates due to the tendency of many Americans to smoke cigarettes. As women smoke more than ever before, these illnesses (once almost totally male phenomena) are becoming more common in women.

The average American believes that it is not manly to cry or complain in the face of pain, so men are expected to bear pain and discomfort stoically. Women, on the other hand, are allowed to cry and "act ill"—but not to the point that it is disruptive. This accepted illness behavior can mask a person's true degree of pain or illness. Learn to assess these levels by gestures such as clenched fists or teeth or rapid breathing as well as by verbal descriptions.

Improving Middle-class American Health Care Practices. A number of considerations by health care providers could improve middle-class American responses to health care:

1. Teach that preventive health care is its own reward (the prize is good health) so that preventive practices will be used more extensively.
2. Respect the cost of health care. People who are materially oriented are cost conscious; they weigh the cost of following your instructions against that of not following them.
3. Respect a future orientation. Making plans for future happenings may be as important as present circumstances.

HISPANIC CULTURE

The term *Hispanic* refers to people who use Spanish as their primary language. There are about 12 million documented persons of Mexican, Puerto Rican, Cuban, or other Spanish-speaking origin in the United States; when added to that is the number of people undocumented or living illegally in the country, the total size of this group of people is close to 19 million or about 9 percent of the total population. This statistic makes Spanish-speaking Americans the second largest minority population in the United States (blacks compose about 12 percent of the total population). By 1990 it is estimated that the Hispanic population will have increased to such an extent that this group will be the largest minority (Anthony-Tkach, 1981).

Cultural Orientations. The largest proportion of the Hispanic population are Mexican Americans. In the Mexican American culture the father is a strong dominant force (a characteristic described as *macho*). He takes pride in his ability to support his family and may work at several jobs or long hours at one job to do so. It may be difficult for a man with this aggressive and unyielding orientation to be ill and accept the almost automatic dependency that comes with not being able to fully care for himself. He may find it difficult to depend on other family people to care for him (and it may be equally difficult for him to allow you to do things for him). When caring for a Mexican American man appreciate that he may expect to direct how things are done, such as when he will go to physical therapy or eat breakfast. You may have to analyze your reactions to his manner carefully so that you neither allow yourself to be intimidated past the point of good judgment or, if you are adverse to being directed so pointedly, rebel against his dominating manner.

The Mexican American woman typically finds fulfillment in her role as a wife and mother; she tends to have a warm and nurturing nature, patterning her life style after the warm mothering she received. Mexican American children may be very lonely when separated from such a loving mother; the mother may be just as lonely, because she is dependent for a great deal of her support and companionship on her children or female friends. No child of any culture should be separated from his mother on hospitalization; parents should be allowed to sleep in a bed next to their child. You may have to intercede for the right of the Mexican American mother to this accommodation, as she needs to be with her child for her own as well as her child's health and, not being a dominant person, may not be sufficiently assertive herself.

Mexican American citizens may have little schooling (only 8 years on the average if they were raised in Mexico). As long as a husband is present, it may be difficult for a woman to work outside her home because of the expected cultural submissive role. If left widowed, her ability to support herself may be very limited.

Children in a Mexican American home are taught to

function in their respective male-female roles early in life. Girls are expected to contribute to housecleaning and the care of other children well before and to a greater extent than girls in average middle-class English-speaking homes. Boys are expected to earn money from outside jobs as soon as possible. This orientation may pose a conflict with education, and you may want to support an adolescent who wants more education than his family sees as important for him. This is particularly true of a child who has a handicap. If a child is limited in the type of work that he will be able to do, education for a job that requires more thinking than physical labor may be the key to his being financially independent.

Boys join with others to form strongly bonded gangs, which serve to allow the boy to practice dominance (which he cannot do at home because his father is so powerful); they are important for self-esteem, and upon hospitalization a boy may be as distressed that he has been removed from his gang as from his family. Ask who is the primary caregiver at health visits. In a family with many children some may be raised by aunts or uncles in order to relieve the primary family of the financial burden.

The majority of Hispanics are Roman Catholic and feel strong bonds to the church. Not being able to attend mass or speak with a priest because of a hospitalization may be very difficult. Prior to surgery or following the announcement of a major illness they may be very anxious to speak to a priest. An old Spanish belief is that being out of favor with God is what causes illness, so subconsciously the person may feel that he needs to see a priest not only to benefit his soul but also to heal his body.

Health Problems. The average age of Mexican Americans (24) is slightly lower than that of the average United States citizen (30). This means that in an area of concentrated Mexican American population more health care facilities for children and young adults are needed than are facilities for care of the older adult. Also, Mexican American women tend to have their children at a young age, and adolescent pregnancy is a high risk state because the adolescent's body is still immature.

Nutrition problems, especially vitamin and protein deficiency, may be present. Mexican Americans do not tend to eat a large amount of meat compared with other cultures; they ingest adequate protein, however, by mixing sources of incomplete protein (beans and rice, for example). A family trying to become more Americanized may modify the diet to omit one source of incomplete protein. When Mexican Americans are hospitalized, check to see that they are eating a balanced diet, especially in terms of protein and iron.

Due to less food intake in Mexico than in the United States (for every child 1 to 4 years of age who dies in the United States, 23 die in Mexico, largely from malnutrition) (Anthony-Tkach, 1981) the height and weight of Mexican American children may plot below the average on charts standardized for United States' children. Parasitic infections (round worms) are commonly found in children from Mexico; stool for ova and parasites is generally tested as a routine screening procedure with children who are recently from Mexico or who have visited recently in Mexico.

Mexican Americans tend to be present, not future, oriented. They may omit routine childhood immunization or other preventive practices such as decreased cigarette smoking or consistent exercise.

A major problem that arises in the delivery of health care to Mexican Americans is a communication problem due to the language difference. Families tend to be very close-knit and so it is common for a member of a family, particularly the mother, not to have much exposure to people outside the family or to those who speak English. Many families use a school-age child as an interpreter at health visits, a practice that may be unfair to the child because of the emotional strain due to the seriousness of the health history that he is translating and the hours that this practice causes him to lose from school. It is important to remember that Mexican Americans have a strong family orientation; letting a member be taken away from the group when hospitalization is necessary may be very difficult. A person used to having close support people around him may be very lonely at separation, particularly if communicating in English is difficult. On the other hand, when such a person is discharged from a hospital, in most instances locating someone to care for him until he is ready for full self-care again will be easy, because family members feel such a strong bond for each other.

Illness may be perceived as the result of external forces. A person who believes that he is not responsible for his illness may not participate in efforts to stay well or return to health. Some believe that illness can be caused by "mal ojo" or someone who is envious of them and looking at them with an evil eye; they believe that such illness is difficult to treat because it has been caused by an unnatural force, and so they may not seek professional health care until the problem becomes severe (a baby has had diarrhea for days) because they believe a physician can be of little help with this type of illness. It is easy to discount this type of belief, but it is in reality only an exaggeration of other widely held superstitions like never walking under ladders and knocking on wood.

Mexican American men tend to be very stoic in the face of pain (macho). Women may be very expressive—crying loudly, punching pillows, screaming at people around them. It may be difficult to appreciate that persons acting in these opposite ways have a similar amount of discomfort.

Folk Medicine. The delivery of health care in Mexico is a less structured system than that of the United States; there are few physicians for the total population. Many drugs are available without prescriptions; a local pharmacist, rather than a physician, may serve as the main health care source for many Mexicans.

In Mexico many people first seek help from a member of the family. Such a family member is termed *el que sabe* (he that knows). During an illness this person's approval of therapy may be crucial; if it is not given, the ill person may not comply with therapy. Outside the family structure are *yerbero* (herbalists) who grow and instruct people in the use of herbs or cures; another advice source is healers known as *curandero* who heal by the use of herbs or diet. Other healers are *espiritualistos* who can treat supernaturally caused illnesses and *brujos* who can not only revoke evil spells but turn them around onto others. For many people, turning to a *yerbero* or *curandero* is preferred to professional health care because these people may not charge a fee, only accept donations or an exchange of goods or services. Relating health problems to them is not difficult because there is no language problem.

Improving Mexican American Health Care Practices. A number of considerations by health care providers would improve responses of Mexican Americans to health care:

1. Respect the role of *yerberos* and *curanderos.* Disparaging remarks about such people does not strengthen the person's feelings about professional health care; rather, such a practice tends to demonstrate how little you value the culture of the person you are trying to help.

2. Since Mexican Americans are family oriented, they may be unable to make a decision about therapy such as whether they should have an x-ray without first consulting the family. Allow time for this exchange of information to take place (call the next day to set up the appointment rather than making it on the spot) unless, of course, the person's health would be jeopardized by a delay. It may be very difficult for an individual in a family to do such things as change to a new diet or increase his daily exercise (especially for women, because of male dominance). Try to incorporate the entire family in care so that all members agree to the decision.

3. Take time to record a good health history; the use of an interpreter increases the normal length by at least half. Do not shout to try to make a person who does not understand your language understand you (a common habit). This does not help the person understand any better; it only allows the confused message to reach him in a louder tone of voice.

Mexican American Health Care Providers. Many agencies are actively recruiting Spanish-speaking health care providers in order to better meet the health needs of Hispanics. Unfortunately the number of Hispanic health care providers still remains at a lower number than desired. Part of this difficulty results from the cultural value that a woman's place is with her family and children rather than in a health care setting. Hispanic nurses, translators, and nursing assistants can be extremely important members of a health care team, especially if they bring from their culture a warm and caring approach to people. When working with Mexican American health care providers, be aware that if family responsibilities conflict with work responsibilities, their family may take precedence. Mexican American women are used to conceding to males; you may have to support them at team conferences to prevent their agreeing to the wishes of male members instead of making known their views. When working with male Hispanics, be aware that they may expect to be dominant; you may have to make it clear to male orderlies or aides that your authority is greater than theirs. It may take time to establish a relationship with them that is interdependent and not dependent.

BLACK CULTURE

The black culture in the United States has arisen primarily from African heritage. A smaller number of the 12 million blacks are immigrants from Caribbean islands such as Haiti, Bermuda, or Nassau. Due to problems of education and discrimination, as many as 40 percent of all black families are low-income families; a great many of the problems that black families encounter, therefore, are those associated with extreme poverty.

Cultural Orientations. Middle-class black families tend to be two-parent families, and both parents work in order to earn enough money to maintain a middle-income home. Often one of the parents is a professional. As with any family with two working parents, it may be difficult to schedule routine health maintenance visits or to provide care for an ill child at home. Children may feel pressure to achieve (most plan on a college education) to prevent the family from "slipping backward" in status. Family duties tend to be shared equally as both parents are providing financial support. Children are asked to assume household chores and child care as part of their contribution to the household.

Religion is an important aspect of most black families' life style. Free time for the whole family may be very church or religion oriented, with the family's church not only serving as a spiritual resource but as a recreational and social one as well. Services may concentrate on the singing of gospel songs, a musical form of prayer. The patient who is hospitalized may feel a real need for this type of prayer, and such a religious practice should not be prohibited in a hospital environment; it would not raise the noise level of an average hospital unit any more than the sound of a television set.

Lower income black families tend to be extended in structure (grandparents or aunts or uncles living in the house also) and are often single-parent matriarchal or woman-dominant families (a mother with her daughter and grandchildren). Single-parent families may depend on government programs for income; lack of schooling may make securing a good income difficult. A male friend may frequently visit and serve as a role model for children and as a very important support person for the family.

Many poor black mothers are very young, so the grandmother of the child may be the primary caregiver. Time orientation for lower income families tends to be present oriented; when money has to be stretched from day to day, there is little incentive to think about ways to use money in the future or a future life style.

Blacks tend to eat small meat portions in comparison with northern Europeans. A typical dish consists of pork products boiled with greens (collards). Their diet, known as soul food, tends to be high in sodium and low in iron; it may be deficient in vitamin C due to the loss of vitamin C in boiling. When caring for a black who is hospitalized and not eating well, ask if missing his usual diet is his problem. The taste of institutional cooking is very bland and unappetizing to people used to soul food.

Health Problems. Blacks tend to be more prone to develop tuberculosis and hypertension (high blood pressure) than other groups. The infant mortality of blacks is higher than the average rate (probably due to influences of poverty). For people living in poor housing, lead poisoning (from children eating lead-based paint that has chipped off walls and windowsills) is also high. Sickle cell anemia (distortion of the red blood cell structure that governs oxygen transport) occurs in approximately one out of every 400 black Americans. About one out of every eight black Americans carries the trait of sickle cell anemia (have no symptoms but carry a recessive gene for the disease so their children may inherit the disease). Sickle cell anemia reaches a crisis state if the person should develop a low oxygen level in his blood or become dehydrated. Any person with the disease is at particular threat when he develops a fever with profuse sweating or a respiratory illness because these may cause dehydration or decreased oxygen levels.

Many black Americans also have lactase deficiency, an inability to digest milk because they lack the enzyme lactase. Drinking milk tends to lead to diarrhea and nausea. Lactase deficiency begins to be apparent by school age. Remember that lactase deficiency may exist when a child or adult says that he does not like milk.

Black Americans generally accept illness as an unwanted but acceptable phase of one's life. They welcome health care for the treatment of physical illness; because of their present orientation they may be less receptive to preventive health practices such as immunization programs. Some people may be suspicious and unaccepting of mental health services (afraid that a white therapist will change their thinking to "white thinking").

Folk Medicine. Most black Americans depend on professional health care providers for the full extent of their health care. Older women in a family may be consulted before a health agency visit is arranged. Wearing herbs or amulets around the neck as a preventive measure is not uncommon. Be certain not to remove this type of charm; disrespecting its meaning to the person is the same as disrespecting the person himself.

Measures to Improve the Delivery of Health Care to Black Americans

1. A young mother may have little experience in judging illness. Provide educational opportunities based on a philosophy of "Let me help you learn how to do this better next time," not "You didn't do a good job this time." No one wants to come for health care and be criticized for shortcomings.

2. If poverty is a problem, the cost of health care must be carefully considered. Poor families may not have reliable transportation and returning for follow-up visits may be very difficult if the health care facility is not located close to community transportation systems.

3. The black population is intensely proud of its heritage and of being black. This is evidenced by the popular slogan "Black is beautiful." Be certain in giving instructions that you do not ask a person to violate a value important to him as a black American. Not only will your advice not be followed, but his respect for you will be lost.

4. Inner-city black Americans often speak a dialect unique to their particular area. Learn the cadence and common words, but do not attempt to imitate it. Trying to speak as they do may be misinterpreted as mockery.

5. Encourage greater problem solving and participation in health decisions. Encourage active participation in health care in order to achieve optimal wellness levels.

NATIVE AMERICAN CULTURE

Native American beliefs and values are difficult to categorize as they vary from tribe to tribe and in different sections of the country. In all there are over 600,000 native Americans in the United States. The bulk of this population is in the southwestern states.

Land on which native Americans live was granted to them by the United States in various treaties. Unfortunately great portions of it are waste land that was of little value to settlers moving west and unsuitable for farming. In the 1800s, under a major government project to redistribute the land of native Americans (The Dawes Act), each native American adult was granted an individual portion of land with permission to sell it after 25 years if he so chose. Many native Americans did sell their land at the end of the time period; this left many without either property or money, as they had no source of income without land to farm. Also attempted in the 1800s was an educational project to assimilate native Americans into the general culture. Unfortunately this project taught children about a culture that was not applicable to their own way of living; it left many younger native Americans with a poor estimation of themselves and little respect for their own culture.

Cultural Orientations. The native American culture tends to be matriarchal; the oldest woman in the tribe is often the person who must give approval for action. Kinship ties are strong and often confusing unless you know the family well. A cousin, for example, may actually have been raised as a brother. Remember this when a native American is hospitalized in a section of a hospital where visiting is restricted to family members. A native American may have many "brothers" who all have family status and want to give emotional support.

Traditionally, native American children are raised to be stoic in the face of discomfort or pain. When caring for a person with this tradition, you should offer medication for pain rather than wait for the person to ask for it. Even young infants may adjust to bearing pain without the usual outward signs; do not depend on a baby's crying to let you know that he is in distress.

The time orientation of native Americans tends to be present. They may live a less structured day with less regard for punctuality or rituals than others. This lack of structure may interfere with a health regimen in which medication must be taken at certain time intervals. Future planning may not be a priority.

A native American may avoid making eye contact while speaking as a sign of respect for the other person. Be certain that you do not interpret this cultural variation as disrespect, inattentiveness, or guilt.

Health Problems. Poverty is a problem of many native Americans living on reservations, so measures to promote health such as care during pregnancy or immunizations for children may be lacking. The infant mortality of native Americans is above average, owing to the poverty of reservation life. Health problems that occur frequently are tuberculosis, diabetes, and alcoholism.

Native Americans' religious rituals and health care beliefs are closely associated. People may wear charms to ward off harm; removing one without permission might be very offensive to the person or his family. Many native Americans accept prescriptions and follow a plan of care well but use their own tribal rituals or healing methods in addition. Healing may be aided by the use of prayer ceremonies, herbal applications, or the application of a substance such as cornmeal on or about the bed. Folk medicine practices of this type are thought to be beneficial because of the concept that health is the result of a balance between man and nature. Illness is caused by an imbalance of some kind in which evil thoughts or actions may be involved, and it is thought that remedies other than a physician's prescription are more suitable to correct this type of imbalance.

Improving Health Care for Native Americans

1. Native Americans are concerned with the harmonious relationship of man and nature. They respect and preserve life around them and expect their privacy and life style to be respected in return. They will return loyalty to health care providers who show respect for their needs but may give little cooperation to someone who does not make an effort to understand what is important to them and why.

2. Health care for native Americans is provided free in native American health service facilities. Although such facilities offer high level care, people may resent the little choice of care available to them.

3. Emotional problems of native Americans are increasing in incidence (both the suicide and homicide rate for native Americans is higher than the average rate). Be sure to offer emotional as well as physical care.

4. Native Americans may believe very strongly in home remedies or herbal cures. Knowing what remedies the person is taking may avoid medication toxicity as a result of his being given the same herb in medicine form.

5. Native Americans tend to use touch less than some other cultures. Assess whether a patient wants this type of support or would prefer a close but not touching presence.

CHINESE AMERICAN CULTURE

The largest numbers of Chinese Americans are concentrated on the West Coast; large cities on the Eastern Coast have fewer numbers. Because there is such a concentration of Chinese Americans in cities, less cultural assimilation may take place than happens with other immigrants.

Cultural Orientations. The Chinese American family tends to be a patriarchal (father-dominated) extended one. Obedience and respect for elders are strongly stressed. Older Chinese Americans are cared for by family members as a rule, and fewer health care facilities, extended care centers, or nursing homes are used. Even those families that at first seem nuclear in structure (only mother, father, and children) are apt to maintain strong psychological bonds if not close physical bonds to an extended family.

Chinese Americans believe that people are responsible for their own lives and welfare and encourage family members to be independent and responsible for self-care. Education is highly valued; the ability to think and reason is regarded as superior to physical ability.

Health Problems. Chinese Americans who immigrated to the United States in the 1930s and 1940s have retained their cultural orientations so strongly that they may still rely more on traditional Chinese practices than on professional health care. Traditional practices of Chinese medicine are based on the belief that health can exist only when two opposing energy forces (Yin and Yang) are balanced. Yin is viewed as a female force (also emptiness and cold). Yang is a male force (also warmth and fullness). If the Yin force should overpower the Yang force, the person may develop Yang-dominated diseases such as gastrointestinal disorders. If the Yang force should overpower the Yin one, Yin-dominated diseases such as dehydration may result.

The importance of balancing Yin and Yang forces is stressed in meal preparation. Meals must be balanced with both hot and cold food (Yin and Yang opposites). If the person's illness is perceived as a "hot" one, he may be reluctant to eat what he perceives to be hot foods and vice versa. Ask Chinese Americans who are eating poorly what foods they think might make them feel better. Help them speak to the dietician or arrange for a family member to bring in meals that will meet any dietary restrictions present and at the same time provide the kind of food that the patient prefers.

Chinese Americans may also believe very strongly in herbal therapy. Ask as part of a health history if the person is taking any home remedies to avoid the possibility of their physician's prescribing the same compound in a medication. Ingesting both sources of a drug may lead to toxicity.

Although acupuncture is not used a great deal in the United States, many older adults or those of any age who are unhappy with health care delivery practices may rely on an acupuncturist as their primary health care provider. Acupuncture is the placing of long slender needles into the skin at designated points on the body. Energy flow from the needles follows body meridians or lines to specific body parts, initiating changes in the body part. Acupuncture appears to be a method of anesthesia by the principle of distraction (and is used in China for many surgery procedures very effectively). It is well documented as a means of pain relief in susceptible individuals.

Many of the health problems of Chinese Americans are related to poverty (malnutrition and dental caries) and crowded living conditions (tuberculosis).

The Chinese American diet is so different from the typical northern European diet (small meat portions, many and varied vegetables) that Chinese Americans may have a great deal of difficulty eating institutional food; they may develop constipation if they discontinue the large amount of natural bulk and fiber foods that their diet normally provides.

Improving Health Care Delivery for Chinese Americans

1. Chinese Americans rely strongly on the advice of senior family members. They may need time to consult with such members before they can make a health care decision such as choosing between two alternatives for therapy.

2. Chinese Americans may not make eye contact during an interview. This shows respect for the other's position and importance and is a compliment, not avoidance of the issues.

3. People who spend the majority of their time in a close-knit community structure may learn little English. In order not to offend you by telling you that they do not understand what you are saying, they may nod and appear to agree with you. Ask a family member to help you assess the degree of understanding. Make a note in the nursing care plan that the person's nod may be a respectful "I'm listening," not "I'm understanding."

4. Chinese Americans may have had a bad experience in the past with a health care provider who disregarded their strong need for family contact or some aspect of their diet. You may have to demonstrate by a consistent caring attitude that you are going to respect these needs before you gain the cooperation of such patients.

APPALACHIAN CULTURE

The Appalachian region of the United States is the region from western New York to northeastern Mississippi; the core of this area is West Virginia, eastern Kentucky, and eastern Tennessee. Although many people in this region enjoy middle-class status, at least 20 percent of people live at a poverty level.

Cultural Orientations. Families in the Appalachian area tend to be extended; they are patriarchal, with sharp distinctions between men's and women's work and responsibilities. Men make the final decisions on health care, as they do in all areas of family life. Family ties and loyalty are very strong; there may be stiff opposition between two families, and they may have difficulty sharing a waiting room at a health care facility if the rivalry between the two groups is intense. People from the region may be antagonistic toward a new health care provider until she proves herself trustworthy. People do not join groups readily because of this intense suspiciousness of other people; organizing activities such as an exercise program or a diabetic teaching group might therefore be ineffective in this region.

People are very family oriented. It would be regarded as a loss of face if for some reason a child had to be raised by relatives.

Time orientation tends to be in the present; when money must be stretched from day to day, it is difficult to look ahead at what will happen tomorrow. Education is not stressed; many adults leave school after the eighth grade to help with the family farm (the soil in the area is poor, and crops are grown only at a great investment of time and energy).

Health Problems. Many men in Appalachia are coal miners; they spend long hours underground in cramped and sometimes unsafe locations. Their wives are left to take full responsibility for child care for long periods of time during the day if work shifts are extensive. For the young mother (and girls tend to marry in their adolescence) this degree of responsibility may lead to unwise health care decisions. If she is home alone without transportation, she may be unable to bring an ill child to a care facility as soon as she would like; she may neglect preventive aspects of care such as immunizations due to transportation difficulties. Pride in being able to make a living despite poor soil makes people unwilling to accept charity; therefore, while they cannot afford to pay for care, they will not accept it if the service is free.

Because of the long exposure to coal dust which is irritating to lung tissue, men have a high incidence of sarcoidosis (black lung), a debilitating lung disease. They may have other physical disabilities from accidents working in unapproved and unsafe "punch" mines. As many families exist at a poverty level, portions of meat in the diet may be small; overall the diet may be deficient in protein and iron. Meat is often boiled with vegetables and thus vitamin C may be lost.

Measures to Improve Health Care Delivery for Appalachians

1. Appalachian citizens do not as a group accept outsiders well. Be sure you are accepted by the people you care for before you begin to make changes. Otherwise you will confront a poor or absent compliance level.

2. Arrange health care services to fit the times of the day when men are home from work. Otherwise women have no transportation available to bring them for health care visits.

3. Appalachian people often are not enthusiastic in affect (facial expression); although they give warm loving care to infants, they may not make physical contact with other family members as readily as other cultures. This is not a measure of noncaring but a cultural variation where touch is not seen as necessary to convey affection.

4. Appalachian people often demonstrate a firm sense of pride in their ability to be independent; unable to pay for health care, they may barter with crops. Unwilling to accept charity, if an exchange gift is refused, they may not return for future care. They may resist available government supplements so strongly that they live at a poverty level more intense than other cultural groups around them who accept these forms of help. Respect the pride that this form of living offers them, even if you disagree with it.

SOUTHEAST ASIAN CULTURE

During 1980 as many as 14,000 people from Southeast Asia arrived in the United States each month. They came primarily from Indochina, Vietnam, Cambodia, and Laos. The beginning of their journey consisted of crossing 900 miles of the South China Sea in rickety, practically unseaworthy boats.

Cultural Orientation. Men are the decision makers in Southeast Asia. Education levels are generally extremely low for both men and women. It is difficult for most people to learn English as the dialects of these nations and their language structures are so different from English that it is difficult to transpose the two. Time orientation is the present. Time, as a whole, is not an important entity; Laotians in particular may arrive an hour late for appointments as a form of respect for the person setting the appointment.

Health Problems. People from Southeast Asia have the problems of people from all poor nations: malnutrition, tuberculosis, dental caries. They often have few immunizations, and eye and ear disease may have left them with vision and hearing handicaps. There is a high incidence of parasitic and hepatitis B infection. Many are lactase deficient and have difficulty digesting milk; ingestion of milk as a dietary staple will lead to chronic diarrhea and dehydration.

Hospitals in Southeast Asia are informal; when a person is hospitalized, his family accompanies and stays at the hospital with him. Therefore, the concept of limited hospital visiting hours is poorly understood; it may be desirable to arrange less structured visiting hours for people whose cultural orientation is so different from that of middle-class Americans.

Hand-me-down clothing may be poorly accepted, as it is commonly believed that the bad luck of a person remains in his possessions. Diapers are not used with infants. Charms such as small bells may be hung around the neck for good luck.

Southeast Asians do not use touch extensively and actually may find a common motion such as rumpling a child's hair intrusive and destructive. Fears and anxieties may be rarely mentioned; present fears or problems that seem serious to you may not appear so to the person who has experienced the distress of traveling a great distance to a new home.

Changing Cultural Concepts

In the 1800s when there were a large number of immigrants from many different countries coming into the United States, the United States was viewed as a giant cultural "melting pot" where all new arrivals gave up their native country's traditions and values and became "Americans." Any behavior that was not like that of middle-class Americans was viewed as strange and inferior and a mark that one was a new immigrant or had lower socioeconomic status.

Today the idea that America ever was a melting pot is being questioned; in addition, it is being stressed that retaining cultural values and traditions is not only acceptable but preferred. Retaining ethnic traditions strengthens and enriches family life; it provides security to younger family members to realize that they are one of a continuing line of people (have a past and will have a future).

It is important not only to respect people's cultural differences but to help people to share their cultural beliefs with you and other health care providers so that they can be known and honored. As a nurse you will have the opportunity to meet many people who hold different cultural values from your own. Respecting cultural differences is as important in giving holistic care as respecting individual traits or characteristics, as important to include in planning as any other element of care.

UTILIZING NURSING PROCESS

Briar Aldaves is a patient hospitalized for a fractured tibia. She has a cast in place on her right leg. She will be on bedrest for three days, then gradually be allowed to learn crutch walking.

In planning care for her, you make an attempt to include some culturally important aspects in her care, as follows:

Characteristic to be Respected	*Implementation*
Importance of family orientation; male dominated culture	Consult with husband regarding aspects of care
Importance of present time orientation	Talk mainly of current problems (bedrest) rather than future care at home
Importance of including Mexican American foods in diet	Speak to dietician about avoiding milk as lactose deficiency may be present

On the third day of Mrs. Aldaves' hospitalization, you read the following nurse's note in her chart: "Mrs. Aldaves discovered crying. Stated she feels as if she is being treated as a second-rate person whose opinions are unimportant (husband is asked for more input about her health than she is). She is concerned about how she will manage at home because she has a two-month-old child to care for and sees this as difficult with crutches; concerned that bone healing is taking place more slowly than necessary because she has had so little milk to drink."

After reading the note, you wonder what could have gone wrong. You set out deliberately to respect Mexican American cultural preferences in her care, yet it is these very things that seem to be making her unhappy. Complete the Questions for Review; then read the solution to this nursing care plan problem, which follows the Questions.

SUGGESTED READINGS

Anthony-Tkach, C. Care of the Mexican American patient. *Nursing and Health Care* 11:424, 1981.

Bailey, F. E., et al. Socio-economic factors and their effects on the nutrition and dietary habits of the black aged. *J. Gerontol. Nurs.* 8:203, 1982.

Becerra, R. M. Knowledge and use of child health services by Chinese Americans. *Health Soc. Work* 6:29, 1981.

Betz, C. L. Faith development in children. *Pediatr. Nurs.* 7:22, 1981.

Bhanunathi, P. P. Nurses' conception of "sick role" and "good patient behavior": A cross cultural comparison. *Internat. Nurs. Rev.* 24:20, 1977.

Bullough, V., and Bullough, B. *Health Care for the Other Americans.* New York: Appleton-Century-Crofts, 1982.

Carpio, B. The adolescent immigrant. *Canad. Nurse* 77:27, 1981.

Cheung, L., et al. The Chinese elderly and family structure: Implications for health care. *Public Health Rep.* 95:491, 1980.

Dahl, J. Transcultural communication on depression with Chinese nurses and physicians. *J. Psychosoc. Nurs. Ment. Health Serv.* 21(2):14, 1983.

Davis, M., et al. A model for cultural assessment of the new immigrant. *Canad. Nurse* 77:22, 1981.

Delgado, M. Hispanic natural support systems: Implications for mental health services. *J. Psychosoc. Nurs. Ment. Health Serv.* 21(4):19, 1983.

Drakulic, L., et al. The East Indian family in Canada. *Canad. Nurse* 77:24, 1981.

Fanning, J. A. Culture. In C. C. Hanes and D. H. Joseph (Eds.) *Basic Concepts of Helping.* New York: Appleton-Century-Crofts, 1980.

Green, M., and Solnit, A. Reactions to the threatened loss of a child: A vulnerable child syndrome. *Pediatrics* 34:58, 1964.

Grosso, C., et al. The Vietnamese American family . . . and grandma makes three. *M.C.N.* 6:177, 1981.

Guerra, F. A. Hispanic child health issues. *Child. Today* 9:18, 1980.

Kalisch, B. J., et al. Minority nurses in the news. *Nurs. Outlook* 29:49, 1981.

Leininger, M. *Transcultural Nursing.* St. Paul, Minn.: Masson Publications, 1979.

Martinez, R. *Hispanic Culture and Health Care.* St. Louis: Mosby, 1978.

Meleis, A. The Arab American in the health care system. *Am. J. Nurs.* 81:1180, 1981.

Mitchell, A. C. Barriers to therapeutic communication with black clients. *Nurs. Outlook* 26:109, 1978.

Muecke, M. Caring for Southeast Asian refugee patients in the USA. *Am. J. Public Health* 73(4):431, 1983.

Pickwell, S. M. Primary health care for Indochinese refugee children. *Pediatr. Nurs.* 8:104, 1982.

Primeaux, M. Caring for the American Indian patient. *Am. J. Nurs.* 77:91, 1977.

Rocereto, L. V. Selected health beliefs of Vietnamese refugees. *J. Sch. Health* 51:63, 1981.

Schafft, G. Health care for racial and ethnic minorities and handicapped persons. *J. Long-term Care Adm.* 8:37, 1980.

Shutin, S. Nursing patients from different cultures. *Nursing 80* 10:78, 1980.

Spector, R. *Cultural Diversity in Health and Illness.* New York: Appleton-Century-Crofts, 1979.

Thomas, A., and Ches, S. *Temperament and Development.* New York: Brunner/Maxe, 1977.

Tripp-Reimer, T. Retention of a folk-healing practice (Matiasma) among four generations of urban Greek immigrants. *Nurs. Res.* 32(2):97, 1983.

White, E. H. Giving health care to minority patients. *Nurs. Clin. North Am.* 12:37, 1977.

QUESTIONS FOR REVIEW

1. Mr. Jack's heritage is Native American. He tells you that he comes from a large family, which you analyze as extended in structure. In planning care for Mr. Jack in the hospital, which factor would you plan for?
   a. Restricting visitors to reduce the noise level.
   b. Organizing nursing care at times other than visiting hours.
   c. Asking the hospital "visitor program" to see him to prevent loneliness.
   d. Spending increased time with him yourself to prevent loneliness.

2. You view Mr. Jack as poor because he describes his home as a "dirt floor" house. Considering Mr. Jack's family structure, in which way might he view you as "poor"?
   a. You do not practice his religion.
   b. You own only one student nurse's uniform.
   c. You are unmarried and live alone.
   d. You stated you value honesty.

3. Mr. Jack is hospitalized with pneumonia. He insists on turning his bed since he believes that facing the North Star while he sleeps will make him heal faster. You best response to this practice is to:
   a. Allow the change as long as you can still view his face from the room doorway.
   b. State the hospital disapproves of moving beds to discourage him.
   c. Ask the physician to explain that bed position makes no difference.
   d. Explain yourself that curing infection and bed position are unrelated.

4. Miss Crawford is a black American whom you visit at home. You are concerned that she does not eat enough vegetables. She states that she is preparing "makings" for dinner. You are unfamiliar with this term. In light of this what would your best response to the situation be?
   a. "I hope you eat that with a vegetable."
   b. "I wish you'd eat more spinach and corn."
   c. "Black cooking always sounds exciting; can I have your recipe?"
   d. "I don't know what makings means."

5. Miss Crawford has a mole on her wrist that is growing. She states that before coming to the hospital to have it removed she wants to have the "evil taken from it" by a voodoo doctor. Your best response to this would be:
   a. Encourage her to make both appointments for care promptly.
   b. State that you thought voodoo doctors were found only in bad movies.
   c. Explain that a growing mole is a danger sign of cancer.
   d. State that voodoo doctors are not licensed physicians.

6. Mr. Wojoynsiak is of Polish heritage. He is angry on hospital admission because so many people have asked him how to pronounce his name. Your best response to him would be:
   a. "Polish names *are* pronounced strangely."
   b. "No one ever says my name correctly either."
   c. "I'll mark in the nursing care plan how to say it correctly."
   d. "Why don't I call you Mr. Wojo? Then I can't say it wrong."

NURSING CARE PLANNING SOLUTION

The error made in Mrs. Aldaves' care plan was in assuming that she was Mexican-American. Rather, her husband is a Mexican-American; she is English-Irish, considers herself an equal to her husband, and would have listed milk as a favorite beverage if asked.

This mistake is a common one—jumping past the step of assessment to rely on stereotyping or assuming that people's names or appearances reflect their cultural patterns. In order to truly meet Mrs. Aldaves' needs, you need to return to a reassessment step and work through the process of analysis, planning, implementation, and evaluation.

11. LEVELS OF HEALTH

OBJECTIVES

Upon mastery of the material in this chapter, you should be able to:

1. Define health according to the World Health Organization.
2. Describe the health belief model.
3. Define the wellness-illness continuum.
4. Describe wellness behavior.
5. Describe levels of health and the implications of these for nursing.
6. Identify the common expectations that accompany the sick role.
7. Describe common reactions to health and illness in different age groups.
8. Describe effects of illness on the individual, the family, and the community.
9. Describe the interrelated effects of illness, the ill person, and the circumstances present at the time of illness.

TERMS

The terms important for an understanding of this chapter are shown below and defined in the glossary:

health
high-level wellness
illness
sick role
sign
symptom

One of the most difficult concepts to define is that of wellness, because what one person defines as feeling well another may view as feeling ill. It is equally difficult to define disease or illness for the same reason.

In 1947 the World Health Organization (WHO) stated in its constitution a definition of health as "a state of complete physical, mental, and social well-being and not merely the absence of disease or infirmity." It is important to note that, according to this well-accepted definition, in order to be in good health, it is not enough that a person is free of any type of physical symptoms of disease; he also must feel good about his present state (mental and social well-being).

Although the World Health Organization definition is widely accepted, it is also criticized as being too ideal. If, for example, you consider the large number of people who have some type of refractive error of vision (lack of physical well-being) or who find themselves shyer than they would like to be in large crowds (lack of mental and social well-being), there are very few people who fulfill the definition of being completely well.

By this definition, it is even less easy to categorize people such as children born with a congenital deformity of a finger who, despite this one handicap, function in school on an equal basis with their peers; or men who have recovered from myocardial infarctions (heart attacks) and have returned to their former occupations and family roles. These people do not have complete physical, mental, and social health; neither are they ill, because they function as well people and, in most instances, want to be treated as well people. Figure 11-1 shows an older man recently discharged from the hospital who considers himself a well person.

Dubos has advanced a more theoretical method for looking at health and illness. He summarizes his philosophy by saying that "perfect health . . . is an illusion. Complete freedom of disease and from struggle is almost incompatible with the process of living." He views the search for health and the process of maintaining it as an ongoing process (Dubos, 1979).

Dunn views health and illness not as entities that can be easily separated from one another but as ends of a continuum or opposite ends of a scale. By this theory at any point in time a person may be at high-level wellness at the upper end of the scale or at any intermediate points of low-level wellness, minor illness, or severe illness, until his death, which is at the opposite end of the continuum (Dunn, 1961). Due to the wide scope of nursing practice today, nurses care for people at all points on the wellness-illness continuum (Fig. 11-2).

HEALTH

Health is a dynamic, ever-changing state; it is achieved only if a person can adapt successfully to changing situations in his internal and external environments. It is important that health care providers try to restore

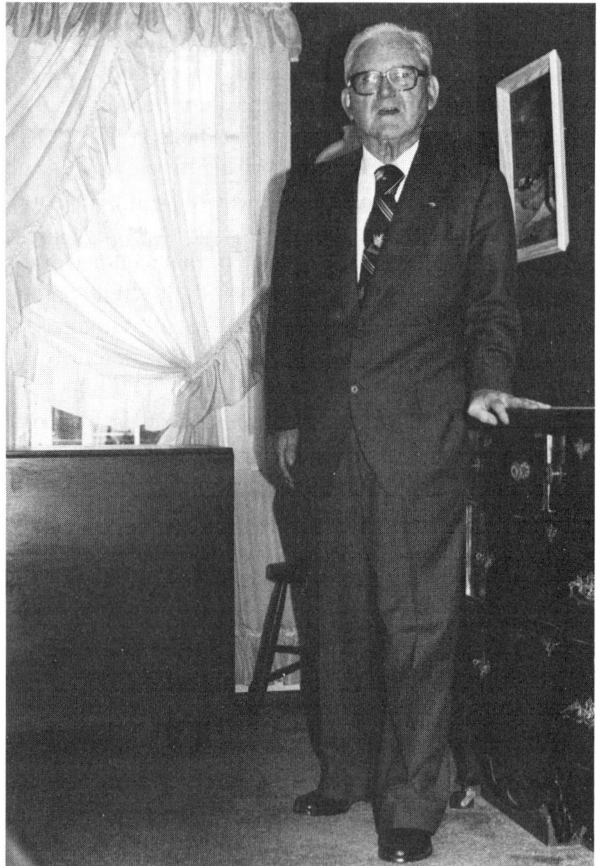

FIGURE 11-1. This older man walks more slowly and sees less well than he once did; however, he considers himself a well person.

Continuum	Points of nursing contact
High level wellness	Teaching classes on normal childbearing, nutrition, safety, coping with stress School health settings Mental health settings Assisting with annual health examinations, health maintenance visits
Low level wellness	Ambulatory care settings, industrial health settings Hospital admission for minor surgery, counseling settings
Minor illness	Emergency care settings, home care, ambulatory care settings Extended care facilities Half-way houses
Serious illness	Acute care settings Hospital admissions
Death	Intensive care settings, home care Hospice care, extended care settings

FIGURE 11-2. The wellness-illness continuum (left column) and points of nursing contact (right column). (Modified from H. Dunn, *High Level Wellness.* Arlington, Va.: Beatty, 1961.)

people to an optimal level of health, as a person who is truly well not only feels well physically but also feels good about his accomplishments and relationships in life and is able to take actions to keep himself well. Table 11-1 contrasts wellness behavior with illness behavior. It is interesting to compare the actions of patients you care for or your own actions with those of the table to see if you and others manifest more wellness or illness behaviors.

Helping people to achieve an optimal level of wellness is an important nursing concern. You can expect, for example, to see Bob Fisher, a 15-year-old recently diagnosed as having diabetes, brought back to a state of glucose-insulin equilibrium or a state of physical health by his physician's interventions. (This is not an easy accomplishment; it requires a great deal of professional judgment and analysis.) Before it can be said that Bob is optimally well again, however, he needs to learn to administer daily insulin injections himself; to balance periods of activity and rest; to conform to certain dietary restrictions; and to reestablish his self-image from "I am a diabetic" to "I am a 15-year-old able to live a normal life." Without these measures he will not be independent and will be unable to demonstrate many of the wellness behaviors shown in Table 11-1. It is a mark of a professional nurse to take this extra step: To complement medical care by moving the level of health in people cared for beyond low-level wellness.

As another example, Mrs. Rodrigues is a 65-year-old woman you care for because she is hospitalized for a persistent urinary tract infection. You can expect her physician to be able to cure this infection by the use of antibiotics, but before you can consider that she has returned to high-level wellness you need to be certain that she has adequate support people (many older persons do not), that she is returning to a community where the environment is safe for her, and that she will take some measures to prevent the reoccurrence of urinary tract infection such as good perineal hygiene and a high daily fluid intake. The concern for establishing optimal health levels is one of the factors that makes a nurse such an important member of a health care team. It is what raises the quality of health care from adequate to superior.

The Health Belief Model

Rosenstack is a social psychologist who has proposed a model for analyzing a person's health behavior, called a *health belief model.* By this model you can assess a person's perception of his susceptibility to and the se-

TABLE 11-1. ASSESSMENT OF WELLNESS AND ILLNESS BEHAVIOR

Area of Assessment	Wellness Behavior	Illness Behavior
Family life	Is an active, contributing member of a family. Takes measures to protect against fire and hazards in home (has a fire alarm; uses proper size fuses; has a fire extinguisher in kitchen). Arranges a set time daily for members to "touch base" with each other. Shares feelings with family members and encourages time to share feelings with them.	Depends on the family to provide for his needs or is in opposition to family. Maintains unsafe living quarters. Operates as a "loner" in respect to other family members.
Self-responsibility	Is able to say no without feeling guilty. Can problem solve on daily problems. Can delay immediate rewards for future greater rewards. Does not spend time worrying about problems that are out of his realm to solve. Rarely takes medication other than vitamins or oral iron. Maintains weight within 15% of ideal weight for age and height. Drives defensively and with the use of a seat belt.	Is afraid to say no for fear of being disliked. Is unable to solve problems without extensive aid from others. Is unable to delay immediate satisfaction. Becomes frustrated over problems that are out of his realm to solve. Depends on medication for stimulant or depressant effects. Is over- or underweight by more than 15%. Expects other drivers to respect him; avoids use of seat belts and car seats for children.
Mood	Finds it easy to laugh. Has more "good" moments than "bad" moments. Expresses anger, fear, sadness, and happiness easily and in constructive ways. Has no nervous habits such as biting fingernails.	Exhibits a sad, angry, or inconsistent mood quality most of the time. Allows outbursts of emotion to interfere with daily interactions or contains emotions. Exhibits nervous mechanisms.
Sexual role	Finds fulfillment in sexual role. Takes responsibility for reproductive life planning.	Finds his sexual role unfulfilling. Unwilling to consider the consequences of sexual relationships.
Life style	Maintains a life style that is fulfilling to himself and those important to him.	Maintains a life style that is detrimental to himself or caring others.
Self-esteem	Views himself as a worthwhile contributing person. Tries to role model measures of good citizenship.	Feels he is less than others; that his suggestions would not be well received by others.
Future outlook	Able to make future plans and set realistic goals for himself.	Makes few future plans; goals are unrealistic for situation or capabilities. Talks or plans about ending life.
Personal care	Is responsible for self-care. Does not smoke. Limits alcohol consumption to none or during social interaction. If a woman, does monthly self breast examinations, and has a Pap test done every 3 years. If a man, does monthly testicular self-examinations; if over age 45, has a yearly prostate gland exam. Avoids or uses protection to guard against loud noise levels to prevent hearing damage. Keeps immunization level up-to-date. Is aware of incidence of dental disease, uses good techniques of oral hygiene, and has a yearly examination. Uses little salt in foods; eats a diet high in uncooked fruits and vegetables. Includes basic 5 food groups in meal pattern every week. Plans for and achieves adequate rest and sleep.	Depends on others for self-care or neglects self-care. Smokes over a pack of cigarettes a day. Drinks excessively or alone. Does not carry out self-examination techniques or does them only sporadically. Exposes himself to excess noise levels. Neglects suggested immunizations. Brushes teeth infrequently, does not use dental floss, eats many sweetened foods, neglects a yearly examination. Neglects to eat one or more of 5 basic food groups. Maintains an inconsistent or inadequate pattern of rest and sleep.

TABLE 11-1. (CONTINUED)

Area of Assessment	Wellness Behavior	Illness Behavior
Work or school practices	Achieves at work or school setting. Has few absences. Usually enjoys the work he does. Feels financially secure (or has an active plan for achieving security). Is able to accept constructive criticism. Rarely feels tired or fatigued.	Totally involves himself in school or work to the detriment of other life facets or finds work or school requires more concentration or effort than he can expend. Is absent frequently. Lives "beyond his means" and does not see a route for improving this. Reacts defensively to criticism. Feels chronic fatigue and lack of energy.
Social contacts	Has at least 1 person he can identify as a loyal, dependable friend. Plans social contacts for both how much he enjoys the association and the importance of the contact to the other person. Can occupy himself during a time span when he is alone. Enjoys touching and being touched by other people.	Has few friends or no friends. Tends to make social contacts for business or because of "obligations," not enjoyment. Resists being alone or is bored if others are not around. Resents others touching him; rarely spontaneously touches.
Recreation	Maintains a consistent program of moderate physical effort recognizing age and capabilities. Regularly walks or bicycles instead of taking car for short errands. Does anaerobic or muscle toning exercises at least 2 times weekly. Climbs stairs of 1 flight rather than uses elevator.	Maintains a recreation program that is too intense or not consistent. Rarely walks or exercises. Never uses stairway even to walk down.
Community awareness	Is an active, contributing member of neighborhood and community; works at one or more community improvement projects a year, and belongs to at least one community organization such as church or political group. Votes regularly; is well informed of local, national, and world events. Knows neighbors and is considerate of their property and needs. Recycles articles to limit environmental pollution; supports programs that encourage clean air and water. Prevents crime by supporting police authority.	Is poorly informed and does not participate in community or national issues or concerns.

riousness of an illness, the modifying factors present, and the likelihood of his taking action concerning the problem (Rosenstack, 1974).

SUSCEPTIBILITY TO AND SERIOUSNESS OF ILLNESS

Whether a person sees himself as someone prone to illness or resistant to it is influenced by his culture, knowledge, and emotional makeup. Almost everyone in a program of nursing finds that when she begins to learn about the incidence and signs and symptoms of many diseases she believes she has some of these illnesses (you are at the age where the peak incidence of the disease falls and you have two of the symptoms). It is a frightening time and only passes when you learn more about the illness (you do not have the other eight symptoms of the illness) or a health care provider assures you that you are not ill. Many people you will care for constantly view themselves as having illness or being very susceptible to illness. Remember that haunting uncomfortable fear that you lived with during the time you were worrying that you had every illness you read about. It will allow you to be empathetic to individuals who constantly live with this level of dread and prevent you from labeling such people hypochondriacs and ignoring them. This diagnosis may be correct for them (they are not ill, only worried about being ill); but while they may be incorrect about the condition, they are not incorrect about the *fear* that accompanies the belief that one is ill. It is very real and needs to be dealt with.

People who have poor self-esteem tend to see themselves as more susceptible to illness than people with high self-esteem. A child always described by his parents as stringy and pale rather than tall and fair may grow up thinking of himself as weak and more prone to illness than a brother or sister. The amount of responsibility a person must assume also influences how ill a person sees himself as being. A student nurse, for example, may quickly categorize herself as ill at the first signs of a cold and excuse herself from class and laboratory experience. In another year's time, working as a nurse in a busy hospital unit when there are many people depending on her presence, she will continue to work with the same symptoms, categorizing herself as well. Mothers of young children function in the same way, rarely categorizing themselves as ill, even though they have the same degree of an upper respiratory infection as the children they keep home from school.

MODIFYING FACTORS

Factors that may modify a person's perception of susceptibility to illness or seriousness of illness are increased knowledge of the disease due to television announcements or pamphlets, advice from friends or family members, prior contact with the disease, age, intelligence level, and level of support people present. These modifying factors can cause the person to see himself as more or less susceptible to illness or to categorize the illness as more or less serious, depending on the individual advice he receives.

A woman who is pregnant discovers that her gum line bleeds as she brushes her teeth. At first she thinks there could not be anything wrong: "I'm young and healthy." Then she hears a television announcement that bleeding is one of the seven danger signals of cancer. She starts to worry that she has oral cancer. She will persist in this worry until she receives assurance from a health care provider that bleeding of this nature is not uncommon during pregnancy, and since she does not have other symptoms of oral cancer (a lesion that does not heal, loss of weight), she does not have the disease.

LIKELIHOOD OF ACTION

Whether a person will take action to prevent illness by taking sensible steps such as stopping smoking or having a yearly health appraisal depends on the perceived *benefit* of this type of action compared to the perceived *barriers* to such actions. The woman who is concerned she may have oral cancer wants to consult a health care provider, but if the health care facility is not on a public transportation line and she does not have a car, she may not go. Many women with signs of possible genital disorders (unexplained vaginal bleeding) delay going for care until symptoms are severe because they dislike pelvic examinations. A man who knows he should stop smoking to benefit his lungs may not do so because he enjoys smoking too much to give it up.

Health Belief and Nursing

Figure 11-3 depicts the health belief model. Nurses play a major role in helping people monitor wellness by

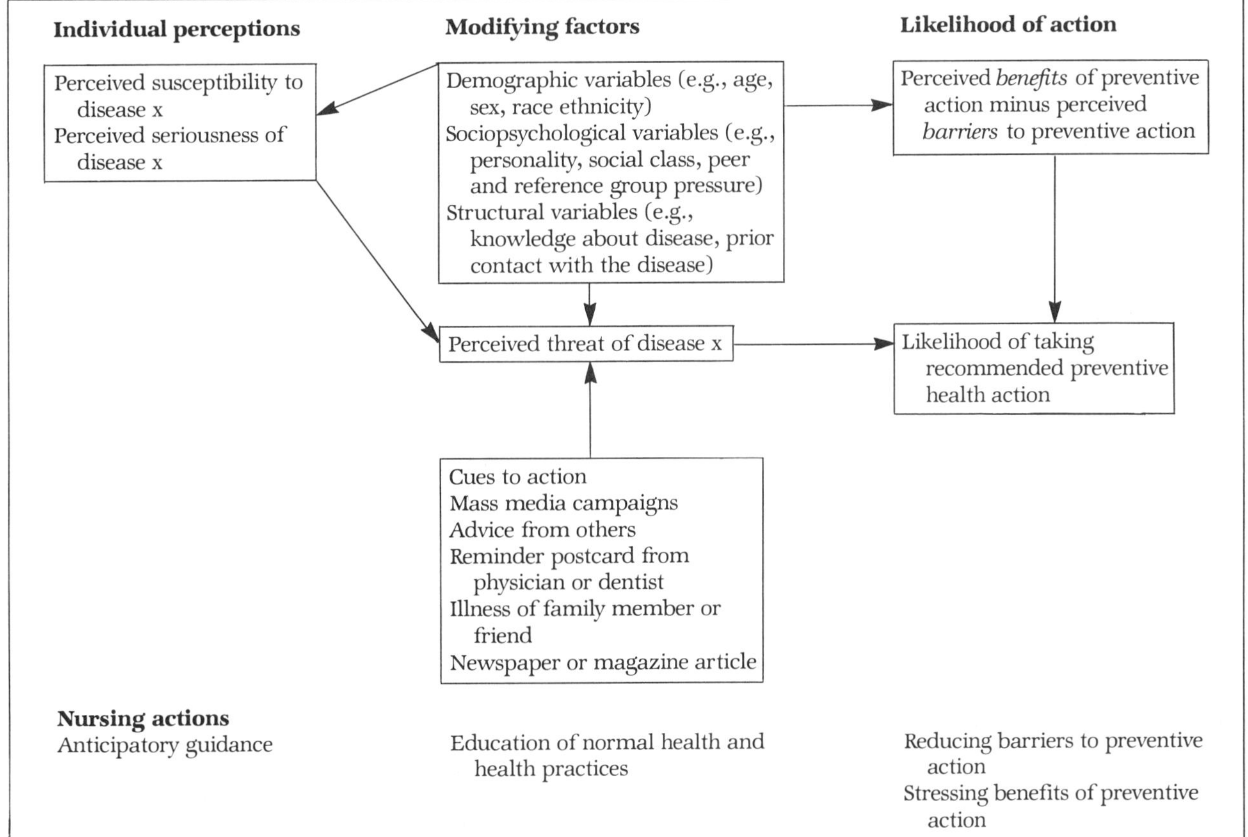

FIGURE 11-3. The health belief model. (Modified from I. Rosenstack, Historical Origins of the Health Belief Model. In M. H. Becker (Ed.), *The Health Belief Model and Personal Health Behaviors.* Thorofare, N.J.: Charles G. Slack, 1974.)

supplying them with correct information about illness so that the person's perception of it is accurate and by helping them to overcome the barriers that are preventing them from maintaining wellness.

LEVELS OF HEALTH TODAY

How healthy are people today? Is the average life span increasing or declining? What are the diseases that cause death?

So that questions such as these can be answered, statistics are compiled by the health services of countries and the World Health Organization. Such statistics are used to predict trends in disease so that increased risks to people can be determined and corrected. *Morbidity* statistics are statistics of the incidence of disease; *mortality* statistics refer to the incidence of death. One mortality statistic that is used as an indication of a nation's overall health is its infant mortality or the annual number of deaths of infants less than one year of age. This statistic is used because it reflects the health of women during pregnancies as well as the immunization status and the sanitary and housing conditions of a country. Infant mortality for the United States for the years 1960 through 1983 is shown in Table 11-2. Although this rate has shown steady improvement in recent years, room for improvement is clearly indicated.

Table 11-3 shows the mortality for all ages in the United States in 1983. The leading causes of death are shown in Table 11-4. Based on statistics, the U.S. Department of Health, Education and Welfare (1981) set a number of health goals it hopes to accomplish by the year 1990. These are:

1. To continue to improve infant health and to reduce infant mortality by at least 35 percent.
2. To improve child health, foster optimal childhood development, and reduce deaths among children ages one to 14 years by at least 20 percent.
3. To improve the health and health habits of adolescents and young adults and to reduce deaths among young people ages 15 to 24 years by at least 20 percent.
4. To improve the health and to reduce deaths among people ages 25 to 64 years by at least 25 percent.
5. To improve the health and quality of life for older adults and to reduce the average annual number of days of restricted activity due to acute and chronic conditions by 20 percent, to fewer than 30 days per year for people aged 65 and older.

TABLE 11-2. INFANT MORTALITY (PER 1,000 LIVE BIRTHS): UNITED STATES 1960—1983

Year	Rate
1960	26.0
1965	24.7
1970	20.0
1975	16.1
1980	12.8
1981	12.3
1982	11.4
1983	11.0

Source: From National Center for Health Statistics, *Monthly Vital Statistics Report* Vol. 32, No. 5. Hyattsville, Md.: U.S. Department of Health and Human Services, Public Health Service, August 1983.

LIFE EXPECTANCY

At the turn of the century the average life expectancy of a newborn infant was 47 years. Health statistics for the United States show that infectious diseases such as typhoid fever, smallpox, tuberculosis, diphtheria, measles, and whooping cough (pertussis) were major killers. Today, due to improved sanitation, immuniza-

TABLE 11-3. MORTALITY (PER 1,000 POPULATION) BY AGE: UNITED STATES, 1983

Age	Number
Under 1 year	4,153
1—14 years	1,637
15—24 years	4,181
25—34 years	4,928
35—44 years	5,866
45—54 years	12,369
55—64 years	28,783
65—74 years	46,965
75—84 years	52,785
85 years and over	37,809

Source: From National Center for Health Statistics, *Monthly Vital Statistics Report* Vol. 32, No. 5. Hyattsville, Md.: U.S. Department of Health and Human Services, Public Health Service, August 1983.

TABLE 11-4. MORTALITY (PER 100,000 POPULATION) FOR LEADING CAUSES OF DEATH: UNITED STATES, 1983

Cause of Death	Rate
Diseases of heart	329.4
Malignant neoplasms	189.0
Cerebrovascular diseases	68.6
Accidents	39.6
Chronic obstructive pulmonary diseases	27.6
Influenza and pneumonia	23.0
Diabetes mellitus	14.8
Chronic liver disease and cirrhosis	12.0
Suicides	11.9
Atherosclerosis	11.3
Homicides	9.0
Causes of mortality in early infancy	8.9
Nephritis and nephrosis	8.0
Congenital anomalies	5.6
Septicemia	5.2

Source: From National Center for Health Statistics, *Monthly Vital Statistics Report* Vol. 32, No. 5. Hyattsville, Md.: U.S. Department of Health and Human Services, Public Health Service, August 1983.

tion programs, housing, and nutrition, these diseases are largely erased (smallpox is extinct), and the life expectancy of a newborn female infant is 77 years; a male infant, 70 years (U.S. Department of Health, Education and Welfare, 1981).

PREVENTION OF ILLNESS

Keeping people well is as important an aim for nursing as helping people to become well again following illness. Certainly not all illnesses are preventable, but based on present knowledge a number of risk factors have been isolated. If these risk factors are kept to a minimum, a person should expect to have a longer life expectancy. Each year, for example, at least 350,000 people die from heart and lung diseases related to cigarette smoking, 100,000 people die as the result of accidents, and 200,000 people die following the misuse or abuse of alcohol. Quality of life as well as life expectancy can be improved by following a few common rules for keeping well at each age level.

The Infant

As mentioned, the infant year is the most hazardous year in life under the age of 65. The most serious threats to infant health during this time are *low birth weights* and *birth defects.* Infants born with a low birth weight have difficulty initiating respiratory and cardiac functions; if they survive the battle of immaturity, they may be left with residual effects of mental retardation or neurological or motor function problems. A low birth weight infant can be born to any mother, but the incidence is higher in adolescent pregnancy, in mothers with no prenatal care, poor nutrition, and low economic status, and in those who smoke, ingest alcohol, or use addictive drugs during pregnancy. The causes of many birth defects such as heart defects are still unknown, but the incidence of serious defects can be reduced by prenatal care, reducing environmental hazards, and identifying parents at risk for inherited defects.

Healthful practices for the infant year are:

Take care of the health of women before their babies are born.
Encourage routine health examinations and counseling.
Teach the need for immunization and proper nutrition.
Encourage a strong parent-child relationship.

The Child

Accidents are the chief cause of death in children. The major diseases of schoolage children are tooth decay and periodontal (gum) disease. In many children problems of overweight (obesity), high blood pressure (hypertension), high blood cholesterol, and lack of exercise are already present.

Healthful practices for schoolage children are:

Keep immunization status current.
Encourage good eating habits and exercise to maintain ideal weight.
Encourage dental hygiene and care.
Promote safety by the use of automobile seat belts and supervised play time activities.
Provide enriching experiences for mental growth as well as physical growth.
Participate in health screening programs.

The Adolescent and Young Adult

Although the death rate has been declining in recent years as a whole, it has actually increased for adolescents. The increase in death is due to violence: automobile accidents, suicide, and murder. While the incidence of many diseases is declining, the incidence of sexually transmitted diseases such as gonorrhea, syphilis, and herpes II (genital) has risen to epidemic proportions in this age group.

Healthful practices pertinent to this age group are:

Learn to drive safely both motorcycles and cars.
Learn the safe use of firearms.
Do not begin to smoke cigarettes.
Learn the wisdom of avoiding unnecessary drugs including marijuana and alcohol.
Learn good nutrition.
Develop responsible attitudes toward sex to prevent unwanted pregnancies and sexually transmitted illnesses.
Learn effective patterns for coping with stress.
Learn effective patterns of relating to others.

The Middle-Aged Adult

Among adults the incidence of heart disease, cancer, and cerebral vascular accident (stroke) rises, and death from these diseases becomes more frequent than death from accidents. Alcohol misuse, depression or anxiety, and periodontal disease are common.

Healthful practices for this age group include:

Have periodic health examinations.
Adopt sound nutrition and exercise habits to avoid obesity and high cholesterol level (high cholesterol levels may contribute to the formation of cardiovascular disease).
Reduce or stop smoking and alcohol consumption.
Utilize preventive health services such as high blood pressure screening clinics to identify illness at its first appearance.
Perform self-examination such as breast self-examination for women and testicular self-examination for men.
Be safety conscious, particularly regarding the use of automobiles.
Learn effective patterns for coping with stress.
Seek to control contamination of the environment with toxic substances.

The Older Adult

The number of people in the older age group of the population is growing yearly; by the year 2000 nearly 20 percent of the population will be over the age of 65 years. Most older adults want to continue their customary life style as long as they can. Helping them to do this despite interferences from heart and vascular disease, joint diseases such as arthritis, and hearing and sight impairments is a major nursing responsibility.

Healthful practices for the older age group include:

Stay active. Retirement should not mean being sedentary, simply not performing previous work.
Utilize health care services before conditions become acute or serious.
Continue to eat regular, nutritious meals.
Be alert to the possibility of drug interaction (a danger when one is being treated for more than one disease process).
Make needs known to others.

STAGES OF ILLNESS

Whether illness occurs rapidly as it does with appendicitis or food poisoning or whether it develops gradually as usually happens with pneumonia, the person experiencing the illness generally passes through three stages: a stage of transition, a stage of acceptance, and a stage of convalescence (Parsons, 1951).

Stage of Transition

The stage of transition begins with "symptom awareness": The person experiences some type of discomfort such as pain or perhaps nausea that alerts him that he is becoming ill. A *symptom* is an awareness experienced by the person such as feeling pain (a subjective finding). A *sign* is something that can be detected by observation or examination, such as seeing the person cringe when he bears weight on his foot (an objective finding). The intensity of the symptoms or signs apparent and the meaning of them to the person determine how soon he moves to the next phase of illness. If pain is severe, for example, the person will probably seek help more quickly than if the pain is a nagging, barely perceptible type. Dizziness is an example of a symptom that people often ignore for a long time as not important, when in fact it could be a symptom of very serious cardiovascular or neurological disease.

The second phase of this first stage is "confirmation of illness." This may entail checking with others as to whether they think the symptoms could be important or if that person notices any additional signs of illness. It is important to remember as a student in nursing that this is a normal, second phase of illness; it means that neighbors, family, and friends will ask you to confirm their illness for them, and because you are a student in nursing, they may rely very heavily on your answers. Be certain to begin your answers in these instances with "I'm a *beginning* student" so that the person realizes that your opinion represents that of a friend at this point more than it represents a professional opinion. Later, as you become more experienced, your answers can be based on a higher level of knowledge about illness.

Stage of Acceptance

A stage of acceptance begins when the person realizes that he is ill enough to seek health care. Many times people visit ambulatory health care settings not because they believe they are ill enough to seek care but because someone close to them feels that they are. They may use your opinion for confirmation in these settings, the same as your friends do: "I get a headache almost every morning just after I wake up. Do you think that's serious?" "My doctor told me to keep on working, yet the medicine she gave me makes me so sleepy I'm afraid to drive. Do you think I should mention that to her?" "I feel so tired lately all I do is sleep. Is there anything anyone can do for me?"

The range of signs and symptoms that people can report this way is almost endless. Table 11-5 lists signs

TABLE 11-5. SIGNS AND SYMPTOMS THAT SHOULD ALWAYS BE REFERRED TO A PHYSICIAN FOR FURTHER EVALUATION

Sign or Symptom	Possible Importance
Pain	Cells are being deprived of oxygen
Tingling, numbness of extremities	Interference with circulatory or neurological function to extremities
Loss of sensation of a body part	Interference with neurological functioning
Loss of motor function of a body part	Interference with neurological functioning
Bleeding	Cells will be deprived of oxygen
Loss of weight	Destruction of body's ability to maintain cell function
Edema (swelling from collection of fluid in subcutaneous tissue)	Compromised circulatory or kidney function
Loss of consciousness	Severe impairment of neurological function
Change in bowel habits	Presence of obstruction; danger to cell nutrition and function
Persistent symptoms such as nausea, shortness of breath, or cough	Specific pathology related to body organ; persistent symptoms reflect serious level of disruption
Break in skin that does not readily heal	Leaves a portal for infection to body
Change in a mole or other skin lesion	Reflects abnormal growth; sign of cancer

and symptoms of illness that, as categories, always suggest serious pathology and should be reported to a physician. In addition to this guide, which is helpful to use until your knowledge of disease pathology increases, would be any symptom or sign that worries a person so much that it increases his level of stress or makes it difficult for him to function.

THE SICK ROLE

Once a person has an illness confirmed by health care personnel, he typically assumes a "sick role" or the role that everyone more or less expects of an ill person. Parsons (1951) has identified four major elements of the sick role:

The person is not held responsible for his illness. This is a common philosophy accepted by most people and if you believe it yourself (that the person who develops pneumonia had no control over getting it), you may have some difficulty working with people who do not fit this common pattern, who *were* in fact responsible for their illnesses (the person who attempted suicide and now is very ill). A parent whose child ran into the street and was injured may be unable to take care of the child the way you would like, because the parent's behavior is affected by the realization that by not being sufficiently careful, he may have been responsible for the child's injury. People who are the exceptions to the rule in these ways need compassionate and understanding care to move forward from a sick role to a well role again. They may be so guilt-ridden by causing their illness that they have difficulty complying with medical care. This philosophy of not being responsible is not held by all people, obviously; some may believe that illness is the result of a person being out of favor with God and that people are always responsible to some degree for illness.

The person is expected to seek health care. During the stage of transition a person uses many home remedies for signs and symptoms; as he enters the stage of acceptance, he is expected to rely more heavily on health care personnel recommendations. When a person comes for medical care, you should ascertain what remedies he has tried; some of these may actually have worsened the signs and symptoms of illness rather than improved them.

It is easy to criticize people who wait until an illness becomes severe before they see a health care provider for help. Such delays in seeking care, however, usually stem from such things as lack of finances (the person could not afford care or transportation to care); fear (worrying that he might have heart trouble seemed better than knowing that he had heart trouble); or lack of knowledge (he did not realize that a symptom such as numbness of the fingers could be serious). The amount of dependence on home remedies is culturally influenced: Mexican Americans, for instance, may rely heavily on folk medicine and so seek professional health care later than people without a folk medicine network. In many instances, people who seek medical care late are people with more health problems than the original one or with secondary problems such as lack of finances. In order to reach high-level wellness again they may need help from a variety of health care services; otherwise, the next time they are ill, they may neglect early health care again and become more ill because of again waiting longer than necessary.

The person is excused from normal social role responsibilities. People who are ill are not expected to report to work; they are excused from school classes and household responsibilities. This reaction is so expected that we often criticize those who continue to work while they are ill. The reason why someone breaks this pattern needs to be explored because it may reveal that the person is under greater financial or social stress than normal, situations that need to be remedied as much as the illness if high-level wellness is to be achieved. Because people expect to relinquish responsibility as a consequence of being ill, they may be surprised (and suspect you are wrong) when you say to them on the day following surgery, "It's important for you to be out of bed, Mr. Jones. Let me help you walk the length of the hallway." This is a statement that you will be making often because early ambulation after surgery stimulates circulation and respiration and therefore prevents many complications. Remembering that as part of the sick role people expect not to be asked to do many things helps you to present this information in a positive and supportive manner.

Cultural influences may reverse this pattern. A Mexican American man, for example, tends to maintain a "macho" or strong front. Even when very ill, he may maintain that he feels few symptoms and continue normal activities.

The person is expected to want to get well and cooperate to do so. Knowing that most people accept this philosophy indicates that the average person will take medicine as prescribed and perform exercises and other therapies. Since there are exceptions to every rule, you will meet some people who do not want to get well. A woman who lives alone and is visited by few friends may find a week's stay in a hospital a stimulating and socializing experience for her and be reluctant to leave or get well. A child who is not doing well in school may find a hospitalization experience the excuse he needs for not having to face what is happening in school; he may be reluctant to return home where he will have to deal with the problem. A person who believes that illness is caused by his poor relationship to God may feel that no active response on his part will help so takes none. People who do not appear to want to get well again in these ways pose a nursing challenge. In addition to therapy for their immediate illness they need help for the problem that makes it less than appealing for them to get well again. Otherwise, they may continue to view themselves as ill or begin unsound health practices in order to become ill again.

Stage of Convalescence

As a person's physical symptoms lessen, he becomes ready to leave his sick role and return to health. A person recovers fastest when he is psychologically ready to do so at the same point that physical readiness is reached. Recovery may be delayed if he is psychologically ready to perform self-care but his body is still too weak to allow this (he could overdo and become more ill); or if, although physically there is no reason that he could not return to his former role, he is still not mentally prepared to do so.

REACTIONS TO ILLNESS

In addition to his willingness or unwillingness to adopt a sick role, a person's reaction to illness depends on the interplay of the illness, the individual, and the circumstances present at the time of illness.

The Illness

The severity of illness influences how a person reacts to it in one of two ways: It may make a person seek help immediately or delay seeking help as long as possible. A woman who discovers a lump in her breast, for example, may phone her physician immediately or use a "what I don't know can't hurt me" philosophy and proceed with normal activities as if she were not aware of her illness.

The body part affected may also make a difference as to how soon a person seeks health care. A facial lesion, for example, may bring someone promptly to a physician because the person is self-conscious about his appearance. A urinary tract infection, however (presenting with symptoms of pain and frequency of urination), may be ignored for some time; because the illness is discernible only to the individual, he receives no confirmation of illness from his friends and so moves more slowly through the first stage of illness. If a person thinks of body systems such as the genitourinary tract as "dirty" or "not nice," this may also prevent the person from seeking medical help, in the hope that the illness will go away by itself and make it unnecessary for the person to consult health care personnel about his problem.

ETIOLOGY OF ILLNESS

Illness can arise from a variety of causes; differing causes typically offer different signs and symptoms and patient reactions.

Altered Defense. Altered defense systems of the body result in the body's being unable to protect itself against invading organisms such as bacteria, viruses, or fungus. The marks of an infectious illness are an abrupt onset, increased temperature (fever), inflammation (redness and swelling), and pain. Altered immunological responses may also lead to allergic responses.

Metabolic Disease. Many diseases are caused by an imbalance of hormones or enzyme-regulating mechanisms. These illnesses typically present with a slow onset and with symptoms that tend to be vague in nature such as dizziness, loss of weight, or blurred vision—symptoms that may be disregarded for a long time before the person seeks help.

Altered Growth. Altered growth of body tissue leads to birth defects in newborns, and tumor growth in people of other ages. In some instances tumors are confined and limited in size (benign); others are malignant and extend rapidly to cause destruction of surrounding tissue (cancer). Altered growth disturbances tend to present with subtle symptoms but eventually produce symptoms of obstruction: pain at the point of compression, deficiency of flow in front of the blockage, and a potential for build-up and blow-out behind the blockage.

Trauma. Trauma in the form of burns, bruises, or lacerations can be a cause of illness. Trauma occurs suddenly and requires a person to act quickly to seek adequate help. If a person underestimates the seriousness of a traumatic injury, he may not seek help soon enough, and a minor injury may become serious.

Chromosomal Disorders. Some illnesses are passed from generation to generation due to the transmission of imperfect genes. Chromosomal disorders such as Down's syndrome, a mental retardation syndrome, are evident at birth. Nursing assessment of all newborns is important to help detect these types of illnesses.

Nutrient Disorders. Many illnesses are caused by interference in absorption, transport, or utilization of nutrients from the gastrointestinal tract. Such illnesses stem from a variety of causes but all have common symptoms of loss of weight, nausea, vomiting, and diarrhea. It is easy for people to disregard the seriousness of these types of illnesses and not seek help until the body stores are depleted to a point that makes cell repair difficult.

Psychosocial Disorders. Abnormal stress can lead to illness processes that interfere with reasoning or ability to function. People with mental illness may seek health care late because they are not aware of the extent of the illness or they fear that health care personnel will not respect their illness as there are no physical signs present.

Individual Variables Influencing Health

A person's ability to adjust to any stressful situation (the toaster breaks, the car does not start, a school class is cancelled) will influence his ability to adjust to or accept an illness situation. Some health problems are related to stress; a person's inability to combat stress can lead directly to illness (stomach ulcers are an example of this). Other individual variables include the following.

AGE

Certain illnesses are age related. Adults, for example, rarely contract measles (rubeola) or whooping cough (pertussis). They have either received adequate immunization against childhood diseases or contracted these diseases as children. Arteriosclerosis (hardening and thickening of the arteries to the point that there is interference with blood flow) is a condition associated with older age and is found only infrequently in younger persons.

SEX

Diseases that affect reproductive function such as uterine or testicular tumors are obviously diseases dependent on sex. Other illnesses have a tendency to occur more often in one sex than another. Lung cancer and cardiovascular disease, for example, are seen more often in men than in women (although they are increasing in incidence in women due to increased cigarette smoking).

MENTAL STATUS

In order for a person to seek health care, he must realize that he is ill. People who are mentally retarded often have difficulty relating the nature of their symptoms to the people caring for them and may be more ill than those who can express their needs adequately. Likewise, people whose perceptions are distorted by mental illness may become very ill before they make someone aware of their symptoms.

PHILOSOPHY OF LIFE

A person's philosophy of life helps to determine the point at which he seeks help for problems. A high school athlete, for example, trying to project an air of "can't be beaten" may make light of a symptom such as a painful knee that another person would immediately seek help for (Fig. 11-4). An individual who derives little fulfillment from daily life and receives little attention from the people around him may find satisfaction in the attention he receives when he is ill and so over a lifetime spend more time than the average person in illness care.

FIGURE 11-4. A team member may not report a leg injury, fearing peer ridicule or responsibility for team defeat.

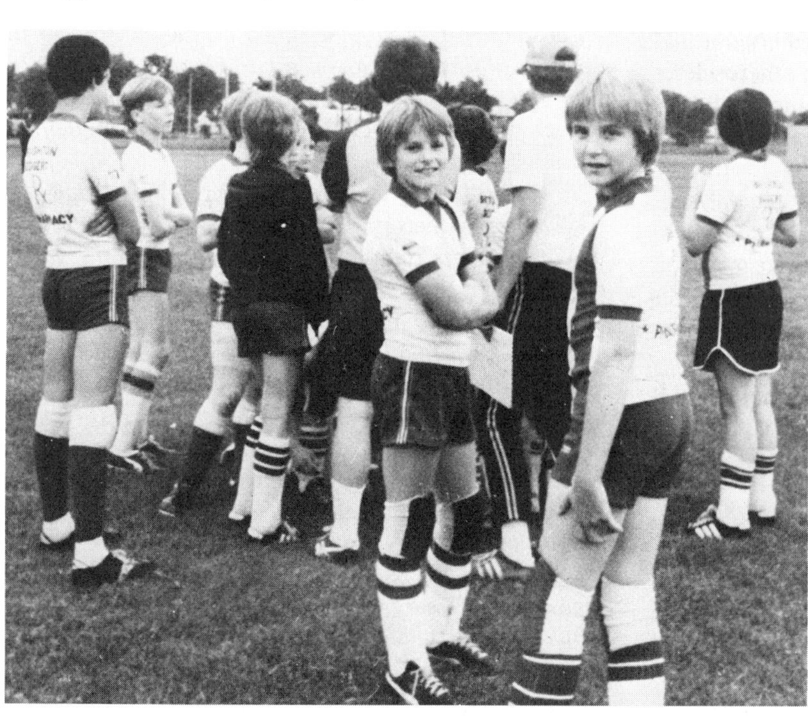

PHYSIOLOGIC RESPONSE SYSTEM

If a body's response systems are not functioning at their optimum levels, a person will become ill more often and perhaps have a more difficult time recovering from illness than the person whose body defenses are functioning normally. People with lowered blood clotting ability, for example, suffer greater effects from open lesions than those whose blood clotting mechanisms are functioning well; those people with less than normal ability to combat infection contract diseases more easily and have a more difficult time recovering from them.

TOTAL BODY HEALTH

A person who is in ill health from one cause has a greater tendency to develop a second illness than the person who is free of illness. This means that in all nursing care you must not only be concerned with carrying out the procedures that will most quickly allow a person to return to wellness again but also take measures to guard against additional illness. People who are confined to bedrest, for example, are more prone to develop pneumonia (infection of the lung alveoli) because of the stasis of fluid that occurs in the lungs from little body movement than is the average ambulatory person.

PAIN THRESHOLD

Pain is felt at different levels by different people. Those people with a low pain threshold feel pain before others do; what the average person interprets as nagging pain, they may perceive as sharp and intolerable pain. Any illness involving pain, therefore, is a more serious illness for these people than others. Pain often appears worse to people when they are under stress, so relieving stress aids pain tolerance.

PAST EXPERIENCE

A person's past experience with disease can influence greatly how he reacts to illness or health care. If a person has had positive experiences in the past (when he contracted an illness, therapy was successful, and he recovered without complications), he will probably perceive his chances of recovery and the quality of his health care as good. On the other hand, if he has had an unfortunate outcome from a previous illness, he may view himself as a person with poor healing ability (or worse than usual luck). A person with this mental outlook may not participate well in his own care. His attitude is, what's the difference, I won't get well anyway. He needs careful planning for care that will meet his individual special needs.

Circumstantial Variables Influencing Health

Equally important in determining how ill a person may become or his reaction to illness are the circumstances present when the illness occurred.

ECONOMIC STATUS

Economic status may influence the type of illness a person develops. If a person lives in a crowded housing situation due to low economic status, contagious (infectious) diseases such as upper respiratory infections tend to spread rapidly from person to person due to the close contact. A diet rich in meat (which contains saturated fat) may lead to an increased incidence of atherosclerosis (fatty deposits along arteries, which lead to obstructed blood flow); as meat is an expensive food item, people who have a higher financial status may be more prone to this illness (heredity may play a large part in the development of atherosclerosis also). Economic status may also influence how soon a person contacts health care personnel or whether he receives routine health guidance. If minor illnesses are not detected by screening programs, major illnesses may develop. Lack of finances can lead indirectly to illness if it results in neglect of preventive health care.

SUPPORT PEOPLE

A person's support people are those people who care about him and offer him counsel and help when needed. A person uses support people during the transition stage of illness to help him confirm that illness exists. The person with few such people around him may allow himself to grow increasingly ill before he seeks confirmation of illness. One reason that people work hard to become well again is that they know people important to them are depending on them to regain their health. The person without adequate support people may lack this stimulus to become well again.

CULTURE

Cultural influences affect how long a person depends on home remedies before he turns to medical care (native Americans may feel very strongly that tribal custom is superior and more dependable than a strange physician's therapy). Culture also influences how long a person uses his immediate family for confirmation of illness (Spanish-speaking Americans tend to be very family-oriented and turn to health centers for care later than many others). Cultural patterns blend quickly in busy cities, and stereotyping as to expected behavior may lead you to wrong assessment. Assess each patient you care for individually as to cultural patterns to avoid this type of mistake.

SEASONAL VARIATIONS

Respiratory infections tend to occur more frequently in the wintertime as do bone injuries related to skiing and ice skating. Summertime brings an increase in drownings and minor illnesses such as insect bites and poison ivy.

SAFETY PRECAUTIONS

Whether safety precautions were present or not at the time of an injury can influence the extent of an injury (whether a construction worker had a hard hat on or not, for example). Nurses working in industry or school settings have important responsibilities to see that safety precautions are reinforced to limit or prevent injuries.

A Sick Role Model

Rosenstack (1974) also designed a sick role model to demonstrate how people react to illness and whether they can be expected to comply with health care. This model, modified to include nursing actions, is shown in Fig. 11-5.

In the first stage a person is influenced by his level of motivation to become well, the value of having the threat of illness reduced for him, and his faith in the outcome of health care. The nursing role at this point is anticipatory guidance so that people appreciate that optimal wellness not only makes them feel well physically but allows them to be optimally productive so they have motivation to seek health care.

In the second stage of the model, modifying factors such as the attitude of health care personnel and the cost of care come into play. Nursing actions during this time center on coordinating or role modeling comprehensive care for individuals so they are not "turned off" by measures necessary to make them well again.

In the third phase, a person's likelihood to comply with his regime of care can be predicted. The nurse's role

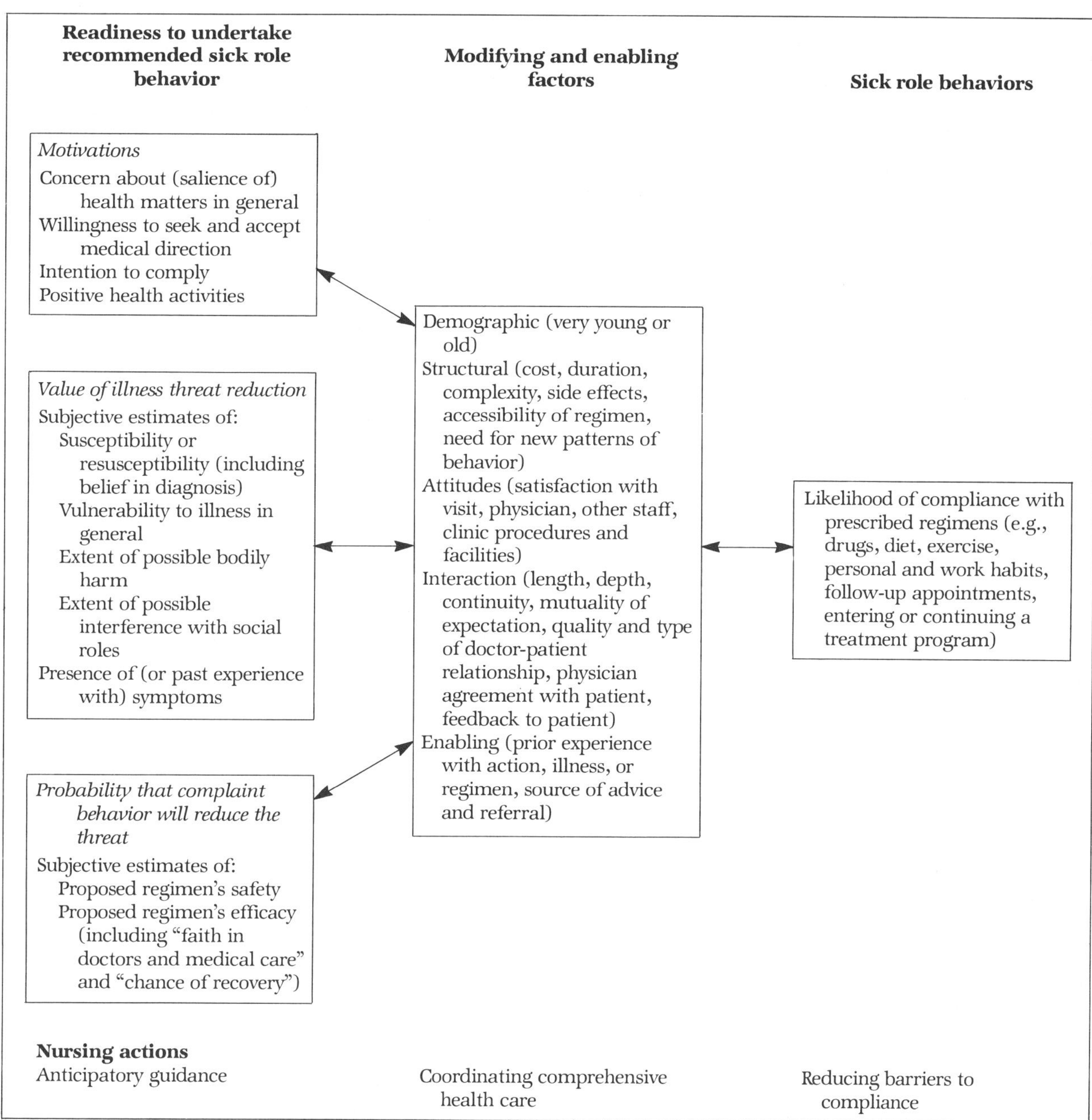

FIGURE 11-5. Sick role model. (Modified from I. Rosenstack, Historical Origins of the Health Belief Model. In M. H. Becker (Ed.), *The Health Belief Model and Personal Health Behaviors.* Thorofare, N.J.: Charles G. Slack, 1974.)

during this time is to make compliance nonstressful by reducing barriers to compliance.

GRIEF AS A REACTION TO ILLNESS

Illness means different things to different people and individual people react differently to it. A reaction of grief, however, is a common reaction that can be seen to occur to some extent in almost all people, no matter what disease is present. People typically grieve when they recognize that they are ill because although we usually associate grief with death, it also occurs with any loss. Being sick stimulates such a reaction because the person loses his concept of himself as a well person.

Denial and Shock

The first phase of a grief process is a feeling of shock (surprise) or denial (inability to accept what is happening). This reaction occurs because even though the person knows that he has symptoms of an illness (pain, shortness of breath), he is still surprised to learn that he has an illness severe enough to need treatment (he had hoped that his physician would tell him that his symptoms meant nothing, that he was worrying for no reason). The more serious the treatment (hospitalization for three weeks, intravenous fluid administration, perhaps), the more likely this reaction is likely to occur, because the distance between what the person hoped would be the outcome and the actuality is so great.

People with this initial reaction to illness are poor problem solvers (they are too surprised to be able to put facts together in the proper order so that they make sense) or are not yet ready to acknowledge that a problem exists. Sometimes this reaction to illness is shown in a response such as a person saying to you, "Is it all right if I smoke?" after you have just finished explaining that he cannot because he has oxygen turned on in his room and oxygen supports combustion. He heard you but he was so stressed that he could not process the information. Repeat information that you offer under such circumstances as often as necessary to be certain that it has been heard and comprehended.

Anger

Following a phase of shock or denial, a person usually enters a phase of anger. In the first phase of the grief process he was saying, "This can't be happening to me." Now he is saying, "It isn't fair that this is happening to me." This is because very few people view any gain in being ill and do see many problems. The illness may mean loss of a position, pain, embarrassment, personal handicap, loss of confidence. People who are angry are sometimes difficult to care for; if they are unable to confine their anger to the fact that they are ill, they may find themselves angry at you or some other health care provider or a procedure or activity you wish them to do (angry at you because the orange juice on their breakfast tray is faintly sour). It is hard not to respond to anger with equal anger (replying to the person that you are not responsible for sour orange juice and it is unfair of him to be angry). It is necessary not to meet anger with anger, however, in order to help the person work through this phase of his reaction to illness. It is often helpful to approach a person who seems to be displaying anger out of proportion to the situation with a statement such as "You seem too angry to be angry just over orange juice. Would you like to talk about any other things you're angry or worried about?"

Bargaining

Bargaining is a subtle phase of grief and one easily missed unless you are aware that it happens. It is putting conditions on how ill a person agrees to become. A statement such as "If I get through this surgery I'll go to church every Sunday" or "I don't mind having diabetes, just so I can go on vacation as I always do in July" are bargaining statements (trying to arrange a better situation for themselves through a promise or a condition). Listen to such statements but, as a rule, do not point out the fallacy of them; continued time will allow the person to move to the next step of grieving.

Depression

As people move away from denial (they can no longer reject the fact that they are ill because their symptoms are growing so acute), anger (being angry is not helping symptoms), and bargaining (also ineffective; they *are* becoming worse, not better), they eventually arrive at a stage of really admitting to themselves that they are ill. This stage is comparable to moving from a stage of transition in sick role behavior. The reaction that may accompany the realization of illness is often depression or an overwhelming feeling of sadness. In many instances, the person's outward behavior during this time appears as a setback in the process of his acceptance of the disease. While he appeared to be accepting a disease diagnosis well, he is now often crying and unhappy. What has happened is that this is the first time he has truly accepted his diagnosis—a change from feeling "It isn't fair that this could be happening to me" to "This is happening to me."

People who are depressed do not problem solve well and they may regress to earlier behavior patterns. This is particularly evident in children (a child who was fully toilet-trained reverts to bed-wetting).

A secondary reaction very common during this phase is a feeling of fear. Fear causes people to overreact to situations or have difficulty putting daily events in proportion. Having to eat breakfast an hour later than normal because of a diagnostic test is seen as a major inconvenience, while in ordinary circumstances the change in routine would be accepted casually.

Once a person begins to accept the fact that he is ill, he often asks more questions about his illness, the drugs that he is receiving, or the diagnostic tests that he is having done than he did before. In some instances it seems as if the person is being overly critical of his care (or you) when this happens. Remembering that this is a manifestation of the stage of depression of a grief reaction will prevent you from overreacting and thinking that a question is a criticism of you or your care. It alerts you to the fact that this is a healthy sign that a stage of acceptance is being reached.

Answer questions during this phase accurately but without long involved explanations as the person cannot necessarily process a long explanation due to his high stress level; try to determine what the person is actually asking (a question such as "Have you taken care of many people who have had heart surgery?" may mean "Did any of them die?" "Will the doctor take much blood?" may mean "Will I have enough blood left if someone takes any more?") Many times you can determine the real question by asking "Are you worried about that?" (the subject mentioned) after you complete your first explanation.

People who are very fearful or sad at this stage may appreciate being told about the coping mechanism of facing only one day at a time (or one diagnostic test at a time) and not worrying about things that are not immediate concerns. This is a technique used successfully by people trying to combat alcoholism or drug habituation and it usually works well with any person under a high level of stress.

Acceptance

Acceptance is the final stage of a grief reaction. Arriving at this stage is a change from "This is happening to me" to "It's all right this is happening to me." If, after diagnostic tests, a person's illness is found to be a minor one that will leave him with no permanent disability, he passes quickly through this stage and returns to his former mental image of himself as a well person. If the illness is found to be one that will leave the person with a permanent handicap or will be fatal, it may take him years or until close to his death to work through to this stage. Before he reaches this final stage, he may regress back to previous stages. Once a person accepts the fact of his illness in this final way, he is able to fully participate in planning his care and participate in self-care. Because many people take a long time to reach this stage (some never reach it), each person needs to be evaluated individually as to his self-care capabilities. Being certain that people understand as much as possible about their illness plays a big role in helping a person reach this final stage.

LIFE SPAN CONCEPTS AND ILLNESS

Illness is always systemic to some degree. This is important to remember when making assessments of a patient and planning care. There is no such thing as a person with just a fractured tibia, for example. Because all illnesses have some systemic aspects, such an injury is accompanied by the hazards of immobility and represents a threat to the person's body image and social capabilities.

The Infant

Infants have little understanding of the seriousness or type of illness. Infants born with handicaps such as a missing arm begin to perform motor functions with one arm without any degree of frustration, unlike an individual who had full motion function and then lost it.

Despite the infant's disregard for illness, illness is always serious in infants because with limited body reserves they may not be able to combat it effectively. Also, if the illness causes the infant to be separated from his primary caregiver through hospitalization, the separation may lead to permanent psychological damage in terms of the infant's ability to relate to people (the infant's grief reaction at the separation is so strong that it interferes with the development of his sense of trust). Illness in an infant may affect the mother's confidence in herself as a mother (she may feel that she should have recognized the illness sooner) and interfere with her ability to care for the child.

The Toddler and Preschooler

Children are developing independence (autonomy) during the toddler period and learning a sense of initiative or how to do things during the preschool period, so that any illness that interferes with the child's ability to explore his environment or make free choices is frustrating to him. Bedrest is a therapy that is particularly difficult to enforce at this age, and children may actually "rest" better if allowed to sit up in a chair rather than actually be confined to (and continually squirming in) bed.

Children during the preschool period are just beginning to distinguish between "good" and "bad." They may become very confused about why they are ill or about painful procedures such as injections; the child does not understand why he is being subjected to such punishment when he was not "bad."

The Schoolager and Adolescent

Schoolage children are learning a sense of industry or how to do things well. They often have difficulty accepting an illness that removes them from school for a period of time or allows them to fall behind their peers' progress. Adolescents are extremely body conscious and may have a difficult time accepting an illness that will leave an alteration in body appearance. The strong need of the adolescent for independence may make following a plan of care a difficult task.

The Young Adult

Because the young adult is concerned with establishing a career, a home, or a family, any illness that sidetracks him from his goals may be particularly difficult to accept. Young adults are often impatient with therapies that do not act immediately; they may need more than one explanation of why a certain therapy is necessary before they are willing to carry it out.

The Middle-Aged Adult

Middle-aged adults are at the peak of their careers and well into child rearing. Some illnesses that occur at this time in life are the result of the strain and stress of home or work life; illnesses that take a person away from work or work responsibilities may be most difficult to accept during this time of life.

The Older Adult

Most older adults are concerned with being able to take care of their own needs as long as possible. Many of them may be reluctant to go for health care at the first sign of illness because they do not have the cost for medical care or they worry that, once hospitalized, they will never be allowed to return home but be transferred instead into an extended care facility or nursing home. Helping older adults to maintain function and have their wishes for housing or care respected are major functions of nursing.

ILLNESS AND THE FAMILY

Illness has important consequences for others in addition to the ill person; the effect of illness reaches out and interferes with family function as well. Some changes that may have to be made due to an illness in a family member relate to roles (someone different may have to cook, houseclean, or care for children), financial support (another family member may have to become the chief money provider), and caregiving (someone may have to care for the ill member).

Some people do not go for health care at the point that they first recognize they have illness symptoms because they do not want to disrupt family life (a mother wants to remain at home to care for children; a father wants to take the family on vacation before he reports for a health check). Trying to anticipate what family effects will occur from one member's illness helps you to anticipate possible problems that may arise with care when the person returns home.

ILLNESS AND THE COMMUNITY

Illness in an individual often reaches beyond the immediate family into the community. When a person is unable to attend work because of illness, his co-workers are asked to perform his work; this may place added stress on the persons performing the extra work and possibly cause illness in others. If an ill person holds a position such as mail or milk delivery, his absence may affect the quality of communication and food supply for the community. Looking beyond the individual at possible community effects helps you to appreciate the possible meaning of the illness to an individual and aids you in planning his care with him.

BASIC ASSUMPTIONS OF ILLNESS AND HEALTH

Because so many factors influence the extent of illness and people's reactions to illness, it is difficult to make generalizations about reactions. The following five assumptions are those that tend to be universal.

1. *Illness is always a stressful situation.* This is an important fact to keep in mind, for it is easy to assume that because an illness seems minor to you, the person's perception of the illness will be the same. This is not necessarily true; what you think of as a minor illness, another may think of as major. No matter how minor, illness is always a stress; the person will not be able to function effectively again until stress is alleviated.

2. *Coming for health care presents a stress situation.* Many people, after realizing that they have an illness, resist coming for health care. They fear injections, surgery, loss of privacy, and that their wishes or opinions will be disregarded in favor of a planned program. Nurses play an important role in lessening this fear.

3. *Health care involves expense.* Even if a person has health insurance, there invariably are some expenses not covered by such a policy that the person must pay himself. Subscribing to such a policy may be difficult for some people as they feel they would like to spend the monthly insurance payments in other ways. Even if all illness expense is borne by insurance payments, additional expenses such as extra baby sitters, food for a special diet, transportation to and from the hospital, loss of work hours or position occur. Health care is a service and consumers today are asking more than ever before for quality care to justify the expense.

TABLE 11-6. FACTORS THAT MAKE IT EASIER FOR PARENTS TO ADJUST TO A HANDICAP IN A CHILD

Factor	Rationale
Support people are available.	Caring for such a child is a series of crises during which support people become very important.
A strong marital bond exists between the parents.	A marriage partner can serve as the strongest support person.
A good relationship exists between the child's mother and maternal grandmother.	The mother has been loved and can love the child.
The handicapped child is other than a firstborn.	The mother has had practice "mothering."
The family lives close to shopping, schools, and transportation.	The family is not isolated.
The family has a supportive religious faith.	Secondary support systems are important in times of stress.
The parents were told of the child's disability as soon as possible.	The sooner people are aware of a problem, the sooner problem solving can begin.

Source: From C. U. Battle, Chronic physical disease: Behavioral aspects. *Pediatr. Clin. North Am.* 22:525, 1975.

TABLE 11-7. MODIFICATIONS OF BATTLE'S CRITERIA TO ADULTHOOD

Factor	Rationale
Support people are available.	Support people play vital roles in sustaining the strength of someone during a chronic illness.
A strong marital bond exists between the ill person and spouse.	A marriage partner can serve as the strongest support person; if the handicapped person is not married, close friends or family members can fill this role.
The person has a number of close friends he relates with easily.	The person can give and receive love and so encourages support people.
The person lives close to shopping, schools, and transportation.	The person can be more independent than if he were isolated.
The person has a supportive religious faith.	Religious affiliations can serve as sources of strong support.
The person was told of his illness as soon as possible.	The sooner a person is aware of a problem, the sooner a problem can be solved.

4. *Good health leads to improved health; poor health leads to worsening health.* A healthy person is able to remain well because he is able to take advantage of eating a nutritious diet, of exercising properly, and of good self-esteem so he is able to cope with stress effectively. The person who begins to feel ill may fail to be able to do any of these things, so his symptoms grow more and more severe or a second illness begins to compound the first. Helping people to move toward high-level wellness and to achieve interventions against illness at the first opportunity is an important nursing responsibility.

Mrs. Fisher, 50 Years Old

Area of Assessment	*Wellness Behavior*	*Illness Behavior*
Family life	Is a mother to three children; wife to husband. Views role as nurturer and protector. Insists on family eating meals together and doing one activity together as a family each week. Encourages children and husband to discuss their problems with her.	Does not share her concerns with other family members.
Self-responsibility	Can problem solve household and work problems. Able to postpone immediate needs for future rewards.	Is 20 pounds heavier than ideal weight. Admits to having difficulty saying "no" to people.
Mood	Describes herself as "serious."	Has little sense of humor; tends to keep emotions to self so "things run smoothly at home." Bites fingernails.
Sexual role	Enjoys being a mother. Sexually active. Is postmenopausal; no reproductive life planning measures needed.	Wishes she were a man at work because "men don't always have to be so tactful." Is rarely active sexually due to busy work schedule and family demands.
Life style	Maintains a life style fulfilling to herself.	Life style is criticized by family. They would like her home more, particularly on weekends.
Self-esteem	Sees herself as a worthwhile contributing person.	Has regrets that her one daughter recently had a child out of wedlock; feels "embarrassed" about discussing this. Feels family does not appreciate her contributions.
Future outlook	Makes short-term plans without difficulty.	Has no plans for what life will be like after children are grown.
Personal care	Takes responsibility for self-care. Does monthly breast self-examination. Is aware of a good diet and provides this for herself and family. Sleeps 8 hours a night.	Smokes a pack of cigarettes daily. Drinks a glass of wine nightly to "fall asleep." Has not been for a Pap test since birth of youngest child 12 years ago. Has not had a dental exam in 4 years.

Work or school practices	Works as a buyer for the children's clothing section of a department store. Enjoys her work, especially short trips she must make to New York City. Feels financially secure because of her husband's position (an accountant) as well as her own. Feels she can take criticism well.	Reports feeling fatigued for the last month. Worries about unpaid bills.
Social contacts	Has a friend she has known since high school she says is her "best friend." Entertains at least once a month (friends or neighbors). Enjoys touch and touching.	Does not enjoy being alone; turns on television to "interrupt the silence."
Recreation	Swims twice a week.	Has no program for exercise. "Too busy" to take time.
Community awareness	Votes regularly; is a member of a community action group for smoke abatement. Knows neighbors and meets socially with them.	Never registered to vote. Considers neighbors unfriendly.

5. *It is better care to keep individuals well than to restore wellness after they have become ill.* Only in recent years have health care providers accepted this tenet. Doing so has shifted the accent of health care to promotion of health and prevention of illness. Today a major role of health educators is keeping people from becoming ill by teaching them to monitor their own health.

CHRONIC ILLNESS

An illness becomes chronic when it persists for a period of time. Adapting to chronic illness is usually more difficult than adapting to short-term illnesses because the number of changes that must be made are compounded when the illness begins to stretch over a period of months or years rather than weeks.

Battle (1975) has identified a number of factors that, when present, make adapting to the birth of a handicapped child easier to accept. These are shown in Table 11-6. Although these factors were identified as being pertinent to the child with a long-term illness, they can be used as evaluative criteria to help determine how easily a person may be able to adapt to a chronic illness that occurs with adulthood. Modifications of Battle's criteria to adulthood are shown in Table 11-7.

Parents of children with long-term handicaps report that a common emotion they experience is "chronic sorrow" (they remain frozen in the depression stage of grief, unable to move on to the stage of acceptance). This sorrow becomes most intense at points in the child's life that otherwise would have become milestones (the day he would have started to a neighborhood school, would be applying for a driver's license, would be receiving first communion, and so forth). Families of people with adult handicaps or chronic illnesses do not pinpoint this feeling as markedly but special family occasions tend to provoke a feeling of exceptional sadness for "what might have been." Planning care for people or families when chronic illness is present is sometimes difficult because it is difficult to plan and look forward to happenings when it is still more enjoyable to look back to a point before the illness.

UTILIZING NURSING PROCESS

Mrs. Fisher is a 50-year-old woman you see in an emergency room. She has come for care because of abdominal pain. Although she first noticed the pain 10 days ago, she felt she had too many home and work responsibilities to "be sick." Her family (a husband and three children) finally convinced her that she needed a health assessment.

To establish whether Mrs. Fisher demonstrates more wellness than illness behaviors, you compare her actions to those representative of a well person as described in Table 11-1.

Based on the above inventory, a nursing care plan on Mrs. Fisher might read as follows:

ASSESSMENT

Problem: Health maintenance.

Subjective: Patient has had no routine health maintenance measures such as dental care or Pap test. Has no regular exercise program; little ability to reach out to her support people; fatigued for last month; pain for 10 days yet no health agency contact.

Objective: 20 pounds overweight; dark circles under eyes; bleeding cuticles from nail biting.

NURSING DIAGNOSIS

Health maintenance deficiency related to family and work responsibilities.

LOCUS OF DECISION-MAKING

Patient.

SHORT-TERM GOAL

Patient will organize home and work responsibilities to provide time for self by six months' time.

Criteria: Patient will state she feels less pressure from conflict in three life areas.

NURSING ORDERS

1. Discuss importance of maintaining own health in the light of family and work responsibilities.
2. Ask patient to list advantages and disadvantages of work to help her determine if work is worth the conflict it causes to family.
3. Ask patient to list ways that she could provide time for herself every week.
4. Teach health monitoring measures so that she will be more aware of responsibility she owes herself.

SUGGESTED READINGS

Ahmed, P. I., and Coelho, G. V. (Eds.). *Toward a New Definition of Health: Psychosocial Dimensions.* New York: Plenum, 1979.

Aiken, L. H. (Ed.). *Health Policy and Nursing Practice.* New York: McGraw-Hill, 1981.

Balog, J. E. The concept of health and the role of health educators. *J. School Health* 51:461, 1981.

Battle, C. U. Chronic physical disease: Behavioral aspects. *Pediatr. Clin. North Am.* 22:525, 1975.

Campbell, J. D. Illness is a point of view: The development of children's concepts of illness. *Nursing Digest* 4:56, 1976.

Collier, P. Health behavior of women. *Nurs. Clin. North Am.* 17:121, 1982.

Diekelmann, N. Wellness: Approaches and resources. *Nurs. Pract.* 5(5):41, 1980.

Dubos, R. *Mirage of Health.* New York: Harper & Row, 1979.

Dunn, H. *High Level Wellness.* Arlington, Va.: Beatty, 1961.

Eggert, G., et al. Caring for the patient with long term disability. *Geriatrics* 32:102, 1977.

Galton, L. Questions patients ask about health and how you can answer them. *Nursing 77* 7:54, 1977.

German, P. S. Delivery of care to older people: Issues and outlooks. *Top. Clin. Nurs.* 3(1):1, 1981.

Gelein, J. L. Aged women and health. *Nurs. Clin. North Am.* 17:179, 1982.

Gleit, C. J., et al. Nursing diagnoses for healthy individuals. *Nurs. Health Care* 2(8):456, 1981.

Gilson, B. S., et al. The sickness impact profile: Development of an outcome measure of health care. *Am. J. Public Health* 65:1304, 1975.

Hazard, M. P. Keeping the well-elderly well. *Am. J. Nurs.* 83(4):567, 1983.

Higgins, S. H. Your patient's illness is a family affair. *RN* 39:48, 1976.

Keller, M. J. Toward a definition of health. *A.N.S.* 4(1):43, 1981.

Lederer, H. D. How the sick view their world. *J. Social Issues* 8:4, 1952.

Moyer, N. D. Health promotion and the assessment of health habits in the elderly. *Top. Clin. Nurs.* 3:51, 1981.

Parsons, S. T. *The Social System.* New York: Free Press, 1951.

Rose, M. A. Problems families face in home care. *Am. J. Nurs.* 76:416, 1976.

Rosenstack, I. Historical Origins of the Health Belief Model. In M. H. Becker (Ed.), *The Health Belief Model and Personal Health Behaviors.* Thorofare, N.J.: Charles G. Slack, Inc., 1974.

Rushmer, R. *National Priorities for Health.* New York: Wiley, 1980.

Shamansky, S., and Clausen, C. Levels of prevention: Examination of the concept. *Nurs. Outlook* 28:104, 1980.

Smith, J. A. The ideal of health: A philosophical inquiry. *A.N.S.* 3(3):43, 1981.

Symposium on women's health issues. *Nurs. Clin. North Am.* 17(1):111, 1982.

Taylor, C. Caring for the chronically ill—one day at a time. *Nursing 78* 8:59, 1978.

Tichy, A. M. Wellness, the worker and the nurse. *Occup. Health Nurs.* 29(2):21, 1981.

U.S. Department of Health, Education and Welfare. *Living Well.* Washington, D.C.: Public Health Service, 1981.

World Health Organization. *Constitution. Chronicle of WHO.* Geneva: World Health Organization, 1947.

QUESTIONS FOR REVIEW

1. Mr. Jones is a 27-year-old man who slipped on the ice walking to work and fractured his tibia. Immediately he had sharp pain in his leg and was unable to bear weight on it. He was taken to the emergency room of a local hospital for care. When a person comes directly for medical care in this way, what stage of illness has he *bypassed*?
   a. Stage of convalescence.
   b. Stage of transition.
   c. Stage of acceptance.
   d. Stage of "sick role."

2. People who become ill often experience a grief reaction. What statement by Mr. Jones would best reflect that he is experiencing the first stage of grief?
   a. "This can't be happening to me."
   b. "It isn't fair this is happening."
   c. "I'm angry at my bad luck."
   d. "I'm worried about getting better."

3. Mr. Jones is admitted to the hospital. If he says the next day, "Get me out of here safely and I'll never complain again," what stage of grief does this statement reflect?
   a. Transition.
   b. Depression.
   c. Bargaining.
   d. Acceptance.

4. The following day Mr. Jones tells you that the care in the hospital is the worst he has ever seen. Based on the fact that he may be experiencing anger as a stage of grief, what would be your best answer?
   a. How many hospitals have you been in before?
   b. You seem angry; is there anything worrying you?
   c. The hospital is hiring a lot of new people to make it better.
   d. I bet your leg is hurting and that is the trouble.

5. The major cause of death in Mr. Jones' age group (young adult) is:
   a. Heart disease.
   b. Accidents.
   c. Lung disease.
   d. Burns.

6. An expected behavior of Mr. Jones as he manifests a "sick role" is:
   a. He should continue to work until he is exhausted.
   b. He should avoid health care.
   c. He should state that pain is his worst symptom.
   d. He should want to get well again.

7. People who seek health care *later* than normally:
   a. Should be assumed to be mentally ill.
   b. Often have multiple problems.
   c. Must be recognized as uncooperative.
   d. Can be assumed to have high pain thresholds.

8. Which of the following is thought to be important in the acceptance of a handicapped child by a family?
   a. The child is the firstborn.
   b. The family was told as soon as possible about the handicap.
   c. The family doesn't live near a crowded shopping area.
   d. The family has strong political convictions.

12. THE IMPACT OF STRESS ON HEALTH

OBJECTIVES

Upon mastery of the material in this chapter, you should be able to:

1. Explain the concept of body homeostasis (homeodynamics).
2. Describe the concept of stress according to Selye.
3. List four areas from which stressors can arise.
4. List cognitive, verbal, motor, and psychological reactions to stressors.
5. Describe methods to help people cope and adapt to stress.
6. Describe the concept of crisis and the technique of crisis intervention.
7. Describe the concept of burnout.
8. Describe possible consequences of poorly handled stress such as alcoholism, drug dependence, and violence.

TERMS

The terms important for an understanding of this chapter are shown below and defined in the glossary:

adaptation
anxiety
ataraxy
coping
crisis
general adaptation syndrome (GAS)
homeodynamics
panic
stress
stressor

Stress is a double-pronged word that can refer either to a threatening experience (illness, pain, a flood, a child leaving for school, pressure of trying to achieve in school) or to the physical and psychological changes that occur in people who encounter threatening events. In order to keep the terms separate here, threatening experiences are referred to as just that (or as stressors) and *stress* is used to refer to the internal physical and psychological body happenings that occur following such experiences.

Although for centuries people have been aware that stress exists and is superimposed on all illness, it was not until 1936 that Hans Selye first identified and described the phenomenon of stress. He termed this body reaction a *general adaptation syndrome* (Selye, 1976).

GENERAL ADAPTATION SYNDROME

A person faced with a threatening happening can be seen to move through definite stages of a general adaptation syndrome (GAS) response in order to return to a state of homeostasis or balance.

The first stage is one of an *alarm reaction*, a period in which the body prepares defenses against the happening. Almost immediately following the alarm state comes a *stage of resistance*, in which concrete body changes occur to maintain homeostasis or body balance. In most instances, these adaptive changes are enough to cope with the threat. If the stage of resistance is unusually prolonged or the threat unusually severe, the body eventually loses its ability to maintain resistance and enters the third *stage of exhaustion*. Actions that occur during these stages are shown in Fig. 12-1 and discussed following the explanation of the concept of homeostasis.

It is important to remember when analyzing a stress response that it is manifested at different levels in different people. Happenings that are viewed as threatening by one person may not be interpreted that way by another, and physical changes vary at least slightly from person to person (some people notice severe perspiration as a response; others notice mostly trembling and weakness).

Homeostasis

Homeostasis is a state of physiological balance; the efforts of the body are always aimed at trying to achieve such a state. *Homeodynamics* is a more recent term used to denote homeostasis; it was coined to imply that even in balance the body is never static but producing new cells and rearranging fluids to maintain balance. *Steady state* is another term often used to denote a balance of both psychological and physical forces. *Stability* may also be used to denote mental or behavioral balance.

Restoration of Homeostasis

Coping is the immediate response of a person to a threatening situation. *Adaptation* is the final response

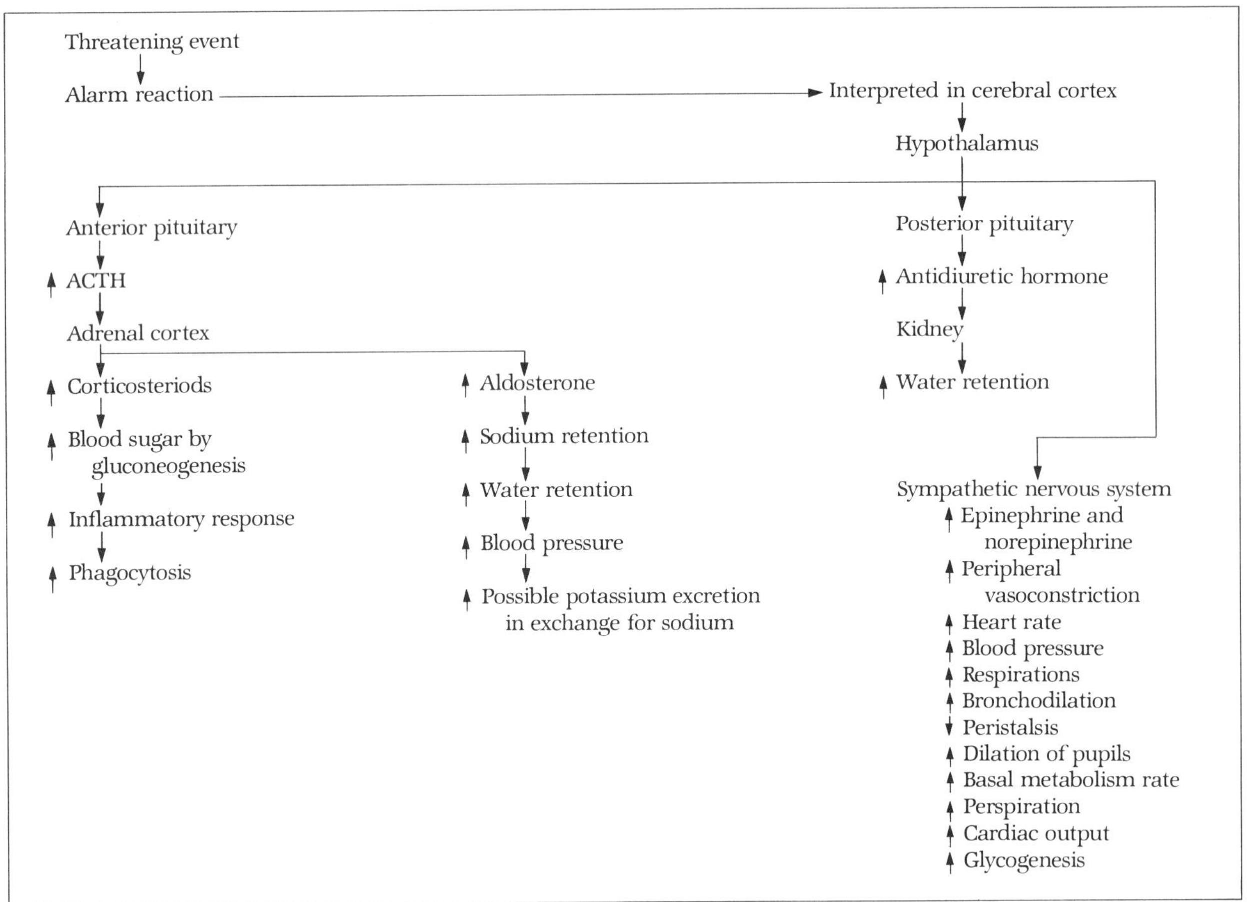

FIGURE 12-1. General adaptation syndrome. (From H. Selye, *The Stress of Life*. New York: McGraw-Hill, 1976.)

or change that occurs from the assault. If your bank makes an error in your account, for example, your first response may be telephoning the bank (coping); your adaptive response may be to change banks. In order to understand this process, it is helpful to examine factors basic to every adaptive response.

Immediate adaptive measures are involuntary. Endocrine, neurological and psychological adaptive responses swing into action without any conscious thought. Except through special training (biofeedback), a person is unable to halt these processes any more than he is able to consciously start them.

Adaptation is most complete if adequate time is present. A person who is suddenly subjected to massive lung alveolar damage, for example, has a more difficult time adjusting to the limited amount of air exchange space present than the person who develops alveolar damage slowly such as the person with chronic emphysema (overinflation of the alveoli). As a rule, then, people in emergency situations are less able to think rationally and plan for their own care than people in more controlled or expected settings.

Adaptation is a whole body process. This is noticeable from both a physiologic and psychological standpoint. A person with a threat to one body part (his foot is trapped under his car) reacts systemically (blood pressure increases, peripheral vasoconstriction occurs, heart rate increases); and although only one part of his body is injured, the whole body image of the person may be altered (he sees his whole self as less now that one foot is injured). It is important to remember when assessing the extent of an injury that adaptation is a whole body process—that although only a small amount of the person's body is actually injured, the body is reacting as if the injury were total.

Adaptive responses have limits. Physiologic responses are limited to the resources the body has to call on. Psychological responses are limited to the creativity, support, and past experiences that the person has available. When such resources are exhausted, outside intervention is required, or death or permanent injury can result.

Adaptation depends on negative feedback. A body regulates itself by always selecting a neutral or balanced state. If a hormone level rises too high, for example, the body acts to reduce it to a normal level again; if a hormone level falls too low, an action is begun to raise it again. By this principle, adaptive responses do not move into action until called upon. While some adaptation begins with anticipated or projected threat, a person can do little to prepare for danger except to be in the best physical and emotional state possible.

Adaptation differs in degree and kind from person to person. Just when you think you know how everyone is going to react to a certain circumstance (surgery, childbirth, adolescence, retirement) a person comes along with a new and unexpected response. The different ways that people use to adapt are as varied as the number of people you care for.

Adaptive responses are egocentric and exhausting. A person whose body energy, both physical and psychological, is involved in adaptation does not have the energy to reach out to give support to another (and often is not even aware that the other person needs support). Parents whose child is mentally retarded, for example, may become so engrossed in their own adaptive response to this problem that they offer no support to each other; over a period of time they may drift apart as they engage in fewer activities in common due to their involvement with themselves and the child. The reaction may be so egocentric that a person is unaware that others around him want to help him (he feels lonely and deserted in the midst of family and friends).

Adaptive responses may cause overcompensation. "Rebound" effects are examples of this. A person has a low blood glucose level, for example, and so, by a physician's order, you administer glucose intravenously to him. His pancreas begins to produce increased insulin to regulate the increased glucose present; in a few minutes the increased amount of insulin present moves all the new glucose out of the person's bloodstream and the person has an even lower blood glucose level than he had before the intravenous supply was administered. Psychologically, a student criticized for handing in a paper with typographical errors may spend so much time on a second typing that he has no time left to complete other assignments.

Adaptive responses may be inadequate or inappropriate. Although the purpose of adaptive responses is to bring the body back into homeostasis, such responses will not always be adequate without some assistance. Interventions initiated in emergency situations often take the form of "running ahead" of what the body is trying to do and giving it the help it needs to achieve effective adaptation.

In some instances, adaptive responses actually complicate therapy. Following severe hemorrhage, for example, vasoconstriction occurs in all peripheral circulation, not just at the hemorrhaging site. Vasoconstriction makes it difficult to insert an intravenous needle, and administering replacement fluid to reestablish blood volume is actually hampered by the adaptive response. A person using the psychological defense mechanism of reaction formation (acting in the opposite way from their true feelings) may lead people to think he is adjusting well to the incident when actually he needs a great deal of support and time to talk about what the issue means to him.

The Alarm Reaction of the General Adapation Syndrome

When a threat is received by a sensory nerve receptor (you burn your finger), the impulse is first carried to the spinal cord where a circuit initiates muscular action to cause you to withdraw from the acute stimulus (pull back your finger from the flame). The impulse then continues to the cerebral cortex of the brain for refinement and conscious awareness (I am burnt and in pain). Psychological events register initially in the cerebral cortex. The cerebral cortex conveys the danger sensation to the autonomic nervous system through the hypothalamus and brain stem. The autonomic nervous system is divided into sympathetic and parasympathetic systems. The sympathetic system acts to increase or stimulate body function, the parasympathetic system to stabilize or keep the body functioning over a long course of time. Continued or long-term threat, for example, generates such parasympathetic responses as increased gastric acidity in the stomach and symptoms of ulceration (peptic ulcer).

With impending or actual threat the sympathetic nervous system causes an increased heart rate and vasoconstriction of peripheral blood vessels in order to pool blood in the central body core so that it is available for vital organs such as the heart, liver, kidneys, and brain. This combination of events (increased heart rate and increased central blood volume) increases the blood pressure. Basal metabolic rate increases, so sweating increases to decrease the temperature. Pupils dilate to allow for increased vision.

In order that the body will have adequate oxygen for optimal cell function, respiratory tract bronchi dilate to allow more air to enter the lungs. Gastrointestinal action is temporarily halted because digestion is at the moment not an important function and would utilize a great deal of body energy possibly needed elsewhere.

The hypothalamus, in addition to communicating the impending danger to the autonomic nervous system, alerts the pituitary gland to the threat, and secretion of antidiuretic hormone by the posterior pituitary gland begins. Antidiuretic hormone (ADH) stimulates the kidney to conserve water (which is necessary for cell metabolism). The anterior pituitary gland secretes adrenocorticotrophic hormone (ACTH). ACTH stimulates the adrenal gland to secrete cortisone and aldosterone. Cortisone mobilizes glucose for cells, in order to provide energy to function, and aldosterone stimulates the kidney to retain sodium, which leads to still more water retention. These hormonal changes occur a little more slowly than do other autonomic nervous system responses but tend to sustain their effect longer.

A person in an alarm state appears pale, and his skin will feel cold due to vasoconstriction; he is breathing rapidly; he may be sweating profusely (diaphoresis). He may sit down suddenly and put a hand over his heart as he senses it pounding and racing. The average person remains in a state of alarm for only a few minutes; the body does not have sufficient resources to maintain a person long in this state of overproduction. A state of alarm is also termed a "fight or flight" reaction, as this is what the person is posed to do: Challenge the threat or run from it, whichever action will result in safety for him.

Stage of Resistance

The stage of resistance immediately follows the alarm reaction. The body begins to be more selective in its response if the danger is still present; it begins to return to normal function if the danger is past. If the danger encountered, for example, is one of air pollution, the lungs are the body organ selected to deal with the threat. Coughing will occur as a means of removing from the body the noxious fumes or dust in the air. This reaction will persist until the air is again clean or the person becomes exhausted and cannot endure coughing any longer. If the threat is a psychological one (a person is criticized for an accomplishment such as a term paper), the intellect is assigned the primary body response. The length of the response (resentment, anger, acceptance of criticism) will last until the episode is over and the importance of it resolved. Activity in a stage of resistance and the length of the stage will therefore be extremely varied depending on the threat. A nursing role during this time is to support the body system involved to ensure that it has the strength to withstand the threat (administer a drug to make coughing more effective, guide a person to use constructive rather than destructive outlets for anger).

Stage of Exhaustion

The stage of exhaustion occurs at the point that the body's strength and resources have been used and can no longer be called on. The body can maintain vasoconstriction for only about 20 minutes, for example. At that point vasodilatation occurs, and vital organs are deprived of a good blood supply as blood suddenly returns and pools in the peripheral circulation. Blood pressure falls, which may keep pulse and respirations at a rapid rate in order to maintain blood pressure. Eventually the heart cannot continue to expend so much energy, so pulse rate slows; with this second physiological point of exhaustion the blood pressure will drop still further. The ultimate consequence of this stage of exhaustion would be death as the last of the body's resources deteriorated and failed. Psychologically, the stage of exhaustion occurs when a person feels that he is too exhausted to mentally "fight" any longer. A legislator, for example, may struggle for years to have a bill on increased Social Security benefits passed, but after a long series of disappointments he may simply stop trying. He expresses this as "I've had it" or "I'm too tired to fight it any longer." Nursing responsibility for the person at a stage of exhaustion is to provide support for body processes that are failing. For mental exhaustion it consists of finding a support person or group to take over the problem and carry out the problem solving for the individual who has become exhausted. A stage of exhaustion has a variable time interval; its length depends on the amount of support and at what point it is reached.

Whether a threatening event is great enough to lead to a stage of exhaustion depends on the nature of the event, the possible perception of the event, the number of events that occur at the same time, the duration of the event, the support people available, and the person's past experience with the same or a similar event.

NATURE OF THE EVENT

Obviously a virus of an extremely virulent strain has greater potential to cause harm than a virus of a less malignant strain. An event such as missing a bus probably causes less stress than losing a job. A fall from a stepstool is probably not so serious as a fall from a scaffold. Identifying the stressor precisely is important in trying to establish the effect that it will have on the person in terms of threat.

PERCEPTION OF THE EVENT

Perception of the event or what the event means to the individual person is as important as the actual virulency of the event. This is a subjective area and therefore differs a great deal from one person to another. No matter how simple the event may seem to you, if the person says that it is the most terrible thing that ever happened to him, you have to proceed as if the event were of that seriousness. Because it is being interpreted as an extremely frightening event by the person, his body will react with an extreme stress syndrome response.

NUMBER OF SIMULTANEOUS EVENTS

Almost everyone can manage one threatening event after another, as long as there is an intervening time to allow the person to regroup and stabilize resources. No one can function well when such events closely follow one another or when more than one occur at the same time. The person who had just learned that he has appendicitis, for example, should be able to cope with (immediately adjust to) his diagnosis (a normally complication-free procedure). He might not be able to cope, however, if at the same time he learned that he was being evicted from his apartment or failing in school, or that his car had been stolen.

This is why you sometimes cannot imagine why a person is so upset about a problem that to you seems so small and easily solvable. The problem *is* small, but superimposed on a series of others it becomes the "straw" that is one too many problems to deal with. Illness often creates simultaneous problems because the person with an illness almost automatically develops accompanying financial difficulties (he has physician and hospital costs to pay); work-related worries (he is letting down other people at work; perhaps he will be replaced); home-related problems (who will watch the children, feed the dog, mow the lawn); and personal stresses (he feels helpless, vulnerable, defeated).

DURATION OF EXPOSURE

While the body adjusts quickly to threatening events (within seconds it is prepared to fight or flee from the event), it cannot maintain its defenses indefinitely. If the threatening event continues for a prolonged time, the person's ability to adjust to the problem decreases. Everyone has had the experience of having a bad headache. It is painful, but if taking a mild analgesic such as aspirin makes it quickly go away, it is not a difficult experience. However, when a headache persists, although the pain remains at the same level, it seems more intense to the individual. A person waiting to hear if a bank loan will be approved, for his physician to tell him of a diagnostic test result, or for results of a physical examination can wait comfortably for a short time interval; he will grow increasingly stressed as the waiting period grows longer and longer.

SUPPORT PEOPLE AVAILABLE

Support people are a necessary factor in adjusting to stress. Availability does not necessarily mean physical presence; closeness in terms of being able to provide support is more important than geographic proximity. A woman may derive more support from talking to her husband who is a truck driver and three states away than from her sister who is standing by her bedside.

EXPERIENCES WITH A SIMILAR OR LIKE EVENT

If a person has successfully adjusted to an event once before, his ability to do so again is usually better than if the person is adjusting to the event for the first time. He is strengthened by the knowledge that he handled the situation successfully once before. People who live along rivers that flood every spring think of flooding as an announcement of spring, for example; a newcomer to the neighborhood may be overwhelmed by the sight of water in his basement.

If, on the other hand, the person's experience with coping the first time the event occurred was not good, his reaction to a second occurrence may be more intense (he feels defeated before he begins) than the person who is experiencing the event for the first time. Learning people's past experiences with similar or like events is important information to obtain at a health history in order to try to estimate the meaning of the present event to the person. Reminding people that they coped successfully with a similar event in the past may be the bridge they need to feel secure in their ability to face the event again.

PSYCHOLOGICAL ADAPTATION

Although the general adaptation syndrome theory explains the physiological happenings that occur with stress, it does not explain the psychological changes or reactions that also occur.

The psychological manifestation that occurs with a threatening event is termed *anxiety.* Anxiety differs from fear in that anxiety occurs in response to an *unknown* threat (a feeling that something not yet defined is happening); fear occurs in response to an *identified* event.

A mild degree of anxiety as a result of a stimulus is not necessarily harmful. An actress with stage fright as she waits in the wings for her cue, for example, may notice that when she steps on stage, she gives a sharp and stimulating performance (all her defenses are functioning to her advantage). If her anxiety becomes too great, however, the reaction is no longer therapeutic (desirable) but harmful (she becomes so anxious that she is unable to walk on stage).

Anxiety is often classified as mild, moderate, severe, and panic. These categories are shown in Table 12-1.

Psychological Coping Mechanisms

The secret of reducing anxiety to the lowest desirable limit lies not in avoiding stress necessarily (it is a basic part of living and so realistically unavoidable) but in coping with a threat so that it is manageable. Various coping mechanisms that people typically use are approach (fight), withdrawal (flight), or inaction.

APPROACH

Approach mechanisms may be anticipatory (getting a vaccination against a disease, studying for an exam) or in response to a real threat (screaming, hitting, punching). The latter approaches to threat are usually helpful if the threat is a physical one such as an attacker, because the person has a feeling of being in control or commanding his circumstances.

WITHDRAWAL

Withdrawal is pulling back from (avoiding) a threatening situation. People very typically use this response when confronted with illness: A woman notices a lump in her breast but avoids going for a physical checkup, thinking, "What I don't know won't hurt me." Although discretion is the better part of valor in some circumstances, withdrawal may give a person a sense of loss of control, making it more difficult to solve his problem as the problem seems to be in charge of him.

INACTION

Inaction is more than simply not doing anything; it is a conscious action. If, for example, you are debating about entering a competition or not, doing nothing solves the problem if the deadline for submitting the entrance form passes; the decision as to whether you will enter or not no longer has to be made. This type of response is not necessarily the best one, but it is a system that many people use (for better or worse). It relieves people of feeling responsible for their actions because they can feel that the decision is ultimately not made by them but by an outside force (the competition rules committee).

TABLE 12-1. ANXIETY CONTINUUM

State of Anxiety	Physical Symptoms	Psychological Symptoms
Panic ++++	Screaming Running Gross motor activity	Details distorted Perceptual field disrupted Awareness of environment reduced Disintegration of personality organization Feeling of extreme terror
Severe anxiety +++	Trembling, nausea Dizziness, hyperventilation Impotence Heart palpitation	Focus only on small detail or scattered details of problem Not aware of whole; connections between parts cannot be determined
Moderate anxiety ++	Increased heart rate Increased respiratory rate Muscular tension Perspiration	Perceptual field becoming narrowed Still able to concentrate on one area well Connections between parts can still be perceived
Mild anxiety +	"Butterflies" or gastric discomfort	Broad sensory perception Can discern connections between parts readily Attention focused on activity Energy and motivation are generated
Well-being	Relaxation	Able to reason with normal problem-solving ability Experiences happiness
Apathy (ataraxy)	Fatigue	No demonstrable response or evidence of motivation or desire

Methods of coping can be further divided into cognitive, verbal, and motor responses.

Cognitive Responses

A cognitive response is a thinking or planning response. It is as a rule a high-level response that is helpful, although, if it involves dreaming or fantasy formation, it can be very destructive.

GAINING INCREASED KNOWLEDGE

Fear of the unknown is, as a rule, more intense than knowing exactly what *is* the threat. Gaining increased knowledge about an illness generally decreases anxiety as it circles or confines the illness. Patient education, then, is not only imparting knowledge; it is helping a person add to his ability to cope with a threatening situation.

PROBLEM SOLVING

Problem solving is thinking through the threatening event and using specific steps to arrive at a solution. Steps in personal problem solving are the same as those that comprise the nursing process, which is a problem-solving format: assessment of the situation, analysis or definition of the true problem, planning or choosing alternatives, carrying out the solution, and evaluation as to whether the solution was successful in solving the problem. People who are good at problem solving do it so quickly that they are not aware of the steps. People poor at problem solving carry out the steps poorly or not at all.

STRUCTURING

Structuring is arranging a situation so that threatening events do not occur: A person who feels threatened by change remains in one job all his working life despite low pay to prevent having to face change; an instructor who is uncomfortable with questions says he will take them only at the end of class, then consistently runs out of time so he never has to answer questions. Structuring of this kind is destructive as it allows no room for growth; such a person can be overwhelmed the day an event breaks through his shield. On the other hand, if a person schedules a physical examination in his yearly routine so that he will not develop a severe illness, such structuring represents a productive coping mechanism.

SELF-DISCIPLINE

Self-discipline (self-control) is internal structuring or arranging facial expression and manner to convey a sense of being in charge or control, no matter what is happening externally. Self-discipline is a good reaction in that it prevents a person from panicking and doing anything harmful or nonproductive in a threatening situation. It can be harmful if it delays the beginning of problem solving or gaining new information. It also may prevent the person from receiving the support he needs from those who care about him (he seems so strong, taking it so well); it may actually alienate his support people if he seems cold and unconcerned.

DREAMING

Many people relive and think through threatening experiences not during the waking hours but while they are sleeping, through dreams. Many people sleep fretfully their first night in a hospital not just because the bed is strange but because their minds are reviewing the threat of hospitalization and they dream frequently. People who are admitted to a hospital following a traumatic experience such as a near-drowning or being in a fire can be expected to have nightmares as part of their cognitive method of handling stress.

FANTASY

Fantasy or day dreaming is reworking a threatening experience by replaying it and having it end differently. People may imagine themselves rushing into the street and stopping the car that hurt their child when in fact they stood frozen at the curb unable to move. They may imagine that a physician the day after surgery will say, "I was wrong. Your heart is absolutely all right." Fantasy reactions of this kind are helpful in that they can lead to problem solving: "If I had run into the street, I might have been hit too and be of no help to my child now; what I really should have done was hold her hand at the curb"; or "The surgeon isn't going to say that I'm all right, but if he only says I can continue to work, I can accept that as good news." Fantasies can be destructive if they are so time consuming that the person spends more time in a fantasy world than in his real one ("If I were Superman, I could have lifted the car right off the street"), thereby repressing more helpful responses.

PRAYER

The use of prayer is a very individual response; for some it is a conditioned response, for others a well-thought-through process. Prayer is reaching out for support; it involves identifying the problem in order to describe it in prayer (please help me, I am failing this course) and suggesting solutions (what I need is to pass a test on Friday). These are the first two steps of problem solving; if it leads into action (studying material for Friday's test), it is a therapeutic technique aside from its special meaning for an individual.

SUPPRESSION

Suppression is the conscious action of putting a problem aside (I won't worry about that today; I'll deal with it tomorrow). Suppression relieves stress only temporarily because it does not face the problem. With illness-related phenomena "putting off until tomorrow" does not change the symptoms or solutions; it only prevents the person from concentrating on them.

Verbal Responses

Verbal responses are often the first responses to a threatening happening. Like cognitive responses, they can be helpful or a hindrance, depending on the situation and the length of time they are used.

TALKING

Most people after a threatening event have an intense need to talk about what happened to them: It was a frightening experience to fall off a scaffold. Talking about it limits the size of it and makes it measurably less fearful: It was a 12-foot scaffold, not a 12-story building. At social events people often talk about their hospital or surgery experiences. Don't discourage people from talking about traumatic events; a person is thereby building a fence around the experience, framing it, and once he has done so, it will never again be so threatening to him.

CRYING

Crying is a pressure release mechanism when an event is so intense that cognitive function cannot yet manage the problem. It can occur in response to either pain or pleasure as well as to a sad event. Crying is sex-related and culture-related: Women tend to cry more easily than men; some cultures view crying as acceptable, some do not. People feel most free to cry when they are with others who they know care about them. After being hurt by a friend's remark, you may show no reaction on a long bus ride home but break into tears as you enter your own home. A patient may not cry about a happening in front of you on your first contact with him; he may do so at a third or fourth contact as he starts to perceive you as one who cares about him. Crying is therapeutic as a release valve; it can become destructive when it interferes with beginning a more long-lasting response.

LAUGHING

Laughter is another pressure release mechanism not unlike crying. It serves the purpose of releasing enough tension to let the person begin to think constructively about the problem. It is not unusual to see the relatives and the patient himself in an emergency room following a severe injury laughing over some small incident (the person's wife wore her good dress and her bedroom slippers to the hospital). Both laughter and crying occur most readily in the presence of people one cares for and is comfortable with, so seeing a person laughing or crying may aid your assessment as to whether the people with him are truly his important support people. Laughter, like talking, helps to build a fence around a situation; after laughing about what happened, the situation will never again be so frightening. There is an old saying that if someone in an emergency room is laughing about what happened to him, he is all right. That may not be true from a physical standpoint, but such a response can be psychologically therapeutic.

SCREAMING

Screaming is a response to fright (a person putting his hand on you as you walk along a dark hallway) or intense frustration or anger (the telephone company keeps billing you for someone else's calls). It is a useful tension-reducing outlet. Screaming becomes destructive at the point that it becomes hysteria or uncontrolled, as when the person is unable to stop screaming. Contrary to many movie scripts, the cure for relieving hysteria is not pouring water on the person's head or slapping his face. Rather it is reducing the tension around him by moving him to a quiet environment and giving assurance that the threat is over. By releasing the anxiety, you release the need for such an anxiety-reducing outlet.

VERBAL ABUSE

Verbal abuse is a conditioned response to a threat: A person hits his thumb with a hammer and says, "Damn!" Most adults confine this type of abuse to stress-producing objects such as their nonstarting car, their lost keyring, or the snow outside, but at times they may respond in this way to people if they see them as being the cause of their threatening situation. Some people may confuse the messenger with the message and verbally attack the person who tells them for instance, that their blood report is abnormal. Verbal abuse is a tension-release mechanism; when you are subject to it, try to categorize it with laughing or crying to keep it in perspective (yesterday when you told a woman that her doctor wanted her to stay in the hospital another day, she cried and you felt sympathetic; today when a woman shouted obscene names at you for the same message, you became angry). Although the method of anxiety release is different, the reason for the response is the same—and just as healthy. Remembering this helps you from becoming emotionally involved (the attack of obscenity *was* unfair; you were only serving as a messenger); responding in kind is not therapeutic or at least better left unsaid.

Motor Responses

Motor responses are also immediate responses to threat; for some people they work effectively in the first few minutes before they assemble a more long-acting cognitive response.

HITTING AND KICKING

Hitting and kicking are basic instantaneous reactions to physical threat. Adults are conditioned so that no matter how much you hurt them during a procedure (such as giving a painful intramuscular injection) they do not respond in this way. Children, however, especially preschoolers, may hit and kick in such situations since they do not have the internal control of adults. Such children are not "bad" for exhibiting such behavior; they simply haven't matured enough to learn better coping strategies.

Some people hit and kick at walls or wastepaper baskets to relieve tension. Although such behavior is not constructive, it may be an extremely effective method of relieving anxiety for some people as long as they do no damage to themselves or the objects. This behavior will often help a person move on to cognitive coping techniques. Gross motor behavior of this type is destructive if it is the only coping mechanism used.

TOUCHING

Families bind together in emergencies and crises. People reach out to each other for comfort and support. Most people only touch others they care about or are comfortable with. Assessing a person's ability to respond to touch from visitors helps you to determine whether the truly important support people are present. Be careful to consider cultural variations in touching, however, as this does vary greatly. Do not take the telephone advertising slogan "Reach out and touch someone" lightly. Touch can be conveyed by someone's voice as well as by actual skin contact. A person talking on the telephone to a person meaningful to him is not carrying on idle conversation, no matter how much it may sound that way; he is being comforted by knowing that someone he cares about is concerned about him.

RUNNING

Running is another motor reaction to an alarm state. It is not often seen, but sometimes a person is admitted to the hospital in severe shock from blood loss because his first response to a threat was to run rather than to seek medical help. The person is so involved in this response that he is unaware that he is bleeding or even that he had been cut or injured.

HYPERVENTILATION

Hyperventilation is deep and rapid respirations. An increased respiratory rate occurs as part of the sympathetic nervous system's response to threat; hyperventilation is an extension of this normal expected response. Intense or prolonged hyperventilation will lead to an electrolyte imbalance (alkalosis) as the person exhales more carbon dioxide than normally. To relieve hyperventilation, encourage the person to concentrate on something else such as counting to twenty; it is very difficult to slow your respiratory pattern as long as you are thinking about it. Breathing into a paper bag may be necessary to restore the carbon dioxide level.

Unconscious Defenses

Psychological defense mechanisms were first identified by Sigmund Freud who termed such defenses *mental mechanisms* (Freud, 1946). They are the working of the unconscious mind to protect or shield the person against threat. Psychological defense mechanisms can be thought of as delaying actions like verbal and motor mechanisms. They provide a time span for the shock of the threat to become less intense, so that the cognitive, verbal, and motor coping strategies will not be overwhelmed by the assault. Remember when you recognize these defenses that they are not conscious mechanisms; you cannot change the person's response by merely telling him he is reacting negatively or in an unhelpful way to the situation. When the threat is less intense and his anxiety level is lower, he should be able to move to a conscious coping mechanism that will eventually solve the problem.

DENIAL

Denial consists of blocking out the awareness of the threat. It is the normal first stage of grief or reaction to extreme loss. A person returning from the cemetery after the burial of a husband or wife may think, "It was a nice funeral; I should tell [the person who was just buried] about it." The mind has blocked out the fact that the person has died to keep the hurt within controllable limits. People following a heart attack may deny that they are ill to the point that they do not take their medicine or attempt to limit their exercise and so increase the likelihood of suffering a second heart attack or delaying recovery.

RATIONALIZATION

Rationalization is substituting an acceptable situation for a threatening one. Rationalization sounds as if it is constructive reasoning because it contains half truths. A football player, for example, who has just been told that he can never play again may say that it is just as well because he will be less likely to develop skin cancer from being out in the sun so much. It is true that exposure to sun can cause skin cancer but the reduced likelihood of his getting cancer is a minor consequence of an otherwise threatening event. He concentrates on it in order to make giving up a life's work more acceptable.

INTELLECTUALIZATION

Intellectualization consists of explaining the course or effects of a condition or the details of a threatening event with no reference to personal involvement. A person with multiple sclerosis, a neurological handicapping condition, may make many television appearances to educate the public about the symptoms of multiple sclerosis; it seems as if she is very well adjusted to being ill until you realize that she never talks about what it feels like to her to have multiple sclerosis. She is intellectualizing to shield herself from having to examine those feelings.

IDENTIFICATION

Identification is taking on the characteristics or behavior patterns of another. Children use identification (becoming like their parents or an idol) to adapt to growth changes.

REACTION FORMATION

Reaction formation is acting in opposition to one's true feelings. An insecure person, for example, often acts very aggressively and projects a secure, threatening manner.

REPRESSION

Repression is the unconscious exclusion of an idea from consciousness. With denial, when reminded of the event, the person remembers instantly that the event did occur. With repression, the person has suppressed the event to such an extent that he no longer can recall the event and may insist that it never happened. When an event is repressed in this way, anxiety may increase and become the substance of dreams (a person who was injured by falling has recurrent dreams of falling) or an unexplained dread or fear (walking near an open window, the person begins to have symptoms of a stress response; he cannot account for the anxiety he feels as he does not remember falling from a height). Repression is utilized when the situation that occurred was so repulsive or frightening that the person does not dare allow it to surface because he would be overwhelmed by guilt or fear.

PROJECTION

Projection is transferring one's thoughts to another. A patient has just been told that he has a fatal illness; when you walk into his room, feeling happy and cheerful, he says, "You must feel sad." It is as if he is looking through his own feelings and so everyone seems to participate in them.

COMPENSATION

Compensation is substituting one activity for the activity one really wants to do. The person with a deformed leg who subconsciously wants to be an athlete works to become a spelling champion. Compensation is healthy up to a point. However, a person may spend every waking hour memorizing spelling words at the expense of being a well-rounded person; or a person may achieve the ultimate in his substitute activity (wins an important spelling contest) but the victory is a hollow one because it really has no meaning for him (despite how good he is, he is not what he really wants to be). A lifetime pattern of compensation that ultimately leaves a person feeling very inadequate may be the reason that some very successful people at the height of their careers suddenly commit suicide.

REGRESSION

Regression is adopting behavior that was comfortable and acceptable at an earlier point in life. An example is a person who, after surgery, becomes increasingly dependent on other people to take care of his needs; or a preschooler who comes into a hospital toilet-trained and by the third day begins bedwetting. Returning to an earlier comfortable time in life offers the feeling of security that was present at that time in contrast to the insecurity of the present situation.

SUBLIMATION

Sublimation is the transformation of unwanted sexual or aggressive drives into socially acceptable pursuits. Punching a punching bag after being fired from a job (rather than the person who fired you) represents sublimation.

INDICATIONS THAT A STRESS STATE IS BECOMING ACUTE

People who are reaching a point of exhaustion in their coping strategies begin to evidence typical behaviors. The better you know a person, the easier it is to recognize these as they may be subtle responses (but it is also easier to treat them as unimportant because they are not unlike the person's usual behavior).

Accentuated Use of a Particular Behavior Pattern

Structuring is an effective way of controlling stress because it does not allow any surprises to impinge on the person's life. As a person feels less and less in control of his situation, he may depend more and more on structuring or repeating a behavior. A patient, waiting for the results of a laboratory test, for example, washes his hands, returns to his bed, gets up to rewash his hands, looks at a magazine for a minute, rewashes his hands. He knows that his hands are not dirty (and neither is this behavior comparable to the psychotic activity of Shakespeare's Lady Macbeth); repetition of an activity that the person is comfortable with keeps his mind off the results of the test. You may find yourself engaging in similar behavior for a few minutes before an important exam: counting the number of pencils you brought, checking that your pen works, rememorizing your student number.

Disorganized Behavior

Acute or severe stress may lead to an inability to think or to organize clearly. If you gave the person mentioned above, for example, a menu for the next day and asked him to check off what foods he wanted for breakfast, he might start to get a pencil out of his bedside stand, then stop, unable to recall what he was intending to do. If you gave him two tasks to do, you might come back in a few minutes and find that he has done neither; he was unable to organize his thoughts enough to establish priorities and therefore did nothing. It is difficult to evaluate disorganized behavior in people you do not know well, because some people normally function in a less organized manner than others. Poor organization hinders functioning, however. Disorganization that disrupts normal functioning is suspect for a high stress level. Students may demonstrate such behavior if they have too many assignments due on the same date, working for a minute on a term paper, changing to work on a chemistry assignment, changing yet again to study for an examination, and getting none of the assignments completed effectively.

Change in Activity from Usual Pattern

A frequent area in which people change activities is personal hygiene. When a person who is usually meticulous in hygiene neglects her make-up or bathing, she is probably under a high level of stress. A safe and cautious driver who receives two speeding violations or reports two "near accidents" in a week is another example. On first contact with people it is difficult to assess them as you are not familiar with their normal routines. Friends and family often comment on such changes. Do not routinely attribute these changes to the patient's physical illness; his stress from trying to face the fact of the illness may be causing the behavioral changes. For example, loss of appetite or excessive eating are responses to stress that are easily recognized by family members (QRS 12-1).

> **☐ QUICK REFERENCE STOP 12-1: NUTRITION**
>
> 1. People under stress may experience chronic nausea or anorexia (loss of appetite). Monitor the intake of such individuals not only for total quantity but quality to be certain the person is not just "grabbing a bite" but maintaining a nutritious pattern.
> 2. Other people under chronic stress eat constantly as a coping mechanism. Help such people to find another manner of rewarding themselves to help prevent obesity.

With an increased stress level a person's tolerance for other forms of stress (a loud television set, hair torn by adhesive tape, a thoughtless remark) is lowered. Everyone has had the experience of "snapping" at another person over something that ordinarily would not upset them. It is evidence of the degree of stress present.

Decreased Sensitivity to the Environment

An increased stress level may also decrease the person's awareness of his surroundings: A woman does not notice food burning on the stove; a man drives past his usual thruway exit. There is an association between accidents and stress due to this phenomenon. Childhood poisoning can also be related to stress: A mother under stress may neglect to put away a bottle of medicine she has just used, an action that she would normally be very careful to do.

Misinterpretation of Reality

Misinterpretation of reality involves a person's misunderstanding what he is told (only hearing what he wants to hear) or reading into a person's reaction that reaction he expects or wants to see. A person may be told by his physician that although his red cell count looks good, his white blood cell pattern is suggestive of leukemia. A few minutes later when you ask him about his laboratory report, he may say that he was told that the report showed that his red blood cell pattern is healthy (he did not "hear" the illness part of the report). Because of this phenomenon you invariably have to repeat instructions you give to people in an emergency situation. Such times are not optimal for patient education beyond necessary pertinent instructions.

Psychosomatic Symptoms

Psychological stress may lead to physical stress such as symptoms of nausea and vomiting, heartburn, headache, or diarrhea. Physiological reactions to threat are often similar; many experience stomach sensations and usually develop a headache, so these symptoms are helpful in identifying the syndrome as a stress manifestation rather than as a part of their primary illness. Such stress phenomena may worsen a primary illness and confuse a person's diagnosis until identified correctly.

Poor Memory

People under stress may not be able to recall even such basic information as their ages or names. They have difficulty remembering to take medicine; they cannot be counted on to remind you when a treatment is due or when you must turn off a heat lamp or heating pad. They may forget return appointments for follow-up care unless they are carefully written down for them.

Lessened Self-Esteem

A person who is overtaken by stress feels as helpless as someone standing in the middle of a railroad track with a locomotive racing toward him. The closer the locomotive gets to him, the more he realizes that he should be doing something about it, yet the less he is able to do. The realization that he is doing nothing causes a loss of self-confidence. For a period of time following intense stress people do not perform at their usual level until gradually they regain confidence in themselves to regulate their lives again.

Quick Reference Stop 12-2 explores some of the latest research findings in the area of stress related to illness.

CRISIS SITUATIONS

In the Chinese language the word *crisis* is symbolized by a character which means both danger and opportunity. Crisis can be defined as a situation of combined danger and opportunity or as a point of time at which a person is being threatened intensely; the outcome of the situation can be either improved functioning or reduced functioning. Caplan (1964) has identified the concept of

☐ QUICK REFERENCE STOP 12-2: RESEARCH
The Patient in Stress

Stress is a fact of everyday life but certainly is more pronounced during illness and/or hospitalization. Nurses are constantly seeking to identify stress-producing factors so that they may intervene, wherever possible, to help alleviate the stress present. The samples of stress-related research cited below exemplify some of the endeavors nurses have made to help advance knowledge in caring for the patient in stress.

WHAT DO HOSPITAL PATIENTS FIND STRESSFUL?

In order to help identify the kinds of stresses groups of patients and individual patients might be experiencing, the Hospital Stress Rating Scale was developed. It is a 49-item questionnaire that nurses can administer to patients they are caring for. The nurse can plan individualized interventions for her patients based on the answers. (Meissner, 1980).

SHOULD PATIENTS BE PREPARED IN ADVANCE FOR THREATENING PROCEDURES?

According to the results of a study of 84 children, the answer is yes. Specifically, in this study it was found that providing sensory information—what the child would see, hear, and feel during a procedure—was more likely to reduce the stress associated with the procedure than being told factual information or being told nothing at all. (Robinson et al., 1982).

WHAT SPECIFIC COMFORT MEASURES HELP ALLEVIATE DISTRESS IN CHILDREN?

According to Triplett and Arneson (1979), previous research has demonstrated that young children experience stress during hospitalization which can prolong recovery from illness. Nurses, therefore, need to identify and utilize measures to alleviate such stress. This exploratory study utilized a sample of 63 children to assess the effectiveness of verbal and tactile comfort measures to alleviate stress in the children. The results clearly demonstrated that touching is the method of choice in comforting young children, especially those under six months of age. The researchers concluded, however, that both verbal and tactile comfort measures can minimize distress. It was suggested that nurses make efforts to obtain information from parents of hospitalized children to determine how individual children react to stress and what comfort measures are usually effective. Further study was recommended.

SUGGESTED READINGS

Meissner, J. E. Measuring patient stress with the Hospital Stress Rating Scale. *Nursing 80,* 10:70—71, 1980. Report on the Hospital Stress Rating Scale developed by B. J. Volicer and M. W. Bohannon Burns, copyright 1975 by AJN Co. and originally cited in *Nurs. Res.* 24:45, 1975.

Robinson, J. E., Kirchoff, K. T., and Endress, M. P. Sensory information can reduce children's fear of threatening procedures. A report of a study presented in *Nursing 82,* 12:24, 1982.

Triplett, J. L., and Arneson, S. W. The use of verbal and tactile comfort to alleviate distress in young children. *Res. Nurs. Health* 2:17, 1979.

crisis and steps that are helpful in reducing a crisis state to an acceptable level (crisis intervention).

Crisis is prolonged stress; it occurs when a person's usual coping mechanisms do not effectively alleviate a feeling of stress. No matter how acute, a crisis state lasts no longer than six weeks; at the end of this time a period of psychological exhaustion is reached, and the person does something to alleviate the problem. Unfortunately, the person's actions may not be therapeutic or in his best interests. Crisis intervention is initiating secondary and tertiary coping strategies that will resolve the stress situation. Successfully resolving a crisis situation enriches the person's ability to problem-solve in a subsequent crisis.

Maturational Crises

A maturational crisis is an expected crisis that accompanies major changes in maturing; it is a situation that can be anticipated. Toddlerhood, for example, with its insistence on independence and doing everything for oneself, may be viewed by a mother as a crisis situation: She enjoyed the rocking, cuddling, and holding that being the mother to an infant involved; she finds allowing a child to play by himself on the floor upsetting and lonely for her. It is a rare parent (or adolescent) who does not view as a crisis situation the slammed doors and stomped feet as an adolescent expresses his independence. Many people think of arriving at middle age as a crisis; many older people who have outlived their support people find that retirement is a crisis period.

Fortunately, maturational crises can be anticipated. Primary preventive measures (anticipatory guidance) can be initiated to help people learn how to manage maturational situations. Parents need to understand that independence and autonomy are desirable characteristics and need to be strengthened, not opposed; the change is not threatening if prepared and planned for.

Situational Crises

Situational crises are unpredictable life events such as loss of a job, death of a loved one, birth of an imperfect baby, financial failure, environmental disasters such as fire and flood, and illness. Situational and maturational crises are compared in Table 12-2.

Rating Events As to Level of Stress

Although events are individualized and mean different things to different people, they can be categorized to some extent in terms of their level of stress. Common life events and their stress values are shown in Table 12-3. If a person's total score from the table is 150 to 199, the person has mild stress; up to 37 percent of people with this level of stress will become physically ill. A score between 200 and 299 points reflects a medium stress level; up to 51 percent of people in this category will become ill as soon as two weeks. A total score over 300 reflects a high stress level; 79 percent of the people in this group will become physically ill.

TABLE 12-2. DIFFERENTIATION BETWEEN MATURATIONAL AND SITUATIONAL CRISES

Type	Definition	Examples
Maturational	An expected event caused by the process of maturing	Toddlerhood Beginning school Adolescence Marriage Middle Age Retirement Death
Situational	An unanticipated event	Environmental disruptions such as flood, fire, tornado Divorce Illness

It is interesting to score your own life style using the figures in the table. If you are a student away at school, you are probably experiencing a change in living conditions (25), a change in residence (20), a change in number of family get-togethers (15), a change in social activities (18), a change in recreation (19), a change in church activities (19), a change in financial status (38), responsibility for a loan less than $10,000 (17), and beginning school (26). This totals 197 points. If even one other factor is present such as a change in sleeping or eating habits, you would be categorized by this measure as being under medium stress. You need not only to gain experience in helping others to deal with stress but to apply these techniques to yourself so that you can cope with the stress load that a college or school experience places on you.

Stages of Crises

A crisis can be divided into three stages. The first stage begins when the threatening situation is first perceived; the person begins to experience anxiety and tension. In this stage he attempts to use common coping or adaptive mechanisms to solve the problem; his usual coping mechanisms fail, however, and the stress continues. For example, a woman who is a poor housekeeper plans an important dinner party for Saturday night. In order to have her house spotlessly clean for this type of event, she typically asks her sister to help her clean house on Saturday morning. In this instance, she learns that her sister is unexpectedly out of town. She thinks of the important people coming to her home in a few hours; her primary coping mechanism has failed; she is facing a crisis situation. Fig. 12-2 shows diagrammatically how a crisis situation is resolved by a primary coping mechanism; Fig. 12-3 shows how a crisis continues when a primary intervention fails until a secondary mechanism is employed. In this instance, a secondary mechanism the woman might use would be asking a neighbor to help her.

Most people are capable of utilizing a primary coping mechanism to solve life situations; most are capable of formulating an alternative or secondary solution. If the

TABLE 12-3. SOCIAL READJUSTMENT RATING SCALE FOR LIFE CHANGES

Rank	Life Event	Mean Value
1	Death of spouse	100
2	Divorce	73
3	Marital separation	65
4	Jail term	63
5	Death of close family member	63
6	Personal injury or illness	53
7	Marriage	50
8	Fired at work	47
9	Marital reconciliation	45
10	Retirement	45
11	Change in health of family member	44
12	Pregnancy	40
13	Sex difficulties	39
14	Gain of new family member	39
15	Business readjustment	39
16	Change in financial state	38
17	Death of close friend	37
18	Change to different line of work	36
19	Change in number of arguments with spouse	35
20	Mortgage more than $10,000	31
21	Foreclosure of mortgage or loan	30
22	Change in responsibilities at work	29
23	Son or daughter leaving home	29
24	Trouble with in-laws	29
25	Outstanding personal achievement	28
26	Wife beginning or stopping work	26
27	Begin or end school	26
28	Change in living conditions	25
29	Revision of personal habits	24
30	Trouble with boss	23
31	Change in work hours or conditions	20
32	Change in residence	20
33	Change in schools	20
34	Change in recreation	19
35	Change in church activities	19
36	Change in social activities	18
37	Mortgage or loan less than $10,000	17
38	Change in sleeping habits	16
39	Change in number of family get-togethers	15
40	Change in eating habits	15
41	Vacation	13
42	Christmas	13
43	Minor violations of the law	11

Source: From T. H. Holmes and R. H. Rahe, The social readjustment rating scale. *J. Psychosomatic Res.* 2:214, 1967.

secondary solution fails, a person may be incapable of designing a third alternate without outside intervention. Fig. 12-4 shows diagrammatically what would happen if in the example above the secondary coping mechanism was also ineffective (no neighbor was available to help out). People cannot maintain mental health in the face of constant unresolved crises. Being present to supply tertiary coping mechanisms is a prime nursing responsibility.

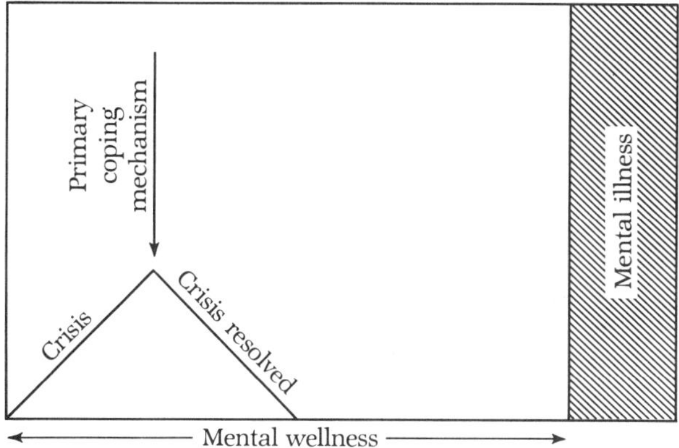

FIGURE 12-2. A crisis situation is resolved by a primary coping mechanism. (From G. Caplan, *Principles of Preventive Psychiatry.* New York: Basic Books, 1964.)

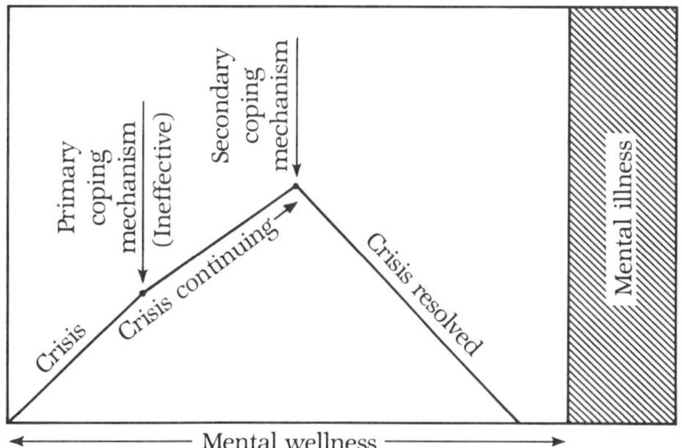

FIGURE 12-3. A crisis situation continues when a primary intervention fails until a secondary mechanism is employed. (From G. Caplan, *Principles of Preventive Psychiatry.* New York: Basic Books, 1964.)

Factors Influencing Ability To Solve Crises

Whether people can manage crisis situations by themselves or need help in doing so depends on three main variables: their perception of the event, the type and availability of support people they have to call upon, and the ways of coping or managing stressful events that they have found successful in the past (Caplan, 1964).

PERCEPTION OF THE EVENT

Perception of an event is a very individual response based on the person's cultural and individual values. A person who dreams of his son becoming an Olympic track star, for example, may perceive his son's broken leg as the ultimate disaster; another parent may view the same injury as a minor happening in a lifetime of raising active children. Do not evaluate an event in terms of how serious (or not serious) *you* think it is. It is the person's perception of the seriousness that will affect his ability to handle the situation.

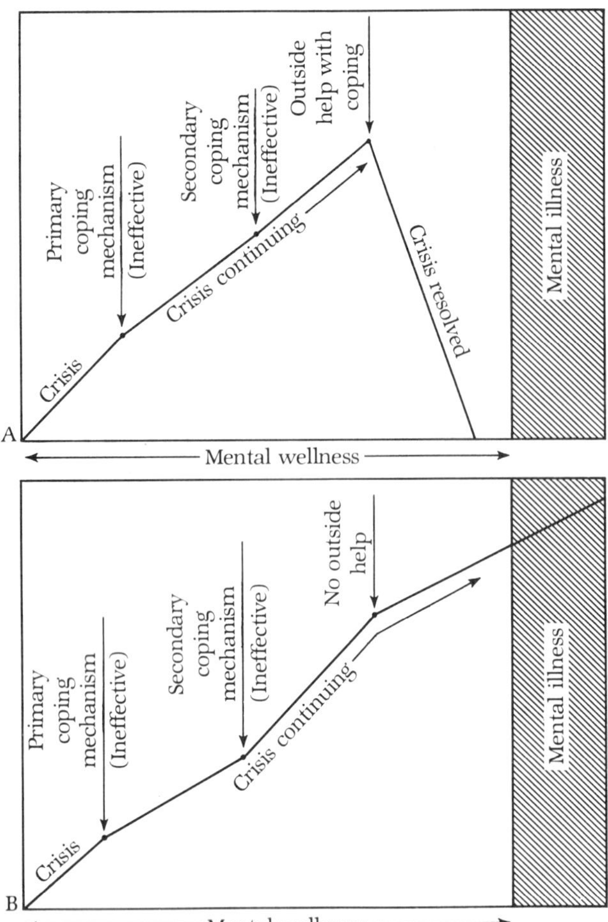

FIGURE 12-4. A. When a person's coping mechanisms fail, outside or tertiary intervention is necessary to solve crisis. B. With no outside intervention, the crisis remains unresolved and may result in mental illness. (From G. Caplan, *Principles of Preventive Psychiatry.* New York: Basic Books, 1964.)

SUPPORT PERSONS

Support people are those who play a significant part in giving counsel or guidance to others in times of stress. In order to be effective support people they must be capable of this function and available when needed. Parents are the traditional support people for a child, spouses for each other; many young adults depend on their peers as their critical support people. Support of this nature can be nonverbal; a person sitting quietly by an ill person's bedside may be offering more emotional support than a very vocal one. Helping people to contact their support persons is an important nursing responsibility; serving as an advocate when the person's usual support system has failed him is equally important.

COPING MECHANISMS

The more experience a person has with resolving crises, the better at it he becomes. In some instances, however, the situation is unique and a person's usual coping mechanisms are inadequate for the problem. Everyone, no matter how experienced, has the potential for facing a seemingly unsolvable crisis. Reminding a person of ways that he has coped successfully in the past helps to give him confidence that he will survive this present assault as well. Helping him to think through the steps of crisis intervention so that he can best use his coping mechanisms is an important nursing responsibility.

If the resolution that a person makes to a crisis situation is realistic (results in acceptance of what is inevitable, strengthens interpersonal ties, or renews equilibrium), it is an *adaptive* resolution. The person has not only resolved a crisis but enriched his ability to deal with future crises. If the resolution is inappropriate to reality (results in lasting interpersonal disturbances or in newly formed neurotic or psychotic syndromes), it is *maladaptive* (Caplan, 1964). Figure 12-5 illustrates the two possible outcomes of a crisis situation depending on the perception of the event, the presence or absence of support people, and the coping mechanisms utilized (Aquilera, 1982).

PERSONALITY TYPES AND STRESS

Friedman (1974) has identified two different personality types, the type A person, who is usually hurried and preoccupied with time, goals, and achievement, and the type B person, who operates at a slower rate and is concerned more with interpersonal relationships.

People with a type A personality are more apt to develop cardiovascular disease than those with a type B personality. This is probably because those with type A personalities are always under at least mild stress due to their urge to meet deadlines and goals. Mild stress maintains blood pressure at a constant elevated level due to vasoconstriction and increased aldosterone secretion by the adrenal gland (aldosterone holds sodium which holds an increased level of water or volume in vessels). People with a type A personality need to identify adequate coping mechanisms early in a stress process to avoid the consequences of major stress on an already taxed system. Characteristics used to identify people with type A personalities are listed in the box on page 215.

CRISIS INTERVENTION

Crisis intervention is a problem-solving technique consisting of a five-step process.

Identifying the Problem

Identifying a problem is often more difficult than it would appear because your own evaluation of what is or is not a problem tends to cloud your judgment. Remember that what is important to the person with the problem is the important assessment. One way to identify this is to ask which of all your problems worries you the most? If there were just one thing I could do for you, what would you like it to be? As long as a problem is nebulous (something is wrong), the person cannot begin to solve it. Once it is clearly identified (*this* is wrong), half the problem solving has been achieved.

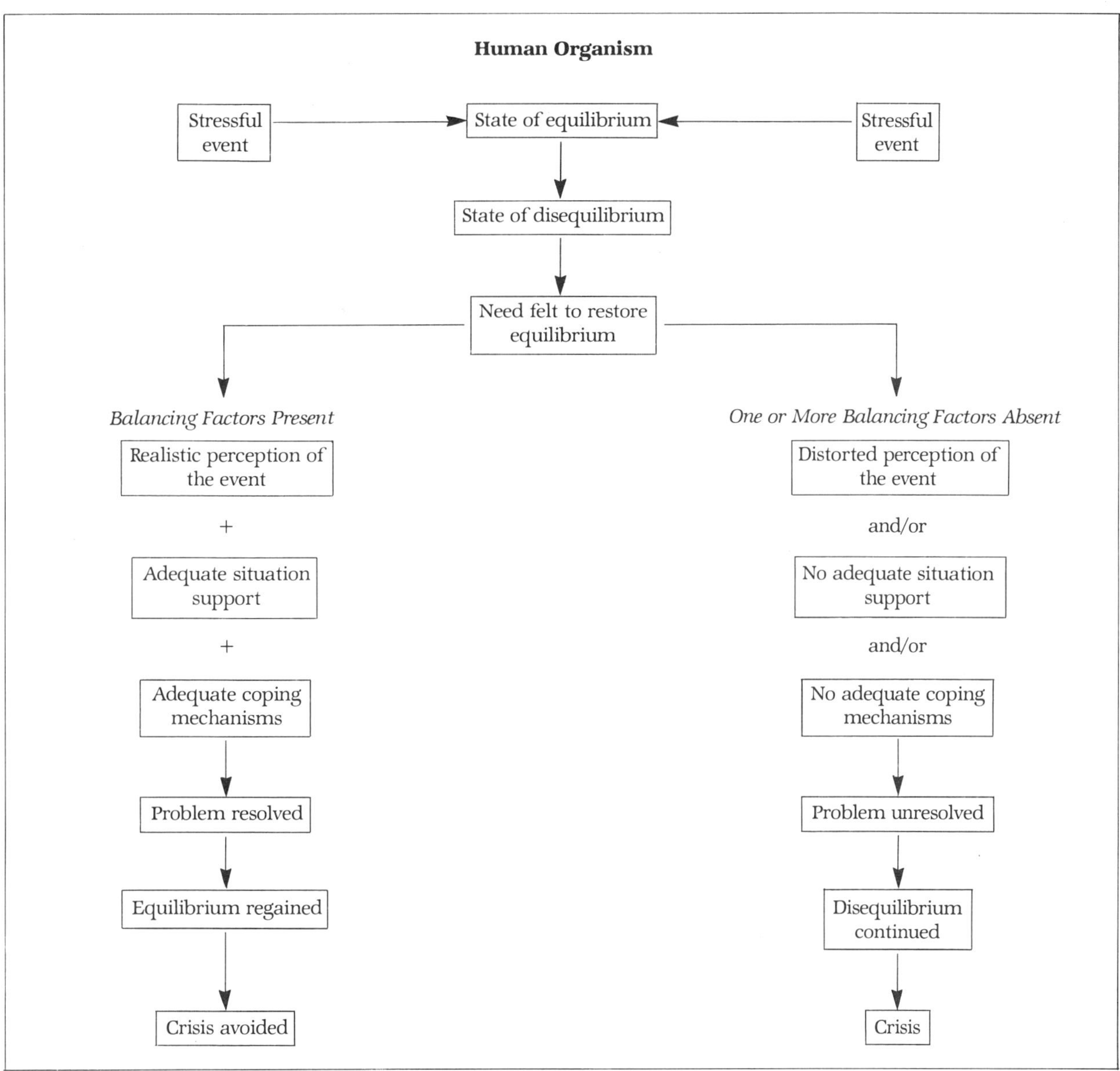

FIGURE 12-5. Effect of balancing factors in a stressful event. (From G. Caplan, *Principles of Preventive Psychiatry.* New York: Basic Books, 1964.)

Characteristics of Type A Personality

- Aggressive, ambitious, unable to delegate authority
- Possesses intense physical and emotional drives
- Concentrates on career and has no hobbies
- Experiences a chronic sense of time urgency
- Preoccupied with deadlines
- Exhibits excessive competitive drive
- Takes little satisfaction from accomplishments
- Obsessed with numbers
- Obsessed with money
- Presents as self-assured and self-confident
- Measures self by number of achievements
- Insecure about status
- Restless during leisure time and guilty about relaxing

Source: From M. Friedman and R. Rosenman, *Type A Behavior and Your Heart.* Greenwich, Conn.: Fawcett Publications, 1974.

Listing Alternatives

The only alternatives that people can choose to resolve any situation are those that they are aware of. A major aspect of problem solving for nurses, then, is to help people to think of or to supply for them additional solutions to their problems. The more alternatives to a problem a person can list, the better the chance that he will find an appropriate solution. It is important to simply list alternatives at this point, not rate or examine them.

Choosing from Among Alternatives

Before people select an alternative, be certain that they have thought through the "what would happen ifs" of the choices. Michael D'Amore, for example, is a young adult who is a medical student at a local university. He has a wife and two children. He works part-time as a laboratory assistant; his wife works full-time as a waitress in order to meet expenses. His wife has recently been hospitalized for a broken tibia suffered in a fall on their slippery front steps. You meet with him to help him think through how to solve the child-care problem while his wife is hospitalized (five to seven days). The solution that he has devised is to ask his mother to care for the two children three days a week. Alternate solutions you work out together are: Notify his school that he will be absent for a week due to an unforeseen circumstance; ask a neighbor who occasionally baby-sits for them if for one week she will do so full-time; pay a professional baby-sitting service for one week; ask a high-school girl in the apartment downstairs to be absent from school and baby-sit for him.

Spending time to think through the "what would happen ifs" in each solution helps to identify the best one. If he asks his mother to baby-sit, for example, the fatigue of caring for two young children might be too exhausting for her; by the end of the week he would be even more frustrated at learning that he had hurt her. Paying a professional baby-sitting service seems beyond his financial reach. In conscience, he could not ask a high-schooler to lie in order to work for him. Taking a week off from medical school would jeopardize his ability to finish the semester. Asking the neighbor to baby-sit during the day and the high-schooler in the evening, with his mother helping out one afternoon, is the solution he selects for the problem.

The alternatives that people choose from the choices available to them differ greatly from person to person, depending on their values and what is or is not important to them. Another person with different values might have no difficulty asking a person to lie for him; a less dedicated one might have no hesitation disrupting a school program.

Implementing the Plan

Some people are best at planning; some at doing. People who problem-solve best are a combination—both talkers and doers. In some instances just talking about a problem is so therapeutic that no action is necessary, but as a rule follow-through is an intrinsic part of the process. Some people need to be urged to carry out the plan they have agreed to as best; those for whom planning is a chore need to be urged to think through the situation one more time before they act, to find a balance between planning and implementation.

Evaluation

Evaluation is a step often forgotten in problem solving; one assumes that because he has planned well and carefully the solution will work. Sometimes obvious factors are overlooked, however, so unless you check that the solution was adequate to solve the problem, problems may go unsolved. Suppose when you ask Mrs. D'Amore as you care for her the following day how the baby-sitting plans worked out, she replies, "Terribly. The neighbor we were counting on to help us is in St. Louis baby-sitting her grandchildren this week." The best laid plans are not always effective solutions. Assuming the D'Amores are still interested in your help, you need to return to identifying new alternatives, perhaps something you missed before. For example, what about *Mrs.* D'Amore's parents? You do not know whether they are available to help out because they have not even been mentioned.

Evaluation is necessary because it sets the stage for further problem solving and offers the reward of knowing that your thought processes are effective. The better you feel about your ability to problem-solve, the easier it is because no alternative on a list seems beyond your capabilities to use successfully. Evaluation produces a feedback loop that strengthens problem-solving ability or leads back to reassessment. Nursing process is a problem-solving technique and has the same basic format.

LIFE SPAN CONCEPTS AND CRISIS INTERVENTION

Practical methods to deal with crises are listed on page 217. The ability to problem-solve and use effective crisis intervention techniques changes with different life stages.

The Infant

Infants have special needs to feel secure and well loved. They depend completely on people to fill these needs and to supply basic food and shelter. Only toward the end of the first year of life does any degree of problem-solving ability become apparent: Learning the concept of permanence, that articles exist out of sight, is the beginning of identifying a problem and realistic perception.

The Toddler and Preschooler

Toddlers and preschoolers learn elementary problem solving. Their perception of an event is often distorted due to lack of experience, however, and they may evaluate it differently from an adult. They have little experience with devising coping strategies or listing alternatives and have few useful coping mechanisms in their repertoire. Everyone has watched a toddler kick a toy that would not work; this action represented the only solution that he could devise.

The Schoolager and Adolescent

Children who are allowed to problem-solve for themselves develop a great deal of skill by the end of the adolescent period. A child who develops a firm sense of initiative in the preschool period enters the school-age period equipped to creatively list solutions and alternatives. As he learns a sense of industry, he develops confidence in his ability to persist with a task and repeat it if

Methods to Deal With Crises

1. Help the person to recognize his individual stress level, a level that differs from person to person. Because he works next to someone who is not upset by some condition does not mean that he will not be annoyed or upset. On the other hand, if a situation does not annoy a person, he should not feel that he has to react to it just because a partner does. Help people to understand and accept individual differences.
2. Help the person to learn to change those things (make external changes) he cannot accept and to learn to accept (change internally) those things he cannot change (termed attitudinal or behavior changes). Trial and error is often required to determine the difference between the two categories. Often a total change is not necessary; a modification in himself or the event will make the difference.
3. Help the person to reach out for support. People under threat are often so involved in the problem that they do not realize that people around them want to help. Often in a stress situation the people closest to someone are under as much threat as the first person and are no longer able to offer support. Call on second or third level support persons for help.
4. Help the person develop a habit of reaching out to give support when others are in threat. Survival is a collaborative function of a social animal; a favor offered now can be called in when he is in need at a later date.
5. Help the person to face the situation as honestly as possible. A test that must be taken, a paper that must be written does not go away by ignoring it, and the knowledge that such a task still must be faced may be more wearing than the actual task. As a rule, knowing exactly the nature of the threat is less stressful than a shadow-haunting, something-is-out-there feeling. On the other hand, people should not be urged to face intense threats such as their own death until they have had time to mobilize their defenses.
6. Help people not to rush decisions or final adaptive outcomes. Many times following the death of a husband a widow will sell her home and most of her furniture and move to a small apartment or a daughter's house. She realizes later when she is able to think more clearly that her home and furniture had more meaning to her than she believed. As a rule, major decisions of this type should be delayed at least six weeks after the event; six months is an even better time interval.
7. Help people anticipate life events and plan for them to the extent possible. A good deal of health teaching with mothers of small children should focus on helping them learn about what to expect of their child before he becomes a toddler, a preschooler, an adolescent. Anticipatory guidance will not totally prepare a parent for the child's new moods or the number of slammed doors he will hear over the next few years, but at least he will recognize the behavior as normal.
8. Alert people that accidents increase when people are under stress. A person worrying about his illness is more apt to have an automobile accident or burn himself on a hot stove than a person who is under less stress.
9. Action feels good in crises. Doing something brings a sense of control to the feeling of hopelessness and disorganization. Action often is so satisfying that people do things such as write threatening letters or make hurtful remarks that they later regret. Help a person to channel this energy into a therapeutic action (going for a long walk) rather than one that could be hurtful.
10. Encourage people to verbalize their reactions. Nothing limits the extent of a threat more than being able to describe it specifically.
11. Encourage people to seek clarification or gain more knowledge about a threatful event. Often knowing more about something makes it more specific and thus less threatening.

necessary until it is well done. As an adolescent he develops a sense of identity and learns what works for him because he has an understanding of who he is for the first time. Adolescence is a stormy time for crisis intervention, however, because it is an egocentric period and perception of an event may be blurred to very narrow dimensions (Fig. 12-6). Also, the typical adolescent depends very strongly on other adolescents rather than adults for support people. Because his support people are no more experienced in coping than he is, problem solving may not be successful. Not being able to problem-solve successfully is a threat to identity; as achieving identity is a strong adolescent task, a threat to identity to an adolescent calls for problem solving.

The Young and Middle-Aged Adult

A major change which the young adult must face is that he must problem-solve not only for himself but for a family and young children as well. The young adult period is often thought of as a wellness period and it

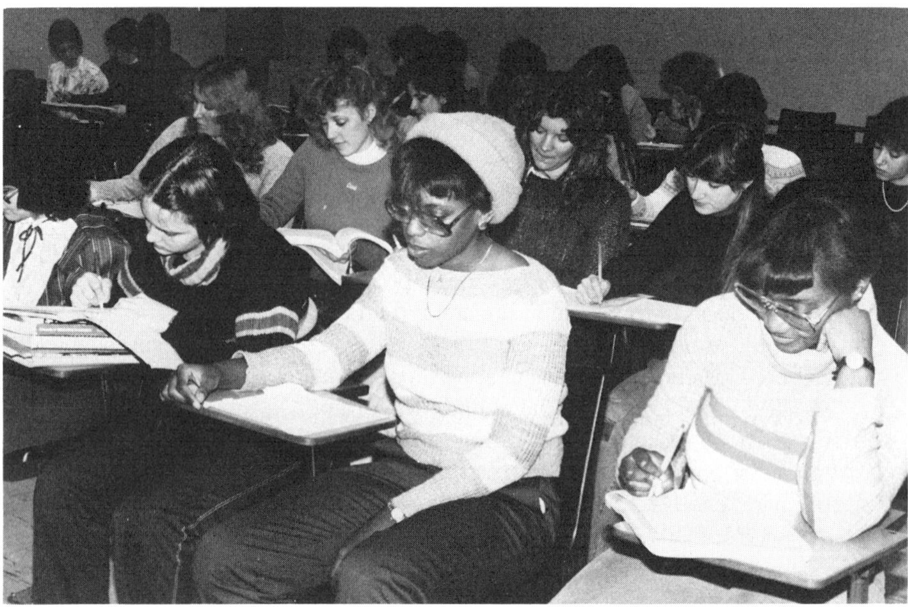

FIGURE 12-6. Social and academic pressures of school may be a constant source of stress for those children and adolescents who have not developed an adequate ability to cope with crisis.

usually is in terms of physical health, but it can be a period of considerable psychological stress. It requires good problem-solving ability to balance pressures from school, work, family, financial worries, and increased responsibility for self-care (Fig. 12-7).

Middle-aged adults can be expected to have the best problem-solving ability in view of their years of experience in problem solving, mature perspectives on problems, and both older and younger support people around them.

The Older Adult

Although the older adult is in the best position from an experience standpoint to be an effective problem solver, if he has limited financial means or health difficulties, his capacity for problem solving may be limited. Never dismiss the ability of the older adult to problem-solve for himself, however. In many instances, older adults can achieve the most clever solutions to problems of any age group; they offer examples you do not want to miss as role models.

USING BIOFEEDBACK TO COUNTERACT STRESS

Biofeedback is a process by which a person can control his involuntary muscles, skin temperature, heart rate, and blood pressure through extensive conditioning (Fig. 12-8). Biofeedback has particular implications for patients who would be affected greatly by stress: A person with heart disease could be taught to prevent his heart rate from rising under stress or to bring it quickly back to a normal level. People who suffer from back pain because of constantly tensed back muscles could be conditioned to relieve the muscle tension causing their pain. Biofeedback cannot be utilized by everyone because it requires the person to play an active role in his treatment (which not all people wish to do); it is a supplementary therapy for individual persons.

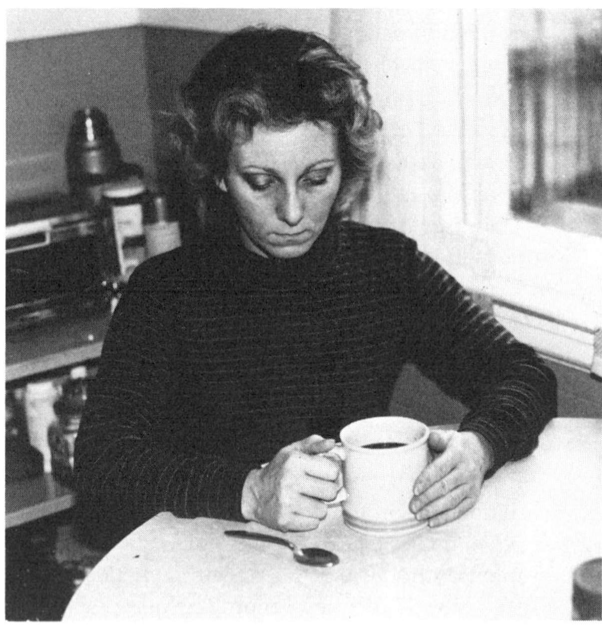

FIGURE 12-7. Stress may come from a variety of sources. The adult must learn to balance these pressures.

EFFECTS OF UNRESOLVED CRISIS SITUATIONS

People cannot function effectively under constant stress; they cannot function well if they cannot use crisis intervention measures well even for short-term stress.

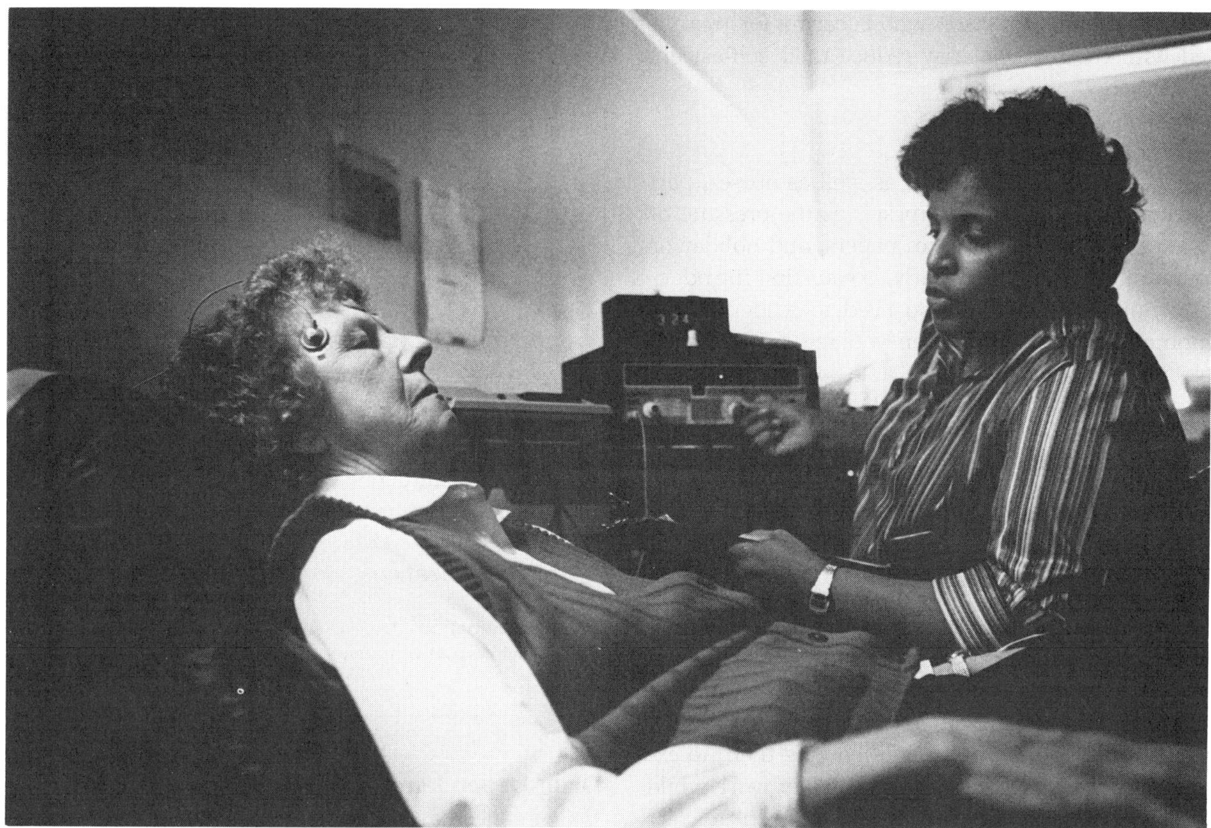

FIGURE 12-8. Use of a biofeedback machine for stress reduction. A patient's pulse rate can be determined by the monitor.

Burnout

Burnout is a popularly used term to refer to the third stage of the general adaptation syndrome when the stress process is work-related. It is described as a syndrome of physical and emotional exhaustion involving the development of a negative self-concept, negative job attitude, and loss of concern and feeling for people (Pines and Aronson, 1981).

Nurses are particularly prone to burnout as nursing is both physically and psychologically tiring. It is physically tiring because of the amount of lifting, turning, positioning, and walking that is necessary. If changes in shifts are involved and a nurse's circadian rhythm (day-night rhythm) is disrupted, fatigue is greatly increased. It is psychologically tiring because in order to empathize you must "live inside another" for a while. Taking on another person's worries and concerns can leave a person as drained as if the worries and concerns were physically heavy.

Nurses who are experiencing burnout begin to show some typical behaviors. These include intellectualization and distancing and detachment (Maslach, 1976). Distancing and detachment result in increased illness, absence from work, and "caring" but not "caring for" behavior (much time is spent socializing and record keeping but little in direct patient care). This creates job dissatisfaction among peers because they must take on the extra work (and so leads to burnout occurring in them as well). It increases the feeling of burnout in the original person because part of the enjoyment of nursing comes with being actively involved in caring for people and this is the phase that she is unintentionally neglecting.

If a person is using intellectualization as a coping strategy, she tends to dehumanize the people she cares for, referring to them by disease condition or room number rather than by name. This effectively limits interaction (if surgery is not successful on the patient in room 209, it is less traumatic than if surgery is not successful on Mr. Bryant, who is depending on returning to work to support his wife and three children).

Physical symptoms of people with burnout are extreme tiredness (physical and mental exhaustion); increased minor symptoms of illness such as sore throat, headache, or nausea; and a feeling of sadness or apathy. People identify themselves according to the work they perform; when a person's work is no longer interesting, he begins to view himself as uninteresting, develops low self-esteem, and becomes noncreative.

Burnout is potentially damaging to work situations in that it is contagious (the person projects sadness and despair and soon everyone he works with begins to feel the same way). It can be personally damaging if the person resorts to the use of alcohol or drugs to regain a feeling of his old self. It can be detrimental to patients who already feel low self-esteem because of their illness;

if they sense that the person who is caring for them is bored with the work, it may reduce their self-esteem even further.

PREVENTING BURNOUT

Burnout may occur in students as well as nurses, particularly near the end of a semester as the pressure of evaluation, examinations, term papers, and holiday or vacation plans closes in. As early as your first introduction to nursing, therefore, you need to recognize the phenomenon of burnout when you see it in friends, instructors, or yourself and be able to institute some interventions toward preventing it. A number of measures are effective:

Avoid burned-out people. Burnout is contagious; don't expose yourself to people with the syndrome any more than you would to those with a physically infectious disease. This may involve changing the person you usually ride to school with, asking to be shifted to a new clinical assignment group, or going to lunch with a different person than normally. If such arrangements cannot be managed, let the person know that you think they have a burnout problem and that you must protect yourself from acquiring it by not allowing them to express their negative feelings about school or work while you are with them. This second approach helps to alert the person to her problem so that she can begin to institute change in herself.

Maintain your physical health. It is easy in the rush of school to avoid common health practices such as balancing adequate sleep and exercise and eating a nutritious diet. A common nutritional deficiency of young adults is iron deficiency anemia (inability of red blood cells to form adequate hemoglobin to carry oxygen to cells). Be certain that your diet includes iron-rich foods such as meat and green leafy vegetables. If you feel increasingly tired (out of proportion to your activity level), a visit to a health care provider for health evaluation is in order. Physical exhaustion can quickly lead to psychological exhaustion, as you become increasingly unable to complete what you have planned to do.

Do something new and different. Boredom and routine are the route to burnout. At least once a week do something different (drive to school by the scenic route rather than the quickest route, change your study time to morning rather than evening, experiment with a new laundry soap).

Do something nice for yourself. Working without reward is another route to burnout. If you do not receive rewards for what you do from people around you (and hardly anybody does), reward yourself with such things as time to read a good novel, setting up an aquarium, an afternoon trip to the sea shore. Do not make a habit of rewarding yourself with food: rewards of this kind can lead to weight gain and decreased self-esteem (what you are trying to avoid) because of your altered appearance.

Profile of an Adolescent with a High Risk for Drug Abuse

Has no close family relationships
Has close friends who use drugs
Currently smokes cigarettes
Sees marijuana use by mother or father
Does not currently practice any religion
Feels he was raised poorly by mother or father or both
Currently uses alcohol at least weekly
Sees sibling use of hallucinogens or intravenous amphetamines
Sees regular use of tranquilizers or sedatives by mother or father
Has a low self-esteem
Is not active in sports, school activities, or community organizations

Source: From D. B. Lauria, et al., The epidemiology of drug abuse with some comments on prevention. *Pediatr. Ann.* 2:11, 1973.

Drug Dependence as a Reaction to Stress

Use of drugs has always been a means of relieving the feelings of stress. When a person takes a drug so often that physical disturbances (withdrawal symptoms) occur when he discontinues the drug, he is said to have a *physical drug dependence.* When a person prefers the state of mind induced by a drug to a drugfree state, he is said to have *psychic drug dependence.* Withdrawal (no longer taking such a drug) results in a craving for the drug that is so strong the person may confine his total life efforts to obtaining more of the drug. In many instances, both psychic and physical dependence exist simultaneously.

Characteristics of People Who Become Drug Dependent

Every person has the potential for developing drug dependence at the point where his usual coping mechanisms fail if he then chooses a drug as his next coping strategy. A person who has a low threshold for frustration, a greater than normal fear of failure, or feelings of inadequacy, or who is more attuned to pleasure-seeking behavior than the average person, is more apt to become drug dependent than the average person; this person may choose drug relief as his first or second coping solution. Some people are inadvertently led into drug dependence seeking to "know themselves better." This is an immature method of problem solving but appeals to adolescents who do not have an adequate level of problem-solving ability yet. Other people become drug dependent because they continue to take a medically prescribed drug longer than recommended. The above box shows characteristics of adolescents who are prone to become drug dependent. It is helpful to learn the symptoms of drug dependence so that you can recognize it and act to help the person change his method of coping rather than continue with such destructive behavior.

Characteristics of Drugs That Cause Dependence

Drugs that can cause dependence are those that provide desirable or pleasant states of mind. Central nervous system depressants such as alcohol, narcotics, barbiturates, and tranquilizers; central nervous system stimulants such as amphetamines and cocaine; and the hallucinogens are the most commonly abused or dependence-causing drugs.

CENTRAL NERVOUS SYSTEM DEPRESSANTS

Opiates. The opiate drugs diamorphine hydrochloride (heroin), morphine sulfate, hydromorphone hydrochoride (Dilaudid), codeine sulfate, and meperidine hydrochloride (Demerol) are the most abused narcotics. Heroin is such a strong opiate that it is only available illegally (it is a Schedule I drug, too powerful to be medically prescribed). Opiates can all be injected subcutaneously, intramuscularly or intravenously. Narcotics act on high control brain centers to produce a feeling of euphoria (a perfect state) that eliminates the desire to seek additional gratification from any source. A person's feeling of well-being can be so complete that he neglects eating or self-care.

Withdrawal symptoms from opiates are restlessness, alternating chills and warm flashes, sneezing and yawning, muscle cramps of the abdomen and lower extremities, vomiting and diarrhea, and a severe craving for the drug. In the extreme, symptoms may result in cardiovascular collapse. Physical dependence on opiates continues for about ten days after withdrawal; psychic dependence may last a lifetime.

Opiate withdrawal can be achieved by gradually reducing the dose of drug or by substituting methadone hydrochloride, a synthetic opiate. Methadone is taken orally; by eliminating the need for injected opiates in the body, it allows the person to function normally in society. Withdrawal programs must be supplemented by psychotherapy or counseling so that the person can learn better coping mechanisms, or he may return to drug dependence at a later time when he again faces a high level of frustration.

Alcohol. Alcohol is the most frequently abused drug in the United States. This occurs because it is easily available and, taken orally, has an easy route of administration. Alcohol is absorbed from the stomach at a rate of 10 ml per hour; if taken in quantities greater than this, it leads to symptoms of intoxication (overdosage). Figure 12-9 shows the influence of alcohol consumption on hand coordination.

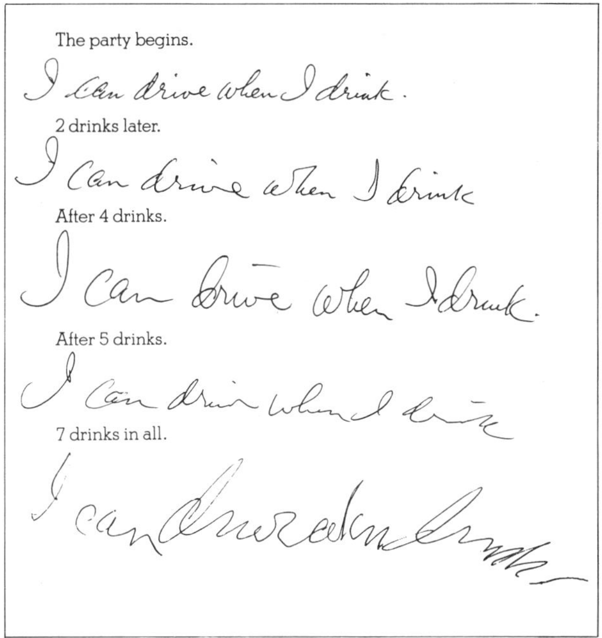

FIGURE 12-9. Influence of alcohol on handwriting. (From The House of Segram, New York, 1973.)

Although many people consider alcohol a stimulant because one of its effects is to make people more uninhibited, it is actually a central nervous system depressant (the uninhibition occurs because upper motor center control is lost as the system is depressed). Symptoms of alcohol use are loss of memory and ability to concentrate and incoordination for fine motor tasks and speech; an excessive amount leads to stupor, or deep sleep. The drug causes diuresis (increased urinary output) because it acts to depress antidiuretic hormone secretion from the pituitary.

People with alcohol dependence may fail to eat properly because they feel no need for physical gratification over and above alcohol consumption. It also interferes with the metabolism of vitamin B6, so the person may become deficient in vitamin B6. Alcohol has a destructive effect on liver cells and over a period of years can cause complete liver cell dysfunction (cirrhosis). In addition, alcohol and many prescribed drugs are synergistic—that is, their effects are increased when taken in combination. The use of alcohol under these circumstances causes unsafe drug administration.

Alcohol withdrawal symptoms are anxiety, tremors, hallucinations (seeing bugs, spiders, etc.), convulsions, or cardiovascular collapse. Withdrawal symptoms last five to seven days; psychological dependence symptoms may last a lifetime.

Barbiturates. Barbiturates are sleep medicines (hypnotics); they are also used for their calming effect in smaller doses. They may be medically prescribed for people under stress in order to help them achieve sleep and hopefully feel better enough the next day to handle

☐ **QUICK REFERENCE STOP 12-3: PHARMACOLOGY**
Tranquilizers

Definition: Medications to reduce anxiety without impairment of conciousness and to control overt behavior, perception, and mood.

Major Tranquilizers (ataractics or neuroleptics)

Use	*Example*	*Action*	*Side Effects*
Used to treat psychotic manifestations	Haloperidol (Haldol)	Depress CNS	Hypotension Depression

Minor Tranquilizers (anti-anxiety or anxiolytics)

Use	*Example*	*Action*	*Side Effects*
Used to treat mild to moderate anxiety often on an ambulatory basis	Chlordiazepoxide hydrochloride (Librium)	Depress CNS	Drowsiness, dizziness
	Diazepam (Valium)	Depress CNS	Drowsiness, ataxia
	Hydroxyzine hydrochloride (Atarax, Vistaril)	Depress CNS	Drowsiness, dizziness, dry mouth

their problems. Barbiturate intoxication symptoms are similar to those of opiates: incoordination and difficulty with concentration. Excessive dosages lead to coma and respiratory depression.

Withdrawal symptoms from barbiturates are tremors, anxiety, insomnia, and generalized weakness. Extreme symptoms are convulsions and cardiovascular collapse. About eight days are necessary for complete withdrawal. Barbiturate withdrawal is exceptionally dangerous because of the danger of convulsions that may lead to aspiration.

Tranquilizers. Tranquilizer dependence has a strong psychic as well as physical basis. Withdrawal symptoms are anxiety, insomnia, and possibly gastrointestinal distress. Diazepam (Valium) and chlordiazepoxide hydrochloride (Librium) withdrawal may result in convulsions similar to the effect of withdrawal from barbiturates.

At one time tranquilizers were considered a harmless type of drug, certainly very effective in relieving the manifestations of severe stress, and so were widely prescribed. Today their use is much more controlled as the strong drug dependence that occurs with them has become well recognized. Quick Reference Stop 12-3 shows the use, action, and side effects of major and minor tranquilizers.

Marijuana. Marijuana is made from the leaves of the hemp plant *Cannabis sativa.* Hashish is a stronger product made from the plant resin. Although both marijuana and hashish can be eaten with food, they are most often inhaled through smoking. The effect of them is depression of upper cortical centers and a feeling of well-being and relaxation. Judgment is slowed and ability to use recent memory appears to be lessened. Both forms produce psychic dependence; physical dependence can occur if extremely high dosages are involved. The chief physical withdrawal symptom is hyperactivity. The active ingredient of marijuana (THC) is currently being administered to persons receiving cancer chemotherapy to lessen the amount of nausea and vomiting that usually occurs with the administration of these drugs.

CENTRAL NERVOUS SYSTEM STIMULANTS

Amphetamines. Amphetamines are used by people to stay awake (truckdrivers, college students, night workers, for example) and for appetite control for rapid dieting. The person begins to develop tolerance for the drug and so takes more and more to achieve the same effect, causing possible drug dependence to occur.

The effect of amphetamines is one of elevated mood, lack of fatigue, and increased alertness. The person may feel capable of performing physical feats never before tried; he may push himself to a point of physical exhaustion; he may feel no need for food and so become malnourished. Amphetamine usage is particularly dangerous as the exhaustion produced may be so severe that cardiovascular collapse may occur. The main withdrawal symptoms are psychological craving and long periods of sleep.

Cocaine. Cocaine is supplied as a white powder which is usually consumed by sniffing; it is then absorbed across the mucous membrane of the nose. It can also be injected intravenously. Effects are similar to those of amphetamines—a sense of well-being and great energy—and they occur very rapidly. Chronic use of cocaine may result in weight loss and insomnia. The nasal mucosa may become necrosed (dead tissue formation) due to acute local vasoconstriction. Cocaine does not appear to cause physical dependence; it produces strong psychic dependence.

HALLUCINOGENIC AGENTS

Hallucinogenic agents are a number of drugs that cause altered visual or auditory perceptions. Frequently used drugs are lysergic acid (LSD), dimethyltryptamine (DMT), mescaline, dimethoxymethylamphetamine (STP), and phencyclidine (PCP). People experiencing hallucinogenic episodes report colors more intense than ever seen before, sounds more beautiful than ever heard before, or sights or sounds that do not exist. A person may have such a distorted perception of reality that he may attempt to walk into traffic or ignore some other dangerous situation. Although these drugs do not have severe withdrawal effects, LSD and PCP both have flashback phenomena: Months or even years later the person may experience a recurrence of the hallucination he experienced at the time the drug was taken. Although still disputed, LSD may be capable of causing chromosomal breakage or the offspring of an LSD user may be genetically damaged.

As ill people are all under stress to some degree depending on the seriousness of their illness (and the person's perception of the seriousness), ill people are always potentially at risk for drug dependence. Educate people when they are well that drug dependence is not a useful coping mechanism; it does not solve problems, and because the person needs money to continue to supply himself with the drug, it causes additional problems and actually increases rather than relieves frustration.

Suicide as an Effect of Stress

Suicide is a leading cause of death in the adolescent and young adult age group. In its simplest context, suicide is an adaptive mechanism in response to crisis that people use when no other solution appears acceptable to them.

The crisis that initiates suicide is always loss: the death of a close friend or relative or loss of a prized possession, self-esteem, or a sense of future (acquiring a debilitating illness). Sometimes it is difficult to document the loss because no one associated with the person appreciated the meaning of the event to him (his parents thought the girlfriend who said goodbye was just another girlfriend; their son felt her departure as loss of an extremely meaningful relationship).

Factors To Assess To Determine Lethality

Whether a person truly means to commit suicide and will probably attempt it is a difficult situation to assess. Before you begin to work with people who are experiencing loss (and illness is always a loss of the former self to some degree), you should be familiar with the concept of suicide as an adaptive mechanism and the ways of determining whether a suicide attempt is likely.

SUICIDE PLAN

The cliché that a person who talks about suicide does not commit it is *not* true. Listen carefully to people who are giving you clues that they are planning an attempt ("Are these pills dangerous? How many would it take for a person to kill himself with them?" "How much fluid do you have to lose before no one can stop you from dying?"). A person who can describe a definite plan (he has a gun and ammunition at home; the first time he is alone he plans to use them) is very capable of suicide.

AVAILABILITY OF SUPPORT PEOPLE

People who have someone to reach out to rarely commit suicide. People without a support system are at high risk. Remember that psychological support is what is important. Because a person lives in an intact family it does not follow that he has really close support people available.

HISTORY OF PREVIOUS SUICIDE ATTEMPT

If there are other instances of suicide among close friends or in the same family, the more easily a person may choose suicide as an adaptive mechanism (he knows it will work). If the person has attempted suicide before, the chances that he will attempt it again are higher than for the average person. The lethality of the former attempt should be assessed carefully: An adolescent who swallows a bottle of aspirin 15 minutes before she knows that her mother is expected to arrive home from work and then lies down on the living room couch in plain view represents a different problem than the teenager who swallows the same amount of aspirin 15 minutes *after* the parent leaves for work. The first is probably an example of acting-out (attention-calling) behavior; the other is a very serious suicide attempt. Unfortunately, some children who plan insincere attempts have disastrous outcomes because on that particular day the person they counted on for rescue changes his pattern of behavior and does not check on them as they anticipated.

AGE AND SEX

Suicide is highest in adolescents and young adults; the incidence rises sharply again after middle age (due to loss of youth). Although women *attempt* suicide more often than men, men are more effective and successful at achieving it.

PRESENCE OF DRINKING AND DRUG ABUSE
Use of alcohol and drugs decreases impulse control. The person using drugs may be more prone to act on impulse and so commit suicide than the person who does not use these substances.

DEPRESSION OR CHANGE IN ATTITUDE FROM SADNESS TO HAPPINESS
A person who is extremely sad (depressed) often cannot think well enough to plan a suicide attempt (he feels numb). However, he may shortly think of suicide; should he decide to commit suicide, the decision may give him so much satisfaction that his mood becomes elevated and he appears quite content and happy. This change in mood is often interpreted as an indication that the person is past a point of suicide when it actually implies that suicide is imminent.

SOCIAL ROLE
There is a high incidence of suicide among people in helping professions such as medicine and social work. This occurs because a sense of loss or failure at not being able to make some one better leading to loss of self-esteem is not an uncommon feeling.

IMMEDIATE DANGER SIGNS
Listed below are lists common observations in adolescents who subsequently committed suicide. Being alert to these preliminary warning signs can help you assess whether the possibility of suicide exists. All major cities have suicide prevention centers or "hot lines" which provide counseling for the person who feels that he cannot stop himself from killing himself. Working at such a center could be a nursing role. Knowing the availability of such a service in your community is a nursing knowledge *must.*

Danger Signs that may be Indicative of Potential Adolescent Suicide

Becomes increasingly isolated.
Gives away prized possessions.
Recent loss, expecially a parent or boy or girl friend.
Statements such as "No one cares about me. It would be better for everyone if I were dead. How many aspirins do you have to take to kill yourself?"
A sudden elevation of mood following a depression; this could be misconstrued to mean that the teenager is improving when actually he may be experiencing a sense of relief that the decision to die has been made.

Source: From N. Hart and Sr. P. Prophit, Adolescent suicide. *Pediatr. Nurs.* 5:22, 1979.

Violence as an Effect of Stress

Violence is yet another manifestation of stress. As stress increases yearly due to the pressures of contemporary life, the incidence of child, spouse, and older adult abuse also is growing. The most extensive research in this area has been done by Kempf and Helfner (1972) in regard to child abuse. Many of the situations that give rise to child abuse are also associated with violence in any age group.

Child Abuse

Child abuse should be suspected whenever a child's injury is out of proportion to the history of the injury: The parent says the child bumped his head on the coffee table but he is unconscious from a severe head injury; the parent says the child woke up from his nap with a burn on his hand but she is unable to account for how it happened.

Abuse of a child is frequently associated with the use of alcohol and drug dependence because these agents reduce impulse control. Three factors are present when abuse actually occurs:

1. *A special child.* In many instances of child abuse, a parent abuses only one child in a family of several or a child that is special in some way: The parent may not have formed a close attachment bond with the child at birth (premature infants are at high risk for child abuse, as they are generally separated from parents at birth due to hospitalization); the child may be more intelligent or less intelligent than the other children; he may have a physical handicap; he may have something as simple as different hair color than the other children.

2. *A special parent.* In order to abuse, a parent must have the potential to do so. In most instances, the parent himself was abused as a child and so is utilizing the parenting techniques he saw demonstrated as a child. In terms of development, such a parent did not develop a sense of trust (ability to love and be loved) as an infant and so is unable to gain a sense of intimacy and love as an adult.

3. *A special situation.* Even though the first two criteria for abuse are present, abuse does not actually occur until the third factor is added. The precipitating event is some form of stressor. This may be something as seemingly small as rain on a picnic or a plugged toilet (the perception of the event, not the event itself is the important factor). With the third element in place, the necessary triad is present and the abuse occurs: beating, starving, burning, for example.

Suspected child abuse must be reported in most states or you could have your nursing license revoked. Know the legislation concerning this in your own state, not only to protect the children you care for, but to learn your legal obligations.

Spouse Abuse

Spouse abuse usually involves battered women although the battered person could be a husband as well. As with child abuse, the abusing spouse is special (has the potential to abuse); the spouse abused is viewed as special (deserving of being treated this way); and a certain level of stress must be present (a burned dinner, the purchase of an expensive article of clothing, a difference of opinion on child-rearing). Spouse abuse has far-reaching consequences the same as child abuse, as a child raised in this environment learns that such behavior is expected and so the pattern may continue into the next generation. Women who are battered have such low self-esteem that at some point they begin to believe, as do their husbands, that they are deserving of such treatment. With this mental set, they are not only helpless to break the pattern but unable to leave the situation, because they cannot imagine themselves as being strong enough to survive on their own.

Spouse abuse, like child abuse, should be suspected when a person has injuries out of proportion to the history of the injury. Most major cities have shelters where an abused spouse can live temporarily. Learn where these facilities are in your community.

Older Adult Abuse

Older adult abuse occurs when the same three identifying factors are present. The abusing person is generally a child of the older adult although it could be a caregiver. He or she has the potential for abuse or never formed a strong sense of trust or intimacy. The older adult is particularly prone to abuse as he may have limited financial resources, physical limitations, and perhaps limited rental resources. Conditions that lead to abuse may be crowded living conditions or desire for the older person's income. Abuse may be tolerated by the older adult because he has little contact with people outside his family to whom he can turn for help and he is unable to live on his own.

Abuse in all age groups is destructive not only to the person being abused but to the abuser and the people who are helpless to intercede with the abuser. In most instances, the abusing person is not pleased with his behavior; he simply knows of no other coping mechanism and needs help to learn an effective method. Most major communities have "hot lines" or organizations where people with the potential to abuse can seek counseling when they feel their stress rising above tolerable levels. Learn these numbers in your community for ready reference. People who watch helplessly when abuse occurs are people with poor self-esteem; the longer they allow the situation to continue, the lower their self-esteem becomes. They as well as the actual abuser need counseling to feel good about themselves again and move in a more productive manner in the future.

Accidents as Related to Stress

Home and automobile accidents rise in proportion to the degree of stress a person is experiencing. The person focuses on his problem to such a degree that he blocks out everyday protective steps he otherwise would have taken.

Caution people who are ill that illness is a stress at least to some degree and that they must observe particular caution to prevent accidents at this time. Emphasize that medicine must be replaced in a high-level or locked cabinet after use, not left on a low counter where a child could reach it. A person already ill and under stress should not be subject to the additional stress and guilt that would occur if he accidentally poisoned his child. Be certain that ill persons plan adequate rest periods for themselves so that they are not so fatigued that their judgment is impaired.

Stress Occurs to Everyone

Crisis situations exist at some time for everybody. Helping people to react to such situations in healthy ways is a primary route to helping prevent mental illness. Learning steps of crisis intervention is not only professionally helpful in that you are capable of helping people resolve crises, but it also enables you to help yourself regulate stress and cope with it better in your personal life (Fig. 12-10).

FIGURE 12-10. Be alert for signs of stress. In this instance, a woman awaiting hospital admission is evidently anxious as she picks at her nails.

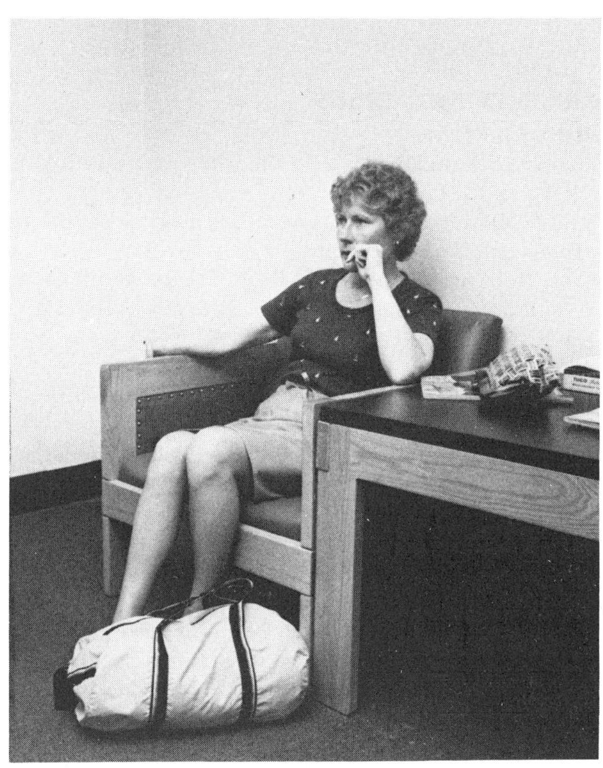

UTILIZING NURSING PROCESS

A month after you help Mr. Rodrigues with his child-care problem, you meet him again on an outpatient basis. He is being seen in an ambulatory clinic for severe abdominal pain. He is diagnosed as having a peptic ulcer (erosion of the stomach lining due to high concentrations of hydrochloric acid associated with chronic high stress levels).

You formulate a nursing care plan for him as follows:

ASSESSMENT

Subjective: States he has to put in 24-hour days to meet the demands made on him by both home, school, and work commitments. Notices severe pain daily as he reaches the end of the day with work or studying still undone.

Objective: Drums fingers on counter top as he talks about problem; glances at watch, frowns frequently.

NURSING DIAGNOSIS:

Anxiety related to difficulty balancing home, work, and school commitments.

LOCUS OF DECISION MAKING

Patient.

GOAL

Patient will have decreased anxiety about commitments by one month.

Criteria: Patient will state he has less abdominal pain; feels more relaxed.

NURSING ORDERS

1. Urge patient to discuss problems with support people, particularly wife (tends not to do so to protect her from worry).
2. Urge patient to establish priorities so that he does not try to accomplish all tasks at the same level.
3. Discuss ways he has been a successful problem solver in the past to help improve self-confidence.
4. Assure him that clinic staff is available and willing to serve as support people and to offer problem-solving assistance at the point that he feels a need for such help.

SUGGESTED READINGS

Stress and Crisis

Aquilera, D. C., and Messick, J. M. *Crisis Intervention* (4th ed.). St. Louis: Mosby, 1982.

Aquilera, D. C. Coping with stressors: A life cycle approach. *Fam. Com. Health* 2:1, 1980.

Byrne, M. L., and Thompson, L. F. *Key Concepts for the Study and Practice of Nursing* (2nd ed.). St. Louis: Mosby, 1978.

Caplan, G. *Principles of Preventive Psychiatry.* New York: Basic Books, 1964.

Dacko, M. The key to coping when everything happens at once. *RN* 45:40, 1982.

Davidhizar, R. E. The instructor's responsibility in reducing patient stress. *Nurs. Health Care* 3(5):273, 1982.

Epting, S. P. Coping with stress through peer support. *Top. Clin. Nurs.* 2:47, 1981.

Freud, A. *The Ego and the Mechanisms of Defense.* New York: International Universities Press, 1946.

Friedman, M., and Rosenman, R. *Type A Behavior and Your Heart.* Greenwich, Conn.: Fawcett Publications, 1974.

Garfield, C. A. (Ed.) *Stress and Survival.* St. Louis: Mosby, 1979.

Green, C. P. Assessment of family stress. *J. Adv. Nurs.* 7(1):11, 1982.

Jacobson, S. E. Psychosocial stresses of working women. *Nurs. Clin. North Am.* 17:137, 1982.

Jasmin, S. J., et al. Keeping your delicate balance: The art of managing stress. *Nursing 81* 11:52, 1981.

Johnson, J. W. More about stress and some management techniques. *J. Sch. Health* 51:36, 1981.

Knowles, R. D. Dealing with feelings: Managing anxiety. *Am. J. Nurs.* 81:110, 1981.

Sandroff, R. When you must inflict pain on a patient. *RN* 46(1):34, 1983.

Scully, R. Stress in the nurse. *Am. J. Nurs.* 80:912, 1980.

Selye, H. *Stress without distress.* Philadelphia: Lippincott, 1974.

Selye, H. *The Stress of Life.* New York: McGraw-Hill, 1976.

Shrewsbury, J. Painting: A coping device for preschool children. *Matern. Child Nurs. J.* 11(1):11, 1982.

Smith, M. T., et al. Reducing the negative effects of stress. *Am. J. Nurs.* 79:1953, 1979.

Stillman, S. M., et al. Helping critical care nurses with work-related stress. *J. Nurs. Adm.* 10:28, 1980.

Thomas, V. M. Hospice nursing—Reaping the rewards, dealing with the stress. *Geriatr. Nurs.* 4(1):22, 1983.

Tierney, M. J., et al. Stress: Type A behavior in the nurse. *Am. J. Nurs.* 80:915, 1980.

Burnout

Clark, C. C. Burnout: Assessment and intervention. *J. Nurs. Adm.* 10:39, 1980.

Gortner, S. R. Strategies for survival in the practice world. *Am. J. Nurs.* 77:618, 1977.

Hagemaster, J. N. Job stress vs. nurse burnout: Are you caught in the middle? *Occup. Health Nurs.* 31(6):38, 1983.

Johnson, S. H. Preventing group burnout. *Nurs. Manage.* 13(2):34, 1982.

Lavandero, R. Nurse burnout: What can we learn? *J. Nurs. Adm.* 11(11—12):17, 1981.

LeMaitre, G. D. A physician speaks out on burnout. *Am. J. Nurs.* 81:1487, 1981.

Maslach, C. Burned out? *Human Behavior* 5(9):16, 1976.

Pines, A., and Aronson, E. *Burnout: From Tedium to Personal Growth.* New York: Free Press, 1981.

Sanders, M. M. Stressed? Or burnt out? *Canad. Nurse* 76:30, 1980.

Shubin, S. Burnout: The professional hazard you face in nursing. *Nursing 78* 8:22, 1978.

Storlie, F. J. Burnout: The elaboration of a concept. *Am. J. Nurs.* 79:2108, 1979.

Thomas, J. Supervisors get burned-out, too. *Nurs. Manage.* 13(5):47, 1982.

Trotter, C. W. What can we do about nursing staff burnout? *MCN* 7:153, 1982.

Yee, B. H. The dynamics and management of burnout. *Nurs. Manage.* 12(11):14, 1981.

Alcohol

Bachman, J. G., et al. Smoking, drinking and drug abuse among high school students: Correlates and trends. *Am. J. Public Health* 71:59, 1981.

Bissell, L., et al. The alcoholic nurse. *Nurs. Outlook* 29:96, 1981.

Booth, P. G., et al. Nurses with drinking problems. *Nurs. Times* 77(39):1676, 1981.

Dains, J. E. Stigma management with the alcoholic. *J.E.N.* 7(5):204, 1981.

Dowell, P. M. Alcohol and pregnancy: A review of the literature 1968—1980. *Nurs. Times* 77(43):1825, 1981.

Effinger, J. M. Women and alcoholism. *Top Clin. Nurs.* 4(4):10, 1983.

Engs, R. C. Responsibility and alcohol: Teaching responsible decisions about alcohol and its use for those who choose to drink. *Health Educ.* 12:20, 1981.

Gaerlan, M. Understanding the physiology of alcohol abuse. *Canad. Nurse* 76:46, 1980.

Jaffe, S. First hand view of alcoholism recovery. *Am. J. Nurs.* 82:578, 1982.

Marks, V. L. Health teaching for recovering alcoholic patients. *Am. J. Nurs.* 80:2058, 1980.

Powell, J. J. The tragedy of fetal alcohol syndrome. *RN* 44(12):33, 1981.

Price, J. H., et al. Alcohol abuse in the elderly. *J. Gerontol. Nurs.* 8(1):16, 1982.

Svitlik, B. Helping the alcoholic patient on the road to recovery. *J.E.N.* 7(5):199, 1981.

Abuse

Anderson, C. L. Abuse and neglect among the elderly. *J. Gerontol. Nurs.* 7:77, 1981.

Bahr, R. T. The battered elderly: Physical and psychological abuse. *Fam. Comm. Health* 4:61, 1981.

Cline, F. W. Understanding child abuse. *Nurs. Pract.* 3:36, 1978.

Cohen, J., et al. Maltreatment of children—The tragedy of yesterday and today. *Int. Nurs. Rev.* 28(4):105, 1981.

Falcioni, D. J. Assessing the abused elderly. *J. Gerontol. Nurs.* 8:208, 1982.

Gray, C. C. Wednesdays and Thursdays child—the abused child. *J. Sch. Health* 50:105, 1980.

Helberg, J. L. Documentation in child abuse. *Am. J. Nurs.* 83(2):236, 1983.

Hendrix, M. J. The battered wife. *Am. J. Nurs.* 78:650, 1978.

Kempf, C. H., and Helfner, R. E. *Helping the Battered Child and His Family.* Philadelphia: Lippincott, 1972.

Luther, S. L., et al. Child sexual abuse: A review. *J. Sch. Health* 50:161, 1980.

Nalepka, C., et al. Nurses' and physicians' recognition and reporting of child abuse. *Issues Compr. Pediatr. Nurs.* 5(1):33, 1981.

Westra, B., et al. Children of battered women. *Maternal-Child Nursing J.* 10:41, 1981.

Drug Dependence

Arras, B. Confessions: Why we nearly lost Miss Mitchell. *RN* 45(2):62, 1982.

Dell, D. D., and Snyder, J. A. Marijuana: Pro and con. *Am. J. Nurs.* 77:630, 1977.

Jefferson, L. V., et al. Help for the helper. Confronting a chemically-impaired colleague. *Am. J. Nurs.* 82(4):574, 1982.

Mann, C. Hooked: The story of one RN's battle with drugs. *RN* 45(6):45, 1982.

Pradhun, S. N., and Dutta, S. N. (Eds.). *Drug Abuse: Clinical and Basic Aspects.* St. Louis: Mosby, 1977.

Ray, O. S. *Drugs, Society, and Human Behavior* (2nd ed.). St. Louis: Mosby, 1978.

Reed, M. T. The dependent nurse—drugs or alcohol. *Nurs. Times* 79:12, Jan 19, 1983.

Rivers, W. L. Is there a relationship between drug use and academic achievement? *J. Sch. Health* 51:171, 1981.

Tennant, F. S., Jr., et al. Children at high risk for addiction and alcoholism. *Pediatr. Nurse* 5:26, 1980.

Suicide

Crumley, F. E. Adolescent suicide attempts. *J.A.M.A.* 241:2404, 1979.

Fuller, E. Caring for the suicidal patient. *Patient Care* 4:101, 1980.

Guze, S. B. Early recognition of depression. *Hosp. Pract.* 16:87, 1981.

Hart, N. A., and Prophit, Sr. P. Adolescent suicide. *Pediatr. Nurs.* 5:22, 1979.

Hemman, S. P., et al. Depression, suicide and the young child. *Emerg. Med.* 13:60, 1981.

Knowles, R. D. Handling depression through positive reinforcement. *Am. J. Nurs.* 81:1353, 1981.

Macdonald, N. Nursing care study—Depression: An unhappy ending. *Nurs. Mirror* 154(10):45, 1982.

Newnes, C. Adolescent suicide: A cry for help. *Nurs. Mirror* 154:16, 1982.

Papa, L. L. Responses to life events as predictors of suicidal behavior. *Nurs. Research* 29:362, 1980.

Sedlock, S. Are you listening? *Crit. Care Nurs.* 1(4):25, 1981.

Valente, S. Suicide in schoolaged children: Theory and assessment. *Pediatr. Nurs.* 9(1):25, 1983.

Whiteworth, R. A. The ethics of suicide intervention: Seen as a nursing problem. *Can. J. Psychiatr. Nurs.* 23(1):12, 1982.

QUESTIONS FOR REVIEW

Mrs. Smith is the wife of a patient you see in an emergency room. She is anxious and unable to function at work due to concern over her husband's illness.

1. A crisis situation of this nature lasts only a set time. This time interval is:
   a. Two weeks.
   b. Six weeks.
   c. Three months.
   d. Six months.

2. To assess Mrs. Smith accurately, it is important to know that of the four factors listed below, the *least* important in determining whether a crisis situation will arise is:
   a. Past experience with coping.
   b. Involvement of family members.
   c. Perception of the event.
   d. Presence of support people.

3. You analyze whether Mrs. Smith is using projection as a psychological defense mechanism. This is defined as:
   a. A return to a less complicated time of life.
   b. Transferring your thoughts to another.
   c. Substituting one action for another.
   d. Repressing the thought from memory.

4. Reaction formation is another psychological defense mechanism. It is defined as:
   a. Acting the opposite way of your true feelings.
   b. Excluding an idea from the conscious mind.
   c. Substituting one activity for a desired activity.
   d. Adopting behavior that is appropriate for another life stage.

5. To plan care, you need to recognize a general adaptive syndrome (GAS). In the first stage of a GAS, which of the following effects occurs?
   a. Respiratory bronchi constrict.
   b. The heart rate slows.
   c. Intestinal peristalsis increases.
   d. Aldosterone secretion is increased.

6. A psychological response to threat you must plan for is anxiety. Anxiety is defined as:
   a. A state of feeling threatened by an unknown assault.
   b. Nervousness and tenseness.
   c. A response to an identified event.
   d. An unconscious manifestation of fear.

7. Implementation will be influenced by whether a maturational crisis is present or not. Which of the following groups of happenings represent maturational crises?
   a. Toddlerhood, marriage, divorce.
   b. Adolescence, middle age, retirement.
   c. Illness, starting school, adolescence.
   d. Marriage, a flood, death.

8. To assess a level of stress, you evaluate a child abuse situation. Child abuse generally occurs when three factors are present. Which factor below is *not* an important factor?
   a. Special child.
   b. Special situation.
   c. Special adult.
   d. Special drug use.

IV. NURSING AS A DYNAMIC FORCE

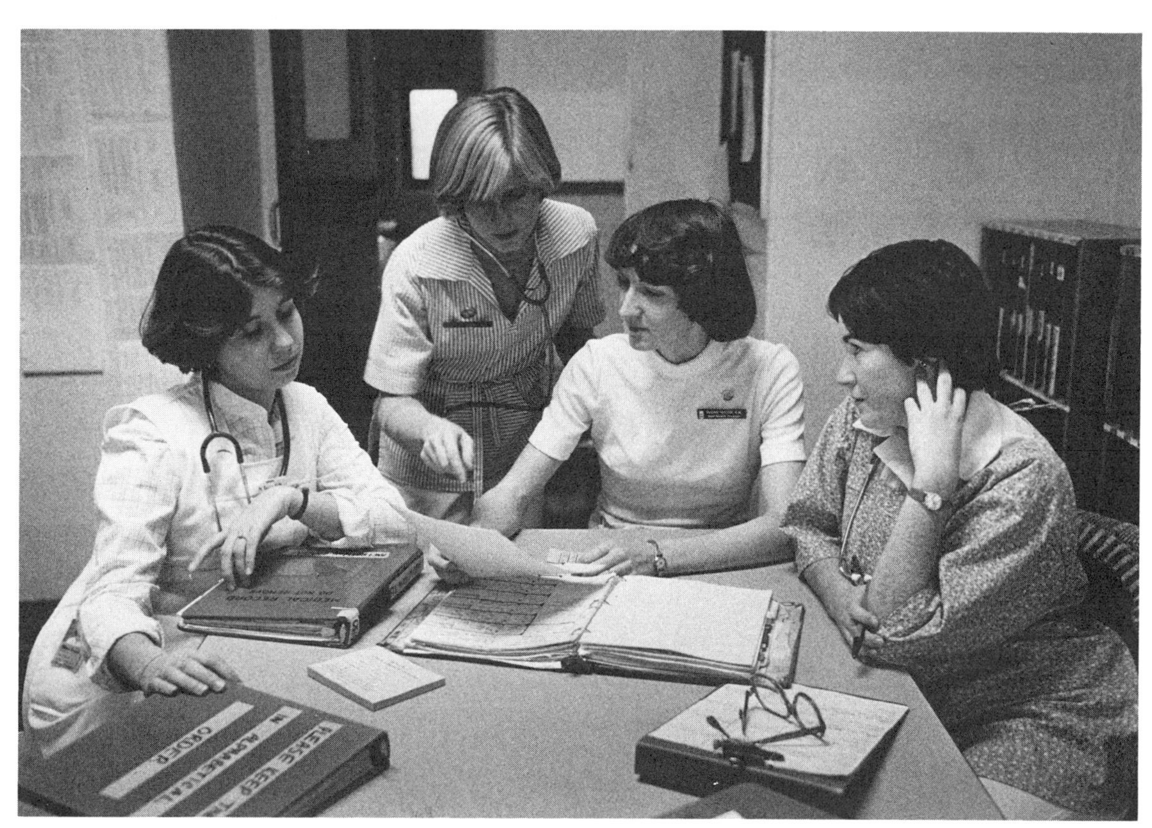

13. THE NURSING PROCESS

OBJECTIVES

Upon mastery of the material in this chapter, you should be able to:

1. Define the nursing process.
2. Describe the five steps of the nursing process.
3. Describe the three component phases of assessment.
4. Compare the terms *objective and subjective data; positive and negative findings.*
5. Describe the importance of maintaining a neutral attitude for the unbiased collection of data.
6. Describe nursing diagnosis and its three required components.
7. Describe the difference between a nursing and a medical diagnosis.
8. Describe the advantage of developing standardized nursing diagnoses.
9. Identify the meaning of the term *locus of decision making.*
10. Describe three components of goal setting.
11. Describe the components of an effective nursing care plan.
12. Compare the format of a nursing care plan and a problem-oriented record.
13. Discuss areas in which care can be implemented.
14. Describe the purpose and process of evaluation.
15. Describe the steps of reassessment if evaluation demonstrates that the patient goal has not been reached.

TERMS

The terms important for an understanding of this chapter are shown below and defined in the glossary:

analysis
assessment
evaluation
implementation
planning

The amount of knowledge that a person must have in order to function as a professional nurse today is ten times greater than it was five years ago and as much as 100 times greater than it was twenty years ago. This increasing amount of knowledge, new technical innovations, and the increased expectations of consumers of health care combine to make nursing a more complex and challenging field every day.

In order for nursing care to be designed and implemented in a thorough manner that ensures quality at all stages, it must be done by a *process* or an organized series of well-thought-through steps. So that nursing care can be consistent from one nurse to another, all nurses need to learn the nursing process.

Nursing process is a form of problem solving, or using the scientific method, to organize nursing care. It consists of five separate steps: assessment, analysis (nursing diagnosis), planning, implementation, and evaluation (Fig. 13-1).

ASSESSMENT

Assessment can be defined as the systematic collection of information in order to establish a data base for a patient. It is necessary in order to identify patient needs or problems and to individualize care.

A man, for example, who supports six people, who is self-employed as a plumber, and who earns income only when he is physically able to work, may view being hospitalized for an illness as a major disaster in his life. A man who lives by himself in a poorly heated apartment and derives his income from a monthly pension that continues whether he is sick or well may consider a hospital experience a welcome break in an otherwise dull existence. Normally, a schoolage child is unhappy at learning that he will be hospitalized. A particular child whom you care for, however, might view hospitalization as exciting, as something that no one else on his block has done. The cast on his arm may represent a badge of courage and give him special status among his friends.

Although these people share similar circumstances (they are all hospitalized), they perceive the event differently—as a major problem, a minor inconvenience, no problem, or a benefit, depending on the specific person and specific circumstances. Assessment is the means whereby you determine not only a person's state of health or illness but the type of person he is and, therefore, what this experience means to him at this time in his life. Assessment lays the foundation for identifying health problems and a plan for care, so the effectiveness of nursing care ultimately rests on the effectiveness and thoroughness of assessment.

Assessment information is gained from three sources: the history, the physical examination, and auxiliary data such as laboratory, x-ray, and consultation reports as well as discussion with other health care providers. These sources are shown diagramatically in Figure 13-2.

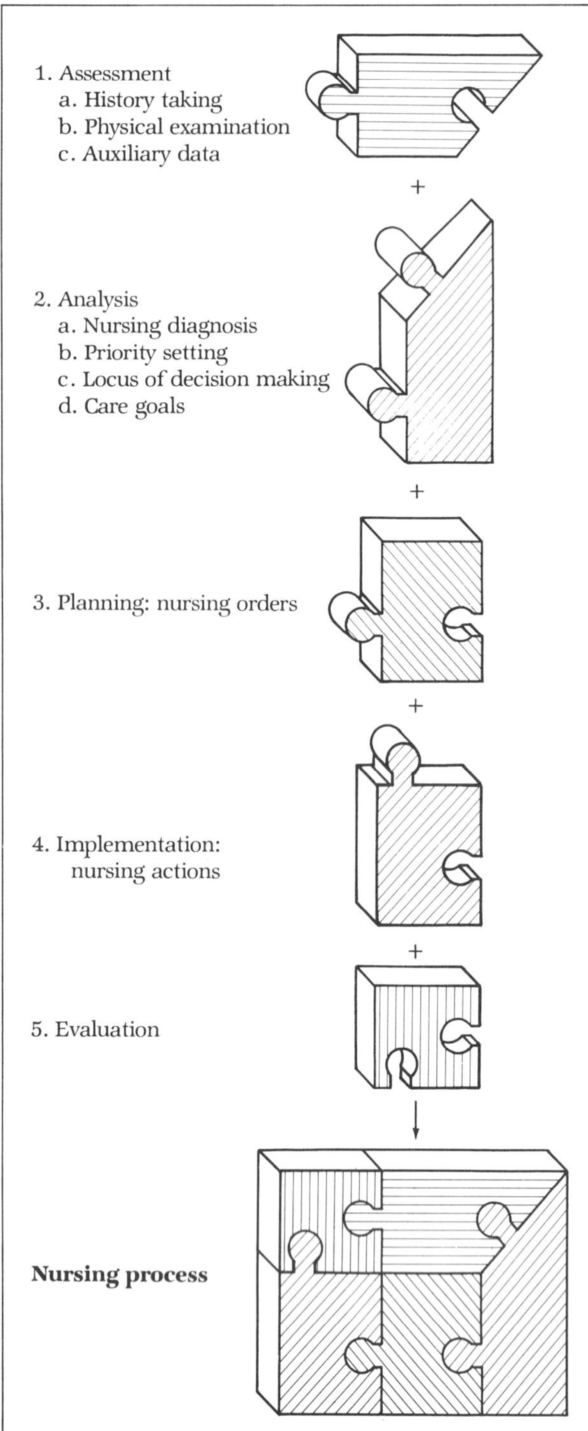

FIGURE 13-1. Steps of the nursing process.

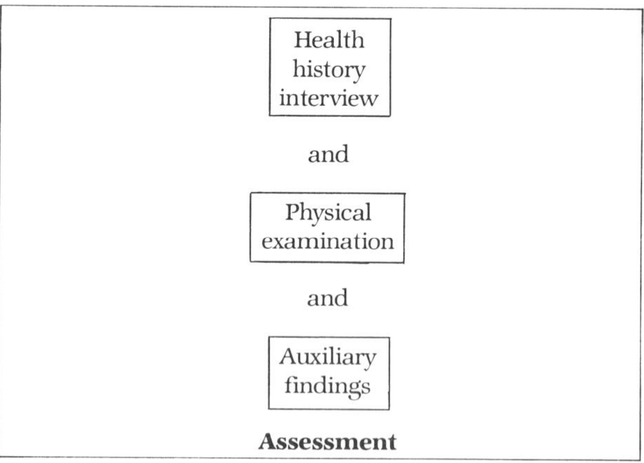

FIGURE 13-2. Nursing process: assessment.

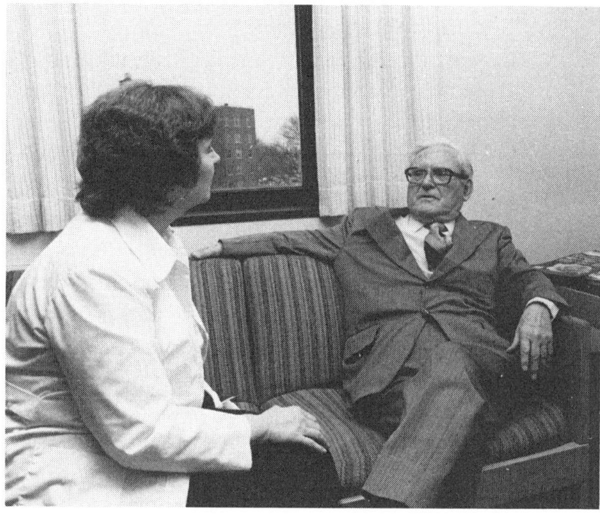

FIGURE 13-3. Health interviewing is an important part of assessment. Initial rapport is built during this time and a data base is established.

Health History

The techniques of interviewing or history taking to establish a person's full health-illness pattern are discussed in detail in Chap. 18. Basically, it consists of collecting information by a question-and-answer process. Fear of illness brings critical stress to people; good techniques of interviewing are necessary to make sure that the information obtained is not distorted or incomplete (Fig. 13-3).

A total data base for a health history consists of the chief concern (the reason that the person is being seen at a health care facility or being visited in his home); history of present illness (a detailed description of the chief concern); family profile (information on the family structure and function); past health history (ways the person has been ill in the past); family health history (incidence of illnesses that appear frequently in the family); and a review of systems (questions pertaining to all body systems). If the patient is a child, a large part of the health history is concentrated on the mother's pregnancy and the child's birth and neonatal history (the first 28 days of life).

Interviewing is supplemented by observation: If a woman looks worried as she talks about her baby but smiles and looks relaxed as she talks about her older child, the worried look should alert you to elicit additional information in this area, even though the woman reported that both children were well and that she knew of no problems they were having.

Physical Examination

The information gained from the health history gives guidance as to what body parts need special or detailed assessment on physical examination, although a full data base requires a thorough physical examination of all body parts. Physical examination must be done by a systematic approach so that data are not missed, in order to determine whether data obtained by the interview are confirmed or contradicted. Techniques of physical examination are detailed in Chap. 19. Basically they consist of using four techniques of assessment: inspection (looking with your eyes); palpation (feeling with your hands); auscultation (listening with your ears); and percussion (listening for the sounds that dense and less dense body parts make as they are struck by your examining fingers).

Auxiliary Data

Nurses are often the first people to see the results of laboratory, x-ray, or consultant reports, as such records are returned from other departments of the hospital to the patient unit to be filed in the patient's chart. In an ambulatory health care setting the nurse is often the person who telephones these departments to ask for reports of blood or culture specimens. Knowing the normal values of common tests and reports helps you to speed important information on to the appropriate health care provider. It adds yet another complementary area of information to your store of knowledge of the person you are caring for, the ways that he is ill, and what unmet needs he has that you should supply for him. Common laboratory tests and the collection of blood, urine, and culture specimens are discussed in Chap. 20 (see also App. G).

Types of Data Obtained

Data collected by interview, physical examination, and auxiliary sources are generally divided into subjective and objective data and positive and negative findings.

SUBJECTIVE DATA

Subjective data are those aspects of the history reported by the patient (or a parent or spouse) that you cannot directly observe or measure: the patient stating that he has pain, for example (only he knows whether he really has pain or not; you have no way to confirm it). It is a category synonymous with the word *symptom* (a finding that the patient experiences). Listing information as subjective does not give it any less credibility or status than other data; it is not saying that the pain does not exist, only that you can not measure it.

OBJECTIVE DATA

Objective data are those findings that *can* be documented by observable or measurable means. It is information synonymous with the term *sign* (a finding that can be observed). Information is often listed as subjective or objective depending on how it was obtained. A mother saying that her child is a "picky" eater is giving you subjective information; your watching a child eat nothing for meal after meal unless it is prepared in a special way is an objective finding (you observed it happening). A person saying that he has pain is providing subjective data; your observation of him wincing as he squeezes your hand is objective.

POSITIVE FINDINGS

A positive finding is a subjective or objective finding that denotes a deviation from the normal suggesting illness. It is sometimes a confusing term because it seems that a positive (right) finding should be used to indicate a healthy finding, not an ill one. The term stems from medical usage, however, and as physicians tend to look for illness, not health, a positive finding indicates a sign of illness or discovery.

NEGATIVE FINDINGS

A negative finding is one that indicates no deviation from the normal. Negative findings are used to "draw a fence around" or determine the extent of an illness. A person with a broken radius, for example, will have positive findings of pain and swelling at the site of the fracture and loss of motor function distal to the fracture (three classic findings in all fractures). He will be asked if he has numbness or tingling in his fingers; his fingers will be palpated for warmth and good blood circulation to ascertain whether nerves or blood vessels have been affected. With a simple fracture, sensation and circulation are not affected; the fact that nerve integrity and circulation are present is listed as a negative finding to demonstrate that the injury is just a simple fracture (a fence has been put around it; its boundaries have been established).

Scope of Data Collection

In order to estimate the person's ability to assume care of his daily health needs or to cope with a stress to his health, the information can be further divided into that which is supportive and offers strength to the person and that which potentially impedes his ability to function.

DISABILITIES

Disabilities are those characteristics that are detrimental to high-level wellness. They are usually identified in psychological, sociological, motor, and sensory function areas. Other terms for disabilities are limitations or weaknesses. Some examples are:

Psychological
- Finds it difficult to adjust to change
- Little success with past coping strategies

Sociological
- Few financial resources
- Fixed income

Motor function
Inability to grasp with right hand
Unsteady on feet
Sensory function
Hard of hearing
Needs glasses for good vision

ABILITIES

Abilities are activities or functions that the person does well. It is easy to neglect collecting this type of information in the assessment process, as one tends to think of assessment as looking for illness. However, assessment of patient abilities is necessary to estimate how well the person will be able to deal with illness or to maintain health. Other terms used to describe these functions are capabilities and strengths. Some examples are:

Psychological
Intelligent
Creative
Sociological
Intact family
Strong support people
Motor function
Has daily exercise program
Good muscle coordination
Sensory function
Intact sense of hearing and vision

Environment

People do not exist as islands but as parts of families and communities. Evaluating the environment of an individual is important, therefore, and should be included as a basic part of assessment. The details of family and community assessment are discussed in Chap. 7.

Health Care Provider's Reactions

Yet another aspect of assessment is your own reactions to the patient and his support people, because personal reactions can interfere with care unless they are identified and modified. Mrs. Jones, for example, is a patient you care for who has totally different ethical and moral beliefs from yours. Your first reaction might be to avoid her as she is different from you. Identifying this reaction helps you to be certain that you are not unconsciously neglecting your patient and, by so doing, leaving her vulnerable to danger from inadequate care.

Verifying Data

In many instances data obtained from one source should be confirmed by data from a second source. If a patient states that his heartbeat is irregular, for example, you should confirm this by listening to the person's heart yourself. At other times a piece of monitoring equipment will be in constant use to record a person's heart or respiratory rate. It is good practice to periodically check these findings personally instead of relying solely upon equipment for assessment. As a nurse you frequently are the member of the health care team who knows a patient best. Learn to judge when one finding truly documents an illness or when, based on your personal knowledge of a patient, another finding would be important. Suppose you take a patient's temperature and find that the thermometer indicates that his temperature is normal. The patient, however, is breathing rapidly, perspiring freely, has a flushed face, and feels warm to your touch. Common sense tells you that the temperature recorded by the thermometer needs reassessment as other findings tend to dispute it.

Communication of Information Obtained

Assessment information should be communicated to the proper members of the health care team so that they can be kept aware of current patient status. In addition to this, assessment information is used to write a nursing care plan and as the basis for your organization of nursing care.

Attitude of the Assessor

Assessment is a process of getting the facts. After facts are collected, they will be weighed for importance and analyzed; if sufficient facts are not obtained, everything else fails. Assessing from a neutral or objective standpoint is important so that you do not misinterpret what is being said. Do not make value judgments or generalize (such as assuming that a person dressed in poor clothes will not be a good historian or that all older people have poor memories). Assessment is like a picture puzzle; obtain all the pieces first before you begin to put the pieces together.

ANALYSIS

Analysis is the study of assessment data to identify the patient's health care needs and to select goals of nursing care based on your interpretation of the data (Fig. 13-4). This step also includes making a nursing diagnosis of patient problems identified as being within a nurse's expertise to manage. Those problems that can best be managed by other health care providers (physician, occupational therapist, dietitian) are referred to the appropriate people for a solution.

Defining a patient's health care needs varies, depending on your concept of optimal health. A health problem might be recognized because of a sign (vomiting); a symptom (nausea); a syndrome or frequently associated findings (failure to thrive); a psychological problem (anxiety); a social problem (inadequate housing); a demographic element (high incidence of tuberculosis in the community); or a risk factor (association of heavy smoking with development of lung cancer). If you define optimal health as the ability of the body to perform all body functions, you would list needs in terms of malfunctioning body systems (e.g., inability to digest food, inability to regulate blood flow). If you define optimal health as the ability to perform self-

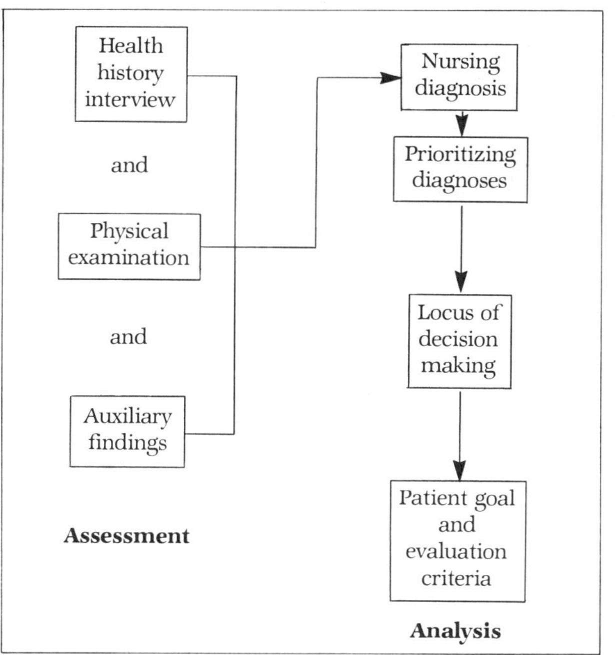

FIGURE 13-4. Nursing process: analysis.

care, you would list needs in terms of the factors limiting this ability (e.g., inability to feed self, inability to communicate). If you define optimal health as the ability of the body to adapt or adjust to new situations, you would list needs in terms of impediments to adaptation (e.g., increasing anxiety, inadequate respirations).

A very common method of determining needs is by Maslow's hierarchy of needs (Fig. 13-5). A need according to Maslow (1970) is defined as an *unmet desire.* A person will usually persist in need-attaining behavior until an unmet desire is fulfilled (when you are thirsty, for example, you will seek a drinking fountain, a sink, or a dispensing machine in order to relieve your thirst).

Maslow determined that certain needs are more important than others; everyone seeks to have these important needs met first. These first-level needs are physiologic and include oxygen, food, elimination, temperature control, sex, movement, and rest. A great deal of nursing care is aimed at helping people meet these basic needs. After these needs have been met, people seek safety and security; then love and belonging, self-esteem (feeling good about yourself), and lastly self-actualization (a feeling of being all that you can become). Nursing care is focused on first-level needs, but must include attention to needs at all levels of Maslow's hierarchy, because if a need such as self-esteem is not met, eventually the first-level needs may be unmet (a person who does not feel worthy cannot hold a job and then will have difficulty affording housing and food—his first-level needs. Table 13-1 lists priority rankings of subgroupings within Maslow's levels of needs. Within the category of physiologic needs, for example, oxygen is ranked as more important than cleanliness.

TABLE 13-1. PRIORITY RANKING OF MASLOW'S SUBCATEGORIES OF HUMAN NEEDS

Physiologic needs
Oxygen, circulation
Water-salt balance
Food balance
Acid-base balance
Waste elimination
Normal temperature
Sleep, rest, relaxation
Activity, exercise
Energy
Comfort
Stimulation
Cleanliness
Sexuality
Safety needs
Protection from physical harm
Protection from psychological threat
Freedom from pain
Stability
Dependence
Predictable, orderly world
Belongingness needs
Love and affection
Acceptance
Warm, communicating relationships
Approval from others
Unity with loved ones
Group companionship
Self-esteem needs
Sense of value, usefulness
High evaluation of self
Adequacy
Self-reliance
Goal achievement
Mastery and competence in skills
Independence
Endurance
Esteem-from-others needs
Recognition
Dignity
Appreciation from others
Importance, influence
Reputation of good character
Attention
Status
Dominance over others
Self-actualization needs
Personal growth and maturity
Awareness of potential
Increased learning
Full development of potential
Improved values
Religious, philosophic satisfaction
Increased creativity
Increased reality perception and problem-solving abilities
Less rigid conventionality
Less of the familiar, more of the novel
Greater satisfaction in beauty
Increased pleasantness
Less of the simple, more of the complex

Source: From C. Campbell, *Nursing Diagnosis and Intervention in Nursing Practice.* New York: Wiley, 1978. P. 15.

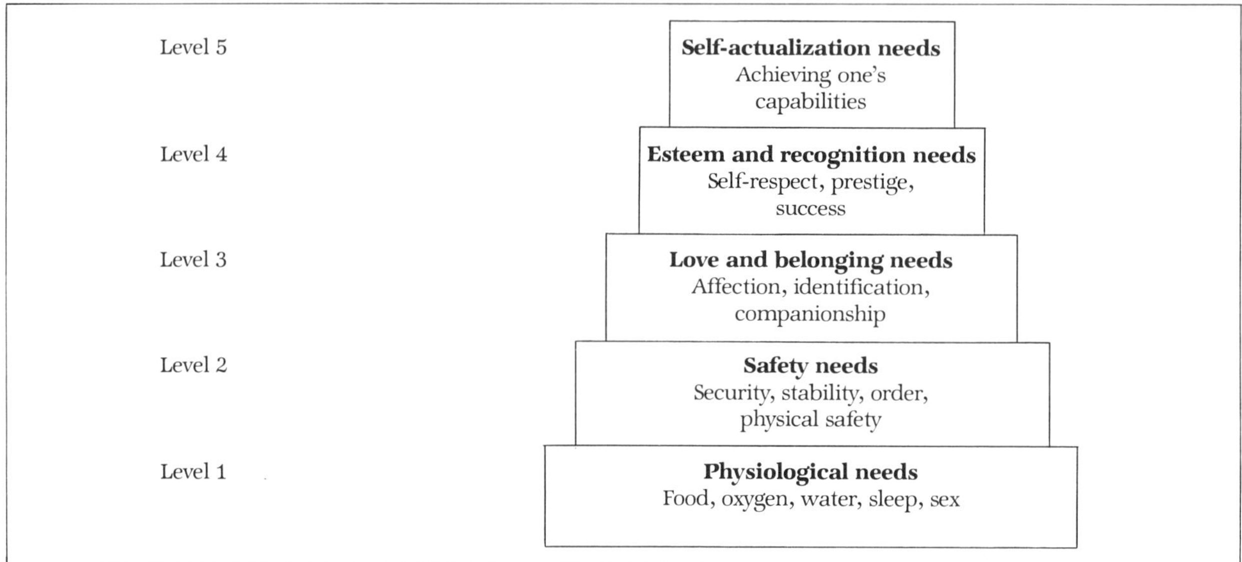

FIGURE 13-5. Maslow's theory of the hierarchy of needs. (Adapted with permission from A. H. Maslow, A Theory of Human Motivation, in A. H. Maslow, *Motivation and Personality* (2nd ed.). New York: Harper & Row, 1970. Copyright © 1970 by Abraham H. Maslow.)

Remember that listing a person's assets is as important as listing his needs, because a plan of care is influenced as strongly by those areas in which he does well as those in which he has difficulty.

Organizing Data

It is helpful to group data into general categories such as those shown in Table 13-2 so that they may be examined more readily and problems or diagnoses properly extracted. Plotting data in terms of these categories helps to view problems in a holistic or comprehensive way. People are not able to block out one part of their life from another; all areas overlap. The extent of any problem in any category depends on data supplied by the other sections. Checking each category for each problem helps you to assess the seriousness of a problem: The social section assures you that the patient has strong support people who will help him weather a good deal of disappointment; in the psychological section a woman reports feeling "not herself" but abnormal findings in the laboratory and physical examination sections indicate that this is not strictly a psychological problem. If a problem overlaps many of these areas, it is probably more serious than a deficiency in only one area. Examining a problem in terms of these categories helps to identify gaps in data. You should always have nutrition data, for example, because people, no matter how ill, have to eat; if you are missing data in this area, you have an incomplete data base.

TABLE 13-2. AREAS IN WHICH PATIENT PROBLEMS MAY BE IDENTIFIED

Comfort
Education
Emotional support
Elimination
Environmental concerns
Exercise
Health maintenance
Hygiene
Nutrition
Prevention of illness
Recreation
Sleep and rest
Social interaction
Safety
Spiritual comfort
Stimulation
Support of physiological functioning

Stating a Nursing Diagnosis

A *nursing diagnosis* identifies an existing problem that a nurse is qualified and licensed to resolve (the patient is worried about having anesthesia for surgery) or potential health problems (the person is a heavy smoker; smoking is associated with the development of lung cancer so he has a potential for developing this disease). In its best form a diagnosis should include a description of the health problem (fear), the etiology or cause of the problem (fear of anesthesia for surgery) and the defining characteristics or signs and symptoms that document the need (trembling hands, insomnia, expressed fear). These three components are referred to as a PES format (Gordon, 1979).

THE PROBLEM

The problem should be stated as clearly and concisely as possible. In order that nurses can be as consistent as possible in the use of terms, the 4th National Conference on Classification of Nursing Diagnoses (Kim and Moritz, 1982) has recommended a number of broad diagnostic categories that can be commonly used (Table 13-3). This list is incomplete as to the

TABLE 13-3. ACCEPTED NURSING DIAGNOSES

Airway clearance, ineffective
Bowel elimination, alterations in
  Constipation
  Diarrhea
  Incontinence
Breathing patterns, ineffective
Cardiac output, alterations in: decreased
Comfort, alterations in: pain
Communication, impaired verbal
Coping, ineffective individual
Coping, ineffective family
  Compromised
  Disabling
Coping, family: potential for growth
Diversional activity, deficit
Fear
Fluid volume deficit
  Actual
  Potential
Gas exchange, impaired
Grieving
  Anticipatory
  Dysfunctional
Home maintenance management, impaired
Injury, potential for
Knowledge deficit (specify)
Mobility, impaired physical
Non-compliance (specify)
Nutrition, alterations in
  Less than body requirements
  More than body requirements
  Potential for more than body requirements
Parenting, alterations in
  Actual
  Potential
Rape-trauma syndrome
Self-care deficit (specify level: feeding, bathing/hygiene, dressing/grooming, toileting)
Self-concept, disturbance in
Sensory perceptual alterations
Sexual dysfunction
Skin integrity, impairment of
  Actual
  Potential
Sleep pattern disturbance
Spiritual distress (distress of human spirit)
Thought processes, alterations in
Tissue perfusion, alterations in
Urinary elimination, alteration in patterns of
Violence, potential for

Source: From M. J. Kim and D. A. Moritz (Eds.), *Classifications of Nursing Diagnosis: Procedures of the Fourth National Conference.* New York: McGraw-Hill, 1982.

TABLE 13-4. ROLES OF NURSES

Role	Activity
Advocate	Speaks for patient to help him achieve goals. Keeps patient informed of his health status. Encourages self-participation in planning and care.
Comforter	Provides measures to keep patients free of both physical and psychological discomfort.
Community liaison	Refers patient to appropriate resources for optimal care.
Counselor	Provides opportunities for patients to explore and problem-solve concerns.
Health provider (for health maintenance, prevention of illness, restoration of health, acceptance of inevitable death)	Provides primary, secondary, and tertiary preventive measures to promote wellness.
Health educator (for promotion of health)	Provides information on principles and techniques of health care to aid people to remain well.
Protector (against environmental hazards, psychological threat, physical threat)	Provides environment conducive to optimal health. Reduces stresses to maintain body integrity. Encourages patient to accept care.
Supporter, psychologically (provide for emotional support, spiritual concerns, stimulation, stress or anxiety relief)	Provides opportunities for developing self-esteem.
Supporter of physical functions (circulation, elimination, exercise, hygiene, nutrition, recreation, respiration, sleep and rest)	Provides assistance with normal physiological body functions.
Supporter of sociological interactions (social contacts and relationships with family, health care providers, other support people)	Aids patient in establishing social contacts so that he can form a support network.

number of possible problems, however, so you are not restricted to these categories. A typical nursing diagnosis might list a problem as "Breathing pattern, ineffective." The signs or symptoms of such a problem might be dyspnea (difficult breathing), shortness of breath, tachypnea (rapid respirations), fremitus (noisy breathing), cyanosis (blue tinge to skin), or nasal flaring. The etiology of such a problem might be pain, anxiety, or neuromuscular or musculoskeletal impairment. Nursing diagnoses, possible etiologies, and defining characteristics (signs and symptoms) accepted by the 4th National Conference on Nursing Diagnosis are included in Appendix C for easy reference.

It is important to remember that a nursing diagnosis identifies a problem that is within nursing's expertise and areas of care. Table 13-4 lists areas of care which a nurse supervises or manages. Check that a diagnosis you have identified falls within these categories to assure yourself that it is a nursing problem. Yet another method of checking is to refer to Quick Reference Stop 13-1, What a Nursing Diagnosis is *Not* (Little, 1976).

A nursing diagnosis is never a medical diagnosis (diabetes); a diagnostic test (low white blood count); a piece of equipment (a respirator); a problem for the nurse (patient weighs 200 pounds and is difficult to turn); or a healthy response (anger at learning that an illness will be fatal). These examples *are* problems, but they are not statements of nursing diagnoses. Diabetes, for example, is a disease that leads to an alteration in carbohydrate metabolism. The nursing diagnosis (the problem that can be dealt with by you as a nurse) is a potential rise in blood sugar level. Likewise, the nursing problem concerned with a low white blood count is the patient's increased susceptibility to infection related to a low white blood count. The problem concerning a piece of equipment is not the equipment but the reason the person needs the equipment: inability to regulate respiration, for example. The nursing problem of the person who is difficult to turn may be inadequate regard for proper nutrition which has led him to weigh 200 pounds. Anger is a normal stage of grief; in this instance the problem that a nurse could alleviate might be the person's inability to communicate with members of his family as a result of his anger.

☐ QUICK REFERENCE STOP 13-1: ADVOCACY
What a Nursing Diagnosis Is *Not*

A nursing diagnosis is *not*:

A medical diagnosis	A medical diagnosis is a disease; a nursing diagnosis is the patient's *response* to disease. Pneumonia is not a nursing diagnosis; pain related to frequent coughing might be.
A laboratory test or test result	Low hemoglobin level, for example, is a laboratory test result; the nursing diagnosis may be fatigue, related to decreased number of oxygen-carrying red blood cells.
A piece of equipment	A respirator, for example, is not the problem. The problem may be fear related to dependence on a respirator.
A nursing problem	A nursing diagnosis should be patient centered. Patient refuses to eat is not a nursing diagnosis. Lack of knowledge of the importance of good nutrition could be a nursing diagnosis.
A healthy response	Nursing diagnosis is used in wellness settings. A nursing diagnosis would *not* be: well 18-year-old female (that is a medical diagnosis). A response such as anger at learning that an illness will be fatal is a healthy response since anger is a normal stage of grief.

THE ETIOLOGY

The etiology of a problem is the environmental, sociological, psychological, physiological, spiritual, or other factor that is the cause of the problem. By common usage, the etiology of a problem is stated as *related to* rather than *due to* these factors (anxiety *related to* fear of anesthesia for surgery rather than *due to* fear of anesthesia for surgery). If the etiology of a problem is definitely known (the patient states that the reason his hand is shaking so much is that he is afraid of anesthesia), it can be stated as anxiety *due to* fear of anesthesia for surgery, but the wording *related to* is considered less legally binding and for most nurses is becoming the standard statement format.

It is important that the etiology be identified because the plan for intervention to solve a problem differs greatly, depending on its cause. Relieving anxiety due to fear of anesthesia for surgery, for example, will require education about the safety of current anesthetic agents. Perhaps you would want to ask the anesthesiologist to discuss this with the patient. Anxiety due to inadequate finances to pay a hospital bill might require consultation with the hospital financial staff about supplementary income sources. Anxiety about child care might require consultation with other family members or the hospital social work department. Anxiety about inability to perform self-care after going home might require consultation with the hospital discharge planner or the person's physician.

When establishing the reason for a problem, it is helpful to examine the general categories of why problems occur. Health problems generally arise because a person has an unmet need and cannot see a clearcut way of meeting it; the patient recognizes two or more ways to meet his need and requires help deciding which method to choose; the patient knows how to meet his need but some obstacle prevents his doing so; or the patient is unaware that a need exists and is making no effort to meet it. Listing the cause of the unmet need reveals the true problem and gives direction for planning care.

SIGNS AND SYMPTOMS

Signs are observable indicators (wincing, a measured increased temperature) or *objective information.* Symptoms are factors reported by the patient (he has pain; he feels warm) or *subjective information.* Signs and symptoms are listed to document that the need identified is not just a "hunch" or a fleeting impression but one that actually exists.

Differentiating Medical and Nursing Diagnoses

A medical diagnosis is invariably a statement of disease; a nursing diagnosis deals with people's responses or actions relating to their illness. They are derived from the same knowledge base (either a nurse or physician skilled in health interviewing could have obtained the data base); they are always complementary. A medical diagnosis remains the same throughout the course of a patient's illness. Pneumonia, for example, may be the medical diagnosis of a patient from the moment the illness is confirmed (a stage where he is very ill) until he is discharged from a health care agency (a stage where he is well again). During this time he may have had several nursing diagnoses such as pain related to frequent cough, fluid loss related to increased body temperature, and fear related to loss of finances. Medical and nursing diagnoses differ because physicians and nurses interpret assessment data in terms of their special areas of care.

Standardizing Nursing Diagnoses

The nomenclature of medicine is so standardized that a diagnosis of an illness represents not only the name of the illness but its origin and a standardized series of care steps as well. The diagnosis of pneumonia, for example, implies infection; antibiotic, fluid replacement, and close assessment of temperature, pulse, and respiration rate are necessary; the problem, its causes, and basic care measures are implied by the one medical term (pneumonia).

Attempts to standardize nursing diagnoses should bring the same uniform use of terminology to nursing care. It took medicine more than 300 years to standardize diagnoses to this point; it will probably take some time before nursing diagnoses are so standardized. Any attempt at standardization, however, increases nursing science to some degree.

Common Errors in Stating Nursing Diagnoses

Nursing diagnoses should be clearly stated so that they are guides to nursing action, not detours to confusion. Each diagnosis should contain only one problem (inability to feed self and concern about this are two separate problems).

TABLE 13-5. MISTAKES TO AVOID WHEN WRITING A NURSING DIAGNOSIS

1. Writing in terms of needs instead of problems (for example, "needs to increase fluid intake" instead of stating the specific problem or response demonstrated which makes this a concern).
2. Using the words *due to* rather than *related to,* which could be legally hazardous.
3. Reversing the two-part statement by putting the contributing factors first (for example, "odors in the room causing inability to eat meals" rather than "inability to eat meals related to odors in room").
4. Writing a response that is not necessarily unhealthful (for example, if a patient has just lost his job and is expressing anger, the anger is not necessarily unhealthful and therefore may not be a problem for nursing diagnosis).
5. Writing an unhealthy response in such a way that it cannot be changed (for example, stating that the problem is "related to inability to speak due to a complete laryngectomy").
6. Writing two parts of a statement which say the same thing (for example, "inability to have bowel movement related to constipation").

Source: From M. Mundinger and G. Jauron, Developing a nursing diagnosis. *Nurs. Outlook* 23:96, 1975.

Problems should include not only present concerns but also risk of future problems as well. They should be stated specifically so that the goal of therapy can be determined: Anxiety from growth and developmental concerns is a poor statement; anxiety related to lack of menstrual cycle at age 16 gives a guide to action. Be certain when analyzing to diagnose a problem not from your perspective but from that of the patient. If you are a very neat person, for example, the inability to carry out normal housework may impress you as a serious problem; not being able to hold a book to read may be more important to the patient.

Mundinger and Jauron (1975) have compiled a number of common pitfalls to avoid when writing nursing diagnoses. These additional reminders are shown in Table 13-5. Checking a nursing diagnosis against this chart is another way of determining whether your diagnosis is in good form.

Prioritizing Nursing Diagnoses

A person normally has one medical diagnosis. He may well have six or seven nursing diagnoses. Obviously all these cannot be dealt with immediately and with the same intensity. You can initiate only a certain number of actions simultaneously; an excessive amount of intervention would overwhelm the patient.

Priority setting is giving preference to one item over another competing item. Determining which need is most important and, therefore, must be met first is important when dealing with health problems because health problems occur in such a variety of forms; they may range from life-threatening events to minor complaints. Obviously, life-threatening needs must be dealt with first. Because people are more than flesh and blood, problems that interfere with integrity, dignity, and self-esteem must be considered as potentially life threatening as physiological problems such as respiratory and cardiac deficiencies. With children, problems that interfere with growth and development are priority problems because of the serious effect such problems may have on the person's life if they are not alleviated.

Other factors that help to establish priorities are the individual *values* of the person (if it seems like a serious problem to a patient, it *is* serious, despite the fact that it does not seem so to you); *cost* (the price of solving a problem may make it undesirable to resolve it at a particular time); *policy* ("red tape" governs many solutions); and *time* (neither the person nor you has the time required for the problem's solution).

Using a hierarchy of needs such as Maslow's is a helpful method for establishing priorities: Basic needs must be met before security needs; security needs before love and belonging needs; love and belonging needs before self-esteem needs; self-esteem needs before self-actualization needs in most instances. Always take into consideration the patient's view of the situation. The problems that he feels are most important should be given priority, with the obvious exception of life-threatening events such as difficulty with breathing or cardiovascular function.

Locus of Decision Making

The next step of analysis consists of identifying the people who will aid with goal setting and devising a plan of care. In some situations the individual is unable to participate in decision making, and nursing care decisions are made without patient input; the locus of decision making is the nurse. In other instances the patient is capable of making his own care decisions; the locus of decision making is the patient. In yet other instances decision making will be shared by the patient and nurse (or the family and nurse).

The locus of decision making is the nurse when a patient cannot participate in planning his care because he is unconscious in a life-threatening situation or because he is an infant. There are few instances when a patient exists without support people around him, however, and it is important to include these people in decision making. Thus, the locus of decision making is seldom strictly with the nurse.

In ambulatory and health care settings a person is often able to exercise full control in meeting his own health requirements. A patient admitted to a health care facility for diagnostic testing or while recovering from illness, for example, is able to make those decisions necessary for health care independently. People are able to participate in their own care only after they are aware of the options available to them. Among the different ways that a person could use to lose weight, for example, would be to diet by himself, join a weight reduction club, marry a nutritionist who would keep him on a diet, lock his refrigerator door, or have surgery to wire his jaw closed. You should suggest such alternatives to people; they may then be able to make their decisions regarding what course to follow.

In some instances the person needs some help in narrowing down the selection. After discussing the alternatives, you and he reach the following conclusions: He has tried many times before to lose weight by himself; he may not be a person who can do this alone. Marrying a nutritionist does not seem like his life style. Locking the refrigerator is not a viable alternative in reality. Surgery is an extreme measure. Joining the weight reduction club, therefore, seems the best choice. A locus of decision making shared between the patient and nurse is the most common form. It is the basis of family-centered care, of thinking of people within the context of their total environment.

Goal Setting

A goal is a destination you want to reach. This destination determines the method (nursing interventions) you will use to get there (to cross an entire country, you will probably not walk; to cross an ocean, you will need a boat). In their best form goals are patient centered; they are the expected patient outcomes of care. Be certain when stating goals that you are not stating a nursing action, but a patient behavior (patient will double fluid intake within 8 hours, not I will give 8 ounces of fluid) (Fig. 13-6). A goal should be precisely stated so that everyone caring for the patient can readily under-

FIGURE 13-6. A nursing diagnosis must be a problem within the expertise of the nurse to manage. In this instance, the locus of decision making is the patient. The goal is a patient behavior: The patient will increase his fluid intake within 24 hours.

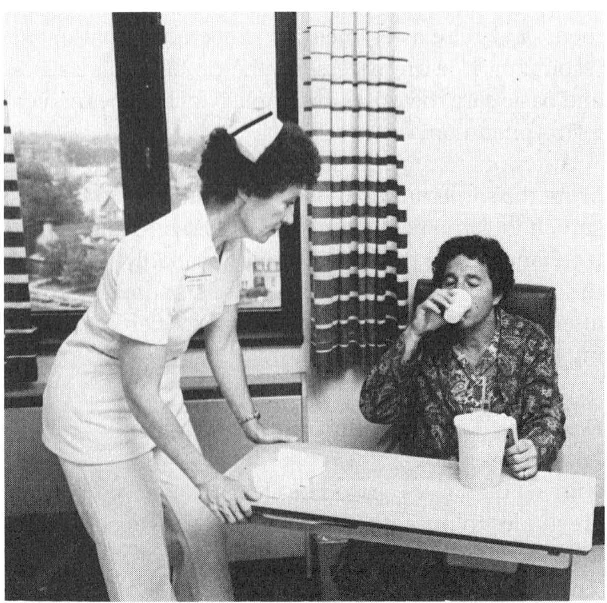

stand it (not simply increased exercise but exactly what exercises he should do).

Accompanying the statement of the goal should be the specific criteria or means by which the goal will be measured. If a goal is that the patient will be free of pain in 20 minutes, the criteria for that goal would be that the patient can walk without limping and will state that he is pain free in 20 minutes. If the goal is that the patient will be ambulatory by the third day following surgery, the criterion by which you would measure that might be that the patient can walk the length of the hallway three times daily.

Another term for a goal is an objective. Goals in nursing concern the condition or behavior of the person at a point of accomplishment; they are the outcome or *behavioral objectives.* In their best form the desired behavior is determined (the patient will change his own dressing); any qualifying circumstances are listed (the patient will change his own dressing using sterile technique); and the time frame within which the objective will be realized is stated (the patient will change his own dressing using sterile technique following one week's instruction).

Since you must be able to measure whether a goal is reached, be certain that the wording of a behavioral objective is measurable. Verbs such as *know, appreciate, understand,* and *enjoy* are difficult to measure. Verbs such as *list, apply, voice, demonstrate,* and *describe* are measurable. Most instructors supply to students at the beginning of a course a list of behavioral objectives (the behaviors you are expected to manifest at the conclusion of the course). If you were given such a list, examine it. You are sure to discover the verbs *list, describe, discuss, compare, contrast, analyze, synthesize,* and *demonstrate.* These are used in preference to terms such as *know* or *understand* (terms you would probably think of first if asked what is expected of you), because they can be so much more easily measured.

SELECTING GOALS

A goal must be realistic for the individual patient. This means that you must consider the patient's preferences, capabilities, and limitations in goal selection. It would be unrealistic, for example, to set as a goal that the patient will consume three servings of meat daily if the patient is a vegetarian. In this instance the goal might be stated as follows: The patient will consume three servings of iron-rich foods daily. Goal setting that is not realistic is exemplified by the old vaudeville joke of the man who asked if he would be able to play violin after his surgery; when assured that he could, he answered, "That's great. I couldn't play before."

Be certain that a selected goal is realistic in terms of what truly can be accomplished. Be certain also that your time frame is realistic. You cannot expect tissue to heal faster than is physiologically possible; you cannot change the way that people feel about having an illness or their knowledge of their illness overnight.

TABLE 13-6. FACTORS TO CONSIDER BEFORE SETTING A PATIENT GOAL

What is a proper locus of decision making?
What is the level of growth and development of the patient?
What environmental influences will affect outcomes?
What is the patient's physiologic status?
What are the patient's personality patterns?
What is the availability of resources/equipment to achieve goal?

Table 13-6 lists factors to consider in goal setting. Be certain that a goal reflects an outcome that is within a nurse's ability to supervise or accomplish. A goal such as "will have surgery for cholecystitis (gallbladder disease) on Monday morning" is a physician's goal. "Will demonstrate knowledge about anticipated surgery by Monday morning" or "will state reduced fear of surgery by Monday morning" are nursing goals.

LENGTH OF GOALS

Goals are either long-term or short-term. There is no definite time interval that makes a goal long- or short-term. The terms reflect the comprehensiveness of the goal rather than any time span. Short-term goals are those steps that lead to fulfillment of the long-term goal. Tissue healing takes place in about seven days, for example, so a long-term goal related to this physiological process might be seven days. Resolving grief takes about six weeks, so that time span is appropriate for a long-term goal for grief resolution.

Establish long-term goals first, then fill in short-term goals as necessary. If you want to fly from New York to San Francisco (long-term goal), in the morning you will go from New York to Chicago, in the afternoon from Chicago to San Francisco (short-term goals). If a long-term goal for a patient is "Learn to transfer self independently from bed to bedside chair," short-term goals might be "Voice advantages of independent movement" and "Increase muscle strength in upper arms by exercise" (so that his arms will be strong enough to lift his body weight).

PRIORITIZING GOALS

Like nursing problems themselves, goals should be listed in order of priorities (importance). For optimal health it is important for a person both to breathe adequately and to feel good about himself. If the situation requires that one goal be achieved first, obviously breathing should be given priority. Some people may need help in recognizing that one goal is more important than another. Otherwise they may try to meet the easier of two goals and never achieve the degree of health they want for themselves. If a person has two goals—to change his own dressing and to work independently outside his home—he has to be able to accomplish the first one before he can effectively achieve the second one.

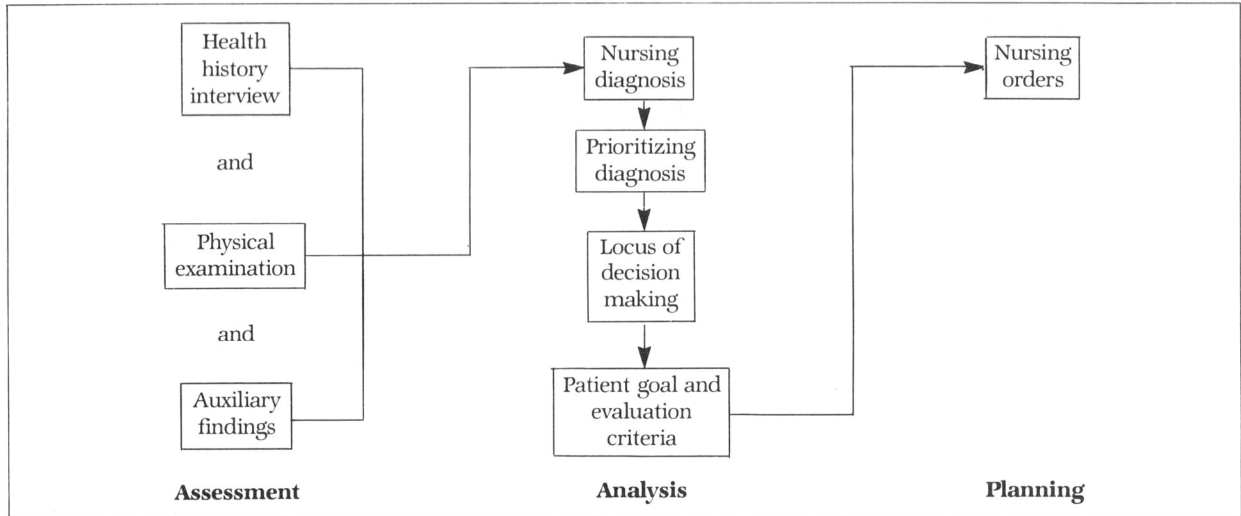

FIGURE 13-7. Nursing process: planning.

Remember when prioritizing problems and goals that aside from life-threatening situations what is most important for you may not be most important for the patient and vice versa. To be truly well the patient has to be in charge of his own life and make decisions about what kind of life he wants it to be.

PLANNING

Once short- and long-term goals are established, the next step in the nursing process is to design, in consultation with the patient or as an assistant to him, the strategy of how these goals will be reached. Plans are often called *nursing orders* (Fig. 13-7).

Suppose the long-term goal is "Increase muscle strength in upper arms." Your detailed plan might be (1) Ask M.D. for approval for muscle-strengthening exercises. (2) Secure trapeze and frame from central supply for over bed. (3) Instruct patient to lift upper body off bed 5 times, 4 times a day for 2 days, increasing number to 20 times, 4 times a day. (4) Secure bar bells with 10-pound weight from central supply. (5) Instruct patient to lift bar bells 5 times from supine position, 5 times a day; increase to 20 times, 5 times a day.

Plans are individualized and never static. If by the third day the plan is not acceptable to the patient or does not fit into the schedule of other procedures, it should be changed. If the patient is a child, the process might be introduced not as exercises but as a Simon Says game that someone plays with him 4 times a day. Nursing orders should be definite steps of action that a nurse can take and should be listed in consecutive order.

It is important in detailing plans to state whether the activity is one that the patient will carry out independently (will take full responsibility for progress), whether he will need to be reminded to do it, whether he will need some assistance with it, or whether it will have to be done for him. This prevents plans from failing because the nurse who relieves you thought that the patient was initiating the action while the patient was waiting for her to initiate it.

Do not make plans that are unrealistic. If it is impossible in the person's total plan of care for him to do muscle-strengthening exercises four times a day (there are too many other procedures that he has done during the day), muscle-strengthening exercises may never get done. It might be better, therefore, to specify one time a day when they should be done thoroughly and well.

Utilizing Other Health Care Providers

When planning activities for patients, consider whether or not you are actually the best person to carry out the plan. The exercises mentioned above, for example, might be better supervised by a physical therapist. They also could be supervised by a nursing aide, the patient's spouse, parent, or friend, or a hospital volunteer. Using auxiliary people often makes the difference between the success or failure of a plan of care. You are only one person in a team of health care providers; delegating activities is often necessary.

Be certain when delegating a portion of a plan of care or when asking for aid with a plan of care that the person who will assume responsibility for the plan understands how it fits into the total program of care and, if the activity is aimed at meeting a short-term goal, what the ultimate goal is that you and the patient are striving to achieve. Be certain that the person is one whom the patient will be able to work with; otherwise the goal will not be met (Fig. 13-8).

Assess progress periodically. Nothing is so confusing for people as to have a multitude of caregivers working with them when each caregiver is working in isolation from all others. You always need to know, for example, what a physical therapist, dietitian, or occupational

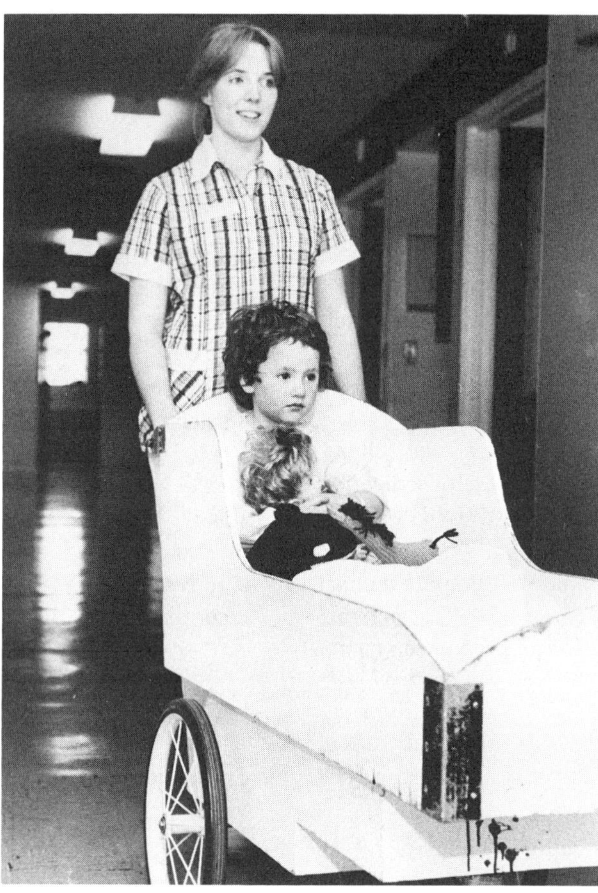

FIGURE 13-8. Planning frequently involves utilization of other care providers. Here the nurse uses a buggy cart to wheel a child for a physical therapy treatment. Note the child's facial expression and the way she clutches a security object, her doll. The nurse as primary care giver and support person will remain for the treatment, and future planning may further involve the nurse in this aspect of care.

therapist is trying to accomplish and incorporate it into the total plan of care for the patient.

A Nursing Care Plan

A nursing care plan is a written direction for action so that all nurses who care for a patient can accomplish it consistently. It encourages comprehensive, individualized care; it is important for communication between caregivers, evaluation of care, and planning of holistic care. It promotes patient satisfaction by preventing the patient from having to repeat the same information to different caregivers. It aids in keeping well people well and helping ill persons return to health again in optimal time.

Two formats can be used to record a nursing care plan. One is the traditional method of keeping this plan separate from the nursing notes on the patient's chart in a desk card file or separate nursing planning book. The other format is to use problem-oriented recording which incorporates the plan in charting. Problem-oriented charting guarantees that the plan and goals are kept current because they are constantly being reviewed. It also makes the nursing care plan a permanent part of the chart, which is important for continuity of care. If a person is readmitted to a health care facility at a later date, by looking at his old chart you can tell clearly what goals were established for him and what plans were effective and what plans were not the last time he was cared for. Nursing care plans kept separately from the chart are often treated as only temporary measures and destroyed at a person's discharge from the health care agency.

An advantage of keeping nursing care plans separate from the chart is that they are available for consultation even when the patient chart is temporarily in another department such as x-ray. It is a worksheet, so it is usually written in pencil so that it can be revised and updated as the patient's condition and needs change.

Every nursing care plan should include at least seven parts:

1. The nursing diagnoses that were identified.
2. The etiology and documentation for these diagnoses (signs and symptoms present).
3. The locus of decision making.
4. The goals and time frame for completion of the goals established for each nursing diagnosis.
5. Criteria by which success or goal achievement will be measured.
6. Nursing orders.
7. The rationale for nursing orders. This may be included as a separate category of information or incorporated into the nursing order statement. (Nursing order: Allow patient to take own medication. Rationale: To raise patient's self-esteem.)

An example of a care plan for Paul Parravano, 25 years old, is shown in Nursing Care Plan 1. He is a student in medical school who is having difficulty managing with the stress of school, a family, a shortage of finances, and the recent death of a brother. He is admitted with a medical diagnosis of peptic ulcer, which is an erosion of the stomach lining. Pain is caused because hydrochloric acid irritates the area of erosion. Pain can be eased by keeping the stomach constantly coated with a neutralizing agent such as an antacid and reducing stress, as stress increases the secretion of hydrochloric acid.

Other problems that might be identified from this example might be financial difficulty, reduced school attendance, lack of knowledge of disease condition, lack of knowledge of bland (ulcer) diet, or incomplete resolution of grief related to brother's death. Notice how these nursing diagnoses all differ from the medical diagnosis of peptic ulcer. The first nursing diagnosis relates directly to the disease pathology and the parenthesis (M.D.

NURSING CARE PLAN 1
Paul Parravano, 25 years old

Nursing Diagnosis	*Goal*	*Criteria*	*Nursing Orders*	*Rationale*
Pain related to mucosal erosion (M.D. confirmed).	Patient will have relief of pain in 1 hr.	States he is free of pain; evidences relaxation.	1. Educate on importance, purpose, and technique of antacid administration.	1. To increase compliance.
			2. Provide prescribed antacid (Maalox) by bedside.	2. To decrease stomach acidity.
			3. Allow patient to assume responsibility for self-medication of 30 ml every 1/2 hr.	3. To increase self-esteem.
			4. Prepare a chart so that patient can keep record of own medication administration.	4. To respect self-control.

Assessment—Signs and Symptoms: Sharp discomfort in upper midabdomen particularly just prior to meals; pain increased on palpation at abdominal midline.
Locus of Decision Making: Shared.

Nursing Diagnosis	*Goal*	*Criteria*	*Nursing Orders*	*Rationale*
Low self-esteem related to difficulty with school program.	Establish improved coping measures for handling stress by return to school.	Voices positive view of capabilities.	1. Offer experiences such as taking responsibility for self-medication, selecting diet, timing of procedures.	1. To increase immediate self-esteem.
			2. Identify and help him to recognize aspects of life where he does achieve (good father, husband, neighbor?).	2. To improve self-esteem.
			3. Determine if goals for self regarding school accomplishment are realistic or whether modification of goals may be indicated.	3. Plan for retention of self-esteem.

Assessment
Subjective: States he has doubts he is good enough for school program although he scored high in qualifying exams.
Objective: Nonsmiling; sad-appearing when describing school difficulty.
Locus of Decision Making: Shared.

confirmed) is used to assure other caregivers that this is an established diagnosis, not one still being investigated.

Nursing care plans are vital to continuity and quality of care. Be certain that they are complete; all information necessary for care must be included to prevent gaps in care. Be certain that they are written in a brief enough form to be easily comprehended and therefore usable. A nursing care plan that is incomplete or written in a hard-to-read style will not be used. Carrying out nursing care without consulting a plan is like sailing without a compass: nondirectional and ineffective.

PROBLEM-ORIENTED FORMAT

Some people prefer to write nursing care plans in a SOAP format (see Chap. 17 for a complete explanation of this format). This form simply changes the order in which items are recorded. The above problems would be presented as follows.

PROBLEM
Pain related to mucosal erosion (M.D. confirmed).
(S) Subjective findings: States he has sharp discomfort in upper midabdomen just prior to meals.
(O) Objective findings: Tenderness on palpation at abdominal midline.
(A) Assessment: Moderate pain; enough to interfere with normal functioning.
(P) Locus of decision making: Shared.
Goal: Relief of pain in 1 hour.
Criteria: States he is free of pain; evidences relaxation.
NURSING ORDERS
1. Educate on importance, purpose, and technique of antacid administration.
2. Provide prescribed antacid (Maalox) by bedside.
3. Allow patient to assume responsibility for own medication administration of 30 ml every 1/2 hour.
4. Prepare a chart so that patient can keep record of own medication administration.

PROBLEM
Low self-esteem related to difficulty with school program.
(S) States he has doubts he is good enough for school program although he scored high in qualifying exams.
(O) Nonsmiling; sad-appearing when describing school difficulty.
(A) Patient with low self-esteem related to distressing life event.
(P) Locus of decision-making: Shared.
Goal: Establish improved coping measures for handling stress by return to school.
Criteria: Voices positive view of capabilities.
NURSING ORDERS
1. Offer experiences that will improve self-esteem (taking responsibility for self-medication, selecting diet, timing of procedures).
2. Identify and help him to recognize aspects of life where he does achieve (good father, husband, neighbor?).
3. Determine if goals for self regarding school achievement are sensible or whether modification of goals may be indicated.

Nursing care planning is done not only with ill people but also with well people to help them keep well. Nursing Care Plan 2 is a care plan for a 12-year-old being seen for a yearly checkup at a health maintenance clinic.

IMPLEMENTATION

Once nursing orders have been carefully planned, the initiation and completion of the actions that were

NURSING CARE PLAN 2
Jill, 12 years old

Nursing Diagnosis	*Goal*	*Criteria*	*Nursing Orders*	*Rationale*
Knowledge of health promotion deficit related to age.	Maintain well health status.	Maintains height and weight on growth chart. Voices progress in school; relates well with friends.	1. Ask Mom about plans for menstruation education.	1. Plan for age-appropriate health education.
			2. Mark for dT immunization at next visit.	2. Plan for routine immunization.
			3. Mark for interview separate from Mom at next visit as she is nearly an adolescent.	3. Respect self-esteem and developmental level.

Assessment: Happy child; doing well in school. Height and weight at 50th percentile on growth chart. Active in swimming program in school. Family intact; all members well.
Locus of Decision Making: Shared with patient.

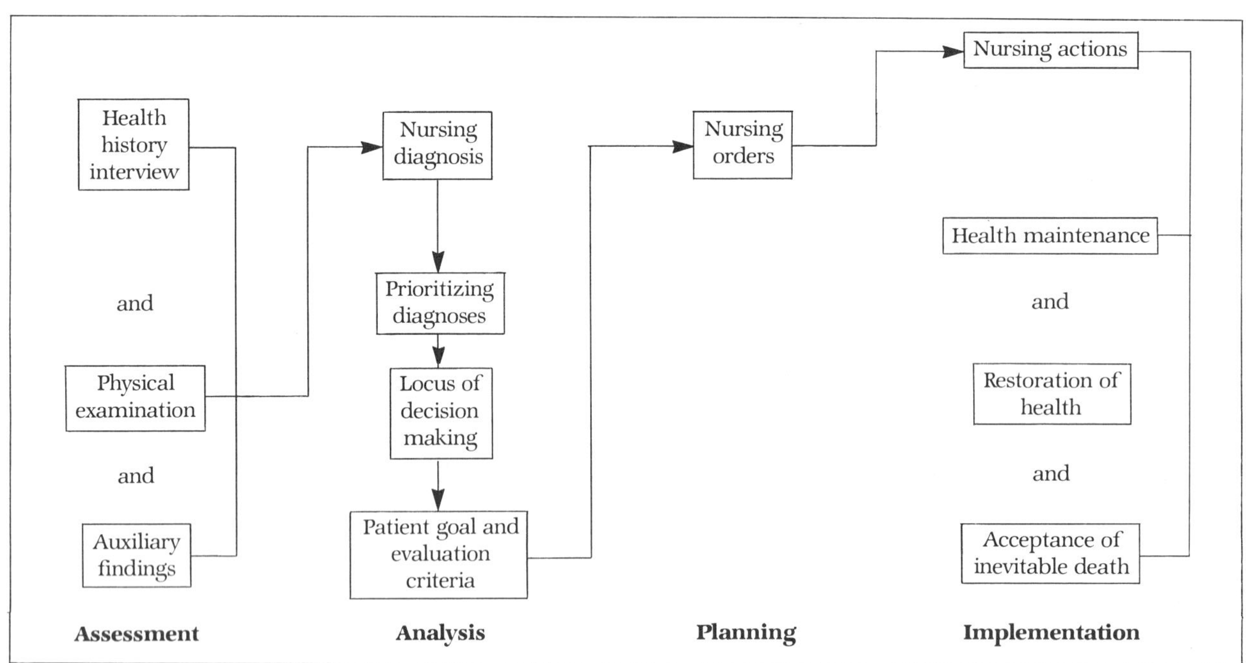

FIGURE 13-9. Nursing process: implementation.

specified to accomplish the established goals should follow smoothly and naturally (Fig. 13-9).

Possible nursing actions vary widely, depending on the age and condition of the patient, the setting, and current patient status. Table 13-7 shows factors that must be considered in implementation. Areas of nursing implementation are discussed below.

HEALTH MAINTENANCE

Health maintenance is wellness care (helping well people keep well). Nurses working in community settings concentrate heavily on this type of implementation. Assisting with health examinations and helping people choose nutritious diets are examples of this type of implementation.

HEALTH PROMOTION

Health promotion is action to encourage health. Teaching people to reduce smoking and demonstrating better methods to handle stress are examples of promoting health. This area is sometimes termed anticipatory guidance.

PREVENTION OF ILLNESS

Prevention of illness is a second line of defense against illness. Giving prescribed immunizations and helping a person to maintain a weight reduction program are examples.

Restoration of Health

Once a person has been ill, many different measures or forms of therapy may be necessary before he can return to health. Such actions could include providing comfort and hygiene measures, carrying out specific treatments such as changing a dressing, and health teaching.

REHABILITATION TO OPTIMAL HEALTH

Rehabilitation is helping a person whose illness has left him with a permanent disability to achieve his full potential (another term is tertiary prevention). It may include such activities as teaching how to carry out self-care activities with one hand or preparing teaching aids to help improve memory.

ACCEPTANCE OF INEVITABLE DEATH

Another area of health care is aiding those patients who cannot return to health again to accept the fact that death is inevitable and helping them and their support people to prepare for it. Implementation calls for a sensitivity to the patient's feelings, sensitive counseling, and support.

Nursing Roles

Nursing actions in implementation can be categorized as dependent, interdependent, or independent.

DEPENDENT ACTIONS

Dependent actions are those actions done under the direction of a physician. Administering medications, for example, is only done under the direct order of a physician. This is a legal matter: Administering a medication without an order will be interpreted as prescribing medication, a role that is outside the legal definition of nursing. A dependent action carries with it no less responsibility than others.

INTERDEPENDENT ACTIONS

The best care for a patient is often determined at a conference with another health care provider as to

TABLE 13-7. CONSIDERATIONS FOR ALL IMPLEMENTATIONS

Always based on scientific principles and theory	Utilization of scientific principles and theory assures safety and effectiveness of implementation.
Always are individualized	Modifications for growth and development, temperament, and current circumstances are made.
Always are holistic	Total person and response is considered.
Always provide for patient to be safe	Patient is identified correctly. Correct body alignment and position are maintained. Body integrity and function are maintained.
Always provide for patient comfort	Gentle technique is used. Reassurance and instruction are included. Self-esteem and self-control are protected.
Always provide for patient privacy	Privacy is considered to respect dignity and personal worth.
Always provide for patient participation	Patient is consulted in terms of preference and goals.
Always include a supportive component	Support in the form of acceptance and understanding is offered.
Always include an educational component	Health teaching is an independent action always included in care.
Always include an evaluation component	Evaluation for effectiveness and efficient use of time and resources is carried out.
Always include documentation of care and patient status	Record keeping and reporting ensures consistency and continuity of care.

what would be the best method to achieve a goal. Patients with burns, for instance, frequently need necrotic (dead) tissue cut away (debrided) from the burned area. This is a procedure that is unpleasant for all concerned because of the pain involved. Traditionally, debridement was done by the physician while the nurse acted as support person (making the physician the "heavy," the nurse the "angel of mercy"). Today, you and the physician may decide to rotate the "good" and "bad" roles or to share both the responsibility and the reward of care. An educational program is another example of a responsibility that might be shared equally between physician and nurse for optimal care.

INDEPENDENT ACTIONS

An independent action is one recognized as needed because of nursing's unique body of knowledge. In a patient who is short of breath, for example, a physician may order that oxygen be administered. You not only place an oxygen mask over the patient's nose and mouth but place him in a Fowler's position (upright in bed) and begin to count his respiratory rate every 15 minutes to assess whether improvement in respiratory function occurs. These independent actions support and complement the patient's medical regime and contribute to his progress and well-being.

Types of Implementation

DIRECT CARE

Many nursing activities are done singly in a one-to-one nurse-patient relationship. This includes such nursing responsibilities as providing comfort and hygiene, good nutrition, assisting with exercise, sleep, and elimination, and providing education and psychological support. Such implementation involves the use of psychomotor skills, teaching, and counseling.

SUPERVISION OF CARE

At times, rather than give direct care, your nursing role is to supervise care given by others. For example, you will determine based on the patient's condition whether it would be better for the patient to be completely or partially bathed; an aide will actually give the bath. Supervising care involves being certain that no matter who is actually carrying out the procedure, it will be done consistently and with good technique. Supervising health care aides is time consuming as it must include both education of the aide on the importance, purpose, and skills of the task and evaluation when the aide reports the outcome and patient response to the procedure. There are legal implications with regard to supervising health care personnel. A person is entitled to quality care whether it is supplied by you or supervised by you. When supervising others, you must be certain that the care the person receives is equal in quality to that which you would have given yourself.

COORDINATION OF CARE

A major nursing role with most patients is coordination of care. A patient who is going to have surgery, for example, must have the time for surgery scheduled with the operating room of the hospital, have a visit and evaluation prior to surgery by the anesthesiologist, and have an electrocardiogram, x-rays, and blood and urine specimens obtained before surgery; a special diet will be begun immediately afterward. As a coordinator of care, it would be your responsibility to see that arrangements for all these different aspects of care are made and that results of studies are reported appropriately.

REFERRAL

After defining a problem your nursing action might be to refer the problem to the person best able to provide the care. You might ask a nutritionist, for example, to talk to your patient about his special diet. You might refer education or care to a nurse specialist—nurse clinician. Referring the patient to the most appropriate person to carry out a therapy assures you that it will be done in the best way possible.

TEACHING
Teaching is always a prime nursing interaction. At times it is a primary action—educating a person about his disease, his medication, or other therapy he will have to continue himself after he returns home. At other times the teaching is done with the patient's family (helping a mother to learn muscle-strengthening exercise for her child) or extends into the community (helping children in the child's classroom adjust to the fact he will use a wheelchair). Patient education always is a basic step accompanying procedures so that the person understands what the procedure involves and any cooperation that is necessary for it.

COUNSELING
Counseling is also always a prime nursing interaction. While teaching consists of supplying answers or information, counseling involves helping the person to find out the answers himself. For instance, you may supply a number of alternative solutions to a problem, but the person himself will decide which alternative fits his situation.

COMFORTING
Comfort is a sensation of being not only free of physical pain but free of psychological stress as well. Interventions to promote comfort should be included with every procedure of care as a person cannot be described as well so long as he does not have comfort.

PROTECTION
A nurse serves as a patient's first line of defense against illness or complication from illness because a nurse is the member of a health care team who spends the most time with a patient and invariably knows him best. Measures of safety and protection should always be incorporated in every nursing procedure.

SUPPORTING
Support means that you are sensitive to a person's feelings and ready to assist him as necessary to maintain psychological well-being. It is yet another action that is a constant accompaniment to nursing care. Support may be accomplished by verbal praise (you're doing well; you look much better today); by acknowledging that feelings such as anxiety, hostility, anger, or sadness are expected and acceptable (this must be very difficult for you; you look as if you feel sad); by responding nonverbally such as by holding a person's hand during a painful procedure; by comforting a person by a touch to the shoulder or hand, sometimes by just being nearby (a comforting presence).

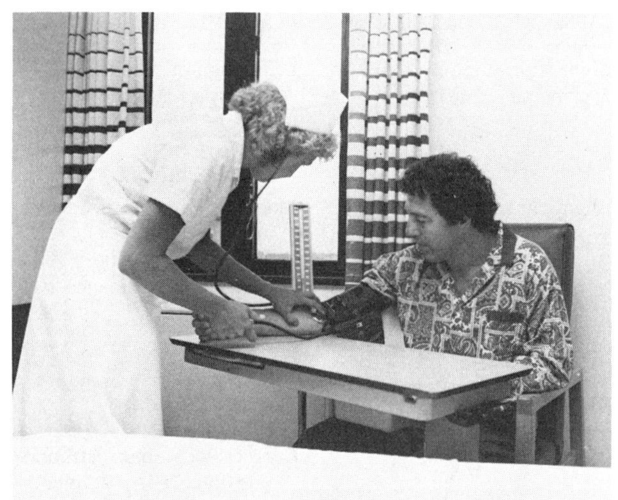

FIGURE 13-10. Accurate measurement of blood pressure is a psychomotor skill; it is learned by practice.

PSYCHOMOTOR SKILLS
Psychomotor skills (combined mental and motor skills) are required for many nursing care procedures such as bathing a patient, changing a dressing, regulating an intravenous infusion, giving an injection, taking a blood pressure (Fig. 13-10). This type of skill requires your knowing the principle behind the procedure, the correct steps to take, and the correct order of them; it is followed by reassessment of patient condition and recording of the procedure and patient observations. Psychomotor skills are learned by practice and increased knowledge of the effect and importance of such care. Areas that require psychomotor skills are providing comfort, assisting with elimination, exercise, hygiene, nutrition, recreation, sleep, and rest, and supporting physiologic functioning.

ANTICIPATORY GUIDANCE
Anticipatory guidance is a form of health teaching. It is "looking down the road" or into the future to try to identify what interferences with health are likely to occur. With this knowledge the person is forewarned what danger is ahead and can adjust his life style to prevent the health problem. Instructing a mother at a well-child visit that her two-month-old baby will probably turn over during the next month and therefore will no longer be safe sleeping in a bassinet is an example of this type of guidance.

Implementation and Nursing Process
Implementation of nursing care is to many people the only step of the nursing process that they are aware of because it is the step that is most visible. It is only one step out of five, however, and must be integrated with other steps in order to be effective.

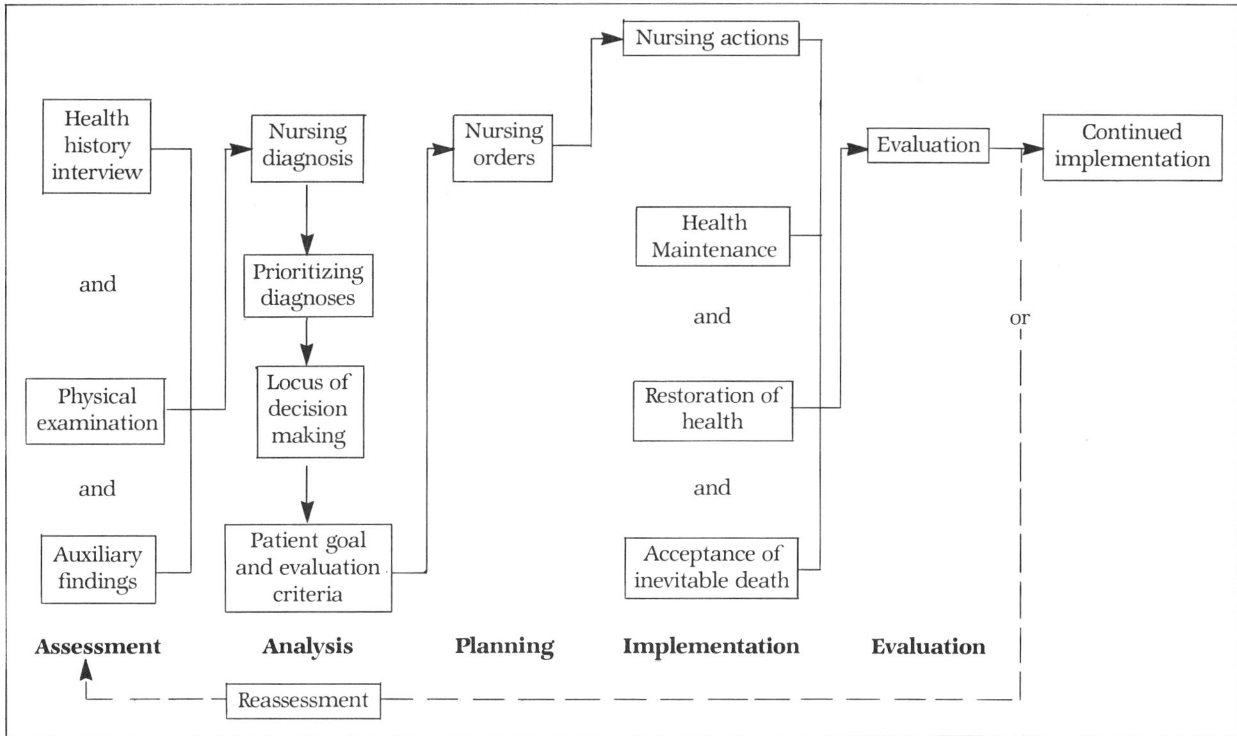

FIGURE 13-11. Nursing process: evaluation.

EVALUATION

Evaluation is the final stage of the nursing process. Following implementation of nursing care, goal criteria are assessed to see if the goal was reached, and a decision is made whether implementation should continue as it is (care is optimal) or needs to be changed in some way (it is not optimal for various reasons).

The step of evaluation makes nursing process a fluid ongoing process, which it must be because nursing deals with people who are ever-changing. If evaluation shows that the plan was not successful, you must return to the assessment step and begin reassessment. Perhaps you will discover that something was omitted in assessment and that is why the problem has been unresolved; perhaps the fault will be found in some aspect of analysis or planning.

The step of evaluation, therefore, leads either to continuation of care or to reassessment and a new plan of care. This is shown diagrammatically in Figure 13-11.

Utilizing Evaluation

Evaluation is an easy step in the nursing process to take lightly because one tends to think that in the light of the careful planning that was done, the implementation of care will be ideal. As patient conditions change, however, an implementation that was ideal for one day may no longer be optimal the next day. Suppose need for nutrition was a nursing diagnosis, for example. The first day a patient is in a health care facility he may receive his nutrition as a liquid nasogastric feeding; after a week he may begin to drink clear fluids, two days later a soft diet, still another day later a regular diet. He may progress from your feeding him (first by a nasogastric route, then by a spoon) to needing some help to feed himself, to not only independently feeding himself but selecting the foods he will eat. Obviously a plan of nutrition that was ideal at the beginning of his hospital stay will be very out of date and meaningless by even the third day. Evaluation detects this and allows and guides change.

Evaluation of Objectives

To evaluate care, compare the person's progress with the goals you established during the analysis phase. Ask if the goals were reached or if not reached, is progress being made toward them. It is important to always include criteria for measurement when establishing goals so that this final evaluation step can be readily accomplished.

Include the patient's evaluation of progress as well as your own. You may feel that the implementation being carried out is very satisfactory; the patient may not find the implementation satisfactory at all. The patient is the ultimate judge of whether progress is satisfactory; if he is not pleased, changes have to be planned and made.

Reassessment of Data Base

At times progress is not satisfactory because some condition, belief, or circumstance was missed in the original assessment. Suppose, for example, that you failed to learn on your initial interview that a patient's brother was left with a permanent arm deformity following a fracture of his arm as a child. Your patient is admitted to your hospital setting with a broken leg. Immediately, you set goals with him to be free of pain, learn self-care within the limitations of a cast, and increase calcium intake to aid in bone healing. By the next day all three goals are reached, yet the patient is still visibly worried and concerned. Merely changing implementation without reassessment will not improve the situation. If progress or goal attainment is not optimal, you must return to the first step of the process, assessment, and work through the steps again. Reassessment, in this instance, will lead to the missed information; a new nursing diagnosis (anxiety related to fear of poor outcome); a new goal (express belief in positive outcome in one week); and new implementation (ask M.D. to spend time giving reassurance). Hopefully, evaluation will then reveal satisfactory goal achievement.

Reassessment of Goal and Criteria Setting

At times when evaluation reveals that a goal was not obtained, examining the goal will reveal that it was set too high or too high for the time interval allowed. Stating that a patient will indicate that he is continuously free of pain within an hour after surgery, for example, is a pleasant-sounding goal but not a realistic one. Even after being administered analgesic medication, a quick movement such as turning over quickly in bed or coughing or sneezing will cause pain. A more realistic goal would be for the patient to be free of distressing pain within one hour following surgery. In the same manner the goal may have been set appropriately but the criteria for measuring it may have been selected wrongly. Ask: Is this truly a sensible goal? Are the specified criteria the best way of measuring the goal attainment? If a goal is that the patient will have full return of arm function in one week, the criterion could be: Patient states full function has returned. A better criterion may be: Patient is completing all written school assignments without difficulty. From a practical standpoint, however, you might find the second criterion hard to assess as you do not have access to these assignments; the first might be the better choice since it can be evaluated fully.

Reassessment of Nursing Orders

At still other times evaluation does not reveal goal attainment because the nursing orders were not sufficiently clear to enable every nurse who saw them to interpret them in the same way. Avoid words like "frequently," "large amount," and "increase fluid intake." Give more specific instructions such as "every 15 minutes," "250 ml," and "increase fluid intake by 100 ml daily" so that there will be no misunderstanding of orders.

Reassessment of Implementation

Evaluate whether implementation has been consistent. Occasionally, time and staff restraints interfere to make the best plan unrealistic in actual practice. An alternate method of implementation may have to be chosen to increase success. Mrs. Jones, for example, has difficulty mothering her child and needs role modeling of ways to hold an infant securely and feed him successfully. You would like to do this role modeling yourself to ensure that it is demonstrated consistently and thoroughly. Unfortunately, you know that you will not always be available at the times that Mrs. Jones will visit her child. You meet with three nursing assistants and review with them the aspects of care that you are particularly concerned be demonstrated and stressed. When various caregivers are supplying care, you need to evaluate whether the implementation is consistent and the best for the circumstances.

Individual Evaluation

Evaluation is most often an individual process (you observe by yourself a patient's progress). Observations are both subjective (the patient states he feels better) and objective (his blood pressure has been normal for two days).

Group Evaluation

At times a nursing team or a total health care team participates in evaluation. A group conference or team conference increases the validity of observations (five people all confirm that although the patient states that nothing is worrying him, he looks and acts worried). Brainstorming among group members can often create a solution to a perplexing problem that one person alone cannot accomplish. Such conferences also serve to increase the ability of group members to identify problems and evaluate progress, thus making it a learning process for everyone in the group.

Tools of Evaluation

Evaluation may be done informally by observation or with the use of a standardized report form or checksheet. The more definite measures of outcome you can state, the more certain you can be that a goal has been reached. Stating that a person appears comfortable, for example, is not as good an evaluation statement as saying that not only does he appear comfortable but he has not asked for any medication for pain for the past eight hours and walks on an injured foot without any evidence of a limp or "guarding." Saying that a person appears to be free of fever is a weak evaluation; stating that his body temperature is 98.6F is a definitive measure.

Discharge Evaluations

An important section of every patient's chart is the final nursing summary or discharge evaluation. This should include a statement on the status of progress toward each goal established and if this status is not full goal attainment, plans for continuation of care.

A discharge summary is important for nursing audit purposes and for establishing a baseline for progress before a patient returns home from a health care facility or is discharged from a community nurse's care. An audit is a periodic assessment of health care facilities and of the quality of the care provided for accreditation or certification purposes. If a patient is readmitted to the health care facility or later requires additional community health home care, this summary will serve as an important source of data.

NURSING PROCESS AND EXAMINATION FOR LICENSURE

In order to be credentialed as a registered nurse, you must, at the completion of your nursing program, successfully pass a national licensing examination (the National Council Licensure Examination for Registered Nurses or NCLEX-RN). Such an examination is designed to test your ability to function safely in the practice of nursing.

Such examinations are commonly called state board exams, because although the examination is a nationally administered one, each state specifies the level of performance that it considers to be a passing grade.

Since 1982 licensing examinations for registered nurses are directly structured on the nursing process format and test your ability to assess, analyze, plan, implement, and evaluate for safe nursing care. A basic philosophy incorporated into the examination is the concept that man is a holistic and unique being who should have input into his own health care. Nursing functions tested are your ability to make adequate assessments of patients and initiate appropriate action; identify health needs and resources of persons you care for; help people maintain life and health, cope with health problems, and return to full recovery from illness. In order to acquire these skills, you need a background in basic human needs, coping mechanisms people commonly use, normal growth and development concepts, effect of age, sex, culture, ethnicity, and religion on health needs and care, actual and potential health problems of people, and ways that you can assist people with health maintenance and participation in their own care, recognizing the correct locus of decision making for care.

Nursing process is not, then, just a convenient method of organizing and planning nursing care. Being able to use it consistently is a requirement of being able to practice as a registered nurse.

UTILIZING NURSING PROCESS; AMBULATORY SETTING

Nursing process is applicable in both ambulatory and impatient settings and with both well and ill people.

Assessment

You have derived the following from your assessment of a child seen in an ambulatory setting and have categorized the data as subjective or objective.

She is crying because she says that her left eyebrow hurts.	Subjective
She has an open two-inch laceration on her left eyebrow.	Objective
Her mother tells you that she is worried that the cut will leave a permanent scar.	Subjective
The child's hemoglobin level determination is normal (12 mg/100 ml)	Objective
The child has an old keloid scar (an overgrowth of tissue) on her finger.	Objective
The mother states that a neighbor told her that sutures (stitches) cause keloid scars.	Subjective
The mother is crying.	Objective
She refuses to allow her daughter to have sutures.	Subjective

Analysis

From this assessment information two nursing diagnoses might be identified.

1. Problem: Discomfort, pain.
   Etiology: Related to laceration of left eyebrow.
   Signs and symptoms: Crying and holding hand over left eyebrow.
2. Problem: Parental concern.
   Etiology: Related to fear of scar formation from sutures.
   Signs and symptoms: States that she is worried; refuses to have stitches put in place; wrings her hands; crying.

The laceration is a medical diagnosis, not a nursing diagnosis. The hemoglobin level is both a normal finding and a diagnostic test, not a nursing diagnosis; the information is used to support the fact that the pain is from a small laceration (blood loss was not great or the hemoglobin value would be decreased). The fall itself is not a nursing diagnosis; it documents the etiology of the pain.

Locus of Decision Making

The mother is capable of fully participating in planning of care and a 12-year-old child is old enough to have specific ideas about her care; both are stressed because of the recent injury, however, and are not at their problem-solving best. The locus of decision making for the interaction then is shared between the nurse and patient-parent. If the child were older, the locus would be shared with the nurse and her; if the mother were not distraught, the locus might be totally with her.

Priority Setting

Pain is always considered to be a priority problem as it is difficult for a person to focus on anything else until it is relieved.

Establishing Goals

A short-term goal for the first problem identified (pain) might be: Patient will have decreased pain within 15 minutes (the time for a common analgesic to be effective). A long-term goal might be: Relief from the pain through healing of the laceration. The criterion for evaluation of the first goal would be: Patient reports that pain has lessened or disappeared; for the second: Skin area appears well healed.

A short-term goal for the second problem (parental concern) might be: Acceptance of sutures as treatment for facial lacerations within one-half hour. The criterion would be: Allows physician to place stitches. A long-term goal might be: Expresses confidence in health care personnel rather than neighbors' judgment concerning health problems by next visit in 10 days. The criterion for evaluation would be: Expresses satisfaction with care at time of return visit.

Planning (Nursing Orders)

Plans or nursing orders for the first problem might consist of:

1. Apply cold compress to forehead for 15 minutes to help relieve pain.
2. Assure patient that pain will be lessened by analgesic administration.
3. Ask M.D. for analgesic order to further relieve pain.
4. Administer analgesic upon receiving medication order.
5. Ask in 15 minutes following analgesic administration if pain relief is achieved.

Nursing orders for the second problem might consist of:

1. Inform M.D. of mother's reluctance to have stitches set.
2. Ask M.D. to discuss importance of stitches in reducing scar formation.
3. Reaffirm M.D.'s advice regarding the effectiveness of stitches in reducing scar tissue.

Implementation

Placing a cool towel for comfort is an independent nursing action; discussing the reason for sutures is an interdependent function; administering the analgesic is a dependent function. Some measures (teaching about sutures) are educational; some are therapeutic (relieving pain). Including all these actions makes the plan comprehensive.

Evaluation

Suppose at the end of one-half hour the mother still refuses to allow the physician to put in sutures. Your criterion for one short-term goal has not been met. To determine why, you need to return to assessment to determine at what step the plan was not adequate.

Suppose on reassessment you discover that the real reason the mother does not want sutures is that her medical insurance does not cover ambulatory care costs and she therefore cannot afford to have care. This does not change the problem (the mother still refuses to have sutures), but it does change the etiology of the problem, which will change the plan of action from education to helping the mother achieve some form of financial aid.

UTILIZING NURSING PROCESS: INPATIENT SETTING

Mrs. Smith is a 70-year-old woman you care for. Her medical diagnosis is arteriosclerosis, a disease that hardens and narrows the arteries and thereby reduces blood flow. Distal body parts may not receive enough blood and so have symptoms of decreased circulation (coldness, pain).

While you care for Mrs. Smith, you make the following observations:

She states that she feels worthless because of her illness.	S
Her feet feel cold to your touch.	O
She states that she has pains in her feet.	S
She says that she doesn't ever feel like walking.	S
There is edema (excess subcutaneous fluid) present in both ankles.	O
She sits for long hours in a chair by the window of her room.	O
She has an order for aspirin 10 grains every 4 hours for pain.	O

Analysis

Nursing diagnoses based on the above information might be:

1. Problem: Discomfort, pain.
   Etiology: Related to cell anoxia from reduced circulation.
   Signs and symptoms: She states that she has pain.
   Her feet feel cold; edema is present.
2. Problems: Decreased self-esteem.
   Etiology: Related to diagnosis of chronic illness.
   Signs and symptoms: She states that she feels worthless.
   She sits immobile in a chair; rarely ambulates.

Locus of Decision Making

The patient is able to participate in her plan of care. Lowered self-esteem, however, limits the ability of people to make decisions; for this reason the decision making would be shared. Later, when the patient arrives at a point where she can accept her illness better, the locus of decision making might be patient-centered.

Priority Setting

Reducing pain is always a priority need (it is difficult for people to focus on other needs as long as it is present) and should be listed as the priority problem. Once discomfort has been relieved, helping the woman to feel better about her whole self will be easier.

Establishing Goals

The short-term goal for the first problem (discomfort) might be: Patient will have reduced discomfort within one-half hour. The criterion for evaluation would be that she states that she feels more comfortable. The long-term goal might be: Patient will increase circulation to distal parts to reduce discomfort. The criterion would be that she ambulates at least three times daily a distance of 20 feet.

The short-term goal for the second problem (decreased self-esteem) might be: Patient will work at one interesting project daily. A long-term goal might be: Expresses satisfaction in herself as a person in spite of chronic illness by the time of hospital discharge. The criterion for evaluation for both goals would be her stated sense of well-being.

Planning (Nursing Orders)

Nursing orders for the first problem (discomfort) might be:

1. Administer pain medication every 4 hours as needed to prevent pain from becoming acute.
2. Urge patient to wear warm slippers and use lap robe to increase warmth in extremities.
3. Teach importance of ambulation to increase circulation.
4. Urge patient to walk width of room 3 times daily to increase circulation.

Nursing orders for the second problem (decreased self-esteem) might be:

1. Investigate interests she enjoyed before illness such as knitting, painting, etc.
2. Encourage self-care to the extent possible to increase self-worth.
3. Ask her to help sort central supply orders every afternoon as contribution she could make to unit functioning to increase self-worth.

Implementation

Nursing measures to be carried out here are both independent (finding a task she can do) and dependent (administering a medicine). Some are diagnostic in nature (investigating previous interests), some therapeutic (providing warmth), and some educational (teaching about the importance of walking). Knowing that a plan includes many different components helps to assure you that it is comprehensive in scope.

Evaluation

After all the above measures have been carried out, it will be important to determine whether Mrs. Smith now feels more comfortable and better about herself. If evaluation does not show such changes, you have to return to the first step of the nursing process and elicit further information to discover why your interventions were for some reason not adequate.

VALUE OF THE NURSING PROCESS

The examples in this chapter describe simple problems so that the steps of nursing process can be separated and examined readily. The test that nursing process is applicable to all situations and settings is that the process works equally well with complex patient problems. It is the essence of nursing care. Learning to work within its framework is necessary in order to move from simple beginning-nurse concerns to those of the professional nurse of today.

SUGGESTED READINGS

Aspinall, M. J. Nursing diagnosis—the weak link. *Nurs. Outlook* 24:433, 1976.

Atkinson, L. D., and Murray, M. E. *Understanding the Nursing Process.* New York: Macmillan, 1980.

Auld, M. G. Nursing in a changing society. *J. Adv. Nurs.* 4:287, 1979.

Baer, E., et al. Taking a health history. *Am. J. Nurs.* 77:1190, 1977.

Bailey, K., et al. An innovative approach to the nursing process. *Nurs. Adm. Q.* 6:71, 1982.

Bower, F. L. *The Process of Planning Nursing Care: A Model for Practice* (2nd ed.). St. Louis: Mosby, 1977.

Bullough, B., and Bullough, V. *Expanding horizons for nurses.* New York: Springer, 1977.

Byers, V. *Nursing Observation* (3rd ed.). Dubuque, Iowa: W. C. Brown, 1977.

Campbell, C. *Nursing Diagnosis and Intervention in Nursing Practice.* New York: Wiley, 1978.

Chinn, P., and Deitch, C. *Child Health Maintenance: A Guide to Clinical Assessment* (2nd ed.). St. Louis: Mosby, 1979.

Cunningham, C. A. Professional nursing practice in the hospital setting. *Superv. Nurse* 11:26, 1980.

Dalton, J. M. Nursing diagnosis in a community health setting. *Nurs. Clin. North Am.* 14:525, 1979.

Decker, F., et al. Using patient outcomes to evaluate community health nursing. *Nurs. Outlook* 27:278, 1979.

Dolan, M. B. Humans are fragile: Handle with care. *RN* 44:34, 1981.

Eichelberger, K. M., et al. Self-care nursing plan: Helping children to help themselves. *Pediatr. Nurs.* 6:9, 1980.

Farrell, J. The human side of assessment. *Nursing 80* 10:74, 1980.

Field, L. N. The implementation of nursing diagnosis in clinical practice. *Nurs. Clin. North Am.* 14:497, 1979.

Forman, M. Building a better nursing care plan. *Am. J. Nurs.* 79:1086, 1979.

Gordon, M. The concept of nursing diagnosis. *Nurs. Clin. North Am.* 14:487, 1979.

Gray, J. W., et al. Care plans in long-term facilities. *Am. J. Nurs.* 80:2054, 1980.

Hagar, L. The nursing process: A tool to individualized care. *Canad. Nurse* 73:38, 1977.

Harris, R. B. A strong vote for nursing process. *Am. J. Nurs.* 79:1999, 1979.

Henderson, V. A. Preserving the essence of nursing—a technological age. *J. Adv. Nurs.* 5:235, 1980.

Henderson, V. The nursing process—is the title right? *J. Adv. Nurs.* 7:103, 1982.

Huckabay, L., et al. The nursing care plan problem. *J. Nurs. Adm.* 10:35, 1980.

Inzer, F., et al. Evaluating patient outcomes. *Nurs. Outlook* 29:178, 1981.

Jones, P. W. A terminology for nursing diagnoses. *Adv. Nurs. Sci.* 2:65, 1979.

Joseph, L. S. Self care and the nursing process. *Nurs. Clin. North Am.* 15:131, 1980.

Kim, M. J., and Moritz, D. A. *Classification of Nursing Diagnoses.* New York: McGraw-Hill, 1982.

King, C. Refining your assessment techniques. *RN* 46(2):42, 1983.

Lamonica, E. L. *The Nursing Process: A Humanistic Approach.* Reading, Mass.: Addison-Wesley, 1979.

Leslie, F. M. Nursing Diagnosis: Use in long term care. *Am. J. Nurs.* 81:1012, 1981.

Little, D., and Carneveli, D. *Nursing Care Planning* (2nd ed.). Philadelphia: Lippincott, 1976.

MacKay, C., and Ault, L. D. A systematic approach to individualizing nursing care. *J. Nurs. Adm.* 7:39, 1977.

Majesky, S. J., et al. Development of a research tool: Patient indicators of nursing care. *Nurs. Res.* 27:365, 1978.

Malasanos, L., et al. *Health Assessment* (21st ed.). St. Louis: Mosby 1981.

Marriner, A. *The Nursing Process: A Scientific Approach to Nursing Care* (3rd ed.). St. Louis: Mosby, 1983.

Maslow, A. H. *Motivation and Personality* (2nd ed.). New York: Harper & Row, 1970.

Mayers, M. G. *A Systematic Approach to the Nursing Care Plan* (3rd ed.). Norwalk, Conn.: Appleton-Century-Crofts, 1983.

McCloskey, J. C. Nurse's orders: The next professional breakthrough? *RN* 43:99, 1980.

Mezey, M., et al. The health history of the aged person. *J. Gerontol. Nurs.* 3:45, 1977.

Miller, S. L., et al. Identification of health problems at well elderly clinics. *J. Gerontol. Nurs.* 7:159, 1981.

Moore, K. R. What nurses learn from nursing audit. *Nurs. Outlook* 27:254, 1979.

Mundinger, M., and Jauron, G. Developing a nursing diagnosis. *Nurs. Outlook* 23:96, 1975.

Nichols, E. G., et al. Do nurses really use standard care plans? *J. Nurs. Adm.* 10:27, 1980.

O'Driscoll, D. L. The nursing process and long term care. *J. Gerontol. Nurs.* 2:34, 1976.

Price, M. R. Nursing diagnosis: Making a concept come alive. *Am. J. Nursing* 80:668, 1980.

Rawnsley, M. M. Toward a conceptual base for effective nursing. *Nurs. Outlook* 28:244, 1980.

Roeder, M. A. Patient care plans and the evaluation of nursing process. *Superv. Nurse* 11:57, 1980.

Sedgwick, R., et al. Family health assessment. *Nurse Pract.* 6:37, 1981.

Spitz, P., et al. Bedside assessment—special considerations. *Nursing 78* 8:70, 1978.

Sundeen, S., et al. *Nurse-client Interaction: Implementing the Nursing Process.* St. Louis: Mosby, 1976.

VanMaanen, H. M. Improvement of quality of nursing care: A goal to challenge in the eighties. *J. Adv. Nurs.* 6:3, 1981.

Wessells, V. G., and Nicholls, M. E. *Nursing Standards and Nursing Process.* Wakefield, Mass.: Nursing Resources, 1977.

Williamson, J. A. Mutual interaction: A model of nursing practice. *Nurs. Outlook* 29:104, 1981.

Yura, H., and Walsh, M. B. (Eds.). *Human Needs and the Nursing Process.* Norwalk, Conn.: Appleton-Century-Crofts, 1983.

Yura, H., and Walsh, M. B. *The Nursing Process* (4th ed.). Norwalk, Conn.: Appleton-Century-Crofts, 1983.

QUESTIONS FOR REVIEW

1. Mr. Jones is a patient whom you care for. Interviewing Mr. Jones for information on his past illnesses represents which step of the nursing process?
   a. Assessment.
   b. Analysis.
   c. Implementation.
   d. Evaluation.

2. A nursing diagnosis should include which three factors?
   a. Problem, etiology, signs and symptoms.
   b. Need, implementation, criteria for evaluation.
   c. Problem, time limit for resolution, etiology.
   d. Objective information, subjective information, problem.

3. When you take Mr. Jones' pulse as part of the physical examination, this represents which step of the nursing process?
   a. Assessment.
   b. Analysis.
   c. Implementation.
   d. Evaluation.

4. Assessment data consist of what three parts?
   a. Interview, laboratory tests, negative findings.
   b. Interview, physical examination, positive findings.
   c. Positive findings, disabilities, laboratory tests.
   d. Physical examination, laboratory data, interview.

5. Which of the following represents a *negative* finding?
   a. Skin is intact.
   b. A bright red rash is present.
   c. Edema (swelling) is present.
   d. Skin feels dry and is cracked.

6. Which of the following is a *subjective* finding?
   a. Patient walks unsteadily.
   b. Patient states that he feels dizzy.
   c. Patient has an abrasion on his knee.
   d. Patient sat down suddenly after walking.

7. Which of the following is a *positive* finding?
   a. Patient's height and weight are normal for age.
   b. Patient states that his appetite is good.
   c. Patient drinks his coffee black.
   d. Patient states that he is frequently nauseated.

8. Which of the following is an *objective* finding?
   a. A mother feels that her child is nervous.
   b. The child states that he worries over school.
   c. The child's weight is below normal on a height-weight curve.
   d. The child's teacher reports that the child bites his nails.

9. Which of the following would be an appropriate nursing diagnosis?
   a. An intravenous infusion of blood.
   b. Fear related to loss of job.
   c. Hepatitis related to liver infection.
   d. Low red blood count related to bleeding.

10. When you make Mr. Jones' bed, this reflects which step of the nursing process?
    a. Assessment.
    b. Implementation.
    c. Analysis.
    d. Evaluation.

11. Goal setting for Mr. Jones should include which three factors?
    a. Goal, criteria, time limit.
    b. Behavioral objective, expected outcome, etiology.
    c. Short-term goal, long-term goal, evaluation criteria.
    d. Objective, evaluation component, stress factor.

12. Mr. Jones has pain. When you ask him if the medication you gave him relieved his pain, which step of the nursing process does this represent?
    a. Assessment.
    b. Analysis.
    c. Planning.
    d. Evaluation.

13. To review terms pertinent to the nursing process, locate the terms the following statements represent in the following word maze.
    a. An identified problem that is within the realm of nursing to resolve.
    b. The systematic collection of data in order to identify a patient need or problem.
    c. An unmet desire.
    d. The cause of a problem.
    e. Type of information that can be documented.
    f. Giving preference to one item over another competing item.
    g. The aim of what you hope to achieve.
    h. Examining goal criteria to see if a plan was successful.
    i. The study of assessment data to reach a conclusion as to what needs or problems are present.

B M X P B A N O R T V E F T B X W M
K E P R I O R I T Y S E T T I N G P
M V T M V R S B Q C D W X M A D C Y
W I M V R B E V A L U A T I O N L T
N T O O V K T T Q P D N A K C A D K
L C N U R S I N G D I A G N O S I S
Y E E U S C O E Y F J L K G Y I R M
P J E Q Y A L M P M R Y Z G B C S K
Z B D N V L O S T E K S M F J X I N
D O V Y W Q G S Z W M I B N O L Y S
W X U P M M Y E R H N S T N P Q Z U
L A C T E Z P S H D N L L K O D X N
M A R T E P W S W R U T V G U R S A
T P W S G H T A P B C X R U H F W B

14. THE ROLE OF THE NURSE IN ADVOCACY AND CHANGE

OBJECTIVES

Upon mastery of the material in this chapter, you should be able to:

1. Describe the concept of advocacy as it relates to health care.
2. List general principles of advocacy.
3. Describe the role of the nurse as a patient advocate.
4. List principles for initiating change.
5. List principles of effective leadership.
6. Describe effective strategies for working with groups.
7. Describe the role of the assertive nurse.

TERMS

The terms important for an understanding of this chapter are shown below and defined in the glossary:

advocacy
advocate
assertiveness
change
leadership
trial period

An advocate is a person who works with or on behalf of another person or system to bring about a positive change in that person's or system's condition. It is an enjoyable role in that an advocate is a person involved with improving existing conditions. It is a responsible role as one change often leads to other changes; the full scope of any change must be anticipated or the change may become destructive. People act as advocates through effective leadership and often through group work. Some nurses are hired for specific advocacy positions such as speaking for people with certain handicapping conditions as a lobbyist in Washington or speaking for any person in a specific health care agency who feels that his rights as a patient have been violated. All nurses, as they plan how to best help a person to remain well or return to optimal wellness, fulfill an advocacy role.

Advocacy does not happen by chance; it never happens if taken for granted. It occurs through well-organized, well-thought-through steps of planning and action, like any other phase of nursing care.

THE ART OF ADVOCACY

People often need help with making decisions about their health care or support for decisions they have made. They may also need help obtaining health care services from a large bureaucratic system. Whether you are helping a person to improve his health or to find the appropriate service in the health care system, a number of general rules concerning advocacy always apply.

1. Assume that everyone is doing the best he can in any circumstance. If you are a naturally assertive person who would readily pick up a telephone and register a complaint about some injustice someone has inflicted on you, it may be surprising to learn how many people are not willing or able to do so. Sometimes the reluctance to do this is culturally based; many times it is because illness has left the person too fatigued or too stressed (problem solving becomes very difficult under stress). Assuming that a person is doing the best he can allows you to meet him at that point and not read more or less into his actions.

2. When acting as an advocate, do not get angry or defensive. Assume that the people you are contacting on behalf of a patient are also doing the best they can. Getting angry prevents you from seeing both sides of a problem and therefore limits your problem-solving ability.

3. Be certain that the person really wants what he says he wants. Mr. Smith, for example, a patient you visit in his home, tells you that he wants to lose weight but cannot because his wife continues to cook high-calorie foods for him. This seems like a good situation for advocacy by speaking to Mrs. Smith about her cooking habits. The next time you visit Mr. Smith you notice not only that he has not lost weight but that he is angry with you, because in fact he enjoys his wife's rich cooking more than he wants to lose weight.

4. Encourage people to be their own advocates if at all possible. If a person's problem is that her return date to a clinic is at such a time that her husband would have to take time off from work to drive her there, you could call the clinic and ask to have the appointment changed. But encouraging her to do this herself—perhaps helping her to find the correct number and standing by while she calls—not only solves the problem (the time of the appointment is changed) but also demonstrates to her that she is not helpless against a large system. The next time she has a problem with health care delivery, she will remember that she was successful this time and be more likely to take action on her own.

5. Follow lines of authority. You will quickly turn people against you and the person for whom you are speaking if you bypass them and go to their supervisors to get some action (Fig. 14-1). Such a maneuver tells a person that you did not think that he was worthwhile talking to; his first reaction when his supervisor sends you back to him so action can start is likely to be that he does not find you worthwhile to talk to, and your advocacy actions will be ineffective.

FIGURE 14-1. Effective advocacy requires following lines of authority.

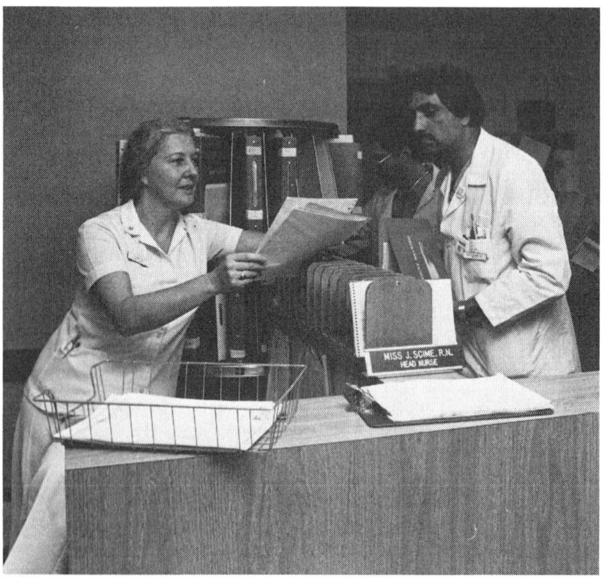

6. Be certain when you obtain a commitment from someone on behalf of a patient that you obtain the name and title of the person making the commitment. If you do not do this, you have no recourse if the commitment is not honored. All you have to refer to is a nameless voice's promise.

7. Do not allow yourself to be "triangled"—to be caught between the person on whose behalf you are speaking and the person to whom you are speaking. This could happen, for example, if Mrs. Jones, an older adult you are caring for, tells you that her daughter wants her to live with her, but Mrs. Jones wants to return to her own apartment. You intercede for Mrs. Jones with her daughter; in the end both Mrs. Jones and her daughter perceive you as working against them because they both choose yet a third alternative: Mrs. Jones will go to a nursing home until she is well again. It is difficult to predict when a triangle will develop but being certain that people know all their alternatives from the beginning is the best way to avoid this problem.

8. Be certain that financial arrangements are clear. More misunderstandings occur from money matters than any other cause. Do not arrange for a patient to visit a clinic or for a second medical opinion without being certain that the patient is informed of any direct charges involved.

9. Do not win battles and lose wars. Insisting that a person must do what you want in one instance may cause him to be less receptive to your future, perhaps more important, advocacy efforts.

Common Areas for Individual Advocacy

One of the areas in which you can act as an advocate is helping a person to make decisions about such health care questions as should he get a second doctor's opinion; who is a good cardiovascular physician; should he continue to use an over-the-counter medicine. Another area is protecting him from invasions of his rights as a health care consumer.

RIGHT TO A SECOND OPINION

Even if the situation involves a medical or surgical emergency, a person has the right to ask for a second opinion about his state of health or treatment. Many people worry that if they do this, their first physician will be so angry that she will refuse to care for them any longer and they will be left without a physician. The right to a second opinion is a commonly accepted right. People can be assured that a legitimate physician will honor the right of people to seek a second opinion without anger (and may actually appreciate it, on occasion, as a way of evaluating her own care and assuring the person that she is treating him in the best way possible).

RECOMMENDING A PHYSICIAN

It is common practice, when a person asks you to recommend a physician, to give the person the names of three physicians. This practice prevents the person from blaming you if he does not like the new physician (and many times a physician you like will be viewed differently by another person because of a personality difference) and alleviates the problem of a physician being accused of using you as a friend of hers to solicit patients for her (a physician's code of ethics does not permit her to solicit patients).

If you do not know three physicians who practice the specialty the person is looking for, you or he can telephone the local medical association for this information.

SELF-MEDICATION

Many people choose to take over-the-counter medication rather than visit a physician for a medicine prescription. The danger of self-medication is that a patient will unwittingly take an over-the-counter medicine that masks his disease symptoms but does not cure the disease (Fig. 14-2). He thinks he is getting better, but he is actually growing worse and becomes seriously ill before he stops self-medication and visits a health care provider.

Taking over-the-counter medicine at the same time as prescribed medicine may cause drug interactions and untoward drug effects. You may have to act as advocate by asking people's physicians to prescribe less expensive medicine so that they will take what is prescribed rather than use over-the-counter medication.

QUACKERY

Quackery is the use of discredited or unproven methods or devices to diagnose or treat illnesses. Some products sold as "sure cures" are useless but at least harmless; others may actually be lethal or increase the symptoms of a person's illness.

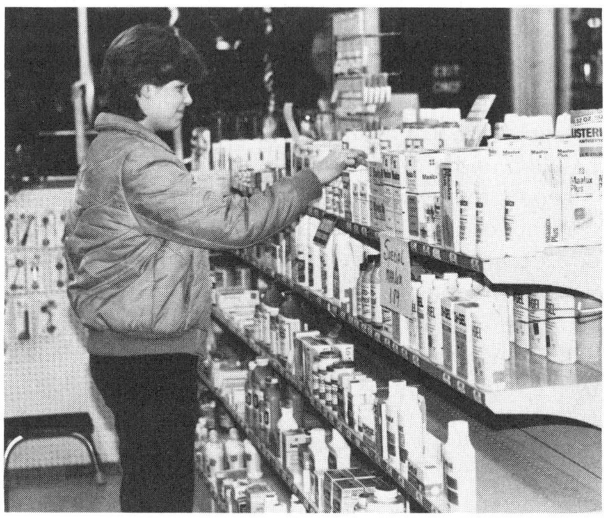

FIGURE 14-2. Over-the-counter self-medication, available in staggering amounts, can mask disease symptoms.

Older or ill individuals are prone to quackery because they may not be sufficiently motivated or do not have transportation to go to a legitimate health information source. People with limited money are prone to quackery because the person promising the new method convinces them that they are getting a bargain for their money. Fraudulent methods are most apt to be associated with treatments for arthritis, cancer, hearing loss, and obesity and with food supplements, beauty aids, and psychotherapy.

Common practices that are helpful in recognizing fraudulent health care methods are:

1. Such a person often uses a special or secret formula or machine.
2. He may promise or imply quick and easy cures.
3. He may advertise, using case histories and testimonials from his patients.
4. He refuses to accept tried or proven methods of medical research.
5. He often claims that the medical community is persecuting him and is afraid of his competition.
6. He claims that his methods are better than surgery, x-rays, and medically prescribed drugs.

You may need to inform people about fraudulent practices and urge them to depend on a proven health care provider in order to save their money and to prevent them from growing more ill waiting for a false cure. If you are unsure about whether a product is being advertised correctly, the Federal Trade Commission, responsible for the control of advertising information, will answer questions for you about the possibility that a claim is misleading. If products are sent through the mail, the possibility of mail fraud will be answered by the post office. The Federal Food and Drug Administration (FDA) is the government agency concerned with the ingredients and labeling of products; they will answer questions concerning the safety of drugs and medical devices. The Better Business Bureau is yet another organization that can provide information on an agency's or business's reputation. If a physician is involved, the American Medical Association will answer questions as to credentials and specific area of practice. A state Professional Licensing Service will supply this information concerning nurses.

SUPPORTING A PATIENT DECISION

Some people are able to make difficult decisions but then have difficulty remaining committed to such decisions without support from someone. Patients need to know that health care providers will support their decisions; otherwise, they may not have the necessary incentive to solve their problems. Mrs. Royce, a 24-year-old patient hospitalized for a fractured tibia, has three young children at home for whom she must provide child care during the length of her hospital stay. The decision that Mrs. Royce makes regarding her children—to have a different neighbor care for them each day—may not be the decision you would like her to make (more continuity of care would seem to be wiser). But as long as the arrangement is short-term and all the caregivers will give safe care, your role at the point that the decision is announced to you is to support Mrs. Royce's solution. She already feels inadequate because she cannot care for the children herself; she should not have to cope with derogatory comments regarding her decision-making ability.

PATIENT RIGHTS

Advocacy for individuals many times consists of being certain that individual or civil rights are being respected. In a health care agency this means that the admission procedure is limited in time and forms. It means that intravenous therapy is started in the person's left hand if possible so that his dominant hand is free. It means being certain that roommates in inpatient settings are compatible (that a person susceptible to infection is not placed with a patient who is coughing and sneezing; that a woman whose baby has died at birth is not placed with a woman who has just delivered a healthy child). It means that instructions are given in a way that is clear and easily understandable (possibly involving an interpreter). It involves seeing that hospitalizations are kept to a minimum and for as short a time span as possible.

These are examples of small issues, perhaps, but they are rights that are easily violated unless someone works to protect them by active advocacy.

INTRODUCING CHANGE

As an advocate you may need to introduce new and different ways of doing things. Although this may be an interesting activity, it is often one of the hardest tasks you have to do. Toffler (1970) in his often quoted book *Future Shock* stresses that the rate of change a person is experiencing is often more distressing than the direction or scope of the change. In planning change, then, it is important not only to be certain you know what exactly it is you want to change but also to establish a sensible rate for the change to take place.

Why People Resist Change

Even the smallest change brings about at least temporary uncertainty and some loss of self-confidence. A person who always drives to work one way, for example, feels some insecurity if one morning he must take a detour.

Change requires energy, both mental and physical (the person has to think through a different route, perhaps locate a road map). Due to other factors in his life, a person may have little energy to expend on changing.

Another facet that interferes with change is fear of failure: A person may read the road map incorrectly or not plan enough time and be late for work. The effort to take the new route—to change—may be too great because the chance at failure is more than he is ready to take.

Change is often most resisted when a person's interpersonal relationships are interrupted. It is easier to change methods of doing things or types of equipment used than to change friends. If a person was unable to stop for coffee and chat with friends at his usual restaurant because of the detour, this deprivation of interpersonal contact might be the factor that would make the change intolerable.

People accept changes imposed on them less willingly than changes that they participated in. The person forced to drive a different route to work may be extremely upset if his first notification of the change is a road sign saying "Detour." He is apt to be less upset if he was informed in advance that the change was going to occur or if he participated in a committee that devised the detour route.

Change Strategy

Change can be instituted with least resistance by following a few rules. Stewart (1959) proposes six steps for initiating change.

IDENTIFICATION

Identification means that a person must feel a need for change (identify with it) before he will successfully change. Suppose that you want to introduce a play program for children on a nursing unit. First you would introduce the nurses on the unit to the concept that psychological scarring may occur in children if the hospitalization experience consists solely of painful procedures with no consideration for normal growth and development activities such as play. Once the nursing staff realizes that they may not be giving the best care because they have been neglecting this important aspect of a child's health, they have identified with the problem and are in a condition to act on it.

For another example, a patient must realize the importance of incentive spirometry (inhaling on a plastic device that registers his depth of inhalation; deep inhalations fully aerate the lungs and prevent pooling of respiratory secretions and possible infection) before he will do this technique independently without reminding by the nursing staff (Fig. 14-3).

REASSURANCE

People affected by a change should be shown ways that the outcome of the change will be beneficial for them

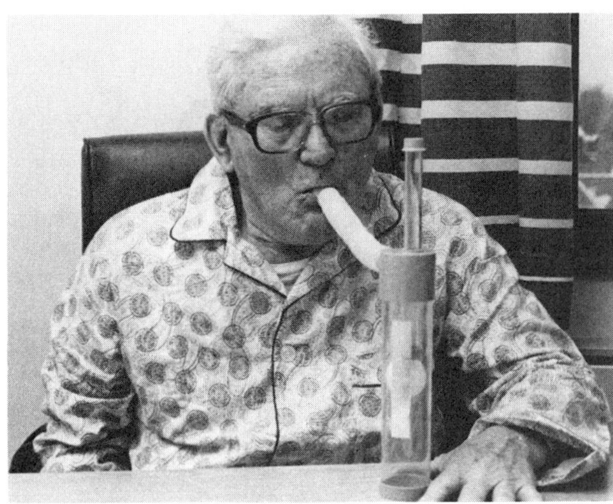

FIGURE 14-3. A patient, realizing the importance of incentive spirometry, begins to do this technique independently. Note his high level of concentration as he undertakes his new task.

and given an explanation of how everything will work after the change.

Participating in a play program, for example, will mean that each nurse will have to transport the children she cares for to the playroom daily. Although this will involve careful coordinating of her care (finishing all procedures before the child leaves his room for the playroom), it will give her additional time to spend with critically ill children. This will increase both the quality of care and her personal satisfaction, as she will not be so hurried with the care of critically ill patients.

As a second example, the person who is to learn incentive spirometry probably needs reassurance that the exercise will not interfere with the right of his wife to visit or cause him any pain or additional expense.

COMMUNICATION

Communication of the change may be done by many means: a printed explanation, audiovisual material, individual or group verbal presentations. The method of communication depends on what is to be changed; one method or many methods may be utilized. As a rule, never use printed or audiovisual materials without being present to answer questions about them and to clarify any misconceptions. A simple statement that you felt was very clear may be misinterpreted by people who are so anxious about change that they misread the meaning of words.

Communicate the need for, process of, and date of change as early as possible. Letting an informal communication channel (a grapevine) carry the information first is dangerous, as the message delivered by this route may convey misleading information. Worrying about unknown change is more stressful than knowing exactly what change is to be implemented, even if you do not like the change.

PARTICIPATION

Participation involves helping people who are involved in change to plan for it. In the play program example, for instance, staff members need to agree among themselves the hours that the playroom will be open, how they will alert play staff or volunteers to a child's special needs, who will return the child from the play area, and so forth. It is important that people's ideas on a project be aired; otherwise a person may feel that his way of doing something is so much better than the method being imposed on him that he does not want to cooperate with the change. Once the idea is aired, you can either show the person why the idea is not superior or use it if it really is better.

Once you ask for group suggestions in decision making, you are bound to use some of the suggestions; otherwise people in the group will think that you asked for their input only to flatter them, not because you really thought that they would have important contributions. Feeling that they have been used badly, people may offer resistance to a plan that they otherwise would have accepted.

If there are no choices or decisions to be made about some aspects of the new project (the fire department code specifies where the playroom must be located, for example), do not ask for suggestions in this area. Try to find areas where decisions can be made and accept suggestions in this area. The person having incentive spirometry could decide when he wants to use the device but not how he will use it (there is only one right way) or what brand of apparatus he will use (the hospital only purchases one model).

MUTUAL INTEREST

Mutual interest means that people understand not only how a change will affect them but how it will benefit people around them as well. Seeing that a change will affect a larger sphere than their own may increase acceptance (encouraging an "everyone-is-in-the-same-boat" type of feeling or pleasure at participation in the greater good).

FOLLOW-THROUGH

Follow-through is an evaluation step to see if change truly occurred or not. In many instances, people use a new system or method of accomplishing something for a short while and then, because the change involved extra energy or participation for them, revert to the original way of doing the task. Follow-through enables you to recognize such situations. In these cases the change must not have met people's needs in the way that was expected, or return to the former behavior would not have occurred.

Rules for Initiating Change

Table 14-1 lists several rules that generally facilitate change. Such rules may have to be modified, depending

TABLE 14-1. BASIC RULES TO FACILITATE CHANGE

1. Appreciate that change is always difficult.
2. Recognize that some people can accept change easier than others; it is a very individual characteristic.
3. Change is accepted best if it comes from within a group. When first joining a group, do not attempt to initiate any change until you are accepted by the group—a time interval of about six months for a new staff nurse.
4. Disrupt interpersonal relationships as little as possible by a change. Change in this area is the hardest to accept.
5. Be agreeable to compromise. Although compromising on an issue may cause you to lose a battle, it may allow you to win a war.
6. Be alert to the use of trial periods. People may not be willing to try a new system if they have to maintain the change indefinitely. They may agree to change for a short time period, (a trial period of four to six weeks) on the condition that at the end of the period whether the new system is superior to the old system will be evaluated. People agree to this type of arrangement because they are certain that the new system will not work. If you truly believe that the new system is better than the old, however, a trial period is on your side. By the end of the trial period people may like the new way of doing things so much better that there will be no question of changing back.

on the size of the change to be made and the willingness and the ability of the people concerned to make the change.

LEADERSHIP

An advocate must be a leader because a leader is in a prime position to initiate change. The personality structure of some people seems to make them natural leaders. Leadership techniques, however, can be learned by anyone, so that even if leadership is not your natural inclination, at the point that you need leadership ability to effect change, you can call on it.

Leadership ability is different from authority or power in that people follow the direction of someone in authority or power because they *have* to; they follow a leader because they are influenced to *want* to follow. People with little authority (student nurses or beginning staff nurses, for example) can change few things because of their position; however, their opinions can influence those with power.

Types of Leadership

There are at least three distinct styles of leadership: autocratic, laissez-faire, and democratic.

Autocratic leadership is a directive style; the leader makes decisions for a group with little consultation or input from the group. This style of leadership is invaluable in emergencies when there is no time for group decision making; under usual circumstances, however, autocratic leaders often generate group dissatisfaction. Such a technique of leadership may lead to a decision for change, but because the majority of people had no participation in the decision, the change may not be maintained.

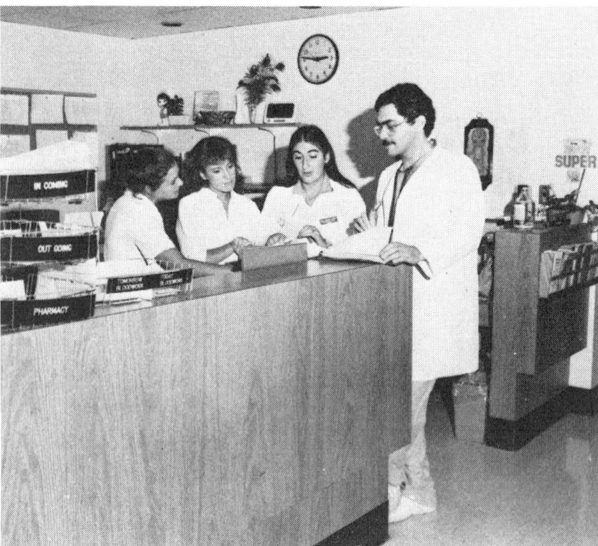

FIGURE 14-4. Democratic leadership allows the group to participate fully in decision making.

Laissez-faire leadership is a nondirective style; the leader serves more as a resource person than as a true leader, strengthening and encouraging people in the group to make decisions and to function more or less independently. In terms of change, if the proposed change is a difficult one, the decision for change is likely not to be made.

Democratic leadership presents information or options to a group and then allows the group members to fully participate in decision making (Fig. 14-4). With democratic leadership you must be certain that members are well informed on issues so that they can make informed decisions. All members of the group have a moral commitment to abide by the decision of the group, even though it is a decision they may not personally like.

Some basic principles of these three leadership styles are shown in Table 14-2.

WORKING WITH GROUPS

As an advocate you will often implement change through a group. People join some groups for social, recreational, or educational reasons. At other times a person is part of a group because of a work or school association. Health care providers automatically become members of planning groups for improved or continued health care.

Although at first glance all members of a group may appear to be the same, if the actions of people in a group are analyzed, specific roles can be detected. Some members, for example, always present new ideas to the group (the initiators). Others serve as clarifiers,

TABLE 14-2. BASIC PRINCIPLES OF LEADERSHIP

1. Be certain that people understand why and what it is that you want them to do. People do not change blindly, but only if they understand exactly what is at stake.
2. Be certain that people have the capability to do what you are asking (have enough energy, equipment, resources available to them).
3. Be certain that you are not asking people to do something that contradicts their personal values. People may temporarily act in opposition to their personal value system but they will not continue to do so.
4. Be certain that what you are asking is not contradictory to the aims or goals of the organization to which people belong. If your plan changes the goal of the organization, a person may leave the organization rather than remain with a structure that no longer fulfills the goals he joined it for.
5. Give the same considerate and respectful care that you give to patients to the people you work with.
6. Role model the actions you want changed. No one respects or follows a person who asks, "Do what I say, not what I do."
7. Reward people for change. If the change you are going to initiate is to improve nursing care, the reward will be improved job satisfaction. Pointing out how successful the achievement has been and how better care has resulted ensures that people see the value of change and sets them up to accept further change (after a period of time has elapsed, as too rapid change is difficult to accept).
8. Know your subject area. You cannot begin to solve problems or offer suggestions that will work if you are not familiar with what has been tried before and whether it was successful.
9. Believe in your ideas. Work through a problem until you believe in your solution; once you believe that your solution is good, you will project that attitude.
10. Be open to suggestions. Even the most experienced person could miss an easy solution or idea about an individual problem.
11. Think through "what-would-happen-ifs" before you present your ideas to others. People do not follow a leader a second time who led them down a wrong path a first time.
12. Do not feel that you have to do everything yourself. Leadership means effectively getting the job done, not doing it yourself to the point that you are so busy nothing gets done well.
13. Do not be afraid to admit mistakes. Leaders are human, not perfect.
14. Do not be reluctant to try again. And again. And again. And again.

restating or interpreting others' comments so that everyone clearly understands what has been said. Others serve as gatekeepers ensuring that everyone has an opportunity for speaking. Someone else may act as a standard setter, keeping the group functioning properly (adhering to procedure). Yet other members of the group participate as information seekers (asking questions to learn more about a topic), while still others are information givers or resource people for the group.

If you are going to attempt to initiate change in a group, try to identify which members fulfill these roles. The gatekeeper and clarifier are assets to you, as they ensure that everyone is heard and understood and no one is led to believe that you are pulling wool over their eyes. Information givers are your asset as long as the information they are contributing is not contrary to what you believe to be true. The standard setter will ensure that you come prepared to the meeting and if the group has rules of parliamentary procedure that you follow them.

Members of a group interact differently, depending on the age or stage of the group. When a group first forms, members tend to be cautious with each other (feeling each other out) as rules of conduct are clarified (smoking will or will not be allowed, for example). A newly formed group often does not achieve its full potential because all the strengths of its members have not yet been identified; give a new group time to mature and its members time to adjust to each other before you expect peak performance from it.

As a group matures, members become more relaxed with each other, and procedure in the group often becomes less structured (minutes are not formally read and voted on any longer; procedures are not discussed because everyone is familiar with them). A fully mature group functions easily and accomplishes goals readily. It may find itself functioning at less than its optimal potential, however, because members may not push each other to achieve but only to do that which is most comfortable for themselves or others in the group. It is difficult for a new member to enter an established group because so much interaction is taken for granted that the new member is easily confused and feels shut out. Some groups mature past their prime as they stray from their original intent or the original intent is accomplished and the group no longer has any reason to exist. If a group organized to raise funds to construct a playground continues to function after the playground is built, the group may find itself duplicating playground supervision personnel activities. Recognizing when to discontinue a group is just as important as knowing how and when to organize or maintain a group.

Group Content and Process

Group *content* refers to those things that are said in a group; group *process* refers to those things that are done in the group (what items are allowed to be discussed, who speaks to whom, nonverbal communication, for examples). To be effective a group must have both good content and process. A group that has poor content (perhaps a member is not speaking to the others or speaks to them rudely) will also usually have poor process (people put their chairs far apart, structure a meeting to end before needs are met, or refuse to honor a suggestion from a member). Assess both content and process since low levels of these are associated with poor output or accomplishment.

Although groups differ greatly as to size and purpose, a number of basic rules for working with groups can be identified. These are shown in Table 14-3.

ADVOCACY AND CHANGE

The following is an example of how you might use advocacy to initiate change.

On a nursing unit where you work, you notice that people who are on bedrest tend to develop breakdowns in their skin from the constant pressure of their body weight. You know this condition can usually be prevented if patients are turned side to side or front to back every 2 hours during each 24-hour period. When Mrs. Royce, the 24-year-old woman with three young children at home, returns from surgery for repair of a badly fractured tibia, you are worried that due to improper positioning during the next 5 days she may develop areas of skin breakdown. If this happens, her hospital stay will have to be extended. You are particularly concerned because it is important for Mrs. Royce to return home as soon as possible to provide care for her 2-month-old baby.

You realize that if Mrs. Royce is to return home on time, the nursing staff on your unit must adhere strictly to the policy about turning patients. As Mrs. Royce's advocate, you must bring in factual data supporting your premise that turning patients every two hours will prevent skin complications. You find three recent journal articles and a textbook that documents the importance of frequent turning in preventing decubitus ulcers (areas of skin breakdown due to lack of oxygen in the cells because of the constant pressure exerted on them).

TABLE 14-3. BASIC RULES FOR WORKING WITH PEOPLE IN GROUPS

1. Clarify the goals of the group. Groups move at the speed of the slowest member of the group, and slowness may result from poor ability to understand concepts or poor ability to accept change.
2. Help members to find common ground on which to relate to each other. Groups whose members have a common interest work best.
3. Help members to see other members' good points by statements such as "That's a good idea, Mary" or "Thank you for calling that to my attention, Chris." Groups work best if members respect each other.
4. Let group members know in advance what they are going to be responsible for discussing at a meeting so that seeds of solutions can start to grow even before the meeting.
5. Encourage a productive group tone. The tone of a group is set by the most responsive or the least responsive member of the group, depending on who is the more dominant personality. (One group will be very active because everything seems exciting; another group will do nothing because everything seems boring). To reset a group tone, try to bring out qualities in other group members that will make them appealing people to follow.

The next step would be to ask for suggestions from the nursing staff as to how turning patients every two hours could be accomplished (the unit actually has five patients that need this type of care). Various members point out that it takes two people to turn someone like Mrs. Royce because of her heavy cast and there never seem to be two of them free at once. Someone else suggests that Mrs. Royce does not like to face the wall and will not lie on her right side. Yet another says that the hospital will have to hire more people for an effective solution to the problem.

As a group leader it is your role to help the group understand that a problem exists: Decubitus ulcers are occurring; people are developing secondary illnesses in addition to their primary illnesses, a situation that should not occur (the step of assessment). The group can do something to prevent this from happening and by so doing improve their nursing care (reassurance). Everyone understands why turning is effective: By limiting pressure on any body area to less than two hours, lack of oxygen to cells does not occur (communication). All the possible solutions are aired by the group and clarified (participation). The overall effect of the change could be that more nurses will ask to work on the unit because of the sense of pride in care evidenced by the nurses there (mutual interest). Finally, you need to see that the formulated plan is actually carried out (follow-through).

If you are an autocratic leader, you will select one solution and announce that that is what everyone must do. If you are a laissez-faire leader you will let everyone try independently the solution she thinks is best. If you are a democratic leader, you allow the group to discuss the solutions proposed and possible problems (turning does not need two people if good body mechanics are used; the hospital cannot hire additional people) and allow the group to vote on several suggestions or agree to try the solution favored by the majority.

Suppose the decision is to try the following plan: Ordinarily, everyone on the unit helps to supervise and distribute meal trays; now, two people will be designated to turn patients every 2 hours in exchange for mealtime supervision. At the end of a month the number of skin breakdowns that have occurred using this system will be compared to the incidence of skin breakdown during the last month when no program of active prevention was being tried. The results of the comparison will determine whether the program should be continued, discontinued, or modified.

This solution may or may not be the best one that could have been devised, but if the staff of the nursing unit accepts it and agrees to carry it out, it is probably a system that will prevent any further skin breakdown. Instituting this type of change is an example of how a nurse always serves as a patient advocate; how good leadership and change skills are incorporated in everyday care. This solution would also fulfill the criteria of a minor research project and demonstrates how nursing research is easily incorporated into care.

Many people think of the term *advocacy* as being limited to the act of protecting consumer rights. This example does in fact protect patient rights: The first right of a patient in a hospital is the right to considerate and respectful care.

THE USE OF ASSERTIVE BEHAVIOR

Assertiveness is the art of making your rights or feelings known to others while at the same time not infringing on others' rights or feelings. Assertiveness is an ability you need to have as an advocate; it is an ability you need to help people develop so that they can speak for themselves.

As the majority of nurses are women and in the past assertiveness has not been considered a feminine characteristic, many nurses are not used to assertive behavior. True assertive behavior is appropriate for persons of either sex; it merely means that a person lets other people know what is important to him and what he needs in order to feel good about himself and continue to be a helping person. It means that he refuses to allow unrealistic demands to be made of him.

A major step in developing assertive behavior is looking inside yourself and examining your strengths and weaknesses (the things you do particularly well and those you typically need some help or support with) and identifying those things that are important enough to you that you are willing to devote some effort to maintaining or achieving them. The second step is making these things known.

A number of common behaviors of people result from lack of ability to use assertive behavior.

1. *Griping behavior.* People who spend time "griping" or telling their friends how things should be run or how they should be treated better are using withdrawal rather than assertive behavior. Assertive behavior would involve telling the people who can effect change about the problem, not reciting grievances to friends.

2. *Angry outbursts.* Angry outbursts are the result of small agitations building up until they can no longer be contained and must be exposed. People who use this technique need to learn to express their feelings of resentment when small issues annoy them. Clearing away the resentment step by step by speaking up about these issues (assertive behavior) prevents feelings from reaching destructive limits. Angry outbursts are not effective strategies because often a person says things he later regrets (I quit! I hate you!).

3. *Loneliness.* Part of being assertive is telling people when you need them, either to help you with some problem or simply for socialization and enjoyment. A person who is unable to do this may find himself alone, because no one appreciates how much he would have liked to have had someone with him.

4. *Depression.* Depression, or a feeling of extreme sadness, can be the result of never letting others know what it is you want (so never receiving what you want). A simple statement such as "I don't want to cook this evening" or "I'd like to choose where we go for a change" are assertive statements that can lift a person's spirits dramatically because they say "I have a right to decide about my life; my ideas are as good as yours."

5. *Fatigue.* Although fatigue may arise from physical causes, it also may be a symptom of depression. Once fatigue begins, it is very difficult to be assertive because assertive behavior requires a certain amount of energy, and energy is what the fatigued person lacks. Using assertiveness on a day-to-day basis helps to prevent depression.

The above behaviors result from lack of use of assertive behavior; the behaviors described below interfere with people using assertive behavior.

1. *False modesty.* False modesty is a belittling response to a situation. Suppose, for example, you are a new nurse and are wearing a new uniform that you know is good design and looks well on you. A fellow nurse tells you that your uniform looks attractive. The assertive person acknowledges such a compliment with a response such as "Thank you. That's nice of you to say that." Such a response says that you are grateful for kindness. A false-modesty response would be, "This old thing? I don't even like it." Such a false-modesty response implies that the person who made the compliment does not have good judgment (she thinks you look nice; you perceive your uniform to be old and unattractive) and that your judgment is also in doubt (otherwise why would you be wearing an old distasteful uniform?) Such a response is therefore belittling to both parties involved and does not respect the feelings of either.

2. *Lack of self-esteem.* A person with good self-esteem feels that his ideas are good (or at least as good as everyone else's), and he is capable of independent actions. Suppose as you arrive for work one morning a physician is standing by the nursing station demanding, "Whose crazy idea was it to chart temperatures in red ink?" The red ink was your idea. The person with good self-esteem (able to be assertive) would probably say, "It was *my* idea" (because you know your ideas are good and therefore it isn't really a crazy idea) or "It's my idea and I don't think it's so crazy." The person with poor self-esteem would probably just agree that the idea was a bad one and promise not to chart in red ink again. This type of behavior prevents change from happening because people must have confidence in a person's ideas before they will change to them.

3. *Aggression.* Aggression, in contrast to assertiveness, is forcing your ideas onto others without respect for their rights or feelings. Assertive behavior has developed a bad reputation in some instances because some people who act aggressively defend their actions by saying that they were only being assertive. Examples of aggressive behaviors would be to respond to the woman who complimented your uniform with "Thank you. That's the first sensible thing I've ever heard you say" or to the demanding physician, "I'll chart temperatures in any color ink I please. Who do you think you are?" Aggressive behavior invariably backfires. The admiring nurse, for example, following your retort, will probably not talk to you again; the shouting physician, who really did not care about the color of ink you used, may counter with aggression or at least you will feel a strain in your relationship that may interfere with your working together in the future.

One way to measure whether a response to a situation is assertive or aggressive is to ask yourself: Do I feel good about the outcome of the situation? Did I protect or stand up for what I believe in? Did I avoid hurting anyone's feelings?" If your answers to these questions are all yeses, your response was assertive. If any of your answers were no, then you crossed the line into either nonassertive or aggressive behavior.

Assertiveness is a necessity for advocacy because you need it to break through the "red tape" of policies or procedures that are preventing you from carrying out the best nursing care possible. Be certain to remember that if you teach a patient to be assertive in order that he can have more input into his own care, he will practice this new strength with you as well as other caregivers. Appreciate this new assertiveness as an indication of the success of your teaching, not opposition to your care.

ADVOCACY AND LIFE SPAN CONCEPTS

Although principles of advocacy never change, the types and individual actions of advocacy vary, depending on the life stage and ability of patients.

The Infant

Infants are always in need of advocacy because they cannot speak for themselves. Helping a mother to better understand infant care or to get to know her baby better are indirectly areas of advocacy for the infant.

Most women in the United States deliver their infants in hospitals. However, because some maternity divisions of hospitals are set up and managed with a certain coolness and adherence to routine rather than to mothers' preferences, more and more women are turning to home births. There is an inherent risk in this practice as, at a time in life that is the most hazardous (birth), the infant does not have quick access to the emergency resuscitation care he may need. If nurses advocated for warmer feeling tones in maternity divisions (birthing rooms that simulate a home setting rather than a surgical suite, family members present during labor and birth, open visiting hours for fathers and siblings, rooming-in so that the infant can remain constantly with the mother rather than in a central nursery, support for breast-feeding), this trend away from hospitals could be reversed, and the number of newborns saved from mental retardation or death at birth could be increased. Home births are a controversial issue; however, the nurse who believes that this type of birth is best should not feel intimidated about advocating the practice.

Another alternative advocated by many nurses is the use of Birthing Centers, midwife (nurse with advanced education and skills) staffed facilities either freestanding (out of hospital) or hospital-based but separate. There are over 300 such licensed, short-stay homelike centers in the U.S. providing comprehensive service for women anticipating a healthy pregnancy and birth. These centers are equipped to provide emergency resuscitation of the newborn, and hospital transport service as needed.

Mothers who want to breast-feed may need support from a nurse if their own mothers feel that they should formula feed. They may need help in learning to speak with health care providers about other care practices they believe in as the infant grows older (whether they want to use a pacifier or not, use commercial baby food or make their own).

Since infants are vulnerable to harm, a nurse serves as a constant advocate or protector of the child in terms of ensuring that he is given safe medication dosages and being cared for in an environment free of lead-based paint and free from abuse or neglect. Speaking up against child abuse is not only a moral obligation but a legal requirement as well in most states.

The Toddler and Preschooler

Toddlers and preschoolers may need someone to speak for them to allow them to exert their new independence (pointing out that knocking over a vase on the coffee table is not because a child is a "terrible two" but because he is adventurous, a characteristic that will serve him well in life). They may need help in being allowed to participate in the type of messy play they enjoy (play dough, mud pies, finger paint). Decision making is a beginning skill of the preschool child. Children this age need this skill protected so that they are not reluctant to use it and can master decision-making skills.

The Schoolager and Adolescent

Schoolage children and adolescents often need advocacy for their right to self-care. Separating a child from his parent while you take a health history and allowing the child to describe his own disease symptoms are common ways of doing this. Many values of adolescents differ from those of their parents. An adolescent may need an advocate to speak to his parents about his educational goals (his parents want him to go to college, while he wants to work as a mechanic; a girl's parents want her to go to a school of nursing, while she wants to be a journalist), social values (sex before marriage; living in his own apartment; working a part-time job), and personal values (attending or not attending church; being a vegetarian or not).

It is most important for the adolescent to learn to advocate for himself; only when he can do this is he truly mature.

The Young and Middle-Aged Adult

Young and middle-aged adults are, as a whole, self-supporting and independent and in the best position to be self-advocates. Even people who are able to do this well for themselves on a daily basis, however, may have difficulty with self-advocacy when they present themselves for health care. The average person has so little knowledge of his body's processes or alternatives to care that he may be unable to use his usual problem-solving ability in this new, strange jargon-filled atmosphere. You can advocate best for people in a health care setting by always keeping in mind how little you knew about the role of your endocrine or neurological system before you first took a course in anatomy and physiology; how difficult it was to recognize the meanings of medical words until you learned to recognize the Latin stems and prefixes that form so many of them; how few alternatives you knew about different ways to do procedures until you studied them. This awareness will help you to recognize a medical explanation that is too technical for the layman to comprehend or an explanation that, because it does not match the individual circumstances, must make no sense to the person hearing it.

The Older Adult

As people live longer and longer, older adults are remaining independent longer than ever before. For older adults with a physical handicap, however, there are many points at which a person needs an advocate (helping him with health care finances, living arrangements, stimulation, maintaining old friendships). A growing concern among this age group is abuse by children or caregivers. As with child abuse, abuse of this age group is a legally reportable situation in many states. At a final life stage many older adults need an advocate to help them plan the type of death they prefer (right to die at home with no heroic measures being taken, for example).

The Handicapped Individual

People with a handicap, whether there is a physical problem that prevents them from usual mobility or an interference with mental or psychological function that prevents adequate reasoning or problem solving, may need advocates to protect their rights. Frequent problems that handicapped individuals may need help with are living conditions (is an institution or their own home the best place for them), education (should they attend a special school or be "mainlined" with children without handicaps), nutrition (who will select and buy food for them), and recreation-social activities (why can't they swim in the "Y" pool; why can't they serve on a planning board for community health needs).

Advocating for handicapped persons is a process that continues throughout the handicapped person's age span as his needs change, depending on different life stage accomplishments.

ADVOCACY AND NURSING

Advocacy as an independent or separate role for nurses has been disputed in the literature, as there may be people better prepared to fulfill a full-time advocate role. Advocacy as an intrinsic part of nursing care is not disputable; it is a basic requirement of quality nursing planning, and is always included as a part of nursing care.

SUGGESTED READINGS

Abrams, N. A contrary view of the nurse as patient advocate. *Nurs. Forum* 17:258, 1978.

Ahmed, M. C. Taking charge of change in hospital nursing practice. *Am. J. Nurs.* 81:540, 1981.

Balik, B., et al. Developing a community-based parent education support group. *JOGN Nurs.* 10:197, 1981.

Brosnan, J., et al. Stressed but satisfied: Organizational change in ambulatory care. *J. Nurs. Adm.* 10:43, 1980.

Douglas, L. M., and Bevis, E. O. *Nursing Management and Leadership in Action* (3rd ed.). St. Louis: Mosby, 1979.

Gadow, S. Advocacy nursing and new meanings of aging. *Nurs. Clin. North Am.* 14:81, 1979.

Kohnke, M. F. The nurse as advocate. *Am. J. Nurs.* 80:2038, 1980.

Kraus, I. Hospitals need humanism. *Hospitals* 53:84, 1979.

Lobb, M. O. Seating arrangement as a predictor of small group interaction. *J. Nurs. Adm.* 7:163, 1982.

Lundborg, L. B. What is leadership? *J. Nurs. Adm.* 12:32, 1982.

Max, C., et al. Breaking the silence: A group project with the institutionalized elderly. *Geriatr. Nurs.* 2:56, 1981.

McWeeny, M. C. The patient's right to learn or not to learn. *Nurs. Adm. Q.* 4:83, 1980.

New, J. R., et al. Guidelines for introducing change. *J. Nurs. Adm.* 11:17, 1981.

Robb, S. S., et al. Advocacy for the aged. *Am. J. Nurs.* 79:1736, 1979.

Rowe, E. L. Take a chance on change! *Nurs. Leadership* 4:21, 1981.

Sampson, E., and Marthas, M. *Group Process for the Health Professions.* New York: Wiley, 1977.

Searl-Varga, S., et al. Working with a mother's group. *Canad. Nurse* 77:36, 1981.

Smith, C. S. Outrageous or outraged: A nurse advocate story. *Nurs. Outlook* 28:624, 1980.

Spradley, B. W. Managing change creatively. *J. Nurs. Adm.* 10:32, 1980.

Stewart, N. Nothing is as permanent as change. *Nation's Business* 47:33, 1959.

Toffler, A. *Future Shock.* New York: Random House, 1970.

Travdel-Korenchuk, D., et al. Nursing advocacy of patients' rights: Myth or reality? *Nurse Pract.* 8(4):37, 1983.

Walsh, S. Parents of asthmatic kids (PAK): A successful parent support group. *Pediatr. Nurs.* 7:28, 1981.

Wichita, C. Everyone wins when you push patient power. *RN* 43:50, 1980.

QUESTIONS FOR REVIEW

1. Advocacy is defined as:
   a. Speaking on behalf of another.
   b. Anticipating another's needs.
   c. Taking advantage of fortunate happenings.
   d. Defending another's actions.

2. Mr. Jones, a patient you care for, says he wants a second medical opinion before he has surgery. As his advocate you would tell him that:
   a. Asking for a second opinion is an insult to his physician.
   b. Second opinions are usually honored only in emergencies.
   c. Second opinions are honored only if a language problem is present.
   d. A second opinion is a reasonable request.

3. Miss Smith, a secretary you see at lunch, asks you the name of a good dentist. Your *best* action would be:
   a. Tell her the name of your dentist.
   b. Tell her that you are not allowed to recommend physicians or dentists.
   c. Give her the names of three dentists who you know are equally good.
   d. Ask her to look in the yellow telephone pages.

4. Miss Smith is currently seeing a dentist who repairs cavities by a new "multi-micro-wave technique." An action that would suggest that this dentist is practicing quackery is:
   a. He participated in a community dental survey last year.
   b. He also uses regular repair procedures.
   c. He asked Miss Smith to write a testimonial of his ability.
   d. He told her that she would have to come for several visits.

5. You are a new staff nurse and want to change the method used to take temperatures on your unit. Which of the following statements is true concerning change?
   a. The rate of change is not important; only the scope of the change.
   b. Changing social relationships is not important.
   c. Unplanned change is best because it occurs so suddenly.
   d. Change requires both mental and physical activity.

6. Which of the following would be your best approach to instituting the change in temperature-taking?
   a. Tell everyone by your third day on the job what needs to be changed.
   b. Begin by telling the director of nurses and work down to your fellow nurses.
   c. Ask an outside expert to come in and order the change.
   d. Wait about six months to try to change the procedure.

7. Leadership is an important ability to use for advocacy. A laissez-faire type of leadership is:
   a. Authoritarian.
   b. Nonproductive.
   c. Only useful with children.
   d. Nondirective.

8. Which of the following would demonstrate the best leadership ability in terms of changing a temperature-taking procedure?
   a. Suggest a trial period of one year after which time you will evaluate the results.
   b. Plan to continue to take temperatures the old way yourself to demonstrate a contrast between systems.
   c. Belittle anyone who does not agree that your new system is better.
   d. Be prepared to admit you are wrong if the new procedure is not effective.

9. A general principle of advocacy is:
   a. Advocate for what is good for people, not for what they necessarily want.
   b. Do not win battles and lose wars.
   c. Encourage people to use advocates, not advocate for themselves.
   d. Use anger as it is an effective problem-solving technique.

10. You are criticized by the director of nurses for trying to institute change on your hospital unit. Which of the following reflects an assertive response to this criticism?
    a. I'm sorry; I thought it would be all right.
    b. No one can tell me what to do or not to do.
    c. I won't do it again.
    d. Exactly what is it that you are objecting to?

V. THE NURSE AS AN EFFECTIVE COMMUNICATOR

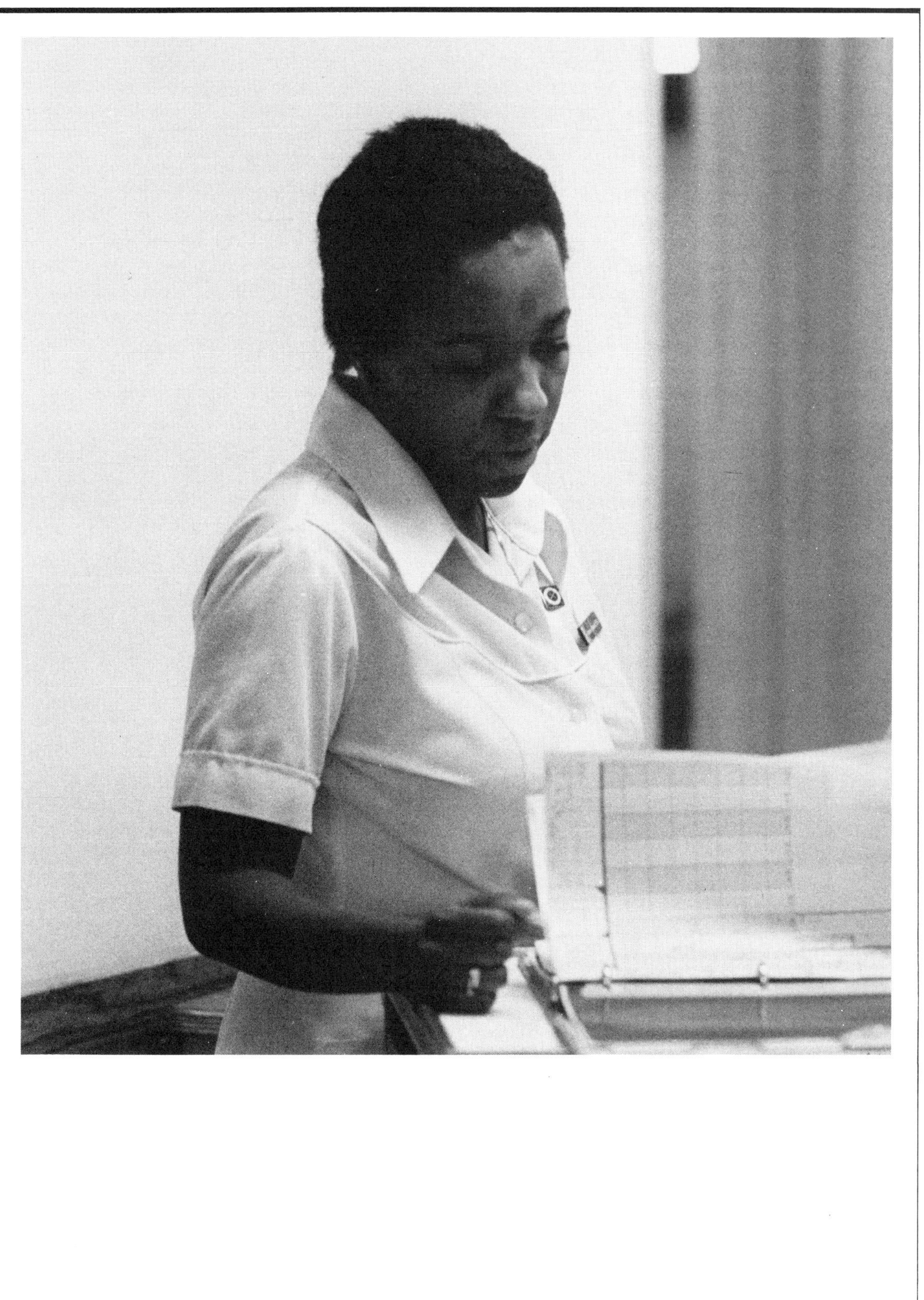

15. THERAPEUTIC COMMUNICATION

OBJECTIVES
Upon mastery of the material of this chapter, you should be able to:

1. Describe the process of effective communication.
2. Contrast the concepts of therapeutic and nontherapeutic communication.
3. Describe techniques that promote effective communication.
4. List factors that can block communication.
5. Describe five levels of communication.
6. Describe how communication affects nurse-patient relationships.
7. Apply the nursing process to give safe and planned care to a patient whose care involves principles of therapeutic communication.

TERMS
The terms important for an understanding of this chapter are shown below and defined in the glossary:

aphasia
decoder
dialect
dysarthria
empathy
encoder

Communication is the exchange of ideas between two or more persons. Although it is an activity that nearly everyone participates in every day and more or less takes for granted, it is an actual process, more than just the simple art of conversation. It is important to nursing because it can make or break a nurse-patient relationship.

NONTHERAPEUTIC AND THERAPEUTIC COMMUNICATION

Communication as a process can be divided into two major categories: nontherapeutic (casual, everyday conversation) and therapeutic (helpful and constructive).

Nontherapeutic Communication

Nontherapeutic communication is identified by its lack of structure or planning (one is not forming sentences carefully to be certain that the intent of the words is not misunderstood) and lack of deliberate purpose other than as a social activity (one is not trying to achieve any results or change of behavior by the activity). Dinner conversation is generally nontherapeutic communication. The average person, not in a helping profession, communicates this way most of the time.

Therapeutic Communication

Therapeutic communication is an interaction between two people that is planned (you deliberately intend to elicit the true way a person feels about a situation), has structure (you will use specified techniques of wording your questions or responses that will encourage the response from the person that you wish to elicit), and is helpful or constructive (at the end of the interaction you will know much more about the person than you did at the beginning of the exchange, and hopefully the person will know more about himself: the beginning of problem solving or coping behavior).

In school catalogues and recruitment advertisements nurses are invariably pictured with a piece of equipment such as a stethoscope or a syringe in their hands. This image of the nurse as someone skilled in the ability to handle complex equipment and complete involved physical care is perpetuated because these activities photograph better than a nurse quietly talking with a patient. In actual practice, however, this second, less recognized role of a nurse as a skilled communicator is the more frequent one; it is a skill that accompanies all physical care.

If you ask people what was the most important thing a nurse did for them when they were ill, they are most apt to give answers like "She seemed to understand how I felt; I liked that"; "She told me I was doing well"; "She came and talked to me when everyone else seemed to be too nervous to do that"; "She was always there—and something about her manner always let me know that as long as she was there, I'd be safe."

In many instances there is no cure for the people you care for: no surgery, no medication, no physical remedy available to help them. In these instances you still have something to offer them: support through therapeutic communication by your words or a nonverbal communication technique such as touch. Learn as a beginning practitioner how to incorporate this type of communication into care. It is the aspect of care that is often the most valued, most appreciated, and most helpful of all the care you offer.

Assessment, implementation, and evaluation cannot be carried out without effective communication ability. What, then, are the components of effective communication and how are they applied to nursing care?

COMMUNICATION AS A PROCESS

Communication as a process can be broken down and diagrammed according to its essential components: the encoder, the code, the decoder, and the response or feedback (Fig. 15-1).

The Encoder

The encoder is the person who originates a message. He experiences a desire to share a thought or feeling with someone else (cognitive processing) and molds this thought or feeling into a form suitable for transferring it from his mind to theirs (a code). Communication can be ineffective if the person omits cognitive processing or speaks without thinking, chooses the wrong words for the message, or accompanies his spoken words with a facial expression, tone of voice, or gestures that are inappropriate for the message. A common example would be a mother telling a preschooler to put her buckle shoes on with the buckle on the outside. In this example, the mother has encoded or designed a message including only a verbal (put the buckles on the outside) component.

The Code

The code is the message that is conveyed and the medium or system used to convey it. Although this usually involves a simple spoken system, messages can also be conveyed by a painting, poem, or novel; Morse code, braille, computers, television, audio tape, and the telephone are all media for transmitting messages. Communication is often ineffective because the person chooses the wrong medium for the message (a lecture with a high proportion of technical words when a drawing with carefully labeled parts would have made the message much clearer; making a telephone call when confronting a person directly would have been more effective) (Fig. 15-1D). The simple instruction about shoes followed by actually handing them to the child would seem to be an appropriate message and a correct medium for transmission.

The Decoder

The receiver of the message not only receives it (hears it, reads it, views it) but interprets it or *decodes* it (cognitive processing). People interpret messages in light of their store of knowledge. Messages may be misinterpreted if a receiver's store of knowledge is so different from that of the sender that the message has a different meaning. Messages may also be misinterpreted (decoded wrongly) if the person misses part of the transmission, such as missing the wink accompanying the spoken words that would have let him know the sender was joking and not serious. Under stress, people tend to narrow their ability to receive information to a small area of concern. When you are dealing with someone who is extremely anxious, you may find that although you gave excellent instructions (both sender and message components of communication were adequate), he did not "hear" you (did not receive or could not interpret the message due to his anxiety) (Fig. 15-1C).

In the above example of the shoes, the preschooler from her limited store of knowledge might take the shoes and walk outside the house to put them on, because she interprets the message to mean that she should put the buckles on outside the house, not on the outside of her foot.

The Feedback or Response

Feedback is the reply that the decoder returns to the sender that acknowledges that the message has been received and interpreted. This could be a spoken statement, a nod of the head, a facial grimace or even the sudden slamming of a telephone receiver. With feedback the roles of sender and receiver become reversed and another communication cycle is beginning (the receiver is now sending). Communication can be ineffective if people do not offer feedback (the message was not understood or not acknowledged as such) or if feedback is offered before the message is fully interpreted (acting before thinking). When you are caring for people with sensory handicaps such as vision or hearing difficulties, you may need to change your usual feedback mechanisms in order to be understood, as a nod of the head or a quiet response may not be received.

LIFE SPAN DIFFERENCES AND COMMUNICATION

The way a person communicates as a newborn differs a great deal from how he communicates as an adult. Being aware of the extent and common characteristics of communication at differing age levels aids your ability to communicate effectively.

The Infant

One of the first responses an infant makes at birth is to cry. A first cry is important because it assures everyone

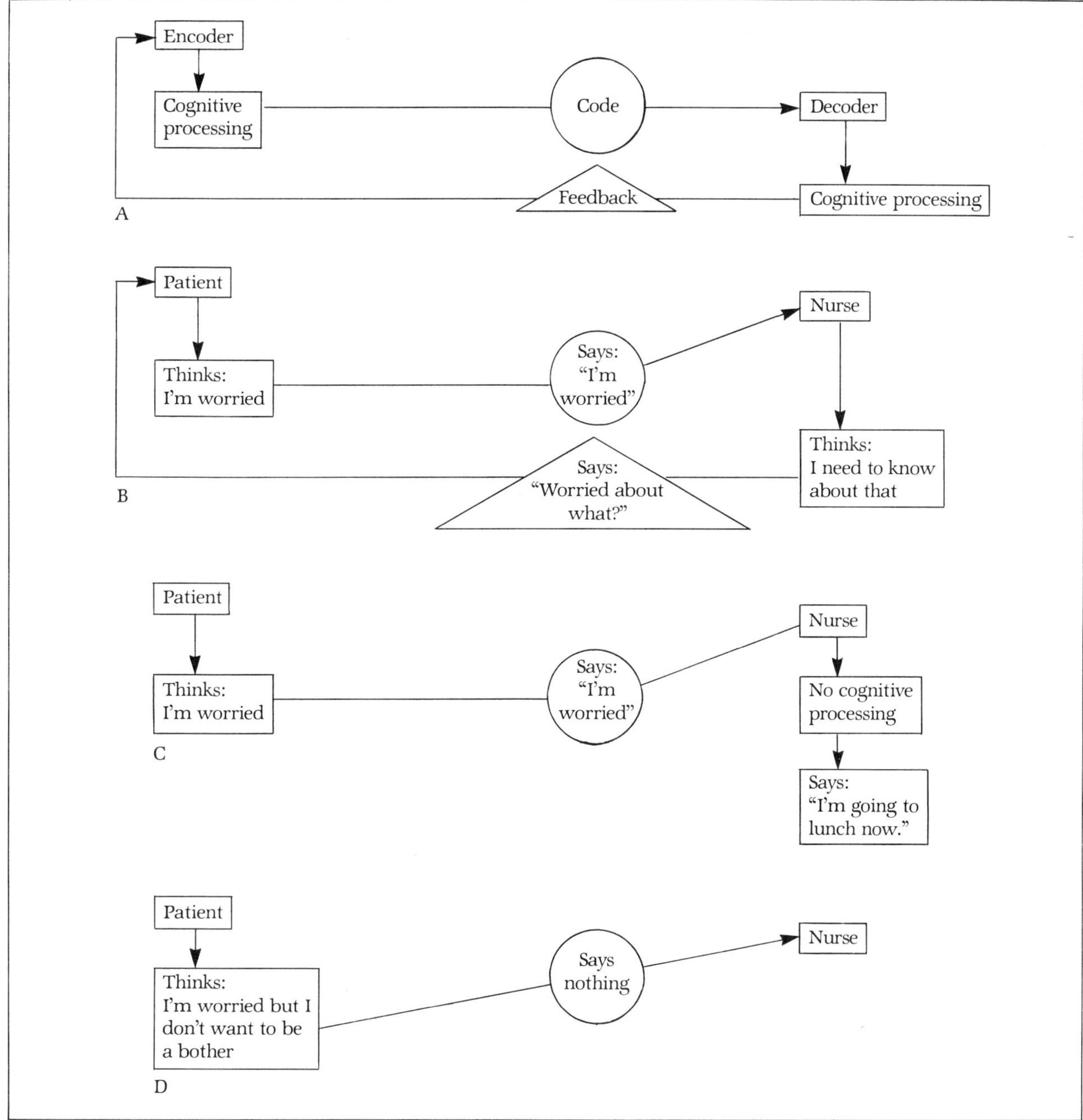

FIGURE 15-1. Communication as a process.
A. The process. (From D. Berlo, *Process of Communication*. New York: Holt, Rinehart & Winston, 1960.)
B. Example of effective communication.
C. Broken communication since feedback does not take place.
D. Broken communication; no code sent.

present that the infant is breathing well and that the hardest adjustment to make at birth has been accomplished (the sound of crying is made by air passing over the vocal cords). A first cry also announces to the mother that the birth is real and is important in stimulating active mother-child interaction (a code is initiating feedback).

During the first 2 months of life an infant cries in response to discomfort (cold, hungry, wet, lonely). His response to these body discomforts is total: not only does he cry, but he kicks his legs and thrashes his arms as well. Many new mothers comment that their newborns have bad tempers because they often seem very angry and get very easily upset. They are usually referring to the phenomenon that the child responds with his total body to stimuli. They may need some reassurance that this is normal newborn behavior and that he will discontinue gesturing wildly with every need as soon as he learns a more refined communication system.

By 6 to 8 weeks of age an infant begins to make a dovelike or cooing sound. This is a spontaneous response; it does not have to be provoked by first speaking to the infant. Even infants who are hearing impaired make this first spontaneous communication. An important happening at this same time is the ability of the baby to form a "social smile" in response to someone smiling at him. This nonverbal communication draws people to him as he now is so much fun to play with. At the same time he differentiates his cry: He begins to cry differently when he is hungry from when he is in pain or lonely. This is an item you always should ask about when assessing two-month-old behavior because it not only lets you know that the infant has met an important milestone of language development but also gives you some indication of the mother-infant relationship: A mother who has spent an average amount of time and concern with her child can tell the difference in his cry; a mother who has spent less time or emotional energy may not yet be able to. Mothers report that care of the infant becomes much easier after this point because since they can interpret messages adequately, their feedback is appropriate.

By six months of age infants can make one-syllable sounds such as "oh," "ooh," or "da." They use this "language" to talk to people who approach them. By nine months the child usually says his first clear word: "da-da" or "ma-ma." Infants typically say "da-da" before "ma-ma" as the *D* sound is easier to articulate. By one year of age an infant typically says two words besides ma-ma and da-da (ball, here, go, dog, or brothers' or sisters' names). He uses his words repetitively; he may walk over to the dog and saying "dog" walk back again in a very few minutes to repeat the word as if exploring the wonderment of this new cognitive activity.

The Toddler

Language development of the child from 1 to 2 years of age consists of not only the acquisition of new words but also the knowledge of word structure. A familiar word which toddlers learn and use frequently as a way to express autonomy is "No!" often accented by a temper tantrum or foot stomping. By 2 years the child should be able to put together a two-word sentence with a noun and verb: Me go; Daddy drive; Tony come. This is a cognitive milestone because it means that the child is not merely mimicking words but has reasoned through the system and purpose of the language he hears around him and can encode a verbal message. It is an important milestone for children to reach because it suggests that they have good hearing ability and adequate intelligence and have had sufficient parent-child interaction for this important association to have taken place.

By the end of the toddler period, a child may have as many as 900—1,000 words in his vocabulary.

The Preschooler

Preschoolers use language to help them explore and discover the world. They ask between 300 and 400 questions a day, mostly how, when, and why questions

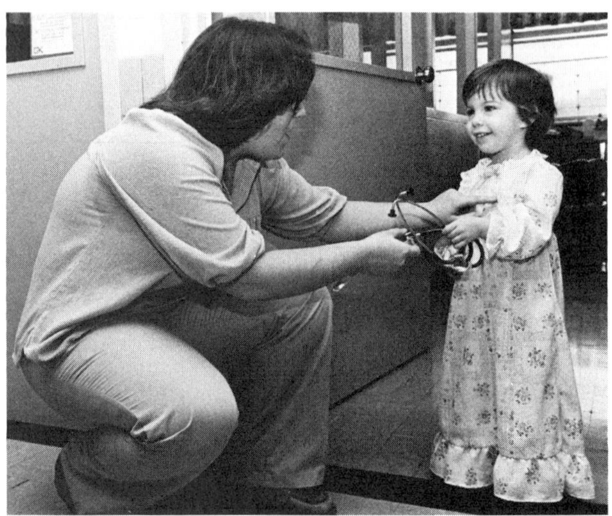

FIGURE 15-2. Preschoolers ask 300 to 400 questions a day. They need explanation of equipment and procedures.

(Why is grass green? Why do dogs wag their tails? How do bees know where flowers are?) (Fig. 15-2). The parent of a preschooler typically describes him as "all questions" or "never quiet." Some preschooler questions are difficult to answer because they require philosophical or scientific explanations that are not easy to communicate at that level (why is green green; why is grass green; why not red or blue). When you care for preschoolers their barrage of questions may appear threatening or it may be difficult for you to both concentrate on what you are doing and answer all of them thoughtfully. Appreciate that they are a part of normal development and not an interrogation of your ability or intentions.

Preschoolers typically pass through a period of "bathroom language," using such words as "shit" to demonstrate annoyance. This illustrates cognitive development—the child has learned that words have more than one usage—and is extremely attention getting. If you wish to discourage this type of language usage, ignore it (if it does not evoke attention, the novelty quickly fades) or correct it by offering the child a more socially acceptable word ("Do you know what I say when I'm angry? I say, "Oh fudge"). Censor the word, not the child; appreciating that words can have double meanings is a big step in becoming an adequate encoder and decoder of messages.

The Schoolage Child

The schoolage child meets other important milestones in communication ability when he learns to read at about 6 or 7 years and when he learns to operate a computer at 8 to 12. Once a child begins to read, he develops both a spoken vocabulary and an expressive one. A person's expressive vocabulary refers to those words he understands the meaning of yet never uses in conversation, such as *inebriated.* Schoolage children imitate the language they hear spoken around them; they do not have better grammar or word usage than is demonstrated to them.

The Adolescent

Adolescents use only a very small portion of their total expressive vocabulary in speech. Deliberately limiting their spoken vocabulary to slang helps them to identify with their group and to separate themselves from adults and smaller children. It is important to remember when you are talking to adolescents that they have a much larger vocabulary than the words that they use; trying to limit yourself to their demonstrated word usage would impede almost any explanation you wanted to give them. Some adolescents who habitually use a very limited vocabulary have difficulty communicating effectively when they need to use more words. They may solve this problem by remaining silent, keeping their anger at being misinterpreted inside themselves until it erupts in a series of slammed doors. As a group adolescents need to be counseled that talking about a problem never makes it worse and almost automatically puts a fence around it and makes it contained and solvable.

Adolescents typically pass through a phase of using words with sexual connotations to punctuate strong statements. This is part of achieving a sense of identity and showing that they are ready to enter the adult world. Try to limit the setting (I don't like to hear that; could you not use that word while I'm here?) as an effective way of containing the problem if it bothers you. Censor the word, not the child. Especially if he is ill, he needs to demonstrate that he is almost adult and up to facing the therapy or consequences of his illness.

The Adult

Adult language patterns vary considerably, depending on culture and work settings. If you are from a home where English grammar was stressed, the range of incorrect usage you hear from seemingly well-educated people can be distressing. If you dislike four-letter words, it can be unpleasant to hear other people using them as common expletives. As a rule, do not correct adult language patterns unless you suspect that, like the adolescent and the preschooler, the person is using the pattern as an attention-getting mechanism (then limit the setting: "If we're going to get anything accomplished here, it's going to have to be without that word"). Nothing interferes with communication more than one person censoring the other's use of words.

When angry or in pain, many patients use language extremely rich in profanities. You can use this in a positive way to help you assess the level of the anger or pain by the number and kind of words the person uses. You may need to reassure a patient who has displayed his pain in this way and apologizes later that expressing emotions is not, as a rule, a bad procedure; if it is helpful to him, it is not upsetting to you. On the other hand, you have rights too, and if this behavior is offending you to the point that it interferes with care, verbalize your discomfort. Do not feel you must be the only one who has to adapt.

The Older Adult

You may notice that older adults begin to develop a slower speech pattern than they used when they were younger. If arteriosclerotic changes (narrowing of arteries) are limiting oxygen supply to brain cells, loss of recent memory may result (they may be able to remember their first-grade teacher's name but not what they ate for breakfast). This is frustrating when it occurs; detecting this language pattern (stories are all from the past, none from the present) is important because it alerts you to the need to employ extra safety precautions (the person may not remember that he is not to eat anything because he is going to surgery, for example).

Some older adults are unable to give feedback to your questions due to neurological impairment. People who have cerebrovascular accidents (strokes) and have lack of blood flow to the speech center may be unable to produce the correct word. If you ask them which color bedroom slippers they want, for example, they may think "yellow" but say "road." The connection between yellow brick road is stronger than the connection between slipper and yellow. This is termed *aphasia* (aphasia can also mean an inability to speak from other causes). Aphasia in any form is a very frightening experience. Repeating the correct word for the person or asking him to tell you something else about the object to help you identify it may be helpful. In all instances a therapeutic statement such as "I appreciate this must be hard for you" and a projection of having endless time to discern the correct word are needed.

Dysarthria is a problem in speaking that results in difficulty with articulation. This can also occur in older adults who have had cerebrovascular accidents, due to lack of muscle control. Patience is needed to decipher the correct word. Also, be aware that people who cannot use their tongue and lip muscles well to form words may have difficulty chewing and swallowing and may need to be observed closely while eating to prevent aspiration.

LEVELS OF COMMUNICATION

Every conversation that you engage in does not (and should not) have the same depth level. Throughout a day a person may use as many as five levels (Powell, 1969).

First Level: Cliché Conversation

Cliché conversation is "pleasant chatting" (comments such as "Have a nice day") between people who think that their relationship will not extend beyond a very superficial one. It is important when meeting a patient for the first time that you introduce yourself not only as to name but as to position and function (as a student nurse who is going to take care of him; as the nurse who is in charge of the unit; as the nurse who will be visiting him in his home once a week). This information will lead the patient to move the conversation from the cliché level to a deeper more meaningful level.

Second Level: Fact Reporting

Fact reporting is simply stating facts about oneself (I'm 40; I work as an accountant; I had surgery yesterday for a hernia repair; I still have a lot of pain). Fact reporting is necessary for you to understand a person but it does not enable you to understand him well as it does not tell you anything about his feelings or needs. A person can only move from this level to a higher level of communication when he feels that he can trust you.

Third Level: Shared Personal Ideas and Judgments

When a person knows you well, he is able to share ideas (I always wanted to be an astronaut) and judgments (this is too hard for me; I am going to have to practice more). This level of communication exposes a person to loss of self-esteem if his views are not respected. This level is the beginning of therapeutic interaction.

Fourth Level: Shared Feelings

Sharing feelings is a difficult level until you truly trust another because feelings are very tenuous, fragile concepts, easily destroyed and crushed by inept or uncaring hands. Listen for an expression of feelings from patients (It's terrible to turn 40; I'm frightened to live alone; I'm worried that two days after surgery, I still have pain). These admissions are much more than a person telling you how he experiences his world; the person is demonstrating that he trusts you and the depth of the relationship that he has established with you.

Fifth Level: Peak Communication

The fifth level of communication is a sense of "oneness" or being able to know what the other person is experiencing without it actually being voiced. This type of communication sometimes occurs spontaneously in high intensity situations but generally arises out of long-term relationships. You will notice it especially between older adults: Mr. Henry visits his wife daily in the hospital and sits almost soundlessly beside her bed all the time he is there; when he leaves, however, she says, "He makes me feel so much better." An outsider may view Mr. Henry as unsupportive (how can he be helpful when he says almost nothing), but by using fifth level communication he has communicated better than other visitors who talked the entire time they were there.

NONVERBAL COMMUNICATION

"Actions speak louder than words" is an old saying but still a very true one. In all situations what people communicate nonverbally is at least as important as the words they actually speak. Nonverbal communication is expressed in a variety of ways.

A Feeling of Genuineness

Genuineness means being yourself. People will have difficulty trusting you (and therefore cannot move to a deep relationship with you) if you change your behavior from one day (maximum patience, absolutely unflappable) to the next (short-tempered and impatient). They have to spend energy every day testing to see who you are that day. The way to achieve a feeling of genuineness is not to try to be what you are not. The insecurity that comes from pretending to be different manifests itself as negative feelings such as aggressiveness or a blasé, bored attitude.

A Feeling of Warmth

Warmth is an innate quality, and some people manifest it more spontaneously than others. Basic ways that warmth is demonstrated are eye contact, using a gentle tone of voice, listening attentively, approaching the person within a comfortable space of 3 to 4 feet (closer may be threatening; farther away may be interpreted as distancing), and using touch appropriately. Warmth is a quality that you display best when you know another person well. Activities that help you to know a person better (taking a health history, talking to him about his work or family and how he feels about his present situation) not only help you to plan care for the person but allow you to be increasingly comfortable with the person and deepen your relationship (Fig. 15-3).

A Feeling of Empathy

Empathy is the ability to actually put yourself in another person's place and experience a feeling as he is experiencing it. At first it might seem that empathy requires you to have experienced all the situations of the people that you are caring for, or to have been told by a doctor, for instance, that you have cancer or are going to be blind. You do not need to experience all these things, however, to develop empathy, because you have experienced the common emotion of these situations in other ways. If you have hoped for something very strongly and then not attained it, loved someone and not had the emotion returned at the same level, lost someone or something that was so important to you that you felt actual pain, you can feel empathy for people who have received a disappointing diagnosis or are unhappy for other reasons. Empathy can be an emotionally draining experience; when you "put on the other's emotions," you experience them at the same depth. People who are capable of empathy are the best support people in any circumstance, because they can

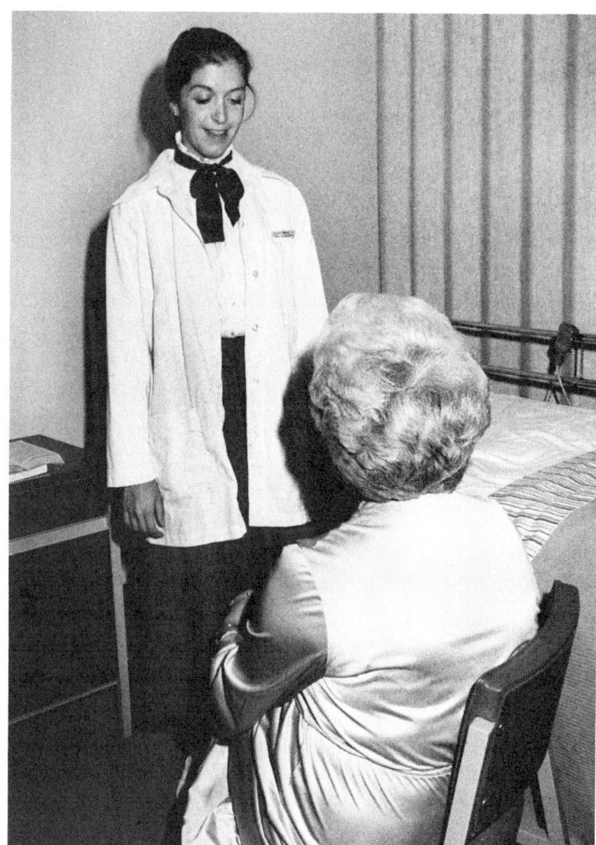

FIGURE 15-3. Nothing communicates as genuinely as a feeling of warmth and caring. Here a student nurse beginning preplanning meets a patient for the first time.

anticipate a person's reactions or fear. Nurses who are capable of empathy need to surround themselves with good support people so they have refueling resources at the times they need them.

Use of Gestures

People vary a great deal in the amount of gestures they use to accompany their spoken words. This is culturally influenced but also an individual trait. Do not assess emotion by its accompanying gestures; some people wave their arms wildly describing an everyday happening, while others would use that degree of expression only when in extreme distress. Be aware that your own gestures are always being read by others. A statement that you approve of something is contradicted by placing your arms across your chest in a disapproving stern gesture.

Body Posture and Gait

People who feel good about themselves typically assume an upright body posture and walk rapidly and surely; those who are depressed tend to slouch and move more slowly and timidly; those who are threatened tend to either draw back or act aggressively. People who are in agreement with you usually maintain eye contact with you as you speak to them; very depressed or insecure people do not (they feel inferior to you). People too angry to deal with you also do not meet your gaze. Facial expression is also important. The meanings of clenched teeth, frowning, and smiling are easily interpreted by everyone.

General Appearance

The way a person dresses often suggests the importance of what he is saying. People who have good self-esteem tend to maintain good body hygiene in dress and appearance. People who are depressed may not feel that the effort involved in these activities is worthwhile. Personal hygiene is a variable phenomenon, however. It is difficult to ascribe much meaning to this characteristic on your first contact with a person (what you see as ill kempt may be well kempt for the particular person; what you think of as well kempt may not be as well kempt as the person usually is).

Be aware that your impression of how people dress registers very strangely on your subconscious. Do not let an unconscious dislike cause you to draw back from someone with an eye patch, unclean clothing, or dirty fingernails or who uses obscene language. Preparing to give nursing care is not the same kind of activity as evaluating whether you wish to invite someone to dinner.

Use of Touch

Touch is the most intimate and meaningful of nonverbal communications. When words are sometimes inadequate, touch rarely is. Learn to use touch such as clasping a patient's shoulder or squeezing a hand to accompany reassuring words or in place of words as a strong support signal (I am here; I understand; it's all right to be afraid). On the other hand, be aware that some people enjoy being touched more than others. Due to individual preferences or cultural variations, some people do not like you to use this nonverbal signal with them. Assess people individually for the technique appropriateness.

Use of Humor

People who incorporate humor into their conversations are invariably spoken to more than those who do not. Some people have a natural knack for finding humor in any situation; others do not instinctively have this quality and need to cultivate it. People who are able to laugh at their own mistakes (Do you believe I could have dropped an entire tray of equipment that way?) are usually very nice people to have around, because their laughter at themselves suggests that when you make a mistake they will be able to laugh at it the same way (or at least not be angry about it). Be careful of the use of humor with people who are fatigued or ill, however. They may be looking for a firm support person to be with them more than a person who is amusing. You can often measure a patient's progress by noting the first time postoperatively that he responds to you with a humorous statement.

Use of Distance

Although it is affected by cultural and personal variables, the distance you place yourself away from a person may indicate your feelings toward him or the type of conversation you want to engage in with him. A person generally considers the space directly surrounding him as *his* space. He likes it crossed only by people who know him well or by those with whom he is very comfortable having body contact. This is termed *intimate* space. It is a distance up to eighteen inches from the body (Hall, 1966). Any time that you touch a patient you violate this distance; if he allows this without protest, you can be sure that the person sees you as safe, protective, and helpful and actually welcomes an action such as a backrub or the administration of an injection to ease pain. Sometimes you will notice in a heated discussion that one party will move aggressively into this space and the other person will automatically step back to protect the space. It is necessary to invade intimate space to whisper. People who greet each other with a light cheek kiss typically invade this space (and take people not used to this cultural gesture very much by surprise).

The distance from 18 inches to 4 feet is sensed by most people as *personal* space. This is the usual distance at which you stand from someone to speak to them; it is a comfortable hand-shaking distance. When you stand by the side of a patient's bed or sit next to a person in his home, you are within this space. A normal voice level is all that is necessary to convey messages. It is a concerned, I-care-about-you distance, but not as invasive as intimate space for most people.

The distance between 4 feet and 12 feet is termed *social* space. Conversation spoken at this distance is readily heard by others. No touching is possible. It is a work or business-conducting space, a teacher—class distance. Notice how uncomfortable everyone in a classroom becomes if an instructor asks a personal question from this distance (Would you see me after class? You're failing this course). The instructor has used social space to ask a personal question and it is perceived as inappropriate. Remember this if you talk with a hospitalized patient from the door of the room. "How are you today?" from the doorway is a social question; the answer will probably be "Fine, thank you," the response almost all people are taught early in life. Asked from a personal or intimate distance, the person's response might be "I'm still terribly short of breath. Is this ever going to get better?"

Distance beyond 12 feet is *public* space. To communicate from this distance you would have to shout; privacy is not protected at all. Waving to a friend in a hallway or across a parking lot is an example of public space communication.

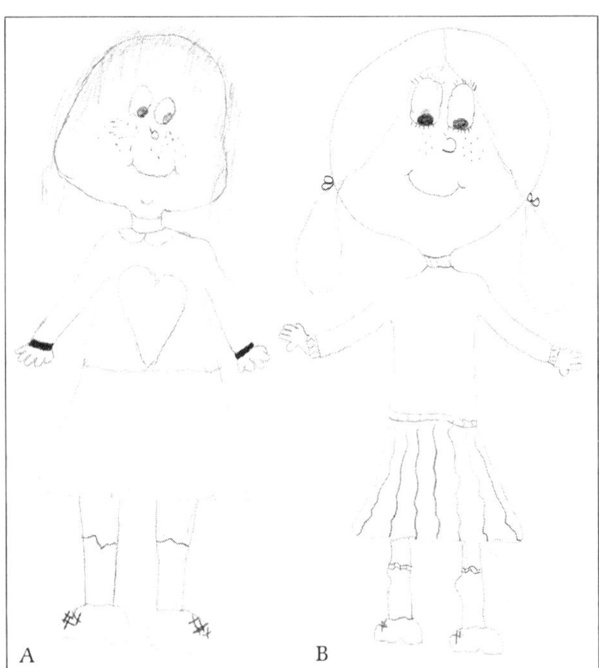

FIGURE 15-4. A. Drawing by a child hospitalized for heart surgery. Notice the prominent heart. B. Drawing by the same child 6 months after successful heart surgery. Her attention in this drawing is focused on her eyes because she has just learned that she might need glasses.

Most people perceive speaking on the telephone as social or personal space. The tone of voice and the words used help to differentiate which area of space they perceive it to be. A message such as "Have I got news for you!" suggests social space; "Can you keep a secret?" brings it into intimate space.

Use of Drawings

A useful nonverbal technique to discern how children feel about a frightening experience is to ask them to draw a picture of what happened to them or a picture of themselves. Figure 15-4A, for example, is a picture drawn by a 10-year-old hospitalized for heart surgery. Notice how prominently she drew her heart. Surely she realizes that she cannot survive if something happens to her heart; it is so all encompassing in her body. Figure 15-4B is a drawing made by the same child of herself 6 months later after she returned home following successful surgery. Notice that her attention in the second drawing is focused on her eyes (she just learned that she might need glasses).

A child's use of colors may be a clue as to mood (happy children tend to use bright colors; depressed children use black or dark colors). A child with good self-esteem usually fills the full page; one with less than this crowds his drawing into a corner. These observations are very variable, however. A child may have had only a black crayon to draw with and may have been saving the rest of his paper for a second picture.

Use of Music

The type of music that people prefer to listen to often conveys their mood. The better the person feels about himself the more apt he is to choose music that has a lively quality; if he is sad, he is more apt to choose a quieter, more comforting type.

GENERAL FACTORS THAT CAN INTERFERE WITH EFFECTIVE COMMUNICATION

Since so much of nursing care is influenced by verbal communication (discussing with a person how he would like a dressing changed; discussing with another nurse how she usually completes a procedure), it is important to communicate clearly. In emergency situations your actions may be the direct result of verbal instructions such as "Give 2 ml of epinephrine." It is important, if you want to communicate clearly and avoid miscalculations, to be able to recognize common situations in which communications can be distorted.

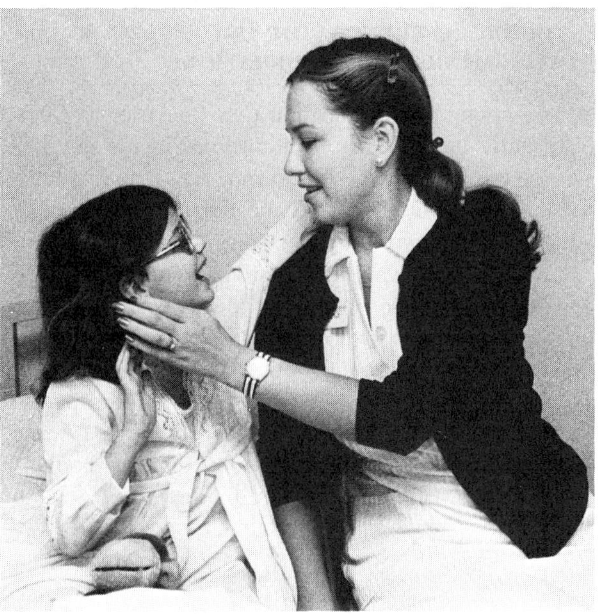

FIGURE 15-5. Touch is an effective means of communication when hearing or sight is impaired.

Personal Factors

Personal factors have a strong influence on whether communication is effective. If you relate well to another person, it is easier to communicate clearly.

Age and Developmental Level

Age and developmental levels influence communication because these factors influence vocabulary so greatly. A 3-year-old, for example, may not have the vocabulary to explain the way his knee feels (he has heard the word "ache" but only in connection with headaches; he does not know that knees can ache as well). Early schoolage children have difficulty describing the blurriness they experience as they try to focus on a blackboard with less than perfect eyesight and sometimes are in need of glasses for a long time before anyone realizes the problem. The ability to describe inner feelings such as anger, sadness, or fear is an ability that comes only with adulthood.

Intellectual Level

Intellectual level, like age, can influence vocabulary size and ability to both encode and decode messages. It can influence the number of languages a person speaks, reading ability, and the depth of explanation that a person is capable of receiving.

Physical Factors

Physical factors such as speech defects and hearing impairment can interfere with the transmission and reception of a message (Fig. 15-5). When people are distracted by such sensations as fatigue or pain, they may have reduced ability to transmit or receive messages correctly.

Emotional Factors

Emotional factors such as anxiety, anger, grief, and excitement interfere with communication because in such emotional states the person's concentration is so intense that he cannot make his wants known clearly or hear clearly what is said to him. In emergencies emotional factors are always present; good communication in emergency situations calls for extra concern and effort.

Social Factors

A person's culture or ethnic background may interfere with communication: Some people are taught by their culture not to express their feelings, either good or bad; some learn not to criticize authority figures (and health personnel are authority figures) even if they are certain that the criticism is justified; and others use a great deal of facial expression and hand gestures to accompany words. This may be threatening to the person whose culture resists a show of emotion or feelings.

Environmental Factors

Environmental factors that can interfere with effective communication include temperature extremes and excessive noise. These are unfortunately not uncommon environmental factors in a busy health care facility and can be present in a person's home as well. Everyone has had the experience of having to shout to make themselves heard over environmental noise such as rattling dishes or has felt too exhausted from an extreme environmental temperature to have the energy to maintain even casual conversation (see QRS 15-1).

☐ QUICK REFERENCE STOP 15-1: PSYCHOLOGICAL CONSIDERATIONS

Therapeutic communication may be easier to carry out early in the morning than later in the day because by the end of day you may feel that you have listened to enough people and do not want to take the time to draw out a person's story or concern. Make a habit of varying the order in which you care for the patients so you do not always end care with the same person, who consequently is the patient with whom you are most apt to be nontherapeutic.

Do not worry about an occasional nontherapeutic response that presents itself out of habit. If your overall manner is one of a helping person, this manner will override many slips of the tongue.

SPECIFIC BLOCKS TO EFFECTIVE COMMUNICATION

Communication patterns between two people typically proceed from a superficial to a deeper level unless problems such as personal and environmental factors interfere. Sometimes communication remains at a superficial level because one person is blocking the process by poor communication technique. It is helpful to record a conversation you have with a patient (or a friend) who attempts to tell you about a problem to see if you unconsciously use any blocking techniques.

Changing the Subject

Changing the subject when someone mentions a subject that is uncomfortable for you is so easy and almost second nature that unless you listen for it you may not even be aware that you do it. Suppose, for example, as part of a health interview you ask a prospective mother "Have you been pregnant before?" and she replies, "My first child was stillborn." She has introduced an emotional topic. You feel that if she talks any more about that subject, she may start to cry. You do not know what to do if she cries, so without thinking, your next response is, "Well, let's talk about the diet you're going to have to follow with this pregnancy."

Changing the subject to avoid discussing a topic may make *you* feel more comfortable, but it does not make the person feel any better about the topic and may actually make her feel worse (if the topic was too intense for you to handle, how can she ever resolve how it has left her feeling?) In addition, you have announced that a fact-finding level of information is all that you are interested in, that you do not wish to engage in a level of communication where feelings can be shared.

Offering False Reassurance

False reassurance is reassurance given without adequate facts behind it (also termed premature advice). Such reassurance not only is ineffective (it does not reassure because it is not factual) but can also be harmful in that it reveals you as shallow and unresponsive to the person's problem. In the example above, if the patient says that she hopes that her present pregnancy will not end as tragically as the first and you say, "Don't worry, no one has such bad luck twice," you have given false reassurance. It is not true that no one has such bad luck twice. No one is likely to trust a person who treats worries so callously.

Giving Your Personal Opinion

In some circumstances giving a personal opinion may be helpful, but these instances are very few. Suppose that in the above example the woman concerned about her pregnancy says, "I'm trying not to worry," and you say, "When I'm worried, I go for a walk. Try that; it always works for me." Your response is not helpful because it is a statement of what solves *your* problem, not the woman's, and it may be harmful because it implies that her problem in your mind is so trivial that it can be brushed aside with a simple solution. When she takes a long walk and still feels worried, she may feel a loss of self-esteem because what works so easily for you does not work for her. Solutions that work for you may not be appropriate for others. Do not impose personal opinions or values on others if you want a relationship to move to a deeper level than fact finding.

Telling People How They Should Feel

It is easy from an outsider's standpoint to think that you know how people should feel and to tell them what you believe. The woman who is worried about her pregnancy, for example, says, "I'm worried," and you say, "Don't worry." It is clearly not possible to change people's feelings about their circumstances by such a simple answer. All your reply does is tell the person that you consider her concerns foolish. She may be reluctant to discuss any other feelings she has, afraid that they will also be treated lightly. You have limited communication to a fact finding level.

Technical Jargon

When you first enter a school of nursing, you are exposed to many unfamiliar medical terms that at first make no sense to you. The more you grow used to the Latin stems from which these terms are derived, the easier medical jargon becomes to decipher; after a time you may not make clear distinctions between medical language and terms that you can expect everyone to understand. Using medical terms that people may not understand blocks communication because a person may be reluctant to tell you that he does not understand the term (you are using it as if he ought to understand it) or may misinterpret it. If you respond to the woman who is worried that she may have difficulty with her pregnancy with a statement such as "Being gravid is a strain on everyone," you not only have supplied trite information, but also have used a term not in general use. *Gravid* is Latin for *pregnant*, but the woman may interpret it as a complication of pregnancy (you expect her to develop gravid—whatever that is—and so this pregnancy will probably also go badly). To communicate effectively, listen to any explanation you give a patient to be sure that you would have understood it prior to your first day in a school of nursing.

Inattentive Listening

No one talks very long to someone who is not listening. Everyone has had the experience of being excited about telling a story only to find that no one was listening. Such a experience is disappointing and frustrating.

Listening, like speaking, is not passive but active. Be aware that your body posture conveys to a great extent whether you are listening (sitting, not standing, to convey that you are not on the run; leaning slightly forward, not backward). Nodding, maintaining eye contact, and stopping all other activities are strong indications that you are attuned to what is being said. In some instances it is necessary to repeat part of what the person said, interject an appropriate "uh-huh" or "m-m-m," or make a direct statement (I'm listening, go on) to assure a person that you are listening.

Be certain when you are listening to your tenth or twentieth patient that you do not exhibit "end-of-the-day" listening behavior. To be therapeutic, you have to give everyone's concerns the same attention that you would have given if they had been your first patient encounter of the day.

Table 15-1 lists Ten Commandments of Good Listening that are helpful to remember to improve listening technique.

TABLE 15-1. TEN COMMANDMENTS FOR GOOD LISTENING

1. *Stop talking.* You cannot listen if you are talking.
2. *Put the talker at ease.* Help him fell that he is free to talk. This is often called a permissive environment.
3. *Show him that you want to listen.* Look and act interested. Do not read while he talks. Listen to understand rather than reply.
4. *Remove distractions.* Do not doodle, tap, or shuffle papers. Would it be quieter if you shut the door?
5. *Empathize with him.* Try to put yourself in his place so that you can see his point of view.
6. *Be patient.* Allow plenty of time. Do not interrupt him. Do not start for the door or walk away.
7. *Hold your temper.* An angry man gets the wrong meaning from words.
8. *Go easy on argument or criticism.* This puts him on the defensive. He may "clam up" or get angry. Do not argue; even if you win, you lose.
9. *Ask questions.* This encourages him and shows you are listening. It helps him to develop points further.
10. *Stop talking!* This is the first and last because all other commandments depend on it. You just cannot do a good listening job while you are talking.

Source: From K. Davis, *Human Relations in Business.* New York: McGraw-Hill, 1957.

Showing Disapproval

People do not come for health care to be criticized; they come to learn more about how to stay well or how to become better again. If they receive criticism from a health care provider they may not reveal their main problem because they do not want it criticized in the way you responded to their preliminary statements.

Suppose the woman above says, "I never drink milk." It is important for a woman to ingest adequate amounts of calcium (found most readily in milk) during pregnancy because the entire fetal skeleton has to be formed during this time. Knowing this, you respond to her, "That's not right. You should drink a quart of milk a day." This response discourages the woman from telling you any more about her diet (neither does she eat much protein) and you miss this important information because she will not expose herself to your criticism again.

Be aware that nonverbal disapproval (frowning, sighing) can be just as detrimental to communication as spoken disapproval. On the other hand, this does not mean that you should show approval of wrong actions. Merely listen to them with no action or comment, and make a mental note of them. At the end of your interaction, introduce the changes in behavior that you wish to see ("Let's plan some ways you can include more calcium and protein in your diet during pregnancy").

Not Showing Approval When Warranted

Every student has had the experience of completing a difficult assignment and receiving only criticism from a teacher; no comment that aside from the area she was unhappy with the bulk of the assignment was done well. This is because the instructor assumed that the student would do a good job; no reward is given for meeting minimum criteria. From the other side of the desk, however, it would have been satisfying—and offered motivation to continue to do well—to have heard the words "good job."

When discussing health care problems with patients, it is easy to forget that what you accept as common behavior may take a greal deal of effort for the person to accomplish (for instance, patients should cough and deep breathe after surgery, but many do not because it causes sharp pains). Giving people praise for things they did well encourages them to tell you more about themselves and to try other things. If a topic is difficult for a person to talk about, telling them that you appreciate that it is a sensitive topic for them helps them to continue to discuss it.

Being Defensive

In the same way that people who come for health care do not enjoy being criticized, neither does the average health care provider. If a person makes a critical remark, therefore, it is easy to respond with a defensive comment. The woman who is concerned about her pregnancy, for example, may say, "I always have to wait so long to see a physician at this clinic." It is easy to reply, "No one forces you to come here, you know." This type of response implies to the patient that no complaining is welcome. Indirectly it tells her that any complaint of hers is out of line. Try to respond instead to such criticism with a supportive comment such as "I appreciate it makes a long day for you."

No health care agency is perfect; neither is any health care provider.

Cliché Advice

Cliché advice is meaningless, unhelpful, and too general. Although statements such as "Rome wasn't built in a day" and "You have to walk before you can run," are true, these statements are so general that they do not really have meaning for any situation. Each person considers his problem unique and resents being given advice that is so general.

Topping Off

Topping off is minimizing the speaker's views by telling a better story. A person tells you he has a headache; you say, "You should feel the one I have." A person says he has a problem; you say, "You want to know what problems are, work here a while." This type of response implies to the patient that his problems are inconsequential. He will not be likely to tell you any more about himself after being so treated.

TECHNIQUES THAT ENCOURAGE THERAPEUTIC COMMUNICATION

A number of techniques are effective in deepening communication patterns and relationships. These techniques can be learned if they are not a spontaneous part of your present communication pattern. You need practice using them so that you do not sound contrived and false.

Attentive Listening

The importance of attentive listening cannot be over stressed. Making it clear that you are hearing and concentrating on what another is saying indicates that you have respect for the person and value what he has to say. A person who feels valued is much more apt to confide his feelings and concerns than the person who feels that you consider him inferior.

Reflection

Reflecting is another technique, like attentive listening, that is so simple that it is easy to discount its importance. Reflecting is restating the last word or phrase a person has said to you when there is a pause in the communication. A patient says, for example, "I'm worried," and then stops. You repeat the last word: "Worried?" The person, assured that you are listening and interested, will generally enlarge on his statement: "Yes, I'm worried about not being able to have any more children after this surgery."

Clarifying

Clarifying consists of repeating a statement a person has made so that you and he can be certain that you have correctly understood what he said. This is particularly helpful if a person has been describing a series of symptoms that he has noticed or a series of actions he has taken. You would clarify his statements by saying, "Let me see if I understand this. You said that you always get the pain first in your chest. Then it spreads to your arm. Then you notice the shortness of breath." If you are not quoting him correctly, the person will interrupt and restate the problem.

Paraphrasing

Paraphrasing is restating what the person has said not only to assure him that you have heard correctly (as in clarifying) but to help him explain what he has been trying to say. In clarifying, you repeat the person's exact words; in paraphrasing, you retain the meaning of the words but repeat them in a clearer or more condensed form. The patient says, for example, "My wife and I don't talk about our problems much." A paraphrasing statement might be, "You're telling me that your wife and you haven't discussed this surgery. Is that right?" Ask for confirmation that your paraphrasing is correct; otherwise you may find yourself putting words in people's mouths.

When the topic a patient is describing to you is embarrassing or emotionally laden (a man discussing a sexual problem such as impotence, for example), he might use such vague terms that the explanation becomes difficult to follow. Paraphrasing an explanation of this type into street language lets him know not only that you understood him but that if he can describe his problem better with words more common to him, it is acceptable to you.

Perception Checking

Perception checking is a step beyond paraphrasing: In paraphrasing, you are documenting a statement or fact reported to you; in perception checking, you are documenting a feeling or emotion. The patient states, for example, "I'm not at all worried about surgery. I know I have a good doctor. I mean, what could happen? I know I'm going to be all right." You say, "Although you're telling me you're not worried, the number of times you've said it makes me wonder if you really are worried. Are you?"

Always ask for validation that your perception is correct; you should not put ideas into people's minds or words into their mouths. As a rule, a person is not ready to deal with an emotion until he can admit that he is experiencing it. When you bring an emotion out "on the table," it can often be confronted and dealt with for the first time. The person loses his reluctance to admit his worry because you have implied that it is acceptable to feel concern.

Focusing

Focusing is helping a person to center on a subject that you suspect is causing him anxiety because he comments about it indirectly or else completely avoids mentioning it. You can help a person to focus on a subject by repeating something that he said ("You mentioned that it isn't easy being a father and that you feel tired all the time.") or by mentioning the avoided topic ("You haven't said a word about how your wife feels about the surgery. Is that a problem?").

Once a subject is brought up for discussion, the average person will respond to it. As long as it is avoided, he will never face the problem and begin to solve it.

Open-ended Questions

A pointed or direct question asks for a specific fact; it implies that all you are interested in hearing about is that one fact. A direct question, for example, is "Do you take aspirin when you have a headache?" An open-ended question is one that is not limited to a simple answer but invites a wide variety of responses. It says to the person, "Tell me as much as you know about the situation; I have a lot of time to listen." An open-ended question might be: "Tell me what you do when you have a headache." The person might answer by describing not only the amount of aspirin he takes but the use of a cold towel, going home from work, closing his eyes to stop the flashing lights he experiences. Three or four times the amount of information has been elicited.

Open-ended questions are not effective if the topic is a difficult one for the person to describe (he has difficulty responding yes or no; a paragraph of material is impossible) or if the person is naturally shy or defensive about the subject (he knows that he has not been doing the things you told him to do and would rather not admit to all his faults if he can avoid it).

Most communication with people is a combination of direct and open-ended questions. Listen carefully the next time you are asking someone to explain something to you to see if you make use of mostly direct (information limiting) questions or open-ended ones.

Supportive Statements

Supportive statements let a person know that you accept him or his behavior or at least appreciate that he has dealt well with unfortunate circumstances. The patient, for example, makes a statement such as "My wife left me while I was in Viet Nam." Not only was such an experience undoubtedly difficult for the person at the time, but it is difficult now for him to talk about it because describing it revives the hurt and anger he experienced. Such a statement deserves a comment such as "That must have been a difficult experience." The average person takes this response to mean that you want to discuss the topic, and encouraged by your expression of empathy, he may elaborate on the situation.

Silence

If you ask a person a question and he does not respond immediately, it is natural to quickly ask another question. This is a social custom that allows you to back off from sensitive areas so that a person is not put into the awkward position of having to discuss a difficult topic. Silence, however, is an effective therapeutic technique. If you ask an emotionally laden question ("Are you worried?") and the person does not answer immediately, allow a period of silence to pass. Because you did not hurry to fill in the silence, the person may respond by hurrying an answer (to fill in the silence); when he does this, he answers spontaneously and often more openly or more uninhibitedly than usual. In other instances, he may answer the question deliberately and cautiously and, because he has had a length of time to answer, will offer more information than normally.

COMMUNICATION SITUATIONS THAT REQUIRE SPECIAL SKILLS

Some patient care situations require special skills in addition to therapeutic communication techniques to promote communication.

The Shy Person

The amount of verbal communication people use varies culturally and individually. Some people talk excessively when they are nervous; others completely stop talking. It is difficult to assess how a person feels about situations (whether he is really psychologically ready for surgery, if he really understands the long-term effect a disease is going to have) if he is not giving you much verbal feedback. When someone answers all of your questions with a simple yes or no, never elaborating on any point, there is a tendency to feel that the person is reacting this way because he does not like you and to therefore draw back from him. That is, however, an insecure behavior, not a therapeutic one. In most cases, once a person feels that he really knows you and can trust you, shyness will fade. A therapeutic response, therefore, is not to back off but to maintain an active relationship despite the lack of feedback. This does not necessarily involve talking to him but checking on him frequently, remaining in the room while a physician examines him, helping with the Bandaid after a technician draws blood, or sitting with him for a few minutes while a medication takes effect.

People who are verbal reach out to secure the help they need from people around them. Shyer people are more apt to have their needs unrecognized and need to have a nurse bring support to them by pursuing a relationship that at first seems very one-sided.

The Angry Person

It is difficult to work with angry people because you feel yourself being pulled into their anger. The typical response to anger is to imitate it (if they are radiating anger as tight-lipped silence, you say nothing; if they shout at you, you shout back at them). These are not therapeutic responses, however. In working with angry people, make a point of not allowing yourself to be drawn into their anger. On the other hand, acknowledge that it is all right to be angry (do not suppress it in them). Help the person to focus his anger so that he can better understand it and begin to deal with it.

Ask the person to define what it is he is angry about. Feeling angry at the entire health care delivery system is frustrating anger because you cannot begin to handle the whole system; defining that what you are really angry about is one nurse's actions establishes a base for resolving the problem. If the person is using silence as a method of maintaining anger, suggesting possible reasons for the anger may be helpful: "I know Doctor Smith was just talking to you. Are you angry about something she said?" "I know you were asking about crutch-walking. Does it have something to do with that?" Few people, when the subject they are angry about is out in the open, can resist describing the extent of their anger. Be aware, too, that when you ask someone to explain their anger, you ask for the emotion and the distress that accompany anger to be expressed also. If you are the object of the person's anger, you are committed to listening to the angry opinion.

Keep anger from affecting you by reacting to the explanation, not the tone or force of it. Keep any response a tone gentler and quieter than that used with you. Help the person to focus his anger (being angry at the physical therapy department seems justified based on what he is saying, but being angry at you does not; not eating dinner or shouting at his wife are not constructive responses). Focusing anger implies that it is all right to be angry but it limits it and allows the person to be constructive in other areas (eating dinner and visiting with his wife). Censor, if necessary, the way that the anger is expressed, not the right to be angry. If more people honestly offered angry opinions instead of keeping them contained, the incidence of psychosomatic illnesses and perhaps hypertension would probably be much lower.

Do not back away from angry people. They are very close to losing control of themselves. They need your support, not your avoidance.

The Demanding Person

Nursing has few equals in job satisfaction (provided that salary and other working conditions are adequate) because the average person is grateful for everything you do for him. It is often upsetting then to discover a person who is not grateful for or even satisfied with your attempts to make him comfortable or to help him. This is another type of patient who is easy to back away from.

Demanding behavior generally stems from insecurity or fear (he is so afraid that something will happen to him while you are out of the room that he constantly finds more for you to do to keep you there; or so afraid of unplanned happenings that he structures things so that nothing unexpected can happen). Give more, not less of yourself, to counteract this response. When you have proven yourself dependable, the person will not feel so insecure, and the need to be demanding usually fades. Withdrawing from such a person may increase the insecurity and the demanding behavior. Ask "is there anything else I can do?"

The Sexually Aggressive Patient

Sexually aggressive behavior stems from the same cause as every other aggressive and demanding behavior—insecurity. It may be most pronounced in the patient who worries that an illness or surgery will interfere with sexual function.

A patient with this degree of insecurity may need counseling to help channel his coping response into more a socially acceptable behavior. He needs factual information as to the true extent or effect of his illness. Set limits as necessary to make giving care acceptable to you. Censor the action, not the person. Be aware that sexually aggressive behavior can occur in both men and women.

The Person with a Language Barrier

Language barriers can be a large impediment to communication. It is not unusual in any nursing care setting to encounter a patient who has a different primary language from your own; in other instances, the person's speech may be limited or difficult to understand because of an accent or dialect; in still other instances, the person speaks your language but his use of words is so different from yours that your words have different meanings.

Most people who do not speak English have a support person who can serve as interpreter. If visiting hours in the facility where you practice are very limited, you may need to investigate the possibility of allowing such a person to remain for longer time periods to ensure good communication. Anticipate the instructions you will need to give the patient (cough, deep breathe, turn, save urine) and ask the interpreter to write these out using your own language. Post these conspicuously in the patient's room or on the nursing care plan so that everyone giving care can become familiar with them.

Most health care facilities have a list of people who will serve as translators as needed by patients; many times you can contact such a person by telephone to ask for a specific word you need to know. In the event that you need to give instructions and there is no translator present, do not be self-conscious about using hand gestures to express the action you want.

Everyone has a tendency to shout at people who speak a different language as if the loudness of your voice will increase the possibility of the message's being understood. Instead use gestures or draw a picture of what you expect (a person lying in bed; an arrow; a person sitting up in a chair for "I'm going to help you sit up for the first time after surgery"). Allow the person ample paper and a clipboard to draw pictures of what he wants; supply a group of pictures for the preschool child so that he can select from the stack the one he wants.

Be certain when you are speaking to people who are translating to their own language that you speak slowly and use common words that can be translated literally. A statement such as "I really goofed this up" cannot be translated.

The Unconscious Patient

Hearing is the last sense lost with unconsciousness and the first sense regained with consciousness. Always be aware that people who do not respond to you may be able to hear and interpret anything you say. Never say anything to an unconscious patient or within his hearing that you would not say if he was fully alert. Use nonverbal communication such as touch to accompany your words to better convey your message.

The Hearing-impaired Person

"Hearing-impaired" is a more accepted term today than "deaf"; it is always preferable to "deaf and dumb" (which implies that hearing-impaired people are not as intelligent as others). When communicating with a hearing-impaired person, check whether he uses a hearing aid; if so, be certain that it is turned on. Face him when you speak so that he can follow your lip movement. Use hand gestures as necessary to convey your message or write out the instruction. If you have difficulty understanding his message, ask him to write it for you. Use common sense about how loud to raise your voice to facilitate communication. As a rule of thumb, at the point that privacy is lost, it is time to resort to a written or sign language form of communication. Most large cities have a person who can translate requests into sign language.

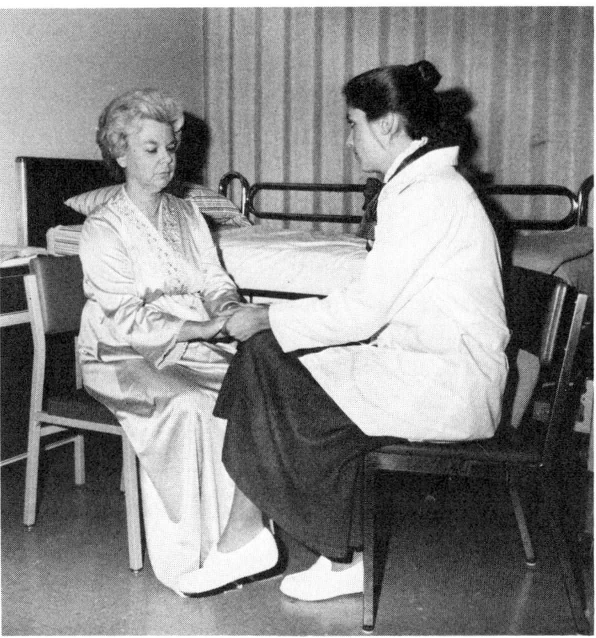

FIGURE 15-6. Nonverbal communication and touch can be as effective as spoken words in establishing a nurse-patient relationship.

The Vision-impaired Person

When speaking to a person with impaired vision, remember that you cannot rely on nonverbal communication techniques such as hand gestures. A statement such as, "Take a piece of gauze about this long," without an accompanying hand gesture is meaningless. Never touch a person who cannot see you without speaking to him first so that you do not startle him unnecessarily.

COMMUNICATION AND THE NURSE-PATIENT RELATIONSHIP

Communication is a primary way to establish rapport with people. Rapport means a sympathetic or harmonious relationship, which is a good description of what the nurse-patient relationship should be (Fig. 15-6). Several phases of a developing relationship can be identified; both you and the person with whom you are forming the relationship behave in certain ways during different phases. It is helpful to be aware of these phases because relationships grow tense or out of syncopation if one member moves on to another phase before the other or if one member wants to terminate the relationship before the other.

Phase I: Initiation

Initiation, the first phase of a relationship, is a get-acquainted time. It is a time when, sometimes unconsciously, your chief activity is to find out as much as possible about the other person to determine whether you can learn to trust him. If for some reason at the end of your appraisal you realize that you cannot trust the person, the relationship will never be a secure one and will probably progress no further.

Many of the questions that you ask in taking a nursing history are aimed at helping you get to know about a person you will be caring for (name, where he lives, what he works at, steps he took when he realized he was ill). The first time that you care for a patient you may recognize that he is asking you similar questions (Are you from this city? How long have you been a student? What do you think of the president's new bill on Social Security?). You observe a person very carefully during this phase of a relationship to determine his physical and mental capacity; he also observes you. As a rule, when you are answering questions about your status or giving an opinion you are not engaging in therapeutic communication; that is always patient not nurse centered. Offering this type of introductory information, however (name, rank, and serial number) is therapeutic in that it allows the patient to become acquainted enough with you that he feels secure with you.

The initiation phase of a relationship may last for only several minutes. If the person with whom you are trying to form a relationship is reluctant to form deep relationships (because he has been hurt recently by a destructive relationship), it may take months. During this phase, no matter how long it lasts, it is important to demonstrate honesty and sincerity, as these are important foundations for establishing trust. It often seems that it might be desirable to exaggerate your level of knowledge in order to build confidence in yourself when you are meeting a person you are going to care for. Unless you are an extremely skilled bluffer, however, this approach is faulty because the person can generally sense your pretense. How can he trust you when you say you know how to administer an injection if the first time you met you lied to him? As a rule, it is better to simply admit that you do not know the answer to a question such as "How long does it take epiphysitis to go away?" (and maybe that you do not even know what epiphysitis is), as that demonstrates honesty. Adding "but I'll ask and find out for you" not only demonstrates sincerity but encourages further questions (is therapeutic).

Patients may also try to bluff during this phase of a relationship. They may describe a symptom such as pain as "nothing" although they are clenching their teeth while they are saying it. You may need to remind such patients that you cannot evaluate their conditions clearly unless they are honest with you.

Occasionally, a patient will test a nurse's sincerity about helping him by asking for many small items that require an extra trip to a supply room or an extra minute's time spent with him. Supplying these items and extra moments is time well spent because it promotes sincerity. Once a person is certain that you are dependable and he can rely on you, you are ready to move to the second phase of a relationship.

Phase II: Working Phase

The second phase of a relationship is time spent working constructively together. In family relationships this is time spent repairing a house or raising children; in a nursing relationship it is time spent helping the person to maintain his well health or, if he is ill at the initial contact, helping him return to wellness. The working phase of a relationship is an enjoyable phase as the pressure and strain of getting acquainted are replaced by the enjoyment of mutually completing a task.

Phase III: Termination

Terminating relationships is something that people do not often actively think a great deal about because the act of saying goodbye is always a little painful if the relationship has been meaningful. Nurse-patient relationships tend to be short-term, however (days to years), so in almost every nurse-patient relationship this third phase is important to consider. In many instances you should plan for termination at the establishment of the relationship or actually set goals for termination at the same time that you set care goals.

Separation is a time when the two people in the relationship have to think about how they will have to change when they no longer see each other regularly. Termination of the nurse-patient relationship usually means that the patient will do more for himself. Also, it is necessary to consider who will provide the emotional support you have been giving. In most instances at the time that a nurse-patient relationship ends (the person is being discharged from a hospital or no longer needs weekly visits from a community health nurse in his home), the person is able to provide his own self-care, and the people around him who were unable to function as support people while he was so ill, because they were too frightened and too much in need of support themselves to give support, are now ready to assume their former roles. It is important that the termination of the relationship be considered well enough in advance that if the person is not able to care for himself or cannot identify emotional support persons, you can help him locate people to provide care and support.

It is important from your own standpoint that you spend some time thinking about terminations with patients before they actually occur so that if the relationship was extremely satisfying for you, you will not be left with a feeling of loss at the end of the relationship. In some instances you need to locate additional emotional support for yourself when a meaningful relationship ends; otherwise you find yourself feeling drained and burnt out and unable to begin a new patient relationship as enthusiastically as you would like to. Be certain on termination that you do not offer more than you can give following a relationship. A promise such as "I'll call you once a week to check on your progress" makes it easier to terminate a relationship, but if you then cannot follow through with the promise, it may result in your feeling guilty and the patient's feeling betrayed.

A person skilled as a nurse can initiate a relationship with a patient quickly and, using therapeutic communication skills, deepen the relationship to a true working one in a short time. She has done her work well when both she and the patient are satisfied on termination.

PROCESS RECORDING

Process recording is a method of examining how effective you are at therapeutic communication. After your next patient interaction (or discussion of a family problem) take a few minutes and write down in the left-hand column on a sheet of paper a statement made to you. In the middle column write what you thought on hearing the statement. In a third column write your response to the statement. Try to record both statements and responses verbatim or as close to the actual words used as possible. You should be able to recall accurately about three minutes of communication.

Examine your responses to each statement. Ask yourself did I encourage the other person to tell me more or block him from doing so? Were my responses supportive or critical or trite? Did I use open-ended questions or closed direct ones? Did I check perceptions or just assume that I understood correctly what was told me?

The average person uses few techniques that are therapeutic. If a family member tends to be authoritarian, process record an interaction with him; you may find he uses none, which is why you find it so difficult to talk with him. You cannot help people if you cannot learn what it is they need help with. A nurse must develop an above-average level of communication ability.

The following is a record of an interaction between a nursing student and Mr. Sandoz, a 22-year-old patient seen in a hospital setting. He is diagnosed as having a stress-related peptic ulcer; he is a medical student at a nearby university, married, with two children.

TABLE 15-2. EXAMPLE OF PROCESS RECORDING

What Patient Said and Did	What I Thought and Felt	What I Said and Did
	I felt anxious meeting a new patient because I assumed he knew more about his illness than I did. On the other hand, I thought he'd be understanding because he was so close to my own age.	I walked into his room and said, "Good morning."
He was sitting up in bed holding his hands over his abdomen. He said, "Get me something for this pain" without even looking up at me.	I felt attacked. As if he thought I should have done something sooner—but I had just gotten there.	I asked, "What kind of pain are you having?"
He said, "I need a student nurse like a hole in the head. Is there anyone else around?"	Now, I really felt attacked.	I said, "I can get you something for pain, Mr. Sandoz. I just need to know what kind of pain you have."
He said, "Hydrochloric acid is carving a hole through my stomach. It feels like someone is boring a hole through my stomach. It hurts like hell. Is that enough explanation for you to get me something?"	I felt angry that he insisted on putting me down so.	I said, "It certainly is. And I appreciate that if I had pain like that I wouldn't want to answer questions either." I left to find my instructor and get him something for pain.
		I returned in 15 minutes and said, "I have an injection for you, Mr. Sandoz."
He said, "Damn! Do you always take so long to do something?"	I was getting really angry.	I said nothing. Just checked his ID band and gave him the injection in his deltoid muscle.
He asked, "Could you get me my Mylanta now?" (his antacid).	Getting angrier at his demanding tone and threatened because I didn't know whether he could have any then.	I said, "I'll have to ask."
He said, "Any chance you could do that in a hurry?"	Really angry.	I said, "Are you always so demanding?"
He turned on his side so his back was to me, clenched his teeth, and pushed his hands against his abdomen again.	I realized that my criticism was unfair because he was in pain but it was too late to take it back.	I said, "I'm sorry. I know you're uncomfortable."

TABLE 15-2 (CONTINUED)

What Patient Said and Did	What I Thought and Felt	What I Said and Did
He shouted, "I am not *uncomfortable*! I am in a damn lot of *pain*! Could you help me out in some decent way?	I realized I was in over my head. I thought I'd limit any interaction with him so he couldn't make me so angry again.	I said nothing. Just left to check on whether he could have some Mylanta.
		I returned with a medicine glass of Mylanta for him.
He said, "Do you know if Dr. M. is still in surgery?"	Threatened again because I didn't even know how to find that out.	I said, "I can find out for you," handing him the medicine glass.
He said, "And then hand me that book on the chair over there, will you?"	Trying to concentrate on not growing angry at his demanding tone, yet I had medicine I had to give safely.	I said, "Let me see your ID band first."
He turned his wrist over, frowning. Said, "If I don't get to that book today, I might as well cash it in."	I thought: I am tired of him telling me to hurry and that comment was just another way of his doing that. That I had things I was responsible for doing for him and wanted to get to those.	I said, "Do you want to try some breakfast?"
He said, "In half an hour. For now, just hand me the book."	Getting angry again. And concerned that his food on his breakfast tray would be cold in half an hour. (And a little concerned about the extra work of getting him warm food again.)	I said, "Don't you even want to try some breakfast now?"
He said, "I'd like to try not failing out of school. Hand me the book so I can do that."	I "heard" what he was saying concerning the book for the first time.	I said, "Failing out of school?"
He said, "That's what's happening to me. I hurt like hell and I'm in this lousy hospital and because of that I'm failing school. My wife is working in a restaurant at a job she hates with high school kids watching my kids so I can do this—and I'm blowing it! I can't ask her to serve scrambled eggs all her life! I can't afford to repeat a semester just because my stomach is bleeding—I'm really blowing this! You still want to know if I want to eat breakfast?"	I didn't. And was surprised how one quick response on my part had brought out so much emotion. I also knew I was in over my head again (but in a nice way).	

EVALUATION

My overall interaction with Mr. Sandoz would have been better if I hadn't been caught so off guard in the beginning. I had thought that he was going to be a person who had a lot of common interests with me (student-student, medicine-nursing, same age group). His initial response to me seemed so much more intense because I had expected such a different one. Stereotyping expected behavior less would have helped me to accept him better.

My responses to Mr. Sandoz were adequate up to the point that I became angry. I should have answered his comment, "Do you always take so long to do something?" with a supportive one such as "I know it's hard to have pain." (Once I heard a nurse answer that question for a patient with "Believe it or not, sometimes I take longer," and all of us laughed and I think the patient felt good about being able to appreciate something funny, but I'm glad I didn't try humor here. Silence was inadequate but at least not irritating.)

If I had been more sensitive to what he was saying (and less angry) I would have noticed that after I gave the injection Mr. Sandoz actually became nicer to me (*asking* could you get me my Mylanta, not just demanding it). I was too angry to notice his change in behavior though, so I cut off his preliminary attempt to interact with me by criticizing him (are you always so demanding?) My supportive statement (I'm sorry. I know you're uncomfortable) was ineffective after the criticism.

In the final interaction I was so concerned with my own needs (not to grow angry and get my work done) that I completely missed what he said about why the book was important ("I might as well cash it in"). Fortunately, when he said "failing school," I got my mind off my problem and onto his and was able to produce a therapeutic response for him. By the time he had finished describing all the things he was worried about I couldn't imagine why I was worried about warm food (and could see why he wasn't).

I'm aware that a patient should not have to describe something with the impact of driving a truck over me before he can get my attention. Better listening (and thinking while I'm listening) would make me "hear" better and be able to be more helpful sooner in this type of interaction.

SUGGESTED READINGS

Adamson, L. S. Strategies for nurse-patient communication. *Superv. Nurse* 11:44, 1980.

Almore, M. Dyadic communication. *Am. J. Nurs.* 79:1077, 1979.

Beanlands, H. E., et al. Nurse, do you hear me? *Canad. Nurse* 77:41, 1981.

Carr, R. M. Perfect communication. *Nursing (Horsham)* 12:136, 1982.

Cosper, B. How well do patients understand hospital jargon? *Am. J. Nurs.* 77:1932, 1977.

Dreher, B. Overcoming speech and language disorders. *Geriatr. Nurs.* 2:345, 1981.

Duldt, B. Anger: An alienating communication hazard for nurses. *Nurs. Outlook* 29:640, 1981.

Garant, C. Stalls in the therapeutic process. *Am. J. Nurs.* 80:2166, 1980.

Goodykoontz, L. Touch: Attitudes and practice. *Nurs. Forum* 18:4, 1979.

Hall, E. T. *The Hidden Dimension.* New York: Doubleday, 1966.

Hames, C. C., and Dayle, H. J. *Basic Concepts of Helping: A Wholistic Approach.* New York: Appleton-Century-Crofts, 1980.

Heineken, J., et al. Confirming, not disconfirming: Communicating in a more positive manner. *M.C.N.* 8(1):78, 1983.

Henrich, A. P., et al. Responding to patients' concerns. *Nurs. Outlook* 29:428, 1981.

Hurtt, B. L. 'Take my hand.' *Geriatr. Nurs.* 3(3):162, 1982.

Jungman, L. When your feelings get in the way. *Am. J. Nurs.* 79:1074, 1979.

Kepler, T. L. Mastering the people skills. *J. Nurs. Adm.* 10:15, 1980.

Knable, J. Handholding: One means of transcending barriers of communication. *Heart Lung* 10(6):1106, 1981.

Langland, R. M., et al. Effects of touch on communication with elderly confused clients. *J. Gerontol. Nurs.* 8(3):152, 1982.

Latimer, J. Learning to listen. *Nursing (Oxford)* 1:1186, 1981.

Leung, J. K. Staff/patient relations: A touching moment. *Nurs. Mirror* 153(12):36, 1981.

Lynch, J. The simple act of touch. *Nursing 78* 8:32, 1978.

O'Brien, M. J. *Communications and Relationships in Nursing* (2nd ed.). St. Louis: Mosby, 1978.

O'Sullivan, A. L. Privileged communication. *Am. J. Nurs.* 80:947, 1980.

Powell, J. *Why Am I Afraid to Tell You Who I Am?* Chicago: Peacock Books, 1969.

Seaman, L. Affective nursing touch. *Geriatr. Nurs.* 3(3):163, 1982.

Sklar, C. When nurses fail to communicate. *Canad. Nurse* 77:47, 1981.

Truesdell, S., and Wood, T. Communication: Key to efficient patient care. *Nursing 77* 7:52, 1977.

Wahl, P. R. Therapeutic relationship with the elderly. *J. Gerontol. Nurs.* 6:260, 1980.

Wiedenbach, E., and Falls, C. E. *Communication: Key to Effective Nursing.* New York: Tiresias, 1978.

Wlody, G. S. Effective communication techniques. *Nurs. Management* 12:19, 1981.

QUESTIONS FOR REVIEW

1. Mrs. Smith states that she is short of breath. Which of the following would be the most therapeutic response from you?
   a. Everyone feels that way sometimes.
   b. Thinking of something else is a nice distraction technique.
   c. Short of breath?
   d. Don't worry; I'll get you something for it.

2. Mrs. Smith says, "I'd like to go home soon." Which of the following responses would probably *not* be a therapeutic communication?
   a. There's no place like home.
   b. You'd like to go home?
   c. I'm listening.
   d. Why would you like to be home?

3. Which of the following statements by Mrs. Smith represents the highest level of communication?
   a. I'm 40 years old.
   b. Being short of breath makes me scared.
   c. I hate rain; rain makes my breathing worse.
   d. My dream is to live in a big house with pillars out front.

4. You and another nurse have worked together for 6 months. Which of the following situations represents the highest level of communication between you?
   a. You can argue with each other and be friends afterward.
   b. You are able to tell her how you feel about her patient care.
   c. She can tell you about her future hopes.
   d. You can tell what patients she is going to ask to care for before she asks.

A patient asks you if you have ever cared for anyone with his disease who is now gone. Match the communication technique in the left column with an example of it in the right column.

5. Paraphrasing	a. Who is now gone?
6. Reflection	b. You're asking me if I've ever cared for anyone who has died.
7. Perception checking	c. Are you asking me if I think you will die?

8. You ask John, a 10-year-old, how he is doing in school and he doesn't answer immediately. Your most therapeutic response might be:
   a. Change to a more comfortable subject for him.
   b. Allow a space of silence.
   c. Assume school is an emotional topic for him.
   d. Demand he answer you.

9. Mr. Jones states that he has pain. Which of the following represents a *supportive* statement?
   a. I'll hold your hand if it helps.
   b. You said you have a lot of pain.
   c. It must be hard to always have pain.
   d. Take your mind off it by deep breathing.

10. Which of the following is the most *empathetic* statement to Mr. Jones' statement that he has pain?
    a. I've had pain myself.
    b. I'm sorry you feel so bad.
    c. I can appreciate it's difficult to have pain.
    d. Everyone has to have some pain sometime in life.

16. HEALTH TEACHING: TEACHING-LEARNING STRATEGIES

OBJECTIVES

Upon mastery of the material in this chapter, you should be able to:

1. List principles of effective teaching-learning.
2. List teaching strategies that are helpful in health education.
3. Describe factors that promote or hinder effective teaching and learning.
4. Describe behavior modification as a learning mode.
5. Describe the learning behaviors of people at differing points in the age span.
6. Describe effective use of teaching aids in health education.
7. Apply the nursing process to give safe and planned care to a patient whose care involves principles of teaching-learning.

TERMS

The terms important for an understanding of this chapter are shown below and defined in the glossary:

behavior modification
learning
learning style
teaching

Health teaching is an independent nursing action which accompanies all nursing care. It is a primary nursing responsibility and probably the most frequently used of nursing implementations. At times health teaching is a formal procedure (teaching a community group of mothers-to-be about breast-feeding); at other times it is a one-to-one process (preparing a person for what to expect in surgery). Health teaching is also done informally by spontaneously answering a person's question about an effect of a medicine or assuring a mother that her child does eat enough even though his eating consists of snacks rather than sit-down meals. Whether teaching is conducted with a group or with a single person, formally or informally, the principles of effective teaching and learning are the same.

THE ART OF TEACHING

Teaching is more than presenting information to people. It is presenting information in order to increase another's knowledge or insight. Stated another way, before teaching has taken place, learning or grasping of content must have taken place. Conversely, before learning takes place, teaching in some manner must have occurred. Teaching is inseparable from learning; you must first acquire the knowledge yourself and then impart it to another.

Principles of Teaching

A person who has reached the point of being a student in a school of nursing has had exposure to teachers for 12 to 15 years. Everyone can remember having one teacher whom they categorize as bad, hopefully one or more they categorize as good, and many others whose skill would be categorized as average. Despite this long-term exposure to so many teachers, the average person has little idea what it was that made a teacher good, bad, or average. In order to learn to be a health teacher, it is important to look at the principles of good teaching and to begin to incorporate them in your care.

Know the Subject. "A teacher learns more than his students" is an old educational truism. In order to teach a subject effectively, you must know it thoroughly. You must be able not only to present information to another but to answer his questions about the subject as well. This means that to present an hour's class on a subject such as breast self-examination you may need to read and prepare at least twice that length of time, perhaps 10 or 20 times longer. Because health care is a rapidly changing field, you cannot do this preparation just once; you have to constantly read new articles and research studies to be certain that what you thought was current information has not become obsolete. Learning is hard work and requires good teaching; teaching is hard work because it requires learning.

Know Your Learning Audience. The teaching techniques you will use will differ, depending on whom you are going to teach. If you are going to teach preschoolers to improve their health, you might choose to use puppets as a teaching aid and tooth brushing as a prime example of an area in which they could participate in their own health improvement. If you are going to teach the same subject—how to improve self health—to a group of business executives, it is not likely that your clever puppet and tooth brushing presentation would be well received. Conversely, a discussion on how to prevent heart attacks that might be well received by the businessmen would not hold preschoolers' attention. Knowing your audience—how many people will there be, what is their background, what are their interests—is the only effective way to be certain that you plan teaching strategies effectively.

Know Yourself. Teaching involves a multitude of techniques: lectures, small group discussion, role playing, audiovisual aids. It could concern any topic imaginable. Identify the teaching strategies that are right for you and topics that are comfortable for you. This does not mean that you are limited to these areas, just that when you move outside these areas you will probably need to prepare yourself better than normally for teaching. You may need to admit to a patient that the area of concern is one that you are not familiar with, so he does not interpret your discomfort as discomfort with him but with a teaching area.

Assess Individual Learning Styles. Not all people learn best in the same way. Some need to see a visual image before they can grasp a concept; for others that would not be necessary. Learn a variety of teaching techniques so that you can adjust teaching to a patient's individual learning style. Being able to establish rapport—individual harmonious relationships—in teaching is the basic reason why some teachers are rated good when most are average (Fig. 16-1).

Define Teaching Goals. Teaching goals serve as guidelines to help you select from all you know about a subject, the parts that you are going to teach and determine the order in which to teach them. If you are going to teach a patient to crutch-walk, for example, your goals with the businessman who is going to return to work in a 12-story office building would probably include how to walk safely on wet rain-soaked pavement, how to maneuver elevator doors, and how to carry a briefcase with crutches. If the person is a homemaker with two small children, your goals would probably include suggestions on how to carry an infant safely and how to walk up and down stairs. Setting goals allows you to isolate pertinent material so that you do not overwhelm people with too much material or give them too little for adequate learning.

Incorporate Principles of Learning in Teaching. Teaching is not effective unless learning occurs. Being aware of principles of learning (discussed below) helps you to organize teaching and choose teaching methods that are effective.

Provide an Environment Conducive to Learning. Learning can take place any time, any place, and under any circumstances. If a concept to be grasped is difficult, however, it is learned best in an environment that is free from distraction with suitable learning materials. A great deal of health teaching can be incorporated informally into care, such as talking to a person about the importance of turning frequently to protect against

FIGURE 16-1. Establishing rapport is the beginning of a teaching experience.

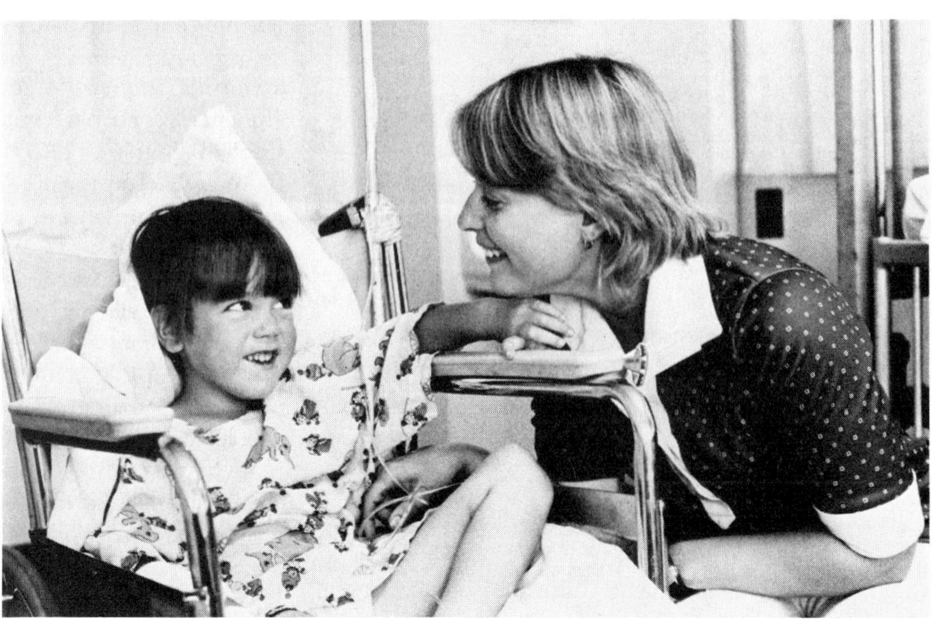

pressure areas while you give a bath and assess skin condition. Other areas of teaching, such as how to give a self-injection, are best done in a sit-down session, concentrating on the procedure for a half hour. Keep teaching time periods short. Divide material into segments so that a person does not grow bored but finds each period attention holding. Include teaching as a definite priority goal in nursing care plans; reserve space for it and give it the same priority as other care.

Be Consistent. Nothing is more confusing when you are learning a skill for the first time than to have a person tell you two or three different ways to do it. Choose one method that you think would work best for a person and then consistently stress that method. Alert other health care providers to the method you have taught so that they can reinforce consistently. After a person has learned a skill, you may suggest alternate methods if he is interested, but trying to learn the basic skill and the alternative actions at one time can be overwhelming.

Recognize That Nonverbal Teaching Is as Effective as Verbal. People watch your facial expressions and your gestures as much as they listen to what you say. To make a teaching point, be certain that a nonverbal statement is not contradicting a verbal one.

Acknowledge That People May Learn More Than You Teach. The store of human knowledge continues to grow because students take the knowledge they gain and improve on it. It is probable that the first man who noticed that round objects roll better than flat or square ones could not envision that in the future every family would own an individual vehicle rolling on round wheels. It is not unusual to teach a person how to change a dressing one day and the next day have the person show you a way to do it that is more economical or neater. Do not be threatened by this. It is not a statement that you did not teach well; it is a consequence of having taught so well that your student continued learning after you left.

Teach Principles, Not Do-as-I-say Actions. Teaching a person the principle behind why he is doing something gives him reason to do it. It promotes self-care and self-esteem because it allows him to modify and change to an alternate method as long as the principle is fulfilled.

Teach What People Should Do, Not What They Should Not. As a rule of thumb, teaching from a positive standpoint makes learning more enjoyable. Teaching what foods a person will be able to eat, not what foods he will be unable to eat, what activities he will be able to participate in, not what activities he cannot do, is the best approach. Some negative things must be presented, of course, but try to put your stress on achievement, not restriction. A person with recurrent seizures, for example, must never swim alone because if he suffered a seizure while swimming alone he would probably drown. You can stress that such a restriction is not really a restriction: No one should swim alone as anyone could develop abdominal cramps while swimming alone and drown. Health care information is information to last for a lifetime. Thinking of it in a positive way makes it applicable to lifetime use.

Be Specific. Be certain that your instructions are explicit so that when the person is home alone he can follow them accurately. Do not tell people to drink "a lot" or to do something "a few times every day." A person's "lot" may be 1,000 ml different from your conception of "a lot"; his "few times a day" may be two while you meant six or eight. State the instruction specifically as to what you want: "Drink an eight-ounce glass of water four times a day."

Teach From the Simple to the Complex. Before you could begin to learn to read, first you had to learn the names and the sounds of alphabet letters. Once you had all those fundamentals grasped, you actually learned to read in a matter of seconds.

Many times before you can teach a person what he must learn to get well again, you must review how his body functions when he is well as well as provide information on the way he is ill. Many people have little idea about body anatomy or physiology. You often have to begin with this basic level and gradually work up to the more complex to make the complex material comprehensible.

Use Leveling. Leveling is a technique for breaking up a great deal of information into segments so that a person is exposed to a section at a time and not overwhelmed by the total amount of information to be learned. A person recovering from a serious respiratory illness, for example, is going to have to learn breathing exercises, some weight reduction activities, some hypertension reduction precautions, a medication schedule, and special steps to take if he should develop extreme shortness of breath. What will be taught first could be decided on the basis of what interests him the most, what will show him the best results (immediate reward) first, or an easy-to-learn to difficult-to-learn order. Information is also said to be leveled if it is arranged from the most simple to the most complex.

Leveling is a technique that is effective because it moves the person's learning progressively forward. It is a useful technique in situations other than formal teaching: it can also be used to impart sad or stressful information to someone. It is often necessary to break down bad news into small segments (level it) so that the person is not exposed to the entire message at once when it would be too traumatic or stressful for him to accept. As an example, you would not say "Mrs. Jones? This is the nurse from the intensive care unit calling.

Your husband is dead," but "Mrs. Jones? This is Miss Smith, a nurse from the intensive care unit calling. You know that your husband has been very ill since last Thursday and all of us hope that when people are so ill they will get better again. When people are as ill as your husband though, that doesn't always happen. (pause) Half an hour ago your husband had a second heart attack. It's very difficult for a heart to stand that much insult. I'm sorry that I'm the person who has to call you with such bad news. (pause) Everyone did everything possible. He said he loved you and to say goodbye. But he has died."

A leveled message allows the person hearing it, by connecting the clues along the way (intensive care unit, some people die, second heart attack, bad news), to expect the end of your message before you reach it. It is a communication device that you have heard used often, but you probably were never aware of it as a technique. For example, a dentist may have said to you: "You should have cleaned your teeth better. If you don't clean teeth well, you develop holes in them that have to be filled. (Bottom line: You have cavities that need filling.)

Leveling is employed spontaneously with practice. At first it takes some plotting to sense, by looking at the person's face, when he is ready for you to move to the next level. As you become proficient at this technique, you will realize that you rarely need to deliver the bottom line as the person interrupts to say it for you: "You're calling to say he's dead, aren't you?" "You're telling me I have cavities, aren't you?" You need to develop this technique for breaking down information into small segments so that you can therapeutically deliver stressful information to people in the way that will allow them to accept it best.

Include Evaluation As a Final Step of Teaching. Since teaching has not been successful unless learning takes place, the only way to know if teaching has been effective is to test or evaluate if learning occurred. Structure the time and method of evaluation when you first establish a teaching plan.

THE ART OF LEARNING

Learning is a two-step process: acquiring new knowledge and then changing behavior based on the new knowledge. Learning has taken place when the change in behavior is measurable.

Types of Learning

Learning is not only a double process but it involves more than one type of activity. Learning the mathematic formula necessary to manufacture plastic, for example, is a different type of learning than learning how to skateboard. Learning to be kind to animals is yet another type. Before beginning teaching, evaluating the prominent type of learning you wish to occur helps to set goals and design teaching strategies.

COGNITIVE LEARNING

Cognitive learning is a change in the person's level of *understanding* or *knowledge.* Learning the principle behind why a particular medicine must be injected into a muscle, not subcutaneous tissue, is cognitive learning. Cognitive learning requires adequate intelligence and attention span. It can be gained through exposure to any teaching technique but is usually learned through lectures, reading, and audiovisual aids.

PSYCHOMOTOR LEARNING

Psychomotor learning is a change in a person's ability to perform a *skill.* Actually learning to hold a syringe and draw up medicine and inject it into muscle is an example of psychomotor learning. Psychomotor skill acquisition depends on muscle and neurological coordination. It is usually mastered best through exposure to demonstration and redemonstration.

AFFECTIVE LEARNING

Affective learning is a change in a person's *attitude.* It is the most difficult area to teach as it is the most difficult area in which to effect change. You may successfully teach a person the reason for and the skill of giving a self-injection, for example, but you may never be able to teach him to *like* giving a self-injection. Affective learning is gained best through role modeling, role playing, or shared-experience discussions.

Learning and Life Span Concepts

The learning ability and consequently teaching techniques used differ, depending on a person's age and developmental level.

THE INFANT

An infant learns by exploring his environment with his senses. He learns best from the person who is his primary caregiver because it is this person whom he most wants to please. There are few health care points that you teach infants as such; any that you do teach must be presented not as a structured activity but as a game or an amusing or attractive activity for the child.

As a rule, do not try to change an infant's routine of care while he is ill (unless it was the routine of care that was making him ill). He needs the assurance of knowing what is coming next as much as possible while he is ill.

THE TODDLER

Remember that children during the toddler period are developing a sense of autonomy or learning to be independent. Trying to teach a two-year-old a new activity such as eating a new food or brushing his teeth may be met with a sharp "No!" as the child exerts this new independence. The retort does not mean that the activity is not appealing to the child, merely that he is aware that he does not have to do everything anyone wants him to do. Toddlers sometimes resist a change in routine because they need rituals in order to feel secure.

THE PRESCHOOLER

Preschool children are very interested in learning; it is the main developmental task of the period. Provided that instructions are geared to their still small vocabularies, they "soak up" new methods of doing things. Because they are so imaginative and uninhibited, they will freely redemonstrate a skill to you.

They are very frightened, however, of intrusive procedures (rectal temperature taking, bladder catheterization, nasopharyngeal suction). They typically remove Bandaids minutes after application to check on the condition of the skin underneath (that it has not disappeared); they worry that any blood removed is the last they have. Teaching this type of procedure or explaining to the child why it is necessary calls for clear explanations.

Preschool children ask many questions about equipment and procedures. Keep explanations short; a preschooler's attention span rarely exceeds 5 minutes. Listen to your vocabulary; would you have understood the words you are using when you were that age?

THE SCHOOLAGE CHILD

Schoolage children enjoy short projects that offer an immediate reward. They learn best if a procedure is broken down into different stages, therefore, and presented as several short procedures rather than one long one.

Schoolage children are used to learning things and accept learning a new procedure or new information as just another experience in a busy day. The "staying power" of schoolage children is notoriously short, however; the ability to continue to perform at the level taught tends to decrease sharply if learning is not reinforced. Be certain that a backup person in the home knows the health care information so that they can reinforce it or carry out a procedure of care as necessary.

Toward the end of the schoolage period children become very interested in doing only those things that their friends are also doing. Asking a child to do something after school (come home and do breathing exercises) that is different from what all his friends are doing (stopping at the playground) may be interpreted as unreasonable by him. Modify a teaching plan as necessary to help him fit what he must learn into his school and social schedule or your teaching will be very short-lived.

Schoolage children thrive on rules or the "right way" to do things. Be certain that if two or more people are going to be involved in teaching that you teach consistently. It is frustrating for a schoolage child to not have a "right way" to do something.

THE ADOLESCENT

The adolescent, struggling for identity, likes to learn things separately from his parents. He can be responsible for his own self-care as a rule; if he understands how the new actions he has been taught will directly benefit him, unlike the schoolage child he will continue to carry them out conscientiously after he returns home. He has a strong need to be exactly like his friends, however; he will not continue any action that makes him different or conspicuous in front of his friends.

Adolescents are very present oriented; they learn procedures and new information best if they can see how it will immediately benefit them. They learn poorly if the only benefit of new information presented to them is something that will happen in the future. Rotating insulin injection sites, for example, prevents "pock-mark" formations in the skin when the person reaches about thirty. Given this information, an adolescent tends not to rotate injection sites, because the benefit is not relevant to him. An explanation such as "Rotating injection sites will ensure insulin absorption and dependability and allow you to play basketball this season" (an equally true statement) is a better adolescent motivator.

THE YOUNG ADULT

Young adults are careless about their health (an it-can't-happen-to-me attitude). They may not be interested in learning much about an illness (what I don't know can't hurt me). They may return to a health care agency several times with complications from not following instructions before they are convinced of the importance of the information. Young adults who live by themselves or in college dormitories may work very hard to learn a new technique or procedure if it will allow them to continue to live independently. Be certain to locate a backup person for anyone living alone to help reinforce or be a person to call on if they need extra guidance or support. Some young adults are unable to name a support person they would truly trust to be a backup person (their friends have no more experience than they do); they rely on health care personnel to act in this position for them.

THE MIDDLE-AGED ADULT

Many middle-aged adults have to be taught a new life style (eat less, maintain a regular exercise program, decrease alcohol intake). These are difficult areas to change because not only is the person you are talking to affected but other family members and perhaps people at work as well. Some middle-aged adults who think of themselves as old are reluctant to change, thinking it is only for another couple of years at best. They need a realistic appraisal from their physician that middle age is not old and that modifications made at this stage of life can allow them to reach older age.

THE OLDER ADULT

The average older adult is like the young adult, anxious to learn new techniques or procedures if learning such information will allow him to remain independent and not have to move into a child's home or an extended care facility. He will practice long beyond the attention span of a younger person, devising measures to modify a procedure so that he can manage it despite lesser sensation in one hand or poor vision. This results from a lifetime of problem solving skill (Fig. 16-2).

People with the intense desire to remain independent need support in their effort. Their support people may need some reassurance that it is desirable for the person to remain independent—that driving across town to check on an older adult daily may be more inconvenient than it would be if the parent moved in with them, but independence at any life stage is important.

Be certain that an older adult does have a support person who can serve as his backup in health care as necessary. Be certain that you carefully assess vision and hearing ability before beginning health teaching; in an effort to remain independent, an older adult may lead you to believe he sees or hears slightly better than he does.

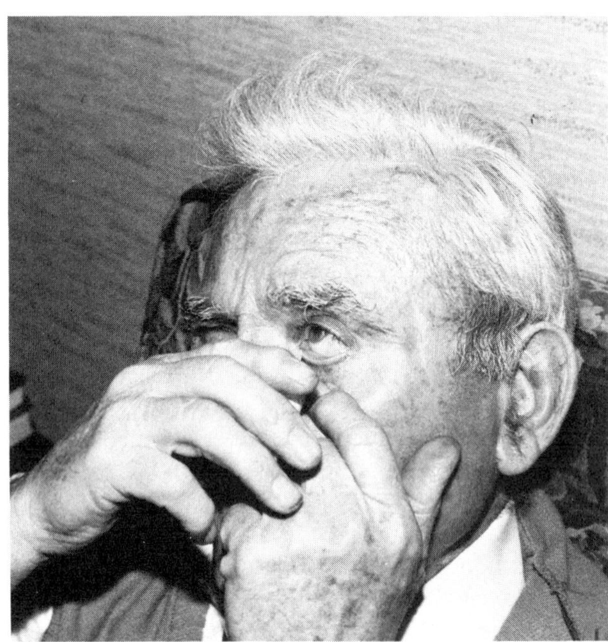

FIGURE 16-2. This older man with a chronic eye condition is learning to instill eye drops. Teaching him to tip back his head while he does this would probably be your next teaching goal.

Principles of Learning

No matter what type of learning is to be the predominant one stressed or the age of the person being taught, the same principles of learning apply.

Learning Occurs Only When a Person is Ready to Learn. Interferences with learning may be physical (pain, chills, hunger) or psychological (fear, anxiety). When a person learns that he is going to have his leg amputated, he is not apt to be ready to learn the technique of crutch-walking immediately; his level of anxiety is far too high. It is important to remember this rule when people are beginning oxygen therapy. You must teach people and their visitors that oxygen supports combustion and that lighting a cigarette near an open oxygen outlet could cause an explosion. However, people with oxygen being administered and the people who care about them may not "hear" your instructions about smoking in such situations; they are so nervous and anxious (times when they enjoy a cigarette) that it is not unusual to watch a visitor shake a cigarette out of his pack even as he is nodding that he understands your instruction about not smoking. When oxygen is being administered, you must recheck that your instruction was understood as well as heard.

Learning Occurs Most Quickly If the Person Can See How the New Information Will Benefit Him. Sixteen-year-olds learn how to drive a car very quickly because they grasp readily that being able to drive will immediately enlarge their world. A person who is dying may not be interested in learning a new procedure as he cannot conceive how he will ever use the new knowledge. On the other hand, he may be very interested in carrying out the procedure so that he can maintain self-care as long as possible. Make a habit of including in your introduction of new information the benefits of learning it (learning coughing before surgery results in less respiratory complications and a shorter hospital stay following surgery).

Learning Occurs Best if Rewards, Not Penalties, are Offered. Notice the amount of shoulder patting and back slapping that a coach engages in the next time you watch a basketball or football game; a minimum amount of criticism is used. When you have been exposed to it for a long time, health information or a procedure may seem so simple that when a person, exposed to the information or techniques for the first time, grasps it, it is easy to overlook the fact that this is a big accomplishment for that individual and neglect to acknowledge it. Give positive reinforcement immediately as this makes it more effective than if it is delayed. If you must criticize the way a task was done, first compliment the person on some aspect he did well and then explain about the part that needs improvement (overall, you did a good job; there's one thing, though, we ought to talk about . . .). This increases self-esteem and allows him to feel good enough about himself that he can accept the criticism. Never be reluctant to praise in public; always criticize in private.

People Learn Best by Actively Participating in Learning. Lecturing is not as a rule an effective teaching method for health care because lecturing does not involve the person deeply in learning. If you have a long procedure to teach, such as how to draw up and inject insulin, break down the procedure into steps and teach them one by one (see box below). Teach and demonstrate drawing up the medicine, then allow the person to participate by practicing the skill. Next teach the actual injection: Demonstrate and again, as soon as possible, allow the person to practice (Fig. 16-3). Breaking up a procedure this way allows the person to be actively involved as soon as possible and immediately makes learning more meaningful. Most nursing students feel that an academic subject that has an accompanying laboratory experience will be a more interesting class for them than one that does not have "hands-on" experience.

Learning Takes Place Best in a Nonstressful and Accepting Environment. No one wants to take a chance redemonstrating a procedure or asking a question if he feels that his actions or opinions will not be respected. Not everyone learns at the same pace; not everyone is

TEACHING PLAN: BOB EVANS, 16 YEARS OLD
Insulin Preparation and Injection

Goal: Patient will learn self insulin injection technique in 1 week.
Criteria: Patient will state correct principles and demonstrate correct technique of self injection.

Cognitive Aspects	*Psychomotor Skills*	*Affective Aspects*	*Teaching Methods*	*Time Frame*
Function of insulin as a regulator of body carbohydrate; importance of balance between insulin and glucose.		He will need to take insulin for his lifetime.	Lecture flashcards. Film: "I'm a Diabetic too."	By Tuesday
Importance of sterile technique, types of insulin, equipment necessary.	Handles syringe, needle and vial with sterile technique. Withdraws insulin from one vial.		Demonstration-redemonstration	By Wednesday
Technique of mixing insulins; principle of withdrawing short-acting first.	Mixes two types of insulins in one syringe with sterile technique.		Demonstration-redemonstration	By Thursday
Importance of rotating injection sites; injection technique.	Identifies acceptable injection sites and system for rotation of sites; injects insulin.		Diagram of rotation sites. Demonstration-redemonstration.	By Friday
Total process of preparation and insulin injection.	Mixes short-acting and long-acting insulin in one syringe and injects, using good technique.			By Saturday
Evaluation				
Can achieve mastery (85%) of information on adolescent series flash cards.	Can redemonstrate mixing and injecting of insulin with safe and aseptic technique.	Voices confidence in own ability. Subjectively demonstrates a positive cooperative attitude.		

TEACHING POINTS

Learning Style

Intelligence above average by school IQ report. Was shy at first contact; still doesn't verbalize concerns well unless asked directly (a raised eyebrow best clue he is puzzled). Responds well to verbal praise; appears to learn best by actually doing (hands-on activities). Mother states he will act bored when insecure; very negative reactions to criticism (door slamming, sulking for hours).

Important Points for Consistency

1. Teach to inject with a no. 25 3/8-inch needle at 90-degree angle.
2. Teach to use 2 deltoid and 2 anterior thighs for injection sites (talking about using abdominal sites made him visibly shudder).
3. Do not teach to add extra bubble of air to syringe (not an IM injection).
4. Keep insulin being used at room temperature.
5. Always draw up short-acting insulin first.

Support Person to be Taught

He wants his father to be his backup person. Mother's job takes her out of town about three days a month. Apparently good relationship between him and Dad.

Teaching Strategies

1. Reward with verbal praise.
2. Allow him adequate "hands-on" practice.
3. Ask for concerns or questions.
4. Keep atmosphere positive. Information has to last him a lifetime.

interested in learning in the same order; no one can learn under stress especially if the learning atmosphere is the factor that is causing the stress. People do learn from "top sergeants"—and sometimes rapidly, just to be free of the situation—but the learning experience has so many unpleasant memories attached to it that they do not tend to retain the learning. Health teaching is too important (a person's life depends on it) to be presented in a way that will lead to its being quickly discarded.

People Learn Best Those Things That Hold a Particular Interest for Them. Everyone is more interested in certain things than in others. When a person has a disease such as diabetes mellitus, for example, he needs to learn about insulin injection, diet, and signs and symptoms of high and low blood glucose levels (hyperglycemia and hypoglycemia). The person who enjoys cooking may be most interested in the diet information (or least interested because he does not want to change the way he cooks); the person who enjoys mathematics may be most interested in determining how he must balance intake and utilization of glucose; the person hoping to return to work quickly may see insulin administration as the key to this and be most interested in this area. As a rule of thumb, presenting information in the order that most appeals to a person makes learning easiest. Learning occurs best when a person is motivated to learn.

Learning Ability Plateaus. People learn to a point of saturation; learning and interest in learning halts at that point and does not continue until the material learned is thoroughly digested and understood. Pushing a person to learn when he is at a plateau level is ineffective because he simply is not ready to learn more at that time. Wait until the information is processed; at that point the person will be interested once more.

A TEACHING PLAN

The knowledge necessary for a person to keep himself well or to safely care for himself when he is ill should be marked in a patient's care plan; this is the minimal amount of information that must be transmitted before the nurse-patient contact can be safely terminated. In most instances a teaching plan will include much more information than just this basic knowledge.

Steps in Developing a Teaching Plan

The first step in developing a teaching plan is to assess the patient's current level of knowledge, his ability to learn the new knowledge, and your ability to teach the new knowledge.

ASSESSMENT OF CURRENT KNOWLEDGE

To learn how much the person currently knows about the area in question, you need to first ask him some questions to determine his level of knowledge and then assess implementation. If you are designing a teaching plan to teach a new mother the basic skills of infant care before she brings her newborn child home from the hospital, you first need to know how much she already knows about infant care (Fig. 16-4). If this is her first child, she will most likely admit that despite the pamphlets she read during pregnancy, she does not feel

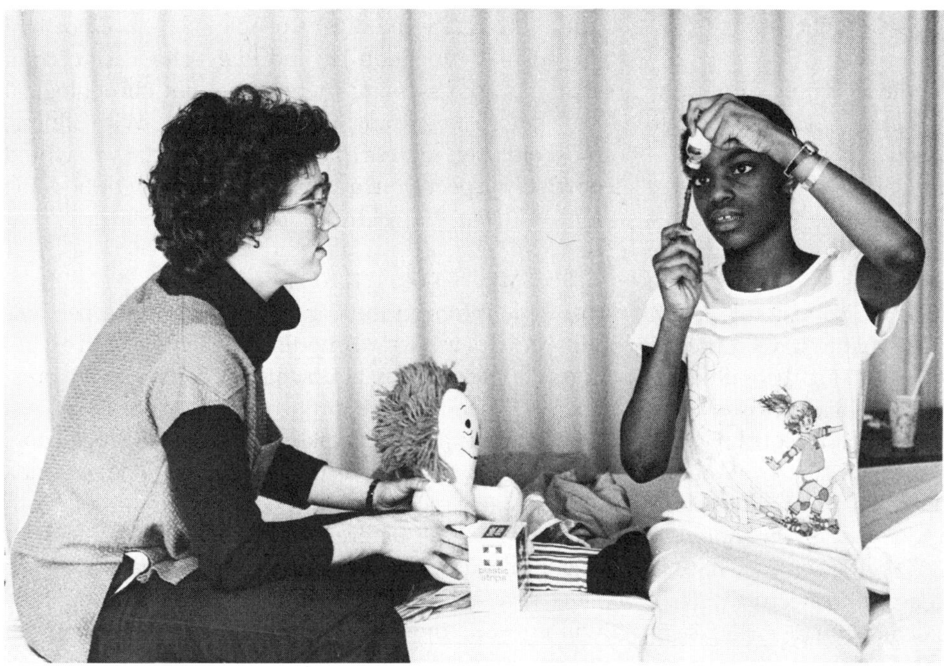

FIGURE 16-3. A 13-year-old girl withdraws insulin from a vial. She will next learn to inject the insulin into Raggedy Andy's thigh, then her own.

FIGURE 16-4. A nurse assesses how much this new mother knows about infant care.

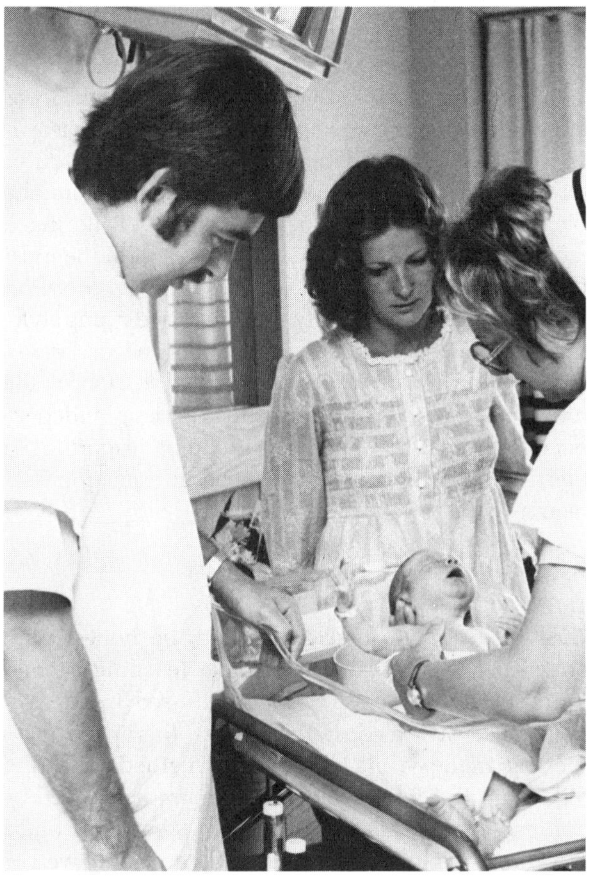

overly confident about any aspect of care and would like you to at least review them. If, on the other hand, this is the woman's sixth child, there may be only one or two points (answers to questions, actually) that she needs help with. Do not stereotype, however. A mother having her first newborn may have spent the last four months caring for her sister's newborn and be very experienced and confident about her care; a woman having her sixth child may not have had a baby for five years and may feel like a first-time mother.

The same assessment is necessary to determine how much a person knows about an illness. Some illnesses (hemophilia, a bleeding disorder, for example) are hereditary; the person may have lived with someone with the illness for years and may know more about what home care problems occur with the illness than you do; on the other hand, what he knows about the illness may be accompanied by so many "old wives' tales" that he needs a great deal of teaching in order not to be hampered by half-truths or unnecessary restraints.

ASSESSMENT OF PHYSICAL CAPABILITIES

If a procedure such as medicine administration or a dressing change (psychomotor skill) will be necessary for care, assess the person's physical ability to perform them. It will be frustrating for both you and the person if you expect a performance above what the person's physical limitations allow him to do. Assess in particular vision and hearing ability and right or left hand dominance; these are important considerations for determining not only whether the person can accomplish the procedure but also how you will present and demonstrate material to him.

ASSESSMENT OF PSYCHOLOGICAL OR EMOTIONAL CAPABILITIES

People may have more difficulty learning about any aspect of their care if it is somewhat distasteful to them. The person who uses food as comfort, for example, may have trouble learning about a restrictive diet because it conflicts with the way he likes to view food. A person with a urinary or bowel disorder may have difficulty learning about these illnesses if he thinks of these parts of his body as "dirty" or distasteful. People with a reproductive tract illness may have difficulty discussing and asking questions about their illness if they were raised to avoid discussion of sexual functions.

Be aware that some people still unconsciously equate illness with punishment. A person who believes that he deserves his illness may not be ready to learn measures that will make him better (he does not feel he should be better or is not worthy of being well). You may have to take some measures to increase self-esteem or give a lesson on bacterial infection before you plan disease or therapy education.

ASSESSMENT OF LEVEL OF EDUCATION

A person's level of education alerts you to the level of vocabulary you will need to use to teach. It alerts you to reading level if you are going to rely on pamphlets or other reading materials as a means of teaching. It also subtly alerts you to a person's overall experience in life: That a person has attended college away from home suggests that he can independently problem solve—otherwise, he would not have survived college; a person who left school at 16 and then worked so conscientiously that he is now an important member of a corporation has had a similar life experience. This may be helpful information to you in planning overall care as well as health teaching. In either instance, you know that you are dealing with a person who is used to problem solving; rather than being told the best way to arrange a medication schedule, such a person might feel most comfortable designing a schedule independently and just checking the completed form with you.

ASSESSMENT OF ATTENTION SPAN

The attention span of an individual and his capability to comprehend concepts and perform psychomotor skills differ a great deal depending on age. In general, the younger the person, the more attention getting you must make your presentation.

Some older adults' attention spans are also short. Evaluate each individual separately, however; just as some 4-year-olds respond at the level of 10-year-olds, some 90-year-olds are more aware of sound health care practices than the average 20-year-old.

ASSESSMENT OF INTELLECTUAL CAPABILITY

Intellectual capability may in many instances be inferred from educational level, but not necessarily. There are many intelligent people who have not had any formal education beyond high school. Be certain that you are assessing mental age, not chronological age, before beginning health teaching. With illness, most children regress at least slightly; what you would normally expect from a 10-year-old may not be possible for an *ill* ten-year-old.

ASSESSMENT OF LIFE STYLE

Life style refers to the common pattern of a person's life. You may have to modify a teaching plan to accommodate working hours, habits, diets, and the presence or absence of support people. Do not teach a night worker, for example, to take medicine four times a day; teach him to take it four times a night. Do not expect a child to carry medicine to school; help him to space out the time intervals before and after school. Do not advise a long-distance truck driver to take antihistamines for sinus headaches (they tend to make people sleepy); he will not take them, or worse, will take them and fall asleep on a highway at 50 miles an hour.

The more you know about a person, the easier it is to teach him because you can more readily see the problem through the person's eyes and adjust a therapeutic plan of care for him.

ASSESSMENT OF LEARNING STYLE

Some people learn well from verbal descriptions. Other people have to see a statement in print before they can fully comprehend it. Still others are very visually oriented; if they see a picture or a diagram of something, they grasp the explanation almost immediately. This is a person's learning style and it differs from person to person. Few people are aware of their learning style so they are unable to tell you what it is. After working with them for a period of time, you should be able to detect the way they learn best. Tailoring a teaching plan to a learning style will result in the most effective learning situation.

Parents can often identify their child's learning style. Listen for such comments as "stubborn" or "won't listen to a thing"; they probably refer not so much to the child's learning style as his need to experience independence. They let you know that it will be important to determine the child's learning style in order for your teaching to be effective.

ASSESSING YOUR STRENGTHS AND LIMITATIONS

When formulating a teaching plan, be honest with yourself. If you feel uncomfortable teaching a child about surgery by clever puppets dressed in surgical scrub suits, you may do better to avoid this approach to teaching; in the wrong hands such a method can sound so flat that the child is left feeling more frightened by the presentation than comforted (children rely strongly on feeling tone to assess when things are going well or not). Attempting to use a teaching method with which you are uncomfortable may cause persons of any age to interpret your insecurity as evidence that there is something wrong with them, not with the method.

Some health teaching involves giving instructions in areas of care that may be personally embarrassing for you (instructing a member of the opposite sex how to obtain a clean catch urine, for example). If you do find yourself about to give instructions that you are not comfortable in presenting, proceeding blindly may not result in effective teaching because the person may be so embarrassed by your discomfort that he or she cannot concentrate on the instructions. Do not be reluctant to ask for help from someone skilled in health teaching to review with you the best way to present a technique or to role model the teaching for you. In doing this type of teaching, nothing serves you so well (as in any patient contact) as honesty. Admit to the patient that you are not used to giving this type of instruction to men (or women). This approach will probably evoke from the person a response that he is not used to having anyone talk to him about it. Once you have found common ground (this is not the most comfortable discussion for either of you), you have a basis for effective health teaching. Honesty also allows the person to know that your discomfort is not from lack of knowledge on the subject (he can trust what you are saying) and not from a fault of his (the subject, not the person is the disturbing factor).

Assess your level of knowledge. Do not try to teach what you do not know. A person can only learn from your teaching if you not only present material well but also can answer any questions he has about the material. Anyone who is not sure of an area of information tends to gloss over it. Health-related questions become easier to answer the more you teach. On the other hand, no matter how well prepared you are, you will not know the answer to all questions. *Nothing serves you so well as honesty.* A reply that is a bluff ("Well, what most people in your circumstances do is . . .") easily destroys your credibility. The patient suspects you are bluffing and not only is this point lost but your entire teaching strength is in question (how can he be certain that your information on diet and exercise was accurate?). An answer of "I don't know" is not helpful but at least is credible; an answer of "I don't know but I'll find that out for you" is a professional health teaching answer. It both maintains credibility (no one asks you to be perfect, only helpful) and obtains the adequate information.

PREPARING PATIENT GOALS

Learning goals should reflect the type of learning desired: cognitive, psychomotor, or affective. It is not necessary (and often overwhelming) for a person to learn everything about his illness in the first day or week following his diagnosis. Information on how to stay well does not need to be presented in one setting. In many instances, you teach part of the information needed and another nurse in another setting such as a community health nurse might teach the remainder. Quick Reference Stop 16-1 summarizes some of the nursing research carried out to find out what patients need to learn and what the best teaching method might be.

Setting patient goals helps to establish time guidelines. Be certain that goals are consistent with the person's ability to learn and that the time frame is appropriate. State teaching goals as behavioral objectives, the activity you expect the person to demonstrate when he has learned the new knowledge—not "Mr. Jones will understand the importance of a low-salt diet" but "Mr. Jones will eat a low-salt diet." (Learning is a two-step process involving not only gaining new information but then acting on the information.)

DETERMINE TEACHING STRATEGIES

Although you have been watching teachers teach for the greater part of your life, you may not be aware of the strategies of teaching they have been using. Strategies of teaching are most effective when they are intermixed and when they are selected in response to the individual person to be taught.

Lecture. Lecture is the most efficient and time-saving method of offering information to both individuals and large groups. A lecture method, however, does not allow for active participation (other than active listening), and is usually effective only in short well-structured time spans.

Demonstration. Demonstration is actually performing a procedure such as a dressing change or instillation of eye drops so that the person can see clearly how the procedure should be done. Never demonstrate a procedure unless you are certain that you are comfortable with the steps of it and any equipment to be used. If you stop in the middle of the demonstration to ask yourself, "What do I do next?" or have to say, "Before you do this, you really should put on gloves, don't do as I just did," the poor technique demonstrated may be the lesson learned, not the good technique you wanted to show. Be certain that you have all the supplies you need before beginning. "Pretend I have a catheter" is not effective demonstration. The purpose of demonstration is to actually show how the procedure is done; having to imagine steps of it is little different from reading about it.

Redemonstration. To know if a person has truly grasped your demonstration, ask him to redemonstrate the procedure to you. Redemonstration is best if it immediately follows demonstration and the person can immediately mimic your motions. Praise the effort

☐ **QUICK REFERENCE STOP 16-1: RESEARCH**
Patient Teaching Goals

Patient teaching is an important component of nursing care. But how do nurses know what patients need to learn and what the best teaching methods might be? A number of studies have been carried out to help nurses determine the answers to these questions.

ASSESSING THE NEEDS OF THE LEARNER—WHAT LEARNING NEEDS DO PATIENTS HAVE?

The interview technique was utilized with a small sample of 15 hospitalized patients to determine what and how much patients really wanted to know about their illnesses and/or treatments. Data from this study indicated that most patients want to know specific facts about their illness. The researchers caution, however, that each patient should be assessed individually for his/her learning desires and needs (Barrett and Schwartz, 1981).

Lauer and co-workers (1982) investigated the learning needs of cancer patients, in particular, to determine if there was a difference in learning needs for the patient as perceived by the nurse and by the patient. The nursing literature is abundant with recommendations for teaching cancer patients various kinds of information related to their illness, treatment, and so on. These researchers sought to validate the usefulness of this information to the patients. Questionnaire and interview technique was utilized to determine how important nurses and patients rated specific learning needs. The results of the study revealed that nurses rated "general information" items, such as self-care, diagnosis, and treatment plan, as significantly more important than the patients did. "Nurses identified 'dealing with feelings' as the area patients wanted the most information about, but the patients ranked this much lower" (p. 16). Patients apparently wanted the most information about "minimizing the side effects of therapy."

CAN PATIENTS REALLY COMPREHEND THE READING MATERIALS WE GIVE THEM?

Written materials are often used in patient education. Yet, it seems, the appropriateness of these materials for patients may often be in question. Mohammed (1964), in a classic study, investigated a population of patients attending a diabetic clinic. She found their abilities inconsistent with the reading levels of printed education materials available to them. Written material was found to be primarily at the eighth grade reading level while the population was found to have an average of 6.8 grades of schooling. The comprehension and learning achieved under conditions of such discrepancy certainly are questionable. The researcher concluded that written teaching materials need simplification and individualization for each patient.

SUGGESTED READINGS

Barrett, N., and M. D. Schwartz. What patients really want to know. *Am. J. Nurs.* 81(9):1642, 1981.

Lauer, P., Murphy, S. P., and Powers, M. J. Learning needs of cancer patients: A comparison of nurse and patient perceptions. *Nurs. Res.* 31(1):11, 1982.

Mohammed, M. F. B. Patients' understanding of written health information. *Nurs. Res.* 13(2):100, 1964.

to redemonstrate, even if the redemonstration is not of the quality you would have liked to have seen. No one likes to be put on the spot and if you show disappointment, the person may not be willing to expose himself to you again by a second demonstration. Be aware that there are many different ways to do almost everything. The person does not have to follow your motions exactly as long as any modification or adjustment he makes is still within the principle of what he must do to make the procedure safe and effective. An effective way to correct a wrong action is to say "That's one way of doing that; what usually works better, though, is . . ." or "You could do it that way, but as a rule most people find it easier to . . ." This type of criticism is fairly nonthreatening, since you first acknowledge that the person is doing well before correcting him.

Discussion. Discussion is a shared learning experience where the person asks questions about particular concerns and you answer them based on his individual circumstances; or you ask him questions about some problem, such as how he anticipates managing some aspect of his care, and together you work out a solution. At the beginning of health education a person may ask very few questions because he does not yet know enough about his illness to realize what his problems will be. As his knowledge increases, so does his ability to project and modify information given to him to his own life style.

Role Modeling. Role modeling is demonstrating a certain attribute or aura that you want the person to learn. Be certain when you are health teaching that you are radiating the attitude you want the person to learn. Showing frustration at getting a bubble out of medicine in a syringe demonstrates that giving injections is frustrating; a bored attitude toward diet instruction implies that nutrition information is boring. Is that what you mean to teach? Actions speak louder than words. The person subtly picks up your role modeling cues sometimes more readily than he does your spoken message.

Visual Aids. "A picture is worth a thousand words" is not an idle quotation but a very realistic one. It is surprising how little the average person knows about such things as where his body organs are located. If you are going to be doing teaching concerning body parts, it generally helps to have an anatomic illustration that shows the location of the particular body organ you are going to discuss. Figure 16-5 shows internal abdominal contents as an example of such a drawing. Copyright laws prohibit anyone from copying this type of illustration for group distribution but you can do so for use as an individual teaching aid.

Preschoolers know the names of common body parts such as hand and foot but may never have heard the terms *wrist* or *abdomen* used before and therefore may not be certain where the wrist ends and the arm begins or where the abdomen ends and the chest begins. Use an illustration that is helpful in identifying body parts or show a preschooler where he will be washed prior to surgery or where he will have his stitches after his surgery. Preschoolers dislike intrusive procedures; a finger placed on the abdomen is more threatening than a finger pointing to a drawing of this kind.

FIGURE 16-5. An illustration showing body parts appropriate for health teaching.

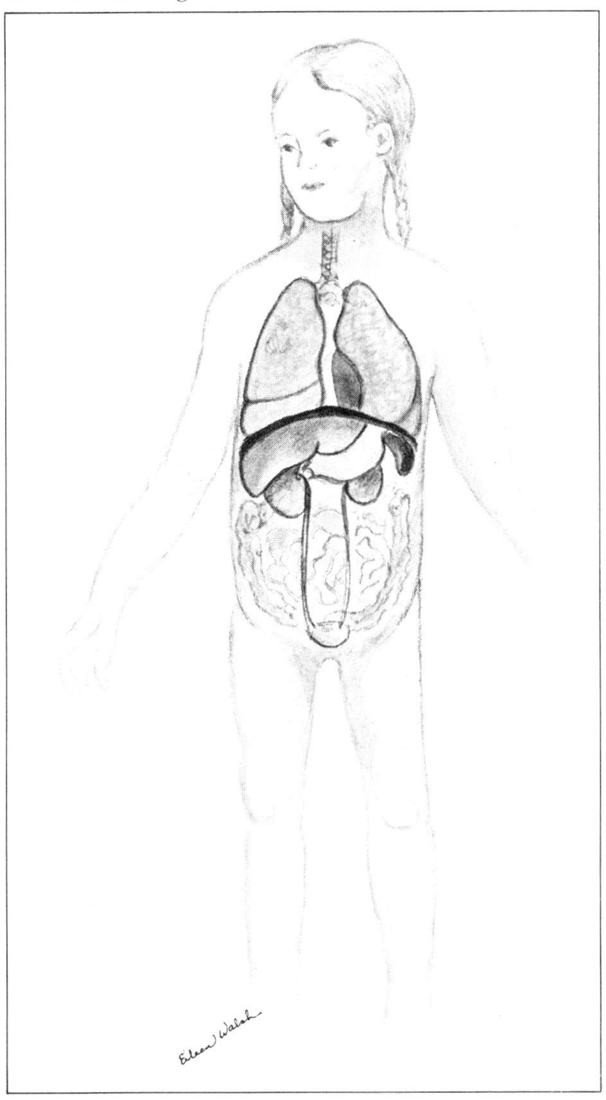

Do not be afraid to draw a picture of a heart, a kidney, a bladder, or any other organ to make a point about anatomic structure. The person you are teaching is more interested in understanding the procedure or the reason for the health maintenance measure that you are explaining than he is in criticizing your art work (and very likely does not know anatomy well enough to be able to tell that your drawing is distorted).

Pamphlets. Pamphlets are helpful teaching aids because they usually contain brief, easily understood informational material and are often clearly illustrated with cartoon characters to make them enjoyable. Do not judge a book by its covers, however. Carefully read any pamphlet before you offer it to a patient to be certain that you agree with the information included in it. Medical advances happen so quickly that a pamphlet only a year old may contain a gross inaccuracy in the light of subsequent knowledge.

Because a pamphlet has some statements in it that you do not agree with or that do not apply to your patient does not make the pamphlet unusable. Simply cross out the information that would be contradictory before offering it to the patient. If the information would be frightening, delete it completely so that the person cannot possibly read it; some people deliberately read what you tell them not to, afraid that you are protecting them from bad news or not being totally honest with them. Do not be misled into believing that because you give someone a clever pamphlet, they will necessarily read it and learn from it. What appeals to you as a learning method may not appeal to everyone.

Learning Games. For memorizing certain kinds of information, such as what foods are high or low in potassium or sodium, the use of flash cards is a helpful learning action. Children enjoy playing board games set up like Monopoly (instead of rolling dice, you pull a card with a question on it such as "Where is insulin produced in your body?" If you can answer the question correctly, you advance a designated number of spaces on the board). Children learn information quickly this way because the reward for learning is so immediate. Having the parent play the game with them educates the parent at the same time.

Word scrambles are easy games to originate. The word scramble in Figure 16-6, for example, deals with activities that are important for a person to do after

M	B	Q	R	J	K	B	C	A	Z	T	D
E	Y	N	C	G	F	O	W	B	H	J	L
K	O	S	P	I	A	C	R	F	S	D	X
U	F	M	G	Y	B	V	I	L	P	T	C
S	Q	I	R	J	S	F	D	W	H	N	G
T	K	L	W	M	C	H	E	A	J	Q	K
E	X	E	R	C	I	S	E	L	E	G	S
B	M	C	Q	O	R	N	P	K	P	S	T
R	J	K	Z	U	J	K	B	M	B	Q	R
T	D	N	C	G	B	C	R	E	Y	N	C
K	P	R	D	H	T	K	E	U	F	G	B
Y	V	U	T	H	N	L	A	T	K	R	J
M	B	Q	R	J	K	B	T	U	R	N	X
C	A	Z	T	D	E	Y	H	C	M	H	B
N	C	G	F	O	W	B	E	F	S	A	D
H	J	L	S	K	P	T	N	R	Y	V	O

FIGURE 16-6. A patient teaching project: Activities important to do after surgery. The patient can locate in the maze *cough*, *deep breathe*, *turn*, *exercise legs*, and *walk*, which will help improve his blood circulation and respiration, and *smile*, which will help improve his outlook.

surgery. Solving this type of maze is not necessarily an activity limited to children. Adults admitted for elective surgery are both bored and anxious preoperatively. Time spent on such an activity passes a little time in addition to reminding them that there are important things for them to do after surgery.

In a hospital setting patients are assigned to different nursing care units according to their medical diagnosis (all people having chest surgery are placed on the fourth floor, bone surgery on the third floor, and so on). On any nursing unit, therefore, while the people you care for differ greatly, the conditions they are admitted for may not. Learning games (flash cards, word scrambles, crossword puzzles) pertaining to particular areas of diagnosis can be duplicated and used with many people.

Video Tapes, Slides and Films. Many health care agencies have videotape playback equipment or slide or film projectors that you can use to show a short tape, film, or slide presentation as part of a health education program. As with pamphlets, be certain that you have viewed the material first before showing it; be certain to check that the vocabulary used is appropriate for your individual patient or audience.

Nursing Textbooks. Textbooks can be helpful teaching aids if you use pertinent portions. Be aware, though, that nursing textbooks cover not only prevention and treatment of illness but complications of illnesses as well. If you leave a textbook with a pregnant woman, for example, so that she can read what normal birth consists of, when you return, you will probably discover that she has also read (or at least looked at the photos) of the section on complications of childbirth and may be frightened that any or all of them may happen to her. It is realistic for people to know that pregnancy or illness can have complications, but learning about them in detail with illustrations may generate too much stress for the patient. It would be better to make a copy of the information that you want the person to read with acknowledgement of the source. Again, be aware that by copyright laws you cannot distribute copies to an entire class but it is permitted on an individual basis.

Written Instructions. Even though a person knows his medicine administration schedule or the foods he must include in his diet every day, he will probably be more likely to remember to take the medicine and eat more of the foods if he has this information in a written form as well. Memory plays tricks on all of us; information that we have completely memorized may be forgotten by the time we need to recall it.

Help people to prepare as many reminders as they need to continue taking medicine at home. It is well documented that people take medicine well as long as physical symptoms are present; at the point that the medicine administration becomes routine, they stop taking it (Mattar, 1975). With illnesses like hypertension where few symptoms are present, their time of compliance may be as short as three days. Give them a reminder chart for the refrigerator door or the bathroom mirror. Knowing that medicine is important is often not enough; a memory aid is often necessary to transfer knowing into doing.

Supplies. If you are working in a nursing unit where many people are admitted for the same type of illness or surgery, you find yourself teaching the same information over and over. To avoid having to reorganize equipment or instructions each time, put together a basket or box of supplies that contains all the information and equipment needed to teach a particular task. This ensures that the teaching will be done (no excuses like "I didn't have time to get equipment together") and is economical in that everyone on a unit is not using separate equipment. It also helps to make sure that everyone is teaching the same information. Nothing is more confusing to people learning a new skill than to be taught two different principles for doing it or two different approaches to the problem.

Resource People. Many health care agencies have specific persons who are available for health teaching about specific subjects (diabetes, colostomy care, respiratory exercises). Utilize such people as appropriate because they know all the "tricks of the trade" for teaching that particular skill. Remain nearby and listen to what they teach for your own information and so that you can answer any questions the patient asks after this person leaves. There is some controversy as to whether designating certain people as specific teachers (a diabetes teaching nurse, for example) is a good educational device. It is good if it results in all people with diabetes learning how to live with their illness in the best possible way. It is not good if the patient grasps the idea that it takes an expert to tell him about his care (if care is so complicated, how can he possibly learn it?), or if nurses adopt the philosophy that only the "expert" can teach a particular subject, that they have no responsibility for education in that area. Health teaching is a part of nursing care, and it is unfair to a patient to be told that his questions cannot be answered until the following day because that is the only time the appropriate person is available to answer them.

Evaluation

Evaluation or assessing whether teaching has been effective is the final step of teaching. In most health teaching situations evaluation takes place at follow-up visits by assessing whether the person is remaining as well as you have tried to teach him to be or has been able to return closer to wellness by following the techniques you taught him ("the proof is in the pudding" type of evaluation).

There is some advantage to asking people questions before and after teaching to assess their knowledge and to prove to yourself that you are an effective teacher as well as to assure yourself that the person has safely learned new health care measures. Demonstration of a change of behavior or attitude, however, is the real proof that learning has taken place.

If you are conducting a formal type of in-service program, ask people to rate the program as to whether it was helpful to them on a scale of one to ten. This type of evaluation not only allows you to evaluate your teaching ability but can be important documentation if you have to defend expenses or time spent on such a project.

EDUCATION OF SUPPORT PEOPLE

It is good practice to be certain that someone in the household other than the person you are teaching has the necessary information or can perform the required skill. This is necessary so that on a day that the primary person does not feel well (develops a bad cold perhaps), someone else can temporarily continue his care. Let the patient, as a rule, choose who this person will be. The individual that you assume is a patient's chief support person (husband, wife, mother, father) may not be the person he perceives as the most reliable choice and therefore not the one he wants as his health care backup. This person, when identified, needs as much information about why the health measure is important as the patient. If diet modification is necessary, be certain that you speak with the person who will prepare the food. A person cannot modify his diet if the person cooking for him does not prepare the appropriate food.

BEHAVIOR MODIFICATION

Typically learning takes place best with positive reinforcement (a person tries to understand a new procedure, you praise him, he tries even harder to master it). Behavior modification is a term used for a system aimed at *erasing* some form of behavior that interferes with health functioning. It was designed to help mentally ill persons erase socially unacceptable behavior; today it has many uses, including discouraging people to continue smoking cigarettes. The basic premise of behavior modification is that the person is rewarded for healthful behavior, while unhealthful behavior is ignored or not rewarded. The person trying to stop smoking, for example, is not scolded or criticized for smoking; this action is simply ignored. Healthful behavior (going an hour without a cigarette, then 2 hours, and so forth) is praised. Children may respond best to behavior modification if in addition to praise they receive a tangible reward such as a star on a chart or an extra privilege of some sort for good behavior.

A behavior modification program must be discussed with the person before it is begun because no behavior can be modified, just as no new behavior can be learned, until the person truly wants a change to occur. You might want to ask the person to sign a learning contract so that you can be certain that you both agree on the method to be used. Many people are able to use self-rewards to reinforce a behavior modification program (using the money they would have spent on cigarettes for the week for some activity they enjoy such as a concert or an article of clothing they otherwise could not have afforded; rewarding themselves for an afternoon of efficient studying or housecleaning by reading a novel or seeing a movie).

Behavior modification is a technique that must be used with common sense and concern so that people are not being manipulated more than they are being helped to achieve a more healthful life style. It is a legitimate device to use in helping an adult to decrease activities such as cigarette smoking, or to enable a hyperactive child to limit his frantic, driven behavior so that he can sit still long enough to eat a meal or learn in school. It can be helpful in encouraging people of all ages to do as much self-care as possible.

Trying to modify beliefs or values by behavior modification is unethical and a reason that behavior modification is often criticized as a learning technique. It is a technique for learning that you should be familiar with, however, as it does have application to health education.

INFORMAL TEACHING

A nurse should be able to do both formal and informal teaching. In a day's time you may do much more informal teaching than formal. Telling a patient who has said he is not hungry that his body needs more fluid and that if he would at least try to drink something it would help him get better faster is an example of this type of teaching.

Be careful that you do not equate informal teaching with disorganized, extra, or unnecessary teaching. It is just as important as formal teaching, but it is conducted in a less structured way. Informal teaching requires you to follow teaching and learning principles (know your subject, recognize individual learning styles, provide an effective environment, limit time span, etc.) just as with more formal teaching (Fig. 16-7). Sometimes informal teaching occurs so spontaneously that it is easy to be unaware of it. Often it occurs in response to a question such as "How long will I have to take this medicine?" If you answer "For 2 weeks," you are just answering a question. If you say "For 2 weeks because . . ." you are teaching. Helping a postoperative patient cough and deep breathe is performing a psychomotor skill. Telling a patient why it is important to cough and deep breathe as you do it is teaching. Table 16-1 lists types of care that should be accompanied by informal teaching.

FIGURE 16-7. Informal teaching is always included as a part of care. Here a nurse is not only helping a patient improve her personal appearance but is explaining how the active arm movement of brushing hair will increase range of motion.

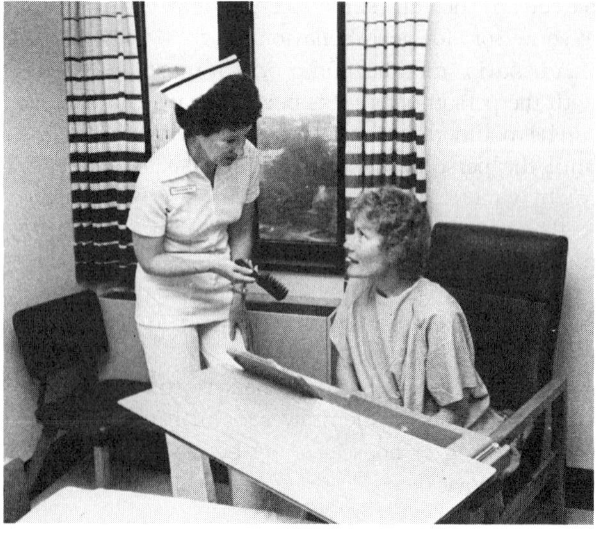

TABLE 16-1. INCORPORATION OF INFORMAL TEACHING IN CARE

Activity	Type of Teaching
Medication administration	People should know the type, and action, and any expected side effects of all medication they are taking. Present medicine not by saying "Here is your pill" but "Here is your Lasix, medicine to help your kidneys remove fluid from your body. You'll notice you start to urinate more by late afternoon."
Vital sign measurement	When taking vital signs such as blood pressure, temperature, and pulse, tell people what normal levels are: "Your blood pressure is 120/70. That's normal."
Any procedure	Always tell people the purpose and principle of procedures, not "You need to drink a lot of fluid," but "You need to drink a lot of fluid because . . ."
Dressing changes	Dressing changes provide an opportunity to teach the danger of introducing infection with an open wound. The person may not have to change this dressing, but everyone applies many Bandaids to small cuts.
Mealtime	Provide information about nutrition: "I know you're not hungry enough to eat the entire sandwich, but could you try the meat? Meat is high in protein and that's important for healing."
Hygiene	Emphasize the necessity of good perineal hygiene to decrease the possibility of urinary tract infection.
Physical assessment	Explain aspects of self breast examination and self testicular examination and describe "normal" findings as both education and reassurance.
Positioning	Teach the hazards of immobility and how change of position and ambulation increase circulation and respiratory function.
Sleep	Teach that sleep is a healing therapy and should not be considered a waste of time.
Bowel elimination	Many people are concerned about their intestinal elimination pattern because they do not appreciate that their pattern is normal. Teach that elimination patterns vary; there is a wide range of "normal."

SUGGESTED READINGS

Bernau, K. M., et al. Integrating parent education into the hospital setting. *M.C.N.* 8(1):13, 1983.

Berni, R., and Fordyce, W. *Behavior Modification and the Nursing Process* (2nd ed.). St. Louis: Mosby, 1977.

Campbell, A., et al. Teaching expectant fathers how to be better childbirth coaches. *M.C.N.* 7(1):28, 1982.

Cosper, B. How well do patients understand hospital jargon? *Am. J. Nurs.* 77:1932, 1977.

Danis, D. M. After instruction: A comprehensive approach. *J.E.N.* 7(3):114, 1981.

Donatelli, N. Patient education programs. *Nurs. Manage.* 12(11):21, 1981.

Eaton, S., et al. Discussion stoppers in teaching. *Nurs. Outlook* 25:578, 1977.

Ford, D., et al. Closed circuit TV . . . high quality instruction to the bedside. *Nurs. Manage.* 14(1):19, 1983.

Fuhrer, L., and Bernstein, R. Making patient education a part of patient care. *Am. J. Nurs.* 76:1798, 1976.

Furlong, B. Setting the stage for learning. *Am. J. Nurs.* 82:300, 1982.

George, G. CEU feature article: If patient teaching tries your patience, try this plan. *Nursing* (Horsham) 12(5):50, 1982.

Gilliland, M. M. What patients can teach you about your patient teaching. *Nursing* (Horsham) 11(12):52, 1981.

Guinee, K. *Teaching and Learning in Nursing.* New York: Macmillan, 1978.

Gulko, C. S., and Butherus, C. Toward better patient teaching. *Nurses' Drug Alert* 1:49, 1977.

Jones, P., and Oertal, W. Developing patient teaching objectives and techniques: A self instructional program. *Nurse Education* 11:3, 1977.

Kohut, S. Guidelines for using interpreters. *Nurs. Digest* 4:55, 1976.

Kratzer, J. B. What does your patient need to know? *Nursing 77* 7:82, 1977.

Leighton, A. Ten steps to better patient teaching. *RN* 39:76, 1976.

Levin, L. S. Patient education and self-care: How do they differ? *Nurs. Outlook* 26:170, 1978.

Loughrey, L. Dealing with the illiterate patient . . . you can't read him like a book. *Nursing* (Horsham) 13(1):65, 1983.

Mattar, M. E., et al. Pharmaceutic factors affecting pediatric compliance. *Pediatrics* 55:101, 1975.

McClurg, E. Developing an effective patient teaching program. *A.O.R.N. J.* 34(3):474, 1981.

McHugh, N. G., et al. Preparatory information: What helps and why. *Am. J. Nurs.* 82(5):780, 1982.

Mitchell, A. Barriers to therapeutic communication with black clients. *Nurs. Outlook* 26:109, 1978.

Pohl, M. L. *Teaching Function of the Nursing Practitioner* (4th ed.). Dubuque, Iowa: W. C. Brown Co., 1982.

Pugh, E. Dynamics of teaching-learning interaction. *Nurs. Forum* 15:47, 1976.

Redman, B. Curriculum in patient education. *Am. J. Nurs.* 78:1363, 1978.

Schrankel, D. Pre-operative teaching. *Superv. Nurse* 9:82, 1978.

Sklar, C. When nurses fail to communicate. *Canad. Nurse* 77:47, 1981.

Talarico, D. Four basic steps to successful patient teaching. *Canad. Nurse* 74:22, 1978.

Williamson, K., and McCray, N. Putting together a patient education program that works. *RN* 40:53, 1977.

QUESTIONS FOR REVIEW

1. Learning takes place most rapidly if the topic:
   a. Is brand new.
   b. Has specific benefit for the person.
   c. Is review information.
   d. Concerns an action not an idea.

2. Learning takes place most effectively in a patient you are teaching if, after he redemonstrates a procedure, you respond by saying:
   a. You did well.
   b. You'll have to improve.
   c. There is a penalty for not improving.
   d. You're an average learner.

3. If you are asked a question for which you do not know the answer while health teaching, your best response is generally to:
   a. Reword the question into one you can answer.
   b. State that you do not have time to answer questions.
   c. Suggest that the person find out the answer independently.
   d. State that you do not know the answer.

4. A person will probably learn a skill best if:
   a. He is actually allowed to practice it.
   b. He has it demonstrated to him three times.
   c. He is shown a photo of someone performing the skill.
   d. He is criticized for not learning well.

5. You demonstrate a procedure and then ask the person to redemonstrate it to you. Which age group probably will do this most spontaneously?
   a. Preschool.
   b. Schoolage.
   c. Young adult.
   d. Middle-aged adult.

6. You ask a nurse clinician to talk to your patient about respiratory exercises. While she does this, your best action would be to:
   a. Avoid listening so that she will not be nervous.
   b. Listen so that your teaching is consistent with hers.
   c. Avoid listening so that you do not have a 2-on-1 situation.
   d. Listen to correct anything she says that is wrong.

7. If you are preparing to demonstrate a skill using sterile gloves, your best technique would be:
   a. Ask the patient to pretend that you have gloves when you do not.
   b. Demonstrate poor technique to contrast with good.
   c. Ask the patient to tell you his learning style.
   d. Demonstrate the technique step by step with gloves.

8. Which of the following is the best instruction for a person who will need to do "blow-type" exercises daily when he returns home?
   a. Do more exercise than before you were ill.
   b. Do 20 "blow-type" respirations four times a day.
   c. Exercise to a point of fatigue.
   d. Do many "blow-type" respirations each day.

9. Which of the following represents a behavior modification technique?
   a. Giving a child a piece of candy for sitting still for 10 minutes.
   b. Taking away television watching privileges for running.
   c. Giving the child extra homework for talking in class.
   d. Not allowing a child to play outside for rude behavior.

17. DOCUMENTATION OF NURSING CARE

OBJECTIVES

Upon mastery of the material in this chapter, you should be able to:

1. Describe the purposes of keeping accurate patient records.
2. Describe the component parts of a source and a problem-oriented patient record in an in-service setting.
3. Describe the meaning of the acronym, SOAP.
4. Compare traditional and SOAP nursing notes.
5. Compare the steps of POR charting and the nursing process.
6. Explain the purpose and content of a data base and progress notes.
7. Describe the component parts of a patient record in an ambulatory setting.
8. Describe the legal considerations of charting.
9. Describe the role that the patient's chart serves in hospital and nursing audits.

TERMS

The terms important for an understanding of this chapter are shown below and defined in the glossary:

audit
charting
documentation
nursing Kardex
nurse's notes
patient record

If one person could remain with a patient constantly during a health agency visit or hospitalization and supervise every aspect of his care, written records would probably not be necessary. This does not happen, however; in any 24-hour period a person admitted to a hospital may have contact with his private physician, as many as three house staff physicians, three nurses (three nursing shifts), a dietician, possibly a nursing student, a medical student, a physical therapist, an occupational therapist, a physician consultant, a respiratory therapist—the list is almost endless. If the patient returns home and is readmitted to the hospital a month later, the only person who sees him who cared for him on his previous admission may be his private physician. Because of the number of people a patient is exposed to at every health care visit, and so that there is legal documentation of care, accurate, thorough records must be kept. This is the only way that quality care can be achieved and continued.

DEFINITION OF A PATIENT RECORD

If a person is well, a patient record is the documentation of his capabilities and disabilities. If he is ill, it also describes factors that have been altered by the present illness, the rationale or justification for care he is receiving, and his response to that care. It is a confidential record intended to be shared with no one but health care providers and the patient himself.

PURPOSE OF A PATIENT RECORD

There are at least eight purposes for a patient record.

Aid to Diagnosis

The information recorded in a patient record on a person's first contact with a health care setting establishes his state of health or illness (termed a data base) and serves as the basis for determining both nursing diagnoses and a medical diagnosis of illness. Nurses may obtain and record the information necessary for a comprehensive data base or may restrict their information gathering to that necessary for establishing nursing diagnoses.

Documentation of Continuity and Justification of Care

If a patient was admitted to a hospital with a burn on his hand and if notes were not written describing the size and condition of the burn in the days to follow, 4 days later, when you first encountered the patient, you would not know if healing was taking place or not because you would not know how the burn looked immediately after it occurred. If it is established that the burn is not healing, the physician would not be able to change to new therapy if he did not have documentation of what treatment had already been tried and apparently was ineffective. Nurses contribute a great deal of assessment and evaluation information and often are the most thorough recorders of this type of information in patient charts.

Effective Communication Between Health Care Personnel

Documentation of care allows health care providers to know what others are doing. One physician (a dermatologist, for example) can see what medicine another physician (concerned with the patient's gastrointestinal problem) has prescribed for treatment. This information prevents the second physician from prescribing the same drug (so that the patient is unknowingly taking twice the usual dosage of a drug due to the double prescription) or from prescribing a drug that interferes or neutralizes the action of another (tetracycline, for example, a drug that might be ordered by a dermatologist for acne therapy, is neutralized by many antacids the person might be taking as ordered by his second physician).

If you were attempting to plan the best way to make a patient comfortable, a well-written chart should tell you what measures were tried before and were ineffective; you could then proceed without having to repeat everything. A chart containing the information that Billy, a 2-year-old, eats best if he sits at a small table rather than from a tray over his bed or that Susie, a 1-month-old, sleeps best on her abdomen eliminates the necessity for everyone on a nursing staff to learn these preferences by trial and error, promotes continuity of care, and hopefully prevents overlapping or inadequate care.

Legal Documentation of Care

All health care agencies are required to keep records by state law and by accrediting agencies. In many instances a patient's record is admissible as evidence in court. When charting, assume that the next time you see what you have written will be 5 years later on a 5′ × 8′ screen in the front of a courtroom and ask yourself did you describe your care fully? Can what you have written stand alone? Is it so clear that it will still be understood at a future date? Does it read as something you could defend at a later date?

Documentation for Research

Patient records serve as the basis for health statistical studies (how many people were seen for tetanus infections last year, how many babies were born last year) and for research on improvement of patient care (how many people who received a certain medication last year truly noticed improved symptoms after receiving it). Patient records are analyzed to see if health care facilities are adequate for the community (the number of births in the community has risen considerably; perhaps more hospital beds are needed?) and to determine if health care patterns are changing or remaining static (more people were seen in ambulatory settings last year than ever before). Thorough documentation of nursing care and patient response adds greatly to the usefulness of patient records as sources of research data.

Documentation for Education

All health care disciplines use patient records as a source of examples of patient care or response for student education. Remember when using patient records for class assignments or reports that these are confidential records with which you are dealing. Never use the patient's full name (abbreviate the name as "Mr. B." or "John S.") or information that would distinctly identify the patient in any other way (word your description as "this patient works for a large corporation" rather than "for IBM").

It is important to keep names confidential because you can be found guilty of slander if you convey derogatory information concerning another verbally, and of libel if you convey derogatory information concerning another in writing (see Chap. 4). The fact that an illness is present can be interpreted as derogatory information because it implies that the person is less able to function efficiently than one who is totally well. Hospital records or reports cannot be given to other health agencies or health care providers without the consent of the patient.

There is much discussion today as to how much access a person should have to his own health record. In the past it was felt that a patient should never see his record because he might encounter a medical term he did not understand, misinterpret it, and cause himself undue fear. The term *idiopathic*, for example, means "without cause." A physician who states that a person has idiopathic hypertension means that the person has high blood pressure for which he has not yet located the cause. A patient reading this diagnosis, however, might associate *idiopathic* with *idiot*, conclude that his illness will reduce his intellectual capabilities, and worry unnecessarily.

Patient access to records varies among states and health care agencies (QRS 17-1). Today many people feel that patients have a right to read their health records just as students have a right to examine their school records. In some health care agencies this patient right is accepted so strongly that patients fill in their own admission data form or supply their own data base of information by punching answers to computerized questions, contributing directly to their record's construction.

Documentation for Audit

Audit, a procedure designed to increase the quality of health care, is required of all Joint-Commission-Accredited hospitals. Patient records are reviewed and the quality of care given a patient as documented in the record is evaluated. An audit may be done on an agency-wide basis where many phases of care are studied; it may be a nursing audit where only aspects of

☐ **QUICK REFERENCE STOP 17-1: ADVOCACY**

A hospital record (the folder, the pages) belongs to the health agency. In many states the *content* of the record, however, belongs to the patient or can be seen by him. In all states a patient's lawyer can gain access to the record's contents by permission of the patient. Occasionally a patient wants to see a consultant's report recommending a certain procedure before he will sign permission for the procedure. As he needs to do this before he can sign informed consent, this type of report is generally shown to him from the record.

Learn your individual state and agency policy on patient accessibility to records so that you can keep patients informed as to their rights. A helpful pamphlet for patients is *Obtaining Your Own Health Record*, U.S. Government Printing Office, Washington, D.C.

nursing care are evaluated. It may be concurrent (studying what is currently being done) or retrospective (studying what previously occurred). An audit is a valuable contribution to improving the quality of care because if it is discovered that a problem is occurring repeatedly (16 patients developed infections following one type of surgery), the cause of the problem can be discovered and measures to improve care identified and instituted. Audit review can act directly to improve your care because the necessity for recording your care makes you consider thoroughly the measures that you should take. An important point to remember when charting is that audit reviewers are not mind readers. If you did a procedure but did not document that you did it, at the time of the audit it will be assumed that the procedure was not done. Think while you chart.

Individualization of Care

Charting the response of a patient to care or the explanation you gave for a procedure enables you to devise care that meets a patient's individual needs. Thinking about how a particular patient responded to a procedure leads you to think of ways you could make that procedure more acceptable to him; it has made you a more effective nurse and improved your level of care.

A TRADITIONAL PATIENT RECORD

Traditional patient records are also termed *source records*. They are divided into sections according to aspect of care (medical, nursing, dietician sources).

A traditional patient record for a hospitalized patient generally consists of the following divisions:

1. An information sheet (also called a personal data or admission sheet).
2. A face sheet (often called a vital signs or graphic sheet).
3. A physician's order sheet.
4. A progress note or history sheet.
5. Nurses' notes.
6. Laboratory and diagnostic findings.
7. Consult sheets.
8. Consent forms.
9. Medication records.

Information (Personal Data) Sheet

An information sheet is typically either the first or last page of a patient record so that it can be readily located. It includes information such as the patient's full name, address, telephone number, birth date, sex, marital status, religion, occupation, name of physician, insurance coverage, nearest relative, date and time of admission, diagnosis or reason for admission, and the hospital reference number assigned to the patient.

This information is generally obtained by a secretary in the admitting or reception department; in an emergency situation it may be your responsibility to elicit the information. When you complete a health interview at the beginning of a hospital admission or at an ambulatory visit, you should check that this information has been obtained. It is essential for differentiating among people with like names (there may be four Mary Smiths in the hospital at the same time; birth date and home address information is necessary to keep laboratory data correct for all four people). A woman's maiden name is also helpful for this type of differentiation.

The remainder of this sheet is often used to list information such as allergies. These also should be marked in red print on the cover of the chart, the Kardex (the use of this file is explained later in the chapter), and in the nursing care plan. There may be space provided on the bottom of this sheet for the person's physician to record a final diagnosis at discharge before the chart is filed in the record department of the agency. A typical information sheet is shown in Figure 17-1.

Face (Graphic) Sheet

Most health care agencies record patients' vital signs (temperature, pulse, respirations, blood pressure) in graphic form (Fig. 17-2) on a sheet at the front of the chart. This sheet serves as a quick reference for determining these vital parameters of health and often quickly illustrates a pattern or change. In Figure 17-2 pulse, temperature, and respirations are all plotted on the same scale, temperature level indicated by °C and pulse and respiration rates by X and •. Because pulse rate in an adult is normally 70—80 beats per minute and respiratory rate is normally a much lower number such as 16—20 per minute, even though the same symbol is used for both, there is no confusion. This method of overlapping graphics is frequently used to consolidate space, and if at first confusing, it will be-

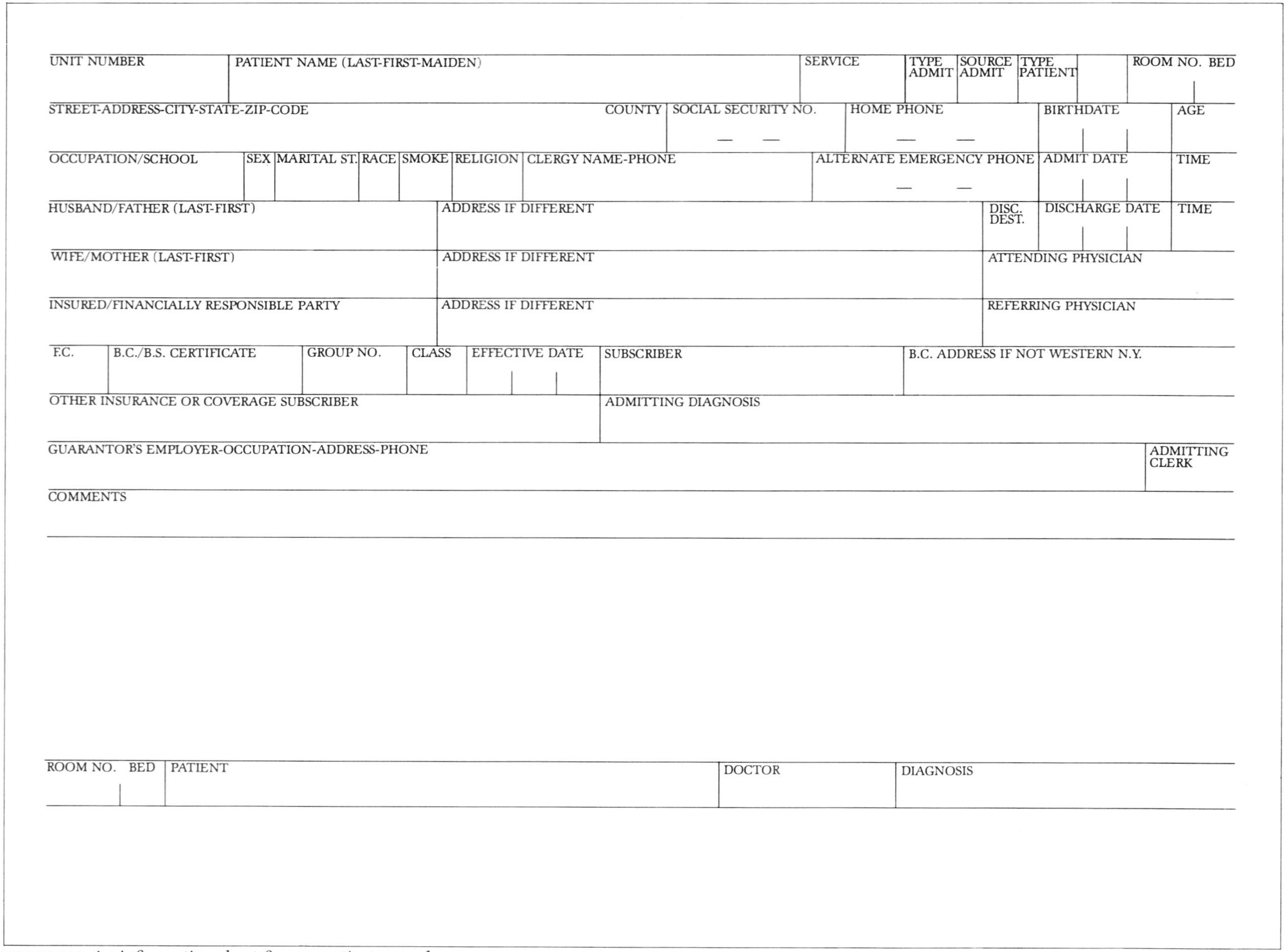

UNIT NUMBER | PATIENT NAME (LAST-FIRST-MAIDEN) | SERVICE | TYPE ADMIT | SOURCE ADMIT | TYPE PATIENT | | ROOM NO. BED

STREET-ADDRESS-CITY-STATE-ZIP-CODE | COUNTY | SOCIAL SECURITY NO. | HOME PHONE | BIRTHDATE | AGE

OCCUPATION/SCHOOL | SEX | MARITAL ST. | RACE | SMOKE | RELIGION | CLERGY NAME-PHONE | ALTERNATE EMERGENCY PHONE | ADMIT DATE | TIME

HUSBAND/FATHER (LAST-FIRST) | ADDRESS IF DIFFERENT | DISC. DEST. | DISCHARGE DATE | TIME

WIFE/MOTHER (LAST-FIRST) | ADDRESS IF DIFFERENT | ATTENDING PHYSICIAN

INSURED/FINANCIALLY RESPONSIBLE PARTY | ADDRESS IF DIFFERENT | REFERRING PHYSICIAN

F.C. | B.C./B.S. CERTIFICATE | GROUP NO. | CLASS | EFFECTIVE DATE | SUBSCRIBER | B.C. ADDRESS IF NOT WESTERN N.Y.

OTHER INSURANCE OR COVERAGE SUBSCRIBER | ADMITTING DIAGNOSIS

GUARANTOR'S EMPLOYER-OCCUPATION-ADDRESS-PHONE | ADMITTING CLERK

COMMENTS

ROOM NO. BED | PATIENT | DOCTOR | DIAGNOSIS

FIGURE 17-1. An information sheet from a patient record.

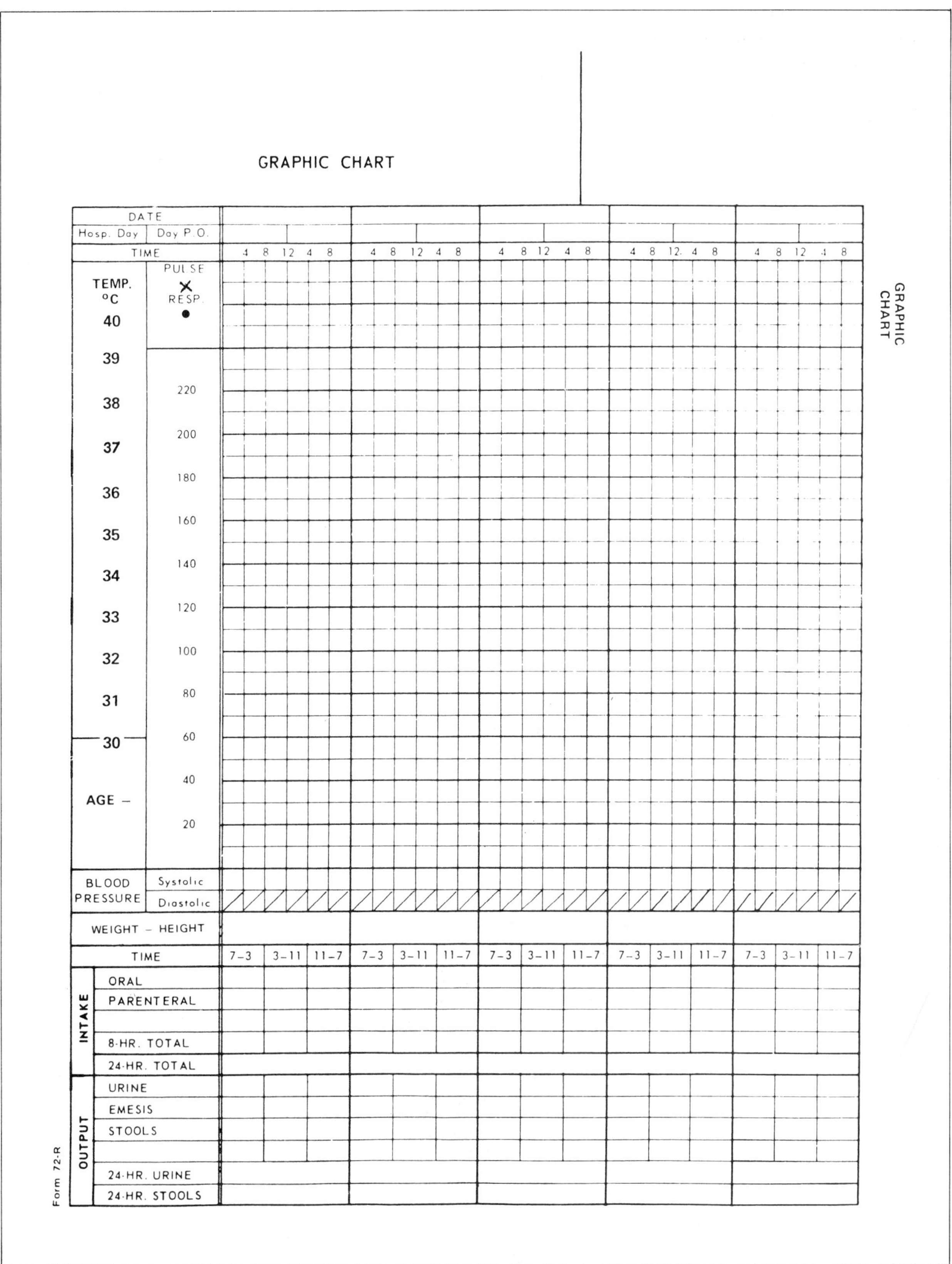

GRAPHIC CHART

DATE
Hosp. Day | Day P.O.
TIME | 4 8 12 4 8 | 4 8 12 4 8 | 4 8 12 4 8 | 4 8 12 4 8 | 4 8 12 4 8

TEMP. °C: 40, 39, 38, 37, 36, 35, 34, 33, 32, 31, 30
PULSE ×
RESP. •
220, 200, 180, 160, 140, 120, 100, 80, 60, 40, 20
AGE –

BLOOD PRESSURE: Systolic, Diastolic
WEIGHT – HEIGHT
TIME | 7–3 | 3–11 | 11–7 | 7–3 | 3–11 | 11–7 | 7–3 | 3–11 | 11–7 | 7–3 | 3–11 | 11–7 | 7–3 | 3–11 | 11–7

INTAKE: ORAL, PARENTERAL, 8-HR. TOTAL, 24-HR. TOTAL
OUTPUT: URINE, EMESIS, STOOLS, 24-HR. URINE, 24-HR. STOOLS

Form 72-R

GRAPHIC CHART

FIGURE 17-2. A face sheet indicating temperature, pulse, respirations, blood pressure, weight, height, and fluid balance.

come clear with usage. In Figure 17-2 blood pressure is recorded as a number (100/70) in the space just below the graph scale; it might be required to be graphed on another form.

The bottom half of this sheet is typically used to record all fluid the patient took in a day's time (input) and all fluid excreted (output) so that there is quick reference for this information also.

Physician's Order Sheet

Every order of a physician for a patient must be put in writing. So that these stand out clearly, a separate sheet in the chart is provided. In many agencies this page is constructed with carbon-copy sheets attached to it so that medication orders do not have to be recopied for pharmacy (an action that not only saves copying time but prevents copying error).

The date and time the order was written must be noted beside the order; the writing must be in ink and signed by the physician. After an order has been written, the physician uses some signaling method (attaches a metal clip to the chart or places it in a special section on the desk) to indicate that there is a current order in the chart. The nurse in charge of the unit, ward clerk, or primary nurse reads the order and then initiates it (for example, requisitions medication from pharmacy, sees that the nurse caring for the patient begins a new therapy). She then draws a line through the order (but not obliterating the writing; the order must still be easily read) and signs her name and title and the time and date. She draws a line across the page to indicate that all orders up to that point have been noted and are in the process of being carried out (Fig. 17-3). Once an order has been so marked, the physician cannot change or add anything to it. To correct the order (for instance, to change a drug dosage), the physician must cancel the first order and write a second (Fig. 17-4). Although this procedure is paper consuming, it eliminates the risk that you would not notice the change of order after it was crossed off and continue to administer the incorrect first order.

Be aware of the "flagging" system at the health care agency where you practice (Fig. 17-5) so that you do not inadvertently remove a "flag" that marks a new order,

FIGURE 17-3. A physician's order sheet. The line drawn across the page signifies that all orders up to that point have been noted.

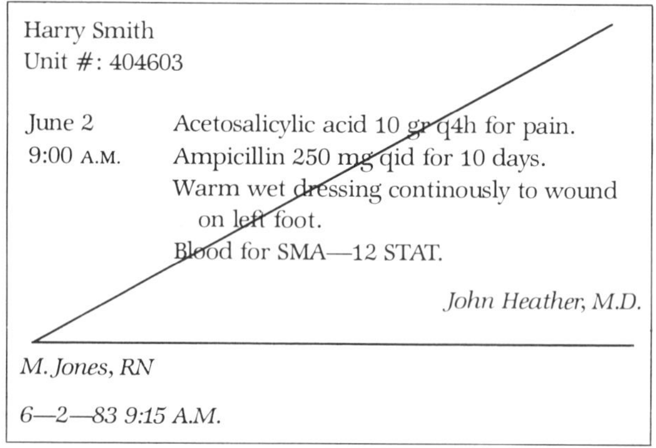

Harry Smith
Unit #: 404603

June 2 9:00 A.M.
Acetosalicylic acid 10 gr q4h for pain.
Ampicillin 250 mg qid for 10 days.
Warm wet dressing continously to wound on left foot.
Blood for SMA—12 STAT.

John Heather, M.D.

M. Jones, RN
6—2—83 9:15 A.M.

FIGURE 17-4. Record of a change in a physician's order.

June 2 10:00 A.M.
Cancel acetosalicylic acid 10 gr q4h for pain.
Change to acetosalicylic acid 15 gr q4h for pain.

John Heather, M.D.

FIGURE 17-5. A nursing unit desk area. That a new order has been written in the chart is revealed by the "flag" on the top right corner.

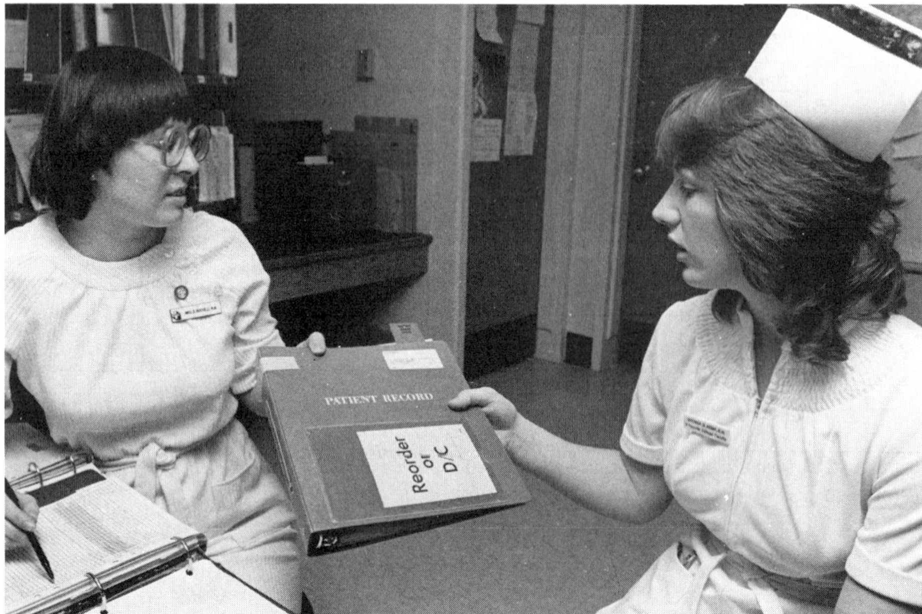

TIME	TEMPERATURE				APR	RESP, 1		BREATH SOUNDS	SUCTION				BP	COLOR	ACTIVITY	TESTS					
	ISO	ISC	HOOD	AX		RATE	TYPE	2	PD	ETT/TR	ORAL	NASAL		4	5	HEMA TEST	D-STIX mg %	SPEC GRAVITY	CLIN TEST	LABSTIX	[illegible]

RESPIRATORY 1

- A — APNEA
- P — PERIODIC
- R — RETRACT
  - 1 - MILD
  - 2 - MODERATE
  - 3 - SEVERE
- G — GRUNT
- F — FLARE
- C — CRYING
- S — SHALLOW
- N — NORMAL

BREATH SOUNDS 2

- A — ABSENT
- B — BILATERAL
- D — DIMINISHED
- E — EQUAL
- CL — CLEAR
- C — CONGESTED
- R — RALES
- U — UPPER
- L — LOWER
- RT — RIGHT
- LT — LEFT

SUCTION 3

- PD — POSTURAL DRAINAGE
- S — SMALL
- M — MEDIUM
- L — LARGE
- CL — CLEAR
- G — GREEN
- Y — YELLOW
- W — WHITE
- B — BLOODY
- F — FROTHY
- T — THICK
- CY — CLOUDY
- ETT — ENDOTRACHEAL TUBE
- TR — TRACHEOSTOMY TUBE

COLOR 4

- A — ASHEN
- C — CYANOTIC
- D — DUSKY
- J — JAUNDICE
- M — MOTTLED
- P — PINK
- PL — PLETHORIC
- PP — PALE
- AC — ACROCYANOSIS
- CC — CIRCUMORAL CYANOSIS

ACTIVITY 5

- A — ACTIVE ___
- A+ — ACTIVE C STIMULATION
- I — IRRITABLE
- T — TWITCH
- Q — QUIET
- L — LETHARGIC
- N — NONREACTIVE
- J — JITTERY
- C — CRYING
- S — SLEEPING

POSITION 6

- RT — RIGHT SIDE
- L — LEFT SIDE
- A — ABDOMEN
- B — BACK
- HE — HEAD ELEVATED

STOOL 7

- S — SMALL
- M — MEDIUM
- L — LARGE
- GR — GREEN
- Y — YELLOW
- BR — BROWN
- SO — SOFT
- P — PASTY
- F — FORMED
- MEC — MECONIUM
- SDY — SEEDY
- LO — LOOSE
- W — WATERY
- WR — SEEDY WITH WATER RING

FORM 40

FIGURE 17-6. A flow sheet.

interfere with the charge nurse's organization for care, or delay the start of patient therapy.

In emergencies or special circumstances a physician may give a verbal or telephone order. Such orders are added to this page by the nurse who accepts them followed by a note such as "Telephone order by Dr. Heather."

Progress (History) Notes

In a traditional chart system there is a series of pages where the physician, a physician assistant, or nurse practitioner records an admission history, physical examination data, and daily (or as often as necessary) notes on the patient's progress and response to therapy. It is an informative sheet for you to read as it not only describes the patient's current health problem but his past illnesses and family-related health problems as well.

Flow Sheets

Flow sheets are pages set up in checklist form so that only a small notation is necessary to describe an event rather than a narrative paragraph. Blood pressure, respiratory rate, and neurological symptoms for example, are often recorded on this type of form (Fig. 17-6). Do not discount such sheets as "work sheets." They are as much a legal document as other forms in the chart.

Consult Sheets

At any point that a physician specialist or other health care provider is asked to contact the patient and offer an opinion as to care or therapy, she records observations or suggestions on a separate consult sheet. Health care personnel such as physical therapists, occupational therapists, dieticians, psychologists, and discharge planners use this type of form. It can be assumed that a consultant's suggestions will be incorporated into the patient's plan of care, but before any of these suggestions are carried out, they must be formally written by the physician writing orders for the patient on the separate physician's order sheet.

If the patient has surgery, included in this section will be the anesthesiologist's summary and the summary of care given in the operating and recovery rooms before the patient returned to the patient unit.

Laboratory Results

Results of diagnostic or laboratory studies typically are returned to the nursing unit on small colored sheets of paper (perhaps a different color for each hospital department), which are usually pasted into the appropriate section by the unit secretary (Fig. 17-7). These pages should be examined by you daily as they are as informative as the physician's progress page in documenting changes in patient condition. When you first begin to examine patient records, these pages seem confusing and difficult to interpret because you are unfamiliar with common laboratory studies and their results. There is a tendency to dismiss them as not important (or because they take too much work to appreciate). As you learn more about pathology and a laboratory study's significance, however, you will come to recognize

FIGURE 17-7. A laboratory report chart sheet.

CHEMISTRY 1

TEST	ACTUAL	ADULT NORMAL
☐ BUN (UREA N)		5-25 mg%
☐ GLUCOSE FASTING		70-110 mg %
ELECTROLYTES:		
☐ CO_2 *		24-32 meq/L
☐ CHLORIDE		98-109 meq/L
☐ SODIUM		135-155 meq/L
☐ POTASSIUM		3.6-5.5 meq/L
☐ KETONE BODIES		
☐ GLUCOSE 2 HR. P.P.		
☐ GLUCOSE TOLERANCE F		
½ HR. GLUCOSE TOLERANCE		
1 HR. "		
2 HR. "		
3 HR. "		
☐		

DATE

NURSE'S SIGNATURE

WRITE → ADDRESS IF OUT PATIENT

NAME

ADDRESS

ADMISSION NO.

DOCTOR

TEST	ACTUAL	ADULT NORMAL	TEST	ACTUAL	ADULT NORMAL
☐ CALCIUM *		9-11 mg%	☐ BILIRUBIN 1 MIN.		0-.2 mg%
☐ PHOSPHORUS *		2.5-4.8 mg%	☐ BILIRUBIN TOTAL		.2-1.0 mg%
☐ CREATININE		1-2 mg%	☐ CHOLESTEROL		150-250 mg%
☐ URIC ACID		M: 2.5-7.0 MGS% F: 1.5-6.0 MGS%	☐ SALICYLATE LEVEL		
☐ TOTAL PROTEIN		6.2-8.5 gm%	☐ UREA CLEARANCE		60-125%
☐ ALBUMIN		3.5-5.6 GM%	☐ CREATININE CLEARANCE		75-125 ML
☐ GLOBULIN		1.3-3.2 GM%	☐ BSP		0-5%
☐ ELECTROPHORESIS SERUM			☐ THYMOL		0-5 units
☐ CEPH FLOC		0-1 plus	☐ Icterus Index		0-6 Units

* DIFFERENT NORMALS FOR CHILDREN

DO NOT WRITE IN ABOVE SPACE

E 03660

CHEMISTRY 1

REV. CODE 403 | DEPT. 3

DATE

the importance of this data. In some instances it is a nurse's responsibility to add these returned slips to the chart; therefore, you will be the first to recognize a sudden change in a patient's condition or learn a patient's diagnosis. Do not begin a negative relationship with data that will later become a mainstay for you in planning nursing care.

Consent Forms

On admission to a health care agency people must sign consent forms which grant permission for health care. Additional consent is necessary for procedures that involve special risk (a lumbar puncture, an immunization, anesthesia, for example). A person's signature on these forms means that he has received a full explanation of the procedure including its risks; this is called *informed consent*. This type of consent must be witnessed; the person witnessing the signature signs on a line beside or under the patient's signature.

Further aspects of consent including when patients are eligible to sign such forms are discussed in Chap. 4. You need to be aware what procedures in your practice area require special consent (this differs from agency to agency) and to ensure that the consent is present before such a procedure is performed.

Medication Records

A separate record details the time, amount, type, and route of all medication administered to the patient (QRS 17-2). These pages may be kept as part of the chart or kept separate on a medication chart and then added to the chart at the time of discharge before the chart is sent to the record room. Remember that even if the page is kept separate from the remainder of the chart for convenience in administration of medications, it *is* a part of the chart. All the legal implications that apply to the chart in general apply to this loose sheet as well. Specific use of this sheet is discussed further in Chap. 29.

Nursing Notes

In a traditional record system documentation of nursing care is entered on a separate sheet in a narrative format. General guidelines for nursing notes are shown in Table 17-1. At least eight categories of information concerning patient care are recorded:

1. Assessment of both physical and psychosocial factors noted during care. This includes information such as evaluation of sleep, nutrition, physical findings, body functions, level of comfort, sense of personal dignity and worth, knowledge of illness, and the patient's own role in care (see QRS 17-3).
2. Assessment of the patient's environment. This includes such assessment as safety factors provided for the specific patient.
3. Documentation of procedures or care accomplished as dependent and interdependent nursing action or done under the supervision or in cooperation with a physician. Removing sutures would be an example of this type of action.
4. Documentation of care done as independent nursing action. Many measures that you initiate are not ordered but are dictated by your knowledge of the patient's condition. Sitting a person upright who is short of breath, for example, is an independent action that should be documented.
5. Response of the patient to care. This is documentation of effectiveness of therapy and aids the physician and other nurses in determining whether care should be continued or changed. It includes such information as whether the patient felt relief after a medication for pain was administered.
6. Documentation of procedures done by other health care personnel. In order that there is documentation of all stimuli that affect a person, you need to record procedures that you assisted with as well as those you carried out alone. Assisting a house staff physician to change a dressing, assisting the respiratory therapist with deep breathing exercises are examples of this type of information.
7. Documentation of visitors or other people who made contact with the patient such as a physician, clergyman, family member. This information documents the extent of the patient's support system. With stress, support people become very important and whether

☐ QUICK REFERENCE STOP 17-2: PHARMACOLOGY

Be certain that medications are recorded immediately after administration so that a second caregiver will not repeat the administration and cause a drug overdose. Record the site of intramuscular or subcutaneous injection so that injection sites can be rotated and good absorption from sites can be maintained. Because medication records are often checklist sheets, do not discount their importance. They are a legal record just as other more formal chart pages.

☐ QUICK REFERENCE STOP 17-3: NUTRITION

Because a person has been *served* a well-balanced diet is no guarantee that he is *eating* a well-balanced diet. Record specifically what people eat, not that they "ate well" or "ate poorly," to document nutritional intake.

Intravenous fluid is usually recorded as fluid intake; blood products (plasma, packed red blood cells, white blood cells) are usually not recorded as fluid intake. Learn each agency procedure for correct recording.

TABLE 17-1. GENERAL GUIDELINES FOR CHARTING NURSING NOTES

1. Each page in a chart should be labeled with the patient's name and unit number. Make a habit of looking for this before you begin charting (and adding it, if it is not there), because this prevents you from recording information on the wrong chart and will identify the page should it be torn from the chart. Such information is usually available on a "charge-card" plate and easily added to all chart pages.
2. Record the *patient's* action or response, not *your* action. A statement such as "Patient taken to surgery; bath given; taken to dayroom for remainder of morning" documents *your* action (and possibly that the elevators in the building work) but it is not patient centered. "Patient states he is less anxious about surgery than yesterday; skin is intact, but pale" are patient-centered statements.
3. Record a note only *after* care has been given; do not anticipate what you will do. When you actually start to do it, the situation may be so different from what you anticipated that your note will no longer be true.
4. Information recorded should be as accurate as possible (250 ml, not a "large amount"; 10:15 A.M., not "mid-morning"). Brevity is important but not at the expense of leaving out important information. A statement such as "ate poorly," for example, is brief, but is also unclear. Did you mean the person does not use his hands to hold a spoon well, did not eat nutritious food, or ate only a small amount? "Drank 40 ml of orange juice for breakfast" is longer but also clear and accurate.
5. Use consecutive lines when charting. This prevents an irresponsible person from adding information at some later point to your notes. If you do not use a full line for some reason, draw a line to the margin so that information cannot be added in the blank space.
6. If you should make an error in recording do not erase. Draw a single line through the error (do not scratch it out) and write the word *error* above it with your initials; following that, enter the correct information to show that you are responsibly changing the record (Fig 17-8).
7. Sign a nursing note with your first initial and your full last name followed by your title. Most schools of nursing use the school initials followed by S.N. for student differentiation. A student from Jamison University would sign her name N. Smith, J.U.S.N.
8. Record observations in a positive manner. "Patient has no complaints" may imply that you think ill people are cranky, complaining people; "patient is in a good mood, laughing with relatives who visited" is a much more professional statement. You do not have to use full sentences; just be certain that information is not so curtailed it becomes confusing.
9. Do not *interpret* people's statements or actions, merely *record* them as facts. Patient states he has "nagging pain" is better than "patient has low-grade pain." His definition of "nagging pain" may not be low-grade pain and you have led his physician into thinking that he is much more comfortable than he is. Do not make medical diagnoses. "Wound is infected" is an interpretive or diagnostic statement; "wound appears erythematous with clear serous drainage" is a factual one.
10. Chart in ink. Ink prevents the record from being changed or distorted by an irresponsible person. Some agencies designate different colored inks for different nursing shifts. Write legibly. Many people will be reading your information. Use professional terms (sanguinous drainage, not bloody drainage).
11. Use abbreviations only as appropriate. Appendix E lists common acceptable medical abbreviations. Do not use so many abbreviations that your recording is more perplexing than efficient to read. Do not use ditto-marks as they may be misinterpreted as to what they represent.

June 2 10:00 A.M.	Patient appears worried; states: "I hope I don't have pain." Walked to ~~playroom~~ desk area and back to bed. error: S.A. Short of breath from exertion.
	S. Ashley, J.U.S.N.

FIGURE 17-8. Correcting an error on a nursing note.

they are actively present or not affects psychological well-being.

8. Education supplied to the patient or his support people. Often a nursing implementation includes teaching the person or a family member how to perform a procedure for himself. Documentation of this instruction is as important as documenting "hands-on" care. A nursing note written in a narrative format will be found at the end of the chapter followed by one written in a problem-oriented record format.

ADMISSION AND DISCHARGE NOTES

A nursing note always begins with an introductory paragraph indicating the time, method of arrival, and description of the patient at the time of arrival at the patient unit.

A discharge note must include the time and method of discharge, instructions, medications, or equipment given to the patient, and the patient's overall response and appearance at discharge (see QRS 17-4). The name

☐ QUICK REFERENCE STOP 17-4: COMMUNITY CONSIDERATIONS

On hospital discharge, if a patient is to be followed by a community health nurse in his home, you need to write a referral detailing what care will be needed. Give information that will be helpful to the community health nurse (patient cannot swallow capsules, grows depressed easily, has strong support people) in addition to specifying the physical care needed (dressing changed, catheter irrigated). Your communication is a link between two agency health records; it becomes a part of both records and is a legal document. Offering this type of information prevents the second agency from having to "reinvent the wheel."

of the person to whom children are discharged must also be included.

PROBLEM-ORIENTED RECORDING

In 1969 Lawrence Weed (1971) devised a new system for patient charting in which information is categorized according to patient problems. Because this system was first used almost entirely by physicians, it was called problem-oriented medical recording (POMR). Today it is used by all health care providers and has come to be known as problem-oriented recording (POR) or a problem-oriented system.

With this system all health care personnel utilize the same pages of information rather than each being confined to a separate section. This increased sharing of information hopefully leads to more comprehensive care, less overlapping of care, fewer gaps in care, and increased education and understanding of other health care provider roles.

A POR Chart

In a POR chart the information sheet, face or graphic record, laboratory sheets, consult forms, and flow sheets are the same as those used in a traditional chart. Two types of divisions differ: data base and problem list.

DATA BASE

A person's data base is the sum of all the health information gathered on him by interview, physical examination, and assessment of laboratory/diagnostic tests. In a traditional chart this information is dispersed through physician's history and progress notes, consultants' notes, and nursing notes. In a POR chart it is presented as one section. This material could be gathered and recorded by either a physician or a nurse.

PROBLEM LIST

Following the collection of a data base, health problems of the patient are analyzed and listed on a separate sheet. A problem is defined broadly as a situation that is less than optimal health. It may be a physical, psychosocial, demographic, developmental, or environmental concern. A problem can be developed by any health care provider. This list is kept at the front of the chart and is added to as additional problems occur; when a problem is solved, it is marked as inactive.

When a problem is identified, it is given an assigned number; it is always referred to by both name and number. When a problem is resolved, its number is not reused. This allows that number always to refer to that specific problem; if the problem should recur, it is reactivated under that number. In addition to problems that are active (currently exist) and inactive (have been resolved), potential problems (the person is a heavy smoker which may eventually lead to lung damage) may be listed as well.

Shown below is a problem list of Robert Smith, a 23-year-old, which was started when he was born:

Number	*Problem*	*Date Identified*	*Inactive*
1	Newborn	5/20/60	6/20/60
2	Health maintenance	6/20/60	
3	Forehead laceration	8/16/62	8/23/62
4	Acne	2/5/73	5/10/77
5	Dizziness, loss of weight (diabetes mellitus)	3/15/76	
6	Acting out behavior	6/15/76	9/20/79
7	Heavy smoker	6/15/76	
8	Fractured tibia	9/8/83	
9	Knowledge of diabetes, lack of	9/8/83	

Most people consider the risk of the newborn period as enough of a health threat to represent a health problem, and it is listed first in the problem list above. The newborn period typically lasts for 1 month, so at the end of the first month (6-20-60) this problem was marked inactive. The second problem, health maintenance, was established as a problem at one month of age when the patient came for his first health maintenance visit. As health maintenance is always necessary, it is never a resolved problem.

The third problem was a transient one—a forehead laceration when the person was two years old. This was healed within a week and was then marked inactive (8-23-62). The fourth problem, acne, arose when the patient was 13 and was marked inactive when the patient was 17.

The fifth problem originally was listed as the symptoms that were first identified—dizziness and loss of weight. As the problem was further evaluated and a medical diagnosis was established, the initial problem designation was changed to diabetes mellitus. It is important to remember that you do not have to know what causes a problem to add it to a POR list; any threat to health that you recognize should be noted.

The sixth problem, acting-out behavior, was identified during adolescence. This refers to attention-getting behavior such as reckless driving and shop-lifting (knowing you will be seen and recognized). It is not an unusual occurrence with adolescents with a chronic disease as they fight to establish an identity. With greater maturity, this behavior faded and when the person was 19, the problem was considered resolved.

At the same health visit that acting-out behavior was identified, the potential problem of heavy smoking was noted also. This has not improved and remains an open problem.

Most recently, when this person was seen at a health care facility for a fractured tibia following a car accident, in the initial interview it was determined that he understands very little about diabetes. Lack of knowledge related to diabetes, and the fractured tibia were both added to the list of problems at that time.

Knowing a person's total problem list is helpful in planning comprehensive care. For example, the last time Mr. Smith was diagnosed as having an illness he manifested erratic and attention-getting behavior. You therefore should question him more carefully than the average patient to ascertain what a new threat to his body image may mean. Will he need more help than the average patient in resolving his feelings about this latest problem? Knowing that he has diabetes is important. Diabetes is a metabolic disease in which people have difficulty regulating glucose in their body. Before he receives an intravenous infusion (usually glucose) prior to and during surgery for his leg, the physician needs to know about this problem so that he can administer fluid safely. The information that Robert is a heavy smoker is important for the anesthesiologist to know before he administers an anesthetic to him.

A patient will have the problem for which he was hospitalized added to his master problem list at the end of hospitalization. His hospital chart will note subproblems relative to this hospitalization. Frequently identified problems of hospitalized patients are pain, anxiety, allergies, lack of support people, and lack of knowledge of illness. At the end of a hospitalization any of these that remain current (new allergies identified; lack of support people that continues) are added to the master problem list along with the main reason for hospitalization (fractured tibia).

A problem list is sometimes referred to as the table of contents for the chart. It has wide-reaching implications and uses in planning comprehensive nursing care.

Nursing Diagnosis

In order to plan nursing care it is necessary to determine which of the problems listed for a patient can be managed by a nurse (nursing care problems). These are the problems for which, as a nurse, you would be designing care and writing progress notes. Nursing care problems are also termed nursing diagnoses.

In the problem list health maintenance (keeping people well), lack of knowledge related to diabetes, and the potential problem of being a heavy smoker are all problems easily within the realm of nursing expertise. Defining nursing problems comes with increased knowledge of nursing. The process for doing this is described in Chap. 13.

Progress Notes

A progress note on each item on a problem list is written at the time the problem is first identified and then as often as necessary to add new information or document the care and therapy being carried out for the problem. In their best form, all progress notes are written on the same page so that all health care providers can be aware of the actions of all others.

In acute care settings progress notes might be written as frequently as every 15 minutes; in a long-term care facility or a home health agency, as infrequently as daily or once a month. Progress notes are written in a standard format. Listed first is subjective information, then objective information, then a statement of assessment (or conclusion as to the extent of the problem at that moment), and finally the plan of care. Because the first letters of these four divisions spell out the word SOAP, writing progress notes is often referred to as SOAPing.

Subjective information refers to information that cannot be observed or factually proven (that told to you by the patient such as the symptoms of his illness or the way that he feels about a happening).

Objective information is material that can be factually documented such as physical examination findings and laboratory test results. A patient stating that he has pain is a subjective symptom; your noticing him wince as he steps on his feet is objective data.

In a note written at the time a problem is identified, an assessment statement includes not only the problem but the conclusion as to why the problem exists to the best of your knowledge (not pain, but pain related to a surgical incision). Thereafter, assessment statements describe progress (patient with less pain than yesterday; patient with increasing level of pain over the past four hours).

The planning section traditionally includes three types of plans: diagnostic information still needed, therapeutic procedures to be initiated, and educational measures. Remember that POR recording was first devised as a medical model. Physicians usually require diagnostic information (a new blood test, for example); nurses may not. In contrast, a physician may not see an educational need; nursing almost always does. Do not feel that all three types of plans should always be included. The following box illustrates a progress note page completed by health care providers in several areas.

POR and Nursing Process

When nurses first began to use a POR format for charting, there were questions as to how the nursing process, the method by which nurses organize care, could be fit into a medical format. In actual practice it is not a problem, only a matter of understanding the basis for the two systems. Nursing process is the *method* by which nurses assess, plan, implement and evaluate care; POR is simply a method by which you *record* that care.

Nursing process begins with assessment consisting of an interview, the information from which is charted as subjective data, and a physical examination and interpretation of laboratory data, which are recorded as objective data. The second step of the nursing process, analysis, is recorded as assessment. An additional step of the analysis phase is setting a locus of decision-making, and goals and criteria for measuring goal

Progress Notes

Cindy White
No. 609021

Problem: Burn, 2nd degree, dorsum right hand.

S: States she has no further pain on movement.

O: Well-granulated surface; culture report negative.

A: Healing within normal limits.

P: Continue current treatment.

H. Melium, M.D.

Problem: Nutrition, related to burn, 2nd degree, dorsum right hand.

S: States eating is difficult because of dressing on hand; never "really hungry."

O: Fluid balance adequate; eating complete protein only once daily.

A: Patient with protein intake decreased from diet prescription.

P: 1. Repeat food preference history.
2. Consult with nursing staff on teaching importance of protein intake and suggestions to increase protein intake.

B. Hallahan, Dietician

Problem: Fear, related to poor cosmetic appearance.

S: States she is worried burn is going to become scar; important to her because she plays guitar part time in a nightclub and scar will show; asking to have dressing reduced in size so it looks better. Pleased she can move hand well; asking if she can begin playing guitar.

O: Dressing changed with sterile vaseline gauze and dry sterile Kerlix. Pink granulating area 1 cm diameter present; debrided of 1/2 cm area of necrotic tissue at burn rim, scant bleeding. Cried at sight of undressed burn.

A: Patient with increasing anxiety over long-term effect of burn as immediate pain and immobility become less.
Goal: Patient will accept possibility of altered hand appearance in 1 week.
Criterion: Patient will voice ability to adjust to possible altered appearance.

P: 1. Consult with M.D. if future cosmetic surgery is anticipated.
2. Consult with M.D. if guitar playing can be begun.
3. Change dressing with 5 strips vaseline gauze and one layer of Kerlix to reduce size.
4. Teach importance of occlusive dressing to keep burn free of microorganisms.
5. Give reinforcement for things she does well to encourage self-esteem and better acceptance of one negative aspect of life.

J. Smith, R.N.

Problem: Whirlpool therapy, related to burn, 2nd degree, dorsum right hand.

S: States therapy time (11:00 A.M.) interferes with only time her mother can visit. Wants to discontinue therapy.

O: Whirlpool therapy for 20 minutes followed by range of motion exercises. Granulating surface present; range of motion within normal limits. Uncooperative with range of motion exercises due to time spent on them.

A: Patient with good hand mobility; uncooperative attitude.

P: 1. Consult with M.D. on projected length of time therapy is needed.
2. Consult with nursing staff for a better time for therapy.
3. Propose that range of motion exercises be incorporated in nursing care.

R. Brown, Physical Therapist

success for patient care. Physicians do not routinely chart goals as there is only one goal for medical care: complete restoration of health and function. There is no provision in a SOAP note for this.

In order to adapt SOAPing to nursing care and planning, you must add this category. Following assessment in which you state the person's problem, add the goals and criteria that you and he have selected for his care. The importance of goal setting is discussed in Chap. 13. This is the only adaptation necessary when nurses use a SOAP format and one that is easily made.

The next step of the nursing process is planning (recorded as planning, separating out diagnostic, therapeutic, and educational aspects). Evaluation, the last step of the nursing process, would be recorded as a second progress note at the time of the evaluation.

OTHER CHARTING METHODS

Ambulatory records contain many of the same forms used with hospitalized patients: an information sheet, a face sheet, a progress sheet, laboratory and diagnostic sheets, and consult sheets. There is generally not a separate page for nursing notes. Nursing assessments and observations are added to the physician's progress notes.

THE NURSING KARDEX

Kardex is the brand name of a secretarial filing system but has come to be used to refer to any quick-reference, temporary recordkeeping system used to record information pertinent for patient care. Such a system usually consists of an index card set into a flip-type file that is kept on the nursing unit desk.

In contrast to the patient's record, this is a temporary, not a permanent record; it is not a legal document. Cards are generally filled in with pencil rather than pen so that they can easily be erased and changed as the patient's condition and plan of care change. They are destroyed at patient discharge.

Information recorded on such a system typically is the patient's name and unit number, current diagnosis, diet, activity allowed, treatments and medications ordered (medications may be kept on a separate medication Kardex by the medication area), family contacts, and nursing care plan (Fig. 17-9). Information recorded on a Kardex is confidential; it serves as a means of quick reference for coordinating nursing care. The charge nurse generally refers to this quick-reference system to take report and give report to the next nursing shift. Although it is a nursing tool, physicians are welcome to consult it as needed. Many physicians regularly use it to refresh their memories before approaching a patient.

Computers and Recording

Most major medical centers are introducing a computer system in order to schedule efficiently the procedures of patient admission and discharge, billing, and routing of laboratory requests and results. In many centers, recording of nurses' notes is now computerized. In the future, instead of learning *charting*, nurses will learn how to chart information on computer disks.

A major advantage of using a computer system is that it prevents a nurse from having to enter the same information in several different places (onto a flow sheet, Kardex, nursing care plan, and nurse's note). A nurse thus has more time to spend with patients as she spends less time in record keeping. In addition, a computer system can serve as a "reminder" center to announce when a procedure such as a medicine dose is due for administration or when a patient who is prone to skin pressure breakdown is due to be turned and repositioned.

Computers are able to eliminate the paperwork for nurses involved in physicians' prescription writing. With a computer, if a physician writes a prescription for care or medicine directly onto a terminal, errors that arise through copying (and poor handwriting) are eliminated. Telephone orders are another common cause of error in prescriptions. A home terminal for a physician would eliminate this problem. If a STAT or emergency order was written, the computer could immediately write the order into the nurses' Kardex, pharmacy, or laboratory. Absolutely no time would be lost since it is not necessary to wait for someone to be free to transcribe the order.

In order to write nursing notes, you would "sign-on" to the computer with a computer code that is specifically reserved as yours. The computer would not accept information from a person who is not registered in this way in order to prevent irresponsible or unscrupulous persons from "playing" with information in a health record, making a change in the information, or with-

FIGURE 17-9. A Kardex, the flip-type organizer by the nurse's left hand.

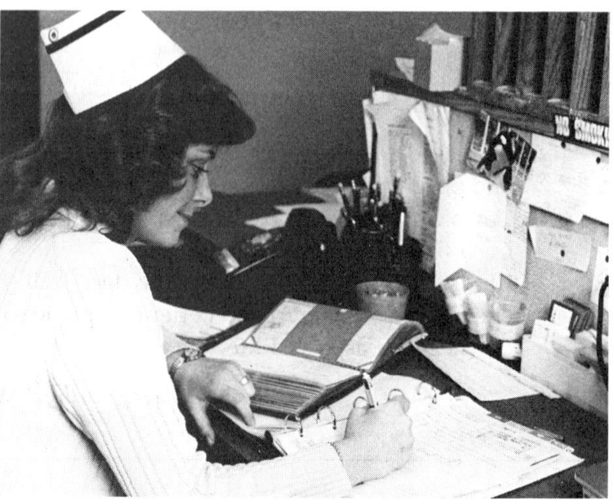

drawing confidential information from the system (violating the patient's right to privacy). You would next be asked by the computer screen what function you would like to do. By pushing a code key you would indicate that you wanted to record in a patient chart. In one computer system currently in use, information is fed into the system by touching a lighted pen to the screen rather than by using a keyboard. This makes computer access equal for everyone, not just those who can type well.

In response to your reply, the computer would ask you which patient's chart you would like opened. You would indicate the patient name, and the computer admission/discharge status line would supply you with the patient number and medical diagnosis.

In most systems, the computer asks you to confirm the patient's name that it shows you. This is comparable to double checking that you have the right patient chart before you record any information in a noncomputer system. In order to enter a patient's initial interview and assessment information efficiently, the computer would supply you with a list of common assessment terms such as "tired-appearing," "jaundiced," and "obese." To add a term to the chart, you would merely touch it on the screen with a lighted pen. If the patient were atypical with unusual symptoms, you could use the keyboard to print in this information. After you formed your analysis from this information, you could construct a nursing care plan by again lightly touching phrases on the screen such as "bedrest," "encourage fluid," or "reassure family."

If you were unfamiliar with the patient's condition and so had difficulty planning care, the computer would supply for you a "standard care plan" for that patient condition. Using your patient assessment information, you could then modify this plan with the same few pen strokes.

Once a care plan has been constructed, it would immediately be printed out for you to use as a worksheet for the day. At the end of the day, recording nursing notes would require only the same few pen touches. The computer could then, on your command, take the information you recorded in a nurse's note and use it to update the care plan. The nurse's note shown at the end of this chapter is written in both a traditional (left column) and a problem-oriented (right column) form. In contrast to these, a computer form would be difficult to show because writing such a note requires no effort other than writing four dots on the paper.

In addition to eliminating paperwork, a computer can be helpful by reminding you of what patient care needs to be initiated. If a throat culture has been ordered, for example, the item would stay on the screen "in process" until you recorded that it was obtained. A computer would print a reminder of what medications were due at 10 o'clock, 11 o'clock, and so on, and remove it from the screen only when you indicated that the medication had been administered.

DISADVANTAGES OF COMPUTER CHARTING

Because computers are still an innovation in health care settings, many people meet their use with suspicion. One problem that can occur is the marking of "completed" into a computer by a nurse who anticipates that she will complete an action but then does not actually carry it out. The computer continues to carry the action as completed. The same situation arises in nursing notes, however, if you anticipate that an action is completed before it actually is. Actually, what can be written into a computer can be erased more easily than penned notations.

One of the major problems guarded against when writing a patient chart is to prevent anyone from adding information to or deleting information from it as it is a legal record. You need to ask a hospital administration that is considering buying a computer recording system what safeguards are built into the system to "write/protect" charts or to prevent anyone from adding anything to the chart after it leaves your control.

An additional problem can occur if only one terminal is available at a nurses' desk, causing you perhaps to spend time waiting to get "on-line" to record your information. Recording a note thus becomes as time consuming as actually writing it.

Computers (hardware) and the programs that make them adaptable to health care settings (software) are currently being devised and improved. It is important that nurses have input into these systems so that the programs developed fulfill the promise of eliminating paperwork for nurses, thereby freeing nurses for more patient care time, rather than merely change the nurse's action from writing to computer programming.

NURSING CARE PLANS

A nursing care plan is another means of recording the plan of care for a patient. This material is generally kept in the nursing Kardex or a separate chart form or notebook; using POR recording eliminates the use of a separate filing system for these as nursing care planning is included in the plan of each progress note. Nursing care plans are considered part of the permanent record and a legal document in many health care facilities. Construction of nursing care plans are discussed in Chap. 13 as they are part of the nursing process.

CHARTING AS NURSING RESPONSIBILITY

Writing nursing notes is considered by some nurses as a time-consuming, unrewarding part of their job. Writing *good* nursing notes should not be boring; it is not unrewarding because it contributes so strongly to the coordination of quality care. It is certainly an art and a challenge. In all instances, being able to do it well is a requirement of a well-qualified nurse.

Nursing Note: Narrative and POR Forms

Mary Jones
No. 100000012

November 18, 1983

3:00 P.M. Patient awake; states she has "sharp pain in back of head"; had lumbar puncture this A.M. and was out of bed immediately afterward. Appears pale; intravenous fluid 5% D/W infusing into left hand at 10 gtts/min.

3:15 P.M. Tylenol 10 gr given p.o. for pain.

3:30 P.M. M.D. visited; removed intravenous fluid from hand and wrote order to give 100 ml fluid every hour for next four hours. Pt. states headache is "better, but still there."

4:00 P.M. Ate dinner of small salad; 4 oz. milk. Lying flat in bed.

5:00 P.M. Urged to drink more fluid. Refused. States "Just not thirsty." Headache "getting worse."

6:00 P.M. States headache is like "hammers pounding inside me." Refusing to drink fluid. States "I'm nauseated from the headache." Asking for something stronger for pain.

S. Ashley, J.U.S.N.

6:00 P.M.

Problem 1: Discomfort, pain

S: Stated she had "hard pounding pain" at 3 P.M.; some relief—headache "better but still there"—after administration of Tylenol 10 gr at 3:15 P.M. By 5 P.M. headache was again "growing worse"; by 6 P.M. it was like "hammers pounding inside me."

O: Had lumbar puncture this A.M. and was out of bed immediately afterward. Tylenol 10 gr given p.o. at 3:15 P.M. Patient appears pale. Lying flat in bed.

A: Patient with severe headache following lumbar puncture; unrelieved by Tylenol administration.
Locus of Decision-Making: Shared between nurse and patient.
Goal: Patient will have pain relief in 20 minutes following analgesic administration.
Criterion: Patient will state she is pain free.

P: Dx: 1. Consult M.D. for stronger pain medication.
Rx: 2. Encourage additional pain relief measures such as cool towel to forehead, dim lights, quiet environment, flat position.
Ed: 3. Teach to lie flat following next lumbar puncture for 8 hours to prevent "spinal headache."

Problem 2: Fluid volume, deficit, potential.

S: States "I can't drink anything, I'm nauseated from the headache."

O: IV fluid (5%D/W) discontinued at 3:30 P.M. by M.D. 100 ml fluid infused. Order for fluid intake changed to 100 ml p.o. q1h. Has taken only 4 oz (120 ml) in 3-hour time span since IV was discontinued.

A: Patient in need of high fluid intake but unable to comply because of nausea.
Locus of Decision-Making: Self.
Goal: Patient will increase fluid intake following relief of nausea.
Criterion: Patient will ingest adequate fluid intake to 100 ml q1h.

P: Dx: 1. Consult M.D. if he feels an antiemetic would be helpful.
2. Ask patient what are favorite fluids (include Jello and Popsicles).
Rx: 3. Obtain favorite fluids from diet kitchen.
4. Offer small amounts of fluid (30 ml) q1/2h rather than large amounts.
Ed: 5. Teach importance of good fluid intake following a lumbar puncture to reduce headache reaction.

CONTRASTING NARRATIVE AND POR NURSING NOTES

Narrative nursing notes used in a traditional record system are written in chronological order (what happened at 9 o'clock, what happened at 10 o'clock, and so on). POR recording focuses instead on the time sequence of happenings, an analysis of the patient's condition, and the plan and goal of care.

The preceding nursing note describes a patient, Mary Jones, who was hospitalized for diagnostic tests, including a lumbar puncture (a needle inserted into the spine's cerebral spinal fluid space for the purpose of withdrawing fluid for analysis). A complication that may occur following a lumbar puncture is a severe headache if the person does not remain flat in bed for at least 4 hours after the procedure. Drinking a large amount of fluid afterward also helps to prevent headache as it causes the amount of fluid that was removed to be replaced more quickly.

SUGGESTED READINGS

Austin, E. How your nursing notes can rob your patients of benefits. *RN* 41:58, 1978.

Barbiasz, J. E., et al. Nursing documentation: A format not a form. *J. Nurs. Adm.* 11(6):22, 1981.

Blount, M., et al. Documenting with the problem-oriented record system. *Am. J. Nurs.* 78:1539, 1978.

Bower, F. L. *The Process of Planning Nursing Care: A Model for Practice.* St. Louis: Mosby, 1977.

Broadwater, S., et al. Before you say "data collecting—ugh" read this. *Nursing* (Horsham) 12(4):50, 1982.

Butters, S., et al. Computerized patient care data: An education program for nurses. *Nurse Educ.* 7(2):11, 1982.

DiCiancia, P. The transfer summary—an essential link when transferring a person from a CCU to a ICCU or a general unit. *Superv. Nurse* 12:36, 1981.

Donaghue, A. M., et al. Some do's and don'ts for giving reports. *Nursing* (Horsham) 11(11):117, 1981.

Dopson, L. Just for the record. *Nurs. Times* 78(12):479, 1982.

Eggland, E. T. Charting: How and why to document your care daily—and fully. *Nursing 80* 10:38, 1980.

Gamberg, D., et al. Outcome charting. *Nurs. Manage.* 12(10):36, 1981.

Gluck, J. The computerized medical record system: Meeting the challenge for nursing. *J. Nurs. Adm.* 9:17, 1979.

Gohen, A. G. The use of computers/data processing in staff development. *Hosp. Top.* 61(1):6, 1983.

Hofing, A. L., et al. The importance of maintenance in initiating change: An experience with problem-oriented recording. *J. Nurs. Adm.* 9:45, 1979.

Krikorian, J. Quality control enhanced by chart review. *Hospitals* 53:97, 1979.

Laing, M. Flow sheets: Meeting the charting challenge. *Can. Nurse* 77(11):40, 1981.

LaMartina Herberg, J. Documentation in child abuse. *Am. J. Nurs.* 83(2):236, 1983.

Lee, G., et al. ED nursing SOAP notes. *J.E.N.* 7(5):216, 1981.

Mancini, M. Documenting clinical records. *Am. J. Nurs.* 78:1556, 1978.

McCloskey, J. C. Nurse's orders: The next professional breakthrough? *RN* 43:99, 1980.

O'Brien, M. J. *Communication and Relationships in Nursing* (2nd ed.). St. Louis: Mosby, 1978.

Pritchard, K. Computers. Possible applications in nursing. *Nurs. Times* 78(11):465, 1982.

Schreiner, R. L., et al. Improving care: Neonatal charting forms in the newborn special care unit. *Perinat./Neonat.* 3:13, 1979.

Sklar, C. You and the law: Problem-oriented recording—could there be a problem? *Can. Nurse* 78(5):47, 1982.

Weed, L. *Medical Records, Medical Education and Patient Care: The Problem Oriented Record as a Basic Tool.* Cleveland: Case Western Reserve, 1971.

Yura, H., and Walsh, M. *The Nursing Process: Assessing, Planning, Implementing, Evaluating* (4th ed.). New York: Appleton-Century-Crofts, 1983.

QUESTIONS FOR REVIEW

1. The following is a narrative nursing note. How many *mistakes* can you find in it?

September 18, 1983 (7:00—3:30)

7:00 A.M.	Patient complaining of pain in right foot. States pain is sharp and penetrating. Foot feels cold to percussion.
7:30	Demerol 50 mg.
8:00	Breakfast taken poor. States "I hate this place. I'm glad I'm going home tomorrow."
8:30	Bath given. Two red areas evident on back. Massaged. Lotion applied. I made bed and talked to her.
9:00	Up to wheelchair; daughter visited for 15 minutes.
10:00	Complaining of pain in foot. I think real problem, however, is loneliness.
2:00	Returned to bed. States toes feel numb and cold.
3:00	In bed. States toes feel numb and cold.

Mary Smith

2. The following is a problem-oriented nursing note. How many *mistakes* can you find in it?

Tracey Burns
Problem: Pain in left knee

S:	Temperature: 100°F. States "My knee is no better and I'm bored." Limps when walks.
O:	Mother states, "I think the swelling is less than yesterday." Left knee feels warm to touch; appears erytematus; aspirin given once during morning; child refused it at noon.
A:	6-year-old with no improvement in pain. Goal: Patient to have pain in right knee reduced to acceptable level.
P:	Therapeutic: Ask M.D. if she could be out of bed more to go to playroom. Education: Educate about pill taking.

S. Ashley, J.U.S.N.

VI. NURSING ASSESSMENT

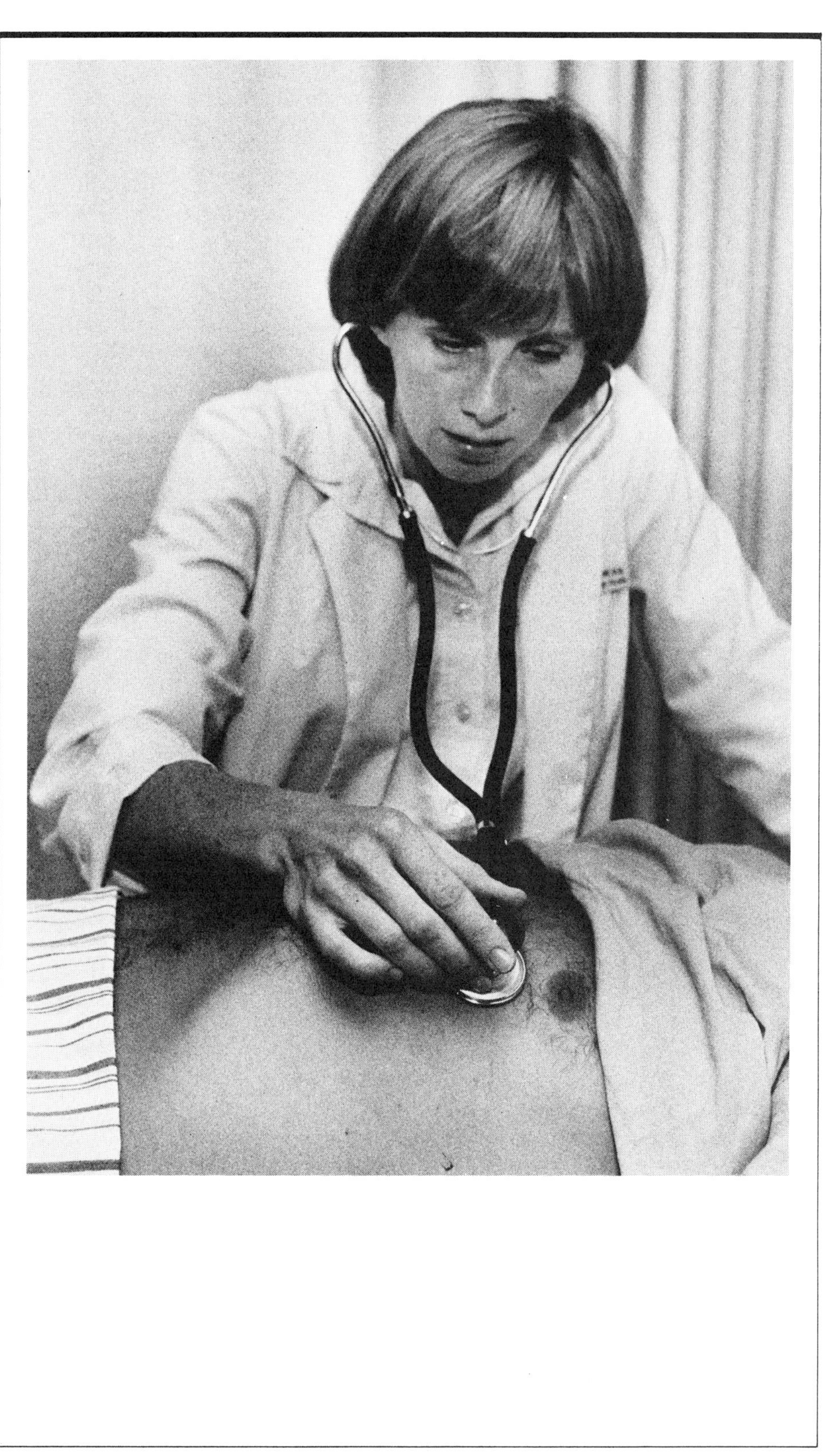

18. ASSESSMENT BY INTERVIEWING MEASURES

OBJECTIVES

Upon mastery of the material of this chapter, you should be able to:

1. Describe the importance of health interviewing and establishing a comprehensive data base.
2. Describe the difference between a nursing history and a comprehensive data base history.
3. List the sections of a comprehensive data base.
4. Describe the components of each section of a comprehensive data base.
5. Describe the sections and components of a return-visit interview.

TERMS

The terms important for an understanding of this chapter are shown below and defined in the glossary:

complete health history
comprehensive data base
nursing history

Comprehensive health assessment consists of three separate parts: a health interview, a physical assessment, and evaluation of diagnostic/laboratory data. In your experience as a consumer of health care, you probably have been more aware of the physical examination and laboratory procedures than interviewing, because these tend to be intrusive and frightening and remembered longer. If you watch a hospital-centered television program, you invariably see little time spent in interviewing but a considerable amount spent performing physical examinations, since physical examination tends to catch the audience's visual attention and interest more readily.

In actuality, interview, physical examination, and laboratory information are three equal prongs of assessment. The interview, in fact, lays the foundation and gives guidance as to what body parts should be given special consideration during the physical examination and what specific laboratory studies are needed.

In order for a person's health history to be complete, information concerning any present illness, family profile, past illnesses, illnesses that are prominently found in the family, pregnancy history, and the functioning of body systems (termed a *review of systems* [ROS]) must be obtained.

OBTAINING A DATA BASE

Information gained from a complete health history combined with information gained from a physical examination and laboratory data form a person's health/illness data base. Obtaining such a data base is necessary for determination of nursing and medical diagnoses, nursing care planning, and implementation. In many settings the nurse's interview serves not only as the basis for a nursing diagnosis but as an aid in helping the physician establish his diagnosis (most physicians agree that up to 80 percent of diagnoses can be made by history alone).

If you are responsible for collecting information for a complete data base, you will be eliciting the information necessary both for nursing and medical planning and for additional health care providers such as the dietician, physical therapist, and psychologist. In some instances you are not responsible for collecting all the information needed for the patient's comprehensive data base. This data will be collected by a physician, a medical student (often referred to as a clinical clerk), a nurse practitioner, or a physician's assistant. In these instances you must review the data base to be certain that information important for planning nursing care (a nursing care history) was asked; if not, you need to obtain this information independently.

Information necessary for planning nursing care is discussed further in Chap. 19. Table 18-1 reviews the important elements of the nursing care history for adults and children.

TABLE 18-1. INFORMATION PERTINENT TO A NURSING CARE HISTORY

1. Demographic information: name, age, sex, marital status (for adult), nickname (for child), family composition.
2. Patient's knowledge of his present illness (if child, parents' knowledge), plan of care (medications, therapy) or diagnostic procedures scheduled, current immunization level, allergies, medication currently being taken. If patient is a child, how does he describe present illness?
3. Past experiences with illness and hospitalization; expectations of this hospitalization. If patient is a child, has he had past experiences with separation (has he ever been to camp? Stayed overnight with a friend?) Has he heard of a relative who died in a hospital or of his illness (could he think that he has come here to die?) Has he had past experience with swallowing pills? What was prenatal history? Are there any significant health problems?
4. Educational and intellectual capabilities.
5. Occupation, economic level, and life style, (if child, of parents).
6. Cultural and religious heritage; language spoken (if not English, who in the family would be a contact person?).
7. Achievement of developmental task and abilities for age group. If patient is a child, how much self-care can be accomplished? School success?
8. Family structure and interaction; living accommodations, presence or absence of support people.
9. Usual health practices; usual methods of coping with stress.
10. "Day history" including nutritional, sleep, elimination, hygiene, and recreational history. If patient is a child, what is bedtime ritual? What is favorite toy? Does he have enuresis (bedwetting)? Are there television programs his parents do or do not like him to watch?

THE HEALTH INTERVIEW

Because a complete health history involves at least eight separate portions or sections and includes happenings from all the years of a person's life, it is lengthy. A thorough history takes a minimum of a half-hour to obtain; it may require more than an hour. Because of the length involved, it may not be possible to obtain a complete history in one setting.

Some agencies supply a data base or nursing history form on which to record this information. There is some danger in using such a form for interviewing because it almost automatically limits you to asking a series of direct questions (How old are you? What is your address? Where do you work?). The average patient responds poorly to this type of interviewing because it makes him feel as if he is being treated in a very routine, computerized way. It is better when taking a comprehensive health history to ask for the necessary information in your own words and record it on a blank piece of paper. This allows you to be yourself and not controlled by a form and allows the patient to elaborate on those aspects he wants to stress rather than answer routine questions.

Take notes as necessary during an interview. Note taking is not distracting to patients; it is, in fact, complimentary. It implies that you consider what they are saying as important. Tell the patient that you will be doing this.

The sections of a comprehensive history are introduction, chief concern, history of present illness, past medical history, family medical history, and review of systems. If the patient is a child, the past medical history is expanded to include pregnancy, birth, and neonatal history. Such a complete history is obtained on a first patient visit to a health care facility. Sections of the interview are generally asked in the order listed above, as with this order transition from one section to another seems to flow smoothly. There is no specific order in which questions must be asked, however. If a person wants to discuss information about a later section first, the order should be changed to accommodate the individual circumstances.

It is important in this type of interview to alert the patient to transitioning between sections so that he knows that you are shifting the topic. If you omit a transition statement such as "I can understand why that concerns you; now the next thing I'm going to be asking you questions about is the ways you've been sick in the past," it is easy to frighten a patient. If you have been asking questions about the person's present cold, for example (information for the history of present illness portion) and then suddenly ask if the person has ever been hospitalized (information for the past health history portion), the person may assume that you think he is so ill that he needs to be hospitalized, when all you were doing was moving on to another interviewing section.

Introduction

Before a person will discuss intimate data about himself, he has to know who you are and that it is important for him to answer such questions. Think how much more readily you tell a nursing school roommate things about yourself than you tell a friend of your mother. This is because having a person you will be working with closely know a great deal about yourself is a help to you; having your mother's friend know these things might or might not be to your advantage.

Letting a patient know exactly who you are so that he understands that you are an important member of a health care team will increase the amount of information that person will supply about present and past health. Always begin any interview, therefore, in which you intend to obtain in-depth information by introducing yourself with your name and title ("Hello, I'm Arlene Smith, a registered nurse") (Fig. 18-1). People like the courtesy of being certain that you know who they are, so follow this with a question to obtain that information: "Are you Mary Jones?" Ask people what they prefer to be called: "Is it all right if I call you Mary?" If the patient is a

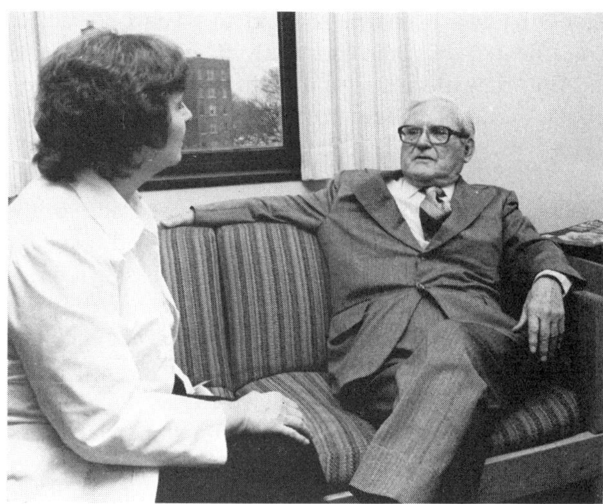

FIGURE 18-1. A formal interview is conducted to obtain a comprehensive data base.

child, ascertain the name and relationship of the person to whom you will be talking: "Is this Eric? Are you his mother?" If a mother is with a child, ask who is his primary caregiver. It is difficult to obtain a complete health history without talking to this person. If you are a student nurse, introduce yourself as such. As a student, not knowing something (you do not recognize the name of a common illness or medication) is readily understandable. If you allow a person to believe that you are more experienced, not recognizing such a thing interferes with your credibility and your relationship.

Explain the purpose of the interview with a simple statement: "In order that I can get to know you well and plan care, I'm going to be asking you questions about yourself and your health." This type of introduction almost automatically establishes this interview as more than casual conversation and deepens the meaning and input from the patient.

When charting a health history, after entering identifying information on the patient (name, age, sex), indicate the source of the history and an indication of that person's reliability (History source: self, some instances of poor memory for recent events noted; history source: mother; good reliability).

Chief Concern (CC)

A chief concern is the reason that the person has come to the health care agency for care. Traditionally, physicians have always called this section of an interview the chief complaint, as physicians are chiefly interested in eliciting a physical sign or symptom. Today since a person may seek medical care for psychological concerns as well as physical ones (nursing always was concerned with both aspects of care), this section of the history in medical as well as in nursing circles has become known as the chief concern. Because it implies unhappy, hard-to-satisfy people, *complaint* is a term best forgotten in both professions.

Ascertain the person's chief concern by asking such questions as "Why did you come to the hospital today?" Do not ask "What brings you to the hospital today"; the answer may be "The number 9 bus brought me" or "My sister drove me," amusing exchanges perhaps but rarely helpful.

Most people respond readily to this question with a description of pain, loss of vision, constant nervousness, etc. If the visit is an ambulatory one for health maintenance, the person may answer "It's just a routine checkup." To elicit a chief concern, follow this with a question such as "Is there anything you are particularly worried about or concerned about that you wanted to ask about today?" The answer to such a question is rarely no.

A chief concern is charted in the patient's exact words and surrounded by quotation marks. Often you could improve on the statement, but do not do so. "Pain in my gut" is proper wording for a chief concern statement if that is how it was voiced. "Pain originating in the left lower quadrant of the abdomen and radiating to the midline" would sound more professional but would be your wording, not his, and should not be used.

You will then explore this chief concern, as explained in the section, History of Present Illness, below. Following the exploration, ask about a second concern. Explore that and ask for a third, fourth, fifth, and so on, until you have asked for one more than the person gives you.

The reason for this is that in ambulatory settings a person must explain to the clinic or office receptionist why he is making the appointment. People learn that if they mention reasons such as routine checkup or constant nervousness, they will be given an appointment perhaps as much as a month in advance. However, if they mention a symptom that calls for acute therapy (vomiting or eye pain), they will be given an immediate appointment. When you say to the person, "What is the reason you are here today?" he will describe this "ticket-in-the-door" or almost made-up symptom. Only when you say, following your first exploration, "Is there anything else that concerns you?" will he tell you why he is there (he is so fatigued that he cannot seem to get through a day and is worried that he has heart trouble). This is not deceit on the part of the patient but an attempt to gain satisfaction from a health care delivery system that can be difficult to deal with.

This same principle applies to interviewing at hospital admission. Although a parent is admitting a child because he is actively wheezing from an asthma attack, the fact that the child is not doing well in school may be their chief concern with this child. Asking about problems in addition to the stated ones may reveal a true chief concern and be the way to truly meet health care needs.

It might seem as if a chronological order of question asking, beginning with pregnancy, then past medical history, and working your way forward to present illness, would be a more organized manner to collect health data. The chief concern is the reason that the person has come to the health care facility, however. Think of yourself with a terrible headache, riding a bus to a busy doctor's office or a hospital, having to wait in a waiting room, and when you do get to see a health care provider, having to supply information from the time you were a child. You want to talk about your headache first and only after you have thoroughly described it will you be willing to discuss anything else. So it is with everyone.

Information about a person's chief concern helps to guide the physician into a diagnosis and alerts you to immediate nursing care necessary (a person who reports he feels warm or has symptoms of an infection needs his temperature taken as an independent nursing action; a person who is short of breath may need to be seen more quickly than one without respiratory distress).

History of Present Illness (HPI)

A history of present illness is a narrative account of the chief concern. There are six questions that you need to ask to identify the problem and describe it fully.

Duration. The length of time that the problem has existed is its duration. This information separates chronic from acute illnesses. It not only helps to pinpoint the cause of a symptom but also gives information as to the person's reaction to stress (how long he coped with the problem before seeking help).

Make a habit of asking people to express time in terms of hours, days, months, and years rather than with statements such as "a long time." Such statements can be misleading: Your idea of "a long time" may be 30 days; to an 80-year-old patient "a long time" may mean 30 years.

Intensity. Intensity refers to the strength of the person's symptom. If the symptom is pain related, the intensity may be described as nagging, tearing, crushing, piercing, cutting, dull, etc. Note carefully the adjective the person uses to describe the intensity and quote it exactly in your notes. "Crushing pain," for example, is the description that people spontaneously use to describe the pain of a heart attack. In contrast, no one ever uses that term to describe the pain of appendicitis. Asking if pain is enough to disrupt the person's usual activity is a good indication of how intensely a symptom is felt.

If the symptom is concerned with vomiting or diarrhea, the intensity refers to the amount or volume of the vomitus or liquid stool. Ask the person to estimate a commonly known measure such as a cupful or a teaspoonful. Terms such as "a lot" or "a little bit" may mean different things to you and the patient.

Frequency. The frequency of a chief concern is how often the symptom being described occurs. Ask the person to commit himself to a definite time (every day, constantly). If he is a stoic person and says "I have it a lot," he may mean he has pain constantly; if he is less than stoic, his "lot" may mean once a month. To avoid misinterpretation and over or underestimating the frequency of a symptom, you need to elicit a definite time frame.

Description. Description refers to the appearance of the symptom: its sequence, location, color, and odor. Sequence refers to any change over time (at first, it seemed like heartburn; now it is pain that is sharp and crushing and radiates down an arm). Location means the body part affected. Ask the person to point as exactly as possible to the body part affected rather than using a term like "over my liver" or "in my stomach." Many people actually have little idea where these organs are located and may give you wrong information by using these terms. Small children sometimes answer "yes" to any question put to them so that if a parent asks a 4-year-old if the reason he does not look well is because he has a stomachache, the child may answer yes. When you ask a child to point to the place where his stomach hurts, he usually points to his umbilicus. A preschool child, pointing to any other location on his abdomen, must be taken seriously as he has responded so untypically for his age group in pointing to a place of actual pain.

After determining the exact point of discomfort, ask if the pain radiates or travels to any other point. This is important to the physician in diagnosing an illness such as gallbladder disease, which typically has this pattern of pain.

Color, odor, amount, and consistency of any discharge are important in defining its nature and need to be detailed if the symptom involves any form of body discharge or drainage.

Associated Symptoms. Associated symptoms are symptoms that occur at the same time as the chief concern. Rarely does a symptom occur as an isolated event and it is the combination of symptoms (syndrome) that allows the physician to establish a specific diagnosis. The symptom that people report as a chief concern is not necessarily the most serious or most diagnostic one but the one that is most upsetting to them. Vomiting, for example, is distressing to most parents. They report it as a chief concern in children very frequently. They may not report other things they have noticed as well (a stiff neck, irritability, fever) until asked if any other symptoms are present. The stiff neck, irritability, and fever, however, are the clues that point to the diagnosis (these three symptoms are highly suggestive of meningitis or infection of the spinal cord). The vomiting will need care but is not as diagnostic as the other symptoms. Knowing specific associated symptoms to ask for comes with additional clinical knowledge of disease pathology, but asking a question such as "Are you ill in any other way?" may reveal the other symptoms of a syndrome.

Person's Actions. It is important to ascertain two aspects of the person's activities in connection with his chief concern. The first is what was happening or what was the person doing at the time of the initial symptoms (had anything unusual happened at or near the time of the initial occurrence?). A man who is being seen with a bothersome, oozing rash on his hands who relates that it occurred just after he returned from a hiking trip, for example, is probably reporting a reaction to something he encountered on his trip such as poison ivy; if the rash happened at the time that he began taking penicillin for an upper respiratory infection, he is more likely describing a drug reaction. This information is very often important for his physician's diagnosis.

The second kind of activity about which you need information is what the person has tried to do to alleviate the symptom. This not only gives some clue as to the strength and cause of the symptom (drinking milk made stomach pain disappear), but it also tells you a great deal about the common sense of the person and his ability to cope with illness. If the mother of a child seen for vomiting, for example, tells you that she had the child lie on the sofa and drink some plain tea, her action may not have been very therapeutic for the child's illness, but it indicates that she is a different type of mother from one who answers, "I didn't do anything. I'm helpless when anyone is sick." In the first instance the woman will readily comprehend your or the physician's instructions for care, get a prescription filled if required, administer it accurately, and call you or the physician for further help as needed. The second person will need more instruction before she is ready to take her ill child home and may need frequently spaced call-back times arranged in order to cope with illness. There are many women who are good mothers to well children but who are not yet ready to proceed to the higher developmental step (or need some help in proceeding to this step) of taking care of an ill child; some men are excellent husbands to a well wife but are not able (or need help in being able) to care for an ill wife. This type of question alerts you to this important fact.

Asking about a patient's actions may also reveal mistakes that he made in self-care (giving adult doses of aspirin to one-month-old infants, using outdated medicine from the medicine cabinet, not being aware that puncture wounds from rusty nails are excellent places for tetanus infections to begin). The interview is not the time to correct a person on something he has done wrong, but discovering these areas and incorporating them into your health teaching at a later time will help patients to take more appropriate action the next time that they or their families are ill (see Quick Reference Stop 18-1: Pharmacology).

☐ QUICK REFERENCE STOP 18-1: PHARMACOLOGY

In history taking document not only the kind but the amount and times of medications a person is currently taking. Sometimes you discover an individual who is taking medicine unwisely—that prescribed for another family member or outdated medicine from the medicine cabinet; sometimes you discover that people are receiving wrong doses—giving adult doses to infants. Educating people about these unsafe practices will make them wiser health care consumers in the future.

Be certain to ask about over-the-counter medications or home remedies as well. Unsafe administration in these areas can be equally dangerous.

Patient/Family Profile (PP or FP)

Traditionally, family profile data were collected at the end of the interview, the thought being that a person would not reveal this intimate type of information until he was very comfortable with the interviewer. This does not prove to be true, however, and leaving this type of information to the end of an interview results in interviewing in the dark and only turning on the light at the very end, as you cannot really "see" the person without this information.

In addition, if a person has psychosocial problems (a family depends on him and he is hospitalized; he is worried not only that he cannot pay for this hospitalization but that his family will have to move out of their apartment as well), he usually wants health care personnel to know them. If you already have serious problems, the last thing you want is for someone not to recognize that these exist and send you home with additional bills and problems.

Introduce this category of information by a statement such as "Before I ask you things about ways you've been sick in the past, I want to ask you questions about yourself and your family." Elicit information on the following elements:

Identifying Data. Identifying information is often collected by a secretary or receptionist prior to your seeing the patient; if it has not been previously obtained, you need to obtain it. It is information necessary for individualizing care and to clearly differentiate a chart as belonging to a specific Mary Smith, John Jones, and so forth. This information is full name, address, birth date, age, sex, marital status, religion, occupation, name of attending physician, and insurance coverage or method of payment for health care; it is recorded on the information sheet in a patient's records. Be certain that this information is recorded prior to the time you see the patient. If not, be certain that these particulars are obtained when you seek family profile information. Many people are sensitive to being asked about how they will pay their health care bill (cash or third party payment), worried perhaps that they will receive a different quality of care if their method of payment is in doubt. From your standpoint the answer to the question is immaterial: You are merely documenting facts, and will provide quality nursing care no matter what the method of payment. It is information for billing purposes and hospital room assignment (some insurance policies pay only the cost of a semiprivate room; people with these policies typically want to be assigned to a semiprivate care setting and you may discover they have not been placed appropriately). Explain the reasons for your questions as needed.

Family Pattern and Structure. How many people live at home? How many people are dependent on this person? Who does this person go to when he has problems (who are his support persons)? What is his overall life style (student, nine-to-five executive, homemaker). If the patient is a child, who is the primary caregiver? What is the child's position in the family? This information is important for planning therapy and in the instance of a child to be certain that you are speaking to the person best informed to report his usual health patterns.

Living Arrangements. Does this person live in a single home? Apartment? Upstairs? Downstairs? If the patient is a young child, are there any sources of peeling paint (windowsills, garage areas) that he could possibly be eating (which could cause lead poisoning because of the lead contained in paint, which can result in extreme neurological damage)? Whether a person lives upstairs or downstairs may be important if he has to be careful of how many stairs he walks up daily after he returns home or if he will have difficulty getting out of the house to buy groceries or get enough exercise. Is the home or apartment convenient to stores, church, transportation?

Occupational History. Occupational history includes not only what the person is working at now but past occupations. This is important both in terms of his illness (if he worked with asbestos in the past, he has a greater-than-average potential for developing lung cancer) and also in telling you about the person as a whole such as his degree of responsibility, his level of stress, and sometimes demeaning events in his life such as the recent loss of a job. It also strongly suggests financial level.

Occupations of parents are important if the patient is a child. Parents exhausted from stressful working conditions may find that therapy for a child such as doing exercises to strengthen a child's muscles is difficult for them; other parents may find this stimulation an enjoyable part of their otherwise routine day. A woman who works all day at a nursery school with 4-year-olds may do very well with her own 4-year-old at home in the evening because she is so familiar with children of this age; on the other hand, her own 4-year-old may be one too many for her to deal with effectively on some days. You cannot begin to help with such problems if you are not aware of them; that is why occupational history is included in an interview.

Educational History. Ask adult patients the highest level of schooling they attained. If the person did not complete high school (the minimum level of schooling accepted by most people), ask the reason. Many older people had to leave school to support their families during the Depression; this is a different situation from the person who chose to drop out of school because he was having so much difficulty with the curriculum. The second person may need more detailed instruction to understand his illness or the procedures that he must continue to perform after he returns home.

If the patient is a child, ask him what grade in school he is in. Is it an appropriate grade? Does he participate in extracurricular activities? Is he happy in school (contrary to popular belief, most children report that they like school)? Knowledge of how a child is doing in school tells you a great deal about what his illness will probably mean to him as it indicates his hopes for the future, his present self-esteem, and how supportive his friends are apt to be if he is ill.

Cultural and Religious Heritage. It is dangerous to stereotype people; at the same time, a person is influenced by the culture around him and his religion. His diet in particular is strongly influenced by culture or religion, as is his concept of what is adequate therapy and what he expects from health care. This information is therefore included in a comprehensive data base.

Economic Status. Economic status is generally closely associated with occupation. Ask the patient about finances: Do you have enough money for the things you need? How will this illness affect family resources? Determine whether additional resources such as food stamp programs could be utilized and probably should be suggested. Many people do not like to discuss their financial situation. Preface such questions with "Medical care or hospitalization is expensive . . ." so that the person realizes that your intent is to assist him if necessary.

Past Medical History (PMH)

The ways that a person was ill in the past may have influenced the way he is presently ill or the level of health that he now maintains.

Childhood Illnesses. Ask about childhood illnesses—mumps, measles, German measles (rubella), chickenpox, rheumatic fever—separately from other illnesses as many people do not consider these as illnesses but as normal consequences of childhood. Most adults are not sure which of these diseases they have had; it is important to know if women of childbearing age have had rubella, as contacting this disease during pregnancy can lead to fetal damage. Because rheumatic fever can result in heart disease, it is important to obtain a history as to treatment and outcome if this illness is reported.

Immunizations. If the patient is a child, ask for dates of immunizations to see if there are common diseases to which he could be susceptible. Immunizations recommended for children are shown in Table 9-16. Most adults are not aware of what immunizations they have had. Information important for adults is rubella immunization if the woman is of childbearing age and the most recent tetanus immunization if a break in the skin is present (tetanus immunization lasts for 10 years, then should be repeated; rubella immunization is theoretically only needed once in a lifetime).

Allergies. Ask about allergies or sensitivities to food, insects, respiratory irritants such as pollen, and medications or drugs. If allergies are present, ask what happens when an allergic attack occurs. This description is important for the physician in evaluating whether a true allergy exists. Some people, for example, state that they have an allergy to penicillin because the last time they took some they developed diarrhea. Diarrhea is an unfortunate side effect of penicillin, not an allergic response to it. In all probability, such a person will be administered penicillin if he needs it for his present illness or one in the future. (Whether it will be ordered is a physician's decision; you just record for him the symptoms that patients report as allergies.)

When recording, make out a separate list of allergies (usually in red for emphasis) to be attached to the front of the patient's chart and the Kardex (a separate charting form kept on the nursing desk—see Chap. 17). If a dietary allergy is reported, be certain that the dietary department is notified if appropriate.

Serious Illnesses. Serious illness is a broad category. If the person reports a serious illness such as pneumonia, heart trouble, kidney trouble, ask for the date and treatment given and any complications from the experience. This information is important not only because it may relate to the present illness (which may be a recurrence, not a new illness) but because it offers clues as to the person's acceptance of health care, his satisfaction with health care providers, and his expectations of recovery from the present illness. A person who had a poor outcome from surgery previously may resist doing breathing exercises because of a "what's-the-difference?" attitude. He may need a better-than-average explanation of his surgery, as he may be more concerned about outcome than the average person; the stress of worry limits people from "hearing" explanations.

Hospitalizations and Surgery. Since some surgery is done on an ambulatory basis (tonsillectomies, sutures for lacerations, herniorrhaphy), a person may have had surgery and not been hospitalized, so these two categories of information must both be included. Document date, place, and attending physician if surgery is reported. As with major illnesses, these categories yield information not only about health problems but also about how the person feels about health care and his expectations from hospitalizations and health care providers.

Accidents and Injuries. Since many people do not consider accidents as illnesses and since such incidents may not have involved surgery or hospitalization, you must ask about them separately. Ask about poisoning separately, as some people think only falls or auto accidents are "accidents" and do not respond about poisonings. As a rule, accidental poisoning does not occur over 5 years of age. If the person was older at the time of the poisoning, think of it as a possible suicidal gesture or attempt. Asking about accidents is extremely important when the patient is a child; ask yourself if you are possibly listening to a history of child abuse. Such a history usually includes accidents more severe than the history warrants—frequent burns and abrasions. (See Chap. 12 for a discussion of child abuse.)

Health Habits. Health habits is a category of information that generally reveals potential health problems of the individual. Ask about smoking, alcohol consumption, any medication currently being taken (prescription, over-the-counter, or home remedy). Document the number of cigarettes or amount of liquor consumed (to ensure that a person's explanation of being a "social drinker" or "occasional smoker" corresponds to your conception of these terms). Documenting medications is important because the medication may be masking symptoms of illness (or actually causing a symptom). Many women do not consider birth control pills as medication; ask about these separately. Adolescents and young adults should be asked if they experiment with drugs of any kind. Most persons answer this type of question honestly if it is prefaced by a statement such as "Many people your age experiment with drugs. . . ."

Also document the person's general health care habits. When was his last routine health examination? Pap test (for women)? Chest x-ray?

Obstetric/Gynecological History. If a patient is a female over 10, ask about age of first menstruation, frequency and duration, and any difficulty associated with menstrual cycles such as cramping or heavy flow. Also note the date of the last menstrual period.

Ask about pregnancies of women past puberty. Document the dates and types of deliveries and weights of babies; include miscarriages and therapeutic abortions. This information tells a great deal about the woman's overall health and life style.

Prenatal History. If the patient is a child under 18, ask for a detailed description of his prenatal history. Begin a prenatal history with an open-ended question to the mother such as "How was the pregnancy?" This encourages the mother to tell you about either physical or psychosocial problems. If you ask "Did you have any problems during pregnancy?" it almost automatically limits the mother to describing physical health problems and puts the burden on her to know what was a problem during pregnancy.

Ask about the prenatal care she received. Statistics show that mothers who receive prenatal care have better pregnancy outcomes than those who do not. Some physical complications of pregnancy that are significant and may have an effect on the child are vaginal bleeding, falls, x-ray, swelling of face or fingers, high blood pressure (hypertension), poor nutrition, rashes, excessive weight gain, medication taking, smoking, and alcohol consumption. As important as physical health during pregnancy is the mother's psychological acceptance of the child and pregnancy. Many instances of child neglect and abuse occur because the mother did not want the pregnancy and never accepted the child during pregnancy. Ask if the pregnancy was planned. This is sometimes an awkward question. One nonthreatening way of asking the question is to give alternatives: "Some pregnancies come at a good time, some don't; how was it with this one?" If the mother replies that she was looking forward to or had planned on becoming pregnant, that is the information that you want.

Many women do not want a pregnancy originally, but accept it as it progresses and, by birth, want the baby very much. If the woman says the pregnancy was not planned, ask her at what point in pregnancy she felt the baby move and offer her the possible alternatives that could have occurred at that time: "Some women feel differently about wanting a baby after they feel the baby move; some don't feel any different. How was it with you?" The average woman answers "Once I felt the baby move, I knew that everything would be all right."

Labor and Delivery History. Ask about the method of delivery (vaginal or cesarian birth); where did the birth occur (hospital, home, or birthing center); any problems the mother was aware of; and length of labor. Ask about the baby's condition at birth (Did he cry immediately? Was any special equipment used with him? Any special delivery room care given to him? Does the mother remember his Apgar score?). Did the baby go to a regular nursery or a special care nursery? Was there any blueness (cyanosis) or yellowness (jaundice), both problems at birth that can lead to long-term effects on intelligence and overall health? Did the mother and child go home together in 1 to 3 days if it was a vaginal delivery, 7 to 10 days with cesarian birth? What was the baby's birth weight? A defective parent-child bonding relationship is important to elicit. Ask how the person felt about being a new parent.

Family Health History

A family health history (FHH) is taken to establish whether there are inherited diseases in the family. Ask the patient about the health of siblings, children, parents, and both sets of grandparents. If a disease is present or a member is deceased, ask about the date and care of the illness and the cause of death. Ask if heart disease, high blood pressure (hypertension), kidney disease, mental illness, mental retardation, diabetes, cancer, tuberculosis, convulsions, anemia, or symptoms like the patient is presently experiencing have occurred in any family members such as aunts, uncles, or cousins. It is helpful when charting a family health history to draw a family pedigree such as the one shown in the history record at the end of this chapter.

Day History

Information about a patient's nutrition, elimination, sleep, recreation, development, interpersonal interactions, and sexual activity can be elicited best not by direct questions (to which the person may try to give the "right" answers) but by asking the person to describe a typical day of his life. If the person is not specific about a period in his day, ask individual questions for more detail. Table 18-2 lists nutritional, sleep, elimination, interpersonal interaction, developmental task, and sexual information that you need to obtain. If any of this information is not reported spontaneously, it must be elicited by individual questions.

A person's sexuality—how he feels about himself and his female or male role—is as much a part of him as other more frequently discussed topics such as nutritional or recreational habits. People coming for health care may well have a sexually-related problem as their second chief concern and are greatly relieved that sexuality is a topic you explore with them along with others.

When charting, information obtained from a day history is often separated into individual categories such as nutritional, sleep, recreational, sexual, and developmental sections so that a person reading the history can discern quickly information pertaining to a specific category. See Quick Reference Stop 18-2 for a key to taking down nutritional information in the day history.

Review of Systems

A review of systems (ROS) is the final category in a health history. It is a double check to be certain that information was not missed. Introduce this section by saying that to finish you are going to review the person's health status from his head to his toes to be certain that nothing was missed. Although a review of systems seems lengthy when reading about it, it is not as time consuming as it seems in actual practice. If a person

TABLE 18-2. INFORMATION GAINED FROM DAY HISTORY

A. Nutritional history

1. 24-hour recall of a well day (be certain that snacks as well as sit-down meals are described). How much fluid is consumed daily (when well)? For breast-fed infants, ask for length of time at breast and how many times they are fed daily. In formula-fed infants how formula is prepared and amount and times of feedings. Regulating fluid is necessary for many dietary regimes; you need a baseline of overall consumption of fluid as well as food. Include alcohol consumption as fluid.
2. Who cooks (you cannot change the diet of a non-cooking household member until you speak to the person who cooks)? What seasonings are regularly used (monosodium glutamate, celery or garlic salt are all high sources of sodium)? How is food usually cooked (foods fried in saturated oil add a great deal of cholesterol; boiled vegetables lose a great many vitamins)?
3. Is food eaten largely in planned settings or mainly as snacks? (Diet planning is harder, as a rule, if the person relies on many snack foods.)
4. Is there any difficulty eating (poor-fitting dentures, difficulty swallowing)?
5. Food allergies? Likes and dislikes?
6. How many meals are eaten out daily? Weekly? (If a special diet is planned as therapy, a person who eats a great deal at fast-food restaurants may have difficulty following it. A person who takes his lunch to school or work may need some help in planning a packed lunch that is compatible with the diet plan.)
7. Are any vitamins or vitamin supplements taken?

B. Sleep history

1. Total hours of sleep each 24 hours; sleep rituals.
2. Any sleeping difficulty such as insomnia, frequency of urination? In children sleep-walking (somnambulism) or bed-wetting (nocturnal enuresis)? Does child sleep by self or with parents or sibling?
3. Has pattern changed recently? (Stress changes sleep patterns; this may reflect concern about illness.)
4. Is medication regularly taken to induce sleep?

C. Recreation history

1. What hobbies are enjoyed? Being able to work at a hobby may be as important to the person as being able to continue his job.
2. How much physical activity (jogging, rollerskating, playing touch football) is enjoyed daily? An illness that limits physical activities may be felt more keenly by an active person than a sedentary one.

D. Elimination history

1. What is the usual pattern of bowel movements? What is urinary frequency? Has this changed recently?
2. Is anything used to aid bowel movements (laxatives, roughage in diet, enema)?
3. Are there any problems with voiding (frequency, greater or lesser amount than usual, burning, irregularity of flow such as stopping and starting)?
4. Is person independent in these areas?

E. Hygiene history

1. Is a bath or shower preferred? Frequency of these (daily, weekly)? Is any help needed with these (when well)? How often is hair washed?
2. Any sensitivity to soaps, skin-care preparations?
3. How often are teeth/dentures brushed or flossed? Is help with this necessary (when well)?

F. Interpersonal interaction history

1. Who lives at home? How do these people interact with each other, particularly husband-wife interaction. Do they eat together or as each arrives home? Who gives psychological support to whom?
2. If the person is a child, does the parent describe time for holding, rocking, or playing? Can the parent name the child's favorite activity or toy? (Remember that the quantity of a relationship is not as important as its *quality*. A working mother may describe more mother-child interaction than a mother who is home with her child all day but does not actively relate to him; an aged parent may live with one child, but in an emergency would phone another child for help.)

G. Developmental milestones

Developmental milestones are discussed in Chap. 9. Review this chart, then determine if milestones in childhood are being met. Ability to complete tasks of daily living (dressing self, eating independently, etc.) is a standard used for adults.

H. Sexual history

1. Is the person sexually active? Is his present sexual relationship satisfying? Is a form of birth control being used? Is infertility ever a concern?
2. For males, is impotence (inability to achieve an erection) or premature ejaculation a problem?
3. For females, is achieving orgasm a concern? Does she have pain on coitus (sexual relations)? (If sexual history seems out of context at this point because of the person's life style, the information can be elicited with the review of systems information at the end of the interview.)

☐ QUICK REFERENCE STOP 18-2: NUTRITION

When taking a nutritional history, be certain to ask about snack foods as well as those eaten at formal meals. If you do not know the ingredients of a dish a person mentions (sauerbraten, for example), ask the person to describe it (sauerbraten is veal).

Therapy for almost all illnesses involves some form of nutritional therapy. Only if a change in diet is based on the foods or method of preparation that is acceptable to a person and fits into his budget will the new diet be followed and be effective as therapy.

acknowledges any symptom you ask about at this time, evaluate whether this symptom should be described in this section when you chart the history or listed as a chief concern. The fact that you often decide to record information gained in this review as a chief concern documents the importance of this double-check system built into the end of a health history.

Do not get into the habit of conducting your ROS, not as part of the interview, but when you begin your physical assessment (when you are examining the person's eyes, asking if he ever had any eye disease, and so on). This is sometimes suggested as a means of shortening the time spent gathering initial assessment data, but it may confuse patients (if you are looking at someone's eyes and ask if he has ever had eye disease, he may think you see something wrong with his eye). Perhaps you save a fraction of a moment's time but you may frighten a patient needlessly by your carelessness in not separating interview questions from physical assessment actions.

Table 18-3 shows questions to ask when conducting a review of systems for an adult and for an infant or young child.

Conclusion of Interview

If a person is especially concerned about a symptom (he is very worried he may have cancer), he may not easily report this worry (perhaps if neither he nor you mention it, it cannot be so). Ask at the end of an interview as a final check for thoroughness (to be certain you have not missed anything) "Do you have any questions? Is there anything else you'd like to ask about or mention?" (Fig. 18-2).

TABLE 18-3. INFORMATION TO OBTAIN FOR A REVIEW OF SYSTEMS

System	Adult	Young Child
General health	Height, weight (any recent weight gain or loss?).	Height, weight (any recent weight loss?).
Neuropsych	Convulsions; fatigue, anxiety, weakness, depression.	Convulsions.
Head	Head trauma, headache, dizziness (vertigo).	Shape; fontanelles; trauma.
Hair	Changes in texture, color, distribution or loss.	
Eyes	Difficulty with vision; wears glasses or not; eye disease (glaucoma, cataracts, infection). Date of last vision examination.	Ability to follow a moving finger; difficulty with vision; eye infections.
Ears	Difficulty with hearing; wears hearing aid or not; ear disease (infection, dizziness, discharge). Date of last hearing examination.	Infections; discharge; difficulty with hearing.
Nose	Nose bleeds (epistaxis); difficulty breathing; discharge (rhinorrhea); loss of smell; sinus problems.	Bleeding; discharge.
Mouth	Difficulty with teeth; wears dentures, braces, or retainers; lesions or irritated points in mouth. Date of last dental examination.	Number of teeth present; cavities; last dental examination.
Throat	Difficulty swallowing; infections, hoarseness; documentation of streptococcal infection (streptococcal infections can lead to glomerulonephritis and rheumatic fever).	Infections; difficulty swallowing.
Neck	Stiffness; swollen nodes.	Masses; stiffness.
Chest	Discharge or masses in breasts (both male and female); if female, does she do monthly self-breast examinations? (See Chap. 19 for technique.)	Symmetry.
Respiratory system	Cough (raises sputum or not); pain; wheezing, shortness of breath; infections. Date of last chest x-ray.	Frequent colds; coughs.
Cardiovascular system	Chest pain, high blood pressure (hypertension); edema in extremities; past heart disease, extreme fatigue on exertion. Date of any ECGs (electrocardiograms) taken.	Any heart murmurs; shortness of breath; cyanosis.
Gastrointestinal system	Appetite, vomiting, nausea, diarrhea, constipation, hemorrhoids, jaundice (yellowing of skin, a symptom of liver disease); change in bowel habits; blood in stools.	Vomiting; diarrhea; constipation.
Genitourinary system	Frequency, pain, blood in urine; incontinence. For females, vaginal discharge; itchiness (pruritis); infections, sexually transmitted disease; pain on coitus. For males, prostate problems; sexually transmitted disease; sexual difficulty such as impotence or premature ejaculation.	Difficulty with urine stream; pain on voiding; frequency.
Back	Pain, stiffness, history of spinal injury.	
Skin	Rashes, changes in moles or other lesions.	Birthmarks; rashes; eccymotic marks.
Extremities	Pain; stiffness; swelling of joints; history of trauma, fractures, varicose veins.	Fractures; stiffness, swollen joints.
Hematological system	Anemia; transfusions (any reactions to transfusions and reason for).	
Endocrine system	Thyroid disease; diabetes.	

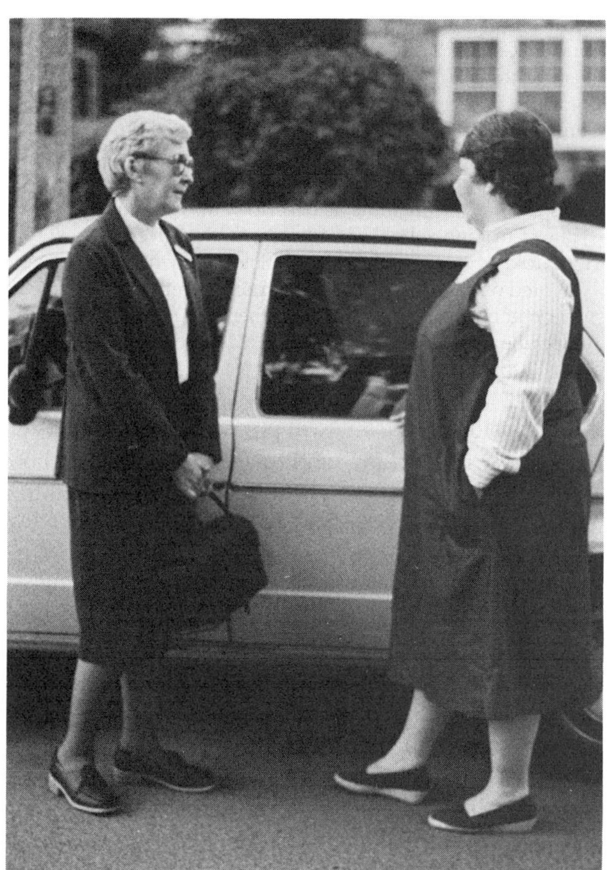

FIGURE 18-2. "I just remembered to tell you this." Note the client left her home and approached the community health nurse just as the nurse was about to leave. Her concern probably *is* important information for the health history.

RETURN VISIT INTERVIEW

Once a person has had a comprehensive data base history recorded, subsequent ambulatory or hospital visits require only an updating of information. The following are areas that need to be updated on subsequent visits:

1. *Introduction.* An introduction of who you are and what you will be doing is important if it is the first time the patient has seen you. Although this may be the person's tenth visit to the health care facility, he cannot have confidence in you without being able to identify who you are.

2. *Identifying data.* People move frequently; check their addresses. Family patterns change in relation to marriage or divorce or death. Check the person's name to see it it is still accurate. Adjust the patient's age according to the birth date.

3. *Chief concern.* Whether a first visit or a subsequent one, ask for one more chief concern than the person gives you.

4. *History of present illness.* Explore chief concerns according to the same six steps used with a first visit: duration, frequency, intensity, description, associated symptoms, and patient action.

5. *Interval history.* An interval history is a description of events that happened since the person was last seen at the health care facility. Include both physical happenings (illnesses, accidents, surgery, hospitalizations) and psychosocial happenings (moves, occupation changes, school changes, marriage, financial changes).

6. *Day history.* It is helpful to record a day history to update nutrition, elimination, developmental level, and life style information.

7. *Conclusion.* Ask if there are any further concerns you should discuss.

HEALTH HISTORY INTERVIEWING

Interviewing for a health history is a time-consuming task. Establishing a comprehensive health history and updating it by thorough return visit histories, however, are essential for comprehensive health care. A nurse skilled in interviewing technique who can elicit a comprehensive history makes a very real contribution to health care. Such interviewing is becoming a nursing responsibility in many settings and a skill you need to acquire to fulfill your role as a health care provider of the future.

Charting a Comprehensive Data Base History

Below is a sample recording of information gained from a comprehensive data base history interview. Recording a health history follows the techniques of charting described in Chap. 17. It should be succinct but detailed enough to be meaningful.

IDENTIFYING DATA

Mary Jones, 18 years old, white, female. Source of information: self; good reliability.

CHIEF CONCERN

"Always tired since starting college 1 month ago."

HISTORY OF PRESENT ILLNESS

Mary states she felt well until a month ago; now so tired she has to miss afternoon classes 3 out of 4 days a week to go back to dorm room to lie down. No days when she feels "really good" although weekends are better. Too early in semester to know her grades but states work is not too hard or frustrating for her. Has noticed joint pain and warmness in shoulders, knees, and elbows (different joints on different occasions) over the past month. Last week had pink rash on abdomen (gone now); has had a painless "bump" since yesterday (size of a pea) on right elbow. Her action has been to take over-the-counter vitamin and iron compound daily (she thinks she might have anemia).

FAMILY PROFILE

Lives in a second-story dormitory room with a roommate on campus (200 miles from home). She is on a full-tuition scholarship for outstanding scholarship through hometown American Legion. Gets along well with roommate (goes to her with problems). Went to camp when younger, and was an exchange student for 6 months last year in Germany;

states she is not homesick. Has two younger brothers (14 and 12); parents supportive of her college education; write frequently. Finances are not a problem; parents send money as needed.

Occupations: Worked last summer and until 1 month ago as cook in hotdog stand; now full-time college student.

PAST MEDICAL HISTORY

Childhood illnesses: Had mumps at 12 years; knows she had a rubella immunization and tetanus immunization when she was 16.

Serious illnesses: None.

Hospitalizations and surgery: Appendectomy at 8 years in Morristown General Hospital. No sequellae.

Accidents and injuries: Fell from tree at 7 years; no loss of consciousness; no sequellae.

Ob/gyn: First menstrual period at 12 years; last menstrual period 2 weeks ago. Usual cycle 30 days; period 5 days in length; moderate flow; slight cramping.

Allergies: None known.

Health habits: No smoking; alcohol consumption several beers each Saturday night; birth control pills daily; iron and vitamin supplement daily.

DAY HISTORY

Recreation: No physical activity now because of fatigue; played varsity basketball in high school; rode bicycle almost daily until 1 month ago.

Nutrition: Eats in college cafeteria 3 meals daily; includes 5 basic food groups daily.

Sleep: Sleeps 10 hours a night plus 1-hour nap in afternoon because of fatigue (former pattern was 8 hours a night, no naps).

Sexual History: Not sexually active now; was for 2 years in high school. "Too tired" is reason for change in pattern.

FAMILY MEDICAL HISTORY

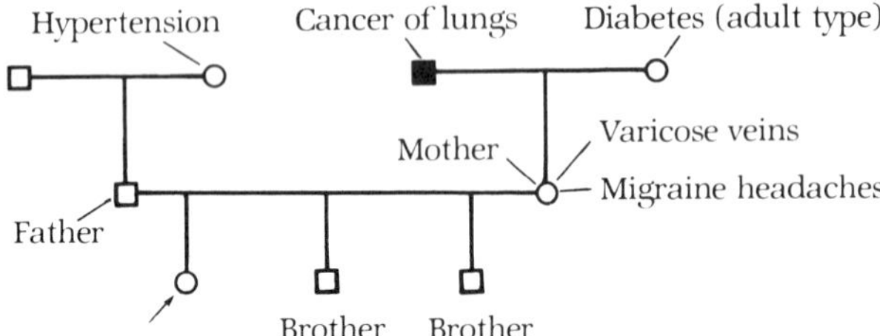

↗ = patient ☐ = living male

■ = deceased male ○ = living female

REVIEW OF SYSTEMS

Height 5′ 4″; weight stable at 110 lb for past 2 years.

Head: No headaches, no trauma.

Neuropsych: No convulsions; no dizziness.

Eyes: Wears glasses for reading; last vision exam in June, 4 months ago; no eye infections.

Ears: No infections; no drainage or pain; no difficulty with hearing.

Nose: No nosebleeds, discharge, or difficulty breathing.

Throat: Very sore throat in July; patient not seen by M.D. but had "high" fever with this, was "very ill"; throat was very red.

Mouth: Still wears retainer following removal of braces 3 months ago; no known cavities; last dental check 3 months ago.

Neck: No masses, stiffness.

Chest: No masses; discharge from breasts; does not do monthly self-exam. No chest x-rays taken.

Respiratory system: No cough or shortness of breath.

Cardiovascular system: No past heart disease, pain, or edema; no ECGs ever taken.

Gastrointestinal system: No vomiting or diarrhea; appendectomy as described in PMH.

Genitourinary system: No difficulty with voiding; no vaginal discharge.

Back: No stiffness or pain.

Extremities: Pain in joints as described in CC. "Flat feet" diagnosed in high school; no treatment ever given.

Hematologic system: Had iron deficiency anemia 2 years ago; treated with Feosol tablets for 6 months; return blood results were good; no follow-up since then.

Endocrine: No diabetes or thyroid difficulties.

Skin: Rash as in CC.

This history lists a series of physical symptoms (swollen joints, rash, fatigue) and psychological ones (school stress). Rash, swollen joints, joint nodules, and fatigue suggest rheumatic fever, which can lead to heart disease. Notice how the patient reported fatigue as her main symptom. Only by asking for associated symptoms were other symptoms of the syndrome elicited. Rheumatic fever invariably follows a streptococcal infection. Notice that the patient did not report the sore throat in connection with the illness but it is revealed by a thorough review of systems.

If the medical diagnosis is rheumatic fever (the physical assessment for such a patient is shown in Chap. 19), the therapy will involve a lengthy hospitalization and possibly even more weeks of convalescence at home. The implication of this for the patient (she may lose her scholarship, fall behind in school) or what the illness will mean to her is revealed by the history. At the same time, it also indicates that she is a person with strong support people (her parents at home; her roommate at college) and has a good chance of coping effectively with this type of stress.

Health history interviewing becomes easier as you learn more about common disease syndromes and expected therapy. The above example illustrates, however, that no matter how experienced the interviewer, thoroughness is the key to success. Even if you did not recognize the syndrome as you read the history or would not have recognized it if you were the interviewer, a physician reading it would have established the suspected diagnosis with no difficulty. When you become experienced in the care necessary for people with this syndrome, you will be able to begin to plan nursing care based on individual needs gained from the history.

SUGGESTED READINGS

Adamson, L. S. Strategies for nurse-patient communication. *Superv. Nurse* 11:44, 1980.

Baer, E., McGowan, M., and McGivern, D. Taking a health history. *Am. J. Nurs.* 77:1190, 1977.

Block, G., Nolan, J., and Dempsey, M. *Health Assessment for Professional Nursing: A Developmental Approach.* New York: Appleton-Century-Crofts, 1981.

Chinn, P., and Leitch, C. *Child Health Maintenance: A Guide to Clinical Assessment* (2nd ed.). St. Louis: Mosby, 1979.

Davis, B. D., et al. Social skills training . . . in nursing . . . the patient profile interview. *Nurs. Times* 78(42):1765, 1982.

Eggland, E. How to take a meaningful history. *Nursing 77* 8:77, 1977.

Garn, S., and Clark, S. Problems in the nutritional assessment of black individuals. *Am. J. Public Health* 66:262, 1976.

Haggard, B. A. Coping with anxiety about patient interviews . . . Pre-operative interviews. *A.O.R.N. J.* 37(2):195, 1983.

Jolly, J. D. Through a child's eyes: The problems of communication with sick children. *Nursing* (Oxford) 1:1012, 1981.

Kesler, A. Pitfalls to avoid in interviewing outpatients. *Nursing 77* 7:70, 1977.

Kress-Golub, E., et al. Teaching history-taking and interviewing skills to PNPs. *Pediatr. Nurs.* 7(1):41, 1981.

Marcus, A. C., et al. Non-participation in telephone follow-up interviews. *Am. J. Public Health* 73(1):72, 1983.

McBride, M. M. Can you tell me where it hurts? *Pediatr. Nurs.* 3:7, 1977.

Mengel, A. Getting the most from patient interviews. *Nursing* (Horsham) 12(11):46, 1982.

Mezey, M., Rauckhorst, L., and Stokes, S. The health history of the aged person. *J. Gerontol.* 3:47, 1977.

Murray, R., and Zenter, J. *Nursing Assessment and Health Promotion Through the Life Span* (2nd ed.). Englewood Cliffs, N.J.: Prentice-Hall, 1979.

O'Brien, M. *Communications and Relationships in Nursing* (2nd ed.). St. Louis: Mosby, 1978.

Snyder, J., and Wilson, M. Elements of a psychologic assessment. *Am. J. Nurs.* 77:235, 1977.

Stanford, D. All about sex . . . after middle age. *Am. J. Nurs.* 77:608, 1977.

Zimney, L., et al. Patient telephone interviews. *J. Community Health* 6:35, 1980.

QUESTIONS FOR REVIEW

To review your knowledge of health interviewing match the descriptions in the left column with the corresponding terms from the right column.

1. The first section of the history asked for following an introduction
2. The section of the history that best reveals nutritional patterns
3. An area to ask about in eliciting the history of past illness
4. A pattern revealed by a day history
5. A description of a patient
6. Another area to ask about in eliciting the history of past illness
7. A personal statistic necessary to obtain
8. A topic to help you evaluate intellectual capabilities
9. A question to ask to help you establish financial status
10. A neurological area to always include in a review of systems
11. An area of information to ask about in a day history
12. A quality relating to chief concern to explore
13. A second quality relating to chief concern to explore
14. Another area to ask about in eliciting the history of past illnesses
15. Another personal statistic necessary to obtain
16. A third area relating to chief concern to explore
17. A question to ask concerning pregnancy
18. A type of disease to ask about in a family health history
19. An assessment area to always ask for in a review of systems
20. A second assessment area to always ask for in a review of systems
21. The last category of information asked about
22. Important fact for a patient to know about you in addition to your name
23. An area of a person's profile that influences diet and health care

a. occupation
b. patient profile
c. description
d. intensity
e. day history
f. hearing
g. seizures
h. age
i. chief concern
j. vision
k. culture
l. duration
m. allergies
n. surgery
o. sex
p. title
q. length
r. education
s. review of systems
t. sleep
u. nutrition
v. hospitalizations
w. heart

19. ASSESSMENT BY PHYSICAL MEASURES

OBJECTIVES
Upon mastery of the material in this chapter, you should be able to:

1. State the purpose of physical examination.
2. Describe the four techniques used in physical examination.
3. Describe the usual pattern of physical examination.
4. List the components of physical examination for each body system or part.
5. Describe modifications of technique depending on the person's age group.
6. Describe the importance of body measurement as a part of physical examination.
7. Describe how physical examination is incorporated into patient assessment as part of the nursing process.

TERMS
The terms important for an understanding of this chapter are shown below and defined in the glossary:

auscultation
inspection
ophthalmoscope-otoscope
palpation
percussion
sphygmomanometer
stethoscope

Physical examination is a prong of nursing assessment that complements information gained from a health interview and auxiliary laboratory sources such as diagnostic test information.

The extent of the physical examination varies in different circumstances. Like the interview, sometimes only a single segment is required to get the information you need; at other times you need to do a total physical assessment. In all instances it is helpful to know the technique of physical examination so that it can be incorporated as an intrinsic part of the assessment step of the nursing process.

NECESSARY EQUIPMENT

A number of items are necessary for complete physical assessment: a stethoscope, a tongue depressor, ophthalmoscope, otoscope, a sphygmomanometer, a tape measure, and a reflex hammer.

A stethoscope is used to listen to heart rate and to assess blood pressure and breath and abdominal sounds. Because these are frequent physical assessment determinants, you should purchase one early in your school or nursing career. The important thing to look for in purchasing a stethoscope (Fig. 19-1A) is that the diaphragm (the flat surface through which sound is transmitted to your tympanic membrane) is small enough to fit easily over a brachial artery in the antecubital space (inner elbow) where you place it to assess a blood pressure level; this size is also small enough to place on a small infant's chest to listen for heart sounds. A good stethoscope also has a bell-shaped portion for transmitting sounds. The diaphragm transmits high-pitched sounds best, the bell low-pitched sounds. The ear pieces should fit comfortably in your ears, and the rubber tubing should be no longer than 18 inches; longer rubber tubing at first appears to have an advantage in that it will reach farther, but breath sounds become muffled if the tubing is too long and become hard to hear. As a rule, do not purchase a stethoscope advertised as a "nurse's stethoscope." These instruments are not very sensitive and will not meet your needs as you become more skilled at auscultating.

Do not bend the tubing of the stethoscope sharply to carry it in your pocket; this may break the resiliency of the tubing. On the other hand, do not carry it across your shoulders; This "Hollywood" look that places the instrument next to your hair is inappropriate for those who really know how to use a stethoscope.

An ophthalmoscope-otoscope (Fig. 19-1B) is an instrument composed of a base (which contains batteries) with exchangeable head pieces. With the ophthalmoscope head in place it is an instrument used to examine the internal structure of the eye. With the otoscope head in place it is used to examine the tympanic membrane; this head also provides a ready light source for examin-

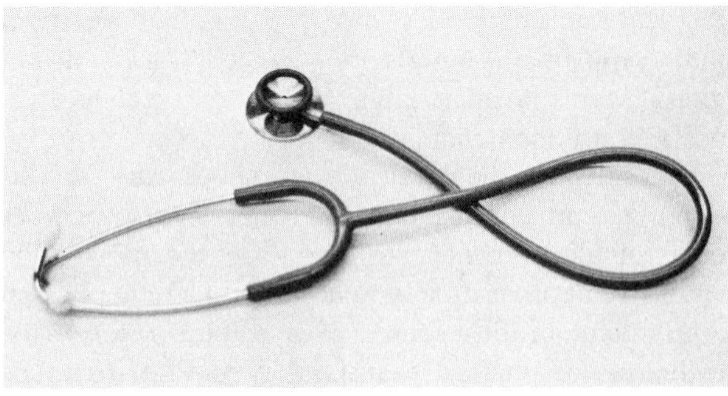

A

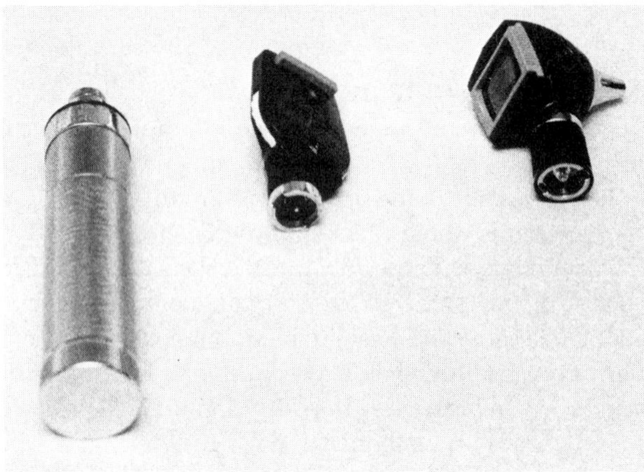

B

FIGURE 19-1. Equipment used in assessment. A. Stethoscope; sound is heard through the diaphragm or bell. B. Ophthalmoscope-otoscope. Notice that these are exchangeable head pieces that fit on a single base.

ing the mouth and checking pupillary responses to light (a pen light can also be used for this purpose). Ophthalmoscope-otoscopes function by batteries that either need to be replaced periodically or to be recharged after use. After using one, be certain always to turn it off to preserve battery life. These instruments are used both for routine eye-ear examinations and for emergencies such as cardiac arrest to check pupillary response. An emergency when minutes are important for life saving is not the time to discover that someone has been careless with battery life.

A sphygmomanometer is the technical name for the instrument used to measure blood pressure; the common name is a blood pressure cuff. Cuff sizes vary a great deal from child to adult; the importance of cuff size is discussed in Chap. 31. The tape measure is used to determine the size of body parts such as head circumference; the tongue depressor is used to view the posterior throat; and the reflex hammer is used to elicit deep tendon reflexes.

During a complete physical examination you must expose every body part. To protect against chilling and to provide for modesty, do this by exposing body parts individually and only for the amount of time necessary for the examination. Use a patient gown or a drawsheet as a drape as necessary.

Be certain that the temperature in the examining room is comfortable. Be certain to provide privacy. If a treatment room is used for examination, be certain that the paper table cover is changed between patients to avoid possible spread of illness.

RESTRAINING FOR PHYSICAL ASSESSMENT

You can assume that adults will cooperate in placing themselves in whatever position you require in order for you to inspect body parts unless they are very short of breath or in some other way unable to comply. Small children may not cooperate and they need to be restrained during the examination of body parts such as nose, throat, and ears. This is done not only to enable the examiner to see well but also to ensure that the instrument used will not accidentally injure the child.

In many instances you will need to restrain a child while a physician carries out a physical examination. Parents can be asked to do this if they wish. As a rule, do not ask parents to restrain with any procedure where the child will be hurt—parents are protectors and comforters—but a simple examination is not a hurting procedure, and their participation is often helpful.

Everyone has the right not to have another person touch his body unless he permits them to do so (legally, this is assault and battery). Always inform people what you are going to do during a physical examination: "Next let me look at your throat," etc. If some action will feel momentarily uncomfortable (deep palpation of the abdomen, for example), offer fair warning: "You'll feel pressure for a minute." (See QRS 19-1).

TECHNIQUES OF PHYSICAL EXAMINATION

Physical examination involves four separate techniques: inspection, palpation, percussion, and auscultation. These techniques are carried out in the above order, with the exception of examination of the abdomen where the order is inspection, auscultation, palpation, and percus-

☐ **QUICK REFERENCE STOP 19-1: PSYCHOLOGICAL CONSIDERATIONS**

Most people have a degree of apprehension at the thought of a physical examination because of fear that illness in some body part will be discovered, discomfort at having their bodies exposed, and worry that some procedure will hurt.

As you examine body parts, explain what you are doing ("next let me feel your abdomen . . .") so that there are no surprises for the person. Protect modesty by means of cover sheets, gowns, and closed room doors.

sion. Palpating the abdomen before auscultation may obliterate bowel sounds.

Inspection

Inspection is examining with your eyes. Because it is the first technique used, it is easy to disregard its importance and move quickly to the second step. Inspection yields a great deal of information, however, about significant physical features and general health.

Smelling is a lesser-used but practical second phase of inspection. Be alert to body or breath odors of people you care for or examine, as some disease processes present with distinctive odors that are important as an aid in diagnosis. Important odors to be familiar with and their significance are shown in Table 19-1.

Palpation

Palpation is examining by touch. It can be either light or deep. The tips of your fingers are most sensitive to texture, vibration, consistency, and contour; the back of your hand is most sensitive to warmth. During a physical examination you should touch all external surfaces of a person's body to ascertain that the person has normal texture, contour, and movement. Use light palpation before deep palpation or people may tense muscles and make light palpation difficult.

If a person has a sensitive or painful body part, palpate that part last; if you examine a tender body part first, the person may be unwilling to allow you to touch other parts for fear he will experience additional pain.

TABLE 19-1. SIGNIFICANT BODY ODORS

Odor	Possible Cause
Breath odors	
Alcohol	Implies recent ingestion (important if coma or neurological symptoms are present as the cause of the abnormal functioning).
Camphor	Mothball ingestion.
Halitosis (bad breath)	Poor dental hygiene, lung infection; foreign body in respiratory tract.
Burnt rope	Marijuana use.
Sweet	Acidosis (seen with a person with diabetes in coma).
Body odors	
Stale urine	Incontinence; poor kidney functioning leading to uremia.
Sweat	May imply fatigue has been so great lately that the person has not maintained his usual hygiene regimen.
"Spoiled" fruit	Wound infection.
Sweet	*Pseudomonas* infection.
Urine odors	
Maple syrup	Protein metabolic conditions.
"Musty or mousey"	Phenylketonuria or a protein metabolism disorder.
Ammonia	Urinary tract infection or poor hydration leading to concentrated urine.
Stool odors	
Putrid	Fat in stool from inadequate fat absorption.

Percussion

Percussion is the assessment of a body structure by determining the sound that you hear in response to striking the part with an examining finger (Fig. 19-2). Dense body areas such as bone have a dull flat sound; those filled with air such as the lungs are resonant. If an organ is stretched (a distended bladder), it has a hyperresonant or low hollow sound. An organ stretched to an even greater point of distention has a *tympanic* or an extremely hollow ringing sound. These sounds and the body locations where they can be elicited are shown in Table 19-2.

Auscultation

Auscultation is listening to sounds that are either discernible to the ear (wheezing or heavy breathing) or, as in

FIGURE 19-2. Percussion of a body part. One finger is held straight and struck by the tip of another.

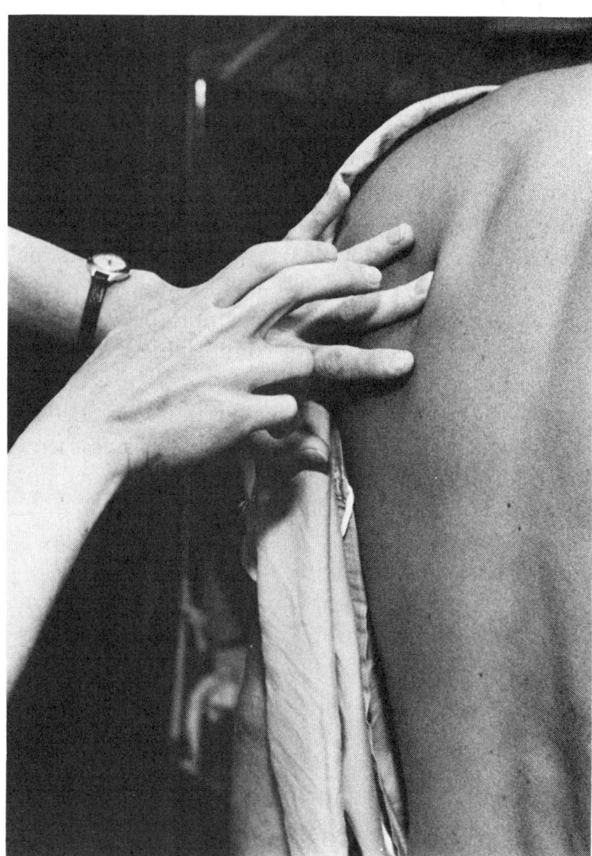

TABLE 19-2. PERCUSSION SOUNDS AND THEIR LOCATIONS

Sound	Body Site
Flat or dull	Over bone
Resonant	Over air-filled space such as the lung
Hyperresonant	Over body cavity distended with air such as inflated lungs
Hollow	Over body cavity filled with fluid such as bladder
Tympanic	Over body cavity distended with fluid such as distended bladder

most cases, made louder by means of a stethoscope. Always listen for four qualities of sound: the duration, the frequency, the intensity (loudness), and the pitch (high or low) (Fig. 19-3).

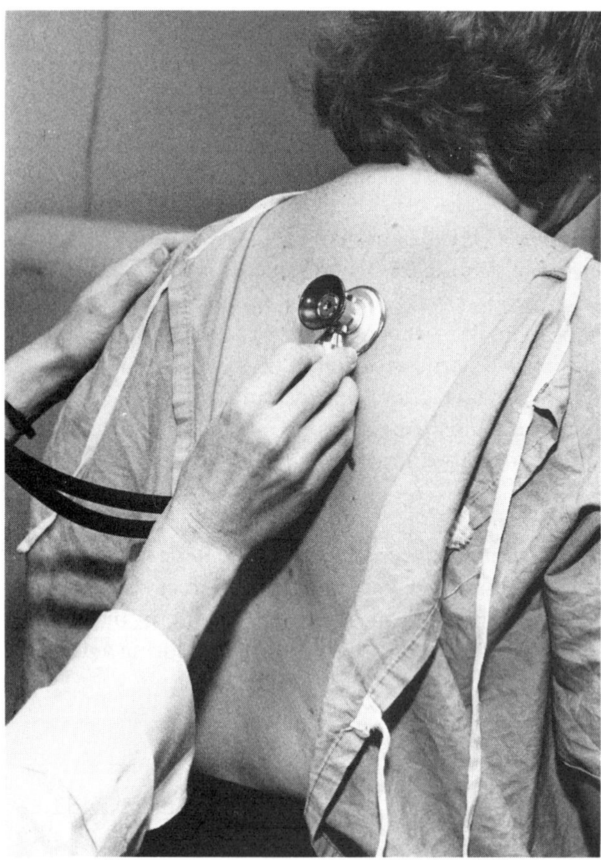

FIGURE 19-3. Auscultation is done by means of a stethoscope.

SEQUENCE OF PHYSICAL EXAMINATION

A physical examination may be done in any order, but to ensure that you are thorough, you should develop a system that you always follow. Traditionally, this proceeds from head to toe; you should examine each body part thoroughly before moving on to the next. In infants and young children, if a full examination is to be done, it is important to begin with the heart and lungs, because if the infant cries, findings in these areas are difficult to assess over the sound of crying.

General Appearance

Physical examination always begins with inspection of general appearance in order to form a general impression of the person's health and well-being. Is the person's height and weight proportional? Does he appear tired or rested? What is his color—pale? yellowed (jaundiced)? cyanotic (blue)? What is his state of cleanliness or dress? (Depressed people often do not dress meticulously.) Does he walk and sit with confidence or uncertainty? Is his posture normal? (People in pain assume abnormal postures for relief.) Are lesions or symptoms of specific illness present? Does he appear comfortable or in pain? Is his breathing distressed or easy?

A general appearance assessment is necessary to alert you to specific body areas that need detailed assessment. Table 19-3 summarizes areas to assess for general appearance and possible implications.

TABLE 19-3. ASSESSMENT FOR GENERAL APPEARANCE

Category of Assessment	Possible Findings
State of health	Appears well (energetic, good color, easy respirations). Appears ill (loss of energy, tired, coughing, heavy breathing).
Stature and gait	Stands erect; walks purposely and with good balance. Has stooped posture; walks with a limp or imbalance.
Weight and body proportion	Weight is proportionate to body. Appears over- or underweight; head or extremeties are out of proportion to trunk.
Dress, grooming, and personal hygiene	Neatly dressed; hair and body clean. Inappropriately dressed for situation or weather; sweaty or dirty skin surface. (Be aware of possible cultural influences and economic restraints.)
Manner	Person is cooperative although faintly nervous. Person is angry, threatening, crying, flat or unresponsive.
Level of consciousness	Person is alert; responds to questions appropriately. Person cannot be roused except by painful stimuli.

Mental Status Assessment

A mental status assessment is made early in the examination as a complement to general appearance information. Additional information is gained on mental status throughout the patient contact.

Assess the person's orientation—his awareness of who he is, where he is, and the date. Assess the appropriateness of his behavior and mood (hostile, frightened, relaxed). Remember that expressing emotions as a rule is a healthful step; a person angry at being ill is probably acting normally. On the other hand, a person who has every reason to be angry or frightened but appears relaxed and smiling may be manifesting abnormal behavior. If the person is to have a complete physical examination, you can expect him to be slightly nervous; most people are concerned that some procedure will hurt them or some illness they are not aware of will be discovered.

At some point in the examination ask questions that test recent memory (how did he feel when he woke up in the morning?) and distant memory (did he have any childhood diseases?). Mental status assessment is summarized in Table 19-4.

TABLE 19-4. ASSESSMENT FOR MENTAL STATUS

Assessment Criteria	Possible Findings
Mood	Person appears content or happy. Person appears sad, angry, depressed or too happy for situation.
Orientation	Person knows the time, date, and place and who he is. Person does not know these facts or perceives them falsely.
Memory	Person can recall both an immediate happening and a long-term one. Person cannot recall recent, distant, or both types of events.
Concentration	Person answers appropriately to questions such as does he have pain on elbow movement. Person repeatedly asks for questions to be restated or ignores questions.
Cognitive ability	Person's response to a question such as "Would you bend your elbow?" is to carry out the action. Person does not comprehend the simple term *bend* or acts inappropriately, such as stating that all his joints are controlled by radio signals and no longer bend.

Body Measurements

Height and weight measurements are important determinants of health. With chronic illness the body expends so many nutrients combating the destructive process of the disease that normal height and weight may not be maintained. Conversely, overweight (obesity) may be the cause of illnesses, particularly those of the heart and lungs.

WEIGHT

Adults and children over 2 years should be weighed on standing scales, in street clothes (no shoes), or if in the hospital, in a patient gown or robe. If the person is going to have serial weights taken (weighed every day or several times a day), it is important that he wear the same clothing every time he is weighed so that any discrepancy in weight is truly a difference in body weight and not a weight change due to more or less clothing. The weight should be taken at the same time each day (preferably before breakfast) on the same scale.

Until they can stand well, infants are weighed on a sitting or infant scale. Because diapers can be very heavy in proportion to total body weight, infants are weighed nude. Always keep a sheltering hand over an infant on an infant scale (hovering but not touching), as infants squirm readily and there is danger of falling (Fig. 19-4). Cover both infant scales and adult scales with paper before weighing to prevent spread of illness from one person to another.

Scales measure in either pounds or kilograms, depending on the measurement system that the health care agency chooses to use. Most people want to know their weight, and if it is measured in a metric number, you often need to convert the number into pounds and ounces. To convert from kilograms to pounds, multiply by 2.2.

To assess whether a person's weight is average for his height, compare his weight to a standardized height-weight table. Tables with adult, child, and infant values are shown in Appendix D for easy reference. In the standardized scale for children, all weights between the 10th and 90th percentiles are considered normal (statistically, a range of weights that includes two standard deviations from the mean or the 50th percentile). As important as the fact that a child's weight falls between the 10th and 90th percentile on a growth chart is the fact that over a period of time his weight follows one of the percentile curves—that he is not at the 80th percentile

FIGURE 19-4. Infants are weighed nude on an infant scale. The nurse's hand hovers (but does not touch) for safety.

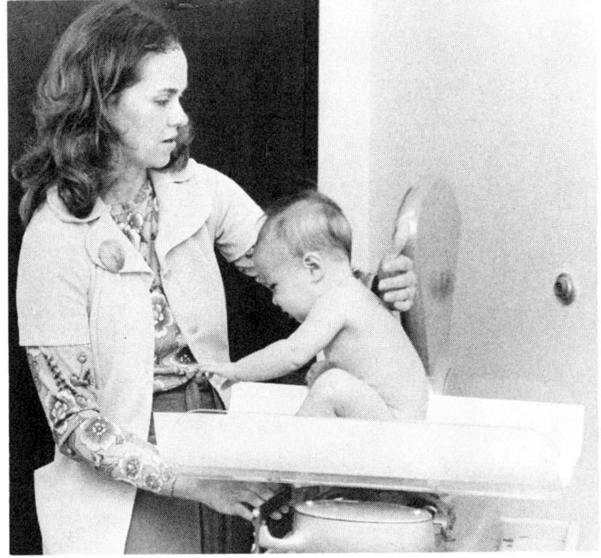

the first time you weigh him and a month later at the 40th percentile. Although both readings are within the normal range, they reflect a weight loss that needs investigation as to its cause. Gaining weight in the same way can be equally serious.

HEIGHT

The height of adults is used to calculate the normalcy of weight. In children it is as good a determinant of health and normal nutrition as weight.

To measure height, be certain the person is standing straight with his head level. Using the measuring bar of a standing scale is adequate as long as you check first that it is not bent; placing a flat object such as a clipboard on the person's head in a horizontal position and reading height at the point that it touches the measuring tape on the back of the scale or a flat wall surface is acceptable (Fig. 19-5).

Until they can stand securely (about 2 years of age), infants are measured lying down on a measuring frame. Align the infant's head snugly against the top bar of the frame and ask an assistant to secure it there. Straighten the infant's body (knees are difficult to straighten in infants because they always keep them flexed) and hold his feet in a vertical position; bring the foot board up snugly against the bottom of the foot (Fig. 19-6). Parents can help you restrain infants for height measurements because it is a painless procedure.

Plot height measurement for children on a height graph. Height and weight should follow the same percentiles. Height-weight charts have been standardized for "typical" United States' children, so there will be variation from child to child. The important thing to look for is a consistency of measurements over time.

A child is defined as having a failure to thrive syndrome (medical diagnosis) if his height or weight falls below the third percentile on a standardized growth

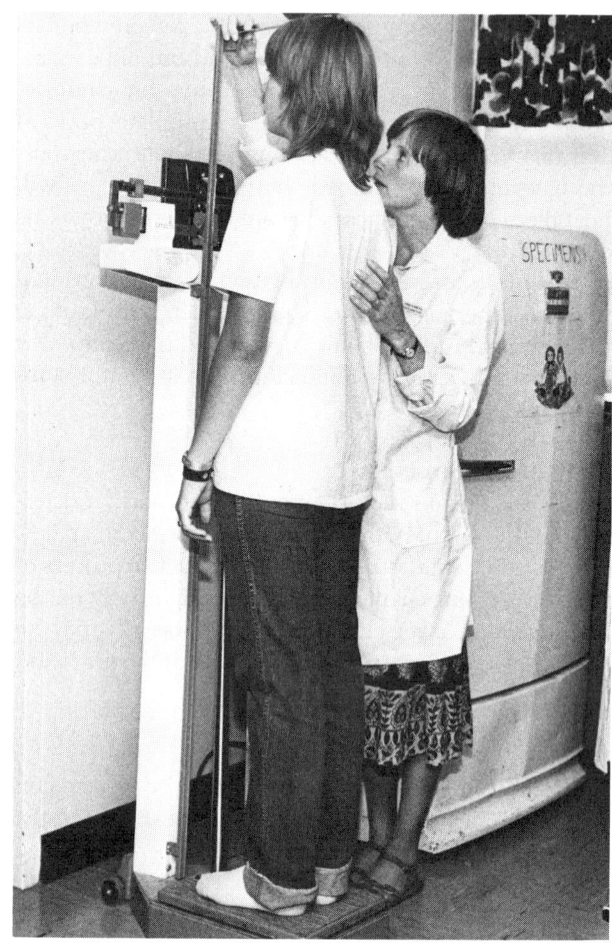

FIGURE 19-5. Measuring height using the measuring bar of a standing scale.

FIGURE 19-6. Measuring an infant's length on a measuring frame. The infant's head must be snugly aligned against the top bar and the legs straight.

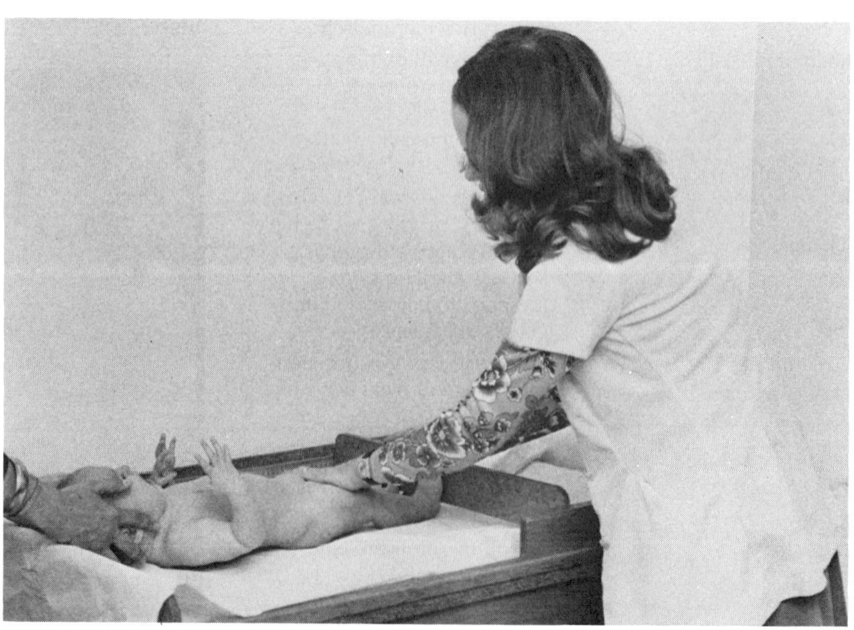

chart. Any height or weight in this category definitely needs to be reported so that its cause can be investigated.

Low Birth Weight Infants. Low birth weight infants are infants with a birth weight below the normal level. Low birth weights occur under two different sets of circumstances: (1) a premature birth, in which case the infant is small but healthy and usually "catches up" in growth by the end of the first year; and (2) an inadequate growth period in utero, caused by inadequate nutritional intake. Infants in the latter category are termed *small for gestational age,* and in most cases do not have "catch-up" growth. A gestational age growth chart is used for differentiating these two groups of infants (Fig. 19-7). The length of the mother's pregnancy (in weeks) is plotted against the infant's birth weight to determine whether his weight is appropriate for gestational (pregnancy) length.

HEAD CIRCUMFERENCE

Head circumference is measured at birth and routinely on physical assessment until 1 year of age (many health care agencies measure routinely until 2 years). Head growth occurs because the brain is growing, so head circumference is an important determinant of brain growth and neurological function. A head circumference measurement is made by placing a tape measure around the head just above the eyebrows and around the most prominent portion of the back of the head (the occipital prominence) (Fig. 19-8). Babies generally push any object away from their heads, so although the technique of head circumference measurement is simple, it is not always easy to carry out. Measurements should be

FIGURE 19-7. A Gestational Growth Chart, showing classification of newborns by birth weight and gestation age and by neonatal mortality risk. (From F. C. Battaglion and L. O. Lubehenco, A practical classification of newborn infants by weight and gestational age. *J. Pediatr.* 71:161, 1967.)

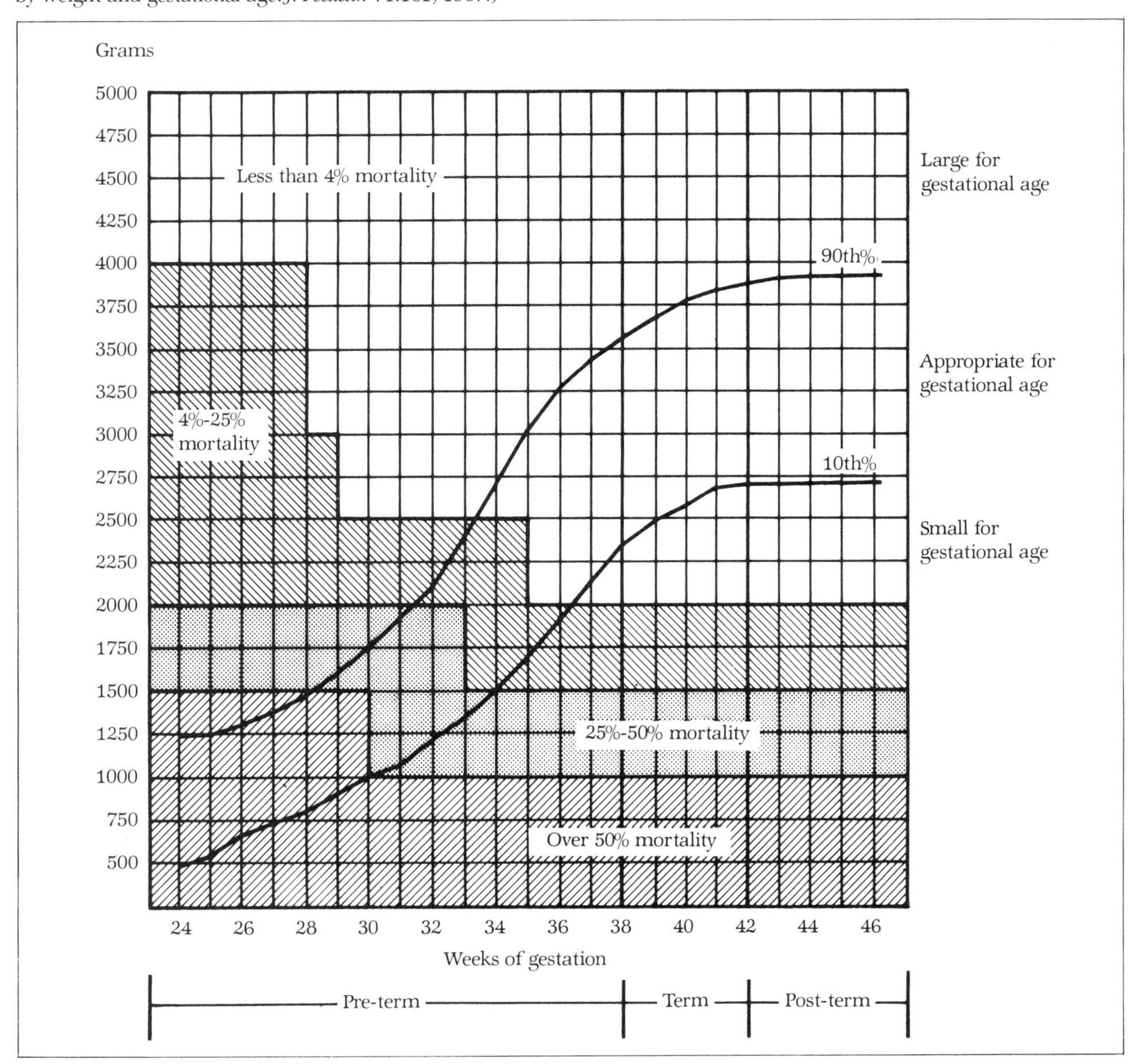

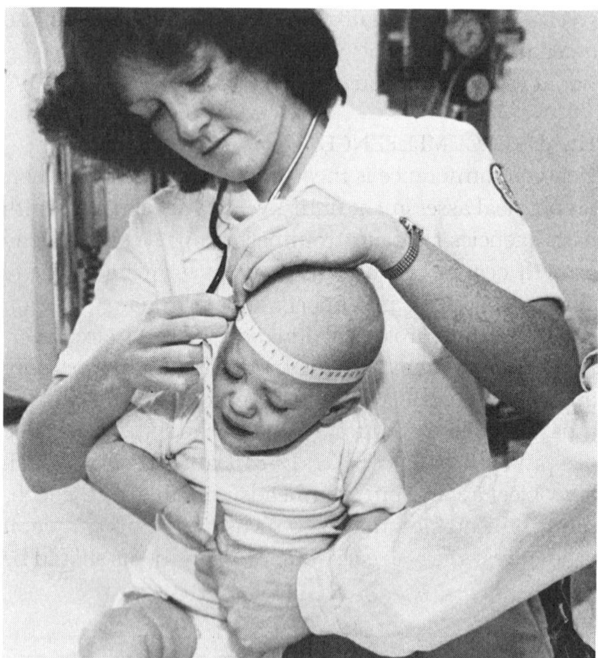

FIGURE 19-8. Measuring head circumference. The tape measure is placed around the head just above the eyebrows and around the occipital prominence at the back of the infant's head.

plotted on a standardized graph. Head circumference should correlate well with the child's length (if length is in the 40th percentile, head circumferences should be also). If measurements of head circumference plot at different percentiles over time, this should be reported as it implies that brain growth is in some way abnormal and needs investigation.

CHEST AND ABDOMINAL CIRCUMFERENCE

Measurements of chest and abdominal circumference are not done routinely on physical examination, but only when specific pathology warrants such measurements. The measurement of chest circumference is made at the nipple line; the measurement of abdominal circumference is made at the level of the umbilicus. Using these markers as points of measurement so that everyone places their tapes at the same place ensures that serial readings will be accurate. If serial readings are to be done as frequently as once a day, mark the exact place on the skin externally and posteriorly with a dot of a ballpoint pen for even greater accuracy.

Vital Sign Assessment

Vital signs refer to temperature, pulse, respiration, and blood pressure. These signs indicate the state of *vital* bodily functions (heart and lung function, metabolic rate). Measurements are recorded not only with complete physical examinations but in many other instances of care because of the important information they provide. Techniques of these measurements and the nursing responsibilities that accompany them are discussed in Chap. 33.

Skin Assessment

Skin assessment is not done separately but as different body parts are examined. Assess color, texture, turgor (the amount of fluid in body tissue, assessed by lifting a ridge of skin and assessing whether it immediately falls back into place or not), and the presence of any lesions. (Table 25-1 summarizes common skin lesions and their causes). Be certain that you examine the person's total skin surface. Remove and replace as necessary Bandaids and other dressings that could hide important findings. Be careful that you do not contaminate skin incisions or in some way introduce infection to a bandaged area.

Skin assessment is further discussed in Chap. 25 (see QRS 19-2).

Assessment of the Head

To examine the head, first place your hands on the top of the person's head and slide your fingers over the skull, assessing for irregular configurations or tenderness. Most people have a prominent occipital outgrowth; do not mistake this natural head contour as an abnormality. A normal-sized head is termed *normocephalic;* if abnormally large, *macrocephalic;* if abnormally small, *microcephalic.* Assess the texture and cleanliness of the person's hair. People who are well nourished usually have hair of good texture; poorly nourished people tend to have dry, brittle hair. If hair is exceptionally oily, it may mean that the person has been too fatigued or depressed to wash it. If a serious protein deficiency is present, hair loses its color. Baldness is a familial trait which results in hair loss from large portions of the head (it can occur in both men and women). Patches of hair loss (alopecia), on the other hand, suggest a fungal infection or possible drug reaction. It is a finding that needs investigation as to its cause.

The Infant. In infants you should palpate the skull for the presence of fontanelles—the places where the occipital, frontal, and parietal bones fuse (the anterior fontanelle) and where the occipital and parietal bones fuse (the posterior fontanelle). The anterior fontanelle is 3 to 4 cm in diameter and diamond shaped; it remains palpable until 12 to 18 months of age. The posterior fontanelle is 1 to 2 cm in diameter and triangularly shaped; it closes at about two months of age.

Although there is no bone at these skull locations, there is a thick membrane covering the space. A fontanelle should feel neither tense (which would indicate increased pressure such as blood or cerebral spinal fluid inside the skull) or depressed (a reflection of decreased body fluid as could happen with dehydration). When a baby cries, cerebral pressure does increase, so with crying fontanelles will feel tense, and sometimes even the fluctuation of a pulse is present. In newborns suture

□ **QUICK REFERENCE STOP 19-2: NUTRITION**

The diet a person typically ingests influences body health and growth and is reflected in physical assessment findings.

Low protein diet	Protein is necessary for cell growth and repair. Assess for normal height and any unhealing lesions. If protein intake is greatly reduced, edema occurs due to fluid leaving the vascular system to equalize osmotic pressure in subcutaneous tissue.
Low iron diet	Iron is instrumental for red cell growth. Assess body areas that best reflect color of blood in capillaries: lower conjunctivas, nail beds, lip color, facial color.
Low carbohydrate	Carbohydrate builds body fat and provides energy. Assess weight in proportion to height; assess for muscle mass that demonstrates person is active physically.
High carbohydrate	Excessive carbohydrate in a diet causes obesity and excess dental decay. Assess weight in proportion to height; assess condition of teeth. Assess blood pressure as it often increases with obesity.
Vitamin deficit	Vitamins are essential for cell growth and repair. Assess for lesions that are not healing, particularly at corners of mouth or mucous membrane of mouth.
Low sodium diet	People are prescribed therapeutic low-sodium diets to reduce body fluid as the presence of sodium attracts body fluid. Assess for edema and blood pressure.

lines where the skull bones touch are also palpable; they feel like protruding ridges under your fingertips.

Newborns have very irregular skull contour because the pressure of birth caused "molding" or overriding of skull bones to occur. This molding lasts for 1 to 2 weeks after which normal symmetry is regained.

Pressure of birth may also cause edema of the outer layer of scalp tissue so extensive that it appears as a goose-egg-shaped swelling. This is termed a *caput succedaneum.* It is a transient finding; the edema will be absorbed by 1 to 2 weeks of age.

Children's hair should be examined with special care. A child with *kwashiorkor* (a protein deficiency disease) develops zebra-striped hair—hair strands with alternating dark-colored and light-colored sections. The dark color forms during periods of good protein intake, the light during periods of protein deficit. Examine hair carefully for small white-yellow sand-sized particles attached to hair strands—the eggs (nits) of pediculi (head lice). Nits cling and cannot be readily removed from hair by running your fingers the length of the hair. Pediculi spread easily in schoolage children due to the sharing of combs and towels in school. The child may have recent scratch marks on his scalp and generally states that he feels "itchy." Since a prescription shampoo is necessary to kill and remove pediculi and nits from hair, notification of a physician of the finding is necessary.

Examine the scalp for round circular areas (perhaps weeping in the center, crusting and scaling on the edges) that would suggest *tinea capitis* (ringworm), a fungal infection. Like pediculi, fungal infections are spread readily among schoolage children, and a prescription is necessary to cure the condition.

A final scalp problem encountered in children is seborrhea (scaling, greasy-appearing, salmon-colored patches). This occurs most frequently in infants (commonly referred to as "cradle cap"). Increasing the frequency of hair washing to once a day will effectively reduce this problem.

Assessment of the Eyes

Observe eyes, lids, and lashes for redness (erythema), which suggests infection. Common ones are conjunctivitis (called "pink eye" by parents; an infection of the thin conjunctiva that covers the eye) and a hordeolum or sty (an infection of the gland that lubricates an eyelash). Both conditions require an antibiotic for therapy.

In addition, observe whether the eyes appear to be in good alignment. *Strabismus* is the term that denotes that eyes are not aligned evenly. If an eye is always turning in, the condition is called *esotropia;* if it always turns out, *extropia.*

One way to detect whether eyes are in good alignment is to ask the person to look directly at the light of your otoscope. If the person's eyes are in straight alignment, the light reflex on the pupils of both eyes will be equal (Fig. 19-9). This is called Hirshberg's test. A second method is a cover test. Ask the person to focus on an object about 4 feet in front of him. Hold a 3 × 5 card over his right eye while you count to 10. When you remove the card, watch the eye for movement. If the person has poor

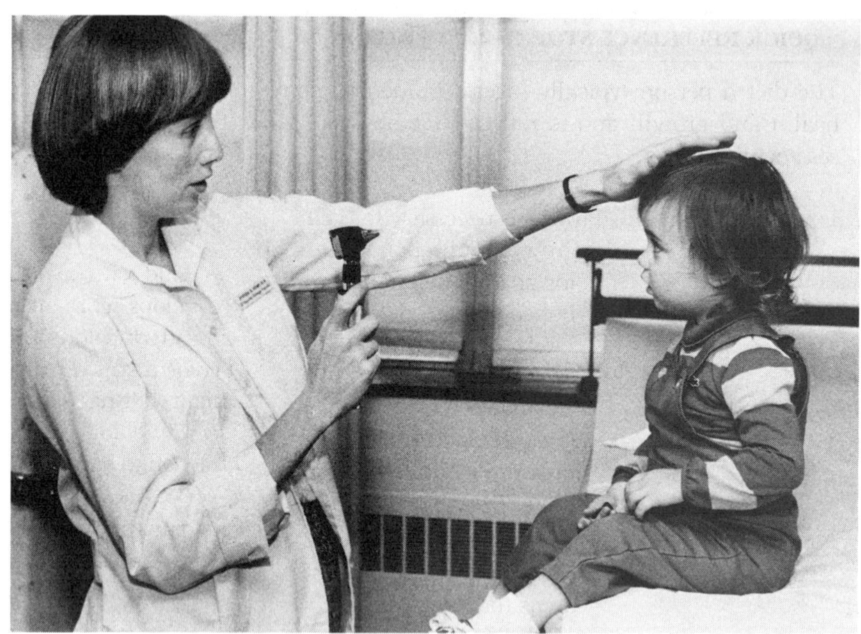

FIGURE 19-9. Testing for good eye alignment by Hirshberg's test. The child is asked to look directly at the light of the otoscope; the light reflex on the pupils of both eyes will be equal if the eyes are in straight alignment.

eye alignment, during the time the eye was covered it will have "drifted" out of alignment; when the card is removed and the person refocuses on the designated object, his eye moves back into alignment.

Inspect the sclera (white) of the eye for spots of hemorrhage (called subconjunctival hemorrhage) or yellowing (jaundice). Black individuals often have a slight yellowing of the sclera and small black spots on the sclera; do not mistake these for abnormal findings. A common finding with middle-aged adults is yellow patches on the sclera (pinguecuela). These are fatty deposits, do not interfere with vision, tend to be transient, and are not important unless they concern the person because of appearance.

Palpate the eye globe with eyelid closed to assess for tenseness. A serious eye disease in older adults is glaucoma (increased intraocular pressure); this causes the eye globe to feel unusually tense.

Determine whether, when the person closes his eyes, his eyelids completely cover his eyes (edema or neurological illnesses may make eyelids too short to do this) and whether, when the person opens his eyes, the lids retract far enough that they do not obscure vision. When a lid obscures vision, the condition is termed *ptosis;* it generally denotes neurological involvement. Be certain that you do not mistake normal oriental lid creases for abnormal findings. The difference in western and eastern eye creases are shown in Fig. 19-10.

Examine the inner lining of the lower eyelid (the conjunctiva) by pulling the lid down slightly with a fingertip. The mucous membrane of this space should appear pink and moist. In persons with anemia it often appears pale; with allergy or infection it may appear unusually red and irritated. Assess the location of eyes in relation to the nose (not unusually wide or narrow spaced) and the relationship of the globe to the socket (neither sunken nor protruding from the socket). Ab-

FIGURE 19-10. The difference between western (A) and eastern (B) eye formation. The extra inner fold of tissue is an epicanthal fold.

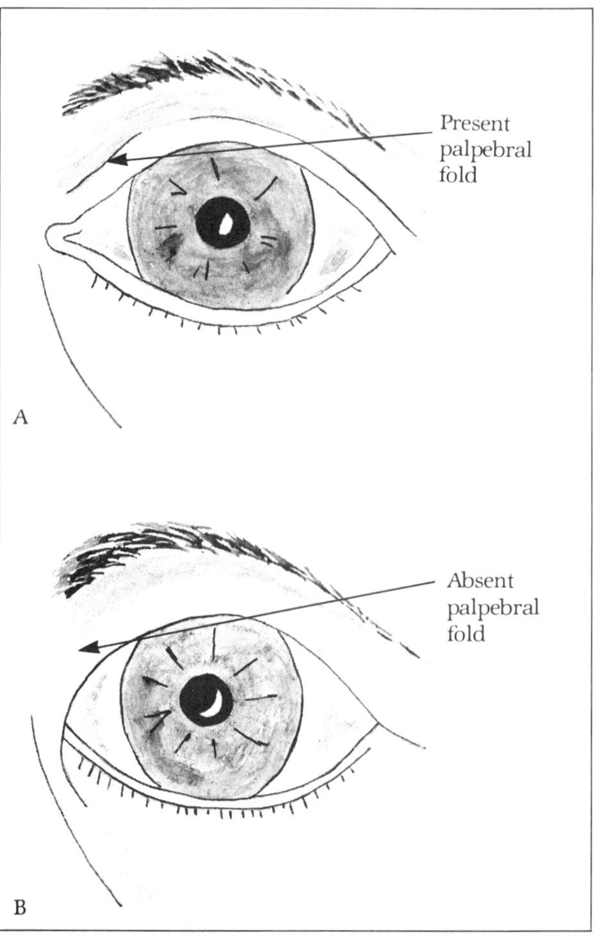

normalities in these areas occur in chromosomal or metabolic illnesses.

To inspect the inner structures of the eye, you need to use an ophthalmoscope head. If the cornea, aqueous humor, and vitreous humor are all clear (no cataract, no infection or tumors present), you will have an unobstructed view of the retina when you shine the ophthalmoscope light directly into the pupil. If the retina is intact, it will appear as a bright red circle in the pupil (a red reflex). (This occasionally appears in colored photographs because the flashbulb initiates the reflex.) Observe at the same time if the pupil constricts (reduces in size) in response to your light. This should occur in response to a light shining directly on a pupil (direct constriction); also in response pupil constriction will occur in the opposite eye (consensual constriction). Ability of the pupil to constrict indicates that the third cranial nerve is intact. The two tests (red reflex and pupil constriction) are included as part of a routine examination. The fact that the pupils are equal in size and react to light is usually recorded as PERL (pupils equivalent, react to light).

In order to inspect the retina more closely, you need to turn the dial on the ophthalmoscope head to focus and magnify the retina until you can see the optic disc and arteries and veins that supply it in close detail (Fig. 19-11). Normally the margins of the optic disc are regular, and there should be no indication that it is swollen (this is papilledema, a severe sign of increased intracranial pressure) or compressed (occurs with glaucoma or increased intraocular pressure). The veins and arteries to the optic disc should be inspected: If these are unusually narrow, systemic hypertension is suggested; if copper colored, arteriosclerosis is suggested. If hazy patches that look like cotton are present, edema with infiltration around the vessel has occurred (often seen in people with diabetes) (Fig. 19-12).

FIGURE 19-11. Looking through and focusing the dial on the ophthalmoscope head to see the optic disc and the blood vessels that supply it.

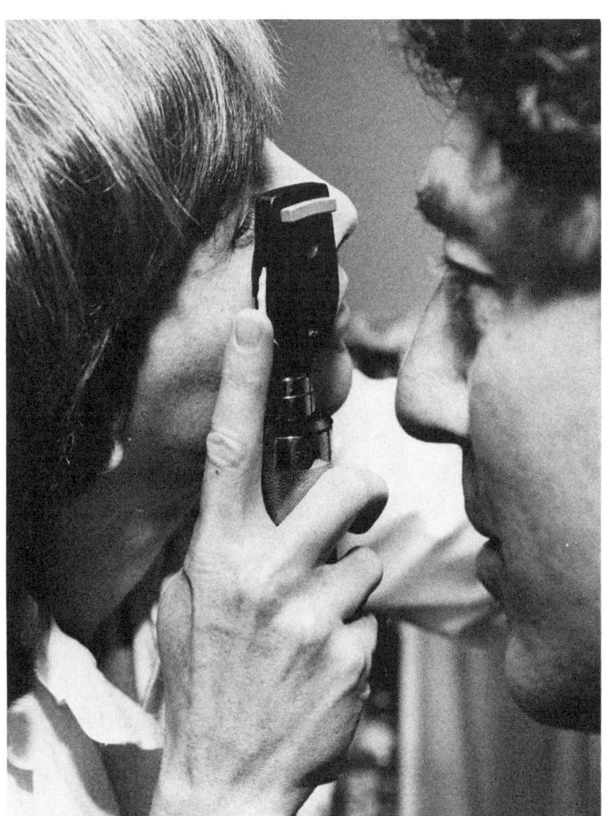

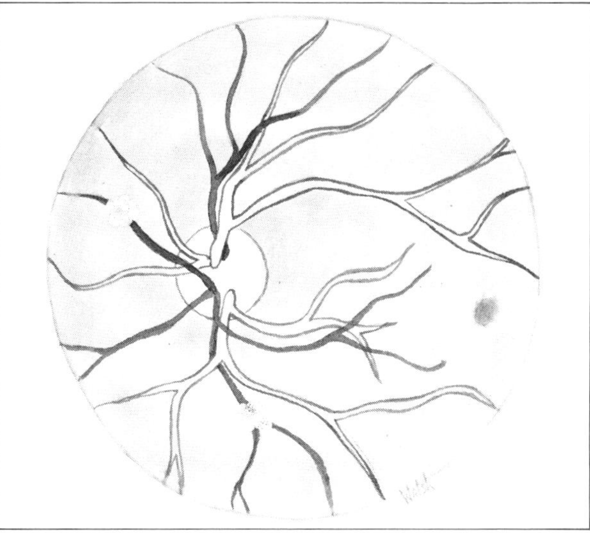

FIGURE 19-12. An optic disc and the blood vessels supplying it. The cloudlike patch on the right, would be seen in persons with diabetes mellitus.

To view a retina with an ophthalmoscope, you must bring your right eye into line with the person's right eye, his left eye in line with your left. Examination of the retina in detail is not routinely done with health assessment but only if specific indications exist. It takes hours of practice to be able to identify all the possible eye ground changes that could be present.

A final test of neurological intactness performed routinely with physical assessment is asking the person to follow your finger or a light through the six cardinal fields of gaze (Fig. 19-13) and to follow the light as you move it in toward his nose (accommodation). The ability to do this indicates that the third, fourth, and sixth cranial nerves are intact. If accommodation is present, this action is added to PERL when it is charted to make it PERLA. When a person looks directly sideways to follow a light, it is not unusual for his eye to quiver slightly for a few seconds; this is called *nystagmus.* Nystagmus elicited on direct lateral gaze is normal; if you notice it at any other time, it is highly suggestive of serious neurological disease.

The Infant. Newborns often have a small bright red spot on the sclera (a subconjunctival hemorrhage) because the pressure of birth has ruptured a small conjunctival blood vessel. This is normal and will fade in 7 to 10 days time as the blood is absorbed.

Infants can easily be tested for a red reflex, but children up to 3 months of age cannot follow across the

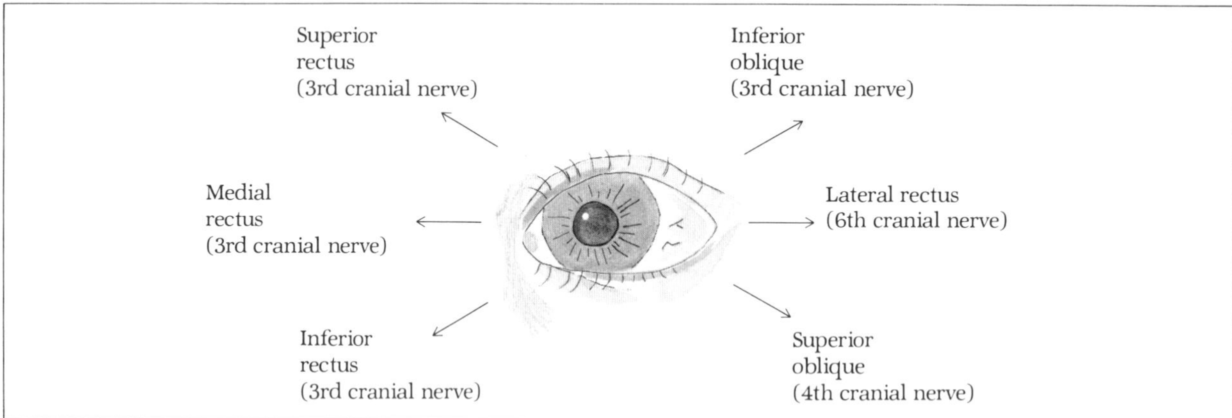

FIGURE 19-13. The six cardinal fields of gaze.

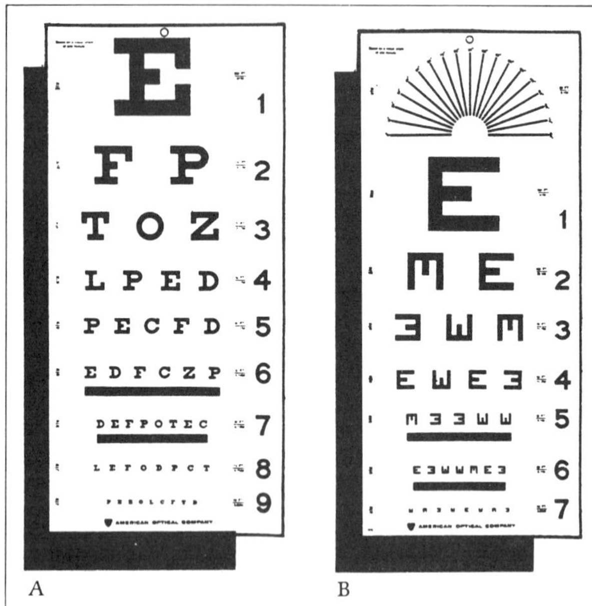

FIGURE 19-14. A. The Snellen Eye Chart. A reading of 20/20 is normal for adults. B. The E Chart. To use, ask the person to point to the way in which the E faces. (Courtesy American Optical Corporation.)

midline and so cannot follow a light into all six positions of gaze. Even a newborn, however, can follow a bright light for a short distance.

TESTING VISUAL ACUITY

During any health assessment observe the person for signs of poor vision such as squinting, cocking his head to one side to focus better, or closing one eye to see better. The only true measurement of a person's vision, however, is to test it using a standardized eye chart.

The usual chart used for testing visual acuity is the Snellen Eye Chart (Fig. 19-14A). The person should stand 20 feet from the chart, and there must be good light so that letters are easily visualized.

Ask the person to hold a 3 × 5 card over his right eye and, beginning at the top of the chart, to read as far as he can. Repeat with the second eye. In order to "pass" a line on a Snellen chart, a person must read the majority of the letters on the line correctly. Record his visual acuity as 20 (the distance in feet he stood from the chart) over the number corresponding to the last line he read correctly. The adult with normal vision standing 20 feet away from a chart can read the 20-foot line correctly, or has 20/20 vision. Preschool children normally have 20/50 vision; children up to nine years of age typically have 20/30 vision. Do not equate these normal changes in eye development with poor vision.

People need to be referred for further vision testing if their vision is less than that described above or they have greater than a two-line difference in the tests of the two eyes. If a preschool child sees 20/20 with one eye and 20/50 with the other, both eyes test within the normal range but the difference in the ability to focus eyes can lead to *amblyopia* (lazy eye) in children under 8 years of age. Amblyopia is suppression of central vision in an eye to avoid blurry vision caused by the difference in ability to focus; if not treated early in life, it can lead to loss of vision in the poorer eye.

For children too young to know the alphabet or people with language barriers, the E chart is used (Fig. 19-14B). When recording the results of vision testing, be certain to record results both with corrective lenses and without.

Assessment of the Nose

Observe the nose for flaring of the nostrils (a sign of need for oxygen). Look at the mucous membrane of the nose for color (it should be pink; pale suggests allergies; redness suggests infection). Note and describe any discharge. Document that the septum is in the midline (displaced septums such as those that occur after facial blows can interfere with respiration and make nasal intubation in emergencies difficult). Press one nostril closed with gentle pressure and ask the person to inhale; repeat on the opposite side to assure yourself that both sides of the nose are patent (no *choanal atresia* or no membrane obstructing the posterior nares exists). Palpate the areas over the frontal and maxillary sinuses for tenderness, a symptom of sinus infection (Fig. 19-15). Sense of smell can be assessed by asking the person to identify a familiar odor such as chocolate or an orange.

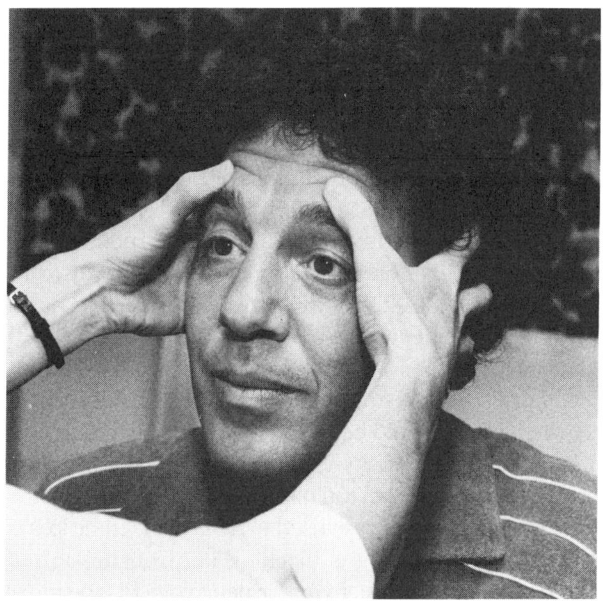

A

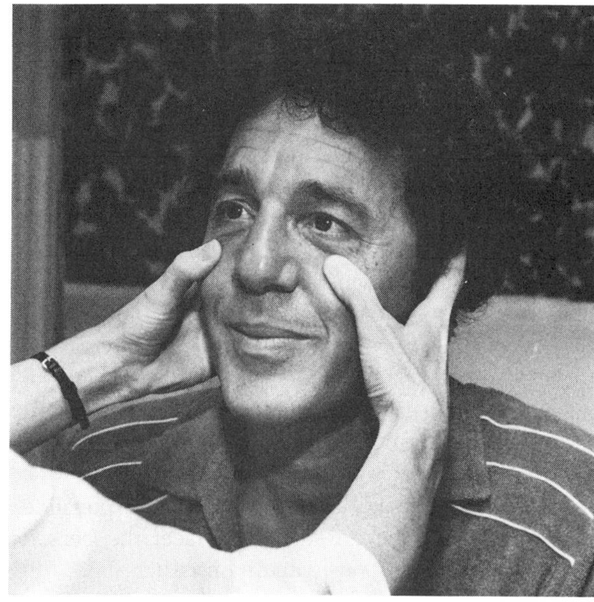

B

FIGURE 19-15. Assessment of frontal (A) and maxillary (B) sinuses.

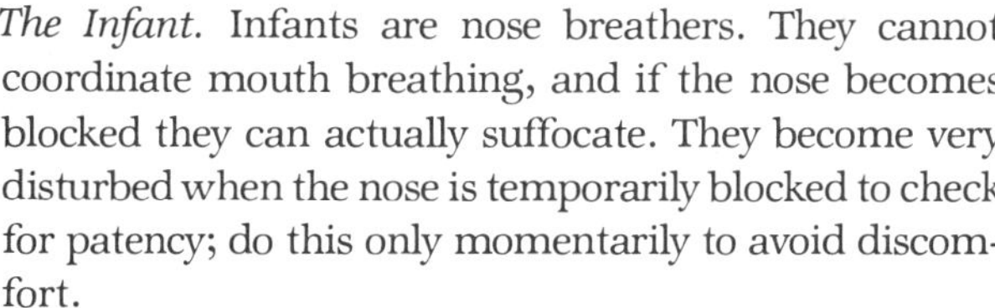

The Infant. Infants are nose breathers. They cannot coordinate mouth breathing, and if the nose becomes blocked they can actually suffocate. They become very disturbed when the nose is temporarily blocked to check for patency; do this only momentarily to avoid discomfort.

Assessment of the Ears

Observe ears for proper alignment. In the average person a line from the inner canthus of the eye to the outer canthus and then to the ear will touch the top of the pinna of the ear. Ears set lower than this are associated with chromosomal disorders. Observe the opening to the ear canal for any discharge. Touch the pinna and watch for evidence of pain (a sign of external canal infections).

To examine the ear canal, the canal must first be straightened. This is done by pulling the pinna gently up and back in an adult, down and back in a child under two years. When inserting an otoscope tip into the external ear canal, always rest the instrument on your hand (Fig. 19-16). In this position, if the person should move his head suddenly, the otoscope will move with him, and there is no danger that the plastic tip will scratch the canal (see QRS 19-3). Otoscope tip sizes vary; use the smallest size possible that still gives you adequate visibility (a 3 is a typical adult size).

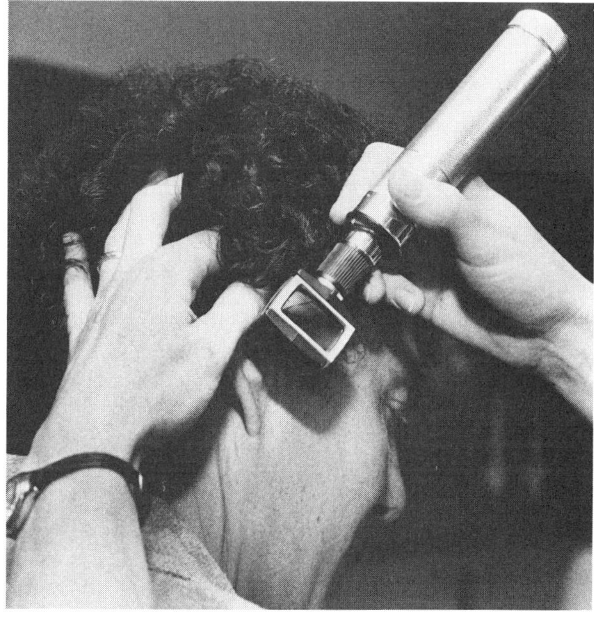

FIGURE 19-16. The otoscope is rested on the examiner's hand to prevent injury if the person moves his head.

Inspect the sides of the canal and the tympanic membrane, and locate landmarks on the surface of the membrane. The outline of the malleus of the inner ear will be evident through the translucent membrane (Fig. 19-17). The color of the membrane itself is pearly gray; if the tension of the membrane is normal, you should see a cone of light—the light reflex in one of the lower corners of your view (either 5 or 7 o'clock).

If ear infection is present, the membrane appears reddened and often bulging forward so that you cannot discern the malleus, and the cone of light is absent; if there is fluid in the middle ear, you may be able to see bubbles of air through the membrane. With chronic middle ear disease (serous otitis media), the tympanic membrane may retract; the malleus is extremely prominent, and the cone of light is again missing. If the membrane is torn, the jagged edge and opening to the middle ear are discernible.

☐ **QUICK REFERENCE STOP 19-3: SAFETY**

1. People who have a swollen and inflammed epiglottis can have acute respiratory arrest if they are gagged with a tongue blade (the motion makes the epiglottis rise and obstruct the airway). *Never place a tongue blade in the back of the throat of a person with symptoms of epiglottitis* (fever, crisp, barky cough, reddened and inflamed throat).
2. Use good technique when using an otoscope to examine an ear canal. Rest your hand between the instrument and the person's head to prevent the otoscope tip from scratching the canal or tympanic membrane.
3. Examining tables in treatment rooms are narrow. Never leave an adult who is not fully responsible or a child alone on such a surface; the person could fall and seriously injure himself.

Many people have wax (cerumen) in their ear canals (this appears as a dark-brown glistening substance). The outward movement of cerumen removes any dust or foreign object that enters the ear.

The Child. Children should be restrained well while their ears are examined. Although painless unless an infection is present, an ear examination is an intrusive procedure and very frightening for the preschool child.

TESTING AUDITORY ACUITY

Hearing acuity is assessed throughout the physical examination by observing the person's responses to your questions or directions. Observe for signs of hearing impairment such as leaning toward you to hear better or turning one ear toward you to form a better hearing surface. To test hearing more accurately, hold your watch a distance away from the person and ask him to cover one ear and tell you at what point he can hear the watch ticking; compare this with your own hearing. Repeat with the second ear. An alternate method is to whisper a number or word a short distance away from the person and ask him to repeat it for you. This has an advantage in that you have proof that the person heard you.

Children over 3 years and adults who have a suspected hearing deficit should be tested with formal audiometry (not included in a routine examination) to establish their level of hearing. If a person has a known hearing loss, the Weber and Rinne tests are used to determine if the loss is conductive (something is blocking the transmission of sound waves to the inner ear) or neurological (the inner ear is unable to receive the waves). These tests are described in Table 19-5.

Assessment of the Mouth and Throat

Assess the external appearance of the lips; look for symmetry and color. Ask the person to smile and to frown to evaluate the mobility of facial muscles. Count the number of teeth present and assess their condition (number missing, cavities present). Inspect the gum line (gingivae) for redness, tenderness, and edema, symp-

FIGURE 19-17. Looking through the otoscope, the malleus of the inner ear is evident through the translucent tympanic membrane. A cone of light is seen at 5 o'clock.

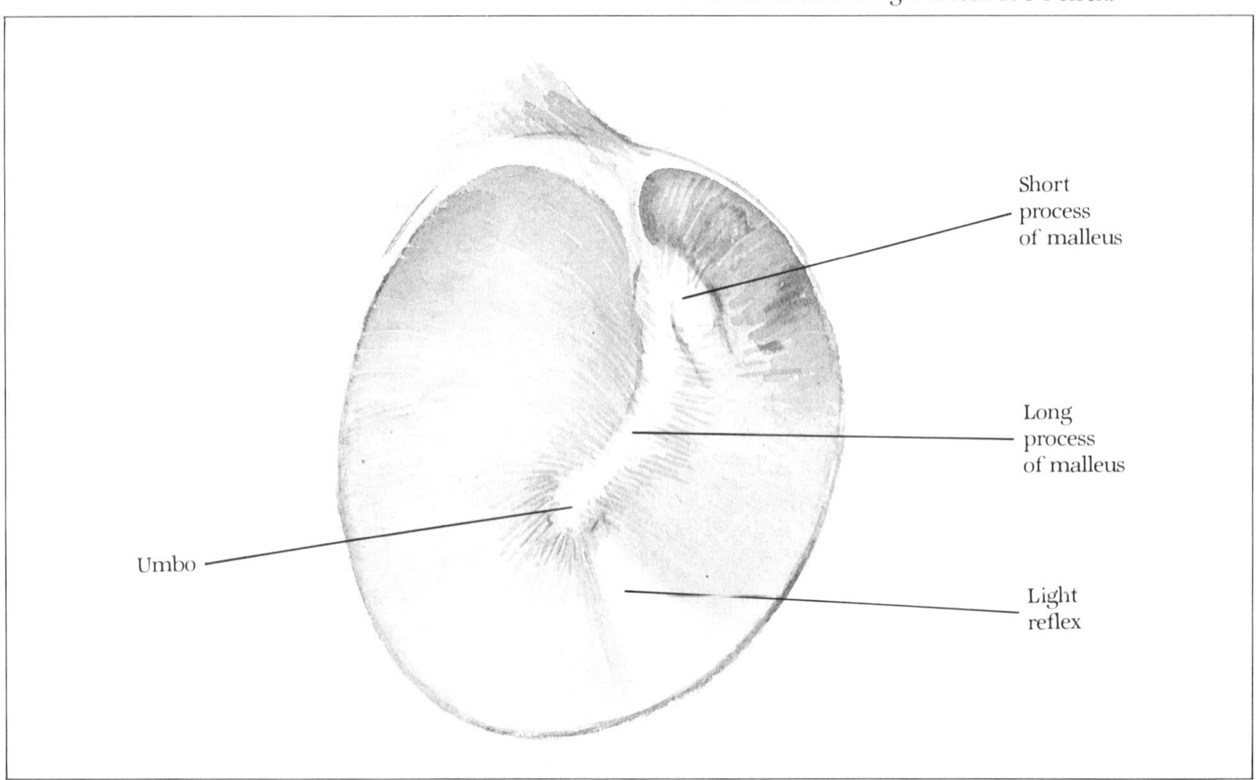

TABLE 19-5. TESTS TO DIFFERENTIATE CONDUCTIVE AND SENSORINEURAL HEARING LOSS

Test	Procedure	Implications
Weber	Strike a tuning fork against your hand or thigh to cause it to start vibrating. Hold the stem of tuning fork against the top of the person's head along the midline. Ask the person which ear he hears the sound in best.	If hearing loss is conductive, the person will hear the sound better in the damaged ear (because there is reduced air conduction, bone conduction is intensified).
Rinne	Strike a tuning fork against your hand or thigh to cause it to start vibrating. Touch the stem of the tuning fork against the bone just in back of the person's ear. When he says he can no longer hear it vibrating, bring it forward and hold it directly opposite the ear. Ask the person if he can hear it in that position.	If conductive hearing loss is present, the person will not hear the sound after it is brought forward (bone conduction is more effective than air conduction).

toms of periodontal disease. Periodontal disease is the leading dental problem in adults; it leads to loss of teeth and nutritional problems if unrecognized and therefore untreated. Inspect the buccal membrane and palate for color (pink) and the presence of any lesions. Ask the person to stick out his tongue and assess for midline position and no fasciculations—trembling. Slight fasciculations may be normal in older adults but not in younger persons. Inspect the area under the tongue for lesions; this and the lips are the areas that are common first sites for oral cancer. A person's tongue normally appears smooth and moist. With dehydration present, it often appears roughened and dry. *Geographic tongue* is a term for the rough-appearing tongue surface that often accompanies general symptoms of illness such as fever; it may also occur normally. Using a tongue depressor to press down on the back of the tongue, inspect the posterior throat for redness or drainage, and ascertain the uvula is in the midline. If difficult to see tonsillar tissue at the sides, ask the person to say "Ah." Tonsillar tissue differs a great deal in size but should not be reddened or have pus in the crypts (indentations).

It is important that you do not depress the tongue of anyone who has epiglottitis or inflammation of the glottis. Symptoms of this condition are a sore throat and a barky cough. If a swollen, inflamed epiglottis occurs due to pressure of a tongue blade, it can obstruct the respiratory tract so completely that the person is immediately unable to breathe (see QRS 19-3).

Infant and Child. In the child compare the number of teeth present to the number appropriate to his development level (see Chap. 9). You may need to use a tongue blade to help move the child's tongue out of the way in order to allow you to view teeth. After gagging a child in order to view the back of his throat, always turn his head sharply to the side so that he does not choke on any saliva that accumulated in his mouth while you were examining his throat, as he is less able to manage this than an adult. Tonsillar tissue in children is bigger in proportion to their throats than in adults (it reaches its peak size at six years of age and then atrophies). Many preschool children therefore appear to be "all tonsils." As long as the tissue does not appear reddened or tender, you can assume it is probably normal for the age.

Assessment of the Neck

Assess the neck for symmetry (the trachea should be in the midline; any deviation suggests lung pathology). Observe the outline of the thyroid gland; this also should be symmetrical. Press on the right side of the gland to cause it to be more prominent on the left; palpate the left half to discern any nodes (areas of hardness). Repeat on the right side (Fig. 19-18). A thyroid node needs investigation: It may be only an innocent transient cyst; alternatively, it may be the first indication of thyroid malignancy.

Palpate the area in front of the ear (location of the parotid gland) and the sides of the neck for lymph node chains. (Fig. 19-19 shows the location of lymph node chains.) Normally no lymph nodes are palpable in

FIGURE 19-18. To palpate the thyroid gland, the examiner stands behind the person, presses on one side of the gland to cause it to be more prominent on the other, and palpates the prominent side.

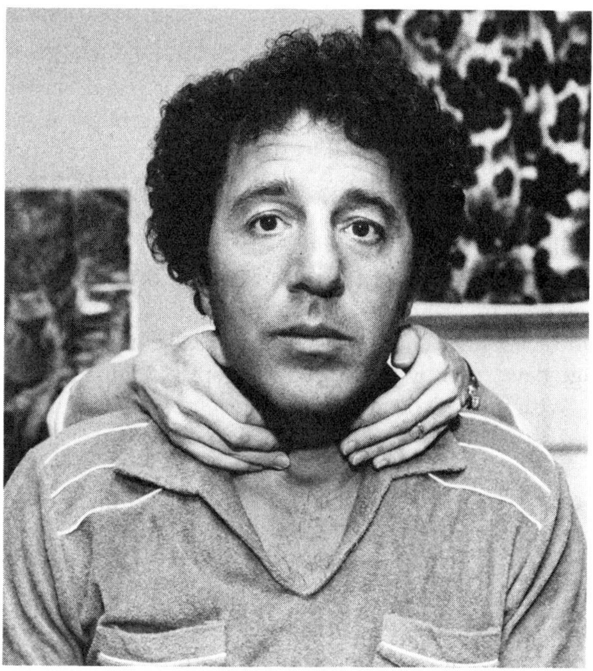

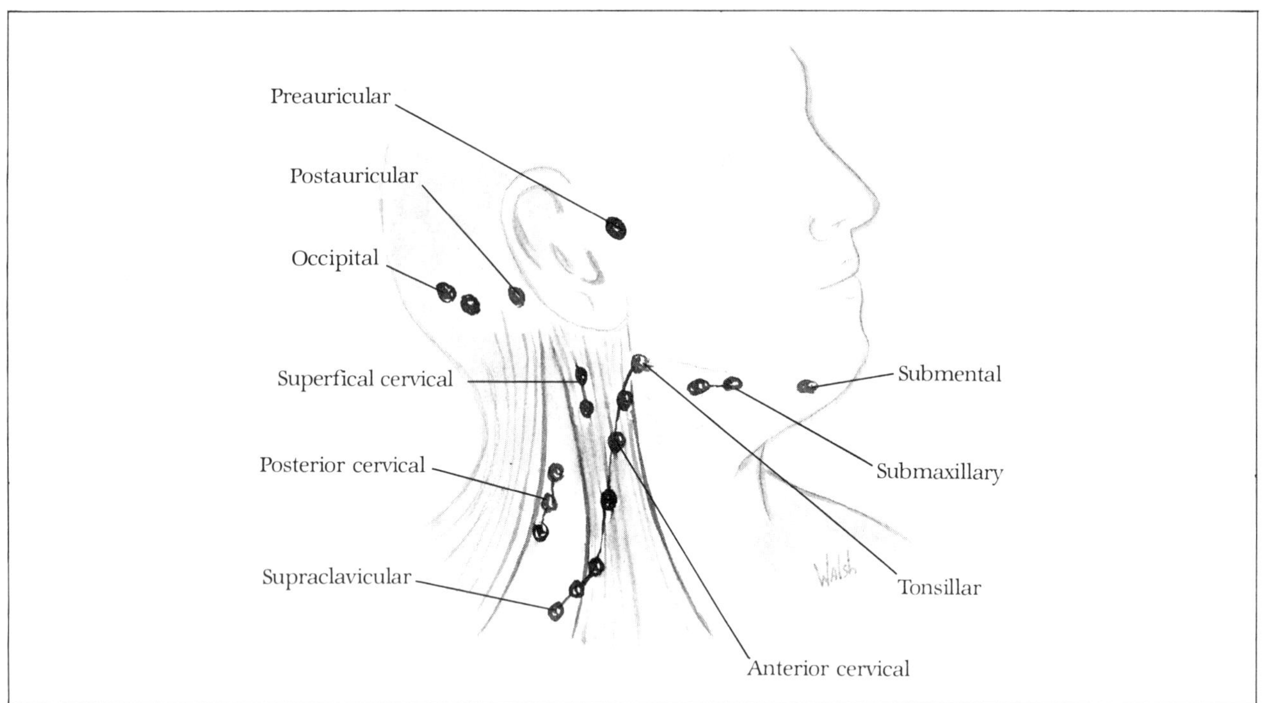

FIGURE 19-19. Location of lymph node chains in the head and neck.

adults. Preauricular and postauricular nodes may be palpable following ear infections, postoccipital nodes following scalp infections. Submental nodes generally denote a tooth abscess. Palpable submaxillary, anterior, and posterior cervical nodes follow throat infections.

Ask the person to move his head (or possibly move it for him) through flexion (touch chin to chest) and extension (raise chin as high as possible), and turn it right and left (rotation). Pain on forward flexion is an important sign of neurological (meningeal) irritation. Difficulty moving a neck into other positions is more often a result of joint limitation due to changes of aging; for older adults with arthritic cervical vertebrae changes, these movements can be very restricted and painful.

The Infant and Child. Infants and children up to adolescence do not need their thyroid gland palpated, as the incidence of thyroid difficulties in this age group (except for congenital hypothyroidism) is small. Observing that the anterior neck appears symmetrical and has a full range of motion and that lymph nodes are not abnormally enlarged is adequate. The presence of palpable lymph nodes the size of peas (termed "shotty" nodes) in the postcervical chain is a normal finding in preschool and school-age children, since almost all children of this age have recently had an upper respiratory infection.

With infants the ability to control the head should be assessed. Lay the infant supine and pull him to a sitting position. A baby less than four months will let his head lag backward as you do this; it is righted only as he reaches a sitting position. After 4 months of age he should bring his head up with him (no head lag) if his neuromuscular coordination is adequate for his age. This is a simple test but important in terms of the information it yields on overall neuromuscular control.

Assessment of the Chest

For ease in specifying the location of chest pathology, the chest is divided in sections by imaginary lines drawn through the midclavicle, midmammary, and midsternum points on the front; the midaxilla on the side; and the midscapula on the back. Pathology is localized in terms of these lines (abnormal lung sound heard at left midaxillary line, etc.). Other helpful means of locating pathology is by the suprasternal notch, the ribs, and the spaces between them called *intercostal spaces.* Intercostal spaces are numbered according to the ribs immediately above them (Fig. 19-20).

Inspect both front and back surfaces of the chest for symmetry of appearance and motion. Assess the proportion of anterior to lateral diameter (normally 1 : 2). People with chronic lung disease develop a broad (barrel) chest or one more rounded than normal. This and other chest abnormalities are shown in Fig. 19-21.

BREAST EXAMINATION

Breast examination is important in both sexes because although breast cancer is typically thought of as a woman's concern, it can occur in men as well. Inspection of breast tissue is easiest if the person sits on the examining table, arms at the sides, with both breasts exposed. Inspect for symmetry, although it is not unusual (and normal) for a woman to have breasts of slightly unequal size. This finding is important only if the difference has recently occurred.

Inspect for edema, erythema, wrinkling, retraction, or dimpling of the skin; all suggest that a tumor is growing in deeper layers of the tissue. Erythema occurs

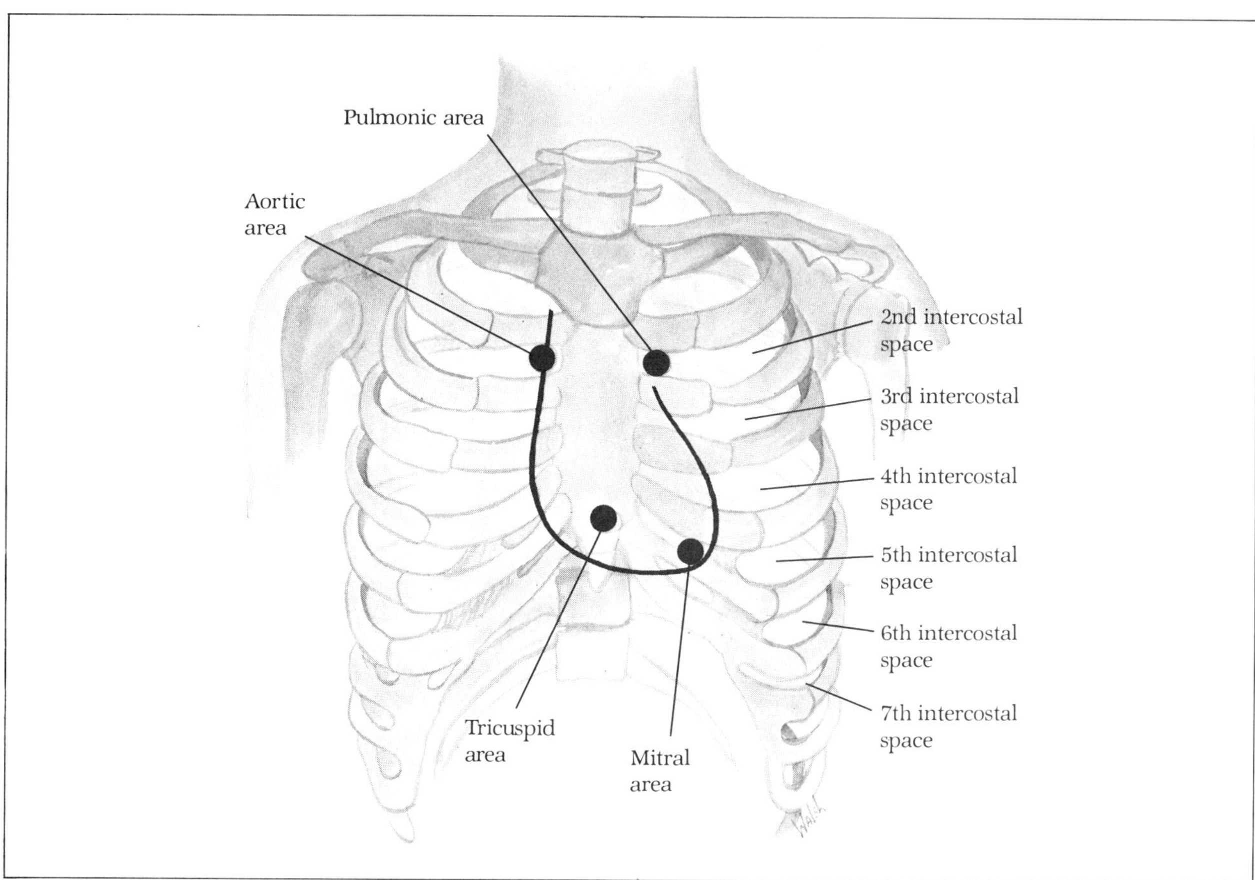

FIGURE 19-20. Intercostal (between ribs) spaces are numbered according to the rib they are immediately below. The points to which the sounds of the heart valves radiate and can be heard best are termed the listening posts of the heart. They are shown as black dots.

from inflammation due to rapidly growing tissue; edema from the blockage of lymph channels due to tumor pressure. Breast edema makes the skin appear not only swollen but pitted (an orange-peel effect) (Fig. 19-22). Note any nipple discharge or "pulled" nipple placement as another way to detect edema.

With the person's arms at the sides to take pressure off breast tissue, palpate well into each axilla as breast tissue extends quite far and also to assess axillary lymph nodes. Normally, no nodes should be felt. Palpate the breast itself with the person lying down with the arms raised and placed beside the head, as this spreads out breast tissue; begin at the nipple and palpate outward in a spiral effect. The lower edge of each breast feels hard; do not mistake this or rib prominences underneath for more than they are.

Women should inspect their own breasts monthly on the day following the end of the menstrual period. This time not only serves as a marking point but is a time when hormonal influences on breast tissue are at a low ebb, and breast tissue is normally not swollen or tender. Postmenopausal women should specify a certain day each month (the first day, the last day, etc.) for self breast examination. Teaching this to women is a major health teaching responsibility of nurses. Never neglect this health teaching rule; every woman should assume the responsibility of self breast examination as an independent self-care task. Another option is for a life partner to assume the responsibility for her. The American Cancer Society's technique of breast examination is shown in Fig. 19-23.

Many preadolescent boys develop hypertrophy of breast tissue due to increased hormonal influences (termed gynecomastia); they are generally concerned and need reassurance that it is normal for their age and will fade as soon as androgen becomes the dominant hormone. Adolescent girls are generally concerned that breast tissue is inadequate or that breast growth is uneven. They need assurance that not all women have completely symmetrical breast tissue.

LUNG ASSESSMENT

Assess the rate of respirations and whether respirations are easy and relaxed or if accessory muscles are necessary for effective ventilation.

On the anterior chest lung tissue extends from above the clavicles to the sixth or eighth rib. On the posterior chest lung tissue is as low as the tenth to twelfth thoracic vertebra. A person's right lung has three lobes; the left only two. It is important when assessing lung tissue that you attempt to evaluate all five lobes as lung disease can be specific for a lobe or involve the entire lung.

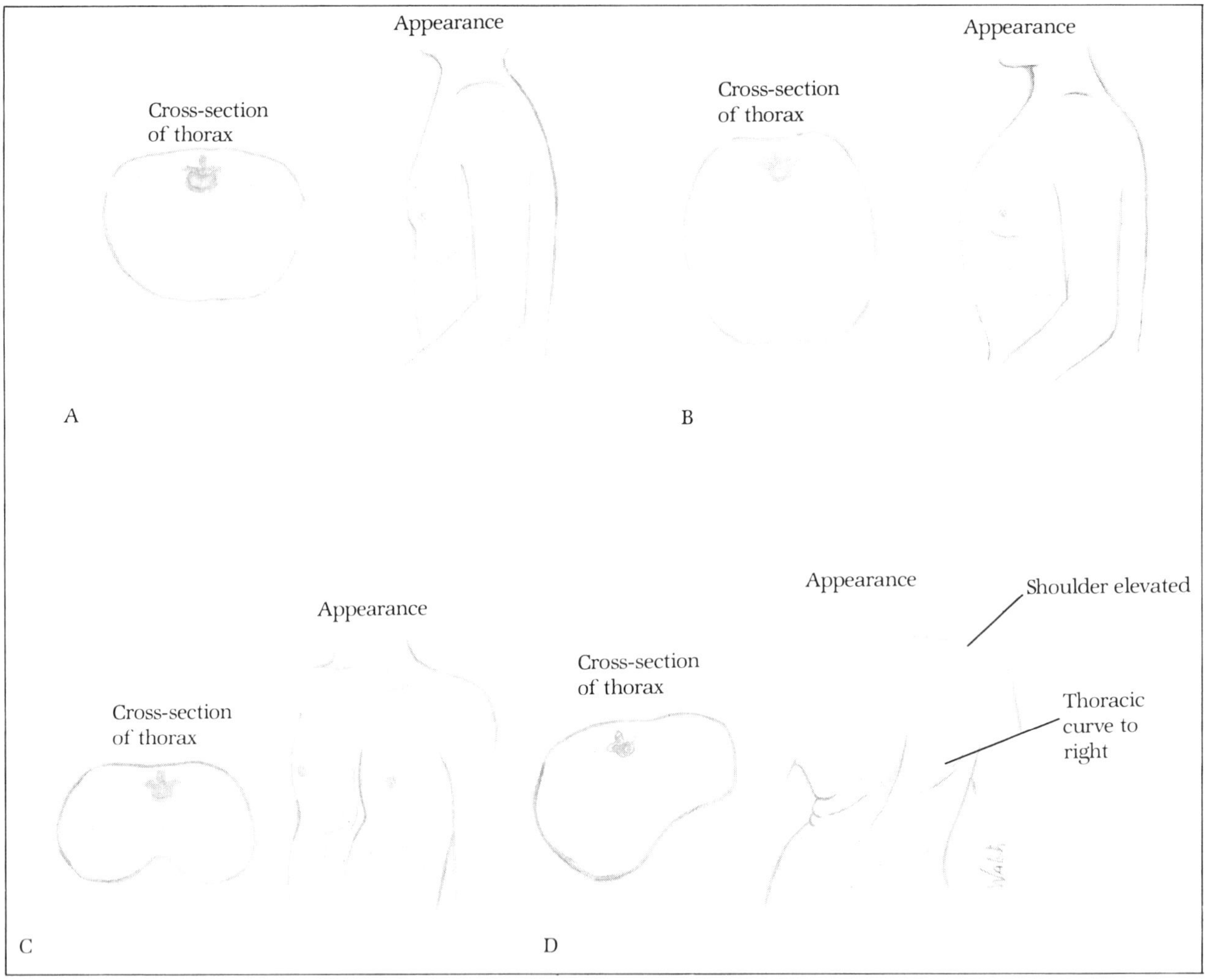

Cross-section of thorax
Appearance
A
Cross-section of thorax
Appearance
B
Cross-section of thorax
Appearance
C
Cross-section of thorax
Appearance
Shoulder elevated
Thoracic curve to right
D

FIGURE 19-21. Chest abnormalities that can be assessed by inspection. A. Normal adult chest. B. Barrel chest. C. Funnel chest (pectus excavatum). D. Thoracic kyphoscoliosis.

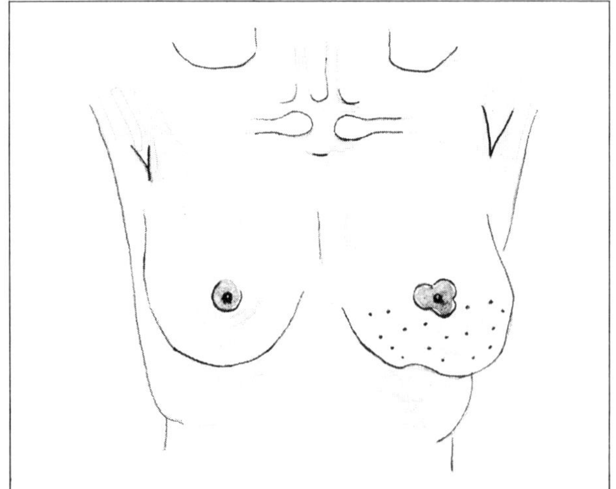

FIGURE 19-22. Breast edema. The skin appears swollen and pitted (orange-peel effect).

Begin lung assessment by percussing lung tissue. Normal lung sounds are resonant; overexpanded lungs sound hyperresonant; and lungs filled with fluid due to cardiovascular disease sound dull. The lower anterior lobe of the right lung will sound dull, as liver covers it on the anterior surface below the fourth or fifth intercostal space.

Diaphragmatic expanse (the distance the diaphragm descends with inhalation) indicates an estimate of lung volume. Establish this by asking the person to take in a deep breath and hold it; percuss the location of the bottom of the lungs (the percussion note changes from resonant to flat at this point). Next ask the person to expire fully and momentarily hold that position. Percuss upward to locate the expired or empty lung position (the percussion note changes from flat to resonant). The difference between these two points is the *diaphragmatic excursion*. In the average adult this distance is 3 to 5 cm; it will be decreased in people with poor lung compliance such as occurs with respiratory illnesses.

Auscultate breath sounds by listening with the dia phragm of a stethoscope over each lung lobe while the person inhales and exhales (preferably with his mouth open). Listen both anteriorly and posteriorly; compare left side to right side for equal findings. Normal breath

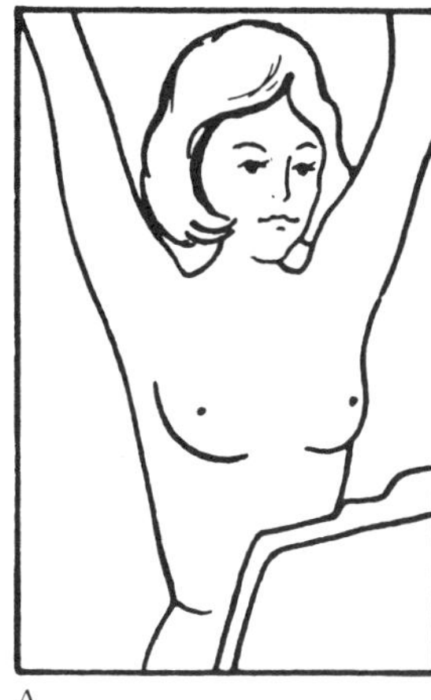

A

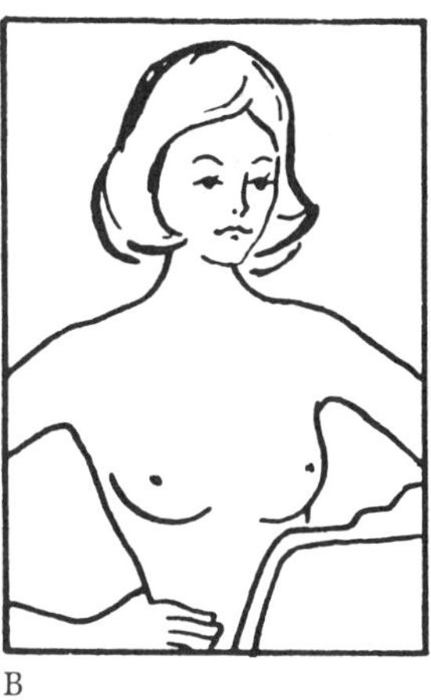

B

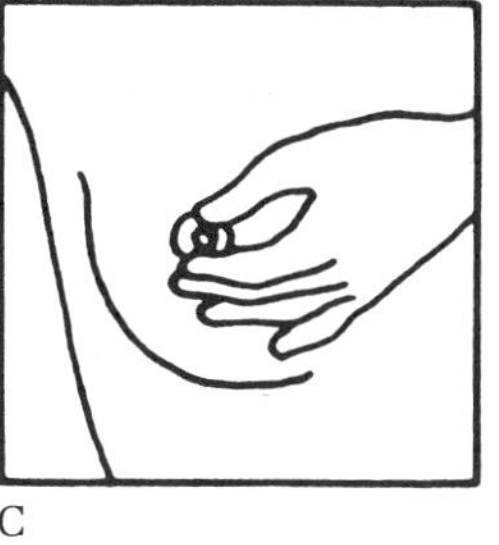

C

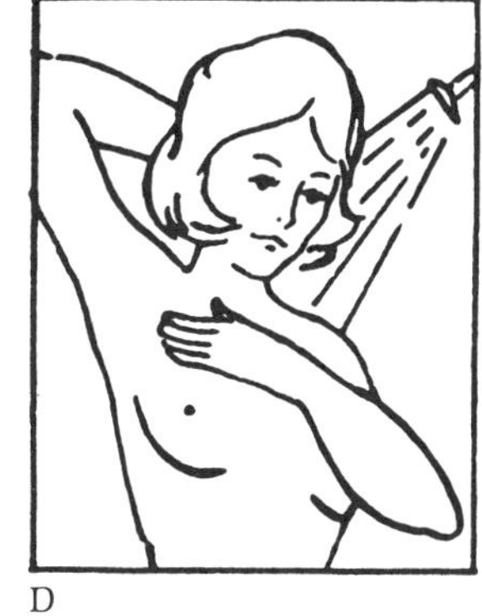

D

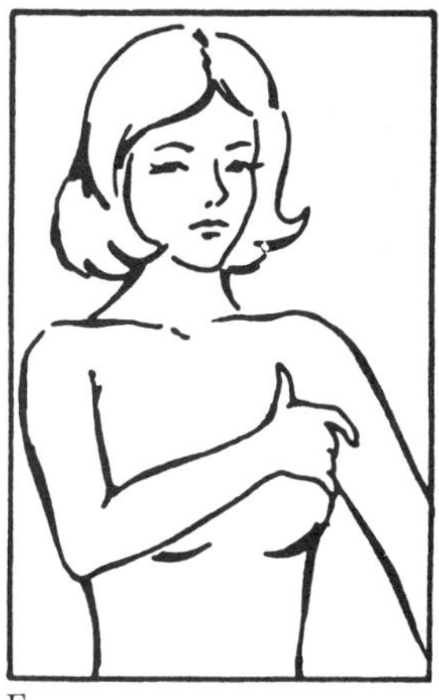

E

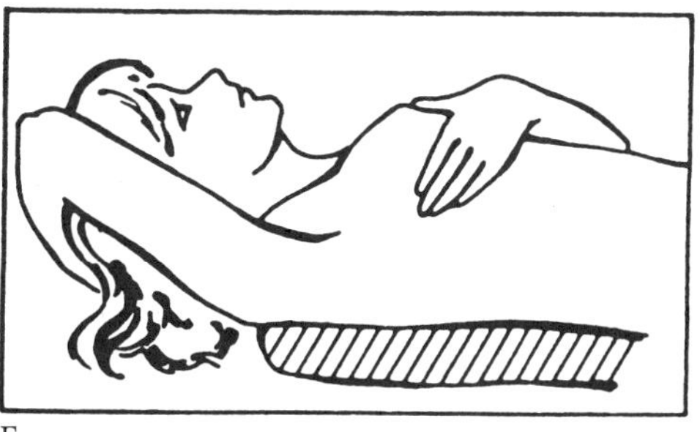

F

FIGURE 19-23. Breast self-examination. Step 1: Inspection. A. In front of a mirror. Look for any change in the size or shape of the breast, puckering or dimpling of the skin, or changes in the nipple. B. Inspect in three positions: (1) with arms relaxed at sides; (2) with arms held overhead; and (3) with hands on hips, pressing in to contract the chest muscles. Turn from side to side to view all areas. C. Nipple examination. Gently squeeze the nipple of each breast between your thumb and index finger, looking for any nipple discharge. Step 2: Palpation or feeling. D. In shower or bath. Fingers will glide over wet soapy skin, making it easier to feel any changes in the breasts. Check the breast for a lump, knot, tenderness, or for any change in the consistency of normal breast tissue. To examine your right breast, put your right hand behind your head, with the pads of your fingers of your left hand held flat and together; gently press on the breast tissue using small circular motions. Imagine the breast as the face of a clock. Beginning at the top (12 o'clock), make a circle around the outer area of the breast. Move in one finger width; continue in smaller and smaller circles until you have reached the nipple. Cover all areas including the breast tissue leading to the arm pit. Reverse the procedure for the left breast. At the lower border of each breast, a ridge of firm tissue may be felt. This is normal. E. Underarm examination. Examine the left underarm area with your arm held loosely at your side. Cup the fingers of the opposite hand and insert them high into the underarm area. Draw fingers down slowly, pressing in a circular pattern, covering all areas. Reverse the procedure for the right underarm. F. Lying down. While lying flat, place a small pillow or folded towel under the right shoulder. Examine the right breast using the same circular motion as was used in the shower. Cover all areas. Repeat this procedure for the left breast. Press firmly but gently while examining your breasts, rolling the tissue between your fingers and the chest wall. (Courtesy American Cancer Society, New York State Division, Inc., East Syracuse, New York.)

sounds are slightly longer on inspiration than expiration. Table 19-6 describes normal breath sounds as well as adventitious sounds you may hear which would reflect illness.

The Infant. Infants cannot breathe in and out on request, so you must listen as they breathe normally. Try to listen to breath sounds early in an examination because if the child cries they are difficult to hear clearly over the sound of crying.

HEART ASSESSMENT

Heart assessment begins with visual inspection to see if there is a point on the chest where the heartbeat can be observed. This point represents the location of the left ventricle or the point where the apical heartbeat can be heard best (Fig. 19-24). In adults this is generally the fourth or fifth intercostal space at the midclavicular line. This point is called the point of maximum impulse (PMI) and is observable in about 50 percent of adults.

Percuss the left side of the chest to discern the left side of the heart. Percussing in from the axillary, the sound will become dull as the heart is identified. If the heart is farther to the left than normally, it suggests an enlarged heart. Normally the percussion note changes from resonant (percussing over lung) to flat (percussing over heart) midway between the midaxillary and midmammary line.

There are five main points at which you should auscultate heart sounds. Although these are not the anatomical locations of heart valves, they are the listening points to which the sounds of the valves radiate and can be heard best (see Fig. 19-20). Table 19-7 describes normal and abnormal heart sounds that may be heard on auscultation. Abnormal sounds are heard best if you listen with both the diaphragm and the bell of the stethoscope.

In order to understand heart sounds, you need to recall heart physiology. The first sound heard (S_1) is that of the mitral and tricuspid valves closing and the ventricles contracting (described as a "lub" sound). The second sound (described as a "dub" and termed S_2) is made by the closure of the aortic and pulmonary valves and atrial contraction.

TABLE 19-6. BREATH SOUNDS HEARD BY AUSCULTATION

Sound	Interpretation and Description
Vesicular	Soft, low-pitched sound heard over the periphery of the lung; inspiration is longer than expiration. Normal.
Bronchovesicular	Soft, medium-pitched sound heard over major bronchi; inspiration equals expiration. Normal.
Bronchial	Loud, high-pitched sound heard over trachea; expiration is longer than inspiration. Normal.
Rhonchi	A snoring sound made by air moving through mucus in bronchi; normal.
Rales	A crackle (like the crackle of cellophane) made by air moving through fluid in alveoli; abnormal; denotes pneumonia which is fluid in alveoli.
Wheezing	A whistling sound on expiration made by air being pushed through narrowed bronchi; abnormal; seen in people with asthma or foreign-body obstruction.
Stridor	A crowing or rooster-like sound made by air being pulled through a constricted larynx; abnormal; seen in infants with respiratory obstruction.

FIGURE 19-24. The nurse auscultates the location of the left ventricle (4th or 5th intercostal space at the midclavicular line), termed the point of maximum impulse (PMI).

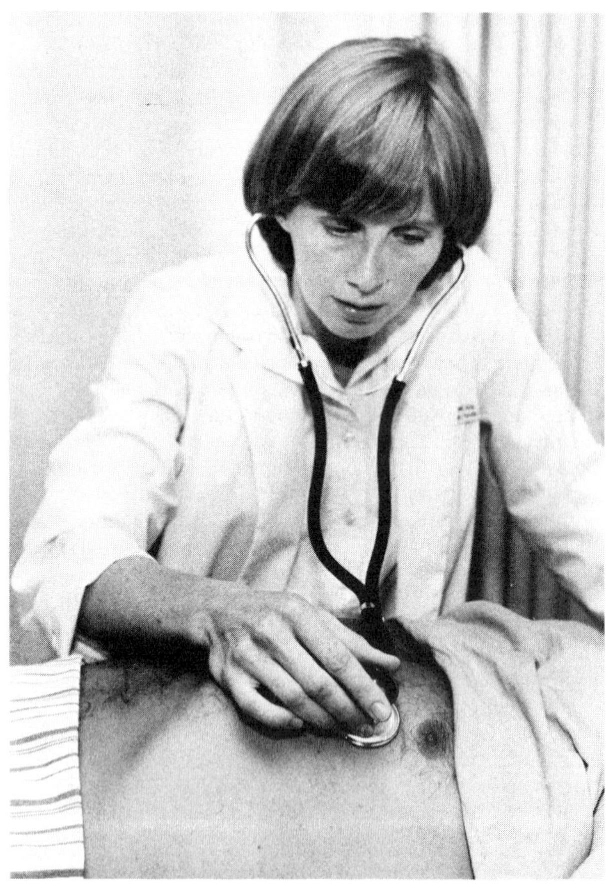

TABLE 19-7. HEART SOUNDS HEARD BY AUSCULTATION

Sound	Cause
S_1	Closure of the tricuspid and mitral valves with the beginning of ventricular contraction (systole)
S_2	Closure of the pulmonary and aortic valves with the beginning of atrial contraction (diastole)
S_3	Rapid ventricular filling
S_4	Abnormal filling of the ventricles

With inspiration and the normal resulting increase of pressure in the lungs, the pulmonary valve tends to close slightly later than the aortic valve. This is termed *physiological splitting* and will be heard as "lub d-dub." As long as this is associated with inspiration, it is a normal finding. Fixed splitting implies that there is always difficulty with pulmonary valve closing and suggests pathology.

At times a distinct third heard sound (S_3) may be heard due to rapid filling of the ventricles. This sound should be investigated but it is not necessarily a serious finding. If a fourth heart sound (S_4) is present (Table 19-7), this generally denotes heart pathology as it indicates abnormal filling of the ventricles.

A heart murmur is indicated by the sound of blood flowing with difficulty or in a different pathway within the heart (a swishing sound more than a murmur) and can be either innocent (functional) or pathogenic (organic). If a heart is pumping with abnormal force, there may be a palpable vibration termed a *thrill*. Palpate the precordium (area over the heart) for evidence of a thrill (feels like the sensation of a cat purring) or a *heave* (a definite outward chest movement), which also denotes a struggling heart. If you hear or palpate any accessory heart sounds or movements, try to describe them with reference to Table 19-8. All additional heart sounds needs further identification and investigation as to their cause. Determining the cause of an abnormal heart sound requires a cardiac specialist. Determining that an abnormal sound exists, however, and securing proper referral is an important nursing role.

TABLE 19-8. DESCRIPTION OF ACCESSORY HEART SOUNDS

Reference Point	Information to Establish
Location	At which listening post did you hear the sound most distinctly?
Quality	Would you describe it as blowing, rubbing, rasping, musical?
Intensity	*Murmurs* are graded according to the following criteria: Grade 6: So loud it can be heard with a stethoscope not touching the chest wall; has a thrill. Grade 5: Very loud but must touch stethoscope to chest to hear; has a thrill. Grade 4: Loud; may or may not have a thrill. Grade 3: Moderately loud; no thrill. Grade 2: Quiet but easily discernible. Grade 1: Very quiet; difficult to hear.
Timing	When in relation to S_1 and S_2 did you hear it? A sound superimposed between S_1 and S_2 is a *systolic* murmur; one between S_2 and the next S_1 is a *diastolic* one. Innocent murmurs (functional, denoting no pathology) are usually systolic (there are exceptions to this); pathologic murmurs are more apt to be diastolic.
Pitch	Would you describe the sound as high or low pitched?
Radiation and thrills	Is there an accompanying thrill? Does it radiate so that it can be heard at another location such as the back of the chest?

Assessment of the Abdomen

The abdomen is divided anatomically into four quadrants. The quadrants and the organs that lie within them are shown in Fig. 19-25. To assess the abdomen, first inspect the surface for symmetry and contour. An adult abdomen is gently depressed; a newborn abdomen is slightly protruberant. Note any skin lesions or scars.

Auscultate the abdomen for bowel sounds before palpating, as palpating may alter bowel movements (peristalsis) and therefore disturb bowel sounds. Bowel sounds can be heard in all quadrants of the abdomen. They are high "pinging" sounds that occur normally at time intervals of about 5 to 10 seconds. If a bowel is distended, they occur more frequently; if the bowel is blocked so that there is no movement of contents, they will be absent. Listen for a full minute before you conclude that no bowel sounds are present.

Listen along the middle of the abdomen over the aorta for a bruit or the sound of blood passing through an irregular space. A *bruit* is a swishing or blowing sound that occurs if there is an outpouching of the aorta (an aneurism), a condition that can be congenital or occur with aging.

Palpate the abdomen in a systematic order such as right lower quadrant, right upper quadrant, left lower quadrant, left upper quadrant. Palpate first lightly, then deeply. If the person has indicated that any portion of his abdomen is tender, begin assessment at the farthest point and work toward the tender area. If no tenderness is present, the order of palpation is unimportant as long as it is thorough. Ascertain whether any area is tender by watching the person's face while you palpate; observe for "guarding" or the person tensing his abdominal muscles to keep you from pressing deeply at that point. Note any hard area or mass.

By palpating from the right lower quadrant to the right upper quadrant, your hand will "bump" against the lower edge of the liver 1 to 2 cm below the right ribs. On the left side the lower edge of the spleen may be discernable. A liver or spleen larger than this is suspicious of disease. Liver, spleen, and bladder size can all be documented further by percussion.

The Child. Children's abdomens are often "ticklish" and they may tense or "guard" their abdominal muscles as you begin to palpate, making it difficult for you to

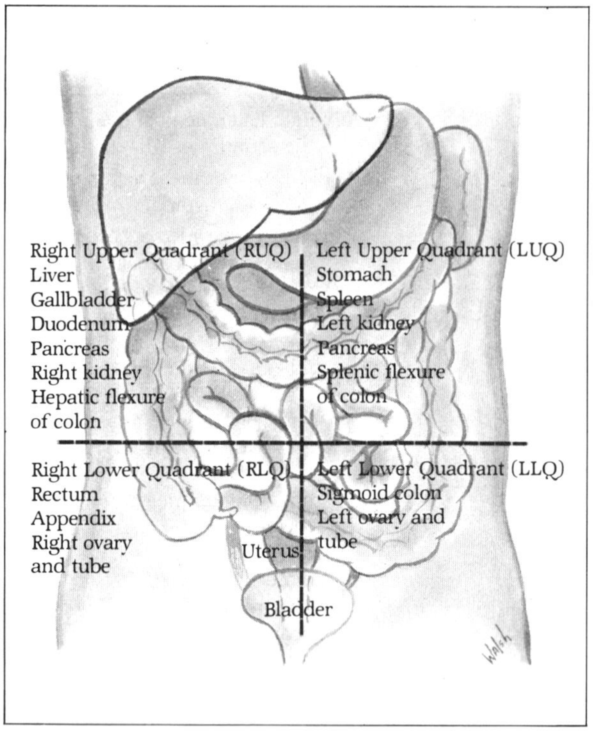

Right Upper Quadrant (RUQ)
Liver
Gallbladder
Duodenum
Pancreas
Right kidney
Hepatic flexure of colon

Left Upper Quadrant (LUQ)
Stomach
Spleen
Left kidney
Pancreas
Splenic flexure of colon

Right Lower Quadrant (RLQ)
Rectum
Appendix
Right ovary and tube

Left Lower Quadrant (LLQ)
Sigmoid colon
Left ovary and tube

Uterus
Bladder

FIGURE 19-25. The four quadrants of the abdomen and the organs that lie within them.

palpate deeply. Distract the child by asking him a question about home or school to help him relax.

Assessment of Female Genitalia

Inspection of external female genitalia and assessment of femoral nodes is included in every complete health assessment. Internal examinations may be performed, depending on any symptoms present. An external examination consists of inspecting for hair configuration (an inverted triangle), presence of vaginal discharge, or vulvar irritation.

ASSISTING WITH AN INTERNAL PELVIC EXAMINATION

Women need careful preparation for internal pelvic examinations because most women find such examinations uncomfortable both physically and psychologically and are worried that they will be painful. Provide a draw sheet as a drape during the procedure to protect modesty; ensure an uninterrupted examining site. Although an internal examination can be done with the woman lying supine in bed, they are generally done on a treatment room table. The woman empties her bladder and lies supine on the table surface with her legs raised in the table stirrups (a lithotomy position). The examiner stands or sits at the foot of the table. Equipment necessary for a pelvic examination is a sterile glove for the examiner, a speculum, and necessary culture equipment.

The examiner first palpates the Skene's and Bartholin's glands at the vaginal outlet (these may be swollen and tender if infection is present). The hand is then introduced into the vagina and the woman is asked to bear down as if she is moving her bowels. This will reveal the presence of a cystocele (an outpouching of the bladder into the anterior vaginal wall), a complication that may occur following childbirth if the vaginal wall was weakened at the time of the birth.

Next the examiner inserts a vaginal speculum into the vagina. If speculum blades are made of metal (disposable ones are plastic), they are usually warmed

FIGURE 19-26. A speculum separates the vaginal walls and allows observation of the position and appearance of the uterine cervix.

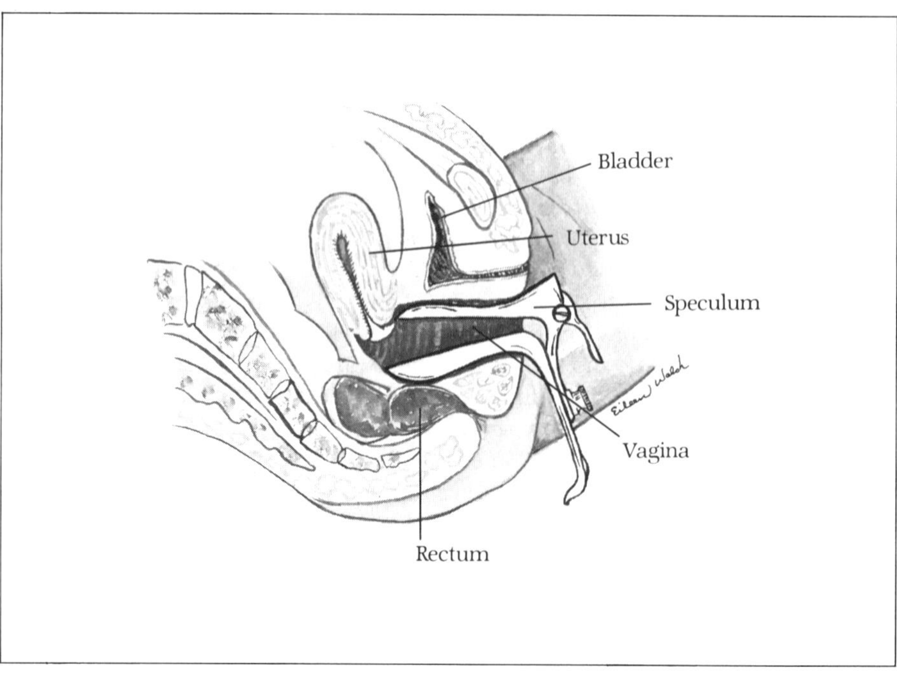

first by holding them under warm running water. Never use oil or a cream as a lubricant, as these can interfere with smears or cultures that will be taken. The position and appearance of the uterine cervix can be observed with the speculum in place (Fig. 19-26).

Following observation, a gonorrheal culture is done by swabbing the cervix with a sterile cotton applicator and then transferring this to a special culture medium. Three Papanicolaou (Pap) smears (for cervical cancer) are obtained: one by a moistened cotton applicator inserted into the endocervical canal; another by a small wooden spatula which is pressed against the cervix and rotated; for the third, a scraping is taken from the posterior vagina next to the cervix. Material obtained is transferred to a glass slide. As the speculum is withdrawn, the sides of the vagina are inspected for color and the presence of any lesions.

A bimanual (two-handed) examination is then performed to determine the size and placement of reproductive organs. One of the examiner's hands is placed on the woman's lower abdomen; two fingers of the other hand are placed vaginally. The vagina, cervix, uterus, and ovaries are palpated for size, consistency, and placement by compressing them between the two hands.

Lastly, the posterior wall of the vagina is palpated by placing one finger in the vagina and one in the rectum and compressing the tissue between them.

If the woman relaxes during a pelvic examination, it is not painful; all she feels is pressure. If she is unable to relax, it can be very uncomfortable. If she has hemorrhoids (distended veins at the rectum), the last examination may be painful for her.

Explaining what the examination will consist of is helpful to aid women to relax; telling them to take deep breaths is helpful (it gives them something specific to do, momentarily taking their concentration off their lower abdominal muscles and relaxing them). Just having you stand at the head of the table and be on "their side" is extremely helpful in keeping the fear of pelvic examinations to a minimum (which in turn relaxes muscles) (see QRS 19-4).

☐ QUICK REFERENCE STOP 19-4: HEALTH TEACHING

Physical examination is a good time for health teaching about body function and care because the person's attention is centered on his body during this time. The teaching point might be an explanation of how to do breast self examination or self testicular examination or a response to something that the person expresses concern about, such as reassurance that the presence of a supernumerary nipple is normal.

The Child. Children under puberty do not have internal pelvic examinations unless specific symptoms are present, as the incidence of disease in this period is minimal.

Assessment of Male Genitalia

Inspection of male genitalia is best done with the man standing. It consists of observing the distribution of hair (male pubic hair has a diamond-shaped distribution), lesions of the penis, appearance and placement of the urethral opening, and ability of the foreskin to retract if the man is uncircumcised (Fig. 19-27). *Hypospadias* is a term for a urethral opening located on the inferior or ventral (under) surface of the penis; *epispadias* denotes a urethral opening on the superior or dorsal (upper) surface. Both these conditions need to be identified. If more than a slight deviation is present, repair is usually initiated before school age. Such a urethral placement may interfere with fertility and self-image.

The scrotum should be inspected for size and the presence of testes. In most men the left testis is slightly lower than the right, so the scrotum does not appear truly symmetrical. Palpate to check that testes are both

FIGURE 19-27. Assessment of male genitalia includes determination of the ability of the foreskin to retract in uncircumcised males.

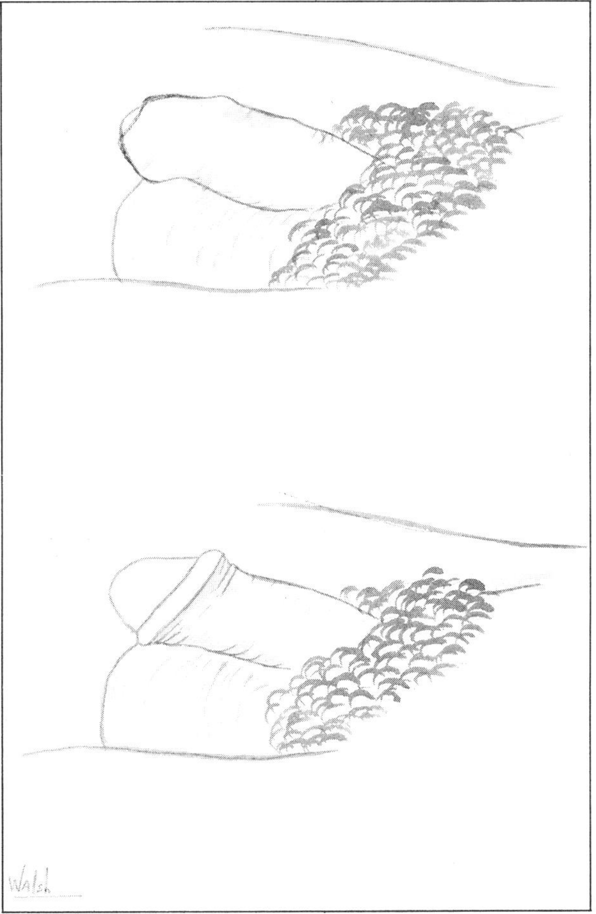

present by placing one hand over the top of the scrotum at the inguinal ring and then palpating the testis on that side. This hand position prevents the testis from slipping up into the inguinal ring and appearing to be absent on palpation. Any swelling or mass in the scrotum needs to be identified. The most likely cause of such a condition is a hydrocele or a fluid-filled sac; it could represent a serious finding such as testicular cancer. Boys (starting at puberty) and men should be taught to do testicular palpation every month. Suggest selecting a certain day each month (the first day, the last day, etc.) and doing it in the shower, as after a warm shower scrotal skin is most relaxed. The man should roll each testicle gently between thumb and fingers to assess for any hard lumps or nodules, any change in consistency, or difference in size. The epididymis at the rear of the testicle feels like a strong cord; he needs to be familiar with the feel of this and also the fact that in most men one testicle is slightly larger than the other and hangs a little lower in the scrotal sac so that he does not think these findings are abnormal.

If the man does heavy lifting, he is prone to inguinal hernia formation (outpouching of intestine into the inguinal ring). He should include a simple hernia assessment following testicular examination. He should stand in front of a mirror and cough or strain his abdominal muscles and watch to see if there is a protrusion or a visible outpouching of his lower abdomen just above the scrotum.

To assess for the presence of a hernia, you should place your fingertips against the inguinal ring in the groin area and ask the man to cough. If the tendency for a hernia is present, coughing tightens abdominal muscles and forces abdominal contents to bulge against your fingers. This technique may not be used extensively by a nurse in a hospital setting but is helpful for a nurse in an industrial setting or health maintenance facility. Palpate femoral nodes (located in the groin and on the inner surface of the upper thigh) for any abnormalities.

Another major health problem of the male reproductive system is cancer of the prostate gland. The best position for the man to assume for examination of the prostate gland is to lean over the end of the examining table. The examiner inserts a lubricated gloved finger into the rectum and palpates the prostate gland through the anterior rectal wall. Normally the prostate gland feels smooth and firm; any hard nodules may indicate the development of prostatic cancer. The gland is also assessed for size. Hypertrophy may be benign (innocent), but if it is discovered, the man needs further assessment. In many older men, it can cause urinary difficulty if it exerts pressure on the urethra, and abnormal growth of any body organ may be an indication of malignant (cancer) growth.

After the examining finger is withdrawn, stool on the examining glove is tested for the presence of blood (a symptom of rectal cancer, another major health problem of adult males).

The Child. The reproductive system examination in male infants is limited to palpation of the testes to see if they are descended and assessment of the penis for lesions, inflammation, and a central urethral opening. Prostatic lesions do not occur until later in life and so are not assessed in children.

Assessment of the Rectum

The rectum should be inspected for any protruding hemorrhoidal tissue (distended veins) or fissures. If specific symptoms are present, it is examined further. With a lubricated glove in place, a finger is inserted gently into the rectum and the anterior and posterior walls are palpated. This is an uncomfortable sensation of pressure for many people; if hemorrhoidal tissue is present, it can be painful. If the person bears down while the finger is inserted, this prevents the anus from being so constricted and the feeling of pressure is less.

Assessment of Extremities

Observe extremities for ease of motion, symmetry, and alignment during the entire examination. Move all joints through full range of motion (see Chap. 26). Palpate all surfaces to detect abnormal swellings or tenderness. Ask the person to walk toward you and away from you to assess gait (easy, mobile). Assess peripheral pulses and other tests of peripheral vascular circulation as well as the presence of varicose veins.

The Child. An infant's hips abduct so far that to do external rotation of hips, the knee will rest on the bed.

Assessment of the Back

The back should be observed for symmetry and spinal column contour and alignment. Note any dimpling at the end of the spinal column; this is a common site for a dermal cyst (pilonidal cyst). This is an innocent finding unless it becomes infected or connects to deeper tissue layers. Assess for tenderness along the spinal column by palpating each vertebra.

The Child. Preadolescent and adolescent children (especially girls) have a high incidence of scoliosis (sideways or lateral curvature of the spine). Ask the child 8 to 18 years of age to bend over and touch his toes while you observe his spinal column. If a scoliosis is present, this position magnifies the malalignment and makes it appear more prominent than it is in a standing position.

Assessment of Neurological Competence

People with neurological disease processes require a complete neurological examination, a detailed procedure. A general examination consists only of testing deep tendon and superficial reflexes (involuntary responses to

TABLE 19-9. GRADING OF DEEP TENDON REFLEXES

Grade	Interpretation
4+	Hyperactive; extremely marked reaction; abnormal
3+	Stronger than average, but within normal range
2+	Average response
1+	Less than average response but within normal range
0	No response; abnormal

a stimulus) and general sensory and motor function. These findings complement findings from the mental status assessment carried out during the entire examination.

Deep tendon reflexes test the intactness of the spinal nerve that supplies the particular body area. They are graded according to the scale in Table 19-9. The biceps reflex (Fig. 19-28A) tests fifth and sixth cervical nerves.

The triceps reflex (Fig. 19-28B) tests seventh and eighth nerves. The forearm will move perceptibly if the reflex is intact.

The supinator or brachioradialis reflex (Fig. 19-28C) tests fifth and sixth cervical nerves. The forearm will move perceptibly if the reflex is intact.

The patellar reflex (Fig. 19-28D) tests second, third, and fourth lumbar nerves. The lower leg will move perceptibly if the reflex is intact.

The achilles tendon reflex (Fig. 19-28E) tests first and second sacral nerves. The foot will move perceptibly in response to the percussion tap.

Superficial reflexes that may be tested are the abdominal and the Babinski reflexes. The umbilicus will move perceptibly toward a stroke motion on the abdomen if the eighth to the twelfth thoracic nerves are intact.

A Babinski reflex (Fig. 19-28F) tests first and second nerves. Newborns demonstrate a positive response as a normal finding for the first three months of life.

MOTOR AND SENSORY FUNCTION

In a routine physical examination cranial nerves are not assessed, except for those assessed with the eye and mouth examination. Test general motor ability by asking the person to grasp both your hands and squeeze and to push against both of your hands with his feet as he lies supine. Recall whether gait was adequate or not when you observed him walking.

To test sensory function, ask the person to close his eyes and identify the location when you touch him for at least six points on different body parts.

FOLLOW-UP CARE

Following a physical examination, be sure that all equipment used is returned to its proper place. Clean ear speculum tips with an alcohol swab before replacing them. Be certain that batteries in an otoscope are replaced or recharged as needed. Be certain that the person is comfortable and that you have answered any questions or concerns about the examination.

ASSISTING WITH A PHYSICAL EXAMINATION

In some instances, instead of performing the physical examination yourself, you will be assisting another health care provider such as a physician, a nurse clinician, or a nurse practitioner to perform an examination.

When you are assisting another, offer information as appropriate, such as "You may feel uncomfortable for a minute." Be careful that you do not answer questions that are asked of the patient such as "What did you eat for breakfast?" "What day is this?" Such questions may be memory testing rather than information seeking.

If you restrain parts of the person's body for the examination, do it with a positive approach such as "Let me help you keep your hand still."

USING PHYSICAL ASSESSMENT

Combine aspects of physical assessment with health interviewing to establish a complete patient data base. Use it to complement the questions you ask when a person tells you of some symptom he is experiencing. If a person tells you he has pain, for example, you ask about the duration, intensity, frequency, description, associated symptoms, and patient action including any precipitating activity (history taking). In addition, you will inspect the part in question to determine whether there is redness or swelling present or any break in the skin in the area. Palpate the area for warmth and edema; percuss perhaps to help determine the consistency of tissue beneath the surface area or auscultate for the presence of bowel sounds. Physical assessment techniques strengthen or validate history taking; they help you evaluate whether the problem requires immediate action or is secondary to another patient problem. Keep in mind that some medications can change or influence assessment findings (see QRS 19-5).

You must use physical assessment skills in order to distinguish between normal and abnormal findings. Palpating an abdomen, for example, is a simple procedure. Recognizing abdominal pathology when you palpate it is a second, more complicated step. You only develop this skill by practicing, in order to become familiar with both normal and abnormal findings. You cannot distinguish between normal liver tissue and a distended liver until you have felt both a number of times.

Physical examination can include many other facets and steps in addition to those described above. The techniques described comprise a guide for general assessment at a level that can be incorporated into nursing assessment for more thorough planning of nursing care.

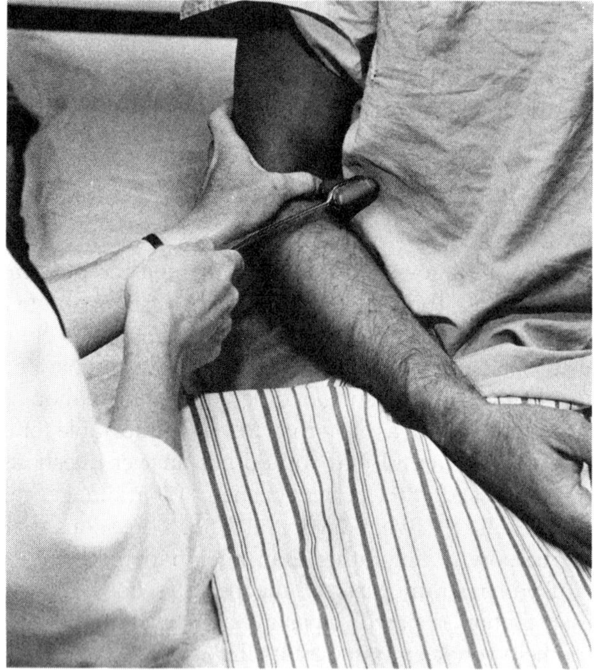

A

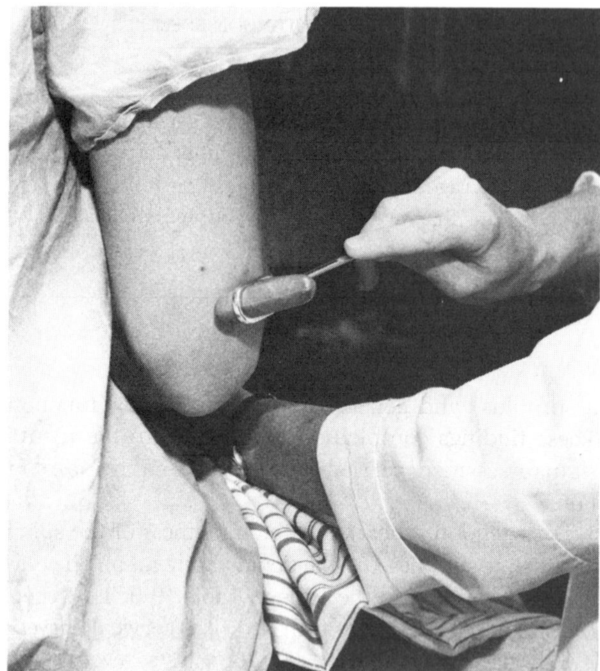

B

C

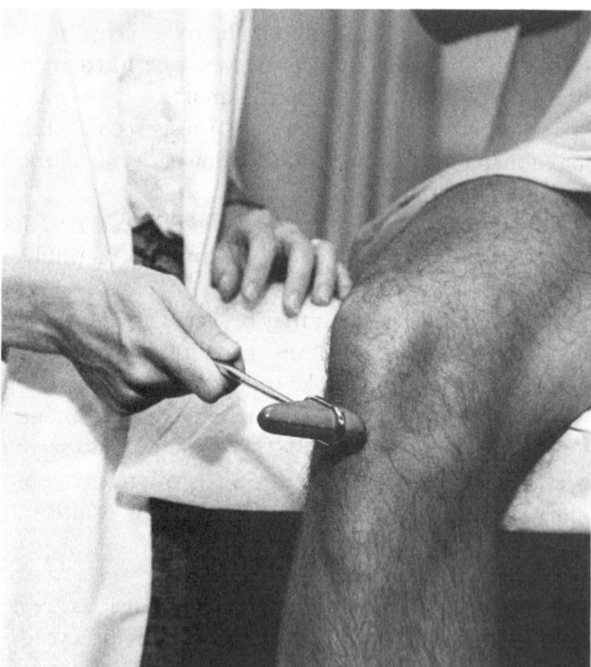

D

FIGURE 19-28. Eliciting reflexes. A. Biceps reflex. Patient's arm should be partially flexed at the elbow. Place your thumb over the biceps tendon; the reflex hammer strikes your thumb. Observe and feel the movement of the forearm. B. Triceps reflex. Flex the patient's elbow. Strike the triceps tendon above the elbow. Observe and feel extension at the elbow and movement of the forearm. C. Supinator or brachioradialis reflex. The patient's forearm should rest in the lap. Strike the radius about 1 to 2 inches above the wrist. Observe and feel flexion and movement (supination) of the forearm. D. Patellar reflex. The patellar tendon is tapped briskly. Observe and feel contraction of the quadriceps, extension at the knee, and movement of the lower leg. E. Achilles tendon reflex. Strike the achilles tendon. Observe and feel movement (plantar flexion) of the foot. F. Babinski reflex. Using your finger or the end of the percussion hammer, strike the sole from the heel to the ball of the foot in an inverted J pattern. The normal response is flexion of the toes; an abnormal response (positive) is flaring of the toes.

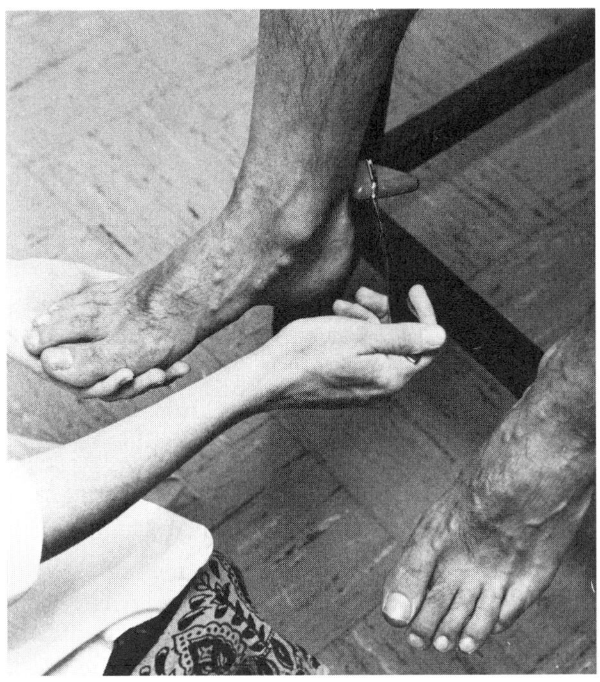

E

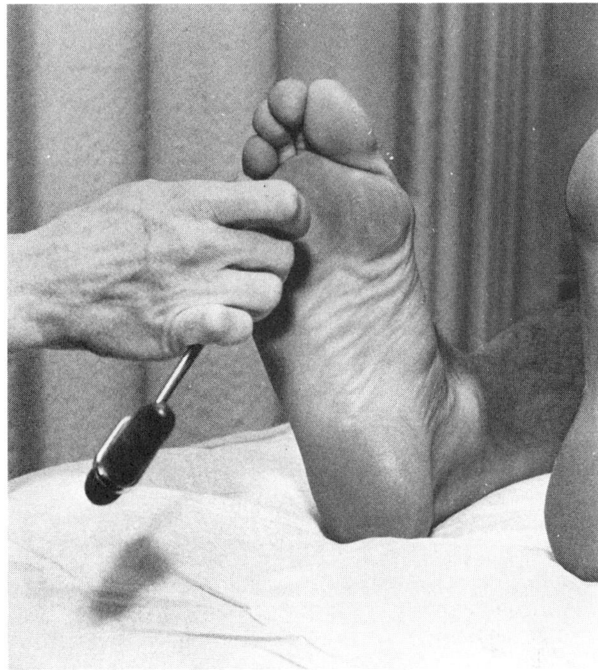

F

LIFE SPAN CONCEPTS AND PHYSICAL EXAMINATION

Techniques of physical examination as well as findings differ depending on the age span involved.

The Newborn

All newborns receive a physical examination immediately following birth and again after the first 24 hours of life. When examining newborns, remember that maintaining body temperature is one of the infant's most difficult tasks. Cover body areas that you are not directly examining. Take newborn temperatures axillary to prevent rupture of rectal mucosa. Take the heart rate apically as peripheral pulses are too faint to be counted accurately. Take femoral pulse to rule out coarctation of the aorta. Include newborn reflexes, head circumference, and an assessment of gestational age (see Chap. 9) as routine parts of the examination. Do not take blood pressure as value is not reliable in this age.

The Infant

Infants are often examined most effectively if the mother holds them during most of the examination. Use an "isn't this fun?" or "this is a game" approach. As a rule, assess heart and lung function first; intrusive procedures such as ear and throat assessment should be done last. Include newborn reflexes until 6 months of age; take heart rate apically, temperature rectally or axillary. Include head circumference for a full year. Do not take blood pressure.

Toward the end of the first year, children become very fearful of strangers. Taking a minute to become acquainted with the child at beginning of the examination helps to counteract this problem.

The Toddler and Preschooler

Both toddlers and preschoolers are fearful of examining equipment. Allowing them to handle items helps to alleviate this fear. Leave intrusive procedures such as genitalia and ear and throat assessment until last.

Include blood pressure as part of routine assessment at 3 years of age; take temperature by rectum or axilla until 4 to 5 years of age. Give generous praise for cooperation (anything short of hysterical screaming or kicking is good cooperation for intrusive procedures). Establish a good rapport with the child's parent, as children this age sense parental trust or suspicion.

The Schoolager and Adolescent

Older children may enjoy having a parent with them while they are being examined or they may resent his presence; give the child the choice. Children often worry about some physical finding such as a mole or supernumerary nipple. Make a habit of commenting on such findings—"You have a mole on your hand; that's normal"—as both a means of reassurance and an addition to history taking.

Schoolage and adolescent children are modest. Protect modesty by careful use of gowns or drapes. Children are usually unaware of what a physical examination includes and whether it will cause discomfort. Offer good explanations so that they are not frightened by the unknown. Begin to include teaching for self breast and testicular examination.

☐ QUICK REFERENCE STOP 19-5: PHARMACOLOGY

Medications that people are taking can influence or change physical assessment findings. Following are specific physical findings to assess for if the patient is taking the indicated drugs.

Drug	*Pertinent Observation*
Antibiotics	Antibiotics may promote growth of fungi infections. Inspect moist damp body areas such as folds of skin, surface of the tongue, beneath foreskin in males, at vaginal surface in women; diaper area of infants.
Anticoagulants	Anticoagulants interfere with blood clotting. Inspect for petechia (small pinpoint red areas) under skin. Assess body parts easily bumped such as knees, over the tibia or the elbow for eccymotic areas. Inspect any laceration (or needle puncture site) to see if bleeding is still present.
Anticonvulsants	Dilantin, a common anticonvulsant, causes hyperplasia or overgrowth of gum tissue as a side effect of the drug. Good oral care—careful brushing and use of dental floss—is necessary to prevent tooth decay under the edematous gingiva.
Diuretics	Diuretics cause loss of body water through increased urination. Assess for skin turgor, moistness of mucous membrane, and sunken eye globes for evidence of dehydration from excessive fluid loss. A diuretic may be prescribed because edema (collection of fluid in subcutaneous tissue) is present. Assess if any edema is present to assess effectiveness of diuretic.
Analgesics	Analgesics interfere with the sensation and consequently the interpretation of pain. A person taking large doses can injure himself such as by a sprained ankle and not be aware of the seriousness of the injury because of the decreased level of pain. Assess specifically for any evidence of pain such as holding a body part stiffly, "guarding" muscles, tense facial expression, inability to perform full range of motion. Narcotic analgesics tend to slow gastrointestinal rate. Listen for bowel sounds.
Antihypertensives	Antihypertensives are prescribed to reduce blood pressure. Assess for blood pressure and also the presence of peripheral pulses to see that blood perfusion to distal sites is adequate.
Cardiovascular drugs	Listen carefully to the heart rate and rhythm; assess peripheral rate and pulses of anyone on a cardiac regulatory drug.
Respiratory regulators	Assess the rate of respirations and listen carefully for adventitious lung sounds.
Chemotherapy	A side effect of almost all chemotherapy is a decrease in leucocyte and platelet counts. Assess carefully for signs of infection (elevated temperature, a skin lesion that is not healing) and signs of poor clotting ability (petechia under the skin; bleeding from a skin lesion).

☐ **QUICK REFERENCE STOP 19-6: COMMUNITY CONSIDERATIONS**

Children receive a physical examination at every well child health care visit; adults at routine health promotion visits. A person being seen by a physician for a specific symptom of illness (a broken finger, painful menstrual cramps, a skin rash) may have only one body part assessed rather than a full physical examination. Do not assume in history taking that when a person says he has recently seen a physician he has had a full physical examination; ask specifically if this was done.

Encourage people to go for health promotion visits so that they have periodic examinations.

The Adult

Adults are familiar with physical examination procedure but are also usually faintly uncomfortable about it because of concern that abnormal findings may be discovered. Be certain to discuss self-care aspects of breast and testicular examination (see QRS 19-4). For thorough assessment, an examination of a man over 40 should include a rectal exam; that of a sexually active woman should include a Pap smear (see QRS 19-6).

The Older Adult

A thorough physical examination may be exhausting for an older adult. If the person is experiencing arthritic changes in joints, assuming different positions may be painful or difficult. An older adult may also become chilled easily if you do not provide for proper draping or gowning.

UTILIZING NURSING PROCESS

Bob is a 16-year-old seen in an ambulatory setting because of chronic fatigue and a recent weight loss. The following is the written report of his physical examination. Be certain in recording physical examination findings that you record what you saw or heard at the time of the examination, not information the patient told you, which is subjective. Physical assessment yields *objective* information.

General Appearance: Thin-appearing white male. Well developed muscularly; height: 5′8″ (70th percentile); weight: 110 lb (40th percentile). Temperature: 98.6° F orally; pulse: 76; respiration: 20.

Mental Status: Nervous mannerisms of chewing on fingernails, rapid speech pattern. Has both recent and past memory recall. Oriented to time, place, and person.

Head: Normocephalic; alert and expressive face. Two "shotty" palpable nodes in posterior cervical chain. Hair lifeless, oily; male distribution.

Eyes: Vision 20/20 on Snellen exam with both eyes. Extraocular muscles grossly intact (follows to six fields of vision); no crusting or erythema present. Pupils react to light and accommodation is present; red reflex present. Eye globe appears sunken; conjunctiva pink but not exceptionally moist.

Ears: Normal alignment; no tenderness present; landmarks of greater and lesser process and light reflex identified on tympanic membrane. Auditory canal clear. Able to distinguish whispered word comparable to examiner (4 feet).

Nose: Midline septum; no crusting or discharge; bilaterally patent.

Mouth: 28 teeth present (no third molar eruption as yet); 1 cavity in left lower first molar; minimal plaque present; Mucous membrane: pink but not exceptionally moist; midline uvula; tonsils present bilaterally and noninflamed; normal sized for age; palate intact.

Neck: Trachea midline; full range of motion present; no nodes palpable in thyroid.

Chest: Symmetrical; no gynecomastia.

Lungs: No adventitious breath sounds to auscultation and percussion. Diaphragmatic excursion: 3 cm.

Heart: Apical pulse: 80; regular rhythm with physiological splitting present. No murmurs.

Abdomen: Bowel sounds present; soft, no tenderness or masses. Liver palpable 1 cm below costal margin; spleen not palpable.

Genitalia: Circumcised; midline urethra. Testes descended.

Rectum: No lesions, no hemorrhoids.

Back: Spinal column straight; no tenderness.

Extremities: Normal gait; full range of motion in all joints. Radial, popliteal and dorsalis pedis pulses present.

Neurological: Biceps, triceps, patellar and achilles: 2+. Motor and sensory function intact.

Skin: Fingernails short and two of them bleeding at distal end (observed chewing on them prior to exam). One cm long linear lesion on right forearm surrounded by 2 cm erythematous area, warm and tender to touch. Slight edema present surrounding area. Yellow drainage can be expressed from lesion.

Impression: 16-year-old male with decreased weight in proportion to height (40th to 70th percentile); evidence of slight dehydration and poorly healing lesion.

This examination of Bob confirms his reported recent weight loss; notice how his hair is described as "oily," a frequent finding in people who have been recently fatigued. It also reveals the additional findings of dehydration (the sunken eyeglobes, the lack of moisture of mucous membranes). Discovery of a tooth cavity is a common adolescent finding but could be serving as a source of infection. The presence of plaque on teeth could reflect the effect of recent fatigue (too tired to bother with regular tooth hygiene). The presence of the scratch mark that is not healing is important because it suggests that the body's nutrients or immunological capacity are deficient in some way. The bitten fingernails suggest that this or some other problem is distressing. In order for Bob to return to a high level of wellness, both physical and psychological aspects must be considered.

Different physical examination findings would have been present if Bob's recent loss of weight were from an innocent cause (deliberately trying to lose weight rapidly to qualify for a wrestling meet or because he was so nervous during a week of exams he ate almost nothing). Physical examination findings are necessary to confirm the history and indicate what laboratory or diagnostic tests are necessary to establish the full disease picture. In Bob's case the presenting picture suggests diabetes. Recent loss of weight, fatigue, and poor healing power are often the first indications that diabetes is present and further investigation by laboratory tests is necessary for confirmation.

SUGGESTED READINGS

Alexander, M., and Brown, M. S. *Pediatric History Taking and Physical Diagnosis for Nurses* (2nd ed.). New York: McGraw-Hill, 1979.

Assessing Your Patients. Springhouse, Penn.: Intermed Communications, 1980.

Assessment tips: Performing palpation. *Nursing* (Horsham) 13(1):68, 1983.

Bailey, P. A. Physical assessment of the elderly. *Opp. Clin. Nurs.* 3:15, 1981.

Bates, B. *A Guide to Physical Examination.* Philadelphia: Lippincott, 1979.

Blackburn, N. A., et al. Honing your respiratory assessment technique. *RN* 43:28, 1980.

Block, G. J., et al. *Health Assessment for Professional Nursing.* New York: Appleton-Century-Crofts, 1981.

Boylan, A. Nursing at the crossroads. 3. Assessment of the patient's physical condition. *Nurs. Times* 78(35):1485, 1982.

Burns, K. R., and Johnson, P. J. *Health Assessment in Clinical Practice.* Englewood Cliffs, N.J.: Prentice-Hall, 1980.

Cannon, C. Hands-on guide to palpation and auscultation. *RN* 43:20, 1980.

Carotenuto, R., and Bullock, J. *Physical Assessment of the Gerontologic Client.* Philadelphia: Davis, 1981.

Cole, P. Breast self examination: An adjuvant to early cancer detection. *Am. J. Public Health* 71:572, 1981.

Cook, L. Renal trauma: Challenging assessment, cautious care. *RN* 46(2):58, 1983.

Cunning, B. R., et al. Well elderly screening clinics: A community clinical experience in health assessment. *J.N.E.* 21(3):38, 1982.

DeAngelis, C. *Pediatric Primary Care* (2nd ed.). Boston: Little, Brown, 1979.

Dickinson, G., et al. Adult arthritis. The assessment. *Am. J. Nurs.* 83(2):262, 1983.

Dunn, B. H. Components of musculoskeletal examination. *Orthop. Nurs.* 1(6):33, 1982.

Ferholt, J. D. *Clinical Assessment of Children.* Philadelphia: Lippincott, 1980.

Freis, P. C. Sounds of a healthy heart. *Issues Compr. Pediatr. Nurs.* 3:1, 1979.

Howe, C. L. Physiologic and psychosocial assessment in labor. *Nurs. Clin. North Am.* 17(1):49, 1982.

Hutchfield, K., et al. Holding children for examination. *Nursing* (Oxford) 1:1003, 1981.

King, R. C. Taking a close look at the eye. *RN* 45:48, 1982.

King, R. C. Checking the patient's neurological status . . . the fine art of giving a physical. *RN* 45(12):56, 1982.

Koeckeritz, J. L. The fine art of giving a physical: Organizing your plan of action. *RN* 44:46, 1981.

Koeckeritz, J. L. The fine art of giving a physical. Assessing the genitalia. *RN* 46(1):53, 1983.

Malkiewicz, J. How to assess the ears and test for hearing acuity. *RN* 45:56, 1982.

Meier, E. M. Evaluating head trauma in infants and children. *M.C.N.* 8(1):54, 1983.

Mitchell, J. R. Male adolescents' concern about a physical examination conducted by a female. *Nurs. Res.* 29:165, 1980.

Moss, J. R. Helping young people cope with the physical examination. *Pediatr. Nurs.* 7:17, 1981.

Murray, M. A. Chest pain, dyspnea, confusion: When should you sound the alarm. *RN* 46(1):66, 1983.

Murray, R. B., and Zentner, J. P. *Nursing Assessment and Health Promotion Through the Life Span* (2nd ed.). Englewood Cliffs, N.J.: Prentice-Hall, 1979.

Nappy, J. E. Churches as setting for teaching physical assessment. *Am. J. Nurs.* 82(8):1235, 1982.

Roberts, S. L. Renal assessment: A nursing point of view. *Heart and Lung* 8:105, 1979.

Sana, J. M., and Judge, R. D. (Eds.). *Physical Assessment Skills for Nursing Practice* (2nd ed.). Boston: Little, Brown, 1982.

Scharping, E. M. Physiological measurements of the neonate. *M.C.N.* 8(1):70, 1983.

Schulmeister, L. Screening for skin cancer: A necessary part of your assessment routine. *Nursing* (Horsham) 11(10):42, 1981.

Schwieger, J., et al. Oral assessment: How to do it. *Am. J. Nurs.* 80:654, 1980.

Sigmon, H. D. Trauma. This patient needs your expert help. *Nursing* (Horsham) 13(1):33, 1983.

Stokes, S. A., et al. Health assessment—considerations for the older individual. *J. Gerontol. Nurs.* 6:328, 1980.

Strange, J. M. The riddle of abdominal trauma: How much damage . . . and *where? RN* 46(3):43, 1983.

Taylor, D. L. Inflammation: Physiology, signs and symptoms. *Nursing* (Horsham) 13(1):52, 1983.

Visich, M. A. Knowing what you hear: A guide to assessing breath and heart sounds. *Nursing* (Horsham) 11(11):64, 1981.

Walleck, C. A. A neurologic assessment procedure that won't make you nervous. *Nursing* (Horsham) 12(12):50, 1982.

Woods, M. E. Assessment of the adult with cancer. *Nurs. Clin. North Am.* 17(4):539, 1982.

Yoos, L. A developmental approach to physical assessment. *M.C.N.* 6:168, 1981.

QUESTIONS FOR REVIEW

1. Percussion, a technique of physical examination, is best described as:
   a. Striking one finger to another to elicit sound.
   b. Feeling deeply, using two hands.
   c. Listening acutely for the report of sound.
   d. Stroking the skin surface lightly to elicit reflexes.

2. In measuring weight, which of the following would be the least important (assuming that a person is going to be weighed every day):
   a. The same scale is used each time.
   b. The person wears the same clothing each time.
   c. The person is weighed at the same time every day.
   d. The same examiner weighs the person.

3. Which of the following best describes the appearance of a normal tympanic membrane?
   a. The malleus is visible through the translucent surface.
   b. The membrane protrudes forward from fluid behind.
   c. The color is dark tan.
   d. The malleus is not distinctly outlined.

4. A head circumference measurement is made from:
   a. Center of the forehead to the base of the occiput.
   b. The hairline in front to the hairline in back.
   c. Middle of the forehead through the parietal prominences.
   d. Just above the eyebrows to the prominent point of the occiput.

5. In assessing vision using a Snellen eye chart, the first number of the vision report represents:
   a. The distance the person stood from the chart.
   b. The distance from which the person could correctly read the chart.
   c. The optic depth of a normal eye.
   d. A Snellen conversion vision factor.

6. Cover testing is a way to assess:
   a. Ability to see in the dark (night vision).
   b. Peripheral vision.
   c. Ability to discern rapid movement.
   d. Eye alignment.

7. Which of the following would you report as a normal lung assessment finding?
   a. Stridor.
   b. Rales.
   c. Rhonchi.
   d. Wheezing.

8. Bowel sounds are heard on auscultation of the normal abdomen. Which of the following best describes the normal frequency?
   a. 1—2 per min.
   b. 5—10 per min.
   c. 30—40 per min.
   d. 60 per min.

9. The heart sound S_1 is made by:
   a. Closure of tricuspid and mitral valves.
   b. Closure of tricuspid and pulmonary valves.
   c. Closure of aortic and pulmonary valves.
   d. Opening of the pulmonary valve.

10. The Babinski reflex is frequently used to assess neurological function. The normal response in an adult is:
    a. Toe flexion.
    b. Ankle moves perceptibly.
    c. Ankle flexion.
    d. Toe hyperextension.

20. ASSESSMENT BY LABORATORY MEASURES

OBJECTIVES

Upon mastery of the material in this chapter, you should be able to:

1. Describe the nurse's responsibility in diagnostic-laboratory studies.
2. Describe the importance of diagnostic-laboratory results in assessment, analysis, and nursing care planning.
3. Describe the care necessary before, during, and after a procedure in reference to blood drawing, electrical impulse, radiographic, aspiration, and endoscopic and nuclear medicine studies.
4. Describe the procedure of venipuncture and capillary puncture for blood drawing.

TERMS

The terms important for an understanding of this chapter are shown below and defined in the glossary:

aspiration studies
bone marrow aspiration
chemistry studies
diagnostic-laboratory studies
electrocardiogram (ECG or EKG)
electroencephalogram (EEG)
electromyogram (EMG)
endoscopic studies
hematology studies
lumbar puncture (LP)
nuclear medicine studies
paracentesis
radiograph (x-ray)
thoracentesis
venipuncture

Evaluation of diagnostic-laboratory studies is the third part of assessment, along with results of an interview and a physical assessment. You use this information to analyze nursing diagnoses and to plan and implement nursing care. Almost every patient, whether ambulatory or in an inservice unit, will have at least one laboratory-diagnostic study because these studies produce so much information about state of health and projected effect of therapy. Laboratory assessment is used even in health maintenance care—for the screening of such conditions as sickle cell anemia and hemoglobin determination (the proportion of oxygen-carrying material in red blood cells to the total number of red blood cells present).

NURSING RESPONSIBILITIES

Nursing responsibility for a diagnostic-laboratory study includes obtaining consent as needed, scheduling the procedure, explaining the procedure to the patient and his support people, preparing the patient physically and psychologically, perhaps accompanying him to the hospital department where the procedure will be done, providing support during the procedure, assessing response to it, and providing after care of equipment and specimens.

Scheduling Diagnostic Procedures

If a number of procedures are ordered, the nurse who copies the physician's order for the procedure or a nursing unit secretary will be responsible for scheduling it with the hospital department involved. In most instances the nurse will never see laboratory personnel at their jobs, but it is her responsibility to record the orders and schedule them in the patient's daily care plan. Scan the list of procedures ordered and ask yourself whether the scheduling is arranged in a pattern that will be the least traumatic to the patient. For example, if blood is needed for both the chemistry and the hematology departments, one venipuncture can be done instead of two and the blood divided into separate chemistry and hematology tubes. If two x-rays are needed (spine and pelvis), they should be taken on the same visit to the x-ray department.

Some studies must be scheduled before other studies or the accuracy of the second study will be questionable. For example, if radioopaque dye (barium) is swallowed for a gastrointestinal x-ray series, it will then be impossible to x-ray the kidneys by radioopaque dye for 3 or 4 days because the kidneys are posterior to the gastrointestinal (GI) tract and the barium there will occlude kidney views. Therefore, a kidney x-ray (intravenous pylogram) must always be scheduled before an upper GI series. Otherwise, 3 to 4 days (the time required for the GI barium to be excreted) will be wasted before a second study can be undertaken. This is costly to the patient (4 extra days of hospitalization) and will delay the start of therapy.

Learning to schedule diagnostic studies well comes with practice and experience. The biggest obstacles to scheduling are radioopaque barium studies and dye injections given intravenously (they distort 24-hour urine collections related to specific gravity, quantity, and possibly to chemical composition while the dye is being excreted in the urine during the next several days; if an iodine-based dye is used, thyroid studies will be distorted for months afterward).

Some patients cannot remain without food or fluid for a long time (people with diabetes or dehydration) and thus cannot have tests requiring fasting scheduled one right after another. Some people may need a rest day free of procedures (threatening events) to protect their mental health. If a battery of diagnostic tests has been ordered, ask, Is this battery as condensed as possible? Will the sequence of procedures be acceptable to this patient's physical and emotional condition and his personality? If the patient is a child, is this schedule acceptable to his support people? (A painful procedure should perhaps not be scheduled on the one day the child's mother has said she cannot visit.)

Obtaining Consent

Additional consent to perform a procedure must be obtained if the procedure carries any risk that would not be present if it were not performed. In order for a person to sign a consent form, he must be informed what the procedure consists of, what risks are associated with the procedure, and what would be the risks to him of not having the procedure performed. In order to be certain that you can explain procedures clearly to people and answer their questions, make every effort to see as many procedures done as you can. If you could not accompany a patient to another hospital department for a procedure, ask the person when he returns what happened to him, and what sensations he experienced, not only to help him work through a possibly frightening situation but also to increase your own knowledge of diagnostic-laboratory procedures.

Explaining Procedure

Laboratory-diagnostic studies vary greatly in technique, from x-ray to blood drawing, dye injection to removing body tissue for analysis (biopsy). The person undergoing the procedure and his support people need a description of the study (you will lie on a table; a physician will inject dye into a vein in your arm; the x-ray machine over your head will take pictures of the dye as it travels through your bloodstream and reaches your kidneys); where the procedure will be done (the treatment room or the x-ray department); any unusual sensations during the study (you will feel a hot flush or pressure); a fair description of any pain involved (the needle will sting); any strange equipment used (an x-ray machine, chest electrodes); the approximate time the study takes (caution support people that although the study itself is done in 10 minutes, the person may have to wait for his turn and thus be gone from the patient care unit for an hour or more); and any special care following the study (nurses will take his pulse and respirations more frequently than usual for the first 4 hours).

Since most diagnostic studies are done at the beginning of an illness, your explanation is being given to a person who is newly admitted to a health care facility or to ambulatory care. The person probably has little knowledge of hospital jargon such as *NPO*, *EEG*, and *serial urines*—terms that patients who have been hospitalized for other episodes of illness are familiar with. Therefore, do not include jargon in your explanation of diagnostic tests. Most people are anxious about undergoing diagnostic studies and appreciate knowing what will happen to them. Be certain that you have evaluated the person's level of understanding well before you begin an explanation so that you do not make the procedure sound simpler or more complicated than it is due to the wrong level of communication. Ask about the patient's previous experience with similar procedures. You may need to clear away some wrong information before the person can relax enough to be receptive to new information.

Some physicians give their patients detailed explanations of what procedures involve; others merely state, "I'm ordering some tests for you," knowing that you will offer full explanations. So that you do not duplicate explanations, ask the patient what his physician told him; fill in gaps and correct misunderstood information as needed.

Children have so little experience with illness that it is often difficult to explain a procedure so that a child will understand. Try to compare equipment and techniques to experiences involved in childhood play or family life. For example, an x-ray machine can be compared to a camera (Fig. 20-1A). Do not refer to procedures as tests; this may lead children into asking what is the "right answer" to the test and cause them to give wrong information to health interviews, hoping to pass the test.

Some persons at a hospital admission are so anxious about being in a strange environment or so anxious about the outcome of the study (it may show that they have a major illness) that they do not take in the explanation of the study. Be prepared to repeat a description of the procedure immediately before the study to counteract this very normal blocking out of input in stressful situations.

If you are unfamiliar with what a procedure entails, do not guess. Most hospital departments will give you a description over the telephone of the specific points they like the patient to know about the study. They appreciate having a well-informed patient because this makes him better able to cooperate—for example, taking deep breaths or lying still for a long time.

Support people need an explanation of the procedure

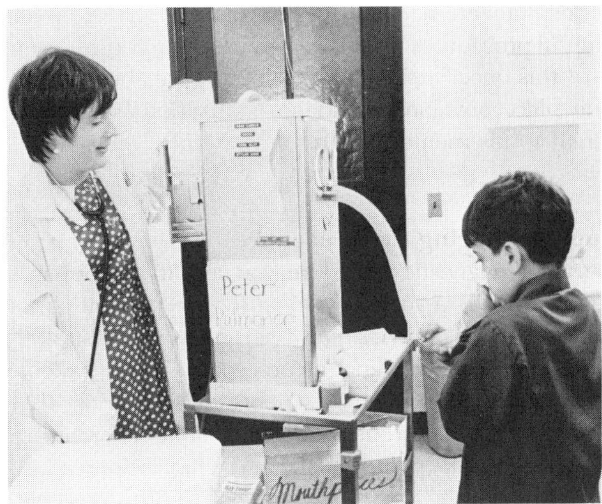

A

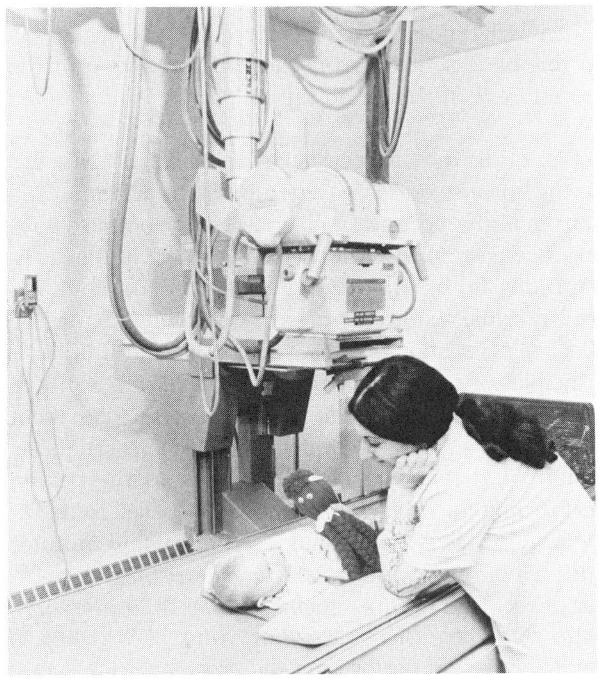

B

FIGURE 20-1. A. All patients need a clear explanation of diagnostic/laboratory procedures. Here a nurse explains to a child what the equipment he will see during a procedure will resemble. B. Any diagnostic/laboratory procedure can be a frightening experience. An infant is shown here with his "security object," an octopus, in the x-ray department.

as well as the patient. A patient cannot relax if his wife is still anxious because she still does not understand what is going to happen.

PREPARATION FOR THE STUDY

Familiarize yourself with the preparation measures for each study. Be certain that patients and support people have a good explanation of the purpose of preparation for the study. Owing to anxiety, people need reminders of things they must do or not do for study preparation. Remove the water pitcher from their room, post an NPO (nothing by mouth) sign on the door and by their bed or a SAVE URINE sign on the bathroom door or whatever else is necessary to ensure compliance with preparation measures. These methods are helpful in reminding people under stress what they would be able to remember without difficulty if stress of the procedure were not intervening (see QRSs 20-1 and 20-2).

☐ QUICK REFERENCE STOP 20-1: NUTRITION

1. Persons having diagnostic studies are often NPO (nothing by mouth) the morning of the procedure. Be certain that the person, if adult, understands this. A helpful measure for a preschool child is to make a sign, "Please don't feed me," and attach it to his front and back.
2. On days that people have been NPO for a study, stress that they try to eat well following the study. Adequate fluid intake for the day is necessary to prevent dehydration.
3. It is possible for patients who have one NPO diagnostic study done each day to become dehydrated. Ask if a rest day isn't necessary to ensure a good food intake.

☐ QUICK REFERENCE STOP 20-2: PHARMACOLOGY

Always be aware of what medications that people going for diagnostic or laboratory tests are receiving. People going for an intravenous pylogram (IVP, kidney x-ray) are kept NPO the morning of the x-ray so there is no mass of food in the stomach or upper intestine obscuring good visualization of the kidneys. A person taking cardiac medication such as digoxin or a person with arthritis who takes aspirin (not enteric coated) probably could take these on the morning of the x-ray without interfering with the study. If it is important not to hold medications this way, ask the diagnostic department or the person's physician for exceptions to rules of this kind.

Before blood drawing, always be aware whether a person is on a medication such as dicumarol to prolong blood clotting. A patient on such a medication needs the blood drawing site compressed firmly following blood drawing to halt bleeding.

Accompanying Patient for Study

When people are admitted to a hospital, one of their biggest fears is to arrive at the patient unit. After they have become comfortable with the health care personnel on the unit, one of their biggest fears is having to *leave* the unit. Thus, although it is not always practical, the average patient appreciates having someone accompany him to a department for a diagnostic study.

Some patients *require* accompaniment for their well-being: patients who are short of breath and need oxygen or other special equipment, who have intravenous fluid infusing that needs monitoring, or who have mental or sensory impairment that would make it difficult to relate to personnel who do not know them well. Children under 12 years of age are never left alone in a strange department because this is too frightening and traumatic for them. Parents should always be allowed to accompany young children to other departments; they are the child's best support people in strange surroundings.

Before leaving the patient unit, check that the person's ID band is securely in place and readily visible despite bandages or restraints. There may be a considerable wait in another department. Ask if the person would like some activity to occupy him, such as reading material or a game. Children should be allowed to take their favorite toy (a security object of unparalleled importance). (See Fig. 20-1B.)

Hallways may be cool. Ask if the person would like a shawl or sweater. Provide adequate blankets for infants and young children. Always provide adequate covering for modesty. Provide restraints as necessary for safeguarding patients in wheelchairs or on stretchers. The use of restraints for this purpose is discussed in Chap. 27.

Before leaving the unit have the patient void for comfort (unless this would interfere with the study). Check proper functioning of intravenous lines and patency of drainage tubes. Check if there is a medication or some other procedure that should be given before leaving the unit for another department in case it will be a long time before the person returns.

Assembling Equipment

If a diagnostic study is going to be done at a patient's bedside or in the unit treatment room, you need to organize the equipment. Most health care agencies use prepackaged sterile disposable equipment so little assembling of equipment is required other than locating or requisitioning the right equipment tray for the procedure. If a procedure will be done in another department, that department will, with few exceptions, furnish the necessary equipment.

Commercially packaged trays of equipment vary from brand to brand. You need to read the instructions and contents of packages before the procedure to be certain that they do contain all the supplies you need. Check whether items such as sterile gloves or antiseptic solutions need to be added.

No painful procedures are done at the bedside with children under 12 years of age. This is done to keep their bedside a safe place for them and to reduce the trauma of hospitalization to one of endurance. Do not set up for painful procedures for this age group at the bedside even "just this once." After "just this once," the child has no safe place any longer and hospitalization becomes a threat to his mental health.

Support During the Procedure

During a diagnostic procedure, you need to function in a trifold role: as a support person for the patient; as an observer of the patient's reactions; and as an assistant to whomever is performing the procedure. To the patient, the support role is the most important. Remember that most people are nervous about diagnostic studies; all are fearful about the pain involved and what the procedure will demonstrate about their state of health. As a rule, the person performing the procedure will inform the patient what step she will be doing next and what the patient will experience as she proceeds. If she neglects to do this because she is concentrating on a step of the procedure, you should do this as part of your support role.

Do not distract with casual conversation. A patient's having to answer casual questions is more annoying than it is therapeutic (and unnecessary because your presence is supportive in itself). Such activities as concentrating on breathing (take a deep breath now and hold it while the needle goes in) or counting may be effective distractions against pain in that they fulfill the principles of gating for pain relief (see Chap. 30).

In your second role, you need to observe the patient carefully for signs of discomfort such as increased pulse, pallor, or dizziness and report these to the person performing the procedure. You may be asked to maintain a flowsheet of vital sign levels every few minutes during a particularly stressful procedure or to remember or record a number such as spinal fluid pressure.

In your third role as assistant, you will be asked to hand the person performing the procedure any necessary equipment not contained in the prepared tray. Be aware what is sterile and what is not so that you do not accidentally contaminate a tray of equipment. When assisting with a procedure being performed on a child, you may also need to restrain a body part. Do this in a positive manner (let me help you hold your arm still) to preserve self-esteem. Techniques of restraints are discussed in Chap. 27.

Most people want to know the results of procedures immediately. In many instances, the results of one study are not enough to pinpoint the exact cause of illness and hence its treatment so the physician may be reluctant to comment on results until all procedures are completed. If he is very anxious about results, let the physician know. Perhaps with a high level of anxiety, the physician will choose to offer midway information.

Do not interpret results of procedures prematurely. Diagnostic results are meaningful only in the context of *all* results.

POST-STUDY PROCEDURES

Following some diagnostic procedures, the person needs vital signs determined frequently to assess for bleeding, might require bed rest for a period of time, needs to drink additional fluid or restrain from drinking, and so forth. The physician often does not order these post-procedure measures. She assumes when she writes "lumbar puncture," for example, that you will not only prepare the person for this, stay with him, and offer support during the procedure, but that you will also keep him in bed for at least an hour afterward and encourage him to drink fluids. If a specimen of tissue was taken during the procedure (biopsy), she will assume that you know an open lesion could lead to bleeding and will frequently assess vital signs. If venipuncture was involved, putting pressure on the site to prevent hematoma formation is understood. If any manipulation involving the airway was involved, common sense should tell you that respirations should be appraised carefully following the procedure. Not appreciating that post-procedure precautions are necessary can turn a simple diagnostic procedure into a complicated hospitalization. Ask, What body part or system was involved in the procedure? What measures should I take to maintain the well-being of that body system or part following this procedure?

Evaluation of Patient

Diagnostic studies are not therapy; they are aids to establishing what pathology is present or documenting the effectiveness of therapy. Therefore, a person cannot expect to feel any improvement in his symptoms, and he may gain additional symptoms related to the procedure, such as a headache or stiffness in some body part. Documenting the patient's response to the procedure is important in determining his overall physical response to intrusive procedures and may help determine the course of therapy and nursing care (a patient who was so anxious over an x-ray that he hyperventilated and became faint will need better than average preparation if a need for surgery is determined). Report post-procedure symptoms immediately so if a complication of the procedure is occurring, therapy to counteract it can be begun promptly (see QRS 20-3).

After-care of Equipment

Disposable equipment should be disposed of immediately following a procedure because body fluids in syringes or on drapes grow bacteria rapidly. Other equipment needs to be rinsed of blood or body fluids and placed in the proper place for sterilization or re-use.

If specimens were taken during the procedure, these need to be labeled accurately and routed to the appropriate department for analysis before any equipment is disposed of. This prevents a specimen being accidentally thrown away, causing repetition of the entire procedure. If the procedure was done at the bedside, check if clean bed linen is necessary. Remove all equipment from the room. Restock supplies as necessary. Make a habit of always leaving a treatment room cleared and ready for the next person. This will assure you that your patient unit is always ready for emergency care.

> **☐ QUICK REFERENCE STOP 20-3: SAFETY**
>
> 1. Evaluate patients carefully before the procedure to determine how much restraint will be necessary. When helping to restrain a child during a procedure use a positive, not a punishing manner.
> 2. When transporting patients to other departments provide adequate restraints for wheelchairs or stretchers.
> 3. Be careful when disposing of equipment trays that contain needles that you do not prick yourself or dispose of a needle so carelessly that a cleaning person could be pricked by it. If you do accidentally prick your finger, allow it to bleed for a minute, then wash the site well with soap and water. Depending on the patient's condition, you may need an injection of tetanus immune globulin.
> 4. Do not leave supplies in a patient's room following a procedure. Some items used, such as the antiseptic for skin preparation, are poisons and could be accidentally swallowed.

Responsibility for Specimens

If a specimen was obtained from a procedure, you must be certain that it is handled correctly and forwarded to the correct department for analysis. Specimens should be transported to the correct department as soon as possible; this keeps specimens from drying out and distorting the analysis.

Specimens must be correctly labeled and accompanied by the correct requisition. Without this information, the specimen cannot be properly processed and the procedure may have to be repeated.

Charting

Although the diagnostic procedure was actually performed by someone else, you need to record the name of the procedure, by whom it was performed, the time, the type of specimens removed and where they were sent, and the patient's response to the procedure in your nursing notes. You may need to mention special considerations in the patient's care plan—such as the fact that although he did not appear nervous, he admitted to being more scared than ever before in his life; thus, other nurses will know his facial expression masks a lot and they will not assume he needs less reassurance than he actually does.

AGE SPAN CONCEPTS AND DIAGNOSTIC-LABORATORY MEASURES

The Infant. The number of tests done on infants are kept to a minimum to reduce the number and extent of painful or uncomfortable procedures so the infant can develop a sense of trust. Parents should be allowed to accompany their child to hospital departments to offer support. Never ask parents to restrain or in any other way to help with procedures that cause pain. Their role should be supportive only.

Infants need to be picked up and comforted following procedures as a basic part of the procedure. Be aware that blood drawing (which can deplete blood stores) and x-rays (which are possibly harmful to bone marrow) should both be kept to a minimum in infants. You may need to help parents understand why these procedures are kept to a minimum or they may feel that their infant's care is being compromised.

The Toddler and Preschooler. Toddlers and preschoolers resist diagnostic-laboratory testing since such testing generally involves some degree of discomfort or pain. Children this age need short explanations of what to expect from procedures. Such explanations should be given close to the time of the procedure so that little time is spent worrying over it.

The Schoolager and Adolescent. Schoolage children are interested in the theory and reason for procedures; they can be convinced to cooperate for a procedure by being promised a look at their x-ray or laboratory report afterward. Be careful when promising children that they can see these results that this is really possible. Otherwise, you will have difficulty obtaining any further cooperation from them. Adolescents may project an air of maturity or sophistication beyond their years in order to remain in control of themselves in the light of frightening procedures. Do not be misled into thinking a child this age would not appreciate an explanation or does not need reassurance during a procedure.

The Adult. Many adults reach middle age without ever having had a severe illness or any diagnostic procedure other than blood drawing. Although they are older than the young adult in the waiting room or bed beside them, they are no more experienced in illness and no more used to terms such as *NPO.* Assess each person individually to find his level of understanding.

The Older Adult. Older adults may have difficulty lying on hard x-ray tables. Blood drawing may be very painful for them due to sclerotic veins. Diagnostic procedures may be exhausting for the older adult and rest days may need to be incorporated into his schedule.

BLOOD-DRAWING PROCEDURES

Analysis of arterial, venous, or capillary blood yields a great deal of information about both health and illness. Thus, almost all people on a hospital admission and many ambulatory patients will have blood drawn. People are anxious about blood drawing because it stings (do not lie—it always hurts to some extent as the needle is inserted) and because many people are a little worried that they need the blood being removed (how can they return to health if you take away a vital substance of health?). They can be reassured that the sting of the needle is temporary and only at the insertion and that the amount of blood taken (1—10 ml) is minute compared with the amount in the body (1,000 ml in a newborn; 7,000 ml in an adult). Low-birth-weight infants (because their entire circulatory system is so small) and patients with severe anemia (because certain blood components are so scarce) will have blood removed only after careful consideration of the need for its removal and may have it replaced immediately by transfusion to maintain a functioning blood level.

Blood may be drawn for analysis from a vein (venipuncture), an artery (arteriopuncture), or capillary (by a finger or heel prick). In establishing a blood clotting time, the earlobe may be pricked and used.

Most blood samples drawn are sent either to the hematology department, where the function or structure of blood cells is analyzed, or the chemistry department, where the plasma or the chemical components of blood are analyzed.

Hematology Samples

A *complete blood count* (CBC) is a frequent laboratory test ordered on a hospital admission or ambulatory basis because it reveals important information about the body's ability to maintain functioning blood components. A complete blood count usually consists of a white blood cell count, white blood cell differential count, red blood cell count, hematocrit, hemoglobin, red blood cell indices, stained erythrocyte scan, and possibly a platelet count. Normal values for these tests are given in Appendix G.

White Blood Cell Count (WBC). White blood cells are important in the body's immunological system. An increased white blood cell count suggests that infection or trauma is present. A decreased count occurs with chemotherapy or with an infection so overwhelming that it prevents the bone marrow from producing new white blood cells.

Differential Count. A differential count breaks down the types and numbers of white blood cells present. Appendix G shows the different types of white blood cells, their action, and normal values. If many immature white blood cells are present, this is often referred to as a "shift to the left" on a laboratory report. It is evidence of rapid regeneration of neutrophils due to acute infection. It can also suggest leukemia, a malignancy in which white blood cells proliferate so rapidly that many remain in immature forms.

Red Blood Cell Studies. Red blood cells are produced in the bone marrow in response to erythopoetin, a kidney enzyme. The presence of red blood cells, therefore, reflects bone and kidney health. In their hemoglobin portion, red blood cells carry oxygen to body cells. Diseases interfering with oxygen transport are always potentially serious. To maintain wellness, a functioning supply of red blood cells must be present for oxygen transport. One test is a gross determination of the number of red blood cells present. *Hematocrit* determination is the concentration of red blood cells in reference to plasma volume. *Hemoglobin* is a specific measurement of the amount of hemoglobin present in red blood cells, reflecting the ability to carry oxygen. Red blood cell indices are ordered to assess the size and hemoglobin-carrying capacity of red blood cells. A stained slide is a method of directly examining red blood cells under a microscope. Iron-deficient anemia is the second most frequently seen nutritional problem in the U.S. (the first is obesity), so routine screening reveals many people to have this type of anemia or to have small (microcytic) red blood cells. Reticulocytes are immature red blood cells; their presence indicates that red blood cells are being produced at a rapid rate, a healthy assessment (see App. G).

Erythocyte Sedimentation Rate (ESR). The rate at which red blood cells settle out of unclotted blood on standing is increased if inflammation is present in the body (probably due to an increase in plasma protein, which causes red cell clumping). A test of ESR is ordered for people with suspected arthritis or joint pain or rheumatic diseases to evaluate the amount of inflammation present. It is ordered frequently since these are commonly occurring diseases.

Sickle Cell (Hemoglobin S). Hemoglobin S is a type of hemoglobin that, in the presence of certain drugs or low oxygen tension, cannot maintain its usual shape and becomes concave or sickled. The sickle cell cannot carry sufficient oxygen. Sickle cell anemia is an inherited disorder.

Caution: The screening test for this condition does not differentiate between the carrier state of hemoglobin S (a person who needs no therapy other than genetic counseling so that he knows he is a carrier) and the disease state (a person who has a potentially life-threatening illness and will need careful health care follow-up). Be careful that you understand the test and its implications before interpreting results.

Bleeding and Clotting Estimations. Many factors combine to initiate and maintain blood clotting (see App. G). Different tests are necessary to pinpoint the exact deficiency or difficulty with clotting.

Blood Chemistries. Analysis of blood for its chemical content also yields important information about the presence of disease and overall health. Appendix G shows the purpose and standard normal values for frequently requested analyses. Normal values vary depending on the test, the method of analysis used, and the patient's age. A patient's value must always be compared with a value accepted as normal. Because normal values are based on a fasting status, blood must be drawn for chemical analysis before a patient eats in the morning. Be certain that the patient understands that this means *all* food, not just breakfast, so he does not eat crackers or some other snack while he waits for a technician to take this blood. Some children must be watched carefully or, not understanding the importance of not eating, they will snack freely during this waiting time.

The tubes used for chemistry samples vary with the type of test being done. Some blood for chemical analysis must not be allowed to clot before it reaches the laboratory and must be placed in a collecting tube that contains a preservative; for other measures clotted blood is necessary. Every department provides lists of this information along with the amount of blood needed for a particular test. Consult these lists before drawing or helping to draw blood until you are familiar with each test.

Sites for Blood Drawing

The site at which blood is drawn depends on the type and amount of blood needed and the age and condition of the patient.

Venipuncture. In adults, venipuncture may be done at the antecubital space in the basilic, median cubital, or cephalic veins or from one of the veins on the back of the hand (dorsal metacarpal, basilic, or cephalic). Even in newborns, these same sites are available and easy for a skilled person to use. The location of these veins is shown in Fig. 20-2. In some instances, it is necessary to use larger veins in infants, such as the jugular or femoral vein. Techniques for restraining an infant for a femoral or jugular venipuncture are shown in Figs. 20-3 and 20-4.

Arteriopuncture. Arteries flow under veins and thus are difficult puncture sites. The radial artery inside the wrist, the brachial artery inside the elbow at the antecubital space, and the femoral artery are sites commonly chosen. The person doing the puncture will palpate the area for the pulse with two fingertips and then insert the needle at a straight 90-degree angle between the palpating fingers. Artery walls are thicker than vein walls so the thrust of the needle must be harder. You can tell that an artery rather than a vein has been entered if the blood return is brighter red and enters the syringe with greater force.

Capillary Punctures. Capillary blood may be used for hematocrit and blood glucose determinations. If blood

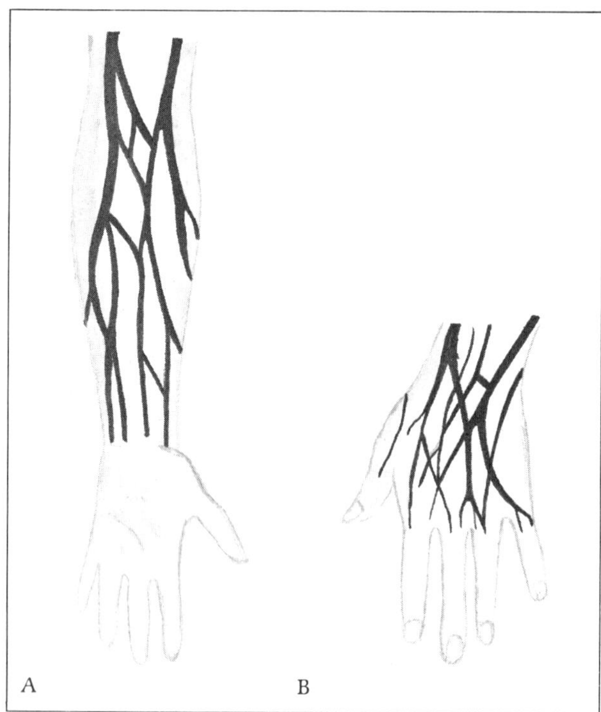

FIGURE 20-2. Common puncture sites. A. Basilic and cephalic veins of the forearm, and brachial vein in the anticubital space. B. Dorsal vein of the hand.

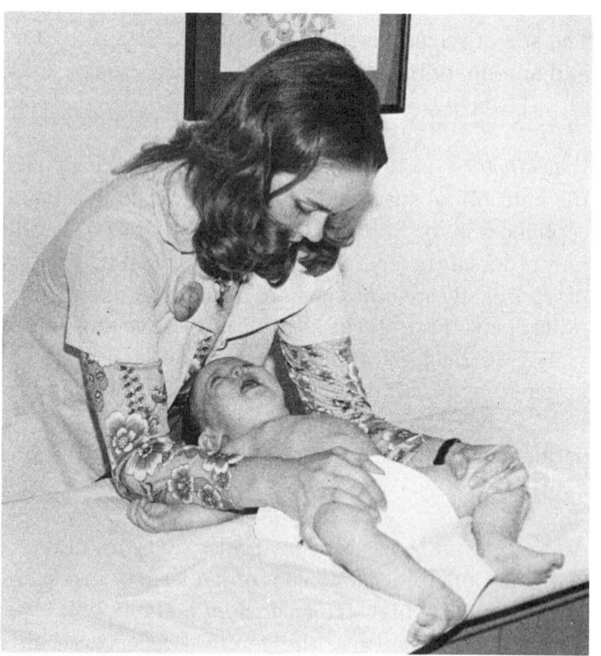

FIGURE 20-3. Restraining for a femoral venipuncture. Notice how the diaper is not removed to protect the puncture site from contamination with urine.

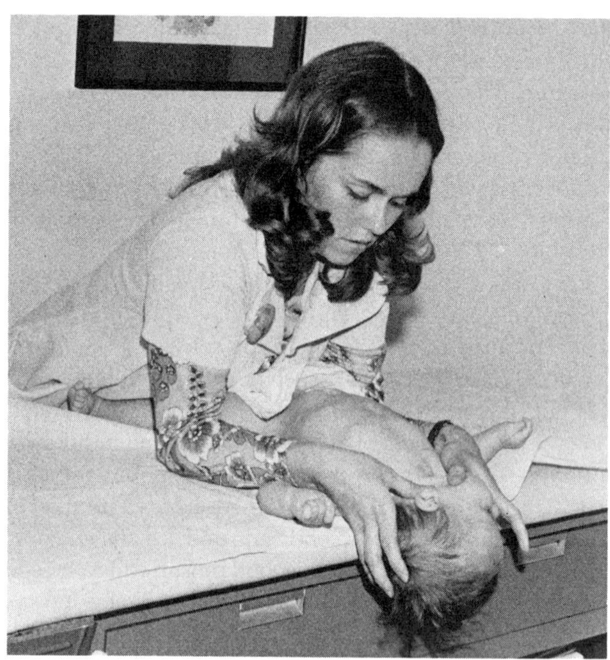

FIGURE 20-4. Restraining for a jugular venipuncture. Notice how the nurse's hand holds the infant's face yet does not cause airway obstruction.

glucose is being monitored in connection with insulin administration, capillary punctures may be done as often as every hour. A heel or finger site is used.

The sting of a blood lancet is just as painful as a needle being inserted for a venipuncture. Therefore, although capillary punctures look simple, they are stressful procedures. Try not to use the fingertips of a person's dominant hand because touching any surface afterward causes pain.

Assisting with Blood Drawing. In some health care settings, nurses draw blood for diagnostic tests; in others you assist a physician, lab technician, or venipuncture technician in blood drawing by explaining the procedure, assembling equipment, offering support, and giving after care to the patient, equipment, and specimens.

You may be asked to apply a tourniquet prior to blood drawing and remove it at the end of the procedure. Apply a tourniquet following the illustration in Fig. 20-5. It should fit snugly enough to cause vein distention distal to it, but not so tight it is uncomfortable. Placing a tourniquet in this way allows you to remove it with one hand. This is important if you are helping to restrain a body part or are holding blood tubes in your other hand.

When preparing people for venipuncture or arteriopuncture, be honest about the degree of pain—it stings at least momentarily.

Check the site afterward to be certain that all bleeding has stopped. Oozing from a venipuncture is rarely enough to cause an important blood loss but can cause an ecchymotic (black and blue) area to form in subcutaneous tissue, which then obstructs the site for future blood drawing for up to two weeks.

As a rule, arterial punctures are used only for blood gas analysis (the level of oxygen or carbon dioxide in the bloodstream). Reasons for blood gas analyses are discussed in Chap. 31. The syringe used to draw a blood gas must be glass and heparinized (draw up 0.5 ml of

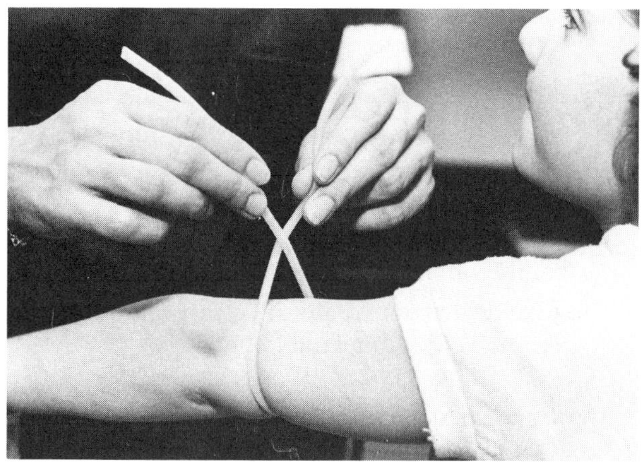

A

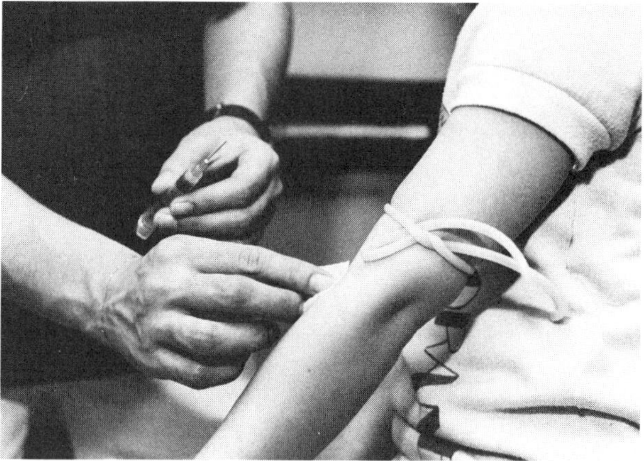

B

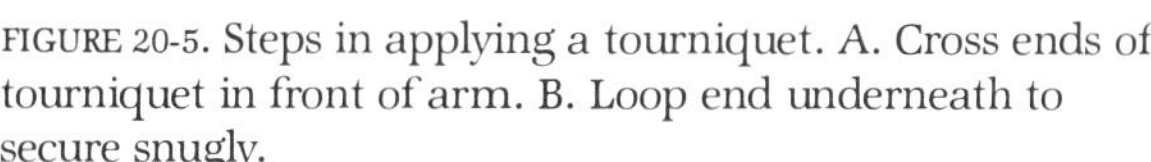

FIGURE 20-5. Steps in applying a tourniquet. A. Cross ends of tourniquet in front of arm. B. Loop end underneath to secure snugly.

heparin into the syringe; pull back the plunger and distribute it through the syringe; empty the syringe again except for the faint amount of heparin that clings to the syringe barrel by spurting the heparin out through the needle). Heparinizing will prevent the blood from clotting while being drawn. The blood syringe is capped and must be placed in ice to keep the gases from changing composition on the way to the laboratory. The specimen must be transported to the laboratory as quickly as possible for analysis.

Keep pressure on an arterial puncture site for 10 minutes following a puncture. The pressure in the arterial system is so great that oozing at the site can cause appreciable loss of blood unless it is compressed long enough following the procedure to effect hemostasis.

Apply a Bandaid snugly to a puncture site if necessary to halt bleeding. For children, Bandaids have value beyond their ability to halt bleeding or shield from infection. They are comforting and a special badge of courage. Apply them liberally.

Technique of Blood Drawing

Until recently blood drawing was a procedure done only by physicians because it carries the possibly fatal risk of air being introduced into a vein or artery. Blood studies for diagnosis and evaluation of therapy have become so common, however, that blood drawing has become a nursing responsibility. Even if you do not actually draw a specimen, you will assist with the procedure frequently in both ambulatory and inpatient settings.

Before blood drawing, assess the point where blood will be drawn for skin lesions or erythema, red and tender areas that suggest infection. Do not penetrate such areas to reach veins; doing so might push microorganisms from the surface lesion into the bloodstream, causing blood infection (septicemia). You cannot penetrate scar tissue or locate veins under hematomas or ecchymotic areas from previous attempts. Determine whether the person is on any medication such as heparin or dicumarol that interferes with blood clotting. If so, more careful compression will be needed to stop blood flow.

Veins become more prominent in a person's hand or arm after a tourniquet is applied and if the person clenches his fist. Be certain the extremity is positioned no higher than the person's heart so blood flow in the part is adequate. Capillary blood flows most freely if the body part is warm; holding a warm compress against a heel or finger for a minute helps greatly.

Assess whether you will need to help the person hold his arm still during the procedure. As a rule, help is needed with mentally confused adults and children under 10.

If a person is having a number of blood tests, you may need as many as six or seven tubes of blood to send to different health care laboratories. This blood can be obtained by only one puncture or one moment of pain for the patient. Do not frighten people unnecessarily by the number of blood drawing tubes or syringes you bring to the bedside.

Blood is drawn with a fairly large needle because blood is viscid and does not move freely through a smaller needle. For adults this is generally a No. 19 or 21 needle; for children and infants a No. 22 or 23. For multiple specimens, the syringe attached to the needle can be unscrewed after filling, a second syringe reattached to the needle hub, and additional blood withdrawn. Blood is then squirted from the syringes into test tubes for the laboratory.

A vacucontainer set may be used. Instead of a regular plunger, such a syringe has a vacuum-filled test tube that slips up next to the needle hub and is punctured by the double-pointed needle. To obtain additional specimens, the test tube barrel is replaced by another test tube.

Techniques for venipuncture and capillary prick are given in Procedures 20-1 and 20-2.

PROCEDURE 20-1
Technique for Venipuncture

Purpose: To remove a sample of blood for analysis from the venous circulation by sterile needle aspiration.

Plan	*Principle*
1. Wash your hands; identify patient; explain procedure to patient.	1. Prevent spread of microorganisms from you to patient. Promote patient safety and well being.
2. Assess patient status.	2. To plan degree of restraint necessary and correct site of venipuncture.
3. Analyze appropriateness of plan, adjust plan to individual patient needs.	3. Nursing care is always individualized based on professional judgment of patient need.
4. Implement care by assembling equipment: alcohol swab, tourniquet, needle (no. 19 or 21); syringe (size determined by amount of blood needed), dry compress or cotton ball, Band-Aid; collecting blood tubes.	4. Conserve energy by organization and preparation.
5. Locate best puncture site (back of hand, anticuboidal space) by observation and palpation. Choose as distal a site as possible to preserve remainder of vein. Place extremity in dependent position.	5. Do not use a site if there are scar lesions present or if you find sclerosis (hardening of vein) proximal to site.
6. Apply tourniquet (Fig. 20-5) so it can be removed with one hand following procedure and it is proximal to venipuncture site. If adult, ask him to make fist. Tapping vein and stroking vein toward heart also help distention.	6. Pressure from the tourniquet will cause compression of venous circulation and distend veins distal to tourniquet. Tensing muscles aids in appearance of veins since it pumps blood into main veins.
7. Cleanse chosen site with an antiseptic using a circular motion. Place thumb distal to puncture site and pull skin taut over site.	7. Prevent introduction of microorganisms at time of puncture. Stabilize vein from rolling.
8. Insert needle, bevel side up, at 30-degree angle, about 1/2 inch distal to point needle will enter vein; decrease angle slightly and push into vein following course of vein. When blood appears in syringe, slowly and steadily aspirate desired amount.	8. See Fig. 1.
9. Remove tourniquet; place dry compress on needle tip; apply gentle pressure and withdraw needle, holding flat to skin surface.	9. To prevent bleeding or hematoma formation at the puncture site.

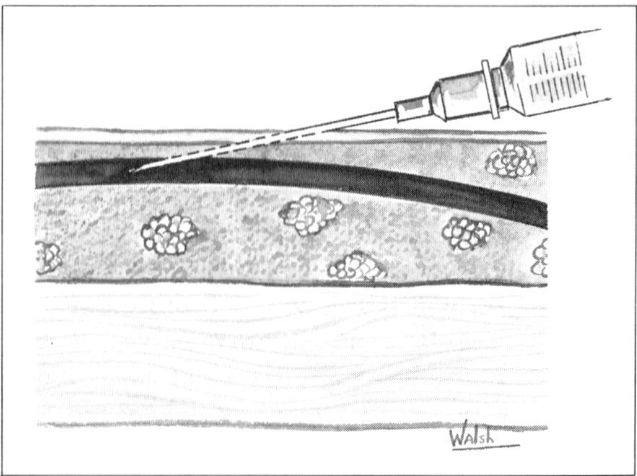

FIGURE 1. Venipuncture. The needle is inserted with the bevel side up.

10. Remove needle from syringe and place withdrawn specimen in suitable container, allowing blood to run gently down the side of the tube. Label appropriately and route to proper laboratory for analysis.

10. Squirting blood through needle or allowing it to fall from height may damage cells. If a preservative is present in tube, gently turn tube several times to mix; do not shake or cells can be ruptured.

11. Be certain that oozing is not present at puncture site. Apply Band-Aid snugly to maintain faint pressure.

12. Evaluate effectiveness, efficiency, cost, safety, and comfort of procedure; record procedure, where specimens were sent, and assessments.

12. Document nursing care and patient status.

13. Plan necessary health teaching, such as need for procedure.

13. Health teaching is an independent nursing action always included in care.

MODIFICATION FOR INFANT OR CHILD CARE

1. Children are extremely frightened by blood drawing. Explain that you are removing only a little and he has a lot left.
2. All young children need restraint for blood drawing as it is so frightening for them. Evaluate whether an older child will be able to hold still for procedure or not. If in doubt, ask for a restraint person to stand by.
3. Band-Aids have a therapeutic value beyond the ability to stop bleeding or shield against infection. Apply liberally.
4. Use therapeutic communication. Do not say "Don't cry, be a big boy." Instead, give the child something to do during puncture, "Say ouch; count to 10 and I'll be done." Praise afterward for good behavior. This is such a frightening procedure than any behavior short of screaming hysterically is good behavior.

MODIFICATION FOR THE OLDER AGE ADULT

Many older adults have sclerotic (hardening) changes in blood vessels that make them roll readily or difficult to pierce. Stabilize veins well before a puncture. Apply pressure for 2 to 3 minutes afterward to prevent oozing from puncture site and inability to use site again.

PROCEDURE 20-2
Technique for Capillary Puncture (Finger Prick or Heel Prick)

Purpose: To remove a sample of blood for analysis from the capillary circulation by sterile puncture.

Plan

1. Wash your hands; identify patient; explain procedure to patient. Pricking hurts as much as venipuncture; give fair warning.
2. Assess patient status.
3. Analyze appropriateness of plan; adjust plan to individual patient.
4. Implement care by assembling equipment: alcohol swab; lancet; collecting capillary blood tube; dry compress or cotton ball; Band-Aid.
5. Fingertips and heels must be warm so blood flows freely; holding the extremity in a basin of warm water or covering with a warm wet washcloth is an effective measure.

Principle

1. Prevent spread of microorganisms from you to patient. Promote safety and well-being.
2. Site must be warm and free of lesions.
3. Nursing care is always individualized based on professional judgment of patient need.
4. Conserve energy by organization and preparation.

6. Select puncture site: tip of finger (Fig. 1); right or left of median artery for heel (Fig. 2).

6. If patient right handed, use his left hand.

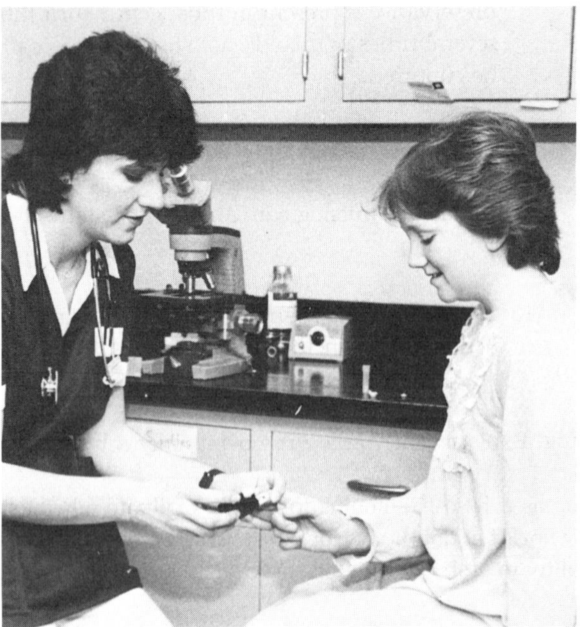

FIGURE 1. Blood analysis by finger prick. Remember that this procedure hurts as much as a venipuncture. Support is just as important.

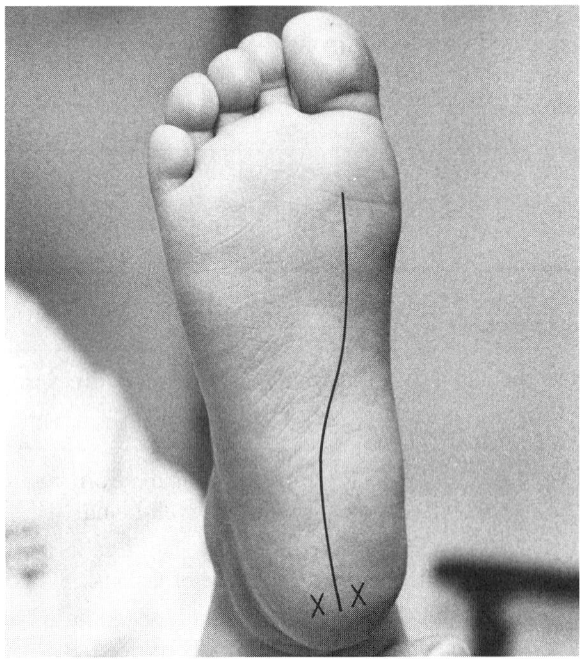

FIGURE 2. Site of capillary heel prick. The incision must be to the right or left of the median artery.

7. Swab site with alcohol; puncture with lancet; wipe away first drop of blood with dry cotton ball.

7. Wipe away first drop so alcohol does not contaminate specimen.

8. Hold heel or finger lower than proximal extremity; touch capillary tube to puncture site and tip to encourage flow. Do not squeeze tissue around site.

8. Capillary action will quickly fill the tube; squeezing causes tissue injury and contaminates specimen.

9. After filling required number of blood tubes, apply dry compress to site to halt bleeding; apply Band-Aid.	9. If tube contains preservative, rotate to mix with blood. Do not shake to injure cells.
10. Label specimen appropriately and route to proper laboratory for analysis.	10. Ensure continuity of care.
11. Evaluate effectiveness, efficiency, cost, safety, and comfort aspects of procedure; record procedure and assessment.	11. Document nursing care and patient status.
12. Plan necessary health teaching such as need for procedure.	12. Health teaching is an independent nursing action always included in care.

MODIFICATIONS FOR INFANT OR CHILD CARE

1. Finger pricks are as painful as venipunctures. Caution child that procedure stings.
2. Allow child to choose which finger you should prick. This encourages active interest in care and independence.
3. With infants, choose heel as site. Do not use center of heel or you may puncture medial artery, obtaining arterial blood and excess blood loss since it is difficult to stop bleeding.

MODIFICATIONS FOR CARE OF OLDER AGE ADULT

Older adults have decreased blood flow in finger tips from arteriosclerosis. Venipuncture may be the only effective method of obtaining blood specimens in this age group.

STUDIES INVOLVING ELECTRICAL IMPULSES

In studies of the brain, heart, and muscle, the strength, tone, and velocity of the electrical impulses present may be evaluated. Most adults are familiar with a cardiogram for study of the heart; they know little about brain and muscle studies. Children need careful preparation for all these studies because they have been warned not to play with electric wires and worry about being burned or electrocuted. They can be reassured that the electricity passes from their body to the machine, not the other way; except for electromyograms, these studies are painless. They are summarized in Table 20-1.

Electrocardiogram

An electrocardiogram (ECG or EKG) is an analysis of the electrical conduction of the heart. It is often done routinely on all people over 40 before surgery. Electrodes (small disks) are attached to the chest and the lower and upper extremities by paste. The ECG machine is turned on and a strip of graph paper emerges from it with the electrical pattern of the heart printed on it (Fig. 20-6).

A heartbeat is initiated in the sinoatrial (SA) node of the right atrium. The charge spreads across both atria, causing them to contract. As the contraction reaches the lower right atrium, it initiates an impulse in the atrioventricular (AV) node and is transferred down into the ventricles by the bundle of His and Purkinje's fibers, causing both ventricles to contract.

When the heart is at rest, it is said to be polarized or charged. As the atria and ventricles contract, they lose their charge or polarization (become depolarized). In the interval between contractions, they become repolarized.

The time of contraction or relaxation can be measured from the length of each segment on the graph paper. The strength of contraction and the completeness of relaxation can be measured from the height of waves of spikes.

Figure 20-7 shows a normal electrographic pattern. The P wave reflects atrial contraction (atrial depolarization). This would be absent if atrial contraction did not occur or the stimulus for contraction arose at a different point than the SA node. The P—R interval (the space between the beginning of the P wave and R point) reflects the time required for a contraction to cross the atria and arrive at the AV node. The QRS interval reflects ventricle contraction (ventricle depolarization). This will be absent or abnormal if ventricle contraction is not adequate or absent. The T wave represents ventricle repolarization. This may be inverted on an electrocardiograph if the heart has suffered lack of oxygen. The S—T segment reflects the time between completion of depolarization and repolarization of the ventricles.

An ECG takes about 10 minutes. If the physician desires a continuous readout of heart activity, a cardiac monitor (which registers a continuous ECG on an oscilloscope screen) can be attached by leads to the patient.

A person must lie still during the procedure so that the leads do not loosen (they are attached only by paste) and so that heart activity does not become so strenuous that it is difficult to decipher a normal pattern. As stated, this is a painless procedure. Privacy is necessary because the person's chest must be exposed for lead placement.

TABLE 20-1. STUDIES INVOLVING ELECTRICAL IMPULSES

		Nursing Considerations		
Study	Purpose	Preprocedure	During Procedure	Postprocedure
Electrocardiogram (ECG, EKG) Setting: cardiology department; can be done by portable machine at bedside Time: 10 min Clean procedure	To evaluate the electrical impulses of the heart by leads (electrodes) attached to chest and extremities. May be read as a paper graph or a display on an oscilloscope.	Good explanation: stress painlessness; electricity flows from pt. to machine; no chance of shock.	Pt. needs to lie still; support as necessary.	Paste used to secure electrodes needs to be wiped away with Kleenex.
Electroencephalogram (EEG) Setting: neurology laboratory Time: 30 min—2 hr Clean procedure	To evaluate the electrical impulses of the brain by leads (electrodes) placed on the skull. Read as a paper graph.	Hair should be free of spray or oily substances so electrode contact will be good. Explain the electrical flow is from Pt. to machine; no danger of shock. Caution that room may be darkened. If agency attaches electrodes by needle, then will feel pin pricks as needles are attached. If sleep will be necessary, keep awake before procedure. Phenobarbital distorts EEG patterns. Question if it should be omitted prior to procedure.	Pt. needs to lie still; support as necessary. May be asked to hyperventilate or watch moving patterns.	Turn on to side; give no fluid until awake if sedative was given. Paste from electrodes will need to be washed away with shampoo. (Older brands of paste need acetone to remove.)
Electromyogram Setting: specialty laboratory Time: 2—3 hr Clean procedure	To evaluate the electrical potential of muscle by leads (electrodes) attached to the muscles to be studied. Read as a paper graph, on an oscilloscope, or phonetically on audio tape.	Good explanation; caution there is some pain from needle electrode insertion.	Pt. will need to relax or tense muscle during procedure.	Pt. may be tired following the procedure due to length.

Electroencephalogram

An electroencephalogram (EEG) records the electrical patterns of brain waves. In adults, an EEG may be made by inserting miniature needle electrodes attached to the recording machine into the scalp. If this technique is used, there will be momentary pain with each needle insertion. With children and many adults, however, the electrodes are attached with paste so the procedure is painless (Fig. 20-8).

Brain waves change on visual stimulation, so the person may be asked to view a moving pattern of jagged lines or swirls as part of the test. Another technique is to ask them to hyperventilate. In certain susceptible individuals, watching a pattern or hyperventilating causes a convulsion. Do not mention this to people during preparation; the fact that it occurs without the person's awareness that it might occur is diagnostic of certain seizure disorders. Mention it to parents if they will be accompanying a child to the department so they are not frightened if a seizure occurs. You can assure parents that personnel in the EEG department are prepared to care for convulsions. Because of the possibility that visual stimulation may cause a convulsion, do not accompany a person to the EEG department unless you are familiar with basic care during convulsions. This is summarized in QRS 20-4.

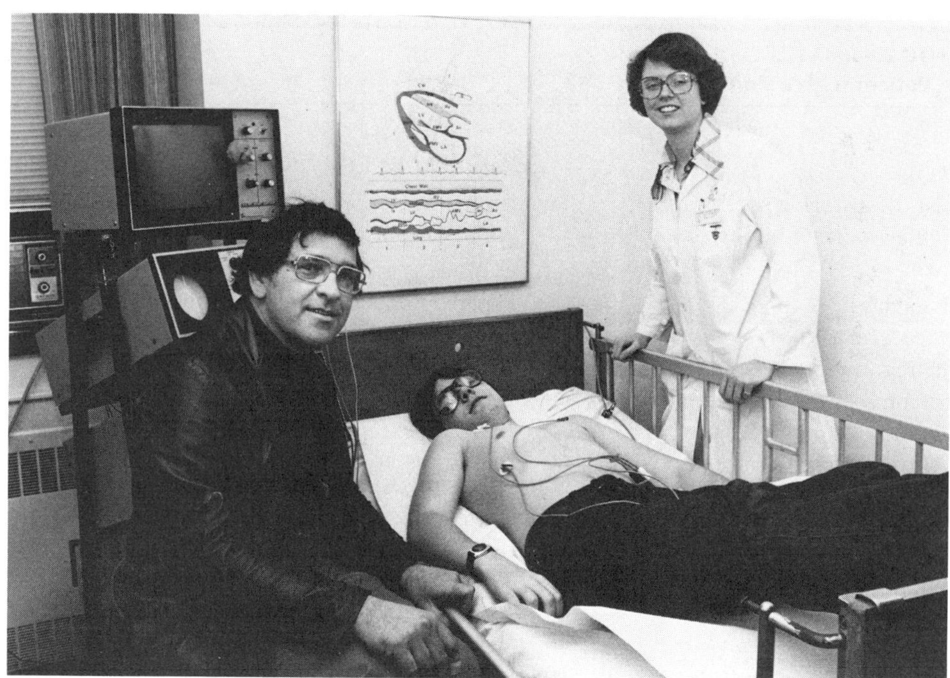

FIGURE 20-6. Recording an electrocardiogram (ECG). The leads are held to the chest by paste. Here an adolescent and his father watch a monitor printout of the son's heart action.

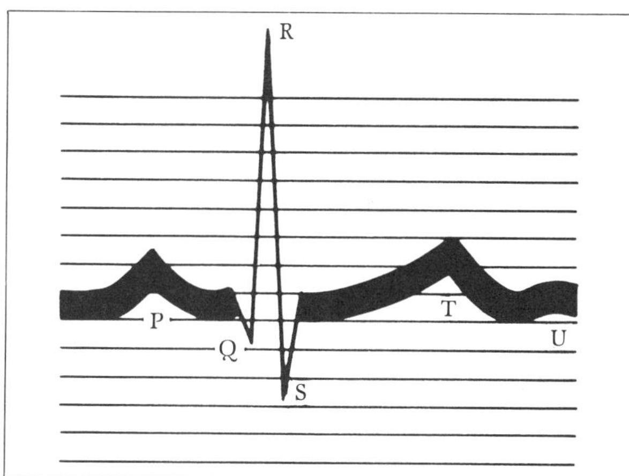

FIGURE 20-7. A normal electrocardiographic pattern.

For some EEG evaluations, a sleeping pattern of brain waves may be required. If so, the person should be urged to stay up late the evening before and awakened early in the morning of the study so he will feel sleepy and be able to sleep during the study. He must actually sleep, not just rest. A sedative to cause the person to sleep may be ordered; this should not be phenobarbital, since phenobarbital causes depressed brain waves and may interfere with the evaluation. If a sleeping pattern is desired, the test will be longer. Caution support people of this so they do not become alarmed by the length of time the study is taking.

Electromyogram

Electromyograms are studies of the electrical potential of muscle. Ordinarily, a muscle has little electrical activity when it is at rest; on contraction, it emits electrical charges that can be picked up on a phonogram as a popping sound or spikes on an oscilloscope screen or graph. To determine muscle activity, leads are inserted by small needles into the muscle (this may be momentarily painful). Muscles may be stimulated by a mild electrical current to contract during parts of the test (this may be mildly uncomfortable).

An electromyogram is often a long test (2—3 hours). Many hospitals do not have the equipment necessary for this procedure and a person must be transferred to another hospital. This increases the patient's fatigue and the length of the procedure because of transfer time.

RADIOGRAPH (X-RAY) STUDIES

X-ray studies direct short gamma waves toward body tissue in order to reveal the density of tissue. Soft tissue such as body organs or muscle do not x-ray well and appear as gray forms on x-ray film. Dense tissue such as bone shows as white space on the film. Empty space such as an empty bladder shows as a black space. As a rule, people need no preparation other than a good explanation of what to expect for a simple x-ray study.

To reveal better soft tissue on x-ray, radioopaque dye (appears as a contrast substance on x-ray) may be injected into the venous circulation and allowed to flow to the body organ to be studied (Fig. 20-9); for the gastrointestinal tract, radioopaque dye is swallowed or administered by enema. Radioopaque x-ray studies are generally time-consuming, since the dye must reach the organ. There is a minimum of pain from the dye injection. Sometimes a thin polyethylene tube is inserted at the injection site and threaded through the venous circulation to the body organ; dye is injected through this tube and arrives undiluted at the organ to be x-rayed.

☐ QUICK REFERENCE STOP 20-4: SAFETY
Nursing Measures for the Patient with a Convulsion

Type of Convulsion	*Description*	*Measure to Be Taken*
Petit mal	Often consists of a staring spell, rapid blinking of eyes, or twitching of an extremity.	Merely observe. Count seconds and include time in your description of the event.
Grand mal	Consists of 4 stages: **aura** warning that convulsion is about to occur (person sees flashing light or hears strange sound). **tonic phase** all muscles of the body contract; jaw closes; breathing temporarily halts. **clonic phase** all muscles of the body contract and relax in spasms; breathing may be difficult. **postictal phase** the person sleeps soundly and is difficult to rouse for about an hour.	Lie person on side to prevent him from aspiration of saliva. Move any object that might harm him (sharp edge of chair, etc.) out of way. Do not attempt to restrain except to keep on side. Restraining could result in muscle injury. An old suggestion for convulsions was to insert a padded tongue blade between the teeth to prevent the person from biting his tongue as jaw muscles contract. This is no longer recommended since the tongue blade may do more harm to oral structures than help. Observe carefully and document time and appearance of convulsion.

General considerations: Remain calm. Convulsions in themselves are not dangerous. They are symptoms of an underlying pathology, not a disease in themselves.

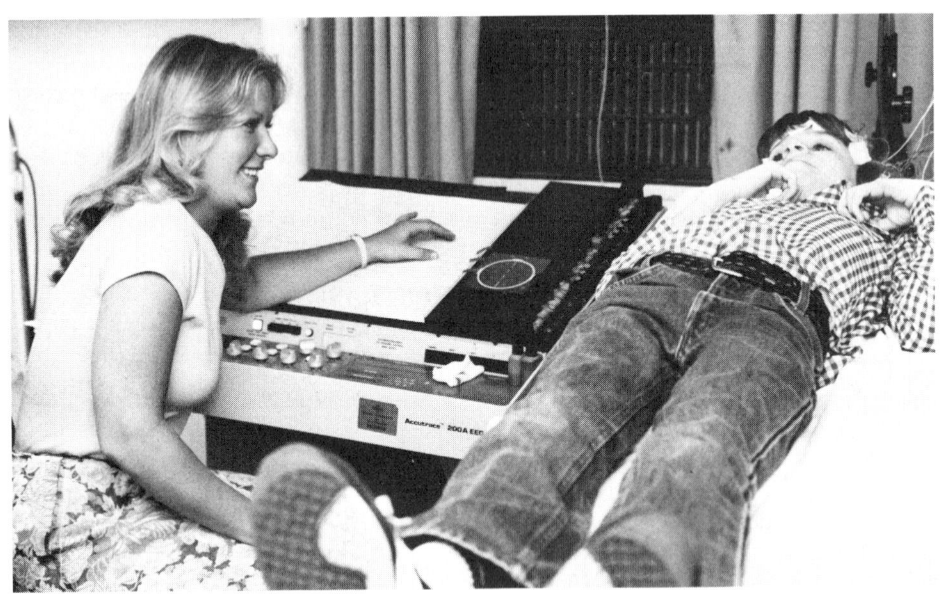

FIGURE 20-8. Recording an electroencephalogram (EEG).

At the time of the dye injection, the person may feel a hot flush, frightening if the person is not prepared for this. Some of these dyes are iodine based; determine whether a sensitivity to iodine exists before this type of study is done. Reactions in a person with iodine sensitivity are summarized in Table 20-2. Common radiographic studies using dye are summarized in Table 20-3.

People welcome having someone accompany them to the x-ray department, since it is often a large department filled with unfamiliar faces. *Do not stay with patients while they are being x-rayed.* In small amounts, x-rays are excellent diagnostic tools. In large amounts, x-rays may lead to infertility and may be associated with the development of blood cancer (leukemia). You cannot afford to stay with a patient even "just this once." You

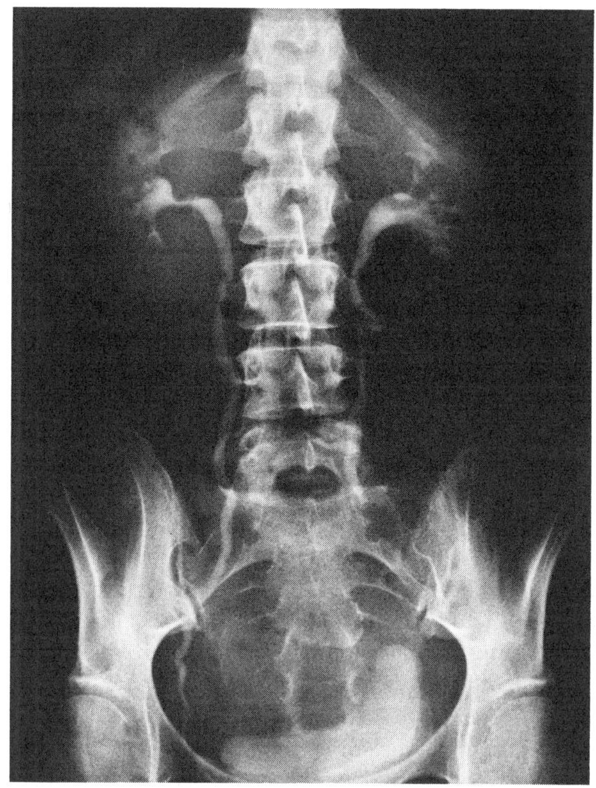

FIGURE 20-9. X-ray demonstration of the use of radioopaque dye to outline circulation in a body organ. Shown here is an intravenous pyelogram (IVP).

want to be a nurse for a long time. Over a long time, "just this once" will expose you to more radiation than is safely recommended. Occasionally a person needs to be restrained while on an x-ray table. Leave this restraint to personnel in the x-ray department or ask for a lead apron for protection.

URINE AND ASPIRATION STUDIES

Urine studies are invaluable diagnostic measures. Collection and analysis of urine are discussed in Chap. 33, as is aiding urinary elimination.

Aspiration procedures are always frightening to patients because they involve the use of needles and some pain. People need good preparation for them; they need a support person with them during the procedure; and they need time to verbalize their anxiety afterward (I am happy it is over; I hope I behaved all right). Because these procedures are so frightening, cooperating during them may be very difficult for the patient.

Aspiration needles are constructed with an inner core (a stylet) fitted into a hollow-bored needle for insertion.

TABLE 20-2. SYMPTOMS OF IODINE SENSITIVITY

Itching
Hives
Lowered blood pressure
Paleness
Wheezing
Unconsciousness

TABLE 20-3. RADIOGRAPHIC STUDIES INVOLVING DYES

		Nursing Considerations		
Study	Purpose	Preprocedure	During Procedure	Postprocedure
Angiocardiogram Setting: surgery or cardiology department Time: 1—2 hr Sterile procedure	To document blood flow through the heart by x-raying passage of radioopaque material through coronary arteries. Dye is injected into distal vein.	Pt. will be sedated to enable him to rest. Assess for iodine sensitivity (dye may have iodine base).	Pt. will need to lie still for extended time on examining table. Will feel a hot flush as dye is administered.	Vital signs are taken frequently. Assess insertion site for bleeding and circulation and edema in leg if inguinal vein was used.
Arteriogram Setting: surgery or x-ray department Time: 1—2 hr Sterile procedure	To document blood flow through arteries at points other than coronary arteries.	Assess for iodine sensitivity.	Same as above.	Same as above.
Arthrogram Setting: x-ray department Time: 1/2 hr Sterile procedure	To visualize synovial and functional status of bones and joints.	Assess for iodine sensitivity.	Joint is washed with antiseptic and local anesthetic is administered; a needle is passed into the joint and dye injected. Pt. will feel sting of local anesthetic; pressure from dye insertion.	Observe injection site for pain or tenderness (signs of infection). Pt. may feel grating sensation for a few days until any air introduced is absorbed. Ice pack may reduce swelling. An analgesic may reduce pain.

TABLE 20-3. (CONTINUED)

Study	Purpose	Nursing Considerations: Preprocedure	During Procedure	Postprocedure
Barium enema or upper GI series	To visualize on x-ray the outline of lower or upper GI tract to detect such abnormalities as tumor or obstruction.	A laxative and a clear liquid meal are given the evening before barium study. An enema is given prior to the procedure. NPO 6—8 hr before either study.	Pt. lies on x-ray table for barium enema; an enema tip is inserted rectally and barium allowed to flow by gravity while x-ray films are taken. For upper GI, pt. drinks liquid barium.	Encourage fluid and activity to aid against constipation. Note at 24 hr whether barium has been passed in stool. If not, may need to ask physician for laxative order or order for cleansing enema.

GI = gastrointestinal.

The stylet provides a sharp tip for easy penetration and strengthens the long thin aspiration needle. Before returning these needles for resterilization after the procedure, be certain you locate both parts of the needle or it will no longer be usable. Common aspiration studies are summarized in Table 20-4.

Lumbar Puncture

The most common aspiration study is a lumbar puncture (spinal tap). A sterile needle is inserted into the spinal canal at the third or fourth vertebral interspace to remove cerebral spinal fluid (CSF) for analysis. Cerebral spinal fluid is formed in the first and second ventricles of the brain, flows into the third ventricle, and then flows through a narrow channel (the aqueduct of Sylvius) into the fourth ventricle. From the fourth ventricle, CSF flows out into the collecting pool at the base of the brain (the cisterna magnum) and on into the subarachnoid space surrounding the brain and spinal cord. It is reabsorbed into the venous circulation by a network of capillaries in the arachnoid membrane.

The pressure of CSF changes if there is a block to fluid flow. If infection is present, the chemical composition of the fluid changes, and red blood cells and the infecting organism will be found.

People need good support for lumbar puncture. There are scare stories about people who had such a procedure done and never walked again because of nerve damage. The chance of this happening is extremely rare. As shown in Fig. 20-10, the spinal cord ends at the first or second lumbar vertebra. Lumbar punctures are made at the third or fourth interspace, which contains CSF but is free of the cord itself. Explain this to people as part of preparation and if necessary draw them a diagram. It is almost as if the spinal cord were designed with a place reserved for the removal of fluid.

Equipment necessary for a lumbar puncture is a spinal needle (2—5 in. long) with syringe, a syringe and needle (No. 25 short) for injection of local anesthesia, sterile compresses, gloves, antiseptic for skin preparation, local anesthesia (Xylocaine), at least three specimen tubes, and a rack or containers for specimens. If a CSF pressure reading will be taken, a manometer and stopcock will be necessary. In most health care facilities this equipment comes prepared as a set.

To separate the vertebrae as much as possible to allow access to the subarachnoid space, the person lies on his side on the examining table and curves his back forward. Infants need to be held in this position (Fig. 20-11A). Older children and even adults may need to be reminded to stay in this position; do this by resting your hands on the back of their necks and knees (Fig. 20-11B).

Figure 20-12 shows the physician preparing to do a lumbar puncture. First she will clean the person's back over the lumbar area with an antiseptic (this may feel cold), place a sterile drape around the area, and then ask you to help her draw the local anesthetic. (The local anesthetic bottle is not sterile, so she cannot touch it with her sterile gloves. Wipe off the top with an antiseptic, show her the label, and hold the bottle so she can inject the needle and syringe into the vial and withdraw anesthetic.) The physician will inject a small wheal of anesthetic into the skin overlying the lumbar vertebrae (this stings a little). Next she will position the long spinal needle through the anesthetized point into the spinal column (the patient will feel pressure).

The physician will know that the needle is in the subarachnoid space by the feeling as it enters the space and by clear fluid flowing from the needle end when she removes the inner stylet. If a fluid pressure is to be taken, the physician will attach the long thin manometer to the spinal needle and change the stopcock direction at the attachment point until fluid flows up into the manometer. She may ask you to read out the point at which the fluid level stops and to *remember* the number. She may ask if you will steady the top of the manometer if you have a free hand. Do not do this if you are restraining a child. Your role as a restrainer is important, and taking your hands away may allow the child to arch his back, a

TABLE 20-4. COMMON ASPIRATION STUDIES

		Nursing Considerations		
Study	Purpose	Preprocedure	During Procedure	Postprocedure
Lumbar puncture Setting: adults, bedside; child, treatment room Time: 1/2 hr Sterile procedure	To remove cerebral spinal fluid from the subarachnoid space for analysis and culture: to measure pressure of CSF.	Assess lumbar area for lesions.	Patient must lie on examining table with back curved. Local anesthetic will be used. Pressure will be felt from needle insertion.	Keep flat for 1—4 hr. Encourage fluid to replace CSF. Check site for leakage or inflammation.
Abdominal paracentesis Setting: adult, bedside; child, treatment room Time: 1/2 hr Sterile procedure	To remove fluid from peritoneal cavity for comfort and analysis and culture of fluid.	Patient must void to empty bladder. Weight is taken as baseline measurement.	Patient sits in semi-Fowler's position. Local anesthetic will be used. Pressure will be felt from needle insertion. Observe for shortness of breath, pallor, fainting, increased pulse. Pressure dressing is applied to site following.	Check dressing for fluid. Assess vital signs every 15 min for 1 hr. Weigh to determine fluid loss.
Thoracentesis Setting: adult, bedside; child, treatment room Time: 1/2—1 hr (depends on length of drainage) Sterile procedure	To remove fluid from the pleural cavity for comfort and analysis and culture of fluid.	Assemble negative pressure drainage bottles, Vaseline-coated compress in addition to procedure tray.	Patient sits upright supported by overbed table. Local anesthetic is used. Will feel pressure from needle. Observe for shortness of breath, pallor, fainting, increased pulse or respirations. Apply air-resistant pressure dressing following.	Observe for vital signs every 15 min for 1 hr. Assess that dressing is airtight.
Bone marrow Setting: adult, bedside; child, treatment room Time: 15 min—1/2hr Sterile procedure	To remove a sample of bone marrow for analysis. Sternum is used in adults; iliac crest in children.	Assess area for lesions.	Patient will lie supine for sternum puncture, prone for iliac puncture. Local anesthetic will be used. Pressure of needle will be felt. Possible pain on aspiration. Pressure dressing applied following.	Observe site for leakage or inflammation. Assess vital signs every hr for 4 hr.

CSF = cerebrospinal fluid.

dangerous move while the needle is in the subarachnoid space.

Cerebral spinal pressure rises if the person coughs or if the internal jugular vein is pressed. The physician may ask you to press on the external jugular vein (be careful to slide your hands under the sterile drape if it extends that far so as not to contaminate the sterile field). She may ask you to read out the increased pressure on the manometer and remember it.

Following the pressure reading, the physician will take samples of CSF for laboratory analysis. She may hand them to you as specimen 1, specimen 2, and so forth. Place them in containers or racks you have premarked. The order of specimens is important because the first sample cannot be sent for analysis of red blood cells (a few may have been introduced by contamination as the needle was inserted) or for culture (some bacteria from the skin may have accidentally been introduced with the needle). You must send the second or third samples for these analyses.

If medicine is to be given as part of the procedure, it is done through the needle at this point. After taking a closing pressure, the physician will withdraw the needle and apply manual pressure to the insertion site for a few

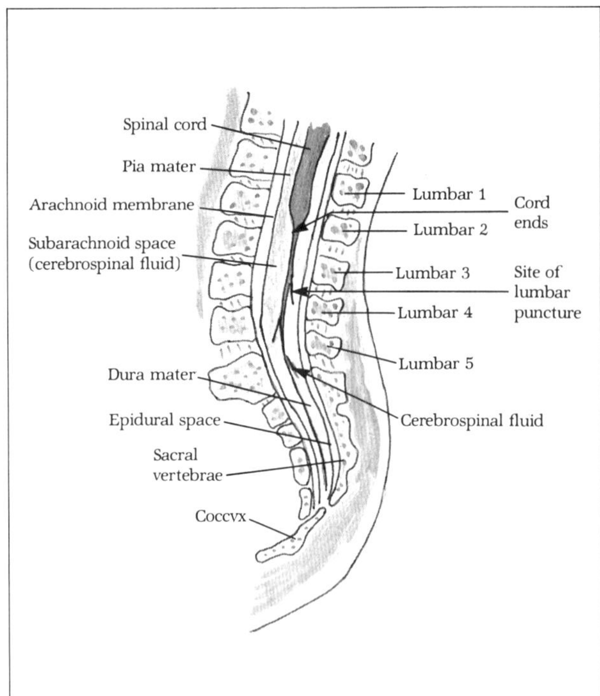

FIGURE 20-10. Anatomy of the spinal cord; notice that the cord ends at the second lumbar vertebra, above the 3—4 lumbar interspace.

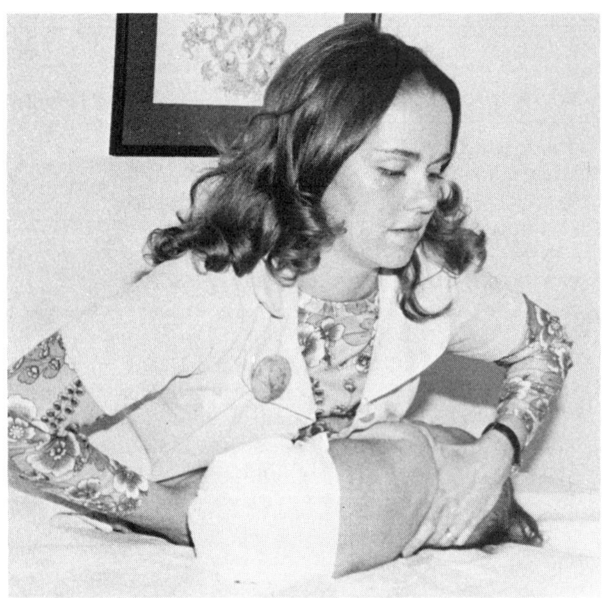

A

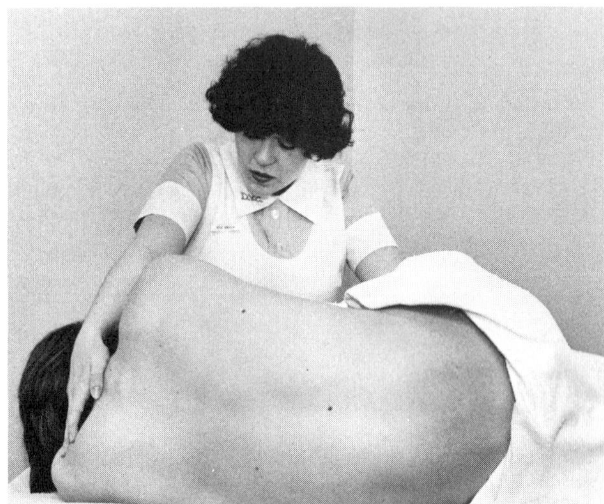

B

FIGURE 20-11. A. Restraining an infant for a lumbar puncture. Turn your head to the side to avoid breathing over the sterile field that will be set up at the puncture site. B. To restrain an adolescent or adult for a lumbar puncture, rest your hand on the back of the neck and knees.

minutes to discourage seepage of fluid. She will apply or ask you to apply a bandage tautly to the puncture site to ensure occlusion.

If any air was introduced at the time of the puncture or if meningeal tissue shifted due to the pressure changes, the person may develop a spinal headache, a severe, penetrating headache often accompanied by nausea and very incapacitating. To prevent this, the person must stay flat in bed for 4 to 8 hours (a flat pillow if one is necessary). Encourage fluid intake to replace CSF as quickly as possible.

In your nurse's notes, record the procedure, the person who performed it, the time, specimens taken and where they were sent, patient response, and post-procedure care given (flat in bed; amount of fluid taken). Normal findings in relation to CSF are shown in Appendix G.

Bone Marrow Aspiration

In bone marrow aspiration, a specimen of bone marrow is removed for analysis. Bone marrow produces blood components. Analysis of bone marrow gives important information concerning structure of blood cells.

In adults, the sternum is often used as a puncture site. In children this site does not contain much marrow. Also, the procedure is more frightening if done at this site. In children, therefore, the bone of the iliac crest is always used for bone marrow aspiration. The person lies on his back for a sternum puncture; prone for an iliac crest puncture.

The area over the bone chosen is washed with an antiseptic (this will feel cold). A sterile drape is placed around the site, and a small amount of local anesthetic is given (this will sting). The large-bored bone marrow needle and stylet is pressed into the bone (this pressure will be felt). The stylet is withdrawn, a syringe is attached to the needle, and bone marrow is aspirated (some persons report this as pain, others as an uncomfortable drawing feeling). Following the aspiration, place a bandage tightly over the aspiration point to keep further marrow from seeping out. Assess the site for the next 3 days for inflammation or tenderness that might suggest infection.

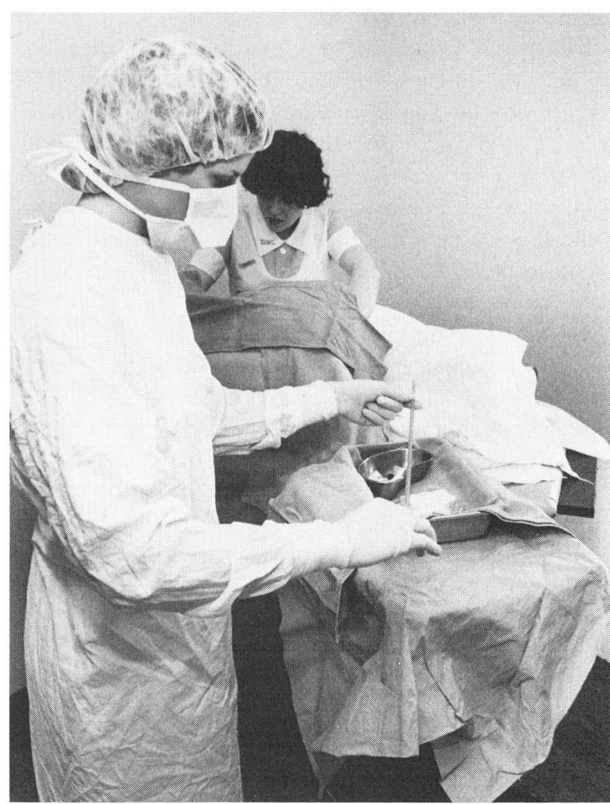

FIGURE 20-12. A lumbar puncture. Here the physician holds the manometer in her hands.

People need good support during bone marrow procedures, which are painful and frightening because of the strong pressure (they may worry their bone is breaking). The procedures are used to diagnose severe blood diseases so the person has reason to be worried about the results of the study as well as the study itself.

Thoracentesis

Thoracentesis is aspiration of fluid from the pleural cavity. Ordinarily, this space has only enough fluid present to lubricate effectively the pleural membranes. With certain disease conditions, fluid collects here; if allowed to collect in great amounts, it becomes a reservoir for infection and may impair lung function.

The procedure is obviously frightening. A person worries that the needle will be inserted not only into the pleural space but further into the lung, collapsing the lung and making breathing difficult. Assure the patient that he is in the hands of a skilled practitioner; offer good support during the procedure.

A person is placed in an upright position bending forward over a bedside table for this procedure (Fig. 20-13A). The area of the aspiration will be cleaned with antiseptic (this will feel cool), local anesthetic will be injected (this will sting), and the aspiration needle will be inserted (this will be felt as pressure). Tubing is attached to the needle, and fluid drained into a negative pressure collecting bottle.

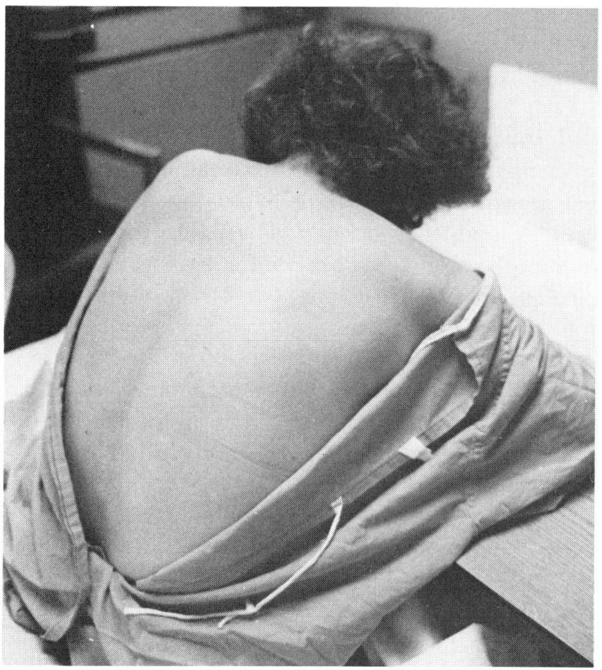

A

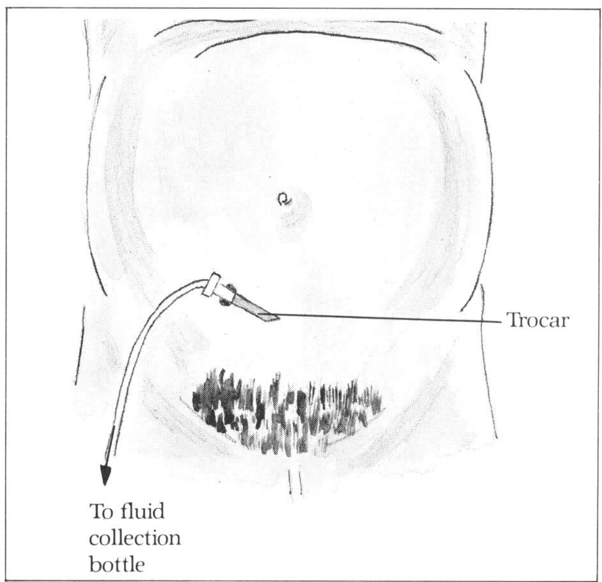

B

FIGURE 20-13. A. Position for a thoracentesis. B. Position for an abdominal paracentesis.

The air in the pleural cavity is at a negative pressure. If left to drain into an open container, instead of fluid draining out, air would flow in, collapsing the lung. The person needs careful observation during the procedure for pulse and respiration rate since removing fluid this way shifts the pressure on the heart and major arteries and varies blood flow.

Following the procedure, a dressing coated with Vaseline gauze is applied tightly to the puncture site. The Vaseline serves to occlude the opening and to prevent air from entering the puncture point, causing a lung to collapse (atelectasis). Vital signs need to be checked frequently (every 15 min for 1 hr or as ordered) to be certain that lung function remains adequate despite the change in chest pressure.

Abdominal Paracentesis

Ordinarily, the peritoneal cavity has no fluid other than that necessary for membrane lubrication. With certain diseases, fluid tends to accumulate in this space. It must be removed so that it does not serve as a reservoir of infection and so it does not obstruct intestinal or stomach function due to pressure.

The person must void before the procedure to reduce the size of the bladder so it is not in danger of being punctured by the aspiration needle insertion. The person is placed in a sitting position so gravity causes the fluid to pool in the lower abdomen for easiest removal (Fig. 20-13B).

The spot chosen for the puncture (a point about halfway between the symphysis pubis and umbilicus) is washed with an antiseptic solution (this will feel cool), a local anesthetic is injected (this will sting), and the aspiration needle will be inserted (this is felt as pressure). Abdominal paracentesis needles are large-bored and are often called *trocars*. Tubing is attached to the needle, and fluid is allowed to drain into an open collection bottle.

Observe the patient carefully during the procedure. The loss of fluid in the abdomen causes the diaphragm to descend and chest pressure to shift, changing blood flow in the heart and major arteries.

Following the procedure, a sterile dressing is applied snugly to the puncture site. Observe this for leakage of fluid afterward. Assess vital signs every 15 minutes for the first hour or as ordered to be certain that circulation remains adequate despite the shifting chest pressures.

ULTRASONIC STUDIES

Ultrasound is a noninvasive procedure that directs high-frequency sound waves toward the body and records the pattern projected as these waves are reflected from body tissue. Sound waves are reflected differently from tissues of different densities, making it possible to distinguish solid tissue such as bone from less dense tissue such as fluid. The pattern of reflection may be viewed on an oscilloscope screen or a photograph may be taken for a permanent record.

Ultrasound scanning does not have the danger of x-ray and thus has no association with infertility or leukemia. It requires no dye or needle injections. A transducer is held over the body part to be studied. In order to assure good contact, a paste is applied under the transducer (may feel cold). No fasting is required for the procedures. Because the procedures are brief, they require no patient sedation (Fig. 20-14). For pelvic studies, the patient may be asked to drink a large quantity of water and then not void so the bladder is distended and the fecal-filled bowel is pushed up out of the way.

Various body organs can be studied by this method, such as the heart, liver, bladder, lung, brain, thyroid, and spleen. The technique has wide use in obstetrics for diagnosis of pregnancy, assessing the health of the fetus during pregnancy, ruling out certain congenital anomalies, and predicting the maturity of the fetus (Fig. 20-15).

Ultrasound studies are done in a special department where the scanning equipment is located. The person must lie still during the scanning procedure (20—30 min). Because the ultrasound waves echo back, these procedures are often also called *echograms*.

FIGURE 20-14. Recording of an ultrasound scan.

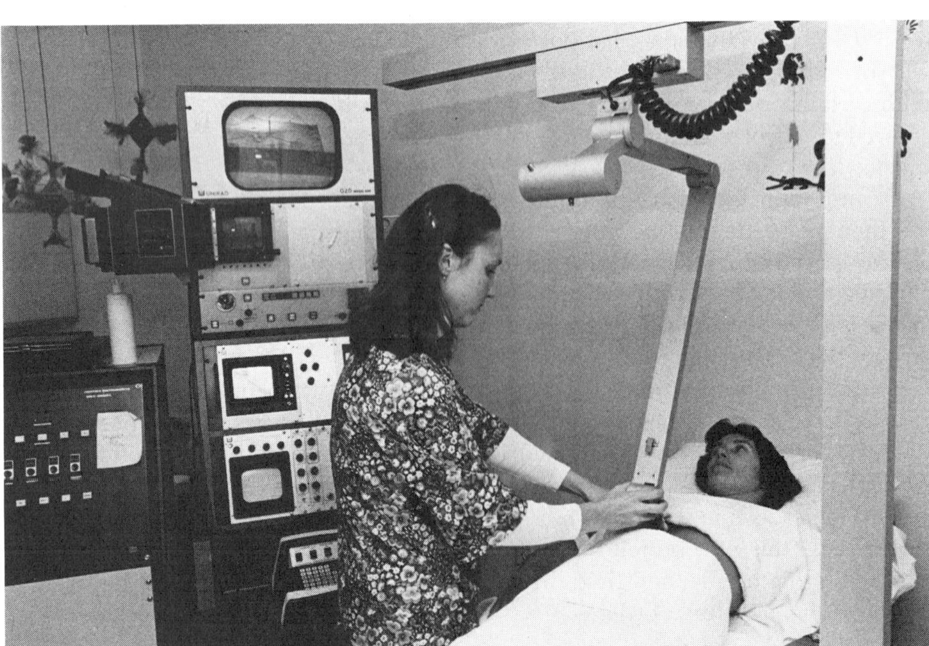

ENDOSCOPY STUDIES

In many instances, direct visualization of a body area offers the most specific information about the disease process present. As a group, these are called *endoscopic studies.* Their specific names refer to the body part examined (Table 20-5).

When first developed, endoscopes were straight metal, stiff instruments, which limited their use. Today, endoscopes are fibro-optic (a flexible, easily maneuvered bright-lighted tube), and thus examinations of this nature are both much more common and more comfortable than ever before.

The procedure is often frightening for a patient. He can easily understand an explanation of the procedure (the physician will extend his head and pass a tube down into his trachea for direct observation), but he is uncomfortable at the thought of someone doing that to him. You can assure a patient he will be in the hands of a skilled practitioner and offer good support during the procedure (Fig. 20-16). During most procedures, the

FIGURE 20-15. An ultrasonic photograph of a 39-week-old fetus in utero.

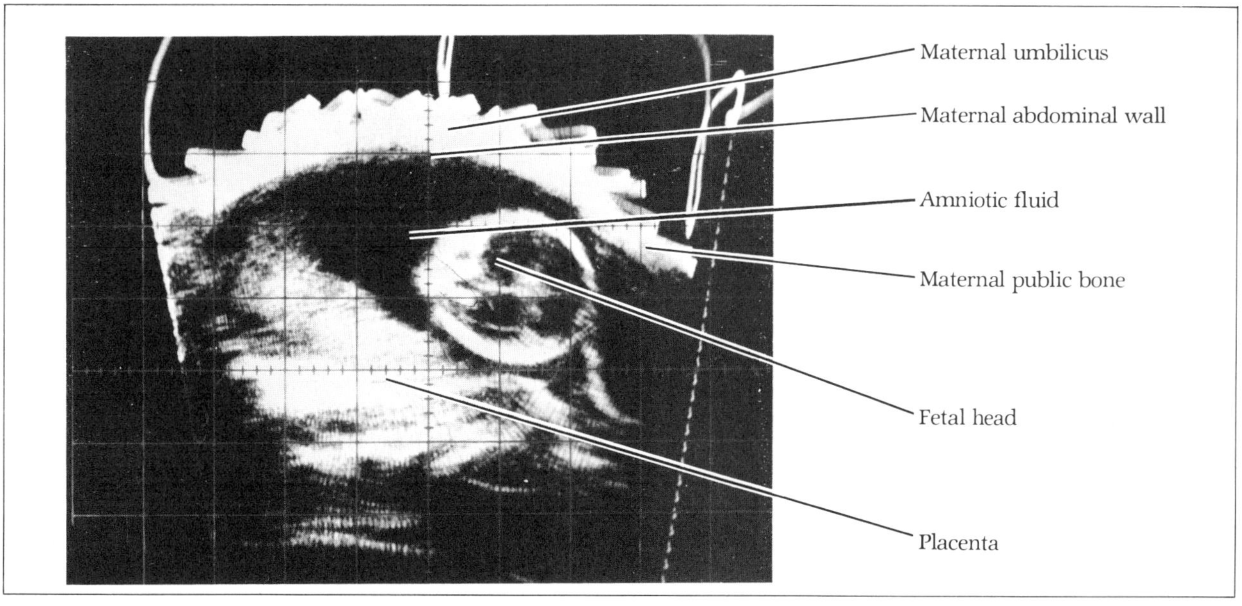

TABLE 20-5. STUDIES INVOLVING ENDOSCOPY OR INTUBATION

		Nursing Considerations		
Study	Purpose	Preprocedure	During Procedure	Postprocedure
Bronchoscopy Setting: surgery or emergency room Time: 1/2 hr Sterile procedure	To evaluate health of tracheobronchial tree by direct visualization; to remove a specimen for biopsy.	Provide good oral care; remove dentures. NPO 6—8 hr. Sedative to help patient lie still may be ordered. Atropine-like drug to dry secretions may be ordered.	Patient is asked to gargle anesthetic solution to anesthesize throat. Positioned on table with head hyperextended. Patient may feel short of breath as bronchoscope is passed. Oxygen by mask may be administered. If the bronchus is washed, saline is introduced into the tube; this feels strange but not uncomfortable; if biopsy is taken, there is a feeling of pressure as tissue is cut.	Observe for respiratory difficulty (edema may occur, closing airway). Take pulse and respirations every 15 min for 1 hr; then every hr for 4 hr. NPO 4 hr (until gag reflex returns). Test first with ice chips. An ice collar may reduce edema. An analgesic for throat irritation may be helpful.

TABLE 20-5. (CONTINUED)

		Nursing Considerations		
Study	Purpose	Preprocedure	During Procedure	Postprocedure
Colonoscopy: (proctoscopy) Setting: surgery or emergency room Time: 1/2 hr Clean procedure	To evaluate health of lower bowel by direct visualization; to remove specimen for biopsy. Proctoscopy involves only rectum and sigmoid colon.	Provide clear liquids day before procedure; laxative given evening before study. NPO 6—8 hr prior to procedure; cleansing enema given morning of study. A sedative may be ordered to relax patient. Have patient void (pressure of procedure might injure a full bladder).	Patient is placed in knee-chest position on table, rectum is digitally examined, then scope is inserted into colon. Patient experiences feeling of having to move bowels from pressure. Air may be introduced into scope to aid visualization. This causes some cramping. (Teach to take deep breaths to relieve.) There is no pain from bowel biopsy since cutting bowel does not hurt. Pressure may occur.	Check vital signs every 15 min for 1 hr, every hr for 4 hr to guard against GI bleeding or trauma. Check next 3 stools for blood.
Cystoscopy Setting: special laboratory or surgery Time: 1/2 hr Sterile procedure	To evaluate health of bladder and urethra by direct visualization; to remove specimen for biopsy; to insert ureteral catheters for further studies.	Assess for signs of urinary tract infection: burning, frequency, blood in urine for baseline data.	Pt. placed in lithotomy position on table; prepped with antiseptic solution; will experience slight pain as cystoscope is introduced into urethra. Placing ureteral catheters causes sharp colicky pain (teach to take deep breaths to relieve). If a biopsy is taken, this is felt as uncomfortable pressure.	Collect serial urines following the procedure until clear. Report bright red bleeding or inability to void by 8 hr. Assess for symptoms of burning, frequency, increased temperature, suprapubic pain (signs of urinary tract infection).
Esophagoscopy, gastroscopy, duodenoscopy Setting: special laboratory or surgery Time: 1/2 hr for gastroscopy; 1 hr for duodenoscopy Clean procedure	To evaluate health of GI tract by direct visualization; to remove biopsy or study digestive enzymes.	NPO 6—8 hr before procedure. A sedative may be ordered to help patient relax. Atropine-like drug may be ordered to dry secretions.	Patient gargles with anesthetic to anesthetize throat. Scope is passed through mouth to esophagus, stomach, or duodenum. If biopsy is taken, pressure will be felt (Fig.20-16).	Observe for respiratory rate as edema of throat may close airway. Delay fluid for 4 hr (until gag reflex is returned). An analgesic may be ordered for throat irritation. Ice chips may be soothing. Report vomiting; test any vomitus for occult blood.
Gastric analysis Setting: adult, bedside; child, treatment room Time: 15—20 min Clean procedure generally; sterile if culture is desired	To analyze gastric secretions for volume, acidity, and content.	NPO 6—8 hr; no anticholinergistic drugs for 12 hr (drugs reduce gastric secretions). No smoking for 1 hr prior (increases gastric secretions).	Nasogastric tube is passed through nose or mouth into stomach (an uncomfortable feeling) and gastric secretions are withdrawn.	Ice chips may soothe throat irritation.

GI = gastrointestinal.

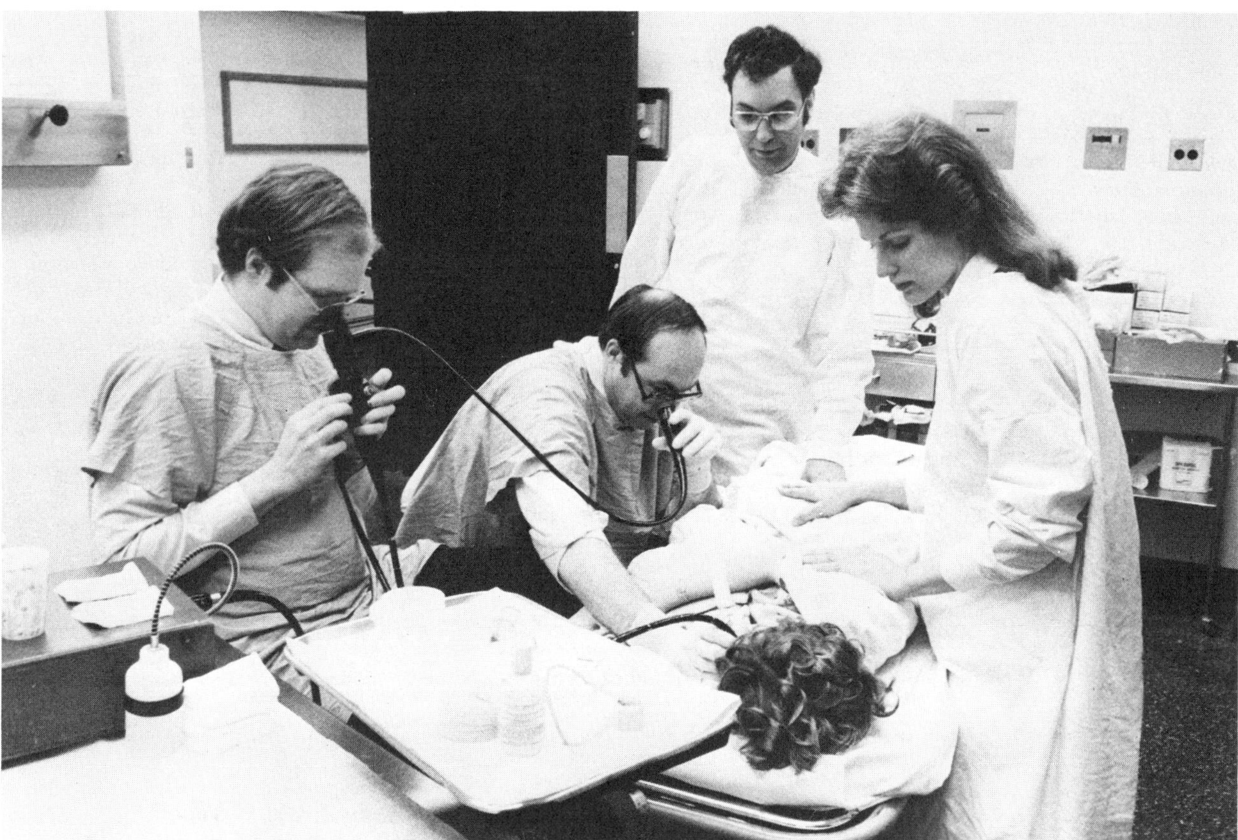

FIGURE 20-16. An endoscopic procedure. The nurse is usually the patient's primary support person during diagnostic procedures.

person lies supine on an examining table. For lower bowel examinations (colonoscopy or proctoscopy), the person is asked to assume a knee-chest position by means of a specially designed table. Observe patients carefully during this procedure to be sure that they do not grow dizzy or short of breath in this head-down position.

Following an endoscopy study, edema or swelling may occur from pressure of the scope. Aftercare consists of close observation to see that edema is not interfering with a vital function or causing discomfort.

NUCLEAR MEDICINE STUDIES

Radiopharmaceuticals are radioactive-combined substances that, when given orally or by injection, flow to designated body organs. The organ dictates the radiopharmaceutical used. When a scintillation machine (a form of Geiger counter) is passed over the organ where the radiopharmaceutical has collected, the pattern of the collected material will outline the organ; it will be produced as a photograph. The names of the studies refer to the body part to be examined, although in the case of gallium, the radioactive substance itself names the study (Table 20-6).

Radioactive-tagged pharmaceuticals pass uniformly through normal tissue; they collect in high concentrations in tissue that is growing more rapidly or abnormally (tumors). Tagged iodine (^{131}I) is frequently used in nuclear medicine studies because it is easy to join with radioactive material. Iodine will go immediately to the thyroid gland when injected intravenously, with the result that so much concentrated radioactivity could accumulate in one site that the thyroid gland could be destroyed. Therefore, especially with children, a blocking agent such as potassium perchlorate is sometimes given before the test. This prevents the radioactive substance from concentrating in the thyroid and protects the gland. Giving a blocking substance is usually your responsibility before the patient leaves the patient unit. *Always check whether or not a blocking agent is required before transporting a patient to the nuclear medicine department.*

People worry that they will be harmed by a radioactive substance. You can assure them that the dose of radiation in these studies is no greater than that employed for diagnostic x-ray so this is not a danger.

Pregnancy is a contraindication to these studies. A breast-feeding mother should discontinue breast-feeding for the time it takes for the substance to be

TABLE 20-6. NUCLEAR MEDICINE STUDIES

Study	Purpose	Nursing Considerations		
		Preprocedure	During Procedure	Postprocedure
Bone scan Setting: nuclear medicine laboratory Time: 30 min—1 hr Clean procedure	To document bone abnormalities such as tumor, infection, or trauma.	Contraindicated in pregnant patients due to radioactivity involved. Sedation may be ordered to ensure that pt. lies still for the procedure.	Radiopharmaceutical is injected into vein; scintillation camera is used to photograph bone after wait for material to reach bone in question.	Turn to side until wide awake; delay fluid until able to swallow well if sedative was given. Pregnant personnel should not care for patient for 48 hr.
Brain scan Setting: nuclear medicine laboratory Time: 30 min—1 hr Clean procedure	To evaluate presence of brain abnormalities such as tumor, abscess, or blood clot.	Same.	Same.	Same.
Gallium scan Setting: nuclear medicine laboratory Time: 30 min—1 hr Clean procedure	To evaluate health of liver, brain, bone, or breast tissue.	Same. A laxative and enemas may be ordered to empty GI tract prior to study if necessary for visualization.	Same.	Same.
Liver scan Setting: nuclear medicine laboratory Time: 30 min—1 hr Clean procedure	Evaluate presence of abnormal tissue in liver tissue.	Contraindicated in pregnant patients. A sedative or laxative may be ordered.	Same.	Same.
Lung scan Setting: nuclear medicine laboratory Time: 30 min—1 hr Clean procedure	Evaluate presence of abnormal tissue in lung tissue.	Contraindicated in pregnant patients. A sedative may be ordered.	Radiopharmaceutical is injected by vein; patient also breathes in radioactive gas. Scintillation camera is used to photograph.	Same.

GI = gastrointestinal.

excreted from her body (times vary depending on the substance used) so the radioactive substance will not be transferred to her infant in breast milk. Pregnant health care personnel should not care for a patient for 48 hours after this procedure to reduce risk of radioactive exposure to a growing fetus.

COLLECTION OF SPECIMENS FOR CULTURE

To culture a specimen means to identify the type of microorganism present in the specimen. Determining culture and sensitivity means that not only will the microorganisms present be identified but also antibiotics effective in eradicating the organisms will be identified. An average of 24 hours is needed for a culture report because the microorganisms must be allowed to grow under laboratory conditions until they reveal themselves. Sensitivity reports take another 24 hours to complete.

When obtaining specimens for culture, one overriding principle prevails—you must obtain the specimen without adding any microorganisms to it. Otherwise, these additional microorganisms may overgrow and conceal the microorganisms infecting the patient.

Most specimens for culture are preserved in a liquid medium. Be certain that the culture tube is kept upright during transport so it does not spill or touch any part of a cotton swab that your hand has touched to obtain the specimen. All cultures should be transported to the laboratory immediately so microorganisms do not dry before they can be grown.

Table 20-7 summarizes common specimens obtained for culture and specific procedures to obtain them.

DIAGNOSTIC-LABORATORY MEASURES AND NURSING PROCESS

Many laboratory studies are done to confirm diagnosis, and others are done to document that therapy is effective.

Learn to assess the results of laboratory reports to add to your knowledge of the patient's condition and to serve

TABLE 20-7. COMMON SPECIMENS FOR CULTURE

Specimen	Special Considerations
Sputum	Furnish a sterile sputum container and tell patient to cough, raise sputum, and expectorate into container. Close top immediately. Urge patient to cough deeply so sputum not saliva from back of throat is obtained. Sputum is raised most easily following a rest period or first thing in the morning. An antiseptic mouthwash should not be used just before obtaining a specimen; rinsing his mouth following this feels refreshing as infected sputum often has a strong aftertaste.
Wound	To culture an open lesion, choose a time just before a dressing change or any wound cleaning. Use a sterile cotton applicator. Dip this into a moist area of the wound and then drop swab into a sterile culture tube. Break off end of applicator your fingers have touched against edge of tube to prevent including this portion of applicator with specimen. If area to be cultured is dry, moisten applicator with sterile water to enable it to pick up microorganisms.
Urine	Urine may be obtained for culture by insertion of a catheter into the bladder, needle aspiration into the bladder, or clean-catch technique. These techniques require understanding of urine elimination processes; they are discussed in Chap. 38.
Blood	Blood cultures are often ordered to be taken at any time a patient's body temperature is suddenly elevated. Assemble equipment so it is immediately available. Normal blood drawing technique except an iodine rather than an alcohol solution is used for skin cleansing and following removal of the specimen, it is sent to the laboratory in the syringe or else the top of the test tube to which it will be transferred will first be held momentarily over an open flame to sterilize it before the blood is added.
Nose	To culture the nose use a special nose applicator (more pliable and smaller than a regular cotton applicator). Use a light to inspect nares to see if there are any collections of mucus; if not, touch application at representative sites in nares, then drop into sterile culture tube.
Throat	To culture throat, use a tongue blade to depress rear of tongue so tonsillar crypts are revealed. Touch a sterile cotton applicator to at least two places on palatine tonsils, especially any areas of pus or inflammation. Use care not to touch uvula, since this will cause the person to gag or vomit. Be careful that the applicator does not touch points in the mouth either during insertion or withdrawal. Drop it into a sterile culture tube.
Stool	Stool cultures may be obtained by asking a person to use a bedpan (or using a diaper from an infant) and then dipping a sterile cotton applicator into the stool mass or by gently inserting the applicator into the rectum until it touches stool. Do not take the specimen from the surface of the stool in a bedpan or diaper or you will actually be culturing that and not the stool.
Vaginal	Vaginal cultures are taken by gently separating the woman's vulva until the vaginal introitus is revealed; gently insert a sterile cotton applicator about an inch; remove it just as gently and drop it into a sterile culture tube. If the woman has a great deal of vaginal discharge, wear a glove on the hand used to separate vulva to prevent contaminating the hand with possibly infected secretions. Be certain to insert applicator far enough into the vagina to culture vaginal, not vulva secretions. Vulvae secretions are generally contaminated by *Escherichia coli* spread from the rectum, which overgrow and conceal other organisms.
Urethral Cultures in males	To obtain a male urethral culture, ask the man to milk secretions found in the urethra by stroking from base of penis to tip (or do this yourself). Touch a sterile cotton applicator to secretions at urethral opening; drop it into sterile culture tube.

as a basic foundation for planning nursing care. Learn common hematology and chemistry values so that you can recognize common abnormalities quickly and immediately begin care based on these facts. For example, if you notice that a person has a hemoglobin level of 5 gm/100 ml (normal is 12—15 gm/100 ml), your analysis would be that the person will undoubtedly tire easily. Hemoglobin carries oxygen to cells; when he exercises, he uses up oxygen faster than when he rests. Your plan of nursing care accordingly should provide for rest periods between procedures; if the patient has to go to another department, he will need a wheelchair; his sleep at night should be protected from interruptions. If a laboratory report tells you that a person's white blood count is very low, it means that he is more susceptible to infection than the average person. Check that his bed is not near a person with an infection; be aware if any nursing aides have colds—if one does, she should not be assigned to care for this patient.

If a laboratory report reveals that a person has a fatal disease, be aware that when the physician talks with this patient that day, she may tell him this. Accompany the physician to give support (for both patient and physician; telling someone this news is not an easy task). Afterward you might provide time for the person to be alone, or you might recognize that the person does not want to be alone—organize your care accordingly.

Being able to use information gained from laboratory results in this way deepens your level of nursing care and individualizes it (see QRS 20-5). Being able to use such information is necessary to nursing process. An example of a problem-oriented record note involving laboratory tests is shown above.

POR NURSING NOTE
Charting Laboratory Procedures

John Derner, Hosp. no. 60920

Problem: Lumbar puncture (diagnostic procedure)

S. Stated, "I hate needles. I think I'll faint if I see it," before procedure. At first did not want to listen to explanation of procedure.

O. Lumbar puncture done by Dr. Smith at 10 A.M. in treatment room. CSF removed clear in color. Opening pressure 66 mm Hg. Specimens sent to laboratory for protein, red blood cells, and culture. Kept flat in bed for 4 hours by encouraging TV watching. Drank 1,000 ml in 4-hour period (orange juice was favorite). No seepage or inflammation at puncture site; dressing intact.

A. A patient concerned with diagnostic procedures who cooperates well if adequately prepared.

P. 1. Determine if other studies are planned.
2. Give good explanation and active support if further studies are needed to reduce apprehension.

☐ QUICK REFERENCE STOP 20-5: COMMUNITY CONSIDERATIONS

Many diagnostic procedures are done on an ambulatory basis, in which the person will be responsible for scheduling the time of his own studies. For example, he might call the ultrasound department to schedule a time for a sonagram on Monday and then call the x-ray department to schedule an IVP on Tuesday and a barium enema on Tuesday. Such self-scheduling has the advantage of allowing a person to arrange studies at a time that are most convenient to him in terms of child care, work responsibilities, or availability of transportation. It has the disadvantage of being exhausting and sometimes frustrating.

Be certain that people have the correct telephone numbers and the correct name of the test they need to schedule. Be certain they have also another telephone number to call if for some reason they are unsuccessful in arranging diagnostic studies. Without such an additional telephone number, the person may give up after the first frustration and never have the ordered studies done.

SUGGESTED READINGS

Altschuler, A., et al. Clean, intermittent self-catheterization. *Crit. Care Update* 6:8, 1979.

Benchimol, A. *Noninvasive Techniques in Cardiology for the Nurse and Technician.* New York: Wiley, 1978.

Bissell, E. A. Diagnostic labels: Do they determine nursing care? *Compr. Pediatr. Nurs.* 3:1, 1978.

Boyd, P. R., et al. Those new tests they're doing—What specimen to get, how to take it and what the results can mean. *RN* 43:43, 1980.

Byrne, J. Hematologic studies. *Nursing 76* 6:15, 1976.

Byrne, J. Liver function studies. *Nursing 77* 7:12, 1977.

Byrne, J. Tips for interpreting the sedimentation rate and reticulocyte count. *Nursing 77* 7:9, 1977.

Chinn, P. L., and Leitch, C. J. *Child Health Maintenance: A Guide to Clinical Assessment.* St. Louis: Mosby, 1979.

Corbett, J. *Laboratory Tests in Nursing Practice.* Englewood Cliffs, N.J.: Appleton-Century-Crofts, 1982.

Dougherty, W. M. Serum bilirubin. *Nursing* (Horsham) 12(11):138, 1982.

Faulkner, P. L. Many diagnostic tests may be unnecessary. *Hospitals* 55:57, 1981.

Fawns, H. T. Vitamin K and blood clotting. *Nurs. Times* 74:1764, 1978.

Fischbach, F. T. *A Manual of Laboratory Diagnostic Tests.* Philadelphia: Lippincott, 1980.

Grimes, J., and Ianopollo, E. *Health Assessment in Nursing Practice.* Monterey, Calif.: Brooks-Cole, 1982.

Gutgesell, M. Practicality of screening urinalysis in asymptomatic children in a primary care setting. *Pediatrics* 62:103, 1978.

Hilton, B. A. Nurses' performance and interpretation of urine testing and capillary blood glucose monitoring measures. *J. Adv. Nurs.* 7(6):509, 1982.

Johnson, J. E., et al. Easing children's fright during health care procedures. *M.C.N.* 5:51, 1980.

Kelber, M. B. Pancreatic enzymes . . . deciphering diagnostic studies. *Nursing* (Horsham) 12(12):65, 1982.

King, E., L. Wieck, and M. Dyer. *Illustrated Manual of Nursing Techniques* (2nd ed.). Philadelphia: Lippincott, 1981.

McHugh, M. K. White blood cell tests; deciphering diagnostic studies. *Nursing* (Horsham) 12:122, 1982.

Markus, S. Taking the fear out of bone marrow examinations. *Nursing* (Horsham) 11:64, 1981.

Murray, B. L., and Wilcox, L. J. Testicular self-examination. *Am. J. Nursing* 78:2075, 1978.

Shearer, D., et al. Preparing a patient for EEG. *Am. J. Nurs.* 75:63, 1975.

Shetler, M. G., et al. Thoracentesis . . . and pericardiocentesis, too. *RN* 43:50, 1980.

Shetler, M. G., et al. Spinal and peritoneal taps: When quick action counts. *RN* 44:50, 1981.

Surr, C. W. Teaching patients to use the new blood-glucose monitoring products. *Nursing* (Horsham) 13(1):42, 1983.

Tilkian, S., M. Conover, and A. Tilkian. *Clinical Implications of Laboratory Tests* (2nd ed.). St. Louis: Mosby, 1979.

Wallach, J. *Interpretation of Diagnostic Tests: A Handbook of Laboratory Medicine* (3rd ed.). Boston: Little, Brown, 1978.

Zucker-Franklin, D. Finding the cause of anemia. *Consultant* 18:163, 1978.

QUESTIONS FOR REVIEW

Mark the following statements concerning laboratory-diagnostic studies true or false.

1. _____ An upper GI series involves swallowing a contrast medium.
2. _____ A finger prick is a painless procedure.
3. _____ A lumbar puncture is made at the third or forth lumbar interspace.
4. _____ The site for a bone marrow aspiration in children is usually the sternum.
5. _____ A therapeutic statement during a procedure is "Be brave."
6. _____ Your chief role during any procedure is assisting the physician.
7. _____ Most blood samples for chemistry analysis are taken by arterial venipuncture.
8. _____ Well-informed people are usually more cooperative during procedures than those less informed.
9. _____ Following a bronchoscopy, the person's gag reflex will be ineffective.
10. _____ Vital signs (pulse and respirations) need to be assessed following an esophagoscopy.
11. _____ A person generally is asked to assume a knee-chest position for a proctoscopy.
12. _____ There is no pain involved in a cystoscopy procedure.
13. _____ A radiopharmaceutical is injected for a brain scan study.
14. _____ Painful procedures in children should not be done at the bedside.
15. _____ Distraction during a procedure by casual conversation is effective.

VII. NURSING PROCESS IN ACTION: SELF-ESTEEM NEEDS

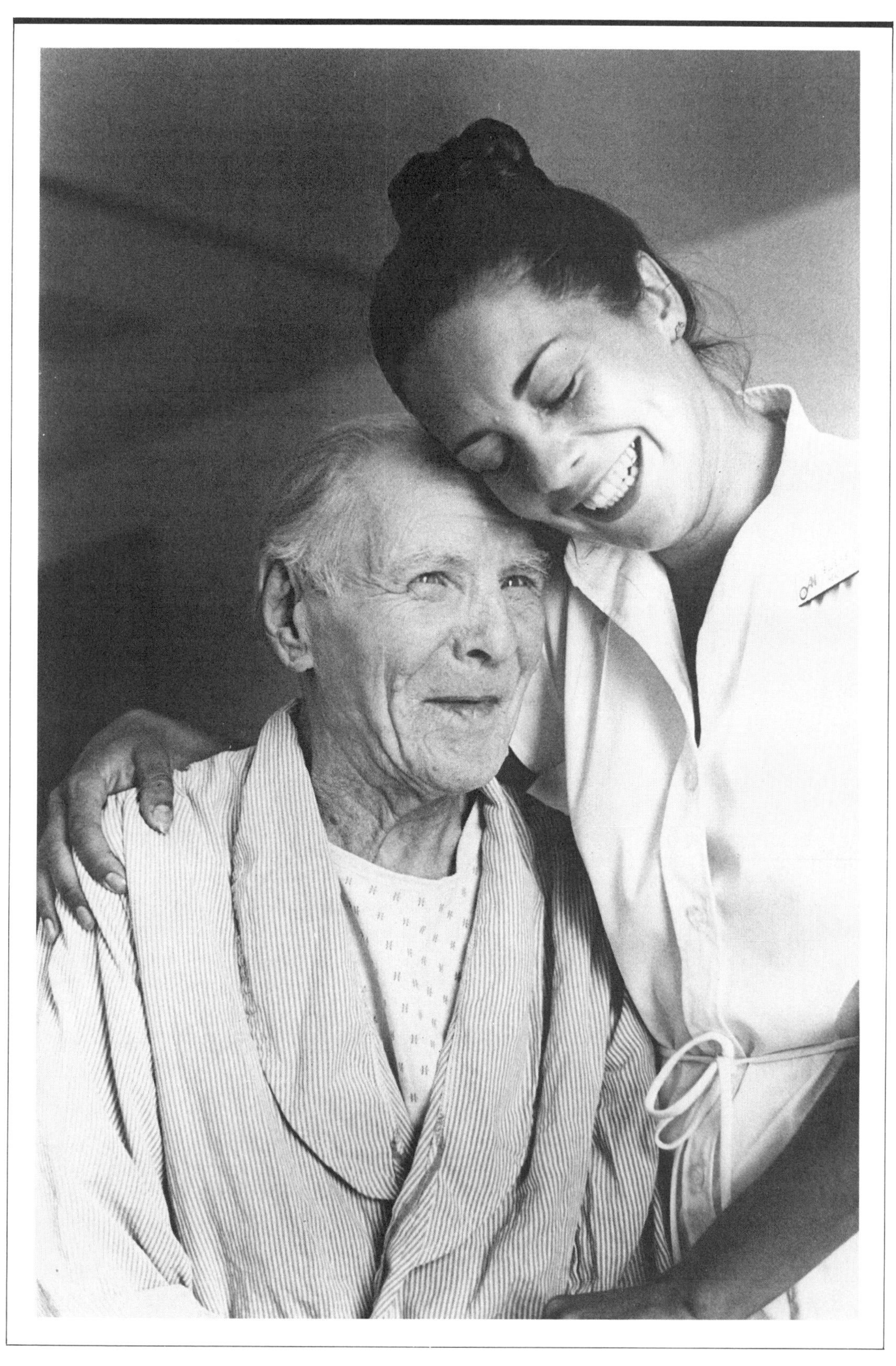

21. THE PERSON AS A SEXUAL BEING

OBJECTIVES

Upon mastery of the material in this chapter, you should be able to:

1. Identify your own attitudes and feelings about sexuality.
2. Describe sexual identity in differing age groups.
3. Describe various measures utilized in reproductive life planning.
4. Describe the human sexual response.
5. Describe nursing interventions for individuals with varying sexual life-styles.
6. Describe normal sexual expressions a nurse may encounter in care.
7. Describe ways to promote sexual development and health.

TERMS

The terms important for an understanding of this chapter are shown below and defined in the glossary:

analingus
anal sex
celibacy
coitus
contraception
cunnilingus
fellatio
fetishism
libido
masochism
masturbation
sadism
sexual dysfunction
sexual identity
sexuality
sexually transmitted disease (STD)
voyeurism

Sexuality refers to a person's maleness or femaleness, including sexual feelings, attitudes, and actions. It is biologically inherited and culturally learned. A person's sexuality encompasses his physical, emotional, social, intellectual, and ethical responses throughout life.

Sexual health is basic to human well-being. As defined by the World Health Organization (1975), "Sexual health is the integration of the somatic, emotional, intellectual, and social aspects of sexual being, in ways that are positively enriching and that enhance personality, communication, and love." Born a sexual being, a child's sexual identity and sexual role behavior evolve from and conform to the societal expectations within his given culture.

You entered nursing with your own feelings and attitudes about sexual health and sexual dysfunction. The subject of sexuality is a sensitive and private one, for you as well as for those in your care.

Sexual gender is the term used to denote chromosomal sexual development: male or female. *Sexual identity* is the sex a person thinks of himself as being (which may be the same as or different from his sexual gender). *Sexual role* is the role he takes (which may or may not be the same as sexual gender or identity).

Sexual gender is set at the moment of fusion of a female ova and male sperm. Ova carry an X or female chromosome. Sperm may carry either an X or a Y chromosome. If the resulting zygote has two X chromosomes, it will develop into a female. If it contains an X and a Y chromosome, it will become male. Therefore, the sperm carries the chromosome instrumental in determining sex.

As a fetus grows in utero, and testerone is secreted by the developing testes, the fetus develops male genitalia and function. If for some reason testerone secretion is suppressed, male development may not occur normally. If a chromosomally female fetus should be subjected to a testosterone-like hormone during pregnancy, a female fetus could be born appearing more male than female.

Sexual identity (feeling male or female) appears to be influenced by psychosocial circumstances, although the amount of testosterone secreted in utero may affect this as well. How appealing a parent makes a sexual role appear influences how a child envisions himself. If a mother makes being a woman seem a second-rate social position and a father makes being a man appear exciting, a daughter may find herself having difficulty accepting herself as a woman and behave with characteristics like those of her more appealing father. A son who can relate better to his mother's kind and caring manner than his father's strict, harsh one may find himself assuming characteristics often regarded as feminine. In an extreme form, a person may truly feel that he is a woman trapped in a man's body or a man trapped in a woman's body and ask to have a sex change operation to make his body correspond to the sex he truly believes is his.

Sexual role is culturally influenced. Traditionally, a woman has been viewed as kind and nurturing; among her duties are rearing children and homemaking. A man has characteristics of responsibility and stability; his duties are to provide for and protect the family. Today sexual roles are interchangeable enough so that women can feel free to accept managerial roles without loss of femininity; men can become househusbands without loss of masculinity. Thus, people can fulfill the roles most satisfying to them rather than those dictated by opinions of family or friends.

LIFE SPAN CONCEPTS AND SEXUALITY

A person's concepts about sexuality and concerns or questions vary with age.

The Infant

From the day of birth, female and male babies are treated differently. People bring girls dainty rattles and dresses with ruffles; on the whole they are treated more gently by parents and held and rocked more than male babies. People tend to buy boys bigger rattles and sports-related jogging suits.

By the end of the first year, differences in play are usually evident. Girls play for longer periods with quiet soft toys, checking back with mother frequently; boys spend more time in gross motor activity, staying away from mother for longer time periods than girls (Fig. 21-1).

FIGURE 21-1. Roughhouse play generally begins earlier for boys than for girls.

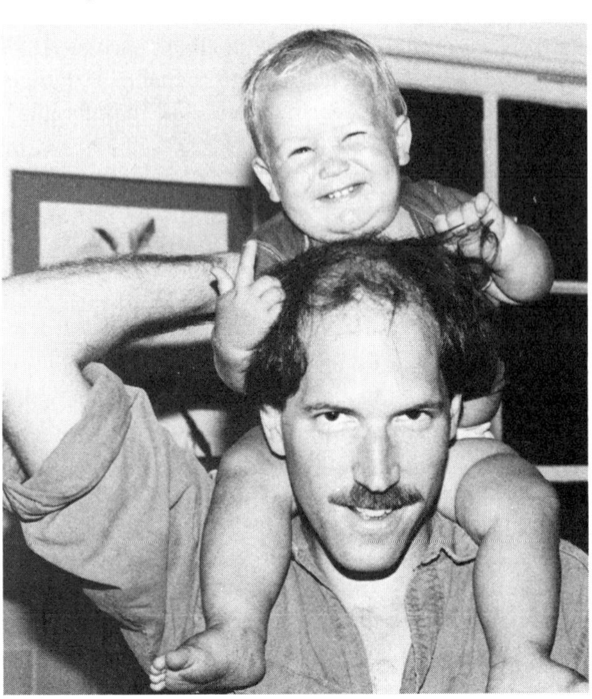

The Toddler and Preschooler

Children can distinguish between men and women as early as 2 years of age. By age 3 or 4 they know for certain what sex they are, and they have absorbed cultural expectations of that sex role. Watching preschool children at play demonstrates this. Girls imitate cooking, washing dishes, and cleaning. Boys go to work with pretend lunch pails or briefcases. Comments such as "What kind of mommy are you going to be, treating a doll that way?" or "Boys will be boys" express approval or disapproval for their actions, and the action is strengthened as apparently right or discarded in favor of action that will bring approval. Sex role modeling also comes from watching family situation programs on television.

If the child lives in a home where both mother and father are kind, loving people, sex role identification progresses smoothly. If one parent does not have a high nurturing capacity, however, it may be hard for the child of the same sex to identify with that person, or because the adult is not a good model, the child perpetuates the poor role.

Preschool children pass through a stage of development where they feel possessive of the parent of the opposite sex. This first love fades as they identify more fully with the parent of their own sex but probably influences their ability to relate heterosexually in later years. Children living in single-parent homes may omit this stage of development if there is no parent of the opposite sex present; they may have difficulty leaving this stage and progressing to same-sex identification for the same reason.

The Schoolage Child

In school, the difference between boys and girls grows wider. There are girls' and boys' activities that are not interchangeable. Teachers often contribute to the difference by expecting boys to be poorer readers, to write less neatly, and to act rougher in the school hallways.

Today girls can play in the Little League or take shop or auto repair courses, and many activities of the school age period are for both sexes.

The Adolescent

At puberty, as the adolescent establishes a sense of identity, or a certain understanding of who he is and what kind of person he wants to be, the problem of final sex role identification surfaces again. Most early adolescents maintain strong ties to their gender group, boys with boys and girls with girls. Some adolescents choose a child of their own sex a few years older as their model of sex role behavior. Parents often worry about this type of attachment and express concerns that the relationship has homosexual connotations. Ordinarily, however, teenagers are just being certain that they understand who they are before they are ready to interact with members of the opposite sex.

The Young Adult

When the young adult moves away from home to attend college or establish his own home, he chooses the way he will express his sexuality along with other life patterns. Many young adults marry with a commitment to one sexual partner. Others establish relationships less binding by legal definitions but perhaps equally binding in concern and support. Many young adults view cohabitation as a means of learning more about a possible marriage partner on a day-to-day basis in the hope that a future marriage will then be stronger and more lasting. The incidence of sexual behavior outside marriage is increasing yearly. Figures are imprecise, but an estimated 50 to 70 percent of young adults engage in sexual activities outside marriage.

Homosexuality or bisexuality may be overtly expressed for the first time. Sexually transmitted disease (STD; disease spread by coitus) is at epidemic proportions in some parts of the country, largely due to the frequent changing of sexual partners in this age adult. When young adults are cared for in emergency rooms or admitted to health care facilities for these diseases, they are usually receptive to health teaching information on how better to prevent such diseases and possibly on contraceptives. They may have questions about sexual practices and their feelings about their sex identity or role.

Many adolescent and young adult athletes are taught that abstinence from sexual activity will increase their muscle strength and stamina (this is false). They may worry that excessive sexual relations early in life will cause them to lose their ability to participate in or enjoy sexual relations later in life (also false). Exactly the opposite is true; the longer and more active a person is sexually, the longer his interest and capacity for sexual activity remains (see QRS 21-1).

Young couples often have questions about reproduction and fertility. If a woman anticipated that she would be able to become pregnant the first month she desired to and then does not, she or her sexual partner may feel a loss of self-esteem. She may need counseling that it takes the average woman 8 to 10 months to become pregnant. She may also need medical investigation of reasons for her not achieving pregnancy. Young mothers may have questions about the appearance of their infant son's genitals. They may be unaware, for example, that the left testis in most males is slightly larger and lower than the right, which allows the testes to slide past each other more easily and results in less pressure with movement. Most parents are aware that masturbation is normal for preschool boys but are unprepared to see it in preschool girls; they need an explanation that it is normal for both sexes as a part of exploring and growing comfortable with one's own body.

☐ QUICK REFERENCE STOP 21-1: HEALTH TEACHING

Many young adults are interested in knowing what is normal sexual response or expected frequency of sexual relations. A commonly accepted rule of thumb is that any act mutually satisfying to both sexual partners is normal. Frequency and type of such activity varies widely within normal parameters.

The Middle-Aged Adult

For many women and men in mid-life sexuality has achieved a degree of stability. A sense of masculinity or femininity and comfortable patterns of behavior have been established. Adults in mid-life have resolved earlier conflicts with mates and have the freedom to satisfy their sexual needs, including the freedom to remain with a partner or return to a single state.

In the middlescent woman, reproductive functioning alters but sexual functioning does not. Menopause is said to have occurred with cessation of menses for at least 1 year. Estrogen levels gradually decrease over a period of about 1 to 7 years with menopause occurring at about 50 years of age.

A woman's response to the physiological and emotional components of menopause is to a degree culturally determined and includes anticipation of its effects. Generally, a woman engaged in a productive, satisfying lifestyle is more likely to progress through this natural biological stage with fewer problems. (See Chap. 9 for further discussion of menopause.)

In the middlescent man, neither reproductive nor sexual functioning alters. However, mid-life is often reported to be the most difficult period of adjustment in a man's life, bringing a need for ego enhancement and reassurance of sexual adequacy. He may find he has sexual dysfunction, such as premature ejaculation or impotence, particularly if he has work or family pressures. The increased incidence of sexual encounters with younger women is seen by many as males' way of reassuring themselves of their attractiveness and virility and denying the fear of aging (see QRS 21-2, 21-3).

As a nurse you need to be aware of the sexual aspects of illnesses and their meanings to middle-aged patients. This period of life has the peak incidence of heart attacks. Patients with coronary disease have many real fears as to how their sexual lives will be affected. Be alert that the man who comments about his need to maintain a reduced activity level at work is also seeking information and direction in other important areas of his life—sex, for one.

Similarily, women who undergo surgery on their reproductive organs, such as a hysterectomy (removal of the uterus), need sensitive nurses to listen to their concerns about the meaning of the experience. For some women the loss of the uterus can be synonymous with

☐ **QUICK REFERENCE STOP 21-2: NUTRITION**

There is a popular belief that Vitamin E increases sexual response in males. Men who are prescribed special diets may ask if a diet of that type contains many vitamins, particularly vitamin E. Although there is little documentation that vitamin E increases sexual ability in men, there is also little documentation that taking amounts of it daily causes any ill effects. Check with a dietician if there would be any contraindication for a person taking vitamin E if you realize that the patient intends to add some to his diet independently.

☐ **QUICK REFERENCE STOP 21-3: PHARMACOLOGY**

Certain medications such as antihypertensives, tranquilizers, and narcotics may diminish sexual responses. Knowing this may occur is important not only to the person taking the medication so he can appreciate this is occurring as an expected response but also to his sexual partner. People who take such medications may need to discuss alternate methods of sexual expression such as mutual masturbation until the medication is discontinued and normal sexual interest or response returns.

the loss of femininity. If both ovaries are also removed (oophorectomy), an immediate surgical menopause occurs. The hormonal changes occurring with the removal of both ovaries must be dealt with openly. Limited hormonal replacement is often a means of simulating the naturally decreasing hormone levels of natural menopause.

The nurse is frequently the care provider who can best communicate to the woman that her sexual satisfaction need not be diminished by surgery on reproductive organs. Voiced or not, the patient may well have such fears.

The Older Adult

Both male and female older adults can enjoy active sexual relationships (Fig. 21-2). Some males in this age group experience less erectile firmness or ejaculatory force than when they were younger, but others discover that they are able to maintain an erection longer. Males remain fertile throughout life and thus need to continue to be responsible sex partners in terms of birth control.

The older woman will have less vaginal secretion present because she has less estrogen following menopause and therefore may need to use a lubricant before sexual intercourse for comfort and enjoyment. Women who have been sexually active throughout their lives seem to have fewer problems.

Older women may have no acceptable partner, since the average lifespan is longer for women. In many retirement communities, the ratio of women to men is as high as 2 : 1. Such women should be assisted in finding individual female and male companionship as well as groups that provide physical contact, social interaction, and intellectual stimulation. Masturbation can provide sexual gratification for persons of all ages.

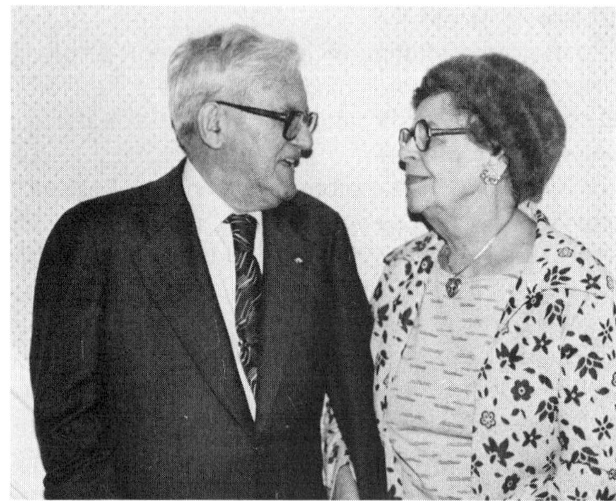

FIGURE 21-2. Sexuality is an important aspect of being alive. Note the obvious love shared by this older couple.

Older adults who live with their children may suffer from lack of privacy for fulfilling sexual relationships. Those who are hospitalized or in long-term care facilities should have sexual needs evaluated along with other care needs; because they are older, needs for sexual expression may be ignored or repressed. Nurses need to advocate that couples share a room and provide for privacy. Unfortunately, lifelong partners are sometimes separated. Even in homes for the well aged, double-bed facilities are rare.

The Handicapped Individual

The handicapped individual has sexual desires and needs but may have difficulty with sexual identity or sexual enjoyment due to the effects of handicapping. Males with spinal cord injury may have difficulty with erection and ejaculation, since these actions are governed at the spinal level. Manual stimulation of the penis or psychological stimulation achieves erection in most men with such lesions so the man can have a satisfying sexual relationship with his partner. Both males and females with handicaps that are interpreted as disfiguring, such as colostomies or mastectomies, may be reluctant to participate in sexual activities, fearing that the sight of the colostomy or the lack of a breast will diminish the partner's satisfaction or enjoyment. The response of a loving partner does much to enhance the body image and feelings of adequacy of his mate.

Sexuality in the handicapped person is a facet of rehabilitation that was rarely emphasized in the past. If a person could accomplish activities of daily living such as eating, elimination, and mobility, he was considered to be leading a normal or near normal life. Today, a sexual relationship is included as an activity of daily living and should be considered in rehabilitation programs as well as more technically oriented activities.

THE HUMAN SEXUAL RESPONSE

It was once believed that the desire for sexual relations was a male concern and that the average female was not interested. However, it is now known that women enjoy sexual relations as much as men and that both men and women have typical reactions to sexual stimulation. Four stages occur in response to sexual stimulation (Masters and Johnson, 1966): excitement, plateau, orgasm, and resolution. To help understand these stages, the internal anatomy of male and female sexual organs is shown in Fig. 21-3.

EXCITEMENT STAGE

The excitement stage is a time of vasocongestion and increasing muscular tension as sexual arousal occurs. In women, vasocongestion causes the clitoris to increase in size and mucoid fluid to appear on vaginal walls as lubrication. The vagina grows wider and deeper. The breast nipples become erect. In men, erection occurs; there is scrotal thickening and elevation of the testes. In both sexes, heart rate, respiratory rate, and blood pressure increase.

PLATEAU STAGE

The plateau stage is reached just before orgasm. In women, the clitoris is drawn forward and retracts under the clitoral prepuce; the lower part of the vagina becomes extremely congested, forming the orgasmic platform. There is increased nipple engorgement. In men, the vasocongestion leads to full distention of the penis. Heart rate has increased to 100 to 175 beats per minute; respiratory rate to about 40 per minute.

ORGASM

Orgasm is a vigorous contraction of muscles in the pelvic area. This violent contraction expels or dissipates blood and fluid from the area of congestion. The average woman has 8 to 15 contractions, 1 every 0.8 second.

In men, muscle contractions surrounding the seminal vessels and prostate project semen into the proximal urethra. These contractions are followed immediately by three to seven propulsive ejaculatory contractions, 1 every 0.8 second, that force semen from the penis.

STAGE OF RESOLUTION

The stage of resolution is the period during which the external and internal genital organs return to a quiet state. This takes about 30 minutes in both men and women. Women are capable of initiating orgasm again almost immediately following the first orgasm; men generally are not capable of this for 10 to 15 minutes, or longer in older males.

Statistics on whether women achieve a stage of orgasm from coitus alone vary from early reports by Freud that women were neurotic if they did not always achieve orgasm through intercourse to findings of Hite (1976) that only 30% of women regularly experience orgasm from intercourse alone. Newer research reveals another reflex, a uterine orgasm, that is achieved by stimulation of a sensitive area on the upper anterior vaginal wall termed a Gräfenberg spot (Perry and Whipple, 1981).

Influence of the Menstrual Cycle

During the second half of the menstrual cycle there is increased fluid retention and vasocongestion in the women's lower pelvis. Because some vasocongestion is already present at the beginning of the excitement stage of sexual response, women appear to reach the plateau stage more quickly and achieve orgasm more readily. Women also seem to be more interested in initiating sexual relations at this time. There is no reason to abstain from sexual relations during menstruation unless the partners find it inconvenient or it causes uterine cramping for the woman.

Influence of Pregnancy

Pregnancy is another time in life when, because of the rapidly growing fetus in the lower pelvic area, vasocongestion of the area occurs. Some women experience their first orgasm during the first pregnancy. Following a pregnancy, many women experience increased sexual desire because the new growth of blood vessels during pregnancy lasts for some time and facilitates pelvic vasocongestion. Occasionally, coitus may be contraindicated during pregnancy if the woman's physician believes that infection of the uterus may occur. Following pregnancy, it is advisable, because of possible infection, that women not resume coitus until the vaginal discharge following pregnancy has ceased (1—6 weeks).

Peak Sexual Response

The peak sexual response in men appears to take place in late teen years. The peak response in women, however, occurs more frequently during the late 30s. This difference in age of peak response has not yet been satisfactorily explained. It may be influenced by men being taught early in life that sexual activity is expected of them and women being taught that sexual activity is not expected of them until after marriage. Possibly women take until their 30s to overcome this inhibition against enjoying or wanting sex. The discrepancy in the age of peak sexual response may account for marital difficulties if the difference is pronounced.

Contraceptives

Because birth control pills contain estrogen and excess estrogen may decrease sexual desire, some women on birth control pills express a lowered interest in sexual

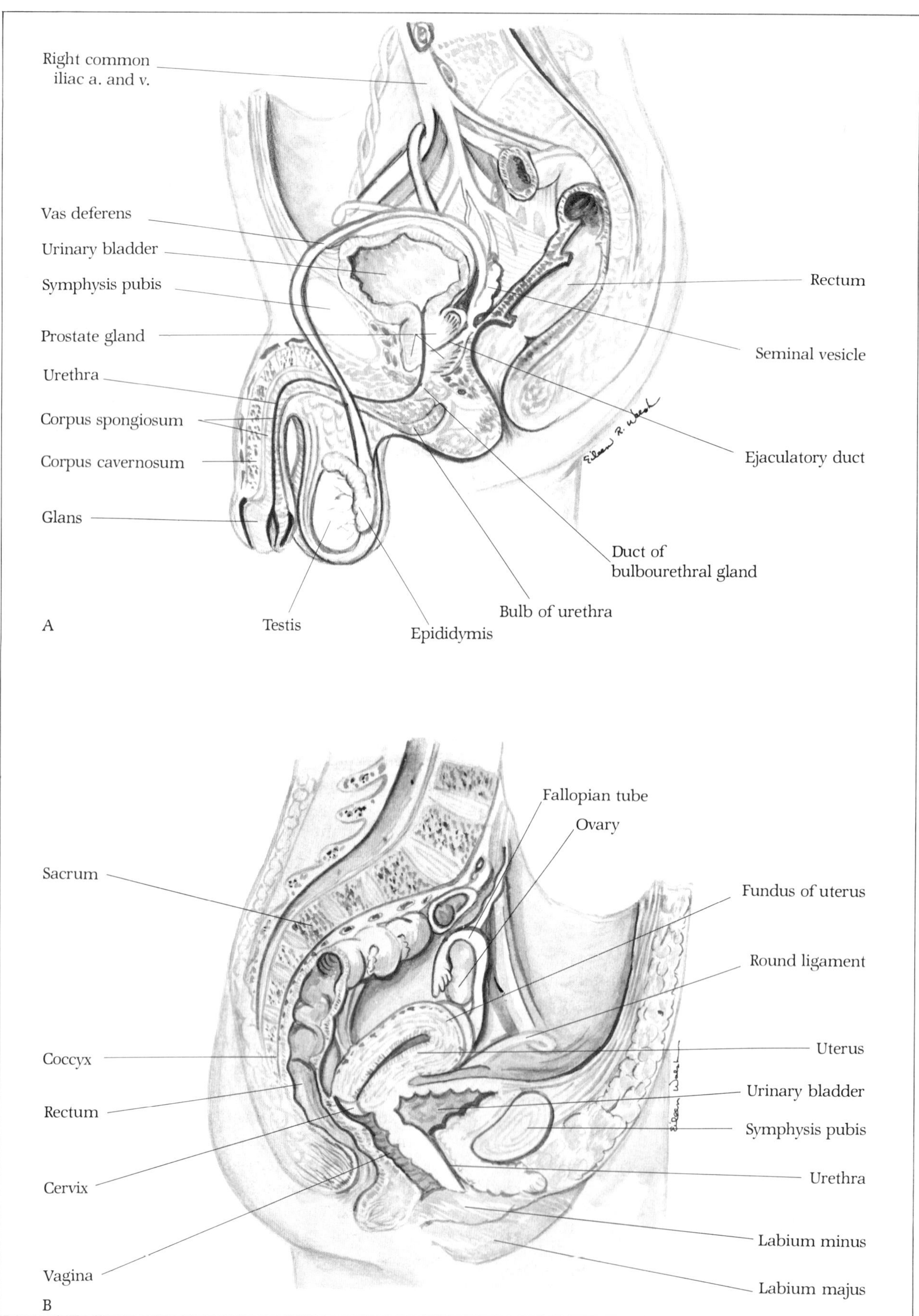

FIGURE 21-3. A. Internal anatomy of the male sex organs. B. Internal anatomy of the female sex organs.

relations. This method of birth control may be unacceptable for the woman since it interferes with her relationship with her sexual partner. Other women find that confidence that they will not become pregnant makes sexual relations more pleasurable for them. Barrier methods of birth control (diaphragm, condom, spermicidal creams) may interfere with sexual expression in that they must be used shortly before coitus to be effective.

Methods of Sexual Expression

A person expresses sexuality by dress, mannerisms, occupation, way of greeting people, and amount of touching in relationships. For example, men greet each other with a handshake; women may or may not shake hands. Women typically touch more (patting an arm, adjusting a sleeve or collar for someone) than do males.

Masturbation

Masturbation is self-stimulation for erotic pleasure; it can also be mutually enjoyable for sexual partners. It offers sexual release, which may be interpreted by the person as overall tension or anxiety relief. Children between 2 and 3 years of age discover masturbation as an enjoyable activity as they explore their body. A child under a high level of tension may become accustomed to using masturbation as a means of falling asleep at night or at naptime. Preschoolers in a hospital setting may masturbate to express their fear of intrusive procedures or to satisfy themselves that all of their body parts are still intact. Preschool children may masturbate without any attempt at concealment because they have not yet been affected by society's view that such activity is private. Depending on the situation, such as on a hospital corridor, distract the child's attention to another activity; this strategy can prevent others from making comments that can be damaging to the child.

Schoolage children continue to use masturbation for enjoyment or to relieve tension but limit such activity to privacy. However, in a hospital setting a schoolage child may assume that he has more privacy than he does, so may be discovered masturbating if you walk unannounced into his room.

Following surgery, a question many adult men are concerned with is how soon will they be able to have sexual relations without feeling pain at their incision line. They may masturbate to erection and orgasm as soon as the first sensation of incision pain has passed in order to test that everything is still in working order much as the preschooler does. It is generally accepted that men use masturbation as a release mechanism; Masters and Johnson (1966) report that women may find masturbation to orgasm the most satisfying sexual expression and use it more commonly than men.

Masturbation is a normal part of sexual expression. Respect closed doors or drawn curtains. Provide privacy as necessary to the person who asks for it.

Nocturnal Emissions

Beginning with puberty, when quantities of seminal fluid form, a boy having an erotic dream can experience erection and ejaculation. This results in a wet circle of semen on sheets (wet dreams). A man reared to consider sexual thoughts as bad behavior may be embarrassed to have you notice such a stain on his bed linen; it is not uncommon for an ambulatory adolescent in a hospital setting to offer to make his own bed in order to avoid this. Check that bed staining is not from enuresis (involuntary urination), which could be due to a urinary tract infection or from some other cause.

Women also have erotic dreams to orgasm but have no accompanying vaginal discharge. Putting these occurrences in perspective helps you to accept them as everyday facts and a part of normal sexual expression.

Erotic Stimulation

Erotic stimulation is the use of visual materials such as magazines or photographs for sexual arousal. Although this is thought of as mostly a male phenomenon because of the girlie magazines on newstands, there is increasing interest in centerfold photographs in women's magazines. Adolescent boys may accumulate stores of such material and use it for sexual arousal with masturbation. Friends of adult males may select this type of magazine for them in preference to one concerned with national news. If a man asks you to bring him a magazine on your way back from lunch, he may be reluctant to suggest this type. Ask for a preference: *Newsweek? Field and Stream? Playboy?* Be aware that such material is a part of daily reading material for a large segment of the population.

Sexual Intercourse

It is generally assumed that a person admitted to a health care facility is too ill or will be hospitalized for such a short period of time that a desire for sexual relations will not occur. In reality, a person admitted to a health care facility for diagnostic studies may not feel ill at all. People who are admitted for conditions such as broken legs, anemia, or infections may be in the hospital for a long time. They may well experience a need for sexual relations or a desire to grant their sexual partner an opportunity to fulfill this need.

Couples who are institutionalized or hospitalized for long periods should be assigned together in rooms. This can occur when both partners are in an automobile accident; it may or may not happen in extended care facilities when an older couple is admitted together for long-term care.

PERSONS WITH ALTERNATE SEXUAL LIFE-STYLES

Sexual gratification is experienced in a number of ways. One's culture determines acceptable forms of sexual expression; what is considered normal varies greatly among cultures. Most individual value systems are closely aligned to the cultural norm, your own included.

In order to make a person with an alternate sexual life-style comfortable in a health care setting, discard a mind set that labels any style good or bad. People with alternate sexual life-styles develop illnesses such as pneumonia the same as people with any other life-style; they may be more likely to develop sexually transmitted diseases (diseases spread by sexual relations). Certain modifications of care may need to be made in order that hospitalization or return to the community can be productive.

The Homosexual

A *homosexual* is a person who finds sexual fulfillment with a member of his own sex. The term *lesbian* refers to homosexual women. People are *bisexual* if they achieve sexual satisfaction from both homosexual and heterosexual relationships. Visiting policies may need to be modified for the homosexual patient in a health care facility if visiting priviledges are ordinarily restricted to only the marital spouse.

Homosexual relationships may be long or short term. This sometimes frequent changing of sexual partners tends to leave the homosexual more exposed to sexually transmitted disease (STD) than the average person. Preventive measures against STD and signs and symptoms of STD are health teaching information that may be needed.

Homosexuality is revealed freely by many patients on a health history. Many homosexuals prefer to use the term *gay*.

The Transvestite

A transvestite is a person who receives sexual pleasure from wearing clothing of the opposite sex. A transvestite may or may not be homosexual. Transvestism as a means of sexual arousal is considered a normal variation as long as the activity does not interfere with normal functioning in other life areas and involves a satisfying sexual relationship. A person may tell you that he is a transvestite because he is concerned with the appearance of a surgical scar that he believes will be disfiguring in the opposite sex clothing he finds enjoyment in wearing.

Female impersonators may be true transvestites or they may be males who have discovered a way to earn a living that is extremely lucrative if done well.

The Transsexual

A transsexual is an individual who, although of one sexual gender, feels as if he is of the opposite gender (a male trapped in a female body or a female trapped in a male body). Such people may have sex change operations so they appear cosmetically as the sex they envision themselves to be. Such operations do not change the person's chromosomal structure, however, so though capable of sexual relationships in his new role (a synthetic vagina or penis is created), the person is not capable of reproduction. The incidence of sex change operations has decreased in recent years because of potential disappointment following the surgery—despite a new appearance, the person realizes that he is still not totally what he wishes to be.

The Fetishist

Fetishism is sexual arousal by the use of certain objects or body parts. Leather and rubber are materials frequently perceived to have erotic qualities. Unpacking a suitcase on hospital admission or packing for a return home may reveal a wardrobe of unusual articles of clothing or photographs that reveal the fetishist's sexual arousal object. Like other alternate sexual expressions, fetishism is considered normal as long as it does not interfere with normal functioning and includes a satisfying sexual relationship with a partner.

The Voyeur

Voyeurism is sexual arousal by looking at another's body. Almost all children and adolescents pass through a stage when voyeurism is appealing; this passes with more active sexual expressions. That some voyeurism exists in almost everyone is illustrated by the large number of R-rated movies shown on television and in movie theaters and by the erotic descriptions in novels. Voyeurism may be practiced to the exclusion of other sexual experiences by insecure people who do not feel confident enough to relate to others on more personal levels.

The Sadomasochist

Sadomasochism is inflicting pain (sadism) or receiving pain (masochism) to achieve sexual satisfaction. It is generally considered that as long as the pain involved is minimal and the experience is mutually satisfying to both sexual partners, the practice is within normal limits.

The Celibate

Celibacy is abstinence from sexual activity. Celibacy is the avowed state of certain religious orders. It is a way of life for many adults and one becoming fashionable among a growing number of young adults. The theoretical advantage of celibacy is the ability to concentrate on the means of giving and receiving love other than sexual expression.

Incest

Incest is sexual activity between family members. It often involves an older male and a young female partner although it may involve an older female and younger male, brother or sister, or same-sex partners. Incest is a deviation from the normal, and incest taboos are common to most cultures. It causes a great deal of guilt and loss of self-esteem in both partners. Incest may be revealed on health history (a young girl worrying that she is pregnant); it may be revealed by a child abnormally anxious for a mother to return home from a hospitalization or by expression of relief that a father is going to be hospitalized. Both the adult and child involved need psychological counseling; the child to improve self-esteem, and the adult to channel sexual expression to less destructive outlets. Nurses and other health care providers are legally responsible to report known or suspected instances of incest involving a child.

Prostitution

A prostitute earns a living by providing sexual pleasure for others. Although prostitutes are typically thought of as female, they can also be male. It is sometimes assumed that a person who earns his living in this way will be provocative in his response to a member of the opposite sex and therefore might be difficult to offer nursing care to. For many prostitutes exactly the opposite is true; they see sex as a business and do not offer any without payment.

Because prostitutes have a high incidence of sexually transmitted disease and, if women, a high pregnancy rate, this occupation needs to be considered in total health assessment. Health teaching about sexually transmitted disease and pregnancy prevention measures may need to be discussed.

COUNSELING THE RAPE VICTIM

Rape is a deviant expression of violence, not passion. As stated by Weinberg (1982), "The sexual expression is one of power and anger, not one of sexual desire or frustration." Persons who are raped need counseling to reestablish self-esteem; rapists need therapy to direct such violent behavior less destructively. Rape victims are seen in emergency rooms for health care. Most women need a female nurse with them during examination following rape if the physician will be male because of their recent bad experience from a male. The sex of the caregiver may not be so important, however, as a caring attitude because it is the uncaring attitude that the patient has been exposed to that has frightened her so. Many cities have rape crisis centers, with a counseling service for victims and sometimes with educational services for health and law professionals or community programs to increase public awareness of the problem.

PROBLEMS WITH INTERCOURSE

During crisis periods—and any illness is a crisis to some extent—people often question their life-styles and beliefs. For this reason, questions about sexuality or sex role may be asked of health care providers. One of a nurse's largest contributions can be to make it clear that such questions or concerns can be discussed. Thus problems of sexuality are brought into the open and made as solvable as other health problems.

Impotence

Impotence is the inability to achieve or maintain an erection. Some causes are physical, such as debilitating disease or drug dependence, and others appear to be psychological, such as doubts about ability to perform or overall masculinity or excessive stress at home or at work. Therapy for impotence depends on the factors involved. Surgical implants to aid erection are possible. If the cause is psychological, sexual counseling may be helpful. In all cases, a loving, supportive partner can help.

Premature Ejaculation

Premature ejaculation is ejaculation prior to penile-vaginal contact. The term is often used also to mean ejaculation prior to the sexual partner's satisfaction. Premature ejaculation is unsatisfactory for both partners: for the woman because she cannot achieve orgasm because of loss of the man's erection and for the man because he has failed to help her achieve orgasm.

Like impotence, premature ejaculation appears most often to be psychologically based. Masturbating to orgasm (where orgasm is achieved quickly owing to lack of time) may be a cause, since it conditions a quicker response. Other possible causes are doubt about masculinity and fear of impregnating. Sexual counseling to help both male and female partners put less importance on performance may be helpful in alleviating the problem.

Failure to Achieve Orgasm

Failure to achieve orgasm can be due to poor sexual technique, concentrating too hard on achieving orgasm, underlying fear, negative attitudes toward sexual relationships, or lack of knowledge of anatomy or the nature of orgasm. Therapy generally consists of instruction for both partners in better sexual techniques and counseling in basic feelings about sexuality.

Dyspareunia

Dyspareunia is pain during intercourse. It can be due to vaginal infection, insufficient lubrication of the vaginal walls, or endometriosis, a condition in which the inner lining of the uterus spreads by way of the fallopian tubes into the peritoneal cavity. It can also be psychological in nature. Therapy is aimed at the underlying cause.

Vaginismus

Vaginismus is involuntary contraction of the muscles of the outlet of the vagina when sexual intercourse is attempted. This muscle contraction prevents penile penetration or causes discomfort with penetration.

Vaginismus may occur in women who have had unfortunate sexual experiences such as rape. It can also be the result of early learning patterns, in which sexual relations were viewed as bad. Sexual and psychological counseling may be necessary to reduce this response.

REPRODUCTIVE LIFE (FAMILY) PLANNING

Family planning is an individual's and a couple's choice. A nurse's role may encompass assessment (health history and physical examination), health teaching, and referral. Independent nursing intervention is usually accomplished as a family planning nurse practitioner, which necessitates advanced education.

The board of directors of the American Nurses' Association has issued the following resolution on family planning*:

It is the responsibility of registered nurses:

1. To recognize the right of individuals and family to select and use such methods as are consistent with their own creed and mores
2. To recognize the right of individuals and families to receive information about family planning if they wish
3. To be responsive to the need for family planning
4. To be knowledgeable about state laws regarding family planning and resources available
5. To assist in informing individuals and families of the existence of approved family planning resources
6. To assist in directing individuals and families of sources of such aids

To each individual and couple, family planning will mean something different, based on early religious teachings, family background, education, and present life situation.

The nurse may need to refer to a specialist the couple who experiences a delay in conception or one with a family history of a genetic disorder. Health teaching about family planning is indicated for those who choose to space their children for developmental (enjoyment and recognition of each child at his own time in the family), economic, or other reasons. A growing number of women are electing to conceive after 30 years of age; career attainment, later marriages, and adult single parenthood by choice account for older first-time mothers. Many married couples choose not to become parents. Many single women choose a lifestyle that includes being an active sex partner, not a mother. Adolescents are more sexually active and at a younger age than ever before. Whether married or single, women can choose an active sex life with confidence that pregnancy can be avoided. Although family planning is a joint decision, the woman frequently assumes responsibility for her own actions, including sexual gratification. Contraceptive methods are summarized in Table 21-1.

*Copyright 1966, American Journal of Nursing Company. Reproduced with permission from the *American Journal of Nursing* 66(11):2376, 1966.

Biological Methods

The biological or fertility awareness method of family planning necessitates a woman determining her fertile period and abstaining from intercourse during that time. The fertile period calculation is based on ovulation, which occurs about 14 days before the end of the cycle (beginning menstrual flow); the egg remains viable for 24 hours and sperm can survive for 2 to 3 days. To effectively use the biological method, a woman must correctly record and interpret her menstrual cycles over a period of months, record her basal body temperature daily, and examine the character of her cervical mucus secretions. (Basal body temperature taken each morning upon arising drops about 0.3°F [0.2°C] 1 or 2 days before ovulation. Following ovulation, there is a temperature rise of 0.7°F to 0.8°F [0.4°C to 0.5°C], which will be maintained for the rest of the menstrual cycle). The biological method may be preferred by those of certain religious faiths as well as others who prefer a nonchemical and nonmechanical means of family planning. Partner commitment is essential.

Hormone Therapy

The use of oral contraceptives requires the woman to take a pill by mouth on a regular basis. Known as *the pill*, oral contraceptives taken consistently and conscientiously provide the most effective method of temporary birth control. However, their use is associated with the greatest number of both serious and minor side effects of all contraceptive measures.

Most pills contain estrogen and progesterone components in a combination form. The estrogen halts ovulation by suppressing the release of the gonadatropic hormones (follicle-stimulating hormone [FSH] and luteinizing hormone [LH]) of the pituitary. The progesterone component changes the consistency of the mucus in the cervix by making it more viscid (thicker) and thus decreases sperm motility and access to the ovum. Progesterone also prevents the lining of the uterus (endometrium) from becoming fully developed, making implantation unlikely. It is this lack of full endometrial maturation that results in decreased flow at the time of menstrual periods. A woman needs to be informed that this change is expected and normal; otherwise, she may think that she is pregnant.

Another oral hormonal contraceptive, low-dose oral progestin, contains only progesterone; it is frequently referred to as the *mini-pill*. Small doses of progestin (progesterone) may inhibit ovulation in some women, but its known contraceptive action is altering cervical mucus and endometrial lining in the same manner as the combination pill. The woman takes the mini-pill every single day. The mini-pill is sometimes prescribed for a woman who has experienced estrogen-excess side effects from the combination pill because the mini-pill contains no estrogen.

TABLE 21-1. SUMMARY OF CONTRACEPTIVE METHODS

Method	Effectiveness Rating	Ideal Failure Rate	Actual Failure Rate	Advantages	Disadvantages
Birth control pills (combination)	Excellent	0.5%	2—3%	Highly reliable; coitus independent; has some health benefits	Side effects; daily use; continual cost
Mini-pill	Very good	1—2	5—10	Thought to have low risk of side effects; coitus independent	Breakthrough bleeding; daily use; continual cost
IUD	Excellent	1—3	5—6	No memory or motivation required for use; very reliable	Cramping, bleeding, expulsion
Condom and diaphragm	Excellent	1	3—5	Highly reliable with no major health risks	Esthetic objections
Condom and foam	Excellent	1	3—5	Highly reliable with no major health risks	Esthetic objections
Diaphragm and cream or jelly	Good—very good	3	15—20	No major health risks; inexpensive	Esthetic objections
Condom	Very good	3	10	Protects against STD; simple to use; male responsibility; no health risks; no prescription required	Unesthetic to some; requires interruption of sexual activity
Cervical cap	Good	3	18—20	Can wear for weeks at a time; coitus independent; no major health risks	May be difficult to insert; may irritate cervix; not FDA approved
Spermicides	Good	3	18—22	No major health risks; no prescription required	Unesthetic to some; must be properly inserted
Rhythm	Poor to fair	13	20—40	No cost; acceptable to Catholic church	Requires high motivation and periods of abstinence; unreliable
Withdrawal	Fair	9	20—25	No cost or health risks	Reduces sexual pleasure; unreliable
Douching	Poor	?	40+	Inexpensive	Extremely unreliable
Breast-feeding	Poor	15	50+	No cost; acceptable to Catholic church	Extremely unreliable
Vasectomy	Excellent	0.15	0.15	Permanent and highly reliable	Expensive; relatively irreversible; possible complications
Tubal ligation	Excellent	0.04	0.04	Permanent and highly reliable	Expensive; relatively irreversible; possible complications

Source: Based on data from Hatcher et al., 1980, and *Population Reports* research reviews (see Suggested Readings). From W. H. Masters, V. E. Johnson, and R. C. Kolodny, *Human Sexuality.* Boston: Little, Brown, 1982.

Hormonal contraceptives are prescribed in 21- or 28-day packages. In using the 21-day combination pill, one pill is taken for 21 days, starting on day 5 of the menstrual cycle. Within 3 or 4 days of stopping the pills, the woman will begin to menstruate. She begins a new series of pills after 7 days off. The first 5 pills in the 28-day dispenser are placebos; the next 20 are the real pills. Here the woman would start a second dispenser of pills the day after finishing the first. Both the 21- and the 28-day container allow the woman to know at a glance if she has missed a day.

Some women experience side effects when using hormonal contraceptives. These may include nausea, weight gain, mild headaches, decreased menstrual flow, breakthrough bleeding (spotting outside the menstrual period), missed periods, depression, and vaginal infections. The pill tends to increase the alkalinity of the vagina, making it more susceptible to yeast and other infections. Side effects are most likely during the first few months of use. Women having side effects should be told that there are many different forms and strengths of pills. They may be able to take another brand without problems.

Serious side effects that should be reported immediately include severe headache, blurred vision, and severe abdominal, leg, or chest pain. Any of these symptoms indicates the need for medical evaluation; use of the pill should be discontinued.

Use of estrogen hormonal birth control is contraindicated in woman with a history of circulatory problems such as thromboembolic disease (blood clots) because estrogen causes increased tendency toward blood clotting. Women with varicosities are prone to vein inflammation and clot formation (thrombophlebitis). Oral contraceptives are not routinely prescribed to women with a family history of cerebral or cardiovascular accident. Also, women at risk for developing circulatory problems with pill use include those who smoke, are over 35 years of age, are obese, or have high blood pressure, high serum cholesterol levels, or pulmonary disease. Since estrogen tends to interfere with sugar metabolism, women with diabetes mellitus or liver disease, including hepatitis, must be individually evaluated for oral contraceptive use. Birth control pills are contraindicated in women with known or suspected breast or reproductive tract malignancy.

Women on hormonal contraceptives should return for an annual health assessment including a pelvic examination and Pap smear. Many physicians recommend that once a year a woman discontinue taking the pill for 1 month to allow for a month of normal ovarian function. Another method of contraception is needed during this month.

When conception is desired, use of the pill is discontinued. Couples should be advised that it may take 6 to 8 months for pregnancy to occur. Otherwise, they may worry unduly about their ability to conceive. If at any time during use of oral contraceptives a woman suspects that she has become pregnant and plans to continue the pregnancy, she should stop taking the pill.

Taken as prescribed, oral contraceptives are the most effective form of temporary birth control. Theoretically, effectiveness is 100 percent; actual effectiveness is between 97 and 100 percent.

Intrauterine Devices

An intrauterine device (IUD) is a small, nonirritating, flexible device that is inserted into the uterus. It is made of plastic, plastic wrapped with wire, or plastic impregnated with a hormone (progesterone). Interuterine devices come in different shapes, such as loop, spiral, T shape, 7 shape, and ring. They include the Lippes Loop, Saf-T-Coil, Copper 7 (Cu 7), Copper T (TCu), Progestasert-T, and vaginal ring.

Although the manner in which an IUD prevents pregnancy is not fully understood, a number of mechanisms have been suggested. The presence of a foreign substance may increase the motility of the fertilized ovum (zygote) through the fallopian tube so that the fertilized egg reaches the uterus before the endometrial lining is ready for implantation. Or the IUD may change the endometrial lining in a way that prevents implantation or dislodges an implanted fertilized egg. Whatever the mechanism, the IUD results in the egg being discharged with the next menstrual flow.

The procedure for IUD insertion is done in an ambulatory setting, physician's office or family planning clinic (Fig. 21-4). The all-plastic IUD can be left in place as long as desired. IUDs containing copper must be replaced every 3 to 5 years, and the Progestasert-T requires replacement every year because copper and progesterone lose their effectiveness in that time. If pregnancy is desired, the IUD should be removed by a health care professional.

The woman should be informed that she is likely to note uterine cramping and spotting (mid-cycle bleeding) for several weeks following insertion. Her regular menstrual flow is likely to be heavier for 2 to 3 months and may continue heavier than before use of the IUD. She should report continued cramping and spotting because they may lead to spontaneous expulsion of the device. Continued heavier menstrual blood loss may result in anemia.

Every woman using an IUD should be instructed to report fever, lower abdominal pain, foul-smelling vaginal discharge, severe cramping, and unusual or excessive blood loss. These indicate infection and necessitate location and removal of the IUD. Infection must be treated with antibiotics to prevent serious complications in the female reproductive tract. Absence of menses must also be reported, since this may indicate pregnancy. Pregnancy requires removal of the IUD.

Contraindications to the use of intrauterine devices include recent or current pelvic infection (cervicitis, endometritis, salpingitis, pelvic inflammatory disease). IUDs are not the contraceptive of choice for a woman with an abnormality that distorts the shape of the uterine cavity. Also, a woman who has an impaired response to infection or impaired blood coagulation response should not be fitted with an IUD.

Properly fitted and retained, the effectiveness of IUDs is about 95 percent. An IUD cannot be felt during intercourse and can enhance sexual enjoyment because it affords spontaneity.

Barrier Methods

DIAPHRAGM

A diaphragm is a dome-shaped rubber disk with a flexible spring rim around the edge; placed correctly, it covers the cervix. It is covered with a spermicidal cream or jelly before insertion. The diaphragm forms a barrier preventing semen from entering the cervix; the spermicide cream or jelly provides further protection by halting sperm movement. Effectiveness of this method is dependent on the combined use of both diaphragm and spermicidal agent.

The diaphragm is initially prescribed and fitted by a physician or nurse practitioner. The woman should be instructed that certain conditions alter the shape of her cervix and require refitting. These include childbirth,

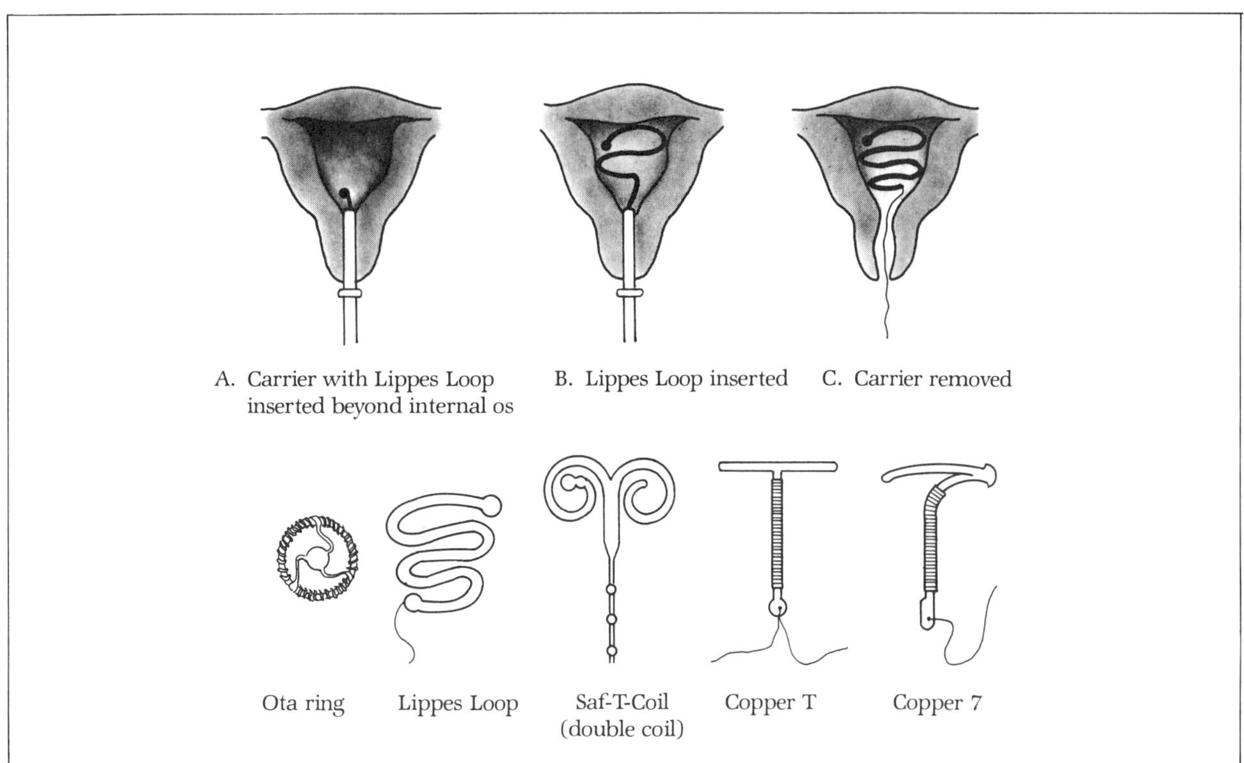

FIGURE 21-4. Insertion of an IUD and several models currently in use.

miscarriage, therapeutic abortion, cervical surgery, and a weight loss or gain of 20 pounds. An adolescent girl may use a diaphragm, but needs to be rechecked as she matures and starts sexual relations.

A woman needs to be instructed and checked in the proper method of insertion and removal of her diaphragm at the time of the initial fitting. Following your directions step by step, have her demonstrate its use. Squeeze about 1 tablespoon of contraceptive jelly from the tube into the dome (concave side) of the diaphragm and spread it inside the cup and around the rim. To insert, use one hand to hold the diaphragm convex side down and press opposite sides of the rim together. Position for insertion is an individual choice—standing with one foot propped up on a chair or toilet, lying on the back (supine), or squatting. Spread the labia with the free hand and insert the folded diaphragm into the vaginal canal, pushing it downward and along the posterior wall of the vagina. Correctly placed, the dome with spermicide inside covers the cervix with the back rim below and behind the cervix and the front rim tucked up behind the pubic bone. The woman can check placement by using her finger to feel the front rim locked behind the pubic bone and the rubber dome covering the cervix (the posterior rim cannot be reached (Fig. 21-5). In place, the diaphragm cannot be felt and causes no discomfort. To remove, place a finger between the anterior rim of the diaphragm and the pubic bone to break the suction. Pull the diaphragm down and out.

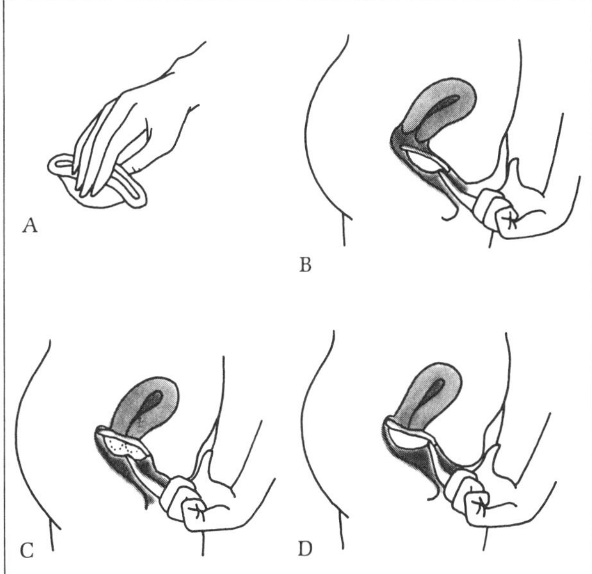

FIGURE 21-5. Proper use of a diaphragm. a) After spermicidal jelly or cream is applied, the rim of the diaphragm is pinched between the fingers and thumb. b) The folded diaphragm is gently inserted into the vagina and pushed downward and backward as far as it will go. c) To check for proper positioning, feel the cervix to be certain it is completely covered by the soft rubber dome of the diaphragm. d) A finger is hooked under the forward rim to remove the diaphragm.

A diaphragm can be inserted up to 6 hours before intercourse because the contraceptive jelly or cream remains active for at least 6 hours. Multiple intercourse requires insertion of additional jelly with a plastic applicator into the vagina; the diaphragm is *not* removed. A diaphragm should remain in place at least 6 hours following intercourse and may be left in place up to 24 hours. A woman must inspect her diaphragm regularly for defects or holes. This can be done by holding it up to the light or filling it with water and watching for a leak. After use, the diaphragm is washed with soap and water, dried, and stored in its case.

A diaphragm cannot be effectively used with a prolapsed uterus (downward displacement) or with uterine retroflexion or antiflexion (posterior or anterior displacement alters cervical placement in relation to the vagina). Insertion of a diaphragm is difficult with poor muscle tone in the vagina or with an intusion on the vagina by a cystocele or rectocele (walls of the vagina are displaced by bladder or bowel). Women with acute cervicitis (inflammation of the cervix) should discontinue use since the rubber and spermicidal jelly may produce additional cervical irritation.

The diaphragm is a safe, highly effective means of birth control if used before every act of intercourse. Its effectiveness rate is about 85—90%. A woman's diaphragm fit should be checked as part of her annual physical examination.

CERVICAL CAP

A cervical cap is a thimble- or bell-shaped cup that looks like a miniature diaphragm with a tall dome. It fits over the cervix and is held in place by suction. It is recommended that a spermicidal jelly or cream be placed inside the cap prior to insertion. Cervical caps are typically made of soft, pliable rubber or plastic in four sizes. A woman must be fitted for one just as she is for a diaphragm (Hastings-Tolsma, 1982).

In theory, the plastic cap can be left in place for up to 4 weeks, the time of the next menstrual period. However, prolonged retention of soft rubber caps produces noticeable vaginal odor after 24 to 36 hours. Thus, it is recommended that the cap be left in place no longer than 24 hours. The cap's main advantage seems to be that it can be used by women who are unable to be fitted for a diaphragm because of poor vaginal muscle tone, cystocele, rectocele, or displaced uterus.

The cervical cap has not been granted Federal Drug Administration (FDA) approval for use in the United States, although it has been widely used in Europe for a number of years. In 1980, the FDA approved the cap for investigational use (Class III); the cap is available only through health providers conducting a FDA-approved study.

CONDOM

A condom (also called a prophylactic, rubber, safe, or skin) is a thin rubber or latex sheath that fits over the erect penis. No prescription is needed for purchase. The condom is one method where responsibility for birth control rests with the man. It is also the only method of birth control that helps prevent the spread of sexually transmitted diseases (STD).

A condom comes rolled in its own foil package (similar to a finger cot but larger in diameter). It is unrolled onto the erect penis with a space left at the end for collecting the semen. Pregnancy is prevented because the ejaculate is deposited in the closed tip of the condom, not the vagina.

To provide effective protection, the condom must be applied prior to penile-vulvar contact since preejaculation fluid may contain sperm. Following ejaculation the penis begins to become flaccid, and the condom must be held in place to prevent leakage as the penis is withdrawn. A new condom must be used for each act of intercourse.

There are no contraindications to use of the condom except for rare rubber sensitivity. Some couples object to its use because it interrupts lovemaking; others incorporate it as part of foreplay with either partner applying the sheath. Some men claim dulled sensation with the use of a condom. Some women report decreased sexual gratification because the man must withdraw promptly following ejaculation.

Use of the condom with each act of intercourse has an efficiency rate of about 90 percent. Combined with the female use of a spermicide it is about 95 to 97 percent effective.

Chemical Methods

The jellies and creams used with the diaphragm are not intended to be used alone. However, there are vaginally inserted spermicidal products intended for use alone. These are sold without prescription as creams, jellies, foams, tablets, and suppositories. Spermicidal agents immobilize sperm in the vagina and change the vaginal pH to a strong acid level, a condition not conducive to sperm survival. Also, by covering the cervical os, they help prevent sperm from entering the uterus.

With an applicator supplied with the product, the woman inserts the spermicidal agent deep in the vagina to the cervical os not more than 1 hour before intercourse (Fig. 21-6). A spermicidal tablet is small and easy to insert. Upon contact with the moisture of vaginal secretions, it dissolves and releases a carbon dioxide foam. A foam-impregnated sponge, when in contact with vaginal secretions acts by creating internal foaming action. Any of these preparations provides protection for only one act of coitus; additional application is required each time.

Spermicidal agents are contraindicated for women with acute cervicitis since their chemical action can cause further irritation of the cervix. There is a degree of vaginal leakage following use; vaginal suppositories with their cocoa-butter and glycerin bases are the most troublesome. Douching (vaginal irrigation) following their use is contraindicated because this decreases the effect of spermicidal action.

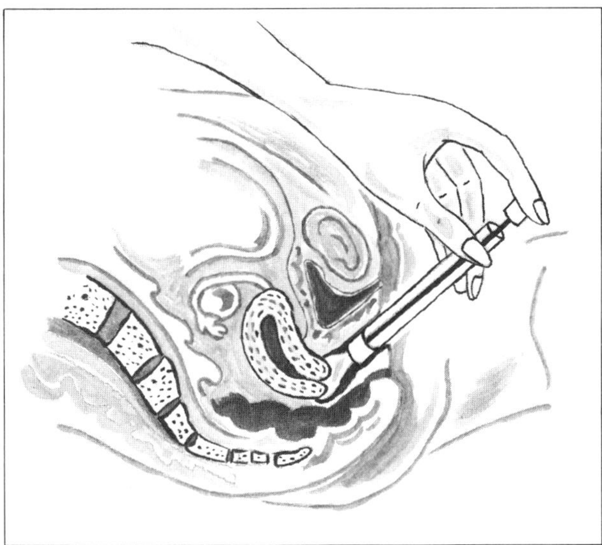

FIGURE 21-6. Vaginal insertion of a spermicidal agent.

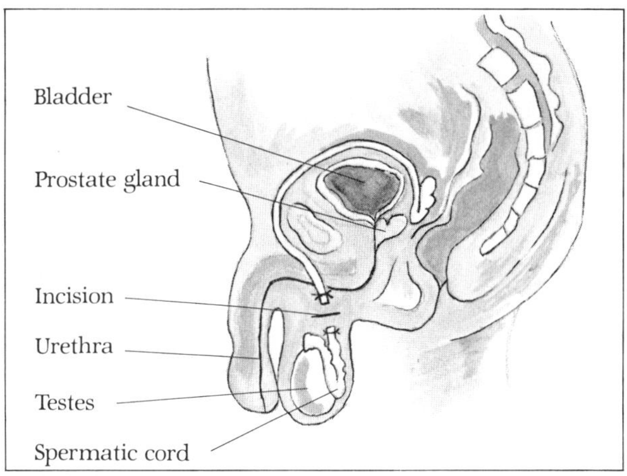

FIGURE 21-7. Placement of a vasectomy.

In family planning, a chemical method is less effective than an oral contraceptive, intrauterine device, diaphragm, or condom. Its effectiveness rate is about 80 percent. It is not the most reliable method for couples who must prevent conception for medical or other reasons.

Sterilization

Both men and women can use sterilization as a permanent means of preventing conception. In sterilization of a male, a small incision is made in each side of the scrotum. The vas deferens at that point is then cut and tied, blocking the passage of spermatozoa. The procedure is called *vasectomy* and can be done under local anesthesia in the physician's office. It is 100 percent effective, although spermatozoa that were present in the vas deferens at the time of surgery may remain viable for as long as 6 months. An additional birth control method should be used until two negative sperm counts confirm sterility (about 8—12 weeks). The man should think of the procedure as irreversible, although techniques of microsurgery make it reversible to a limited extent.

Some men resist the concept of vasectomy because they do not know exactly what the procedure involves. Vasectomy does not interfere with the production of sperm. The testes continue to produce sperm, but the sperm do not pass beyond the severed vas deferens and are absorbed at that point. The man will have full erection and ejaculation capacity. Because he also continues to form seminal fluid, he will ejaculate seminal fluid; it includes no sperm. The incision site for a vasectomy is shown in Figure 21-7.

Following vasectomy, some men form antibodies against sperm. Even if reconstruction of the vas deferens is successful, the sperm they produce do not have good mobility and are incapable of fertilization. Successful reversal of vasectomy procedures is therefore low, about 30 percent.

Sterilization of women generally refers to a surgical procedure called a *tubal ligation*, which occludes the fallopian tubes and prevents passage of the ova into the uterus.

The simplest operation for female sterilization is laparoscopy (Fig. 21-8). Under general or local anesthesia, an incision less than an inch long is made just under the woman's umbilicus. A lighted laparoscope is inserted through the incision. Carbon dioxide is then pumped into the incision to lift the abdominal wall upward out of the line of vision. The surgeon locates the fallopian tubes by viewing the field through the laparoscope. An electrical current is passed through the instrument or a plastic chip is applied to coagulate the tissue of the tube and seal it. The operation is quick; the woman is either kept in the hospital overnight or discharged in a few hours. She may notice abdominal bloating following the procedure for the first 24 hours until the carbon dioxide is absorbed. She may notice sharp diaphragmatic or shoulder pain as some of the carbon dioxide escapes under the diaphragm.

Women need to be informed before the procedure that it will not change their hormone balance and that their menstrual cycle will be unaffected by the procedure. The only change is that the flow of the egg is interrupted and therefore fertilization will not occur.

Although newer procedures can be reversed, tubal ligation should be undertaken only after the woman has decided firmly that she not only does not want children now but also will not want them at some future date.

Abortion

Abortion does not prevent conception, but interrupts an existing pregnancy. In countries such as Russia, Japan, and China, abortion is used as a means of contraception. However, it is not considered a method of birth control in the United States.

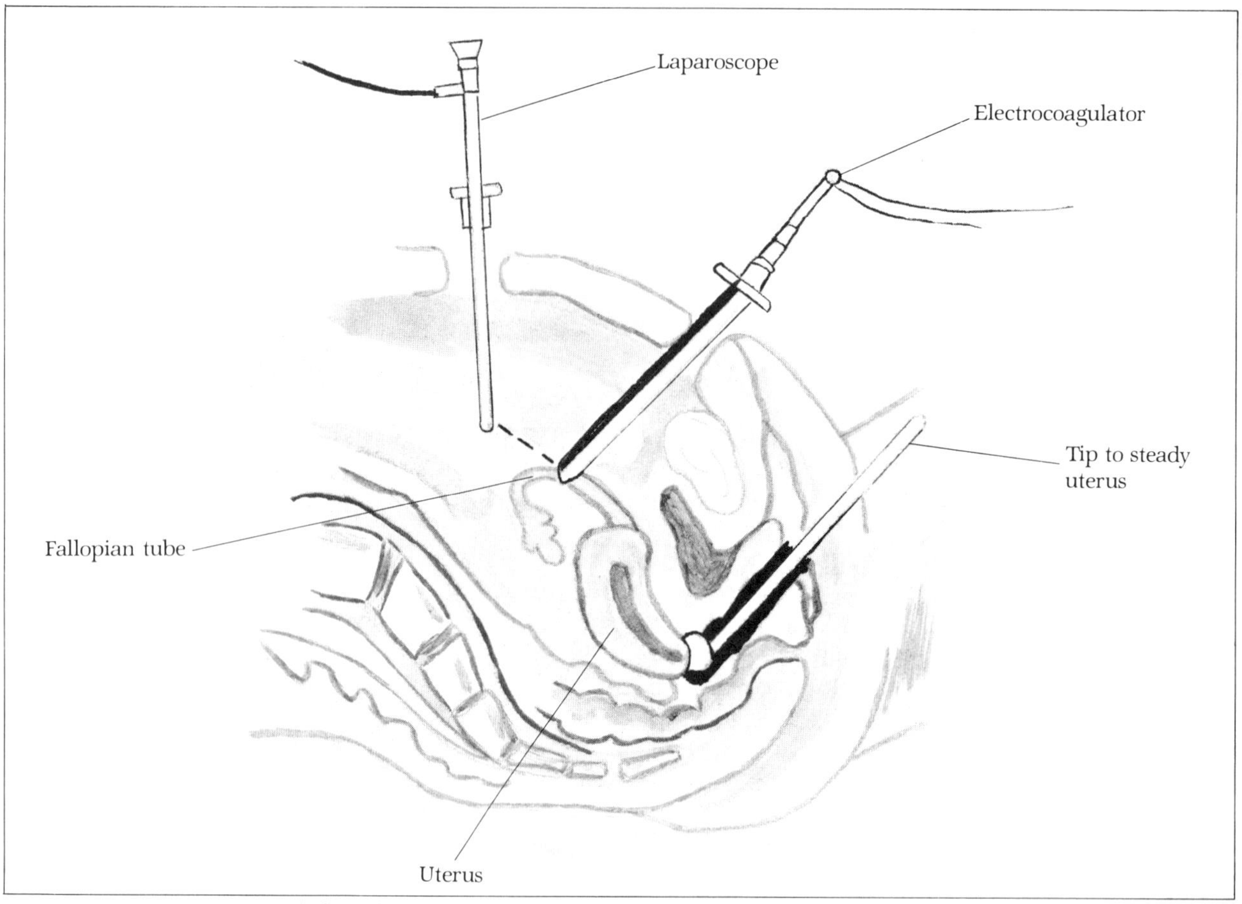

FIGURE 21-8. Laparoscopy for tubal sterilization. The patency of the tubes is destroyed by application of an electrical current. Two small abdominal incisions are used here.

Future Measures of Reproductive Life Planning

The ideal contraceptive—one which is completely safe, reversible, convenient, low in cost, and esthetically pleasing—has yet to be found. Research in the area of female and male fertility continues. In the female, estrogen is responsible for most of the serious as well as minor side effects of oral contraceptives. Low-dose estrogen pills are now available, and a still lower-dose estrogen component is under investigation. Oral progesterone-only pills are in greater use. Long-acting progesterone in the form of a monthly injection continues to be evaluated, as does a slowly dissolving progesterone skin implant. Other hormonal research is investigating a way to block hypothalamic releasing factors, since the hypothalmus signals the pituitary to secrete LH and FSH necessary for ovulation.

The greatest share of research effort and money continues to center on ways to control female fertility through hormonal regulation. Improvements in barrier and spermicide measures are just that: improvements. There is significantly less research in the area of male antifertility hormonal regulation. It is known that testosterone and progesterone inhibit spermatogenesis; however, they act slowly and after use, time is required to return to fertility. Some men equate fertility with potency, which may play a part in research interest and funding. In China, a male oral, nonhormonal antifertility agent has been successfully used for over 10 years.

UTILIZING NURSING PROCESS

Problems of sexuality may not be evident on first meeting a patient as he may not be able to voice a problem in this area of his life until he feels more secure with you. Good follow-through and planning is important with this type of problem because a person may find the courage to discuss it once but then will not be able to do so again. If the problem is ignored or forgotten through a change in caregivers, it will be lost.

Assessment

Sexual assessment is not a routine part of every health assessment. Many people are not able or willing to discuss sexual problems or concerns at a first health assessment. Include sexual assessment, therefore, when it is appropriate—for example, a man following a heart attack is usually concerned about sexual activity; following birth of a baby, most women want to know how soon they can resume sexual relations; or the person offers you a clue from a statement or nonverbal action that this is a concern. Be aware that persons having surgery on their reproductive organs (also urinary tract surgery, in men) will always have concerns, voiced or not.

Health History

The format for a sexual history is shown in Chap. 23 with a comprehensive health status assessment base. Clues that a person may want more information about a sexual concern or that you need to explore this area in depth are often subtle (I'm not the man I used to be; I guess marriage isn't for everybody; Are there sometimes funny effects from this medicine I'm taking?). Telling a seemingly inappropriate sexual joke may be a verbal clue. Nonverbal clues that suggest a person may have some discomfort or a problem with sexuality are extreme modesty, obvious embarrassment at a televised sanitary napkin or douche commercial, or obvious embarrassment in response to a question about voiding or perineal pain or stitches.

Interviewing to obtain a sexual history takes practice and conviction that exploring sexual questions is as important for health as exploring less emotionally involved ones of dietary intake or activity level. Frank admission that you do not understand words that a person is using helps communication; frank admission that you are not always at your best when exploring this facet of a person's life also aids communication because it lets the patient know that his difficulty explaining it is a common reaction.

Physical Assessment

Any change in physical appearance can intensify or create a sexual problem. Observe for changes such as excessive loss or excessive gain in weight, a disfiguring scar from surgery or accident, hair loss such as occurs with chemotherapy, surgery on reproductive organs, inflammation or infection of reproductive organs, chronic fatigue or pain, spinal cord injury (which limits sensation reception and function of reproductive organs), and the presence of a retention catheter.

Observe for normal distribution of body hair (hair on face, arms, axilla, chest, abdomen, and diamond-shaped pubic hair in men; hair on axilla, arms, and triangle-shaped pubic hair in women). Following menopause, women may develop some facial hair owing to less estrogen. Observe for normal genital and breast development. Genital and breast development in adolescents is divided into Tanner stages. Remember that increase in breast size occurs as a normal phenomenon in boys just before puberty. This is most apparent in overweight boys and a concern to them until they receive an explanation that it is normal.

Analysis

The Fourth National Conference on Classification of Nursing Diagnoses accepted two diagnoses in reference to sexual functioning: sexual dysfunction and rape trauma syndrome. The defining characteristics of these diagnoses are given in Appendix C. Another approved nursing diagnosis that could be adapted to a sexual problem is self-concept, disturbance in. In addition to officially approved diagnoses, a nursing diagnosis related to sexuality might be a major problem such as loss of sexual identity related to recent surgery. Analysis to determine whether a sexual need exists should always be considered in long-term illness and in any illness that results in a change of physical appearance or self-esteem.

Planning

Planning for strengthening a person's sexual identity or sexual role behavior may be the planning of interventions that strengthen maleness or femaleness. A male who states men are assertive and women passive needs built into his care plan opportunities for decision making and self-care; a woman who views a woman as one who is well groomed and has her hair washed every day needs time structured for these activities at the same priority level as deep breathing exercises. Planning for these activities must be carefully structured because they are activities that are easy for a busy health provider to omit (see QRS 21-4).

Implementation

Many nursing interventions that are physical in nature—such as stroking, comforting, and needs gratification—are also sexual in nature. Be aware that there are times when holding a person's hand is not appropriate because the person will interpret the gesture not as a nurturing one but as a sexual one. Be aware that in the course of intimate care such as urinary catheterization, bathing, and suppository insertion, you can evoke sexual responses. Thinking of these reactions as healthy responses to intimate interventions allows you to keep them in perspective and not overread or underread their importance.

☐ QUICK REFERENCE STOP 21-4: COMMUNITY CONSIDERATIONS

Sexual expression or relationships may be a topic that a person thought about during a health care facility stay but never felt comfortable asking about or assumed would work out after he returned home. After he returns home, he discovers that it is his biggest concern because all his other problems have been solved. Because sexual needs are part of basic human needs, recognize when this is a problem and help people to ask these questions at health assessments or return health care appointments. In some instances, the nurse may need to take the initiative in addressing sexual concerns.

People who are insecure about their sexual identity may demonstrate acting out or attention-getting behavior such as allowing a patient gown to slip and a woman to expose her breasts or a man his genitals. This is most noticeable in adolescents who have questions about whether their development is progressing normally or not. For example, a girl who has one breast slightly larger than the other (a normal development) might want to be certain that you noticed this in her; a boy who has less penis development than his friends might want to make you aware of what he perceives as delayed development. Other, sometimes less easy to accept acting out mannerisms are fondling of your body by a patient as you assist him into a sitting position or another position in bed. The first type of acting out is normal behavior; the second type may or may not be because it is socially unacceptable. Set limits with such behavior to make the situation acceptable for you; at the same time, recognize the person's extreme need to have help with this phase of his life.

People recovering from illnesses that have affected them in some way (such as arthritis that makes it painful for a woman to lie supine, or respiratory difficulty that leaves a man short of breath on exertion) may ask you about alternate coital positions from those to which they were accustomed or alternate methods of sexual expression such as oral-genital stimulation or anal intercourse. These questions must be answered in the light of the person's limitations and disability but often the person is seeking basic approval that it is all right to be concerned with such things. With your reply showing that concern is all right, he can then ask his physician about specific physical limitations.

Evaluation

How a person feels about himself has a great deal to do with how quickly he recovers from illness, how quickly he is ready to begin self-care following illness, or even how well motivated he is to do those things necessary to remain well. Evaluating whether goals related to sexuality were achieved is important in being certain that the person will be able to accomplish activities in other phases of his life that depend on his being sure of his sexuality or sexual role.

NURSING CARE PLAN

Henry is a 22-year-old male you see in an ambulatory orthopedic clinic. He was to have been admitted to the hospital 2 months ago for revision of scar tissue on his arm but he cancelled his admission the day before surgery. He again cancelled surgery the same way a month ago.

The following is a problem-oriented nursing note from his clinic visit.

Problem: Noncompliance with health care projections.

S. Patient states that he is a practicing homosexual. Reluctant to be hospitalized because he worries his lover will not be able to visit morning of surgery. Also concerned that he may have STD because of high incidence of disease among sexual contacts at gay bar he frequents. Concerned that presence of infection at time of surgery will lessen chances of surviving surgery.

O. No pain or frequency on urination; no urethral discharge. No ulcerations or other lesions present on penis or scrotum. Culture for GC (gonorrhea) and VDRL (syphillis) taken.

A. Patient with anxiety of surgery related to fear of lack of support person and inadequate knowledge of sexually transmitted diseases.

Goal: Patient to receive adequate support during surgery interval.

Criteria: Support person will be allowed to visit in place of family member.

Goal: Patient to be more knowledgeable of sexually transmitted diseases in 2 days time.

Criteria: Patient to be able to cite signs and symptoms and spread of herpes, gonorrhea, and syphillis.

P. 1. Patient to ask clinic-hospital nursing coordinator to clear regulations to allow for visitor of choice day of surgery.
2. Patient has clinic number for back-up if unable to obtain satisfaction by first route.
3. Given pamphlet on sexually transmitted diseases; and signs and symptoms reviewed with him.
4. To return in 2 days for culture reports and presurgery admission blood work. To review signs and symptoms of STD and barrier means of prevention with him at that time.
5. Following surgery and before discharge, nurse clinician alerted to discuss more positive means of approaching problem solving than he currently uses (withdrawing from situation).

SUGGESTED READINGS

Amonker, R. G. What do teens know about the facts of life? *J. Sch. Health* 50:527, 1980.

Ayvazian, A., Contraceptive choices of female university students. *J.O.G.N. Nurs.* 10(6):426, 1981.

Barnard, M., et al. *Human Sexuality for Health Professionals.* Philadelphia: Saunders, 1978.

Bernstein, A. How children learn about sex and birth. *Psychol. Today* 9:31, 1976.

Brick, P. Sex and society: Teaching the connection. *J. Sch. Health* 51:226, 1981.

Burgess, A. W., et al. Youth prostitution. *Am. J. Nurs.* 82:832, 1982.

Calderone, M. S. Children and parents as sexual people. *Health Educ.* 13(6):27, 1982.

Delia, J. E. Contraception for adolescent girls. *Consultant* 21:63, 1981.

Driver, J., et al. Elders and sexuality. *J. Nurs. Care* 15(2):8, 1982.

Dryfoos, J. G. Contraceptive use, pregnancy intentions and pregnancy outcomes among U.S. women. *Fam. Plan. Perspect.* 14:81, 1982.

Falk, G., and U. Falk. Sexuality and the aged. *Nurs. Outlook* 28:51, 1980.
Federman, D. D. Impotence: Etiology and management. *Hosp. Pract.* 82:17:155.
Fiscella, K. Relationship of weight change to required size of vaginal diaphragm. *Nurse Pract.* 7(7):21, 1982.
Fisher, S. G. The sexual knowledge and attitudes of professional nurses caring for oncology patients. *Cancer Nurs.* 6(1):55, 1983.
Godow, A. G. *Human Sexuality.* St. Louis: Mosby, 1982.
Griggs, W. Sex and the elderly. *Am. J. Nurs.* 78:1352, 1978.
Hampton, P. J. Coping with the male patient's sexuality. *Nurs. Forum* 18:304, 1979.
Hastings-Tolsma, M. T. The cervical cap: A barrier contraceptive. *MCN* 7:382, 1982.
Hatcher, R. A., et al. *Contraceptive Technology 1980—1981* (10th ed). New York: Irving, 1980.
Heiman, J., and J. LoPiccolo. *Becoming Orgasmic: A Sexual Growth Program for Women.* Englewood Cliffs: Prentice-Hall, 1976.
Hite, S. *The Hite Report.* New York: Macmillan, 1976.
Hogan, R. M., et al. *Human Sexuality: A Nursing Perspective.* New York: Appleton-Century-Crofts, 1980.
Hyde, J. S. *Understanding Human Sexuality.* New York: McGraw-Hill, 1979.
Kinsey, A., et al. *Sexual Behavior in the Human Female.* Philadelphia: Saunders, 1953.
Kolodny, R. C., et al. *Textbook of Human Sexuality for Nurses.* Boston: Little, Brown, 1979.
Krozy, R. Becoming comfortable with sexual assessment. *Am. J. Nurs.* 78:1036, 1978.
Lion, E. N. (Ed). *Human Sexuality in Nursing Process.* New York: Wiley, 1982.
LoPiccolo, J., and L. LoPiccolo (Eds). *Handbook of Sex Therapy.* New York: Plenum, 1978.
Luria, Z., and M. Rose. *Psychology of Human Sexuality.* New York: Wiley, 1979.
Masters, W. H., and V. E. Johnson. *Human Sexual Response.* Boston: Little, Brown, 1966.
Masters, W. H., and V. E. Johnson. *Human Sexual Inadequacy.* Boston: Little, Brown, 1970.
Mims, F. *Sexuality: A Nursing Perspective.* New York: McGraw-Hill, 1980.
Mims, F. H. Sexual stress: Coping and adaptation. *Nurs. Clin. North Am.* 17(3):395, 1982.
Murray, B. L., and L. J. Wilcox. Testicular self-examination. *Am. J. Nurs.* 78:2075, 1978.
Perry, J. D., and Whipple, B. The Varieties of Female Orgasm and Female Ejaculation. SEICUS report. May—July, 1981*f*.
Phipps, W. J., B. C. Long, and N. F. Woods. *Medical-Surgical Nursing: Concepts and Clinical Practice* (2nd ed.). St. Louis: Mosby, 1983.
Renshaw, D. C. Adolescent sexuality: How to deal with it effectively. *Consultant* 18:72, 1978.
Robinault, I. P. *Sex, Society and the Disabled.* Hagerstown, Md.: Harper & Row, 1978.
Stanford, D. All about sex . . . after middle age. *Am. J. Nurs.* 77:608, 1977.
Stephens, G. J. The creative contraries: A theory of sexuality. *Am. J. Nurs.* 78:70, 1978.
Stockard, S. Caring for the sexually aggressive patient; you don't have to blush and bear it. *Nursing* (Horsham) 11:114, 1981.
Symposium on sexuality and nursing practice. *Nurs. Clin. North Am.* 17(3):343, 1982.
Taylor, R. B. Physical orgins of sexual dysfunction. *Female Patient* 5:61, 1980.
Trimmer, E. When patients ask about the latest and safest oral contraceptive. *Midwife Health Visit Community Nurse* 18(11):484, 1982.
Watts, R. Dimensions of sexual health. *Am. J. Nurs.* 79:1568, 1980.
Weinberg, J. *Sexuality, Human Needs and Nursing.* Philadelphia: Saunders, 1982.
Woods, N. F. *Human Sexuality in Health and Illness.* St. Louis: Mosby, 1979.
Zelnik, M., and F. K. Shah. First intercourse among young Americans. *Fam. Plan. Perspect.* 15(2):64, 1983.
Zilbergeld, B. *Male Sexuality: A Guide to Sexual Fulfillment.* Boston: Little, Brown, 1978.

QUESTIONS FOR REVIEW

1. Susan is a child you care for. When making plans of care for her, at what age would you expect a child to be able to differentiate males from females?
   a. 1 year.
   b. 2 years.
   c. 5 years.
   d. 7 years.

2. Susan's mother asks you about childhood masturbation. Which of the following statements is true concerning masturbation?
   a. It leads to early loss of fertility.
   b. It is practiced by individuals of all ages.
   c. It is less satisfying to women than men.
   d. It is almost exclusively a practice of preschool children.

3. Mr. Jones is a patient whom you care for. In assessing Mr. Jones for sexual gender, which of the following points would you assess:
   a. Temperament.
   b. Hair distribution.
   c. Ability to love.
   d. Stability in work experiences.

4. Mr. Jones' sexual role refers to:
   a. His chromosomal inheritance.
   b. Sex he sees himself as being.
   c. His sexual identity.
   d. His demonstrated sexual behaviors.

5. Mr. Jones tells you he is a practicing homosexual. Which of the statements below is most apt to be true of him?
   a. He is also a transvestite.
   b. He will cry readily under stress.
   c. He also enjoys bisexual relationships.
   d. He is capable of satisfying sexual relationships.

6. In relation to Mr. Jones' sexual feelings and activities, which of the following questions would *not* be assessed?
   a. Is the behavior voluntary?
   b. Does the behavior enhance the self-esteem of both partners?
   c. Does the behavior offer pleasure and gratification?
   d. Is the behavior normal?

7. Mrs. Smith is another patient whom you care for. She is concerned because she does not regularly achieve orgasm. Orgasm or the third stage of a sexual response can be described as:
   a. Extreme pelvic vasocongestion.
   b. Increased vital sign response.
   c. Contraction of pelvic muscles.
   d. Responses preceding erection.

8. Orgasm results mainly from:
   a. Penile penetration.
   b. Clitoral stimulation.
   c. Uterine stimulation.
   d. Sensory arousal.

9. In the patients you care for, in which of the following would you most likely assess concerns about sexual functioning?
   a. Adolescent male following leg surgery.
   b. Young adult woman following childbirth.
   c. Middle-aged man following a heart attack.
   d. Older man with chronic back pain.

10. The following patients are seen at a family planning clinic. Ms. Green had an intrauterine device (IUD) inserted 1 month ago. She calls the clinic and reports that she has had some cramping since insertion and that her present menstrual flow is heavy. She should be advised to:
    a. Come to the clinic as soon as possible.
    b. Consider this normal as her IUD has been newly inserted.
    c. Use an additional method of birth control.
    d. Change her method of birth control.

11. Mrs. Lee visits the clinic to request a prescription for birth control pills. Assessment of which of the following would indicate that hornomal contraception would *not* be the method of choice for Mrs. Lee?
    a. Thirty years of age.
    b. Irregular menstrual cycles.
    c. Varicose veins.
    d. History of cervical infections.

12. Mrs. Brown uses a diaphragm as a method of family planning. She should be instructed to return to clinic to have her diaphragm fit checked under all of the following occurrences *except*:
    a. Cervical infection.
    b. Miscarriage.
    c. Weight change of 20 pounds.
    d. Childbirth.

22. STIMULATION TO PROMOTE DEVELOPMENT

OBJECTIVES

Upon mastery of the material in this chapter, you should be able to:

1. Describe the role of stimulation in everyday life.
2. Describe the effect of sensory deprivation and sensory overload.
3. Using the nursing process, describe ways to increase stimulation (sensory, cognitive, social, or physical) for people in different age groups.
4. Using the nursing process, describe ways to decrease sensory overload by decreasing stimulation.

TERMS

The terms important for an understanding of this chapter are shown below and defined in the glossary:

cognitive stimulation
physical stimulation
response
sensory deprivation
sensory overload
sensory stimulation
social stimulation
stimulation
stimulus

The average person is in constant interaction with both internal environment (body) and external environment (surroundings) by means of the five senses and the central nervous system. Thus, a person can respond to change in environment and, by so doing, meet basic needs. In order for a person to perceive and process stimuli correctly, basic orienting receptors must be intact and the central nervous system must then process the information accurately.

A person orients himself in space through the function of the vestibular mechanism in the inner ear and proprioception (ability to discern the shape of objects, a touch sensation). These functions enable a person to sense if he is upright or not, to maintain balance, and to make smooth, effortless motions against the force of gravity.

A person also orients himself by the use of touch to determine the size, consistency, and surface of objects around him and by the use of visual, auditory, and taste perceptions. For example, auditory receptors perceive not only that a sound is present but also how far the sound source is away.

Sensory stimuli pass through peripheral nerve receptors to the spinal cord. If the stimulus is acute (the person's hand is touching a flame) a synapse at the spinal cord level immediately evokes a motion response that causes motion action (the person jerks his hand back from the flame). The response continues past the synapse to the cerebral center where the stimuli is interpreted (the hand hurts because it has been burnt). Almost everyone has had an experience of having an incoming stimuli misinterpreted (expecting to feel a hot surface, you feel it as hot even though in reality it is cold; you interpret the sound of rustling leaves against the pavement of a dark alley as footsteps when it is rustling leaves). These momentary misinterpretations of stimuli are frightening. People who steadily misinterpret incoming perceptions due to a specific illness or to a sensory overload experience a very frightening world.

RESPONSE TO STIMULI

A *stimulus* is a factor that will be perceived by the sensory receptors. *Stimulation* is the inciting of a person to mental or physical activity through sensory reception and central nervous system interpretation of a stimulus. The stimulus might be social or psychological, such as acquiring a new job or reading a new novel; it might be sensory, such as a loud voice or a flash of light; it might be physical, such as an oncoming car. The response to the stimulus may be emotional (a feeling of pleasure or fright), cognitive (thoughtful), or motor (moving toward or away from the stimulus).

In order to develop and function mentally as well as physically, a person must have stimulation every day, just as he needs food and water every day. He must not be submitted to an overload of stimulation. It is necessary to plan for stimulation needs as part of patient care along with rest, sleep, and adequate nutrition.

A person receiving either too little or too much stimulation will experience sensory alteration and almost the same symptoms: confusion, apathy, loss of time orientation, and extreme fatigue. In adjusting stimulation levels, all four types of stimulation must be considered: sensory, cognitive, social, and physical.

Sensory Stimulation

Sensory stimulation is receiving stimulation through one of the five basic senses—sight (visual), hearing (auditory), touch (tactile), taste (gustatory), and smell (olfactory)—or from muscle (kinetic) or body organs (visceral). Reception of stimulation from the basic senses is important for safety (seeing a red light, hearing a train whistle) and pleasure (smelling perfume or food, tasting a chocolate dessert, hearing music). Kinesthetic sensation allows a person to orient himself in space (you can sense whether you are standing upright or lying down and where your hands and feet are at any given time). Losing this orienting process—as in some neurological or inner ear diseases, or through lack of input—is an extremely frightening and confusing feeling. Body organ (visceral) sensations are important in alerting a person to overdistention of a body organ (the bladder is full, the stomach is distended) by pain transmission. Thus, like the basic senses, the signal system is a protective one.

The importance of sensory stimulation is shown when one of the senses is lost. For example, children who have difficulty seeing may be seen poking their eyes or fluttering their fingers in front of their eyes as if they are trying to evoke all the visual stimulation they can (as if seeing is not just something that allows you to see where you are going but is something that offers an inner sense of enjoyment or accomplishment). When one sense is lost, others become more acute to compensate or fill the need for greater stimulation.

Interferences with sensory stimulation such as blurring of vision, impaired taste, or loss of sensitivity to touch or smell often accompany neurological impairments. People with such disorders need careful assessment for stimulation needs. Over a period of time, repetitious sounds are no longer heard, which means the monotonous sounds of an intensive care unit that at first lead to sensory overload can shortly lead to sensory deprivation. Remember this when planning care; what you hear as sound a patient may not hear at all.

As a person becomes unconscious, the last sense lost is hearing; as consciousness returns, hearing is the first sense regained. This means that many people who cannot speak to you are able to hear and appreciate instructions and the sound of voices; they can be just as deprived without this form of stimulation as those who can tell you their feelings. Touch is a second important sensory stimulation for unconscious persons; they appear to quiet readily to a soothing touch as if they also are able to interpret this action.

Cognitive Stimulation

Cognitive stimulation is the interest or excitement of thought processes. A puzzle, a murder mystery, or a riddle is interesting because it gives pleasure by cognitive stimulation (Fig. 22-1). A class where you are called upon to provide answers or think through a problem rather than listen to a lecture is on the whole a more stimulating class because it requires the mind to work at a different level of thought.

After an illness such as a stroke, people miss cognitive stimulation and reacting to it. They often state as their chief loss, not the inability to move the right arm, but the inability to think so clearly or solve problems so quickly as before illness.

Social Stimulation

Social stimulation is the special stimulation that comes from interaction with other people. It is a combination of sensory stimulation (hearing amusing stories, seeing familiar faces) and cognitive stimulation (thinking about what is said or not said) but goes beyond both to a level of satisfaction or enjoyment not able to be achieved in any other way.

Illness may restrict social interaction if hospitalization or a long period of rest at home is required. Such restriction may be what makes an illness most difficult to bear.

Physical Stimulation

Stimulation that leads to physical activity may be environmental, such as cold that makes you walk quickly; pleasurable, such as learning to ski; or protective, such

FIGURE 22-1. Reading for enjoyment is a form of cognitive stimulation.

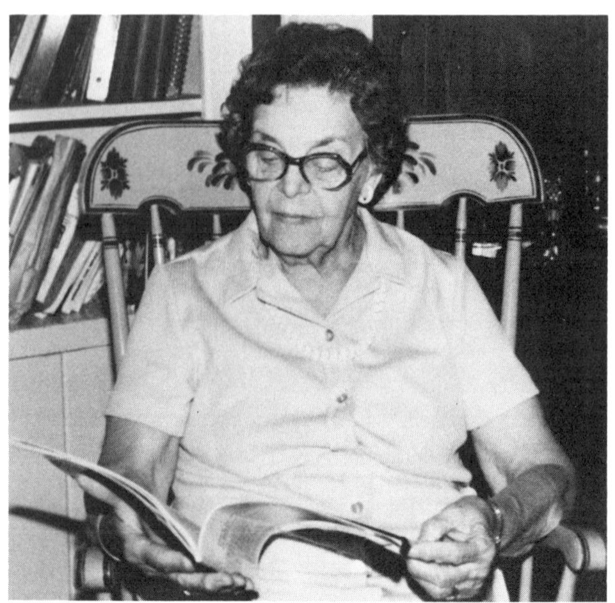

as moving away from danger. Physical activity increases heart rate and body metabolism; it helps to reduce stress and often, although it may leave the person physically tired, it also leaves him pleasantly relaxed. People say, "I feel good after a hard day's work."

SENSORY DEPRIVATION

Sensory deprivation is the condition of being deprived or lacking adequate sensory, social, physical, or cognitive stimulation. People with this condition tend to lose the ability to think logically and may have difficulty orienting to time and space, concentrating on a given task, or even hallucinating (seeing or hearing things not actually there). Space and time disorientation (e.g., unable to remember the day of the week) may be largely the result of sensory deprivation accompanying aging and not of aging in itself. Acute sensory deprivation may remove the ability to function effectively.

Whether sensory deprivation exists or not is a factor to be assessed with all patients. In particular, it needs to be assessed for people in the following circumstances.

Premature (Low-Birth-Weight) Infants. Premature infants formerly were placed in Isolettes for warmth and easy observation. They were fed and cared for appropriately, but touched only as necessary for basic care so that they would not become fatigued and their immature body systems overtaxed.

Hasselmeyer (1961), a nurse researcher, found that all infants, even those born before their estimated birth date, enjoy and need normal stimulation, especially touch. Premature infants handled, stroked, and cuddled in the way the average mother would handle an infant gain weight faster than those who are isolated. Therefore, parents are urged to visit frequently and to touch, talk or sing to, cuddle, and hold their premature infants in order to provide a stimulating atmosphere. If parents cannot fulfill this function (often very ill newborns are hospitalized in a tertiary center a long distance from their home), providing stimulation by stroking and talking becomes the nurse's responsibility.

Children Separated from Their Parents. Children at any age (most noticeably those under 5 years) interact at a deeper level with their parents than with other people around them. When separated from parents, their level of cognitive interaction falls markedly. Infants totally separated from their mothers may lose weight, test lower on IQ scores, and perform fewer motor functions. This syndrome of symptoms is termed *maternal deprivation.* It can result from death or illness of the parent, imprisonment, or divorce. When a child is hospitalized, maternal deprivation always occurs to some extent because the child is separated from the parent. Providing stimulation as a substitute parent is an important nursing responsibility.

Children with a Poor Parent-Child Relationship. Children who have a poor or scanty level of interaction with their parents receive less than normal cognitive stimulation. If this happens to a preschool child, he shows the same symptoms of maternal deprivation as the child whose parent is not actually present. Such *failure-to-thrive children* need a warm, reassuring relationship and cognitive stimulation in order to develop normally.

Adolescents who are having a particularly difficult time relating to their parents manifest a hunger to relate with other adults to fulfill the need for interaction. They may discuss issues with nurses that they can no longer discuss with their own parents.

People on Bed Rest. People on bed rest are unable to secure materials for cognitive stimulation by themselves or to participate in physical stimulation except to a limited degree. A room where walls and windows offer no visual appeal and an air conditioner provides the only sound will give them little sensory stimulation. If no one comes into the room, they can develop social deprivation. Watching television, a common activity for people on bed rest, provides little cognitive stimulation after the first 24 hours since the average television program is aimed at a fourth-grade level. When the novelty is gone, it provides no more cognitive stimulation than a fourth-grade reader.

Simply placing a patient in a wheelchair will not promote stimulation—that act alone does not alter level of stimulation (Fig. 22-2).

Occasionally, a person is placed on bed rest in order to reduce stimulation around him (to rest his heart completely, for example) but the average person is on bed rest only to inactivate one part of the body, such as a fractured bone. Other stimulation must be provided so the person can maintain physical bed rest (without this, he feels bored, and irritable, thrashing and turning instead of lying still). This is particularly true in children. The average mother is aware that her child will receive more rest on the living room couch where he can participate in the family's activities than in a distant bedroom where he constantly calls out for attention or interaction. This principle applies to hospitalized children. A toddler may rest better in his mother's lap in a chair than in bed.

People in Isolation. People who are isolated due to the possibility of contagious illness may experience severe sensory deprivation if everyone who enters the room must gown and mask to enter and if the number of entrances is kept to a minimum. If gloves are part of precautions, the person can experience a significant loss of skin-to-skin contact. Isolation technique is discussed in Chap. 28 (Asepsis). Careful planning must be done to be certain that a person in isolation is not psychologically isolated and that every possible measure to main-

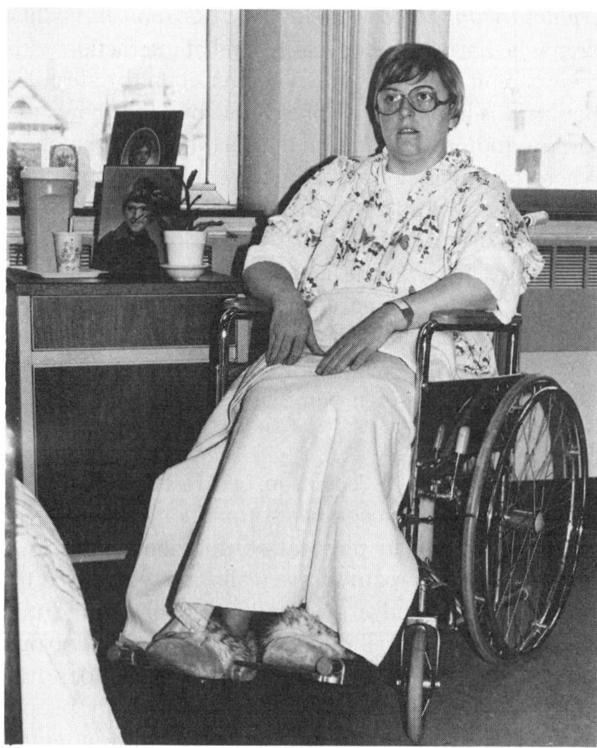

A

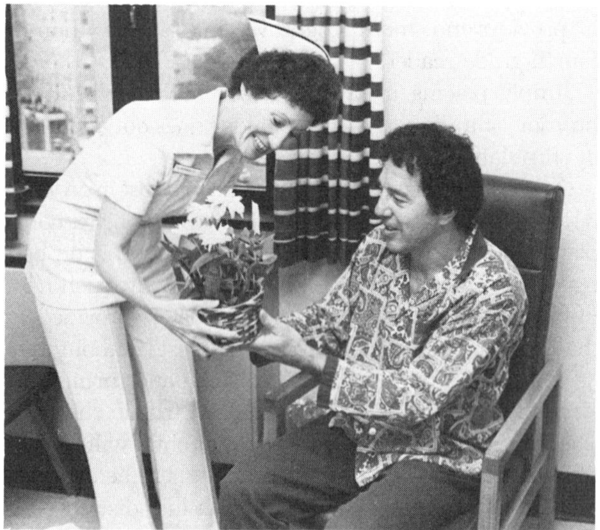

B

FIGURE 22-2. Stimulation may come in many forms. A. To increase stimulation for this woman, wheel her to the day room; provide newpapers and magazines. B. Flowers may be just the thing to brighten any patient's day and provide needed stimulation.

tain sensory, social, physical, and cognitive stimulation is carried out.

People with Sensory Interferences. People with hearing or visual deficits are prone to sensory deprivation. People with forms of sensory nerve loss may lose their sense of touch, taste, or proprioception. If after losing these forms of perception, the person also draws back from interaction with people (aware his loss has become a problem), he may develop social and cognitive stimulation deprivation.

☐ QUICK REFERENCE STOP 22-1: PHARMACOLOGY

Sedatives are medication to induce rest; tranquilizers are to induce relaxation. A person who is receiving a drug such as a sedative or tranquilizer may not possess his usual awareness of stimulation around him and thus suffer from sensory deprivation. Assess this carefully with people on such drugs.

Some people on such medication, unable to process all the stimulation they are receiving, may interpret ordinary stimulation as sensory overload and need their environment controlled by drawn curtains or reduced conversation. Common sedatives and tranquilizers are summarized in Chap. 29.

People with Medication to Reduce Sensory Input. A sedative is a medication to induce rest; a tranquilizer, to induce relaxation. People receiving these medications may be less aware of stimulating factors in their environment. In order not to suffer sensory deprivation, they need definite orientation measures, such as always mentioning the day of the week and the time of the day. At the same time, they may need overly stimulating factors, such as many visitors, reduced so that perceptions can be interpreted clearly and they can rest or relax. See Quick Reference Stop 22-1 for a summary of the use of sedatives and tranquilizers.

Older Adults. Older adults may suffer greater sensory deprivation than younger people if they have a degree of visual, auditory, or taste loss. In health care facilities where large numbers of older adults are cared for, recreation or group therapists are generally employed to reduce problems of sensory deprivation. Nursing care must be coordinated with stimulation programs.

LIFE SPAN CONCEPTS AND STIMULATION

Needs for and sources of stimulation differ over the age continuum.

The Infant

Infants experience the world around them almost entirely by the use of their senses. During the first year infants most enjoy toys that appeal to the senses: stuffed animals of soft velvet or rippled corduroy; mobiles that move and play music; and objects to put in the mouth.

It is obvious how much a baby uses his senses every day, but less obviously, people depend on their senses for exploration and stimulation throughout life.

Senses are well developed at birth. A newborn sees (he will follow an object immediately to the midline of his vision), hears (sound may be slightly muffled for the first hour after birth until fluid in the middle ear drains), responds to touch (a newborn comforts readily by stroking), and can distinguish sweet from bitter tastes and pleasant and noxious odors.

The object that an infant focuses on longest is his mother's face. Thus, having his mother actively holding and talking to him is his best form of visual stimulation. In addition, every infant should have a mobile over his crib for increased visual appeal; his crib should be positioned so that he can see people walking by his door or so that he can see the activity outside his window.

If no mobiles are available, create one from a wire coat hanger, string, or strips of adhesive tape and objects that will suspend easily and are light enough to move from motion of the crib or an air current (e.g., colored paper, cotton balls, colored tongue blades, inflated rubber gloves). Hang the mobile high enough for the infant to see but not reach these potentially dangerous objects. Mothers can create mobiles at home from photographs cut from magazines, sections of egg cartons, or flowers made from tissue. In a health care setting, preparing a mobile for an infant's crib should be part of admission responsibility or routine.

Infants enjoy soft sounds. Always talk quietly when caring for an infant so that he receives stimulation from your voice. In the second half of the first year, infants enjoy mimicking sounds; saying a sound the child has mastered, such as *da-da*, so he'll repeat it is both auditory and cognitive stimulation. At this age infants also enjoy the sound of a music box or record played again and again (both an auditory sensory experience and a reassuring one). Do not feel foolish talking to infants even when you are sure they cannot understand what you are saying ("the next thing I'm going to do is to get some dinner for you and then I'm going to get your medicine for you"). It is the sound of your voice, not the content of your words, that is important.

Infants do not necessarily enjoy the taste of a new food and usually resist new flavors too different from those they are used to. Therefore, though food should have some variety, diet is not the best area in which to introduce stimulating activities to a sick infant.

Infants respond intensely to touch. They quiet rapidly at a gentle touch and grow disturbed at a less than gentle touch. Take time every day when caring for an infant to rock and hold him. Also, be sure that his mother is given the opportunity to do this. Many mothers lose confidence in themselves as mothers when their child becomes ill, feeling they should have prevented this illness. In this state of lowered self-esteem, they may be reluctant to assert themselves and do the things for their child they would have done before he became ill, such as brush away a tear or pick him up to comfort him. If restraints or equipment such as intravenous fluid lines are in place, the average parent is reluctant to touch a child—knowing it hurt the child to have the intravenous line started, they do not want to do anything to dislodge it. You need to suggest that parents pick up children (Why don't you sit in the rocking chair and I'll hand him to you?) or to provide a role model of mothering behaviors while the child is ill. As the child's health improves and the mother's confidence returns, you need to do this less.

At about 3 months of age, infants begin to learn the concept of permanence (that although people may appear in different clothing, they are the same people). By 4 months of age, an infant will register disapproval when you leave him and recognize you when you return if the absence is short. By 10 months of age, the infant is aware that appearances may change but basic things stay the same and he is ready for peekaboo (you disappear, you come back or do not really change). If he pushes an object off the tray of his high chair, he will search for it or expect you to replace it for him. This is not merely play, therefore, but cognitive stimulation (theory testing) for him.

An infant practices the motor skill he is currently learning (turning, sitting, walking) over and over until he has it mastered. Learning basic skills of ambulation appears to be almost driven behavior, so when an infant is deprived of the ability to do them, he needs substitutes that simulate these activities (Fig. 22-3). An infant over 6 months (the earliest age at which he would sit up on his own) needs to be propped or positioned in an infant chair in an upright position unless otherwise contraindicated for a major part of each day. This allows him to see from the position he would normally assume and also aides eye development. It probably also aids in social development because he is able to see more people. The

FIGURE 22-3. An immobilized infant needs stimulation—in this case, a playboard.

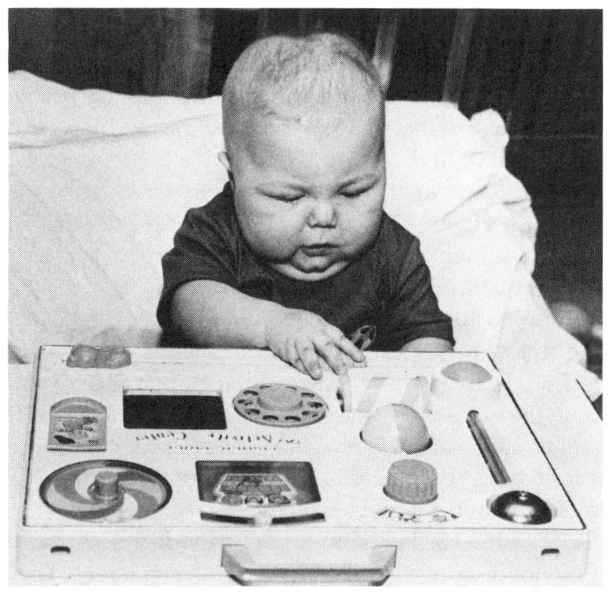

infant learning to walk needs not just to be out of his crib for part of the day but out of his crib walking; the infant learning to creep, out of his crib creeping. Many infants are admitted to health care facilities without shoes, and their walking barefoot in hallways that host many pathogenic bacteria is not advisable. Make slippers for infants out of stockinette (the cotton padding used to cover an extremity before a cast is applied) and adhesive tape. Put a bed sheet on the floor to provide clean creeping space. Many infants are hospitalized for intravenous therapy, and active maneuvers like these are limited when the intravenous line is in place. However, lines tend to infiltrate easily in infants. Take advantage of this misfortune to make the short time interval until the line is restarted an active motor stimulation time.

For social stimulation, most infants react best in a one-to-one situation. Toward the end of the first year, they may become so fearful of strangers that they will cry when anyone but their mother holds them (8-month anxiety). Do not let this reaction deter you from social interaction—the infant does not dislike you; he does not yet *know* you. Spend time with him so he can feel secure enough with you to interact socially.

The Toddler and Preschooler

Toddlers and preschoolers respond to activities that require touch or manipulation. They spend hours leafing through books with colored pictures and listening to nursery rhymes (visual and auditory stimulation). The popularity of dolls scented to smell like blueberries and of scratch-and-sniff books demonstrates children's response to the sense of smell.

A preschool child asks between 300 and 400 questions a day, reflecting his interest in the world and in social stimulation. Preschool children enjoy simple jokes. They like to solve simple puzzles or hidden picture games as forms of intellectual stimulation.

For motor stimulation, the toddler most enjoys objects that he can manipulate, such as boxes to fit inside one another and take out again, trucks to push, and pegs to pound. In a health care setting, you can usually find boxes to fit together (boxes from central supply or plastic vials from pharmacy). For another action toy, blow up a rubber glove and tie it to the crib side for a punching bag; one tied to the foot of the crib serves as a leg exerciser. Figure 22-4 shows a fish tank located in the nurses' station, which provides stimulation for ambulatory toddlers.

Along with the independence that toddlers are learning, they love experiences that offer security. Like infants, they like to hear a favorite record played over and over, the same story read again and again. To an adult it seems as if varied records or stories would be more stimulating, but security seems more important for most children than experimentation.

Social interaction is important to toddlers although they are discriminating with whom they interact. They may venture to meet new friends only if their parent is close by. They enjoy social interaction through puppets, since a puppet is small and nonthreatening. A puppet face can be created on your hand with a marker or pen; a rubber glove blown up and given a face makes a companion for a lonely toddler.

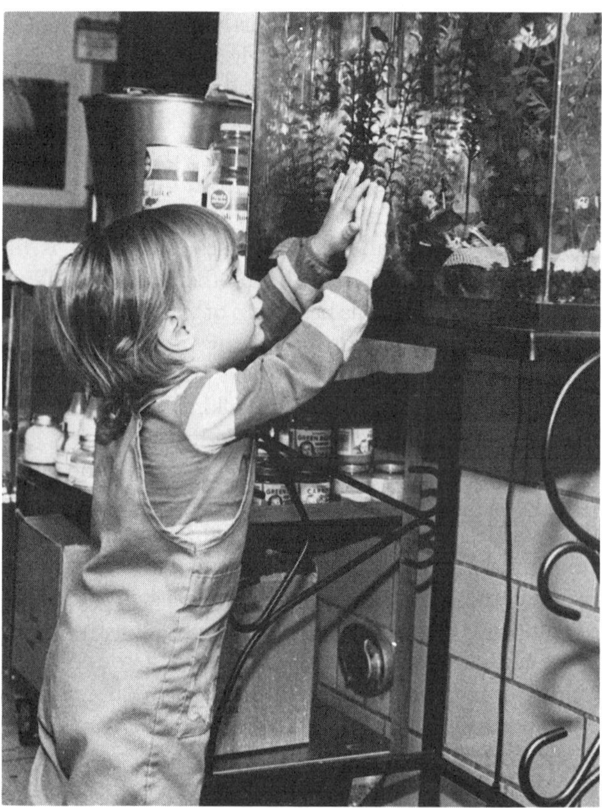

FIGURE 22-4. This toddler is fascinated watching the fish swim. Under the nurse's supervision, she is allowed in the nursing station; note she is dressed in her own clothes.

Remember that toddlers are so new to the world that almost everything they experience is new. If they are in a health care facility, this is probably the first time they have ever eaten a meal in bed, had pain that was not quickly relieved, tasted medicine, had anyone but their mother wash them, or had a dressing bigger than a Band-Aid in place. Thus, their problem may be overstimulation, not stimulation deprivation.

Cognitive stimulation for the preschooler can be achieved by games such as picture puzzles (cut a picture from a magazine into large pieces) or a pencil-and-paper game, such as guessing what things have been added to a drawing (draw a dog or a house or whatever you can draw); ask the child to close his eyes while you add one more thing to the drawing—an ear, a chimney—and then ask the child to identify the new item. If you draw in pencil, you can reverse the game and ask him to identify what item you erase each time. When caring for a preschooler, plan always to have in mind a game of this kind that requires no equipment other than that you have readily available for cognitive stimulation.

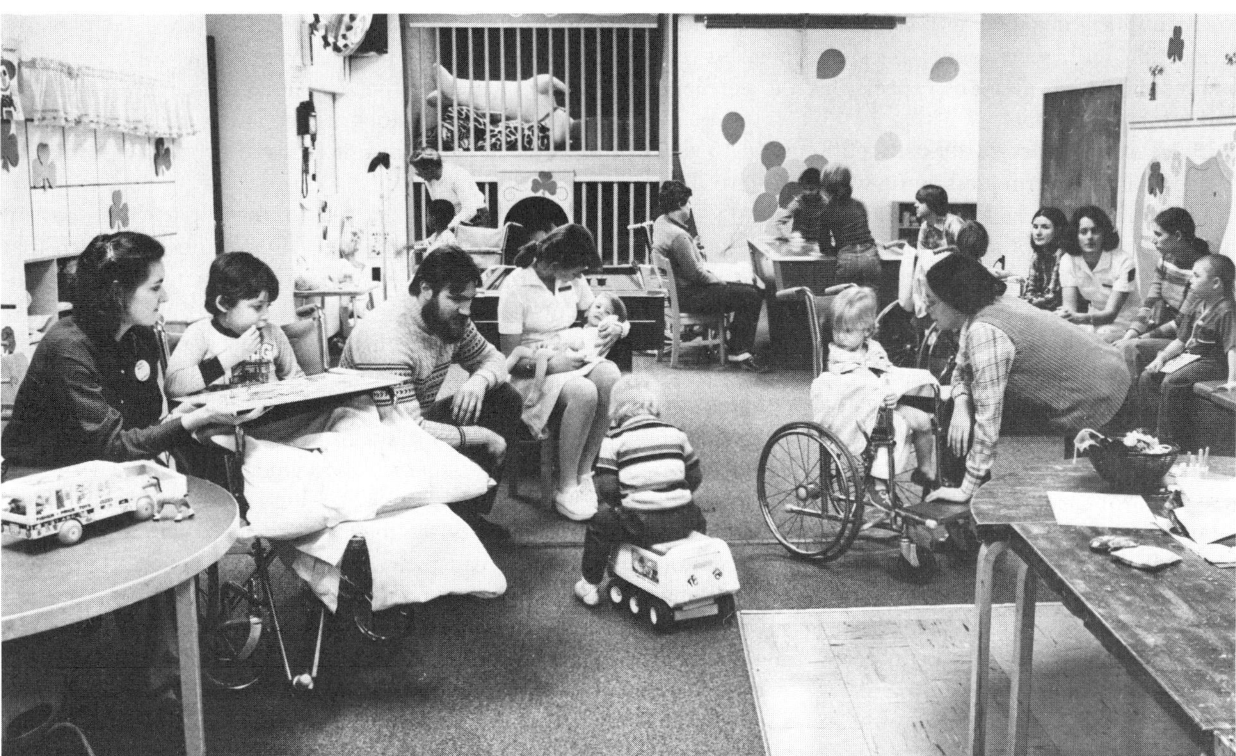

FIGURE 22-5. Young children in a hospital playroom; note the two children immobilized in wheelchairs watching the boy riding the truck.

Manipulative materials such as clay or play dough are excellent for preschooler's cognitive, physical, and sensory stimulation. Preschool children also enjoy finger paint, a basin of soapy water to splash in and make bubbles, or pans filled with dry oatmeal or cornflakes to use as a sandbox.

To increase social interaction, preschoolers are interested in going to other hospital departments to help with errands. Singing along with records can be as cognitively stimulating for them. This is normally an active age for motor accomplishments. Try to incorporate games such as Simon Says as a way not only to gain cooperation for therapy but to give active exercise. Preschoolers are generally sociable. They enjoy activities with other children and can play cooperatively for social stimulation (this is the first age that sharing is possible).

Hospitalized children need to be provided the kind of stimulation found in a playroom. However, the room shown in Figure 22-5 might provide sensory overload for some children.

The Schoolager and Adolescent

The schoolager and adolescent develop eye-and-hand coordination that allows them to read small print (a third-grade task). Learning to read (first-grade level) opens their world and offers endless intellectual stimulation. Anyone who lives with an adolescent knows that hearing stimulation is important to him from the sound level of his stereo or tape deck.

For intellectual stimulation, this age group enjoys paper and pencil games (how many words can you make from *happy birthday*) and, although they may not readily admit it, the challenge of school assignments. Children of this age actively seek stimulating experiences and make it known quickly when the level of stimulation around them is less than expected (I'm bored). They tend to become bored easily because they are accustomed to a constant level of new information on any school day. An adult may not learn one new thing in a routine day. A slow day lying in a hospital bed is felt as even more unstimulating by a child this age than by an average adult.

Schoolagers work at accomplishing a sense of industry or learning how to do things well. They enjoy short-term projects with a visible reward or sense of accomplishment at the end. Therefore, an activity ending in a product (putting together a picture puzzle cut from chart forms or a magazine photo) is more stimulating than an activity that has no visible product (listening to a record).

Games that take little equipment but are cognitively stimulating are pencil-and-paper games, such as ticktacktoe or connecting the dots. Adding an extra item to a drawing is still effective with young school children if the details are kept fine and challenging; picture puzzles are good if the pieces are cut smaller than for a preschooler. Put a time limit on completing a puzzle if the pieces are not small enough to make it challenging.

Doing school homework is strong cognitive stimulation. Although few admit it, most children recovering from an illness enjoy doing homework. It is not only a connection with their friends back at school but also assures them that everyone expects them to get better and return to school.

Children are not ready for competition until 10 years of age. All children regress some when they are ill, so introducing competition (such as a board game) to an ill child under 12 is not stimulating, only frustrating.

Most adolescents enjoy card games. If no deck of cards is available, make one from rectangles of paper and felt-tipped markers (make the deck with the child for added cognitive stimulation).

Part of an adolescent's acquiring a sense of identity is learning about other people and ways that he is like or unlike them. Therefore, the adolescent's search for interaction with other people is almost as driven as the infant's urge to perform motor skills. Allowing the adolescent to interact with others (in a playroom, a visitor's lounge) is crucial in meeting his social stimulation needs. Talking about what being a nurse is like or what being in college is like may be important cognitive and social stimulation.

Adolescents need to concentrate on school assignments for the same reasons as schoolage children. A high school or college assignment tends to be longer and more mentally fatiguing than grade school work so the adolescent may need some help in dividing homework into small segments so that he can accomplish it without becoming fatigued. Homework of this level calls for concentration; he may need periods reserved daily in his nursing care plan for homework (no interruptions allowed). Adolescents enjoy active motion skill games and enjoy having a punching bag (blow up a rubber glove) by their bedside. They like to race wheelchairs (not usually recommended but something you should be aware of).

The Young and Middle-Aged Adult

As people reach adulthood, they develop a sensory stimulation level that is comfortable for them. If some are placed in a noisy factory, a crowded highway with many honking cars, or a room of noisy children, they may become uncomfortable from temporary sensory overload. Others may feel oppressed if they vacation in a quiet spot or find themselves alone in a house. Some people of this age have beginning hearing losses from working in noisy environments or from loud music; they miss a level of sound that others around them are hearing and thus have a constant mild sensory deprivation.

Middle-aged women are prone to chronic fatigue. This symptom needs to be investigated for possible physical causes, although a high percentage of this fatigue may be the result of boredom. Career women with children may actually have too much sensory stimulation and need to cut back in order to not feel oppressed. Although many young and middle-aged adults do not participate in structured, intellectually stimulating programs, they read for enjoyment and work crossword puzzles or sport quizzes. Women who do not work outside the home need to assess their level of social stimulation. Both sexes need to assess their level of physical stimulation, since it tends to decline with middle-age.

Individualize activities to meet particular patient needs. College students may need to be reminded that their time might be well spent reviewing school assignments or working on a report. Talking about present or future career plans is intellectually stimulating to most young adults.

Women who have begun their homes or families are often interested in updating their recipe file if someone brings it in to them. Provide them with women's magazines you find and 3-by-5-inch cards so they can copy recipes to add to their collection. Other women may prefer to read the *Wall Street Journal.*

Many young adults who are out of school have not read a book in a long time (they still think of books as work and not pleasure) and may enjoy beginning a good mystery or romance. Often young adults turn to television for their primary stimulation. Talking about activities they normally participate in (volleyball, swimming) is good social interaction. Be certain when doing this that you are discussing activities that the person is describing, not describing activities interesting for you; that would be cognitive stimulation for you, not the young adult for whom you are caring.

Once careers are established, many adults are work oriented. They like to spend time on projects (a salesman takes time to organize his list of customers; a teacher corrects papers). There is a tendency to tell people not to work while they are ill (relax, rest). However, such activities are stimulating for people and may provide much more satisfaction than an afternoon of lying quietly in bed.

Adults are also community or world oriented. Sometimes students may become so engrossed in school activities or homework that days go by without their reading a newspaper or listening to news. When caring for adults, make a point of knowing about major world news, since discussing it is cognitive stimulation for this age group. Many men and women do not feel comfortable starting a day without reading a newspaper; securing one may be the most appreciated thing you do for them all day. However, reading a newspaper may be much more fatiguing than reading a book or magazine because the pages require such a large sweeping action to turn. People on complete bed rest may need newspapers read to them to reduce the effort of page turning.

Often a person who spends a considerable amount of time away from home or who has many housekeeping or child care concerns at home normally spends little time watching television. Such a person may find television stimulating because he watches programs that everyone else has been talking about but he has never seen before. Many hospitals have volunteers who offer such adult activities as teaching needlepoint or painting or who distribute library books.

The Older Adult

If hearing or eyesight becomes less acute with age, the older adult may become sensory deprived. The food intake of some older adults decreases because their taste sensation fades and foods they once enjoyed no longer taste the same. Fortunately, the pleasure of touch (providing this is culturally acceptable) remains constant throughout life; cognitive ability or ability for intellectual stimulation remains intact. The cat-napping of many older adults is caused not by physical need for increased sleep (the older adult probably needs only 6 hours of sleep in comparison with an average 8 hours for a younger person) but as a result of boredom or lack of stimulation.

Providing stimulation is particularly important for the older adult because if he has some deficiency of hearing or vision, he may not even be aware of the lessened amount of stimulation that reaches him daily. If the person has any motor incapacity, social isolation can occur.

Many older women know how to do needlework such as crocheting or knitting. Participating in these activities provides not only physical stimulation (moving joints of fingers and wrists) but cognitive stimulation (keeping count of stitches or the pattern). It also can offer a sense of achievement, improved self-esteem, and the ability to contribute to the family in a concrete way if the product is something such as a pair of slippers for a grandchild. If patients report such arthritic changes in joints that these skills are difficult, substituting thicker needles or thicker yarn may help; rug punching (making a rug or wall hanging or pillow from pieces of yarn punched through a net canvas) is a needlework skill that may still be possible. Most health care agencies have occupational therapy departments that can furnish supplies for use in this way. Asking an older adult to teach you needlework may at first seem an unprofessional use of your time (you are there to give care not to learn a craft) but being asked to teach something can foster self-esteem, can be cognitively stimulating, and can be very rewarding (provided that you are a good student and actually learn).

Many older adults enjoy games of chess or checkers; these are cognitive stimulation games, since the person has to plan moves. If a health care agency does not have board games available you can construct some from bottle caps, vials, or bottles from pharmacy.

Some older adults have outlived most of their friends. They may find talking to other people their own age more stimulating and enjoyable than any other activity. Remember that it is a *myth* that cognitive function necessarily decreases with aging. Many older adults enjoy playing cards or learning new skills as much as younger people. General principles of supplying stimulation to people in all age groups are shown in Quick Reference Stop 22-2.

SENSORY OVERLOAD

Sensory overload, in contrast to deprivation, occurs when a person receives more stimulation than he can tolerate or process. Such a situation occurs in a room where the lights are too bright or the sound too loud. Every student has had a sense of too much cognitive stimulation or too many assignments due at one time.

People with sensory overload react similarly to those with sensory deprivation (confusion, inability to make decisions, and severe fatigue). Sometimes it is difficult to determine the cause of these symptoms whether these symptoms are caused by sensory deprivation or by sensory overload.

People in Intensive Care Units. The lights in intensive care units are never turned out so that people in such units can always be observed. There is excessive sound (the whir of machines, the buzzing of ventilators, the ringing of alarms, the mix of voices in consultation). Thus, people in intensive care units often sleep poorly. Most intensive care units have no windows so that wall space can be used for monitoring equipment; therefore, night and day are not easily observable. It is easy to become confused as to time and place, and after a time, set routines lead to monotony. Either providing stimuli if confusion is due to monotony or reducing sensory stimulation if overload is present is an important role of nurses in such units.

People Under Stress. One important symptom accompanying stress is reduced decision-making ability. For example, a person under stress may be able to choose between two alternatives but not among three or four. Excessive pressure can make him totally unable to function. Such a person may be able to choose when a room is quiet but not when it is noisy. Reducing environmental stimuli for people under stress is important; they need to use their problem-solving ability to reduce the cause of their stress.

People With Distorted Reality. People whose mental processes are disturbed to such a point that they misinterpret stimuli (they look at your watch and see it as a snake curling around your arm; they misinterpret the clock face as a person watching them) may need stimuli reduced so they are not exposed to so many sights or sounds that they can misinterpret. Such disturbances in perception are termed *delusions* (misinterpreting something that is actually present). If a person's mental processes are even further disturbed, he may see or hear

☐ **QUICK REFERENCE STOP 22-2: HEALTH TEACHING**
General Principles of Stimulation

1. No activity is stimulating forever. Introducing a variety of activities allows a person to choose the activity most appealing to him and to stop it and go on to another before it fatigues or bores him.
2. Activities are stimulating only if they are age appropriate.
3. As a rule, people who are ill tire easily. Balance stimulation activities against a need for rest and sleep.
4. Television has limited value as a stimulating activity; a television set turned on and running is more apt to be contributing unnecessary noise and confusion to a person's environment than stimulation. The exceptions to this are programs designed especially to be educational or culturally satisfying. Do not be surprised to see people on long-term bed rest watching shows designed and produced for preschoolers to teach the alphabet or beginning language development. Although the content of the show is simplistic, the host (or a puppet) speaks directly to the television watcher and often asks questions; this allows a greater degree of active participation than watching a so-called adult show does. Do not underestimate the value of soap operas as a form of social interaction. For the person who watches the show daily, the people in them become their second family and watching may be as stimulating as a telephone call from their first family.
5. Providing a change of scene is invaluable in stimulating a person to think of new things and to be more active physically (the person must walk or transfer to a wheelchair or stretcher to reach the new scene). Taking people to a sunroom, playroom, or recreation room (sometimes called day rooms) daily offers at least twice the stimulation that just getting out of bed to a bedside chair would provide.
6. Orient to time and date by the use of a calendar on which you cross out the dates and a clock that can be seen to supply the time of day. It is easy to lose track of these things when confined to one room day after day. In addition orient by including the date and time in your conversation, "It's 10 o'clock, Mrs. Smith. I'm going to get your medication for you."
7. Look around patients' rooms to see if the bed is positioned in the best way possible (Can the person see into the corridor the way it is positioned? Out the window?). Rotate the pictures on the walls from room to room every week. Post signs made from treatment room paper (rolls of white paper to cover examination tables) to mark holidays and other special events.
8. Mark people with immobilization devices such as casts, traction, or isolation as high risk for sensory deprivation. Try to arrange to have their rooms near the nursing station so they can benefit from the action at this site.
9. If people are not receiving traditional meals (being fed by intravenous or tube feedings), provide socialization with them at what would have been a regular mealtime. Mealtime is for most people a time not only for physical nourishment but for social nourishment in the form of interaction as well. Many health care facilities provide dining room space for patients where they can eat with other patients for the socialization involved.
10. Help people to change to street clothing if at all possible rather than to wear a hospital gown or robe. Changing clothing helps to maintain identity and helps to make the person feel more well. It also helps as an effective orientation to mark the passage of time (It is day; time to wear a shirt and slacks. It is night; time to change to pajamas.).
11. Provide growing plants in rooms. Taking an interest in a plant offers a sense of control and an opportunity to experience change as the plant grows. A philodendrum flourishes with little light and sometimes-forgotten water. African violets are the easiest flowering plant to grow; they bloom best in fluorescent light so often grow well in hospital rooms. For people at home, owning and caring for a pet furnishes this same stimulation.

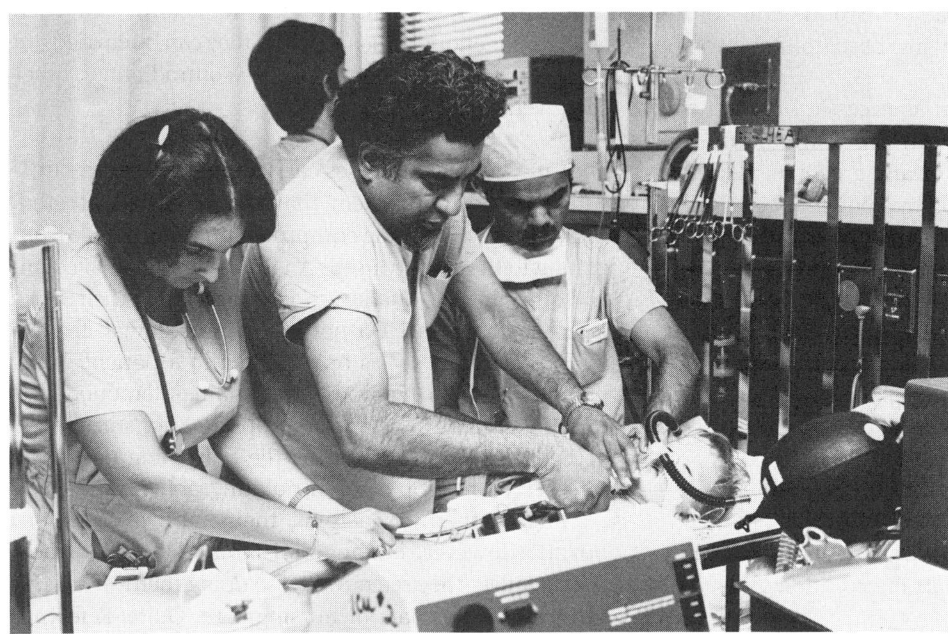

FIGURE 22-6. Reducing sensory overload is an important role of the nurse working in an intensive care setting.

things that only he can see or hear (termed *hallucinations*). With this phenomena, stimuli also may need to be reduced so they do not compete with his mental imagery and increase confusion.

Reducing Stimuli

Make an effort to reduce stimuli to prevent sensory overload by means that reduce sensory, cognitive, physical, and social stimuli (Fig. 22-6).

If bright lights cannot be diminished, consider folding a washcloth across the person's eyes so the room seems darker. Consider the placement of any heart or respiratory monitor in terms of the patient. Some people find it reassuring to be able to see their heart is beating; others find them a needless and disturbing sensory input.

If the level of sound in the room is disturbing to a patient, consider soft music through earphones or earplugs. If a patient is wearing earplugs, post a sign near the bed that says this or another caregiver may seriously misinterpret his level of consciousness. Not all sound can be eliminated or covered up in these ways. Be certain that the person understands the source of the sounds he hears (the high beeping sound is the alarm that regulates the intravenous therapy; the lower beeping is the respiratory alarm). This does not take away the sound but does prevent the person from being frightened by its strangeness.

If a nearby person is disoriented or in sharp pain and thus may call out frequently for help, be certain the person understands the reason. Again, this does not eliminate the sound, but the patient is reassured that he is among people who care. It also prevents his being startled by the sudden distress of a person nearby.

Listen for excessive sound such as the nursing staff laughing in the desk area or people calling out vital sign information rather than meeting at a central point to exchange it. Either eliminate these sounds or transfer a person to a quieter room where he will not notice them.

Eliminate pain and itching if at all possible in a person with sensory overload; such irritation as bedclothes against a tender body joint can be as annoying as excessive noise or light. This small annoyance by itself might barely be noticed ordinarily, but added to all the other stimuli coming at a person it may be the last straw that causes sensory overload.

To reduce cognitive stimuli, reduce the level of worry or concern by always beginning a treatment or answering a call light promptly. Once a person feels confident that you are conscientiously looking after him, he can relax and let things happen more easily. Reduce decision making to a point that it is not stressful. That point differs greatly from person to person. Being able to make decisions allows people to remain in control; the feeling that they have control over their body and environment may be the factor keeping sensory overload from becoming acute. On the other hand, being asked to make decisions may be overwhelming for a person who is ill.

Another cognitive area that leads to extreme confusion is distortion of time. Help people to keep track of time by the use of calendars and clocks. Refer to the day and hour periodically throughout the day.

Be certain that you explain procedures or acts before beginning them. This offers a sense of control and helps to make sense of the stimuli a person is submitted to. Repeat instructions and explanations as necessary; stress reduces people's ability to process information, so many times a person receiving many environmental stimuli will not remember even having been told something before.

Decrease social interaction as necessary by reducing the number of visitors present. Check the number of auxiliary personnel such as cleaning people, clerks, or laboratory personnel who stop by a patient's bed to chat. These people, meaning to be friendly or therapeutic, can add greatly to sensory overload. Be conscious of the importance of support people at a time of stress, however. Worrying about how family members at home are reacting and not being allowed to speak to them may be more stressful than having people clustered around a bedside.

UTILIZING NURSING PROCESS

To establish stimulation needs of patients, use the nursing process to assess and plan interventions.

Assessment. First assess sensory status because sensory stimuli are so important to well being. Can he hear well? See well? Is his sense of touch, taste, and smell intact? Assess intellectual age and ability as well as chronological age; a person functioning at a level below his chronological age, such as a person with mental retardation, may be overwhelmed by normal stimuli. Assess special circumstances or equipment, such as a cast that limits movement or a diagnosis that will probably require a long period of bed rest. Assess the environment for noise and light levels. Ask, How would I feel if I were the person in this situation?

Analysis. A nursing diagnosis of sensory-perceptual alteration related to inability to ambulate or to multiple caregivers is made as an independent nursing judgment. This nursing diagnosis is easy to overlook in the light of other diagnoses dealing with oxygen or circulatory disturbances, but it can interfere with a person regaining true wellness. Because nurses are present with patients for considerable lengths of time, stimulation deprivation or overload may be recognized most easily by a nurse.

Planning. Make specific plans for stimulation so the level of stimulation will be consistent from caregiver to caregiver (not "increase cognitive stimulation," but "play chess with him," "be sure he has a morning paper," etc.). After a week an activity may no longer be stimulating. Thus, a care plan for such activity can never be static. Some plans for restructuring environments, such as changing a patient's room assignment to offer him a change of view or activity after a long stay, call for cooperation from other departments such as housekeeping or admissions. Changing a patient's routine, such as going to physical therapy in the morning rather than the afternoon, calls for cooperation from that department (that might be very inconvenient for them). Plan such changes far enough ahead so that they can be carried out without friction and without contradicting other caregivers' goals or plans.

Implementation. Activities carried out best require little equipment or equipment that can be easily gathered. Time spent assembling equipment prevents people from getting to the activity itself. An important form of cognitive stimulation is talking to people about their likes, interests, or plans. Do not call a nurse away from a bedside because she is only talking to a patient; "only talking" may be her most important interaction that day. Use nursing assistants appropriately for stimulation activities. A caring nature is the only thing needed to interact with people in stimulating activities such as reading to them or helping them with a crossword puzzle. However, nursing assistants will not do these things unless they see nurses also doing them—that this is an important part of nursing care. Quick Reference Stops 22-3, Nutrition, and 22-4, Safety, offer extra guidelines for implementation.

Evaluation. Evaluating whether people have less stimulation deprivation than they would have had if activities had not been introduced to them is difficult. One measure should be increased nursing job satisfaction. Working with and relating to people is necessary for stimulation and brings deep satisfaction to most nurses.

☐ QUICK REFERENCE STOP 22-3: NUTRITION

Most people have strong preferences in foods. As a rule, introducing new and different foods is not a good area to use to increase stimulation, especially if people also have a physical illness that needs adequate protein and vitamins for tissue healing. Encourage people to list foods they enjoy eating and feel good when eating rather than just likes and dislikes so they can be stimulated by food.

☐ QUICK REFERENCE STOP 22-4: SAFETY

People with both sensory deprivation and sensory overload may develop confusion or lack of judgment. A person who is confused cannot safely be left alone to meet his own self-care needs or could injure himself if left alone with equipment such as a heat lamp. Use siderails appropriately to prevent falls. Do not allow self-medication if time orientation is a problem or if a person may forget a dose of medication or take an extra dose due to confusion.

NURSING CARE PLAN

Mrs. Greenberg is a 73-year-old woman hospitalized for 3 weeks for a persistent infection. The following is a nursing care plan for her pertaining to stimulation.

ASSESSMENT

Patient rarely leaves room although she can ambulate freely. Not interested in eating in patients' dining room. Has knitting with her but has difficulty doing it since following pattern takes a long time. Reluctant to make telephone calls because increased costs not paid for by hospital insurance. Has slight hearing impairment.

NURSING DIAGNOSIS

Potential for stimulation deprivation related to length of hospital stay.

Locus of Decision-Making: Shared.

Goal: Patient will not demonstrate symptoms such as confusion or boredom by end of hospital stay.

Criteria: Patient will remain oriented to person, place, and time and participate in activities appropriate for health status and age group.

NURSING ORDERS

1. Do not raise level of voice to address her because of hearing difficulty (this irritates her). Just be certain to face her before you speak. Vision, touch, and taste intact.
2. Encourage ambulation: walk to sunroom morning, afternoon, and evening with her for socialization as well as physical stimulation.
3. Enjoys knitting (has material with her). Provide uninterrupted time for knitting (at least an hour) so she can follow a pattern that requires concentration.
4. Do not encourage to eat in sunroom with other patients. Her niece visits her almost every day at lunch time and provides social interaction for this meal for her.
5. Has friends who have difficulty visiting due to poor bus connections. Encourage her to ask them to telephone her and provide time for this.
6. Enjoys talking about her grandchildren (2 months and 2 years old), has interesting stories about 1977 blizzard in Buffalo she likes to talk about; encourage this. Slightly shy at first but warms quickly on a one-to-one basis.
7. Has no bedside clock. Pull bed forward so she can see wall clock in hallway. Pharmacy is sending up a drug company calendar for over her bed. Post to aid in time orientation.

EVALUATION

Evaluate in 3 days time whether implementation is still current to prevent plan from becoming outdated.

SUGGESTED READINGS

Bassett, C., et al. A 10-week exercise program for senior citizens. *Geriatr. Nurs.* 3(2):103, 1982.

Bazian, M. W., and Clark, H. M. Counteracting sensory changes in the aging. *Am. J. Nurs.* 80:473, 1980.

Belkengren, R. B., et al. Physical fitness from infancy through adolescence. *Pediatr. Nurs.* 8(4):C-I, 1982.

Bell, C. W., et al. Aerobic exercise: Just the prescription for pulmonary patients. *Consultant* 22(10):270, 1982.

Bernard, B., et al. Exercise for children with physical disabilities. *Issues Compr. Pediatr. Nurs.* 5:99, 1981.

Berra, K., et al. The effects of controlled exercise on the client with coronary artery disease. *Top. Clin. Nurs.* 3(2):65, 1981.

Cole, J., et al. Exercise during pregnancy. *Parents* 58(2):39, 1983.

Feibusch, B. G. The socially isolated elderly. *Am. J. Geriatric Nurs.* 2:28, 1981.

George, G. Exercise and coping with stress. *Top. Clin. Nurs.* 4(2):13, 1982.

Glaser, R. M., et al. Exercise program for wheelchair activity. *Am. J. Phys. Med.* 60:67, 1981.

Goldberg, W. G., et al. Movement therapy with the aged. *Nurs. Res.* 29(6):339, 1980.

Gotch, P. M. Incorporating activity into diabetic self-care. *Occup. Health Nurs.* 30:16, 1982.

Hagerty, G. Growing more balmy each day. *Am. J. Nurs.* 80:2173, 1980.

Hahn, K. Using 24-hour reality orientation. *J. Gerontol. Nurs.* 6:130, 1980.

Halfman, M. A., et al. Exercise and the maintenance of health. *Top. Clin. Nurs.* 3:1, 1981.

Hasselmeyer, E. G. *Behavior Patterns of Premature Infants.* Washington, D.C.: U.S. Government Printing Office, 1961.

Hayter, J. Nursing care of the severely confused patient. *Nurs. Homes* 30:30, 1981.

Lindenmuth, J. E., et al. Sensory overload: An approach to nursing care. *Am. J. Nurs.* 80:1456, 1980.

Maring-Klug, R. Reducing low back pain in pregnancy. *Nurse Pract.* 7(10):18, 1982.

Milazzo, V. An exercise class for patients in traction. *Am. J. Nurs.* 81:1842, 1981.

Payton, O. D., et al. Aging process: Implications for clinical practice. *Phys. Ther.* 63(1):41, 1983.

Price, J. H., et al. Physical fitness: Its role in health for the elderly. *J. Gerontol. Nurs.* 6(9):517, 1980.

Sachs, M. L. Nursing therapy for the depressed client. *Top. Clin. Nurs.* 3:77, 1981.

Savitz, J., et al. Diagnosing boredom and confusion. *Nurs. Res.* 30:16, 1981.

Spitz, R. Hospitalism: An inquiry into the genesis of psychiatric conditions in early childhood. *Psychoanal. Study Child.* 1:53, 1945.

Wesser, S. H. When the walls listen. *Am. J. Nurs.* 78:1016, 1978.

Wolf, S. I. Exercise the asthmatic child and PL 94-142. *Pediatr. Nurs.* 6(6):21, 1980.

QUESTIONS FOR REVIEW

To review your knowledge of stimulation needs, unscramble the following words:

1. Too much stimuli in an environment can result in sensory ______________ .	L A V O E R O D
2. An area of stimulation you improve by playing chess with a patient.	O T N I G C E V I
3. Infants particularly prone to sensory deprivation.	T M R R A E P E U
4. To reduce stimuli, if you cannot remove a sound, you should ______________ it.	P X A N E L I
5. People confined in this way are prone to sensory deprivation.	D R E B E T S
6. Every patient hospitalized for a long time needs one of these on his wall.	L N A D A C E R
7. Watching this is not usually stimulating.	E L S O E V T I N I
8. The appearance of someone with either sensory overload or sensory deprivation.	N F E O U D C S
9. A good cognitive stimulating activity for a school age child.	M R K O O H E W
10. An adult age particularly prone to sensory deprivation.	D E L O R

23. SPIRITUAL CONSIDERATIONS

OBJECTIVES

Upon mastery of the material in this chapter, you should be able to:

1. Define the difference between spiritual belief and religion.
2. Describe the major religious practices of the religions of the world.
3. Describe the nurse's role in assessment of spiritual needs and the implementation of fulfillment of unmet spiritual needs.
4. List ways of stating spiritual needs as nursing diagnoses.
5. Describe the concept of spiritual belief as it relates to the life span.
6. Describe methods to include members of the clergy in nursing care planning.

TERMS

The terms important for an understanding of this chapter are shown below and defined in the glossary:

chaplain
religion
spiritual belief

A *spiritual belief* is a belief that a higher power than oneself guides life. When people are ill, they may find their spiritual beliefs either severely shaken or a source of strength. Some people who have few spiritual convictions before an illness may begin to examine their beliefs. People may not voice these concerns because they view them as a personal struggle or a topic you as a health care provider are not interested in discussing. However, in order to view a person holistically and to assess his support system, you need to be as familiar with the spiritual part of a person's life as any other.

Being sensitive to spiritual needs and assisting a person to clarify his beliefs or to strengthen them when he wants help can be an important nursing role.

Religion, in contrast to spiritual belief, means an organized form of worship; a religious person is one committed to the tenets of an organized form of worship. An individual may have a strong spiritual belief but not subscribe to a religion. As a rule, the depth of a person's spiritual belief or religious commitment will serve as an additional support system should he become ill, not the kind of religion. Religion is closely related to ethnic background. When assessing spiritual needs, be sensitive to ethnic as well as religious differences since these are so interwoven.

LIFE SPAN CONCEPTS AND SPIRITUAL NEEDS

The Infant. The infant has little concept of motivating forces beyond his parents. You may be asked to help with the circumcision of a Jewish male infant if he is hospitalized at the eighth day of life; you may be asked to help to baptize (or baptize yourself) a Catholic infant who is in imminent danger of death. Infants are assumed to be of the same religion as their parents unless it is specifically stated otherwise. An infant who learns a good sense of trust is able to develop a better spiritual orientation in coming years.

The Toddler and Preschooler. Children pass through stages of moral development just as they do other kinds of development (Kohlberg, 1963).

Toddlers begin to formulate a sense of right and wrong, but their reason for doing right is centered most strongly in "mother says" rather than "God says." Kohlberg (1963) refers to this as a punishment-obedience orientation. Preschoolers begin to have an elemental concept of a God. This belief in an outside force aids the development of conscience. However, preschoolers tend to do good out of self-interest rather than out of intent truly to do good or strong spiritual motivation.

Children this age enjoy the security of religious holidays (which occur year after year). If they are hospitalized on a religious holiday, they like to celebrate it as they would if they were at home. Time for prayers at bedtime or grace before meals offers the same reassurance to children accustomed to them that a familiar nursery rhyme read over and over does. Ask on a hospital admission if the parent wishes the child to participate in these activities.

The Schoolager and Adolescent. Schoolagers begin to learn about the rituals and meaning behind their religion so it becomes more meaningful to them than to the preschooler. Schoolagers are rule oriented; they expect God also to follow rules (if you are good and pray for something, you should receive it). A child of this age can be confused if such a prayer is not immediately answered.

Almost every adolescent passes through a questioning of the existence of God and the religious practices he has been taught. This is part of forming a sense of identity (establishing a value system that works for him) but may leave him without an important support system at a time in life when he utilizes all support systems poorly.

The Young and Middle-Aged Adult. Young adults may or may not incorporate religious practices into their lifestyle. If they were reared in a religion, returning to old practices after years of shunning them as an adolescent may make them very meaningful. If a marriage has merged two religious practices, values and customs may be questioned more than ever before. A young adult may be distressed at learning that he is going to miss a religious holiday observance more because he wants his children to have the satisfying experience he enjoyed as a child than because he regrets missing it himself.

Middle-aged adults may be active in religious activities and may be worried if illness keeps them away not only because they are missing the celebration but because if they are not fulfilling their responsibilities, the celebration will be incomplete for others as well. Middle-aged adults should have developed a full moral conscience, where they do good deeds simply because they are right to do and they live by internal values of conscience, not by what others expect or ask of them.

The Older Adult. The older adult has a sure concept of what he believes or does not believe. If the person is asked to contemplate death or permanent disability, the presence of a strong religious faith may be the determining factor that helps him accept his situation. If there has been a change in a religious practice (e.g., it is no longer necessary for Catholics to omit meat on Friday), many older adults continue to maintain the practice as they learned it. Many older adults have well-worn religious symbols (tattered Bibles, bent medals, or icons). Respect these articles: the wear testifies to their worth to the individual (Fig. 23-1).

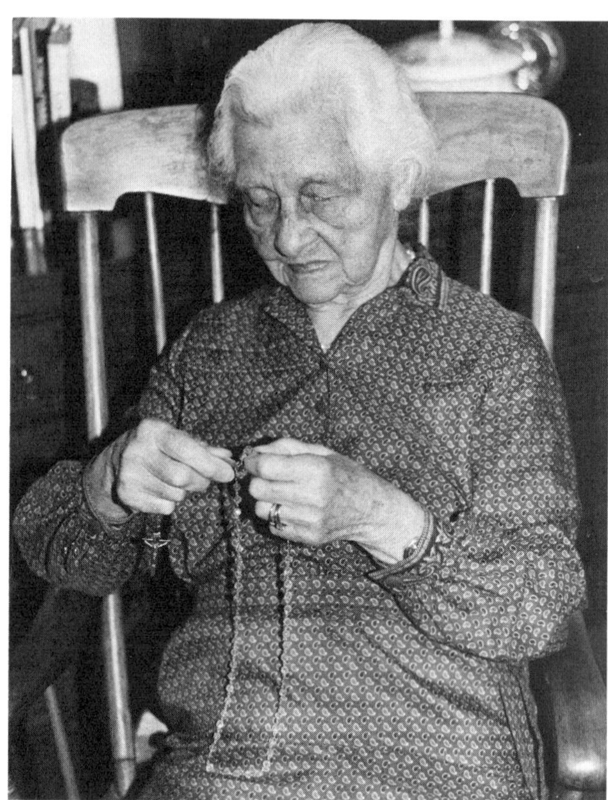

FIGURE 23-1. For over 80 years this woman has said the Rosary daily. Respect her religious practice as well as its symbol.

RELIGIONS OF THE WORLD

The urge of humans to practice religion is as old as humanity itself. Man is thought to be the only creature who comprehends things he cannot see and believes in things he cannot comprehend. It is impossible to know the tenets of all religions, but it is helpful to have some appreciation of common customs and practices of the religions most prevalent in your community.

Faith Healing

Faith healing is healing by belief in the power of God to cure rather than by medical or surgical intervention. Faith healing may be tried as a primary health care experience or as a last resort after usual methods of established medical practice have failed. It is an effective technique for some people, demonstrating the power of mind control over physical processes.

Faith healers as a group have a reputation as people taking advantage of illness to acquire wealth and power for themselves. Intermingled in this group are some sincere people who believe that all healing comes ultimately from a higher source than man himself and who practice conscientiously.

If a person decides to use faith healing, your role is to support his decision after you are certain that he has investigated all his options. Formal health care is a right, not an obligation. An exception to this may be a minor child's health clearly being compromised by avoidance of established medical practices.

Hinduism

Hinduism is an old religion; its origins go back over 8,000 years. God is called Brahma (addressed in prayers as OM). Brahma is referred to as It or That, not He or She. For many sects, It appears as a triad: Brahma to create the world; Vishnu to sustain it; Siva to destroy it and allow its rebirth. Brahma appeared in ten earth forms. As Rama he was the ideal man. Rama is a common name for Hindu children and to die with his name on your lips is a common Hindu death wish. Krishna was another, lovable and popular earth form. Followers of the Hare Krishna Consciousness Movement (followers of Sir Raman Krishna), wearing saffron colored robes with shaved heads, are seen in the United States.

The goal of Hinduism is to achieve union with Brahma. This union is achieved through the common ideals of purity, self-control, truth, nonviolence, charity, and compassion.

The writings of Hinduism are referred to as the Vedas (meaning "knowledge"). A Hindu teacher is a *guru* (addressed as Swami). Although Hindu beliefs are written, he generally teaches orally because Hindu writings are complex and require a one-to-one teacher-disciple relationship to be understood. One common form of prayer is called a *mantra;* it is thought that if repeated enough (chanting), prayer becomes a two-way communication between man and God. Yoga (yoking or joining with God) is a system of exercises for attaining bodily or mental control and well-being. Many people of the Hindu faith use transcendental meditation in connection with ritual prayers.

Eating meat or drinking alcohol is prohibited (even medications with an elixir or alcohol base may be unacceptable for a few sects). All inequalities in life are explained by the doctrine of Karma. By this theory, man creates his own fate. He receives that which he is fated to receive, goes only where led by fate, and finds only as much pleasure or pain in life as he is destined to meet. A person with this philosophy may resist participating in a health care activity because although correct actions can break the justice wheel of Karma, he may feel that fate has greater control over the outcome than he does.

Most Hindus believe in cremation following death. Following death, man (and all creatures) then goes to heaven, hell, or purgatory; he later is born again (reincarnation), in a form depending on the life he has lived and the influence of Karma.

Buddhism

Buddhism is another of the world's oldest religions (over 2,500 years old). The form *Hinayana Buddhism* (the lesser vehicle) is practiced in Southern Asia. Salvation is attained largely by individual example. *Mahayana Buddhism* (the greater vehicle) is practiced in Japan, Korea, and China. Salvation in this form is attained largely by good works.

The prophet is Siddhartha Gautama, known as Buddha or "the Enlightened One." Gautama was born of a wealthy family and cast aside this life to teach the poor and change their conditions. Statues of Buddha are not realistic appraisals but idealistic and symbolic.

Four important truths of Buddhism are that suffering is universal; it is caused by selfish desire; the cure of suffering is the elimination of selfish desire; and the way to eliminate selfish desire is to follow an Eightfold Path of right knowledge, intention, speech, conduct, means of livelihood, effort, and mindfulness. Buddhists abstain from intoxicants in order to keep the mind clear to follow these dictates.

Buddhism has few ceremonies. Almost all males spend a week or two as monks upon coming of age. Monks are strict vegetarians (they harm no living animal). Various levels of vegetarian diets may continue to be followed. Nirvana (peace with God) is the ultimate goal. Enlightenment or reincarnation will help to achieve this.

Islam (Muslim)

Islam is the major religion of the Middle East and North Africa. The spiritual leader is the prophet Muhammad (not considered a savior but a man through whom God spoke). *Islam* means submission to God's will and that is a guiding life goal. God is called Allah. The book of sacred writings is the Koran.

The devout Muslim tries to pray five times a day, always facing toward Mecca (the Holy City). At some time in his life he hopes to make a pilgrimage to Mecca. Ramadan, the ninth month of the Muslim year, is a month of fasting during daylight hours (Muhammad received his first revelation during this month). Pork products and alcohol are prohibited. You may have to alert the dietary department to the fact that a Muslim must space his meals during this special period of fast from sunup to sundown, although as a rule, children, pregnant women, the elderly, and the ill are excused from this practice (see QRS 23-1).

BLACK MUSLIM

Black Muslim practices closely follow those of Islam. The use of pork and alcohol is prohibited. The person may be dedicated to support of black power and to perpetuating black culture.

BAHA'I

People of the Baha'i faith are limited in number but the practices of this faith are so pervasive that treatment of illness is influenced. Alcohol is not permitted; medica-

☐ **QUICK REFERENCE STOP 23-1: PHARMACOLOGY**

1. Fasting may be observed by many people as part of their religious practices. For most people, fasting does not include omitting medicine or water. If the person thinks that taking prescribed medicine while fasting would compromise his beliefs, investigate whether medicine can be administered by another route (subcutaneously or intramuscularly) during this time or if a delay in administration would be safe. Certain drugs such as liquid potassium must be administered with food or they cause gastric irritation; be certain that giving a drug without food will be safe.
2. If a person has stated that he wants to talk to a clergyman, you might want to delay administration of medicine such as a sedative or hypnotic (sleeping medicine) so that the person is not overly sleepy at the time of the clergyman's visit. Preparing oneself spiritually for a threatening procedure such as surgery is as important as any other form of preparation.

tion is used minimally. Various days throughout the year are total fast days. People may ask if fasting would be detrimental to their health or if you would respect a fast day for them. If a fellow health care worker is of this religion, you may have to adjust a work schedule to allow for her not to work on a fast day because when nothing is eaten for 24 hours, one's energy level falls quickly by midafternoon.

Judaism

Next to Christianity, Judaism is the most frequently practiced religion in the United States.

Sacred writings of Judaism are contained in the Torah. A spiritual leader is called a *rabbi.* God is known as YHWH (a name not to be pronounced). Three orientations of Judaism are currently practiced: Orthodox Jews believe in the laws of the Torah as divine revelation and interpret its teachings literally. Reform Jews view the Torah as an ethical guide. The third, *conservative judaism*, is between the other two.

Religious services are held in synagogues or temples, but home services and worship are also extremely important. The Holy Day is termed the *Sabbath* and is observed from sundown on Friday night to sundown on Saturday. Orthodox practitioners hold this day as one for rest and worship. They may refuse to participate in an elective surgical procedure such as a biopsy on the Sabbath.

All male infants are circumcised on the eighth day of life to commemorate God's covenant with Abraham that they are a chosen people. This may be done by a Rabbi in a special ceremony if the child is in a health care facility on the eighth day of life.

Two important holidays observed in the fall are Rosh Hashanah (the Jewish New Year; occurs in September or October) and Yom Kippur (the day of atonement, 10 days later). Orthodox Jews observe a 24-hour fast in the period between Rosh Hashanah and Yom Kippur. Other important holidays are Hanukkah (the feast of lights, an 8-day celebration in December) and Passover (in March or April; a celebration of freedom from bondage in Egypt). The ceremonial meal of Passover is termed the *Seder*; a person may ask if his family can bring in special food such as unleavened bread for him for this occasion.

Orthodox Jews maintain a *kosher diet*: no pork or shellfish is allowed; eating meat and milk together at a meal is prohibited. All meat must be slaughtered and prepared under kosher restrictions. Most health care agencies can readily make arrangements for a kosher diet to be prepared. Be certain to ask at admission how closely the person follows these guidelines because otherwise he might eat almost nothing during a hospital stay. Most Orthodox Jews do not believe in postmortem examinations after death and wish to bury the individual as soon as possible, preferably before sundown on the same day. You may have to speed agency procedures so this can be accomplished.

Christianity

Christian religions can be divided into two main categories, Catholic and Protestant.

CATHOLICISM

Catholicism has several branches but the one most frequently encountered in the United States is Roman Catholic. The sacred writings of Christianity are contained in the Old and New Testaments of the Bible. The savior is Jesus, who is God incarnate. God is viewed as a trinity: God, the father; God, the son; and God, the Holy Spirit (three persons in one God). The spiritual advisor in Catholicism is a priest. Unity with God that will lead to resurrection following death is the ultimate goal to be strived for during life.

Important holidays observed are Christmas (December 25, the birth of Jesus) and Easter (in March or April; the death and resurrection of Jesus).

Baptism. An infant is thought of as being born with original sin or impure until he is baptized. If he should die without being baptized, he cannot go to heaven. If an unbaptized infant is in imminent danger of death, a priest or the agency chaplain should be called to baptize him. If there is no time to call a priest, any adult may baptize the infant by pouring water on his head while saying, "I baptize you in the name of the Father, and of the Son, and the Holy Spirit." Include a statement in the child's record that baptism was performed and tell the family. It is believed that a soul exists from the moment of conception in utero so a dying fetus should be baptized in the same manner. This belief that a soul exists from conception explains why Catholic teachings oppose abortion.

Holy Communion. Holy communion (the Eucharist) is an activity mandated as a memorial by Jesus Christ at the Last Supper during the week before his death. The person is given or has bread placed on his tongue (usually a wafer), the sacrament of the body of Christ (the Host). Some people prefer to fast for at least an hour before communion. This is not usually thought to exclude water or prescribed medication, however. The wafer used for communion dissolves on the tongue without the use of additional water; thus, a person who is restricted to nothing by mouth (e.g., just before surgery) can take communion as long as he is cautioned about the necessity for not eating in any other way.

Reconciliation (Confession). Reconciliation is confessing to a priest sins the person has committed and asking for God's forgiveness through the priest's intercession. Allow privacy for confession to protect the confidentiality of the relationship. Reconciliation may precede the rite of communion or may be initiated independently.

Annointing of the Sick. Before 1963, this rite was termed *Extreme Unction* or *Last Rites* and was administered only to people in immediate possibility of death. Today the rite is more often done any time a person is ill, since the prayers are designed to help the person endure his illness as well as to obtain salvation if he should die. Holy oil is applied to the forehead and the hands and feet; allow this to dry naturally rather than wash it away as respect for the rite.

PROTESTANTISM

The Protestant religions originated as protests against Catholicism. Although some Protestant beliefs are in strong opposition to Catholicism (the belief in sainthood or the immaculate conception of Jesus), many similarities exist. The spiritual leader is generally termed a *minister.*

Protestants celebrate both Christmas and Easter. Attendance at church is not compulsory. Prayer is often more informal. People may be baptized during the first year of life or as adults; if a person should die unbaptized, it would not be of consequence. Major Protestant religions practiced in the United States are Presbyterian, Episcopalian (Anglican), Methodist, Lutheran, and Baptist. Most denominations use wine or grape juice and bread for communion so this may not be possible if a person is required to have nothing by mouth.

Jehovah's Witnesses. All Jehovah's Witnesses are ministers. Each as a minister has an obligation to spread the meaning of his religion to as many people as possible. Blood transfusions are refused, although this is ultimately an individual decision so there may be exceptions. If a child's life is threatened, a court order transferring custody to the state may be obtained to allow the transfusion. Jehovah's Witnesses tend to disregard ceremonies, so the parents of a child may ask that he not participate in a program such as a Christmas or Easter party.

Mormonism. Mormonism is also known as the Church of Jesus Christ of Latter-Day Saints. Once known as a religion that advocated polygamy (a man having several wives), today strict monogamy is practiced. Marriage, procreation, and parenthood are high ideals. Mormons cannot become like God except as a couple.

Unlike most Christians, Mormons believe that the death of Jesus did not atone for the sins of mankind; a man earns his way to godhood by the power of his free will, not by the grace or forgiveness of Jesus Christ. Based on this philosophy, a cross is rarely used as a symbol and Easter has little meaning.

All young adults are urged to spend 2 years as missionaries as a rite of passage into church leadership. Alcohol, tea, coffee, and tobacco are prohibited as clouding clear reason. Procreation being so important, any illness that interferes with the ability to conceive children may be viewed as extremely serious. A chronic illness that would prevent a young adult from fulfilling his missionary requirements may also be viewed as serious. Death, on the other hand, has many positive focuses. Dying to join a former marriage partner may be viewed as setting in motion a progression toward godhood.

The Mennonites and Amish. Both the Mennonites and the Amish require strict observation of religious services and periods of prayer. Alcohol may be prohibited. A show of worldly wealth or possessions is forbidden. If you wear noticeably expensive jewelry or heavy make-up, such a person may have difficulty relating to you.

Christian Scientist. Christian Scientists believe that illness is a fault of the mind or a miscommunication with God. Healing is accomplished not by medical treatment but by prayer and reading by Christian Scientist readers or healers. Smoking, alcohol, and coffee are prohibited; medication, blood transfusion, and diagnostic procedures such as biopsy, physical examination, and x-ray as well as treatment such as surgery may be refused. A Christian Scientist may have difficulty deciding which route he wants to follow—follow the physician's advice and have surgery but feel guilty because he did not have enough faith to refuse; refuse and worry that surgery was necessary. Do not allow your own spiritual beliefs to influence this type of decision. It is the person to whom the problem is happening who must live with it in the years to come, not you. Support, inform, and respect; leave decision-making to him.

Atheists and Agnostics

An *atheist* is a person who denies the existence of God. An *agnostic* is a person who is uncertain about the existence of God. Both atheists and agnostics may have ethics as strong as the person who believes in God.

An atheist or agnostic may be an effective problem-solver because he does not have so reliable a support as the person who believes in God. He may need greater support from you at trying times because he does not have this outside support that the average person relies on to some extent in any crisis.

> **☐ QUICK REFERENCE STOP 23-2: NUTRITION**
>
> Dietary restrictions accompany many religious practices. Ask on health care agency admission if there are any foods such as ham that the person does not eat because of religious practices. A dietician can construct a diet around these food preferences only if she is alerted to the problem.
>
> Although it is no longer necessary, many older Roman Catholic adults still refrain from eating or drinking before communion. Respect this period of fasting as important to the person even though this is no longer practiced by younger church members.

ASSESSING SPIRITUAL OR RELIGIOUS NEED

Check the admission form to see if a person in a health care agency or being seen by a community health nurse gave his religious affiliation, but do not assume that this information is complete. Leaving the section blank does not mean that the patient has no spiritual belief; it may mean merely that he belongs to no structured religion or that he considers this a private matter. Another person may leave it blank because although he is devoutly religious, he does not want the hospital chaplain to call on him. In any event, when someone prints the word *Catholic*, *Jewish*, *Protestant*, or *Islam* on an admission form, it does not tell you the *strength* of the person's religious commitment. Some people offer you clues to the importance of religious practices in their life by bringing religious articles such as a prayer shawl, a rosary, or a Bible with them to a health care agency or displaying them prominently at home.

People may ask you to let their spiritual counselor know that they are hospitalized or they may ask you to give their name to the hospital chaplain. Again, a person's not asking for these services does not mean that he does not need them; he may not know that a chaplain is available or realize how much a visit from a clergyman would mean to him. When you mention that a chaplain is available, preface the statement by saying you routinely offer the information so a patient does not worry that you think he is dying or otherwise in special need of a chaplain.

Be certain to ask as part of a nursing history on admission if there are special religious activities or needs the person wants to observe in a health care agency (e.g., a special diet, time for morning prayers, grace before meals, bedtime prayers) (see QRS 23-2). If this information is not recorded and time planned for such activities, during the time when the person is most ill (and therefore perhaps most in need of solace from his religion) and having most of his self-care needs met by the nursing staff, these needs can easily be neglected.

As a rule, the more stressful life becomes, the more a person needs support people around him. For the person with a spiritual belief, this may be his most important support. People recovering from serious surgery after learning that the diagnosis is poor or that they are going to die are people to whom spiritual support may be extremely important.

The seriousness of an illness is not so important in determining who needs support as is the person's perception of the seriousness of the illness. A person with a minor illness may be extremely distressed and need spiritual support. Offering to call a clergyman for him ("a great many people like to talk to their own clergyman or the hospital chaplain before surgery; would you like me to contact someone for you?") is as important as calling on the anesthesiologist or the physical therapist if their concern centers on fear of anesthesia or concern for painful daily exercises.

THE ROLE OF SPIRITUAL BELIEFS IN CARE PLANNING

A part of plan of care for everyone should include measures necessary to respect or help the patient with religious observations. For example, people who have a clergyman calling daily may need to have their hospital room and bed straightened earlier in the morning than people who will be having no visit (providing other factors are equal). Just as most people dress up to attend church or synagogue, ill persons like to look presentable when their clergyman calls.

Most people appreciate being left alone with their clergyman. This is generally a time for you to excuse yourself rather than carrying out some other activity in the room. Clergymen are frequent hospital visitors and have encountered equipment such as intravenous therapy or even ventilators. Despite this, do not expect a clergyman to be responsible for the patient's condition anymore than you would a family member. If a clergyman is going to administer a rite such as communion to the patient, he may need some help from you to reposition the patient so the patient can swallow easily or at least assurance from you that the rite is not medically contraindicated.

Some patients do not plan on having a member of the clergy visit, but would appreciate being able to visit the hospital chapel daily for prayer. Some may want to attend a service held on Saturday or Sunday in the hospital chapel. Investigate the hospital's facilities for attendance of people in wheelchairs or stretchers at such services. Some are held in such small chapels (niches in hallway walls, actually) that it is impossible to include a person who is less than almost well. Most hospital chaplains are willing to attempt a trial period of holding services in the hospital auditorium or a large conference room where handicapped people can be accommodated. Nurses who value planning for spiritual needs as well as other needs arrange the patient's care (and perhaps free an aide or arrange for volunteer help) to accommodate time in care for religious services.

Allowing people time to say grace before meals if that is their practice before you begin to feed them and time to read a Bible passage before you turn out their light for the night are other common ways of respecting religious practices. Remember that nontraditional meals such as tube feedings *are* meals and a person may wish to say grace as much before this unusual feeding method as he does before a usual meal. A person who is receiving his total nutritional intake by intravenous therapy (total parenteral nutrition) may feel dissatisfaction with this type of feeding not only because of the lack of tasting or chewing food but also because the constant infusion interferes with his practice of saying grace before meals.

Ask parents of small children to write out the grace they wish their child to say before meals or a bedtime prayer they want him to use if they cannot be present at those times. Leave a copy on the child's care plan so everyone can assist him at meals or bedtime.

Be certain when making beds or straightening a patient's possessions that you are alert for religious articles; do not accidentally throw anything important to the person into the laundry. Many people pin a religious symbol to their gown, pillow case, or sheet thinking this will keep it safe. Mark on the nursing care plan that the article exists so everyone giving care can be equally careful (Fig. 23-2, QRS 23-3).

Occasionally, a person may ask you to read a favorite prayer or a passage from the Bible. Listening to a favorite passage this way offers both security and spiritual comfort. Thus, the Twenty-third Psalm remains a constant during illness and also offers specific comfort for them (Lo, though I walk through the valley of the shadow of death, I will fear no evil . . .). Another patient may ask you to remember him in your prayers or to pray with him.

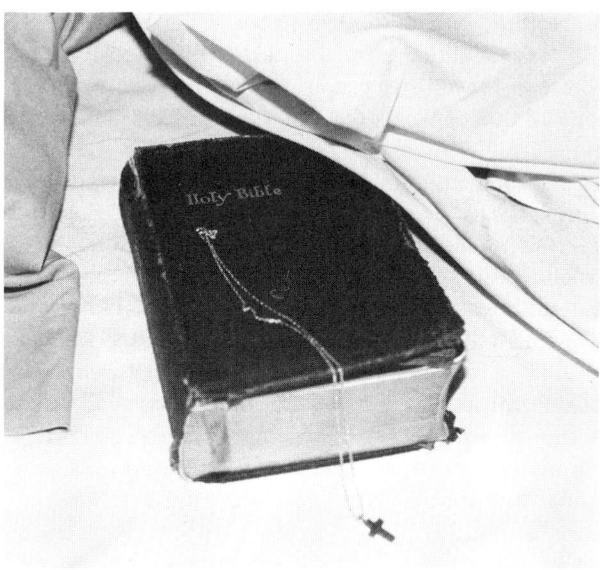

FIGURE 23-2. Use care in handling religious articles. This well-worn Bible means a great deal to its owner.

☐ QUICK REFERENCE STOP 23-3: SAFETY

Be certain when handling patient's possessions that you do not accidentally throw away a religious symbol. Replacing a well-loved article with a new one is never the same.

If a person has such an article with him, write on his care plan what it is and where it is placed.

Requests such as these may be awkward if your religion is different from that of the patient or you have no strong spiritual beliefs. However, reading a religious passage to someone is not generally interpreted as practicing that religion, so there should be no reason not to fulfill the request—just as you would read a letter from a family member or an insurance company to a person who temporarily could not read such material himself. If a patient asks you to do this frequently, it may suggest that he would appreciate a call from a clergyman or chaplain. If you become concerned that any practice compromises you in some way, discuss the matter with your own clergyman.

If you do not normally spend time in prayer, it would be hypocritical to promise that you will include a person in your daily prayers. On the other hand, it might be destructive when a person has revealed such vulnerability to you to tell him that you do not believe anyone listens to prayer. A compromise might be to assure him that you will say a prayer for him this day with no mention of daily prayer. If a patient asks you to say a prayer with him (perhaps before he is taken to surgery or is going to have a painful treatment performed) and prayer is a part of your religious practice, you might say a prayer that is one of your favorites or suggest saying a prayer both of you know together. If your religion and the person's differ to such an extent that you have no common prayer, suggesting that you both pray silently for a moment is another alternative. This is also an alternative if you do not believe in prayer; that you really say nothing in your silence is between you and your conscience, a compromise between patient caring and your own beliefs.

Respecting spiritual beliefs is often done in the role of patient advocate. Examples of this are reminding the dietician that a Muslim patient does not eat pork, mentioning to a doctor that a patient does not believe in blood transfusions (e.g., a Jehovah's Witness), speaking with housekeeping about a native American belief that cornmeal spread around his bed will keep away evil spirits, and speaking with a physician when a Christian Scientist wants to leave the hospital against medical advice because he does not believe in surgery. People have the right to make these kinds of choices based on religious beliefs; the exceptions are when the decision would endanger the life or well-being of a child.

Implementation: Assisting Clergymen

People who have effective spiritual counselors may need help reaching them. People who do not have current spiritual support people may need help establishing a new support system through the chaplain or another source.

Clergymen serve as strong resource people and may be called upon for consultation. Always be aware, however, that clergy other than one assigned as a chaplain are not entitled to confidential information unless the patient has explicitly said that the clergyman may have the information. Information that can be shared with them is limited to the patient's name, room number, age, sex, reason for hospitalization, and any reason they gave for wanting to see their clergyman. In the same way, a clergyman maintains a confidential relationship with his parishioner, and he gains information that he may not share.

Respect for Your Own Beliefs

Occasionally a patient you care for practices a religion with such a strong missionary mandate that he tries to convert you to his religion. Such instances can be awkward; learn to handle them smoothly in the same way you would handle a situation of any patient describing a life-style that does not appeal to you (you care for a drug addict and listen to him describe his life but do not intend to make it yours; a patient makes a sexual advance to you but you continue to give care). If you feel a person's insistence on converting you to his religion is interfering with your care, you may need to establish a relationship with him that includes firm limits—you will discuss religion with him in order to learn more about it, but you already have your own religion. Be careful that you do not handle the situation by spending as little time as possible with the person. A withdrawal technique is a temptation because it quickly solves your problem, but it does not add to the quality of your nursing care or meet the person's needs.

☐ QUICK REFERENCE STOP 23-4: COMMUNITY CONSIDERATIONS

Spiritual needs of people can go unmet after a person is discharged from a health care facility because he is not well enough to travel to his place of worship and no longer has access to the health care facility chaplain. Assess this aspect of a patient's life to be certain that his spiritual needs can be met. Remember that some people use their place of worship for social stimulation and interaction as well, making it doubly important to them.

☐ QUICK REFERENCE STOP 23-5: PSYCHOLOGICAL CONSIDERATIONS

Mental health is as important to people as physical health. Assisting them to locate a spiritual counselor is as important as any physical care measure. Some people are anxious to talk to a spiritual counselor, not so much out of spiritual concern, but because he has good listening skills. Be alert to this use of the clergy, since it is a role that you can fill. Many times if a person can put a problem into words to a skillful listener it becomes half as fearsome as it was minutes before.

Evaluation

When evaluating whether the goals of spiritual needs have been met or not, do not assume that because a person was visited by a spiritual counselor that he is now free of concern. This may be so, but because relief of this nature happens at a cognitive or emotional level, the visitor may not have accomplished this. QRS 23-4 and 23-5 address two other aspects of the spiritual needs of your patients.

NURSING CARE PLAN

Mrs. Jeffrey is a 65-year-old woman you care for. She has been admitted to the hospital for a urinary tract infection. She tells you that she is discouraged about the amount of pain she is having. The following is a source-oriented nursing note you might write on her.

8:00 A.M.	Patient appears tired; ate no breakfast although she had been given a breakfast tray. Stated she had too much pain to be hungry.

8:30 A.M. Codeine 30 mg administered orally. Resting afterward; but reported no real relief from the medication.

9:00 A.M. Observed crying as she spoke on telephone to grandson about the diagnostic tests planned for her. Took tub bath hoping warm water would help her relax; reported feeling no better afterward. Neglected to comb hair; stated, "What's the difference? Nice looking hair won't make me feel better."

9:45 A.M. Visited by hospital chaplain.

10:45 A.M. Sitting up in bed; joking with roommate. Has combed hair and put on lipstick. States, "I'm starting to feel better. Any chance I could have some breakfast?" Asked if chaplain's visit was helpful to her, she stated, "I asked him to come back tomorrow. It's easy to forget what's important to you, isn't it?"

An addition you might make to her nursing care plan based on these observations might be:

NURSING DIAGNOSIS
Spiritual distress related to present illness.
Locus of Decision-Making: Patient.
Goal: Patient to demonstrate increased use of spiritual support people during hospital stay.
Criteria: Patient voices greater peace of mind related to spiritual support.
NURSING ORDERS
1. Save time in A.M. for chaplain's visit. (10:00—10:30 A.M.)
2. Provide support as necessary for diagnostic testing program since it is a stressful time for patient.

SUGGESTED READINGS

Baasher, T. The healing power of faith . . . across a wide range of cultures. *World Health* 10:5, 1982.

Belgum, D. (Ed.). *Religion and Medicine: Essays on Meaning, Value, and Health.* Ames, Iowa: Iowa State University Press, 1967.

Betz, C. L. Faith development in children. *Pediatr. Nurs.* 7:22, 1981.

Burghardt, W. J. Models of church, models of health apostolate. *Hosp. Prog.* 62(5):35, 1981.

Buys, A. N., Discussion series sensitizes nurses to patient's spiritual needs. *Hosp. Prog.* 62:44, 1981.

Damstugt, D. Pastoral roles in presurgical visits. *Am. J. Nurs.* 75:1336, 1975.

Devine, B. A. Attitudes of the elderly toward religion. *J. Gerontol. Nurs.* 6:679, 1980.

Dickinson, C. The search for spiritual meaning. *Am. J. Nurs.* 75:1789, 1975.

Father Bill and the sacrament of the sick . . . an act of faith . . . don't call it the Last Rites. *Nursing* (Horsham) 13(2):68, 1983.

Fish, S., and Shelley, J. A. *Spiritual Care: The Nurse's Role.* Downer's Grove, Ill.: InterVarsity Press, 1978.

Fuller, S. S. Holistic man and the science and practice of nursing. *Nurs. Outlook* 26(11):700, 1978.

Henley, A., et al. Asians in hospital . . . illness and the life cycle . . . some aspects of Hinduism. *Health Soc. Serv. J.* 92(4809):972, 1982.

Highfield, M. F. Spiritual needs of patients: Are they recognized? *Cancer Nurs.* 6(3):187, 1983.

Humphrey, J. B. Recognizing your patient's spiritual needs. *Nursing 77* 7:64, 1977.

Kohlberg, L. The development of children's orientations toward a moral order. *Vita Humana* 6:11, 1963.

Krieger, D. *Foundations for Holistic Health Nursing Practice: The Renaissance Nurse.* Philadelphia: Lippincott, 1981.

Leslie, R. C. *Health, Healing and Holiness.* Nashville, Tenn.: Graded Press, 1971.

Recognizing your patient's spiritual needs. *Nurs. 77* 77(12):64, 1977.

Richards, F. What they believe and why. *Nurs. Mirror* 138:65, 1977.

Shannon, M. Spiritual needs and nursing responsibility. *Imprint* 27:23, 1980.

Shelton, R. L. The patient's need of faith at death. *Top. Clin. Nurs.* 3:55, 1981.

Stang, M. A. Lay-religious collaboration essential in health ministry. *Hosp. Prog.* 62(5):46, 1981.

Stoll, R. Guidelines for spiritual assessment. *Am. J. Nurs.* 79:1574, 1979.

Walker, C. Attitudes to death and bereavement among cultural minority groups. *Nurs. Times* 78(50):2106, 1982.

QUESTIONS FOR REVIEW

1. Religion is defined as:
   a. Organized worship.
   b. A spiritual belief.
   c. An inner trust.
   d. Belief in God.

2. Mr. Stein is an Orthodox Jew. Which of the following foods on his breakfast tray would you question?
   a. Milk.
   b. Eggs.
   c. Bacon.
   d. Oatmeal.

3. The Jewish New Year is termed:
   a. Passover.
   b. Seder.
   c. Hanukkah.
   d. Rosh Hashanah.

4. If a Roman Catholic infant is about to die, he can be baptized by which person?
   a. A priest.
   b. A physician.
   c. A nurse.
   d. Any of the above.

5. An agnostic is a person who:
   a. Does not believe in God.
   b. Is not certain of God's existence.
   c. Believes in a primitive god.
   d. Hates God.

6. People of Islam follow which dietary pattern?
   a. Eat no pork.
   b. Eat kosher meat.
   c. Eat no vegetables.
   d. Eat no shellfish.

7. The prophet of Islam is:
   a. Muhammad.
   b. Brahman.
   c. Buddha.
   d. Allah.

8. The age at which children tend to question their faith is:
   a. Toddler.
   b. Adolescence.
   c. School.
   d. Preschool.

24. GRIEVING AND THE MEANING OF LOSS

OBJECTIVES

Upon mastery of the material in this chapter, you should be able to:

1. Define death.
2. List other losses that may evoke a grief reaction.
3. Describe the physiological changes that occur with death.
4. Describe the stages of grieving cited by Kubler-Ross.
5. Describe the differing perceptions of death by different age span groups.
6. Describe the care of people who have been diagnosed as having a terminal illness.
7. Describe nursing responsibilities for postmortem care.
8. Describe alternatives to hospital environments for dying persons.
9. Describe preparations necessary to make to be prepared to care for people suffering loss.

TERMS

The terms important for an understanding of this chapter are shown below and defined in the glossary:

euthanasia
autopsy
death
hospice
rigor mortis
terminal illness
thanatology

Grieving or mourning is the predictable psychological phenomenon that accompanies a loss. Although this loss often involves death, it occurs to some extent with any illness when the person feels a loss of the former well self. It also occurs in response to the loss of material objects (a person's home is robbed; he loses money through poor investments), valued persons (a child leaves for college; parents retire and move to Florida; a couple is divorced), a loss of self (a person is fired from an important position or loses an election; develops an illness that leads to vision or hearing impairment or a chronic disease such as diabetes or asthma and will never be completely "well" again), a developmental loss (loss of being a child to becoming adult; loss of being single when a person gets married; loss of being responsible only for himself to becoming a parent). Figure 24-1 illustrates two kinds of losses that may be dealt with by some form of grieving.

STAGES OF GRIEVING

Kubler-Ross (1969) has described the stages of grief and observable behavior that occurs with each stage. The following discussion summarizes these stages, but it is important for you to remember that every person will handle his grief in his own way: he may not go through all the stages described, or he may go through them in different order.

Denial

Denial is the first stage of reaction to loss. People often refer to this as a sensation of feeling numb or shocked. It is a basic protective technique to prevent themselves from truly feeling the loss. A person in this stage of grief may be unwilling to talk about the loss because talking about it will make it real; some people will intellectualize the loss, discussing it calmly but without any emotion.

It is sometimes difficult to care for people who are experiencing denial because you want them to move to the next stage and begin to deal with their loss. Do not force people to move quickly out of a stage of denial. This protective stage prevents a person from facing the loss until he has amassed enough coping ability to deal with it. Pushing him past this stage before his coping ability is organized can cause him to be overwhelmed and to adapt unhealthy mechanisms to deal with his loss. In sum, during this time he feels, "This isn't happening."

Anger

Anger follows the stage of denial. The person talks about the unfairness of what is happening (he knows many people who are not as good a person as he is and yet they are well; it is unfair that he is ill). He may overtly demonstrate anger by slamming doors or criticizing health care personnel. He may resist self-care (it is unfair

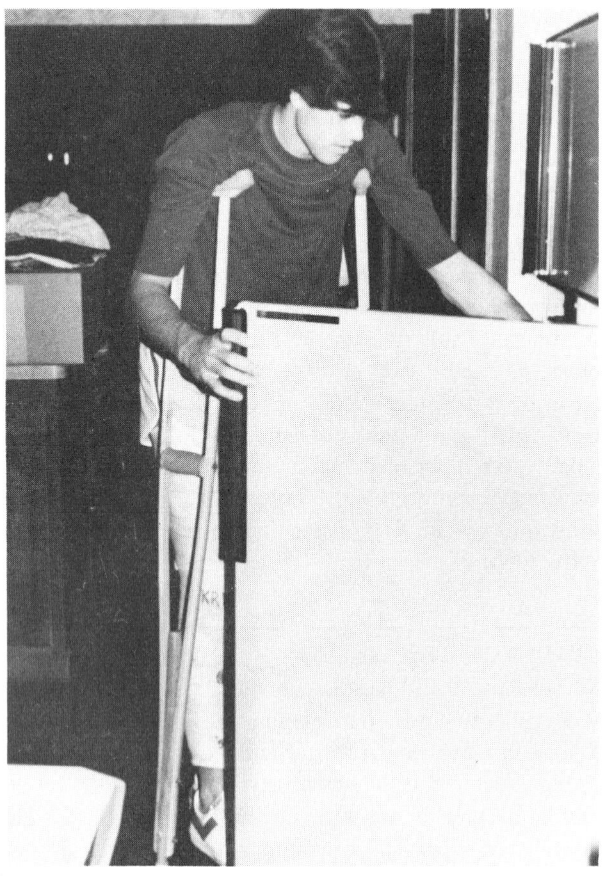

A

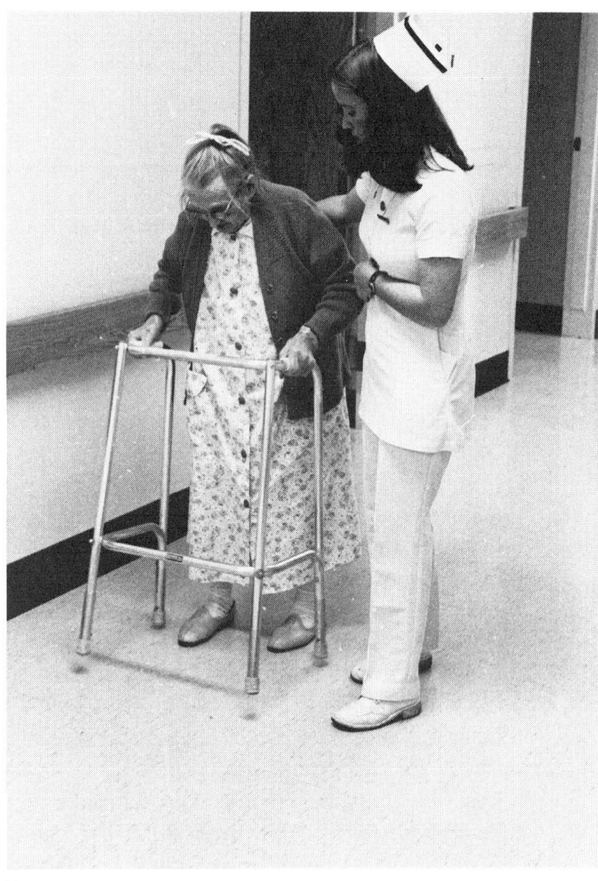

B

FIGURE 24-1. A person will grieve the loss of functioning in his own body. A. This adolescent has a temporary loss of ambulatory function; he must give up many daily activities as well as football for a season. B. An older woman is experiencing a permanent loss of ambulatory function. Here she is learning to use a walker with the help of a nurse.

of you to ask this of him because the entire situation is so unfair).

It may be difficult to work with people who are experiencing anger because they are not receptive to suggestions (if you were really helpful you would take away the primary loss, not offer suggestions for dealing with it). During this time a person feels "It's unfair this is happening."

Bargaining

Bargaining is an intermediate step in grief, a time when the person tries to correct what is happening by making a bargain to be a better person if only the loss will be corrected. For example, a person vows to never drive fast again if only his leg is not amputated, or if the loss will be his own life, that he does not mind dying if only it can be after his children all graduate from school. When people realize that bargaining is ineffective, they reach a very low point in grief. They may need more support when bargaining fails than at any other point.

Depression

A feeling of depression or sadness occurs when the person begins to realize for the first time that this situation is truly happening. This is a change from "No, it isn't happening" to "It's unfair this is happening" to "It's all right if it happens but" to "This is happening and it is happening to me." Crying is the most common sign that this stage has been reached; accompanying loss of appetite and energy, causing the person to neglect self-care, usually occur as well.

On the surface, depression, the most acute point of grief, appears to be a step backward (he had seemed to be accepting a poor diagnosis well; now he is overwhelmed by it). Actually, this is the first time he has appreciated the hurt or the full extent of the situation.

In this stage patients may begin to ask more questions about their care or treatments than they did before. Do not interpret this questioning as criticism. The person is asking because this is the first time he is fully aware of what is happening to him.

This stage of grief requires a great deal of your time and energy because the person is at least temporarily overwhelmed and unable to plan for himself.

Acceptance

Acceptance is the final stage or the resolution of grief. It is a change to "It is *all right* this is happening to me."

How long it takes a person to reach this stage depends on the level of his coping ability and the depth of the loss. It may take 6 months to 2 years for family members to accept a death. A person grieving for his own death may not reach this stage before death occurs.

Anticipatory Grief

Anticipatory grief is mourning or grieving before an event actually takes place. This reaction shields a person from the onslaught of the loss when the loss actually occurs. As a rule, it is a healthful reaction because it blunts the actual pain of the loss. Occasionally, it can be harmful if a parent begins grieving for a child he has been told will die (born prematurely or very ill at some later point in life) and then the child does not die. Without meaning to, the parent may cut off effective relationships with the child during the anticipatory grief stage and not be able to rekindle them effectively later on. Such children are termed *vulnerable children*. They may develop behavior disorders or acting out behavior as they grow older, as if to say, "Notice me, I am alive."

Chronic Grief

Chronic grief is grief that continues past the normal time limit. A person who has been diagnosed as having a chronic illness such as diabetes may find himself feeling sad and unable to make decisions or to feel really good about himself although objectively he recognizes that he is able to do everything he could before he became ill with few exceptions.

Feelings of chronic grief are most apt to occur at holidays or special events (such as weddings, christenings) when the potential of the person is most easily contrasted with what his potential would have been if the loss had not occurred (parents of a retarded child grieve the day their retarded child would have started school). People may need special support during these life crises.

FACING DEATH

Death generally leads to a strong grief reaction, not only in the person who is dying but in his support people and health care personnel as well.

Death is a paradoxical topic in the modern world. Few people speak about it comfortably, but it obviously has great interest because books on the subject rapidly become best-sellers. Although most people make few concrete plans for death, it is the only certainty in life.

When life-styles were simpler and largely rural, death was accepted more commonly and comfortably than today because as a child grew up on a farm, he saw death as farm animals were slaughtered for food; he outlived cats, dogs, and chickens; he saw nests of field mice destroyed by plows or his dog. Families were often extended and medicine less advanced; he watched family members die. Family and friends all gathered at home to mourn.

At the same time, he also saw life: new crops every year, new calves born every spring, new chickens to brood every year. Birth, life, and death were viewed as cyclical. This view was reinforced by religious rituals from earliest times.

Today, a child reared in an inner city with no pets may have little or no exposure to death until he reaches adulthood and his grandparents die. Dying in major cities is done in hospitals; the rites of death are conducted at a funeral home. The event is frightening and hard to accept because it is so out of context with his usual pattern of living. The person is no better prepared to accept the death of a child or of his parents as he reaches middle age—or his own death at any age.

Nurses work closely with people who have been diagnosed as having a terminal illness (an illness for which there is no expected recovery). They are in the best position to give support to a person at this critical point. Yet nurses, too, are often ill prepared to deal with the crisis of death. Preparation for this role in nursing is as important as learning measures that make people well again or help them to remain well.

Life Span Concepts and Death

A person's concept of death varies from age to age as his ability to conceptualize and his past experiences, religion, and family-living concepts increase.

The Infant and Toddler. Infants and toddlers are too young to appreciate death except as the loss of a person who cared for them and the presence of a void in their life. If such a loss interferes with the development of a sense of trust, its implications for the child's ability to ever achieve warm, close relationships will last his lifetime.

The Preschooler. Preschoolers learn about the concept of death when a pet dies or they discover a dead bird or mouse. However, they envision death as temporary and appear to have little adult fear of it. This casualness toward death is sometimes interpreted as heartlessness (a child told that his brother has just been killed in an automobile accident says, "That's too bad," and then asks if he can have his radio). He thinks of his brother as being gone only for a short time so he should take advantage of the situation. This temporary concept is strengthened by children's cartoons, where frequently a character is killed and then immediately revives and goes on with the story.

Preschoolers do fear separation greatly and are stunned by the death of a parent. If a child grasps the concept that he is himself dying, his worry might be that he will be alone and separated. He may need someone to stay with him constantly to assure him that he is not alone.

The Schoolager. The schoolager begins to have additional experience with death so his knowledge of it as a final measure increases. However, he thinks of it as something that affects only adults. He has little of the adult's worry about being accountable for his life or sins so that if he realizes that he is dying, he has sadness from the thought of separation but little fear of not having done all the things he should have done in life. At about 9 years of age, the child fully understands that death is not only permanent but inevitable.

The Adolescent and Young Adult. Although adolescents have an adult concept of death, they also may feel immune to death. Driving at high speed and walking along the ledges of high cliffs reflect this phenomenon. Accepting his own death is difficult as a whole for a young adult; he may deny the symptoms for longer than usual because he believes it is impossible that anything serious could be happening to him.

The Middle-Aged Adult. The middle-aged adult begins to look at death as a real possibility and begins to make concrete plans (writing a will, examining life insurance coverage). The parents of most middle-aged adults die so they are faced with the fact of their own mortality. A youngest child in a family may be startled to realize that with the death of older siblings, he is now the oldest child. A middle-aged adult who was a "junior" becomes a senior when his father dies. Death has caused change in self-image or life role.

The Older Adult. The older adult has more evidence that death is inevitable than other age groups as his peers die. If you ask an older adult what age he thinks of himself as being, however, many of them will answer "40" or "50" (people of 50 often think of themselves as 40; people of 40 as 30). The person who thinks of himself as younger than his chronological years may not be aware of himself as being at an age when death can be anticipated. Being told that he has a terminal illness may be as unexpected as if he were much younger.

Part of the achievement of the final developmental phase in life is achieving a sense of integrity. This is not only feeling good about one's life, but feeling prepared for death. An older adult who is reminded by an episode of ill health that he is vulnerable to death, may spend time discussing his past life (termed *life review*). The person needs a listener in order to be able to do this. It is time well spent for you, as a rule, not only in helping the person achieve a sense of integrity, but in helping you better to understand how history influences people's lives.

Other Factors Influencing Reactions to Death

Since people are individuals, a person's reaction to learning that he or someone he cares about has a terminal illness will be affected by his personality. It is also affected to some degree by factors such as age, sex, and past experience.

One effect of the person's age is the attitude of his support people and health care providers toward his death. Interventions to prolong life are usually more intense for the child or young adult than for a very old adult. On the other hand, a parent may wish almost no interventions used with a child once the impossibility of recovery has been established in order to make death easier for the child, or a family might want everything possible tried for a strong parent even though he is past 80.

Coping Ability. Learning that death is imminent is stressful, and the manner in which people react to it reflects their reaction to other stressful situations. All people move perceptively through the stages of grief, but some more quickly than others because of better coping ability (see Chap. 12). Three factors helpful in successful coping are presence of support people, past successful coping, and correct perception of the event (loss, death).

Information Available to Dying Persons. Usually, the question arises of how soon a person should be told he is going to die and how much information he should be given. This information is part of a person's prognosis, so usually the physician tells the patient. When a person is told depends on how soon he seems ready, the wishes of his family for him to know or not, his overall condition, and the physician's ability to deal with telling him, which is never easy. Most people want to know that they are dying as soon as the physician knows so they can make plans for their estate or care of children. There is sometimes a sense that a person with many responsibilities or much property has a right to know immediately because he has much to settle whereas a person with little property or responsibility can wait longer to hear the truth. However, outsiders have no right to judge the importance of a person's decisions to him.

People give subtle clues when they are ready to face the knowledge that they are dying by statements such as "I don't seem to be getting any better, do I?" or "Do you think my heart condition is a bad one?" Listen for such statements or questions as evidence the person has reached a plateau in his acceptance of his illness and is ready for more information from his physician. You may need to urge a physician to tell a patient more about his poor prognosis than she has done thus far if you recognize that he is seeking this information. Urge such a patient to ask his physician to be frank with him. Families may ask a physician not to tell a patient about his prognosis so that they do not have to cope with the situation, but this is hardly fair to the patient.

Communication Blocks

Four possible communication blocks occur because people may or may not know about their terminal prognosis.

1. *Closed awareness.* In closed awareness, neither the patient nor his family are informed that the patient is dying. Such a situation may lead to the patient making unrealistic plans (registering for a new school year, buying a house, becoming pregnant). It can cause strained relationships between health care providers and the patient because their conception of what is happening is so far apart.

2. *Suspected awareness.* With suspected awareness, the patient suspects that he is dying, but health care providers do not confirm it. Again, this can lead to strained relationships and may cause the patient to lose confidence in his caregivers because he suspects they are not being honest with him.

3. *Mutual pretense awareness.* In this situation, both patient and health care providers are aware of the prognosis but neither mentions it to the other. Such a relationship is easier for the health care provider (although shallow and not therapeutic); it can be very frustrating and unfulfilling for the patient, since he cannot grieve—that would break through the pretense.

4. *Open awareness.* In open awareness, both the patient and health care providers know the person is dying and discuss it openly. This situation allows the patient to grieve and to make appropriate plans. This is the best of the four situations for most people, although it may not be best for everyone. Some people would truly rather not know they are dying and need their wishes respected.

Support People

Support people become very important to a person who is dying. Unfortunately, many people are overwhelmed by the thought of death and their ability to accept it; thus, they are unable to offer support. A person who is dying may day by day find himself more and more alone as his usual support people draw back from him. If no further therapy is being given in a hospital unit, he may be moved to a room at the end of the hall away from the nursing station so that patients who require more time-consuming care can be moved closer. This location is convenient from the aspect of nursing efficiency, but it often increases a person's loneliness—not only are friends and family visiting less but health care providers are visiting less as well. You may need to advocate to avoid such room placement or to include in the person's care plan time for visiting him as primary intervention.

If family are not available as support people, secondary or tertiary support people may be able to give some support. Investigate this with church groups, people from the person's place of work, and organizations such as Parents of Retarded Children or the Cancer Society. Such secondary support groups can be helpful not only to the person who is dying but also to the family, so that they can continue to be effective support people.

Past Experiences

In the past when people died at home and friends and neighbors gathered at the house before and after the funeral, people grew up more prepared to cope with dying because it fell within their previous experience. It is sometimes helpful to remind a person that dying or accepting death of a person who is meaningful to them can be managed because although they have not faced this particular stress before, they have accepted other stresses in life (e.g., not attending the college of their choice, not obtaining a job they wanted, being unable to have any more children). Remembering that he coped with difficulty in the past helps a person to realize that he can cope with the present crisis also.

Life Philosophy

A person's feelings about life influence his feelings about death. A person who believes in life after death may be able to accept death more easily than one who does not (or may have a more difficult time because he is worried about his fate in another life). A person who has been disappointed in his life may view death as a preferred alternative to experiencing more disappointment as he grows older. As a rule of thumb, a person who has a strong religious faith views death as less threatening than one who does not. This means faith, not active church going, which can be a superficial or even social function and not one of faith.

Disease State

A terminal disease provokes many people to extreme anger (they are a better person than others who do not have this disease, so that death is unfair for them). If the disease brings extreme pain, they may come to think of death as a valued release. If therapy or hospital costs are draining the family's resources, a person may view death as a contribution to his family's welfare and so value it.

Preventable death, as from accidents, is generally more difficult to accept than nonpreventable death. It reminds everyone how vulnerable people are to the care or lack of care of those around them. It also confirms that death is inevitable.

THE ONSET OF DEATH

Physiological changes as a person nears death are important in nursing care. Basically, these are changes in slowed metabolism and decreased cell oxygenation; decreased cell oxygenation leads to cell dysfunction and body system dysfunction.

Cardiovascular Changes

As stroke volume of the heart lessens with impending death, the power to circulate blood becomes less. The person develops characteristic appearances because of poor circulation. The skin will feel cool and appear mottled or cyanotic since blood is no longer well oxygenated and not pushed well into distal sites. Just before death, blood will begin to pool in the dependent body parts, making them mottled or purple (the abdomen of a person lying supine will become pale; his back would be purple hued from this dependent collection of blood). Pooling of blood in dependent body parts is the means whereby pathologists can identify the position of a person when he died, a fact sometimes helpful in solving murder.

As circulation fails, absorption of a drug from a muscle becomes virtually impossible. Giving an emergency drug into the muscle of a person with extreme cyanotic mottling would be a useless measure; it would need to be administered intravenously to have any effect.

As peripheral circulation fails, less heat is lost from the body. The person's body may compensate for this by increased perspiration to increase heat loss through evaporation. The person's skin may feel not only cool but damp. You may need to change linen frequently because of this increased moisture on the skin.

Respiratory System

Slowed respiration leads to increased secretions in the lungs or the appearance of rales (the sound of air being pulled through fluid in alveoli). In order to compensate for a few minutes of very slow respirations, a person may take a couple quick or extremely deep inhalations periodically or demonstrate a very irregular breathing pattern. As a deep inhalation is drawn in past accumulated fluid or a lax larynx there may be an audible snoring sound (harsh rhonchi).

Neuromuscular System

Decrease in muscular function leads to severe weakness and fatigue. More and more, the person maintains the exact position in which you placed him. Of particular concern is a general loss of ability to swallow and loss of a gag reflex, so he may aspirate on oral fluid. As the tone of body sphincters is lost, the person may be incontinent of bladder or bowel contents. An often-noticed phenomenon is constant hand movement, a picking at bedclothes that probably represents the loss of upper centers of voluntary muscular control. Neurologically, deep reflexes (achilles tendon, knee jerk, brachioradialis, as well as triceps) are no longer perceptible. A corneal reflex may be tested on a person near death (touching a wisp of cotton to the cornea should cause acute pain and tearing normally) or pressure to the inner canthus of the eye globe (will cause acute pain except in the person who is deeply unconscious).

As a person nears death, he generally begins to demonstrate a lessened level of consciousness although he may remain perfectly alert until seconds before death. Vision apparently blurs because the person tends to turn toward the light. Touch seems to remain intact because the person responds positively to touch and often quiets by a gentle stroking of his forehead or arm; he grasps one's hand meaningfully as if the touch is appreciated and felt. Hearing remains intact. People who have been declared dead and then resuscitated report of hearing exactly what their caregivers said over them during the resuscitation attempt (not always kind remarks). *Hearing is the last sense lost.* For people regaining consciousness following coma or anesthesia, hearing is the first sense regained.

Gastrointestinal System

Digestion slows as total body metabolism slows. The person may notice nausea or revulsion to food from this slowed digestive process. Constipation due to the poor bowel tone and decreased peristaltic action will occur. The person's abdomen will become distended from intestinal flatus. As intake is decreased, dehydration with dry mucus membrane and conjunctiva will occur unless intravenous supplement is begun. The person's temperature will generally rise a degree or so due to this dehydration, further increasing the perspiration noticed on skin.

Modifications of Care Based on Physical Changes

Because body metabolism is slowing, modifications in care for the person who is dying center on carrying out care at a pace that allows the person's slowed body resources to adjust. For example, perfusion of distal body parts is slower, so turning the person suddenly to a new position might overtax his circulation. Turning him gradually will allow his cardiovascular system to compensate. Be certain the person's chest is not compressed by pillows or tight bedclothes because he needs optimal lung expansion. If the person's gag or swallowing reflex is impaired, position him on his side in a Sim's position to allow saliva to drain from his mouth and prevent aspiration. Mouth dryness will lead to cracking and secondary infection and pain; prevent it by frequent cleaning of the mucous membrane with swabs and clear water. If eye conjunctiva appear dry, ask the physician to prescribe moistening eye drops; keep any crusting at eyelids washed away so optimal vision is possible.

Keep skin surfaces from rubbing against one another by supporting pillows and good positioning. Keep skin dry from urine or feces from incontinence. This care prevents painful decubiti ulcers from forming, and you want to avoid pain if at all possible.

Assess for motion or other indications that the person

has pain. If the person is conscious, you may need to ask his physician for an analgesic so he can be comfortable; if he is unconscious (does not rouse except to deep pain stimuli), it is assumed that he is not experiencing pain. Prescribing analgesic medication such as narcotics to people with slowed respiratory function poses an ethical problem—prescribing it will undoubtedly slow respiratory function further and probably hasten death; not prescribing it will allow the person to live slightly longer but the additional time will be spent in pain. The person has a right to participate in this decision. Occasionally a person will have an important reason to want to live one more day (until a son or daughter who lives far away arrives) and will ask not to have pain medication administered even though he is obviously in severe pain.

Remember that hearing is the last sense lost. A person even minutes away from death is capable of hearing everything you say. You may need to remind family members and, on occasion, other health care personnel of this. Continue to explain procedures to unconscious people as if they were conscious because they undoubtedly do hear you. Never make any comment in their presence that you would not make if they were alert.

Continue to use the same gentle touch and nonverbal communication, such as holding a hand or brushing hair from the forehead, as if the person were fully conscious. He may be fully aware of your actions even though he can give no indication of it.

Whether people die with quiet acceptance or fight the final minutes has a great deal to do with their psychological acceptance of death. The person who has his estate in order and has accepted that his death is inevitable generally dies imperceptively. People appear to appreciate having someone with them at the moment of death and will return your hand grasp until their hand relaxes with death.

ENVIRONMENT FOR DEATH

Most people do not think about where they would like to die while they are well. When they have a terminal illness, this can become important. For too long, caregivers offered no choice. Today, a number of alternatives are available. Often, however, people are unaware of these alternatives and of their right to choose.

The Hospital

People who need a great deal of physical care (have a tracheotomy, require nasogastric feeding) generally remain in a hospital because none of their support people have the finances, energy, or skill to care for them at home. For others, being in a hospital assures them and their support people that everything that can be done for them is being done.

When intensive care units were first established, health care tended to be routine, technical in nature, and often dehumanized. A person could easily feel lost in the machines surrounding him. Today, the concept of skilled care as also being individualized and caring is beginning to make the care of dying persons as compassionate as that given to people who will recover.

Home

Many people, particularly elderly adults, prefer to die at home surrounded by their families and possessions. Many parents of young children prefer to die at home because children are not usually allowed to visit extensively in hospitals and want to spend as much time as possible with them. The person's support people must want this as much as the person or the situation will be unworkable.

Both the person and his support people need careful explanations of his illness and the care that will be needed. Time spent talking about arrangements—such as whom they should contact if the person suddenly becomes more ill than usual, how they will manage periodic check-ups, how they will purchase medicine or drugs (Does their insurance cover this?), and how they will schedule their time to have leisure periods. No one can work 24 hours a day caring for an ill family member. Even if they could physically, they should not, because such care will shut them off from friends, work, and outside contacts. When the person dies, they will find themselves very much alone. They must be able to balance the care of the ill person in their lives in order to prevent this from happening.

Overall, home care can be an extremely satisfying experience both for the person who is dying and for the people who care about him as long as it is managed with safeguards for protecting the caregivers' health as well as providing good care for the patient.

Hospices

In 1967, St. Christopher's Hospice in London was opened as a setting for people who wanted to die in a homelike setting while under skilled professional care. Hospices are now available in most major communities. In a hospice, people may have unlimited visitors; even small children and pets can visit freely. People are invited to bring those possessions that will have meaning for them, even to such items as a favorite comfortable chair or favorite dishes. They are urged to choose the degree of pain relief they wish if pain is present and to remain active and involved with the community and family until death.

A basic philosophy of hospice care is that death is an extension or part of life, not a separate entity. Thus, it can be dealt with—not with separate or awkward rituals but with the same warm concern as other situations in everyday life. In order to keep people pain free, a strong narcotic mixture (originally called a *Brompton's cocktail*) may be administered every 4 hours around the clock or may be given not after pain is felt but to keep ahead of pain. Some critics of hospice care argue that such a procedure hurries death. Advocates of hospice care view such a preventive measure in the same light as immunization, differing only in the situation being prevented. Relief from pain affords dignity to the dying.

DEATH

Defining when death has occurred has always been controversial. In early civilization, it was defined as the moment that respirations could no longer be detected. After stethoscopes were readily available, it was defined as the point that cardiac function was no longer discernible. To these two measures was then added a third, lack of body reflexes. By the 1960s, technology had become so advanced that heart and lung function could be maintained by machine for indefinite periods. People then began to seek a better definition of death. It is generally agreed today that death occurs when the brain stops functioning. Therefore, the test appears to be how to measure brain death. An electroencephalogram (EEG) measures the electric currents of the brain. In the average person, an EEG recording will show periodic spikes and waves that reflect active electrical discharge across the brain hemispheres. A person with brain death has a flat EEG or a straight-line pattern. However, an exception to this is people with drug overdose, particularly phenobarbital, and those with severe hypothermia; both conditions may show a straight-line EEG in the presence of life.

In 1968, a committee of the Harvard Medical School issued a definition of irreversible coma including four criteria that is currently used to define death: (1) unreceptivity and unresponsitivity, (2) no spontaneous muscular movement or breathing, (3) no reflex response, and (4) flat EEG.

This definition of death allows body organs to be removed for transplant. The definition is controversial, however, because some people declared legally dead by these criteria have continued to breathe and maintain their heartbeats after having their support systems turned off. Most people fear treating a live person as if he were dead and omitting to give him care. On the other hand, treating a dead person as if he were alive and continuing to give care comes at the expense of others who need that caregiver's time and energy in order to return to health.

Documentation of Death

Signs of death for the person not on ventilatory or mechanical assistance are absence of respirations, no audible heart sounds by stethoscope, no pulse by palpation, no apparent blood pressure, absence of body movement or reflexes, and dilated fixed pupils.

A person must be certified dead by a physician, who signs the death certificate and documents the cause of death. If a person dies at home, a physician may make this certification there or ask to have the person transported by ambulance or rescue squad to a hospital for verification.

Donation of Organ Transplants

In all fifty states, a uniform donor card is accepted as a legal document of a person's desire to donate body organs. In many states there is a space on a driver's license, a form of identification that almost everyone carries, that says whether the person wishes to donate a body organ. The driver's license alone is not a legal document, but it alerts you to look for the donor card.

When caring for people in an emergency room who are comatose or who are admitted in serious condition, look for such a card with the person's identification. People who are scheduled for heart or other high-risk surgery may mention that they wish to donate a body organ if they should not live through the procedure. Mark this information on the person's care plan in a conspicuous place and alert his physician. You want a person to go to surgery thinking that he will arrive safely back in the room because that motivation will allow him to survive surgery. On the other hand, for the person who has a commitment to donate a body organ, knowing that his wish has been properly recorded and will be respected may provide the satisfaction and relaxation that he needs to survive surgery.

When a person who has stated he wishes to donate an organ meets the Harvard criteria of death, life support is maintained until a proper recipient for the body organ is located. Awkward situations can arise when a recipient is waiting for a body organ and a person who has stated he will donate such an organ does not fully meet the criteria (a sense of ghoulish waiting occurs). Except for these rare awkward instances, the donation of body organs gives many people a reason for death and makes death more acceptable.

Postmortem Care

Good nursing care continues after death so that the person's body is aligned properly and that the death is accepted as well as possible by the people important to him. The thought of touching a dead body is frightening to many people at first. Be honest if this is true for you and ask for assistance. You will discover that death does not distort a person as much as you expected and care does not differ greatly from what you would give to an unconscious patient. The major difference is that body heat is lost fairly quickly after death so the person's body feels cold to touch.

Do not be surprised to hear health care providers react to death of a patient with anger, comments such as "I tried so hard and *you* gave up," or crude jokes about death. These reactions are defense mechanisms to help health care personnel cope with death and proceed from the patient's room to the room of another person who still needs their support. Be certain, however, that health care providers around you confine these mechanisms to private places. Witnessing such behavior can be devastating to the patient's family or to other people who are ill if they perceive their health care providers as heartless and uncaring. Sometimes it is necessary to caution other health care providers to be more aware of their effect on others or to explain to families or other patients that a health care provider's brusqueness or apparent callousness was the result of her feeling of loss.

Before beginning any after care, check with family members to see if they want to spend a few minutes with the person or if there are any religious rites they want to complete before his body is moved to the morgue. This is necessary for some people to comprehend death. Some people have special prayers they want to say, and others want to say a final goodbye in privacy.

Check that the patient's bed and room look neat and clean before you ask family if they would like to spend some time in the room. This is particularly important if a final resuscitation attempt resulted in blood-soaked sponges or scattered equipment.

Place the bed in a flat position and turn the person onto his back. Close his eyes and arrange his arms either flat along his sides palms down or bent gently across his chest or abdomen. Replace dentures if they are not in place unless some disease pathology or tubing prevents this being accomplished easily. These actions are necessary in order to place the body in good alignment for a coffin before *rigor mortis* (stiffening of all body parts) occurs and to prevent *livor mortis* (positional hypostasis, or the dependent pooling of blood that occurs after death) from disfiguring body parts. If a hand were placed palm up, the back of the hand would discolor to purple; if a person were left lying on his side, the dependent side of his face would discolor to purple.

Remain in the room with family in case they need your support but be unobtrusive. Some people fear touching a person's body after death, but touch is a strong and intimate communication technique that a family member may appreciate being shown how to use. Role model touching by holding the dead person's hand or brushing hair away from the forehead as if he were still alive. Other family members may seem unable to leave the room or to let go of the person's hand. You may need gradually to separate their hands, saying, for example, "I'll always remember your mother the way she was when I first met her—so full of life and always laughing. I'm sure that's how you think of her too." This will help the person begin to accept the fact that in more than a physical sense it is time to let go. As a rule, crying is helpful; it relieves tension. You may need to say to family members (especially men) that it is all right to cry; however, the absence of tears does not indicate lack of concern. It is not unprofessional for nurses to cry; you can offer support despite tears on your face. A family member's warmest memory of a hospital experience may not be of the skilled care that the person received from nurses but of a nurse who cried as she said goodbye to his parent—the implication being that his parent was so good he affected other people's lives even in death (Fig. 24-2).

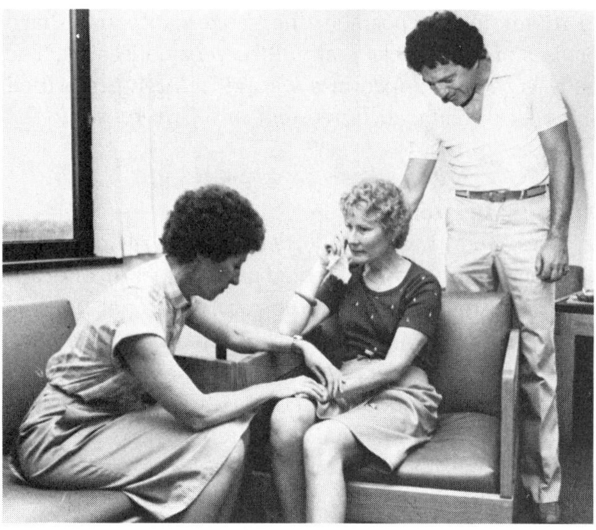

FIGURE 24-2. This family needs time to console one another over the loss of an older family member.

After this last visit, you need to prepare the body for autopsy or for removal to the morgue, where it will be kept cold until transport to a funeral home. All health care agencies have specific procedures, but certain principles always apply.

Remove and list all personal clothing and jewelry. Give these to a family member and ask him to sign the list. This may seem unnecessary in a time of distress, but when upset at the death of someone close, people do not reason or remember well. Later, they may be completely unable to recall taking an expensive ring or watch unless reminded by their signature.

Many people like to have a wedding band or engagement ring left in place rather than removed. Follow your agency's policy; some agencies allow this, and in others, the ring must be removed and given to the family (it can be replaced at the funeral home).

List eyeglasses as valuables. If the person always wore these, the family will probably choose to have them buried with the body.

Handle the body as gently as if the person were still alive because pressure marks will cause pooling of blood and unappealing blemishes on the skin surface. In most health care agencies, a special pack of equipment is available for further care. Two or three cotton balls are gently packed in the rectum by means of a clean tongue blade to prevent loss of feces from the loss of sphincter tone with death. The wrists and ankles are padded with soft cotton pads crossed gently and tied together with gauze. The body is labeled with identification attached to a toe or wrapped with gauze around a lower extremity. Position the chin fully closed by placing a folded towel under it. Do not use gauze strips around the chin to maintain this position; the gauze can cause sharp bruises on the cheeks that will be very noticeable. The body is then wrapped in a shroud (a large preformed sheet) and then transferred to a cart for removal to the morgue.

Autopsy Permission

In cases of homicide, suicide, death within 24 hours after a hospital admission, suspected harmful death, or death in a jail or at home where the person was not under a physician's care, an *autopsy* (examination of the body after death) is required by law, and the next of kin has no decision to make about consent. In other cases, it would be helpful to medical programs or research if an autopsy could be done, and the next of kin is asked to sign a form giving permission for autopsy. Sometimes only one body organ will be examined. People may need reassurance that no one will be able to tell that an autopsy was performed following the funeral director's preparation of the body. Organs removed at autopsy are generally not returned to the body but incinerated at the autopsy site.

Refusing to grant permission for an autopsy is a legitimate right. Do not allow people to be intimidated into signing such forms any more than you would allow a person to be intimidated into signing a form for surgery. Autopsies advance medical science and can be very helpful; on the other hand, the person has every right to refuse without being made to feel guilty.

Effects of Terminal Illness on Families

Sudden death (accidents, homicide, suicide) occurs without any long-term planning. Otherwise, death is preceded by at least some illness, often an illness known to be leading to death for a period of years.

Terminal illness puts a special strain on families because it forces them to deal not only with the person's potential death but also with the thought of their own eventual death. If the person dying is a newborn, it is important that the parents see the child unless they specifically refuse. It was once thought that a mother's grief would be much less if she did not see a stillborn child, although the father was typically allowed to see him. Psychologically, it is very hard to see a newborn for whom a mother has been planning suddenly dead. However, seeing the child allows her to begin a grief process to acceptance and resolution. If she does not see the child, she may continue to grieve and be unable to make a solid relationship with a future child. She may view a second child as a replacement of the first and not a separate child. "Replacement children" tend to feel less well loved than average children because in their parent's eyes they are not so perfect as the child who died (not so pretty, not so well behaved, not so intelligent); the parent's memory has blurred the reality of what really was.

Parents who have had a child die at birth are often advised to have another child right away. Better advice might be for them to wait at least 6 months to a year before another pregnancy, to be certain that they have completed grieving and are ready to accept a second child as a separate person.

If the dying person is a young child, parents may find themselves spending much of their time with the child to the detriment of older children or work responsibilities. Part of this is protective of the dying child, making certain that he is comfortable and not frightened by being left alone; part of it arises from a feeling that if they are there, surely the child will not die this day. Older children in the family may find themselves doing homework and caring for young children at a level well beyond that expected of them before the illness. They may be overwhelmed with jealousy of attention and gifts flowing to the dying child. Almost every child, caught in this situation, wishes the ill child dead. When the ill child does die, the remaining child's guilt may be overwhelming. He may need time to talk about his wish and an explanation that his wish was normal and did not produce death; his brother or sister was dying whatever he wished.

Siblings of dying children need to visit the child in the hospital or home visits need to be arranged so the other children can see that nothing terrifying is happening to the child. Otherwise they come to view death as so frightening that it is why they were kept from seeing the child. Parents may need help dividing their time between the ill child and the well children.

If the dying person is a young adult, family members may have difficulty determining how many decisions should be left to him. He is of legal age, so certainly he can decide whether he wants to die with or without heroic interventions, but the question of whether his judgment is adequate to make this decision arises. Both the patient and his parents need good explanations of proposed care and estimated success of interventions, such as how long death can be delayed by further surgery or chemotherapy. When a decision is made, the family needs support. Family members will live with this decision for many years to come and can only do so in mental health if they think of it as the best possible decision under the circumstances.

If the dying person is a middle-aged adult, families may be disturbed because the dying person is the family financial provider or the caretaker. In many instances, a mother or a father fills both these roles. If the dying person is aware that he is dying, he can actively participate in financial planning and decision-making about future care of children. Families need time to realize that decisions are based not on a statement made at any one moment but on a philosophy of life. Taking time to think through the dying person's philosophy will help them make decisions in the months to come (mother always thought laughter was important, and she would have agreed that spending money for a vacation is important; father believed in education, and he would have insisted on the oldest child remaining in college even though money has become scarce).

If an older adult is dying, families dispersed across the country may find themselves pulled back together again after a long separation. They may find themselves wishing that they had spent more time with family members in recent years and particularly with the dying parent. If decisions about care must be made, they may return to childlike quarrelling because that is how they always dealt with one another. If they have relied heavily on the older adult's judgment, they need support to begin to trust their own judgment even in the midst of such childish behavior. Like all family members, whatever the age of the dying family member, they need time to reassess their own life, goals, and intentions. They came to a health care agency to deal with a parent dying, but they discover they must also deal with their own plans for living.

Effects of a Dying Patient on Other Patients

What to tell other patients on a nursing unit when a patient dies is often a concern. Explanations may be inappropriate—for example, a person going to surgery probably should not be told that another patient just died following surgery; a patient who is extremely depressed may be unable to handle upsetting news of a death. On the whole, however, patients know when someone has died on a nursing unit and telling them about it is not really news but merely confirmation of what they already suspect.

Death of another person on a nursing unit may cause a foxhole phenomenon, the reaction of a soldier when he first realizes that a friend in the same foxhole has been hit by enemy fire. Eventually his feeling will be grief, but his *first* thought may be, "Thank God it got him and not me." A hospital patient may feel guilty for having this same response. A way of working through such guilt is to talk about it with someone. Reassurance from you that the patient who died was very ill is comforting because this explains that death did not occur by chance but was expected.

Other hospital patients and their families may be supportive to the family of a dying patient since they have spent many days together in waiting rooms during therapy. This is particularly true in intensive care units where families are allowed to visit with the patient only 5 minutes out of every hour. The remainder of every hour is spent talking with other families in the unit waiting room. Lasting friendships are often formed from such associations, and comfort from such people may be very meaningful.

THE ROLE OF FUNERALS

Funerals are commonly accepted as a means of helping people to accept the reality of death, to accept the support of people who care about them, and to express emotions and cement memories about the person who has died. For some survivors, funeral planning is so lavish that their actual grieving is prolonged or does not begin until after the funeral. This may be therapeutic in giving them longer to marshall their defenses to accept the fact of death. For others, funeral rites initiate mourning—the funeral makes the death real, not the announcement at the bedside that death has occurred.

Some people who know they are dying plan their own funeral as a way of working through the acceptance of their own death. Others plan a funeral as a way of protecting their family's resources (they would rather their wife save the money and make house payments with it). Sometimes family members use funerals to make up to the person for things owed him in life or as an expression of guilt. Resolving these feelings is better done by therapeutic counseling.

THE USE OF EXTRAORDINARY MEANS TO PROLONG LIFE

Many people are concerned today not only about prolonging life but about the quality of life that can be prolonged. This raises questions such as: If a person can be kept alive for an additional 2 weeks but those 2 weeks will be filled with intense pain, should the measure be undertaken? If a person in an emergency room can be resuscitated after a drowning but would remain comatose and unresponsive forever, how long should resuscitation measures be continued?

In order to prevent extraordinary measures that would prolong life beyond the point desirable, many people today are writing *living wills.* These state that in the event a person is at a disease state from which he cannot recover and he is unable to participate in decisions, no extraordinary measures should be taken to keep him alive; he should be allowed to die.

A living will is accepted as a legal document in California; other states will no doubt begin to accept it in the years to come. The presence of such a document causes complex situations in practice in determining what is a *heroic* measure and what is a *routine* measure. For example, is adjusting intravenous fluid to increase a person's blood pressure heroic or routine? Resuscitation is done routinely in hospitals, but would the person regard it as heroic or routine?

In states other than California, when a living will exists, emergency measures to resuscitate must be undertaken unless you have a specific physician's order not to begin such an action. A stop order must be written and not just understood in order to be legally respected and carried out.

No Code Orders

The term *code* has come to mean a page for cardiopulmonary resuscitation. A *no-code order* means that in the event a person suffers a cardiopulmonary arrest, no emergency care will be initiated for him.

By law, all a physician is obliged to do for a patient is what the average physician would do; she does not have to provide heroic measures beyond that. If a person has determined that he wants no heroic measures such as cardiopulmonary resuscitation, therefore, his physician may write a no-code order.

Be careful when working with this order. A no-code order is a legitimate order, but respect it only when it is written with the same protocol as other physician's orders.

Euthanasia

Euthanasia is the deliberate ending of life of a person suffering from an incurable and painful disease. It also means an easy or painless death. It can be active, by drug administration, or passive, by not offering a heart medication that would prolong heart function further. Euthanasia is an ethical as well as a legal concern. A person in great pain who takes his own life may also interpret his act as one of euthanasia.

Advocates of euthanasia (popularly termed *mercy-killing*) view it as carrying out the person's wishes and place it in the same category as a living will. Opponents of euthanasia consider it to violate Judeo-Christian beliefs and regard it as murder. Physicians see their primary responsibility as prolonging life so euthanasia is outside their ethical code. Nurses see the optimal care of patients as their primary responsibility. An ethical question is whether this philosophy can be interpreted to mean that a nurse carrying out a patient's wish to die is *ethically* performing her duty.

PREPARATION FOR A NURSING ROLE WITH DYING PATIENTS

Before you can offer support to people with any life concern, you need to be aware of your own reactions and feelings. Thus, to offer support to a person who is dying, you need to examine how you feel about caring for someone who is dying.

Fear. Fear is a natural response to death because the phenomenon is strange to you. To overcome this fear, put it into perspective. In nursing you care for many people who have illnesses and experiences you will never have. Thus, caring for people with experiences beyond your own is not really strange, but almost routine in nursing.

People who have never seen someone die are often afraid that the moment of death will be terrifying to watch. Death usually occurs gently, with body functioning gradually lessening until it stops in a painfree, quiet manner. People who have been declared dead and were then resuscitated by heroic measures report that death was not frightening but involved a feeling of exceptional calm and comfort; a number of people have said afterward that they wished they had been allowed to die rather than called back to their body because death seemed so appealing.

Failure. Some people find themselves drawing back from care of dying people because death symbolizes failure to them. Many people who are dying feel health care personnel pulling back from them, which makes them feel failure—they have not been able to keep their body from dying despite everyone's best efforts.

Remind yourself that death is the ultimate outcome for everybody. At the point that death becomes unpreventable, the only failure that can exist is the failure of health care professionals to help the patient to a death with dignity and consideration and free of guilt that he has failed his caregivers.

Grief. One of a person's greatest needs is intimacy and love, a feeling that someone cares and is concerned about him. In primitive times, man envisioned the heavens populated with many gods, probably partly from people's need to be cared for and loved (even if one god grew angry and ruined your grain crop, another would still love you). The loss of anyone you care about evokes grief. Nursing care is so intense that the relationship formed may be closer than you realize until the person is diagnosed as having a terminal illness or dies.

The nurse's grief that accompanies caring for dying people can be broken down into the same stages of grief experienced by the person himself when he learns that he is dying.

DENIAL. A nurse who is using denial may care for a person without mentioning that he has more than a simple illness. This includes omitting the use of such common expressions as "How are you this morning?" because she does not want to hear the answer. Denial may be so extensive that she avoids going into the room unless she has an important procedure. This is both confusing and lonely for the patient, since he misses the normal exchange of conversation and contact.

Nurses sometimes change professions following the loss of a patient to whom they felt close, saying that nursing no longer gives them satisfaction.

ANGER. It may be intense when a young child or a young adult dies, since the death seems so unfair. A person who is angry has difficulty offering effective care. The person perceives herself as giving thorough, comforting care, but you notice sharp abrupt movements that are actually causing pain. Anger clouds judgment for decisions, such as which analgesic would be best to administer. The dying person cannot approach angry caregivers or ask questions. He is left alone and perhaps feels guilty that he has caused this anger. Anger is always destructive. Nurses may notice themselves making poor judgments in their personal lives (not following through on projects, spontaneous buying) because they carry this feeling of anger.

BARGAINING. Caregivers begin to bargain for life the

same as the person does himself. A statement such as, "I hope that Mr. O'Brien dies during the weekend while I'm off" is a bargaining statement. Statements of this kind are easy to miss in your fellow co-workers and easy to interpret as uncaring statements ("I hope Mr. O'Brien dies while I'm not here"). Listening for them helps you to evaluate when a fellow co-worker is having difficulty caring for a particular patient and perhaps needs to change assignments. Hearing you say them should alert you that you are more involved with the person than you perhaps realize. You need to talk to someone about your feelings or ask for help. Remember that when bargaining fails, a person reaches his lowest point. Recognizing bargaining statements in yourself helps you to be prepared for the depression to follow.

DEPRESSION. Nurses who enter this phase may be ineffective caregivers, since depressed people are poor problem-solvers (everything becomes a crisis). A nurse may make unwise decisions in her personal life (drop out of a night school course, file for divorce, etc.) because she cannot effect good problem-solving.

Depression is doubly destructive because when you are depressed your reasoning processes are so slowed that you lose the ability to recognize that depression is the problem. When caring for a patient who is expected to have an amputation or death, monitor your usual behavior to see if you are following your usual pattern. If irregularities occur, assess whether depression has overwhelmed you. When depressed, try to make no major decisions for at least a week to give your perspective time to change or you may find you have made a decision irreversible when you are again able to think clearly.

ACCEPTANCE. The average person can reach a stage of acceptance in grief because he is subjected to few true losses in his lifetime. As a nurse on a unit where many terminally ill persons come for care, you may find yourself facing loss or death over and over. Therefore, a stage of acceptance may never be reached. A caregiver who cannot reach a stage of acceptance is in a stage of depression and cannot function.

To achieve a stage of acceptance, you may need to modify what it is you are accepting. You cannot accept the unfairness of death, but you can accept your ability to offer care that gives death dignity and compassion. Do not compensate by not feeling. This is a dangerous attitude because it blocks your ability to feel happiness, love, and trust. You may need to ask for a temporary change of assignment in order to reestablish your perspective. You may need to concentrate on self-esteem therapy for yourself.

UTILIZING NURSING PROCESS

Nursing process is as applicable to care of patients who are dying as to those whose full recovery can be expected.

ASSESSMENT

It is important to assess persons who are dying for difficulty in swallowing or loss of a gag reflex because at the point that these functions are lost, it is no longer safe for the person to take oral fluid. Assess also the degree of circulatory impairment. As circulation to muscle decreases, intramuscular injections can no longer be absorbed. The threat of decubiti formation becomes greater and greater because oxygen does not reach cells well. Assess circulatory function by blood pressure, pulse recording, and blanching time of fingerbeds.

Assess skin carefully for beginning signs of pressure areas (whitened or reddened areas each time the person is turned). Assess respiratory function (both rate and appearance), since with the slowing of respiratory movement, secretions begin to form in bronchi and alveoli, further decreasing the person's ability to exchange gases at the alveoli-blood interface.

Assess for comfort and the readiness of the patient and his family to accept impending death by both observation and good communication.

ANALYSIS

One of the hardest judgments to make concerning people who are dying is whether they want to know more about what is happening to them or not. It is equally difficult to judge how prepared family members or friends are for accepting death because people mask strong emotions as a defense mechanism. The better the person and his family know you, the more likely they will be to reveal their true feelings around you and the more accurate this judgment will be.

PLANNING

The planning stage of nursing process is easy to bypass when caring for a person who is dying because the care may seem temporary and the setting of long-range goals more academic than practical. No one can anticipate the timing of death accurately, however, so what begins as a seemingly transient interaction may be prolonged.

As a rule, establishing plans that are cut short provides better nursing care than plans that end before death and leave the person with unorganized care.

IMPLEMENTATION

Administering care to people who are dying deserves the same careful attention as that given to people who will fully recover. Be extremely careful that you do not neglect general rules of care such as bed rest. People need to be repositioned every 2 hours; catheterization must be a strictly sterile procedure; injection technique and medication dosages must be accurate. Contracting a urinary tract infection or developing decubiti ulcers causes unnecessary pain; such carelessness in procedures also sets a bad example and causes other health care providers to question your ability and integrity.

Sometimes a conflict in care occurs if turning the

TABLE 24-1. APPROACHES TO COMMUNICATING WITH DYING PERSONS

1. Conversation is a normal means whereby people interact; continue it.
2. Use moments of silence therapeutically. Such moments occur normally just as speech occurs normally. Do not feel you have to chatter to fill quiet intervals.
3. Use the word *death* or *dying* as appropriate. Trying to avoid a word makes interchanges awkward. Statements such as "These flowers are dying," "That's a dead-end job," "I'm dying to try that" may make it acceptable for the person you are caring for to voice for the first time what is happening to him ("I'm dying too; let me tell you about dead-ending").
4. Preserve a dying person's defenses. If he is using denial or bargaining, do not try to push him to the next step of grieving by confrontation. The person will move on to the next step when he is psychologically ready.
5. Many people assume that they will die at night. Therefore, night is "owned" by the dying. A person may talk more freely at night about his fears or his unfulfilled life ambitions than he can during the day.
6. Be supportive, not trite. A statement such as "All of us are dying" is true but not helpful. A supportive statement such as "This must be hard for you" is better.
7. Keep your beliefs about death to yourself. "God works in mysterious ways" may explain death for you but is little comfort to the person who does not envision that as true.

person appears to cause pain and one of your prime goals is to keep the person free of pain. In these instances, it is better to ask for an analgesic to control pain and continue turning as you cannot predict how long the person will live and you do not want additional painful complications to occur. Communicating with the dying person is often one of the most important elements of care that you can give. See Table 24-1 for some approaches.

EVALUATION

Evaluation of whether goals of care were achieved or not helps to strengthen your planning with the next dying person you care for and helps to improve your self-esteem and build confidence in your ability to care for dying people. The care of people who are dying is not simple or easy. Evaluation will reveal discrepancies between the wish and the reality, identifying areas you need to strengthen in order to grow as a health care provider.

NURSING CARE PLAN

Mr. Roberts is a 61-year-old patient who was admitted to a hospital for hepatitis. On the fourth day of hospitalization, he suffered a cerebral vascular accident and became unconscious. Oxygen was deflected from reaching portions of the brain for an extended time interval. His physician has explained to his family that recovery is not expected; the family has asked that no extraordinary measures be implemented to prolong life.

The following is a nursing care plan for Mr. Roberts.

NURSING DIAGNOSIS

State of unconsciousness related to terminal illness.

Locus of Decision-Making: Nurse.

Goal: Patient to remain comfortable until death.

Criteria: Patient demonstrates no signs of discomfort by word or motion.

S. . . .

O. Patient sometimes stirs in response to sound of loud voices in room; quiets in response to grandson's or granddaughter's voice. Winces in response to painful stimuli. Respirations 16 and labored; skin temperature cool to touch and diaphoretic. Pulse 60; Blood pressure 92/50. Lips dry and peeling.

A. Patient with decreased respiratory and circulatory function due to impending death.

NURSING ORDERS

1. Use gentle touch to avoid bruising of skin surfaces.
2. Change position every 2 hours to prevent collection of respiratory secretions and formation of decubiti.
3. Provide oral care every 4 hours.
4. Urge family to visit as desired; apparently comforting to patient.
5. Be cautious of statements made around patient; appears to hear normal conversational levels.

SUGGESTED READINGS

Ames, B. Art and a dying patient. *Am. J. Nurs.* 80:1094, 1980.

Babb de Ramón, P. The final task: Life review for the dying patient. *Nursing* (Horsham) 13:44, 1983.

Bauer, F. L. (Ed.) *Nursing and the Concept of Loss.* New York: Wiley, 1980.

Brockhaus, J. P. Foster care, adoption and the grief process. *J. Psychosoc. Nurs. Ment. Health Serv.* 20(9):9, 1982.

Brown, I. A., et al. Four nurses talk about dying and death in a long term care setting. *Canad. Nurse* 78:30, 1982.

Chee, C. M. A child's right to die. *M.C.N.* 7:81, 1982.

Constantino, R. E. Bereavement crisis intervention for widows in grief and mourning. *Nurs. Res.* 30(6):351, 1981.

Davis, A. To tell or not. *Am. J. Nurs.* 81:156, 1981.

Dimond, M. Bereavement and the elderly. *J. Adv. Nurs.* 6:461, 1981.

Downey, A. M. Living, loving and losing: Implications for health and well-being. *Health Values* 7(1):7, 1983.

Earnshaw-Smith, E. Emotional pain in dying patients and their families. *Nurs. Times* 78(44):1865, 1982.

Flood, D. M., et al. Helping children and their families grieve. *Canad. Nurse* 78:34, 1982.

Flynn, J. B., et al. Unresolved grief in battered women. *J.E.N.* 7(6):250, 1981.

Hine, V. H. Holistic dying: The role of the nurse clinician. *Top. Clin. Nurs.* 3:45, 1982.

Johnson, S. Giving emotional support to families after a patient dies. *Nurs. Life* 3(1):34, 1983.

Johnson-Soderbeig, S. Grief themes. *A.N.S.* 3(4):15, 1981.

Kowalski, K. When birth becomes death. *A.O.R.N. J.* 38(1):57, 1983.

Kübler-Ross, E. *On Death and Dying.* New York: Macmillan, 1969.

Kübler-Ross, E. *Questions and Answers on Death and Dying.* New York: Macmillan, 1974.

Kübler-Ross, E. *Death: The Final Stage of Growth.* Englewood Cliffs, N.J.: Prentice-Hall, 1975.

Kübler-Ross, E. *To Live Until We Say Good-bye.* Englewood Cliffs, N.J.: Prentice-Hall, 1978.

Lambert, V. A., and Lambert, C. E., Jr. *The Impact of Physical Illness and Related Mental Health Concepts.* Englewood Cliffs, N.J.: Prentice-Hall, 1979.

Lattanzi, M. E. Hospice bereavement services: Creating networks of support. *Fam. Community Health* 5(3):54, 1983.

McCorkle, R. Death education for advanced nursing practice. *Death Educ.* 5:347, 1982.

McMahon, M., and Miller, P. Behavioral cues in the dying process and nursing implications. *J. Gerontol. Nurs.* 6:16, 1980.

Miles, G. C. Books to help children understand death. *Am. J. Nurs.* 79:291, 1979.

Miles, M. S. The search for meaning and its potential for affecting growth in bereaved parents. *Health Values* 7(1):19, 1983.

Neki, J. S. Grief . . . different cultures have developed different ways of dealing with it. *World Health* 11:20, 1982.

Ross, H. M. Societal/cultural views regarding death and dying. *Top. Clin. Nurs.* 3:1, 1981.

Schodt, C. M. Grief in adolescent mothers after an infant death. *Image* 14:20, 1982.

Schultz, C. A. Grief at sudden death . . . you can help. *Crit. Care Update* 10(2):9, 1983.

Seidel, M. A. Death education: A continuing process for nurses. *Top. Clin. Nurs.* 3:87, 1981.

Shelton, R. L. The patient's need of faith at death. *Top. Clin. Nurs.* 3:55, 1981.

Simos, B. G. *A Time to Grieve: Loss as a Universal Human Experience.* New York: Family Service Association of America, 1979.

Sperhac, A. M. Sudden infant death syndrome. *Nurse Pract.* 7(8):38, 1982.

Stowers, S. Nurses cry, too. *Nurs. Manage.* 14(4):63, 1983.

Tatro, S. E. Regression: A defense mechanism for the dying older adult. *J. Gerontol. Nurs.* 8:20, 1982.

Toth, S., and Toth, A. Empathetic intervention with the widow. *Am. J. Nurs.* 80:1652, 1980.

Ufema, J. Grieving families: Let your heart do the talking. *Nursing* (Horsham): 11(11):80, 1981.

Welch, D. Anticipatory grief reactions in family members of adult patients . . . with cancer. *Issues Ment. Health Nurs.* 4(2):149, 1982.

Zelauskas, B. Siblings: The forgotten grievers. *Issues Comp. Pediatr. Nurs.* 5(1):45, 1981.

QUESTIONS FOR REVIEW

1. Mrs. Jones is a patient whom you care for. She is scheduled to have a leg amputated tomorrow. Which statement that she makes would make you assess her as in a first stage of grief:
   a. I'm angry this is happening to me.
   b. I hope to go home by tomorrow night.
   c. As long as I can still work, I don't care.
   d. I can't stop crying.

2. What statement best represents the third stage of grief:
   a. I'm angry this is happening to me.
   b. I hope to go home by tomorrow night.
   c. As long as I can still work, I don't care.
   d. I can't stop crying.

3. Miss Smith is a woman you care for who is dying. The most important assessment to make with Miss Smith because she is dying would be:
   a. Estimation of her ability to see well.
   b. Assessment of the temperature of her skin.
   c. Assessment of the softness of her abdomen.
   d. Estimation of her ability to swallow.

4. Miss Smith asks you if she could be cared for in a hospice. A hospice is:
   a. A hospital where nonskilled care is given.
   b. A facility for care of the dying.
   c. A facility where the major goal is to preserve life.
   d. An ambulatory clinic to go to for pain relief.

5. Miss Smith becomes comatose. In planning for her care, which plan reflects the best approach to care:
   a. Avoid the word *dying* even if it causes awkward sentences.
   b. Do not talk in the room because talking is distracting to unconscious people.
   c. Give normal care instructions as she may hear well.
   d. Touch her as little as possible as touch is disturbing to unconscious people.

6. Miss Smith dies. Following her death, you administer postmortem care. What implementation would you use:
   a. Work rapidly to prevent chilling her body.
   b. Position her lower jaw open to stabilize her tongue.
   c. Position her body on her side to equalize blood coagulation.
   d. Handle extremities gently to prevent bruising.

7. Miss Smith's mother asks to see her after she has died. Which of the following would be your best response?
   a. It's better not to do that.
   b. Your daughter does not look like herself any more.
   c. I'll take you into the room.
   d. Do you doubt that she is dead?

8. You evaluate your care of Miss Smith. You notice that you tended to avoid going into her room the last 2 days. This response might be a reflection of which stage of grief:
   a. Denial.
   b. Acceptance.
   c. Bargaining.
   d. Ambivalence.

9. *Death* is a difficult concept to define but the generally accepted definition today is:
   a. No discernible reflex activity.
   b. No heart rate by monitor.
   c. No respiratory movement by stethoscope determination.
   d. A flat electroencephalogram pattern.

10. *Euthanasia* is a term frequently discussed in relation to death. This is:
    a. A person killing himself.
    b. A husband refusing to allow his wife to have pain medicine before death.
    c. A wife killing her husband because he is in pain.
    d. A person killing another because that person asked him to.

VIII. NURSING PROCESS IN ACTION: SAFETY NEEDS

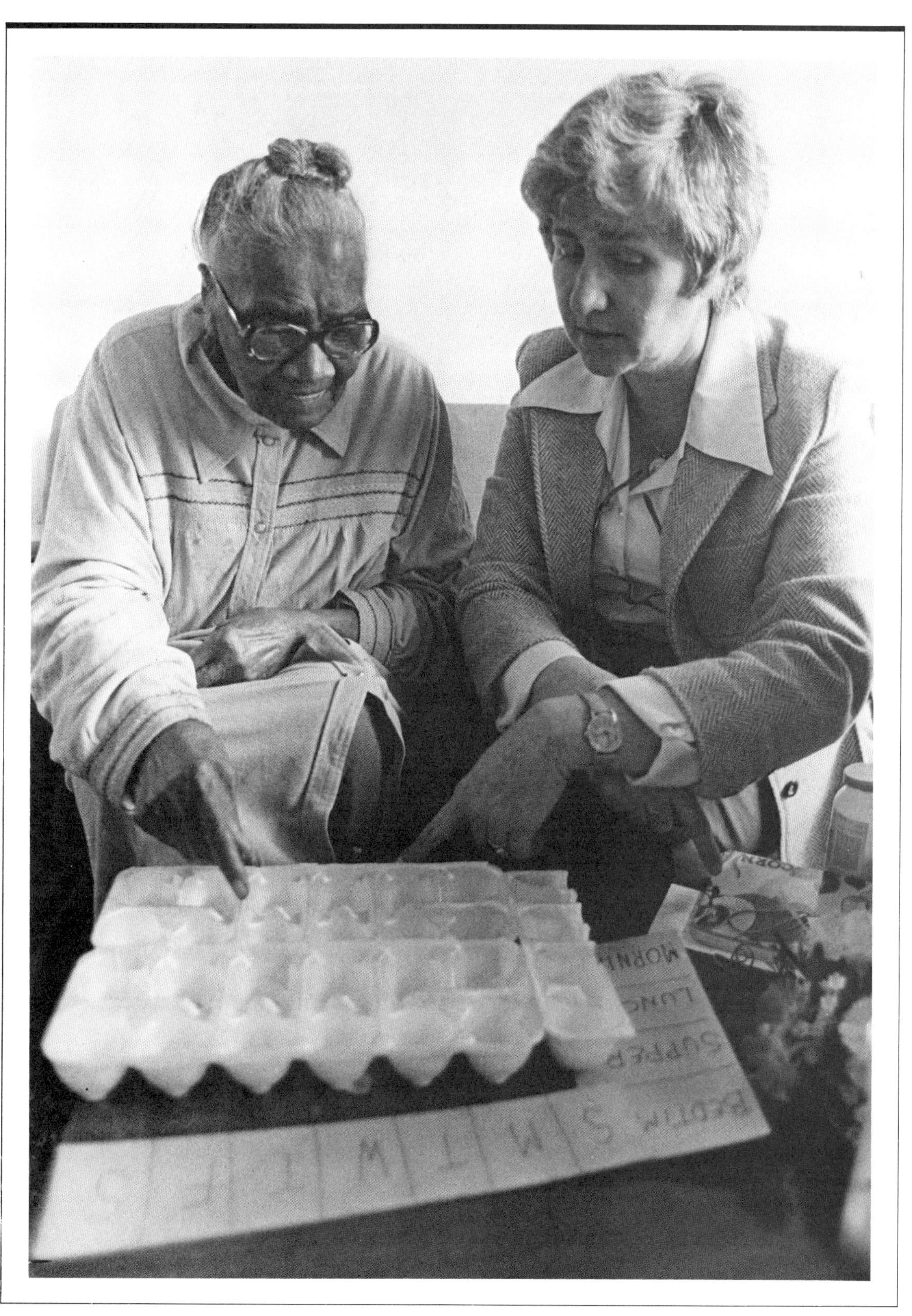

25. PERSONAL CARE AND HYGIENE

OBJECTIVES

Upon mastery of the material in this chapter, you should be able to:

1. List the factors that influence a person's personal hygiene practices.
2. Describe how to give a complete bed bath and how to assist with a bed bath, tub bath, and shower.
3. Describe administration of a backrub.
4. Describe administration of oral care to both conscious and unconscious persons.
5. Describe how to shampoo the hair of a person in bed.
6. Describe normal integument findings across the age continuum.
7. Discuss principles of skin care.
8. Describe preventive measures and common measures of care for the patient with a decubitus ulcer.

TERMS

The terms important for an understanding of this chapter are shown below and defined in the glossary:

caries
comedones
cyanosis
decubitus ulcer
edema
erythematous
halitosis
hygienics
plaque
pruritus
sebum
sordes
turgor

When people are ill, their body resources are needed to combat their illness, not to combat such things as wrinkled bed linen, a backache, or concern at neglected appearance. Some people can tolerate both pain from a surgical incision and a feeling of nausea from an anesthetic, but cannot, in addition, tolerate the lack of hygiene measures.

Providing personal care to patients not only plays a major role in promoting a sense of self-esteem, but adds to patient comfort and safety and aids healing. It also provides a time for health teaching, skin and mobility assessment, and therapeutic touch.

HYGIENE

Hygienics is the science of health and cleanliness. *Hygienic measures* are those measures necessary to promote cleanliness. This is a broad category of actions such as keeping the air and water supply pure and preventing the spread of disease. Nurses play active roles in instituting hygienic measures in their community. *Personal hygienic measures* are those measures that an individual undertakes to keep his body clean and free of disease, such as bathing and hair and oral care.

Increasing Self-Esteem. How interested people are in giving their own personal care has a great deal to do with both their level of energy and their level of self-esteem. Helping a person to appear well-groomed generally aids greatly in improving self-esteem—not only is he aware that he looks better but the fact that you took the time to spend with him proves he deserves care and concern.

Therefore, you reserve time to spend with people doing personal care not because you are concerned about cleanliness alone but because you are concerned about the person as a whole being and how he feels about himself and his ability to face challenges in his coming day.

Providing Comfort and Safety. Bathing protects the surface of the skin by washing away secretions and microorganisms. The skin in a healthy mobile person is a strong, resistant body part that needs little special protection. However, a person who is ill has decreased nourishment ability to all body cells and his skin can become very dry or, if circulatory disturbances are a part of the illness, fluid filled (edema). It is susceptible to breaking and cracking at those points, allowing microorganisms to enter the body, unless it is protected by special care. A breakdown in skin integrity also leads to painful lesions.

Providing Therapeutic Touch. The term *therapeutic* means healing or helping. *Therapeutic touch* serves a purpose over and above merely accomplishing a task such as touching to clean a body surface; touching is an intimate, warm, caring way that people relate to each other. Under stress, many people communicate not so much with words but by squeezing another's hand or putting an arm across his shoulder. Any time you touch a person to give care you subconsciously convey this level of concern and caring. Since bathing requires a great deal of touching, it is a procedure that says to a person strongly: people care about you. This may be the incentive a person needs to carry out the activities that will make him well again.

Providing Health Teaching. Health teaching is an independent action of nurses and should be incorporated into every procedure. Doing personal care may be an opportune time to spend informally discussing ways that a person could improve his overall health through better health promotion measures. Another person may most need a time for relaxed conversation, so you would use personal care time for this and schedule more formal times for health teaching.

Providing Mobility and Circulatory Assessment. A danger of being confined to bed for a long time is that body joints will not only stiffen but form permanent deformities (contractures) and blood circulation will slow to such a point that it clots (forms thrombi) in susceptible locations such as the lower extremities. A common assessment for thrombi in the calf (Homan's sign) and passive range of motion exercises should be incorporated as intrinsic parts of bathing for people on bed rest.

SKIN ASSESSMENT

The skin or integument is composed of two layers: an outer, the epidermis, and an inner, the dermis. Directly under the dermis and closely associated with it is an adherent layer of subcutaneous tissue that supplies the blood and nerve supply to the dermis (Fig. 25-1).

The *epidermis* is a thin layer of tissue composed of two separate types of cells. The outer, dead cells serve as a protection for inner cells. This outer layer contains *keratin*, a protein substance formed by cell compression that makes skin waterproof. Toenails and fingernails are dense keratin material. The inner layer is living cells; *melanin*, the substance responsible for skin color, is formed here. The epidermis has no blood vessels, but fine nerve fibers are interwoven in the cellular levels.

The *dermis* is composed of strong connective tissue and has a rich blood supply. It contains the *sebaceous glands*, which secrete the lubricant sebum into hair follicles, and the shafts of the hair follicles.

The subcutaneous tissue lying just under the dermis has a high proportion of fat cells. It also contains the sweat glands and the base of the hair follicles. Sweat or *sudoriferous glands* are of two separate types. *Eccrine* glands open directly onto the skin surface; through perspiration they help to control body temperature. *Apocrine* glands open into hair follicles rather than directly onto the skin surface. They are found chiefly in the axillary and genital areas, the forehead, and palms of the hands. Secretions from the apocrine glands is stimulated by

FIGURE 25-1. Cross-section of skin layers.

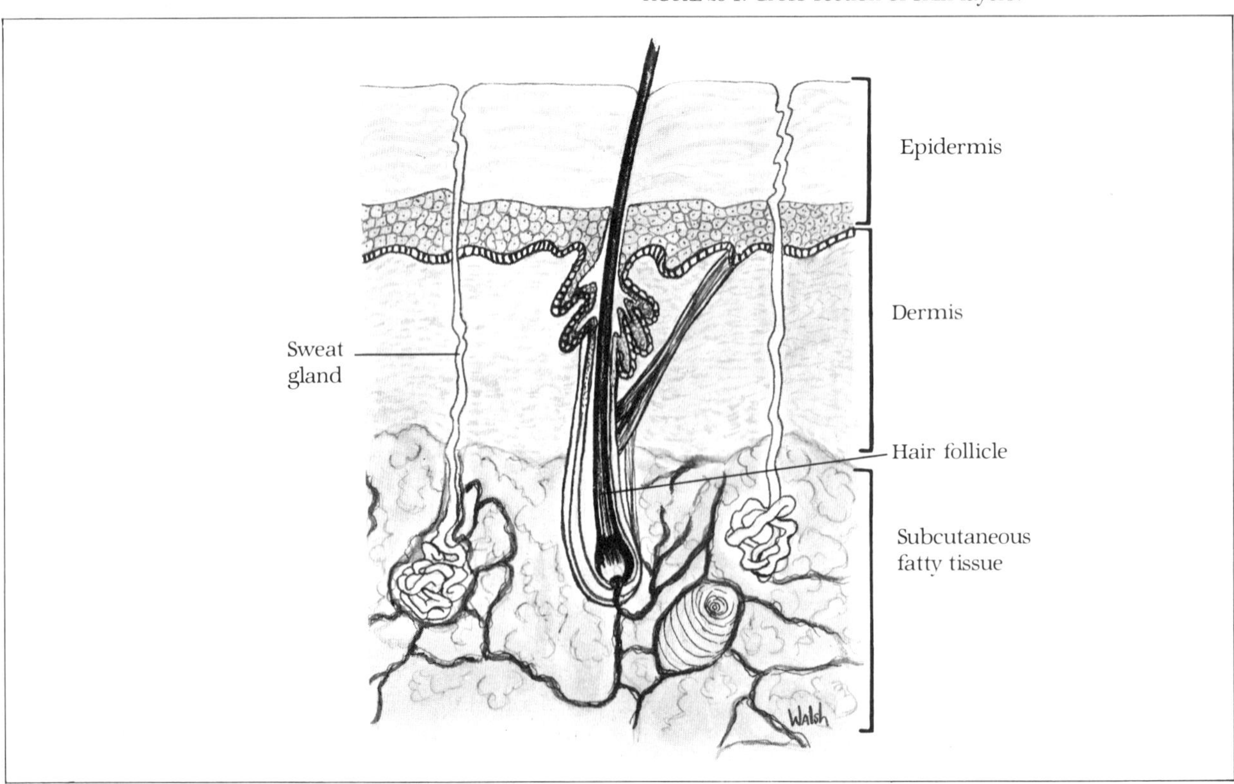

emotional stress; body odor is formed by action of bacteria on apocrine gland secretions.

Mucous membrane is a special integument continuous with the skin that lines the respiratory, gastrointestinal, urinary, and reproductive tracts and forms the conjunctiva of the eye. Periodontal disease is a frequent abnormal condition of the mucous membrane.

Assessing Skin

The integrity of skin must be assessed and guarded by care because the skin is responsible for protection of inner body structures. Sweat has a mild bacteriostatic action and reduces the number of organisms that can remain intact on the skin surface. Skin helps with temperature regulation through evaporation of perspiration. It helps to maintain fluid and electrolyte balance by the elimination of waste products and water. It is a receptor for sensations of pain, touch, pressure, heat, and cold—important to body safety. It aids in the production of vitamin D.

Skin assessment consists of observing the skin for general condition, color, and presence of lesions and then palpating it for temperature, moisture or texture, edema, and turgor.

Skin and mucous membrane are assessed by observation to be certain that no breaks in the skin surface are present. Skin color varies greatly; assess whether it appears correct for an individual. Skin appears pale if a person has a low hemoglobin level *(anemic).* It is yellow *(jaundiced)* if the person's liver cannot convert indirect bilirubin to direct bilirubin; then the indirect form leaves the bloodstream and invades muscle and skin layers. It is blue *(cyanotic)* if there is a decreased amount of unsaturated hemoglobin because oxygen does not reach red blood cells present in arterial blood. It is reddened *(erythematous)* if there is a local inflammation or irritation calling an increased blood supply into the area.

Edema is fluid accumulating in the subcutaneous level. It makes the skin appear pale, stretched, and shiny from the increased tension and fluid level covering the color of the blood vessels. Press on the skin if you think edema is present in a body part. If there is extreme edema at that point, your finger will not only indent the area, but the circle of indentation will remain after you withdraw your finger (termed *putting edema*) (Fig. 25-2).

The back of your hand is best able to assess temperature. A person's skin will feel warm to the back of your hand if either fever is present or there is a local inflammatory process. It may feel cool to your touch if there is decreased circulation to the body part or the environmental temperature is decreased.

Turgor is the degree of elasticity or water present. To test for it, lift a ridge of skin. If the raised ridge returns to its former shape immediately, turgor is normal; if it remains a ridge of skin, turgor is decreased (Fig. 25-3). People with poor hydration have decreased skin turgor. Elderly people tend to have decreased elasticity in their skin, revealed as poor skin turgor.

Skin should appear and feel soft and smooth. It will feel rough if it is dry or has been traumatized by excessive friction or by scratching. Various lesions found on skin or mucous membrane should be documented (see

FIGURE 25-2. Edema. Pressing on the skin leaves an indented area if fluid has accumulated in interstitial tissue. A. Grade 1+: slight pit, normal contours. B. Grade 2+: deeper pit, fairly normal contours. C. Grade 3+: deep pit, puffy appearance. D. Grade 4+: deep pit, frankly swollen. (From R. D. Judge, G. D. Zuidema, and F. T. Fitzgerald, *Clinical Diagnosis* [4th ed.]. Boston: Little, Brown, 1982.)

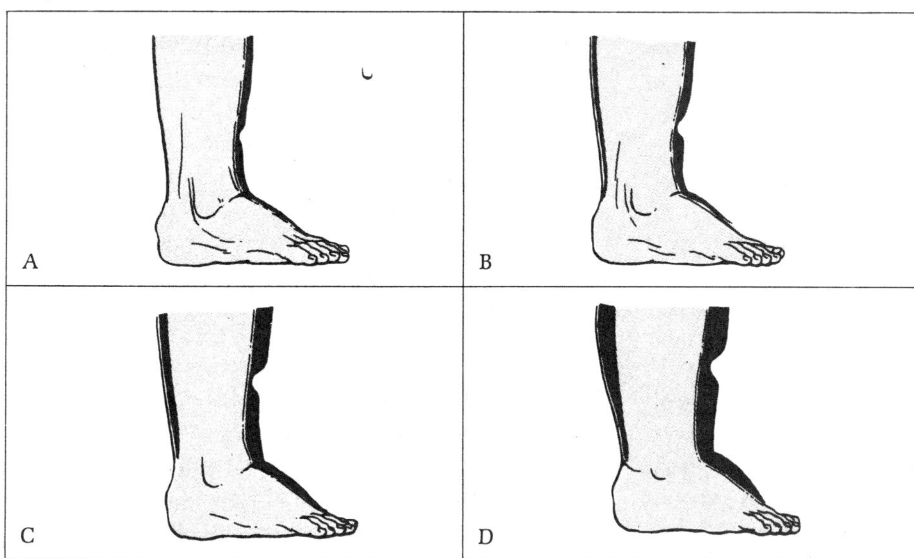

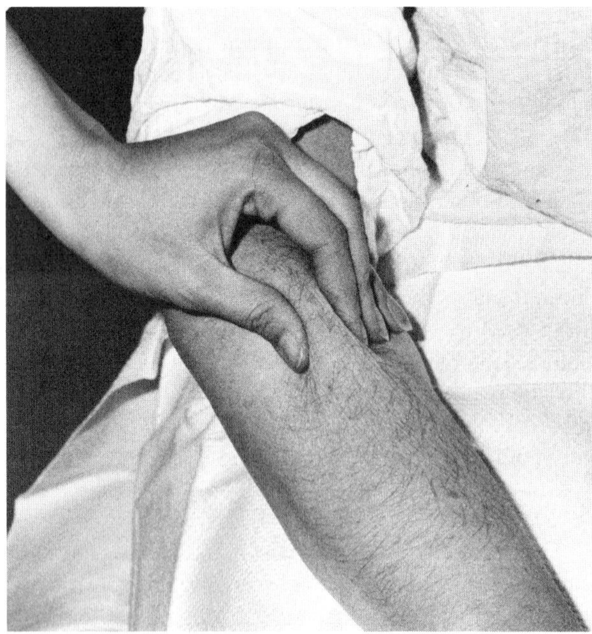

FIGURE 25-3. Poor skin turgor is indicated if skin, after being raised as a ridge (as shown here), remains in this pattern.

Table 25-1). Types of drainage from lesions found on skin that should be documented are summarized in Table 25-2.

Life Span Differences

The appearance of skin and lesions differs with age.

The Newborn. Newborn skin appears ruddy in Caucasian babies because newborns have a decreased supply of subcutaneous fat and the color of blood vessels is more noticeable. Black babies often appear only slightly pigmented at birth; as the skin is exposed to sunlight, the pigment darkens. The back and shoulders of newborns are covered with a fine downy hair called *lanugo* that apparently helps to maintain body heat for the first few weeks of life. This hair is worn away by 2 to 4 weeks of life and does not return. Newborns may have *milia* (small white pinpoint lesions) on their nose or cheeks from unopened sebaceous glands. These disappear by 2 weeks of age as the glands open and drain.

Newborns have fingernails extending over the tips of the fingers at birth, a sign of good intrauterine nourishment. Some newborns need to have these fingernails clipped so that they cannot accidentally scratch their faces.

Infant skin is more prone to environmental contamination than adult skin. This is evident from the newborn rash present on almost all babies in a hospital nursery, an innocent finding that needs no treatment. Newborns are given sponge baths until their umbilical cord drys and falls away at 7 to 10 days of age. A tub bath before this would soak the cord and invite infection.

The Infant. The age at which teeth appear varies with heredity, but the first teeth are generally lower central incisors at about 6 months of age. The presence and condition of teeth need to be assessed beginning at this age. A child develops a new tooth about every month after this until 2 years of age, when all of his deciduous (temporary) teeth are present. During the infant period, babies will develop diaper rash easily if urine or stool is left in contact with their skin for a long period. Infants enjoy splashing in a bathtub for a bath as soon as they can sit steadily. If they cannot have a full bath, they need their face and diaper area washed well to prevent rashes.

The Toddler and Preschooler. Toddlers and preschoolers almost always have one or two black-and-blue marks (ecchymoses) on their skin from bumping against furniture. They may have mosquito or flea bites and excoriations of the skin from scratching at these bites. Children this age are not old enough to leave alone in bathtubs. They can turn on hot water and scald themselves or slip under the water and drown.

The Schoolager and Adolescent. The school child may also have many ecchymoses from rough play. Children lose their deciduous teeth between 5 and 7 years of age. First molars develop at about 6 years of age; second at 12 years; and third between 15 and 25 years. Tooth decay is the chief health problem in school children; most children this age have one or more caries (cavities) that appear as a dark brown spot on the enamel of a tooth.

In adolescence, sebaceous glands produce more sebum, leading to oily skin. Bacteria decomposing sebum in plugged sebaceous glands cause white heads or blackheads *(comedones)* or acne. Acne can be destructive to self-image. From helping with personal care, you may be the person most aware of skin lesions from acne and may need to remind the physician caring for an adolescent with severe acne of this secondary condition so it can be treated.

With puberty, both boys and girls begin to develop thick, curly pubic, axillary, and facial hair as adult hormones become active. Facial hair growth is normal in girls; once female hormones become regulated with maturity, there is less of it. Pubic hair is diamond shaped in females; triangular in males. Many adolescents wash their hair daily. One of the kindest things you can do for many hospitalized adolescents is offer to shampoo their hair; afterward, their whole self-estimation has been improved.

The Young Adult. As women begin childbearing, skin changes associated with pregnancy can be seen. During pregnancy, the pigment on the face and on a vertical line of the abdomen darkens markedly (called *chalasia* and *linia nigra*, respectively). As the woman's abdomen increases in size, abdominal skin expands to form pink or dark red stretch marks (called *striae gravidarum*). They

TABLE 25-1. COMMON SKIN LESIONS

Type	Description	Cause
Angioma: cherry	Bright red small round spots found mainly on trunk surrounded by pale halo.	Apparently caused by aging; of no significance.
Angioma: spider	Fiery red spiderlike lesion found on nose, trunk, or thighs.	Occurs with pregnancy and also as a sign of liver disease.
Crust	Yellow-appearing hardened discharge (scab).	Dried secretion of a ruptured vesicle.
Ecchymosis	Purple-blue mark that passes through green, yellow and brown shades until it fades.	Collection of blood under the skin from bruising.
Excoriation	Linear abrasion (scratch); loss of superficial epidermis.	Usually denotes pruritis is present; and lesion has resulted from fingernail mark.
Fissure	A crack or break in the skin surface.	Seen with fungal infections such as athlete's foot.
Hemangioma: strawberry	Elevated, rough-textured sharply circumscribed area. The color of a dark strawberry. Located in superficial tissue.	A birthmark of unknown cause. Will increase in size during the first year of life; fade entirely by 10 years.
Hemangioma: cavernous	Elevated, purple-red, sharply circumscribed lesion; located in deeper subcutaneous layer.	A birthmark of unknown cause. If the lesion is bumped, it may bleed profusely either internally or externally.
Hemangioma: port-wine mark	Deep purple, flat lesion found most commonly on face or thigh.	A birthmark; unknown cause. Does not fade with growth.
Keloid	Elevated, overgrowth of scar tissue.	Unknown cause although tendency toward keloid formation occurs chiefly in dark-skinned persons.
Macule	Discolored circular lesion flat with skin surface e.g., a freckle.	Found commonly with childhood infectious diseases.
Mongolian spot	Slate gray, macular pigmented area found most frequently on sacral area of back.	A birthmark; unknown cause. Occurs chiefly in black or Oriental children.
Papule	Elevated, pinpoint lesion e.g., a pimple.	Found commonly with childhood infectious diseases such as measles.
Petechia	Pinpoint dark red or purple spot; does not blanch on pressure.	Minute collection of blood under skin.
Pustule	A pus-filled papule.	Found in childhood infections such as chickenpox.
Scale	A flake of epidermis e.g., dandruff.	Dry skin.
Scar	White, shiny, flat lesion.	Fibrous replacement of skin following healing.
Striae gravidarum	White silvery streaks found on abdomen.	Occurs with pregnancy as a result of abdominal skin stretching.
Telangiectasia (storkbite)	Reddened, flat marks at base of neck or on eyebrows.	A birthmark; unknown cause; fades in a week or is covered by hair so is not noticeable.
Ulcer	Circular induration.	Loss of epidermis from injury.
Vesicle	A fluid-filled papule.	Seen with common infections such as *herpes simplex* (cold sores).
Venous star	Bluish, spiderlike lesion found primarily on legs.	Found in patients with increased pressure in legs. Often results with pregnancy.

TABLE 25-2. TYPES OF EXUDATE

Type	Description
Sanguineous	Red; seepage of blood
Serosanguineous	Pink; combination of blood and plasma
Serous	Yellow; seepage of plasma
Rhinitis	Clear watery discharge from nose

remain on the abdomen afterward but turn to white or silver streaks. A person who has had a considerable weight loss may show these same marks. Pregnant women may take tub baths up until a month before delivery and as soon as 4 days afterward. They must be careful not to slip in bathtubs or showers.

The Middle-Aged Adult. During middle age, the skin is less elastic. Wrinkles develop, particularly on the forehead, and skin may feel dry. Many men lose scalp hair. After menopause, many women notice an increase in facial hair similar to that at puberty as estrogen levels decrease.

The Older Adult. The skin of elderly persons tends to be thin, dry, and nonelastic. Hair tends to be thin and dry.

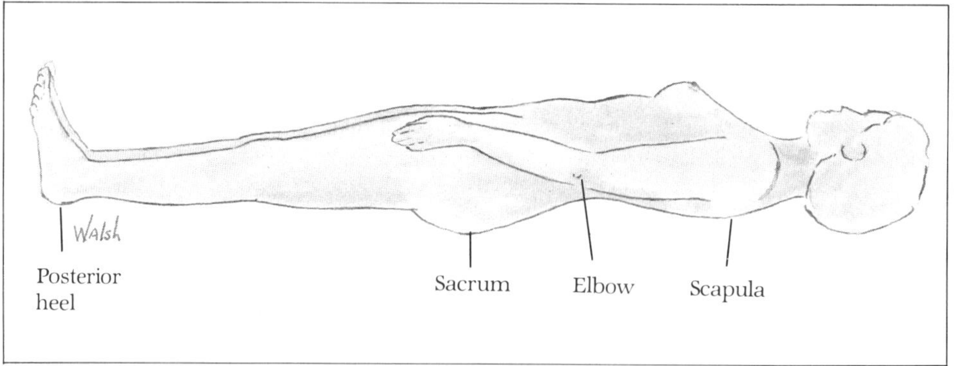

A

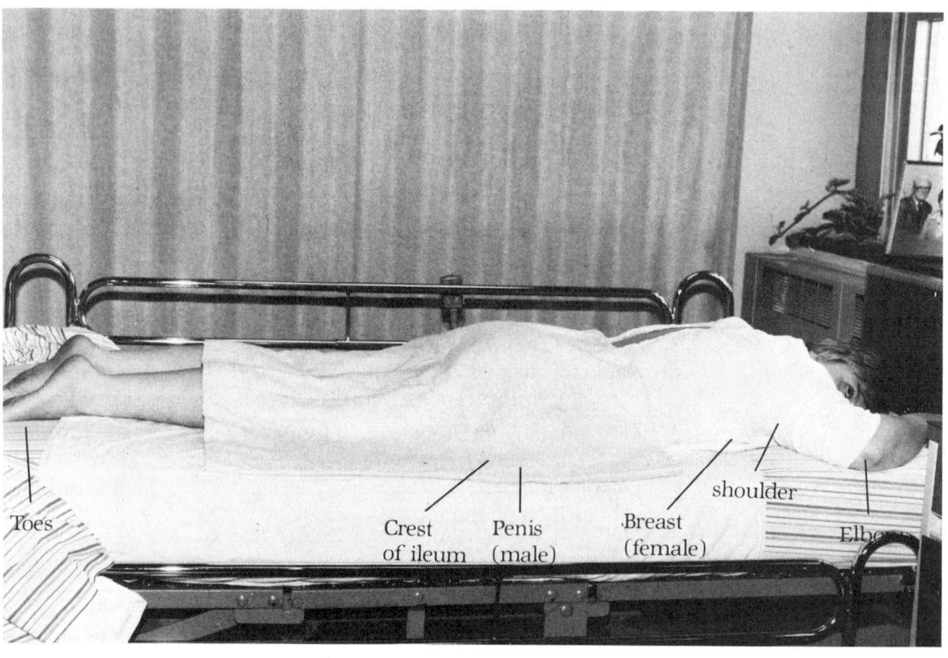

B

FIGURE 25-4. Points where pressure occurs in (A) supine, (B) prone, (C) side-lying, and (D) sitting positions.

Brown *keratotic* spots (termed *age spots*) appear. Fingernails may be brittle and ridged. Owing to poor nutrition or lack of oral care many older people have lost teeth and use partial or full dentures. Soap is drying; use it sparingly with older adults. Be careful that someone with failing eyesight or poor balance does not slip in a shower or bathtub.

DECUBITUS ULCERS AND INTEGUMENT

Decubitus ulcers (commonly termed *pressure sores* or *bed sores*) are areas of cellular necrosis caused by a lack of blood flow to the skin area. Thus, skin cells cannot receive nourishment, waste products cannot be removed, and the cells die. Initially, the ulcer affects only the surface layer of skin, but if it is untreated or circulation is not improved, subcutaneous tissue, muscle, and even bone can be affected.

The principal cause of a decubitus ulcer is *sustained pressure* to a body part. Cell injury can be caused by even low to moderate pressure for a sustained period. Body parts subjected to sustained pressure when a person is supine, prone, side-lying, and sitting are shown in Fig. 25-4. In all instances, the three body sites most likely to be involved are the sacrum, greater torchanters, and ischial tuberosities.

Shearing force is another cause of decubitus ulcers. Shearing occurs when a tissue layer slides past another, kinking or stretching the subcutaneous blood vessels and interfering with the blood supply. Shearing of sacral tissue tends to occur when the head of a patient's bed is elevated more than 30 degrees, causing him to slide toward the foot of the bed. Tissues firmly attached to body structures move with the patient; superficial skin layers tend to cling to the bed linen and not move, causing shearing (Fig. 25-5). Moving a patient up in bed frequently causes shearing in his heels and lower back if these body parts are not lifted off the bed surface when moved. Decubitus ulcers then develop at these sites.

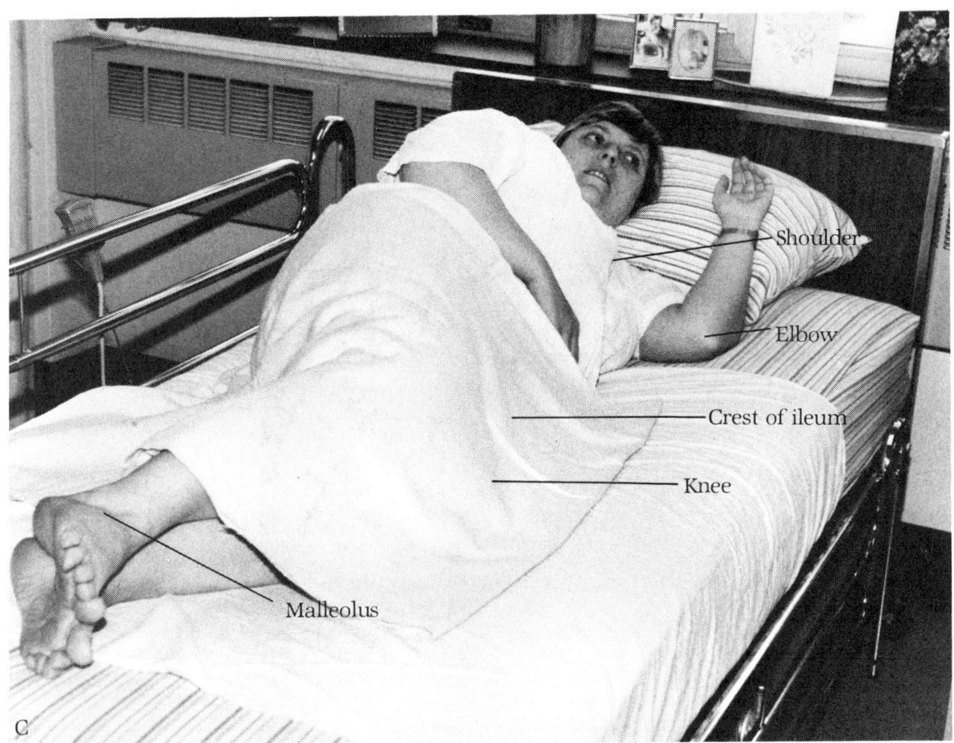

C

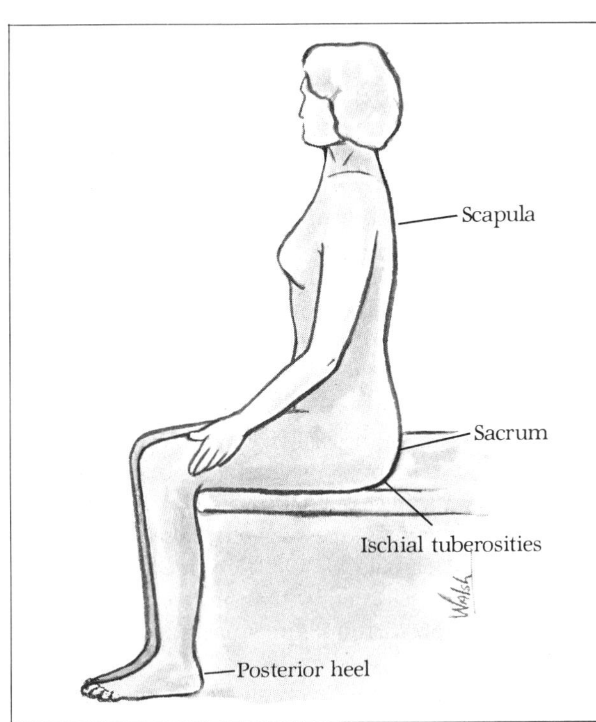

D

Assessing for Decubitus Ulcers

Some patients are more likely to develop decubitus ulcers than others (see QRS-1, Nutrition): postoperative patients because they move little and have already lain for hours in one position during surgery; overweight people because of added weight and pressure; underweight people because they have little protection over bony prominences.

People who are not eating adequately may develop low hemoglobin levels, reducing hemoglobin available to bring oxygen to cells; loss of subcutaneous fat, reducing protection from pressure; and hypovitaminosis and hypoproteinemia, limiting the growth materials available to cells. People receiving drugs to reduce pain may develop pressure areas without being aware of them. People with edema develop poor circulation to cells because the fluid pushes cells further from their blood supply.

If skin remains moist for an extended period, it may break down easily. Likewise, if it becomes too dry, it may crack and become susceptible to infection and injury.

A scoring system for estimating the probability of a patient developing decubitus ulcers is shown in Table 25-3. Rate the patient according to his general condition, mental state, activity, mobility, and whether incontinence exists or not on a scale of 1 to 4. If the patient scores less than 12, he is at risk and needs an active program of prevention measures.

The Development of a Decubitus Ulcer

When blood flow is decreased, at first a skin area appears pale. Then local inflammation occurs and the area appears reddened (erythematous); when you press on it with your finger, it will blanch. If interference with the blood supply continues, the area will turn dusky or blue-gray; it will no longer blanch with pressure. In the next stage of development, the area will blister (separation of the uppermost skin layer) and the skin will denude or ulcerate as the blister ruptures. Infection of

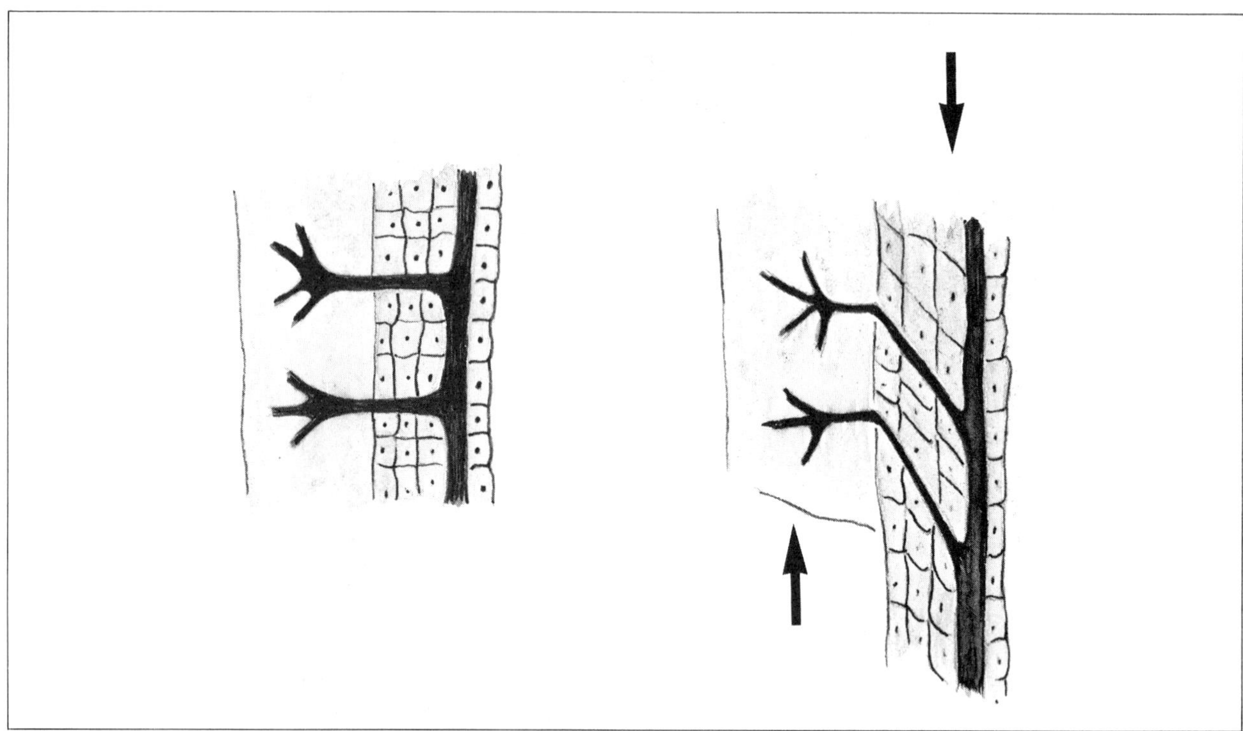

FIGURE 25-5. Shearing force. As shown on the right, when one layer of tissue slides past another, circulation to the outside layer is hampered.

necrotic tissue will occur quickly to destroy cells (Fig. 25-6).

Prevention of Decubitus Ulcers

Prevention of decubitus ulcers involves three actions: prevention of pressure areas, promotion of circulation, and maintenance of skin in a healthy condition.

Prevention of Pressure Areas. People who are on bed rest need to have their position changed every 2 hours; those on air-circulating or water mattresses must also be turned, every 3 hours. Turn a person who must remain in bed alternatively from back to front, and side to side (four separate positions). Sitting in a wheelchair is refreshing, but should be considered a supine position, since it puts pressure on the sacrum just as sitting in bed does (Fig. 25-4).

To be certain that a person is turned every 2 hours you must keep a record. A chart with times and spaces to write in the position maintained for that 2-hour block could be hung by the patient's bed or included as a part of the nursing care plan at the nursing station. Devise a plan that is consistent with the patient's wishes. For example, if a man enjoys watching television between 12 and 2 P.M., be certain that he can see the television set during that time.

Shearing force can be decreased by not raising the head of the bed over 30 degrees for more than short periods of time or by elevating the knee rest of the bed to prevent the patient from sliding down. However, raising the knee rest may lead to blood clotting or hip contractures, so must be used cautiously with patients on bed rest.

A water mattress reduces sustained pressure because of the increased pliability of the mattress surface. An alternating air-pressure mattress reduces pressure by gentle massaging action on the surface touching it. Sheepskin pads are helpful in relieving pressure points since they absorb moisture, keeping skin areas both dry and pressure-free. Gel-filled flotation pads reduce pressure by shifting readily and distributing body weight evenly, as water mattresses do.

If you do not have these aids, you can relieve pressure on a specific area by constructing a bridge. Place a folded towel or a piece of foam rubber on one side of the area where pressure is excessive; place a second towel on the other side. Circulation can flow readily across the bridge (Fig. 25-7). Do not use an inflated rubber ring, which completely surrounds an area and tends to cut off circulation.

People sitting in wheelchairs should lift themselves up off the seat for about 60 seconds every half hour by pushing down on the armrests. This is a fatiguing activity at first and many people omit it unless you remind them to do this. The footrests of the wheelchair should be positioned neither too low (so the seat rubs against the back of the legs) nor too high (lifting the legs off the chair and forcing pressure on the ischial tuberosities).

Any person on bed rest for over 24-hours has high risk for decubitus ulcer formation. Include active measures to prevent decubitus formation in your care plan as an

☐ **QUICK REFERENCE STOP 25-1: NUTRITION**

Nutritional Problem	*Relation to Skin Health*
Person who overconsumes food: obesity	Individual is prone to develop decubitus ulcers due to increased weight exerted on body parts. Also prone to skin irritation due to touching of body surfaces at folds of skin.
Person who underconsumes food: underweight	Individual is prone to develop decubitus ulcers due to lack of adipose tissue to protect bony prominences.
Person who has temporary decrease in nutritional intake	Individual is prone to poor healing of skin lesions and breakdown of skin due to inadequate nutrient supply to cells.
Person who has temporary decrease in fluid intake	Individual may develop poor skin turgor; dry skin may lead to decubitus ulcers, cracking, or peeling.

TABLE 25-3. SCORING SYSTEM FOR ESTIMATING PROBABILITY OF DECUBITI FORMATION

General condition		*Incontinent*[c]	
Good	4	Not	4
Fair	3	Occasionally	3
Poor	2	Usually of urine	2
Bad	1	Both urine and feces	1
Mobility		*Activity*	
Full	4	Ambulant	4
Slightly limited	3	Walk/help	3
Very limited	2	Chairfast	2
Immobile	1	Bedfast	1
Mental state			
Alert	4		
Apathetic[a]	3		
Confused	2		
Stuporous[b]	1		

Source: From D. Norton, R. McLaren, and A. Exton-Smith, *An Investigation of Geriatric Nursing Problems in Hospital.* London: Churchill Livingstone, 1975.
[a]Taking no interest in surroundings or plan of care.
[b]Cannot be roused easily from deep sleep.
[c]Involuntary loss of urine from bladder.

FIGURE 25-6. Decubitus ulcer.

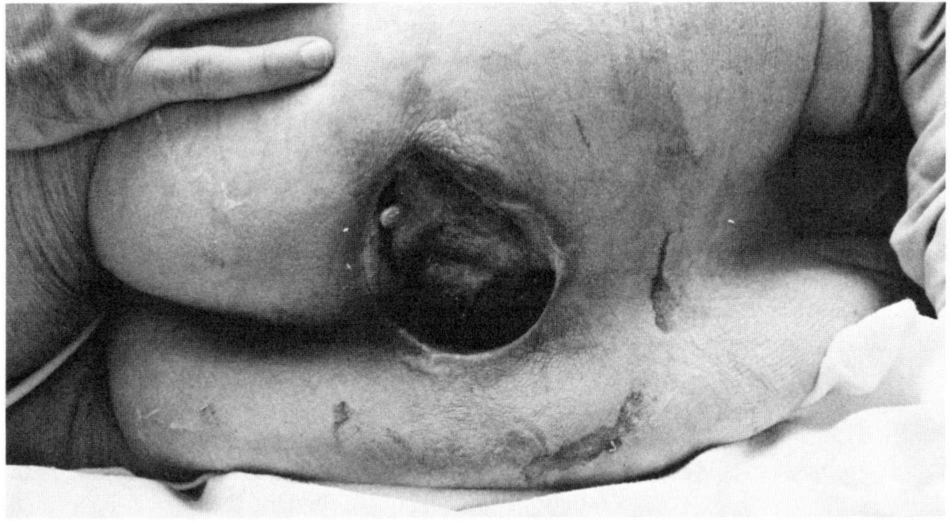

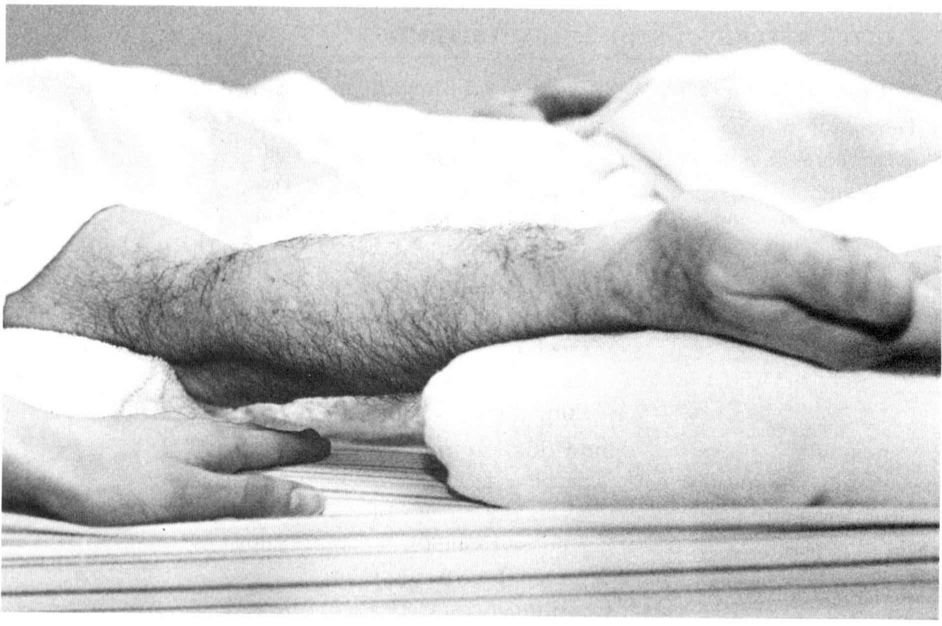

FIGURE 25-7. "Bridging" to relieve pressure from a body area—in this instance, the elbow.

independent nursing action. It is often necessary to call a physician's attention to the high-risk state. The best outcome of surgery or other therapeutic measures will be destroyed if a person cannot return home because of a *preventable* phenomenon.

Promotion of Circulation. Circulation to body parts is stimulated by activity of the part. Asking a person to move body parts, moving body parts through a passive range of motion exercises (see Chap. 26), or giving a backrub with particular attention to the sacral area all aid circulation. When you turn and reposition a patient, always massage bony prominences or any area that appears pale or reddened to increase circulation to that part.

Maintenance of Skin Health. People who are immobile and therefore prone to decubitus ulcers need diets high in protein, calories, and vitamins (see QRS 25-1). This prevents decreased hemoglobin, protein, and vitamin levels, and builds subcutaneous fat deposits. Skin must be allowed to become neither macerated nor dry. Use lotion for a backrub. Do not use alcohol, which dries skin and produces evaporation that causes temporary vasoconstriction, reducing blood flow to an area. Do not use tincture of benzoin, which, although it may toughen the skin surface, causes skin to stick to bed linen and increases the possibility of shearing force with the movement. Frequently straighten linen to keep wrinkles in the bottom sheet from causing pressure lines.

Implementation of Care for Decubitus Ulcers

If an ulcer should develop, it becomes even more important to relieve pressure on the area. Damaged tissue cannot heal unless it receives adequate nutrition and blood circulation for cell repair. Until recently, decubitus ulcers were kept dry and the dressings applied for them were changed frequently, perhaps 2 or 3 times a day. In contrast to this method of care, the usual treatment now is to clean the surface with normal saline, dry it with a sterile gauze square, and apply a self-adhesive transparent plaster dressing *(Op-Site dressing)*, which will remain in place for about 4 days. The moist environment created by such dressings appears to accelerate healing, since it encourages rapid proliferation and spread of granulation tissue. An Op-Site dressing loosens after about 4 days and needs to be replaced. If the ulcer is weeping, the dressing may need to be changed as early as 24 hours. To take the dressing off before it loosens, soak the edges in soapy water to peel it back.

Enzymatic debriding agents such as fibrinolysin (Elase), collagenase (Santyl), or proteolysin (Varidase) may be ordered to dissolve tissue at the site. These products work best if you flush the ulcer surface with normal saline before applying them. Half-strength hydrogen peroxide is another product used to remove tissue. Providine (iodine) may be used for cleansing. Do not use a hexachlorophene-based cleanser, since hexachlorophene can be absorbed into healthy tissue through the ulcer and in large amounts it is toxic to nervous tissue. Debridement or cleaning away of necrotic tissue by a whirlpool bath may also be effective. If necrotic tissue is extensive, surgical debridement may be necessary.

If an involved area is superficial, Karaya powder may be used as a drying agent; it both absorbs moisture and acts as an antimicrobial agent. A 60- or 75-watt bulb in a gooseneck lamp focused on the area for 20 minutes 3 or 4 times a day, with the bulb 18 inches away from the skin surface to prevent a burn, will provide heat treatment. Heat not only acts as a drying agent but causes vasodilatation and thereby moves more blood into the area, improving healing. Sugar may be applied to the ulcer to cause local irritation and thereby increase blood flow in the area. Because glucose is hypertonic, it draws fluid from surrounding tissues, reducing edema, and also destroys bacteria. Dextranomer (Debrisan) is a commercial polysaccharide compound that may be used for the same action. Gelfoam, a sponge impregnated with protein that absorbs moisture, is another agent that may be used to aid granulation tissue formation.

If the ulcer is weeping, a sample of the drainage should be sent for culture so that any microorganisms can be identified and treated. If drainage is present, a person may lose as much as 50 gm of protein every day from this source. Normally, the daily requirement of protein is 60 gm a day for women, 70 gm a day for men. In order to maintain a protein balance, therefore, the person must almost double his normal amount in order to heal the ulcer. Skillful planning is required to provide high protein foods in a form that this patient will eat. A high vitamin C intake to ensure skin integrity and a high iron intake to ensure hemoglobin formation are also important.

Evaluation

Evaluation of methods to prevent or to heal a decubitus ulcer must be done daily. Otherwise, a problem that appeared to be solved might merely change to a different problem. Much nursing research has been done to find the most effective strategies for prevention and treatment of pressure ulcers. Some of these findings are presented in Quick Reference Stop 25-2.

PERSONAL CARE

Meeting hygiene needs involves a number of procedures. To determine when you will carry out such procedures and when the person will do them himself calls for assessing the patient's activity level and a correct locus of decision-making (see QRS 25-3).

A.M. and P.M. Care

Most people enjoy washing their face and hands before they eat breakfast. Most people also need to void (urinate) on first arising. Helping hospitalized patients to freshen up for breakfast is termed *morning* or *A.M. care.*

☐ QUICK REFERENCE STOP 25-2: RESEARCH
Prevention and Treatment of Pressure Sores

The prevention and treatment of pressure sores is a major nursing responsibility. Nursing research has taken great strides in this area. This summary barely skims the surface of research on the prevention and treatment of pressure sores.

1. *Identifying Patients Prone to Pressure Sores.* The tool *Assessing a Patient's Potential for Pressure Sores* developed by Gosnell and reported by Meissner (1980) can be used to assess patients' potential for pressure sores. The tool quickly assesses patients on eight points: mental status, continence, mobility, activity, nutrition, skin appearance, skin tone, and skin sensation. It can be used in planning nursing interventions when specific potentials are identified.
2. *The Side-lying Position.* In positioning patients to prevent pressure sores, the side-lying position is often utilized to keep patients off their back. Traditionally, this position has been defined as extreme hip and knee flexion of the upper leg, with this same leg placed forward of the midline of the body and the neutral lower leg. However, an experimental study by Garber et al. (1982) found that trochanteric pressure was less when the upper leg was placed behind the midline of the body and less flexed positions were utilized. The researchers believe this modified position should reduce the potential for skin breakdown in prone patients.
3. *Pressure Sore Treatment with Topical Insulin.* A number of therapies have come into practice for the treatment of pressure sores. The application of topical insulin was tested with 27 geriatric patients. Data demonstrated no effect in subjects treated as compared with subjects untreated. The authors question the current practice of recommending topical insulin as an effective therapy. They also caution that insulin may be unsafe as topical therapy since it can be absorbed through the ulcer and result in systemic problems (Gerber and Van Ort, 1981).

SUGGESTED READINGS

Gerber, R. M., and Van Ort, S. R. Topical application of insulin to pressure sores: A questionable therapy. *Am. J. Nurs.* 81(6):1159, 1981.

Garber, S. L., et al. Trochanteric pressure in spinal cord injury. *Archives of Physical Medicine and Rehabilitation,* 64(11):549, 1982. Cited in Medical highlights, *Am. J. Nurs.* 83(2):293, 1983.

Meissner, J. E. Which patient on your unit might get a pressure sore? Here's the tool that can tell you. *Nursing (Horsham)* 10(6):64, 1980. Report on the tool *Assessing a Patient's Potential for Pressure Sores* developed by D. J. Gosnell.

☐ **QUICK REFERENCE STOP 25-3: PSYCHOLOGICAL CONSIDERATIONS**

Providing hygiene measures involves intimate contact. Be certain to provide privacy by drawn curtains, closed doors, and use of a bath blanket to reduce embarrassment.

Remember that self-care aids self-esteem. Provide measures as much for this reason as for cleanliness or protection of skin integrity. Allow people to do as much for themselves as possible. Sometimes it would be faster for you to bathe a person than to allow him to do this himself, but resist performing care that he can do himself. Being asked to perform self-hygiene measures may say to him more clearly than anything else that he is getting well again.

Important steps of morning care are shown in Procedure 25-1.

Before people retire for the night, they usually wash their face and hands and need to void. Helping a person prepare for a restful night's sleep is termed *evening* or *P.M. care.* Steps of evening care are shown in Procedure 25-2.

Bathing

Many illnesses increase body temperature. An elevated temperature increases perspiration as the body attempts to cool itself by evaporation at the skin surface. A bath is generally refreshing because it washes away this excess perspiration. The friction in bathing stimulates blood circulation and helps cell oxygenation. The movement of body extremities as they are positioned or exercised during bathing improves tone and preserves joint function.

PROCEDURE 25-1
Morning Care (A.M. Care)

Purpose: Help person prepare for activities of day. Meet physiological need for elimination. Provide clean hands and face before breakfast.

Plan	*Principle*
1. Wash hands; identify patient; explain procedure.	1. Prevent spread of microorganisms; promote patient safety and well-being.
2. Assess patient status; analyze appropriateness of plan; adjust plan to individual patient needs.	2. Nursing care is always individualized based on professional judgment of patient's needs.
3. Implement care by providing privacy by drawn curtains or closed door. Offer bedpan or urinal.	3. Privacy is an important right of most people. Many persons feel need to void on first awakening.
4. Bring bed to semi-Fowler's position if patient condition permits. Place towel, washcloth, soap, a basin of warm water, supplies for oral care: toothpaste, toothbrush, emesis basin and water for rinsing on overbed table convenient for patient. If gown is soiled, provide clean gown.	4. Conserve energy by organization and preparation.
5. Position call signal within easy reach. Leave patient to wash face and hands and complete oral care in private. (Perform care if patient is unable to do this by himself.)	5. Encourage self-care yet arrange for quick contact if unexpected difficulty arises.
6. Return to room to remove equipment and return it to proper place. Arrange pillows, straighten bed as needed. Leave bedside table prepared for breakfast tray. Open curtain or room door.	6. Provide psychological as well as physical comfort. Patient safety is assured by easy access.
7. Evaluate effectiveness, cost, efficiency, comfort, and safety aspects of procedure; record procedure and patient's ability to perform self-care.	7. Documentation of nursing care and patient status. Incorporating assessment into procedure is a work of a professional nurse.
8. Plan health teaching needed such as importance of toothbrushing.	8. Health teaching is an independent nursing action always included in care.

MODIFICATIONS FOR CARE OF CHILD

Children are often confused by an unfamiliar environment when they first awake. Use an unhurried approach until they become used to the setting and you.

MODIFICATIONS FOR CARE OF OLDER ADULT

Many older adults have at least some mild arthritis in body joints on awakening so have pain and stiffness on motion early in morning. They may need some help with self-care during morning hours that later in the day they would be able to perform without difficulty.

PROCEDURE 25-2
Evening Care (P.M. Care)

Purpose: Meet physiological need for elimination. Help provide a restful atmosphere conducive to sleep.

Plan	*Principle*
1. Wash hands; identify patient; explain procedure.	1. Prevent spread of microorganisms; promote patient safety and well-being.
2. Assess patient status; analyze appropriateness of plan; adjust plan to individual patient needs.	2. Nursing care is always individualized based on professional judgment of patient's needs.
3. Implement care by providing privacy by drawn curtains or closed door. Offer a bedpan or urinal.	3. Most people consider privacy an important right. Most persons feel need to void before they can sleep comfortably for the night.
4. Bring bed to semi-Fowler's position if patient condition permits. Place a basin of warm water, soap, washcloth, towel, and supplies for oral care: toothpaste, toothbrush, water for rinsing, and emesis basin on overbed table within patient's easy reach.	4. Conserve energy by organization and preparation.
5. Attach call bell in easy reach; leave patient to wash hands and face, complete oral care. (Do care if patient is unable to do this by himself.)	5. Encourage independence yet arrange for quick contact if unexpected difficulty arises. Privacy is an important right for most people.
6. Return to room to wash patient's back and administer backrub (see Procedure 25-5).	6. A backrub is soothing just before falling asleep.
7. Remove equipment; clean and return supplies to bedside stand.	7. Provide psychological as well as physical comfort.
8. Remove wrinkles from draw sheet; turn and arrange pillow; change draw sheet and pillowcase on bed as needed.	8. Provide clean unwrinkled surface to promote rest.
9. Be certain bed is left in low position. Position bedside stand near to bed; adjust call signal within convenient reach; raise siderails to safety position for night.	9. Provide for patient safety in case patient should get out of bed in darkened room.
10. Ask if the patient has any concerns or questions you could answer for him. Dim lights preparatory for sleeping or provide activity such as reading material or TV control until patient is ready for sleep. Open curtain or room door.	10. Night and darkness are anxiety-producing situations. Therapeutic communication helps to relieve anxiety.
11. Evaluate effectiveness, efficiency, cost, comfort, and safety aspects of procedure; record procedure and patient ability to perform care for self.	11. Document nursing care and patient status. Incorporating assessment into procedures is a work of a professional nurse.
12. Plan health teaching needed such as rest is conducive to healing.	12. Health teaching is an independent nursing activity always included in care.

MODIFICATIONS FOR CARE OF CHILD

Children like to have the bedtime routine they are used to at home carried out in the hospital. They may like to have a favorite bedtime story read to them, to be helped to say prayers, and to have their favorite toy tucked in with them.

Many young children are afraid of the dark and need their overhead light turned on at night.

Many parents sleep in the same hospital room with their child. Offer them a clean washcloth and towel, pillow, and linen for the night. Children do not sleep if their parent is uncomfortable or anxious about a situation.

MODIFICATIONS FOR CARE OF OLDER ADULT

When an older adult is ill, he may be very concerned that he will die. A great many people assume that death will come in the night. An older adult may feel a real need to talk to someone before what he sees as his last night. Provide this by being a supportive presence.

☐ QUICK REFERENCE STOP 25-4: ADVOCACY

If a person has a handicap and mobility is difficult, it is easier from a nursing standpoint to give such a patient a bath in bed. However, many people feel really clean or as if they are returning to health again only if they can take a tub bath or shower. You may need to advocate for a patient to attempt these methods of bathing.

Most patients are bathed in the morning so that they feel fresh for visitors and the rest of the day. Also, observations about any change in their condition can be described early in the day and new interventions begun. However, many children take their bath at bedtime and are most comfortable being bathed in the evening.

You may give a complete bath; a partial bath, in which only the face, hands, axilla, back and perineal area are bathed; or an assisted bath, in which the patient does most of his own care (see QRS 25-4). Types of *therapeutic baths* are a sitz bath, to promote healing of tissue through the application of warm water; a baking soda bath, to reduce the pruritus of a skin rash; a tepid bath, to reduce body temperature; and whirlpool bath, to relax muscle strain or debride injured skin. Therapeutic baths require a doctor's order to perform. They are discussed in Chap. 33 with other examples of therapeutic heat application.

Principles of Bathing. As in other therapeutic heat application, the water used for bathing patients should be pleasantly warm, between 105° and 110°F (40.5°—43.3°C). Estimate the warmth of water by submerging the inside of your wrist into the water. Change water any time it is soiled or too cool. Soap reduces surface tension of water and cleans by fat emulsification. Do not leave the soap in the basin of water while you work. It will dissolve too quickly and the water will become too soapy to be used as rinse water. Rinse body parts well, since soap is drying if it is left on the skin. This is particularly important with infants and elderly patients, who have dry skin.

Always work from clean areas to less clean ones. Use strokes for bathing that are firm enough to clean but are still gentle. Stroking from the distal to the proximal portion of an extremity aids in venous flow of blood and better cell oxygenation. Steps of bathing are shown in Procedures 25-3, 25-4, and 25-5.

Nurses typically speak of bathing a person as if it were the extent of their intervention. However, total nursing care consists not only of bathing, but also of oral care, shaving, hair care, perineal care, a back rub, observing the patient's mood and general physical condition, health teaching, changing the bed linen, straightening the room, and providing stimulation. Steps in total care are shown in Procedures 25-6 through 25-13. These should always be thought of as one integrated procedure. Specific assessments to be made during bathing are shown in the following box.

Assessments to be Made During Bathing

1. Are there any lesions on the patient's skin or scalp? How shall I describe them?
2. Is skin and hair texture, dryness and oiliness normal?
3. Is skin turgor normal?
4. Is there any abnormal body odor?
5. Is any skin surface reddened or more pale than surrounding surface that suggests interference with circulation at that point?
6. Are teeth and gums in good repair?
7. Are there any breaks in the continuity of the skin or mucous membrane that could be a possible entry for infectious organisms?
8. Is Homans' sign (pain in calf of leg on dorsiflexion of the foot) negative?
9. Is there tenderness or sensitivity in any body part that I touched?
10. Is there stiffness in any body part?
11. Was the patient's communication during the bath appropriate to his age and condition?
12. What is the patient's overall mood and level of self-esteem?
13. Is there any finding that is different from what I expected? Different from the last time I bathed this patient that I cannot explain?

PROCEDURE 25-3
Bathing in Bed an Adult Who is Unable to Aid in Care

Purpose: Cleanse the skin. Stimulate circulation by aiding venous return. Promote self-esteem through improved physical appearance. Promote relaxation through soothing application of water. Provide a time for patient mobility, circulatory, and skin assessment. Provide an opportunity for use of therapeutic touch.

Plan	*Principle*
1. Wash your hands; identify patient; explain procedure to patient.	1. Prevent spread of microorganisms. Promote patient safety and well-being.
2. Assess patient status; analyze appropriateness of plan; adjust plan to individual patient needs.	2. Nursing care is always individualized based on professional nursing judgment of patient needs.
3. Implement care by assembling supplies: a basin of pleasantly warm water, soap, towel, washcloth, bath blanket, clean gown, and any personal supplies the patient enjoys such as deodorant or body powder.	3. Conserve energy by organization and preparation (Fig. 1).

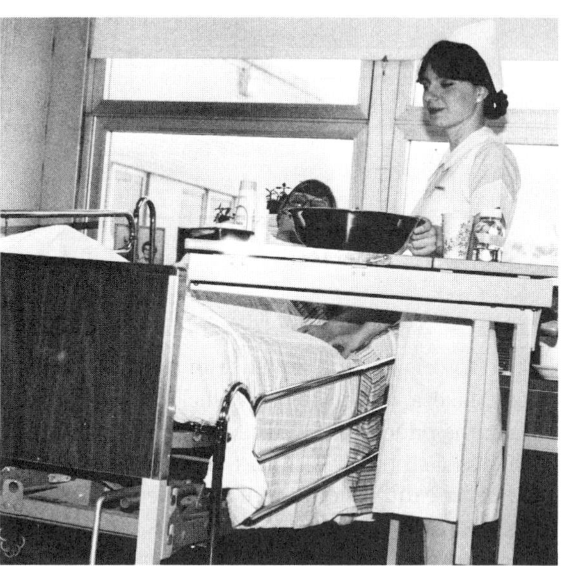

FIGURE 1. A student nurse assembles supplies necessary for bathing. Notice that the bed is in the high position to prevent back strain.

Plan	*Principle*
4. Provide privacy by drawing the bed curtain or closing room door.	4. The right to privacy is highly valued by most people.
5. Raise the bed to a high position; lower the siderail on the side you choose to work from. Offer a bedpan or urinal.	5. Prevent stretching and bending. Allow easy access to the patient for care. Most people prefer to use a bedpan before a bath.
6. If patient's condition allows, place the head of the bed flat. Remove pillow if patient does not object.	6. Easier access to all skin surfaces. Prevent pillow from becoming moist.
7. Loosen the top covers of the bed. Fold spread, remove and place over the back of the bedside chair or foot of bed if it is to be used again. Discard it in a linen hamper or place pillowcase over back of bedside chair to serve as a linen hamper and place it in that if it will be replaced with a clean one. Fold a bed blanket if in place and place over the back of the patient chair or foot of bed the same way.	7. Always fold, not fluff linen so microorganisms are not thrown into the air with linen changing. Keep linen away from uniform when handling it to prevent organisms from touching your uniform. Never put linen on the floor since the floor is contaminated with organisms.

8. Place bath blanket over top sheet. Gently pull top sheet from under blanket, fold and place on chair or discard in linen hamper. Be certain not to expose patient to protect privacy.

8. A bath blanket prevents chilling more than does a top sheet as it absorbs moisture. If no bath blanket is available, use top sheet as substitute bath blanket.

9. Provide oral care (see Procedure 25-11) and if an adult male, assist him with shaving (see Procedure 25-10).

9. Performing these procedures at this point prevents stains on clean linen at end of bath.

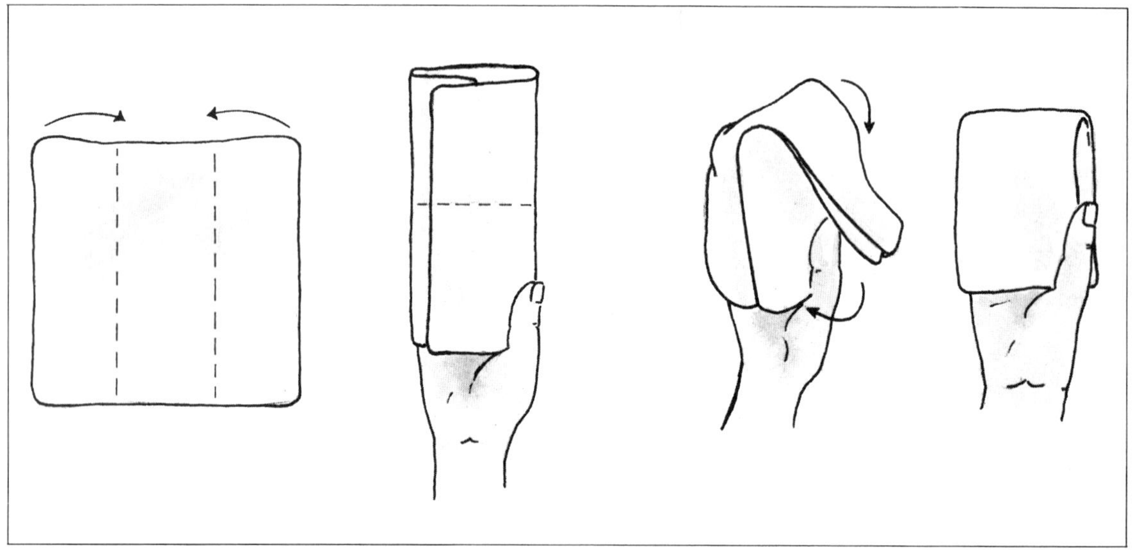

FIGURE 2. Making a mitten from a washcloth. A. Fold washcloth from side to side. B. Tuck far side under near edge.

10. Place towel over the top edge of the bath blanket. Make a mitten for a washcloth and gently wash the patient's eyes, face, and ears with clear water. Wash the eyes from the inner canthus to the outer canthus to prevent any infection in one eye from spreading to other. Always use a clean space on the cloth for the second eye. Dry the face with a gentle patting motion; facial skin is sensitive.

10. Using a mitten technique (Fig. 2) prevents edges of the washcloth from becoming cold or dripping water. Soap is irritating to sensitive facial skin. Never place anything smaller than the corner of a washcloth into an ear canal to avoid scratching and injuring the canal.

11. Assess patient skin condition, patient mobility, mood, and level of self-esteem as you work (see box, p. 484). Remove the patient's gown, being certain not to expose him and cause chilling. Place towel over chest and draw down the bath blanket to below the towel.

11. Ability to incorporate assessment into procedures is a mark of a professional nurse.

12. Rewet washcloth, soap it, and wash patient's neck and chest. Keep towel over chest to protect modesty. Be certain to wash well under female breasts. Rinse and dry area. Apply body powder if needed to decrease skin irritation under breast tissue. Assess range of motion of neck as you clean it.

12. Any area where skin surfaces touch is a potential point for irritation and skin breakdown.

13. Place towel under arm farthest from you (Fig. 3). Wash, rinse, and dry the arm using distal to proximal strokes. Apply any deodorant or powder patient enjoys to axilla. Assess range of motion of extremity as you position arm for procedure. Repeat with second arm.

13. Washing farthest arm first prevents you rewetting dried arm. Stroking from distal to proximal area aids venous return.

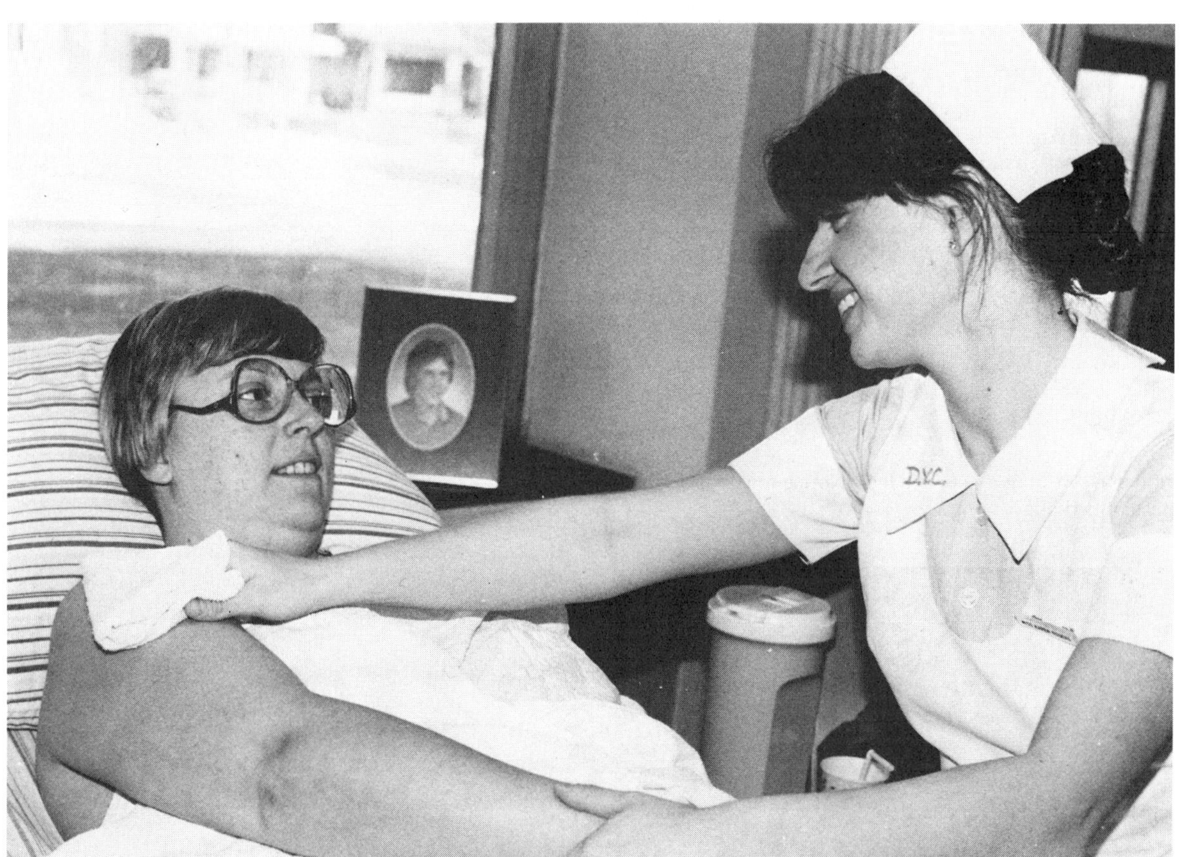

FIGURE 3. Washing a patient's arms. Begin with the farther arm. Place towel under patient's arm as you work.

14. Assist patient to put on a clean gown.

14. Prevent chilling from exposure while you wash the abdomen.

15. Place towel over the abdomen; lower bath blanket to pubis to allow easy access. Wash, rinse, and dry area.

16. To wash legs, fold bath blanket toward center of bed to expose one leg at a time (Fig. 4). Place towel on bed under leg. Flex knee, dorsiflex foot, and ask if patient has pain in the calf of the leg while you have the leg in this position (Fig. 5). If the patient experiences pain this is suggestive of a blood clot in the vein of the leg (Homans' sign). *Do not touch this area further if Homans' sign is positive.*

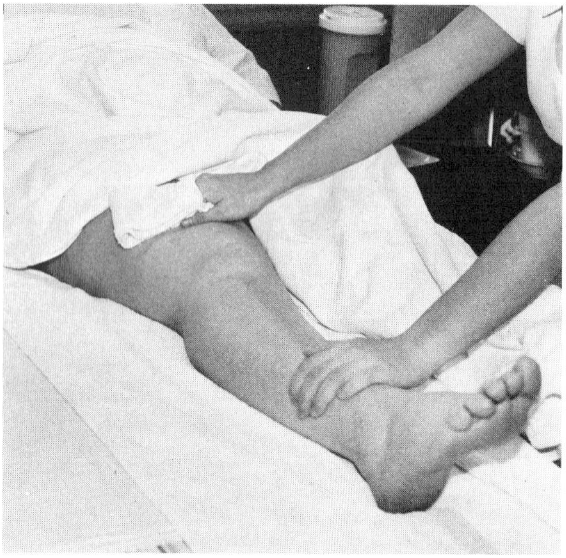

FIGURE 4. Washing a patient's legs. Notice towel under leg to protect bedding.

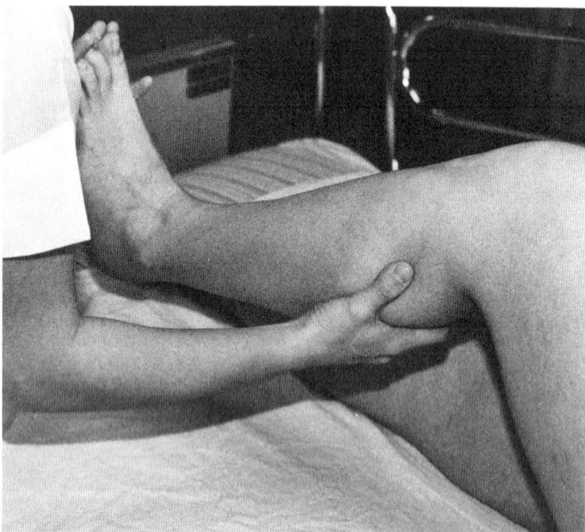

FIGURE 5. Homans' sign will be positive if a blood clot is present in the calf of a leg. Dorsiflex the foot; bend the knee; ask if there is pain.

16. Massaging a blood clot (a thrombophlebitis) may loosen it and cause it to become an embolus. If it should move to the lungs, it would obstruct and cause loss of respiration (pulmonary emboli). Report positive Homans' sign to the person's physician.

17. Wash, rinse, and dry one leg using strokes from a distal to proximal direction. Assess range of motion of the leg as you work. Repeat with second leg.
18. Move towel to bed area at patient's feet. Place basin of water on bed. Place patient's feet in the basin for a few minutes (Fig. 6), remove gently, and dry well. If skin on feet is dry, apply lotion. If you trim toenails, trim them straight across.

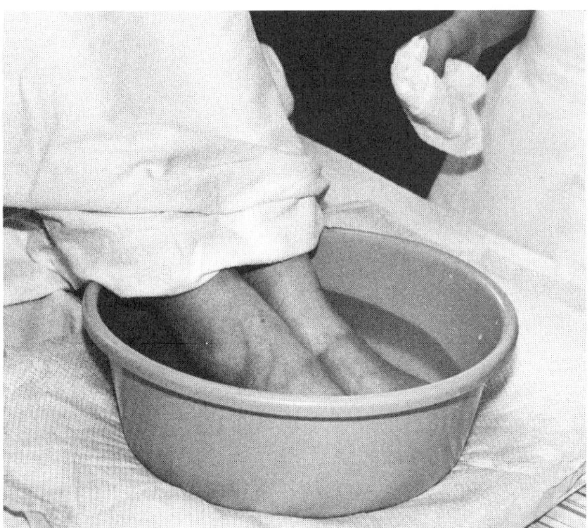

FIGURE 6. Soaking feet for a moment is soothing and softens hardened areas.

18. Soaking softens calluses and aids circulation. Square-cut toenails help to prevent ingrown toenails. Never cut toenails of patients with diabetes or circulatory diseases due to risk of infection with these diseases.

19. Help patient turn to lie on side facing away from you. Wash, rinse, and dry neck, shoulders, back, and buttocks (Fig. 7). Place towel as needed to keep bed dry.

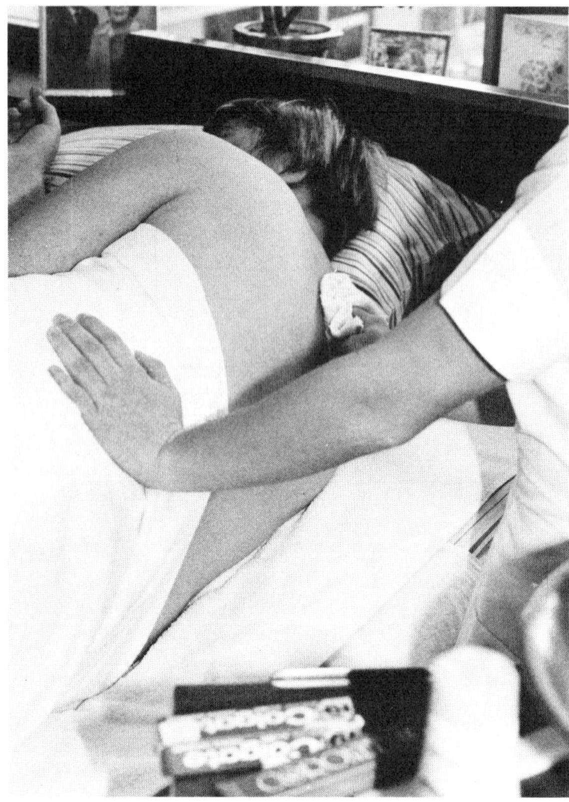

FIGURE 7. Washing a patient's back. Notice the placement of the towel.

20. Complete a backrub (see Procedure 25-6).

21. With patient on back, wash, rinse, and dry genital area or, if patient is able, leave him with basin of water, washcloth, and towel to wash own genital area. If giving care, place a disposable pad under patient's hips and buttocks. If a man is uncircumsized, gently retract the foreskin of penis, and wash. Rinse area and return foreskin to its place. Apply body powder between scrotum and legs as needed to prevent skin contact and irritation. For a female, always wash, rinse, and dry the perineal area with strokes that move from anterior to the posterior area.

21. Washing with anterior-posterior strokes prevents pathogenic organisms from spreading from rectal area to vagina or urinary meatus in women.

22. Help patient to turn onto his side; wash, rinse, and dry the anal area. If there are feces present, clean away with toilet tissue. Provide body powder if needed between buttocks to prevent skin surfaces from contact and irritation.

22. Leaving anal area until last leaves a highly contaminated body area until last.

23. Make bed with clean linen.

23. See Procedure 27-4.

24. Comb, style hair, position patient comfortably. Provide activity for patient consistent with condition (TV, reading material, etc.).

24. Provide a therapeutic environment.

25. Remove soiled linen; empty, rinse, and dry water basin and return it to bedside stand. Hang towel and washcloth to dry. Open curtain or room door.

25. Provide psychological as well as physical comfort. Patient safety is assured by easy access.

26. Evaluate effectiveness, efficiency, cost, comfort, and safety aspects of procedure; record procedure and assessments of patient.

26. Documentation of nursing care and patient status.

27. Plan health teaching as indicated from assessment data such as need for increased exercise while in bed.

27. Health teaching is an independent nursing action always included in care.

MODIFICATIONS FOR CARE OF CHILD

Children generally find the thought of bathing in bed strange and point out that because they have not been out of bed, they are not dirty. Incorporating a talk time or a time for game playing (I'm thinking of something in the room that is red; can you guess it?) into the procedure is a smooth way of making the activity not only acceptable but enjoyable as well. Plan for bathing an infant is given in Procedure 25-5.

MODIFICATIONS FOR CARE OF OLDER ADULT

Many older adults have dry skin; omit the use of soap for bathing to prevent further drying or limit full bed baths to every other day.

Range-of-motion exercises may be difficult to accomplish in the older adult who has arthritic changes. You may choose to do these at a time separate from bathing if they are time consuming and you worry the patient would become chilled.

PROCEDURE 25-4
Assisting a Person with a Bedbath

Purpose: Encourage self-esteem through self-care and improved physical appearance. Provide cleanliness and skin stimulation. Provide a time for patient condition and skin assessment. Provide an opportunity for therapeutic touch.

Plan	*Principle*
1. Wash your hands; identify patient; explain procedure to patient.	1. Prevent spread of microorganisms. Promote patient safety and well-being.
2. Assess patient status; analyze appropriateness of plan; adjust plan to individual patient needs.	2. Nursing care is always individualized based on professional judgment of patient's needs.
3. Implement care by discussing with patient what portions of the bath he would like to do himself to facilitate self-care without unnecessary fatigue.	3. It is difficult for a patient to wash his back or legs while in bed. Most men prefer to shave themselves. Likewise, most persons prefer to give own perineal care.
4. Provide equipment necessary for care: basin of warm water, washcloth, towel, clean gown, and supplies for shaving and oral care. Position them in easy reach for patient. Remove top bed covers and replace with bath blanket.	4. To prevent chilling while giving self-care.
5. Be certain that call signal is in an easily reached position.	5. Patient safety; patient can signal you quickly if he has unexpected difficulty.
6. Provide for privacy; draw curtain on bed or close room door.	6. The right of privacy is highly valued by most persons.
7. Return in about 15 minutes to finish any part of the bath necessary. If water is not still pleasantly warm, replace it with fresh water.	7. People often become more fatigued than they expect when recovering from an illness.

8. Complete back care and make the necessary skin assessments; make bed; clean and straighten room; open curtain or room door; and provide a diversional activity.

8. Incorporating assessment into care is a mark of a professional nurse. Patient safety is assured by easy access. Provide psychological as well as physical well-being.

9. Evaluate effectiveness, efficiency, cost, comfort, and safety aspects of procedure; record procedure and assessments.

9. Document nursing care and patient status. Incorporating assessment into procedures is a mark of a professional nurse.

10. Plan necessary health teaching based on assessment data, such as need for increased movement in bed.

10. Health teaching is an independent nursing action always included in care.

MODIFICATIONS FOR CARE OF CHILD

Young children may need some touching up of body parts washed themselves. You usually need to supervise oral and perineal care to be sure it is done thoroughly.

MODIFICATIONS FOR CARE OF OLDER ADULT

Most older adults pride themselves on their ability to be independent and continue to provide for themselves. Be certain you do not equate old with ill. Evaluate each person independently on his level of self-care and ability to provide for his own hygiene needs.

PROCEDURE 25-5
Giving a Bath to an Infant

Purpose: Cleanse skin. Provide opportunity for therapeutic touch. Provide opportunity for enjoyment of water play.

Plan	*Principle*
1. Wash your hands; identify patient; explain procedure to patient.	1. Prevent spread of microorganisms. Promote patient safety and well-being. Even if infants are too young to comprehend your meaning, they respond to the sound of a caring voice.
2. Assess patient status; analyze appropriateness of procedure based on patient condition; adjust plan of care to individual infant.	2. Nursing care is always individualized based on assessment of patient needs.
3. Implement care by assembling supplies: towel, washcloth, mild soap, basin of warm water, change of clothing, powder or lotion.	3. Conserve energy by organization and preparation.
4. Place towel on bed surface. Lay infant on towel. Assess condition of total skin and scalp.	4. Incorporating assessment into care is a mark of a professional nurse.
5. Wash eyes with clear water, using a different part of a washcloth for each stroke. Wash face with clear water also.	5. Wash from cleanest to most soiled body areas; soap may be irritating to sensitive facial skin.
6. Hold infant in football hold over edge of water basin. Wet hair; lather well with soap and massage scalp. Rinse well by splashing water from basin over hair. Place on towel and dry well.	6. Hair is shampooed daily with infants to prevent seborrhea (cradle-cap) on scalp. Soap may be used as shampoo.
7. If infant is not to be placed in basin of water, lather hands with soap and using hands soap front of infant's body. Rinse with wet washcloth and dry with towel. If cord is still present, prevent it from becoming wet. Pay special attention to body creases to remove accumulated secretions.	7. An infant should not be submerged in water until his umbilical cord has dried and fallen off (7—10 days of age). Wetting the cord encourages infection.

8. Turn infant onto stomach. Repeat soaping, rinsing, drying process.

8. Infants enjoy the feel of warm water. Caution: Infants' skin is very slippery when wet due to its smoothness.

9. If infant may be placed in basin, soap as in steps 7 and 8; gently place in sitting position in basin to rinse. Dry after placing infant back on towel.

10. Apply lotion as needed to any dry skin area. If cord is still present, 70% alcohol may be applied to cord.

10. Infants tend to have dry skin that needs lotion. Alcohol dries the cord and prevents infection.

11. Redress infant; change linen on crib or bassinet.

12. Evaluate effectiveness, efficiency, cost, comfort, and safety aspects of procedure; record procedure and skin and scalp assessments. Return equipment to proper storage.

12. Documentation of nursing action and patient status.

13. Plan health teaching such as bathtime is a time for social interaction—a good time for play as well as achieving cleanliness.

13. Health teaching is an independent nursing action always included in care.

Offering a Bedpan or Urinal

Many people prefer to use a bedpan before their bath. A bed may become soiled when a bedpan is used, so it is wise to offer a bedpan or urinal before giving a bath rather than after you have just changed linen on the bed. The technique of offering a bedpan or urinal is described in Chap. 39 with other aspects of elimination.

Administering a Backrub

The skin on a person's back grows irritated from rubbing against sheets, and his back receives a great deal of pressure if he is in bed for any length of time. Giving a backrub following bathing aids circulation, soothes stiff muscles, and prevents skin breakdown. Steps for a backrub are shown in Procedure 25-6.

PROCEDURE 25-6
Administering a Backrub

Purpose: Stimulate circulation. Improve muscle tone. Relax muscle tenseness. Offer a psychological feeling of comfort and well-being. Provide opportunity for use of therapeutic touch.

Plan	*Principle*
1. Wash your hands; identify patient; explain procedure.	1. Prevent spread of microorganisms; promote patient safety and well-being.
2. Assess patient status; analyze appropriateness of plan; adjust plan to individual patient need.	2. Nursing care is always individualized based on professional judgment of patient's needs.
3. Implement care by assembling equipment: bath lotion or powder and a towel to protect bottom sheet.	3. Conserve energy by organization and preparations. Alcohol, once used extensively for backrubs, is drying to skin, so rarely used today.
4. Bring bed to high position; lower the head rest to a flat position unless patient's condition prevents this.	4. Prevent stretching and bending.
5. Provide privacy. Help turn patient onto his side facing away from you. Place towel on bed beside back to protect bed linen.	5. Privacy is a highly valued right of most persons. Allows best access to observe back.
6. Assess back for lesions, bruises, pressure areas, or break in skin integrity.	6. Incorporating assessment into care is the mark of a professional nurse. Damaged skin is in danger of tissue breakdown and development of decubitus ulcer.

7. Place lotion on hand and apply to back of patient's neck. Place fingers of right hand along right side of cervical vertebrae; fingers of left hand along left side of vertebrae, massage using small circular motions from shoulders to hairline. (Or use one hand, fingers on one side of vertebrae, thumb on the other).

7. Applying lotion to hand first warms it before it touches patient. Small circular massage motions are most relaxing to neck muscles.

8. Apply lotion to hands again and rub back using strokes that move upward at the vertebrae, then out to the lateral aspect of the back and down (Fig. 1). *Be sure to include buttocks as part of back.*

8. Upward strokes along the center back; downward at the periphery is most relaxing.

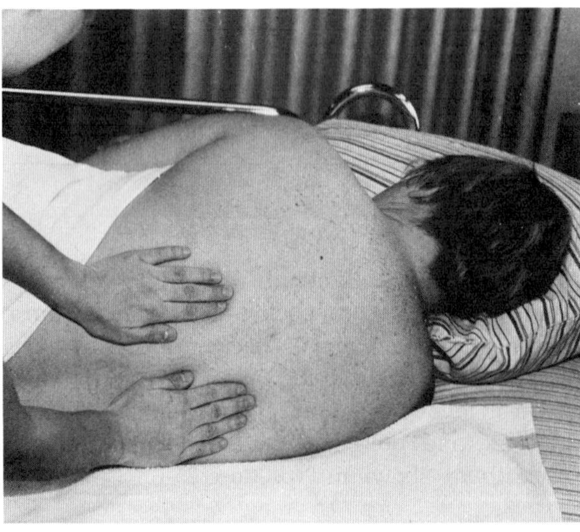

FIGURE 1. Giving a backrub. Stroke upward along the spinal column; downward at the periphery of the back.

9. Rub area at base of spine and shoulder blades with small circular motions to ensure stimulation and good circulation to this area; finish with long relaxing strokes as in step 8.

9. These are prime areas for decreased circulation to occur due to bed rest.

10. Return equipment to proper place; readjust bed linen; position patient comfortably; supply diversional activity; open curtain or room door.

10. Provide psychological as well as physical well-being. Patient safety is assured by easy access.

11. Evaluate effectiveness of procedure; record procedure, any areas of redness, paleness, bruises, or abrasions.

11. Document nursing care and patient status.

12. Plan health teaching such as need to turn every 2 hours while in bed to avoid sustained pressure to body parts.

12. Health teaching is an independent nursing action always included in care.

MODIFICATIONS FOR CARE OF CHILD

Never use alcohol for backrubs for children. It shocks immature nervous systems; inhaling the fumes may cause liver intoxication.

Do not leave bath lotion on a bedside stand where it could be swallowed.

MODIFICATIONS FOR CARE OF OLDER ADULT

As with children, never use alcohol for a backrub. It is too drying for older skin.

Showering and Tub Bathing

Patients who are able to be out of bed usually enjoy taking a tub bath or a shower. These methods are so much more like home bathing that the patient gains a sense that he is getting better and is in control of his body again. Procedures 25-7 and 25-8 describe the steps for assisting a patient with a tub bath or shower.

Hair Care

Brushing hair stimulates the circulation of blood in the scalp and helps sebum move along the hair shaft, lubricating the shaft and prolonging hair life. In addition, hair care improves physical appearance and, therefore, self-esteem.

Women with long hair may like it brushed and

PROCEDURE 25-7
Assisting a Person with a Tub Bath

Purpose: Promote maximum self-care and self-esteem through improved body image. Cleanse the skin. Promote relaxation and improve circulation. Promote return to usual means of bathing.

Plan	*Principle*
1. Wash your hands; identify patient; explain the procedure.	1. Prevent spread of microorganisms; promote patient safety and well-being.
2. Assess patient status; analyze appropriateness of plan; adjust plan of care to individual patient need.	2. Nursing care is always individualized based on professional judgment of patient's needs.
3. Implement care by assembling equipment: soap, 2 towels, washcloth, clean gown or pajamas. Clean bathtub with scouring powder and rinse tub well so no powder remains.	3. Conserve energy by organization and preparation. Prevent cross infection between patients.
4. Run water into tub; bath water should be pleasantly warm to the inner surface of your wrist. Run water before patient gets into tub to assure yourself that the patient will not be scalded by too hot water.	4. Patient safety.
5. Place towel on floor by tub to serve as a bathmat. Help patient to put on robe and slippers and walk to bathtub room.	5. Patient safety.
6. Assist patient into tub as necessary. Use tub rails to prevent slipping.	6. Patient safety.
7. Demonstrate how the bathroom call system operates.	7. Patient safety; patient can contact you quickly if he should encounter unexpected difficulty.
8. Provide privacy. Close bathroom door but *do not lock.* Hang an *in use* or *do not disturb* sign on doorknob. *Never leave an adult not fully alert alone in a bathtub.*	8. An adult not fully alert may slip under the water or turn on scalding water if left unsupervised. Patient safety is assured by easy access.
9. Check on patient in a few minutes by knocking on door of bathroom and asking if he is managing all right.	9. The warmth of a hot bath is often more relaxing and fatiguing than the person expected.
10. Assist the patient from the tub and with drying his back and redressing as needed. Assist to return to his room as needed. Give backrub when patient returns to bed if desired.	
11. Empty bathtub and clean as needed for next patient.	11. Aid other health care providers to perform quality care.
12. Evaluate effectiveness, efficiency, cost, comfort, and safety aspects of procedure; record procedure and assess level of self-care.	12. Documentation of nursing care and patient status. Incorporating assessment into procedures is a mark of a professional nurse.
13. Plan health teaching based on assessment data, such as need for increased self-care.	13. Health teaching is an independent nursing action always included in care.

MODIFICATIONS FOR CARE OF CHILD

1. Provide a bathtub toy if desired such as a rubber duck.
2. Bubble bath may be used as a special treat but not routinely, since it may lead to a urinary tract infection, especially in girls.
3. *Never leave a child under 8 years alone in a bathtub.* He might slip under the water or scald himself by adding new water.
4. A bathtub for a baby is his water basin. Water play (splashing, etc.) is therapeutic in that it is anxiety relieving to children as well as cleansing.

MODIFICATIONS FOR CARE OF OLDER ADULT

Be certain that a bathtub is equipped with safety rails so the older adult does not slip stepping into the bathtub.

PROCEDURE 25-8
Assisting a Person with a Shower

Purpose: Promote and maintain cleanliness and sense of well-being. Allow patient to assist in his own care. Promote circulation. Promote return to usual means of bathing.

Plan	*Principle*
1. Wash your hands; identify patient; explain procedure to patient.	1. Prevent spread of microorganisms; promote patient safety and well-being.
2. Assess patient status; analyze appropriateness of plan; adjust plan to individual patient need.	2. Nursing care is always individualized based on professional judgment of patient's needs.
3. Implement plan by assembling equipment: washcloth, soap, 2 towels, clean gown. Check that shower stall is clean and unoccupied. Place towel on floor as bathmat.	3. Conserve energy by organization and preparation. Prevent spread of microorganisms.
4. Help patient to put on robe and slippers, and walk to shower room.	4. Patient safety.
5. Adjust water temperature; give help as necessary with undressing. Urge patient to use safety railings.	5. Patient safety.
6. Demonstrate how the signal device operates. If you worry that a person will grow dizzy or become too fatigued, place a straight-backed chair in the shower stall so the patient can sit and shower. Some health care agencies have commercial chairs for this purpose.	6. Assure safe patient communication should unexpected difficulty arise. Assure patient safety.
7. Provide privacy by closing curtain or bathroom door. *Do not lock door.* Hang an *in use* or *do not disturb* sign on door.	7. Protect sense of privacy, yet allow safe access.
8. Return in a reasonable time to assist patient as necessary with dressing. Help to return to bed. Return to shower room to discard towel used as floormat. Clean shower for use with next patient.	8. People may become more fatigued showering than anticipated. Leave shower stall safe for next patient use.
9. Evaluate effectiveness, efficiency, cost, comfort, and safety aspects of procedure; record patient activity, skin condition, response to procedure.	9. Document nursing action and patient status. Incorporating assessment into procedures is a mark of a professional nurse.
10. Plan health teaching as needed, such as better body hygiene.	10. Health teaching is an independent nursing action always included in care.

MODIFICATIONS FOR CARE OF CHILD

Many children under school age have never showered so this is a new experience for them. Most children under adolescence prefer tub baths because of the advantage of water play.

MODIFICATIONS FOR CARE OF OLDER ADULT

Remember that exposure to warm water may be more fatiguing than expected. Check frequently or remain with patient if this is a concern.

combed into braids to keep it from tangling if they are on bed rest. Be certain that hair lies flat against the head at the sides so that the woman can rest her head on it in that position.

Shampooing is a procedure that most people enjoy. If the person should not be chilled, you can use a dry shampoo, which clings to the sebum on the hair shafts; as you comb it away, it removes excess sebum and dirt. These shampoos are limited in effect.

A plan for shampooing the hair of a person in bed is given in Procedure 25-9. If blowing hair dry, do not use a heat setting over *low.* Never allow any electrical appliance to come in contact with water.

Black patients' hair tangles easily when shampooed. Comb it while still wet to remove the tangles. If it appears dry, apply some mineral oil or petroleum jelly to make braiding or styling less difficult.

In North America, most women shave the hair from their axilla and legs. You can remove unwanted body hair by shaving or the use of depilatories. Depilatories can irritate the skin; read the instructions well, and test some on a small skin area before applying to a large area.

Most men prefer to shave themselves if they are physically able to do so. Provide adequate light and a mirror. Assisting a person with shaving is shown in Procedure 25-10.

Pediculosis. When combing or shampooing hair, watch for small white particles that cling to the hair shafts and are difficult to remove. Often there are also scratch marks at the hairline, or you notice the person scratching his scalp.

The small white particles are nits or the eggs of hair lice. The pruritus (itching) is from the bite of mature lice. Generally lice are too small to see, but if you detect nits on hair they are present. The physician can order a medicated shampoo, such as gamma benzine hydrochloride (Kwell), to wash them away.

Lice may also occur in the pubic area *(pediculosis pubis)* or on the body *(pediculosis corporis).* Lice are easily transmitted on combs, hats, or towels.

Eye Care

Always wash the eyes first when giving a bath since you work from cleaner areas to more soiled areas. Wiping eyes from the inner canthus outward prevents spreading any infection present from one eye to the other. Always use a clean section of washcloth for the second eye.

Care of Eyeglasses. When you handle eyeglasses, do not put your fingers on either lens; smudges are difficult to see through. To wash glasses, wet the glass by dipping it under running water, then wipe dry with a soft tissue. Do not use hot water; water too hot can melt plastic

PROCEDURE 25-9
Giving a Shampoo to a Patient in Bed

Purpose: Stimulate circulation to scalp; cleanse the hair. Promote self-esteem by increased physical appearance.

Plan	*Principle*
1. Wash your hands; identify patient; explain procedure to patient.	1. Prevent spread of microorganisms; promote patient safety and well-being.
2. Assess patient status; analyze appropriateness of plan; adjust plan to individual patient needs.	2. Nursing care is always individualized based on professional judgment of patient's needs.
3. Implement care by assembling supplies: shampoo, pitcher of warm water, towel, comb, personal equipment for setting or styling hair, and shampoo trough (if not available make one from plastic bag and paper clips). If patient can be moved to a stretcher, do so and bring stretcher up to a nearby sink. Provide privacy with closed curtain or room door.	3. Conserve energy by organization and preparation. Privacy is an important right to most people.

4. Place shampoo trough under head (Fig. 1A) or position head over edge of sink. Place towel over chest.

4. Protect patient gown from water. Protect bed linen from large amount of water used during procedure.

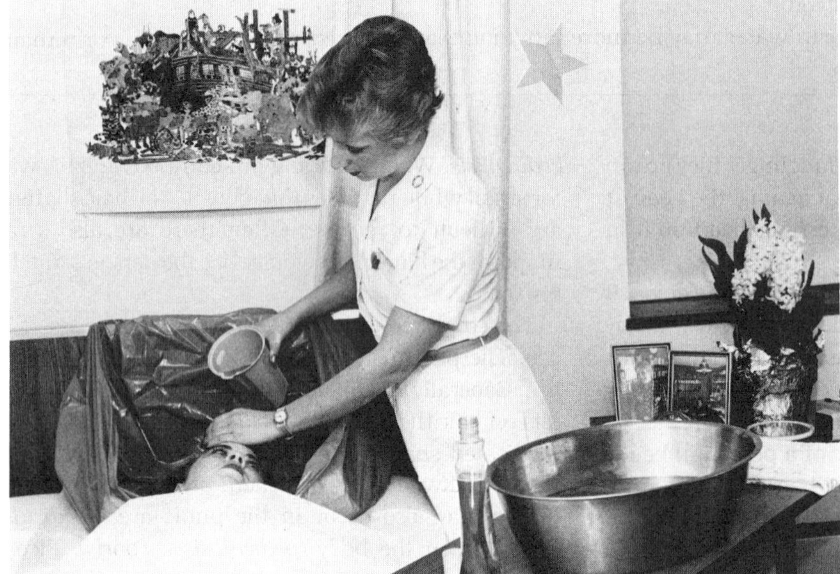

A

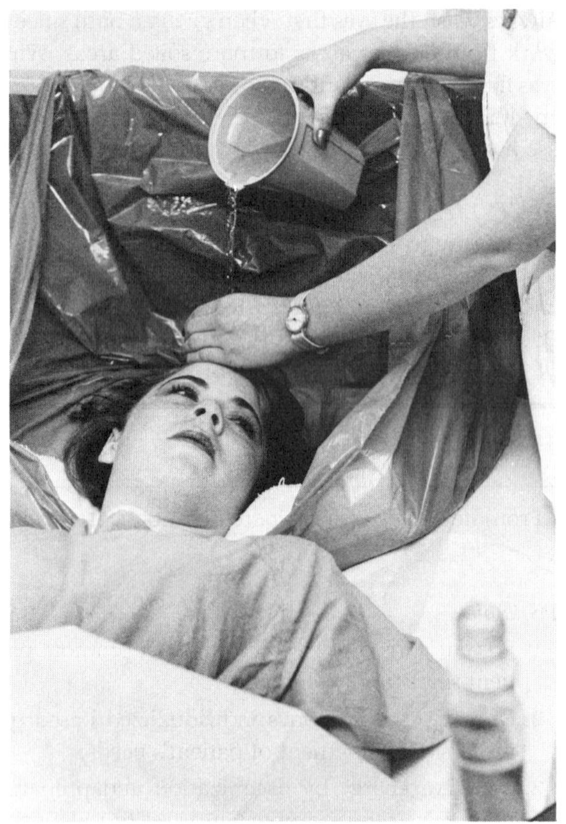

B

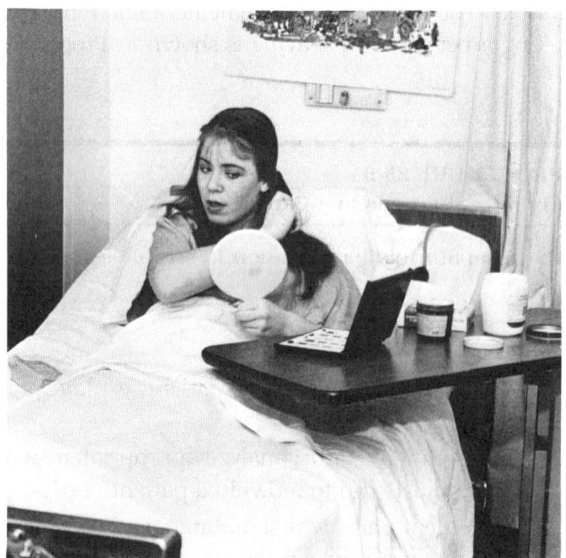

C

FIGURE 1. A. Giving a shampoo in bed. B. Notice the shampoo trough made of plastic. C. Personal care measures enhance self-esteem.

5. Assess condition of hair and scalp. Is hair well-nourished? Thinning? Brittle?	5. Incorporating assessment into care is a mark of a professional nurse.
6. Wet hair by pouring water from pitcher (Fig. 1B) or faucets at sink. Apply small amount of shampoo to hair. Rub in well; massage scalp. Do not allow shampoo to enter patient's eyes.	6. Massage to scalp increases circulation. One frequent reason for shampooing hair is to remove paste following electroencephalogram (EEG) tests. Newer pastes are removed with regular shampoo; older type pastes require acetone. If the shampoo has been ordered to remove pediculosis (lice), you must use a medicated shampoo. Follow directions on bottle carefully for amount to use and frequency of use.
7. Pour water from pitcher or faucet to rinse hair. Repeat shampoo application and rinse again if hair is exceptionally oily.	7. Soap remaining in hair attracts dirt easily.
8. Rub hair dry. Wrap hair in towel while you remove equipment if shampoo trough is used.	8. Prevent chilling.
9. Comb or brush hair into appropriate style (Fig. 1C). Patient may like to have hair blown dry. Never use a *hot* setting for such equipment. Use electrical equipment only *after* you have removed the shampoo trough or are away from a sink. Open curtain or room door.	9. Patients who are receiving medication for pain have decreased heat sensation and can be burned easily. *Electrical equipment always presents a hazzard near water.* Patient safety is assured by easy access.
10. Evaluate effectiveness, efficiency, cost, comfort, and safety aspects of procedure; record procedure and assessments. Return equipment to proper storage.	10. Document nursing care and patient status.
11. Plan health teaching as necessary, such as importance of hygiene for self-esteem.	11. Health teaching is an independent nursing action always included in care.

MODIFICATIONS FOR CARE OF CHILD

1. Newborns and infants always have a shampoo included with their bath. Frequent hair washing at this age prevents seborrhea, a gray, scaly scalp condition of infants.
2. Pediculosis (lice) infections occur frequently in the school population because schoolchildren exchange towels and combs freely. Always assess hair of schoolchildren carefully for nits (eggs of lice).
3. A well adolescent, as a rule, shampoos his hair almost daily. Offering to help an adolescent shampoo his hair may be the action that makes him feel better than any other.

MODIFICATIONS FOR CARE OF OLDER ADULT

1. Many older adults feel chilly quickly because they have less subcutaneous fat than younger persons. Towel dry hair well to prevent chilling following a shampoo.
2. An older adult may have decreased sensation to heat. Use any appliance such as a hair dryer *very cautiously* and only on a low setting.

PROCEDURE 25-10
Assisting a Person with Shaving

Purpose: Promote self-esteem by improving physical appearance. Promote self-care and sense of control.

Plan	*Principle*
1. Wash your hands; identify patient; explain the procedure.	1. Prevent spread of microorganisms. Promote patient safety and well-being.
2. Assess patient status; analyze appropriateness of plan; adjust plan to individual patient need.	2. Nursing care is always individualized based on professional judgment of patient's needs.

3. Implement plan by assembling equipment: mirror, good light source, electric razor or safety razor, emesis basin of warm water, soap or commercial shaving cream, towel, aftershave lotion if desired.

3. Conserve energy by organization and preparation.

4. Bring bed to high position; raise head of bed to semi-Fowler's position if patient condition permits; cover chest and neck with towel.

4. Prevent stretching and bending. Protect bed linen from falling hair.

5. Provide privacy; if patient is going to shave himself, arrange equipment within easy reach (Fig. 1). (Perform procedure if unable to do this by himself.) To shave facial hair, stretch facial skin taut and use short firm strokes with a safety razor; shave in the direction that the hair grows. Rinse razor head in warm water following each stroke. Use gentle but firm motions to clear whiskers with electric razor.

5. Privacy is a highly regarded right by most people. Be certain to use electric razor before you set basin of bath water on bedside stand so there is no danger that the razor will fall into the water and an electrical shock will occur.

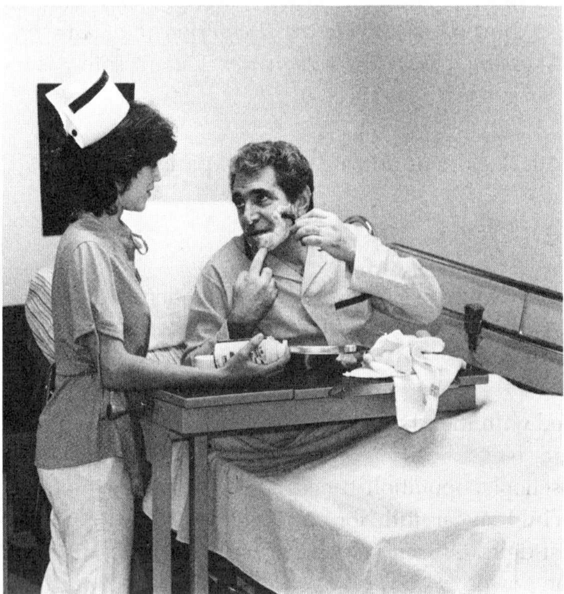

FIGURE 1. This man shaves himself. The nurse assists with supplies.

6. Assess condition of skin. Apply shaving lotion if desired to clean face. Remove towel carefully so you remove hairs with it and they do not fall onto bed.

6. Incorporating assessment in procedures is a mark of a professional nurse.

7. Evaluate effectiveness, efficiency, cost, comfort, and safety aspects of procedure; chart procedure and assessments made.

7. Documentation of nursing action and patient status.

8. Plan health teaching indicated from assessment data, such as importance of a good physical appearance to a sense of well-being.

8. Health teaching is an independent nursing action always included in care.

MODIFICATIONS FOR CARE OF CHILD

Most boys need to shave at least occasionally by the time they are 15. Respect shaving as a rite of passage into adulthood; it may be more important for a boy this age to shave to feel adult than to remove almost invisible facial hair.

MODIFICATIONS FOR CARE OF OLDER ADULT

Shaving is a life-long habit; most older age men enjoy using the razor they have used at home. If you substitute soap lather for shaving cream, moisten facial skin with lotion afterward as soap is drying to older skin.

frames. If the patient will not be wearing his glasses, store them in a case labeled with the person's name to prevent their being broken or misplaced.

Care of Contact Lenses. Contact lenses are small plastic disks that fit directly on the cornea of the eye. To remove a hard lens from a person's eye, separate the upper and lower eyelid of the eye. Exert pressure on the lower eyelid margin and move the eyelid slowly toward the bottom edge of the lens. This will tip the contact lens and it will lift out on the bottom edge (Fig. 25-8).

To remove a soft lens, ask the patient to look upward. Pull down the lower lid and place the tip of your index finger on the lower edge of the lens. Slide the lens down to the inferior aspect of the eye. Compress the lens slightly between your index finger and thumb. This will cause it to bend; air will enter beneath it and then it will slide off easily.

Hard and soft contact lenses should be stored in normal saline or in a commercial solution in marked containers when not in place. Be certain that containers are marked right and left eye lenses. Do not leave lenses in water glasses on bedside stands. Patients have been known to swallow their lenses with the water.

Hard contact lenses cannot be left in place for over 8 to 12 hours, or they will occlude oxygen so completely that the cornea is damaged. Do not allow people to sleep with them in place. Never allow a patient to go to surgery with contact lenses in place; while under anesthesia, he cannot feel pain and could suffer eye damage without anyone being aware of it. Contact lenses should be removed from the eyes of unconscious people for the same reason.

Ear Care

Never insert any object smaller than the corner of a washcloth into an ear canal. Attempting to clean ear canals with small objects may scratch the delicate membrane of the canal or rupture the eardrum. Many people worry that unless they clean their ear canals, ear wax *(cerumen)* will collect. Cerumen always moves slowly outward, bringing dirt and debris with it. Removing it unnecessarily prevents this protective function. If cerumen causes hearing loss, it may be removed by a physician.

Care of Hearing Devices. Persons who have hearing impairment have devices fitted that rest in the ear or just behind it. The battery that operates the unit may be located in eyeglasses, behind the ear, in a shirt pocket, or on a cord around the neck.

Do not allow a hearing aid to get wet while you bathe a patient; remove it before you wash hair. When the device is removed, turn off the power. If the person will not be wearing it for a period of time, store it carefully to prevent damage. Hearing aids are not only expensive but they are important means of communication for people who are hard of hearing.

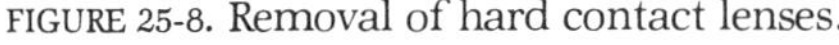

FIGURE 25-8. Removal of hard contact lenses.

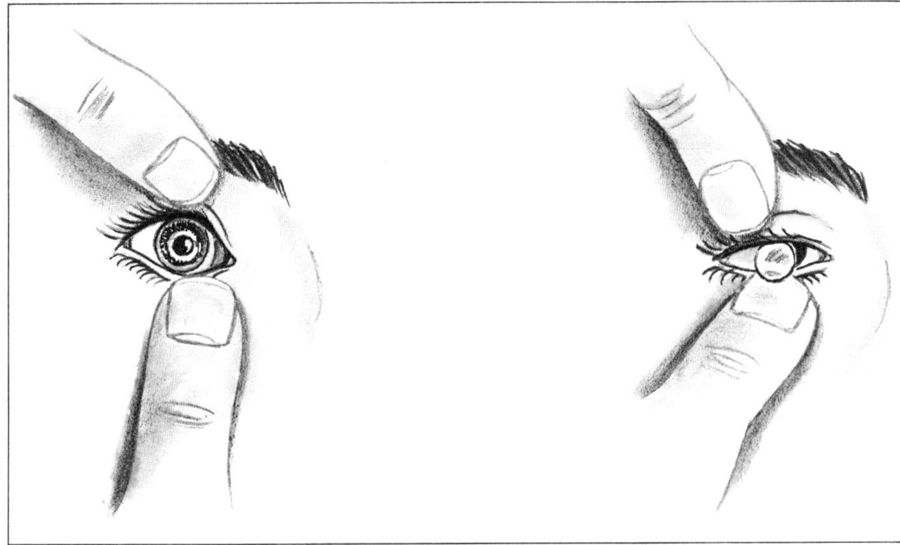

Oral Care

Many times illness interferes with normal nutrition when a patient is not allowed to eat anything or is limited to clear liquids. When people are taking nothing by mouth, the mouth begins to feel dry, rough, and uncomfortable. A person can develop *halitosis* (bad breath) easily or *sordes* (crusts on teeth and gums). Poor oral care over a period of time will lead to periodontal disease and dental decay. Steps in oral care for people able to assist are given in Procedure 25-11. Care of the mouth for an unconscious person and for one with dentures is given in Procedures 25-12 and 25-13. Preventive oral care is discussed in Quick Reference Stop 25-5.

Helping a patient to clean his mouth is a procedure that he generally appreciates. A clean mouth gives a person a feeling of being on the road to good health. Brushing teeth removes not only food particles but also *plaque*, a bacteria-laden film.

PROCEDURE 25-11
Oral Care for a Person Able to Assist

Purpose: Clean teeth and other mouth surfaces. Prevent dental caries and gingivitis. Encourage self-esteem through self-care and improved physical appearance. Prevent dry and cracked lips to reduce possible portals of infection.

Plan	*Principle*
1. Wash your hands; identify patient; explain procedure to patient.	1. Prevent spread of microorganisms; promote patient safety and well-being.
2. Assess patient status; analyze appropriateness of plan; adjust plan to individual patient's needs.	2. Nursing care is always individualized based on professional judgment of patient's needs.
3. Implement care by assembling equipment: toothbrush, toothpaste, glass of water, emesis basin, towel, and mouthwash if desired. Provide privacy with drawn curtain or closed door.	3. Conserve energy by organization and preparation. If no toothbrush is available, cover a tongueblade with a 4 × 4-inch gauze and secure gauze with adhesive tape. It is the brushing that cleans teeth, so no toothpaste is really needed. Privacy is a highly regarded right by most people.
4. Position patient on back with head of bed elevated about 45 degrees. If unable to have head of bed raised, turn patient to side.	4. The greatest danger of oral care is that patient will aspirate (choke) during procedure. Head elevation or side-lying prevents this.
5. Cover front of chest and neck with towel.	5. Protect bed linen.
6. Wet toothbrush with water, place toothpaste on toothbrush. Hand toothbrush to patient or clean all surfaces of teeth (outside, inside, top and bottom) for him. Use firm but gentle motion.	6. Teeth are cleaned by friction.
7. Assess status of mouth—i.e., reddened, bleeding gums, dental caries.	7. Incorporating assessment into care is a mark of a professional nurse.
8. Offer a glass of water to rinse mouth. Hold the emesis basin under the patient's chin so he can spit water into it conveniently.	
9. Many adults floss their teeth after brushing. Flossing technique is shown in Fig. 1.	9. Flossing ensures that all particles of food are removed from between teeth.

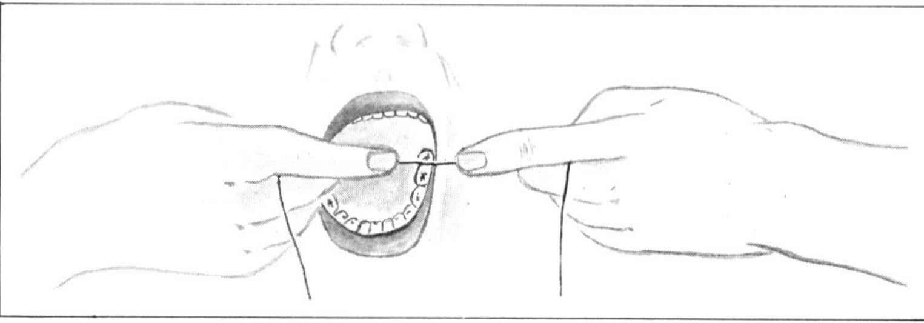

FIGURE 1. Technique of flossing teeth. Floss is pressed between teeth and then rubbed against them to remove plaque.

10. If patient wishes, offer a cup of mouthwash.	10. Mouthwash creates a clean, refreshing taste.
11. Help patient to wipe away any toothpaste or water on face. Clean and return equipment to bedside stand.	11. Provide psychological as well as physical well-being.
12. If lips are dry, apply petroleum jelly (Vaseline) or other salve suggested by the individual health care agency. Open curtain or room door.	12. Dry and cracked lips provide a portal of entry for infection. Patient safety is assured by easy access.
13. Evaluate effectiveness, efficiency, cost, comfort, and safety aspects of procedure; record procedure and assessment.	13. Document nursing care and patient status.
14. Plan necessary health teaching, such as need for toothbrushing.	14. Health teaching is an independent nursing action always included in care.

MODIFICATIONS FOR CARE OF CHILD

1. If a child is wearing braces, pay particular attention to removing food particles stuck to wires.
2. Children under 3 or 4 years of age do not know what the word *rinse* means. They swallow the water. Therefore, *do not offer water or mouthwash to young children who are limited to nothing by mouth.* Wet the toothbrush and brush teeth again to serve as a rinse.
3. Children who wear braces should floss their teeth after brushing to remove food particles from between wires.

MODIFICATIONS FOR CARE OF OLDER ADULT

Many older adults wear full or partial dentures. If they have partial dentures be certain these are removed and remaining teeth are brushed well. Otherwise these will become carious, the partial denture will no longer fit, and another will have to be purchased.

Oral cancer renders its highest incidence in older adults. Always assess under the tongue of an older adult for a lesion of any type to detect this.

PROCEDURE 25-12
Oral Care for an Unconscious Patient

Purpose: Cleanse mouth and teeth. Prevent aspiration. Prevent dental caries and gum disease.

Plan	*Principle*
1. Wash your hands; identify patient.	1. Prevent spread of microorganisms; promote patient safety and well-being. Hearing is the last sense lost and first sense regained with unconsciousness. A patient may therefore be able to hear you although he does not respond to you.
2. Assess patient status; analyze appropriateness of plan; adjust plan to individual patient needs.	2. Nursing care is always individualized based on professional judgment of patients' needs.
3. Implement care by assembling equipment: a toothbrush or wrapped tongueblade (tongueblade wrapped with a 4 × 4-inch piece of gauze and secured with adhesive tape); mouthwash or water, emesis basin, towel, possible glycerin and lemon juice swabs or Vaseline for lip care.	3. Conserve energy by organization and preparation.
4. Provide privacy. Bring bed to high position; position the patient flat in bed, turned to his side. Position back of his head on a pillow so face tips downward and fluid will flow out of his mouth, not back to throat. Place the towel under his head to protect sheets from moisture.	4. Avoid stretching and bending. If swallowing or gag reflexes are not intact, you must allow liquid to flow from back of mouth. Patient would aspirate.

5. Apply a small amount of toothpaste to toothbrush or wrapped tongueblade or merely moisten toothbrush or tongueblade with mouthwash or water; wash surfaces of teeth, roof of mouth, and tongue (Fig. 1). *Never put your fingers in the mouth of an unconscious patient.*

5. An unconscious patient might have a muscle spasm that would cause him to bite your finger. Human bites are as dangerous as animal bites. The friction of brushing, not toothpaste, cleans teeth so no toothpaste is needed.

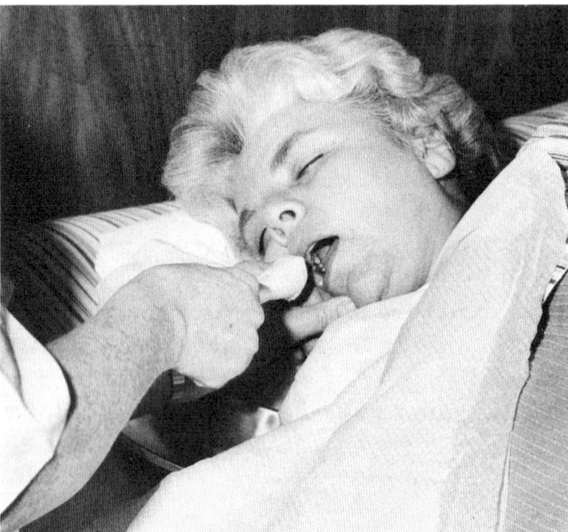

FIGURE 1. Oral care for an unconscious patient. Notice the padded tongue blade used in place of a toothbrush.

6. Assess condition of mouth, teeth, and gingiva.

6. Incorporating assessment into procedures is a mark of a professional nurse.

7. Rinse mouth with clear water using moistened tongueblade or toothbrush. If suction equipment is available, use suction to remove any excess fluid from mouth.

7. Using no more water than clings to toothbrush reduces the possibility of aspiration.

8. Apply petroleum jelly (Vaseline) to lips if they are cracking or dry.

8. Do not use mineral oil. This might drain backward and flow into lungs causing pneumonia. Glycerin and lemon solution may be used but promote dryness in some persons.

9. Clean equipment and return to its proper place. Position patient comfortably on side. Open curtain or room door.

9. Unconscious persons must lie on their side, not their back, to prevent aspiration of saliva. Patient safety is assured by easy access.

10. Evaluate effectiveness, efficiency, cost, comfort and safety aspects of procedure; record procedure and assessment of mouth.

10. Document nursing care, patient status. Incorporating assessment into procedures is a mark of a professional nurse.

PROCEDURE 25-13
Denture Care

Purpose: Cleanse dentures safely to promote oral care and self-esteem. Promote oral health by reducing friction from unclean dentures.

Plan

1. Wash your hands; identify patient; explain procedure to patient.
2. Assess patient status; analyze appropriateness of plan; adjust plan to individual patient need.

Principle

1. Prevent spread of microorganisms; promote patient safety and well-being.
2. Nursing care is always individualized based on professional judgment of patient's needs.

3. Implement care by assembling equipment: container to hold dentures (emesis basin or denture cup), denture cleanser or toothpaste and toothbrush, small gauze square and washcloth. Provide privacy.

   3. Conserve energy by organization and preparation. Privacy is a highly regarded right of most people.

4. Ask patient to remove dentures and place them in the container for you. If he is unable to do this, place gauze square on the front of the denture and remove it by grasping the front teeth between your thumb and finger; pull down gently but firmly to loosen the suction that holds the upper denture in place. Loosen lower dentures by lifting up and out.

   4. Dentures are valuable in cost and convenience. Most people prefer to clean them themselves if they are able. Using a gauze square prevents your fingers from slipping on the wet surface.

5. Soaking dentures in a denture cleanser allows food particles to soak away readily. If a denture cleanser is not available, use warm water and cleanse dentures with a clean piece of gauze or toothbrush and toothpaste. Place washcloth in sink when cleaning dentures so if you accidentally drop them, they will not break.

   5. Never use hot water since excessive heat might melt the denture material.

6. Assess condition of mouth while dentures are removed. Improperly fitting dentures can cause ulcers; chronic irritation can cause mouth cancer.

   6. Incorporating assessment into procedures is a mark of a professional nurse.

7. Rinse the dentures and help the patient rinse his mouth with clear water or mouthwash before he returns the dentures to his mouth. If a person is unable to do this, wrap a gauze square around a tongueblade; moisten it and clean gingiva and roof of mouth.

   7. Provide a clean refreshing feeling.

8. Return equipment to its proper place.

9. If dentures are not to be returned to the person's mouth, they must be stored in a suitable protective container. Dentures are an expensive investment. Do not handle them irresponsibly.

   9. When not in the mouth, dentures are generally kept in a water solution in a covered container. Label the box with the person's name; mark *Important: do not discard* to ensure their safety.

10. Evaluate effectiveness, efficiency, cost, comfort, and safety aspects of procedure; record procedure and oral assessments.

    10. Document nursing care and patient status.

11. Plan health teaching as needed, such as improperly fitting dentures cause ulceration.

    11. Health teaching is an independent nursing action always included in care.

MODIFICATIONS FOR CARE OF CHILD

Children rarely have dentures but they do have retainers, which need similar care. Retainers are plastic molds that continue to hold teeth in good alignment after braces have been removed.

A retainer should be removed daily and cleaned. Use warm not hot water. Do not use commercial denture cleaners on retainers; toothpaste or simply water is adequate and safe.

The chief danger in oral care is that the patient will choke and aspirate the solution used to rinse toothpaste from his mouth. Carefully evaluate whether the person is able to swallow normally before beginning oral care.

Care of Extremities

As people move about in bed, they press their heels and elbows against the bottom sheet to lift and turn their bodies. After only a few hours, elbows and heels can start to feel rough and irritated from this friction. Rubbing lotion into these areas after bathing helps to reduce the irritation present. As you bathe a person, assess the range of motion in his extremities. Including range-of-motion exercises (see Chap. 26) as part of a daily bath not only aids in assessment but increases circulation by planned body movement.

☐ QUICK REFERENCE STOP 25-5: HEALTH TEACHING
Preventive Oral Care

Toothbrushing in children should be started as soon as teeth first erupt (about 6 months). Toothpaste used with children should contain fluoride and carry the seal of the American Dental Association Council on Dental Therapeutics as proven effective in preventing tooth decay. Toothbrushing should be done well at least twice a day. Topical application of fluoride at yearly visits help to ensure good enamel formation. The 20 deciduous teeth are shown in Fig. 25-9.

Diet should be nutritious and high in calcium and phosphorus. It is the action between bacteria and sugar that dissolves tooth enamel. If children are going to eat candy between meals, the candy should be easily dissolved rather than sticky. Eating coarse food such as apples or carrots help to clean teeth; these are good foods to place in a child's lunchbox when it is known that the child will not be brushing after eating.

Adults need to continue good toothbrushing habits to keep their teeth free of decay. Brushing well once a day is more effective than brushing carelessly many times daily. Stimulating gums by massage at the time of brushing helps to improve mouth circulation and prevent periodontal disease. Fig. 25-10 shows the 32 permanent teeth.

Fig. 25-11 illustrates the difference between teeth surrounded by healthy gums and teeth after periodontal disease has developed. Periodontal disease will lead eventually to loss of teeth and difficulty thereafter with nutrition.

When bathing the legs, dorsiflex the foot by bending the top toward the anterior surface and ask the person if he experiences pain at the motion. If the person has pain at this motion, it generally denotes a blood clot *(thrombus)* in a vein. *Never massage the calf area of the leg for anyone who has pain on dorsiflexion.* This could loosen a blood clot and cause it to travel. If it lodged in the heart, lung, or brain, it could be fatal. Pain found in this way in the calf of the leg on dorsiflexion is called *Homans' sign.* It is always a sign of potential danger; report it to the person's physician so the presence of a thrombus can be fully evaluated.

Foot Care. The skin of the feet tends to become dry when people lie in bed for a long time. You may notice *calluses,* hard, superficially dense areas of keratinized tissue caused by a shoe having rubbed. They are not painful although applying lotion is soothing. A *corn* is a keratinized area so deep it is painful. Applying lotion helps to soften these also, but they may be too tender to touch. Submerging a person's feet in bathwater helps to guard the integrity of skin on feet and should be included in the bath of a person on bedrest.

Fissures or cracks between toes are usually a sign of a fungal infection termed *athlete's foot.* Drying the area well is important, but medication is needed for healing. *Plantar warts* are circular, slightly indented painful areas on the sole; this mild virus infection disappears spontaneously after a prolonged period. Preventive foot care is shown in Quick Reference Stop 25-6.

Nail Care. To prevent toenails from growing into the soft tissue at the corner of each nail, toenails should be cut straight across, never rounded. To prevent hangnails beside fingernails, the cuticle of the nail should be softened with oil or warm water and pushed back gently at least weekly.

An infected fingernail or toenail is termed a *paronychia.* A paronychial area is red, swollen, and painful to touch. Report it to the person's physician. Special care, such as an antibiotic, may be necessary to aid healing.

Do not cut toenails of people with diabetes or circulatory problems. Poor blood supply to the feet makes infection such a high probability that such care is generally given only by a podiatrist.

Perineal Care

Accumulated vaginal or penile secretions can cause extensive erythema or excoriation of tissue. If a person is going to wash in bed, let him know that you are leaving this responsibility for perineal care to him by a phrase such as, "Why don't you wash your face and front and between your legs and when I come back I'll do your back."

In a complete bath, include washing genitalia. Do not allow modesty to interfere with thorough cleaning and inspection. In uncircumsized males, retract penile foreskin gently and wash the glans penis with soapy water, being sure to rinse and dry gently and replace the foreskin. A penis reacts to handling by engorgement of capillaries and erection. It is not unusual for a male to experience erection during the process of washing, rinsing, and drying. Put this in its proper perspective, a physiological response to handling, and proceed with care. Using a firm rather than a light touch tends to decrease penile stimulation and reduce the possibility of erection.

When washing the external genitalia of women, always wash from anterior to posterior and change the position of the washcloth for a second stroke to reduce the possibility of carrying contaminants from the rectum to the urethra or vagina. Do not allow modesty to limit your inspection.

Wash, rinse and dry vulva, and gently separate labia to clean between the folds. If a woman is menstruating, and wishes to use a tampon, change this at the time of

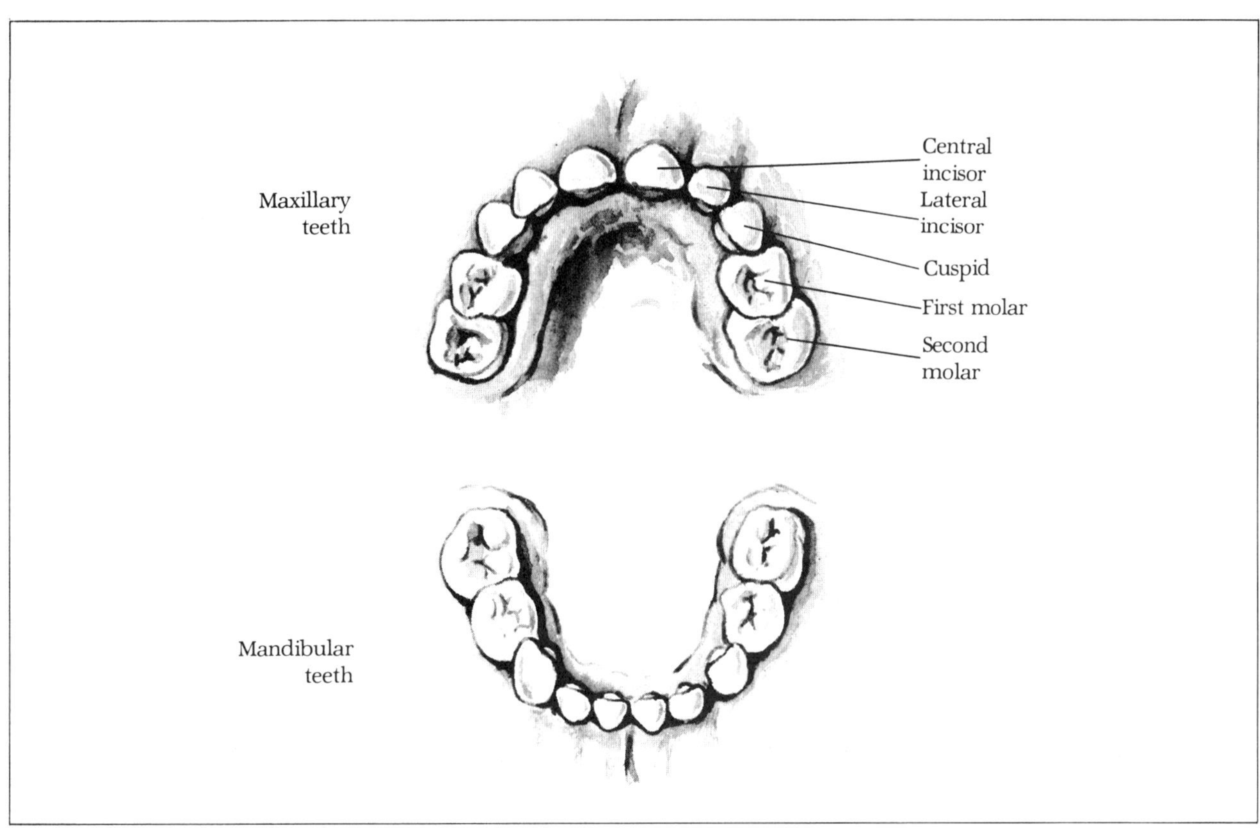

FIGURE 25-9. Deciduous teeth. (Courtesy Department of Medical Illustration, State University of New York at Buffalo, Buffalo, New York.)

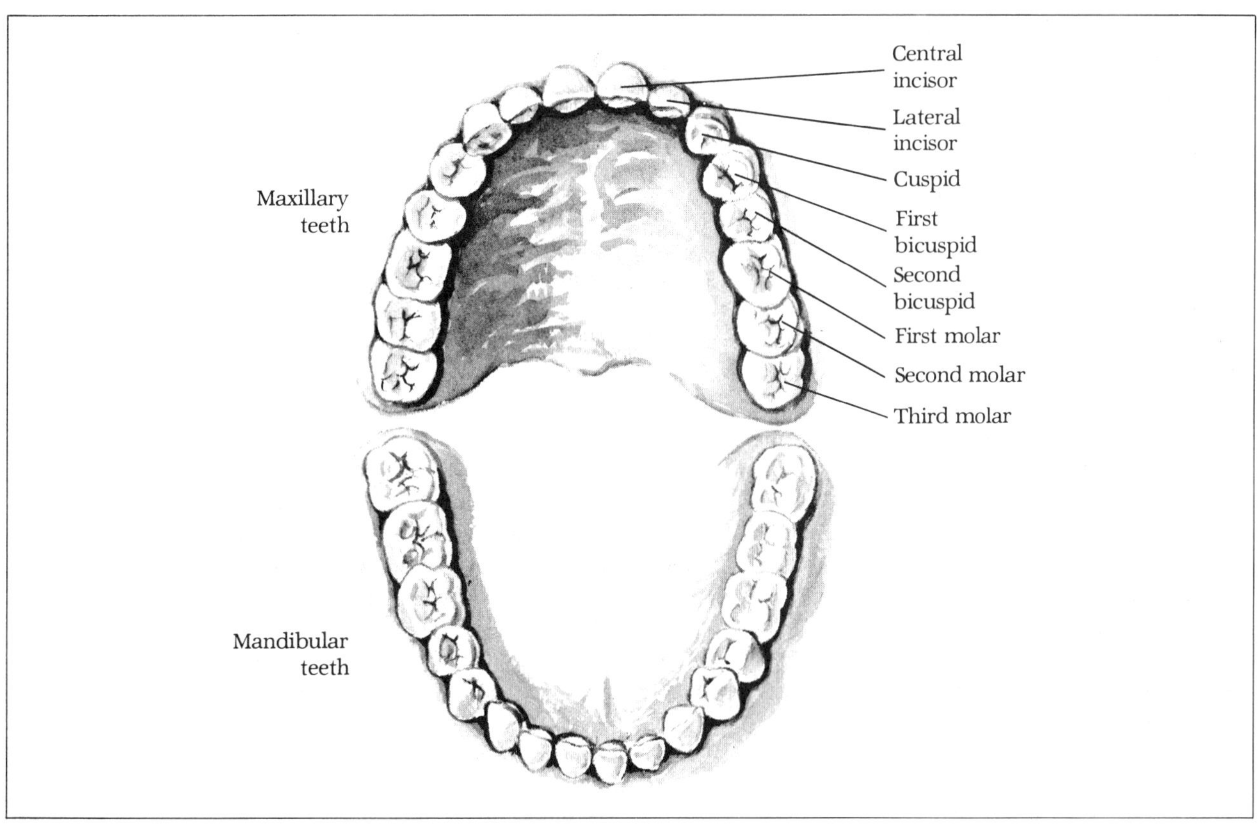

FIGURE 25-10. Permanent teeth. (Courtesy Department of Medical Illustration, State University of New York at Buffalo, Buffalo, New York.)

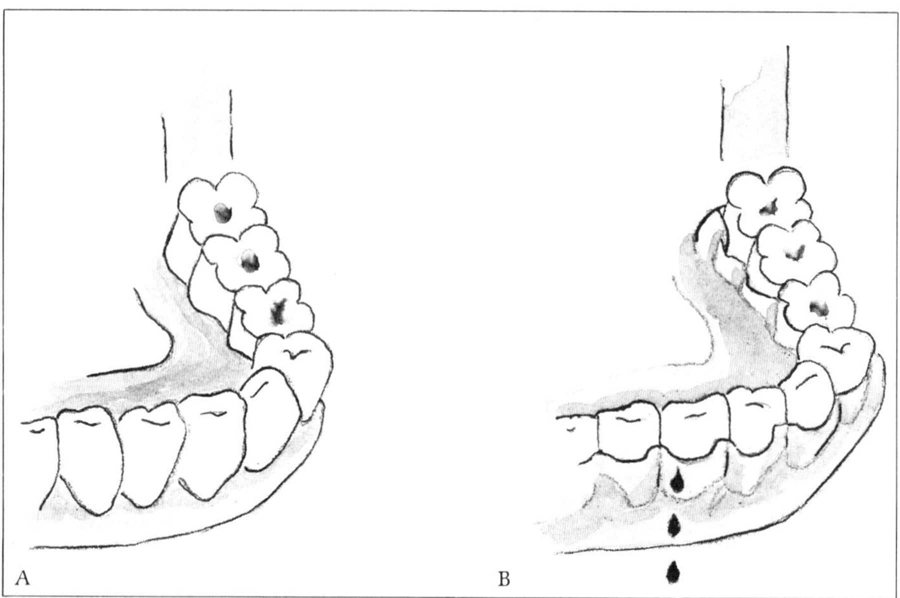

FIGURE 25-11. Comparison between healthy (A) and unhealthy (B) gum tissue.

> □ **QUICK REFERENCE STOP 25-6: HEALTH TEACHING**
> **Preventive Foot Care**
>
> Most foot problems are caused by ill-fitting shoes. Children, in particular, must have shoes fitted so that a thumb's width can be placed between the large toe and the tip of the shoe to provide for growth room. To prevent fungal infection, caution people to avoid walking barefoot in public showers. Always dry feet well after soaking them, particularly between toes. Many older people wear warm socks to keep their feet warm and improve circulation.

the bath. Lay a paper towel on the bed surface and gently remove the used tampon to be disposed of in the paper towel. After perineal cleaning, insert a clean tampon, being careful to touch only the tampon inserter, not the tampon itself. Women should not leave vaginal tampons in place over 4 hours even if bleeding is slight because of the damage of bacterial invasion (toxic shock syndrome). If the woman is going to use a perineal pad for menstruation, change this also at the time of the bath without touching the surface of the pad that will contact the perineum. Menstruation care is considered by many women a private responsibility. Approach the situation with a common-sense attitude: menstruation is a sign of female health, and helping to change pads or tampons part of holistic care.

UTILIZING NURSING PROCESS

The time spent with a patient during personal care may be the longest single interaction with a patient during any day. Therefore, such care must be done with planning and concern.

ASSESSMENT

Whether a patient will need to be given a bed bath or assisted with taking one, or whether he can take a tub bath or shower depends on his medical condition. Assess such items as: Is he allowed to do this as part of his own care or is rest more important for him? Does he have full function of his hands? Is he old enough to wash himself adequately without help? How long has it been since his hair has been shampooed?

ANALYSIS AND PLANNING

Once you know your patient's physical limitations, analyze the best type of hygiene measures for him. If a patient cannot get out of bed, he cannot take a shower. If he will not become too fatigued and has full use of his hands and arms, an assisted bed bath will probably be best. A patient might be well enough to be out of bed for a short time each morning. What would be the best use of this time? To walk to the shower room for a shower? To take a bath in bed now and walk to the sun room later in the morning when his wife is visiting to demonstrate how well he is doing? If a mother of a toddler visits in the afternoon, do you want to delay the child's bath until then so she can give it? Or will you give the bath now and allow his mother free time to read to the child? Does a patient want his bath before or after breakfast? Safety measures to consider in planning hygiene are shown in Quick Reference Stop 25-7.

IMPLEMENTATION

Helping people with personal care is rewarding because people feel appreciably better after a bed bath, a

☐ **QUICK REFERENCE STOP 25-7: SAFETY**

Remember when helping people to take tub baths or showers that there is a great danger of them slipping or falling. Urge them to use safety rails and bathmats. Never leave a child under 8 or an adult not fully alert alone in a bathtub. When assisting a bed patient, be certain that supplies are arranged conveniently so that he does not have to stretch to reach items.

Do not use water and electrical appliances at the same time. This could lead to electrical shock.

Assess a person's capabilities before beginning personal care. Asking more of a person than he is capable of is unsafe physically; asking less than he is capable of is detrimental to self-esteem.

backrub, and having bed linen changed. Performing such care is the essence of nursing. Drugs commonly used in implementation of personal care are shown in Quick Reference Stop 25-8.

EVALUATION

When a person is recovering from an illness, his state of health changes almost daily. Daily evaluation is necessary so that plans continue to be appropriate (see QRS 25-9).

NURSING CARE PLAN

Mr. Smith is a 60-year-old man who has suffered a stroke. He is unable to be out of bed and has almost no use of his right arm and leg; he has lost some use of the

☐ **QUICK REFERENCE STOP 25-8: PHARMACOLOGY**
Drugs Commonly Used in Personal Care

Classification	*Example*	*Action*	*Nursing Considerations*
Antiperspirants	Many well-advertised brands	Reduces amount of perspiration by constricting pores to eccrine glands.	Stings when applied to irritated or freshly shaved skin.
Antiseptic	Alcohol	Cleans skin by solvent action on sebaceous secretions; drys and toughens skin.	Quick evaporation following use leads to vasoconstriction and chilling. Do not use with elderly persons as it tends to dry skin. Do not use with children as fumes can cause liver intoxication.
Antiseptic	Povidone-iodine; Betadine	Mild bacteriostatic agent.	Iodine stains bed linen or patient clothing brown.
Astringent	Many well-advertised brands	Alcohol content causes reduction of pore size.	Offers a fresh, cool feeling.
Bath oil	Nivia	Lubricates skin; prevents excessive drying.	If added to bath water, makes tub surface very slippery and a fall may result.
Bubble bath	Many well-advertised brands	Softens water; provides pleasant aroma to bath.	Use of bubble bath may be associated with urinary tract infection in young children. Do not use routinely.
Dental floss	Many well-advertised brands	Removes plaque from teeth through scrubbing action.	
Denture cleanser	Many well-advertised brands	Cleans dentures by effervescent action.	*Tablets are poisonous. Do not leave on bedside stand after use.*

Depilatory	Many well-advertised brands	Removes unwanted hair.	Read directions carefully. Many brands are not safe for use on facial hair.
Deodorant	Many well-advertised brands	Masks or diminishes body odor from apocrine sweat.	Stings when applied to irritated or freshly shaved skin.
Fibrinolytic debriding agent	Collagenase (Santyl); fibrinolysin (Elase)	Digests necrotic tissue and collagen in wounds, leaving a clean, granulation surface.	Applied topically to decubitus ulcers; use with hexachlorophene, detergents, or acetone solutions decreases action.
Hydrophilic wound cleanser	Dextranomer (Debriasan)	Absorbs toxins from wound that impede tissue repair. Promotes granulation tissue formation.	Supplied as beads. Pour onto secreting wound. Remove by irrigating with saline.
Mouthwash	Many well-advertised brands	Provides a clean oral feeling.	Mouthwash cannot replace good toothbrushing as routine oral care; does not clean plaque from teeth.
Oxidizing agent	Hydrogen peroxide	Oxidization produces a bacteriocidal action.	Usually used half strength (equal parts of hydrogen peroxide and water).
Toothpaste	Many common brands	Acts to remove food particles and plaque from teeth because of abrasive action.	Children should use a fluoride toothpaste to help strengthen tooth enamel.

☐ **QUICK REFERENCE STOP 25-9: COMMUNITY CONSIDERATIONS**

Assess people's living conditions on hospital discharge to see if they will be able to maintain hygiene practices at home. A person who lives in a home where there is no hot water or where the bathroom is upstairs may not be able to take a bath or may become exhausted doing so. People living in rooming houses may have no access to a bathtub.

People who have difficulty leaving home to shop may neglect toothbrushing if they are out of toothpaste. They can subsitute baking soda unlcss they are on a salt-restricted diet. Stress that it is the friction of brushing, not the toothpaste, that makes the difference so they can even brush with water in order to maintain oral care while at home.

muscles of his face. A nursing care plan for him related to hygiene might be as follows:

Problem: Self-care deficit, Hygiene.
Subjective: Patient states, "I can't do anything for myself; I'm a helpless old man. I can't even shave myself."
Objective: Skin on elbows and heels dry and scaling. An erythematic area 2 × 3 in. at base of spine. No break in skin integrity. Has partial dentures; some difficulty rinsing following oral care due to lack of facial muscle coordination.
Assessment: Older adult capable of partial self-care related to medical condition.
Locus of Decision-Making: Shared.
Goal: Patient will complete partial self bath in 1 week's time. (M.D. approval obtained as consistent with medical condition.)
Criteria: Patient to wash own face, chest, right arm, and complete oral care, shaving, and perineal care by self.

NURSING ORDERS

1. Position all equipment on left side of patient.
2. Use electric razor before bath (daughter to bring in). Use before water is provided.
3. Give verbal approval for any self-care activities patient completes to increase self-esteem.
4. Following self-care, complete bath including special attention to back.

5. Massage sacral area to encourage circulation.
6. Apply lotion to elbows and heels for dry skin.
7. Include Homans' sign and passive sign of motion exercises as part of bath daily.

SUGGESTED READINGS

Ahmed, M. C. Op-site for decubitus care. *Am. J. Nurs.* 82:61, 1982.

Barsevick, A., et al. A comparison of the anxiety-reducing potential of two techniques of bathing. *Nurs. Res.* 31:22, 1982.

Berglas, C., et al. Decubitus ulcers. *J. Nurs. Care* 13(4):16, 1980.

Bersani, G., et al. Oral care for cancer patients. *Am. J. Nurs.* 83(4):533, 1983.

Boyd-Monk, H. Taking a closer look at contact lenses. *Nursing 78* 8:38, 1978.

Cameron, G. Pressure sores: What to do when prevention fails. *Nursing 79* 9:42, 1979.

Davis, M. Getting to the root of the problem: Hair-grooming techniques for black patients. *Nursing 77* 7:60, 1977.

DiMascio, S. Debrisan for decubitus ulcers. *Am. J. Nurs.* 79:684, 1979.

Dobson, A. Showers for the elderly. *Nurs. Times* 75(20):841, 1979.

Dodd, M. Self-care for side effects in cancer chemotherapy: An assessment of nursing interventions—Part 2. *Cancer Nurs.* 6(1):63, 1983.

Dyer, E., et al. Dental health in adults. *Am. J. Nurs.* 76:1156, 1976.

Freeman, P., et al. How to get the most out of op-site . . . and avoid those "not so sticky" problems. *RN* 45:36, 1982.

Gruis, M. L., and Innes, B. Assessment: Essential to prevent pressure sores. *Am. J. Nurs.* 76:1762, 1976.

Hilton, D. Oral hygiene and infection. *Nurs. Times* 76(29):1270, 1980.

Jones, E. Prevention of pressure sores: The clinical score chart. *Nurs. Times* 76(13):565, 1980.

Kavchak-Keyes, M. A. Four proven steps for preventing decubitus ulcers. *Nursing 77* 7:58, 1977.

Krieger, D., et al. Therapeutic touch. *Am. J. Nurs.* 79:660, 1979.

Maurer, J. Providing optimal oral health. *Nurs. Clin. North Am.* 12:4, 1977.

Michelsen, D. How to give a good backrub. *Am. J. Nurs.* 78:1197, 1978.

Programmed instruction: Skin rashes in infants and children. *Am. J. Nurs.* 78:1041, 1978.

Schweiger, J., et al. Oral assessment: How to do it. *Am. J. Nurs.* 80:654, 1980.

Sykes, J. Black skin problems. *Am. J. Nurs.* 79:1092, 1979.

Speedie, G. Nursology of mouth care: Preventing, comforting and seeking activities related to mouth care. *J. Adv. Nurs.* 8(1):33, 1983.

Uhler, E. Common skin changes in the elderly. *Am. J. Nurs.* 78:1342, 1978.

QUESTIONS FOR REVIEW

1. You worry that Mrs. Jones may develop a decubitis ulcer. The area of the body most likely to develop decubiti that you particularly assess is:
   a. Calves of the legs.
   b. Thighs.
   c. Bony prominences.
   d. Perineum.

2. The most important reason for the development of a decubitis ulcer is:
   a. Wrinkled sheets.
   b. Sustained pressure on a part.
   c. Constantly wet skin.
   d. An infected scratch.

3. The most important measure you would plan to keep Mrs. Jones free of decubitis ulcer would be:
   a. Turn her every 2 hours.
   b. Apply lotion to her back.
   c. Change her bed frequently.
   d. Handle her extremities gently.

4. To assess if a blood clot is forming in Mrs. Jones' legs as part of morning care, which sign would you elicit?
   a. Homans' sign.
   b. Arterial sign.
   c. Kernig's sign.
   d. Horner's sign.

5. In giving denture care, which of the following is the best procedure?
   a. Use hot water for thorough cleaning.
   b. Put a washcloth in the sink while you work.
   c. Leave dentures out of the mouth for an hour after cleaning.
   d. Never use a commercial denture cleaner.

6. When giving Mrs. Smith a bath, a principle for washing her eyes would be:
   a. Use a mild soap.
   b. Wash from the outer to inner canthus.
   c. Begin by washing the eyes.
   d. Wash the eyes with diluted alcohol.

7. To complete a backrub, the motion of your strokes should be:
   a. Horizontal to the back.
   b. Moving upward along the spinal cord; downward at the periphery.
   c. Short and fast.
   d. Moving downward along the spinal column; upward at the periphery.

8. Bobby is 1 month old. In planning care for him, you would shampoo his hair how frequently?
   a. Once a week.
   b. Only if obviously oily.
   c. Daily.
   d. Every third day.

9. The scalp condition that infants tend to develop is termed:
   a. Scabies.
   b. Seborrhea.
   c. Acne.
   d. Pediculosis.

10. You might choose not to use soap to give Bobby a bath. This is because soap:
    a. Tends to be drying.
    b. Causes diaper irritation.
    c. Tends to cause an oil build-up on the skin.
    d. Is expensive for daily care.

11. Mr. Smith, an older adult you care for tells you he wants to bathe before bedtime rather than in the morning. Your best response to this would be to:
    a. Teach him that morning bathing is more therapeutic to skin.
    b. Stress the importance of not disrupting hospital routine.
    c. Educate him regarding sleep-wake cycles and bathing.
    d. Assess who will be able to assist him in the evening.

12. Mr. Smith is going to shave sitting up in bed. Which statement below describes the best approach on your part?
    a. Offer to shave him.
    b. Place his electric razor beside his basin of water.
    c. Cover the bed with a rubber sheet.
    d. Supply a mirror.

13. Mr. Hasen is unconscious. Which statement below describes the best technique for oral care with him?
    a. Position him supine.
    b. Elevate the head of the bed.
    c. Elevate the foot of the bed.
    d. Position him in a side-lying position.

26. BODY ALIGNMENT AND BODY MOVEMENT

OBJECTIVES

Upon mastery of the material in this chapter, you should be able to:

1. Describe growth changes affecting mobility in people of different age groups.
2. Describe the different types of joints of the human body.
3. Describe range-of-motion exercises.
4. Describe the effects of immobilization on body systems.
5. Describe positions of good body alignment.
6. Describe nursing actions to assist people to increase mobility.
7. Apply nursing process to give safe, planned care to a patient whose care involves principles of good body alignment and body movement.

TERMS

The terms important for an understanding of this chapter are shown below and defined in the glossary:

isometric exercises
range-of-motion exercises
Valsalva's maneuver

The human body is composed of 206 bones and over 600 muscles. These muscles with accompanying tendons and supports coordinate in rhythm to produce smooth movement. When something interferes with this coordination, the effort becomes tiring. If interference is so great that immobility occurs, the total system can be affected (Fig. 26-1). Body movement and exercise are so much a part of everyday life that it is difficult to appreciate how beneficial they are to total body function. Helping people to remain active and encouraging people to return to activity following illness are both major nursing responsibilities.

LIFE SPAN CONCEPTS AND BODY MOTION

The level of activity that people are capable of or interested in differs by age group.

The Newborn. A newborn needs careful assessment to be certain that his musculoskeletal and neurological systems are intact. Examine a newborn for good body proportion—head is one-fourth of body length; when the arms are extended, the hands reach to midthigh. Newborns have a full range of motion in joints; assess with passive range-of-motion positions.

When supine, newborns typically demonstrate an asymmetrical or tonic neck reflex position, in which the head is turned to one side; arm and leg on that side both extend; arm and leg on the other side flex. A tonic neck reflex is present for the first 2 or 3 months of life. Do not mistake this normal newborn reflex for true asymmetrical body alignment.

If the newborn's neck was stretched at birth in a difficult delivery, the sternocleidomastoid muscle on the side of the neck may be torn. A hematoma forms at this point and as it is absorbed with fibrotic infiltration, the muscle on that side will contract. The infant tips his head to that side; it is difficult to manipulate his head into straight alignment. This condition *(torticollis)* needs to be identified early in life so muscle stretching exercises can be initiated. With conscientious exercising, the disability will not be permanent.

Another injury that can occur at birth from a stretched neck is tearing or edema of the cervical nerve roots. This will result in loss of function of the arm on the affected side *(Erb's paralysis).* The infant holds his arm close to the body and with the palm turned downward. Erb's paralysis may be a permanent disability if the nerve is actually torn (nerves generally do not regenerate when torn close to the spinal cord); it will be only temporary if the effect is from edema and compression, without actual nerve damage. Careful early diagnosis allows therapy to begin as soon as possible.

The Infant. Infant development proceeds from proximal to distal parts and from head to toe. To assess development, compare the infant's abilities with a chart show-

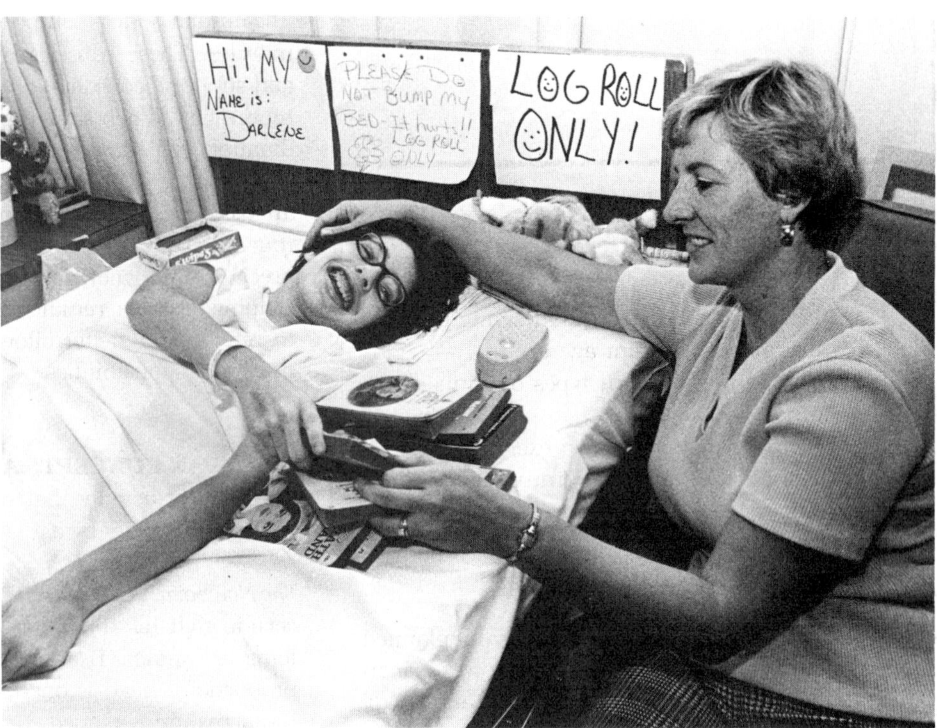

FIGURE 26-1. A schoolage child confined to bedrest. Although bedrest is many times necessary, it has many hazards.

ing normal motor development. Certain milestones—such as ability to hold up head while prone (2 mo), pull to sit without head lag (4 mo); to sit steadily (8 mo); to creep (9 mo); and to walk (12—22 mo)—should always be assessed. Mothers may need to be reminded that motor development is complex and such a seemingly easy task as transferring a toy from one hand to the other takes 7 months to learn.

The Toddler. Children begin to walk between 9 and 22 months. As a toddler, a child walks with a wide-based, unsteady gait. Assess legs carefully for bowleg (genu varum) and knock knee (genu valgum.) These are usually developmental variations in a toddler but need to be documented so that their progression or regression can be watched. Many infants show a flat footprint until their arches mature with more walking practice.

The Preschooler. Preschoolers are constantly in motion and demonstrate greatly improved motor coordination over that of the toddler. This is often the first time that a child suffers a fracture. Any fracture has a possibility of not healing perfectly; osteomyelitis or bone infection may occur, leading to a chronic, disabling injury.

The Schoolager. Schoolage children set the pattern for exercise throughout their life. Children who are not participating in active sports need encouragement to begin a structured exercise program to aid muscle coordination. All children need to be cautioned not to undertake activities such as gymnastics or play on trampolines without supervision because they could injure themselves seriously (Fig. 26-2).

A number of bone diseases can occur in this age group. One of these is an interference with blood supply to the head of the femur (Legg-Calvé-Perthes disease). Another is a slipped epiphysis or displacement of the femur head. Both conditions may require long periods of bed rest before correction is complete. Limping is one of the first symptoms of these conditions. Thus, a limp in a schoolchild must be considered serious until these illnesses are medically ruled out.

A second orthopedic condition that tends to occur in this age group is lateral curvature of the spine (scoliosis). This is best revealed if a child is asked to bend forward at the waist and touch his toes; rotation of the rib cage occurs in this position causing a shoulder hump to become prominent (Fig. 26-3). This condition is more common in girls than in boys, but all children aged 8 to 18 years should be examined for scoliosis. Most states have mandatory screening programs implemented by the school nurse.

The Adolescent. The chief musculoskeletal problems in adolescence are postural difficulties and sports injuries. Posture needs to be assessed at health visits. More effec-

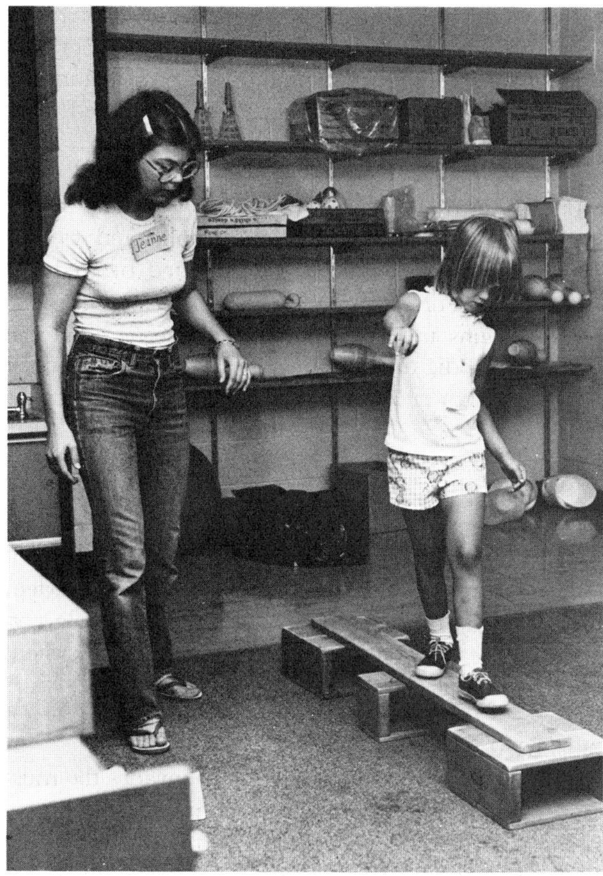

FIGURE 26-2. Assessing balance in a schoolage child. Falls and accidents often happen in this age group from trying to balance on fences or unsteady surfaces.

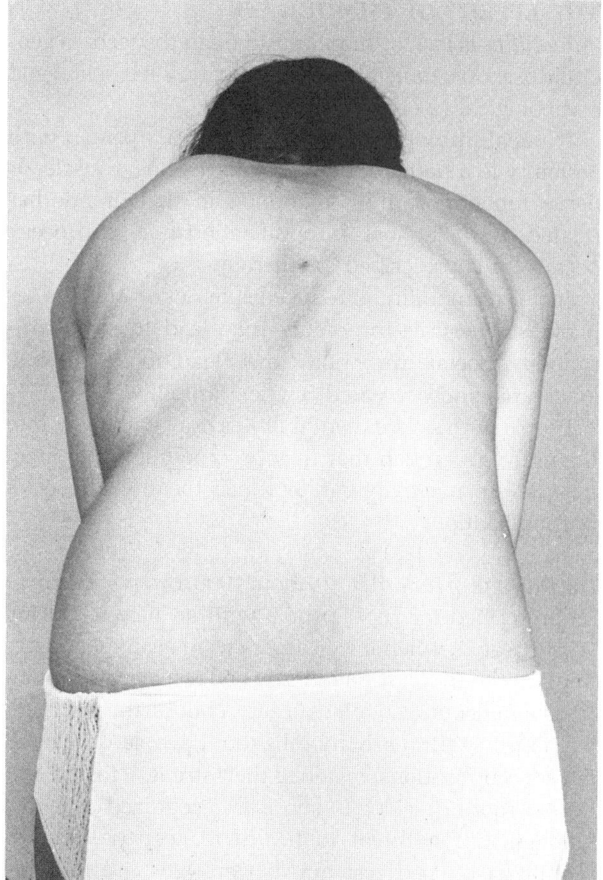

FIGURE 26-3. Scoliosis (lateral curvature of the spine) becomes more obvious if a child bends forward.

tive than urging adolescents to maintain good posture is initiating an active exercise program for them. As teenagers become more comfortable with their bodies, self-consciousness decreases and posture improves.

Among common sports injuries are elbow injuries from throwing and knee injuries from hyperextension in football games. Good follow-up is needed to be certain that the joint receives adequate rest while the injury is acute; adequate exercises are required with knee injuries to return them to optimal joint function.

Children and adolescents are normally so active that even when immobilized by a large cast or traction equipment they are eager to keep busy; thus, they do not experience such extensive damage from immobilization as adults. Your main nursing problem may be finding activities for their time and energy.

The Adult. Adults generally exercise less than they did as children or adolescents. The best exercise program is consistent moderate exercise. Pregnant women should walk at least a city block each day; this increases venous return from lower extremities by the compression action of muscles against veins. Women with young infants are urged to wheel them in a carriage or stroller daily for the stimulation of the experience and the exposure to sunshine, which produces vitamin D.

There is a high incidence of heart attack in males of 40 to 50. The usual therapy for a person who has just suffered myocardial infarction is absolute bed rest to reduce the work on the heart. Do not begin exercise programs for anyone with a heart condition until medically ordered.

The Older Adult. Normal aging results in loss of calcium from bones *(osteoporosis)*, especially in women; some loss of size in muscle *(atrophy)*, and some stiffening and pain in joints *(arthritis)*. A person with these conditions on bed rest is threatened by immobility because some changes that occur with immobility, such as joint stiffening, have already begun.

When the brain is deprived of its blood supply by stroke (CVA), motor, sensory, vocal and cognitive damage all may occur. Patients with these limitations need good body positioning, frequent change of position, and a stimulating environment to regain motor function and return to self-care.

THE EFFECT OF IMMOBILITY

Immobility is lack of motion. Although the term is generally used to denote physical inactivity, it has social and psychological levels as well.

Physical immobilization occurs when a person with an injury to a body part does not have bone, muscle, or nerve function to initiate motion in that or another related part. Physical immobilization may also occur because it is prescribed for therapy.

Social immobility is reduced interaction with other persons. Physical immobility may lead to social immobility. Social immobility may lead to depression, loneliness, and decreased physical mobility.

People with severe mental illness may withdraw into themselves so much that they become physically inactive. Severe inactivity can produce the full effects of immobilization.

The Dangers of Immobility. About 1900, bed rest began to be prescribed for most people with an illness. During World War II, when fewer nurses were available to give total care to so many patients on bed rest, early ambulation was encouraged after surgery, childbirth, and medical illness. With early mobilization, people developed fewer complications, regained their strength faster, and healed more quickly. Today, it is recognized as not a kindness but a threat to health to keep people immobilized on bed rest any longer than is absolutely necessary.

A nurse who understands this and initiates preventive measures from the first day can prevent permanent disability due to immobilization. Many preventive measures are not activities prescribed by the person's physician; they are independent nursing activities determined by nursing orders—such as active exercise programs, frequent positioning, maintaining good body alignment, and providing a stimulating and time-oriented environment.

MUSCULAR SYSTEM

Lack of use causes muscles to atrophy and to lose strength. Muscles need to be stimulated by frequent contraction in order to maintain size and strength. The person begins to look smaller in frame or lighter in weight; periodic measurement of the circumference of the upper arm or leg will reveal the decreased muscle mass.

Encouraging people to do those activities for themselves which their medical condition permits will keep muscles contracting. Incorporating an active exercise program or isometric (pushing, pulling tension without joint movement) exercises into daily care (to the extent permitted by medical condition) is an enjoyable and effective means of keeping the musculoskeletal system from losing mass during immobility.

SKELETAL SYSTEM

If joints are not moved, fibrotic tissue invades the muscle attachments to the joint, making movement impossible thereafter. Fibrotic stiffening of joints was once thought to occur only after a prolonged period of immobility, but it can occur in a week—the average hospital stay. It occurs most rapidly when circulation to the joint is compromised, as with poor bed positioning, edema, venous disease, or bone fracture.

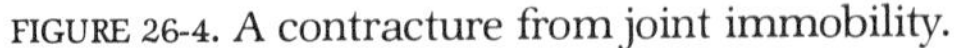

FIGURE 26-4. A contracture from joint immobility.

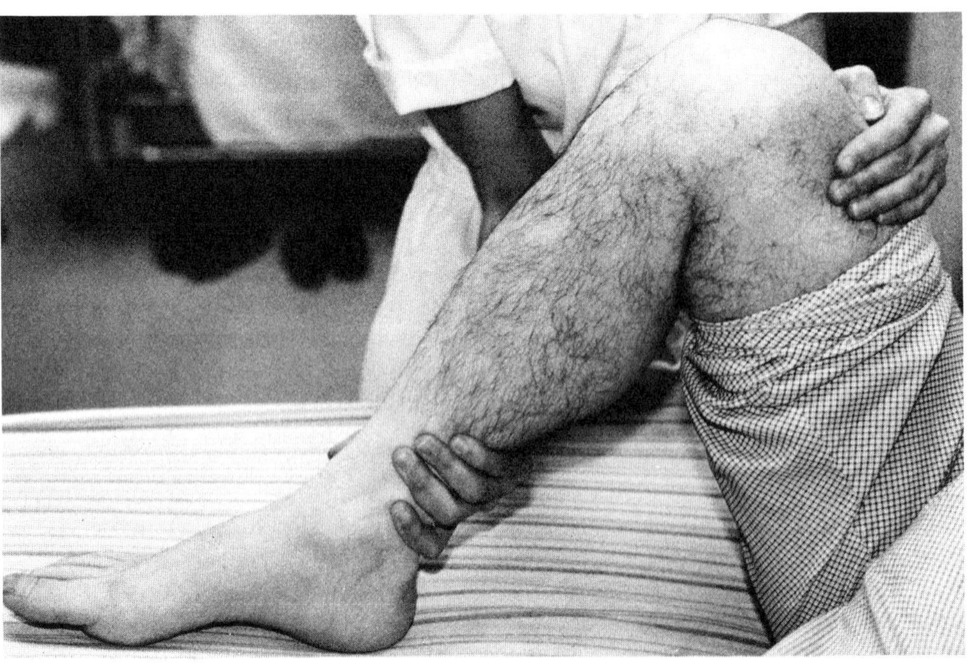

As muscle fibers become infiltrated with fibrous tissue, they shorten, fitting the joint into an abnormal (flexed) angle, or contracture (Fig. 26-4). Flexion occurs because flexors are affected more than extensor muscles. Contractures may be relieved to some extent by extensive exercise or tendon-release operations. They are serious permanent disabilities that must be prevented. Although some cannot be prevented, as a rule, a contracture identifies poor nursing care in terms of maintaining good body alignment and function.

To prevent contracture, a patient should exercise all joints through all their motion capability at least once a day. If the person cannot do this, then you must include passive range-of-motion exercises as part of daily care. Medical condition permitting, incorporating range of motion exercises is an intrinsic part of bathing.

BONE CHANGES

Bone is not a static substance. New cells are constantly being formed *(osteoblastic formation)*, and old cells are being absorbed and need to be replaced *(osteoclastic formation)*. With immobility and reduced pressure and strain on bones by muscles, more cells are absorbed and secreted from bone than are replaced. The bone becomes porous and loses its strength (osteoporosis). High levels of calcium and phosphorus, basic components of bone, move into the bloodstream.

This loss of calcium, measurable by the level of calcium excreted in urine, begins within the first week of immobility. Once weight bearing and normal exercise are resumed, osteoporosis can be reversed. The danger is that a bone weakened by this process can fracture when the person first begins weight bearing (pathological fracture). Osteoporosis is associated with declining levels of estrogen (postmenopausal women) and irregularities of adrenal and parathyroid function.

To prevent osteoporosis, exercises and weight bearing as soon as possible are effective. Increasing calcium in the diet is not effective; extra calcium simply increases the amount the kidneys must excrete.

NEUROLOGICAL SYSTEM

The major threats to the nervous system from immobility are due to compression on nerves, particularly as they press on bony prominences, and lack of stimulation in a restricted environment.

Changing the position of people on bed rest at least every 2 hours so there is no sustained period of pressure and being certain that the person is positioned in good body alignment with no sharp body angles are preventive measures. Nerve damage can occur quickly—in less than 10 minutes—if pressure is intense, such as occurs at the edge of a cast. Special diligence is necessary if such a condition exists (Fig. 26-5).

A person confined to bed has a restricted view of the world. He hears sounds he cannot accurately identify. He may receive little auditory or tactile stimulation.

Dependent on others for care, the person is apt to be bored. When sensory stimulation is drastically de-

FIGURE 26-5. An infant with traction equipment in place. Pressure from this type of equipment can cause serious interference with nerve conduction.

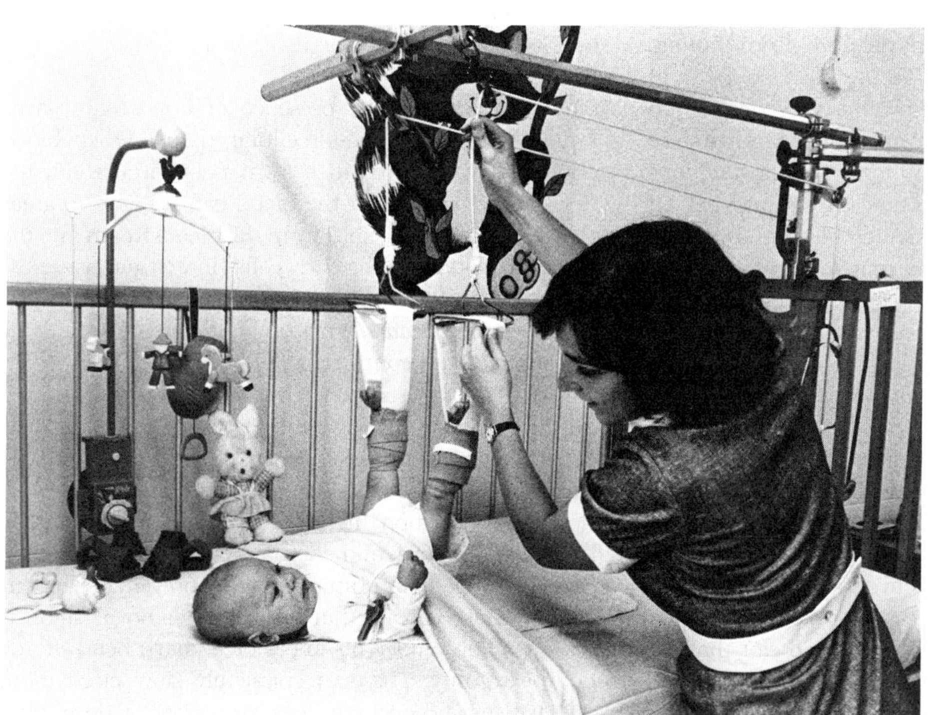

creased, people tend to lose the ability to concentrate, to solve problems, and to remember.

To prevent these effects of immobilization, people on bed rest should be placed so they can see activity in the hallway. A clock to help them keep track of time and a calendar to help them keep track of the date are helpful. Newspapers, books, and a television set help to bring in the outside world. Provide time for discussing events separate from therapy; be aware of whether support people visit or not.

With children, plan a time each day for games such as crossword puzzles or mind-twisters; a part of each day reserved for homework not only keeps a child mentally alert but reassures him that you are pleased with his progress and expect him to return to school. (See Chap. 22 for more stimulation activities).

CIRCULATORY SYSTEM

A person resting quietly in bed appears to be putting the minimum strain on his heart, but the opposite is true. In a sitting or standing position, gravity causes a high proportion of blood (up to 1 L) to pool in the lower extremities. Flat in bed, a high proportion of blood constantly remains in the chest, forcing the heart to work harder to handle the blood being returned to it. Heart rate and output both increase. Raising the head of the bed to a semi-Fowler's position helps to relieve the increased workload on the heart.

Postural Hypotension (Orthostatic Hypotension). When a person rises from a supine to a standing position under normal circumstances, vasoconstriction in peripheral blood vessels occurs, pushing blood into major organs and preventing central blood pressure from falling. Everyone has had the experience of rising too fast and feeling momentarily dizzy before this vasoconstriction effectively stabilized blood pressure. When this response system has not been stimulated for a time, it functions sluggishly or not at all. The first time the person is helped to sit or raised to a sitting or slanted position from bed rest, he will become dizzy and may faint.

Applying elastic stockings to compress leg veins and always helping a patient change from a supine to a sitting or sitting to standing position gradually, not rapidly, help to relieve postural hypotension. Elevating the head of the patient's bed (medical condition permitting) for part of each day or helping a person to sit on the edge of the bed with his legs over the side before he stands helps to prevent postural hypotension. A Circoelectric bed (see Fig. 26-37B), which allows for easily changing position, is also effective in preventing this.

Thrombophlebitis. A *thrombus* is a blood clot that occurs in a vein and is loosely attached to the vein wall; *thrombophlebitis* is inflammation with an accompanying blood clot. Thrombophlebitis is most apt to occur with immobility from circulatory stasis in women following childbirth, older adults, and persons who are dehydrated or have a history of previous thrombus formation. Blood tends to pool by vein valves and then to clot. If the person has narrowed vessels *(arteriosclerosis)* or plaque-lined vessels *(atherosclerosis)*, blood pooling is more pronounced and thrombi are more apt to form. In some instances, the clotting occurs first and then the inflammation occurs; in others, the inflammation may be the primary factor.

The development of a thrombus is serious because clot formation could obstruct blood flow at that point. If the blood clot should break loose from the vein wall, it is termed an *embolus.* If the embolus travels to the lungs, it could obstruct blood flow to the lungs; if it reaches the brain, it could obstruct circulation to vital brain cells, causing a cerebral vascular accident (CVA).

To prevent thrombophlebitis, prevent circulatory stasis. Range-of-motion exercises, elevation of lower extremities on pillows, and elastic stockings are all effective measures. Do not allow the person to lie with a pillow under his knees in a supine position or to sit or lie with his knees sharply bent or crossed. These positions encourage circulatory stasis. A physician may prescribe an anticoagulant to reduce the possibility of blood clotting.

Homans' sign (pain in the calf on dorsiflexion of the foot), is an indication of possible thrombophlebitis formation. Testing for Homans' sign should always be part of daily bathing. If you suspect that thrombophlebitis is present (positive Homans' sign, redness, warmth at the site), *do not massage the area.* Massaging a thrombus may dislodge it, becoming an embolus; an embolus may be fatal if it moves to the heart or lungs.

Edema. Edema is the presence of abnormally large amounts of fluid in intercellular tissue. When blood pools in lower extremities from poor circulation, the hydrostatic pressure of the blood can become so great that it causes fluid to shift from the bloodstream into the spaces surrounding the body cells (interstitial tissue). If edema occurs in body parts below the level of the heart, it is termed *dependent edema.*

The frequent contraction of lower leg muscles in walking helps to constrict and move blood in lower extremity veins. With immobility, vessels dilate, stasis occurs, pressure increases, and the fluid shift occurs.

Edema is dangerous because the fluid presses nerves, slowing conduction; it often gives an uncomfortable feeling of pressure; and edematous tissue breaks down easily, leading to decubitus ulcers. To prevent dependent edema, make certain that the person is not positioned with a pillow under his knees or a sharp bend in any body extremity. These mechanically slow circulation. Applying elastic stockings to compress veins, promoting active or passive exercise, and elevating body parts that are apt to become edematous owing to recent surgery or trauma are all preventive measures.

THE RESPIRATORY SYSTEM

Lying in a supine position increases the work of breathing because the person has to raise his chest muscles against gravity and the diaphragm has to push against abdominal organs. This decreases *vital capacity*, the amount of air exhaled from the lungs after a maximum inspiration. With exercise, a person breathes heavily and deeply, but without exercise, these periodic deep respirations are absent. Body fluids always pool at the lowest point according to gravity. Lying in one position causes pooling of lung secretions in the lower, often posterior alveoli. Stasis of any fluid leads to accumulation of bacteria and infection.

To prevent pooling of secretions, reposition the person in a pattern that assures that he is not in one position over 2 hours time (right side, left side, supine, prone). Asking him to take two or three deep breaths every hour and asking him to cough every hour also help to move secretions. Specific clapping and vibrating therapy to better loosen and move secretions may be ordered (postural drainage; see Chap. 32).

THE GASTROINTESTINAL SYSTEM

People who exercise are apt to have good appetites and can therefore eat a nutritious diet. A person who exercises little may never feel hungry and may eat less and less the longer the period of immobility continues. This eventually leads to undernutrition.

If the person eats little fiber, peristalsis is not so forceful in the intestine, and constipation results. Constipation also occurs because excretion requires contraction of the abdominal muscles. In addition, when a person attempts to use a bedpan, unless the head of the bed is raised enough so that he sits almost upright, the role of gravity in passing stool is lost; the person cannot use abdominal muscles correctly and has trouble defecating using a bedpan. If stool is retained in the colon, additional water is absorbed and it becomes hard and even more difficult to pass.

To prevent loss of appetite in immobilized persons, encourage as much activity as their medical condition permits (Fig. 26-6). Allow them choices of food but be certain that high-fiber foods are included. Provide a bedside commode rather than a bedpan if the person's medical condition permits. Include laxative foods such as prune juice if possible. A laxative or stool softener may be prescribed for the patient to prevent constipation.

THE URINARY SYSTEM

The high level of calcium being lost from bones is filtered and excreted from the body by the kidneys. This high level of calcium in urine may lead to *renal calculi* (kidney stones), which plug the ureters and cause intense pain. Whether calcium remains dissolved in urine or crystallizes into stones depends on the acidity of the urine (the more acid the urine, the less crystallization occurs).

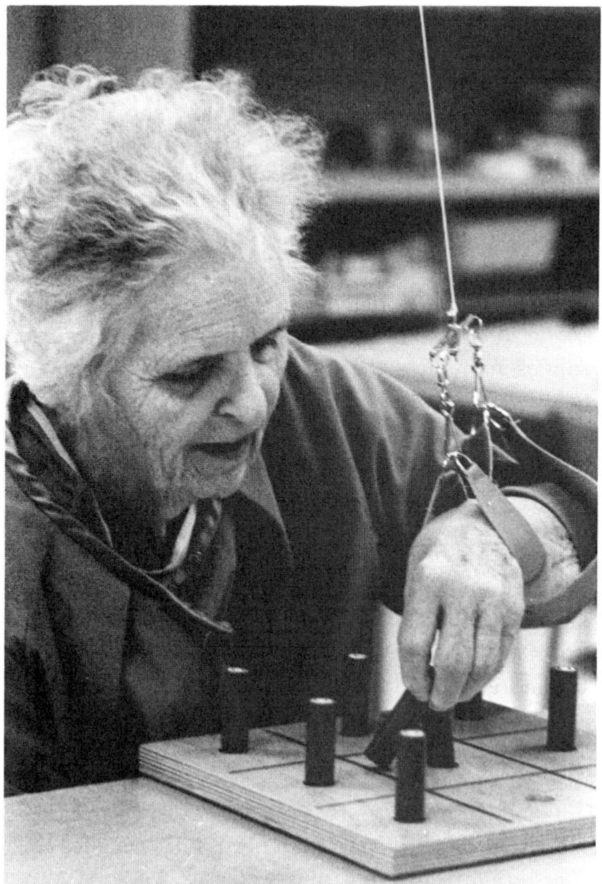

FIGURE 26-6. Activity to the extent allowed is beneficial; here a woman learns to reuse her hand after a cerebral vascular accident.

The normal standing position encourages urine flow through ureters. A flat bed rest position slows ureter flow and leads to relative stasis. Stasis encourages stone formation and infection.

To prevent urine stasis and stone formation, be certain that the person's fluid intake is adequate. Elevate the head of the bed at least part of the day to encourage ureter drainage. Encourage foods that leave an acid residue that will keep the urine acid (pH below 7); such foods include poultry, fish, meat, cereals, and cranberry juice. Increasing activity to keep calcium from leaving bones so rapidly is the best prevention of renal calculi.

In a supine position, the kidney receives more blood than normal so that glomeruli filtrate increases and kidney output or urine volume increases. This means that the bladder of a person on bed rest fills to capacity quicker than that of a person standing. If the person does not void or has lost his ability to perceive a voiding sensation, the bladder overdistends and then loses its tone or ability to empty. Bladder distension or *urinary retention* is serious because an overfilled bladder may develop miniature tears in the mucosal lining, leading to infection aided by the stagnant urine.

To assess for urinary retention, record the time intervals between voidings. Examine the abdomen to see if the bladder is full—a hard mass may be palpated, and a dull sound may be percussed by tapping with fingers just over the pubis if a bladder is full. Sometimes the full bladder does not empty completely; only enough urine empties to reduce the bladder size a small amount *(retention with overflow).* If a person on bed rest is voiding frequently but the amount of urine passed is small (under 100 ml each time in an adult), retention with overflow is a possibility. This voiding pattern can lead to urinary tract infection because of the stasis of ever-present urine.

To prevent urinary retention, allow a woman to use a commode if possible; a man to stand if possible. These natural positions for voiding encourage sphincter relaxation and good urinary output.

METABOLIC CHANGES

Since an immobilized person is not performing much activity, his basal metabolism falls. This means fewer calories are being burned than normal. To balance this, a person's appetite generally decreases.

If a person continues to eat his usual amount of food or eats less but of foods high in carbohydrates or fats, he will gain weight while immobilized. This may prevent him from using a wheelchair effectively or from crutch walking when he is first out of bed.

Negative Nitrogen Balance. Nitrogen is a product of protein breakdown. A negative nitrogen balance exists when a person is excreting more than he is retaining (catabolism exceeds anabolism). It begins about the sixth day of immobilization and even sooner if tissue trauma is the reason for immobilization. Nitrogen is apparently lost primarily from skeletal tissue. This nitrogen loss indicates that the body is no longer in the state best to effect tissue repair because high levels of nitrogen are needed to build new cells. Increasing oral protein intake does not appear to reverse nitrogen loss. However, supplying amino acids by total parenteral therapy (hyperalimentation) is effective.

To prevent a negative nitrogen balance, institute an exercise program for skeletal muscles (to the extent of the person's medical condition) and encourage a well-balanced diet. A diet well balanced among carbohydrate, protein, and fat provides carbohydrate for energy so that protein can be used for cell building and not for energy.

THE INTEGUMENT SYSTEM

The largest threat to the integument from immobility is the development of decubitus ulcers or pressure sores (see Chap. 25). They are caused by pressure to a body part that compromises the circulation. Without adequate nutrients or oxygen being supplied to cells in that part, cells die, leaving large, open draining sores on the body.

Prevention of decubitus ulcers is discussed in Chap. 25. It consists primarily of preventing sustained pressure to any body part by positioning in good body alignment, turning and repositioning at least every 2 hours, massaging to increase circulation, and using devices such as air and water circulating mattresses.

Effects of physical immobilization on all body systems are summarized in Fig. 26-7.

USING BODY MECHANICS FOR SAFE MOVEMENT

Body mechanics refers to optimal use of the body for work, correlating body systems with physical laws to achieve the greatest effect with the least effort.

Center of Gravity. Many nursing activities require working against gravity.

The *center of gravity* in an object is the point where the bulk of the object is centered. In a standing person, this is a point at midpelvis just anterior to the sacrum. A basic rule of body mechanics is that the lower the center of gravity in an object, the greater its stability. A taller person may have less stability than a shorter one.

Support Base. Another basic rule of body mechanics is that the broader the base of the object, the more stable the object. An object is most stable if a line drawn from the center of gravity dissects the center of the base of support. If you lean forward, this line does not dissect the center and you lose stability. If you stoop to recover an object from the floor or lift something, your center of gravity remains over the support base, whereas if you bend to lift something, the center of gravity moves outside the center of the support base and you lose stability (Fig. 26-8).

Increase the size of your support base by spreading your feet a comfortable distance apart (10—12 in.); increase it front to back by placing one foot ahead of the other.

Using Body Mechanics. The back is prone to injury because of its narrow interlocking vertebrae. In lifting or pulling, avoid using back muscles to protect the tenuous vertebrae relationships. Instead, use the muscles of the upper thighs, which are strong themselves and attached to strong pelvic and femur bones. Do this by stooping to lift up objects, not bending.

Muscles of the abdominal wall are also prone to injury. Protect them by taking a breath and pulling them in before lifting or moving a heavy object. This action is sometimes referred to as "setting the internal girdle." It

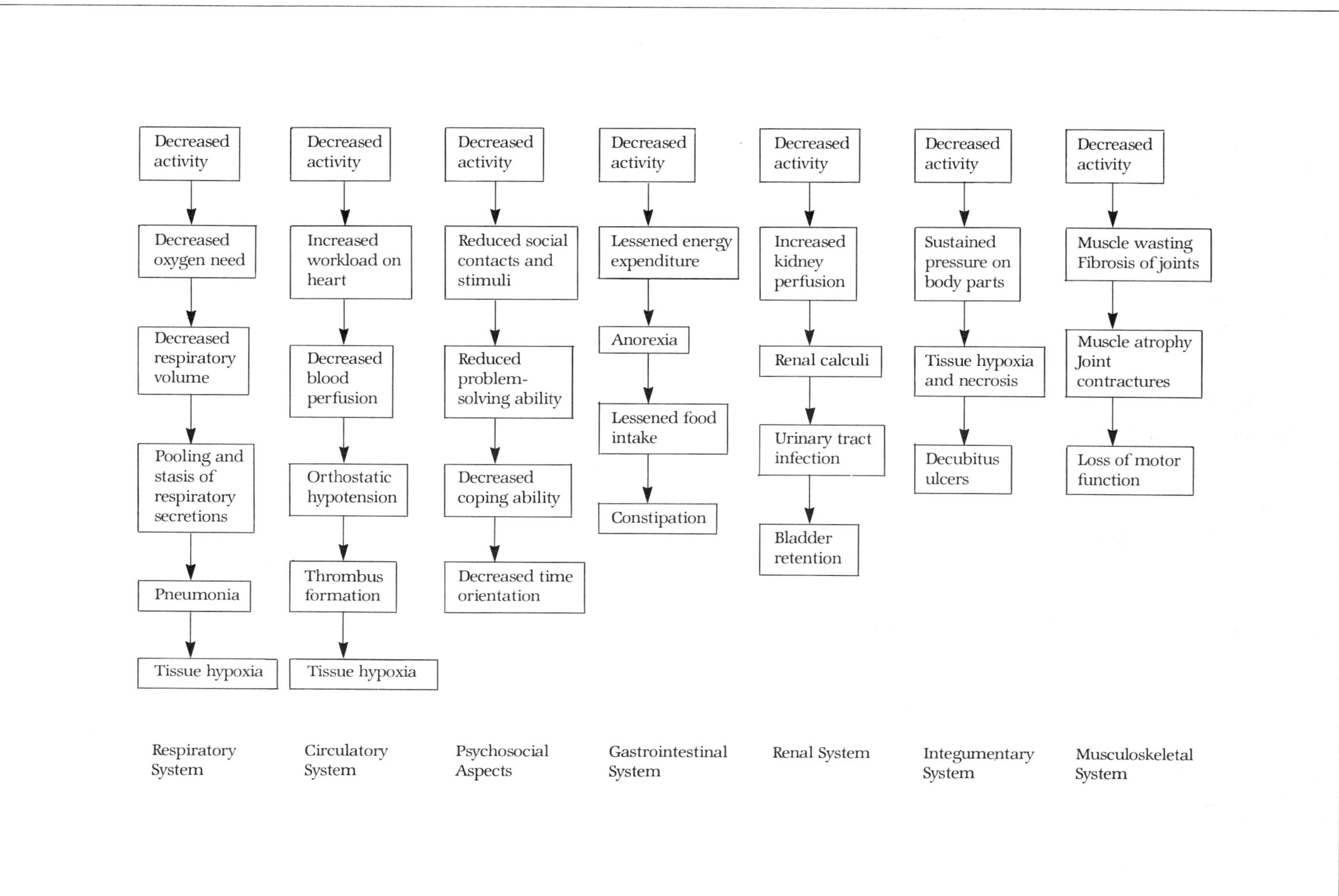

FIGURE 26-7. Effects of immobilization.

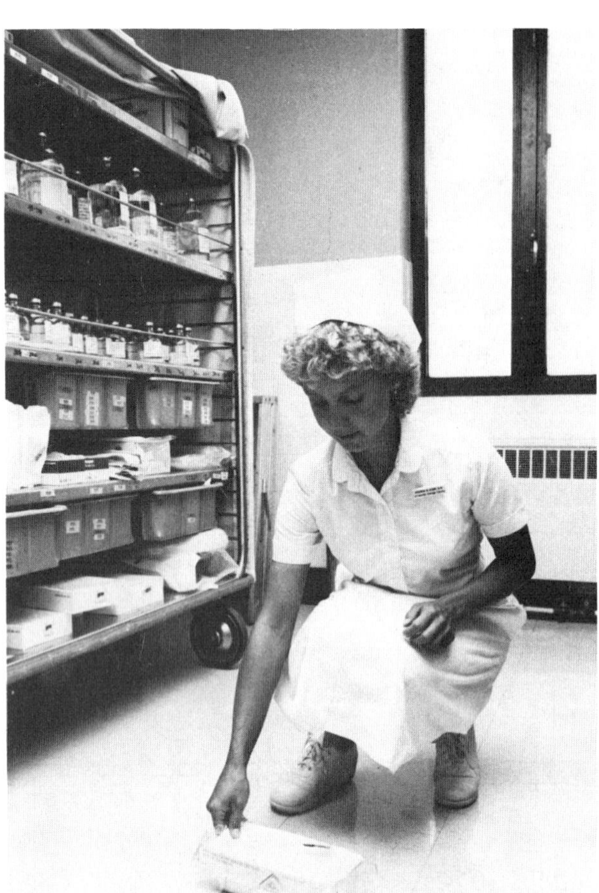

A

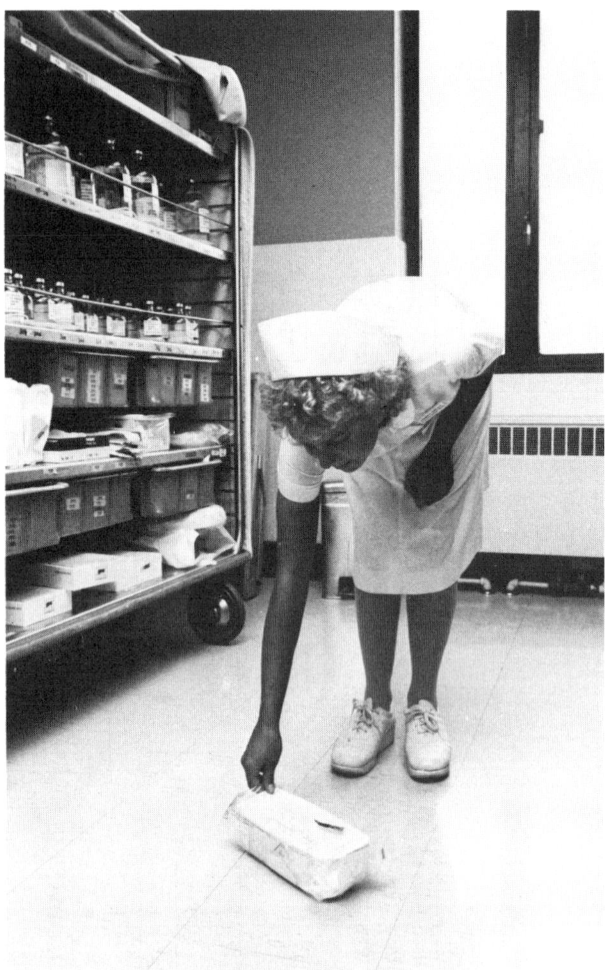

B

FIGURE 26-8. A. Stooping to recover an object from the floor keeps your center of gravity over your support base or makes you more stable. Stooping also makes use of the large thigh muscles and saves back muscles. B. Bending puts the center of gravity outside the base and is not as stable.

protects not only abdominal muscles but also the lower spine (lumbosacral area).

Provide a wide base of support by separating your feet. Bring an object close to your body before attempting to lift it to prevent bending and shifting your center of gravity in front of your support base and losing stability.

BODY ALIGNMENT

Good body alignment keeps strain to a minimum because muscles and joints are kept in positions where they can function efficiently. It also helps prevent muscle contracture from nonuse.

Standing Position. Figure 26-9 shows a standing position of good body alignment. Notice that the feet are spread 10 to 12 inches apart for a firm base; the abdominal muscles are flat; the pelvis is tilted forward; shoulders and hips are at 90-degree angles to the axis of the spine. This position supports body organs well and relieves strain at joints.

Sitting Position. When a person sits, good body alignment must be maintained as well as it was in a standing position. In a wheelchair (Fig. 26-10), the head should be erect, shoulders should be in a straight line with the hips, arms should be supported by the chair arms, and feet should be flat on the chair footrests. The position of footrests on wheelchairs is very important. If these are too high, the angle of the hip is too great; if too low, feet do not touch and plantar flexion of the feet may occur.

Resting Positions. When a person lies down, in order to maintain good body alignment, you must fill in the hollows with pillows or other supports so good alignment can be maintained.

Supine Position. Lying on the back is a supine position. A pillow should be placed under the person's head to

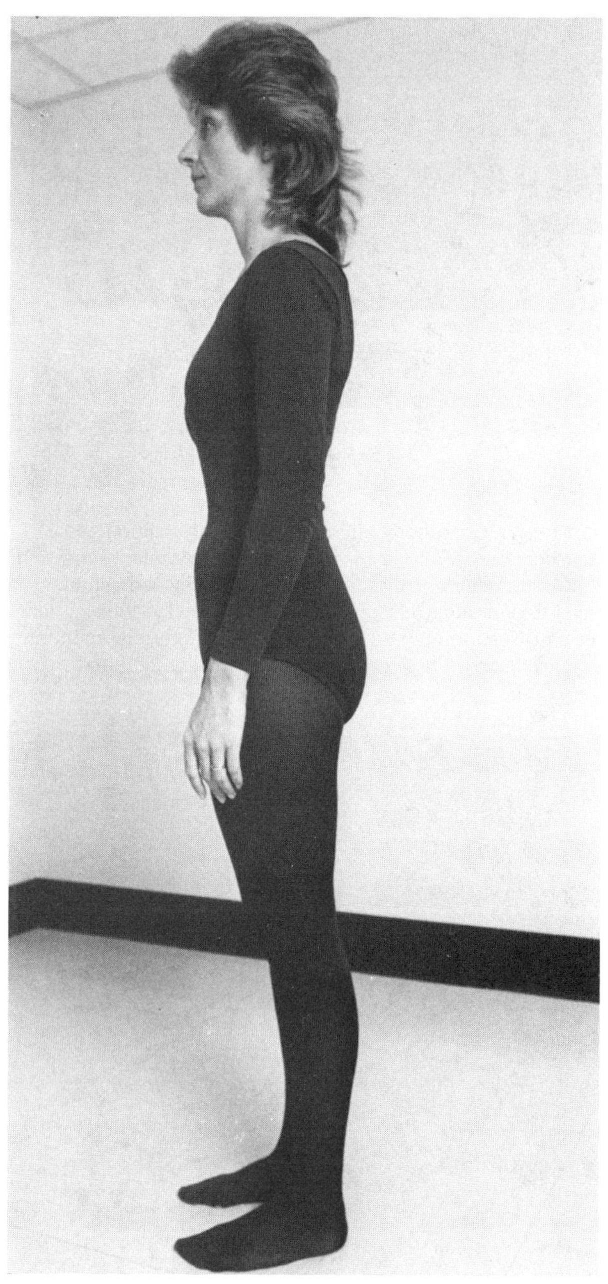

FIGURE 26-9. Good body alignment—standing position.

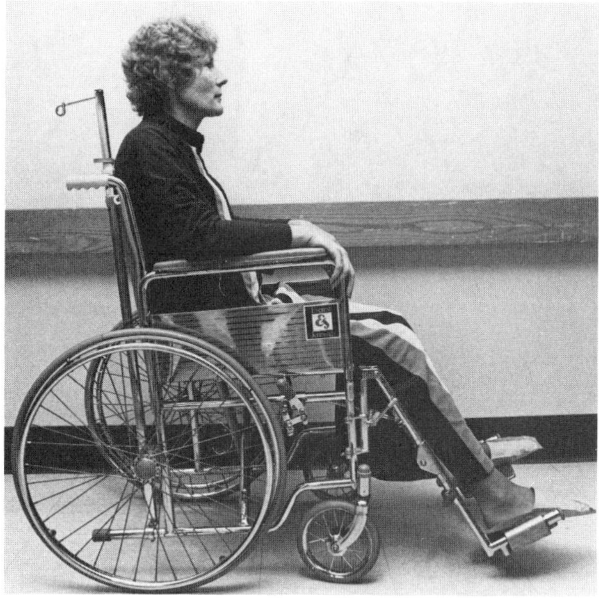

FIGURE 26-10. Good body alignment—sitting position.

prevent the head from falling too far back (hyperextension). A small pillow may be necessary under the knees for good alignment. A pillow or folded blanket under the ankles keeps the heels from rubbing on the mattress and becoming irritated. A blanket roll on the outside of the thigh (a trochanter roll) keeps the leg from turning outward at the hip (external rotation) (Fig. 26-11). A footboard at the end of the bed prevents the feet from bending downward (plantar flexion). Position the arms in a relaxed position at the person's sides. Do not place the arms across the chest or they may interfere with deep inhalations.

Do not place a pillow under the knees of any person with circulatory difficulty or raise the knee position of the bed with such people. Pressure behind the knee could interfere with circulation in the lower extremities.

Fowler's or Semi-Fowler's Position. A Fowler's position is the position in which the head of the bed is raised at a 90° angle; the knees may or may not be elevated. A semi-Fowler's position is the position in which the head of the bed is raised about 45°. With both positions, place a small pillow under the person's head and bulky pillows under the person's arms to prevent the shoulders from rotating forward. A footboard keeps the person from sliding down in bed and plantar flexion from occurring (Fig. 26-12). This is the best position for patients with respiratory difficulty, since the diaphragm descends and allows good lung aeration.

Prone Position. Lying on the abdomen is a prone position. For good body alignment in this position, turn the person's head to the side. Place a flat pad if needed for comfort under his head. Women may feel most comfortable with a pillow under the abdomen to prevent their breasts from pressing on the bed. A pillow under the ankles prevents the feet from straightening too far and keeps them in good alignment; placing the feet over the foot of the bed also accomplishes this. Position the arms over the head in a flexed (bent) position (Fig. 26-13) or comfortably at the sides.

Side-Lying Position. In a side-lying position, use a firm pillow to maintain good head alignment. Elevate the

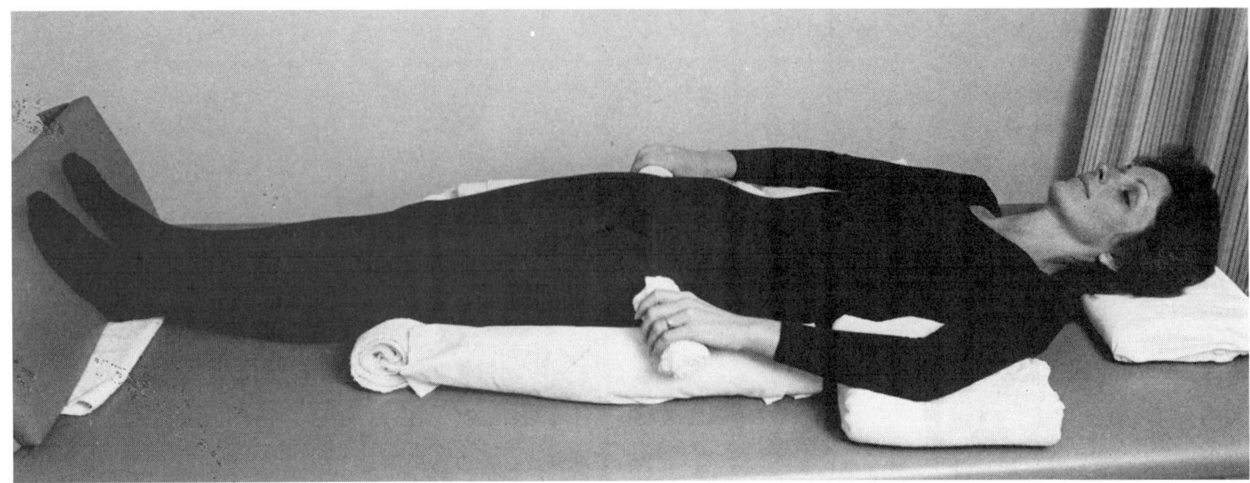

FIGURE 26-11. Good body alignment—supine position. Note the trochanter roll to keep the leg from externally rotating. If the person were to maintain this position for bedrest, a towel folded under her ankles would be needed to keep her heels from rubbing on the bed surface. Hand rolls maintain normal flexion. These can be made from tightly rolled washcloths.

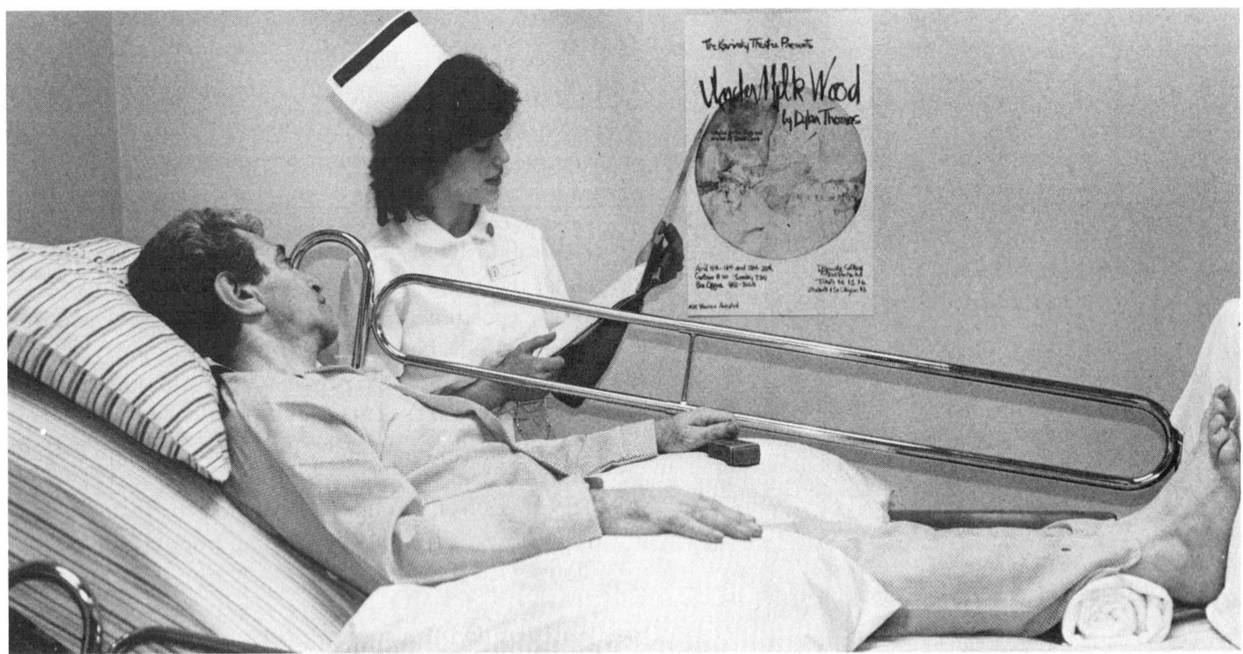

FIGURE 26-12. Good body alignment in a semi-Fowler's position. Notice the foot board and heel roll.

upper arm on a bulky pillow to maintain position. Place a flat pillow or folded blanket between the legs to spread the weight of the upper leg evenly over the lower leg and to maintain position. Fitting another pillow snugly behind the back would help maintain this position.

Sims's Position. Sims's position allows the weight of the person's abdomen to rest on the bed. It is the recommended position for women to use during pregnancy to allow the weight of the uterus to rest on the bed and free blood flow in the vena cava. A pillow is necessary under the head and between the legs as in a side-lying position. The lower arm may be placed in a position behind the person or forward as in a side-lying position (Fig. 26-14).

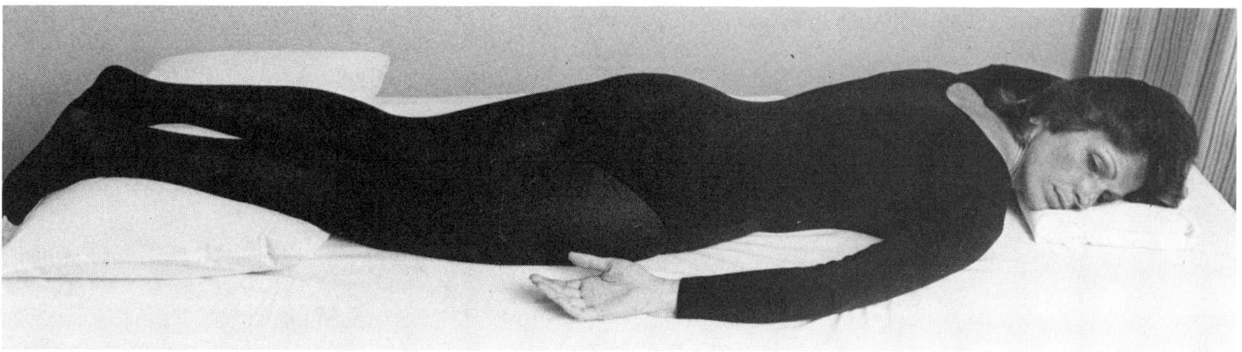

FIGURE 26-13. Good body alignment—prone position.

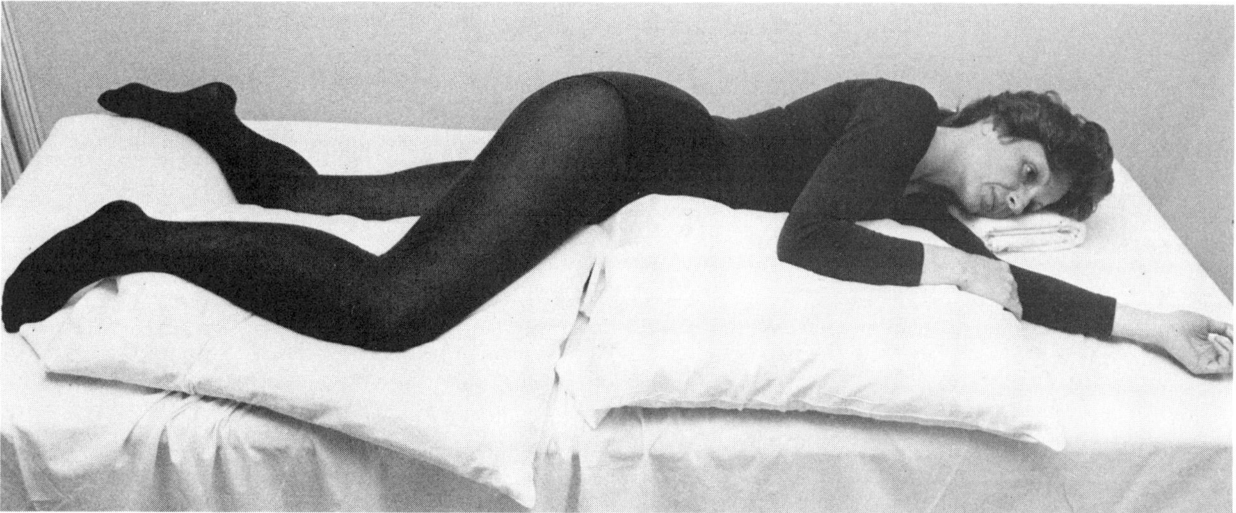

FIGURE 26-14. Good body alignment—Sims's position.

Additional Patient Positions. A number of body positions are used as diagnostic or examining positions. Although people remain in these positions only for the length of a procedure, it is important that comfort and good body alignment be maintained. Limit the amount of time spent in these positions by helping the person take the position just before a procedure.

KNEE-CHEST POSITION. A knee-chest position (Fig. 27-15) is prescribed for pregnant women to aid venous return from rectal veins and relieve pressure from the weight of the uterus on the vena cava. The woman rests on her knees and chest this way for about 15 minutes twice a day. A knee-chest position is also used for some rectal examinations and to promote emergency circulatory changes for women in labor and for some children with heart disease.

In this position, the head is noticeably lower than the pelvis. A small pillow under the head may or may not

FIGURE 26-15. Good body alignment—knee-chest position.

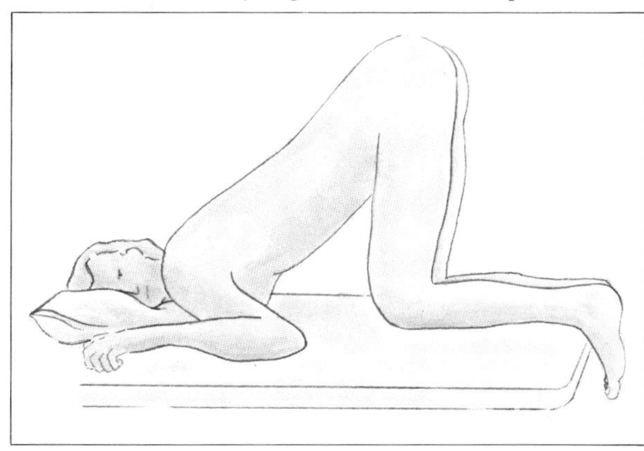

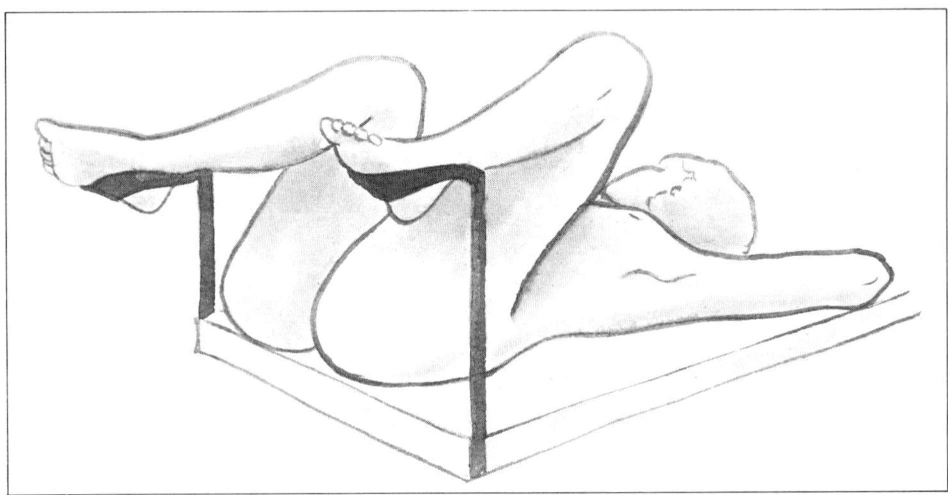

FIGURE 26-16. Good body alignment—lithotomy position.

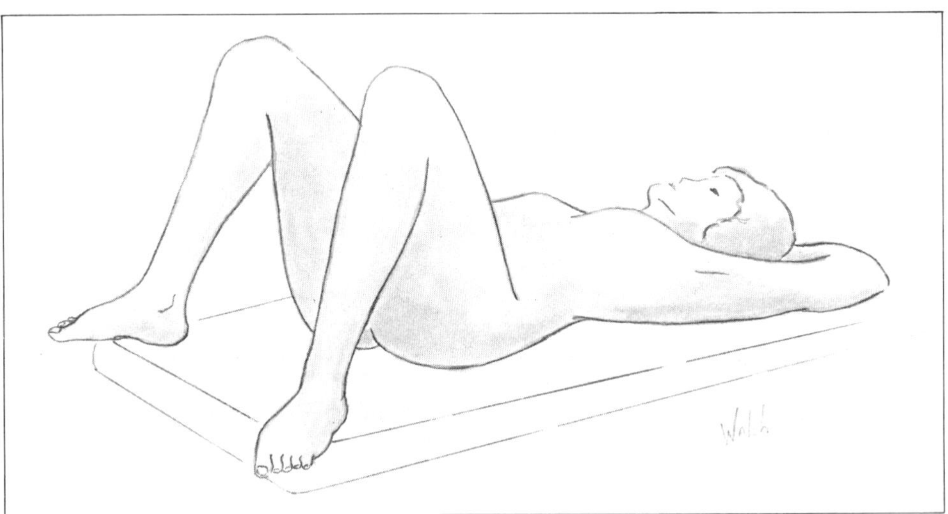

FIGURE 26-17. Good body alignment—dorsal recumbent position.

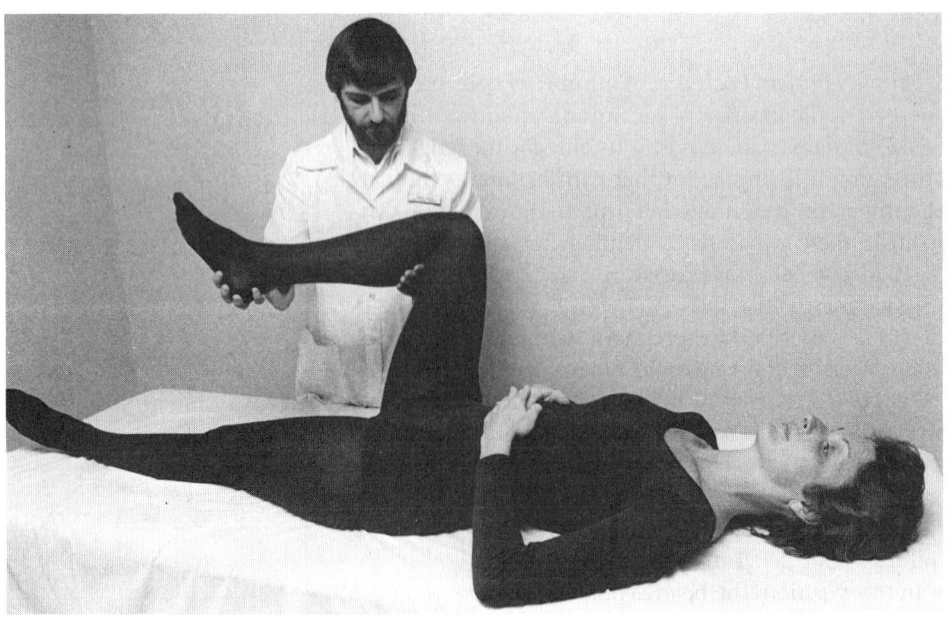

FIGURE 26-18. Support a joint distal to the one that you are moving in range-of-motion exercises.

feel comfortable. People often grow dizzy and lightheaded in a knee-chest position. A pregnant woman using the position should begin with only a few minutes daily and work up slowly to 15 to 20 minutes each time. To rise from the position, roll on the side, stay flat for a minute or two, and then rise slowly in order to ensure good equalization of blood pressure after this head-dependent position.

A knee-chest position is contraindicated in persons with high blood pressure (hypertension), since it would shift additional blood to the head and put great pressure on carotid arteries.

LITHOTOMY POSITION. A lithotomy position (Fig. 26-16) is a supine position with the feet and legs elevated in stirrups. It is used for gynecological examinations and procedures and may be used for childbirth. When placing someone in this position, both legs should be raised simultaneously to prevent strain on back muscles; the same is true when removing legs from the position.

DORSAL RECUMBENT POSITION. A dorsal recumbent position is a supine position with knees flexed and feet flat on the bed. The person can have a pillow under his head or not for comfort. It is used for gynecological or rectal examinations and childbirth (Fig. 26-17).

Aids to Positioning. When positioning patients, secure enough pillows to maintain good alignment. Use rolled bath blankets or towels as substitutes.

A footboard is invaluable in preventing plantar flexion. To bring it close to the person's feet, considerable padding may be needed. Do not move a short person down to the end of the bed; the Gatch bed will then be out of place for his back. If a person is very short and the footboard is not adjustable, a padded cardboard box may be substituted.

Some people need sheepskin padding under bony prominences to reduce pressure. Bed cradles (curved metal hoops) can be positioned to keep bedding off a body part. These are often used to supply a low source of dry heat (see Chap. 33).

RANGE-OF-MOTION EXERCISES

Range-of-motion exercises put joints through their normal planes of motion. These are *active* if the person performs them himself, *passive* if you perform them for him. If the action is shared or a person exercises an injured body part with a healthy one, they are *assistive.* Active range-of-motion exercises minimize both joint contracture and muscle atrophy. Passive range-of-motion exercises help maintain normal joint movement. Make a habit of incorporating passive range-of-motion exercises into patient bathing. Always support the joint distal to the one you are moving (Fig. 26-18).

Each joint in the body is of a specific type and is capable of a specific range of motion. Table 26-1 summarizes types of joints in the human body. Table 26-2 summarizes types of motion that joints can accomplish.

Whether active or passive (assistive), range-of-motion exercises are the same. They are summarized in Table 26-3. General guidelines for performing exercises are the following:

1. Always do motions gently and smoothly.
2. Support the joint distal to the one you are moving.
3. Move joints to a point of resistance, pain, or fatigue only.
4. Establish an order for performing exercises so you always do them consistently and thoroughly.

Neck. The neck is capable of four separate motions. Older adults often have some neck immobility or pain on motion because of cervical arthritis; people who have had whiplash injuries in the past may not have full range of motion in the neck due to resultant stiffness. To assist the patient with these motions, place one hand on the back of the neck for support and, with the other, bend the head forward (Fig. 26-19A). A neck normally flexes far enough forward so that the chin touches the chest; then tilt the head back as far as it will go (extension) (Fig. 26-19B). With a patient in bed, you need to remove the pillow to do this. Another way to accomplish this is not to bend the head, but to lift the shoulders upward, letting the head fall back or extend.

Many people use the term *hyperextension* to describe this position. However, *hyperextension* in reference to neck motion refers to a pathological condition, as in neurological injury.

Next bend the person's head to touch each ear as close as possible to the corresponding shoulder, being certain that the neck is bending and not the shoulder moving upward (Fig. 26-19C). For the last neck motion, turn the chin about 90 degrees, so it comes as much in line with each shoulder as possible (rotation) (Fig. 26-19D).

Hand. Lift the fingers of one hand and support them. Interphalangeal joints are hinge joints. Flex and then extend them (Fig. 26-20A, B). The proximal finger joint (the metacarpophalangeal joint) is a pivot joint and has four motions: flexion, extension, abduction, and adduction (Fig. 26-20C, D). Repeat these motions with all fingers. The thumb has special motion. The interphalangeal joint is a hinge joint, accomplishing flexion and extension. The carpometacarpal joint flexes, extends, adducts, abducts, and has opposition, crossing the palm to touch the fifth finger (Fig. 26-21). If a person loses opposition, he loses the ability to grasp or hold a pencil.

TABLE 26-1. TYPES OF JOINTS IN THE HUMAN BODY

Type	Type of Motion Possible	Example
Hinge	Limited to flexion and extension	Knee
Condyloid	Permits all movements but rotation	Wrist
Pivot	Limited to rotation	First cervical vertebrae
Saddle	Permits all movements but rotation	Thumb to palm junction
Ball and socket	Permits all movements	Hip
Gliding	Allows only gliding or slipping of two surfaces	Vertebrae

TABLE 26-2. TYPES OF JOINT MOTION

Type	Description
Flexion	To decrease the angle of a joint.
Extension	To increase the angle of a joint.
Hyperextension	To extend a joint beyond its anatomic range.
Rotation	To pivot or move around a center axis.
Eversion	To turn the sole of the foot outward.
Inversion	To turn the sole of the foot inward.
Pronation	To turn the palm of the hand downward.
Supination	To turn the palm of the hand upward.
Adduction	To move toward the body midline.
Abduction	To move away from the body midline.

TABLE 26-3. RANGE-OF-MOTION EXERCISES

Body Part	Type of Joint	No. of Motions	Motions to Perform
Neck	Pivot	7	Flexion, neutral position, extension, right and left lateral bending, right and left rotation.
Fingers			
Interphalangeal joint	Hinge	2	Flexion, extension.
Metacarpophalangeal joint	Condyloid	4	Flexion, extension, abduction, adduction.
Thumb			
Interphalangeal joint	Hinge	2	Flexion, extension.
Carpometacarpal joint	Saddle	5	Flexion, extension, abduction, adduction, opposition.
Wrist	Condyloid	5	Flexion, neutral position, extension, abduction, adduction.
Forearm	Pivot	2	Pronation, supination.
Elbow	Hinge	2	Flexion, extension.
Shoulder	Ball and socket	6	Flexion, extension, adduction, abduction, internal and external rotation.
Toes			
Metatarsophalangeal joint	Condyloid	4	Flexion, extension, adduction, abduction.
Interphalangeal joint	Hinge	2	Flexion, extension.
Ankle	Combined hinge and gliding	4	Dorsiflexion, plantar flexion, eversion, inversion.
Knee	Hinge	2	Flexion, extension.
Hip	Ball and socket	6	Flexion, extension, abduction, adduction, external rotation, internal rotation.

Support the hand and forearm for wrist movement. A person who has broken his wrist at some time may always have some stiffness in it and so may lack a full range of motion. A wrist flexes, extends, adducts, abducts, pronates (palm turns down), and supinates (palm turns up) (Fig. 26-22A—F). Many people use the term *hyperextension* to denote extension, but again, *hyperextension* refers to an abnormal position.

Elbow. Support the wrist and upper arm while accomplishing motions of the elbow. An elbow flexes and extends (Fig. 26-23) and also participates in pronation and supination.

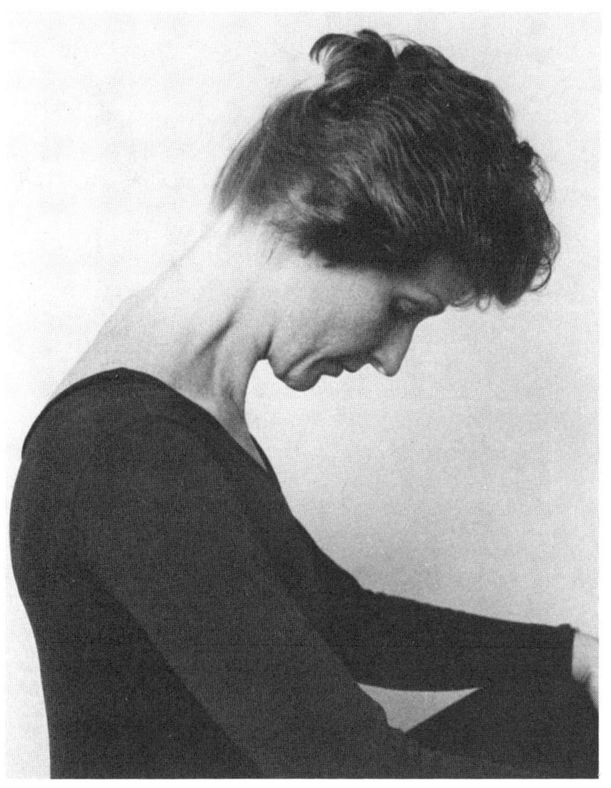

A

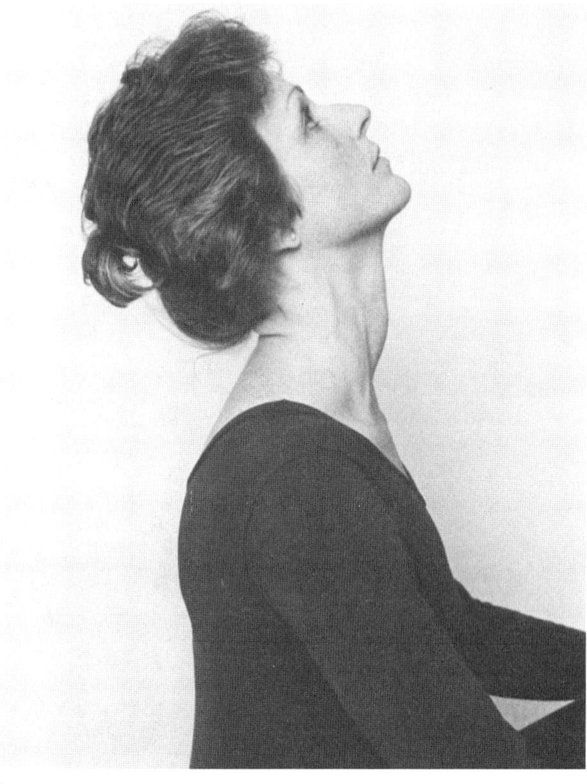

B

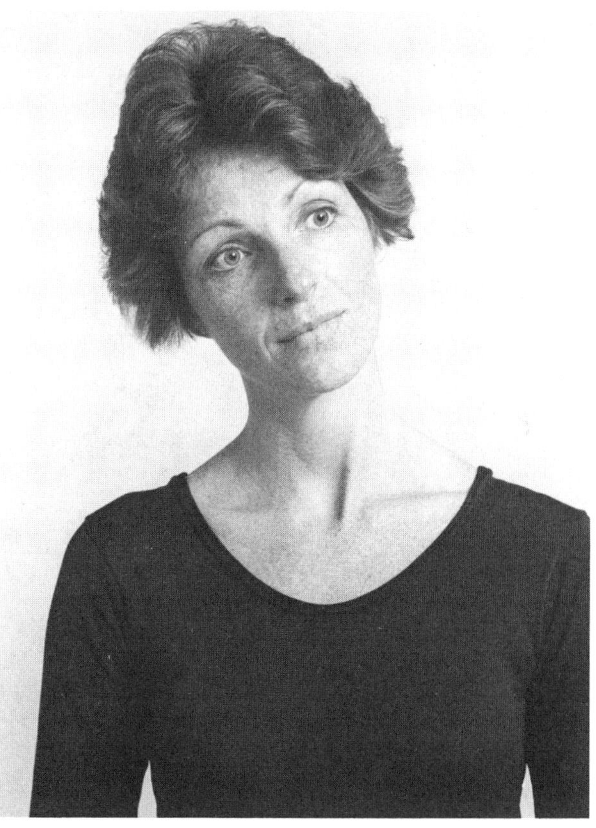

C

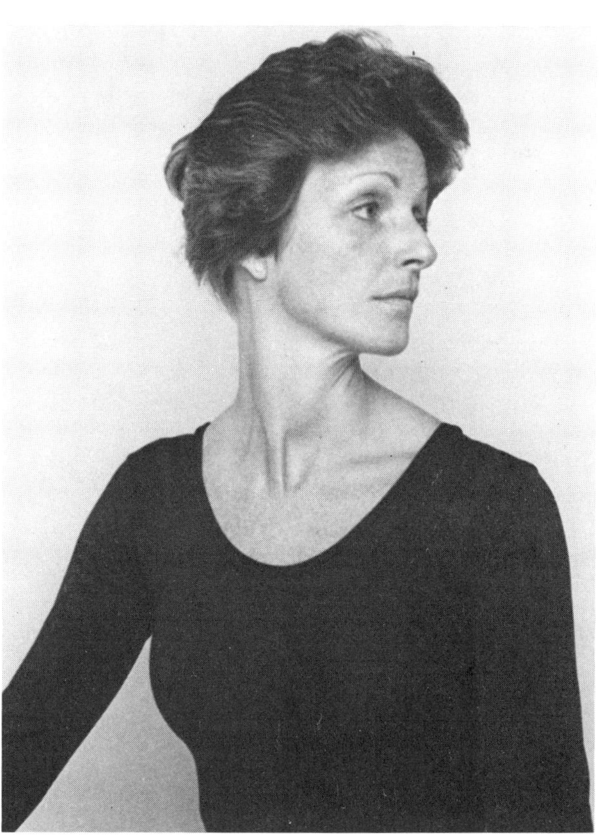

D

FIGURE 26-19. A. Neck flexion. B. Neck extension. C. Lateral bending. D. Left rotation.

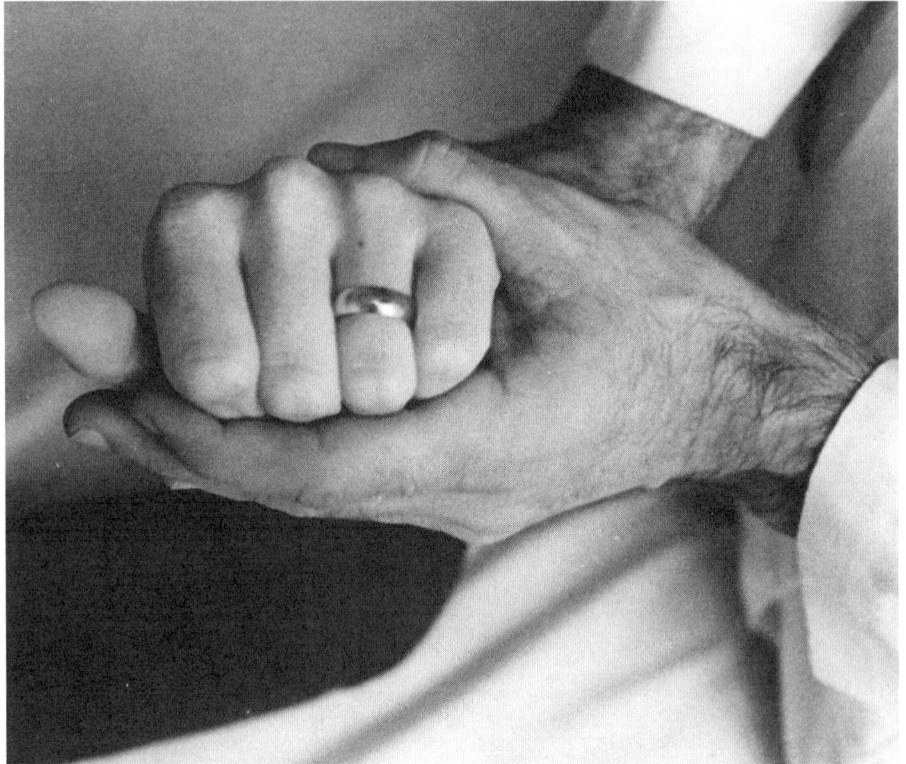

A

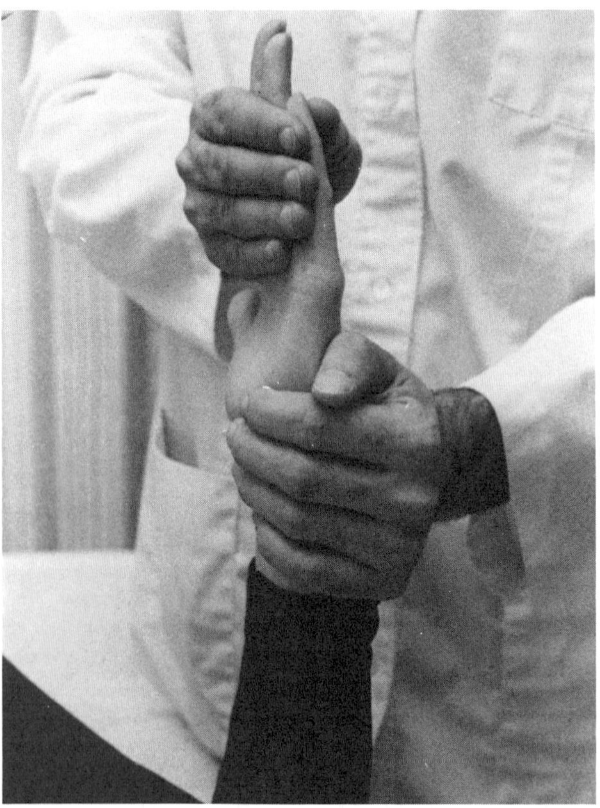

B

FIGURE 26-20. A. Finger flexion. B. Finger extension. C. Adduction of the metacarpophalangeal joint. D. Abduction of the metacarpophalangeal joint.

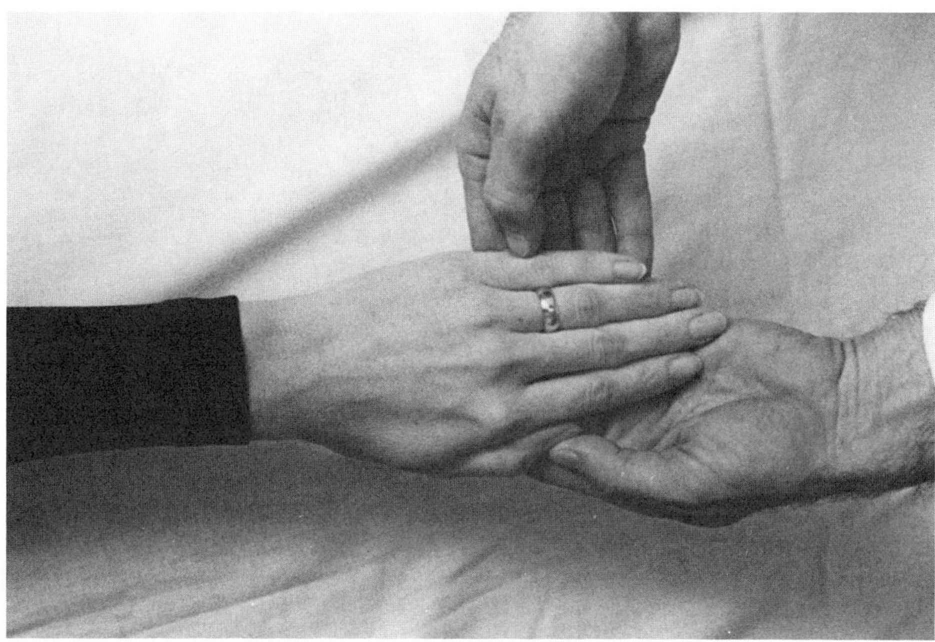

C

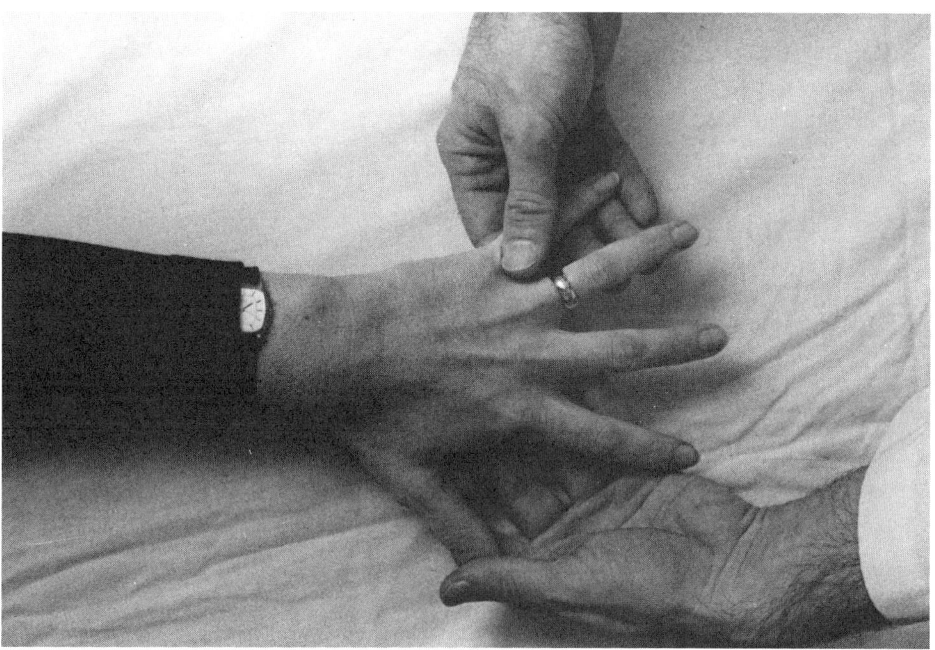

D

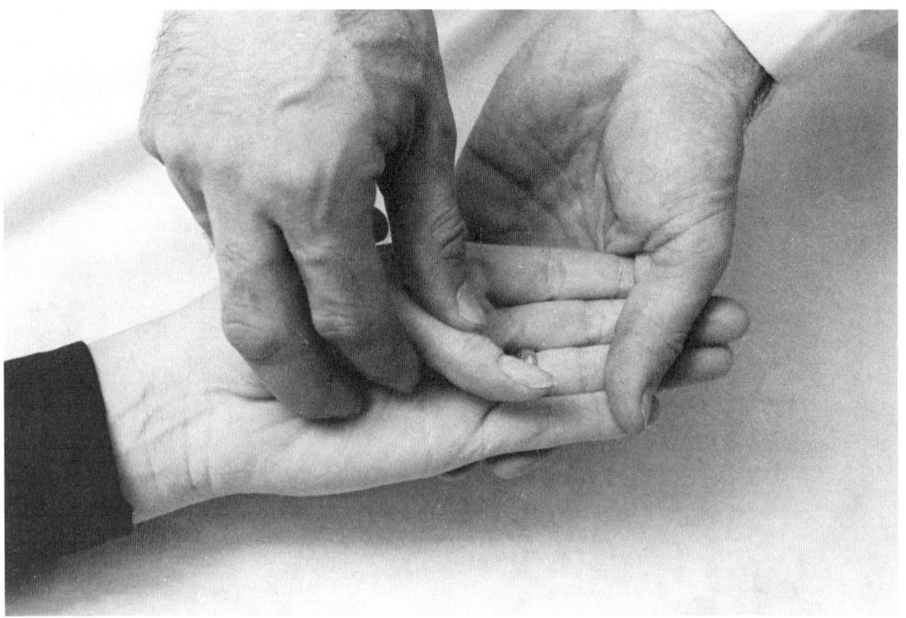

FIGURE 26-21. Opposition of the thumb.

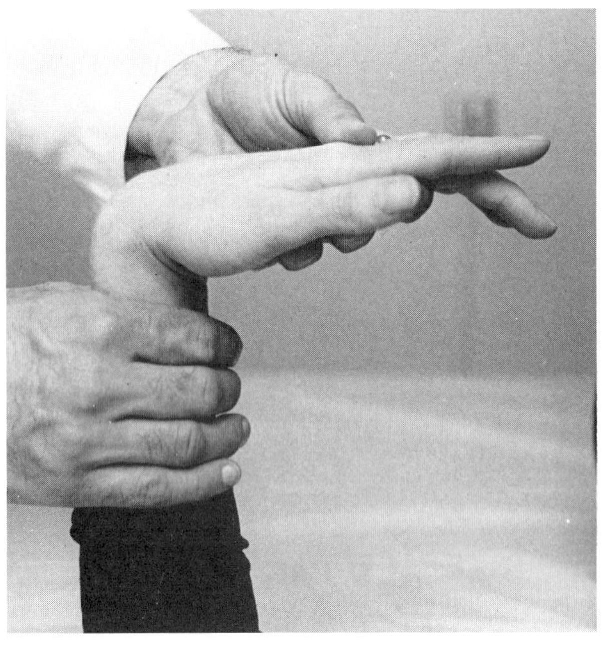

A

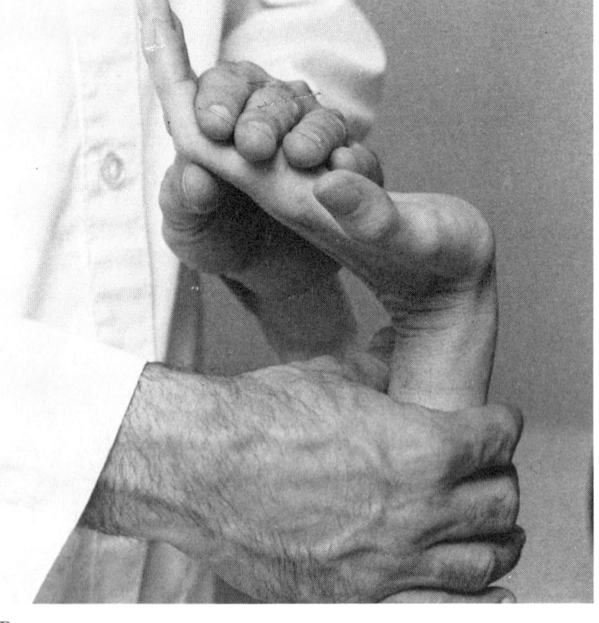

B

FIGURE 26-22. A. Wrist flexion. B. Wrist extension. C. Wrist adduction. D. Wrist abduction. E. Pronation. F. Supination.

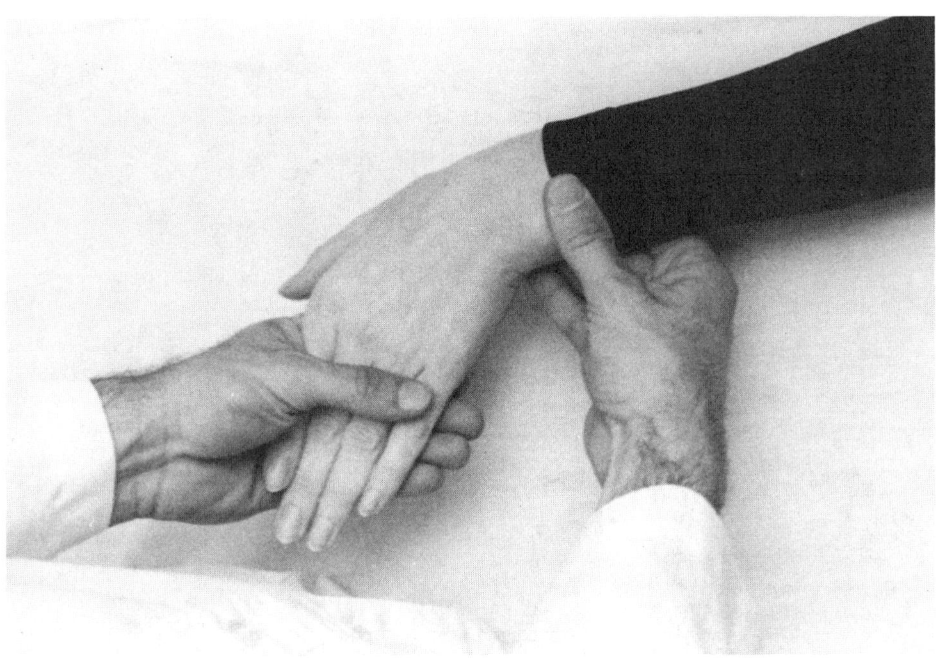

C

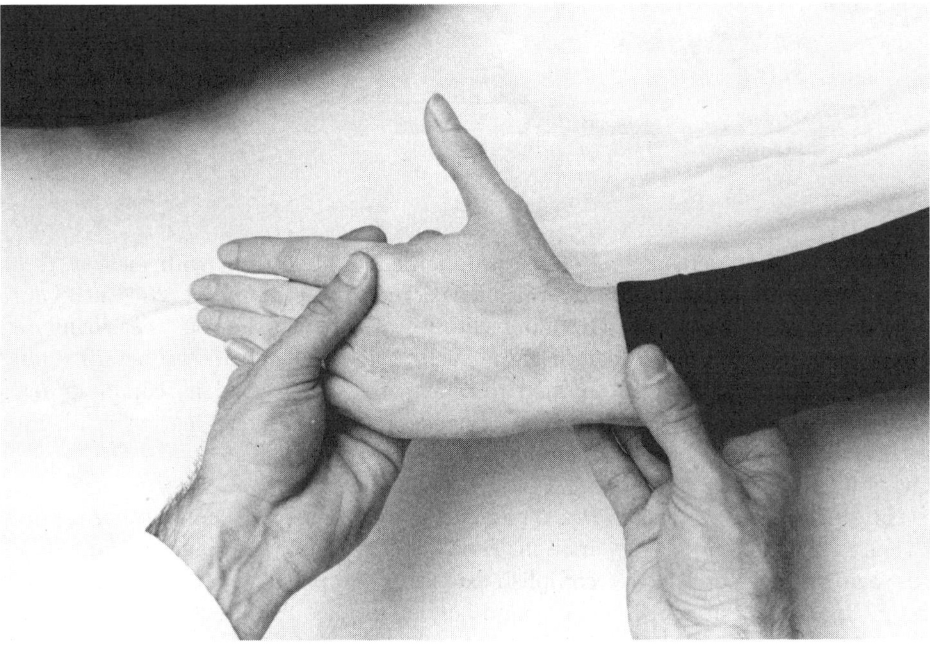

D

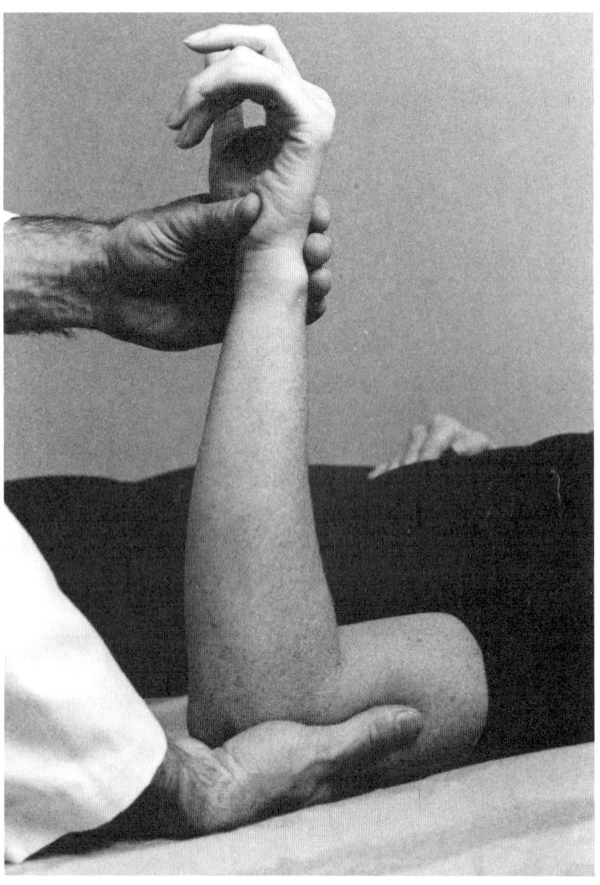

E

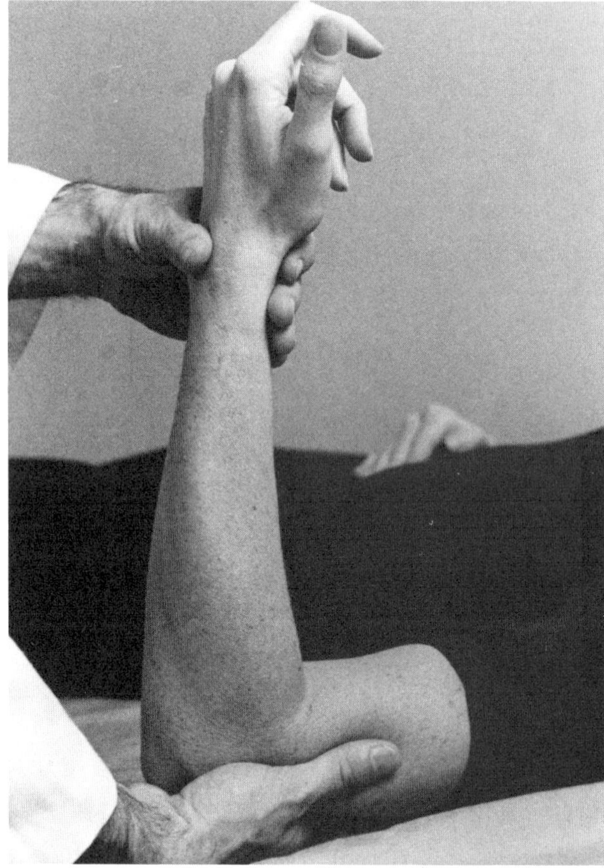

F

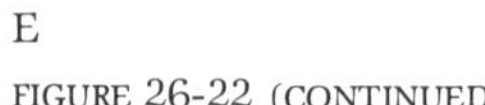

FIGURE 26-22 (CONTINUED)

Shoulder. As a ball-and-socket joint, the shoulder has optimal motion. To flex the shoulder, raise the arm over the head (Fig. 26-24A). To extend the arm, lower it and allow it to move beyond the neutral position. This can be accomplished by allowing the well-supported arm to move downward off the side of the bed or by raising it up off the bed when the patient is lying prone (Fig. 26-24B). Accomplish abduction by moving the arm away from the body to a 90-degree angle (Fig. 26-24C); accomplish adduction by moving it back (Fig. 26-24D). To accomplish external rotation, bend the arm at the elbow, and abduct the shoulder; roll arm up. To accomplish internal rotation, roll it down (Fig. 26-24E, F). Many older people with arthritis have difficulty moving shoulder joints. Move the joint only to the point of resistance or pain.

Toes. The interphalangeal joints of toes are hinge joints with motions of flexion and extension. The metatarsophalangeal joints have the added motions of adduction and abduction (Fig. 26-25).

Ankle. An ankle is a versatile joint capable of plantar flexion, dorsiflexion, eversion, and inversion (Fig. 26-26).

Knee. A knee joint is a hinge joint with the two main motions of flexion and extension (Fig. 26-27). Because rotation is limited at the knee, the knee is easily injured in a game such as football, where a sudden twisting motion forces it to rotate beyond its capability or a hard tackle causes it to hyperextend, tearing cartilage or ligament.

Hip. The hip is a ball-and-socket joint and has optimal motion. Bend the leg up to accomplish flexion. To accomplish extension, the person should lie prone; place your hands under the leg and lift it off the bed (Fig. 26-28A). Bring the leg away from the midline to accomplish abduction and back toward the midline to accomplish adduction (Fig. 26-28B, C). Roll the leg inward for internal rotation; outward for external rotation (Fig. 26-28D, E). A newborn is capable of so much external rotation that with the knee flexed the rotated leg lies flat on the bed surface in external rotation (Fig. 26-28F). Older children and adults have far less mobility in the hip joint than this.

Remember too that the spinal joints flex, extend, and rotate, and should receive daily range-of-motion exercises whenever indicated.

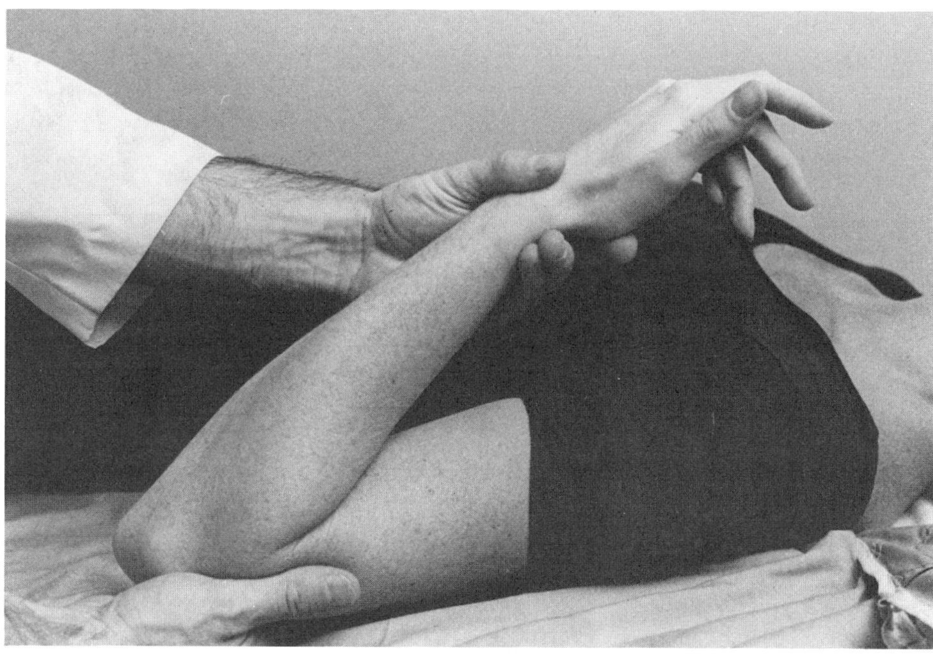

A

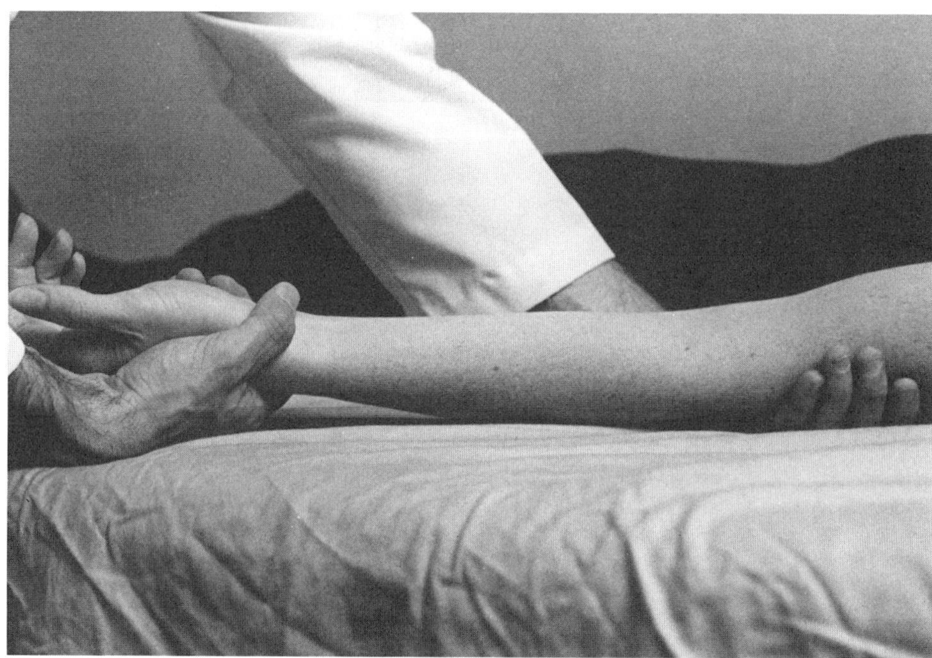

B

FIGURE 26-23. A. Elbow flexion. B. Elbow extension.

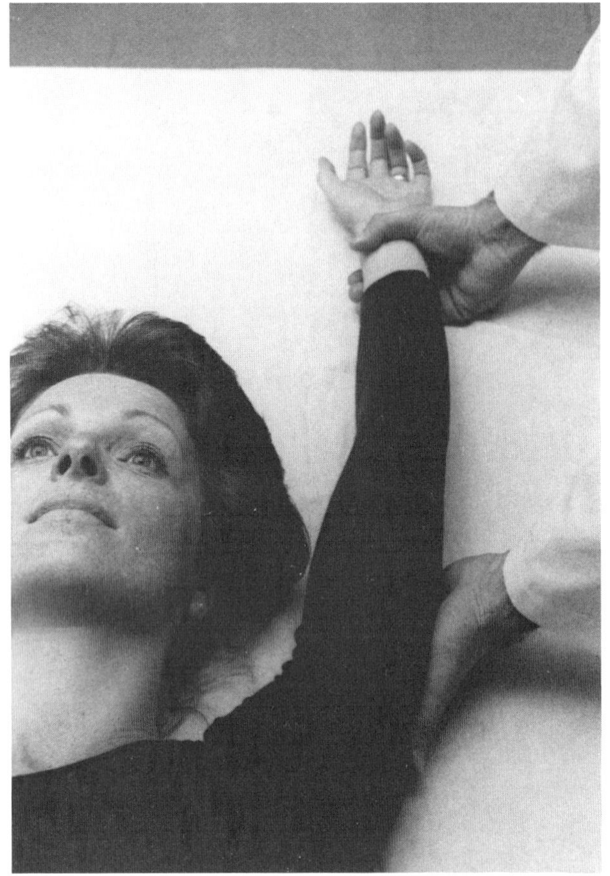

A

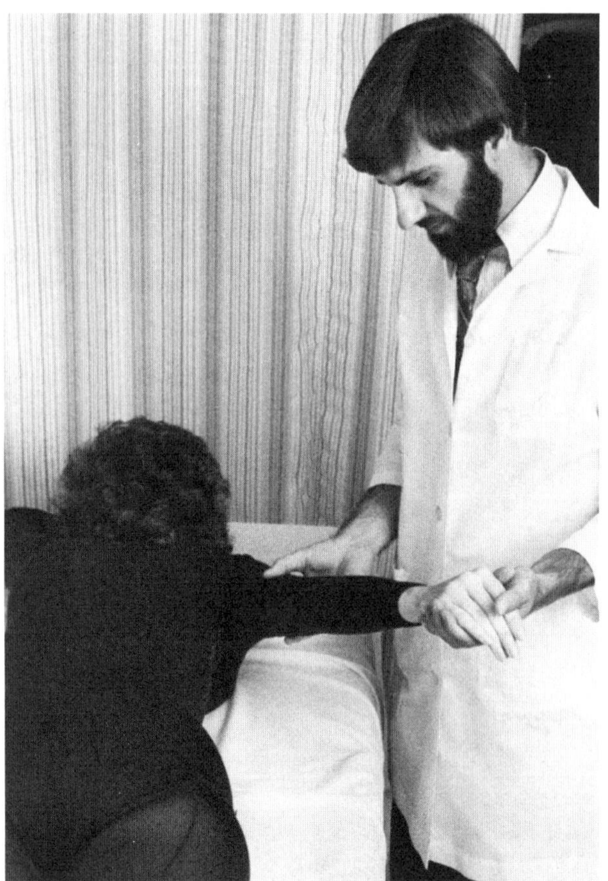

B

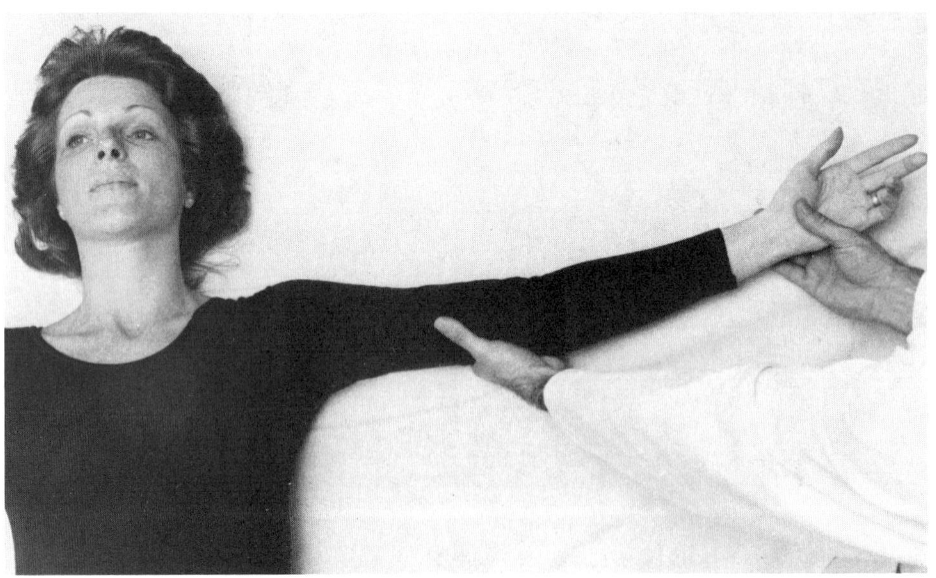

C

FIGURE 26-24. A. Shoulder flexion. B. Shoulder extension. C. Shoulder abduction. D. Shoulder adduction, neutral position. E. External rotation. F. Internal rotation.

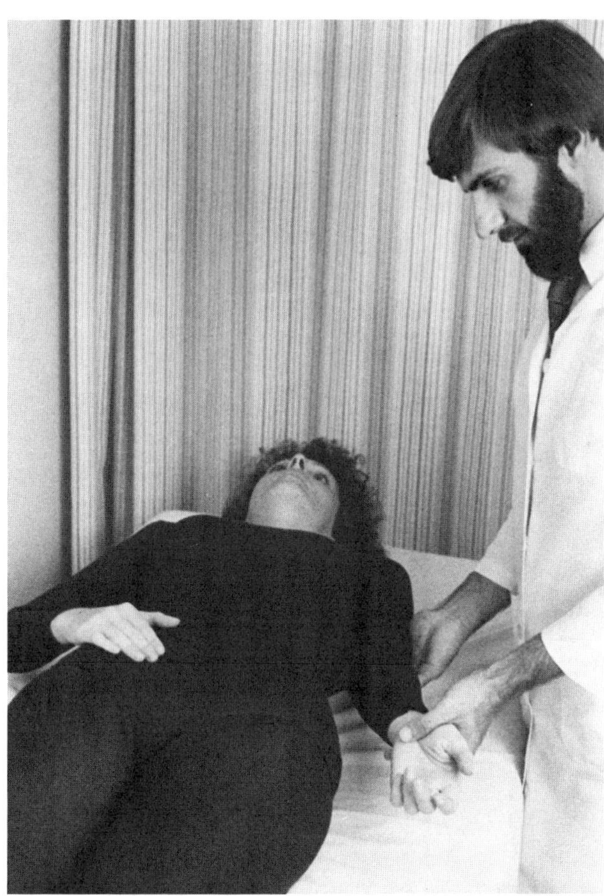

D

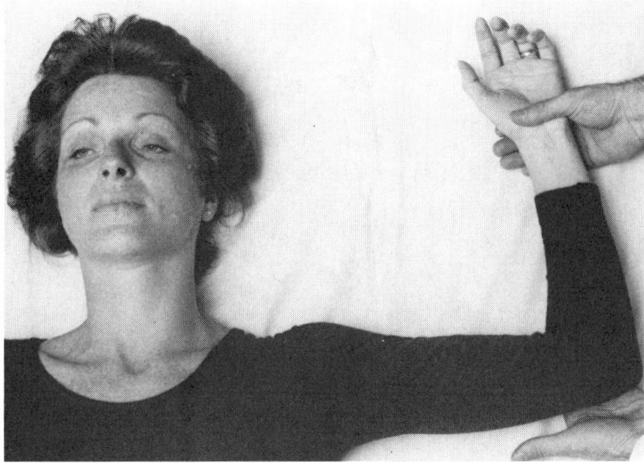

E

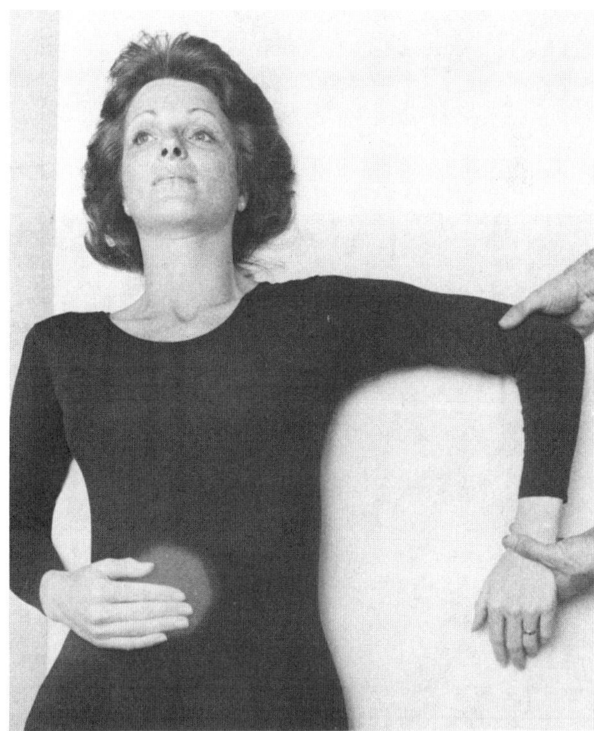

F

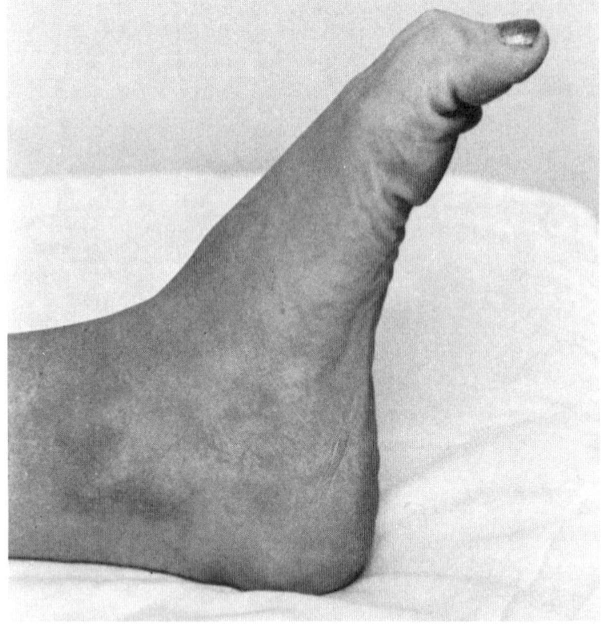

A

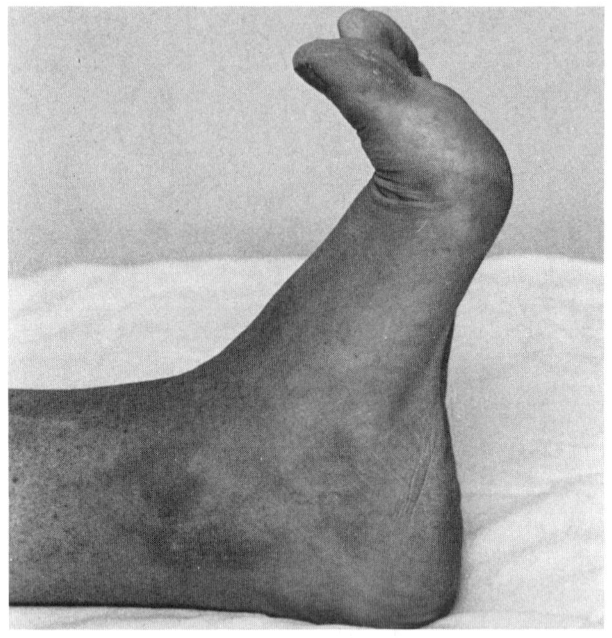

B

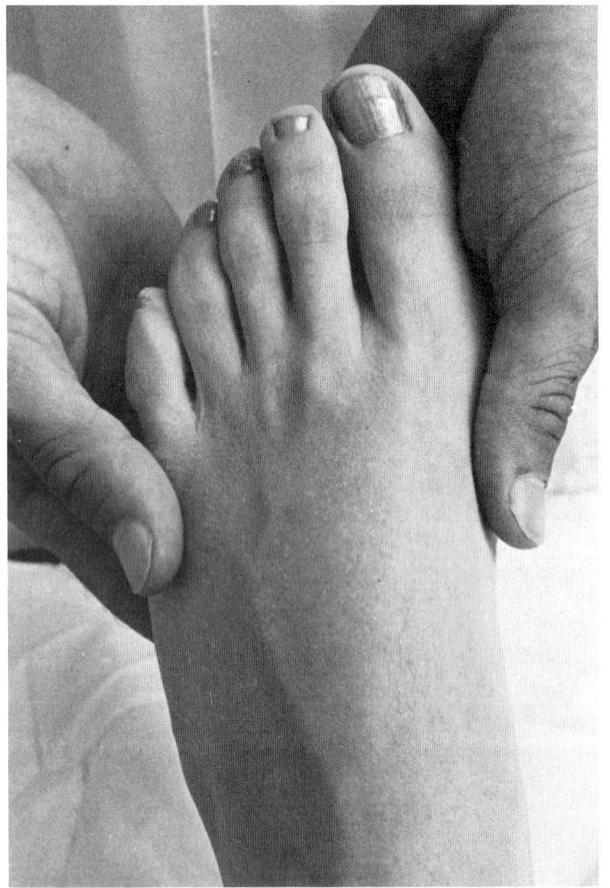

C

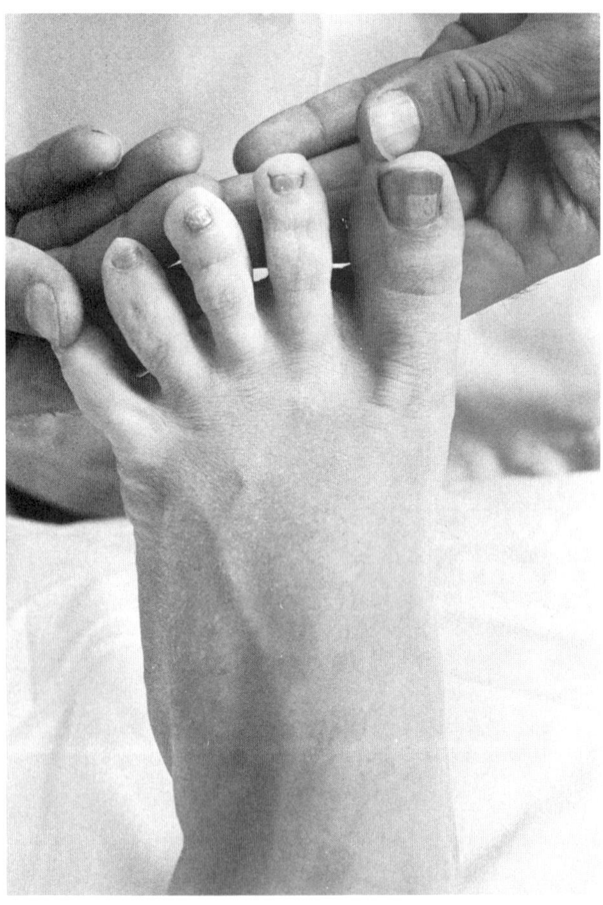

D

FIGURE 26-25. Metatarsophalangeal joint. A. Flexion. B. Extension. C. Adduction (neutral). D. Abduction.

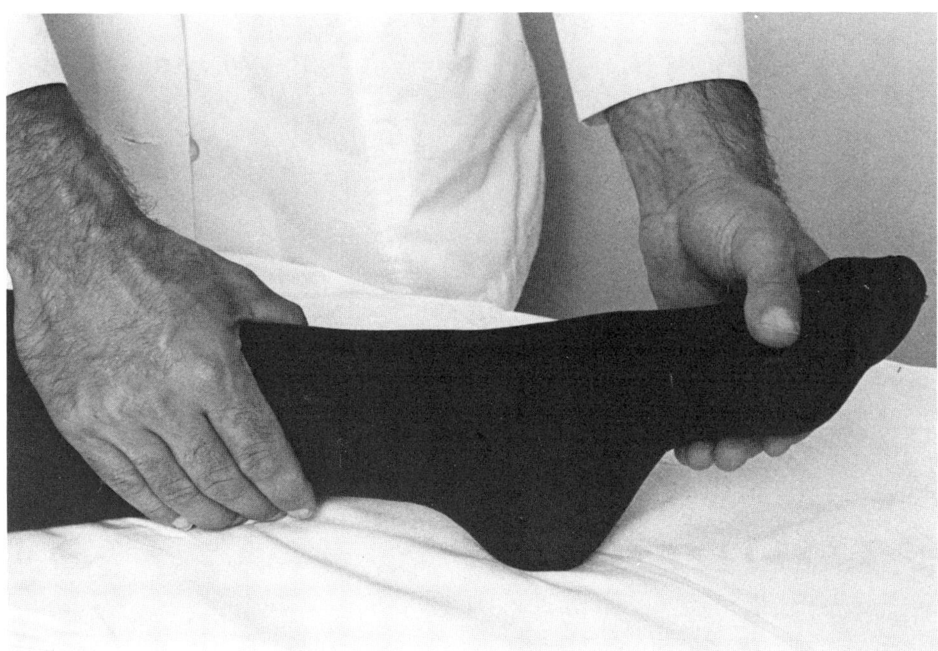

A

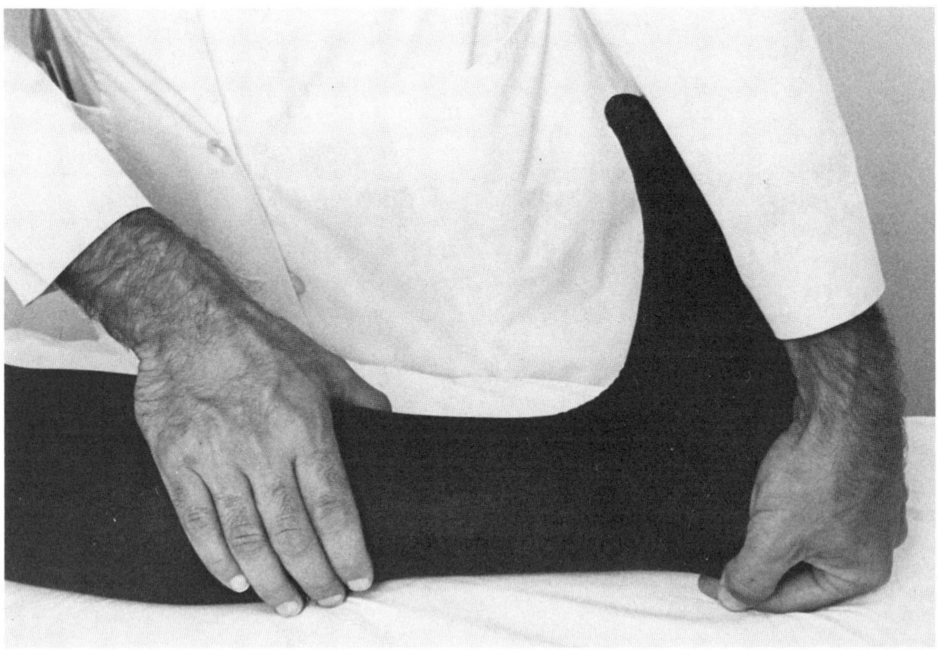

B

FIGURE 26-26. A. Ankle plantar flexion. B. Dorsiflexion. C. Eversion. D. Inversion.

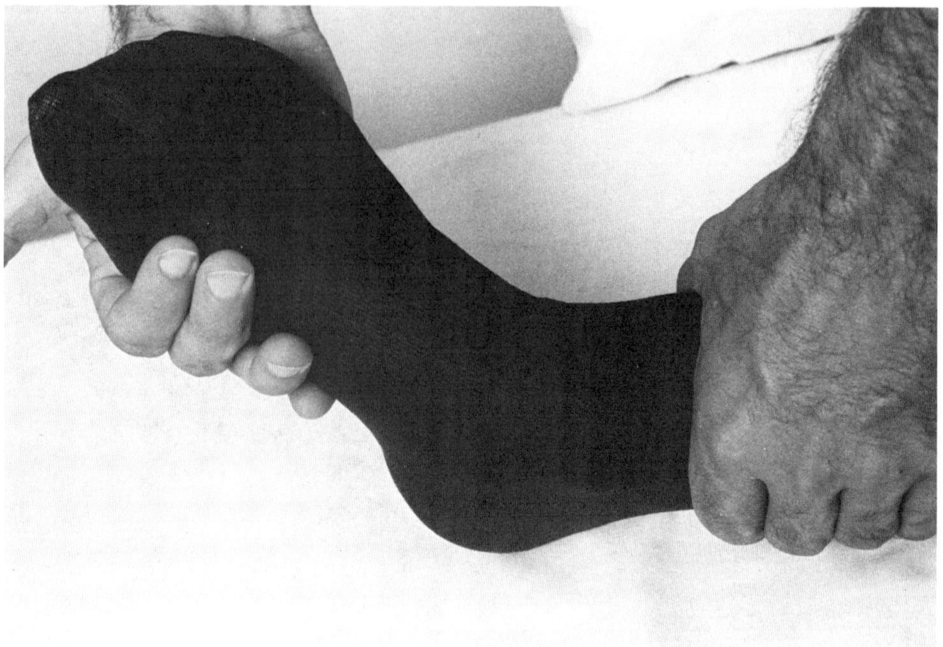

C

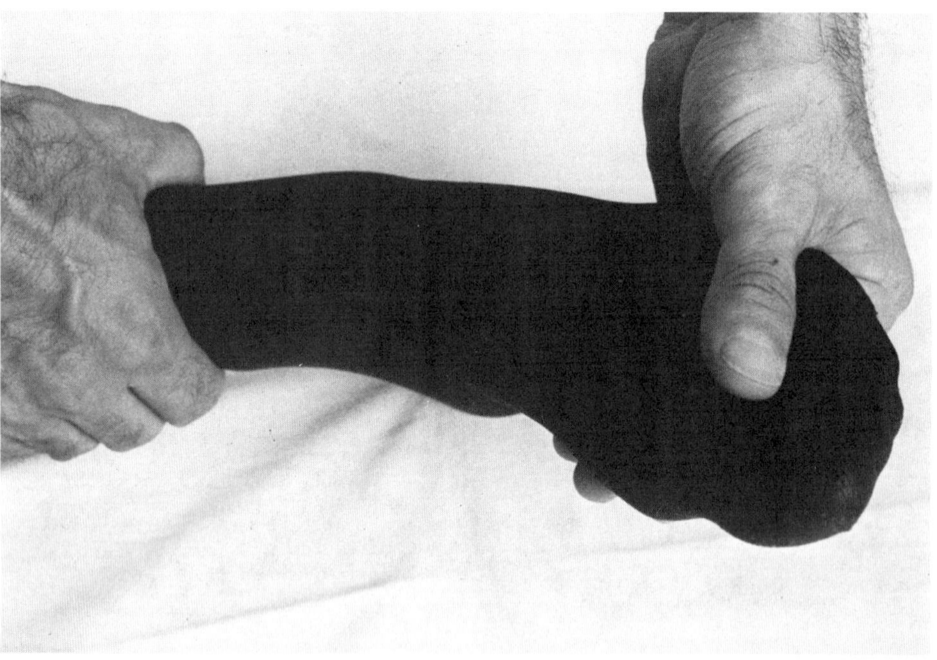

D

FIGURE 26-26 (CONTINUED)

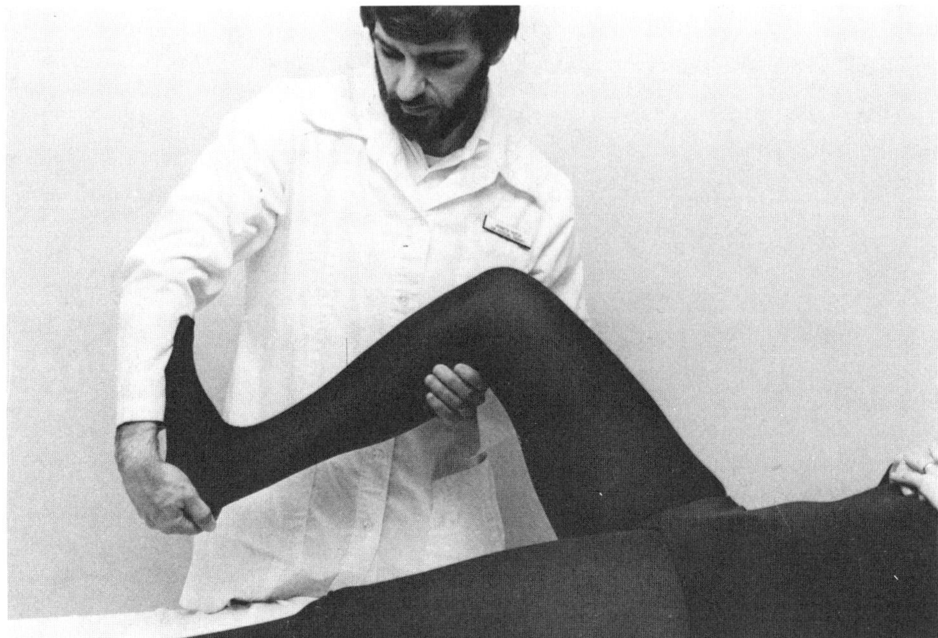

A

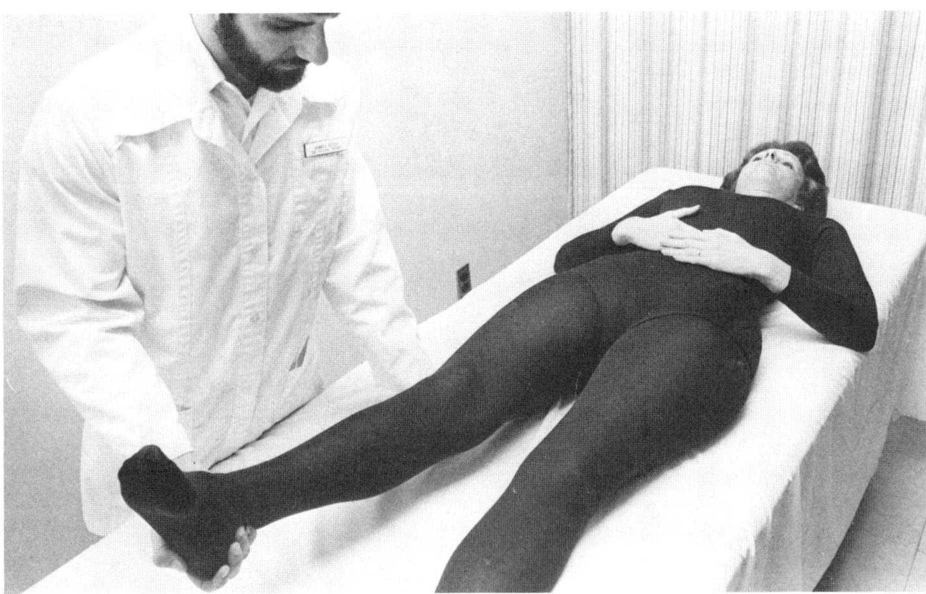

B

FIGURE 26-27. A. Knee flexion. B. Knee extension.

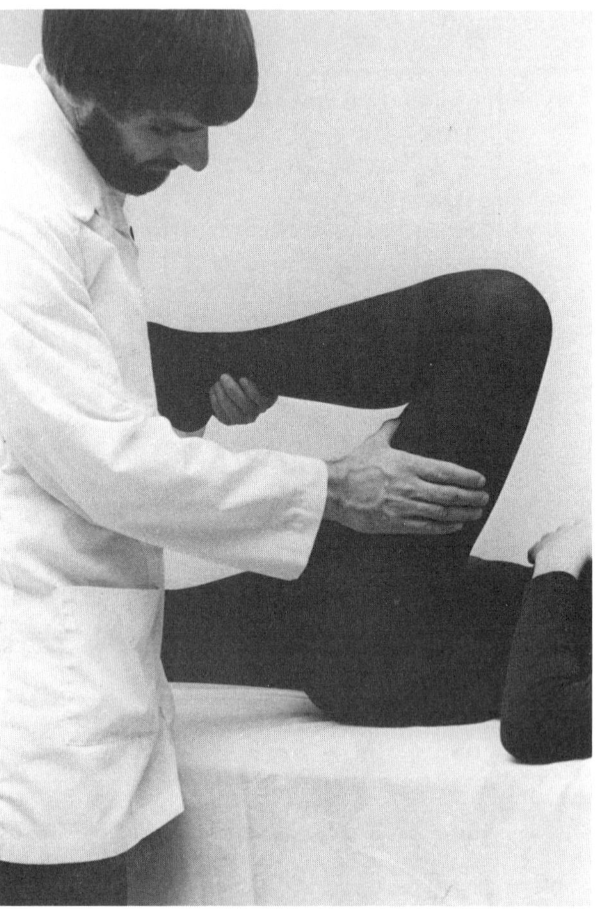

A

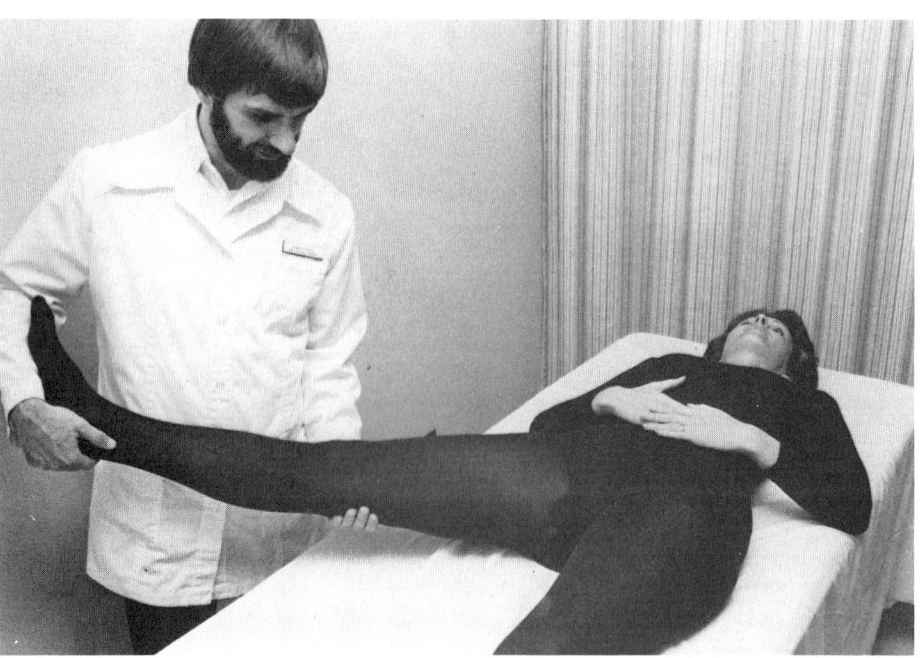

B

FIGURE 26-28. A. Hip flexion. B. Abduction. C. Adduction (neutral position). D. Internal rotation. E. External rotation. F. External rotation in a newborn.

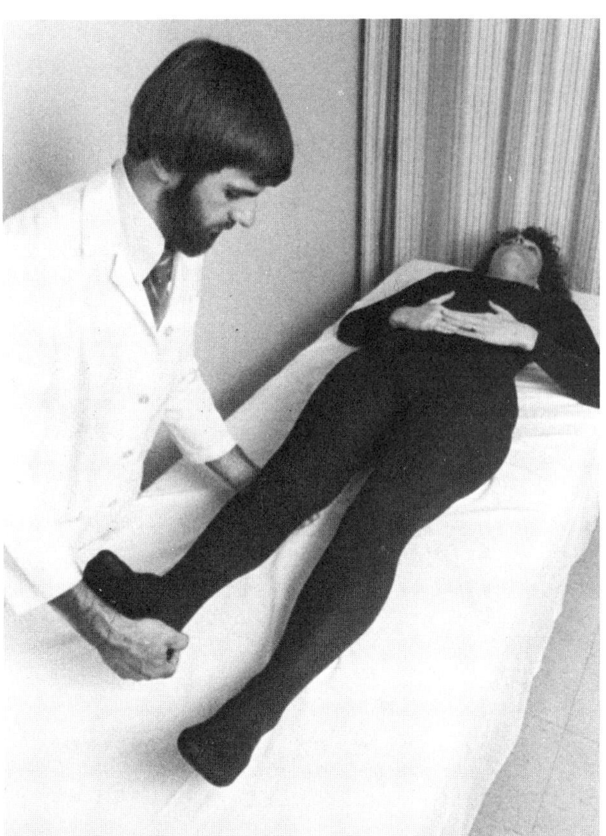

C

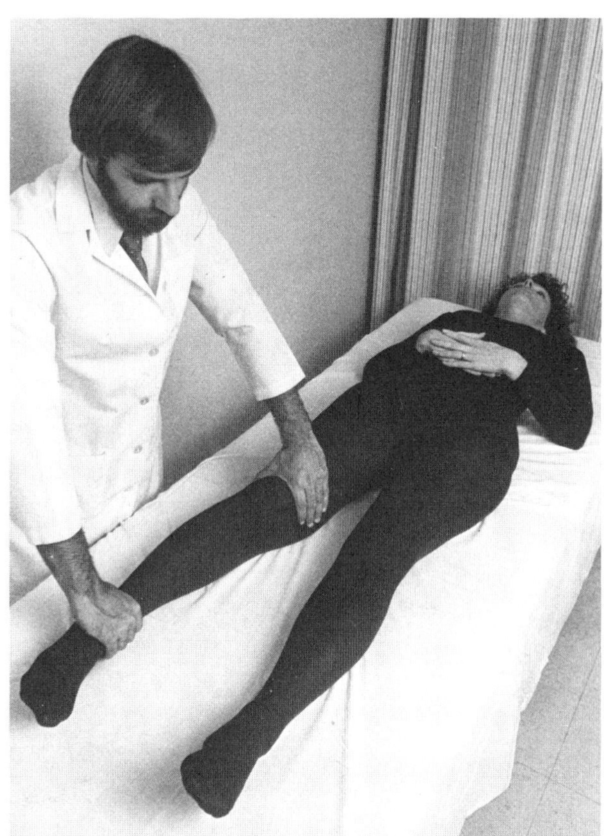

D

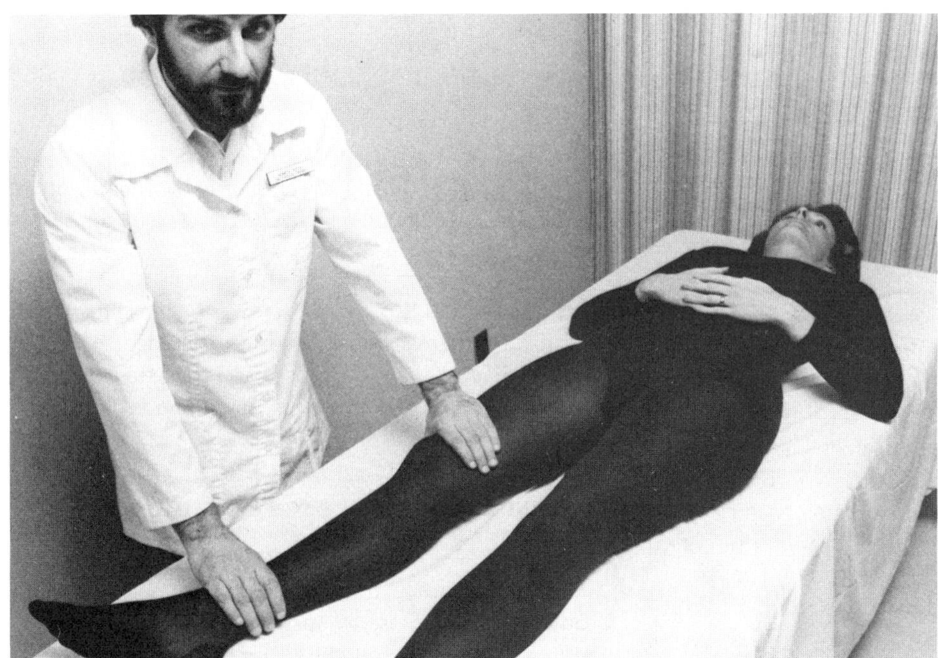

E

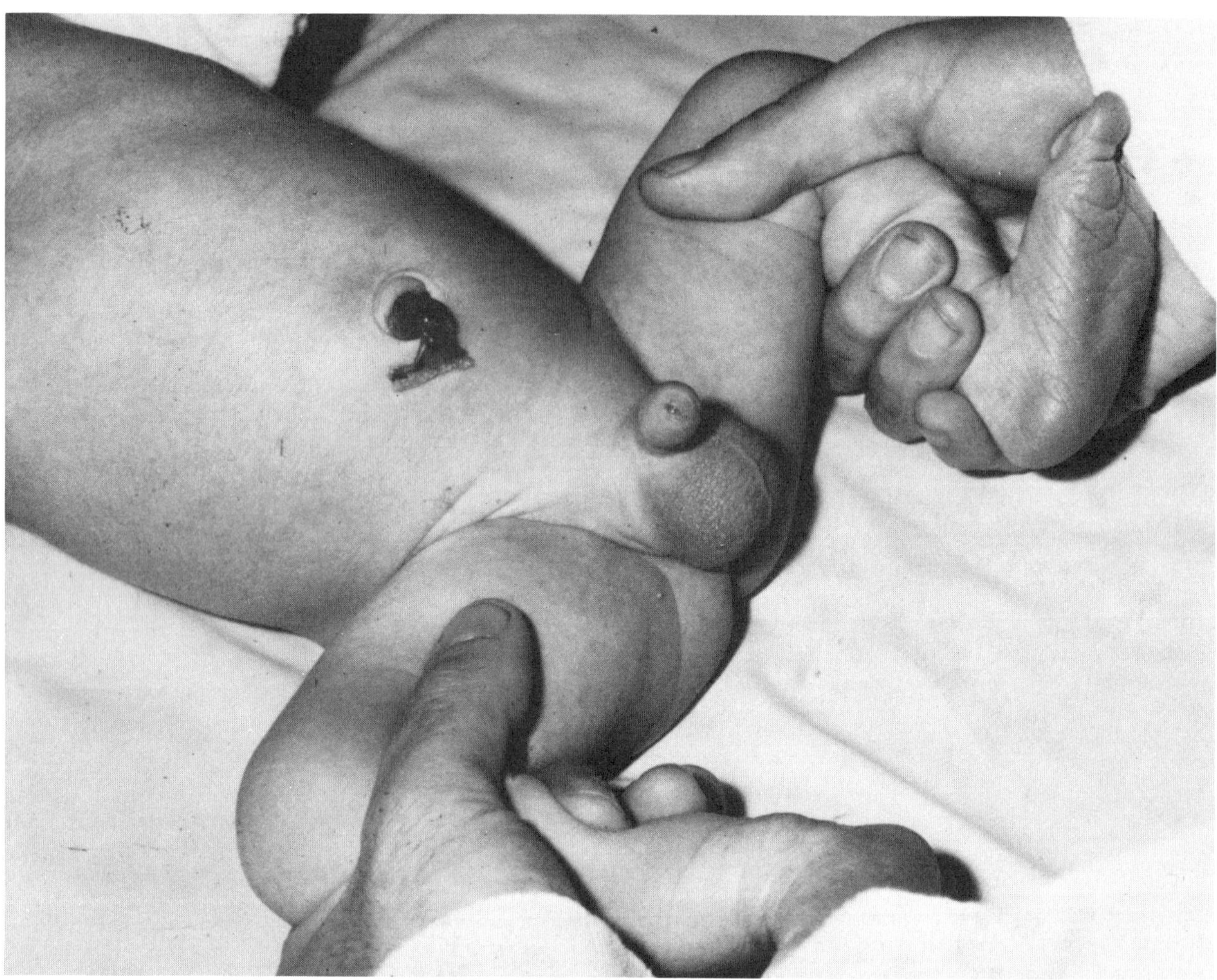

F

FIGURE 26-28 (CONTINUED)

ISOMETRIC EXERCISES

Ordinarily, a muscle contracts so fully that it shortens in length. This is termed an *isotonic* contraction.

If no joint movement is permitted during contraction, and actual length does not change, the exercise is termed *isometric*. Isometric exercise is easily accomplished by a person confined to bed and minimizes loss of muscle strength and size. Isometric exercises are contraindicated for people with cardiac limitations because they increase peripheral resistance and ventricular pressure.

A common isometric exercise is "setting." The person concentrates on a muscle, contracts it, holds it contracted for 10 seconds, and then allows it to relax completely. This works well with abdominal, perineal, gluteal, biceps, triceps, and quadriceps muscles.

Isometric exercise can also be resistive exercise. The person exerts a force against a solid object as if trying to move it or pull it. Pushing against a footboard, locking the hands and attempting to pull them apart, placing the hands on the bed and attempting to lift the hips up, and attempts at lifting or chinning by means of an overbed trapeze are all resistive exercise (see QRS 26-1).

Effect of Exercises. Isometric exercises increase the blood pressure by increasing peripheral resistance so people with cardiac limitations must not be started on these exercise programs until their heart action is stable and

☐ QUICK REFERENCE STOP 26-1: HEALTH TEACHING

Most people are aware that exercise is good for them but think of exercise as push-ups, jogging, or weight lifting. They discount the value of simpler exercise, such as walking across their hospital room, transferring to a wheelchair, or turning in bed. Teach the value of this so that when a person returns home he does not omit exercise entirely, waiting until he is well enough to do what he typically thinks of as exercise.

able to function adequately with the increased arterial pressure. When persons with cardiac disease begin these exercises, they are instructed to breathe out as they exercise so they do not hold their breath.

If a person holds his breath while exercising, the increase in pressure in the respiratory system from the closed glottis results in an overall increased intrathoracic pressure. This pressure causes increased systolic and diastolic blood pressure and decreases venous return and filling of the heart. When exhalation occurs, intrathoracic pressure decreases, and venous return increases greatly. The sudden volume overload on the left ventricle can cause severe tachycardia.

This phenomenon is called *Valsalva's maneuver.* It also occurs if a person holds his breath while straining to pass stool or to move in bed. As long as the glottis is not closed, this increased intrathoracic pressure does not occur. Exhaling ensures the glottis being open.

Exercise Tolerance. Exercise tolerance promotes circulation and respiration. A person's tolerance or optimal exercise level can be determined by measuring his pulse rate. Exercise that makes a person work at about 60 percent of capacity is ideal. To determine an optimal heart rate (termed the *target heart rate*), subtract the person's age from 220 and take 60 percent of this number. Check the pulse rate 10 seconds after completion of exercise to determine whether the pulse rate rises to about this limit.

A person with cardiac limitations is usually not allowed to increase his pulse rate by more than 20 beats per minute, a number that may be below the optimal heart rate by the formula.

AMBULATION

Helping people ambulate is a major nursing responsibility because early ambulation is the best safeguard against the damage of immobility.

GAIT

Gait is the pattern or characteristics of a person's walk. The average person walks by placing his heel on the ground first and smoothly allowing his weight to come forward to the ball of the foot; he keeps his feet parallel; and he shifts his weight easily and comfortably from one foot to the other. As a person shifts his weight, he swings his other foot forward, and the arm opposite the swinging foot moves in the same cadence.

Gait is described in terms of ease, balance, pace (steps per minute), smoothness, and length and width of step. The average person walks at a pace of about 70 to 100 steps per minute. Observing a person's gait and the pattern of wear on his shoes are both good ways to discover his normal pattern.

People with cerebellum brain disease are unsteady as they walk. People with spasticity (upper motor neuron damage) may develop a contracture of the Achilles tendon at the back of the heel, causing plantar flexion of the foot so the person walks on his toes. Older people may walk with small, halting steps due to neurological changes and decreased motion in joints.

HELPING A PERSON AMBULATE

A person who has been in bed for a long time will feel unstable the first few times he is out of bed because of muscle weakness. He may feel dizzy from orthostatic hypotension. Always remain with a person while he walks the first time to be certain he is able to walk unaided and will not fall.

Be certain that the patient is wearing stable shoes. It is better to wear street shoes than soft bedroom slippers that offer little support. Modesty should be protected with a robe over an open-backed or scanty gown. Be certain the person is dressed warmly enough if there are drafts in the hallway.

To help a patient walk, support him by placing one hand under his arm (Fig. 26-29A) and walking with a wide stance for stability. If a person has a weak and strong side, walk at his weak side. Do not hesitate to ask another health care provider to help you, especially the first time a patient is out of bed following surgery or a long illness.

A person unstable on his feet may feel secure if he walks with a straight-backed chair or wheelchair in front of him (Fig. 26-29B). Avoid aids such as a harness around the patient's waist that harm his self-esteem.

Ambulation with Equipment. Following surgery, people are asked to ambulate only hours after they recover from anesthesia. At the time they still have equipment such as intravenous fluid therapy and Foley (bladder) catheters in place. Always safeguard this equipment before helping the person out of bed. A Foley cathether could be clamped; if you do not clamp it, be careful not to raise the drainage bag above the person's bladder or urine will backflow, possibly leading to bladder infection. Provide a portable intravenous pole for easy movement with fluid infusion; be certain that the tubing does not kink or dislodge from a sudden pull on it (Fig. 26-30).

Protection While Ambulating. Occasionally a person may not appreciate how weak he is when he starts to walk. Walking with him allows you to protect him from falling. If he should suddenly feel dizzy, lean him back against your outstretched leg and gently lower him to

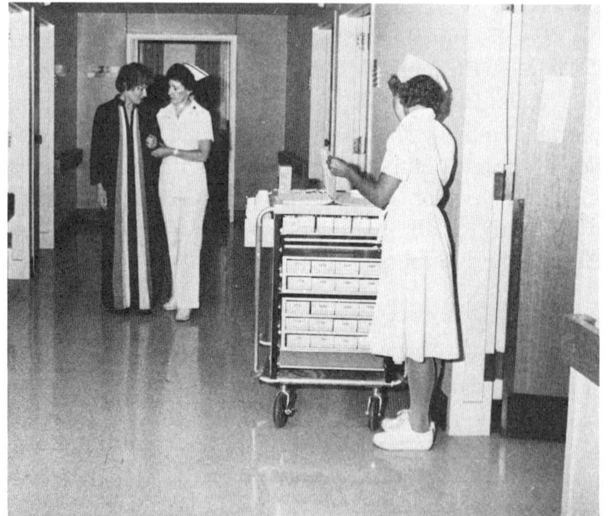

A

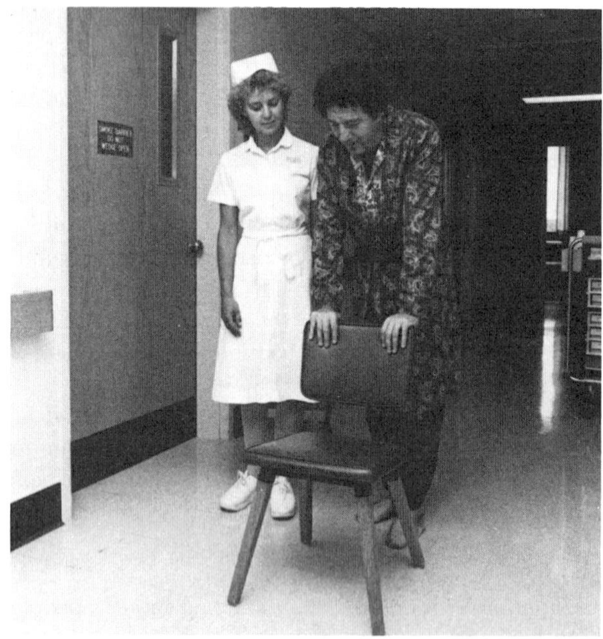

B

FIGURE 26-29. A. Helping a person ambulate. B. Using a straight-backed chair to help ambulation.

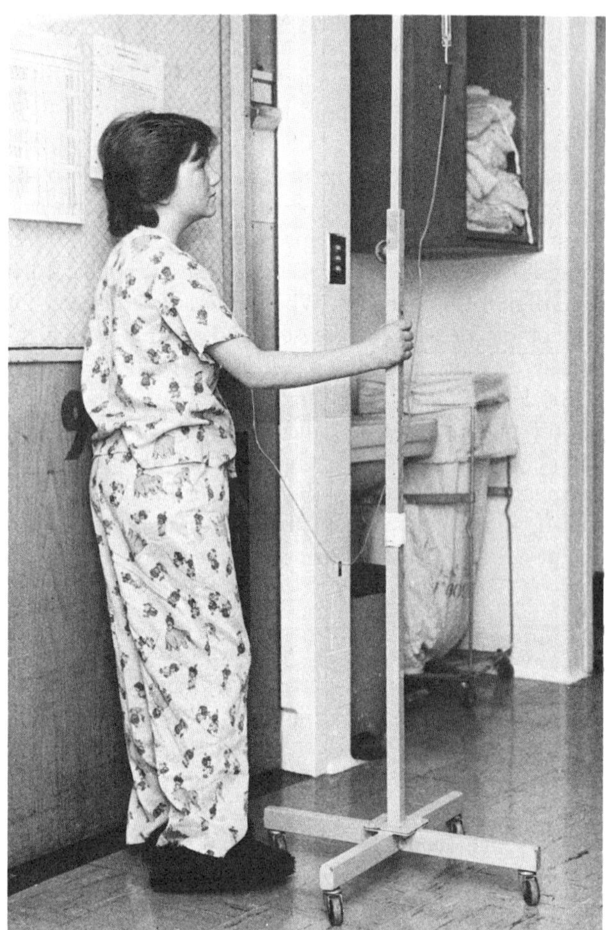

FIGURE 26-30. Many people need to be provided with a portable intravenous pole in order to be ambulatory. Here a schoolager is able to ambulate by herself.

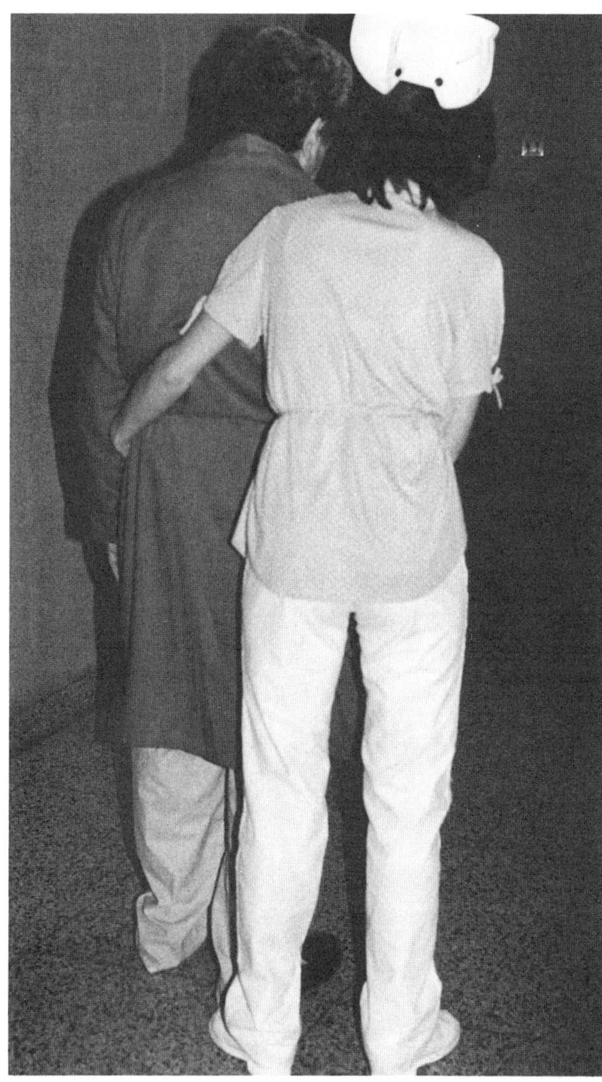

A

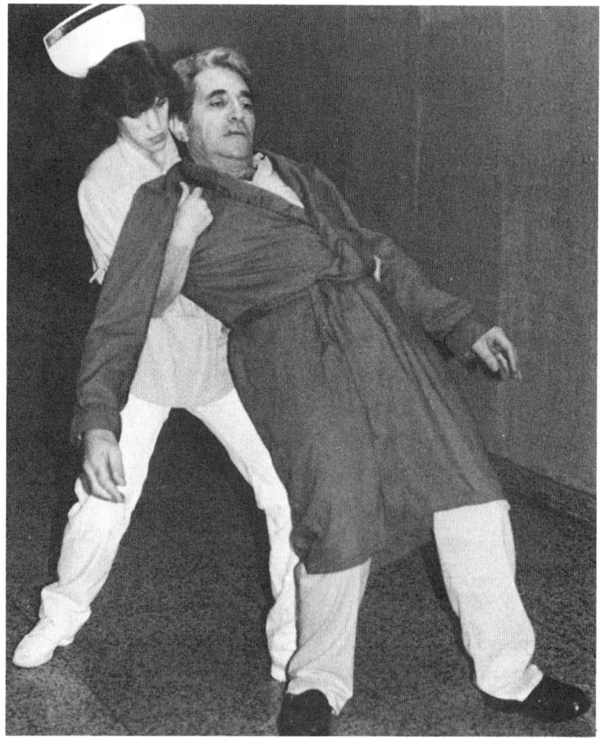

B

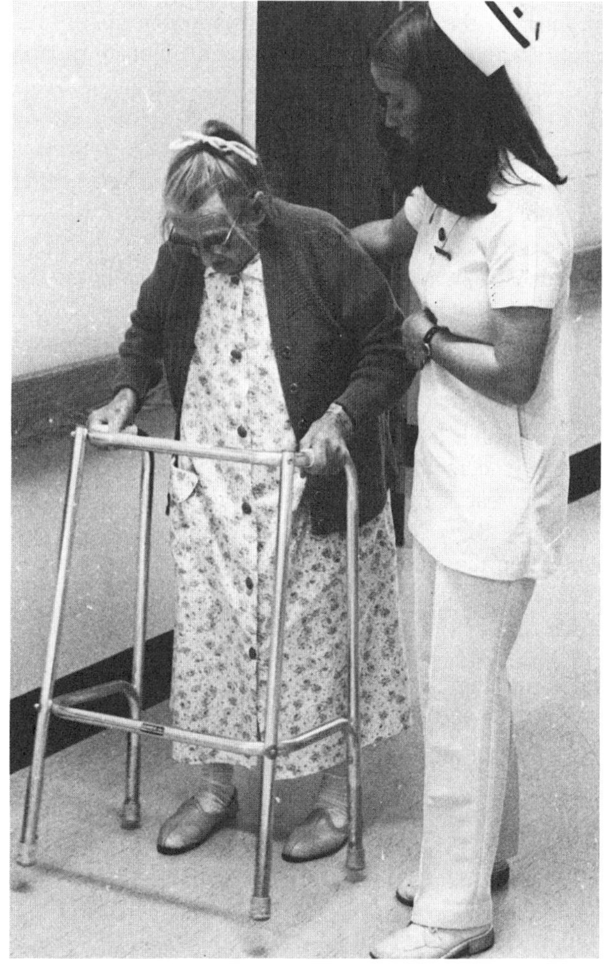

C

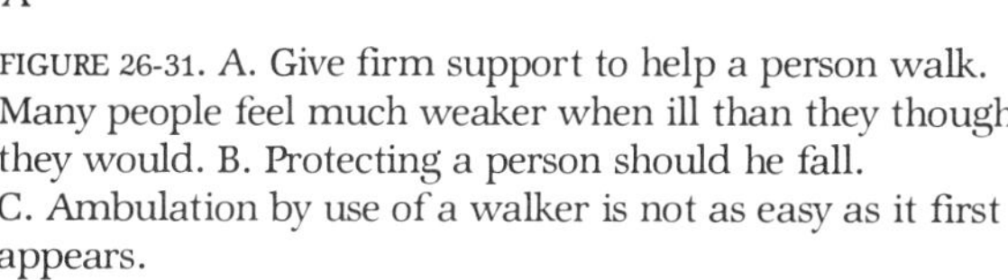

FIGURE 26-31. A. Give firm support to help a person walk. Many people feel much weaker when ill than they thought they would. B. Protecting a person should he fall. C. Ambulation by use of a walker is not as easy as it first appears.

the floor (Fig. 26-31A, B). This situation should rarely happen because your initial assessment of the patient's condition and your unhurried approach to ambulation with time to "dangle" on the side of the bed first prevents it.

USING A WALKER

A *walker* is a metal frame that a person can lean on to maintain a stable gait (Fig. 26-31C). Walkers feel firm and stable because of their wide base. Teach people to pick up the walker to move it, not to push it forward, so that it crosses floor cracks and rugs easily. A person with weak muscle strength in his upper arms may have difficulty doing this. A person may not be able to use one in a small apartment if there is not enough room for its broad base.

CRUTCH WALKING

Crutch walking is prescribed for patients for one of three reasons: to keep weight off one or both legs, to support weakened legs, or to maintain balance. Usually, a physical therapist measures crutch length and gives beginning instruction in crutch walking. You need to be familiar with the measurement of crutches and the supervision of crutch walking in order to give emotional support to the person as he learns and to assess his progress at ambulatory return appointments or during a visit in his home.

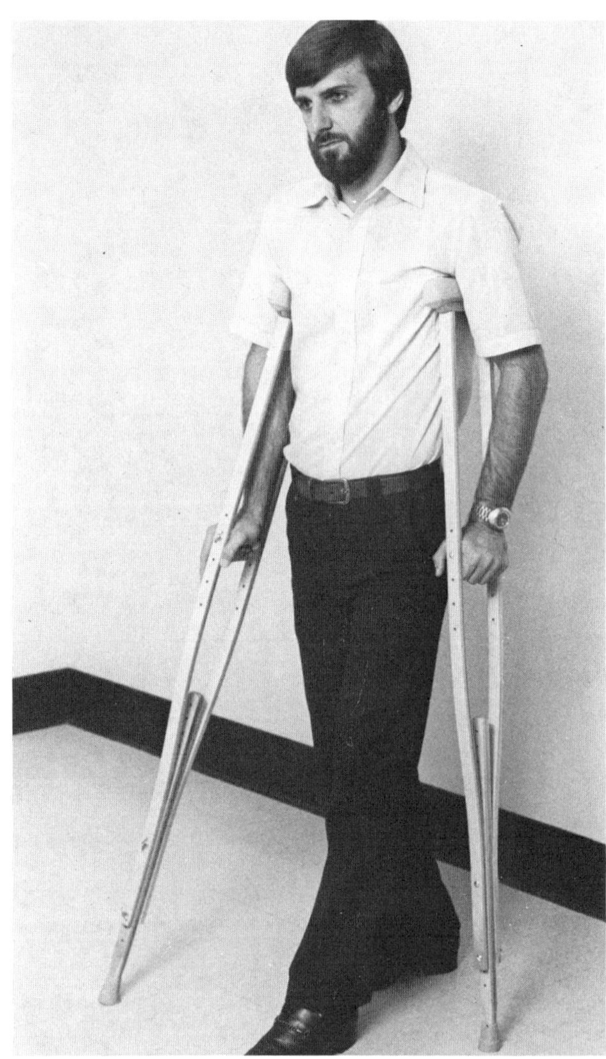

FIGURE 26-32. Crutches fitted so that when the person stands upright, his elbow bends about 20 degrees. Always check to see that crutches have intact rubber tips to prevent slipping and an axilla pad.

Measuring Crutches. Crutches are measured and fitted by a physical therapist. To assess for proper length, ask the person to stand with the crutches wearing the shoes he will use to walk in. With the crutch tip 6 inches to the side of his foot and about 2 inches in front, there should be a 1- to 1 1/2-inch space between the axilla crutch pad and his axilla. Placing two fingers between the crutch top and the axilla is a good rule of thumb to ensure proper crutch length.

When a person stands upright and places his hand on the handrest of the crutch, his elbow should flex about 20 degrees (Fig. 26-32). This means that when he bears weight on the crutch, his body weight will be borne by his arm, not his axilla. Pressure of a crutch against the axilla may lead to compression and damage of the brachial plexus nerves as they cross the axilla, resulting in permanent nerve palsy. Teach people not to rest with the crutch pad pressing on the axilla but always to support their weight at the hand grip.

Two-Point Gait. Two main crutch-walking patterns are used. A two-point gait is a crutch-walking pattern used when the person needs support for weakened muscles or balance but may bear weight on both lower extremities. The person places his right crutch and left foot forward, then left crutch and right foot forward, and so on. Using the crutch opposite a foot provides a wider base of support than would the crutch next to the foot. Caution people to take small steps until they feel confident (Fig. 26-33).

Three-Point (Swing-Through) Gait. A three-point swing-through gait is used when no weight-bearing is allowed on one foot. The crutches are both brought forward. The weight of the body is shifted forward as both legs are swung through the crutches. The person bears weight on his good leg and moves the crutches forward again (Fig. 26-34). It takes strong arm support to bear full weight on crutches this way. Be certain the person is bearing weight on his hands, and not the axillae, as he

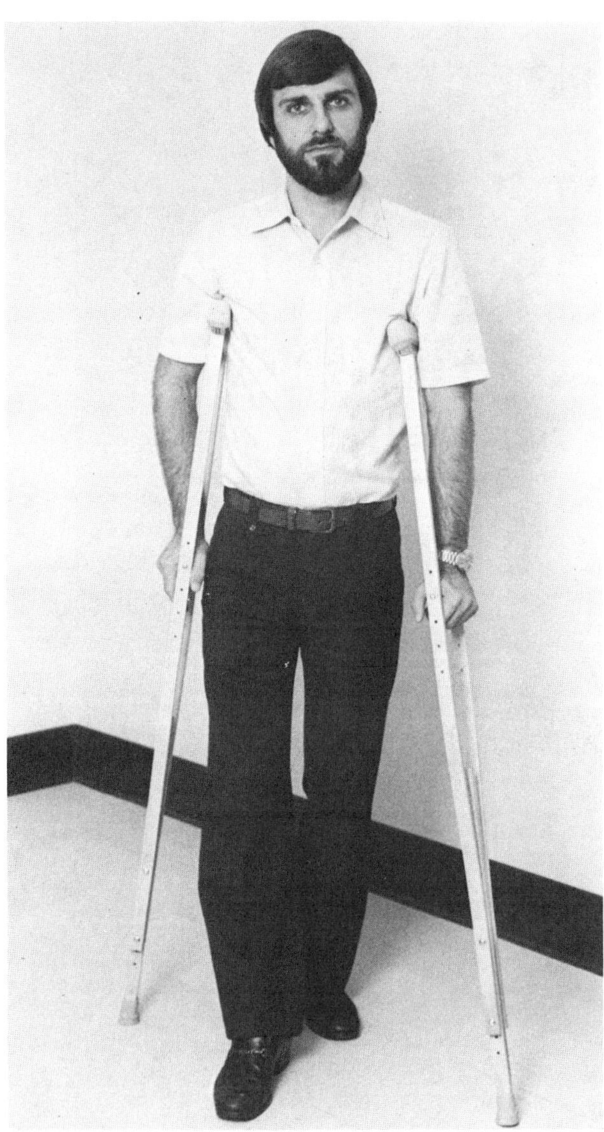

FIGURE 26-33. A two-point gait. Crutch and opposite limb move simultaneously together to provide a wide base of support.

swings through. Some young people use a swing-through gait rather recklessly and need to slow their pace to a safer one.

To walk downstairs, the person places the crutches on the lower step, then swings his good foot forward and down to that step. To go upstairs he places his good foot on the elevated step, then raises the crutches on the step and lifts himself up. To help him remember this pattern, he learns that "angels" (the good foot) go up; "devils" (the bad foot with the crutches) go down.

Canadian or Lofstrand Crutches. A Lofstrand or Canadian crutch is a metal crutch with an armband that circles and supports the forearm to keep the crutch from falling. Because it does not reach the axilla, there is no pressure on the axilla to cause nerve damage. People with neuromuscular disease are the most frequent users of this crutch (Fig. 26-35).

Assisting with Crutch Walking. A person needs strong upper arms and shoulders in order to use crutches effectively without muscle fatigue or cramping. Isometric exercises such as holding muscles contracted for 10 seconds, then relaxing them, and locking the fingers and pulling to separate them are helpful. Pressing on the bed to raise the buttocks off the bed is also helpful.

Always check the tips of crutches to see that the rubber tip is intact and not worn through. The tip prevents the crutch from slipping when it is placed. Be certain that the person places the crutch tips 6 to 10 inches to the side of his foot. This furnishes a wide base for support. Be certain that the person is not resting the crutch in his axilla, compressing the radial nerve.

If the person is going to go home with crutches, he will need to learn to maneuver stairs. Explore with him any problems he anticipates, such as a long walk from where he must park his car to his apartment. If he carries a briefcase to work or books to school, he may prefer to wear a backpack until he is free of crutches so he can leave his hands free for the handrests (see QRS 26-2).

Ask him to clear articles such as throw rugs and small footstools out of the paths at home. If there are small children at home, they will need to keep the traffic areas free of toys. Slippery floors will be difficult to navigate with crutches.

CANES

Canes are helpful for people who can bear weight but need support for balance on an injured leg or foot.

A cane serves as a third point of support for the person. It is the proper length when the handle reaches the height of the greater trochanter of the femur. The person holds the cane in the hand opposite the injured extremity and advances it at the same time. The good foot is then moved forward while body weight is maintained on the cane and the injured foot.

Moving downstairs, the person advances the cane and the injured leg first; then the good leg. To go upstairs, he advances the good leg first, then the cane and injured leg.

Most people prefer simple wooden canes. A person with poor balance may use a tripod (three-legged) or quad (four-legged) metal cane (Fig. 26-36). Check the tips of canes for worn spots that would slip easily. Caution the person to remove throw rugs from places they will be walking, and to beware of smooth slippery floors.

WHEELCHAIRS

Wheelchairs come in child, junior, and adult sizes. The seat and back is made of vinyl. When positioning a

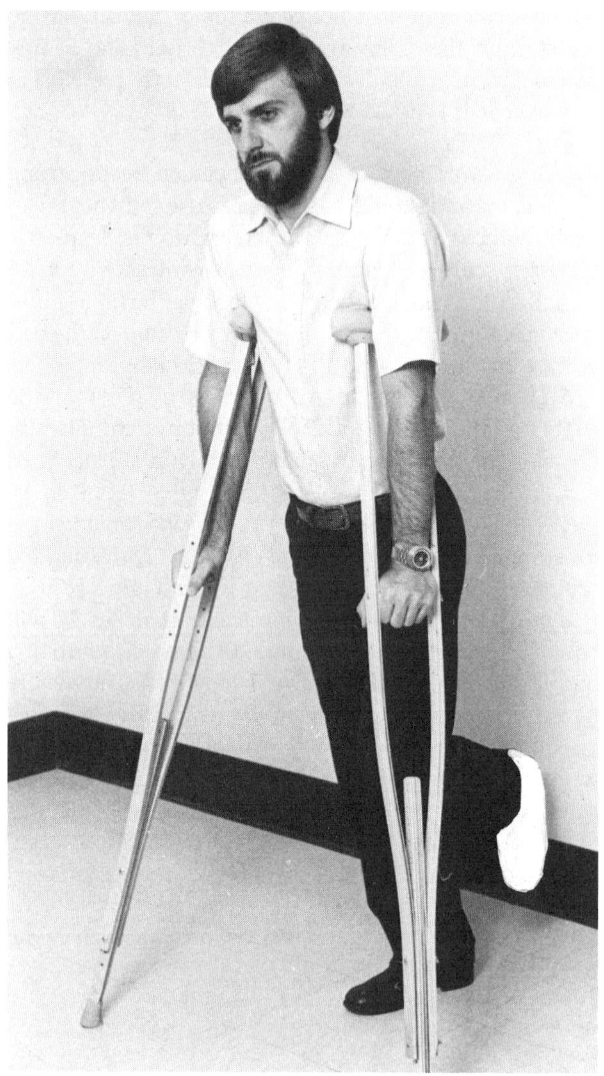

A

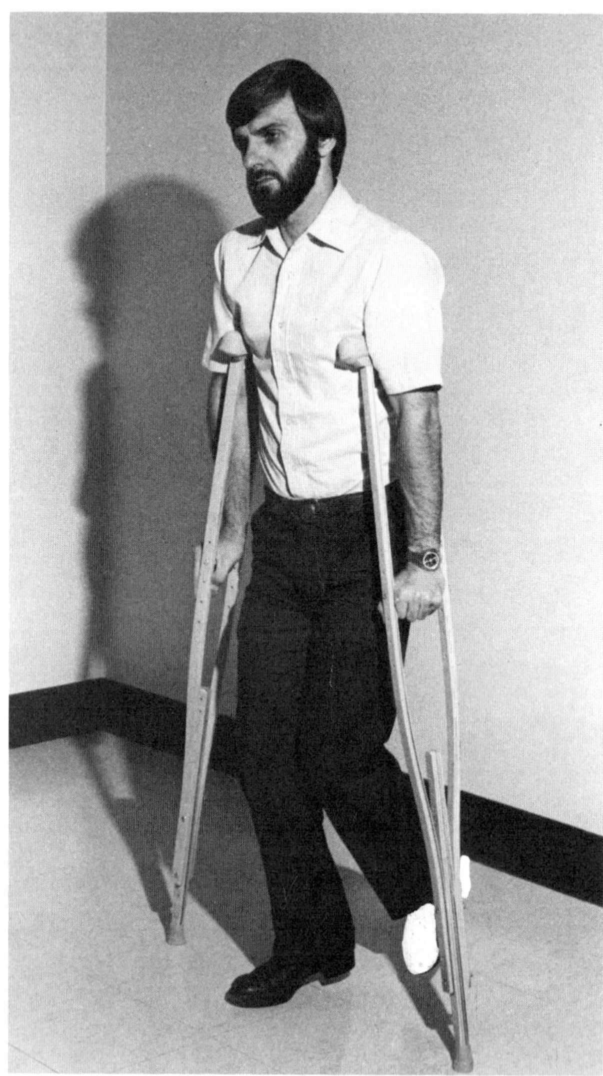

B

person in a wheelchair, provide a pad or blanket on the seat of the wheelchair to absorb perspiration. Assess the height of the footrests. If rests are too high, the person's knee and hip are bent too sharply, impeding circulation. If the rests are too low, the person's feet hang in plantar flexion (footdrop) and can form contractures over a period of time.

The purpose of providing a wheelchair for a patient rather than a bedside chair is to give him mobility to see sights he could not otherwise see. Take advantage of the wheelchair to encourage social interaction or a change of scene that would not otherwise be possible. Some people need a restraint to help them stay in good body alignment in a wheelchair. Use restraints as necessary for safety if you will be leaving the person alone (on use of restraints, see Chap. 27). Be certain that a wheelchair is locked before a person sits in it or stands to get out of it (see QRSs 26-3, 26-4).

STRETCHERS

Stretchers are a means of transportation for immobilized people who are unable to sit in a wheelchair. They are used to transport people to surgery or other hospital departments. They can also be used in the same way as wheelchairs to provide social interaction or a change of scene. The time a person is lying on a stretcher rather than in bed is an ideal time to wash his hair because a stretcher can be brought next to a sink.

Always use safety straps or siderails on stretchers. They are potentially dangerous because they are so narrow; a person could fall from one if not properly protected.

FRAMES

A person who is immobilized may be turned from a supine to a prone position by means of a turning frame,

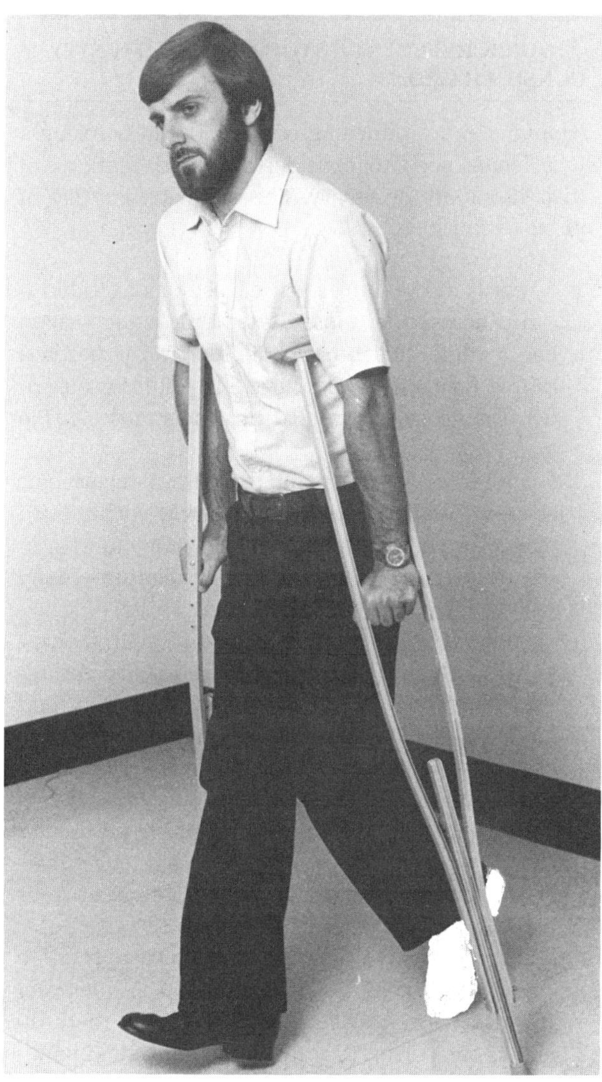

C

FIGURE 26-34. A three-point swing through gait. A. Crutches are advanced with the affected limb held off the floor. B. Weight is taken on the hand grips to lift the body and swing through the crutches. C. The heel of the nonaffected limb makes contact with the floor to complete the pattern; the bandaged foot does not touch the floor. Crutches are then lifted and advanced again.

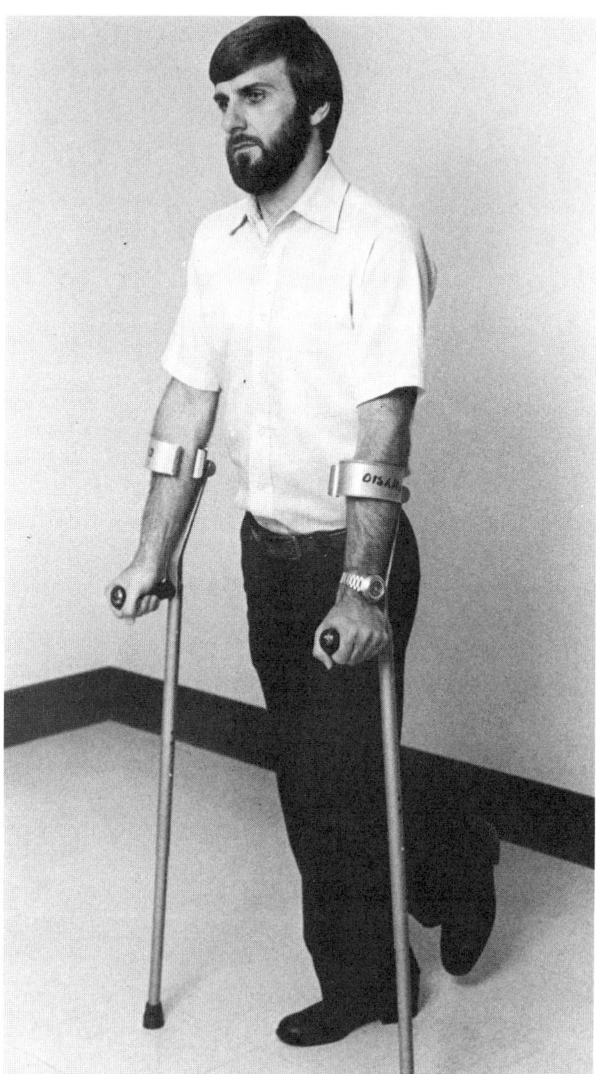

FIGURE 26-35. A three-point gait using Lofstrand crutches.

and from prone to supine the same way. These Stryker or Foster frames have a posterior frame of canvas stretched across steel bars (Fig. 26-37A). The patient rests on this posterior surface. A matching anterior frame is placed over him, and the two frames are locked together. By means of a pivoting device on the ends, the frame is turned so the bottom frame becomes the top, and the person is completely turned from a supine to prone position. The process is reversed to turn him prone to supine.

Although turning frames are designed to be rotated by one person, it is safer to have two people present as the frame is turned. Be certain that safety straps are in place before turning the frame. Give the person a good explanation of what will happen so he can enjoy the new positioning, and not be frightened by it.

☐ QUICK REFERENCE STOP 26-2: NUTRITION

Obese people have more difficulty transferring and supporting themselves on crutches than other people. Urge a diet high in protein and vitamins for healing, without an excessive carbohydrate level to prevent weight gain.

If a person has a broken bone, he needs calcium for healing, but if he is on bed rest, excessive calcium can be detrimental because bed rest leads to loss of calcium from bones and an elevated blood calcium level. Excessive blood calcium level can lead to kidney stones and possible ureter blockage.

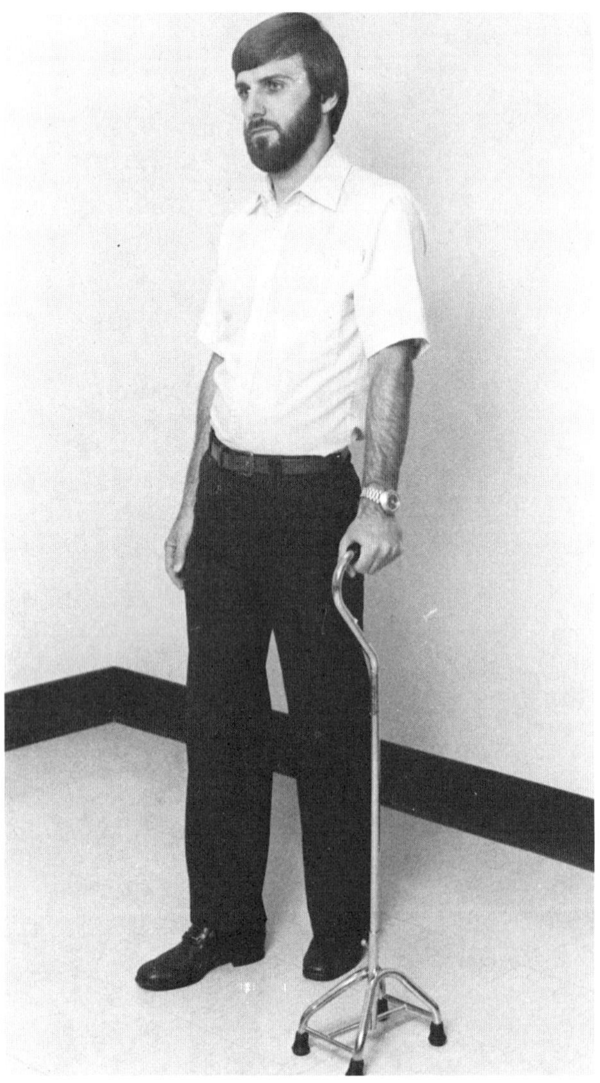

FIGURE 26-36. A three-point (Quad) cane. A cane is held in the hand opposite the injured foot and advanced with it.

CIRCOELECTRIC BED

A Circoelectric bed (Fig. 26-37B) has the features of a Stryker frame except that it is turned electrically rather than manually and is turned in a standing/lying fashion as well as a supine/prone position. As with Stryker frames, do not attempt to use a Circoelectric bed unless you are familiar with its operation. Be certain that safety straps are in place and that both you and patient are fully prepared for the turning.

ACTIVITIES OF DAILY LIVING

Activities of daily living (ADL) is a term originated by physical therapists to denote those activities necessary for independent function. Traditionally, ADL activities include eating, hygiene (bathing; hair, nail, and dental care; shaving), dressing, and body elimination. This

☐ QUICK REFERENCE STOP 26-3: COMMUNITY CONSIDERATIONS

People who are returning home and will be using a wheelchair need to consider what adaptations of their home are necessary. The following is a list of items to consider.

1. *Access to home.* Any local carpenter can build a ramp across the house steps. Unless the person has a motorized wheelchair, the ramp needs a railing for the person to grasp to pull himself upward or to stop himself from moving down too fast.
2. *Living area.* It is difficult to move a wheelchair across a high pile carpet. Covering carpet with plastic is helpful. Throw rugs can tangle in wheels; remove them. Placing furniture along walls allows for increased turning space.
3. *Kitchen.* It is impossible to reach high shelves. Move supplies to bottom cupboards. A mirror angled over stove allows the person to watch food boiling in pots on stove. Stove must have controls at waist height or they cannot be reached. Kitchen tongs are helpful for reaching objects; carry to other rooms as well. Kitchen counters may be too high to work on. Place supplies on a kitchen chair or a lapboard to stir or mix ingredients. Keep floor wax to a minimum; no throw rugs.
4. *Bathroom.* An angled mirror allows a man to shave or a woman to put on makeup. A safety rail by toilet helps transfer. A chair placed in bathtub allows the person to transfer to bathtub. A hand-held shower attachment best provides for self-care.
5. *Safety.* Wall telephone may be too high to use. Be certain person has one to use easily in an emergency and to expand social contacts. A smoke detector on each floor is a wise precaution. A downstairs bedroom is not only safest in case of a fire, but allows the person more self-care ability. Fire departments supply free decals for the bedroom windows of children or those with a handicap. Have him contact local fire department for this safety measure.

☐ QUICK REFERENCE STOP 26-4: ADVOCACY

By federal law, all public buildings must provide easy access for people in wheelchairs. In some small cities, buildings may not be equipped because no one in the city used a wheelchair before. Urge the person to contact his city council about the problem. Free access is a *right*, not a nicety. Advocate for him if his approach is met with less than prompt action.

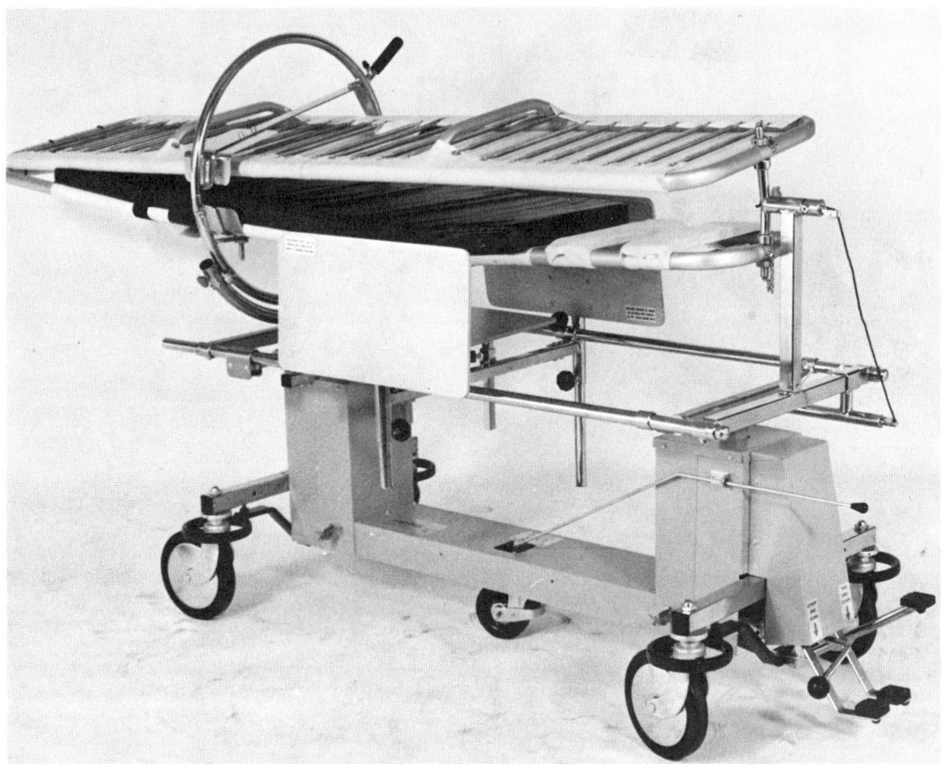

A

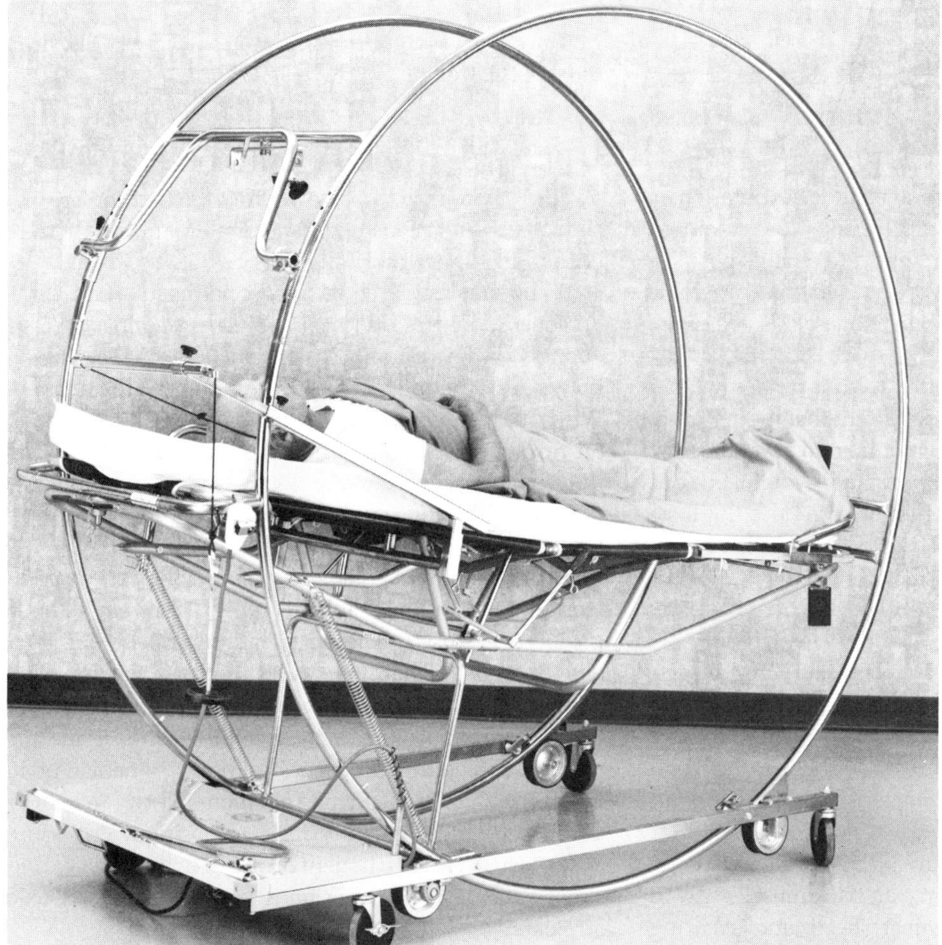

B

FIGURE 26-37. A. A turning frame. B. A Circoelectric bed.

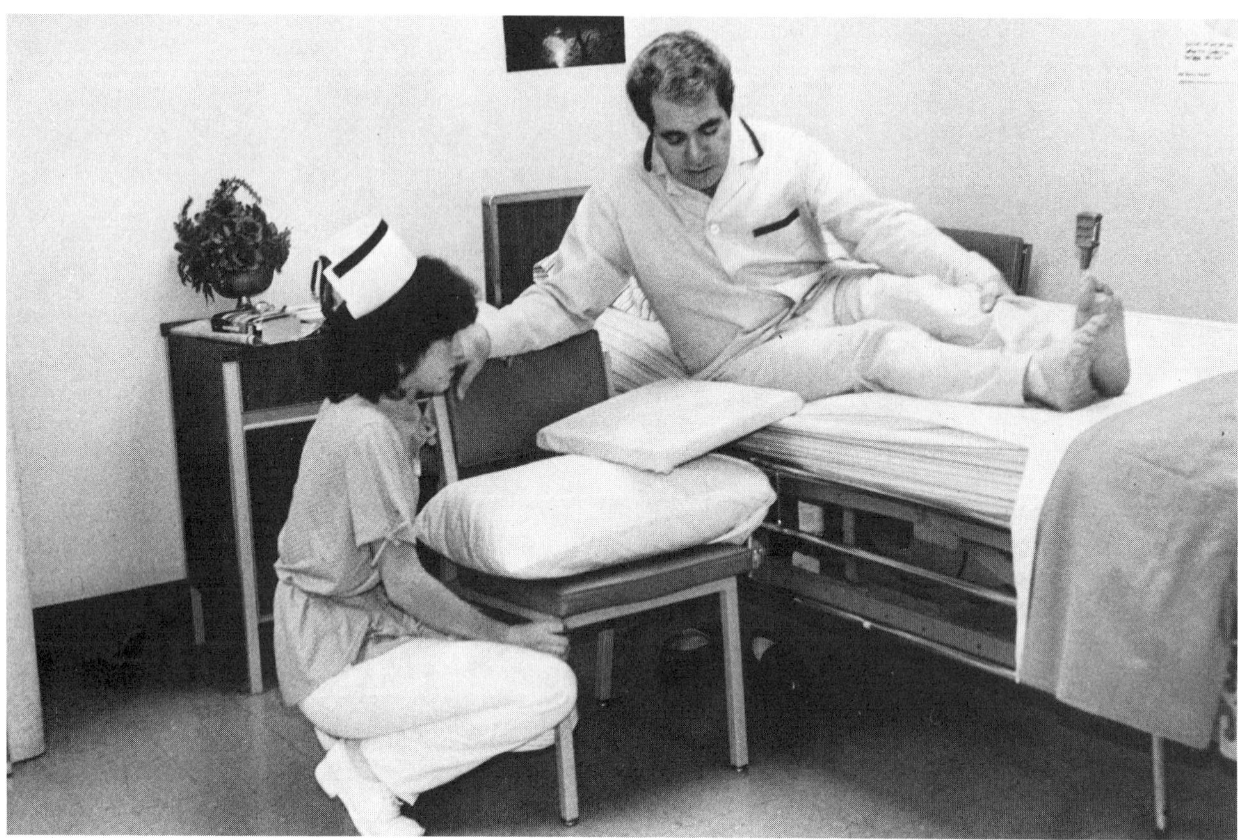

FIGURE 26-38. By use of a small board, a patient who can help himself is able to transfer from bed to chair.

category of activities has come to include ambulation or such activities as the ability to transfer to a chair, to operate a wheelchair independently, to change position in bed, to walk with assistive devices such as braces or crutches, to drive a car, and to help oneself as necessary (Fig. 26-38).

Even with these additions the term is a narrow one. Holistic care of people includes strengthening not only physical functioning but also mental and psychological functioning. A person who can brush his own teeth but does not feel good about himself or who does not have the confidence to relate to people because of his handicap is not fully participating in daily living.

MOVING AND TURNING PATIENTS

Whenever the head of a bed is raised, a person's body tends to slide toward the foot of the bed. Soon, the curve of the bed is at the thoracic level of his back rather than at his buttocks. He is uncomfortable and apt to be in poor body alignment.

When moving people in bed, use good body mechanics so you do not strain your back muscles. Avoid scraping a person's skin against sheets and shearing force by "bouncing" a person across the bed rather than sliding. Always reposition people after moving them to ensure good new body alignment.

To bounce, slide your hands palms up under the person's shoulders and buttocks. Press against the bed enough to cause a gentle rocking motion. As the person's body rises from the rocking motion, move it toward you. With this technique, you are moving the person through air rather than pulling him across the bed. A 100-pound nurse can easily move a 200-pound person by this method with no strain on the nurse's back or friction on the patient's skin.

Immobilized patients need their position changed at least every 2 hours. Establish a schedule so that all body positions are used. Before repositioning people in bed, assess carefully whether you will be able to accomplish it alone. In the presence of a heavy cast or other apparatus, ask for help to avoid muscle strain for yourself and the patient. Procedure 26-1 describes moving a person up in bed; Procedure 26-2, turning a patient in bed; Procedure 26-3, logrolling a person to a new position; Procedure 26-4, transferring a patient from bed to a chair; and Procedure 26-5, transferring a patient from bed to a stretcher.

PROCEDURE 26-1
Moving a Patient Up in Bed

Purpose: To promote good body alignment. To promote a position of comfort.

Plan	*Principle*
1. Wash hands; identify patient; explain procedure.	1. Prevent spread of microorganisms; promote patient safety and well-being.
2. Assess patient status.	2. Nursing care is always individualized based on professional judgment of patient's needs.
3. Analyze appropriateness of plan; adjust plan to individual patient needs.	3. Evaluate whether you will be able to accomplish procedure by yourself. Ask for help as needed to prevent muscle strain on yourself or patient.
4. Implement procedure by bringing bed to high position with head flat.	4. A high bed reduces back strain; a flat bed prevents you from working against gravity.
5. Ask the patient to place his hands on the headboard or siderail of the bed and bend his knees and pull when you say *ready.* Position yourself on the side of bed with a wide-based stance facing the head of the bed (Fig. 1). Place one arm under the patient's shoulders and one under the patient's hips.	5. An informed patient can assist in his own care. A wide-base stance is a stable position.

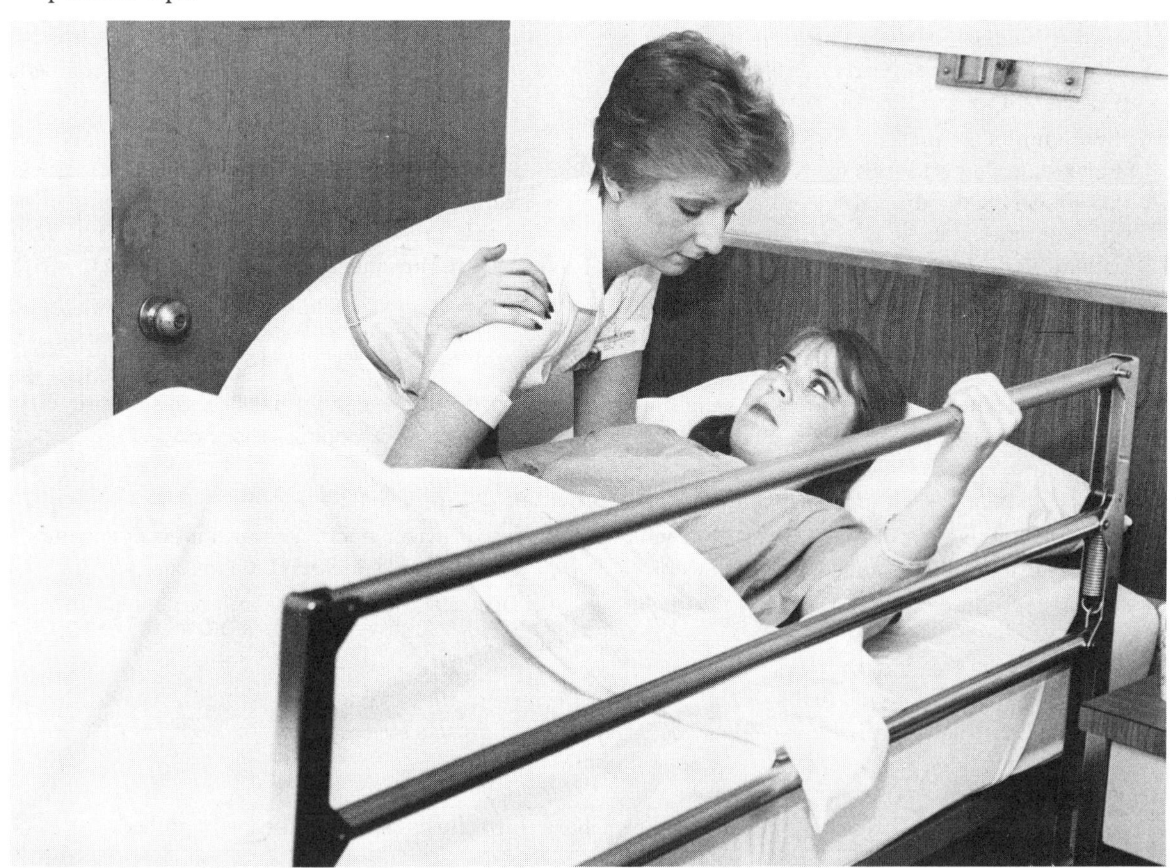

FIGURE 1. Moving a patient in bed who can help herself.

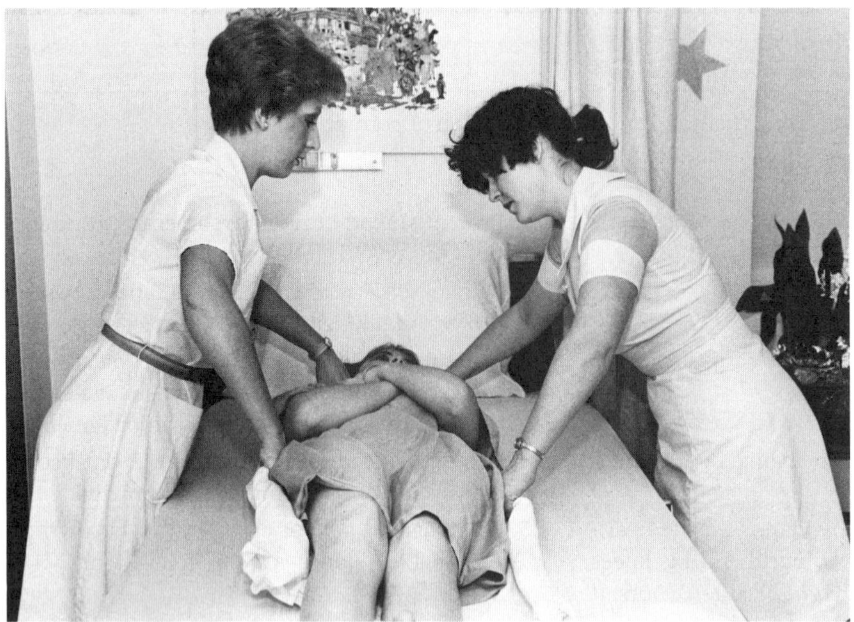

FIGURE 2. Moving a patient in bed who cannot help herself.

6. On your cue, the patient pushes with his heels as you lift his shoulders and hips off the bed and help him slide to the head of the bed by shifting your weight forward to your forward foot.
7. If two nurses are present, each can place a hand under shoulders and hips from both sides of the bed or loosen the drawsheet on the bed, roll it on both sides until it is about 10 in. from the patient, and use it to lift.
8. Check the bed to see it has a smooth surface and sheets have not wrinkled. Straighten appropriately.
9. Reposition patient into good body alignment; provide diversional activity as needed; return bed to low position.
10. Evaluate effectiveness, efficiency, cost, comfort, and safety of the procedure. Plan health teaching such as importance of good body alignment.
11. Record procedure and assessment of findings.

6. Lifting shoulders and hips off the bed reduces friction and so makes movement easier; it prevents shearing force or sliding of subcutaneous tissue compressing tissue blood supply.
7. Rolling the drawsheet strengthens it and prevents it from tearing from the weight. Do not use the patient's axilla to lift; this could put considerable pressure on the radial nerve. Lift, do not slide to prevent sacral pressure. (Fig. 2).
8. Wrinkled sheets can interfere with good circulation.
9. Good body alignment is necessary for prevention of effects of immobilization.
10. Evaluation is the final step of the nursing process. Health teaching is an independent nursing action always included in care.
11. Document nursing care and patient status.

MODIFICATIONS FOR THE CHILD

Children do not slide down in bed as much as adults because of their lighter body weight. A child's weight is often deceptive, however. Ask for help as necessary to avoid muscle strain.

MODIFICATIONS FOR THE OLDER ADULT

If an older adults has arthritic joint changes, he may have difficulty assisting with moving in bed.

PROCEDURE 26-2
Turning a Patient to His Side

Purpose: To ensure comfort and a safe transfer to a new position; to promote good body alignment and change of position; to prevent complications of prolonged bed rest; to turn to a position for increased social interaction.

Plan	*Principle*
1. Wash your hands; identify patient; explain procedure.	1. Prevent spread of microorganisms; promote patient safety and well-being.
2. Assess patient status.	2. Nursing care is always individualized based on professional judgment of patient's needs.
3. Analyze appropriateness of plan; adjust plan to individual patient needs.	3. Evaluate whether you will be able to accomplish procedure by yourself. Ask for help as necessary to prevent muscle strain on yourself or patient.
4. Implement procedure by bringing bed to high position. Provide for intravenous fluid tubing or other apparatus that needs protection during movement. Move the patient to the side of the bed by placing one of your feet in front of the other as you face the bed. Place one arm under the patient's shoulders and one under his hips. By rocking to your rear leg, lift and move him toward you.	4. A high bed position relieves muscle strain on your back. Always lift, do not slide people across bedsheets to prevent skin irritation or damage to subcutaneous tissue. Bouncing or pressing on the bed mattress until a gentle rocking action occurs, then moving the person toward you each time his body rises from the rocking motion is also an effective method of safely moving a patient across a bed surface.
5. If turning the patient to his left side, move him to right side of bed; if turning to right side, move him to left side of bed.	5. Provide room for turning.
6. To turn the patient to the right side, cross the left leg over the right; place the person's arms across the chest. Raise the siderail to walk around the bed.	6. Careful placement of the arms will avoid their being sprained by the weight of the person's body falling on them while they are in a poor position. A siderail protects the patient as he lies near the edge of the bed (Fig. 1).

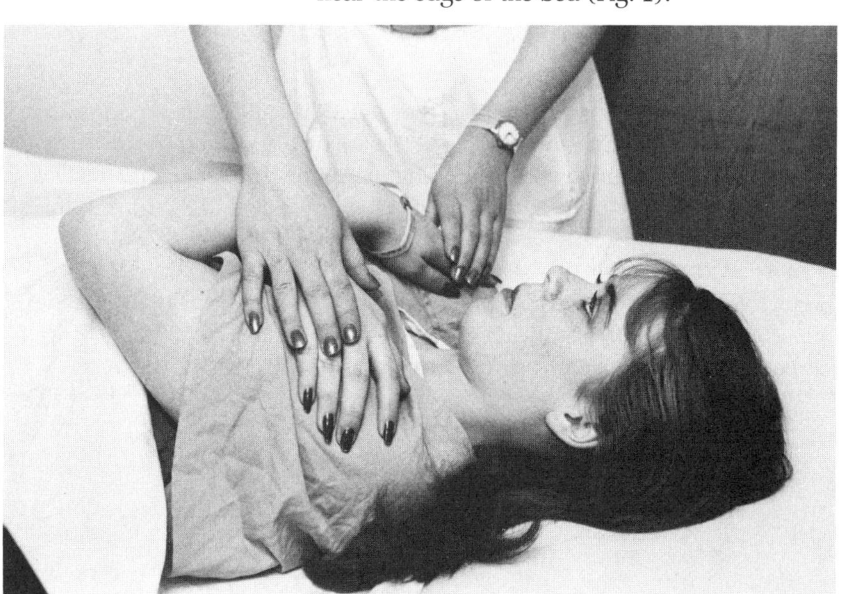

FIGURE 1. Positioning a patient's arms prior to turning her.

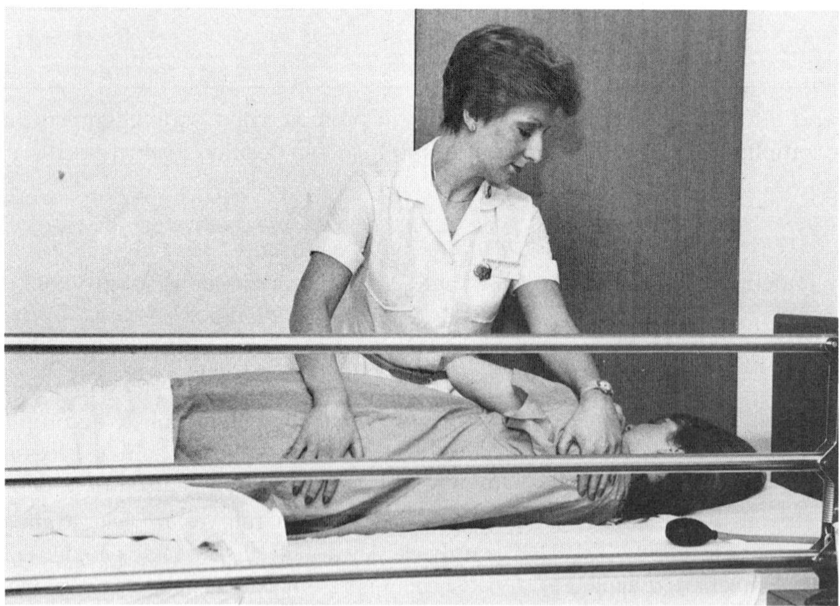

FIGURE 2. Roll a patient toward you to turn her to her side.

7. Stand on the side of the bed toward which the person will be turned. Place one hand on the patient's shoulder and one on his hip and gently roll him toward you (Fig. 2).

   7. Rolling expends little effort for the action accomplished.

8. Evaluate effectiveness, efficiency, comfort, and safety aspects of the procedure; reposition patient with good body alignment; provide diversional activity as needed.

   8. Good body alignment is necessary for prevention of effects of immobilization.

9. Record procedure and assessment of findings.

   9. Document nursing care and patient status.

10. Plan health teaching such as importance of good body alignment or frequent repositioning.

    10. Health teaching is an independent nursing action always included in care.

MODIFICATIONS FOR THE CHILD

Children grow bored with bed rest; they have difficulty lying in a position facing away from the door of the room. You may need to turn the bed after turning the child so that although he is now on his opposite side, he still faces the doorway. Repositioning his TV or playing a game such as "List how many items in this half of the room start with A, B, C, etc." may be necessary to keep him in this position.

MODIFICATIONS FOR THE OLDER ADULT

Many older adults have little subcutaneous fat so there is little protection on iliac crests. They can develop pressure sores easily when lying on their sides. A person who has a hearing loss in one ear may be unwilling to lie on that side since he hears poorly with the good ear resting against a pillow.

PROCEDURE 26-3
Logrolling

Purpose: To turn a patient who must not flex his back while turning; to promote comfort and safe transfer to a new position; to promote good body alignment and change of position; to prevent complications of prolonged bed rest.

Plan	*Principle*
1. Wash your hands; identify patient; explain procedure. *Never attempt to logroll a person with spinal cord surgery or injury by yourself.*	1. Prevent spread of microorganisms; promote patient safety and well-being. To keep a person's spinal column from flexing, two people are necessary. In people with spinal injury or surgery, flexing the spinal column will lead to injury.
2. Assess patient status; analyze appropriateness of plan; adjust plan to individual patient need.	2. Nursing care is always individualized based on professional judgment of patient's needs.
3. Implement procedure by moving equipment, such as intravenous equipment; loosen the drawsheet under the patient and roll it on both sides to about 10 in. from patient.	3. The patient will be moved by the drawsheet to help support his back. Rolling it increases its strength and keeps it from tearing.
4. Move the patient to the side of the bed by moving the drawsheet (Fig. 1). To turn to left side, position left arm close to body; position right arm flexed across chest.	4. Positioning the arms before turning prevents them from being injured by the weight of turning.

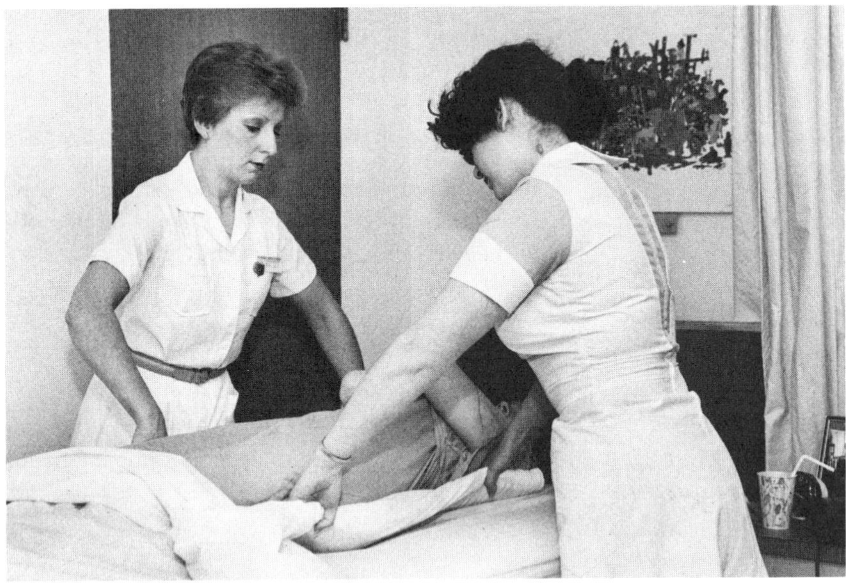

FIGURE 1. Prior to logrolling, move a person to side of bed using drawsheet.

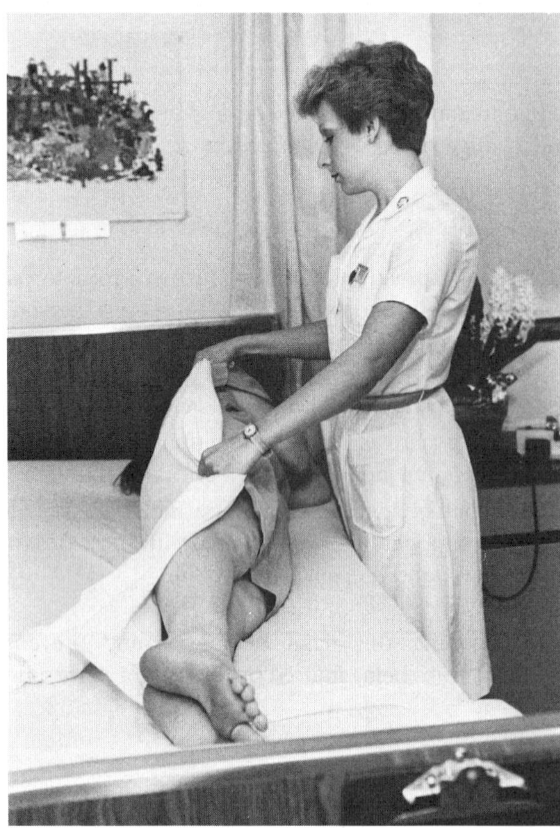

FIGURE 2. Logroll using the drawsheet so that the person's back does not flex.

5. Use the drawsheet to support the person's back and turn to side-lying position. *Both people must turn in unison to keep back straight.*

   5. Using the drawsheet to turn keeps the person's back straight. Stand with two people on one side of the bed or one on each side (Fig. 2).

6. Evaluate effectiveness, efficiency, cost, comfort, and safety of procedure. Reposition in good body alignment; provide diversional activities as desired.

   6. Good body alignment aids in preventing effects of immobilization.

7. Record procedure and assessment findings.

   7. Document nursing care and patient status.

8. Plan health teaching such as importance of frequent turning, need to keep back in a rigid position while turning.

   8. Health teaching is an independent nursing action always included as part of care.

MODIFICATIONS FOR THE CHILD

Children will stay in the position you place them in only if you provide a diversional activity. If a child dislikes one position, choose a special activity for him during that time that is done only at that time to make the position seem special. Children can help to keep their back from flexing while they are turned if told to think of themselves as a stiff robot.

PROCEDURE 26-4
Transferring a Patient from Bed to Chair

Purpose: To provide for a means of transportation to another location; to provide safe transfer without injury to patient or personnel; to provide for a change in body alignment and position.

Plan	*Principle*
1. Wash your hands; identify patient; explain procedure to patient.	1. Prevent spread of microorganisms; promote patient safety and well-being.
2. Assess patient status; assess ID band is in place before removing a person from his assigned bed. Take pulse rate.	2. Nursing care is always individualized based on professional judgment of patient's needs. Assure identification; establish baseline for further assessment of stress on cardiovascular system.
3. Analyze appropriateness of plan based on patient condition; plan modifications as necessary. *Determine if you will need assistance.* Provide for accessory equipment such as intravenous equipment.	3. A patient's condition may have changed so drastically since the last time he was out of bed that this plan may no longer be practical or well advised.
4. Bring bed to low position; bring head of bed to Fowler's position. Place chair or wheelchair close to side of bed facing head of bed. Lock wheels of wheelchair.	4. Using the bed to rise to a sitting position saves you energy. Moving the shortest distance saves both you and the patient energy. *If the person is handicapped on one side, transfer toward strong side.*
5. Support patient's back with one hand; move patient's legs to side of bed. Allow patient to dangle or sit momentarily in this position for a few minutes while you place shoes or slippers on his feet and help him with a robe.	5. People who have been lying flat may suffer from orthostatic hypotension (low blood pressure due to sudden change of position) when brought to a sitting position. Sitting for a moment on the side of the bed helps the circulatory system make necessary adjustments to maintain blood pressure (Fig. 1).

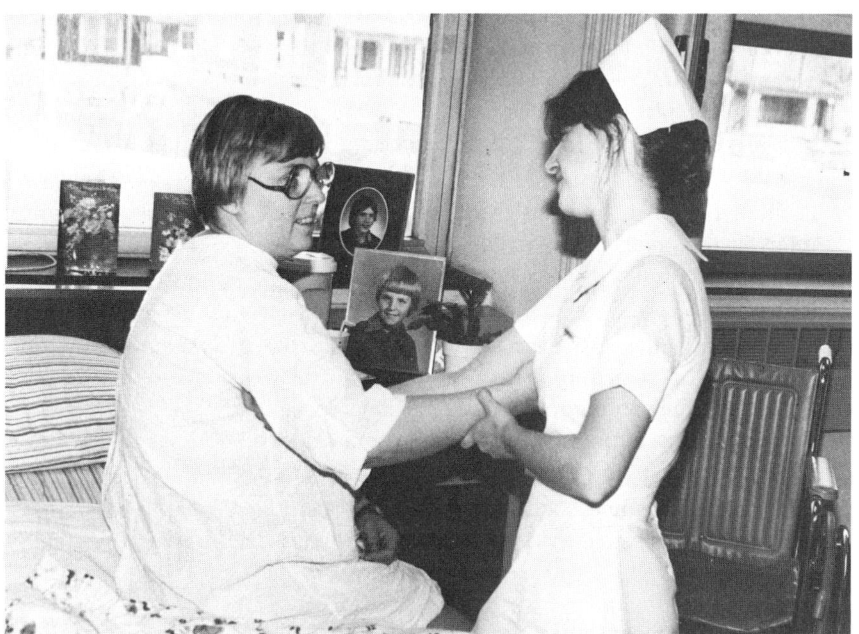

FIGURE 1. Sitting on side of bed (dangling) prior to transfer helps reduce orthostatic hypotension.

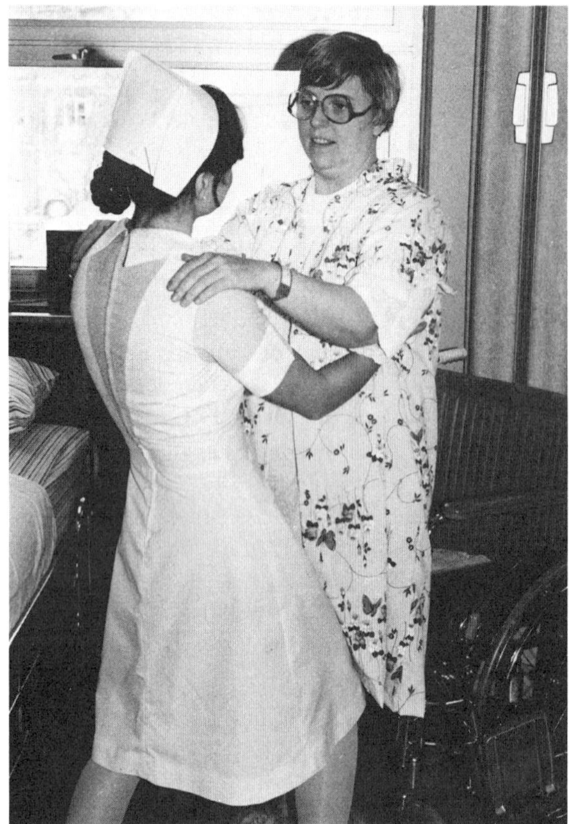

FIGURE 2. Stoop to lift a patient; never bend.

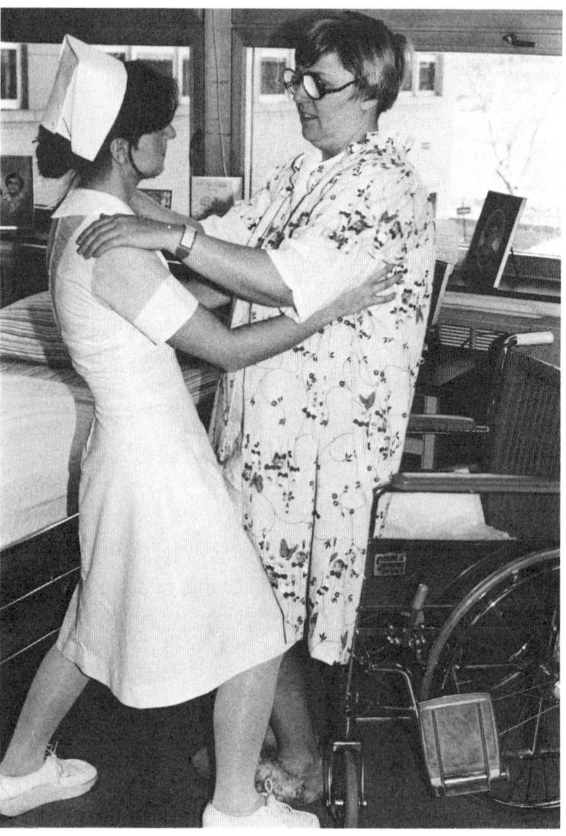

FIGURE 3. Pivot to turn the patient until she is in front of the chair.

6. Stand in front of the patient with a wide base for support; stoop and place your hands around the patient's waist. Press your knees against his knees. Lift upward, pivot to face the chair, lower the person gradually into the chair by stooping, not bending.

6. Stooping protects back muscles. Check before you turn that you will not bump the chair legs with your foot or accidentally bump the patient's legs as you turn. Support at the patient's waist, not under his armpit, to avoid strain on the nerves at the axilla (Figs. 2,3).

7. Position patient comfortably and in good alignment in the chair. Secure safety strap on wheelchair as necessary; provide lap robe as necessary for warmth.

7. Good body alignment prevents some of the effects of immobilization. Some people need a restraint to maintain good alignment.

8. Evaluate effectiveness, efficiency, cost, comfort, and safety of procedure; take pulse 10 sec after sitting in chair to compare with baseline measurement; record procedure and assessment findings.

8. Document nursing care and patient status.

9. Plan health teaching such as need for frequent change of position. Provide diversional activities as necessary.

9. Health teaching is an independent nursing action always included in care.

MODIFICATIONS FOR THE CHILD

Evaluate how heavy a child is before you help transfer him to a chair. Children's weight is often deceptive; ask for help as needed.

MODIFICATIONS FOR THE OLDER ADULT

Older adults are prone to orthostatic hypotension. Allow them to sit on the edge of the bed (dangling) for a count of at least 20 before proceeding further. Older adults may have arthritic knee changes that cause pain on standing. The pain may startle them as they stand, causing them to be unstable on their feet momentarily.

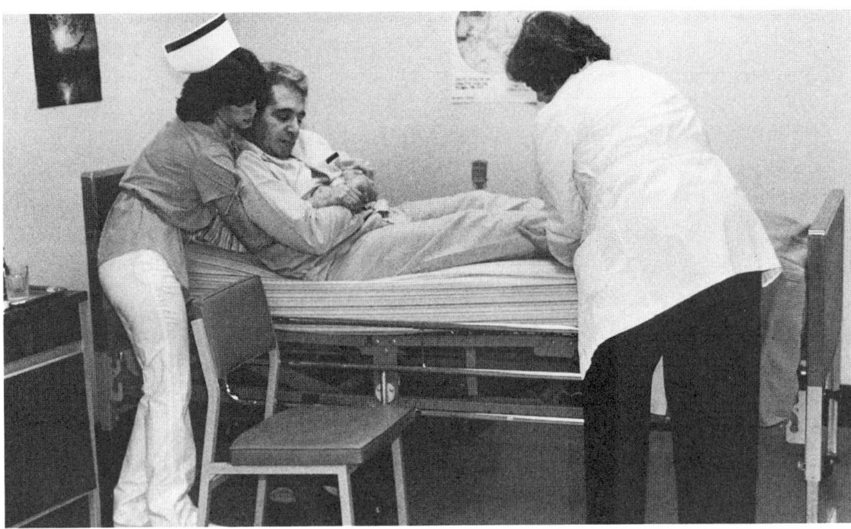

FIGURE 4. To lift a patient into a chair, slide your hands under patient's back and grasp his wrists.

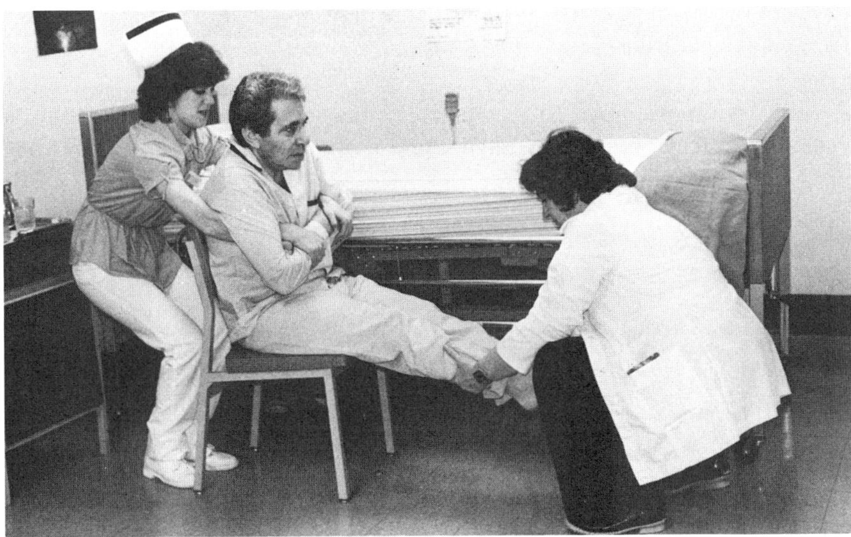

FIGURE 5. Lift together to move him to a chair.

MODIFICATIONS FOR THE PERSON WHO CANNOT BEAR WEIGHT

A patient who is unable to bear weight must be lifted into a wheelchair. The easiest method to do this is by a two-person lift. Move the patient to the near side of the bed and ask him to cross his arms on his chest. Move the wheelchair next to the bed with the back of it toward the head of the bed; lock the wheels. Remove the right armrest if removable; if not, bring the bed height up to armrest height. Stand behind the wheelchair, slide your hands under the patient's back, and reach forward to grasp his wrists. Ask your work partner to stand facing the front of the wheelchair and slide her hands under the patient's knees. On a mutual signal, lift the patient and slide him gently into the wheelchair (Figs. 4,5). Reverse the procedure to return him to bed.

When lifting, use thigh muscles, not back muscles. Be certain that both of you lift together to avoid causing muscle strain to the patient's back.

A person who will always be unable to bear weight will be taught to transfer from a bed to a wheelchair by himself by removing the side of the wheelchair, placing a firm board between the chair and bed (bed slightly higher than chair) and sliding from bed to chair, reversing the process to return to bed again. Some people have such a need to be independent that even though their non—weight-bearing period will be very short, they appreciate learning this self-transfer technique so they do not have to feel dependent on others for even a short time (see Fig. 26-38).

PROCEDURE 26-5
Transferring a Patient from a Bed to Stretcher

Purpose: To allow a change of location without patient or personnel injury; to provide for a means of transportation to another location.

Plan	*Principle*
1. Wash your hands; identify patient; explain procedure.	1. Prevent spread of microorganisms; promote patient safety and well-being.
2. Assess patient status; assess ID band is in place before transferring to another location.	2. Nursing care is always individualized based on professional judgment of patient's needs. Assure identification.
3. Analyze appropriateness of plan; plan modifications of procedures based on individual need. Determine if you will need assistance. Provide caution for dressings, intravenous equipment.	3. If a person can roll by himself, one person can help him transfer; if he cannot do this, you will need assistance.
4. Bring bed to high position; ask the person to move or you and another nurse move him to the side of the bed where the stretcher will be placed. Using the drawsheet is an effective way of moving a patient to the side of the bed prior to stretcher transfer.	4. If not using a drawsheet, lift and move or bounce the person to the side of the bed. Do not pull him across the bed surface to prevent skin and subcutaneous tissue destruction.
5. Move bedside stand away from bed; position stretcher next to bed; lock wheels of stretcher.	5. The greatest danger of transfer is that the stretcher will move and the patient will fall (Fig. 1).

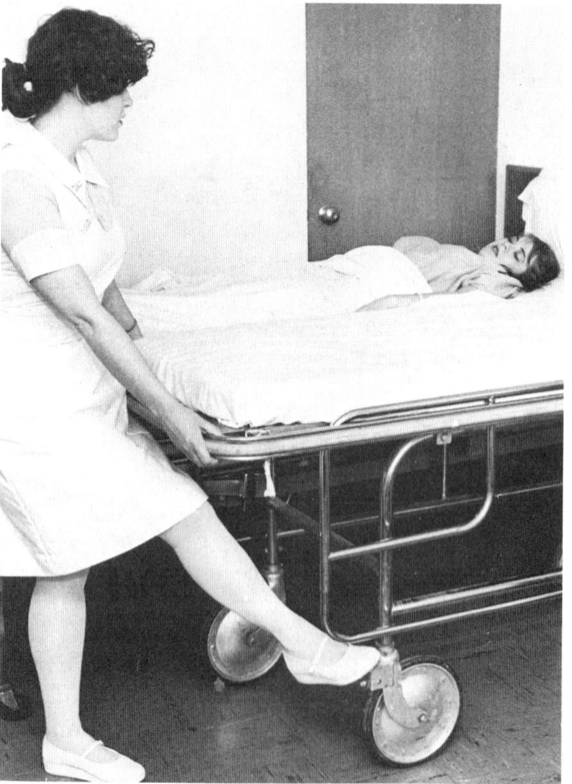

FIGURE 1. Be certain a stretcher is locked next to the bed before transfer.

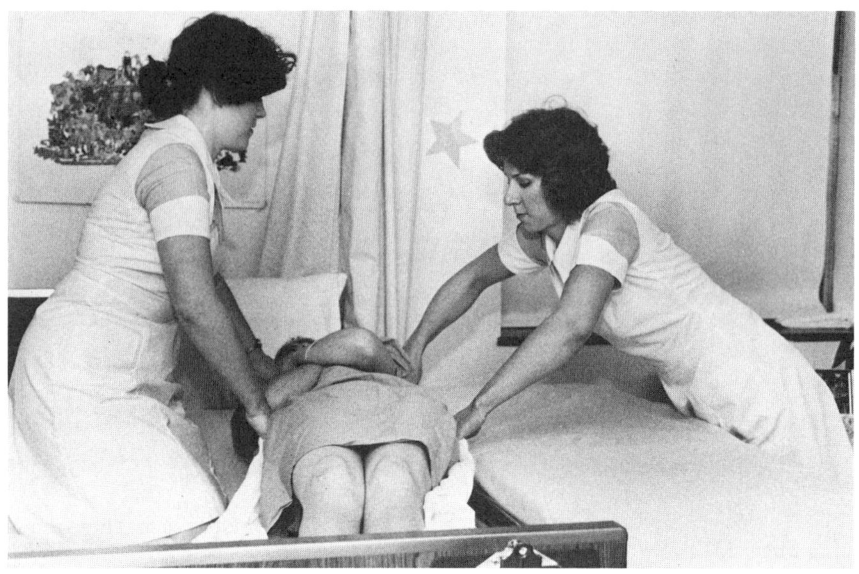

FIGURE 2. Transfer the patient to the stretcher by using the drawsheet. Do not be reluctant to kneel on bed for effective leverage.

6. If person can roll, stand by side of cart and ask him to roll toward you. If he cannot roll, stand by side of cart, reach across it, and move him to stretcher with drawsheet. Press firmly against the stretcher to ensure it will not move away from bed. Protect patient modesty moving top sheet with him.

6. Person assisting you may assist either from same side of cart as you or from across bed. It is not unprofessional to kneel on the bed to be nearer patient for more effective lifting (Fig. 2).

7. Position patient comfortably on stretcher in good body alignment. Provide pillows as needed. Secure *safety strap; raise stretcher siderails.*

7. Stretchers are narrow and a person can fall easily. *Never leave a person on a stretcher unattended without safety straps or siderails in place.*

8. Evaluate effectiveness, efficiency, cost, safety, and comfort of procedure. Record procedure and assessment findings.

8. Document nursing care and patient status.

9. Plan health teaching as needed, such as importance of diagnostic procedure person is being transferred for.

9. Health teaching is an independent nursing action always included in nursing care.

MODIFICATIONS FOR THE CHILD

A bed has a special security meaning to a child as a safe place. Asking him to transfer to a cart, therefore, is not merely moving him to a stretcher but a very threatening procedure for him. If he is to be taken to another department, place his favorite toy or blanket on the stretcher with him if possible for security.

MODIFICATIONS FOR THE OLDER ADULT

An older adult may be reluctant to transfer to a cart because he is afraid he will fall; he knows a fall could cause extreme damage due to osteoporosis. You may need an extra person to assist you just to offer a sense of support.

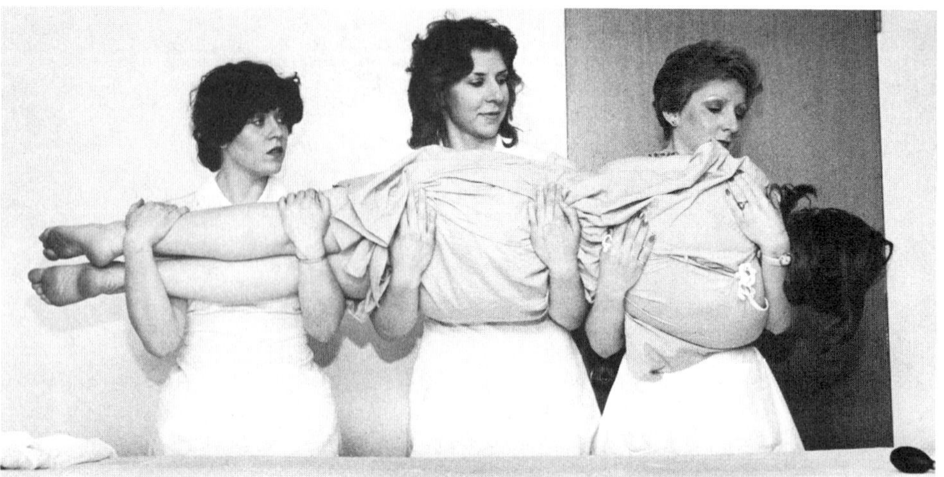

FIGURE 26-39. Three-man lift.

THREE-MAN LIFT

A three-man lift is a means of lifting a patient who cannot help in transferring to transfer to a stretcher. It requires much more energy than rolling the person from his bed to the stretcher utilizing a drawsheet or a simple rolling technique. However, it is a good technique when the bed will not rise to the height of the stretcher or the stretcher will not fit next to the bed, making the easier methods infeasible. It might be necessary when evacuating patients in a fire emergency.

To accomplish a three-man lift, move the patient to the side of the bed by using the drawsheet or bouncing him. One person slides her arms under the person's head and shoulders; the second slides her arms under the person's hips; the third slides her arms under the person's legs. Together, all three roll the person against their chests, lift, and carry him to the stretcher (Fig. 26-39).

Carefully assess the weight of the person being lifted before you attempt a three-man lift. It is never the preferred method of transfer.

HYDRAULIC LIFT

A hydraulic lift is a mechanical device that aids in moving people from bed to chair or chair to bathtub (Fig. 26-40). Models differ, so you must be completely familiar with the type you will use before using it. The lifter consists of a canvas sling that fits under the patient and an extended metal arm that, when attached to the sling, lifts the patient off the bed.

Place the chair parallel to the bed; if a wheelchair, lock the wheels. To place the sling under the patient, turn him to his side away from you, place the sling on the bed, roll him back on top of it. The upper part of the canvas should come to his axilla; the lower part to about mid-thigh. Move the hydraulic lift up to the bed at a 90-degree angle. Fasten the hooks of the lifter to the corresponding openings in the canvas sling. Slowly press on the elevating apparatus that causes the lifter bar to elevate and the canvas sling and person to rise off the bed. Support the person's head and arms as necessary. Raise the person high enough so that his body clears the surface of the bed; swing him gently and slowly until he is positioned over the chair. Release the control on the lifter that allows the person to be lowered into the chair. Remove the attached hooks from the canvas; leave the canvas in place for easy transfer back to bed. Position in good sitting alignment in the chair. Most people are frightened by mechanical lifts because they are big and cold looking. You can assure them that the only part that touches them is the soft canvas sling. Never use a lift unless you are familiar with its operation. Never use one you suspect may be broken or has faulty operation. Hydraulic lifts are an excellent means of increasing mobilization and social interaction for people unable to help with transferring to a chair (see QRS 26-5).

PROSTHESES

A *prosthesis* is an artificial body part. Types of prostheses include glasses, hearing aids, and dentures; however, the term most frequently refers to artificial arms and legs. Prostheses are individually fitted to the contour of the remaining arm or leg and are held in place by plastic or leather straps. People remove them at night for sleeping. Be certain prostheses are placed where they will not be damaged because they are expensive and being without one while it is being repaired would be inconvenient or incapacitating. Inspect the stump of the arm or leg for any area of irritation. If this has occurred, padding on the prosthesis may have become worn and need to be replaced. Encourage people with a leg prosthesis always to ambulate with it in place. If it is not used regularly, the contour of the stump will change and then compression and irritation at the stump will occur when the prosthesis is used. Learning to use a prosthesis is more difficult than it might appear.

UTILIZING NURSING PROCESS

Maintaining good body alignment and proper ambulation techniques depends on using the nursing process.

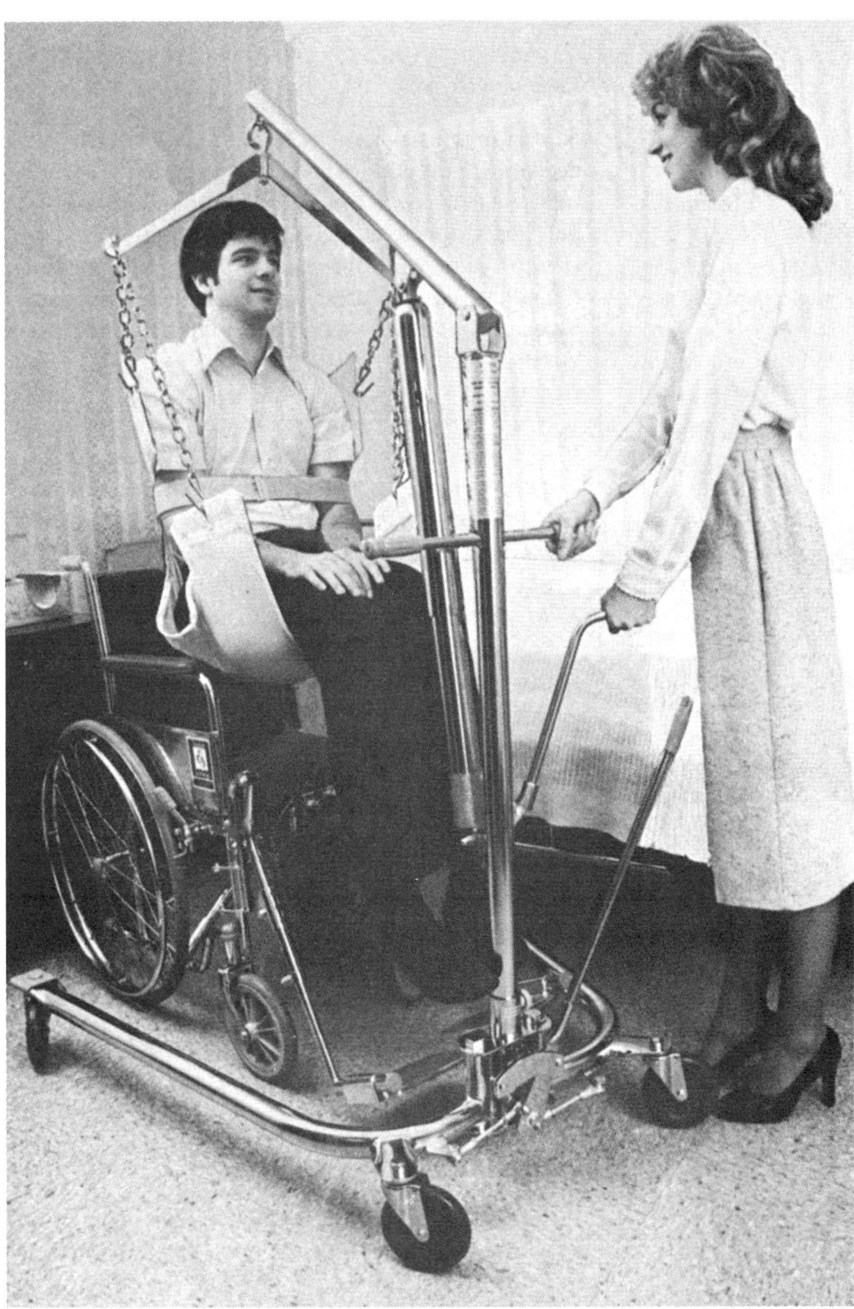

FIGURE 26-40. Use of a hydraulic lift for a patient transfer.

ASSESSMENT

Assess all patients in ambulatory or in-service care for body alignment and effects of immobility. Watch people's gait and posture for ease and coordination.

Ask people if they have any difficulty with muscle or skeletal function as part of a health history. Some people do not mention that they have a limitation of function because it is not a new problem or because they think of it as part of the normal aging process.

Ask people at ambulatory visits to walk for you. Assess their gait, since many neurological illnesses as well as musculoskeletal illnesses are manifested in an awkward, poorly balanced gait. Note carefully whether a child limps or not because a limp in a child is usually a sign of serious bone disease. Watch to see if a baby uses all extremities. Watch whether a child walks with his heel down as he steps. One of the first indications of cerebral palsy may be walking on tiptoes from a contracted or spastic heel cord (Achilles tendon).

Assess for full range of motion. This can be done actively by asking the person to perform range-of-motion exercises or passively by assisting joints through range-of-motion positions. Assess the back of all children 8 through 18 years for scoliosis by asking them to bend forward at the waist. Scoliosis becomes more pronounced with growth and thus must be identified as early as possible so that therapy to prevent further malformation can be started.

People on bed rest may have laboratory and diagnostic studies done to document the effects of immobiliza-

☐ QUICK REFERENCE STOP 26-5: SAFETY

1. When postioning people into good body alignment, never use a pillow under the knees in a supine position. This could compromise lower extremity circulation and lead to thrombus formation.
2. When lifting, always use a wide stance and lift using leg, not back muscles to prevent back strain.
3. Use a high bed position when giving patient care to reduce back strain; be certain to lower bed again for patient safety.
4. When doing exercises, caution patients to breath out. Holding their breath can lead to Valsalva's maneuver or increased intrathoracic pressure and decreased blood supply to the heart.
5. Be careful of shearing force when moving patients to prevent decubiti. Lift or bounce body parts to move them.

tion. The test most frequently ordered is serum calcium to detect how much calcium is leaving bone from inactivity. A normal level of serum calcium is 4.8 to 5.2 mEq per liter.

ANALYSIS

Problems related to inactivity fall into many categories. Common problems relate to the effects of immobility or an inability to accomplish activities of daily living. There might be an acute finding, such as pain on walking or swelling that limits joint function, or a vague finding, such as easy fatigue, the result of muscle disease.

The Fourth Conference on Nursing Diagnosis has accepted the diagnosis of "mobility, impaired physical." It is suggested that patients be rated by functional level to determine their level of impairment. The defining characteristics of this diagnosis and the suggested functional level classification are shown in Appendix C.

The locus of decision-making for people with problems of activity ranges from patient-centered to shared to nurse-centered because the person may have little loss of function (as with a single joint involvement) or nearly total loss of function (as with total body paralysis).

Be certain that goal-setting is done realistically. Complete return of motor function may not be a realistic goal in many circumstances. The realistic goal may be to accomplish modified activities of daily living using left hand. An accompanying goal might be to voice high self-esteem in light of limited function of right arm.

Bone healing is a lengthy process; learning reuse of injured or paralyzed muscles is a lengthy process. Long-term goals for problems related to activity must be

☐ QUICK REFERENCE STOP 26-6: RESEARCH
Patient Activity

Numerous nursing activities are associated with needs related to body movement and alignment. Patient activity needs to be closely monitored and supervised to prevent accidents and complications of therapy and to maintain adequate mobility functions. The research presented below deals with some aspects related to nursing care of patients with these kinds of needs.

1. *Lifting a patient.* In a preliminary study of a small sample of female subjects, Geden (1982) investigated client response to different lifting techniques in moving from bed to chair. Specifically, energy expenditure was studied. Results suggest that utilization of a mechanical lift requires the greatest energy of the client, followed by the assisted technique (nurse and patient), and the self-lift, respectively.
2. *Hazards associated with wheelchairs.* According to Hartigan (1982), prolonged sitting in *collapsible* wheelchairs, designed for transport and not for sitting, has resulted in pressure sores and radial nerve paralysis. Data were obtained from three case studies.
3. *Coronary precautions.* Coronary precautions are frequently prescribed for patients with cardiac problems. The list of restrictions (e.g., bed rest, no very hot or very cold beverages, no stimulant beverages, no rectal temperatures or vigorous backrubs) is designed to prevent vagal stimulation and Valsalva's maneuver, which can alter cardiac rhythm. Kirchhoff (1981) examined research on coronary precautions to determine if evidence supported their continued use. She found, "The only restriction in the list of coronary precautions that is well supported by research is the restriction of stimulant beverages . . . In contrast to the conclusions drawn in this study, a recent national survey of nurses who care for cardiac patients revealed that coronary precautions remain in practice" (p. 878).

SUGGESTED READINGS

Geden, E. A. Effects of lifting techniques on energy expenditure: A preliminary investigation. *Nurs. Res.* 31(4):214, 1982.

Hartigan, J. The dangerous wheelchair. *J. Am. Geriatr. Soc.* 30(9):572, 1982. As cited in *Nurses' Drug Alert* 7(2):15, 1983.

Kirchhoff, K. T. An examination of the physiologic basis for "coronary precautions." *Heart and Lung* 10(5):874, 1981.

supplemented with short-term goals or goals will seem too far away to accomplish successfully.

PLANNING AND IMPLEMENTATION

Because the problems that lead to an interference in activity vary, nursing implementation also varies. Since learning to adjust to a motor handicap is frequently involved, education is a strong component of care. People learning a new life-style need frequent praise and support in order to maintain the program.

Be certain that nursing orders are specific for activity. There is a wide variation in people's definitions of such terms as "increase activity" or "ambulate frequently." Be certain your order is so specific that it cannot be over- or underinterpreted.

EVALUATION

Evaluation needs to be done consistently and conscientiously following injury to the musculoskeletal system so that progress can be documented and new planning and implementation begun as necessary. Quietly resting body parts, an action that seems to many people a therapeutic measure, may not be therapeutic. Evaluation will reveal progress and problems. Quick Reference Stop 26-6 highlights some of the recent findings related to patient movement activities.

SUGGESTED READINGS

Axe, J., et al. Turning your patients—mechanically. *RN* 43:47, 1980.

Beall, M. S. Evaluation of the musculoskeletal system in the pediatric patient. *Compr. Pediatr. Nurs.* 2:1, 1977.

Boots, S., et al. Creative movement and health . . . expressive dance. *Top. Clin. Nurs.* 3(2):23, 1981.

Ciuca, R., and Bradish, J. Passive range-of-motion exercises: A handbook. *Nursing 78* 8:59, 1978.

Ciuca, R., Bradish, J., and Trombly, S. M. Active range-of-motion exercises: A handbook. *Nursing 78* 8:45, 1978.

Cohen, S. Teaching a patient how to use crutches. *Am. J. Nurs.* 79:1111, 1979.

Finn, K. L. How's your post-op ambulation technique? *RN* 42:69, 1979.

Ford, J. R., and Duckworth, B. Moving a dependent patient safely, comfortably. Part I: Positioning. *Nursing 76* 6:27, 1976.

Ford, J. R., and Duckworth, B. Moving a dependent patient safely, comfortably. Part II: Transferring. *Nursing 76* 6:58, 1976.

Frankel, L., and Richard, B. Exercises to help the elderly to live longer, stay healthier, and be happier. *Nursing 77* 7:58, 1977.

Getz, P. A. Preventing contractures: The little "extras" that help so much. *RN* 45(12):44, 1982.

Hirschberg, G., et al. Promoting patient mobility and preventing secondary disabilities. *Nursing 77* 7:42, 1977.

Jones, K. L., et al. *Total Fitness.* San Francisco: Confield Press, 1972.

Jungreis, S. Exercises for expediting mobility in bedridden patients. *Nursing 77* 7:47, 1977.

Long, B. C., and Buergin, P. S. The pivot transfer. *Am. J. Nurs.* 77:980, 1977.

Lynch, T., et al. Metabolic effects of prolonged bedrest: Their modification by simulated altitude. *Aerospace Medicine* 38:10, 1967.

Mock, M. S. Urinary tract infections and the orthopedic patient. *O.N.A. J.* 5:13, 1978.

Needler, W., et al. Movement, music, and remotivation with the regressed elderly. *J. Gerontol. Nurs.* 8(9):497, 1982.

Potter, A. Moving patients easily . . . lever-type action of the Paroll board. *Nurs. Focus* 4(2):14, 1982.

Rantz, M., et al. *Lifting, Moving and Transferring Patients: A Manual.* St. Louis: Mosby, 1981.

Roberts, A. Nervous system. Testing motor functions. Part 2. *Nurs. Times* 78(27), 1982.

Roberts, B. L., et al. Improving balance—Therapy of movement. *J. Gerontol. Nurs.* 9(3):150, 1983.

Ryback, R., et al. Psychobiologic effects of prolonged bedrest. *Aerospace Medicine* 42:529, 1971.

Troyer, H. The effect of short-term immobilization on the knee joint cartilage. *Clin. Orthop.* 107:249, 1975.

Vasey, J., et al. A neuromuscular approach. Get into condition. Part 2. *Nurs. Mirror* 154(18):22, 1982.

Vasey, J., et al. At ease . . . mechanically based concepts about the way to lift do not take into account associated body reactions. Part 3. *Nurs. Mirror* 154(19):28, 1982.

Vasey, J., et al. Handle with care . . . the use of the hands in lifting and positioning patients. Part 4. *Nurs. Mirror* 154(20):30, 1982.

Vasey, J., et al. Easy on the base . . . handling and lifting patients from a relaxed base stance. Part 5. *Nurs. Mirror* 154(21):36, 1982.

Vasey, J., et al. Safety first . . . way to lift and handle patients. Part 6. *Nurs. Mirror* 154(22):44, 1982.

QUESTIONS FOR REVIEW

Mr. White is a patient you care for. He has little use of his left side due to a cerebral vascular accident (CVA).

1. Mr. White is placed on bed rest. In planning care for him, which of the following statements is *not* an effect of bed rest?
   a. His heart output will decrease.
   b. Calcium will be lost from his bones.
   c. His appetite will decrease.
   d. Renal calculi are prone to form.

2. When you help to turn Mr. White, which statement below describes the best use of good body mechanics?
   a. A high center of gravity increases stability.
   b. Do not stoop since stooping tires leg muscles readily.
   c. Bending permits a smooth graceful reach.
   d. Hold an object close to your body when lifting it.

3. You place Mr. White in a Sims's position. The advantage of this position is that:
   a. The weight of his abdomen rests on the bed.
   b. He can remain in this position for 4 hours or longer.
   c. It mimics a wheelchair or sitting position.
   d. It is the best position if he is short of breath.

4. As a nursing implementation, you accomplish range-of-motion exercises with Mr. White. Which of the statements below describes an acceptable approach to these exercises?
   a. Move all joints to their full anatomic potential.
   b. Use a systematic approach or order.
   c. Support a joint proximal to the joint moving.
   d. Do not do passive exercises for patients on bed rest.

5. You transfer Mr. White to a stretcher. Which of the following statements describes the best technique for a transfer?
   a. Check his identification prior to transfer.
   b. Use a drawsheet to move his head.
   c. Kneel on the stretcher to assist.
   d. Assess that the wheels on the stretcher are unlocked.

6. To help Mr. White ambulate for the first time, which statement below describes the best technique?
   a. Walk beside his injured side.
   b. Walk directly behind him.
   c. Allow him to walk by himself to increase self-esteem.
   d. Help him choose his softest slippers for comfort.

7. During the second week of care, Mr. White is allowed to ambulate with a cane. To evaluate your teaching, you would observe that he has learned:
   a. To hold the cane in the hand on his injured side.
   b. To advance the cane with his injured foot.
   c. To use a four-point gait.
   d. To not use a cane outdoors.

27. COMFORT AND SAFETY

OBJECTIVES

Upon mastery of the material in this chapter, you should be able to:

1. Define comfort.
2. Describe characteristics of a safe therapeutic environment.
3. Describe how to make an unoccupied, closed, open, surgical, and occupied bed—isolettes through adult beds.
4. Define the etiology and characteristics of pain.
5. Describe common implementations for reducing pain.
6. Describe the use of restraints as a mechanism of patient safety.
7. Describe nursing responsibility with the use of patient restraints.
8. Describe nursing responsibilities for fire safety.

TERMS

The terms important for an understanding of this chapter are shown below and defined in the glossary:

comfort
therapeutic environment
pain

Comfort and safety are second-level needs in Maslow's hierarchy of needs, coming immediately after primary needs such as hunger, respiration, and circulation. Because a patient may be absorbed in meeting primary needs, a double responsibility falls on the nurse to provide for second-level needs, especially safety.

COMFORT

Besides freedom from pain or irritants, comfort means a sense of well-being. A person cannot feel comfortable if there is physical interference or if he is anxious.

Comfort is difficult to assess because people express feelings of discomfort differently. A baby expresses comfort readily by smiling and discomfort just as readily by crying. Some adults express discomfort quickly; others experience great discomfort before they express it or ask to have it relieved. A person's reaction depends on his background, his culture, his interpretation of his sex role, and his ability to trust you.

People in extreme distress may be in such shock that they have not yet begun to feel what has happened to them and cannot express their discomfort. Children in a strange situation may be so frightened that they say nothing.

Therapeutic Environment

Environment refers to a person's surroundings, external and internal. Environments are *therapeutic* if they are conducive to health and a sense of well-being.

EXTERNAL ENVIRONMENT

A person's home and community must be therapeutic in order for him to remain well. Because hospital patients spend so much time in their rooms, the design and surroundings of the room play a major role in determining how a patient feels about himself.

Ventilation. People who are ill (especially people with nausea) are more sensitive to odors or stuffiness than normally. Hospital rooms should be well ventilated to decrease odor while not allowing a draft from an air conditioner or an open window to strike the bed area. Change soiled bed linen and remove bedpans, urinals, or emesis basins promptly after use from rooms to prevent odors from these sources. If a room is near the kitchen or a food cart, it may smell as if fresh coffee is perking. Be certain that a patient who will not be allowed to have fluid or food is not placed in a room where food odors might tease him.

Temperature. Most people are comfortable at a room temperature between 68° and 74°F (20—23°C). Rooms for newborns may be kept warmer than this because they have little subcutaneous fat and an immature neurological system. Many elderly patients enjoy an environment warmer than 72°F because they, too, have decreased amounts of subcutaneous fat. A person who is ill and thus moves less than usual needs a warmer room temperature than a well person who moves briskly.

Certain sections of hospitals such as the surgery and the delivery suite are kept cool to reduce the possibility of inhalation gases exploding and to be a comfortable temperature for hospital personnel who must wear sterile cover gowns. People going to surgery often need a blanket to keep warm.

People ill at home in cold climates may need to close off unnecessary rooms in order to heat the room they use most. Otherwise, owing to lack of exercise while they are ill, they can suffer hypothermia.

Humidity. Humidity is the amount of moisture in the air. When humidity is high, you cannot perspire freely and thus you feel warmer than when humidity is low. Air conditioning units regulate humidity as well as temperature to maintain a relative humidity of 30 to 60 percent. Dry air without humidity can be irritating to nasal mucus membranes. Cracking of nasal mucosa and nosebleeds typically occur in the first fall days when a heating system is turned on if humidity is not well regulated by the system.

Noise. A high noise level can be psychologically fatiguing. Keeping noise to a minimum on hospital units helps people who are already fatigued from illness to rest effectively. Be certain that you do not create noise by loud talking, laughter, or banging equipment. Remind patients to keep their television sets at a reasonable volume. On children's units a daily nap or quiet time is usually scheduled; adults may need an individual quiet time planned so they do not become extremely fatigued.

Lighting. Bright lighting is necessary to perform nursing procedures safely. Light sources must be adjustable because most people sleep better in subdued light. Bright sunlit rooms, with large windows, though cheerful, allow heat to be lost in winter and to enter in summer; thus, they may not be cost efficient.

Rooms should have a night light that illuminates the floor area for walking safely at night. Many preschool children are too frightened to fall asleep unless there is some light in the room at night.

Environmental Hazard. A person cannot be comfortable if there is an environmental hazard around him, such as electrical equipment with a frayed cord or flammable sponges sitting on a hot radiator. Assess rooms and hospital units for hazards to be certain that a patient's environment is safe for him. Common environmental hazards in a hospital and methods to reduce them are shown in Quick Reference Stop 27-1; common environmental hazards in the home, in Quick Reference Stop 27-2.

INTERNAL ENVIRONMENT

A person's internal environment consists of his body functions and the way he views himself. In order for an environment to be truly therapeutic, a person's self-concept must be positive.

A Sense of Privacy and Property. The rights to privacy and to own property are strongly felt by most people. Even toddlers have a strong sense of what is *their* toy or *their* bed. Protect people's privacy by knocking before opening closed doors. When giving care at a bedside, pull drapes to offer privacy. Do not perform nursing procedures when visitors are present except for noninvasive procedures such as oral temperature taking. If a procedure must be carried out while visitors are present, ask them to step outside the room until you are finished. However, young children may feel more secure when the parent is

☐ QUICK REFERENCE STOP 27-1: SAFETY
Common Health Care Agency Environmental Hazards

Item	*Potential Hazards*	*Item*	*Potential Hazards*
Electrical equipment	Electrical equipment always has the potential for three dangers: electrical shock, fire, and burn. Never use electrical equipment with frayed cords or without a three pronged plug or grounding wire. Never use electrical equipment near water. Closely supervise any patient with heat or cold applications to reduce the possibility of burns.	Poisoning	Many common hospital solutions are poisonous. Never leave anything on a patient's overbed table or stand such as an iodine solution that would not be safe for him to ingest. Never leave medicine in patient units where it could be ingested by another patient or horded and swallowed in a lethal dose. Be certain that medicine in a central medicine area is protected by cabinets or locks.

Falls	Falls are a common hospital accident. Always leave beds in low positions for ambulatory patients; use siderails appropriately, especially following administration of medicines that cause drowsiness. Be certain light in rooms is adequate at night. Make a habit of removing any furniture, suitcases, or stepstools from the path between the room door and bed and bathroom door and bed. Urge people to use sturdy bedroom slippers or their street shoes to avoid slipping. Wipe up spills to keep floors from being slippery. Keep a person's telephone and bedside stand nearby so he does not fall trying to reach them.
Mistaken identity	Accidents involving mistaken identity are always preventable. Never initiate any procedure with a patient without identifying him correctly by asking him to state his name or reading his armband.
New equipment or procedure	The rapid advance of medical technology introduces new equipment or procedures everyday. Insist that a health care agency give you adequate instruction in new equipment or procedures to make your actions safe. Ask for explanations or demonstrations as many times as it takes for you to feel comfortable with equipment.
Emergencies	In emergencies, actions must be taken quickly and safely. Ask for periodic in-service review on cardiopulmonary resuscitation technique; common drugs and dosages used in resuscitation attempts; and actions to take for the person with sudden chest pain, hemorrhage, or a concussion to be certain your actions will be safe in these emergency situations.
Research	In order for research on human subjects to be carried out, the person must consent and it must be approved by an institution's Committee on Ethical Research. Be certain that such permission has been obtained before assisting with research projects.
Psychological health	People can withstand only so much stress or so much change at any one time and still maintain sound mental health. Give anticipatory guidance as necessary so people can be prepared for what is to happen to them. Reduce stimuli so they are not bombarded by so many new sensations that they have difficulty interpreting them accurately.
Infection	Use aseptic technique as appropriate to reduce the number of organisms contacting an individual. Use sterile technique if the person has a break in his skin or a body cavity will be entered.
Nutrition	Be aware of the temperature of foods such as soup and coffee to prevent burns. Position people with their head elevated or on their side prior to eating to prevent aspiration. Do not offer oral food or fluid to anyone without swallowing and gag reflexes intact.

☐ QUICK REFERENCE STOP 27-2: COMMUNITY CONSIDERATIONS

Help people to look at whether their home environment is safe for them or not and to make those changes necessary to reestablish safety. Common problems divided by age group are listed below:

Age Group	*Common Problems*
Newborn	The most common cause of death in newborns is aspiration. Ask: Do parents prop bottles? Keep small parts of toys away from the child's instinctive grasp reflex?
Infant	Falls and auto accidents are common first-year problems. Ask: Do parents always raise cribrails? Remember not to leave the baby on a couch or bed unprotected? Do they use an approved auto seat?
Toddler	Burns and poisoning are common problems. Ask: Do parents turn pot handles on the stove toward the back? Have covers for electrical outlets? Keep matches up out of reach? Keep medicine in a locked cabinet? Resist taking medicine in front of children? Keep poisons such as cleaning agents up and out of reach? Know the number of their local poison control center? Have ipecac (an emetic) on hand?
Preschooler	Auto accidents are a common problem. Ask: Have parents stressed street safety? Not to play between parked cars? To wear a seatbelt while in the car?
Schoolage	Auto accidents, child molestation, and firearm accidents are common problems. Ask: Have parents stressed street safety? Importance of using crosswalks and respecting red lights? Does the child know rules of not talking to strangers or taking presents from them? If there are firearms in the house, are they locked? Has the child been taught firearm safety?
Adolescent	Auto accidents, drug-induced accidents, and drowning are common problems. Ask: Does the adolescent appreciate the danger of driving while under the influence of alcohol or another drug? Can he refuse to ride with someone who is? Some accidents are actually suicide attempts. Has he ever thought of this or tried it? Does he have someone to turn to for advice if his world seems overwhelming for him? Does he appreciate the danger of swimming alone? Can he refuse a "dare" he knows is beyond his physical skill?
Young adult	Motorcycle accidents and sports injuries are common problems. Ask: Does the person appreciate that motorcycles are subject to the same safe driving precautions as automobiles? Does he use protective equipment for sports activities? Not participate beyond his endurance?

Middle-aged adult	Automobile accidents and work injuries are common problems. Ask: Does the person appreciate the danger of driving while under the influence of alcohol or fatigued? Does he use safety precautions at work (hard hat, salt tablets to guard against heat stroke, not using antihistamines if he works with machinery)?	Older adult	Falls are a common problem. Ask: Does the person have adequate light on stairways? Keep stairways clear of clutter? Limit exposure to slippery sidewalks? Resist changing lightbulbs from high stools?

present; ask a child if he wants his parent to stay or not.

People value privacy, but they also value the security of knowing that they are being checked on frequently by health care personnel. As a rule, people like to have their bed positioned in a room so you can see them (and they you) as you walk by the doorway. Following a procedure for care, always reopen curtains or room doors to allow for patient observation.

Be certain when giving care that you respect property. Children bring their favorite toy into a hospital with them. To the child it is a symbol of security, the one normal thing in his world. Many elderly people bring prized possessions with them to the hospital as well. Whatever the age of the patient, always ask before removing anything from a room, "Is it all right if I discard this?" Respecting a person's property is an important way of saying, "You are important to me. I respect you."

A Sense of Control. Few people enjoy the feeling of things happening around them that they cannot understand. Explain what is planned for a patient. If possible, allow patients to choose their order of care or to participate in their care. Knowing that they have some control over what is happening around them allows people to maintain a strong sense of self-worth and control (see QRS 27-3).

Freedom from Pain. Of all the discomfort that a person can feel, pain is the most distressing. Pain is difficult to assess because it is subjective; the person experiencing it is the only one who can accurately report the level of pain he is experiencing.

According to the *gate control theory* of why people experience pain, as soon as the endings of small peripheral nerve fibers detect a stimulus, they transmit it to cells in the dorsal horn of the spinal cord. Impulses pass through a dense, interlacing network of cells in the spinal cord (the substantia gelatinosa) and immediately, a synapse occurs that returns the transmission to the peripheral site through a motor nerve (you touch a candle flame; the impulse travels to the spinal cord and back, and you lift your hand away from the flame). Following this short-circuit synapse, the impulse then continues in the spinal cord to reach the hypothalmus and cortex of the brain. Here, the impulse is interpreted and perceived as pain.

Basically, pain is a protective mechanism. A person who lacks pain perception has to be taught to inspect his body daily to see if injury to skin or muscle has occurred. A person who is anesthesized for care needs your protection until his protective system of pain sensation returns.

The types of injury that can cause pain are lack of oxygen in tissues from decreased circulation, pressure on tissue, external injury, or overstretching of body cavities with fluid or air.

☐ QUICK REFERENCE STOP 27-3: PSYCHOLOGICAL CONSIDERATIONS

A person who does not know what is going to happen to him or has happened to him cannot feel safe. Make a habit of asking yourself, If I were this person, what information would I want to know to feel safe? What happenings would I like to be prepared for so I am not frightened by them? Incorporate explanations of what you are going to be doing and assurance of safety as intrinsic steps of procedures of care. (Surgery is over now. You are back in your room. Your blood pressure is 120/70; that's normal. You are going to have a chest x-ray taken this morning; that is routine before surgery, not because your physician thinks you have a chest problem. This medicine has a side-effect of making you feel lightheaded; don't let it worry you if you notice that. You are going to have an ECG, a heart tracing, done this morning. Do you understand why you are having that? How it is done?)

Assessment of Pain

In order to recognize the level of implementation needed to alleviate discomfort, you need to know the extent and possible causes of the sensation. For most people, discomfort is interpreted by one of the five senses. Assess whether there is anything in the environment that would be disturbing to them. A sixth sense, or awareness that something is wrong, also leads to discomfort. A person who feels insecure, lonely, or anxious, who resents a loss of privacy, or who feels his body or private property is not being respected experiences some degree of discomfort.

Pain stimulates the sympathetic nervous system, activating a fight-or-flight reaction; thus, with discomfort, heart rate and respiratory rate increase and peripheral vasoconstriction occurs. These vital sign changes generally reflect level of discomfort. Other observable indications that pain is present are muscle tension, abnormal body position, strained tone of voice, tense or unusual facial expression, increased perspiration, unusual restlessness, and increased or decreased skin color from changes in vasoconstriction.

In order to determine the severity of discomfort and the extent of the condition causing it, you need to determine the duration, frequency (continuous or intermittent), intensity *(sharp, nagging, burning)*, description (localized to a small area or occurring over a large area; acute, chronic, or intermittent; superficial or deep), associated symptoms, and any action the person takes that alleviates it.

Pain is *acute* if it is sharp, intense, and lasts only a short time. Stubbing a toe leads to acute pain. Acute pain can cause high anxiety because it is so sharp, sudden, and uncomfortable that the person has difficulty coping with its presence. Pain is *chronic* if it has existed for a long time, usually over 6 months. A condition such as arthritis can produce chronic pain. Chronic pain may cause depression or sadness because it is always present and becomes tiring. Pain is *intermittent* if it is interspersed with periods free of pain. For example, pain in the gastrointestinal tract occurs with peristaltic contractions but is not noticeable between contractions.

Persistent pain is not easily relieved. Low-back pain from stiffened vertebrae is often persistent pain. *Intractable* pain cannot be relieved by even the most extreme interventions. A tumor continuing to grow and constantly pressing on body nerves can cause this. *Referred* pain originates at one site, but is perceived at another. In a child, the presence of a hip problem is often detected because of referred pain to the knee.

ANALYSIS OF PAIN

It has been suggested by the Fourth Congress on Nursing Diagnosis that a nursing diagnosis of discomfort be worded as "Alternatives in comfort: pain." Signs and symptoms to document that the problem exists are shown in Table 27-1. When setting a goal of care concerning pain, be realistic. Setting a goal for management of pain at too high an expectation results in disappointment that it was not accomplished and increased concern because a patient may interpret the unmet goal as indicating that a complication has occurred.

TABLE 27-1. COMMON SIGNS AND SYMPTOMS OF DISCOMFORT

Muscle tension
Abnormal body position
Impaired thought processes
Restlessness, pacing, verbal expression of pain, moaning, crying, screaming
Facial grimace, clenched jaw
Pupillary dilation
Diaphoresis
Increased or decreased respiratory rate
Increased blood pressure level
Increased pulse rate

PLANNING

Gating mechanisms in the substantia gelatinosa appear to be capable of halting an impulse at the level of the spinal cord so the impulse is never received at the brain level as pain; a process similar to closing a gate takes place. You can assist gating mechanisms by three techniques: cutaneous stimulation, distraction, and reduction of anxiety.

Cutaneous Stimulation. If large peripheral nerves next to an injury site are stimulated, the ability of the small nerve fibers at the injury site to transmit pain impulses appears to decrease. Therefore, rubbing an injured part and applying heat or cold to the site are effective maneuvers to suppress pain.

Distraction. If the cells of the brain stem that register an impulse as pain are preoccupied with other stimuli, a pain impulse will not register. Distraction or having a person focus on some pattern or action accomplishes this. Telling a child to say *ouch* while you administer an injection is using this technique. It is also basic in prepared or natural childbirth.

Reducing Anxiety. Pain impulses are perceived more quickly if anxiety is also present. Thus, the third technique of gating is to reduce patient anxiety as much as possible. Teaching what a patient can expect of a procedure is a means of achieving this.

Implementation for Comfort

Comfort is more than the absence of pain, and helping a person achieve comfort involves measures beyond simple pain relief.

COMMON ANALGESICS

Analgesics are drugs that significantly reduce or alleviate pain. They limit the ability of the brain cortex to interpret the incoming sensation as pain. A number of commonly used analgesics are summarized in Quick Reference Stop 27-4.

☐ **QUICK REFERENCE STOP 27-4: PHARMACOLOGY**
Common Analgesics

Generic Name	*Trade Name*	*Special Consideration*
Narcotic analgesics		
Opium	Morphine	Strong respiratory depressant (respiratory rate should be over 16 before administration). Decreases gastrointestinal mobility so may cause constipation. Strongly addictive. Constricts pupils.
Opium	Codeine	One-third the strength of morphine; addictive; same side-effects as above, only less in degree. Strong cough suppressant so should not be administered to persons who need to raise respiratory secretions.
Meperidine	Demerol	Antagonistic effect with monoamine oxidase inhibitors. Strongly addictive. Produces mild euphoria.
Propoxyphene	Darvon	Analgesic. Large doses may cause dizziness or drowsiness; has a strong synergistic effect with alcohol.
Nonnarcotic analgesics		
Acetosalicylic acid	Aspirin	Causes gastrointestinal irritation and prolonged bleeding time. Analgesic, antipyretic, and antiinflammatory. Large doses may cause *salicylism*: ringing in the ears, skin rash, hyperventilation.
Acetaminophen	Tylenol	Analgesic and antipyretic. Large doses may cause liver toxicity.

PRECAUTIONS TO USE IN ADMINISTRATION OF ANALGESICS

1. Narcotic analgesics are habit forming.
2. Narcotic analgesics are schedule II drugs under the provisions of Controlled Substances Act 1971; this necessitates extra care in administering and documenting use.
3. Use caution in applying heat to anyone who has received an analgesic; he could be burned easily because he does not feel heat readily.
4. Never give medicine to relieve pain without identifying the pain source. A patient may be developing a new source of pain; giving the analgesic would disguise it and an illness complication could be missed.
5. Never give *just* an analgesic; straighten sheets, offer a backrub, and so forth.
6. Use a positive approach with administration.
7. Give analgesics before pain becomes acute for best results.
8. Use siderails as appropriate after administration since some cause drowsiness.

When administering medicine for pain do not stop with one measure. Follow through with a good explanation of what causes the pain and why the medication will take care of it. A positive approach also reduces anxiety. A statement such as "This medicine will work in a few minutes to take away that pain" is therapeutic. Muscles tightly contracted from apprehension that pain will not go away can lead to increased pain.

Use analgesia adequate for the situation; remember, however, that narcotic analgesics are habit forming. Many times a lesser analgesic will control pain if other measures such as distraction or providing general comfort are used in conjunction with it.

Try to prevent discomfort from becoming acute whenever possible. If a person has had surgery on an arm, for example, edema at the incision site will occlude venous return and cause pain. Elevating the hand and arm on pillows to increase venous return prevents this. Likewise, frequent backrubs or changes of position reduce the possibility that back pain will develop in the person on bed rest. Encourage people to report pain or to ask for medication for pain relief. To admit to having pain is not a lack of character; it is reporting a subjective sensation. Pain free, a person will increase his activity level markedly, which will reduce risks from immobility.

Chronic pain is fatiguing. Provide periods of rest balanced with exercise for the person so that his body resources can support healing.

Include measures that the patient thinks will be helpful. Discomfort is subjective. What the patient thinks will relieve it may be more effective than what *you* think.

Be persistent. There are few instances when discomfort is truly intractable or cannot be minimized by some measure (see QRS 27-5).

☐ QUICK REFERENCE STOP 27-5: PHARMACOLOGY
Comfort and Pain Relief

There is a fine line between too much analgesia for comfort, the right amount, and too little. In order that patients do not become drug dependent, many nurses move quickly to choosing a nonnarcotic analgesic following surgery. You may need to advocate for a patient to have stronger analgesia so that he can be comfortable enough to do deep-breathing and coughing exercises or ambulate well.

EVALUATION

Sometimes your efforts to alleviate discomfort do not work so well as you or the patient hoped they would. Be certain that you follow up within half an hour to be certain that a measure was effective and the patient is truly comfortable now. Document what measures were effective so that another nurse does not have to repeat solutions to find the correct one but can know immediately what will work. Some nursing research findings in the area of pain relief are presented in Quick Reference Stop 27-6.

Establishing a Therapeutic Patient Environment

A patient's room should provide comfort and not distract from well-being. Knowing the specifics for such a room in a hospital allows you to assess or modify a room in a patient's home to fulfill the same requirements.

HOSPITAL BEDS

Providing a hospital bed correct for a patient is a prime consideration in providing comfort.

The Newborn. Well newborns are admitted to bassinets for care (Fig. 27-1). A bassinet has clear plastic sides so the infant is clearly visible. The mattress is a firm pad that can be tilted at the foot or head to different positions.

Ill newborns or those of low birth weight are often admitted to incubators for care. An Isolette has a clear plastic dome for easy observation of the baby. It can be flooded with heat or oxygen to maintain body warmth and good oxygenation of body cells. The infant is cared for by passing the hand through plastic portholes.

The Infant and Toddler. Children used to sleeping in cribs at home should be placed in cribs in the hospital for the feeling of security and for safety. Most children sleep in a crib until they are 3 or 4; some children as old as 5 or 6 may still be sleeping in a crib. The crib in Figure 27-2 is popularly called a climber crib, designed to prevent a toddler from climbing out.

☐ QUICK REFERENCE STOP 27-6: RESEARCH
Pain Relief

Nurses are continuously involved in attempts to relieve patients of pain. Some of the research on various aspects of pain relief is presented below.

Relaxation Technique.
Wells (1982) conducted a small experimental study to investigate the effect of relaxation technique versus routine postoperative instruction on postoperative muscle tension and pain. Postcholecystectomy patients were the sample. Results suggest that relaxation training alters the psychological components of pain, with subjects reporting less distress when relaxation technique was used. No physiologic differences were noted in use of the two techniques.

Lessening Pain with Injections.
Giving injections is one aspect of nursing care that most nurses would prefer to avoid. Lessening the pain perceived by patients receiving injections would certainly make the injection a less stressful experience for both nurse and patient. Levin (1982) studied 138 preoperative patients to determine if allowing them to choose the site of the injection lessened the pain they perceived from the injection. No differences in pain perception were noted. The author suggests that further study is necessary.

SUGGESTED READINGS

Levin, R. F. Choice of injection site, locus of control, and the perception of momentary pain. *Image* 14(1):26, 1982.

Wells, N. The effect of relaxation on postoperative muscle tension and pain. *Nurs. Res.* 31(4):236, 1982.

For an infant, another method is to apply over the top of the crib a *crib net*, a sturdy cotton net that allows you to view the infant while safely keeping him inside. Always tie crib nets to the bottom frame of the crib not the siderail, so that in an emergency, the siderail can be quickly lowered.

When placing an infant in a crib, provide him with some activity such as a music box or a manipulation toy so he has less reason to want to leave his crib.

The Schoolager and Adolescent. School and adolescent children are provided with adult beds in hospitals. Despite this use of adult furniture, rooms can be decorated to appeal to the patients' growth and development needs (Fig. 27-3).

The Adult. Hospital beds are narrower by about 12 inches than regular beds so you can reach across them more easily. They can be raised to a high position from

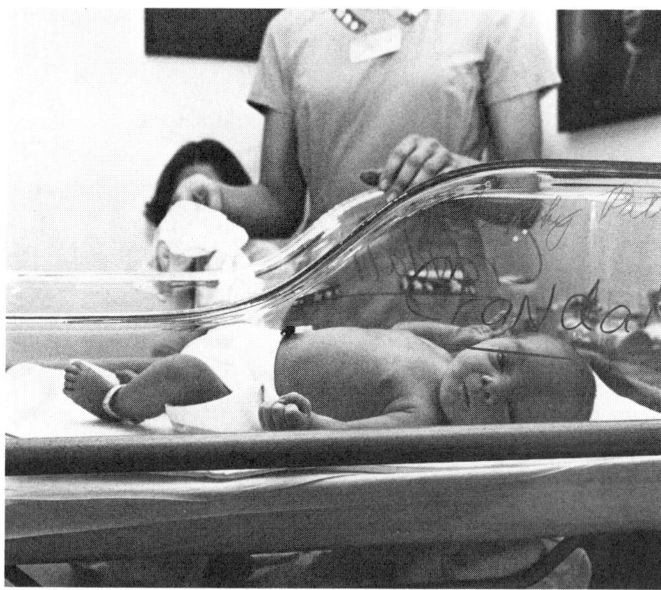

FIGURE 27-1. A bassinet. Bassinets are used only for newborns in hospitals since even babies as young as 2 months are capable of squirming enough to not be safe.

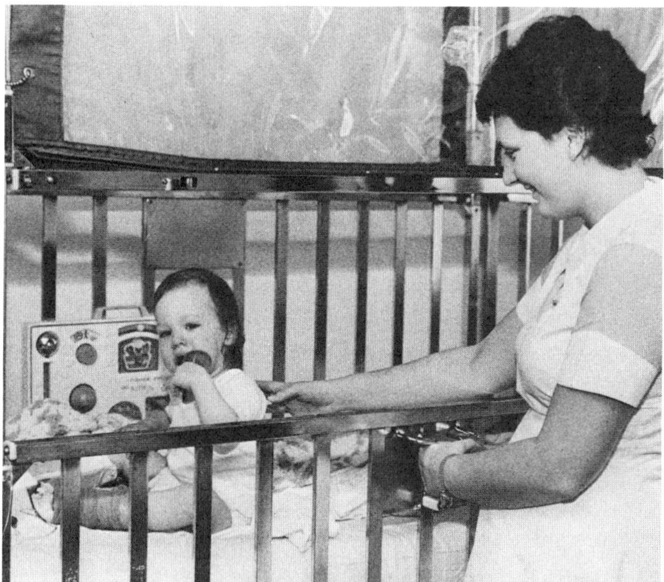

FIGURE 27-2. A preschool age child in a crib. Before leaving a child in a crib always test the siderail to see that it is securely in place. The crib shown here is a climber crib. The additional plastic section prevents this toddler from climbing out of the crib.

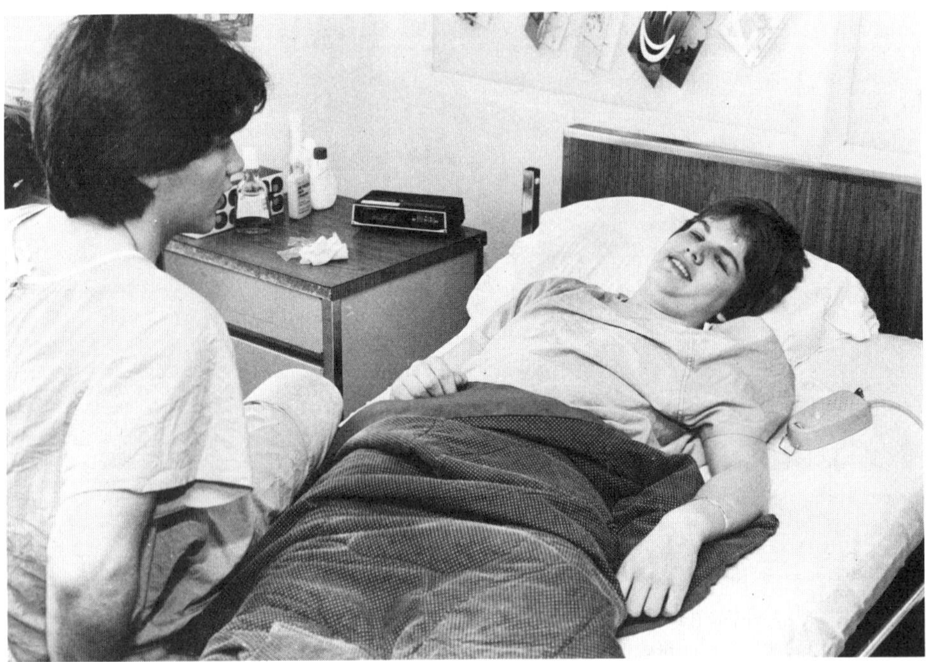

FIGURE 27-3. An early adolescent provided with an adult type bed. Notice the cards from school friends on the wall, which help make the atmosphere appealing to this age group.

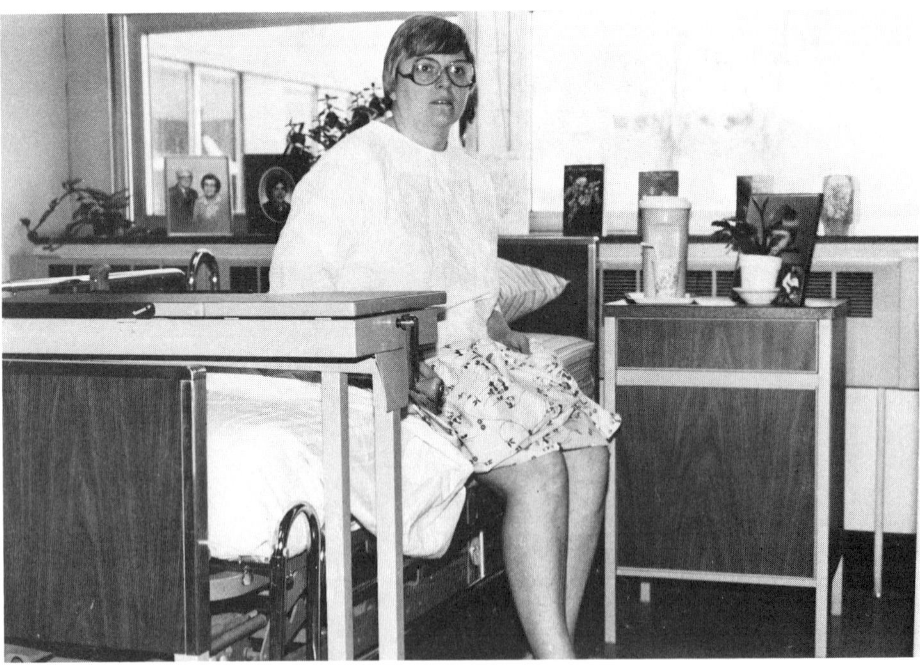

FIGURE 27-4. A bed in a low position. From this position, the patient can get out of bed easily without hurting herself. Notice the overbed table, a convenient surface for you and the patient's needs; the bedside stand provides for equipment storage.

the floor (about 66 cm; 26 in.) for times when care is being given and a low position (Fig. 27-4) so the patient can get out of bed easily without danger of falling. This is accomplished by means of an electric control that you or the patient operates or by means of a crank at the foot of the bed that you operate. If a bed's controls are broken or it cannot be placed in a low position, you must provide a footstool for the patient.

By means of the electric control or by turning a second crank at the foot of the Gatch bed, you can raise or lower the head of the bed or the section of the bed under a patient's knees (Fig. 27-5). Be certain that electric controls are not allowed to get wet to avoid electrical shock. After adjusting a bed with a foot gatch to a position, tuck the crank back in its recess under the bed. Otherwise, either you or the patient may bump it and injure a leg.

A patient who is unable to turn in bed may be placed on a frame or cyclopedic bed, designed to turn to different positions (see Chap. 26, Fig. 26-37B).

MATTRESSES AND PILLOWS

Mattresses of hospital beds or cribs are firm in order to supply good body support and comfortable alignment of the body. Mattresses may be protected by plastic coverings to make them water repellent. Be careful when you are performing a procedure that includes the use of safety pins or other sharp objects that you do not tear the covering and leave the mattress open to damage from water or increased wear. Air-filled, alternating pressure, or water-filled flotation mattresses reduce constant pressure on resting body parts. Use sharp instruments carefully around these mattresses because puncturing will destroy their function. Although not so effective in reducing pressure, corrugated foam pads are frequently placed over standard mattresses because they are less expensive and disposable (Fig. 27-6).

Hospital pillows may also be protected by a plastic covering. Plastic coverings have the advantage of being easily cleaned. Unfortunately, they are also hot, slippery, and uncomfortable.

Pillows are not used in cribs, basinets, or Isolettes. An ill infant young enough to be placed in this kind of bed might suffocate from a pillow.

SIDERAILS

Hospital beds are provided with siderails that extend from the head of the bed at least halfway down the sides of the bed. These are safety devices to remind a patient that he has rolled close to the edge of the bed; they are also sturdy enough to use in turning or getting out of bed. Lower siderails when performing procedures at a bedside so that you do not have to stretch over them and raise them again before you leave. Crib siderails must always be raised to a high position before you leave.

ADDITIONAL ROOM FURNITURE

Every patient is provided with a bedside stand (Fig. 27-7). Traditionally, the top drawer is used by the patient for items such as his toothbrush, loose change, or reading material. Inside, two shelves are used to store hospital equipment. A towel rack on the side or back of the stand provides a space for a towel and washcloth. Both Isolettes and bassinets have storage space built into the bottom so no bedside stand is necessary.

Adults are also provided an overbed table (see Fig. 27-4). These have a flat surface on which to write or place a meal tray. Some overbed tables have storage space and a mirror that can be raised by tilting the surface. The overbed table can be raised or lowered by a crank or other device on the end of the upright portion. A simple lift-out bedtable (Fig. 27-8) is generally used with children because it is less complicated for them to operate.

Every hospital room should have a comfortable chair for a visitor or for the patient to sit in for part of the day. Many rooms are furnished with two chairs so the patient and a visitor can be seated at the same time. Rooms for infants should be provided with a rocking chair so that you or a parent can sit and rock him for a part of every day.

BATHROOM FACILITIES

Private hospital rooms have a bathroom with a toilet and sink off the room readily accessible to the patient. Two-, four- or eight-bed units have a bathroom shared by all the patients in the room. In addition, most hospital units have a central tub or shower room for patients' use.

EQUIPMENT FOR PATIENT CARE

The usual equipment in a hospital room is a water pitcher and a drinking glass, an emesis basin and mouthwash cup, a basin for bathwater, a soap dish, a bedpan, and for males, a urinal. The pitcher and water glass sit on top of the bedside stand; the water basin, emesis basin, mouthwash cup, and soap dish are placed on the upper shelf of the bedside stand; the bedpan and urinal are placed on the lower shelf (see Fig. 27-7). This arrangement is convenient for the patient and fulfills a principle of asepsis, with the cleanest items at the top.

Children under 2 years who are not yet toilet trained do not need bedpans or urinals and may be furnished a potty seat instead. The emesis basin and mouthwash cup are used for toothbrushing and oral care. They are not necessary for the infant under 6 months who has no teeth yet.

Making a Hospital Bed

Although health care agency procedures differ in small details, hospital beds are traditionally and universally made as in Procedure 27-1. Making a bed in this way provides optimum comfort and safety. Because the bed remains neat for a long period of time, it adds to a pleasant environment.

When making a bed, do not shake linen; always unfold it smoothly. Shaking linen stirs up dust and spreads airborne organisms. If a piece of linen falls on the floor,

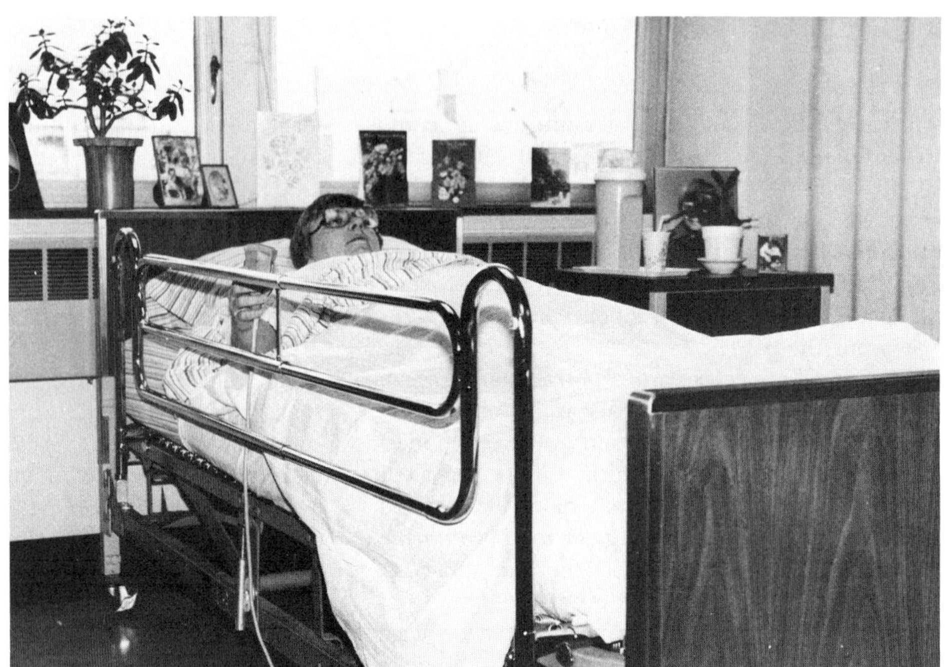

A

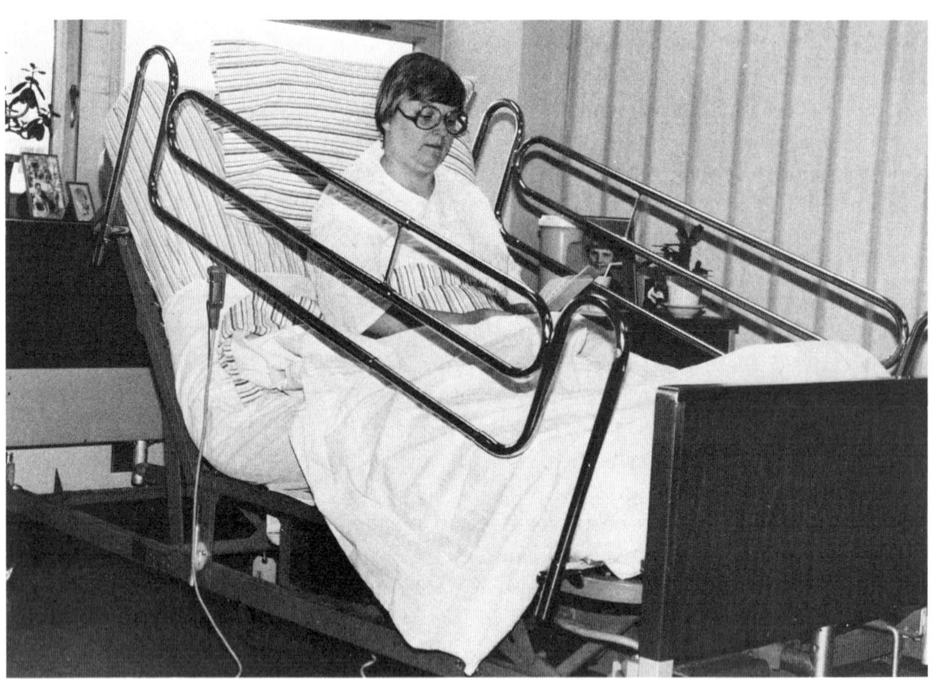

B

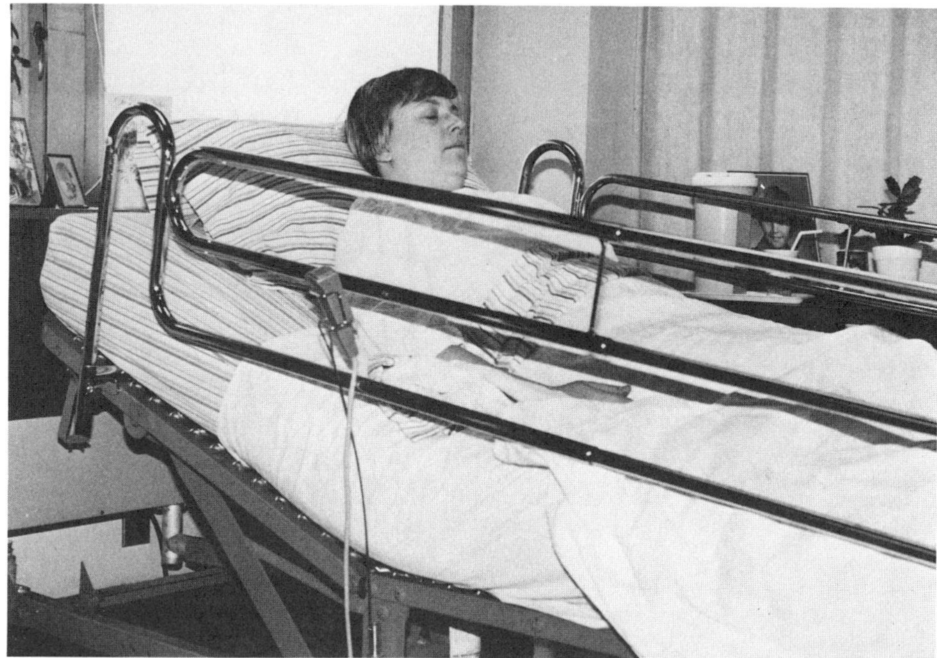

C

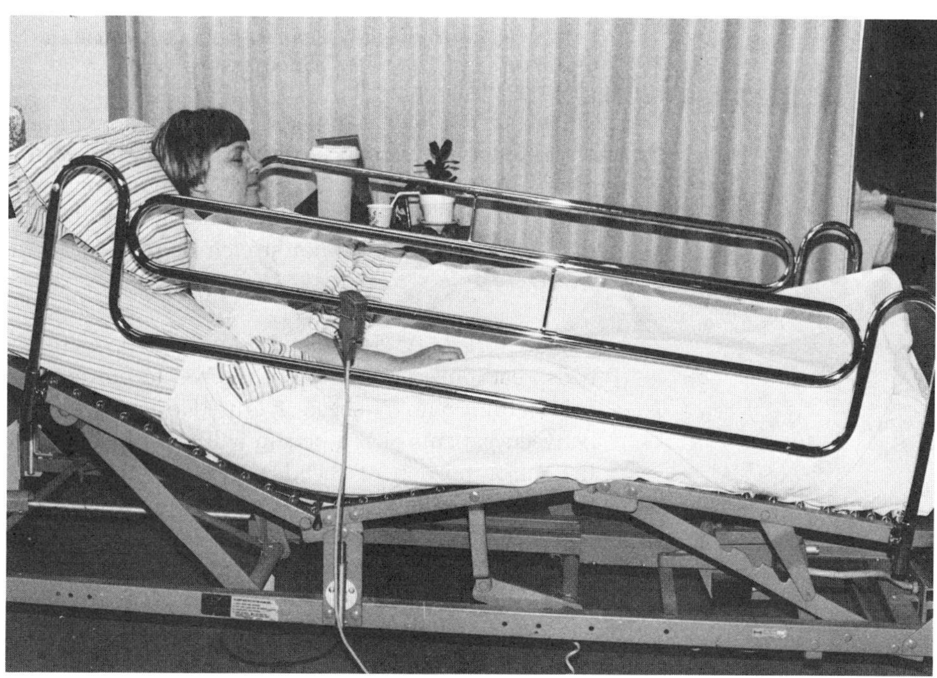

D

FIGURE 27-5. Commonly used bed positions. A. Flat. This position is used for performing most procedures. B. Fowler's position. The headrest of the bed is raised to a 90-degree angle. This position might be used with a patient who has difficulty breathing. C. Semi-Fowler's position. The head rest of the bed is raised to a 45-degree angle. D. Contour position. The headrest of the bed is raised at a 45-degree angle; the knee rest at a 15-degree angle; the foot may also be raised. Patients with a tendency toward blood clotting should not have the knee position raised as in this position since the bend at the knee may lead to clotting.

A Trendelenberg position (not shown) is a position in which the foot of the bed is higher than the head.

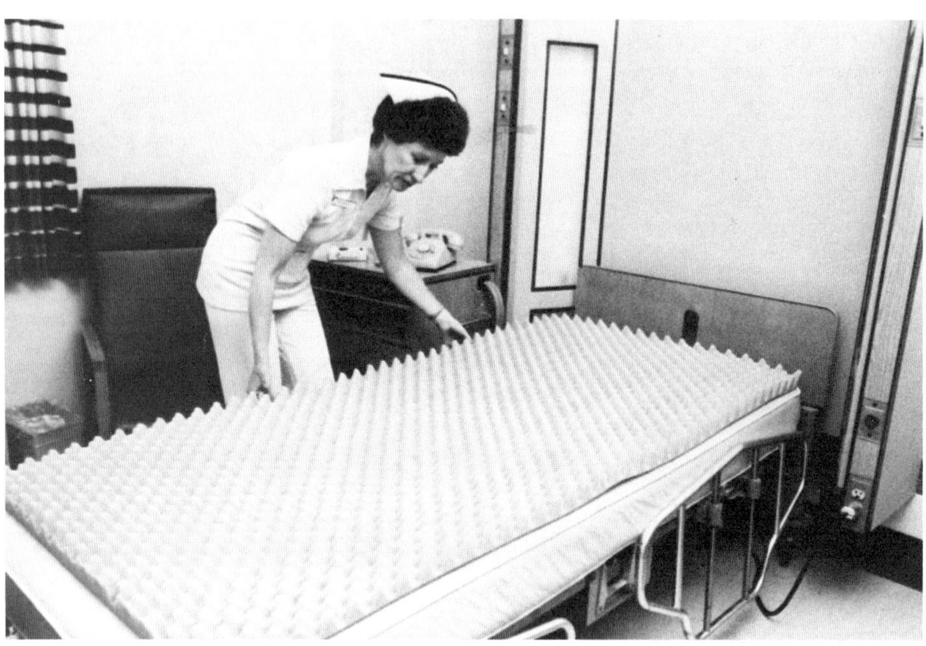

FIGURE 27-6. A foam (eggshell) mattress. After positioning, the nurse covers it with the bottom bed sheet.

FIGURE 27-7. Contents of a bedside stand. Note that cleaner articles are always placed above more soiled articles.

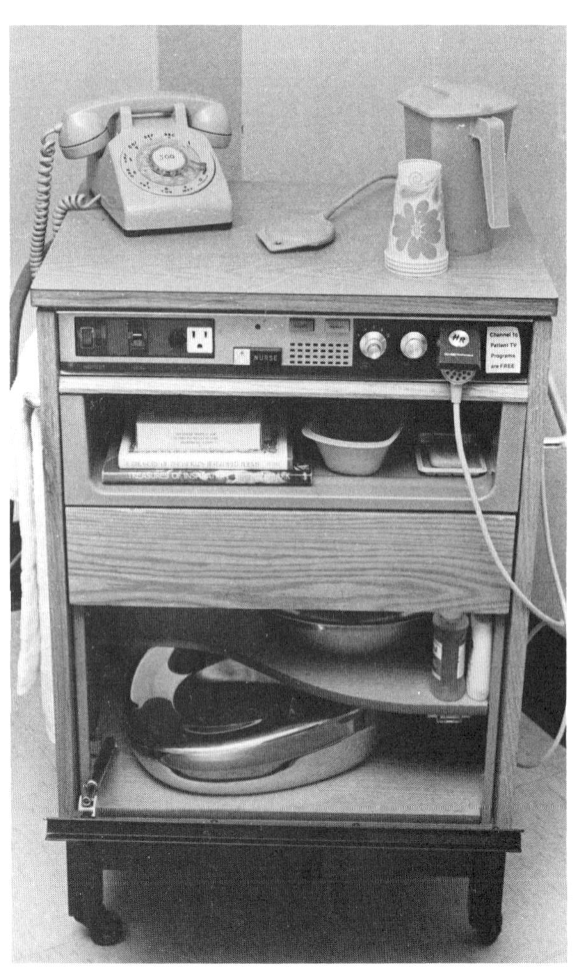

discard it in a linen hamper. Using it after it has been dropped would introduce organisms into the bed that could infect the patient. To reduce strain on your back, use good body mechanics while making beds. Bend at the hips and knees; do not stretch or bend from the waist.

A Closed Bed. A closed bed is one made with the bedspread pulled to the top of the bed to prevent dust from settling onto the sheets. It is used to keep beds clean between patients or if a person will be ambulatory for the major portion of the day. The bed described in Procedure 27-1 is a closed bed.

An Open Bed. A bed is opened when its top covers are turned down so that it is easily accessible to a patient. Steps in making an open bed are shown in Procedure 27-2.

A Surgical Bed. A patient returning from surgery is still sleepy from the anesthetic and may have difficulty turning easily due to a painful surgical incision. Steps in making a surgical bed, one easy to help a patient turn over into, are shown in Procedure 27-3. Such a bed is also used for a patient with a large cast or other circumstance that would make it difficult for him to transfer easily into bed so the term *surgical bed* is not used only for postsurgical patients.

An Occupied Bed. Many patients in hospital settings are unable to get out of bed owing to recent surgery or immobilization with a large cast or traction. You make the bed while such patients occupy it. Steps for this are shown in Procedure 27-4.

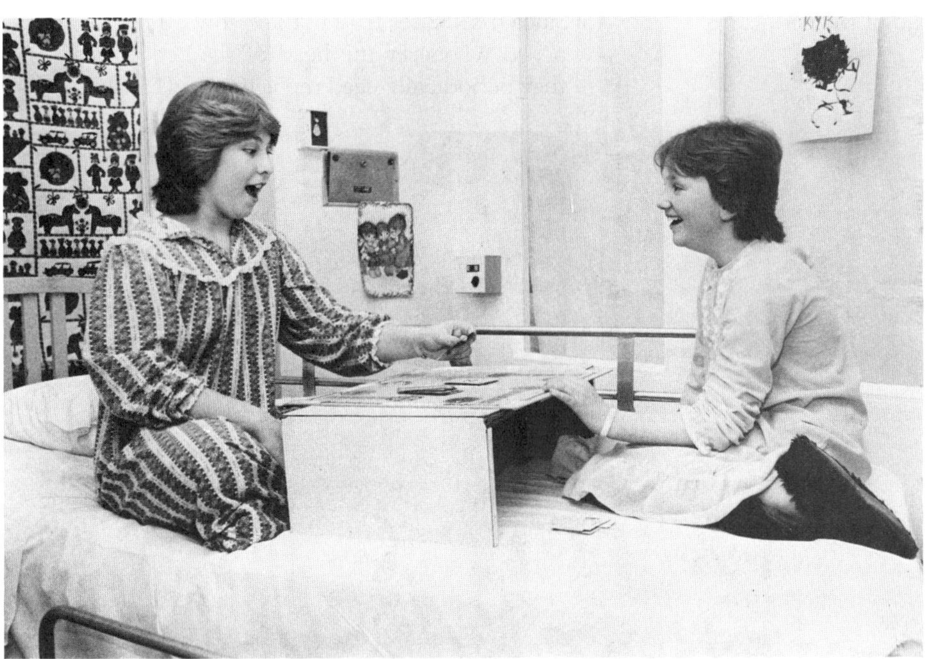

FIGURE 27-8. An overbed table used with children. In this instance, it is being used as a game table.

PROCEDURE 27-1
Making a Closed Unoccupied Adult Bed

Purpose: Create an unwrinkled bed surface with a minimum of energy expenditure. Create a bed that remains free of dust.

Plan	*Principle*
1. Wash your hands.	1. Ensure patient safety from spread of microorganisms.
2. Assess patient situation; analyze appropriateness of plan; adjust plan to individual patient need.	2. Nursing care is always individualized based on professional nursing judgment of patient need.
3. Implement care by assembling necessary supplies. Place them on the bedside stand in the following order: 1 pillowcase, 1 bedspread, 1 top sheet, 1 linen draw sheet, 1 bottom sheet. Optional: 1 blanket, 1 rubber or plastic draw sheet, 1 mattress pad. Plan to work so that you complete half of the bed before you begin the second half.	3. Arranging linen in the order it will be used saves time. Making one side of a bed at a time saves you energy.
4. Raise bed to its *high* position; lower the siderail nearest you; place the mattress flat.	4. Reduce possibility of muscle strain. Ensure firm fit for sheets.

5. Move mattress to the head of the bed.

5. Since mattresses tend to move toward the foot of a bed whenever the head of the bed is raised, they periodically need repositioning (Fig. 1).

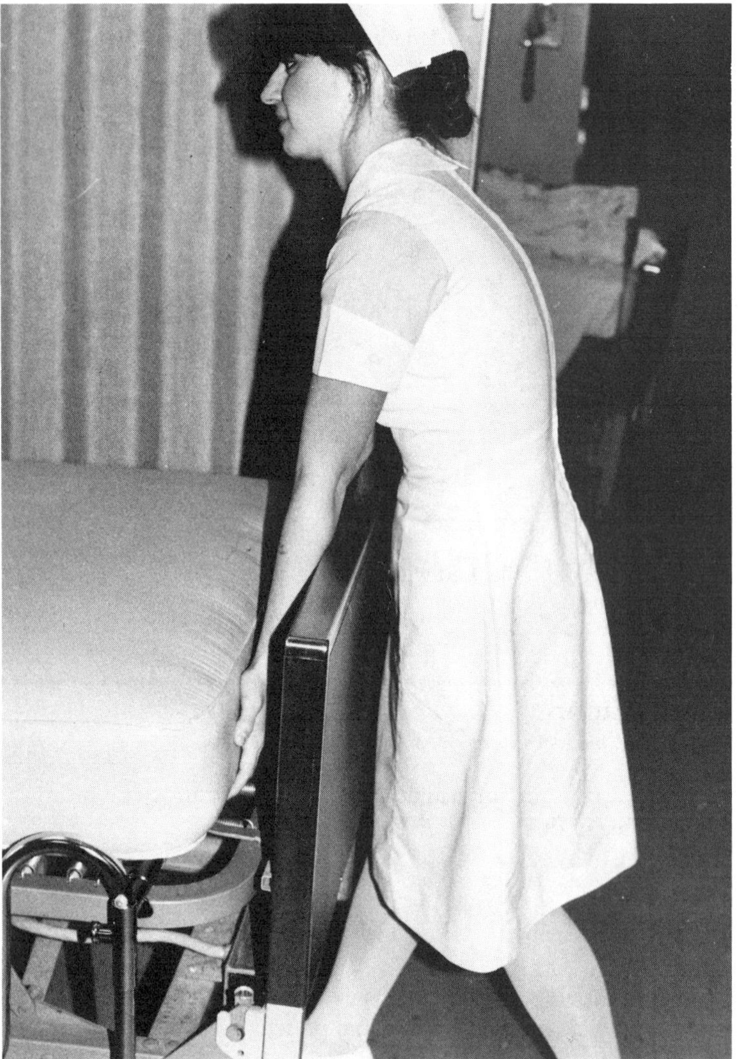

FIGURE 1. Use both hands to move a mattress. Ask for help as needed.

6. Place mattress pad on bed if the mattress is plastic covered.

6. A mattress pad provides comfort and decreases the contact of a plastic-covered mattress near the skin.

7. Unfold bottom sheet so it covers half the mattress nearest you and the rough side of the hem faces down toward the mattress. Bring the lower edge of the sheet even with the bottom edge of the mattress; tuck the upper edge of the sheet under the head of the mattress.

7. If the rough hem were facing up, it might irritate a patient's heels. Tucking a wide band of sheet under the head of the mattress prevents the sheet from loosening when the head of the bed is raised (Fig. 2).

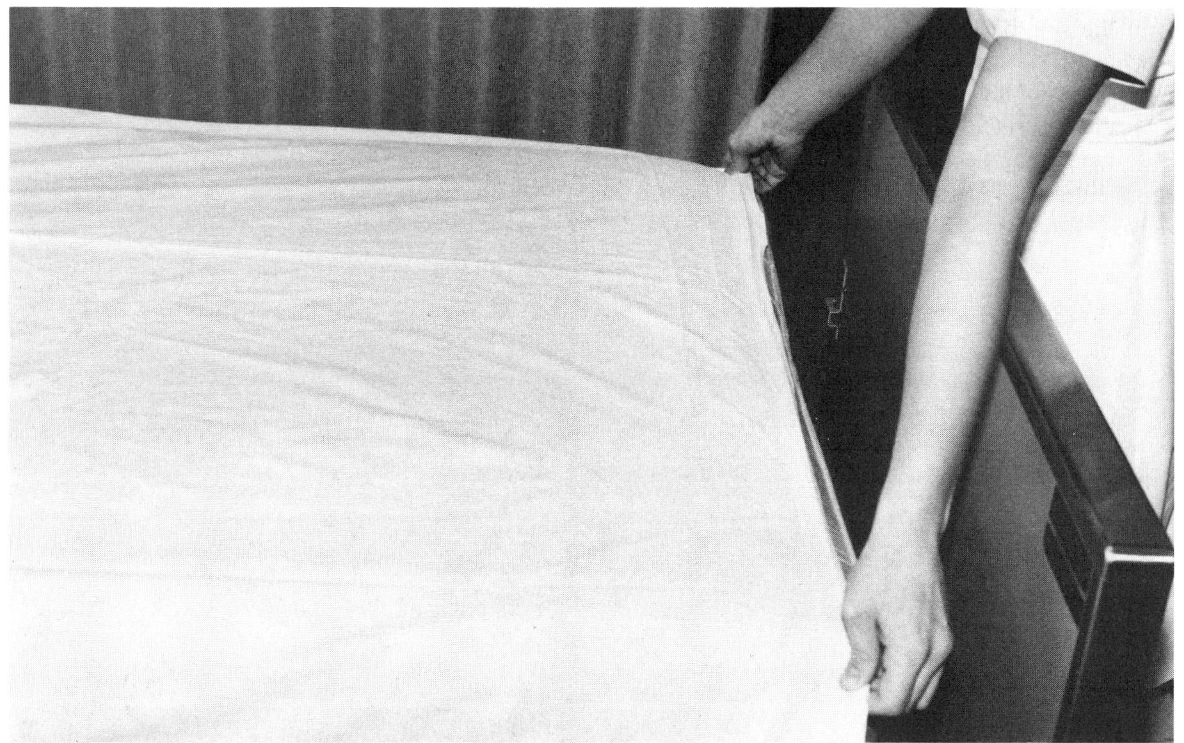

FIGURE 2. The bottom sheet of a bed is placed even with the lower edge of the mattress.

8. If an agency uses contoured bottom sheets, merely pull the puckered corner down over the top and bottom mattress corners. If a contour sheet is not used, you must make a mitered corner on the top corner. To square a corner, after tucking the sheet in firmly under the head of the bed, lift the portion of the sheet that overhangs on the side back over the bed. Hold the sheet against the side of the mattress and tuck in the excess. Bring the folded portion of the sheet back to side of bed and tuck underneath.

8. In order for the bottom sheet to stay in place for an extended period of time, it must be anchored securely at the corner and side (Fig. 3).

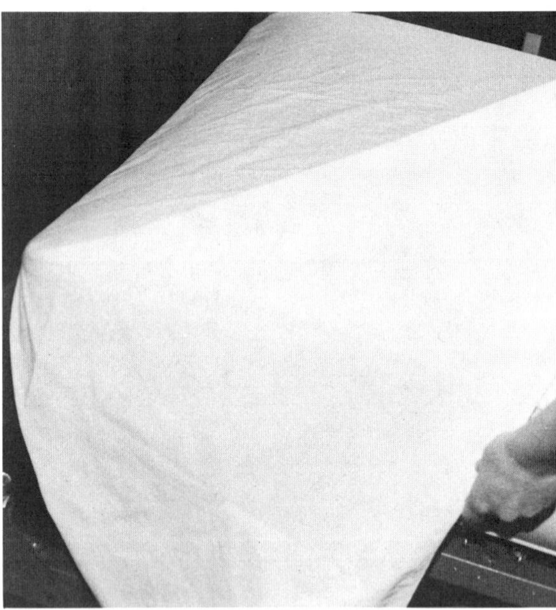

A

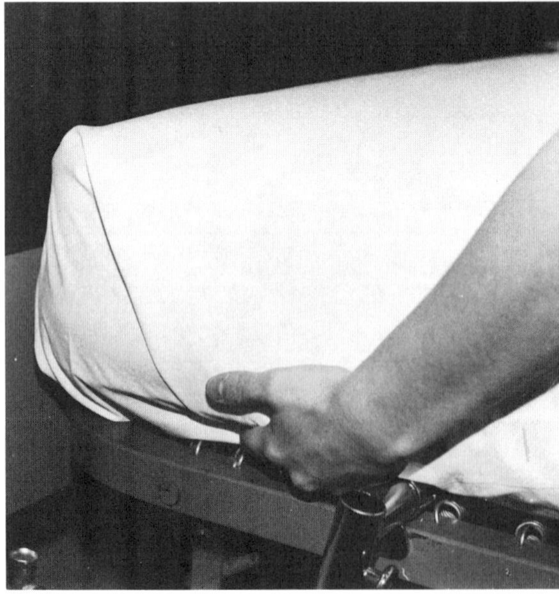

B

FIGURE 3. Mitering or squaring a corner on a bed. A. Tuck sheet in at bottom; fold side back over mattress. B. Bring sheet over side of mattress to complete fold.

9. Tuck in the remainder of the side of the bottom sheet the length of the mattress.

10. Place plastic or rubber draw sheet on bed (optional). Center it so the middle of patient's back will be at top of sheet; knees will be at bottom edge. Place the linen draw sheet (rough hem down) over the plastic sheet.

10. A draw sheet is easy to change if the bed should be soiled. It also can be used to help position the patient in bed.

11. Tuck in the side of the plastic and linen sheets (Fig. 4).

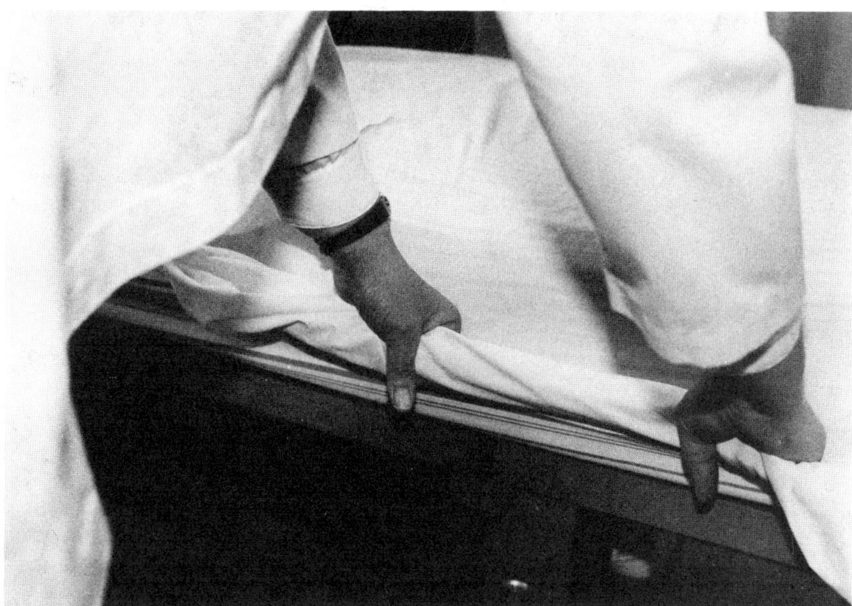

FIGURE 4. A draw sheet needs to be pulled taut and firmly secured under mattress so that it does not pull free and wrinkle.

12. Unfold the top sheet and place it on the bed so the top edge comes even with the top edge of the mattress. Place it so the rough hem is down. Tuck the sheet under the bottom of the bed and square the bottom corner.

12. When the bed is opened for patient use, this top sheet will be cuffed, turning the rough edge up, away from the patient and reducing the risk of irritation to patient skin.

13. Place the blanket (optional) and bedspread over the top sheet (right sides up); bring them even with the top of the mattress, tuck the bottom and square the bottom corner.

14. Walk around the bed to complete the opposite side.

14. Making one side of a bed at a time saves energy since it reduces the number of steps you must take to complete the bed.

15. Fold top linens back so bottom sheet is revealed. Pull the bottom sheet taut, square the top corner and tuck in firmly the length of the mattress.

16. Pull the plastic draw sheet tightly and tuck under the mattress.

17. Take top sheet and bedspread and make a horizontal or a vertical pleat about 2 inches in width at the bottom of the bed. Square the bottom corner. Cuff the sheet over the spread at the head of the bed.

17. Ensure adequate footspace to prevent pressure on feet (Fig. 5).

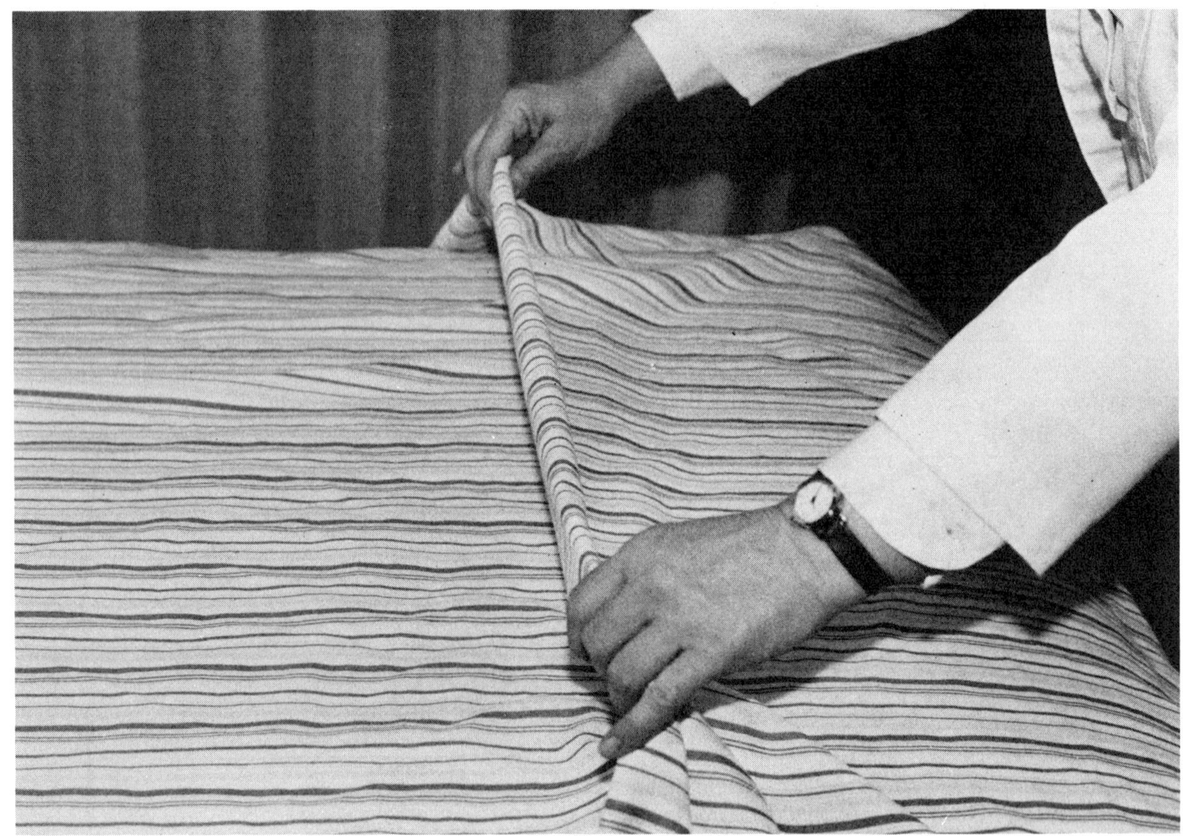

FIGURE 5. A pleat should be placed on top sheets to prevent pressure on a patient's feet. Shown here is a horizontal pleat; if preferred, a vertical pleat may be used.

18. To prepare the pillowcase, put one hand inside the case; grip it at the bottom point; fold the case inside out back onto your other hand.
19. Grasp the end of the pillow with the hand holding the pillowcase and fold the case down over the pillow. If the pillow does not fit snugly, make a pleat along side of the pillow to secure any extra material.

18. Hold the pillow away from your uniform to prevent cross infection to your uniform (Fig. 6).

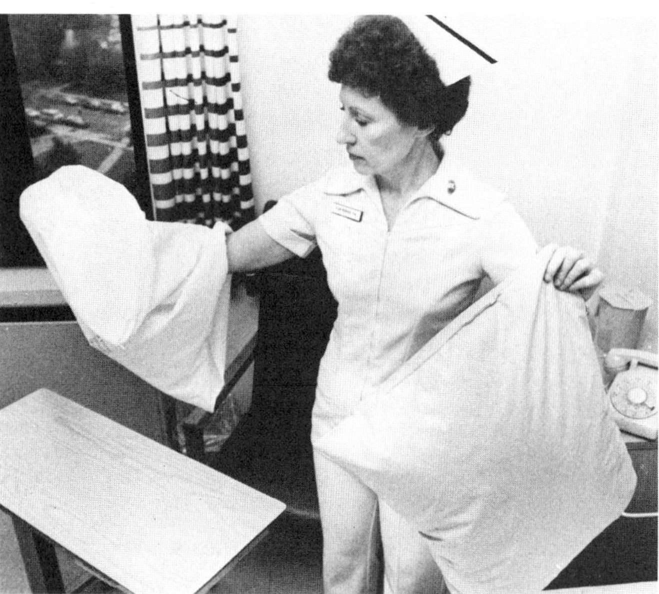

A

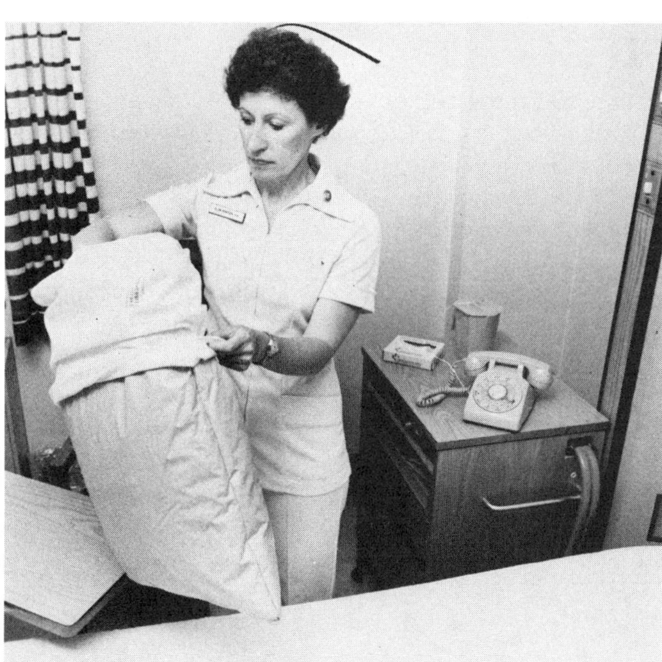

B

FIGURE 6. Covering a pillow with a pillowcase. A. Grasp pillowcase on center crease. B. Pull down over pillow.

20. Place pillow on bed at head of bed on top of spread with the opening to the pillow facing away from the door of the room.

20. Ensure a neat appearance (Fig. 7).

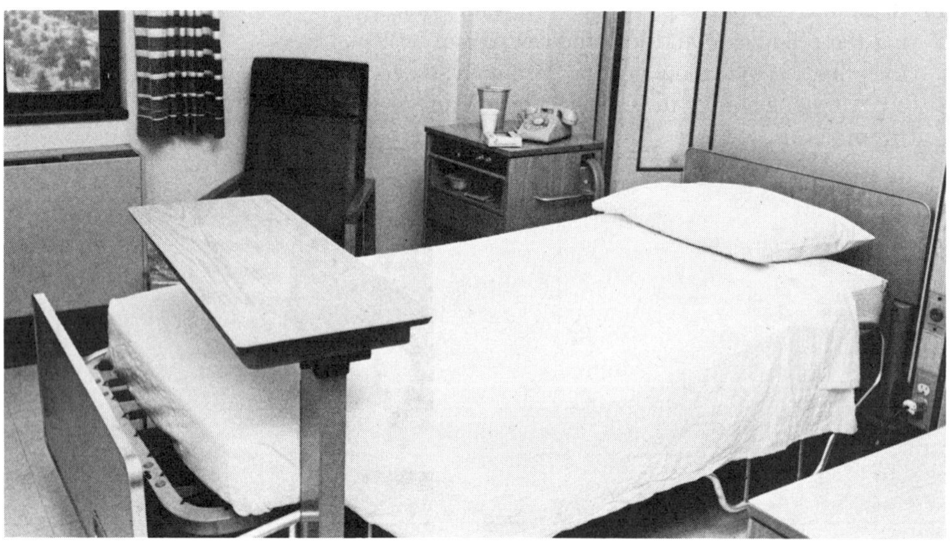

FIGURE 7. A completed closed bed.

21. Straighten other furniture in room. Leave room neat and inviting; return bed to *low position* for easy patient access.

21. Provide psychological as well as physical comfort.

22. Evaluate effectiveness, efficiency, cost, comfort, and safety aspects of procedure.

22. A therapeutic environment requires more than just a comfortable bed.

MODIFICATIONS FOR CARE OF CHILD

1. Both basinet and Isolette mattresses are covered by pillowcases. Place the cover on the mattresss as you would onto a pillow.
2. All cribs have waterproof mattresses so no draw sheet is used. Use a full sheet or draw sheet for bottom sheet; square corners.
3. Place a folded baby blanket at the foot of the bed for a top cover. The blanket may be used for security (touch) reasons as well as for warmth.

MODIFICATIONS FOR CARE OF OLDER ADULT

An older adult may become chilled easily because of reduced subcutaneous fat; you might provide a cotton blanket instead of a top sheet for additional warmth.

Be extremely careful that the bottom bed surface is wrinkle free. A ridge of linen can seriously impair circulation in the older adult.

PROCEDURE 27-2
Preparing an Open Bed

Purpose: To create a bed that provides for easy access.

Plan	*Principle*
1. Wash your hands.	1. Prevent spread of microorganisms.
2. Assess patient condition and analyze appropriateness of plan; adjust plan to individual patient needs.	2. Nursing care is always individualized based on professional judgment of patient need.
3. To convert a closed or unoccupied bed to an open bed, fanfold the top sheet and bedspread down to no more than half the length of the bed.	3. Ensure easy access to the bed (Fig. 1).

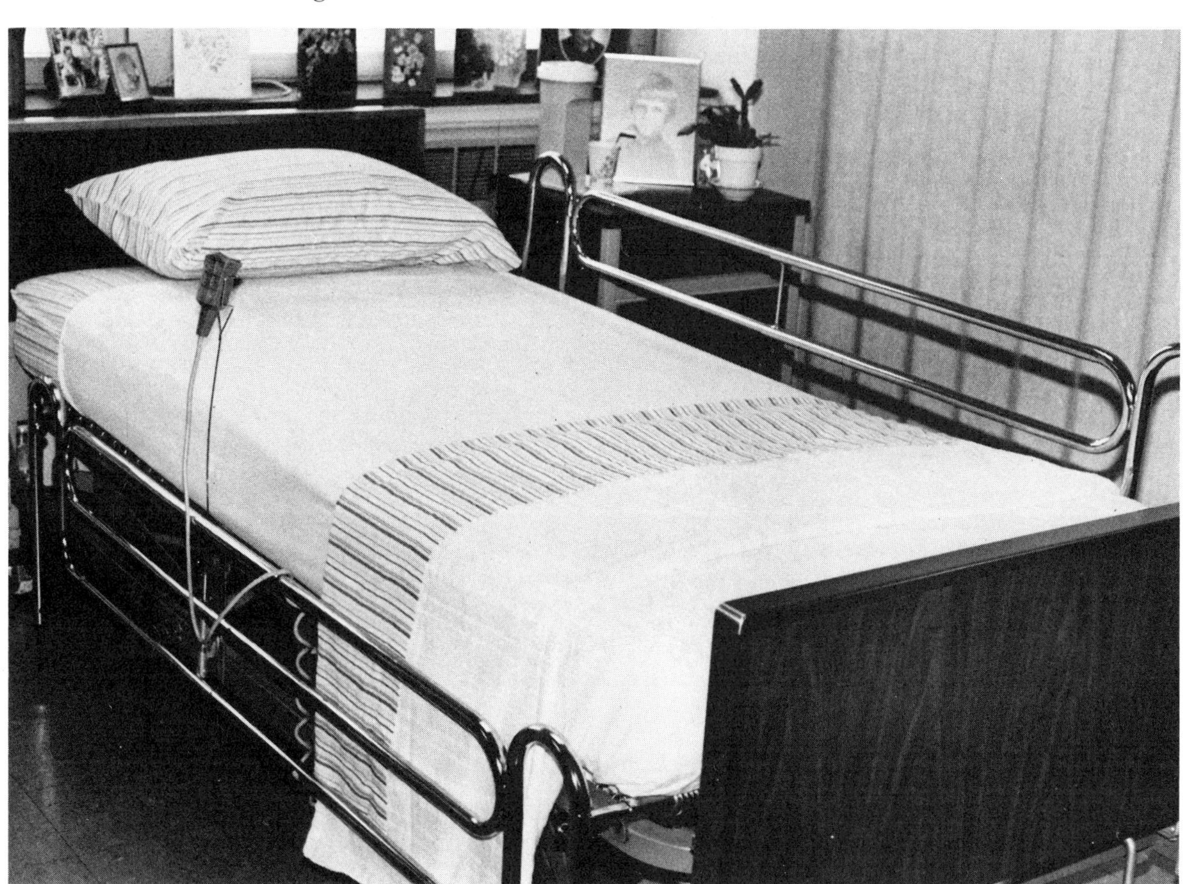

FIGURE 1. An open bed. This bed may be entered easily by a patient.

4. Lower the bed to the low position.	4. Ensure safe and easy patient access.
5. Attach the call bell to the bed or sheet so it is easily available.	5. Ensure safe communication with the patient.
6. Straighten other furniture in the room; leave room neat and inviting.	6. Provide psychological as well as physical comfort.
7. Evaluate effectiveness, efficiency, cost, safety, and comfort aspects of procedure based on individual patient need.	7. A therapeutic environment includes more than a comfortable bed.

PROCEDURE 27-3
Preparing a Surgical Bed

Purpose: To prepare a bed that provides for easy access for the patient who has limited mobility.

Plan	*Principle*
1. Wash your hands. Use all clean linen.	1. To ensure as clean a unit as possible to prevent spread of microorganisms.
2. Assess patient condition. Analyze appropriateness of plan; adjust plan to individual patient need.	2. Nursing care is always individualized based on professional judgment of patient need.
3. Prepare bottom sheet as with closed bed. Do not tuck in top sheet. Instead make a cuff at the bottom and top of the bed by bringing the top sheet up over the spread.	3. A surgical patient arrives at his bed by stretcher. It must be possible for him to slide over into bed easily (Fig. 1).

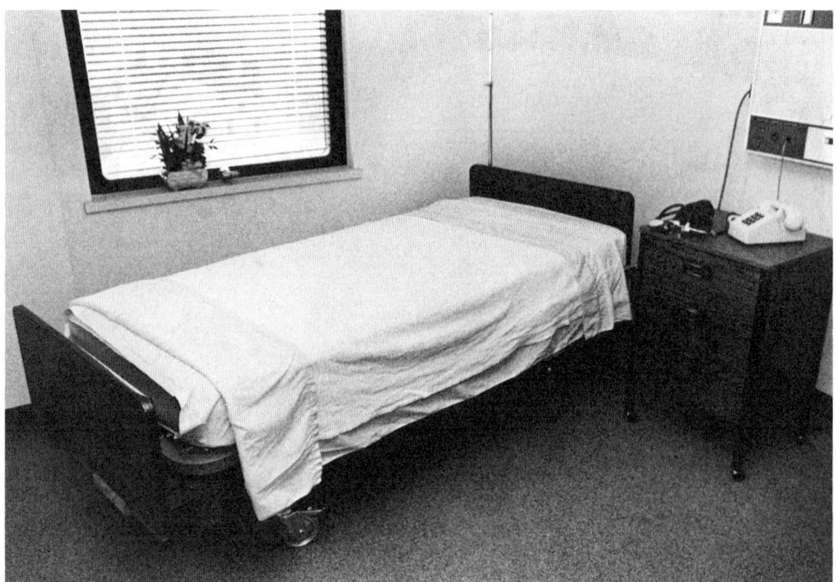

A

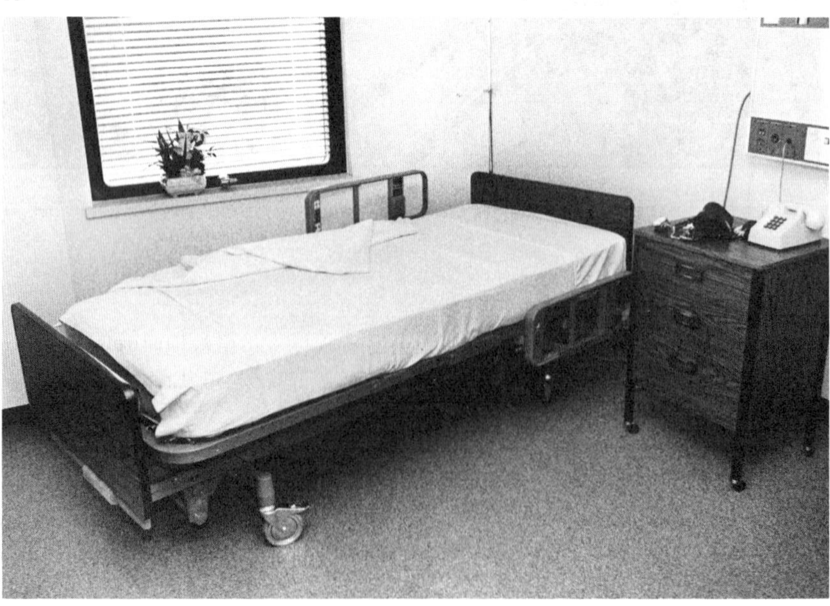

B

FIGURE 1. Making a surgical bed. A. The top sheet is cuffed at top and bottom. B. The top sheet is now fan-folded to the side.

Plan	Principle
4. Fold the corners of the top sheet into a triangle. Fanfold to side of bed away from door.	
5. Place the pillow upright at the head of the bed or on the overbed table.	5. It is unsafe for anesthesized patients to have their head elevated until they are wide awake, to prevent aspiration.
6. Place a disposable pad over the pillow area; place the emesis basin and a box of tissues on the bedside stand.	6. To protect the bed, since many people returning from surgery are nauseated and may vomit in the first few hours following surgery.
7. Make sure no liquids are at bedside.	7. It is not safe for them to drink fluids until they are fully awake to prevent aspiration.
8. Leave the bed in the high position. Push the bedside stand away from the bed.	8. The stretcher will fit snugly against the side of the bed and patient transfer is facilitated.
9. Attach call bell in easily accessible position.	9. Ensure safe communication with the patient as soon as he is awake.
10. Straighten other furniture in room; leave room neat and inviting.	10. Provide psychological as well as physical comfort.
11. Evaluate effectiveness, efficiency, cost, comfort, and safety aspects of procedure.	11. A therapeutic environment requires more than just a comfortable bed.

MODIFICATIONS FOR CARE OF CHILD

1. Top covers are not used in cribs. Merely fold top blanket to foot of crib.
2. Remove not only water from the bedside stand, but all reminders of food or water from the room (out of sight, out of mind).

PROCEDURE 27-4
Making an Occupied Bed

Purpose: Preparing a clean, unwrinkled bed surface with a minimum of energy expenditure while a patient remains in bed.

Plan	*Principle*
1. Wash your hands, identify the patient, explain the procedure.	1. Prevent spread of microorganisms. Promote patient safety and well-being.
2. Assess patient status; analyze appropriateness of procedure; adjust plan to individual patient need.	2. Nursing care is always individualized based on professional nursing judgment of patient's needs.
3. Implement care by assembling supplies: 1 or 2 full sheets, 1 draw sheet, 1 pillowcase, and 1 bedspread.	3. Conserve energy by organization and preparation.
4. Raise the bed to a high position, provide privacy; lower near siderail of bed; lower head of bed to flat position if patient condition allows.	
5. Remove pillow from under head of patient; remove pillowcase. Place over back of chair to serve as laundry bag for soiled linen.	5. Prevent spread of microorganisms from linen.
6. Move mattress toward head of bed.	6. Whenever head of bed is raised, a mattress tends to slide toward foot of bed. Do not attempt this by yourself if patient weights over 100 pounds. Wait until you have help.
7. Check that the far siderail is in raised position. Help patient to move to far side of the bed or turn him to his side facing away from you.	7. Provides half the surface of the bed as a working area.

8. Loosen bottom linen and roll each sheet separately (linen draw sheet, bottom sheet) toward the patient. Tuck each roll as close to the patient's body as possible.

8. If linen is soiled with drainage, cover patient's back with towel or waterproof pad to protect skin (Fig. 1).

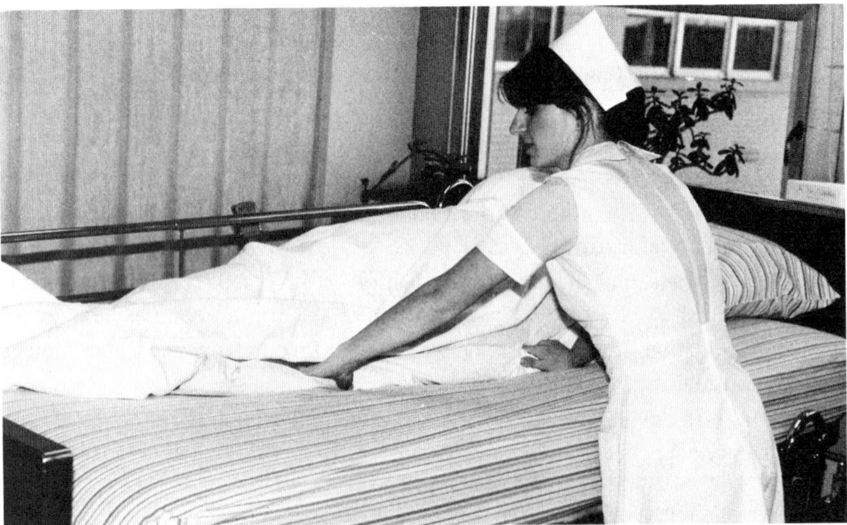

FIGURE 1. To make an occupied bed, roll soiled bottom sheets and tuck them under the patient's back.

9. Place clean bottom sheet on bed as in step 7 of making an unoccupied bed. Tuck the middle edge of the sheet under the roll of soiled linen.
10. Unroll plastic draw sheet and stretch it back over bottom sheet; tuck edge under mattress (Fig. 2).

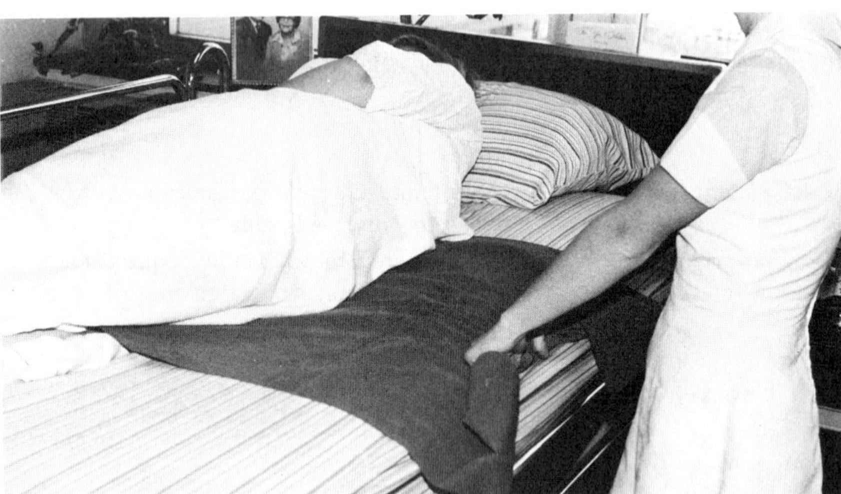

FIGURE 2. After clean bottom sheet is in place, if a plastic or rubber drawsheet is used, unroll it and retuck under mattress.

11. Place clean linen draw sheet on bed. Tuck near edge under mattress. Roll far side and tuck under patient.
12. Place clean top linen on bed as in step 12 of making an unoccupied bed. Remove soiled sheet by sliding it from underneath top covers so as not to expose patient. Raise the siderail.

12. Fully making one side of bed before the other reduces the number of steps necessary for you to take and expenditure of patient energy.

13. Ask patient to move or roll over ridge of tucked linen toward you to clean side of bed.
14. Walk to other side of bed, lower siderail. Fold top linen back so bed surface is exposed but patient is not. Loosen soiled bottom linen, remove from bed, and discard into laundry bag.
15. Pull bottom sheet to proper position and miter corners. Stretch draw sheets into place and tuck under mattress. Finish placement of top linens (Fig. 3).

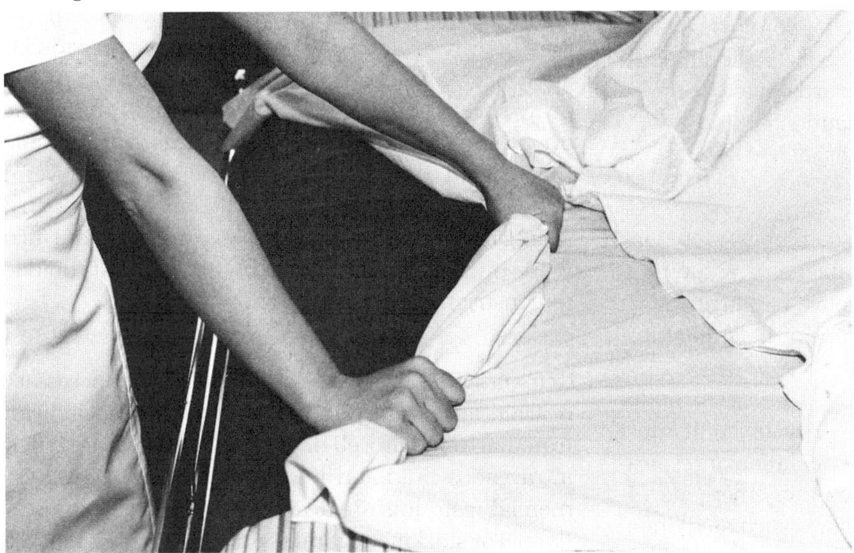

FIGURE 3. After the patient has moved to the far side of the bed, remove soiled linen from the bed and tuck in clean linen firmly.

16. Cover pillow with clean pillowcase as in steps 18 and 19 of making an unoccupied bed. Position patient comfortably; raise siderail; provide diversional activity; return bed to low position.
17. Secure signal device within easy patient reach. Place towel and washcloth in bedside stand; straighten patient unit.
18. Evaluate effectiveness, efficiency, cost, comfort, and safety aspects of procedure; chart procedure and assessments made.

    18. Document nursing action and patient status.
19. Plan health teaching indicated from assessment data such as association between wrinkled sheets and skin irritation.

    19. Health teaching is an independent nursing action always included in care.

MODIFICATIONS FOR CARE OF CHILD

Many children have never heard of anyone making a bed with them still in it. You may need to reinforce your instructions to stay on one side of the bed as you proceed or they will move out of interest in what you are doing.

MODIFICATIONS FOR CARE OF OLDER ADULT

Be careful that bottom sheets are left wrinkle free following a linen change as a ridge of linen can seriously compress circulation in an older adult. Arthritic changes may make it difficult for an older age adult to turn without pain to the opposite side of a bed. Be prepared to assist as necessary.

Beds as Part of Total Environment. When a person is ill and confined to a bed or a hospital room, his bed is only part of his environment. After changing bed linen, always straighten the top of the bedside stand and overbed table. Remove unnecessary supplies from the room and check that items the person will need are readily accessable. Be certain he has an activity to provide stimulation.

SAFETY

A person's safety is closely related to his comfort because he cannot feel comfortable unless he feels safe. In addition to removing environmental hazards, safety includes the use of restraints and fire precautions.

Use of Restraints

People who are not responsible for their own safety may need a form of restraint. For example, a person who is disoriented or delirious might remove bandages or an intravenous fluid line, ending therapy or harming himself.

A restraint must be sturdy enough to not tear under the strength of an average person's resistance; it must not draw tightly enough to restrict circulation or respiration. It must be releasable quickly in an emergency. It should be applied only when measures such as manual restraint prove inadequate.

It is always legal to restrain a person to prevent him from hurting himself or others. Following this immediate action, however, a physician's order is needed to continue the use of restraints because restraining someone unduly is a form of false imprisonment. It is important to document the behavior that necessitated the use of restraint and the type of restraint used.

TYPES OF RESTRAINTS

Manual Restraint. The type of restraint used differs according to the purpose and age of the patient. The fastest form of restraint is to use your hands, manually restraining a body part. You do this while assisting with the insertion of intravenous fluid lines in children or helping an adult remain in one position for a procedure. Be certain when you restrain manually that you never exert more pressure than necessary to achieve the task and that body parts are in good alignment. People under stress are very strong because of the abundance of epinephrine produced by a general adaptation syndrome. Even a 2-year-old under these circumstances may be too strong to restrain effectively without help.

Body Restraints. In some instances it is necessary to keep a patient from getting out of bed or help him stay seated in a wheelchair. The most effective type of restraint in these instances is a vest restraint (Fig. 27-9). These were manufactured originally by the Posey Company of California and are popularly termed *Posey restraints* even though another brand may be used. A vest restraint can pull tight under the axilla and interfere with circulation to an arm; it could put unnecessary pressure on neck veins or arteries, causing decreased cranial circulation. Assess these sites every 2 hours to be certain the vest is not pulling tight or interfering with circulation.

Mummy Restraint. A mummy restraint is a temporary total body restraint for an infant during a procedure. To apply such a restraint, lay the infant in the center of a draw sheet or towel. Fold the left side of the restraint over the infant and tuck the edge under the infant's trunk. Fold the right side of the restraint over the infant's body and tuck under the left side of his trunk (Fig. 27-10). Such a restraint secures an infant firmly while putting no pressure on body parts that could lead to constriction of respiration.

Extremity Restraints. In some instances it is necessary to restrain an arm or leg in order to keep an individual from harming himself or to allow some therapy such as intravenous fluid administration to be effective. Commercial restraints are available. Some agencies use soft flannel or stockinette for this purpose (Fig. 27-11). When making a restraint, tie the restraint to the person's extremity with a *clove-hitch* knot. This is a knot used for centuries to secure the delicate legs of race horses, and it will not draw tight if the person strains against it (Fig. 27-12). Tie the free ends of the restraint to the bottom frame of the bed, *not the siderail*, so that when the siderail is raised or lowered, the person's extremity will not be pulled.

Transport Restraints. Equipment used for transport has safety straps that buckle over a person's body. They also have siderails to prevent a person from rolling off the narrow width of the mattress. Never leave or transport anyone on a stretcher without these restraints in place (Fig. 27-13).

SAFETY RULES FOR RESTRAINTS

The biggest danger of restraints is that they will interfere with circulation. Every 2 hours, assess circulation to the body part distal to a restraint by obtaining a pulse in that part (dorsalis pedis for a leg restraint, radial for an arm restraint, temporal for a vest restraint). Loosen the restraint and assess the skin immediately under it for irritation or erythema. If the restraint is applied to an arm or a leg, move the extremity through a passive range of motion in order to ensure that joint mobility is not being compromised by inactivation.

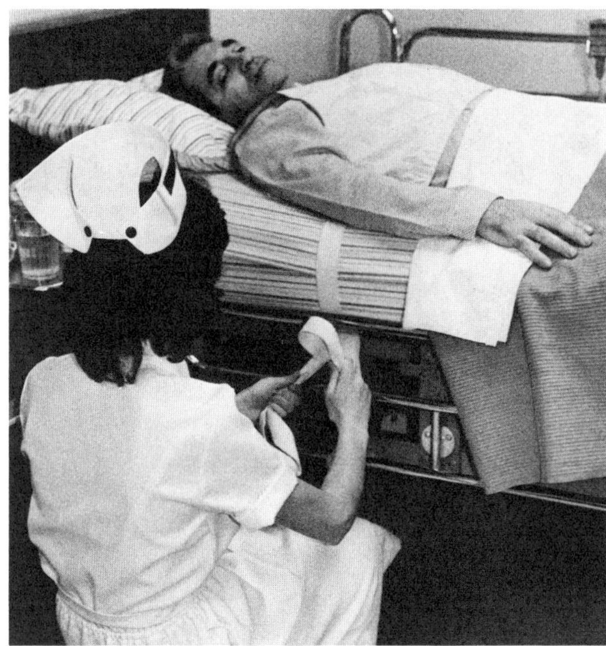

A

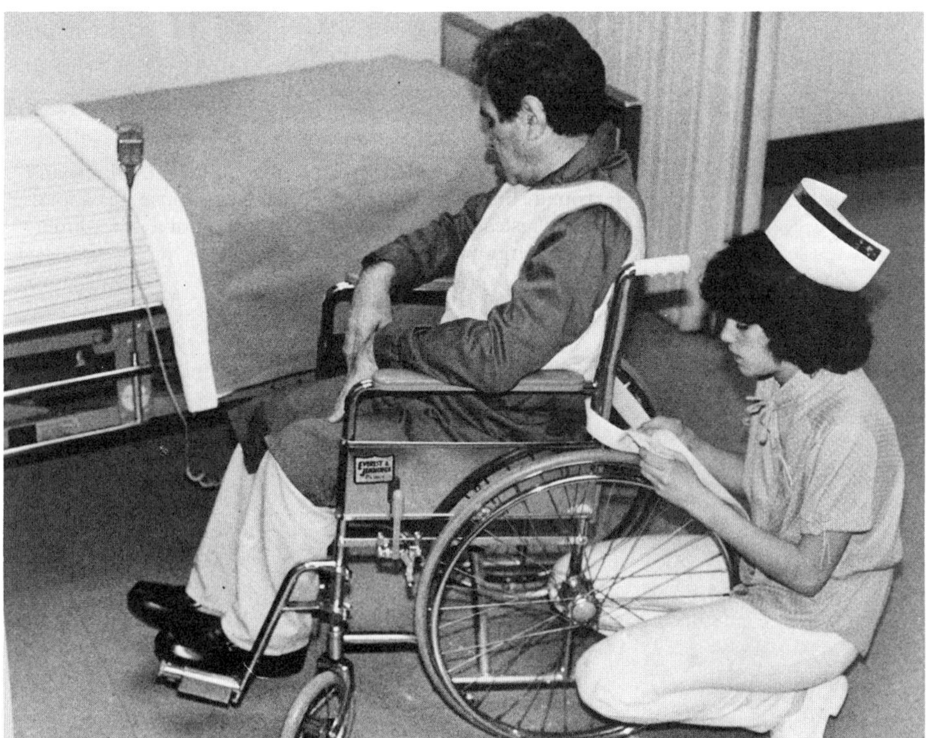

B

FIGURE 27-9. Vest restraint. A. Restraining a patient in bed using a vest restraint. Notice that the nurse ties the straps to the bed springs since these are a movable portion of the bed (when the bed position is changed, the restraint will not pull tight.) B. Using a vest restraint for a patient in a wheelchair. Notice again that the nurse secures the straps using a bow, which can be readily released in an emergency, rather than a knot.

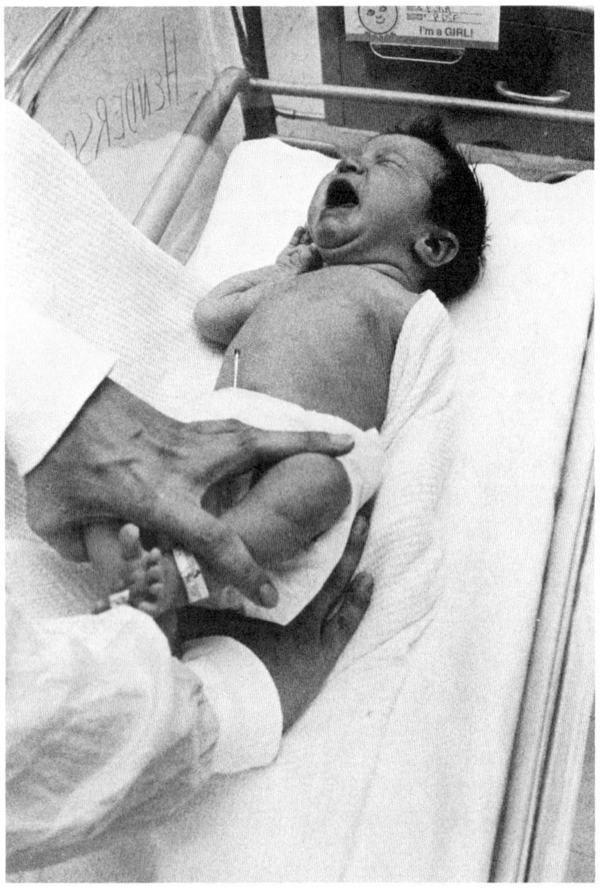

A

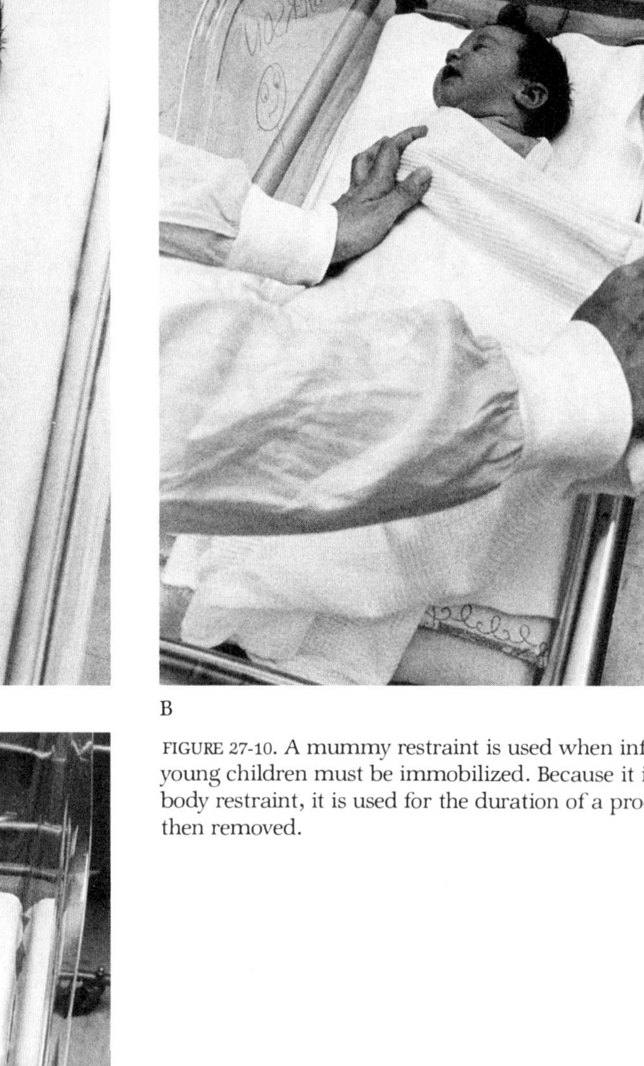

B

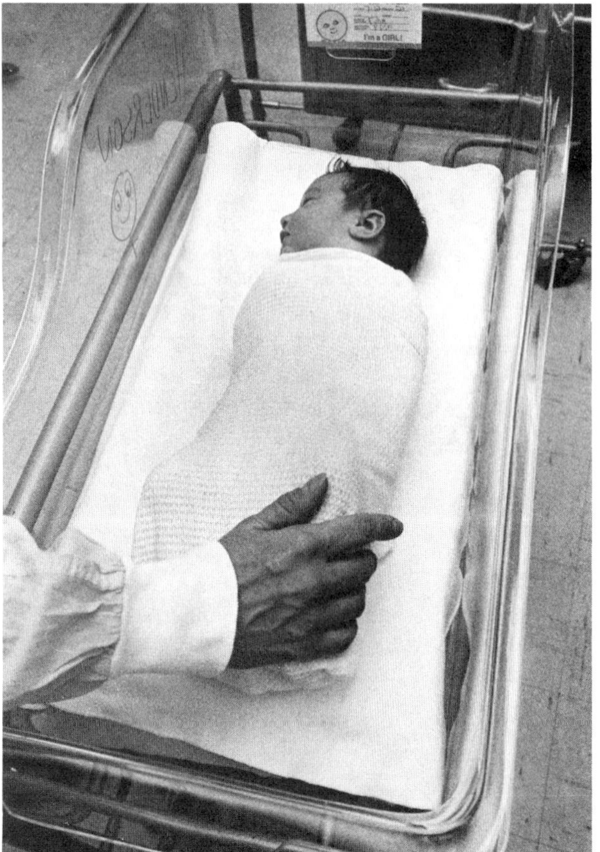

C

FIGURE 27-10. A mummy restraint is used when infants and young children must be immobilized. Because it is a total body restraint, it is used for the duration of a procedure, then removed.

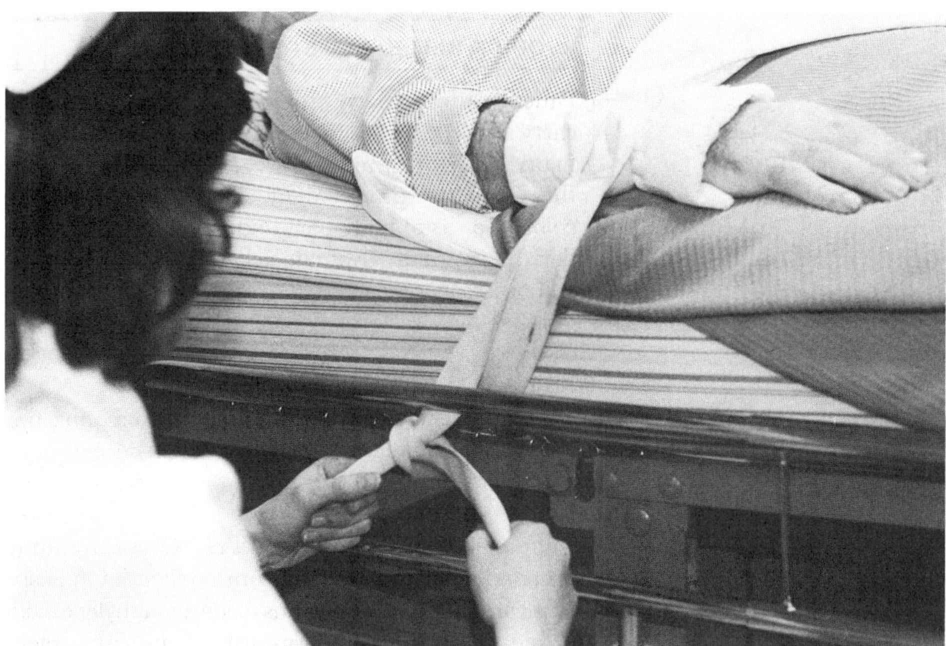

FIGURE 27-11. Restraining an extremity. Here an abdominal dressing pad is used to pad the patient's wrist; the restraint is then secured using a clove hitch knot and tied to the bed springs.

FIGURE 27-12. A clove hitch restraint. A soft strip of cloth is formed in a figure eight (A), with both ends of the cloth on top of the figure eight (B). Bring the loops together and pull the two ends (C) to adjust the loop to the size of the patient's wrist or ankle (D).

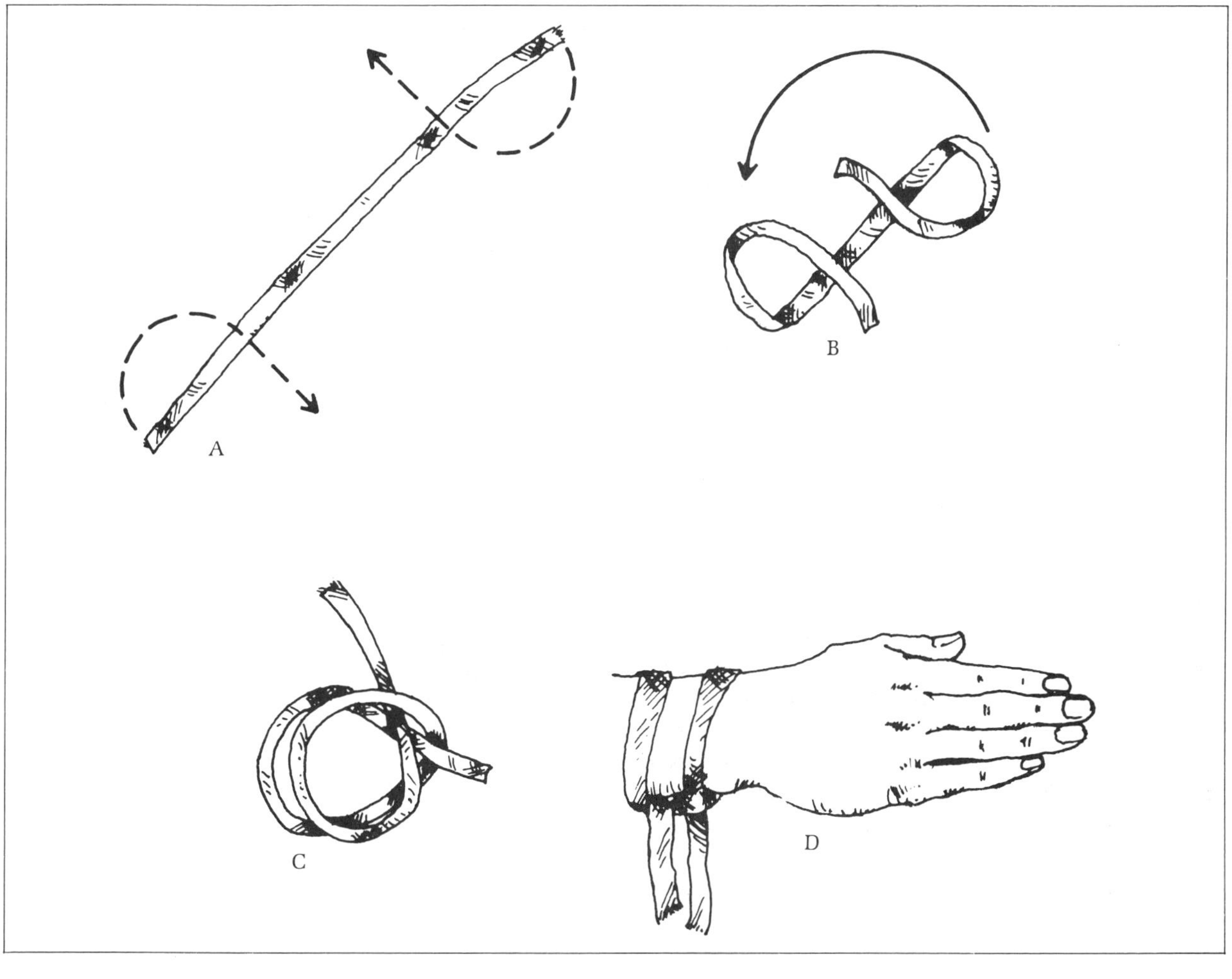

A

B

C

D

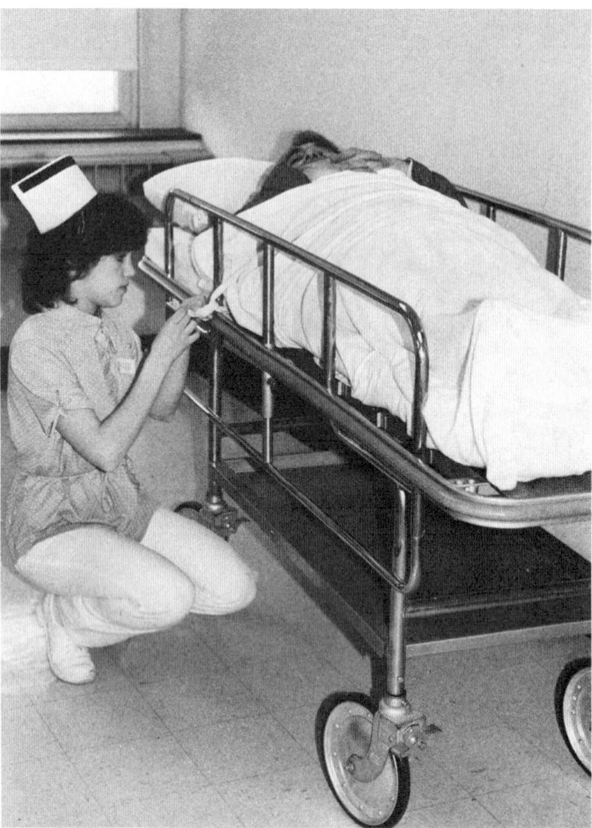

FIGURE 27-13. Use safety straps as well as siderails to protect a patient during transport.

With restraints in place, remember that the basic rule for people on bedrest still applies: they must be turned and repositioned every 2 hours. Massage bony prominences well following turning to be certain that the use of restraints does not lead to skin breakdown.

Tie upper extremity restraints to the *movable* portion of a hospital bed so when the bed position is changed, the restraint will not pull tight.

As a rule, if a health care provider or a member of the patient's family can remain with him, he does not need to be restrained. Always consider this possibility before using restraints in order to preserve self-esteem (see QRS 27-7).

Fire Safety

One of the most serious emergencies that can occur on a hospital unit is fire. Many patients are unable physically to remove themselves from the unit, others are mentally confused or too young to appreciate the seriousness of fire, and many hospital units are located far above ground so fire-fighting equipment and personnel have difficulty reaching the area. As the health care provider who spends the most time with the patient, you are the best prepared to keep him safe should a fire occur.

☐ QUICK REFERENCE STOP 27-7: SAFETY

Patient restraints are protective measures but also carry a risk of occluding circulation or causing nerve injury. Check restraints every 2 hours to be certain they have not drawn tight. Assess the pulse and color of a distal body part and the skin surface under the restraint. Evaluate whether the restraint is still necessary.

FIRE HAZARDS

A number of situations are high risk for creating fire. Whenever these circumstances exist, be on double guard for safety.

Flammable or Combustible Gases. Oxygen, nitrous oxide, and ethylene oxide are commonly used in hospitals; all are flammable. Nitrous oxide and ethylene oxide are anesthetics, limited primarily to use in surgery, emergency room, or dental clinics. When these gases are in use, be certain that adequate signs against smoking are posted. Urge the hospital to use bilingual signs or signs that show a cigarette crossed out. If you have no bilingual sign available or discover that a patient's visitors speak a language for which you have no sign, ask the family interpreter to make a No Smoking sign in that language and hang it prominently on the room door.

Cigarette smoking increases with nervousness or stress. A visitor can forget that smoking is not safe because of his worry and concern. Other people remember not to smoke but flick a cigarette lighter on and off as a means of reducing tension. You may have to remind them that this produces a flame. Be extra cautious about fire on people's birthdays. A visitor who has been extremely careful about not smoking in a room where oxygen is running all week may decide to light candles on a birthday cake, forgetting that it is the flame that will do the damage, not the smoking (see QRS 27-8).

Flammable Liquids. Flammable liquids ignite readily in the presence of an open flame. Those liquids most apt to be hazardous on a hospital unit are acetone and adhesive removal solutions that contain acetone. If you are flaming specimen tubes for blood cultures or a patient is

☐ QUICK REFERENCE STOP 27-8: HEALTH TEACHING

After English, Spanish is the most prevalent language in the United States today. The words *Non Fume* mean no smoking in Spanish. Remember to post them in rooms where oxygen is being used if a patient's visitors speak Spanish.

smoking, do not bring these liquids into the immediate vacinity.

Electricity. All electrical plugs used in hospitals should be three pronged to prevent shocks; no more than one piece of equipment should be plugged into a single outlet. Do not use frayed electrical cords. Be aware how many appliances a patient is plugging into outlets such as radios, electric hair blowers, tape decks, or calculators. Be careful when raising or lowering beds or changing bed positions that you do not trap electrical cords and strip insulation from the cord. Any electrical motor can overheat. Keep bed linen and room curtains away from equipment such as nebulizers so if heating should occur, the cloth will not catch on fire.

Careless Smoking. Careless smoking by patients and health care personnel can lead to fire. To prevent ashes from being tossed directly into wastepaper baskets, provide an ashtray for the patient or visitor who is going to smoke; insist that staff members use them. If no ashtray is available, provide a china bowl from the kitchen. Urge patients not to smoke near bedtime or after they receive a medication such as an analgesic, sedative, or hypnotic because they could fall asleep with a lit cigarette in their hand.

Before you empty patient ashtrays, run cold water over them to be certain no hot ashes could remain or flush the ashes down a toilet.

EMERGENCY FIRE ACTIONS

If a fire should occur on a hospital unit, you need to use common sense for what actions to take and the best order in which to take them. Basically, there are four separate areas of responsibilities that you must address:

1. Keep the patient safe.
2. Keep yourself safe to rescue other patients.
3. Alert others of the fire.
4. Analyze why this fire occurred and help prepare better preventive plans for the future.

The order of first three areas of responsibility depends on the circumstances. The fourth, planning better prevention measures, follows as soon as the hospital is again secure from fire.

Patient Safety. A patient can be injured by open flame or smoke inhalation. He can be indirectly injured if he falls over a piece of equipment or a stairway.

People most often suffer injury from direct flames because linen or their bed catches on fire from careless smoking. The easiest method to extinguish this type of fire is to pour water on it from the patient's water pitcher or smother it with a blanket. Spraying the bed with foam from a fire extinguisher is equally effective, but you could take as much as 5 minutes fetching an extinguisher. Use the patient's call light or telephone or shout to bring assistance.

If the bed is on fire, but the patient is not and you cannot immediately extinguish the fire, remove the patient from the bed by rolling him to the edge of the bed and easing him onto the floor. If a person's clothing is on fire, the worst thing he can do is run; running will fan the flames and increase them tenfold. Give reassurance as you work to prevent this reaction.

If you enter a patient's room filled with smoke, remember that smoke rises. There is always less smoke near the floor than at a standing height. To remove an immobilized person from such a room, ease him to the floor and pull him toward the doorway of the room on your hands and knees. If there is fire in a room but it is not near the bed and smoke is not excessive, remove the patient in his bed. After a patient is removed from a room or fire, close the door to the room. This reduces the oxygen available to the fire and should help limit it.

Your Safety. As basic orientation to any nursing unit, ask to be shown where the fire extinguishers and fire hose are located (Fig. 27-14). Be certain you understand how the wall cabinet where they are kept can be opened and how the extinguisher is activated. Memorize the emergency code number that the telephone operator needs to be told to activate fire procedures.

Learn the route that you should use to evacuate patients from your area if this becomes necessary. Most hospitals have numerous built-in fire walls dividing the building into fire zones. Evacuation routes are determined not just to get to another part of the building, but to get behind a fire wall. What appears to be the quickest way to evacuate your area, therefore, may not necessarily be the safest way; ask about fire walls.

In a fire, electrical connections may burn, plunging the area into darkness. Do not use elevators in a fire. Elevator shafts suck the fire into them because of drafts; also, an elevator may fall the full length of the shaft due to loss of power. If your clothes should catch on fire, remember the rule of fire safety: stop, drop and roll. These three actions smother flames by eliminating the amount of oxygen reaching them.

Alert Others to the Fire. If a fire is a small, self-contained one, you need to alert others that the fire occurred only after it is safely out. In other instances, additional help is necessary.

Most hospitals have a set code number or procedure for reporting a fire. The telephone operator needs this code number or procedure before she will respect your communication. This system is used to prevent a practical joker from alarming people unnecessarily. You must know this code or procedure in order to use it effectively. Be certain you are aware of the locations of fire alarm

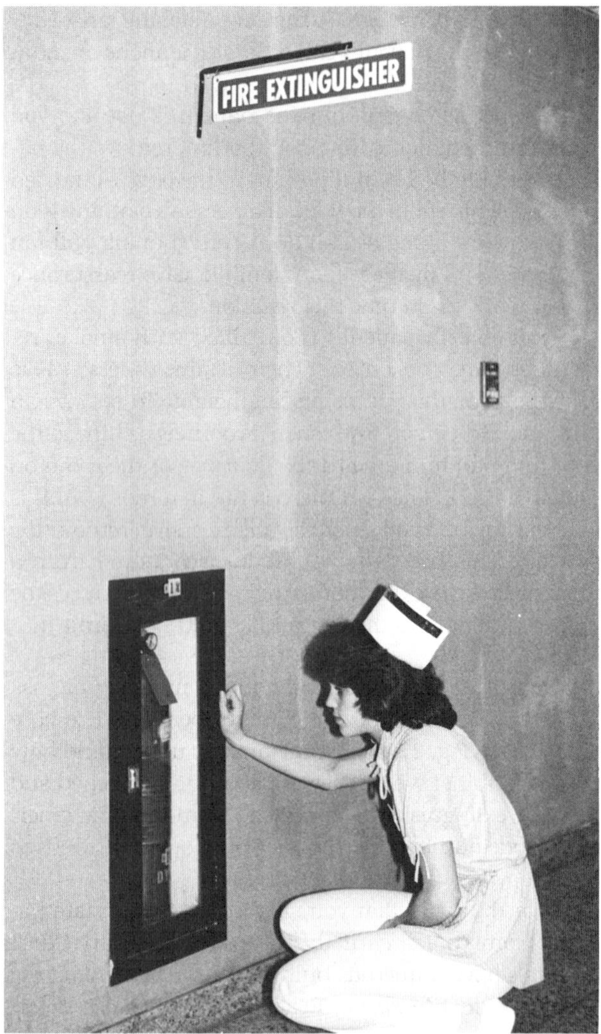

FIGURE 27-14. Knowledge of fire safety is an important nursing responsibility. Know the locations of fire extinguishers or alarms on a nursing unit.

boxes and telephones on the unit. Ask if there is a special way to get a telephone operator from a patient's telephone.

Planning Preventive Measures. Review what happened at the time of the emergency and devise more effective ways to do these things in the future. Unfortunately, fire is such a serious happening that afterward is far too late to restore life and property damage.

Take the time to know safe fire procedure. Insist that any health agency you work for provide in-service training on fire prevention so you and your fellow workers can be prepared to handle this type of emergency.

Evaluation

Comfort and safety must be evaluated for every procedure with patients. Safety precautions are mentioned in Quick Reference Stops throughout other chapters because safety is a basic part of nursing implementation. Quick Reference Stop 27-9 discusses some of the specific research carried out in the area of accident prevention.

□ QUICK REFERENCE STOP 27-9: RESEARCH
Preventing Accidents

Safety is a major concern for the nurse and the patient. Research into this area has attempted to identify why accidents and injuries occur so that efforts can be directed toward prevention.

Patient Falls

Preventive strategies can be developed if we identify the most frequent causes and times of occurrence. Lee and Pash (1983) reviewed 170 reports of falls in one particular hospital. The majority of the patients who fell were over 60 years of age, and more than half the falls were during the late night shift as patients were getting out of bed to go the bathroom.

Staff Injuries

One hospital's records over a year revealed the following: most injuries occur at the bedside or on the patient unit; punctures and strains or sprains were the most frequently occurring injury; most injuries were to fingers, legs, hips, and back; most injuries occurred while staff were handling equipment, assisting patients with transfer activities, or giving medications. The most serious injuries were back and leg injuries, which accounted for 86 percent of all time lost from the job due to injury. The authors suggest that accidents are not always preventable but that in many instances application of body mechanics could prevent the types of injuries noted (Hefferin and Hill, 1976).

Patients' Assaults on Staff

Patients and nurses on a rehabilitation unit were interviewed or given questionnaires by Maagdenberg (1983) to determine if assaults were in some way related to attempts to defend their territory. Patients stated that they "felt anger to the point of assault when nursing staff did not ask permission before touching them" (p. 403). Patients wanted to know in advance what staff planned to do and said they thought staff should ask permission before performing tasks. Few staff had any idea why patients became assaultive. Based on these results, a staff education program on the concepts of personal space and territoriality was conducted. Soon after the course was given, its effectiveness was assessed. A 25 percent reduction in time lost due to injuries resulting from assault had occurred.

SUGGESTED READINGS

Hefferin, E., and Hill, B. J. Analyzing nursing's work-related injuries. *Am. J. Nurs.* 76(6):924, 1976.

Lee, P. S., and Pash, B. J. Preventing patient falls. *Nursing 83* 13(2):118, 1983.

Maagdenberg, A. M. The "violent" patient. *Am. J. Nurs.* 83(3):402, 1983.

NURSING CARE PLAN

Mrs. O'Brien is a 22-year-old woman admitted to the hospital for a surgical repair of a broken tibia. She returns from surgery with a large leg cast. Her physician expects her to have considerable pain for at least 24 hours because of the extensive manipulation needed to set the bone. She has ordered a choice of analgesics: either meperidine (Demerol) 75 mg intramuscularly every 3 hr or acetaminophen (Tylenol) gr x every 4 hr by mouth.

Below is a nursing care plan in reference to pain you might devise for her.

Subjective Assessment: Patient states pain is boring throughout the entire lower half of her leg; continuous in nature.

Objective Assessment: Forehead is wet from perspiration from effort trying to reposition cast to allow for better drying; clenches teeth to talk because of pain; sitting upright, unable to lie back against pillows. Blood pressure, 126/70; pulse, 82; respiration, 22. Cast intact and drying; toes are pink and warm with circulatory return under 5 sec, sensation of touch intact.

Locus of Decision-Making: Shared.

Goal: Patient will have tolerable level of pain by 20 min.

Criteria: Patient will state she is at acceptable level; able to rest in semi-Fowler's position.

NURSING ORDERS

1. Assess neurocirculatory status of toes every hour for first 24 hr, every 4 hr thereafter. Include warmth, nail blanch, color, touch, movement, and subjective report of pain.
2. Keep cast elevated on two pillows to encourage venous return and prevent edema.
3. Turn every 2 hours to decrease pressure points and increase general circulation.
4. Offer meperidine intramuscularly every 3 hr for first 24 hr (unless sleeping) to prevent pain from becoming intense. Record sites administered so sites can be rotated.
5. Reassure that pain is expected following traumatic repair but will decrease in amount daily to decrease apprehension.
6. Encourage patient to discuss accident or surgery to relieve apprehension.
7. Patient feels that keeping wool sock on foot helps relieve pain. Respect the value of this to her.
8. At end of first 24 hr, evaluate need for meperidine every 3 hr and plan method for lengthening meperidine intervals and gradual change to acetaminophen.

SUGGESTED READINGS

Armstrong, M. E. Current concepts in pain. *A.O.R.N. J.* 32(3):383, 1980.

Baker, M. L., et al. Safe or sorry: Exposure to radiation. *Pediatr. Nurs.* 8(4):237, 1982.

Banyard, S. G. New drug-free technique cuts postop pain. *RN* 45(4):31, 1982.

Bedfalls and nursing liability: Legal factors. *Regan Rep. Nurs. Law* 22(11):1, 1982.

Beyerman, K. Flawed perceptions about pain. *Am. J. Nurs.* 82(2):302, 1982.

Booker, J. E. Pain: It's all in your patient's head (or is it?). *Nursing* (Horsham) 12(3):47, 1982.

Boyer, M. W. Continuous drip morphine. *Am. J. Nurs.* 82(4):603, 1982.

Colling, J., et al. Home, safe home. *J. Gerontol. Nurs.* 9(3):174, 1983.

Cooper, S. Common concern: Accidents and older adults. *Geriatr. Nurs.* (N.Y.) 2(4):287, 1981.

Creighton, H. Are side rails necessary? *Nurs. Manage.* 13(6):45, 1982.

DeBlas, M., and Washburn, C. Using analgesics effectively. *Am. J. Nurs.* 79:74, 1979.

DiFabio, S. Nurses' reactions to restraining patients. *Am. J. Nurs.* 81(5):976, 1981.

Dolan, M. B. Controlling pain in a personal way. Sharing. *Nursing* (Horsham) 12(1):144, 1982.

Ellmyer, P., et al. A guide to your patient's safe home use of oxygen. *Nursing* (Horsham) 82(1):55, 1982.

Ford, A. H. Use of automobile restraining devices for infants. *Nurs. Res.* 29(5):281, 1980.

Greenlaw, J. When leaving siderails down can bring you up on charges. *RN* 45(12):75, 1982.

Jacox, A. Assessing pain. *Am. J. Nurs.* 79:895, 1979.

Kustaborder, M. J., et al. Interventions for safety. *J. Gerontol. Nurs.* 9(3):158, 1983.

Lee, P. S., et al. Preventing patient falls. *Nursing* (Horsham) 13(2):118, 1983.

McCaffery, M. *Nursing Management of the Patient in Pain* (2nd ed.). Philadelphia: Lippincott, 1979.

McCaffery, M. Patients shouldn't have to suffer: How to relieve pain with injectable narcotics. *Nursing* (Horsham) 10(10):34, 1980.

McGurie, L. A short simple tool for assessing your patient's pain. *Nursing* (Horsham) 11(3):48, 1981.

McMahon, M., and Miller, Sr. P. Pain responses: The influence of psycho-social cultural factors. *Nurs. Forum* 17:58, 1978.

Melzack, R., and Wall, P. D. Pain mechanisms: A new theory. *Science* 154:971, 1965.

Misek, I. About using restraints—with restraint. *Nursing* (Horsham) 11(6):50, 1981.

Nursing guidelines for the use of restraints in non-psychiatric settings. *J. Gerontol. Nurs.* 9(3):180, 1983.

"Restrain as needed": Nursing judgment required. *Regan Rep. Nurs. Law* 23(3):4, 1982.

Riffle, K. L. Falls: Kinds, causes, and prevention. *Geriatr. Nurs.* (N.Y.) 3(3):165, 1982.

Robbins, D. Ethics and the ED nurse. Pain control: Information, palliation, or toxification? *J.E.N.* 8(1):46, 1982.

Robinson, E. H. Reflections while reading. *Nurs. Outlook* 29(9):525, 1981.

Ruehsegger, D. R., Jr. Radiation exposure levels in an intensive care nursery. *Pediatr. Nurs.* 8(4):244, 1982.

Seigel, H. Assessing an environment for safety first. *J. Gerontol. Nurs.* 8(9):509, 1982.

Shindul, J. A., et al. Legal restraints on restraint. *Am. J. Nurs.* 81(2):393, 1981.

Silman, J. The management of pain: Reference guide to analgesics. *Am. J. Nurs.* 79:74, 1979.

Sklar, C. Safety and accident prevention on hospital premises. *Can. Nurse* 79(1):53, 1983.

Stellman, J. M. Safety in the health care industry. *Occup. Health Nurs.* 30(10):17, 1982.

Thorne, B. P. A nurse helps prevent sports injuries. *M.C.N.* 7(4):236, 1982.

Vadurro, J. F., et al. Reducing the anxiety and pain of childbirth through hypnosis. *Am. J. Nurs.* 82(4):620, 1982.

West, B. B. Understanding endorphins: Our natural pain relief system. *Nursing* (Horsham) 11(2):50, 1981.

QUESTIONS FOR REVIEW

Mr. Jones is a patient whom you care for. You assess his condition to determine what bed position would be more appropriate for him. Match different bed positions in the right column with the correct definitions in the left column.

_____ 1. Semi Fowler's position
_____ 2. Contour positon
_____ 3. Trendelenburg position
_____ 4. Fowler's position

a. Foot of bed higher than head of bed.
b. Head of bed elevated 45 degrees.
c. Head of bed elevated 90 degrees.
d. A flat position.
e. Knee gatch of bed raised; head raised 45 degrees.

5. In making Mr. Jones' bed, you drop a sheet on the floor. Your *best* action would be:
   a. Place it on the bed clean side up.
   b. Discard it.
   c. Don't use it for 24 hours.
   d. Shake it to air it before use.

6. The purpose of putting a draw sheet on a bed is to provide:
   a. An easily changed bottom bed surface.
   b. An extra layer of linen under the patient's head.
   c. An extra layer of linen under the patient's feet.
   d. Padding to protect the patient from the siderail.

7. Mr. Jones has pain. The *best* assessment of pain is:
   a. Mr. Jones' voice trembles as he speaks.
   b. Mr. Jones never moves his right hand.
   c. Mr. Jones clenches his teeth as he speaks.
   d. Mr. Jones states he has pain.

8. When implementing care for Mr. Jones which of the following statements would be best to use as you administer an analgesic to him?
   a. "This medicine doesn't work well unless you lie still."
   b. "Let me position you more comfortably first."
   c. "Thinking about your pain so much doesn't help."
   d. "Fair warning: This is all you can have for pain until morning."

9. Mr. Jones has a wrist restraint applied so he does not destroy his dressing. Such a restraint should be loosened and his circulation assessed:
   a. Every 15 minutes.
   b. At the end of the procedure.
   c. Every 2 hours.
   d. If he has pain in his hand.

10. A wrist restraint should be tied to:
    a. The siderail.
    b. The foot of the bed.
    c. The head of the bed.
    d. The bedsprings.

11. Mr. Jones smokes in bed. As you walk by his room, you see flames on his bed. Your *best* immediate action would be:
    a. Pour water from his water pitcher to put out the flames.
    b. Telephone the fire department from the desk area phone.
    c. Ask Mr. Jones to follow you quietly out of the room.
    d. Pull the fire alarm at the end of the hallway.

28. ASEPSIS

OBJECTIVES

Upon mastery of the material in this chapter, you should be able to:

1. Define medical and surgical asepsis.
2. Describe the concept of a chain of infection and interventions necessary to break such a chain.
3. Describe procedures necessary for initiating medical and surgical asepsis.
4. Define sterilization and list principles of sterile technique.
5. Describe common methods of sterilization and indications for sterilization.
6. Describe reasons, types, and precautions for different isolation procedures.
7. Describe principles and techniques of wound care.

TERMS

The terms important for an understanding of this chapter are shown below and defined in the glossary:

antiseptic
asepsis
autoclave
bacteriocidal
bacteriostatic
clean
communicable disease
endemic
epidemic
infection
isolation
nosocomial infection
pandemic
pathogenic
resident flora
sterile
sterilization
transient flora

Asepsis is the state of being free of pathogenic or disease-causing microorganisms. Using *aseptic technique* means performing a procedure in such a way that you do not spread disease-causing microorganisms.

There are two divisions of aseptic technique, medical asepsis and surgical asepsis. Medical asepsis involves reducing the number of organisms present and preventing their spreading (confining microorganisms to as small a space as possible). Medical aseptic technique is also referred to as *clean technique.* In surgical asepsis an object or area must be kept *free* of microorganisms. It is synonymous with *sterile technique.*

THE CHAIN OF INFECTION

An infection is an illness produced by the action of microorganisms in the human body. Infection results from a chain of reactions or circumstances: existence of a pathogen (disease-producing organism), a reservoir or place for it to grow and multiply, a method of exit from the reservoir, a means of transmission (transportation) to a new site, a method of entering a new body, and a susceptible host or a person vulnerable to the infection. Breaking a chain of infection is a major nursing responsibility. It involves understanding how the chain operates, taking measures to disrupt the chain, and providing health education to reduce people's vulnerability to infection.

The Pathogenic Organism

Because many people are seen at health care agencies for infection, the number of microorganisms capable of causing infections in such institutions is always high. Although a large number of microorganisms exist, surprisingly relatively few are harmful to man. Whether an organism is pathogenic depends on its virulence, the number present, and its ability to live at body temperature and cause human illness.

BACTERIA

Bacteria, a common cause of infection, are categorized according to shape: spherical (cocci), rod-shaped (bacillus), or corkscrew (spirochetes). Bacteria that when stained with a gentian violet (Gram's stain) resist decolorization are termed *gram-positive;* those that can be decolorized again (counterstained) are termed *gram-negative.* Gram-positive and gram-negative bacteria are unlike in nature; many antibiotics are effective against gram-positive strains but totally ineffective against gram-negative strains, and vice versa.

Bacteria differ also in that some grow only in the presence of oxygen (aerobic), others grow without oxygen (anaerobic), and others grow equally well with or without it. Some bacteria are particularly resistant to destruction because they can form spores within their cell that survive despite great heat and drying. When favorable conditions return, the spore reorganizes into a functioning bacteria.

Gram-Positive Cocci. Three of the most commonly encountered types of bacteria are gram-positive cocci.

STREPTOCOCCI. Streptococci are gram-positive cocci. They are found in several types. Alpha-hemolytic streptococci are normal inhabitants of the upper respiratory tract and gastrointestinal tract and are not pathogenic. In contrast, beta-hemolytic streptococci are extremely pathogenic and cause the illnesses strep throat and scarlet fever. They are chief offenders for uterine infection following childbirth (puerperal fever). Some beta-hemolytic types produce a toxin as they grow that may lead to severe heart disease (rheumatic fever) or kidney disease (glomerulonephritis). The term *hemolytic* means that when the organism is grown in a blood medium a zone of blood destruction (hemolysis) appears around the growing bacteria, the method used by a laboratory to identify each bacteria.

STAPHYLOCOCCI. Staphylococci are found primarily on the skin and in the nasal cavity. They cause local skin infections such as boils; they can spread from skin surfaces to cause severe infections in surgical wounds. When inhaled they can be responsible for a particularly resistant form of pneumonia. Staphylococci are, as a group, particularly resistant to antibiotic therapy. Their presence is a constant threat in hospitals because of their high resistance to antibiotics and their presence in surgical wounds.

PNEUMOCOCCI. Pneumococci are a common cause of pneumonia or lung infection. Any person in ill health is more prone to develop pneumonia than the average person. Thus, secondary pneumococci infections are always a threat to a person ill from some other cause.

Gram-Negative Cocci. Most gram-negative cocci are nonpathogenic; they are natural inhabitants of the upper respiratory tract. There are two pathogenic forms. *Neisseria meningitidis* causes a severe infection of the spinal meninges (meningitis), and *Neisseria gonorrhoeae* causes severe and common infection of the reproductive tract (gonorrhea).

Gram-Positive Bacilli. Gram-positive bacteria in anaerobic forms are important causes of infection. When this type of bacteria is spore forming, the organism is termed *clostridium.* Represented by this type are gas gangrene, tetanus, and botulism; they produce toxins as they grow that are so potent they cause potentially fatal infections. They must be guarded against whenever a deep penetrating wound such as a stab wound or dog bite is present because they grow in the sealed deeper area of the wound where oxygen does not reach. Aerobic non—spore-forming bacilli are termed *corynebacteria.* Most of this type exist in nonpathogenic forms in the upper respiratory tract. However, this type is also responsible for the symptoms of facial acne and for diphtheria, a severe throat infection.

Gram-Negative Bacilli. Enteric bacteria, which grow in the gastrointestinal tract and are excreted in feces, tend to be gram-negative bacilli. Important examples of these that cause severe potentially fatal infections are *Salmonella*, *Shigella*, and cholera. A new strain often involved in hospital infection is a *Serratia-Klebsiella* strain.

Spiral Bacteria (Spirochetes). The best known of the group is *Treponema pallidum*, the type that causes syphilis. Syphilis has reached epidemic proportions in some areas of the United States and despite the availability of treatment, appears to be increasing in incidence.

Acid-Fast Bacteria. Acid-fast bacteria are coated with a waxy shell resistant to normal destruction means. Chief among this group is *Mycobacterium tuberculosis*, responsible for tuberculosis, and *Mycobacterium leprae*, responsible for leprosy. Acid-fast bacteria are also resistant to normal antibiotics because of their special protective shell.

ANTIBIOTICS AND BACTERIA

An antibiotic is a drug that halts the growth of or kills microorganisms. Bacteria are complex organisms with a rigid cell wall, a cell membrane, and protein-synthesizing ability. Antibiotics interfere with bacterial growth by dissolving the cell wall, destroying the permeability of the cell membrane so nutrients can no longer enter the cell, interfering with protein synthesis of the cell, or, simulating a nutrient, being drawn into the cell to cause destruction from within. Some bacteria become resistant to an antibiotic because they are able to restructure against it. Owing to the long use of penicillin as an antibiotic, for example, some strains of bacteria produce a penicillin-inactivating substance, making penicillin completely ineffective against them. In order to keep bacteria resistance to a minimum, antibiotics are prescribed only when necessary, never indiscriminately. Many people are not aware that antibiotics should not be used liberally and expect to have one ordered even if they have only minor symptoms. Using procedures that are aimed at keeping microorganisms away from people is always preferable to allowing a person to contract an infection and then treating him with antibiotics. Any measure to this end not only keeps a person free of disease today but safeguards everyone in the future by keeping the use of antibiotics to a minimum. The possibility exists that at the point a microorganism becomes resistant to all known antibiotics and no new one can be devised, there will no longer be a way to combat infections.

An antibiotic is termed *broad spectrum* if it destroys both gram-positive and gram-negative organisms, *bacteriocidal* if it kills organisms, and *bacteriostatic* if it halts the growth of bacteria.

FUNGAL INFECTIONS

Fungi are small plants found in abundance on skin, in the gastrointestinal tract, oral cavity, and vagina. Most fungi do not normally cause disease. They may become pathogenic when the normal bacteria present in these areas are disturbed, pH changes, or a person's natural resistance to infection decreases. Bacterial flora can be disturbed when a person is treated by a broad-spectrum antibiotic that kills many normal bacteria as well as pathogenic ones. The usual slightly acid medium of the vagina becomes more alkaline in pregnancy, so pregnant women are more prone to fungi infections. Any person with a debilitating illness is more prone than usual.

Common fungi infections are *Candida* infections (vaginitis; in the mouth, thrush). Antibiotics are not effective against fungal infections. Special drugs or antifungal agents are necessary to halt such growths.

VIRUSES

Viruses are the smallest microorganisms that cause disease. They consist of only a central structure of nucleic acid and a protein shell. They differ from bacteria in being unable to carry on metabolic processes. They live and reproduce by invading a body cell and then converting that cell's metabolic processes to produce the enzymes they need to survive. Coexisting in cells this way may result in cell necrosis (death), cell hyperplasia (abnormal growth), or no change (a symbiotic relationship). The herpesvirus is an example of a virus that exists inactively in body cells for years; it is activated only when the body's defense mechanisms become less than usual as when under psychological stress or with fever—herpesvirus type I causes the common cold sore or fever blister. Some viruses cause the formation of inclusion bodies (round, densely stained structures) in cells they invade. The presence of inclusion bodies serves to diagnose that the virus is present.

A unique protein called interferon prevents virus multiplication to some degree and appears to prevent the growth of two different virus infections in the body at once. Adrenocortical steroids inhibit the production of interferon, so people receiving corticosteroid medication are susceptible to virus infections. Steroids also decrease the entire inflammatory process so that infection from all microorganisms may be masked. Many childhood diseases (measles, rubella, mumps) are caused by viruses; immunization to these diseases was difficult to devise because in the presence of interferon, the three types of virus would not all grow at once and until this problem was solved, triple vaccines could not be used.

Usual antibiotics are not effective against viruses. Mechanisms to protect people from exposure is their best safeguard.

RICKETTSIEAE

Rickettsieae are miniature, intracellular parasites similar to bacteria but the size of viruses. They are transmitted by insect bites. They cause a systemic febrile illness often associated with a skin rash. Typhus and Rocky Mountain Spotted Fever are the most common rickettsial diseases seen in the United States.

PROTOZOA AND METAZOA

Parasites are organisms that live in an environmental host. They often live in the intestinal tract, and the eggs of parasites are discharged in feces. Protozoa are simple one-celled parasites; Metazoa are large, multicelled structures. Malaria is caused by the protozoa *Plasmodium* and is transmitted by the bite of the *Anopheles* mosquito; amebic dysentery, a very severe diarrhea, is caused by the protozoa *Entamoeba histolytica*. Examples of metazoal infestations are roundworms, pinworms, and tapeworm. Since many parasite infections are spread by feces, good hand washing is an extremely important means of preventing their spread.

Breaking the Chain of Infection

Breaking the chain of infection by destroying microorganisms may be accomplished by use of an antiseptic, a substance to inhibit the growth of organisms on skin; a disinfectant, a substance to inhibit or destroy growth of organisms on inanimate objects; or sterilization, a process to destroy organisms on inanimate objects. Common disinfectants and antiseptics are shown in Table 28-1. Conscientiously administering antibiotics on time in order to maintain a high level of the drug in the bloodstream is a major way that organisms are eliminated inside the human body.

THE RESERVOIR

Bacteria may be aerobic, anaerobic, or both. Thus, reservoirs differ, depending on the organisms present. All need water and food to grow. Most grow best in the dark. Temperature and pH are important. If a person has current immunization status, organisms for that disease cannot use him as a reservoir for growth. Some people serve as reservoirs for microorganisms without showing clinical symptoms. Typhoid fever is an example of bacteria that can be carried in the gallbladder and excreted in feces without the person himself showing any sign of illness.

To break a chain of infection at the reservoir point, change dressings frequently (other factors permitting) in order to limit the extent of moist, warm secretions available. Empty wastepaper baskets or a paper bag you have provided for disposable tissues at least every 8 hours. Toxic shock syndrome, caused by bacteria trapped and held by vaginal tampons, is an example of an infection that can be prevented.

TABLE 28-1. COMMON DISINFECTANTS AND ANTISEPTICS

Solution	Action	Comments
Alcohol (isopropyl or ethyl)	Bacteriocidal	Antiseptic/disinfectant. Can damage plastic; drying to skin.
Chlorine compounds	Bacteriocidal	Disinfectant. May corrode metal instruments.
Formaldehyde	Bacteriocidal	Disinfectant. Toxic to human tissue; fumes are irritating to lung tissue. Action is blocked by presence of protein tissue so clean item well of any organic material first.
Hydrogen peroxide	Bacteriocidal	Antiseptic/disinfectant. Destroys pathogens by oxidizing action; will cause foaming when in contact with protein.
Iodine (iodophor, povidone-iodine, Betadine)	Bacteriocidal	Antiseptic/disinfectant. Stains clothing brown.
Phenolic compounds (hexachlorophene)	Bacteriostatic	Antiseptic. Remains active for a sustained period of time after being applied to skin. Do not use with infants or broken skin or fatal degree of absorption can occur.

PORTAL OF EXIT

Many airborne microorganisms exit from the body in coughs and sneezes. They exit by feces, vomitus, and saliva if they grow in the gastrointestinal tract. They may exit by urine or vaginal secretions. If the organism is present in the bloodstream, it may exit by blood-drawing apparatus. A local infection will drain to the surface and exit by way of the skin.

To break the chain of infection at this point, follow good isolation procedures (gowns, gloves, or mask as appropriate). Good hand washing between patients is crucial in breaking the chain of infection. Always supply an adequate number of disposable tissues so the person can limit respiratory or airborne spread. Be certain the patient has hand-washing facilities to use after changing his own dressing or coughing.

MEANS OF TRANSMISSION

A disease is *communicable* if it can be spread from one person to another. It is *endemic* if it is always present in a population, as is the common cold. It is *epidemic* if large numbers of people over the expected average number are currently affected. A disease is *pandemic* if it occurs over a wide area of the world.

Organisms may be spread by direct contact, by fomites (inanimate objects), by vectors (insects such as mosquitoes or flies), in food and water, or through air currents. Airborne organisms settle onto objects in a room and then are picked up onto fingers or settle onto food and so may also be spread in this manner. These methods of spread are summarized in Table 28-2.

To break the chain of infection at this point, use isolation precautions as appropriate and wash hands between giving each patient care. Provide hand-washing facilities for patients as well as yourself.

PORTAL OF ENTRY

Pathogens enter the human body through breaks in the skin or mucous membranes, the gastrointestinal tract by direct access such as kissing or in contaminated food or objects, and the respiratory system by inhalation.

TABLE 28-2. METHODS BY WHICH MICROORGANISMS SPREAD

Method	Definition
Airborne	Spread by droplets coughed or sneezed into air or suspended dust particles.
Direct contact	Spread by direct contact from one person to another such as kissing, sexual relations, or hand contact.
Vector	Spread by means of an insect such as a mosquito or a flea.
Vehicle	Spread by means of an intermediate object such as contaminated food or water or a contaminated object (a fomite) such as a comb.

Protecting the integrity of skin and mucous membrane, using strict sterile technique in changing dressings of wounds, preparing food and medicine with conscientious technique, and maintaining isolation are interventions to break the chain at this point. Encourage the patient to wash his hands well before eating and after using the bathroom to discourage spread of organisms. Women should wipe the perineum front to back after defecation to prevent organisms spreading from the rectum to the urethra.

SUSCEPTIBLE HOST

No one is totally resistant to infection. The person with weakened immunological defenses, fatigue, poor nutrition, or chronic disease is more susceptible than others. Immunologic defenses are less well developed in the very young, older adults, people on drugs such as steroids or receiving irradiation or chemotherapy, those born with a deficient immunological system, and those who have not received basic immunization series. Psychological stress may reduce body defenses.

Breaking the chain of infection at this point consists of encouraging people to keep their immunization status current, and identifying and giving extra protection through isolation to those people who are highly susceptible to infection. Persons receiving an antibiotic may be high risk for fungal infections because when the normal bowel flora are suppressed by the antibiotic, fungi may overgrow; this is termed a *superimposed infection.*

THE INFECTION PROCESS

The infection process begins in a susceptible host shortly after invasion of the microorganism. However, symptoms of infection may not be present for days or weeks.

The *incubation period* is the time interval between the invasion of the body and the onset of symptoms of infection. During this time the organisms are growing and multiplying. The length of incubation period varies depending on the pathogen. It tends to center on 7 to 10 days but can be longer; tetanus has an incubation period from 2 to 21 days.

The *prodromal period* is the time from the beginning of nonspecific symptoms until specific illness symptoms appear. Nonspecific symptoms include lethargy, low-grade fever, fatigue, and malaise. A person is infectious during this time, but because his symptoms are so vague he does not generally take any precautions against spreading disease. This is why infectious diseases spread so readily through communities if people are not immunized against them. Prodromal stages are generally short, ranging from hours to a few days.

The *stage of illness* is the stage during which specific illness symptoms are evident. Most illnesses have local symptoms relating to the specific body organ affected and systemic symptoms reflecting the entire body. A person with a streptococcal throat infection, for example, has the local symptoms of throat erythema, throat pain and edema, warmth, and difficulty with swallowing. He also has systemic symptoms of fever, headache, enlarged lymph nodes in the anterior neck, lethargy, and perhaps sleepiness and fatigue. Many infections have an accompanying rash on the skin *(exanthem)* or on mucous membrane *(enanthem).*

The *convalescent period* is the time interval between symptoms beginning to fade and the person returning to full wellness and a high energy level. Because fatigue is often an accompanying symptom of infection, the convalescent period is often longer than people expect; it lasts at least a week.

LIFE SPAN CONCEPTS AND INFECTION

People's resistance to infection, the type of infections that occur, and therefore, nursing care vary with age.

The Newborn. Newborn infants are born with antibodies to those diseases for which the mother had sufficient levels of antibodies that crossed the placenta (IgG type). This usually includes measles, poliomyelitis, rubella, diphtheria, pertussis, and tetanus. Even if a mother has had chickenpox (varicella), little immunity to chickenpox is transferred across the placenta. No person with a herpes lesion (cold sore or genital lesions) should be caring for newborns, who have little protection against this common virus. Strict aseptic technique (good hand washing, gowning) is used with newborns to protect them from invading pathogens.

The Infant. The immunization system or ability to produce antibodies is immature for at least the first 2 months of life. This is why immunizations are not begun until after that. As the baby begins to explore his environment, he tends to place any object he can into his mouth. Therefore, any object given to a baby should be clean. Breast-feeding supplies antibodies to the child. If the mother is bottle-feeding, she needs to use a chlorinated water supply, pasteurized or commercially prepared milk source, and clean technique to prepare formula; otherwise, she should sterilize formula for the first 3 months.

Because the eustachian tube in infants is short and more horizontal than in adults, an upper respiratory infection spreads easily to become a middle ear infection.

The Toddler and Preschooler. Toddlers and preschoolers are exposed to more infections than the infant. They may have as many as 10 to 12 colds a year. Children this age have frequent mosquito bites or scratches from playing with cats or dogs that can easily become infected if scratched into open lesions.

The Schoolager and Adolescent. Young school children contact a series of upper respiratory infections as they are exposed to new and different friends in school. Streptococcal infections may cause serious throat infections (tonsillitis). Swimmer's ear, or a fungal infection of the outer ear canal, is a frequent summer infection of school children. Childhood diseases (mumps, measles, rubella) are becoming infrequent as greater numbers of children are immunized against these diseases.

In contrast, venereal diseases are increasing in incidence and are at epidemic proportions in populations with a high number of adolescents or young adults. Venereal diseases or sexually transmitted diseases (STD) are spread by sexual contact. The most common are gonorrhea, syphilis, herpes type II, and pubic lice. A drug-using population tends to contact diseases spread by unclean needles such as hepatitis.

The Adult. Adults contact infections through exposure to fellow workers who are ill. A frequent summer infection is gastrointestinal illness contracted through poorly refrigerated food. Most adults are susceptible to tetanus (lockjaw) because they do not keep their tetanus immunization current; one should be reimmunized every 10 years.

The Older Adult. The older adult may have decreased production of antibodies due to the length of time since he received his primary immunizations. If he has difficulty maintaining good nutrition on a fixed income, he is more susceptible to infection than normally. People with chronic lung disease are more susceptible to lung infection than normally.

MEDICAL ASEPSIS

A nurse always serves as a patient's second line of defense against infection; the first is his own body resources. She does so by the use of medical or surgical aseptic technique.

Medical asepsis is clean technique or giving patient care in a way that never exposes patients (or yourself) to more microorganisms than necessary and that breaks the transmission of bacteria from one location to another. Basic principles of medical aseptic technique, shown in the following box, are guides for action; modification for individual patients is often necessary.

Basic Principles of Medical Asepsis

1. Wash your hands before beginning care on a nursing unit and just before leaving the unit.
2. Wash your hands before and after caring for a patient.
3. Wash your hands after touching obviously contaminated surfaces or material such as diapers, bedpans, or soiled dressings.
4. Provide supplies for patients to wash their hands before eating (and do so yourself).
5. Provide adequate tissue supplies and bags for disposal for patients who are coughing or sneezing so microorganisms cannot be spread by airborne droplets.
6. Do not use supplies used for one patient with another without having them first cleaned or sterilized.
7. Do not spread dust by shaking linen; to dust, use a damp cloth or paper towel to remove dust effectively, not just raise it into the air.
8. Carry soiled materials such as linen away from your uniform so your uniform does not become a source of transmission for microorganisms.
9. Discard or return for recleaning any item dropped on the floor; floors of health care agencies are very contaminated from the settling of bacteria. Do not put soiled linen on the floor to add to the floor microorganism count.
10. Dispose of soiled materials immediately in a covered container away from a patient area. Leaving soiled items in a patient wastebasket is not only aesthetically unpleasing because of its slight odor, but such material can serve as a reservoir of infection.
11. Be aware of what areas on a nursing unit are considered clean (a utility room counter where equipment taken to patient rooms can be assembled) and dirty (sinks, the bedpan flusher, a counter where equipment used with patients is placed to be recleaned). *Do not interchange these areas.*
12. Keep patient care rooms free of extra equipment and supplies. The more articles in a patient room, the more difficult it is for housekeeping to keep it free of dust. On the other hand, do not discourage personal items that have psychological importance to a person.
13. If isolation technique is warranted, observe thorough precautions. There is no concept of *almost* isolation technique. It is black and white; isolation technique or no isolation technique.

Hand Washing

Hand washing, one of the major means of breaking a chain of infection, can easily be overlooked because it is such a simple procedure. Always wash your hands after reporting to a nursing unit and before beginning care to avoid carrying microorganisms from the outside environment into the unit. Wash your hands before caring for a patient and immediately following care in order to prevent spread of infection from you to the patient or from one patient to the next. Wash your hands before changing dressings and after handling contaminated material or equipment such as bedpans or wound dressings.

Hand washing technique is described in Procedure 28-1. *Do not underestimate it as a primary means of infection prevention.* Despite its simple nature, it is extremely effective against spreading and contacting infection (see QRS 28-1).

Whether your hands should be held higher or lower than your elbows during rinsing is debatable. The principle is to let water flow from the cleanest to the more soiled area. Following washing, your hands are cleaner than your arms so elevating hands fulfills this principle. This technique is consistent with surgical scrubbing and allows you to move from one area of a nursing service to another with least difficulty.

Isolation

Isolation or barrier technique is a procedure for limiting the spread of microorganisms. The technique varies, but basic recommendations are always consistent. In general, isolation is best done with a private patient room although strict and respiratory isolation are the only two types where this is absolutely necessary. Provide a table or extra bedside stand outside the door to

PROCEDURE 28-1
Hand Washing

Purpose: To clean hands by use of running water, soap, and friction in order to break a chain of infection from patient to patient, patient to self, self to patient.

Plan	*Principle*
1. Assess proper equipment: a sink with warm running water and soap; paper towels and wastebasket; hand lotion (optional).	1. Running water is necessary to flush away dirt from hands. Water should be warm, not cold because soap is better utilized; not hot because chapping occurs. Soap emulsifies bacteria and removes them better.
2. Remove any ring other than a plain wedding band and pin to shirt or uniform. Push wristwatch 4—5 in. above wrist.	2. It is impossible to clean rings with irregular surfaces by just handwashing; secure it to protect it from being lost. Move your watch to protect it from getting wet and to wash skin surface under it.
3. Turn on faucets and adjust to warm water. Stand back enough from sink so your uniform does not touch edge; not so far that your stance is awkward.	3. Faucets may be controlled by your hands or by foot- or knee-operated pedals. Protect your uniform from getting wet.
4. Wet hands under running water; add soap by pushing dispenser over sink or rinse off bar soap, lather hands with it, rinse again, and replace in soap dish.	4. Rinse bar soap before use to reduce level of surface bacteria present; rinse lather away afterward to not leave obvious soil on soap.
5. Rub palms and ventral surface of fingers together with circular motions; with right hand, grasp side of each finger on left hand and rub lateral surfaces; repeat with right hand.	5. Applying friction to all hand surfaces—ventral, lateral, and dorsal—is the action that cleans. Be sure to include the lateral aspect of the thumb, an area often missed. If a wedding band is worn, lift and wash under the ring.
6. Rub right palm over back (dorsal) surface of left fingers and hand; left palm over back surface of fingers of right hand. Flex knuckles slightly so folds of skin smooth out for more thorough cleaning.	6. Touching all surfaces with a friction motion is the best cleaning motion.
7. Clean fingernails by an applicator end to remove film under fingernails.	7. An orangewood stick or fingernail file is not usually available.
8. Grasp each wrist with the other hand and apply friction in a circular motion.	8. Wrists are considered a part of your hand in hand washing.
9. Rinse hands by elevating fingertips under running water and letting water run from tips of fingers toward wrists. If hands were heavily contaminated, repeat steps 4—9.	9. Running water rinses off soap lather, which contains dirt and microorganisms. Let it run toward wrists to prevent running back toward fingertips, carrying microorganisms from dirty to clean area.
10. Dry hands with a paper towel. Use paper towel to turn off faucets.	10. If paper towel is wet, use a second towel to turn off faucets. Wet objects allow microorganisms to transmit by capillary action. Do not use your bare hand. Faucets are highly contaminated areas; you turned them on before you washed your hands.
11. Discard paper towel in wastebasket. Wipe away excess water from sink edge. Apply hand lotion if desired to hands.	11. Washing hands removes skin oil. Lubricating with a lotion prevents excessive dryness and potential breaks in the skin. Do not leave pools of water on sink brim or floor to become reservoirs of infection.

☐ QUICK REFERENCE STOP 28-1: PSYCHOLOGICAL CONSIDERATIONS

The average patient appreciates that spread of infection is a danger to him in a health care setting facility. It is comforting to hear you say, "*Let me wash my hands* and then I'd like to take your blood pressure."

Be careful what objects you set on a patient's overbed table where his meal tray will sit. Placing a bedpan or soiled dressing on such a surface is not only unsafe in that it could cause direct contamination of food, but also unappetizing.

the room to hold supplies necessary for isolation—gowns, masks, gloves, and bags for removal of supplies from the room. If supplies are not readily available in this way, people will break technique. Having supplies ready also prepares for an emergency, when you need to enter the room both quickly and safely.

In the room, check that the paper towel dispenser is full and there is adequate soap so no one avoids good hand washing for lack of supplies. Provide a bag for disposal of tissues if the person is coughing or sneezing and respiratory secretions are infected. Provide a laundry hamper for soiled gowns so they will not be worn outside the unit and a wastebasket or covered container for soiled gloves and masks.

RESPIRATORY ISOLATION

Respiratory isolation is used to contain the spread of airborne microorganisms. The person being isolated must be kept in a private room; the door of the room must be kept closed. To enter the room, wear a mask over your nose and mouth. Respiratory secretions should be handled with gloves and removed from the room by a double-bag technique. If handling an infant who might drool, wear a gown over your uniform to keep secretions off your uniform. If a person in respiratory isolation must be removed from isolation, he must wear a mask over his nose and mouth.

ENTERIC ISOLATION

Enteric isolation describes precautions used to limit the spread of microorganisms spread by feces. The person is best cared for in a private room with a private bathroom. When giving direct care (touching the patient or his bed), wear a gown. Wear gloves to handle a bedpan. Specimens of feces brought out of the room must be double bagged to protect laboratory personnel.

WOUND AND SKIN ISOLATION

Wound and skin precautions are utilized when a local infection is present. You can walk into the room without precautions other than normal hand washing but in order to give direct care you need to wear a gown, mask, and gloves. Any object that has come in direct contact with the infected area must be double bagged to be removed from the room.

BLOOD PRECAUTIONS

When a person has a disease that is carried by the bloodstream, special precautions need to be taken with blood or objects such as needles and syringes that have entered the bloodstream. Objects need to be double bagged before removal from the room. Be exceptionally careful when handling contaminated needles not to prick yourself; if this should happen, report the incident to unit personnel. You may need antibodies against the disease.

STRICT ISOLATION

A few microorganisms are so virulent that maximum precautions are necessary to limit their spread. With strict isolation, you must wear a mask, gown, and gloves to give care. The person must be in a private room with the door kept closed. All articles removed from the room must be double bagged.

PROTECTIVE ISOLATION

In some instances, isolation is necessary to prevent microorganisms from spreading *to* the patient. A child born without immunological function or one with leukemia who has no functional white blood cells to combat infection is a candidate for protective or reverse isolation. All objects are sterilized or disinfected before they are brought into the unit. To enter the unit you must wear a gown, mask and gloves. Life Island Units, plastic bubbles that surround a patient, are an extensive method of providing this type of isolation.

ENTERING AN ISOLATION ROOM

To enter an isolation room, wash your hands as usual. Following hand washing, put on mask, gown, or gloves. You are not putting on sterile gloves, mask, or gown, only clean ones, so no special technique is needed for putting them on other than seeing that the mask is well fastened over both your nose and mouth and the gown is well fastened in back to protect the back of your uniform as well as the front. However, always putting gloves on with sterile glove technique is a good practice. If you need sterile gloves for a procedure inside the room, take another pair still wrapped and sterile into the room and double glove when you need them.

Organize the supplies you will need for care so that you do not waste time ungowning and regowning. Open the door to the room and take in the supplies needed. Remember that with a gown and mask, the patient cannot easily identify you as a nurse. Introduce yourself by name, purpose, and rank if this is the first time you have met the person.

PROCEDURE 28-2
Entering A Strict Isolation Room

Purpose: To shield yourself from microorganisms present in a room through protective covering.

Plan	*Principle*
1. Wash hands; analyze patient care necessary; plan and assemble supplies needed for patient care to take with you into room and extent of protection necessary.	1. Hand washing is always done preparatory to patient care. Reduce the need to enter and leave the room due to poor organization.
2. Don mask, gown, and gloves in hallway outside room. Turn cuff of gloves up over gown sleeves to maintain uninterrupted expanse of protection for arm.	2. Isolation protection is clean, not sterile, so no special technique is required. To maintain good habits, put on gloves as if they were sterile.
3. If a watch will be necessary for pulse taking, seal it in a plastic bag.	3. Protect your watch from having to be cleaned with a disinfectant that could damage it.
4. Carry supplies necessary for care, open door to room and enter; close it from inside.	4. Since you touch the inside of the door upon entering the room, you cannot exit without full exit procedure.

Wear the gown, mask, and gloves all the time you are in the isolation room unless gown or mask becomes wet or a glove tears. A wet object is no longer protective since moisture spreads microorganisms by capillary action. Therefore, leave the room and change mask and gown and then return. If a glove tears, remove it, wash your hands well, reglove outside the room, and reenter. Technique for entering an isolation room is summarized in Procedure 28-2.

Isolation technique seems time consuming at first, but as you grow accustomed to the procedure, it takes less time. Unless respiratory or strict isolation is in effect (when the door to the room must be kept closed), time spent putting on the gown and gloves can be used for conversation with the patient. This casual approach helps the patient to feel less isolated—he sees you taking extra precautions to care for him but does not see it as an inconvenience. Ordinarily, conversation from a patient's doorway is never considered therapeutic, but it *can* be done in a way that conveys a sense of caring.

REMOVING SUPPLIES FROM AN ISOLATION ROOM

Supplies removed from an isolation room must be double bagged outside the room to keep organisms from spreading. This is done by a person outside the room holding a linen bag or plastic bag (depending on agency policy) while the person inside the room lowers the bag of supplies to be removed into it, being careful not to touch the outside of the second bag or the holder's hands (Fig. 28-1). The outside bag is then sealed and labeled to denote contaminated articles. Double bagging in this way protects everyone who handles the articles removed—people in the laundry, the laboratories if specimens were removed, the janitorial staff.

LEAVING AN ISOLATION ROOM

After double bagging supplies, you may be ready to leave the room yourself. The principle that governs your actions while doing this is to leave all contaminated equipment with the exception of your mask and one paper towel inside the room. To do this, untie the gown ties at your waist level. These ties are considered contaminated because microorganisms settle, making the lower half of any room more contaminated than the half above waist level. Take off your gloves and dispose of them in a wastepaper basket; wash and dry

FIGURE 28-1. A double-bagged procedure is used to remove soiled supplies from the isolation room.

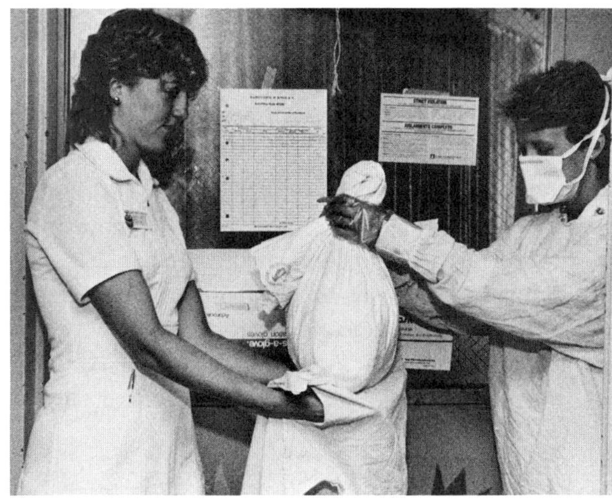

your hands well at the room sink. Next, untie the neck ties. You cannot do this without touching your hair or collar so your hands must be clean to touch this tie. Remove the gown by touching the neckband and folding it forward. Grasp the sleeves by the inside if you need to remove it from your arms; do not allow the outside of the gown to touch your uniform. Discard the gown in a laundry bag in the room. Use a clean paper towel to cover the doorknob while you turn it to leave the room to keep your hands clean. Discard the paper towel into container inside the room or a covered container just outside the room. If a mask is required, untie it just inside the room and discard it in a container immediately inside the room or remove it just outside and discard it into a covered container there. Rewash your hands. Use lotion as necessary to prevent excessive drying from such frequent hand washing. Technique for leaving an isolation room is summarized in Procedure 28-3.

Do not reuse gown, mask, or gloves because reuse probably results in gross contamination of your uniform. Disposing of gown, mask, and gloves after you leave a room avoids tempting another health care provider to reuse any of them.

PROCEDURE 28-3
Exiting from a Strict Isolation Room

Purpose: Leave a room containing virulent microorganisms without spreading such organisms to yourself or the environment outside the room.

Plan	*Principle*
1. Complete patient care and assure patient safety during the time no one will be with him.	1. Establish patient safety and well-being.
2. Damp dust surface areas such as overbed table, window sills, and bedside stand with a moistened paper towel or predetermined agency disinfectant solution.	2. Damp dusting prevents spread of microorganisms by being airborne. Process reduces reservoir of infection in room. In some agencies, this is housekeeping not nursing responsibility.
3. Remove linen supplies from room by placing them in a cloth or water dissoluable plastic bag provided; close top of bag. At doorway to room, slide bag into a second one held by a second health care provider outside room being careful not to touch outside of second bag.	3. This is double-bagging technique. Touching outside of second bag or bringing second bag into room would contaminate it.
4. Second health care provider immediately closes bag of linen and labels as isolation linen.	4. Protect welfare of persons in laundry from contacting microorganisms.
5. Remove disposable supplies such as soiled dressings, plastic dishes, used paper tissues with same double-bag technique.	5. Reduce reservoirs of infection inside room.
6. If removing watch from room, tear plastic bag containing it and spill it out into clean hand of second health care provider or onto accessory table outside doorway.	6. Careful technique protects your watch from contamination.
7. Untie waist level ties of gown; remove gloves by grasping cuffs and peeling forward off hands; discard into covered room container; wash hands; use paper towel to turn off faucets; untie neck ties.	7. Waist ties are very contaminated from being at waist level. Do not touch collar of gown near hair without clean hands.
8. Remove gown by touching only the inside. Discard into linen bag inside room. Remove mask and discard into designated container.	8. Avoid touching most heavily contaminated gown surface with bare hands. Leave contaminated articles inside room.
9. Take clean paper towel and use to turn doorknob to leave room. Close door from outside with your bare hand.	9. Paper towel protects your hand from becoming recontaminated on doorknob.
10. Rewash hands. Apply lotion as necessary to prevent chapping.	10. Additional hand washing assures your hands are clean for a second patient's care.

ISOLATION AND SENSORY DEPRIVATION

Many people do not do well with isolation precautions because they miss the feeling of skin and being able to see the face of the person talking to them. A person in isolation typically has fewer visitors than the average patient because friends and relatives do not want to have to gown to visit. Nursing staff tend to visit the room less frequently also because it is time consuming to mask or gown or glove.

Most difficulties with sensory deprivation in isolation settings can be overcome with careful planning. With good technique, it is not dangerous to enter the isolation room. Orient family and visitors to good isolation technique so they are not reluctant to visit. If visitors seem to be few in number, ask the patient whether they are staying away and could the nursing staff help make them feel more comfortable. Encourage the patient to maintain contact with people important to him by telephone. Written communications can be gas sterilized; if written in pencil they can be steam sterilized and mailed without fear of spreading infection.

Sometimes people in isolation rooms are reluctant to have their family bring items important to them because they fear that at the end of the isolation period, they will have to throw them away. Fortunately, gas sterilization permits almost any item to be taken into an isolation room and sterilized afterward. Most items with hard surfaces need to be washed with a disinfectant in order to be removed from an isolation room. If you have any doubt about the ability of an article to be gas sterilized, call the central supply department and ask whether it can be sterilized or not.

Make a habit of visiting in the room at times other than when you have to give direct care, just as you would with all other patients. This is extremely important for people in isolation to show them that although you are taking precautions to prevent the spread of microorganisms, you are not isolating yourself from them. Fortunately, in most instances antibiotic therapy quickly reduces the number of pathogenic agents present, so that isolation technique except for reverse measures need be in effect for only a few days.

Sometimes people with communicable diseases remain at home. QRS 28-2 lists ways the nurse can help people adjust isolation technique to the home setting.

☐ QUICK REFERENCE STOP 28-2: COMMUNITY CONSIDERATIONS

Few people are confined at home with communicable diseases. However, this occasionally occurs, and wound or skin precautions may need to be carried out in a home setting. Help people adjust isolation technique to the home setting by following a few basic rules:

Hand-washing is an effective means of breaking a chain of infection. Supplying a basin of water and soap outside or in the ill person's bedroom may make hand-washing easier if the bathroom is a hallway away.

Washing linen and clothing separately from the family wash helps to prevent spread of microorganisms to other family members.

Do not allow cats or dogs in the ill person's bedroom. Animals jump on beds and walk on floors, areas apt to be high risk for the presence of microorganisms.

Teach that trying to save money by changing dressings infrequently may prolong the infection by increasing the presence of a reservoir. Teach instead to use a minimum of compresses and change more frequently.

To reuse an isolation gown, hang it from a hook by the neck band so the inside of the gown folds closed. Put it on by touching only the neckband and the inside of the gown. Take it off by (after washing your hands) touching only the inside. A man's shirt or kitchen smock are good substitutes for gowns.

OTHER CONSIDERATIONS

The floor of isolation rooms is considered heavily contaminated because microorganisms settle by gravity. Flat surfaces such as counters or overbed tables become heavily contaminated in the same way. When cleaning in an isolation room, always use a wet dustcloth so dust is not airborne. The floor should always be damp mopped for the same reason.

An object removed from an isolation room must be carefully marked. This protects the personnel who work in the laundry or laboratory from being exposed to microorganisms without their knowledge.

In an isolation room when a gown is required, the long sleeves of the gown cover your watch so you cannot see it for counting the patient's pulse. A corridor clock is often visible; consider this when choosing which room will be the nursing unit's isolation room. If a wall clock is not available, remove your watch and place it inside a plastic bag, seal with tape, and take it into the room with you.

Patients should have a thermometer that remains in the room. If vital signs will be assessed frequently, a sphygmomanometer and stethoscope should be left inside the room. If this is not possible, protect the cuff of the sphygmomanometer by placing a paper towel or a clean patient gown next to the patient's arm. Wash stethoscope, rubber tubing, and bulb of the sphygmomanometer after they are removed from the room with an appropriate disinfectant.

Use disposable supplies whenever possible so that supplies do not have to be disinfected or sterilized for reuse. Discard supplies in double-bagged containers.

TABLE 28-3. SUMMARY OF ISOLATION TECHNIQUES

	Precautions Needed						
Type of Isolation	Private Room	Gown	Mask	Gloves	Blood	Secretions	Excretions
Respiratory (pulmonary tuberculosis, meningitis, pertussis, rubella, rubeola)	x		x			From nose and throat	
Enteric (salmonellosis, shigellosis, typhoid fever, diarrhea of undetermined origin)		For direct care		For direct care			x
Wound or skin (infected surgical or wound incision)		For direct care	For direct care	For direct care		From infected area	
Blood precautions (hepatitis)					x	x	
Strict (smallpox, diphtheria, rabies)	x	x	x	x		x	x
Reverse (protective) (presence of a low white blood count; immunological deficiency)	x	x	x	x			

To transport a patient outside the isolation room, cover a stretcher or wheelchair with a clean sheet to protect it. When the patient returns to his room, discard the sheet used as a cover into his laundry hamper. With respiratory isolation, the patient must wear a mask.

If a person in an isolation room must sign a permission form for care or some other legal paper, cover the overbed table with a clean paper towel. Place the legal document on the clean paper towel. Ask the person to read the document without touching it. Place a paper towel over the bottom of the form below the level of the signature where his hand will rest. Ask him to rest his hand only on the paper towel not the form while he signs. Do not rush him. A signature is legal only if it is informed. *Informed* means that he has had time to read and understand the document he is signing.

Do not take medication cards or medication trays into isolation rooms. Make out a separate card for patient identification, which can be discarded in the room. Use disposable syringes and needles; double bag to be disposed of safely at the medication area.

Be certain that specimens such as urine or sputum are doubled bagged before being brought out of rooms. It is easy to think of specimens as contaminated, but in isolation, the outside of the container is contaminated as well.

Table 28-3 summarizes various types of isolation care and some examples of illnesses that require such care. When you are caring for a patient in isolation, you are responsible that all people entering and leaving the room observe good technique. Microorganisms are not selective.

Good isolation technique is threefold: (1) a well-marked room door so everyone is aware that isolation is being practiced, (2) clearly written instructions as to what precautions are necessary, and (3) ample supplies available so there is no delay in being able to put on the proper apparel for protection.

Reducing the Possibility of Being a Susceptible Host

Antibodies are produced by T cells of the lymphatic system to attack and destroy invading organisms (antigens). People are susceptible to communicable disease if they do not have antibodies against that specific invading organism. Immunization is a means of elevating the level of antibodies present in circulation. It is of two main types: active and passive.

ACTIVE IMMUNIZATION

In active immunization, an antigen has entered the body and provoked the formation of a specific antibody. Natural active immunization occurs when the person contacts a disease. Artificial active immunization occurs when an antigen is administered as an immunization. Whether natural or artificial, active immunization is long-term immunization, as long as 20 years.

PASSIVE IMMUNIZATION

Passive immunization is the administration not of an antigen, but of antibodies. Natural passive immunization occurs when antibodies of the IgG class cross the placenta in utero to the fetus. All newborns are born transfused with antibody protection to the diseases for which the mother has an adequate antibody level. Natural passive immunity is effective only for the first year of life; measles immunity lasts a little longer, which is why measles immunization must be delayed until 15 months. Artificial passive immunization occurs when an antibody serum (gamma globulin immune serum globulin) is injected. This is a quick method of elevating antibody level. However, these antibodies are foreign to the person, and the body begins to reject them fairly rapidly. Passive artificial immunity is effective for only about 3 months.

VACCINES

Immunological material is termed *vaccine.* Vaccines are supplied in a variety of forms.

Antigens. An antigen may be injected as a live form, an attenuated (live but weakened) form, or a dead form. The form chosen depends on the virulence of the agent. All forms produce an adequate antibody response. Some antigens produce a toxin (poison) as they grow, and the symptoms of the disease are caused by the toxin, not the antigen. In these instances, the toxin is injected, generally in an attenuated form called a *toxoid.*

Antibodies. Antibodies are injected in the live form. Antitoxin forms are also available.

Informing people of appropriate immunization schedules and assessing patients' immunized status is considered independent nursing action (see QRS 28-3). The immunization schedule recommended by the American Academy of Pediatrics is shown in Chap. 9, Table 9-16.

Basic Principles of Surgical Asepsis

1. The only object that can touch a sterile object is another sterile object; if touched by an unsterile object, the first object is no longer sterile.
2. Reaching over a sterile field or coughing or sneezing near a sterile field contaminates the field. Do not turn your back to a sterile field since you cannot monitor what is happening to it when it is out of your vision.
3. Any object held below waist level is considered contaminated (bacteria settle).
4. A wet object is no longer considered sterile. Capillary action moves organisms into it.
5. Do not soak transfer forceps in disinfectants as a means of keeping them sterile. Use dry, sterilized forceps only. No disinfectant is strong enough to maintain sterility for any length of time.
6. Any object that will pierce or penetrate below the skin surface must be sterile (needles, catheters, drains). Any dressing covering a broken skin surface must be sterile.
7. The outer inch of a sterile field is *not* sterile.
8. If you have any doubt that an object is sterile, consider it *not* sterile.

SURGICAL ASEPSIS

Surgical asepsis is *sterile technique,* aimed at destroying pathogens or stopping their transmission. This technique is used in surgery, but it is also used whenever you perform a procedure that pierces, penetrates, or contacts a broken skin surface. Basic rules of surgical asepsis are summarized in the box above.

STERILIZATION

An object is *clean* when it is free of pathogenic organisms. It is *sterile* when it is free of all microorganisms and their spore form. *Sterilization* is the technique of making objects free of all microorganisms and spores. Sterilization can be achieved in a number of ways.

Autoclave (Steam) Sterilization. An autoclave is an airtight chamber that uses steam pressure to raise the temperature inside until all microorganisms are destroyed. Before being placed in an autoclave an object is wrapped in double paper or cloth and the date of sterilization is marked on tape holding the wrapper in place. This tape also indicates whether the autoclave reached a true autoclaving temperature or not by turning color when this is reached. When working with autoclaved materials, always check the tape to see that it has colored (Fig. 28-2). Commercial bags or wrappers for autoclaving supplies have a similar autoclave mark.

In order for sterilization to take place, an autoclave must reach a temperature of 132°C (270°F) for 25 minutes. Autoclaving is impractical for plastic or rubber objects because plastic melts and rubber deteriorates at this temperature.

☐ QUICK REFERENCE STOP 28-3: HEALTH TEACHING

Teach that maintaining current immunization status is a person's first line of defense against communicable illnesses. There is no such thing as just measles or only mumps. Childhood communicable diseases can be fatal or result in permanent handicaps.

Gas Sterilization. Gas sterilizers are airtight chambers flooded with ethylene oxide gas. A reduced temperature is used (54—65°C; 130—150°F). The exposure time is longer (45 min to several hours). Objects are wrapped for gas sterilization as for traditional autoclaving and marked with special gas sterilization tapes, which turn from a dark to a light color. Following removal from the sterilizer, items must be given time (at least 20 min) for the concentration of ethylene oxide gas to dissipate into the air.

Gas sterilization has the advantage over steam sterilization that plastic and rubber can be safely

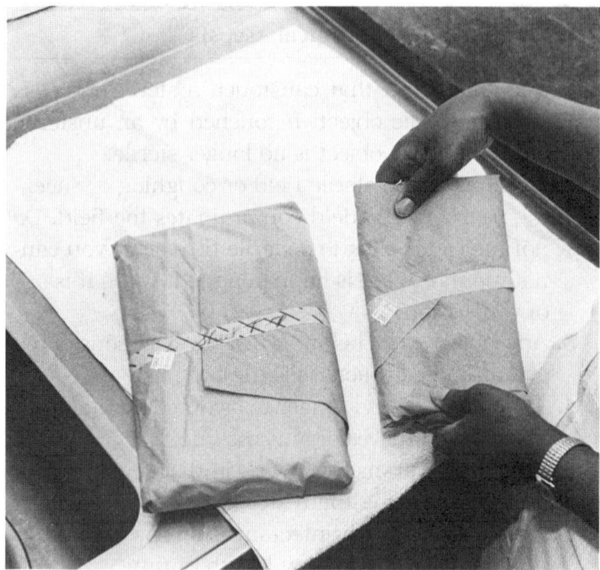

FIGURE 28-2. "Autoclave" tape that has changed color indicates that the contents inside the wrap are sterile. The package on the left has been sterilized; the date on the tape denotes the day of sterilization.

sterilized; the disadvantages are increased cost and the longer time required.

Dry Heat Sterilization. Baking or using dry heat is an alternative method of sterilization. It can be used for metal equipment to prevent the rust that can occur with steam sterilization. However, it requires time and high temperatures (180°C; 356°F for 2 hr or more) and thus is limited in practical use except in clinics or physician's offices, where it can be used as a convenient and low-cost method.

Cold Sterilization. Cold sterilization is soaking the object to be sterilized in a disinfectant solution such as Betadine (iodine) or alcohol. Cold sterilization does not destroy all spores and is never the method of choice to achieve surgical asepsis.

Boiling. Boiling supplies in water has long been accepted as a good method of sterilization because it is practical for home use. However, boiling does not destroy spores, so it is not the method of choice in a health care facility. Boiling at 100°C (212°F) at sea level for 30 minutes is the usually recommended procedure for home use. Water boils at a lower temperature (as low as 83°C; 181°F) at high altitudes; there an object should be boiled about twice as long to achieve the same degree of asepsis.

Ultraviolet Sterilization. Exposing an object to ultraviolet radiation is an effective but impractical solution to sterilization. The object must be directly exposed to the rays (not wrapped) and must be turned so the rays strike all of its surfaces. In addition, prolonged exposure to ultraviolet radiation may be harmful to the eyes so you cannot remain in the area where sterilization is taking place. Ultraviolet sterilization is used primarily to reduce the number of bacteria in the air. It may be used at the entrance of a surgical suite to reduce bacteria being carried into the area or used to disinfect a room following discharge of a patient who had a known infection.

STERILE SUPPLIES

An object remains sterile after sterilization only if it is handled with precautions. When selecting a sterile package from a shelf to use, always check it for intactness of the wrapper, colored autoclave mark, expiration date, and dryness. The importance of these factors is summarized in the following box, Points to Check When Selecting Sterile Supplies.

Many items needed for patient care come in commercially prepared presterilized packages; others are

POINTS TO CHECK WHEN SELECTING STERILE SUPPLIES

1. *Torn wrapper.* Once a tear occurs in the wrapper, the package is no longer considered sterile.
2. *Tampered-with wrapper.* Once a wrapper is opened, the object inside is no longer sterile. A person cannot open a package to see what is inside and then close it again.
3. *Wet wrapper.* If water enters a package it draws bacteria into it, so a package that is wet or has a watermark to show it has been wet even though it is now dry is no longer sterile.
4. *Doubtful contamination.* If you have any question as to whether something is sterile or not, consider it unsterile. Sterility is a black-and-white concept. If you do not know that it is sterile, it is not.
5. *Outdated shelf life.* The shelf life is the period of time a package is considered sterile following sterilization. Most health care facilities accept 4 wk as the maximum time that an object could still be considered sterile. After this time, it must be reprocessed. Commercially prepared articles may have longer dates than this but all dates are carefully marked. Make a habit of putting freshly sterilized supplies away at the rear of a shelf so the older dated packages will automatically move to the front and be used first. Items on an emergency cart (with luck, never used) can become outdated and no longer sterile unless the cart is systematically checked for shelf-life dates.
6. *Colored indicator tape.* An indicator tape that did not turn color means the article was *never* properly sterilized and is not sterile.

wrapped or prepared by the health care agency in its central supply department.

Commercial Supplies. Commercial supplies are packaged and sterilized at the company making the product. Many companies make sterile and unsterile forms of the same items; for example, gauze squares are supplied sterile to use for wound dressings and nonsterile to use for padding under casts. These packages look similar; always check for the word *sterile* on the package if that is the form you need. Do not use the sterile form unless needed because it costs more.

Single items are usually supplied in an envelope-like package that opens by peeling down one side at the top (Fig. 28-3). Be careful when opening that your thumb does not contaminate the object inside. The inside of the wrapper is sterile too, so you can use it as a sterile foundation for other sterile supplies—except the place on the rim where your thumb touched. This is termed using it as a *sterile field.*

Total supplies for certain procedures such as a urinary catheterization or a dressing change may be packaged together in large commercial procedure sets, generally in a cardboard box or tray covered by a plastic bag. Instructions for opening the outer wrapper and a list of the supplies inside are on the outside wrapper. Read the instructions because different brands open differently; note what supplies are inside so you know if you have to add anything for the specific procedure you are undertaking.

Agency-Wrapped Items. An item wrapped and sterilized by the health care agency itself is double wrapped in either a paper or cloth square similar to an envelope. Always open the flap *away* from you first, then the side flaps, then last, the one nearest you. This order of opening prevents you from reaching over the item, which would contaminate the item. You can use the inside of an agency-wrapped package as a sterile field.

Sterile Liquids. Commercially prepared sterile liquids are supplied in glass or plastic bottles or plastic bags that have protective seals. The seal is lifted off for pouring from the container. Medicine is supplied in rubber-topped vials that are entered by a sterile syringe and needle after the rubber stopper has been wiped with a disinfectant such as alcohol. Agency-prepared liquids are supplied in glass bottles with rubber caps. As the cap is lifted, you should hear the release of the vacuum seal; if you do not hear such a sound, the container is unsterile. Be careful when handling the cap of any sterile liquid container not to touch the inside surface of the cap or you cannot recap the bottle again. If you put the cap down to pour, place it inside up so the inside surface is not contaminated by touching an unclean table or countertop (Fig. 28-4).

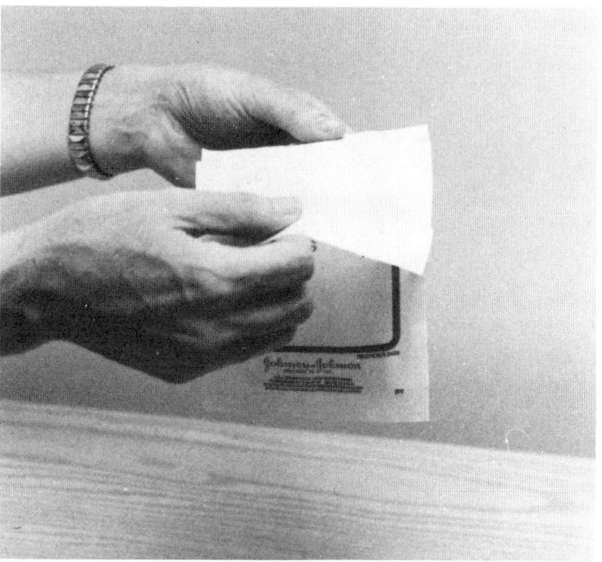

FIGURE 28-3. Open a commercially packaged item such as a sterile gauze square by peeling down one side at the top.

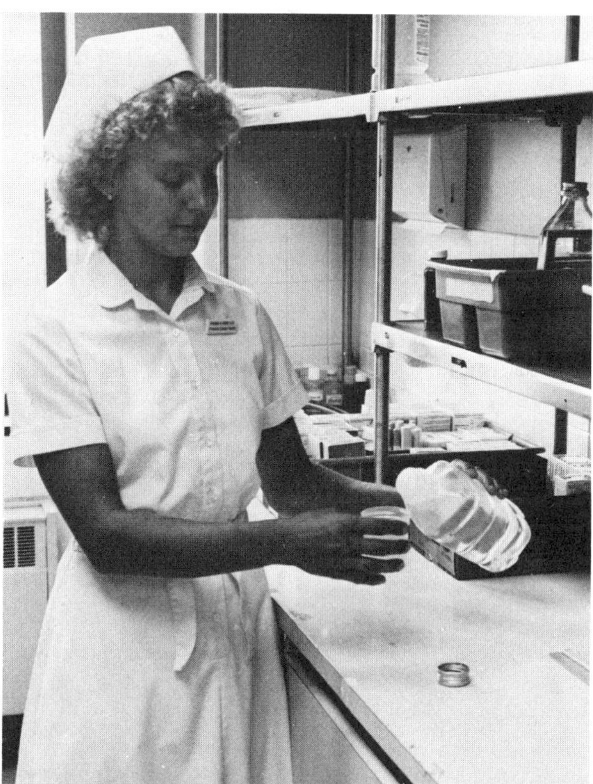

FIGURE 28-4. When pouring a sterile liquid, invert the cap to prevent contamination and place it on a flat surface. Do not allow the lip of sterile containers to touch other surfaces.

ESTABLISHING A STERILE FIELD

A sterile field is a sterile work area. You need a sterile field to contain supplies for various procedures such as changing a wound dressing or bladder catheterization. The surface area must be dry so materials do not become damp; a wet article is no longer sterile. The surface must be at waist level or above. Since microor-

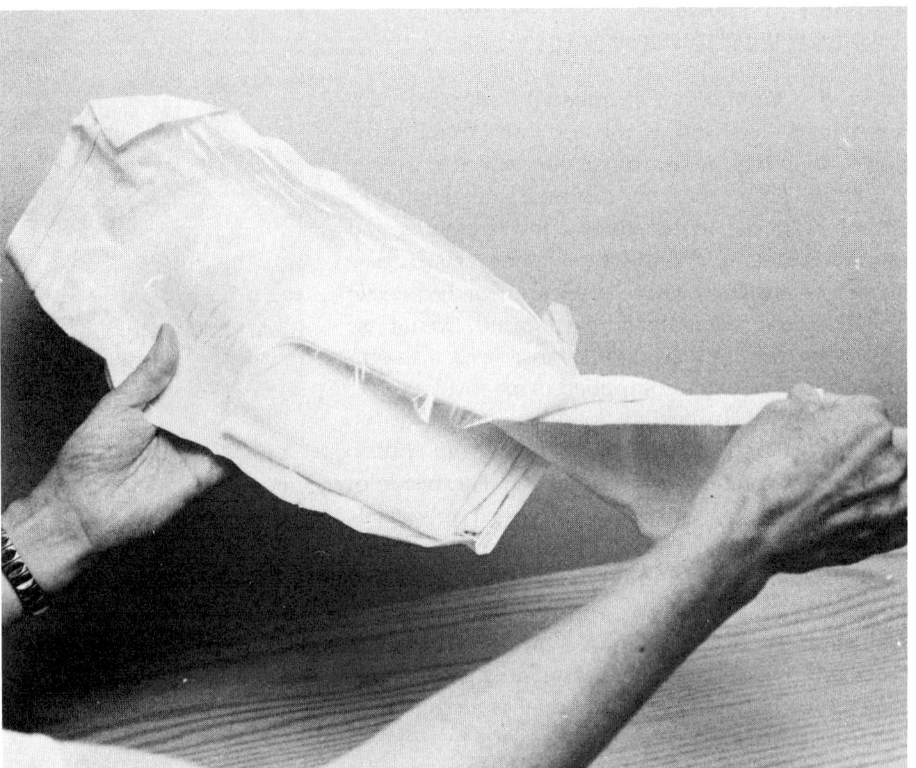

A

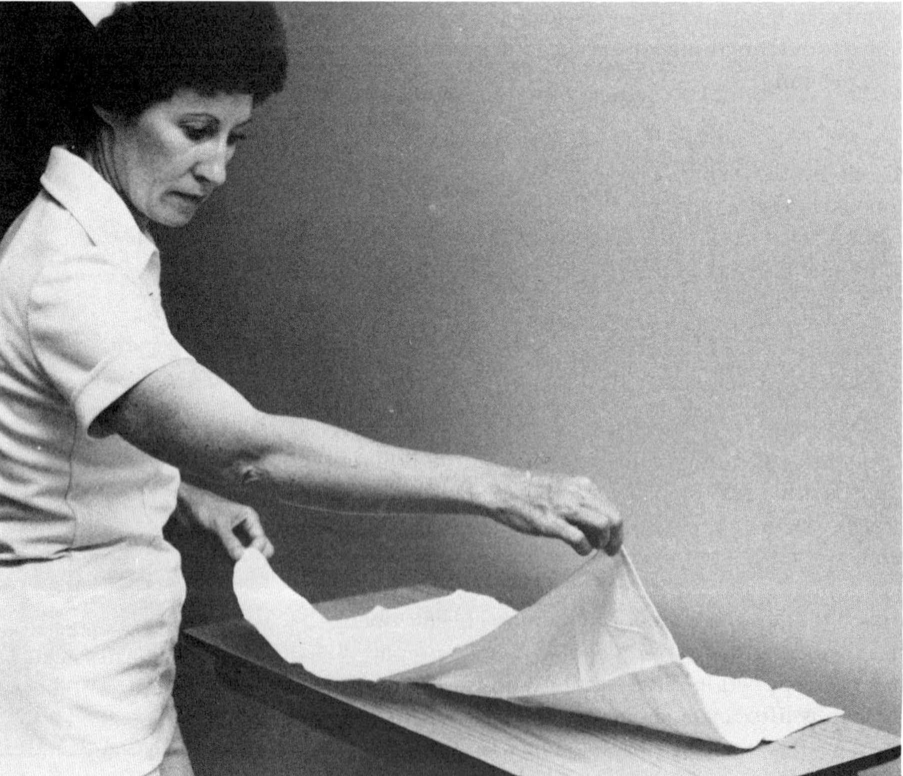

B

FIGURE 28-5. A. To use a sterile towel for a sterile field, unwrap the outer paper; lift the towel out by its corners. B. Place it on a surface such as the overbed table.

ganisms settle, any area below the halfway point in a room has a higher microorganism count than one at waist level or above. For a foundation, you can use a sterile towel. Open it by unwrapping the outer paper, lift the towel out by its corners and place it on the surface selected by touching only its corners (Fig. 28-5). The wrapping of an agency-prepared or commercially prepared sterile package may be fully unfolded to become a sterile field (Fig. 28-6). Because you have touched the corners of the towel or a package wrapper, the outside inch of the field is not considered sterile. Any supply that touches this outside inch will have to be discarded as unsterile.

To add sterile supplies needed for the procedure, either drop them from commercially prepared envelopes—being careful to drop from a 6-inch distance so the unsterile outside wrapper does not touch the sterile field (Fig. 28-7A)—or unwrap an agency-prepared sterile supply package and fold the wrapper back over your hand to prevent it from touching the surface of the field (Fig. 28-7B). An alternate way to add supplies is to place them on the field with sterile transfer forceps. Transfer forceps are wrapped so the handle is easily accessible when unwrapped. Once you touch the handle, this part of the instrument is contaminated. To rest the forceps, place the sterile tip and shaft on the sterile field and the handle off (Fig. 28-8).

FIGURE 28-6. When using any agency prepared or commercially prepared sterile package, the wrapping may be fully unfolded to become your sterile field.

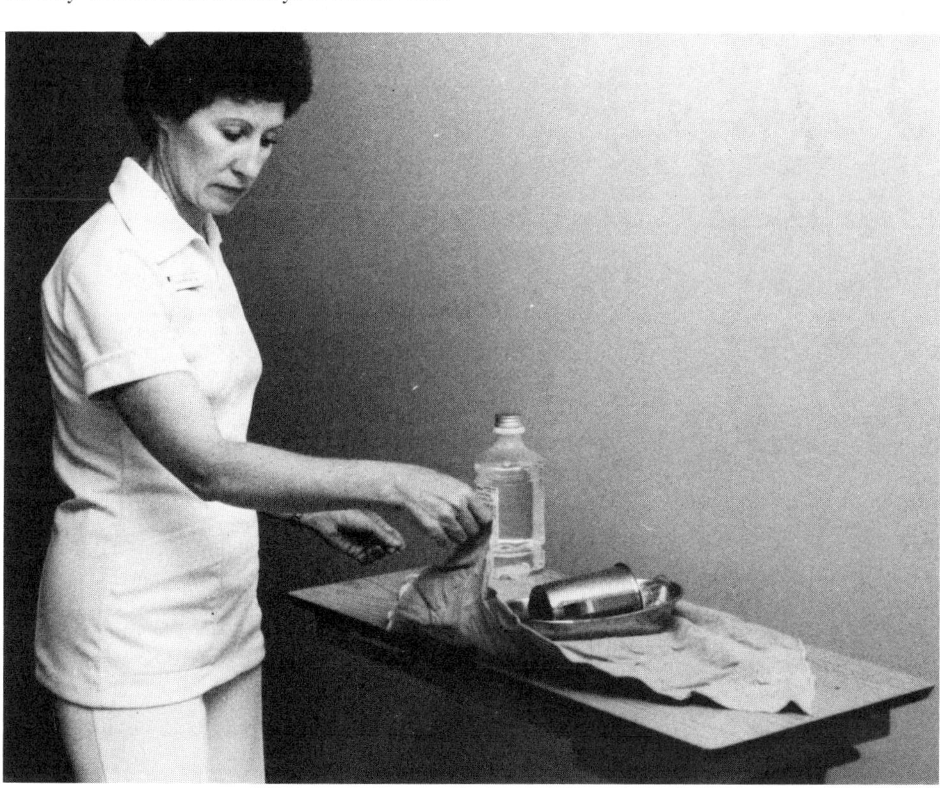

If you need to add a liquid to the field, unwrap a suitable container and place it on the field close to the side (but not on the 1-in. space that is considered contaminated). Open the sterile liquid container and either hold the cap in your left hand so it does not touch anything or place it inside up on a clean surface near by. Read the bottle label three times—as you select the liquid, as you uncap it, just before you pour it—and pour the liquid from a distance of about 6 inches. Do not touch the bottle rim to the sterile container or pour from such a distance that you would splash liquid on the sterile field. Be certain the container into which you are pouring is near the side of the field because reaching across a sterile field contaminates it.

Commercially prepared bottles of sterile liquids may not be resealable. If this is so, the solution not used must be discarded. Agency-prepared bottles with rubber caps and some screw-type commercial types may be reused for up to 24 hours (unless agency policy states otherwise) as long as the bottle lid was not contaminated in the opening or pouring procedure. Mark the time and date the bottle was opened on the label for the beginning of this time period.

Items on a sterile field may be rearranged by means of the transfer forceps. An alternative method would be to put on a sterile glove and arrange supplies manually.

Preparing a sterile field takes only a short time and is good assurance that you are providing supplies to a patient in their sterile state. Remember the black-and-white concept of sterility: if you have any doubt

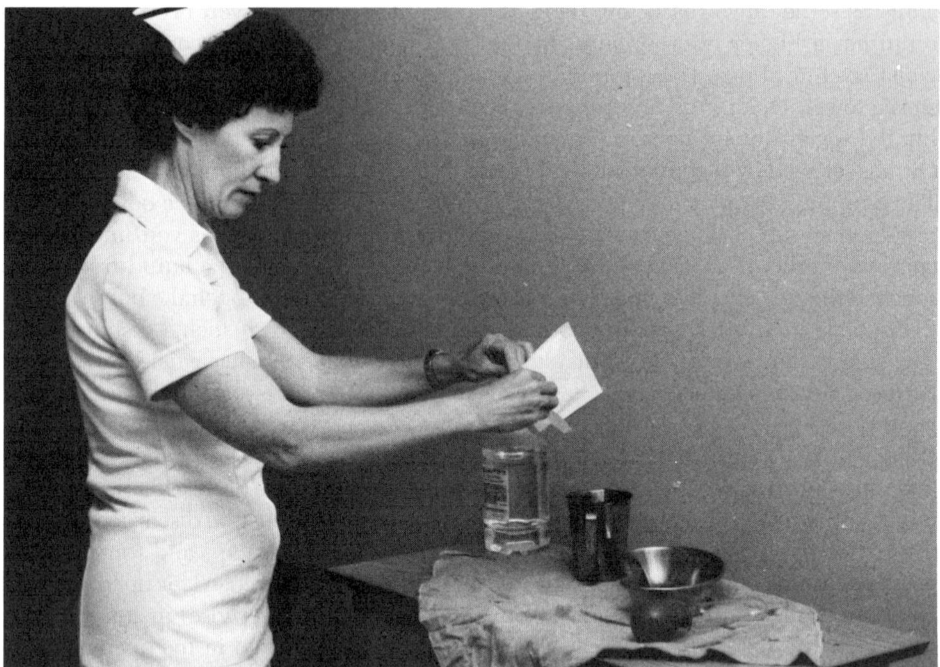

A

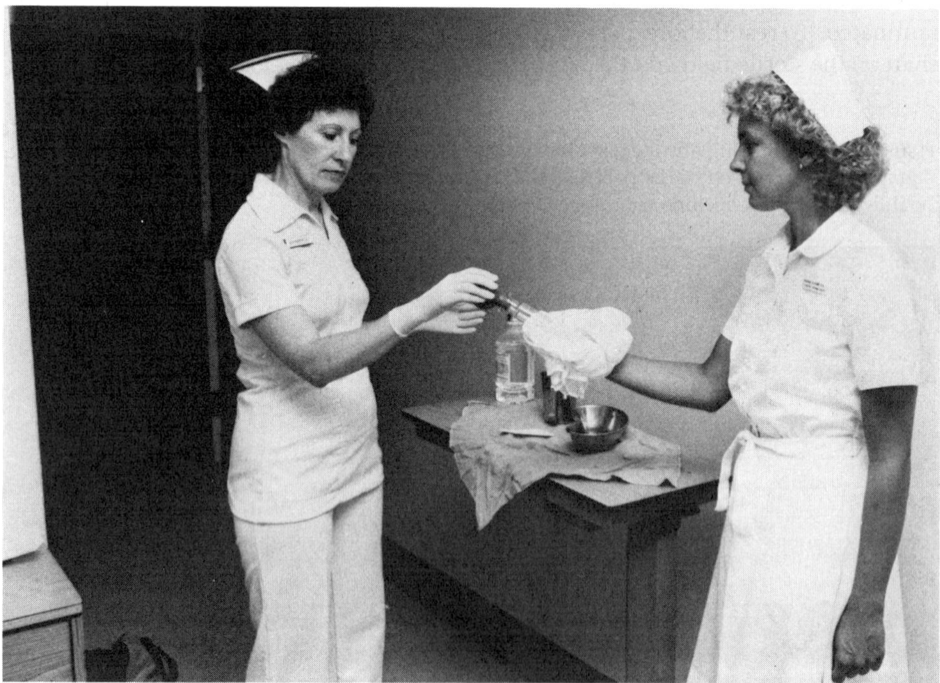

B

FIGURE 28-7. A. Add commercially prepared sterile supplies needed for procedure by dropping them onto the sterile field from about a 6-inch distance. B. Agency prepared sterile supply packages are added by unwrapping and folding the wrapper back over your hand to prevent it from touching the sterile field.

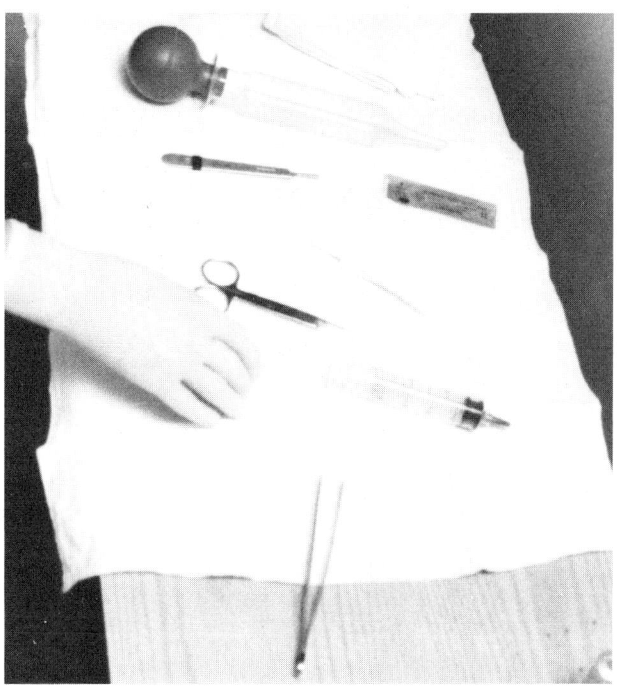

FIGURE 28-8. After use, sterile transfer forceps are placed to rest with the sterile tip and shaft on the sterile field, the contaminated handle off.

that your field has been contaminated, consider it unsterile. The cost of another towel and a few gauze squares to an agency is nothing compared to the cost of an extra week's hospitalization (or a lawsuit) because you introduced microorganisms to a patient through careless technique (QRS 28-4).

STERILE GLOVES

Sterile gloves are worn to handle sterile supplies so that they remain sterile. They must be put on with careful technique so you do not contaminate them in the process; after they are in place you must be certain that you touch only sterile objects. The technique for donning sterile gloves is shown in Procedure 28-4.

☐ QUICK REFERENCE STOP 28-4: SAFETY
Rules for Maintaining Sterile Technique

If you do not know whether an object is sterile, consider it *not* sterile. Otherwise you unknowingly spread microorganisms.

If an object will pierce a skin surface or cover a broken skin surface, always use sterile objects to avoid introducing infection.

Use enough equipment, such as extra sterile gloves or forceps, to change sterile dressings. Trying to make do with less equipment than needed is not cost effective if it leads to a wound infection and added days of hospitalization.

STERILE GOWN

If you will be leaning over or close to a sterile field to assist with a procedure, you need to don a sterile gown as well. Technique for putting on a sterile gown and mask is shown in Procedure 28-5. Observe steps carefully in order to avoid contaminating the gown as you pull it on; be certain afterward that no unsterile object touches the front. The back of a gown is never considered sterile.

WOUNDS

Wounds are breaks in the skin surface. They may be accidental injury, self-inflicted, or surgical. They may be caused by chemical substances such as acid burns, by extreme hot or cold such as sunburn or frostbite, or by radiation. Whatever the source, wounds heal in predictable ways and need safeguards against the introduction of microorganisms.

Wound Healing

A wound healing from side to side is termed *primary intention.* A surgically sutured incision heals this way. A wound healing from the bottom of the wound upward is *secondary intention.* Ruptured blisters heal this way. A wound that becomes infected, has to be opened, and reheal is termed *tertiary intention* (Fig. 28-9).

No matter which level of healing is involved, wounds heal in three well-defined stages. Observing what stage of healing a wound is in helps you to determine whether proper healing is occurring or not.

PROCEDURE 28-4
Sterile Gloving

Purpose: To put on sterile gloves without contaminating the outside of the gloves in order to prevent the spread of microorganisms from your hands to sterile objects (Fig. 1).

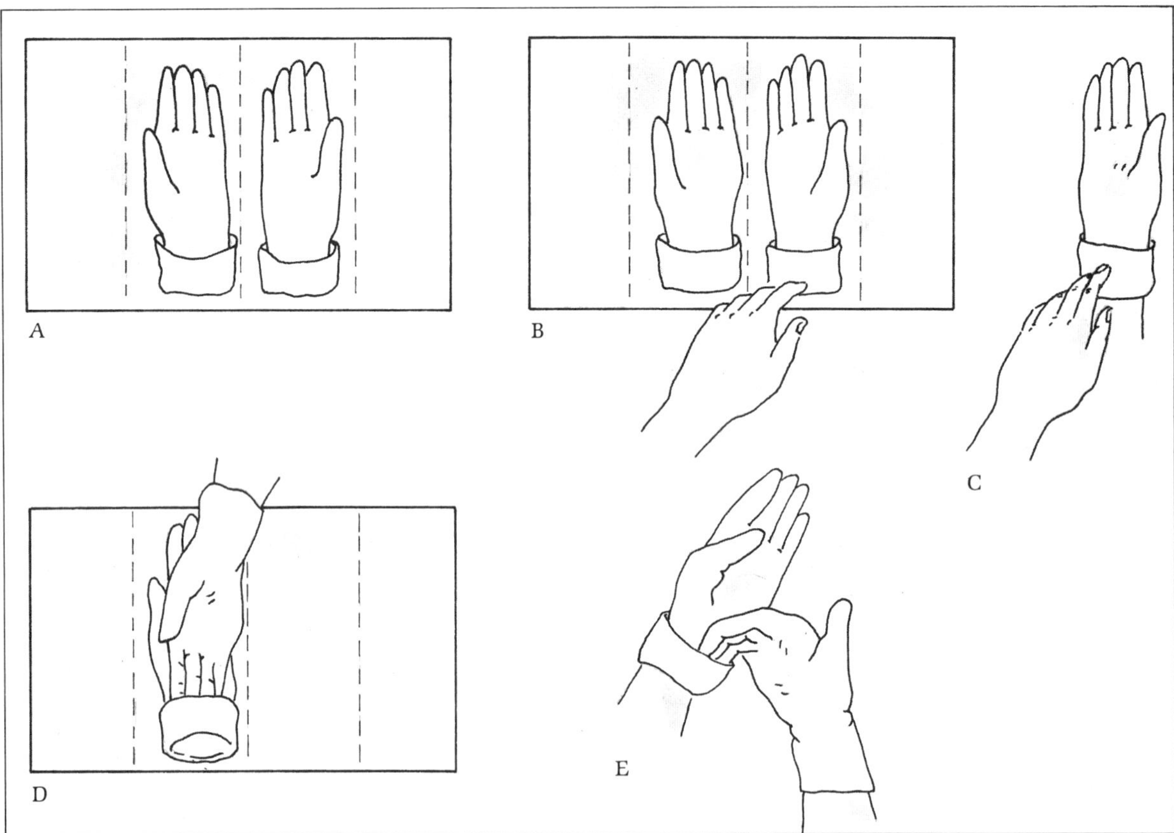

FIGURE 1. Gloving technique.

Plan	*Principle*
1. Wash your hands; be certain that your fingernails are short and you are not wearing a ring with sharp corners.	1. Sharp fingernails or a sharp ring edge might puncture the glove; a torn glove is contaminated and must be removed. Hand washing reduces the number of microorganisms present that could be transferred if a glove did accidentally tear.
2. Select proper size of glove. Clear a flat dry area waist level or higher on which to open glove package.	2. The average woman wears a size 6—7-1/2 glove; the average man, 7—8-1/2. Surfaces waist level or below are considered contaminated; a wet surface will contaminate the gloves by capillary action.
3. Open outside wrapper, flap farthest from you first; flap nearest you last. Open inside wrapper to reveal gloves; place so cuffs of gloves are toward you, right glove to your right.	3. Always open nearest flap last to avoid reaching across a sterile surface. A commercial package may peel open to reveal gloves. With any package, *do not touch any surface of the gloves in the opening process.*
4. Pick up the right glove by the *inside* of the cuff with the left hand; insert right hand into glove. Hold hands high to be careful that you do not touch glove against any nearby object such as a countertop or doorframe.	4. Be certain that your hand touches only the *inside* of the glove so as not to contaminate the glove. Keep your hands above waist level.
5. Resist making any adjustment to the glove at this point; it is difficult to do that without contaminating glove.	5. An adjustment is made more easily after the second glove is in place.

6. Pick up left glove by sliding gloved hand under the folded cuff on glove side. Be careful not to touch bare left hand with gloved thumb of right hand; slide left hand into glove.	6. Sterile surfaces can touch only other sterile surfaces in order to remain sterile.
7. Flip open both glove cuffs by touching glove side. Adjust fingers for comfort and fit by gently pulling on fingers.	7. Elongating the cuff gives you a larger area that is sterile. If you have a sterile, long-sleeved gown in place, flip glove cuffs up over gown sleeves to create a long, continuous sterile expanse.
8. To remove gloves, pinch the first cuff just below the level of the thumb and peel off by touching only glove to glove. Slip bare hand under thumb side of second cuff and peel off touching only underside of glove.	8. Once gloves are used they are no longer sterile. Do not deliberately contaminate your hands against glove surface, which at that point probably has more microorganisms present than your bare hand.
9. Discard disposable gloves in suitable waste container; place gloves to be resterilized in proper container. Wash hands.	9. Do not attempt to reuse sterile gloves. The chance you would contaminate them while trying to replace them is too great to risk.

PROCEDURE 28-5
Putting on a Sterile Gown and Mask

Purpose: To cover your uniform and mouth and nose to prevent the spread of microorganisms from your mouth, nose, or infections to a sterile field.

Plan	*Principle*
1. Wash your hands. Put on mask, being certain it covers both your nose and mouth. Tie strings over your ears.	1. Prevent spread of microorganisms. The mask is clean but not sterile so must be touched before the gown is touched. Be certain it is firmly in place and comfortable because if after putting the gown in place you also put on sterile gloves (and as a rule, you will), you cannot return to the mask to straighten it.
2. Place gown wrap on a flat, clean dry surface above waist level. Open pack with flap farthest away from you first, nearest you last.	2. A surface below waist level is considered contaminated. Open nearest flap last to avoid reaching across the sterile gown.
3. Grasp gown by collar and hold it in front of you being certain that it does not brush the counter or tabletop.	3. The collar of the gown is now no longer sterile. Avoid touching any other part or touching gown to any unsterile surface or gown will be contaminated and unusable.
4. Push right hand into inside of gown sleeve but not so far that it protrudes through gown sleeve. Grasp outside of second sleeve with covered hand and support gown while you push second arm into inside of sleeve.	4. Touch bare hand only to *inside* of gown; hand covered by gown sleeve only to *outside* in order to keep outside of gown surface sterile.
5. Grasp outside of sleeve cuffs by covered hands and tug up over hands.	
6. *Do not tie strings!* Reaching behind you will contaminate gown sleeves against your hair. Wait for someone to tie strings for you. After the ties have been fastened, they are no longer sterile. Do not turn your back to your sterile field.	6. If assisting with gowning someone else, slip hands along the inside back of gown, to locate neck strings and tie them. Tug at bottom of gown hem at center back to straighten back; tie waist level ties. *Touch only the inside of the gown and the ties.*

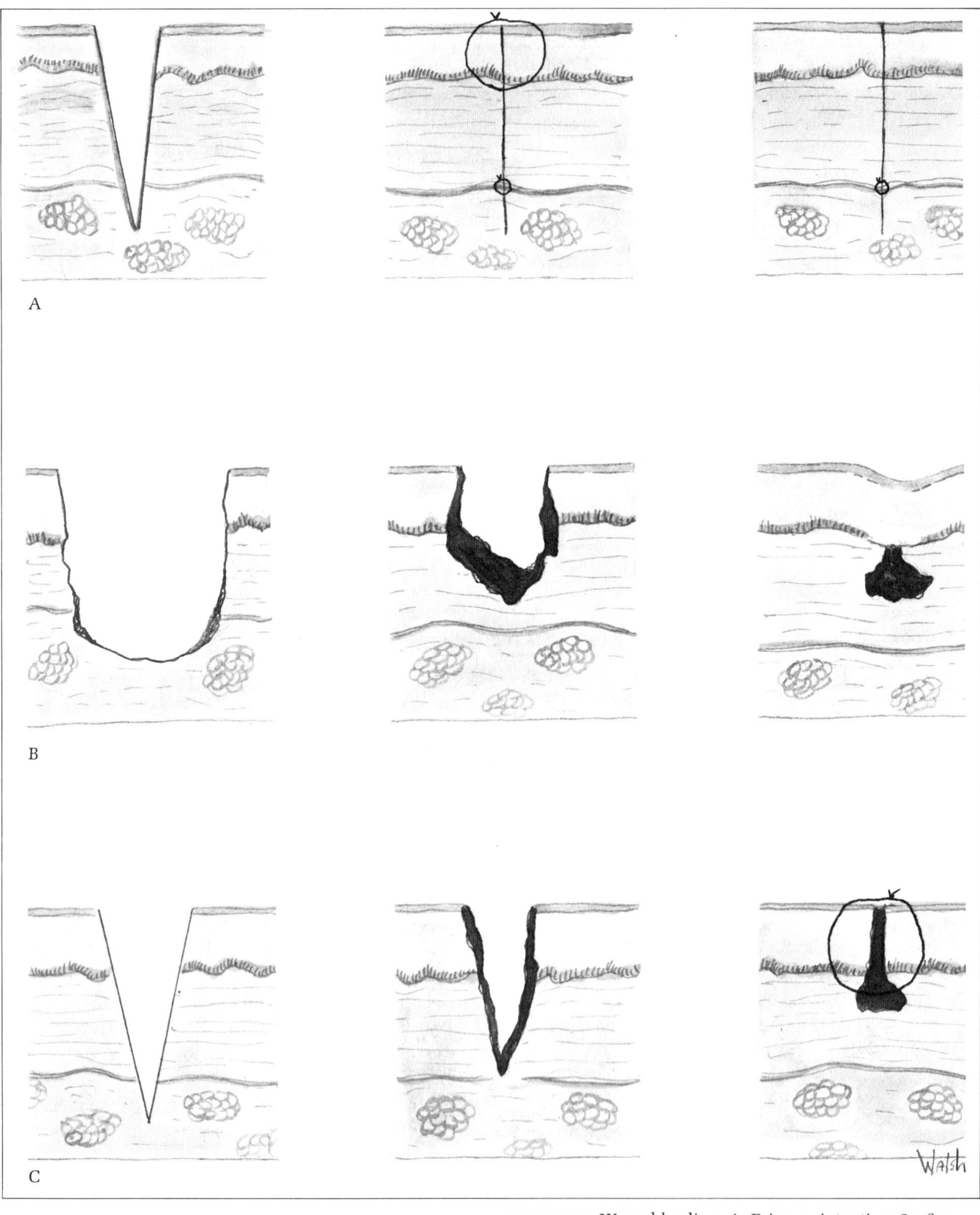

FIGURE 28-9. Wound healing. A. Primary intention. Surface suture is removed; internal suture will dissolve over time. B. Secondary intention. Healing occurs from the bottom and sides. A large scar results. C. Tertiary intention. A clean incision becomes infected and heals, leaving a scarred area.

Stage I: Inflammation. One of the first responses of body tissue to injury is inflammation or the occurrence of redness, heat, pain, swelling, and impaired function of the involved part. Such responses prevent further spread of the injury, begin repair of the injured tissue, and destroy the injuring agent if it is still present. It is local adaptation to a stressful event.

In order quickly to reduce the possibility of hemorrhage from an injury, the initial reaction of blood vessels in the area is constriction. Injured cells at the site begin to release histamine, which dilates local capillaries. This leads to rapid infiltration of leukocytes into the area to fight infection and also slows blood flow because of pooling of blood in capillaries. The increased blood supply in the area gives the symptoms of erythema and warmth to the area. The increased pressure in capillaries causes diffusion of plasma leukocytes, platelets, erythrocytes, and antibodies from the capillaries into the surrounding tissue.

Diffusion of plasma from the capillaries continues to occur at a greater rate than can be explained simply by the increased hydrostatic pressure in capillaries. Therefore, a specific vascular permeability response must also occur, probably as a result of histamine being present. As this continues, swelling begins. Tissue is drawn taut against nerve endings, and dull pain occurs.

Antibodies drain into surrounding tissue, increasing resistance to microorganism invasion. Leukocytes drain into the surrounding tissue and begin to destroy microorganisms by the process of phagocytosis. As the number of leukocytes increases to meet this demand, leukocytosis (a white blood count above 20,000/mm) occurs. A normal white blood count is 5,000—10,000 per millimeter.

Stage II: The Exudate Stage. The second stage of healing forms a seal over the injured area to localize the inflammation, to prevent further loss of fluid, and to protect exposed nerve endings and reduce pain. The seal is formed from the drying of erythrocytes, platelets, and plasma. This dried exudate (clot or scab) will also serve as the basis for tissue repair.

If blood plasma is the chief ingredient, the exudate is clear or yellow, a *serous* exudate. This forms in friction blisters. If large amounts of fibrin are present, the exudate is sticky and yellow; a *fibrous* exudate denotes that a serious inflammatory response has occurred because extensive capillary permeability is necessary for such large protein molecules as fibrin to leave the circulatory system. It is the type of exudate that forms on burns from gymnasium floors. Fibrin exudate is so tacky that surfaces coated with it adhere easily to other surfaces. When fibrin exudate is present, surfaces must be kept separate while they heal or *adhesions* or permanent tissue connections may form.

If the exudate has a small amount of erythrocytes present, it is *serosanguineous.* If a large number are present, it is *sanguineous* or hemorrhagic. Sanguineous exudate denotes that blood vessels in the area did not immediately constrict or that a larger break in blood vessels occurred than if the exudate is fibrinous or serous. Sanguineous exudate is bright red as it forms; it becomes dark brown as it grows older.

If a large number of pyogenic (pus-producing) microorganisms or dead tissue is present, the exudate after a few days may appear thick and yellow (purulent). This occurs from the action of leukocytes or macrophages. The purulent material is formed from a combination of the leukocytes, tissue debris, and microorganisms. The formation of purulent exudate is termed *suppuration* and denotes that microorganisms were present. It is a step beyond simple inflammation. Drying purulent exudate often appears light green in color. Note the color of this exudate because some bacteria emit particular descriptive colors as they grow (e.g., *Pseudomonas* becomes bright green), the way in which they are identified.

Injured mucous membrane, particularly of the upper respiratory tract, produces a thin, watery exudate mixed with mucus. This is termed *catarrhal* exudate. It causes rhinitis or a runny nose.

Often, the type of exudate is mixed. Examples of this are a serosanguineous exudate from a surgical wound (both serous and sanguineous exudates are present) and mucopurulent exudate from the nose (a secondary infection has occurred with a common cold so the exudate is both mucoid and purulent).

Stage III: Regeneration. Healing of tissue continues with clearing away of any injured or useless tissue by the lymph system. New tissue forms either by replacement cells identical with the original cells (granulation tissue) or by fibrous tissue (scar tissue).

The ability of tissue to regenerate or to form original cells depends on the type of tissue. Epithelial (skin), respiratory, osseous, lymphoid, and digestive tract tissue has good regenerative potential—the new tissue will simulate or be identical with the tissue before injury. Nervous, muscular, and cartilage tissue has poor regeneration potential; these types of tissue repair by formation of scar tissue, which is why heart damage is always serious. Another term for scar tissue is *cicatrix.* Although scar tissue covers injured areas that cannot heal by regeneration and is strong and thus difficult to injure again, it is undesirable because it differs in appearance, may cause immobility if it forms at a joint, and cannot perform the same functions as original tissue.

Measures to Encourage Wound Healing

A number of measures encourage wound healing. Some are dependent nursing actions, but many are independent actions.

Limit the Wound. Emergency treatment of burns is immediately to place the burned part under cold water or to apply ice to reduce the temperature of the tissue as quickly as possible and decrease the extent of the burn. Keeping wounds free of destructive organisms is another way to limit the extent of injury. Cleaning a wound in an emergency room to remove surface contamination of grease or dirt accomplishes this. Using strict surgical aseptic technique when performing intrusive procedures so microorganisms are not introduced is another way. Both physical and psychological stress lead to a general adaptation syndrome with possible shunting of blood away from major body organs due to vasoconstriction. Limiting stress may aid healing by reducing effects of a general adaptation syndrome and allowing better blood flow to a part.

Good Nutrient Supply. Excessive edema in an area occludes blood vessels and prevents nutrients from reaching the area. Assess whether anything could be constricting blood flow to or lymph drainage from the site. Elevating an extremity on pillows is often effective in aiding drainage and reducing edema. This also improves comfort; extensive edema is painful from constant pressure.

Good Nutrient Intake. Injuries produce systemic responses because of psychological as well as physical stress. Psychological stress may lead to loss of appetite. Protein must be present for cell regeneration; the B vitamins are necessary for proper protein synthesis; vitamin C has a direct effect on the production of collagen. If the gastrointestinal tract is injured, adequate dietary intake may be a problem since the person may be limited to a liquid or soft diet for a period of time. Make efforts to make mealtime appealing; make food substitutions within the diet prescription as necessary to promote a good intake adequate for healing.

Psychological Stress. Reducing psychological stress has indirect effects on wound healing because a person may be so stressed by the accident causing a wound that he cannot cooperate or participate in his care. Following an accidental injury, a person needs some therapeutic talk time and a person to serve as a listening ear. Similarly, following surgery, patients need time to discuss its impact. Do not discount this time spent listening to accounts of how wounds occurred as idle conversation. Spending time to reduce psychological stress is as important as spending time to reduce physical discomfort.

High Risk Areas. People in poor health from a chronic illness at the time of an injury or surgery heal more slowly than those in good health because nutrients are used for repair processes throughout the body, not just at the injury site (QRS 28-5). Older persons tend to heal more slowly than young people because basic metabolic processes are slower; persons on corticosteroids or radiation therapy tend to have decreased healing properties. Cortisone decreases the inflammatory response and possibly the formation of collagen fibers. In some instances, corticosteroids are given to persons following injuries in order to reduce the inflammatory response and thus to maintain good joint or muscle function.

☐ QUICK REFERENCE STOP 28-5: NUTRITION

People who are in good health are better prepared to withstand and counteract the invasion of an infectious process than people in poor health. People who have wounds need a diet rich in protein and in B and C vitamins to encourage healing.

Health teaching aimed at helping people to include all five basic food groups in their diet is health teaching to aid in maintaining a community free of infectious diseases.

Immunological Potential. People with an intact immunological system are able to ward off infection following injury as long as usual measures to prevent infection at the site are followed. These are strict aseptic technique in surgery or the emergency room and sterile technique in cleaning or caring for the wound. An important immunological measure to assess is tetanus immunization. Tetanus bacilli grow in closed, warm, unoxygenated spaces. Wherever a wound (not a surgical incision) is closed with sutures, assess whether the person has received tetanus immunization within the last 10 years. If not, a booster or tetanus toxoid will usually be administered. If he has never been immunized for tetanus, passive immunity with tetanus immunoglobulin is advised.

Wound Care

Never use anything less than strict sterile technique when changing dressings on surgical wounds. Most wounds have dressings to shield the wound from microorganisms, reduce tension on the wound edges, and absorb drainage from the wound. Dressings have the disadvantage of creating a warm, dark, wet environment over the wound, which invites the growth of microorganisms. Another disadvantage is that the dressing may adhere to the wound and, if not removed carefully, removal can destroy newly healing tissue. Dressings are used less frequently today to allow for surgical incision drying. Decubitus ulcers tend to heal best if kept moist; dressings applied to them, such as Op-Site, are changed as infrequently as every 4 days.

Changing dressings is a balanced responsibility of reducing a reservoir for infection and yet not harming healing (granulation) tissue or introducing new infection. The first dressing change for an incision or wound is ordered by a physician or done by her; subsequent changes are usually made as necessary based on a nurse's judgment. Before changing a dressing, review the surgical note or admission note on a wound so you know the appearance of the incision or wound at first, and the most recent nursing note, so you know its most recent description; then you can make an informed comparison as to appearance. Note any special cleaning agent ordered or any special instructions. The nursing care plan should contain individual patient preferences, such as sensitivity to adhesive tape or size and type of dressing.

The technique for changing and cleaning a wound is shown in Procedure 28-6. The box on page 635, Wound Dressing Technique, describes the possible conditions of old dressings and the sterile equipment you will

PROCEDURE 28-6
Changing a Wound Dressing Using Sterile Glove Technique

Purpose: Replace a wound dressing without introducing microorganisms to the wound; protect the surrounding skin from excoriation; provide for patient comfort; reduce the potential for a reservoir of infection; provide an opportunity for the assessment of the wound.

Plan	*Principle*
1. Wash your hands; identify the patient, explain procedure.	1. Prevent spread of microorganisms; ensure welfare and safety of patient.
2. Assess patient status; analyze appropriateness of procedure. Read chart for presence of drains and special technique required. Plan modifications of care.	2. Some surgeons prefer to change a dressing for the first time after surgery. You must know whether drains are in place so you do not accidentally remove one with the soiled dressing.
3. Begin implementation by assembling equipment: sterile gloves, towel, gauze squares, abdominal pad, cup or basin, and sterile bottle or normal saline. Nonsterile adhesive or nonallergenic tape, plastic bag for soiled dressing.	3. The quantity of supplies differs according to the size of the dressing and the amount of drainage from the wound present. Use nothing but sterile supplies even if drainage from wound is known to be infected so you do not introduce a secondary infection.
4. Provide privacy by a curtain or closed door. Position patient comfortably; remove clothing as necessary to reveal old dressing.	4. Privacy is a highly valued right for most people and also reduces airborne flow of microorganisms. Use a drape as necessary to ensure modesty and prevent chilling.
5. Set up sterile field on flat clean, dry surface (overbed table, bedside stand, or Mayo stand) using sterile towel. Drop needed number of gauze squares and pads onto field. Place sterile basin or cup close to edge of field.	5. Surface used should be waist high. You can use the wrapper of sterile supplies as your field in place of towel. Use a field large enough so that you will not contaminate supplies at the edge of the field.
6. Cut number of tape strips necessary to secure dressing in place at end of procedure and hang from edge of table or stand.	6. Once the new dressing is in place you want to secure it immediately to prevent a portion of the dressing from moving from the wound.
7. Pour appropriate antiseptic solution or normal saline to be used for cleaning wound into cup or basin. Read label three times—basic medication safety technique.	7. Your responsibility for using the proper solution is no less than if you were offering it orally or injecting it parenterally.
8. Remove abdominal dressing pad by loosening tape gently and toward the incision. If dressing is dry, lift it and remove it with your hand, touching only the outer surface; discard it into an open plastic bag. If the dressing is wet, use a sterile glove to protect your hand. If drains are present, remove the inner dressing layer by layer to avoid pulling the drain. Discard gloves with soiled dressing.	8. Pulling tape toward the incision avoids pulling healing tissue apart. Placing soiled dressing in a paper bag prevents spread of microorganisms from it. A wet dressing is presumed to be contaminated; do not expose your hand to microorganisms in case you have a break in your skin. Do not keep glove to use to clean wound as soiled dressing you touched is considered contaminated.

9. If the dressing is adhered to the wound surface, do not pull it away. Pour a small amount of sterile normal saline onto the dressing, wait a few minutes until the adhesion dissolves and the dressing removes easily.	9. Pulling away a dressing that is adherent to the wound surface is painful, dislodges granulation tissue, and harms healing.
10. To wash away any exudate from the wound, put on a second sterile glove, use it to lift a gauze square, dip the square into the basin of cleaning solution, and clean the wound in a circular motion from the center outward or if a linear incision, the center of the wound upward; use a second square to clean center downward.	10. Cleaning from the center of a wound outward prevents you from bringing contamination into the wound. Always use a gentle motion to avoid causing pain or disruption of new healing tissue. Using a sterile glove or capillary action will transfer microorganisms from your fingers to wound as you clean.
11. Pat wound dry with a sterile gauze square, moving from center of wound outward. Remove and discard glove.	11. Microorganisms grow best in dark, warm, moist environments. Drying limits moistness.
12. Replace dressing by applying a new sterile glove, then placing the number of gauze squares needed, and last placing the abdominal pad on top. If drains are present, place a gauze square under each drain so the rubber drain does not rest directly on the skin surface.	12. Rubber may cause excoriation if it is in contact with a skin surface for an extended time period.
13. Tape dressing securely in place. If dressing will be changed frequently, make Montgomery straps or use a gauze wrap so skin will not be irritated by frequent tape changes.	13. Irritation from tape can cause skin breaks and a second portal for infection plus increased discomfort.
14. Replace patient clothing, position comfortably, dispose of supplies used appropriately.	14. Sterile supplies that were opened but not used must be discarded because once open they are no longer sterile.
15. Evaluate effectiveness, efficiency, cost, safety, and comfort aspects of procedure. Record observations.	15. Document patient status and nursing action.
16. Plan health teaching as necessary such as a high protein diet needed to promote wound healing.	16. Health teaching is an independent nursing action always included as part of care.

MODIFICATIONS FOR CARE OF CHILD

Young schoolchildren have little concept of how long it takes healing to occur. They are often surprised that the day following surgery or injury their incision or wound is not already healed. Preschoolers are often worried that a part of their body under a dressing is missing and find it reassuring to see the body part. Knowing what something is like is better than thinking about the unknown. Therefore, do not discourage children from looking at their incision. Even if it looks raw and unhealed, it may look better than how the child envisioned it (a statement true of many adult perceptions of surgical incisions also).

Young children may need to be reminded not to touch the incision line when their dressing is removed. If the child is not toilet trained as yet and the dressing is in an area where it may become wet with urine or feces, consider covering it with a layer of plastic firmly taped in place to keep it dry. Some children have a collodion (a clear sticky substance that adheres like clear nail polish) applied to the incision in surgery. Collodion serves as the dressing and no further care is necessary.

MODIFICATIONS FOR CARE OF OLDER ADULT

The skin of the average older adult is very sensitive to adhesive tape. Use Montgomery straps or nonallergenic tape if at all possible. Healing tends to be slower in the older adult. Be extremely careful not to harm granulation tissue by removing adherent dressings.

MODIFICATIONS USING STERILE FORCEPS

To arrange supplies on a sterile field or to place dressings on a wound, instead of using sterile gloves, you can use sterile forceps. Open these from their sterile package by touching only the handle; place them on the sterile field by leaving the touched handle off the side of the field. If the soiled dressing is wet, use the forceps to lift it away to prevent touching your hand to it. However, the forceps are then contaminated and cannot be used any further to arrange or replace dressings. If the soiled dressing is dry, lift it away with your hand and discard into plastic bag. Use forceps to pick up gauze square and clean wound. Then use them no further. If soiled dressing is dry and no cleaning will be done, use forceps (still sterile) to pick up new dressing and place on wound.

If forceps are used for cleaning and can no longer be used, you can pick up a new gauze square by the edge and place it over the wound. You can do this within the principle of asepsis that the outer rim of a sterile field or compress is not sterile or that the edge touches an unsterile surface. This is not workable if the dressing is complex and needs arranging or layers need careful placement.

If an old dressing is dry and the wound will not be cleaned, you need neither a sterile glove nor sterile forceps but can lift the old dressing away with your hand and also place new dressing by its edge with your hand.

Yet another variation to accomplish wound cleaning is to moisten a sterile applicator by pouring the cleaning solution over it. See Wound Dressing Technique (box below) for a summary of conditions under the above acceptable technique.

MODIFICATIONS FOR CUTTING DRESSINGS FOR DRAINS

In order to cut a sterile dressing, you must use sterile scissors. Drop them on the sterile field and pick them up by touching only the handles. It is difficult to stabilize a sterile dressing with your bare hand, touching only the outer edge while you cut it. It is always easier to use a sterile forceps or glove to hold a compress while you cut it.

In some agencies, it is acceptable technique to wipe the blades of your bandage scissors with 70% alcohol or Betadine before using them to cut a dressing. This solution does not solve the problem of how to avoid contaminating the dressing while you secure it to cut it. As a rule, it is better to open an instrument set that supplies you not only with the scissors but with a pair of forceps as well.

Wound Dressing Technique

Condition	*Equipment Needed Beyond Dressing*
If old dressing is damp, wound will be cleaned; arrangement of new dressing is needed	3 separate sterile gloves or sterile forceps
If old dressing is dry, wound will be cleaned; arrangement of new dressing is needed	2 sterile gloves or sterile forceps
If old dressing is dry, wound will not be cleaned; arrangement of new dressing is needed	1 sterile glove or sterile forcep
If old dressing is dry, wound will be cleaned; no arrangement of new dressing is needed	1 sterile glove, sterile forcep, or sterile applicator
If old dressing is dry, wound will not be cleaned; no arrangement of dressing is needed	Dressing may be handled by edges; no sterile glove or sterile forcep necessary.

need. When changing dressings, make a habit of commenting on incisions that look clean and dry and appear to be healing well. This is important reassurance to the patient that everything is going well.

Patients need a dressing large enough to cover the entire incision and thick enough to absorb plasma oozing from the wound. Dressings larger than necessary are bulky and tend to loosen easily; dressings too small invite infection because the incision is exposed. Common sense and experience help you to select appropriate dressing size and thickness.

You also need to evaluate when a dressing is no longer necessary (wound edges are firmly approximated and no drainage is present). There is a growing trend toward leaving incisions uncovered to reduce moisture at the site; you may need to reassure a person that this is beneficial, since he expects to see a dressing in place.

Provide privacy by a drawn curtain or a closed door for dressing changes, both to provide for modesty and to avoid chilling. Use a bath blanket or a separate drape as necessary. Be certain that you have adequate light for dressing changes so that you can inspect the wound well. Assess the appearance in relation to color of any drainage present, wound edges, increased temperature at the site or not, and presence of sutures and drains (see following box, Observations to Make While Changing a Wound Dressing).

Drains. Drains are placed in an incision or in a stab wound next to an incision if the physician anticipates that there will be exudate or blood oozing from the injury site. Allowing such exudate to leave the area by means of a drain not only encourages the motion of such fluid by capillary action but also controls the drainage away from the suture line so the tissue at the suture line will heal effectively. A Penrose drain (a flat rubber type) will have a safety pin attached to prevent it from slipping back into the incision or to allow it to be located by x-ray if this should happen. Never remove this marker from a drain. If the drain is inserted deeply, a vacuum suction apparatus may be attached to the drain (Hemovac) to increase fluid removal from the site (Fig. 28-10).

Observations to Make While Changing a Wound Dressing

1. Is there any drainage? Describe the color (sanguineous, serosanguineous, serous), consistency (tacky, watery, thick), and amount (ml).
2. Is there any odor? Describe it (sweet? noxious?).
3. Are there any drains present? Document kind and placement.
4. Are the edges of the incision adherent?
5. If an unapproximated wound, is the tissue clean (no necrotic tissue, foreign material) and dry (no drainage)?
6. Is there any reddened area in the area surrounding the wound or incision? Any edema? Any ecchymotic areas?
7. Does the area surrounding the incision or wound feel warm to touch?
8. Is the person satisfied with the state of healing?

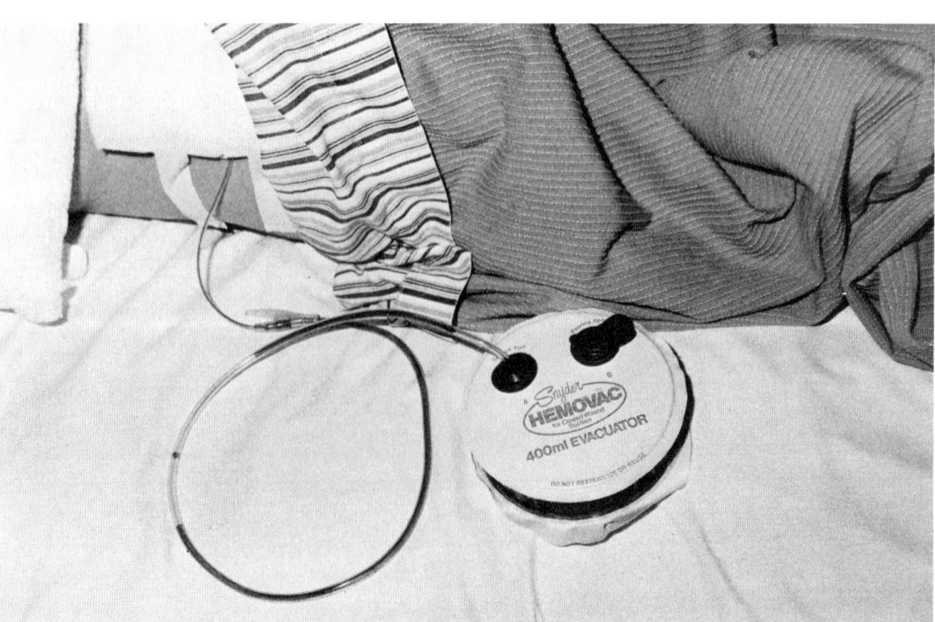

A

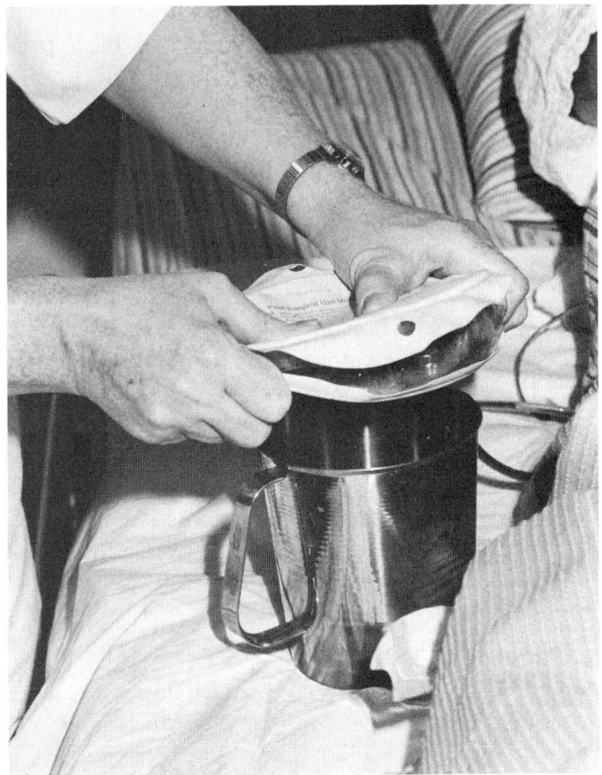

B

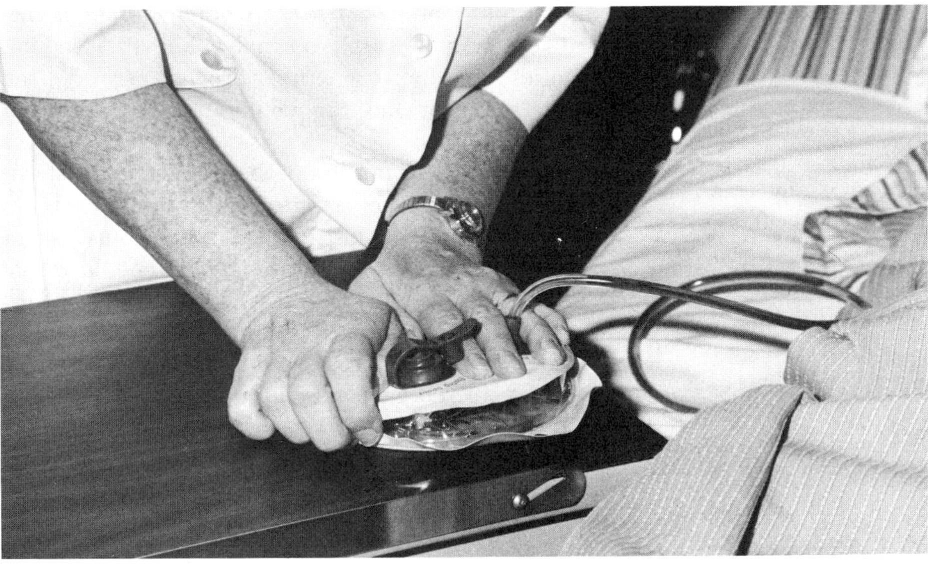

C

FIGURE 28-10. A. Drainage of a deeply inserted drain may be accomplished by use of a vacuum suction apparatus (Hemovac). B. To empty and measure the drainage (usually every 8 hours), open the drain spout on top, invert Hemovac, and squeeze firmly. C. To close, compress Hemovac against a hard surface and again obtain vacuum suction; when firmly compressed, close spout.

A drain may be shortened by a physician at a dressing change or she may leave that responsibility to you as drainage gradually decreases. If you are preparing equipment for this, provide a suture set (forceps and scissors) and a new sterile safety pin on the sterile field to be used to cut and mark a new drain. Drainage is always suspect for infection; when cleaning an incision, always clean the incision line first and then the space surrounding the drain, lifting it away from the skin to be certain that skin immediately under the drain is not becoming excoriated by constant drainage and inviting bacterial invasion.

Debridement. Debridement is cleaning a wound of foreign material or dead tissue at the wound site to discourage the growth of microorganisms. It is usually done by a physician. Cutting dead tissue is not painful but if fresh granulation tissue is touched or cut, it is very painful. If you know that debridement is to be done daily at 10 A.M., offer a prescribed analgesic 20 to 30 minutes before the procedure. Small children may have a sedative administered before debridement to ensure they do not struggle during the procedure or feel extreme pain.

Wounds that have been contaminated with grease or dirt at the time of injury or that are high risk for becoming contaminated may be ordered irrigated with an agent such as hydrogen peroxide, which accomplishes light debridement by oxidizing protein material.

Packing. If an incision becomes infected, it is opened and a packing material such as gauze may be placed in the open wound to keep it from closing readily again. Following surgery on body parts that are difficult to suture, such as the vagina, pressure packing may be placed to prevent oozing from small capillaries.

Always read surgical notes and admission wound assessments to see if packing was placed or not. It should be noted on the front of a patient's chart or some other predictable and easily visible place if packing is in place. Pressure packing is generally left in place for 2 or 3 days and then removed because thereafter it can become a reservoir of infection. If packing is in place, be certain you do not dislodge it inadvertently when changing dressings. Sometimes packing is removed and replaced at each dressing change. When this is done, make a note of it each time. If self-dissolvable packing is used, no removal is necessary. In this case, it should be noted in a prominent place on the patient's chart.

DRESSING MATERIALS

Dressing materials differ according to the type and size of the wound, body location, whether exudate is present or not, and preference of physician, nurse, and patient. Next to the wound is generally placed layers of soft, absorbent squares of gauze (called 4×4s). Such squares are small enough to tuck under drains to prevent the rubber or plastic from resting directly on the skin and causing irritation. They can be cut easily with a v notch with sterile scissors to better fit around drains or catheters present. Sterile obstetrical sanitary pads are also good for absorbing excess drainage.

If the dressing is large, an abdominal pad is used to cover and contain the smaller squares.

Telfa is a special type of gauze that has a shiny, nonadherent coating on one surface. The shiny surface is placed next to the wound. Telfa does not stick to the wound and does not harm granulation tissue when removed. It helps to keep the incision dry, since exudate seeps through the shiny surface and remains held away from the incision.

Vaseline gauze is gauze impregnated with petroleum jelly. It is used to keep a dressing from adhering to the wound and destroying sensitive new tissue.

CLEANSING AGENTS

If a wound is dry, cleaning it with each dressing change is not necessary. If exudate is present, it is generally cleaned away with each dressing change to reduce the warm, moist fluid that can serve as a reservoir for infection. Agency policy helps to decide the cleaning agent to be used; specific cleaning agents may be ordered by the physician for individual situations. Betadine (an antiseptic), normal saline (0.9 sodium chloride) or half-strength hydrogen peroxide (an oxidizing agent) are frequently used solutions for cleaning.

Cleaning agents may be applied to wounds by sterile cotton balls, gauzc squares, or cotton-tipped applicators or may be flushed against the wound by the use of a sterile syringe. If sutures are present, do not use cotton balls; they tear against the rough edge of the sutures and leave wisps of cotton in the wound. Always clean from the center of a wound outward to avoid carrying microorganisms into the wound.

SECURING A DRESSING

Dressings are secured in place by strips of adhesive tape or nonallergenic tape (also called eye tape or paper tape), which is removed and changed each time the dressing is changed, or by binders or bandages that can be removed easily without the irritation of tape.

Adhesive tape holds firmly and strong enough not only to secure the dressing well but also to pull skin toward the wound and thus reduce tension on the incision edges. It is also strong enough to pull across so firmly that this added compression helps to minimize bleeding. The disadvantage of adhesive tape is that it adheres to skin so firmly that it pulls hair and is painful to remove. Pulling the tape in the same direction the hair grows may cause less pain. Tape often leaves a cover of sticky adhesive behind that needs to be washed away; use a commercial adhesive tape remover or acetone. Some people are allergic to adhesive tape and develop tender, irritated skin areas wherever it touches them.

Nonallergenic tape can be placed on the skin on both sides of a dressing to serve as a base for adhesive tape; adhesive tape is used to secure the dressing and then taped to the nonallergenic tape rather than to the skin. This technique is particularly helpful for securing pressure dressings to the face. Tincture of benzoin, which toughens skin, may be applied under adhesive tape to protect skin integrity if frequent dressing changes are anticipated.

Another technique for securing a dressing is to wrap soft gauze or Kerlex around the body part. This avoids tape allergies.

Montgomery Straps. Montgomery straps may be used to decrease the irritation to skin from tape. Montgomery straps are supplied commercially or can be made by folding wide adhesive tape strips lengthwise so the sticky sides touch. A slit is cut near the end of the strips and two strips are taped in place on opposite sides of the dressing. Ties of gauze or cotton umbilical tape are then threaded through the slits and tied as a shoelace over the dressing. (Rubber bands and safety pins also work.) Montgomery straps do not need to be replaced, although the gauze tie might; thus, for the length of the time the dressing will be in place, no adhesive tape removal is necessary (Fig. 28-11).

Butterflies. A butterfly refers to a small strip of adhesive tape or Band-Aid secured tightly on both sides of an incision (Fig. 28-12) in order to pull the edges of the

FIGURE 28-11. Montgomery straps rather than adhesive tape are used to secure a dressing that needs frequent changing.

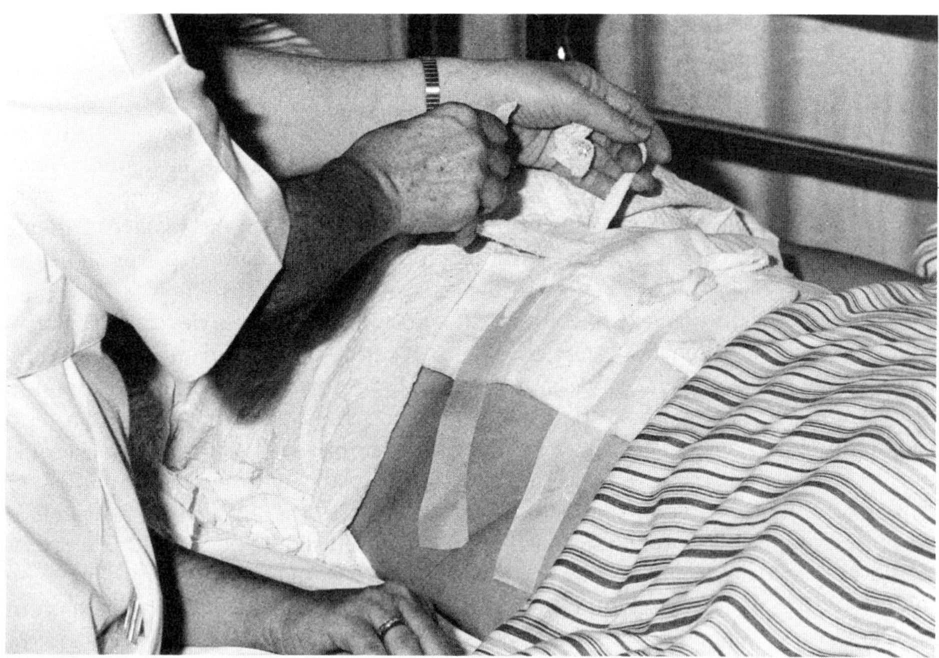

FIGURE 28-12. A butterfly refers to one or more small strips of adhesive tape or a Band-Aid that is secured tightly to both sides of an incision to encourage healing by preventing strain on the incision line.

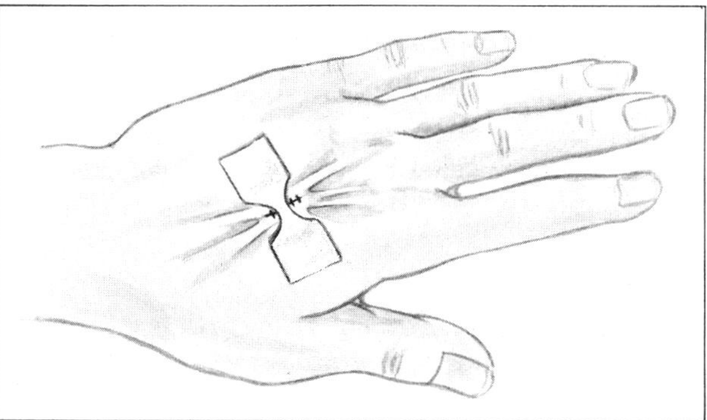

incision close together and encourage proximity and healing. Mothers often use butterflies on small cuts on children, hoping to avoid the necessity of sutures.

Deciding what material to use to secure a dressing is a nursing judgment except in rare circumstances. Always consider a method that will secure firmly but will cause the least skin irritation and discomfort to the patient.

Binders. In order to reduce strain at a suture line, a binder or strip of cloth to wrap around the body area may be ordered. These fasten with safety pins or velcro or are made of many tails that fold over and over (a scultetus bandage). Use of a binder has the temporary advantage of relieving pressure on a suture line; if used for a long period of time, a binder diminishes muscle tone.

Sutures. Sutures are made from a variety of materials—silk, cotton, nylon, catgut, synthetic gut, or metal—and placed in a variety of patterns. Sutures placed internally are made of material that absorbs after 14 or 20 days and do not need to be removed. Skin sutures are generally not absorbable and need to be removed in about 7 days. *Interrupted* sutures are stitches placed with each one completely separate from the one beside it. These may be single threads or *mattress* sutures, in which a double thread runs under the skin for increased strength. *Continuous* sutures are stitches made from one continuous thread; each suture is joined to the next. These may be simple continuous sutures or *blanket* sutures, in which a running stitch is visible. An advantage of interrupted sutures is that if strain to the suture line should cause one suture to break, the incision line will remain intact because the broken one is not joined to any other.

Metal sutures (staples) are a form of interrupted suture. They are easily placed with a staple gun, are interrupted, and are easily removable with a staple remover. People used to thinking of thread sutures after surgery may need some reassurance. Metal sutures are used predominantly with wounds that have increased tension, such as abdominal surgery incisions. They tend to leave less scar than thread sutures.

Sutures are removed 7 to 10 days after surgery—usually by a physician because this is the time the final healing of the wound area is evaluated, although removal is becoming a nursing responsibility. Sterile technique is always used. The suture line is cleaned with an antiseptic before the removal of sutures to reduce the surface bacterial count. Although a thread suture is cut by the knot, a small portion is pulled under the skin with removal; the cleaner this segment is, the less chance there is of contaminating the wound. An advantage of metal sutures is that no portion of the sutures is pulled under the surface on removal. Cleaning the suture line also softens dried secretions present and prevents pain from the tugging action of the suture against the dried material. The technique for assisting with suture removal is shown in Procedure 28-7.

If interrupted sutures are in place, every other one may be cut and removed on one day; if the incision remains intact and is obviously healing well, the remaining sutures are removed the following day. Interrupted sutures are lifted upward by a sterile forceps at the knot and cut with scissors next to the skin on the opposite side. The suture is then pulled by the forceps so that as little as possible of the suture that was above the surface is pulled underneath the skin (Fig. 28-13). Patients may need forewarning that as a suture pulls free, they may feel a faint stinging sensation due to adherent dried secretions under the surface. Patients have sutures removed close to discharge from a health care agency; thus, even though there may be some pain involved in the process, most people view it as a positive step to wellness. If sutures are placed on an ambulatory basis, people need to return to have the sutures out in about 7 days. Sutures must be removed, since after a time the body begins to react to suture material as it does to any foreign body—with an inflammatory or infection response. In a health care agency, the fact that sutures have been placed should be marked in a prominent, consistent place in the nursing care plan or on the front of the patient's chart so their presence is not forgotten on discharge.

After suture removal, a dry sterile dressing is generally placed over the incision. The patient is instructed to leave this in place for about 24 hours and then no

PROCEDURE 28-7
Assisting with Suture Removal

Purpose: To assist a health care provider in removing sutures from a healed incision by supplying sterile supplies. To offer information and psychosocial support to the patient.

Plan	*Principle*
1. Wash your hands, identify patient, explain procedure.	1. Prevent spread of microorganisms, ensure patient safety and well being.
2. Assess patient status. Analyze appropriateness of procedure. Plan modifications of care.	2. A nurse always serves as a patient's advocate and second line of defense against infection.

3. Implement procedure by assembling equipment: sterile suture set, gloves for person performing procedures plus cleansing agent and supplies for dressing change; plastic bag for disposal of soiled dressing.

3. Following suture removal only a small dressing is necessary (often only a single- or double-gauze square); no dressing may be necessary.

4. Provide patient privacy by a drawn curtain or a closed door. Provide a flat dry clean area to open suture set and glove pack.

4. Privacy is a highly valued right of most people; a closed space also limits the spread of airborne microorganisms. Prepare your sterile field waist high or above.

5. Position patient comfortably, remove clothing to reveal incision site; use a drape as appropriate for modesty.

5. People as a rule are nervous about having sutures removed. Position comfortably to reduce muscle strain.

6. Untie tapes or remove adhesive tape *toward* incision; remove top dressing. If dressing is adherent, pour a small amount of antiseptic or normal saline solution onto adherent fibers and wait for fibers to dissolve and dressing to lift easily.

6. Pulling tape toward the incision prevents unnecessary tension on new healing tissue. Lifting away an adherent dressing causes pain and may interfere with new healing tissue.

7. Add a sterile gauze square to field next to suture set. Person removing sutures will pick it up with sterile glove and hold it over disposal bag or wastebasket for you to pour antiseptic over gauze.

7. If the person prefers not to use gloves, she can pick up gauze by forceps from suture set.

8. Following cleaning of the wound, the person removing sutures will use forceps and scissors to do this. Offer fair warning that pulling sutures causes a faint stinging.

8. In some instances, every other suture is removed one day; the remaining sutures the next. Sutures are always cut close to skin surface and pulled so that as little of suture as possible passes under skin surface.

9. Following suture removal, the incision line is covered by a dry sterile gauze square or no dressing. Evaluate effectiveness, efficiency, cost, comfort, and safety aspects of procedure and status of wound at close of procedure. Record observations of wound and suture removal.

9. Documentation of patient status and nursing action.

10. Plan health teaching such as teaching that following suture removal healed tissue is as strong as original tissue so person does not need to favor suture line beyond sensible precautions.

10. Health teaching is an independent nursing action always included as a point of care.

11. Return supplies used to proper site for disposal or resterilization. Leave patient comfortable.

11. Nondisposable instruments should be washed under cold water and returned to be resterilized; disposable instruments should be discarded outside patient room.

MODIFICATIONS FOR CARE OF CHILD

Adults as a rule do not mind suture removal because although it is not entirely a painfree process, they see it as proof they are almost well again and accept it readily. Children are unable to appreciate the meaning of suture removal and need a great deal of support, especially if there are a large number of sutures to be removed. Do not make a habit of bribing children to cooperate with procedures. If you offer a bribe once, you have to offer it again for a second procedure and soon you have no bribe big enough to gain cooperation. Give generous verbal praise for cooperation, a substance you never run out of. With a painful procedure, any action short of hysterical screaming for a young child is cooperation.

MODIFICATIONS FOR CARE OF OLDER ADULT

As a rule, the skin of the older adult does not heal so quickly as that of the younger person. Sutures are more apt to be removed in stages with the older adult to ensure healing has taken place before the final sutures are removed.

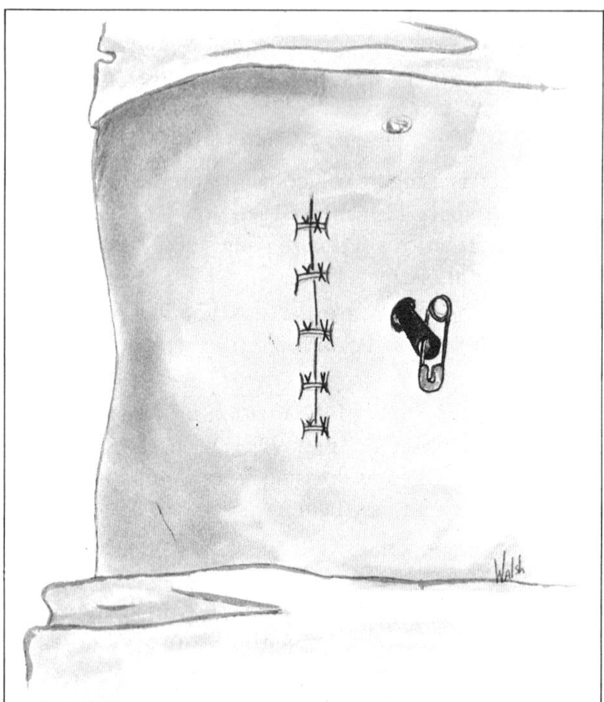

FIGURE 28-13. Interrupted sutures are lifted upward by a sterile forcep at the knot and cut with scissors next to the skin on the opposite side in order to pull the minimum of suture material underneath the skin surface.

further dressing will be needed. He is generally instructed to take showers rather than baths for 2 or 3 more days or until the pinpoints where the sutures were removed have completely healed. If drainage or erythema occurs any time after suture removal, the patient should contact his physician. Such drainage suggests poor healing or possible infection.

Retention sutures are large sutures that are used to anchor and to pull toward the incision line underlying fat and muscle in order to reduce strain at the incision line. Abdominal incisions on obese individuals may have retention sutures or wire covered with short pieces of rubber tubing to keep the suture material from cutting into the skin from the pressure exerted on them. Retention sutures may be left in place longer than the skin sutures; they should be noted separately on the nursing care plan.

AT HOME CARE

Many people are discharged from a health care agency before wound healing is complete and need to change wound dressings at home. Be certain that the person understands the importance of changing a dressing in order to reduce moisture at the site, the technique to use, supplies needed, and where supplies can be obtained.

Irrigations

If a wound is developing symptoms of infection, it may be ordered irrigated with a solution such as hydrogen peroxide, normal saline, or Betadine.

Irrigating solutions should be slightly warm so as not to chill the patient. Warm a solution by setting the bottle of solution in a basin of warm water for 10 to 15 minutes before use. Check the solution temperature by pouring a few drops on the inside of your wrist. Use only sterile solutions and strict sterile techniques for wound irrigations; you do not want to introduce a secondary infection to an already infected area. Technique for a wound irrigation is described in Procedure 28-8.

ASSISTING WITH STERILE PROCEDURES

In some cases you will not be performing a sterile procedure yourself but assisting a physician or nurse clinician with one. As an assistant, you may be asked to set up the sterile field and to add solutions or additional sterile supplies to the field.

You can add new supplies to a sterile field at any time by dropping them from their sterile wrapper. Alternatively, once the person you are assisting has her sterile gloves on, you can open the outside wrapper and let her take the supply directly from the wrapper. When hand-

PROCEDURE 28-8
Irrigation of a Wound

Purpose: To cleanse a wound; to promote healing by providing a warm and clean environment; to apply an antiseptic or debriding agent to a wound.

Plan	*Principle*
1. Wash your hands; identify patient; explain procedure to patient.	1. Prevent spread of microorganisms; promote patient safety and well-being.
2. Assess patient condition, analyze appropriateness of procedure. Plan modifications of care.	2. Wounds that are irrigated are those infected or with a high possibility of becoming infected. There may be painful edema surrounding the wound. Assess whether you should offer an analgesic for pain relief before procedure.

3. Implement care by assembling a sterile field with a sterile bulb syringe or large regular syringe, sterile gauze squares, basin, supplies for dressing change, unsterile basin, plastic bag for disposal of soiled dressing, a waterproof pad for bed, bottle of sterile irrigating solution (about 250 ml), and 2 pairs of sterile gloves.

3. Always use irrigating solutions at a temperature pleasantly warm to your wrist. Warm solution by placing bottle in a basin of warm water 10—15 min before procedure. *Check temperature by pouring a small amount over wrist* to ensure that you will neither chill nor burn patient.

4. Provide patient privacy by a drawn curtain or closed door. Position patient comfortably; place waterproof pad next to patient to protect bed.

4. Privacy is a highly regarded value of most people; providing privacy also halts the flow of airborne bacteria.

5. Establish a sterile field on a flat clean dry surface (overbed table or stand). Add gauze squares, fill basin with irrigating solution.

5. Be certain to place basin close to edge of field so solution will not splash onto field.

6. Remove soiled dressing. If drainage is present, you may want to put on a sterile glove both to protect your hand and to prevent organisms being spread to dressing. Discard dressing and glove into disposal bag. Do not reuse this glove once it has touched soiled dressing.

6. An infected wound requiring irrigation to help healing often has purulent, very contaminated exudate.

7. Place unsterile basin on bed next to patient to collect irrigating solution. Put on sterile gloves. Pull up irrigating solution in syringe and irrigate wound with gentle pressure. Allow solution to flow across wound and collect in basin. Stabilize basin with left hand.

7. Use a gentle but thorough technique to wash but not harm newly healing tissue. Your hand stabilizing the basin is easily contaminated since it is easy to touch the patient's skin. Do not return this hand to the sterile field.

8. Pat the area dry with sterile gauze squares from center of wound to periphery. Discard gauze into paper bag.

8. Patting is more gentle than rubbing. Always touch a wound from the center to periphery to prevent bringing microorganisms into wound.

9. Apply new sterile dressing, being certain to add gauze under any drains present to protect skin beneath from contact with rubber. Apply Montgomery straps since dressing will be changed frequently for irrigations and skin must be protected.

9. Dressing is secured in a manner which allows easy removal at the time of next wound irrigation.

10. Evaluate patient status, effectiveness, efficiency, cost, safety, comfort, and asepsis of procedure; record observations of wound and irrigation. Dispose of equipment or return for resterilization appropriately.

10. Documentation of patient status and nursing action.

11. Plan health teaching necessary such as need for adequate nutrition and rest to ensure wound healing.

11. Health teaching is an independent nursing action always included as part of nursing care.

MODIFICATIONS FOR CHILD CARE

Children are often unable to lie still for the length of time it takes to irrigate a wound. You may need an assistant to restrain or distract the child during the procedure. It is helpful to save an activity a child likes (listening to a favorite sing-along record or being read a favorite story) to be done only during such a procedure. Other children would prefer the time not to be used this way; once the activity that must be done is accomplished, you can interact free of the distraction of the procedure with them.

MODIFICATIONS FOR OLDER ADULTS

Many older adults have decreased sensation for hot or cold. Be extremely careful of the temperature of solutions used with these persons so you do not burn or chill them.

ing supplies this way, peel the wrapper well back so the person does not contaminate her gloves by touching the unsterile outside wrapper.

If you will be adding solutions or medicine to another person's sterile set-up, be aware that legally you are as responsible for the right solution or medicine as the person who accepts the addition. For example, if the person needs some Xylocaine (Novocain) or other medicine contained in a vial, drop a sterile needle and syringe on the sterile field for her to assemble with her sterile gloves. Read the label of the vial you choose three times, and clean the top of the rubber stopper with 70% alcohol. *Show the label to the person who will use the medicine so she has certain knowledge of the type and strength you are offering her.* Hold the vial so that she can puncture the rubber stopper with the needle tip; tap the vial down onto the needle; tip the vial so the syringe can be filled; lift the vial free of the needle when the desired amount of solution has been obtained (Fig. 28-14).

As an assistant, you are often in a better position to notice when a sterile field has been contaminated than the person performing the procedure. Voice these observations and offer replacement sterile supplies. Do not be defensive if an assistant points out a break in technique on your part. Sterility is a concept. Only when absolute sterility is accepted as the standard can the chain of infection be broken.

NOSOCOMIAL INFECTIONS

A *nosocomial* infection is a hospital-acquired infection (*nosocomium* is Latin for "place of care"). Criteria for a nosocomial infection differ, but basically it is an infection that developed after the person was in the agency. It could be an infection of any body system, but the respiratory, urinary, and gastrointestinal systems and skin and subcutaneous tissue are the most frequent sites (Fig. 28-15).

A number of patients are high risk for acquiring nosocomial infections. High-risk criteria are listed in the box on page 646, along with common measures to reduce the possibility of infection in such patients. The development of a nosocomial infection suggests that the person's caregivers did not maintain medical and surgical asepsis as carefully as they might.

A major cause of nosocomial infection is insufficient hand washing. *Transient flora* are bacteria that are recently acquired on hands and can be easily washed away. Even poor hand washing probably removes transient bacteria. *Resident flora* are bacteria found in folds of skin that are difficult to remove since they adhere closely to the skin. Transient flora may become resident flora if they are not washed away. Health care agencies develop resident flora that are resistant to antibiotics and, therefore, result in difficult-to-treat infections. Preventing transmission of these flora to patients is the only safeguard that infection will not occur.

FIGURE 28-14. Adding medicine from a vial to another person's sterile set-up. After cleaning the vial with alcohol, hold it so that the rubber stopper can be punctured with the needle tip; tip the vial in order to fill the syringe; lift it off again free of the needle when the desired amount has been obtained.

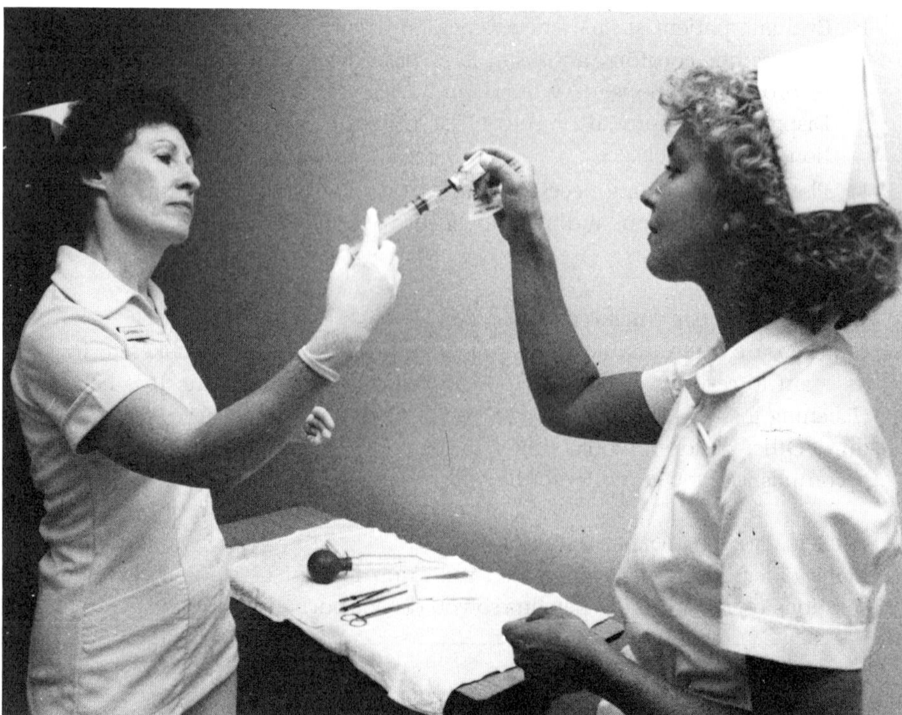

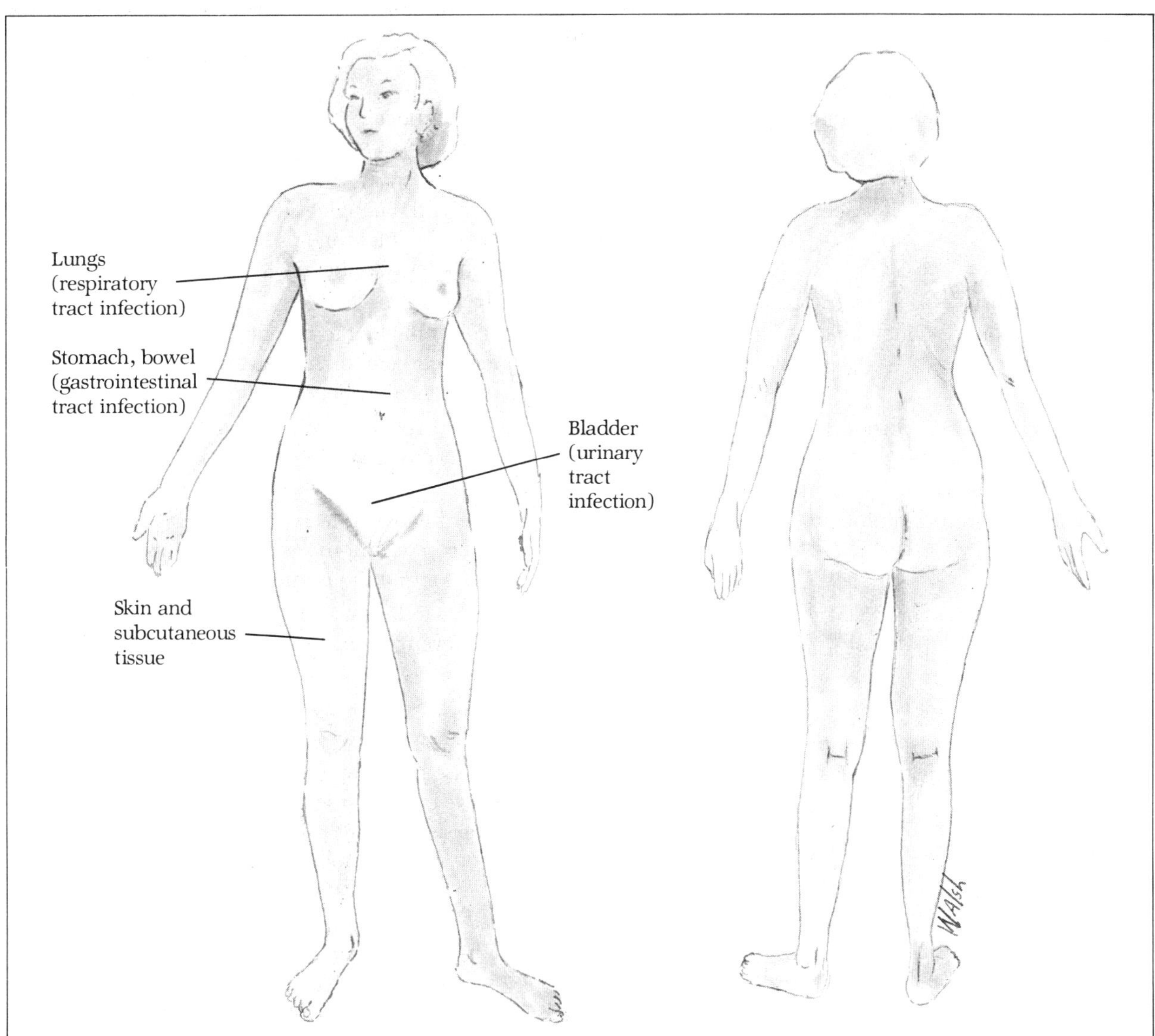

FIGURE 28-15. Most common body sites for nosocomial infections.

INFECTION CONTROL COMMITTEES

Simmelweiss, a physician in Vienna, was the first to document how careful hand washing between patients actually prevented the spread of infection from patient to patient or physician to patient. Florence Nightingale helped to design isolation procedures after concluding that a "hospital should at least do the sick no harm." Today, nurses are a patient's best protector against acquiring a secondary infection while he is hospitalized for a primary illness by the use of conscientous technique.

Every hospital, in order to be accredited by the Joint Commission on Accreditation of Hospitals, must maintain an infection control committee charged with the responsibility of detecting, controlling, and preventing infections within the hospital. An infection control nurse serves an important place on this committee. She is instrumental in seeing that the hospital has active programs to control sources of contamination through effective isolation and sterilization techniques, that transmission of contamination is limited through hand-washing and aseptic techniques, that patients with special susceptibility are adequately protected through reverse isolation or anticipatory administration of antibiotics (prophylaxis), and that everyone is educated to be aware of the danger of nosocomial infections. An infection in a postsurgical patient will extend his hospital stay by about 10 days and increase the cost of his hospitalization accordingly.

UTILIZING NURSING PROCESS

Determining when medical or surgical aseptic measures are necessary is often a nursing decision. In order to make these determinations, rely on nursing process.

ASSESSMENT

Assess every patient seen in ambulatory care or admitted to a health care facility for the possibility that he has a process that could be infectious and therefore com-

People High Risk for Nosocomial Infections and Common Measures to Reduce Risk

Patient at Risk	*Measures to Reduce Risk*
Patient with nutritional deficit	Attempt to make mealtime an attractive and stimulating time of day. Be conscientious with fluid, electrolyte, and vitamin replacement.
Patient with in-dwelling vascular lines	Use careful technique with changing intravenous solutions and tubing; avoid trauma to site; rotate sites with the exception of central insertion lines about every 3 days to avoid phlebitis and infection.
Patient with in-dwelling bladder catheter	Avoid reflux from collecting bag to bladder; maintain good fluid intake; remove catheter as soon as medically advisable; use conscientious perineal hygiene.
Patient who is immunosuppressed	Protect patient from microorganisms by reverse isolation; thoughtful room placement; conscientious hand-washing technique.
Patient on multiple antibiotic therapy	Use conscientious hand-washing technique. Danger of fungal infection growth; keep warm, moist areas that could be reservoirs for fungal growth to a minimum.
Patient hospitalized over 3 weeks	Do not allow technique to lapse no matter how many times it is accomplished; prevent secondary complications to allow for early discharge.
Patient with extremes of age	Both newborns and older adults are more prone to infection than the middle age groups. Observe special precautions.
Patient with underlying disease	A person who must use his body resources to fight a severe illness may not have enough reserves left to combat infection. Use conscientious technique to prevent a secondary infection from compounding a primary illness.

municable, causing increased risk of illness in health care providers and other patients. Clues that special precautions need to be considered are shown in the box, Assessments to Detect Signs and Symptoms of Communicable Disease (p. 647).

Assess every patient as well as to whether he needs extra precautions to protect him against infection. Base this on age, general health, current drug therapy, denuded or broken skin, and the level of immunization present. Remember that immigrants to the United States may never have had a basic immunization series or may be severely underimmunized.

ANALYSIS

In many instances the nurse is the first person to be aware of symptoms of infection or a history of recent exposure to disease. Therefore, making a decision that precautions are necessary becomes an independent nursing judgment. As an example, you change a dressing and discover a purulent thick exudate. You decide this probably represents infection and institute enteric wound precautions to save exposure of personnel and patients to the microorganisms before a physician can visit the patient and order such precautions. You take a wound culture so the microorganisms can be identified. This is an independent nursing judgment based on knowledge of microbiology and the transmission pattern of disease.

PLANNING

Once the need for isolation is decided, be certain that hospital personnel are adequately oriented so that everyone abides by the regulations. This includes not only the nursing staff but other health care personnel such as laboratory technicians and dieticians, many of whom do not appreciate the danger of microorganisms and their role in transmission. Be certain isolation rooms are well labeled and that adequate supplies are readily available for the full 24 hours.

Plan with the patient some ways of passing his time so that he is not bored in isolation. Plan your day with adequate time to spend in isolation rooms, so that a person in isolation is not lonely.

IMPLEMENTATION

Never grow careless about good hand-washing technique. Be certain that your surgical aseptic technique is always strict and conscientious because this is how

Assessments to Detect Signs and Symptoms of Communicable Disease

Assessment	*Possible Importance*
Any body discharge	Many infections reveal themselves by vaginal, respiratory, or wound drainage.
Vomiting and diarrhea	Gastrointestinal illness is often revealed in these ways.
High fever (over 101°F; 38.4°C)	Elevated body temperature is seen in almost all infections.
History of recent exposure to communicable disease	A person may be in the prodromal stage of illness and not yet have signs and symptoms but be infectious.
Elevated leukocyte count (over 10,000/mm)	An elevated white blood count is a body response to bacterial infections.
A systemic skin rash is present	Many childhood communicable diseases have skin rashes (exanthems).
A laboratory report confirms an organism is present	A nurse is often the first member of a health care team to see such reports.

good habits are built. Always put on gloves as if they were sterile; then, when they are sterile, you have no doubt of good technique.

Set up a sterile field to hold adequate supplies. Avoiding this may save a minute but will invariably result in some sterile object brushing against an unsterile one. Always include health teaching about the importance of not coughing over open wounds and handling dressings correctly for patients who will be changing a dressing at home. Nursing research can help you make sound judgments about use of aseptic technique. Quick Reference Stop 28-6 presents some interesting findings.

EVALUATION

Whether personnel on a hospital unit are using good medical and surgical aseptic technique or not is usually revealed quickly by the spread of infections from patient to patient or by a high incidence of infection in patients. This is costly evaluation from the standpoint of any patients or personnel who become infected. Review aseptic techniques periodically with nursing staff so everyone has a good understanding of what is meant by these terms and what is good technique. Practice changing a dressing until your sterile technique is accurate and efficient.

NURSING CARE PLAN

Bob Green is a 16-year-old who is admitted to the hospital with a diagnosis of diabetes mellitus. In addition to this, your assessment reveals that he has an infection of a linear laceration on his right arm and he is allergic to adhesive tape. The following section of his nursing care plan describes his anticipated nursing care related to the arm infection.

NURSING DIAGNOSIS

Inflamed laceration with purulent exudate right forearm related to cat scratch 1 week ago.

Locus of Decision-Making: Shared patient and nurse.

Goal: Signs and symptoms of infection will decrease in intensity by 3 days.

Criteria: Area of erythema, amount of exudate, and pain will be decreased. Oral temperature will be normal (98.6°F; 37.0°C).

NURSING ORDERS

1. Warm sterile normal saline irrigation to right forearm 3 times day (TID) per M.D. order to aid debridement.
2. Wound and skin isolation precautions in effect.
3. Keep forearm elevated on two pillows to increase venous return and reduce edema at site.
4. Administer analgesic (Tylenol 10 gr every 4 hr) as necessary per M.D. order to reduce pain and encourage movement in extremity.
5. Administer ampicillin 250 mg every 6 hr per M.D. order. Patient asking for liquid form because capsules are difficult to swallow; pharmacy to substitute new form if practical.
6. Cover right forearm with dry sterile dressing (2 4-x-4s, Kerlex gauze) between irrigations. Use no adhesive tape to decrease skin irritation.

The following is a problem-oriented nursing note describing a morning's nursing care in relation to Bob Green's infection and how the nursing care plan would be modified to be kept current.

Subjective Assessment: States pain is decreasing in amount; hurts only when he makes a fist or leaves arm in a dependent position for over a few minutes. Refused to take 10 A.M. liquid ampicillin because of aftertaste until parent interceded. States even though capsules were hard to swallow they were better than liquid. States he is annoyed with isolation precautions and wants them ignored.

Objective Assessment: 6-cm linear laceration on right forearm still present; area erythematous and warm to touch 2 cm on all sides. Slight amount of thick yellow purulent drainage on dressing; no apparent odor. Wound soaked 20 min with sterile normal saline compresses. Dry sterile dressing replaced, secured with gauze. Oral temperature 101.6°F.

PLAN

Urge to keep arm elevated to decrease pain and edema. Ask pharmacy to change dosage form of antibiotic back to original capsules. Allow optimal opportunities for decision-

☐ **QUICK REFERENCE STOP 28-6: RESEARCH**

The concept and practice of asepsis carries over into every aspect of nursing care. Wound care and the prevention of infection are only two aspects of nursing care within this all-encompassing topic.

Hand Washing.
Handwashing has been applauded as one of the best means known to prevent the spread of infection. An institutional study conducted by Larson (1982) was undertaken to assess the presence of bacteria on hands of hospital staff members. The hand flora of 21 percent of 103 hospital staff members revealed one or more species of bacteria. "Personnel washing hands fewer than eight times per day were found to persistently carry the same species far more frequently than did those who washed their hands more often" (p. 27). It was also found that 21 percent of 541 nosocomial infections reported over a seven-month period could be traced to and were probably caused by organisms from the hands of hospital personnel. Increased hand washing was found to reduce the number of pathogens on hands.

Hydrogen Peroxide in Wound Care.
According to Bassam and Dudai (1982), irrigation of deep, semiclosed wounds with peroxide could be dangerous. This case study of a 54-year-old man whose wound was irrigated with peroxide provides significant data for nurses to consider. In this man, oxygen emboli, resulting from irrigation of a partially closed wound with 3% hydrogen peroxide, entered the systemic circulation and resulted in temporary shock and coma.

Estimation of Blood Loss.
Nurses are frequently required to assess the amount of blood loss on an item from a patient. Commonly, nurses use adjectives such as *heavy*, *moderate*, and *slight* to estimate blood loss. What do these words mean among different nurses? Do they accurately reflect the amount of bleeding a patient is having? Clough et al. (1981) demonstrated that a majority of nurses had difficulty estimating actual cc's of blood lost and that considerable discrepancy existed among nurses in how they categorized the amount of blood lost by a patient and noted on Chux, peripads, 4-×-4s, and lap pads. This study seems to indicate a need for further nurse education in this area.

SUGGESTED READINGS

Bassam, M., Dudai, M., and Shalev, O. Near-fatal systemic oxygen embolism due to wound irrigation with hydrogen peroxide. *Postgrad. Med. J.* 58(681):448, 1982. As reported in Hydrogen peroxide disaster, *Nurses Drug Alert* 6(12):89, 1982.

Clough, D. H., and Higgins, P. G. Discrepancies in estimating blood loss. *Am. J. Nurs.* 81(2):331, 1981.

Larson, E. L. Persistent carriage of gram-negative bacteria on hands. *Nurs. Res.* 31(2):121, 1982. As cited in C. Isler (Ed.). Nursing press in review. One more reason to wash your hands. *RN* 45(9):27, 1980.

making where he can have choices (perhaps diet selection) so he can better accept areas where in the interest of healing and staff protection he does not have much choice—he must take the antibiotic in one of the two forms; isolation must be maintained. Continue wound care as above. Continue skin and wound precautions.

SUGGESTED READINGS

American Hospital Association. *Infection Control in the Hospital* (4th ed.). Chicago: American Hospital Association, 1979.

Aspinall, M. J. Scoring against nosocomial infections. *Am. J. Nurs.* 78:1704, 1978.

Brubacher, L. L. To heal a draining wound. *RN* 45:30, 1982.

Charnock, A. Research project: One nurse's attack on microorganisms. *Nurs. Mirror* 154(20):41, 1982.

Committee on Infectious Diseases. *Report of the Committee on Infectious Diseases (Redbook).* Evanston, Ill.: American Academy of Pediatrics, 1982.

Creighton, H. Liability for infection control. *Nurs. Manage.* 13(11):42, 1982.

Crow, S. Nurses' compliance with aseptic technique. *A.O.R.N. J.* 37(6):1066, 1983.

Fisher, P. C. Twelve (at least) incredibly simple tips on how you can control infection. *RN* 41:57, 1978.

Freeman, P., et al. How to get the most out of op-site—and avoid the not so sticky problem. *RN* 45:36, 1982.

Gray, M. J., et al. Infection prevention and control in TPN. *Hosp. Top.* 61(1):32, 1983.

Hagan, B. Infection: A convenient myth? *Nurs. Manage.* 13(1):26, 1982.

Hargiss, C. D., et al. Infection control: Putting principles into practice. *Am. J. Nurs.* 81:2165, 1981.

Infection control in nursing care: Legalities. *Regan Rep. Nurs. Law* 22(9):1, 1982.

James, S. M., et al. Breaking the chain of infection. *Nurs. Manage.* 12:29, 1981.

Jenner, E. Infection control nursing: Of microbes and men. *Nurs. Mirror* 154(20):56, 1982.

Jones, C. C., et al. Care of ICP monitoring devices: A nursing responsibility. *J. Neurosurg. Nurs.* 14(5):255, 1982.

Kirkis, E. J. Disposal techniques to confine contamination. *RN* 45(7):87, 1982.

Kirkis, E. J. Tips and tactics to hold microbes at bay for your patient's sake . . . and your own. *RN* 44:139, 1981.

Meshelany, C. M. Post-op wound dressings. *RN* 42:23, 1979.

Nadolny, M. D. Infection control in hospitals. What does the infection do? *Am. J. Nurs.* 80(3):430, 1980.

Nichols, R. L. Techniques known to prevent post-operative wound infection. *Infection Control* 3:34, 1982.

Palakonetz, I. Nosocomial infection: The hidden cost of health care. *Hospitals* 32:101, 1978.

Shamian, J., et al. Infection prevention—A long-term investment. *Dimens. Health Serv.* 59(12):14, 1982.

Taylor, L. An evaluation of handwashing techniques. *Nurs. Times* 74:54, 1978.

Weymont, G. Infection control in the community. *Nurs. Times* 78(7)Suppl:7, 1982.

QUESTIONS FOR REVIEW

1. Mr. Bennett is a patient admitted to a hospital for a respiratory infection. In order to assess his problems accurately, you need to know that in the development of an infection the time interval between the invasion of the organism and the beginning of disease symptoms is which period?
   a. Secondary invasion.
   b. Prodromal.
   c. Incubation.
   d. Pathogenic.

2. Aseptic technique is one you use frequently. *Asepsis* is defined as a state of being:
   a. Free of all microorganisms.
   b. Free of all microorganisms except spores.
   c. Sterility.
   d. Freedom of pathogenic microorganisms.

3. Which of the following represents good hand-washing technique?
   a. Use cool water to avoid chapping your hands.
   b. Use a detergent to wash with.
   c. Turn off the faucet using a paper towel.
   d. Wash and rinse hands three times for thoroughness.

4. Which of the following represents the best respiratory isolation technique?
   a. Wear a gown and gloves to enter the room.
   b. Place the patient in a semiprivate room.
   c. Dry dust all room surfaces daily.
   d. Provide a table for supplies outside the room door.

5. You plan to set up a sterile field. Which of the following represents the best technique?
   a. Place all supplies as close to the edge as possible.
   b. Do not turn your back to the field.
   c. Set up the field below waist level.
   d. Add only clean supplies.

6. To pour a sterile solution into a container on a sterile field, which of the following represents the best technique?
   a. Pour from a height of 18 inches.
   b. Touch the sterile container to the rim of the basin.
   c. Lift the basin off the field with your hand while you pour.
   d. Pour from a height of 6 to 8 inches.

7. To open a sterile package, your best technique would be to first open:
   a. The flap nearest you.
   b. The flap on the lefthand side.
   c. The flap farthest from you.
   d. The flap on the right side.

8. To put on sterile gloves, you should pick up the *first* glove:
   a. By the fingers of the glove.
   b. By the edge of the cuff that will turn inside.
   c. By the side of the cuff that will turn outside.
   d. By using the sterile wrapper to cover your hand.

29. MEDICATION ADMINISTRATION

OBJECTIVES
Upon mastery of the material in this chapter, you should be able to:

1. Describe the difference between a drug and a medication and recognize common effects of medications.
2. Describe the importance of different drug names and sources of drug information.
3. Describe the pharmacodynamics of drug action.
4. List the nurse's responsibility for safe practice with scheduled drugs.
5. Describe how drug administration differs according to age group.
6. Describe differing systems of drug administration.
7. Describe methods for calculating fractional doses of drugs.
8. Describe procedures for drug administration in parenteral, oral, topical, inhalation, and suppository forms.
9. Describe the importance of teaching safe administration of medication for effective self-medication.
10. Apply nursing process to give safe and planned care to a patient whose care involves principles of medicine administration.

TERMS
The terms important for an understanding of this chapter are shown below and defined in the glossary:

adverse effect
antagonistic effect
drug
idiosyncratic effect
medication
pharmacology
pharmacodynamics
pharmacokinetics
pharmacotherapeutics
pharmacy
side effect
synergistic effect
therapeutic effect
tolerance
toxic effect

Drug administration and education of people about the drugs they are taking are primary nursing responsibilities in almost all health care settings. These responsibilities are broad and include knowing the action and correct dosage of the medication, knowing the correct techniques of medication administration, teaching safe medication practices, evaluating the effects of medication, and the correct recording of the medication and patient condition.

A *drug* is any substance that is capable of affecting a person's state of health or ability to function. A *medicine* is any substance that improves a person's state of health or ability to function. Another way to distinguish between the two terms is that a medicine has a therapeutic (helpful) effect whereas a drug may not. Aspirin (acetylsalicylic acid), for example, is a medicine; alcohol is a drug. Despite these differences, in common usage, the terms *medicine* and *drug* are used interchangeably.

Sources of Drugs

Drugs are derived from a variety of sources. Plant derivations are a major category. Digitalis, a drug effective at slowing and strengthening the heart beat, is a drug derived from the foxglove plant. A drug such as iodine (used in thyroid illnesses) is derived from a mineral base. Insulin (used to replace natural insulin in people with diabetes) is derived from an animal source.

Antibiotics such as penicillin and tetracycline are obtained from microorganisms. Synthetic drugs made in a chemistry laboratory are used with increasing frequency. They tend to be economical to manufacture, standard in strengths, and free of impurities.

Classification of Drugs

Drugs are classified according to their specific therapeutic actions or according to the body system on which they act. It is impossible to memorize the action or effect of every drug used today because there are over 25,000 drugs available (Fig. 29-1). It is important, therefore, to recognize the classification of drugs and to be aware of the important precautions and/or guidelines for all drugs in that classification. Common classifications of drugs are shown in Table 29-1.

Drug Names

Drugs may be identified by their generic, chemical, official, or trade (proprietary) name. Learning about drugs often is confusing because drugs may be prescribed or dispensed under a number of different types of names.

The *generic name* of a drug is the original name given to it by the drug company who develops the drug. The *official name* of a drug is the name under which it is listed in one of the official drug publications. The official name may or may not be the same as the generic name. A drug's *chemical name* is a chemical description of its ingredients. A drug's *trade name* is the brand name

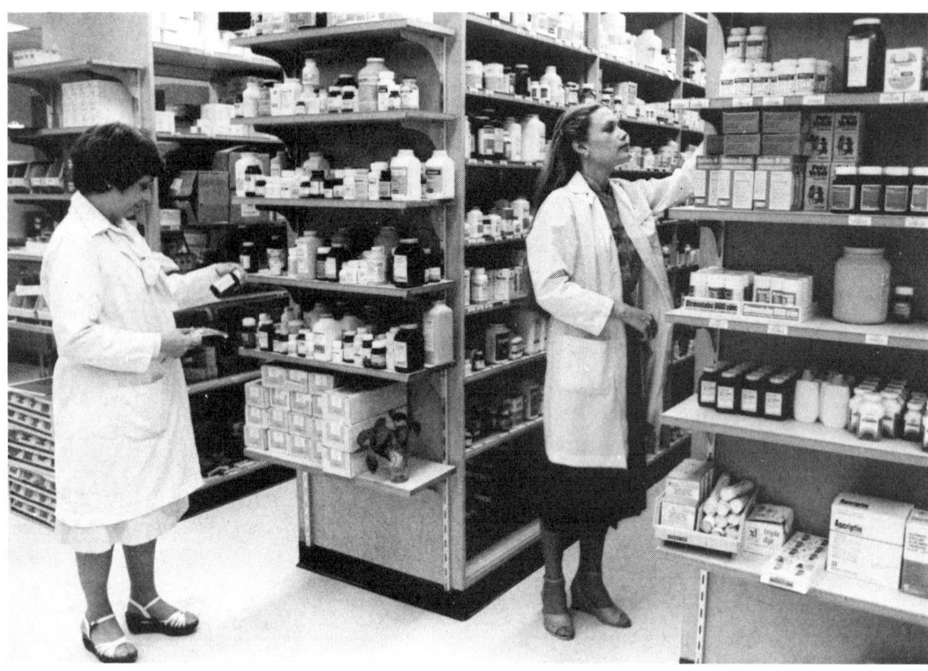

FIGURE 29-1. Learning different types of medications may be difficult because of the number of medicines prescribed.

TABLE 29-1. COMMON CLASSIFICATIONS OF DRUGS

Classification	Action	Special Assessment or Knowledge Needed for Safe Administration
Anti-infectives Example: Polycillin (Ampicillin)	Halt the growth of or kill microorganisms.	Antibiotic therapy may reduce normal body flora and allow overgrowth of fungal infections. Assess warm, moist body areas such as folds of skin, the umbilicus, vulva, vagina, and between toes. Antibiotics are generally administered for 7—10 days. It is important that they be taken for the full course to prevent organisms that have not been destroyed fully from returning to full strength. Allergies to antibiotics are common. Always check chart and ask patient if he knows of an allergy before administration. Antibiotics are most effective if administration is well spaced throughout a 24-hour period. Many oral antibiotic agents need to be refrigerated in order to maintain their effectiveness. Read label carefully.
Antineoplastic agents Example: Methotrexate	Destroy rapidly growing body cells. Used as chemotherapy against cancer.	Because white blood cells are rapidly growing cells, these usually are destroyed as a side effect of antineoplastic agents. Initiate protective measures to guard against infection (reverse isolation). All antineoplastic agents are contraindicated during pregnancy and breast-feeding (lactation). Nausea and vomiting are frequent side effects. An antiemetic may have to be requested to reduce vomiting. Assess level of nutrition. Loss of hair is another side effect. Offer support for insecurity because of altered body appearance and concept.
Antianemic agents Example: Ferrous sulfate (Feosol)	Increase number of red blood cells or increase iron or hemoglobin level.	Patients with anemia often are fatigued easily; space nursing care appropriately to conserve strength. Iron compounds turn stools black and often cause constipation. Teach patients that color change in stools is normal, and constipation can be relieved by adjustments in drug, dose, or time of administration. Iron compounds also may cause gastric irritation. Give with orange juice to increase absorption of compound and decrease irritation.

TABLE 29-1 (CONTINUED)

Classification	Action	Special Assessment or Knowledge Needed for Safe Administration
Anticoagulants Example: Bishydroxycoumarin (Dicumarol)	Reduce clotting ability of blood.	Assess patient for evidence of excessive difficulty with blood coagulation: ecchymotic (black-and-blue) areas, petechiae (pinpoint spots of bleeding), and bleeding gingiva. Firmly compress venipuncture sites used for drawing blood or intravenous therapy to effectively halt bleeding following needle withdrawal. Check that people on anticoagulants are not using aspirin (acetylsalicylic acid) for pain relief because aspirin prolongs bleeding time. (Many people do not think of aspirin as medicine and do not report it in a health history.)
Antihypertensive agents Example: Hydralazine hydrochloride (Apresoline)	Reduce blood pressure.	People on antihypertensives may develop dizziness and weakness when standing (orthostatic hypotension). Caution the patient to rise slowly to prevent this. Assess blood pressure before administration. Many people do not appreciate the seriousness of chronic hypertension and may discontinue the use of antihypertensive medication as soon as they no longer notice symptoms. Teach that long-term administration is important to reduce strain on cardiac and vascular systems even after obvious symptoms disappear.
Antiarrhythmic agents Example: Digitalis (Digoxin)	Regulate cardiac rhythm and rate.	Take apical heart rates of patients on antiarrhythmic drugs rather than peripheral pulses; take rate for a full minute to best detect irregularities. Assess for edema as an indication that heart actions are inadequate to handle incoming venous blood. Caution patients to buy new medication in time to always have a supply at home so they do not run out of a drug on a holiday or vacation.
Analgesics Example: Meperidine hydrochloride (Demerol)	Reduce or obliterate sensation of pain.	Many analgesics are narcotics. Follow specific drug administration regulations for narcotics. Narcotic analgesics have potential for abuse. Assess patients for dependence and tolerance. Some narcotic analgesics lead to constipation. Assess for this. Be cautious about applying heat or cold to people on analgesics because their pain sensation is decreased (for example, they can be burned without feeling it). Assess respiratory rate before administering Morphine Sulfate; do not give drug if rate is below 16.
Anticonvulsives Example: Phenytoin; Diphenylhydantoin (Dilantin)	Prevent or halt convulsions.	Anticonvulsive administration should not be halted abruptly; caution people to plan ahead to maintain an adequate supply at home. Alcohol is synergistic with many anticonvulsives. Caution patients about this. Excess drowsiness often accompanies effective therapeutic levels; regulation of the drug may take time. People need support and encouragement during this time.
Anesthetics Example: Local anesthetic (Lidocaine hydrochloride [Xylocaine])	Prevent pain sensations. May be used for local, regional, or systemic action.	Alert patient to "guard" an area that has been injected by a local anesthetic until sensation returns, or the area could be injured unknowingly. General anesthetics lead to loss of consciousness and loss of body reflexes. Protect patient's airway until gag and swallow reflexes are regained. People receiving spinal anesthesia should remain flat for 8 hours afterward to prevent a spinal headache.
Hormones Example: Insulin	Regulate metabolic processes.	Hormone administration should not be halted abruptly or "rebound" effects can cause major hazards. Caution people to keep a sufficient supply at home so they do not deplete their supply.
Diuretics Chlorothiazide (Diuril)	Increase urinary output.	Assess patient for excessive fluid loss (poor skin turgor, loss of weight). Many diuretics cause loss of potassium. Urge people to ingest foods high in potassium.
Cathartics Example: Bisacodyl (Dulcolax)	Promote intestinal elimination.	Cathartics should not be administered to patients with undiagnosed abdominal pain because the appendix could rupture. Unless otherwise contraindicated, teach people to increase intake of natural cathartics (fiber and fluid).

TABLE 29-1 (CONTINUED)

Classification	Action	Special Assessment or Knowledge Needed for Safe Administration
Hypnotics Example: Flurazepam (Dalmane)	Induce sleep.	Decrease environmental stimuli following administration of a hypnotic to help induce sleep. Many older adults react to hypnotics with confusion. Assess patient's safety if such a reaction occurs. Encourage people to utilize other sleep-promoting measures such as stress reduction or quiet surroundings rather than using hypnotics regularly. Hypnotics may reduce the amount of REM (rapid eye movement) sleep a person attains and leave him feeling unrested in the morning.
Sedatives Example: Phenobarbital (Luminal)	Promote relaxation.	Barbiturates can be used either as sedatives or hypnotics depending on the dosage. Observe scheduled drug procedure with barbiturates. People receiving sedatives may have slowed reaction times. Teach them to avoid situations where sudden judgment would be crucial to safety.
Antianxiety agents (tranquilizers) Example: Diazepam (Valium)	Improve feeling of well-being.	Such drugs may slow a person's reaction time. Caution them to avoid working in areas where instant judgment is necessary for safety. Such drugs have potential for dependence or tolerance. The action of most antianxiety agents is synergistic with alcohol. Caution patients to avoid alcohol consumption.

TABLE 29-2. NAMES OF DRUGS

Name	Definition	Example
Nonproprietary		
Generic	The name first given to a substance when it is developed.	Acetylsalicylic acid
Official	The legal name of the substance or the name as listed in the *United States Pharmacopeia*. This may also be the generic name.	Aspirin
Chemical	The chemical components of the drug.	$CH_3CO_2C_6H_4CO_2H$
Proprietary		
Trade	Name given to the substance by the manufacturer (the trademark name).	Bayer Aspirin, Bufferin, Ecotrin, St. Josephs

under which the drug is marketed. Trade names are followed by the initial ® to indicate that the name is trademarked and cannot be used by another drug company. Names of drugs are summarized in Table 29-2.

Sources of Drug Information

There are many sources of drug information that can be consulted in order to familiarize yourself with the action, route of administration, and range of dosage of a medication. The sources can be categorized as official and auxillary sources.

OFFICIAL SOURCES

The official sources are the *United States Pharmacopeia* (USP) and the *National Formulary*.

The *United States Pharmacopeia* lists drugs by their official names. Also included are a drug's source, its standard strength, and its range of dosage. The first *United States Pharmacopeia* was published in 1820 by order of the Federal Food, Drug and Cosmetic Act in an effort to achieve standardization of drugs.

The *National Formulary* serves much the same purpose as the USP or lists drugs according to their official names and describes their standard ingredients. The USP tends to list drugs in their most simple form. The *National Formulary* tends to include formulas of more complex drugs.

AUXILIARY SOURCES

Official sources of drugs often are not available in health care agencies. Therefore, they are not practical sources of drug information on an everyday basis. Auxiliary sources must be evaluated individually as to year of publication (not over 5 years since publication), credibility of author, and the inclusion of nursing implications in the information provided. The following are commonly available auxiliary sources.

American Hospital Formulary Service. The *American Hospital Formulary Service* is a collection of monographs (descriptions) of drugs published by the American Society of Hospital Pharmacists. Drugs are located in the index by name or by their pharmacologic action. This is a very complete reference and with few exceptions, contains all the information you need to administer medicine safely. It does not give specific nursing actions, however, nursing actions can be surmised from the drug action.

Physicians' Desk Reference (PDR). The *PDR* is published yearly by Medical Economics, Inc. and contains descriptions of drugs by their manufacturers. Drugs are listed according to their brand name, generic name, or therapeutic use. A colored product identification section displays photographs of commonly used capsules and tablets. This section is helpful in the case of a patient who is admitted to a health care agency who does not know the name of the medicine he has been taking. The colored product identification section will aid in identifying the medicine. Diagnostic products are included in the PDR as well. At one time information presented in the PDR was suspect by many health care providers (the thought was that manufacturers might glorify their product descriptions rather than state them honestly); the federal government restricts product descriptions on drugs to only factual information, however, so this is no longer a concern. A second criticism is that the PDR does not list nursing implications of drug administration. Nursing implications can be surmised from the product description.

Package Brochures. Drugs come from the pharmacological company accompanied by a brochure describing the action, range of dosage, and known adverse effects of the drugs. The information in such brochures is regulated by the Food and Drug Administration in order for it to be accurate and trustworthy. This guarantees that the information is not designed to enhance the drug's actions so that it will sell better. In many health care agencies, these brochures are kept in the pharmacy but are available to you on request.

Nursing Pharmacology Textbooks. Nursing pharmacology textbooks list and describe the actions, route of administration, and adverse effects of commonly prescribed drugs. Nursing texts concentrate on tips that are helpful in the administration of the drug (whether it tastes neutral or bitter, for example) and important factors necessary to assess before and after administration of the drug.

Nursing Journals. Most nursing journals (*American Journal of Nursing, Nursing 84*, and *RN*, for example) have columns or frequent articles on medicine administration, concentrating on newer drugs that would not be described in nursing textbooks because of their recent release dates. Like nursing textbooks, these sources concentrate on offering tips of administration that are pertinent specifically to nursing.

DRUG LEGISLATION

In 1906, the Federal Food and Drug Act designated the *United States Pharmacopeia* and the *National Formulary* as the official sources concerning standards of drugs in the United States. Drugs manufactured or sold in the United States must meet the criteria defined by these sources.

In 1938, the original Food and Drug Act was updated further and requirements for safety testing of new drugs before they can be marketed, as well as standards concerning accurate labeling, were included. In 1952, the Durham-Humphrey Amendment limited the dispensing of many drugs as prescription orders only and limited the ability to refill such prescriptions. It allowed for telephone authorization for prescriptions and refills of drugs.

Narcotics and other drugs that have the potential to cause drug dependence are regulated by additional laws. In 1914, the Harrison Narcotic Act was the first narcotic control act passed by any nation. It regulated the importation, manufacture, sale, and use of narcotics and their derivatives.

Although narcotic laws today still are frequently referred to as "Harrison" laws, the first act was amended in 1970 by the Controlled Substance Act. An important portion of this act was the classification of drugs with abuse potential into *schedules* (see Table 29-3). Drugs

TABLE 29-3. SCHEDULES OF CONTROLLED DRUGS: FEDERAL CONTROLLED SUBSTANCES ACT, 1970.

Schedule	Description and Example
I	Drugs that have a high potential for abuse, lack accepted safety measures for use, and have no accepted medical use. Examples: heroin, LSD, cocaine.
II	Drugs that have a high potential for abuse and high potential for psychological and/or physical dependence, but have accepted medical use. Examples: morphine, meperidine, some barbiturates.
III	Drugs with less potential for abuse than those in schedule II and a moderate potential for psychological and/or physical dependence. Examples: Empirin combined with codeine, barbiturates.
IV	Drugs with a low potential for abuse and a limited potential for psychological and/or physical dependence. Examples: tranquilizers, chloral hydrate.
V	Drugs with very low potential for abuse and low potential for psychological and/or physical dependence. Example: cough syrup with codeine.

that meet these criteria are termed *scheduled* drugs. A drug that can be purchased without a prescription is termed an *over-the-counter* (OTC) drug. A drug that needs a prescription in order to be dispensed because it has drug-dependent properties, high or frequent toxic effects, or is a new drug is termed a *legend drug* because it must bear the legend "Caution: Federal Law prohibits dispensing without prescription."

Because scheduled drugs carry a high danger of drug dependence, it is illegal to transfer a drug listed in schedule II, III, or IV to any person other than the patient for whom it was prescribed. It is illegal for any person to possess a controlled substance unless it is obtained by a valid prescription or temporarily held in a person's possession (such as a nurse) during the course of medicine administration. Nurses are required to account for all scheduled drugs administered on separate forms and to keep accurate records of all controlled medicines dispensed to their nursing care unit. Violations of this could result in revocation of a nursing license as well as a fine or imprisonment.

The drug enforcement administration (FDA) of the Department of Justice is the drug-enforcing agency in the United States. Biological products such as vaccines are controlled by the Public Health Service, a subdivision of the Department of Health and Human Resources. The Federal Trade Commission is responsible for regulating the advertising of medicine for the general public.

TABLE 29-4. ROUTES OF DRUG ADMINISTRATION

Route	Description
Oral	Taken by being swallowed; may be in liquid, tablet, or capsule form.
Buccal	Placing a drug against the mucous membrane of the inner surface of the cheek; it is absorbed across the membrane of the mouth.
Sublingual	Placing a drug under the tongue to be dissolved; it is absorbed across the membrane of the mouth.
Parenteral	A drug given by injection that is always in liquid form.
Intradermal	Injection into the dermis; useful for skin or allergy sensitization.
Subcutaneous	Injection into subcutaneous tissue; used with thin, easily absorbed drugs.
Intramuscular	Injection into a muscle; used with thick, poorly absorbed drugs.
Intravenous	Injection into a vein; used for immediate response because step of absorption is bypassed.
Intrathecal	Injection into the spinal canal.
Intracardial	Injection into the heart muscle.
Intra-articular	Injection into a joint cavity.
Topical	Application to the skin.
Inunction	Applied with rubbing to create friction. Liniments are applied this way.
Instillation	Placing a drug that is in solution into a body cavity for absorption across a membrane.
Irrigation	Flushing mucous membrane or skin with a drug that is in solution; useful for local effect.
Inhalation	Application of a drug to the respiratory membrane.

DRUG PHARMACOKINETICS

Four important pharmacokinetic processes are necessary in order for a drug to be used safely by the body: proper absorption, proper distribution, proper biotransformation, and proper excretion.

ABSORPTION

Absorption is the process of a drug being transferred from its point of entry in the body into the bloodstream. Absorption is influenced by the route of administration, the drug solubility and concentration, the acid-base balance of the body, and local influences at the site of administration.

ROUTE OF ADMINISTRATION

Various routes of drug administration are shown in Table 29-4. The poorest route of administration for drugs (unless only a very local effect is desired) is topical application of medicine (application to the skin) because substances are absorbed very slowly and incompletely by this route. It is important to remember, however, that some absorption always does take place from topical application so the number of times a topical application is to be applied as well as the amount to be applied, must be followed as strictly as if the medicine were given by any other more efficient route. Nitro paste, a form of nitroglycerin, is a drug commonly administered by topical application.

Medicine is absorbed across mucous membranes much more efficiently than it is absorbed across skin. Therefore, this method will yield quicker and more certain systemic results. Sublingual administration (absorption from under the tongue) is a route of choice for nitroglycerin, a medicine used to dilate coronary arteries and relieve heart pain due to inadequate oxygen supply to the heart muscle (angina pectoris). Absorption from this area places the drug almost immediately into the subclavian vein and carries it directly to the heart. The buccal (cheek) membrane may be used as an oral, mucosal absorption route as well. Medication also may be administered by way of the rectum and be absorbed by the mucosa in this area. Administration of medication by this route is influenced by the amount of feces present in the rectum. Due to rectal stimulation on insertion, the medication may be expelled before full absorption and benefit can be achieved.

A limited amount of medicine is administered by inhalation in order to be absorbed across the mucous membrane of the respiratory tract. Absorption from either a skin or mucous membrane site is termed *percutaneous administration.*

The efficiency of skin absorption is increased if there is a break in the skin surface or if the area is covered and kept moist after a medicine is applied. The efficiency of mucous membrane absorption is increased if interfering substances (for example, feces in the rectum or thick mucus in the lungs) are removed before administration.

The oral (enteral) route of administration is the easiest and most economical route. Absorption by the oral route is influenced by the presence or absence of food, the amount of stomach and intestinal activity, and whether or not the drug's composition will be altered by gastric secretions. Insulin, for example, is a drug that is inactivated by gastrointestinal enzymes and therefore is ineffective when given orally. A patient with diarrhea may be having very active peristaltic movement that causes all substances, including medicine, to move through the gastrointestinal tract so rapidly that there is no time for absorption.

For more rapid absorption of medicine, and to avoid the problems of gastric emptying times as well as the effect of gastrointestinal secretions, medicine may be administered parenterally (any route that bypasses the gastrointestinal tract). Topical application, inhalation through the lungs, and injection routes are all methods of parenteral administration. The fastest most efficient route of parenteral administration is the intravenous route (into the venous blood) or actually bypassing the entire absorption step and injecting the drug directly into the bloodstream. In emergencies, therefore, when medicine action must be immediate, drugs typically are given by the intravenous route.

Injecting medicine into a large muscle mass (intramuscular injection) is the second most rapid type of absorption that can be achieved. Blood supply to big muscle groups is active and the drug moves quickly from the muscle into the bloodstream. Injection into subcutaneous tissue, subcutaneous injection, is a third injection technique. This technique is often called "hypodermic" because it is *hypo* (under) the *dermis* (skin). Subcutaneous absorption is slightly slower than intramuscular absorption and is therefore used when slower, more continual absorption is desired. Insulin is always injected subcutaneously in order to provide for sustained continual absorption.

SOLUBILITY AND CONCENTRATION OF A DRUG

Medicine is not absorbed as a dry form. It must be put into a solution first. Therefore, absorption will take place more rapidly for those drugs that easily enter a soluble form. Drugs administered orally as liquids are more quickly absorbed than those administered as tablets or capsules because the latter two must dissolve first into a liquid form. Oily based (lipid-based) solutions are absorbed more rapidly from the gastrointestinal tract than water-based forms. In contrast, lipid-based solutions are more slowly absorbed from muscle and subcutaneous tissue than isotonic sodium chloride (normal saline) or water-based ones. This fact may be advantageous. Sus-phrine, for example, a bronchodilator, has an oil base. When injected subcutaneously, it gives long lasting bronchodilatation because it is absorbed more slowly than the same drug mixed with a water base. Keep this principle in mind when preparing emergency drugs. As a rule, oil-based drugs are not used in emergencies because rapid absorption is necessary to relieve the emergency.

Drugs of higher concentrations are absorbed more quickly than drugs of lower concentrations. Be aware of this when you are diluting medicine for the purpose of disguising a bitter taste. Your dilution may change the concentration of the drug and as a result, cause slower absorption.

ACID-BASED COMPOSITION

As drugs dissolve in body fluids, they enter either an ionized or nonionized form. An ionized drug has a chemically electrical charge and is lipid insoluble. Therefore, it will have difficulty crossing the gastrointestinal mucosa. A nonionized form is lipid soluble and diffuses readily across the gastrointestinal mucosa. Most medicine is either slightly acidic or slightly alkaline. As a rule, mildly acidic drugs dissociate most readily into an ionized state in a base medium (the intestine), while mildly alkaline drugs dissociate most readily into an ionized state in an acid medium (the stomach). This means that a drug which is slightly acidic (aspirin, or acetylsalicylic acid, for example) does not ionize well in the stomach; left in the nonionized state, it is lipid soluble and is absorbed rapidly from the stomach and the first part of the duodenum. If a buffer such as sodium bicarbonate is added to the aspirin (some people need this addition to keep aspirin from irritating the stomach lining) the drug will ionize, become lipid insoluble, and will not be absorbed freely until it enters the intestine. A patient or physician chooses which action is desired more: rapid absorption or a more comfortable effect. In actual practice, however, "buffered" aspirin contains very little "buffer" and thus has little effect.

LOCAL INFLUENCES

Before administering any medicine, you need to consider how factors at the site of administration will influence drug absorption. In some instances the route must be changed because of these factors. A nurse, as the one administering medicine, serves as a patient's second line of defense against ineffective drug therapy. The first line of defense is the patient himself. In instances where the patient is unable to make decisions for himself concerning drug administration, responsibility of deciding rests primarily with the nurse.

Topical administration, as mentioned previously, increases greatly in efficiency if there is a break in the skin surface or if the skin is lacerated at the absorption site. Gastrointestinal route absorption will be most effective if the stomach is free of food so that a large surface area for absorption is available. A drug cannot be absorbed if vomiting is present because vomiting will remove the drug from the body immediately. Absorption may also be limited if diarrhea is present due to the increased peristalsis in the intestine that rapidly removes the drug.

Oral mucosal absorption will be effective only if the person will cooperate by holding the tablet under the tongue or against the buccal mucosa. Rectal mucosa absorption will be ineffective if the medicine is placed inadvertently into a mass of fecal material rather than allowed to lie in contact with the rectal wall or if it is expelled before absorption can take place. Absorption across the respiratory tract mucosa will be impaired if large amounts of mucous secretions reduce the ability of the drug to contact the mucosa.

Intramuscular and subcutaneous routes of administration will have poor absorption if there is not a good supply of blood to the chosen site. People in shock, for example, have such low blood pressure that muscle and subcutaneous tissue is poorly perfused and absorption becomes inadequate. The presence of edema (fluid in subcutaneous tissue) also will interfere with absorption (cells are pushed further away from capillaries than normal). Circulation to injection sites can be increased by rubbing the site following injection or applying heat to the area.

Not only is it ineffective to inject medicine intramuscularly or subcutaneously in people with extremely low blood pressure or edema, it is actually dangerous. Because no absorption takes place at the time of injection, no response is achieved. Thus, more and more medicine is generally ordered to be injected. At the point that sufficient blood pressure is restored and normal muscle perfusion begins, the total amount of drug present will be swept into the bloodstream causing a toxic dosage. Drugs placed in edematous tissue tend to cause abscesses (infections) because they cannot be absorbed.

Intravenous administration, as mentioned earlier, actually bypasses the absorption step. (Medicine is delivered directly to the bloodstream.) This route becomes difficult in people with low blood pressure whose veins are barely distended because it is harder to pierce their veins with a needle. Difficulties also arise if there is a skin lesion over the course of a vein that obscures the vein and may cause an infection.

Distribution

Distribution is the movement of the absorbed drug through the bloodstream to the specific site of action. In order for distribution to take place effectively, both blood volume and pressure must be adequate.

Many drugs are carried by the bloodstream bound to plasma proteins (most often albumin). This binding action limits the amount of free drug in the circulation and therefore protects against toxic levels of the drug. A free drug is utilized; the bound drug is released to maintain the functioning level. People with low plasma protein levels (as could happen with vomiting when they are not receiving enough protein or with kidney disease that causes them to lose protein) may not be able to distribute some drugs well or may develop unexpected toxic symptoms because of the amount of free drug not bound in the circulation. Bilirubin, a product due to the breakdown of hemoglobin, is a substance also carried by plasma protein. Bound to plasma protein, bilirubin is harmless. However, in free form, it can leave the bloodstream and enter other body tissues; if it enters brain cells, it destroys their ability to function. This is particularly a problem with newborns who are breaking down proportionately more red blood cells than people at any other ages because of the necessity to convert a fetal form of hemoglobin to an adult form of hemoglobin. If a newborn is receiving a drug such as sulfonamide (a type of antibiotic) that competes for protein binding sites, a large quantity of bilirubin may be left unbound and the child may develop severe mental retardation because of brain cell destruction (kernicterus).

Most drugs, particularly those that are water-based, do not penetrate into the brain and spinal cord as readily as into other body tissues. They appear to be stopped by a "blood-brain barrier." This phenomena is a helpful barrier that protects sensitive brain tissue from assault by potentially harmful agents such as those that might occur from poisoning; it unfortunately may interfere with the distribution of a helpful substance such as penicillin. In some instances, if action on the spinal cord is desired, the drug will be effective if injected directly into the spinal fluid (intrathecal administration). In cardiac emergencies, drugs may be administered directly into the heart (intracardiac administration).

Today it is well accepted that the placental barrier does not prevent drugs from crossing the placenta and entering into fetal circulation; lipid-based drugs in particular diffuse readily into fetal circulation. Pregnant women must be extremely careful not to take any drug (including caffeine, alcohol, and nicotine) without their obstetrician's confirmation that the drug is safe to take during pregnancy.

Biotransformation

In addition to absorption and distribution, a third step that must take place before some drugs can be utilized by cells is biotransformation, or conversion, of the drug into an active, usable form or into a less toxic, more usable form. This step may also be termed *conjugation*.

Other drugs are biotransformed to some extent before leaving the body. Ether is one of the few substances that enters and is excreted from the body in an unchanged form.

Biotransformation is accomplished basically by liver action, although all cells perform biotransformation to some extent. People with liver disease or cardiovascular disease (which causes back pressure on the portal circulation and liver), newborns who have immature livers, and older adults who have some loss of liver function particularly have difficulty with this step of drug utilization. This will result in the buildup of toxic or raw drug levels. Chronic alcoholism causes cirrhosis of liver cells. Therefore, people with cirrhosis have difficulty with the biotransformation of drugs. Chronic alcoholism is a condition not readily admitted to by most people. Because alcoholics may have adverse reactions to medicine, you need to be certain to ask about alcohol consumption on admission to a health care facility or if you are going to supervise a medication program at home. The alcoholic's physician and you should be forewarned of the problems that improper biotransformation may cause.

Excretion

Ultimately, any drug administered to the body must be excreted from the body. Gaseous substances such as inhaled anesthetics are excreted by the lungs (blown off). A minimal amount of medicine is excreted in the intestines as bile combined with feces. Breast milk is a potential route of excretion for drugs and lactating (breast-feeding) mothers must follow the same guidelines they followed during pregnancy concerning drugs. No drugs should be ingested until they are approved by physicians who know the women are breast-feeding.

The main organ responsible for drug excretion is the kidney. Unused portions or inactive portions of drugs filtrate from the kidney glomeruli into the proximal tubules and are excreted in urine. Only a drug in its free form (not protein-bound) can be excreted, so protein binding slows drug excretion. Adequate circulatory pressure must be present in order for glomeruli filtration to occur (blood pressure must be greater than tubular pressure); kidney nephrons must not be diseased.

Newborns, because they tend to have immature kidney function, and older adults, who have some loss of kidney function, are prone to having difficulty with drug excretion. Poor drug excretion can lead to unexpected toxic drug levels despite normal dosages.

FACTORS AFFECTING DRUG ACTION

One important function of taking a medication history on a person you will be caring for is to attempt to assess factors that might lead to interference with the absorption, distribution, biotransformation, or excretion of drugs. A number of factors that influence the action of drugs are discussed below.

AGE

Age plays a major role in drug action because both hepatic and renal function are altered by age extremes (immature in newborns, decreased or with limited function in older adults). Older adults also may have hardening and stiffening of blood vessels, which makes distribution of drugs a major problem.

BODY SIZE

As would be expected, accompanying a larger than average body size is a larger than average number of body cells. Therefore, a larger drug dosage will be necessary to achieve a therapeutic drug level. In people of less than average body size, drug dosages must be appropriately adjusted to smaller amounts or toxic effects will occur.

SEX

Sex has an indirect effect on drug dosage because the average woman is smaller than the average man. A woman's body tends to have a higher proportion of fat cells than a man's body; drugs that are more soluble in fat than water may be more easily distributed in women than men. Women of childbearing age must be careful that they do not ingest drugs that would be harmful to a fetus because most fetal damage takes place in the time before a woman realizes that she is pregnant. Therefore, a woman "expecting to be expecting" must be concerned about drug ingestion.

MEDICATION EFFECTS

The effect that is desired from a drug is termed its *therapeutic effect.* Such an effect may be a local one, a systemic one, or a combination of the two.

LOCAL EFFECT

A *local effect* is just what the name implies: only the body tissue at the site of medicine administration is affected. Cough drops, for example, exert a soothing effect on the mucous membranes of the mouth and throat only; other body surfaces are not affected.

SYSTEMIC EFFECT

A *systemic effect* is a total body effect. In addition to any local effect of the medicine, as the medicine is absorbed into the bloodstream and distributed to distant sites, generalized body effects occur. Epinephrine, for example, is injected into subcutaneous tissue on the upper arm but is circulated throughout the body by the bloodstream to produce effects on major body organs such as the heart (heart rate is increased) and lungs (bronchioles are dilated); any effect at the original injection site is negligible.

SIDE EFFECTS

In addition to the therapeutic effect for which it is prescribed, a medicine may have additional actions or effects, known as *side effects*. Such effects are not usually desirable but are necessary consequences of taking the drug. Acetylsalicylic acid (aspirin), for example, has two effects. It is an analgesic (reduces pain) and an antipyretic (reduces temperature). In some instances, it is administered to make use of both effects as therapeutic ones. If it is administered primarily to reduce a person's fever, however, its antipyretic effect would be its therapeutic effect; that it is also effective in reducing that person's headache (its analgesic effect) is a *side* effect. If it were administered to relieve pain and also acted to reduce a person's elevated temperature, the analgesic effect would be the therapeutic effect; the antipyretic effect would be a side effect. Some medicine cannot be used by specific people. For example, although the medicine's therapeutic effect (increasing the heart rate) would be desirable, the medicine's side effect (increasing the blood pressure) would be detrimental to the patient's overall health.

TOXIC EFFECT

A *toxic effect* is an effect caused by an overdose or an excessive accumulation of medicine. A toxic effect may occur suddenly if the initial dosage given is excessive; it can occur slowly over a period of time if the person has poor excretory or liver function (usual doses of medicine build up in the person's system and reach toxic levels). Digoxin is a medicine that has the effect of slowing and strengthening the heartbeat. A toxic effect of digoxin is a cardiac arrhythmia such as bradycardia. Because bradycardia can occur fairly readily, assessing a patient's pulse is always necessary before more of the drug is administered.

SYNERGISTIC EFFECT

A *synergistic effect* is a complementary effect that occurs when two drugs are administered together and an effect is produced by their combination that is greater than the effect of either drug if given separately (a magnified reaction). This can be a harmful effect. Phenobarbital slows respiratory rate. If a person consumes alcohol (from this point on, think of alcohol as a drug and not as a social beverage, or you can miss its important physiological effects on the body) at the same time phenobarbital is ingested, respiration may be slowed to the point where the person cannot obtain adequate oxygen. This is an example of a synergistic effect.

ANTAGONISTIC EFFECT

An *antagonistic effect* is a lessened effect that occurs when two drugs are administered simultaneously (the resulting action is less than that of either drug given separately). Many drugs cannot be mixed in intravenous fluid or this type of reaction will occur. Always check medications for compatibility before combining them in an intravenous fluid or syringe.

UNTOWARD EFFECT

An *untoward effect* is an undesirable but predictable effect of a medicine. Untoward effects lead to iatrogenic diseases (drug-induced illnesses), such as difficulty with blood formation, or liver, kidney, stomach, or skin damage. Teratogenic (destructive to fetal growth) problems may also be the result of untoward effects.

Chloramphenicol is an antibiotic that is very effective against gram-positive bacteria; unfortunately long-term use of chloramphenicol leads to permanent destruction of red blood cells, making it rarely the drug of choice for infections despite its proven capabilities to destroy microorganisms. Untoward effects of this nature are unfortunate because they limit the use of certain medicines. Side effects and toxic effects, if they can be predicted, are also spoken of as untoward effects.

ADVERSE EFFECT

Adverse effects are unpredictable, detrimental effects of medicine. Such effects generally can be more clearly isolated as allergic or idiosyncratic effects.

Allergic Effects. When an antigen (a foreign protein substance) is introduced into the human body for the first time, the body forms antibodies to counteract or stop the invasion of the substance. In some individuals, the second time an antigen is introduced, the antibody reaction proceeds at a quicker rate and begins an "over reaction" that produces histamine. This is an *allergic* phenomenon. Allergic symptoms may be as mild as the development of a skin rash or be as extreme as severe hypotension and laryngeal spasm that occlude the airway and cause instant death. This severe reaction is termed *anaphylactic shock* and needs the immediate intervention of cardiopulmonary support.

Penicillin is a medicine that is capable of causing this kind of severe allergic reaction in people who are sensitive to penicillin. Before administration, always ask a person if he is allergic to penicillin and double check a record to see if the person to whom you are administering penicillin has any past record of allergy to the drug or its derivatives. A person who has had an allergic reaction to a drug in the past must not receive the same drug again because with the new administration, a fatal anaphylactic reaction could occur.

Idiosyncratic Effect. An *idiosyncratic effect* is an abnormal effect that is caused by individual body responses to medicine. These responses probably reflect undetectable genetic differences in drug metabolism; they cause an over- or under-response to the drug administered.

TOLERANCE EFFECT

A person has developed *tolerance* to a drug when he must take larger and larger dosages of the drug in order to achieve therapeutic effects. Why tolerance occurs is unknown but probably results from increased drug-metabolizing enzymes in the liver. Alcohol is a drug that is well documented for causing tolerance; morphine sulfate, effective for pain relief early in the course of an illness, commonly becomes ineffective over a period of time as tolerance to it occurs.

CUMULATIVE EFFECT

A *cumulative effect* is an effect due to the gradual accumulation of a drug in a person's body because of inadequate liver function (lack of biotransformation ability) or inadequate excretion of the substance. Lead poisoning is an example of a condition that occurs, not because the child eats a great deal of lead at any one time, but because lead is poorly excreted from the body. Thus, a cumulative effect occurs. Cumulative effects lead to toxic effects or sometimes unexplained synergistic or antagonistic effects.

Drug Interaction

Drug interaction is the overall term for an adverse effect that occurs from the concurrent administration of two or more drugs. The interaction may stop the action of a drug at the absorption, distribution, biotransformation, or excretion level of drug action. Antacids that contain aluminum or magnesium will interfere with the absorption of tetracycline, an antibiotic, and make the administration of tetracycline useless. Competition for protein-binding sites will distort the effect of the drugs competing for these sites. Monoamine oxidase inhibitors (a class of antidepressant drugs) compete with the biotransformation of tyramine, a constituent of cheese. People taking these drugs may develop severe symptoms after eating cheese because the tyramine in the cheese is not fully biotransformed. Probenecid's ability to halt the excretion of penicillin is an example of drug interaction at the excretory level. This interaction may be used therapeutically to prolong the retention of penicillin in the body and increase its effectiveness.

There is a possibility that a drug interaction may occur when drugs are mixed in an intravenous solution bottle or in a syringe prior to administration. Sometimes this forms an insoluble precipitate that would cause an embolus when administered. Before mixing any medicines for parenteral administration, you need to check that they are not drugs that interact in this way.

Drug Dependence

Dependence on a drug means that the person feels a physical or psychic need for the drug (drug addiction). If such a drug is withdrawn, the person may have physical disturbance or psychological cravings for the substance. Drug dependence can become a problem when narcotics and barbiturates are administered over a long interval of time.

Timing of Administration

Drugs, as a rule, are absorbed most rapidly from the gastrointestinal tract when the stomach is empty; some drugs are so irritating to the gastric mucosa, however, that they must be timed to be administered with a buffer substance or with food to decrease irritation (see QRS 29-1). A person's circadian rhythm (pattern of sleep and wakefulness) may affect the rapidity of absorption, distribution, biotransformation, and excretion of drugs although there is little practical application of this point at this time.

Environmental Influences

Drugs that achieve a hypnotic (sleep) effect are not effective if other means to promote sleep (dark, quiet, warm room) are not provided at the same time; medication to relieve pain is not effective if other means to relieve pain (elevating an extremity, reducing anxiety due to other factors) are not carried out at the same time. Any drug that influences mood may be more effective if you assure patients that the drug will achieve the effect they desire. (Providing assurance that a tranquilizer will help a patient relax helps him relax and increases the action of the drug.) A principle of drug administration is as follows: Never just give a drug; always follow through with any other measure that will help or complement the drug's effectiveness.

☐ QUICK REFERENCE STOP 29-1: NUTRITION

1. As a rule, medicine is absorbed best from an empty stomach. Taking medicine before a meal, therefore, will result in faster absorption than taking it after a meal.
2. Some medication is irritating to the stomach lining and is best taken with an accompanying solution like milk to coat and soothe the stomach lining. Nausea is a frequent side effect of many medicines. Be conscious of the nutritional intake of people on medicine to be certain that nausea is minimized and is not reducing intake greatly.
3. Most people use mealtimes as reminders of when to take medicine. Unfortunately, some drugs are inactivated by the presence of food in the stomach. Help people to devise other systems to remind them when drugs should be taken (e.g., when they wake up, just before they go to bed, with the 6:00 P.M. news).

State of Health

People with gastrointestinal, renal, or hepatic dysfunction may have difficulty with the absorption, biotransformation, and excretion of drugs. People with cardiovascular illness may have difficulty with the distribution of drugs. The presence of one type of illness may make a drug prescribed for another illness unacceptable. Careful assessment before drug administration is necessary to determine a person's present state of health, which may be constantly fluctuating.

Genetic Differences

Genetically inherited differences can influence ability to utilize drugs effectively. Glucose-6-phosphate dehydrogenase deficiency (G6PD), for example, is a disease found mainly in people of black or oriental extraction. When people with this syndrome ingest a drug such as aspirin (acetylsalicylic acid), their red blood cells begin to lyse (lose their structure). Not enough oxygen is carried to body cells and the person becomes anemic. People with this syndrome need to be aware of the medicines they cannot take; for their protection, you also need to be aware of the medicines they should not ingest.

Psychological Factors

As a rule, if a person believes that a medicine will help him to feel better, he will derive a greater effect from it than if he distrusts its ability to cure him. (This is why people taking noneffective drugs such as Laetrile, for example, often report that the drug is making them feel better.) This effect is termed a *placebo* effect. Administer medicine with a positive attitude ("This should make you feel more comfortable," not "I don't think this will work, but try it.") Remember, however, that sensations of pain or "feeling better" are subjective. If a person does not feel improvement after taking a medicine, perhaps a different type of medicine or a stronger type is needed (due to some effect of absorption, distribution, biotransformation, or excretion).

LIFE SPAN CONCEPTS AND DRUGS

Age is one of the biggest factors that makes drug administration differ a great deal from patient to patient.

The Infant

Newborns, in particular, and all infants have less acceptable injection sites than adults. They have more difficulty with biotransformation and excretion of drugs than adults, so the number of medications given to infants is always limited to the minimum necessary.

Tablets or capsules need to be crushed or opened and mixed with a suitable medium, such as a spoonful of baby food, so the infant may swallow the medicine easily. Unfortunately, some tablets and capsules lose their maximum therapeutic effects if crushed. These types of medication cannot be given safely to infants. If the medicine is in liquid form, it can be drawn into a syringe and administered by placing the syringe (no needle on the syringe) at the side of the infant's tongue and injecting small amounts of the liquid into the infant's mouth. Keep the infant's head in an elevated position while doing this, so that aspiration does not occur. Placing rubber tubing on the end of a medicine dropper and using the dropper to administer liquid next to the child's tongue is a similar technique. Never place a glass dropper in an infant's mouth because he may bite it and break the glass tip. In some instances you might use the needle of a syringe to draw the liquid out of its container; immediately dispose of the needle after you have the medicine correctly measured in the syringe. Remember that walking into a child's room with a syringe and needle may frighten him unnecessarily; also, you could inadvertently inject an oral medication, causing a serious medication error. Omit the possibility of either of these problems with immediate disposal of the needle you use to draw up oral medications.

As a rule, hold an infant or young child on your lap for oral medication administration so you can restrain the child's arms with your free hand (Fig. 29-2). If you

FIGURE 29-2. A toddler receives an oral liquid by means of a syringe (no needle). Notice how the mother restrains the child's arms and upper body.

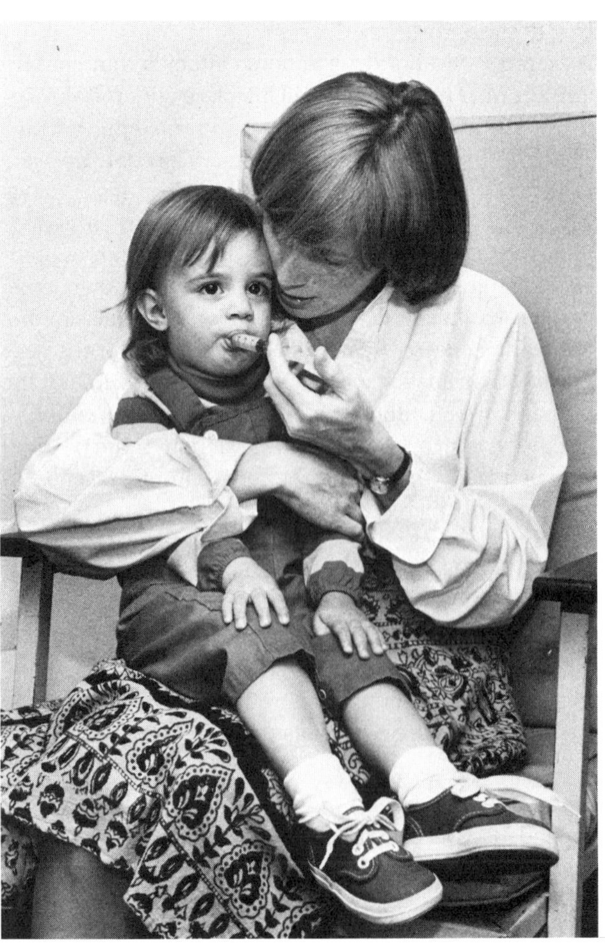

do not do this, even a newborn is capable of knocking your hand and spilling the medication. Provide all crushed tablets in a single spoonful so the child only has to take one bite. (Anyone can get a baby to take one bite of something; no one can be certain of convincing the baby to take a second bite.)

Injection sites in infants are limited because the only acceptable site for intramuscular administration is the vastus lateralis (anterior thigh). The only acceptable subcutaneous injection sites are the vastus lateralis and the deltoid (upper arm). Using other sites, particularly the dorsogluteus (upper outer buttock), prior to the time the child has walked for a year is extremely dangerous. The sciatic nerve occupies such a large portion of the buttock in infants that the chance of causing permanent nerve damage from an injection is too dangerous to attempt.

The Toddler and Preschooler

Toddlers and preschoolers are suspicious that medicine will taste bitter and often reject it even before they taste it. If the medicine does taste bitter, be certain it is in the smallest amount possible and offer something that tastes good after it.

Most children under 3 cannot swallow tablets or capsules because they have not yet developed the physiological coordination necessary to move the tablet to the back of the tongue and swallow. A child over the age of 4 may have the ability to swallow medication but be reluctant because he has never done so before. You can teach the child to swallow medicine by having him practice with a small ice chip or a small, readily dissolvable candy such as an M & M that melts almost instantly at the back of the throat. Practicing with these items is helpful because if a piece of ice or candy sticks halfway down, it will dissolve or melt quickly and not cause pain.

Introducing the use of a straw or offering the child's favorite fruit juice as a chaser after the medicine are ways to encourage interest in swallowing medicine. *Do not bribe children to take medicine.* Be aware that bribes must be increased each time to achieve the same result; soon you will not be able to offer rewards great enough to warrant taking the medicine. Do not allow toddlers to have a choice as to whether or not they want to take medicine. Instead, tell them the primary task ("I have your medicine for you to take") and give them a secondary choice ("Do you want your mother to hand it to you or me to hand it to you?").

Both the toddler and the preschooler mimic adult behavior. Do not act as if the medicine is unappealing to you or the child will refuse it. Never refer to medicine as candy or say it tastes like candy because the child may remember what you said and swallow the entire jar of medicine believing it is candy.

Preschool children strongly fear intrusive procedures. Following the administration of an injection, they need praise for their cooperation (any action short of hysterical screaming is cooperation from preschool children during an injection). They may enjoy giving a play injection to a doll or to you (no needle on the syringe). Reviewing experiences this way offers children a sense of control and greatly relieves tension. State and federal laws require quick disposal of syringes and needles to prevent their use by drug abusers; allowing a preschooler to play with one following an injection is acceptable as long as the syringe is properly disposed of after the play period. Such play is termed *therapeutic* play and a health care agency may supply specially marked syringes just for this purpose.

The Schoolager and Adolescent

Schoolagers and adolescents are very interested in the "whys" of things. Explaining to them what a medicine will do for them is often enough to provoke their interest in taking it even though there may be a bitter aftertaste. Although many schoolagers say they can hold still during an injection, you may need a second person to help restrain them. If this is done with a "Let me hold you to help you stay still" approach, it is not degrading.

Schoolagers and adolescents have notoriously poor compliance levels if they are expected to continue to take medicine on an ambulatory basis. Explaining the importance of the drug and the consequences of not taking it is the best way to ensure continued compliance. Be certain that the administration time of medicine does not coincide with school hours because many school systems do not allow children to bring medicine to school.

Be certain the medicine history of an adolescent obtained during admission contains questions about the use of illegal drugs. The use of such drugs may lead to unusual drug interactions and unpredictable results from administered medicines.

The Young and Middle-Aged Adult

Young and middle-aged adults tend to be impatient with illness and eager to take medicine if it will make them well again. In fact, many people in these age groups ask for medicine in situations that do not warrant it (for example, an antibiotic for a cold). If a medication does not show detectable results immediately, they may fail to continue to take it. Education about the use and abuse of medicine is the best means of helping this age group learn to be a wise consumer of medicine.

The Older Adult

Many older adults have some form of chronic illness that necessitates drug therapy. Many take four or more prescription drugs on a daily basis. In addition, these people may be taking several nonprescription (over-the-counter) drugs. Taking this number of drugs leads

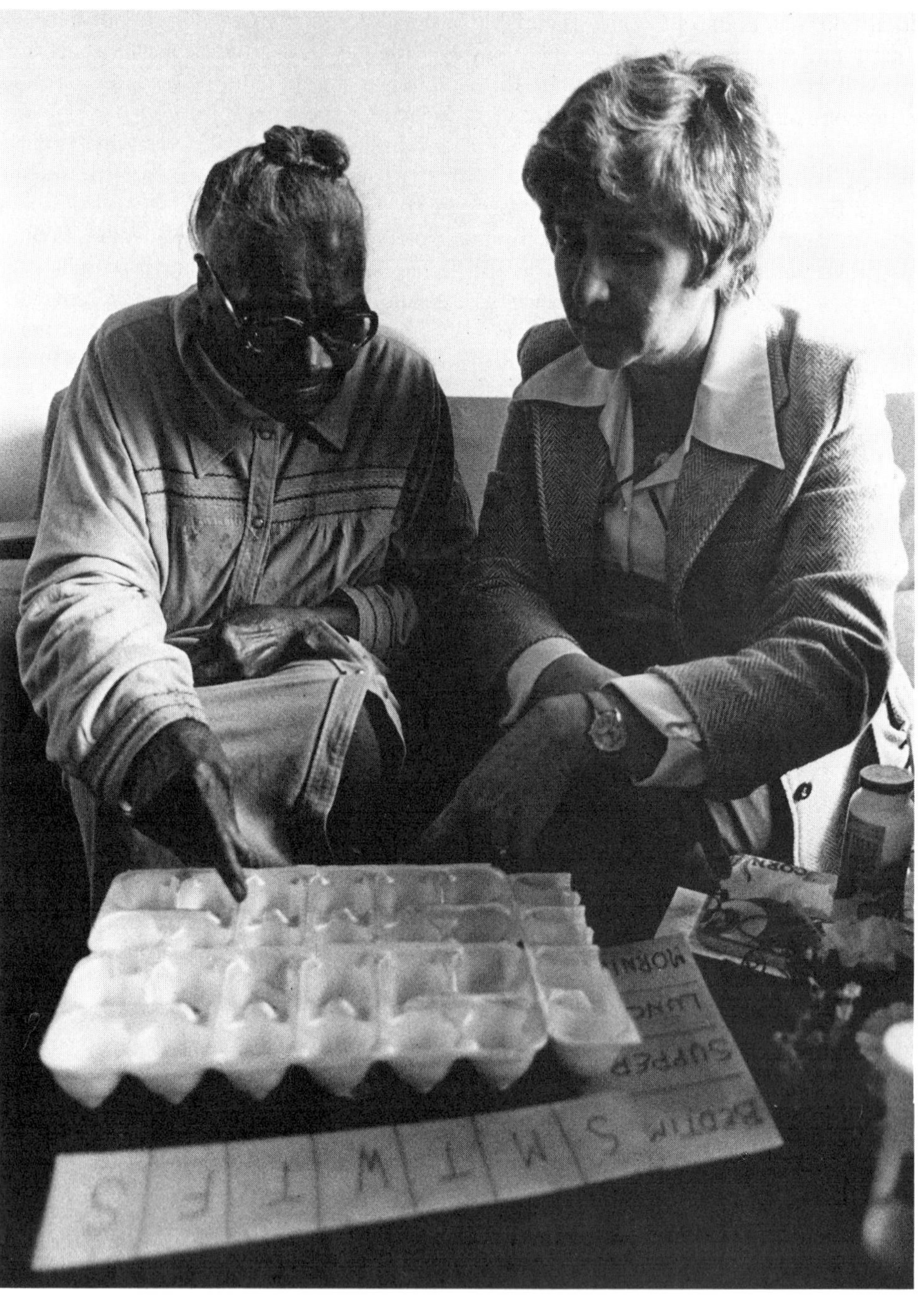

FIGURE 29-3. This egg carton serves as a handy reminder tool to help this woman take medications on schedule.

easily to drug interaction problems or drug administration error.

Other factors may influence the effects of medicine with this age group. Absorption from the gastrointestinal system may be reduced because stomach contents are less acid than in younger people. Distribution may be limited if arteriosclerosis (hardening of the arteries) and lack of strong blood flow are present. Biotransformation may be impaired if liver degeneration exists. This means that toxicity from unchanged drugs may occur. Excretion of drugs may be inadequate if there is kidney degeneration and result in toxic levels of drugs.

Some older adults are prone to idiosyncratic effects of medicine. With administration of a sedative (a medication to induce relaxation), for example, the person may instead become restless, disoriented, and confused.

When helping older adults to learn the medication schedule they will need to follow at home, assess carefully for hearing and visual impairments. If a hearing difficulty is present, the person must have clearly written instructions about medication time and dosage; otherwise he may not hear everything you say and, therefore, fail to follow such a program. If a visual problem is present, the person may need to locate a support person to identify which medication should be taken at what times. If there are only two medications to differentiate, coloring the top of one of the containers with magic marker or placing a tag of adhesive tape that protrudes from the vial's side are ways to aid in the differentiation.

Older adults must also be assessed for memory loss. Almost all people of all ages need a medicine reminder chart to remind them when it is time to take medicine (Fig. 29-3); the older adult may particularly need this type of aid. Commercial containers are available (Fig. 29-4) in which a patient's medicine is separated into divisions in a dispenser box. Each division represents the amount of medication to be taken at a specific time. For example, a person can tell what medicine he should take at 10 A.M. by the pills in that place of the box. He will also know if he remembered to take his 10 A.M. medications by whether or not they are gone from the space. It is not good practice to tell older adults to keep their medicine in a conspicuous space such as the kitchen table in order to remind themselves to take it (as it is not good advice for any age group) because if grandchildren or other young children visit, this creates a potential for accidental poisoning. It is better to post a note "take your medicine" on the kitchen table and keep the medicine itself well out of the reach of children.

Be certain that older people understand the action of each medication they are taking and know about untoward effects for which they should watch. This could help prevent some problems. For example, if they are taking five medicines and develop nausea, they may not be certain which pill is causing the nausea. As a result, they may discontinue taking all five. Some older adults continue to take medicine past the point they need it or take two types that cause the same effect because they do not know which is the correct medicine to stop and which is the one to continue. A medication chart or the color coding of medication bottles may assist in helping people who are taking a multitude of medicine to keep the types straight.

FIGURE 29-4. A commercial medicine dispenser box is divided into separate sections to alert a person when to take medication.

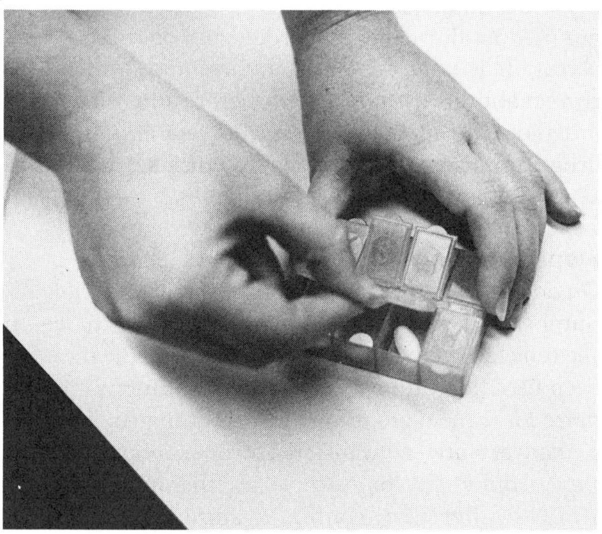

Older adults may have difficulty swallowing large tablets or capsules if they have some neurological or arthritic problems that make swallowing difficult. They may need to crush tablets or capsules. In many health care facilities, jars of baby food are used as the medium to mix crushed tablets, not only for infants, but for people of all ages. Do not refer to this as baby food within the patient's hearing range as it is demeaning to be fed baby food when one is 80-years-old. Call it what it is whether it be applesauce, custard, peaches, etc.

Older adults lose some subcutaneous tissue so they may have fewer subcutaneous injection sites than young adults. If there is muscle atrophy, intramuscular injection sites may be fewer. This may limit the dose and the times that parenteral injections can be administered.

THE PHYSICIAN'S ROLE IN MEDICINE ADMINISTRATION

Only in a few instances such as administration of a potent or experimental medicine when the effects of the medicine are potentially life threatening will the physician actually administer a medication. The chief role of the physician is to prescribe (order) the medication after her assessment of the patient's health and therapeutic need.

Medicine Prescriptions

Medicine may be prescribed by a physician, a dentist, or a veterinarian. In some states a physician's assistant or nurse practitioner working under the guidance of the physician can write prescriptions. It is important when practicing in a health care agency where medical students practice to remember that such students cannot prescribe medication (they must have an order countersigned to make it legal). It is also important to remember that nurses cannot prescribe medicine (nurse practitioners working under the approval of a physician are the exception to this in some states due to newly revised Nurse Practice Acts). Nurses cannot offer someone a medicine as simple as aspirin without it being ordered by a physician. Nurses are not legally able to dispense medicine (a pharmacist's responsibility). This means that nurses are not able to take a stock medication from a hospital pharmacy. They are only able to take the smaller bottle or single dose of medicine prepared by the pharmacist.

A medicine prescription must be written in a standard form to be legal and accepted by a nurse.

Date: 12/4/84
Patient Name: Harry Smith
Address: 16 Court Street

Rx Polycillin 250 mg
T.I.D. P.O.

Dispense: 30 tablets
Sig. T.I.D. × 10 days

Jean Brown, M.D.

FIGURE 29-5. A prescription for an antibiotic is given to a patient in an ambulatory health care setting to be filled at a local pharmacy.

Ambulatory Prescriptions

In an ambulatory health care setting, patients are given medicine prescriptions to have filled by the pharmacist of their choice. A prescription of this type must include four parts. A *superscription* includes the date, the person's name and address, and the symbol Rx (Latin for "take thou"). The *inscription* lists the name and dosage of the medicine desired, as well as the times and route of administration. A *subscription* lists instructions for the pharmacist about how much medicine to dispense and also includes the physician's signature and title. The word *Sig* means "write on the label" (Fig. 29-5).

If the patient is a child, the child's age or weight is usually included so the pharmacist can double check that the dose of the medication is appropriate for age and weight. If the medicine is a controlled (scheduled) substance, the physician's narcotic number representing her right to prescribe controlled substances must be included with her signature. Not all physicians apply for narcotic numbers so not all physicians may be able to write prescriptions for these substances.

Additional information is stated at the bottom of the prescription and includes the number of times the prescription can be refilled as well as whether the physician wants the person to have a specific brand (trade) name of a medication or whether a generic name can be dispensed. (In many instances a generic [no-name brand] drug may be less expensive; in other instances a certain brand name product has a particular added ingredient or flavoring that the physician feels is an important part of the prescription.)

In-Patient Prescriptions

In an in-patient care unit, a physician writes prescriptions along with instructions for other therapeutic modes on a physician's order sheet. This order sheet already contains the patient's name and hospital number, so she writes only the medicine name (proprietary or official name), dosage desired, route of administration, time and frequency of administration, date and time of the order, and her signature (Fig. 29-6).

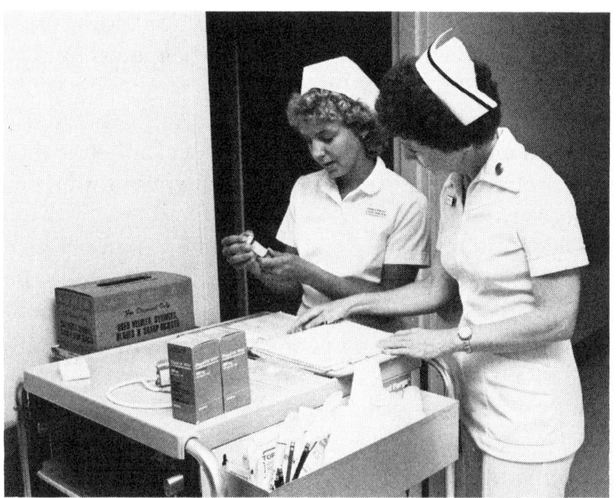

FIGURE 29-6. A medicine prescription for a hospitalized patient is written on the physician's order sheet. Always check a medicine against the original order the first time of administration.

In a health care agency, information that is recorded this way on physician's order sheets is transcribed onto a medicine card or Kardex (the actual working order). The nurse doing the transcribing copies the patient's name, room number, medicine name, dosage, route of administration, and times of administration. She also provides her signature. A typical medicine card is shown in Fig. 29-7A. A medicine Kardex record is shown in Fig. 29-7B.

Common Prescription Abbreviations

At one time almost all information on a prescription was written in Latin so the person receiving the medicine could not decipher what it said. Today, the common belief is that every patient has a right to know (and should know) what medicine he is receiving. A number of abbreviations are used to shorten the writing into as brief a form as possible. These abbreviations are used in all medication orders and on nursing care charts. It is vital for you to understand and use the correct abbreviations so that drugs are administered as ordered. The most common abbreviations used for drug administration are shown in Quick Reference Stop 29-2.

Stop Dates for Drug Prescriptions

On an ambulatory prescription, a physician writes the number of days a patient should take the medicine (or she may tell them to take it until all the medication has been used). Health care agencies have automatic stop dates for some types of medicine that may be harmful if inadvertently administered over a long period of time. Antibiotics, for example, are therapeutic for 7 to 10 days; after that, continued administration of an

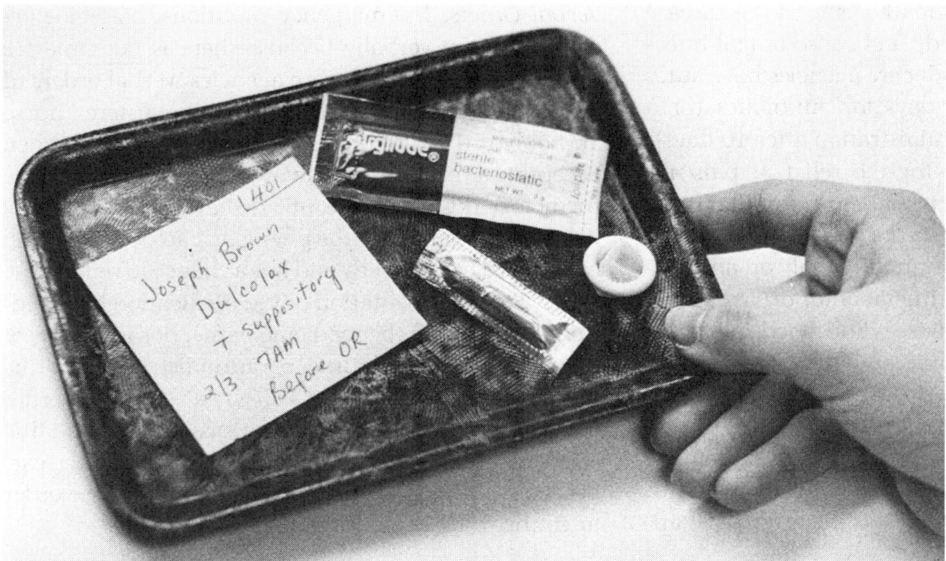

A

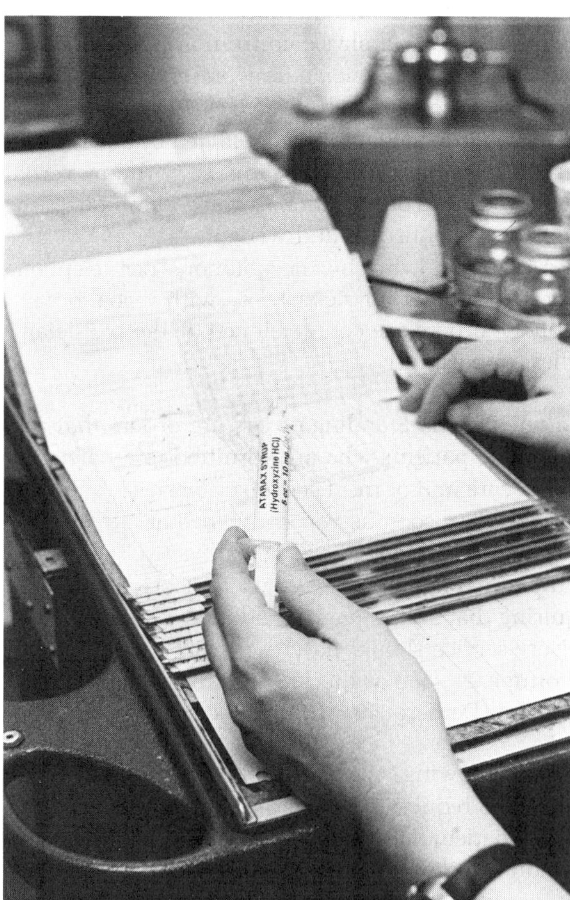

B

FIGURE 29-7. A. A medicine card. B. A medicine Kardex, which serves not only as a record of the medication order, but also as a place to record that the medication has been given.

☐ QUICK REFERENCE STOP 29-2: SAFETY

Abbreviations are used in all medication orders and in nursing care charts. It is vital that you understand and use the correct abbreviations so that drugs are administered as ordered. Following is a list of the most common abbreviations used for drug administration.

A.C. before meals (*ante cebum*).
ad lib freely, as desired.
bid (BID) two times a day
c̄ with
gm gram
gr grain
gtt drop
hr hour
HS hour of sleep (*hora somni*); bedtime
IM intramuscular
IV intravenous
m minim
mEq milliequivalent
ml milliliter
O.D. right eye
O.S. left eye
os mouth
oz ounce
p.c. after meals (*post cibum*)
PO by mouth (*per os*)
prn as required (*pro renata*)
q every (*quaque*)
qd every day
qid (QID) four times a day (*quater in die*)
qod (QOD) every other day
sc subcutaneous
STAT immediately (*statim*)
tid (TID) three times a day (*ter in die*)

antibiotic might destroy nonpathogenic (non—disease causing) bacteria in the body and cause fungal infections. Therefore, most health care agencies have automatic stop dates after 10 days for antibiotics (or a policy to question their administration after 10 days).

Narcotics are necessary for the relief of pain for approximately three days after surgery; after that time, continued administration may lead to drug dependence. Most narcotic orders are used only on an inpatient basis. Anticancer (antimetabolite) drugs destroy cells that grow rapidly. Because white blood cells grow rapidly, anticancer (chemotherapy) drugs destroy appreciable amounts of them. Drugs of this nature, therefore, generally have stop orders that limit them to one-time administration or stop orders that explain the necessity to check a laboratory report for the status of certain cells before another administration is approved.

As a general policy, all drugs are discontinued while a patient is in surgery; they must be reordered following surgery in order to still be considered current orders. Likewise, if a patient is transferred from one service to another (moved from the surgical wing of the hospital to the rehabilitation wing) all orders are cancelled and must be renewed. If a patient was taking medicine at home, he must not continue to take it in the hospital until it is ordered for him. All institutions have policies regarding the handling of drugs a patient brings to the agency with him. In most instances, a family member is asked to return them to the patient's home so he accidentally does not receive an overdose of the drug (for example, if he takes a tablet and the nurse gives him a tablet of the same type). These drugs could also be held in the agency's pharmacy for him during his stay.

After a stop-order time for a medication has been reached, the physician must reorder it in order to continue administration. It is dangerous for some medication, such as phenobarbital, to be stopped abruptly. Therefore, it is a courtesy for the nurse to call stop-order time limits to the physician's attention before the limit expires so that the physician is aware that a medication needs reordering or cancellation. In the course of a busy day, this information is easy to overlook.

Types of Medicine Orders

Types of medicine orders may vary depending on the patient's condition and the circumstances present at the time of the order.

Written Orders. Unless extenuating circumstances exist, all medicine orders must be written. This is because the danger of an order being spoken incorrectly is greater than one being miswritten. An order is more apt to be misunderstood when heard than when read.

Verbal Orders. In emergency situations, medicine orders are given verbally because there is not time for writing. In most health care agencies, verbal orders of this nature only can be accepted by a registered nurse and only if the situation is truly an emergency. When accepting a verbal order, always repeat the name of the medicine, dosage, route of administration, and the name of the patient so the physician can be certain you have heard her correctly and has a chance to rethink the order. For documentation of the medication being administered, write the medicine name, dosage, route of administration, and time of administration on the physician's order sheet and also write "per verbal order of Doctor (name)," followed by your signature and title after the medicine has been administered. At her earliest convenience, the physician countersigns the order to confirm the prescription.

Telephone Orders. Telephone orders are a second type of verbal order. In a limited number of circumstances, distance separates a physician from an order book; in these instances, a physician may prescribe a medicine over the telephone. In most health care agencies, these, like verbal orders, only can be accepted by a registered nurse. The procedure is the same as with any verbal order: repeat the prescription as you receive it over the telephone to confirm it and write it in the physician's order book following by the notation "per telephone order of (name of physician)." As with verbal orders, telephone orders are countersigned at the physician's earliest opportunity.

Standing Orders. Standing orders are orders that will apply to all patients who are admitted to a particular nursing care unit or meet certain criteria. They may be carried out as soon as you confirm that the circumstances under which the order is "active" exist. For example, a physician might write a standing order requiring that all her patients admitted to a labor and delivery service should have a certain medication for discomfort as soon as uterine dilatation reaches a certain point (Demerol 50 mg IM at 3-4 cm cervical dilatation).

When following standing orders, you must be certain that all the requirements for administration exist and that the patient does not have an unexpected contraindication to a medication, such as an individual allergy, that would make the medicine or dose inappropriate. Never think of standing orders as "routine." They call for a great deal of independent nursing judgment.

STAT Orders. The term *STAT* is Latin for "immediately." A STAT order, therefore, is one to be carried out as soon as possible. It is the procedure in most health care agencies for the nurse to record the time the medication was administered and her initials on the physician's order sheet so at her first check back, the physician can see the medication has been given.

PRN Orders. The term *PRN* is Latin for "as needed." A medicine ordered on a PRN basis, therefore, is given only when the patient needs it. Medications typically ordered on this basis are analgesics (pain relievers), hypnotics (sleep-inducing medications), and laxatives (medicine to effect a bowel movement). Knowing when a PRN medication is needed requires nursing judgment and may require consultation with another nurse or the patient to confirm the need. A patient may ask for a PRN medicine or you may suggest it.

A typical PRN order would read: Acetylsalicylic acid 10 grains every 4 hours for pain, PRN. With this order, a patient could have 10 grains of aspirin as frequently as every 4 hours if he needed it for discomfort. Be certain that you do not regard a PRN order in terms of what the patient feels is needed. In the above order, the patient cannot have as much aspirin as he wishes: he can have only 10 grains every 4 hours. Always interpret PRN orders within their limits.

THE PHARMACIST'S ROLE IN MEDICINE ADMINISTRATION

It is the pharmacist's responsibility to furnish medication to an ambulatory patient and to the nursing staff for an inpatient. The medication must be in a form that is both correct for and acceptable to the patient. In many health care agencies, a unit dose system of medicine is used, whereby medicine is prepackaged in the pharmacy. This system provides the amount to be taken at any one time of administration in an accurately and conveniently prepared form. Unit dose systems (compared to an older system where the pharmacist sends a large bottle of medicine to the nursing unit and, when each dose is due, the nurse pours the correct amount from the large bottle) increase the amount of time the pharmacist spends dispensing medicine, but decreases the amount of time the nurse must spend preparing medications. It also decreases medication errors because a pharmacist works undisturbed, whereas a nurse preparing medicine may be interrupted constantly.

The pharmacist has an added responsibility for the control of scheduled and legend drugs in her setting; she safeguards the patient against synergistic or antagonistic effects of medicine. She is an excellent resource for information about medicine and may be the only resource available for determining the action of a drug if it is new and, therefore, not described in any nursing unit references. If you question whether or not a patient should receive a medication based on a change in condition, and the patient's physician cannot be immediately contacted, a hospital pharmacist is an excellent person to contact for a knowledgeable opinion.

THE NURSE'S ROLE IN MEDICINE ADMINISTRATION

The nurse's role in medicine administration is to assess the patient's status prior to medicine administration (to determine whether his condition contradicts the administration), to store medication, to actively administer the medicine, to reassess the patient as to the medicine's effect, and to document or record the administration. Physicians, pharmacists, and nurses all should serve as role models for the safe administration of medicine.

Patient Assessment

Patient assessment prior to medicine administration is always important because a person's state of health may change significantly between the time a medicine is ordered and the time the medicine is administered. Perhaps the medicine is no longer necessary or may even have become unsafe. Morphine, for example, is a narcotic that is excellent for pain relief, however, it has a side effect of slowing respirations. At the time a physician orders it, the person's respiratory rate is 20 per minute (normal); 8 hours later, however, at the time you are about to administer the medication, you assess respirations and find them to be only 14 per minute. Giving the drug at this time, even though it has been ordered, might slow respirations to the point where the patient's oxygen exchange is seriously compromised.

On admission to a health care facility or when beginning care in an ambulatory setting, a medication history should be obtained as part of the person's total nursing history. A medication history should consist of information concerning medicine currently being taken and adverse or allergic reactions to medications. If an adverse or allergic response is reported, ask the person to describe it so the response can be evaluated as to severity (some people interpret side effects of drugs as adverse reactions). Most people do not think of vitamins, laxatives, cold remedies, antacids, or birth control pills as medicine so you need to ask about these specifically.

Ask about the use of illegal drugs as most people do not offer this information spontaneously. Many drugs are synergistic with alcohol or nicotine. Include a person's cigarette smoking and alcohol consumption habits in a medicine history. Vaccines and immunological agents are considered drugs. Ask if the patient has had any recent immunizations prior to the history taking.

If a person describes allergies to drugs, mark ALLERGIC TO (name of drug) on the front of the patient's record and in his nursing care plan. (Most agencies do this in red ink.) Most physicians appreciate if you attach a note to their order sheet that lists these drugs. Never give any medication to a patient without checking these places to see whether or not an allergy has been reported (see QRS 29-3).

In addition, assess swallowing ability, presence of nausea and vomiting, the condition of the most common injection sites (deltoid, anterior thigh, ventrogluteal muscles), and the condition of veins at the most common intravenous administration sites (dorsum of hands and antecubital space of elbow) to determine if medication administration by these routes will be contraindicated. Assess the condition of oral mucous membranes for comfort in taking oral medication.

APPROPRIATENESS OF DRUG

As part of daily patient assessment, include assessment for medicine appropriateness. In the assessment for whether or not a medicine is achieving the desired effect, a comment the person makes might be included ("I feel better since I started on penicillin"). Objective assessment measures may be used such as noticing increased range of motion in formerly stiffened joints.

If the medication being administered is an electrolyte supplement, such as potassium, or a medication that interferes with blood coagulation, you need to know the potassium level or clotting potential of blood before you can administer the next dose. In some instances, the physician's orders state the need to assess a laboratory report prior to administration. In other instances, the physician assumes that your level of knowledge is such that you should independently be aware of the necessity to do this.

Systems of Medicine Administration

The traditional system for medication administration in health care agencies has been a *stock supply system.* With this method, a nursing unit stocks various types of commonly administered medicine in the most common tablet, injection, or liquid strengths. It is the nurse's responsibility to calculate the correct dose of a medicine. At the proper time intervals, a patient's medicine is poured from the stock supply in the nursing unit. Unfortunately, stock supply systems tend to make it easier for a busy nurse to make a medicine error because stock bottles and vials tend to look alike. Stock supply systems are also disadvantageous because they are not cost effective; as medicine is outdated, it must be discarded even though a large amount may be wasted.

A more recently developed system of medicine administration that is rapidly being adopted is the *unit dose system.* With this system, few or no medications are kept on the nursing unit as "stock." Each patient's medicine is prepared in the pharmacy in individual packages. It is labeled and delivered to the nursing unit to be kept in individualized compartments for each patient. Unit dose systems are cost effective because usually only a 24-hour supply is sent to the nursing unit each time. Therefore, no medication is wasted. It has a low error rate because the calculation of correct dosages and amounts is done in the pharmacy and not on the nursing unit. (A pharmacist in a quiet environment whose only job that hour is to prepare patient medicine is much less apt to make a calculation error than a nurse who is preparing medicine as only one of many tasks.) Nurses save time with this method because they do not have to pour and calculate medication dosages. However, nurses still have the important responsibility of making sure that the appropriate prepackaged medicine is correctly administered to each patient. The unit dose system does have a disadvantage that does not occur with the stock supply system. If a dose is dropped on the floor so it cannot be used, or a new medication is ordered suddenly, no medicine is available until the pharmacy sends it to the nursing unit.

In a few health care facilities, self-administration medicine systems are utilized. With this type of system, a person's medications are kept in his patient unit and he takes them by self-administration. Self-administration is not applicable in all settings (a person who is hospitalized may be too ill to take responsibility for self-care); it is a useful method for encouraging people in long-term health care facilities to be responsible for self-care and achieve a feeling of participation in their care. As with all systems of administration, although the patient takes his own medication, the responsibility for seeing that it is taken rests with the nurse.

☐ QUICK REFERENCE STOP 29-3: SAFETY

Any person with an allergy to a drug should be advised to obtain a *Medic Alert* bracelet or necklace so that in an emergency, it will be obvious to his health caregivers that the allergy exists. Always look to see if such an emblem is present before administering medicine to an unconscious patient.

The minimal cost of securing a Medic Alert identifying emblem is tax deductible as a medical expense. To obtain an emblem or more information, write:

Medic Alert Foundation International
Turlock, CA 95380

Storage of Medication

Each hospital unit has a designated area for the storage of drugs. This might be an area in a centrally located wall cabinet or it might be a cart on wheels that rolls from room to room (Fig. 29-8). Medicine storage space should provide areas for drugs that must be refrigerated or kept from sunlight. If a self-administration

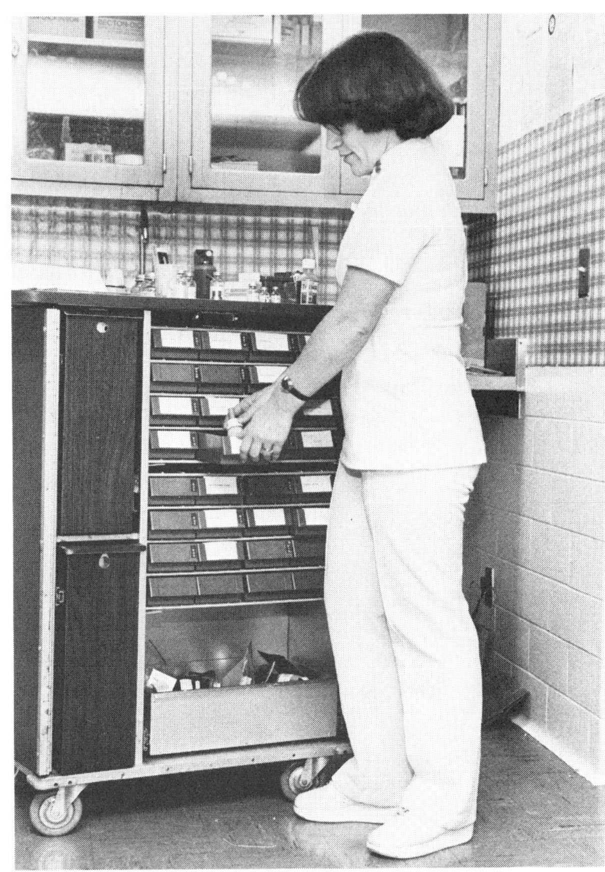

FIGURE 29-8. A medicine cart. Such a cart may be rolled from room to room to administer medicine. There is a separate drawer for each patient.

system is used, the patient's bedside stand or a special cabinet in his room will be used for his own medicine storage area. Separate cabinets are being designed in patient rooms in many new hospitals for use with unit dose systems that keep each person's medication separate. The door to the storage area must be kept locked at all times in order to prevent misuse of drugs.

Narcotics and controlled substances must be kept inside a double-locked cabinet. The keys to the cabinet should be in the possession of one of the designated nurses at all times. Every time a drug is removed from the cabinet, the name of the patient who received the drug, as well as the amount given, the time, and the names of the prescribing physician and the administering nurse, must be recorded in a designated record book. If a drug should accidentally be wasted (an oral tablet is dropped on the floor) or a patient refuses the drug, this information must be recorded also and the drug must be destroyed. Most institutions require that a second person witness the destruction of the medicine (crushed and flushed into a sink drain). Otherwise, the drug must be returned to the pharmacy to be destroyed.

The number of scheduled substances present in the cabinet must be counted at each change of nursing shift by the nurse who will be taking responsibility for these substances during the coming shift and the nurse who has been taking the responsibility and is going off duty. These nurses sign a narcotic drug record stating that they agree with the amount and type of drugs present. If there is a drug or an amount of a drug missing that cannot be accounted for, it must be reported to the nursing supervisor immediately. Storage and recording of the administration of scheduled drugs is under the authority of the federal government and these records are checked periodically as to their thoroughness and credibility.

Administration of Medicine

Administration of medicine consists of the proper preparation of the drug for administration, patient identification, and the actual administration.

DRUG PREPARATION

Medicines are commercially prepared in various forms. In order to prepare for the administration of medicine, you need to become acquainted with these differing forms. Table 29-5 summarizes them. Drug preparation consists of many steps including gaining knowledge about the drug, assessing drug appropriateness, calculating or confirming the dosage and amount, and preparing the drug.

Drug Knowledge. Before you can safely administer a drug, you need to know the classification or type of drug, range of safe dosage, method of administration, expected therapeutic effect, and known side effects and symptoms of overdose (toxicity). This information can be read in any standard drug reference. This step must not be overlooked.

Drug Appropriateness. You need to know the age and condition of the patient for whom the drug is intended (can he swallow a tablet? does he have acceptable injection sites?), his history of past response to the drug (has he had any untoward effects?), and his total plan of care. The total plan of care is important so you can appreciate how this one drug fits into his total therapy and what complementary procedures are needed with its administration (for example, darken room lights or put up side rails of bed).

Calculating Fractional Doses of Drugs. In a unit dose medication system, medicine comes prepared from the pharmacy with the correct dose. (If 50 mg of a medicine is desired, 50 mg of the drug is prepackaged for you and ready to be administered.) With stock medication systems (which are rapidly becoming obsolete), each dose of a drug must be calculated individually just before administration. (The bottle label says each ml contains 125 mg of the drug; if you desire 90 mg of the drug, how many ml will you administer?) In

TABLE 29-5. PREPARATION OF DRUGS

Type of Preparation	Description
Aqueous solutions	A medicine dissolved in a water base.
Syrup	A medicine dissolved in sugar and water (used to give a soothing, pleasant taste to medicine).
Suspension	Water is added to the dry drug form. Because the ingredients tend to separate, suspensions must always be shaken prior to use.
Emulsion	A suspension with an oil base.
Magma (milk)	A soluble suspension with a water base.
Spirit (essence)	A concentrated alcoholic solution of volatile substance. Because it is always a potent solution, the usual dosage will be small in amount.
Elixir	An aromatic alcoholic and potent preparation. The usual dosage will be small in amount.
Tincture	A potent solution with an alcoholic base. The usual dosage will be small in amount.
Tablet	A compressed, powdered drug that may be covered with an enteric-coating (causing it to dissolve in the intestine, not the stomach.).
Capsule	A drug encased in a gelatin form to disguise its taste or to allow for absorption in the intestine rather than the stomach.
Time-release capsules (spanules)	Capsules that contain a drug in a form that dissolves slowly to provide the drug's effect over a long time span.
Lozenges (troches)	A flat tablet held in the mouth to be dissolved.
Powders	A medication in a noncompressed form that must be mixed with a solution such as water before administration.
Powder, effervescent	A powder that foams as it is mixed with liquid. The foaming action disguises the taste of the drug.
Ampule	A sealed glass container that holds a single dose of medicine and is used for parenteral administration.
Vial	A glass container of medicine with a rubber stopper top. It is used for parenteral administration in single or multiple doses.
Suppository	A drug combined with a glycerin or cocoa butter base for rectal or vaginal insertion. The base melts at body temperature and releases the drug.
Ointment	A drug combined with an oil base to be used for external application.
Lotion	A drug combined with a water base to be used for external application.

emergency situations or with drugs that are not common enough to be supplied in every strength you need, you still have to calculate the correct dose just prior to administration, so you need to be able to do this with not only extreme accuracy, but with an acceptable degree of speed.

Systems of Weights and Measures. There are two systems of measurement currently in use in the United States: the *metric system* and the *apothecary system.* In order to calculate drug dosages, you must be familiar with both of these systems. At home, people make measurements with household containers, so in order to give people instructions about medicine taking at home, you must be familiar with household equivalents as well. Table 29-6 shows common weights and measurements.

METRIC SYSTEM. The metric system is a fairly new system of measurement, invented by the French in the 18th century. In the metric system, the *meter* is the basic unit of measurement for length, the *liter* is the basic unit of measurement for volume, and the *gram* is the basic unit of measurement for weight.

The metric system is easy to compute because it is a decimal system. The *meter* (m) is divided into *decimeters* (dm), 0.1 m; *centimeters* (cm), 0.01 m; and *millimeters* (mm), 0.001 m. The relationship of these is summarized in Table 29-6. All people admitted to a health care agency have their height measured in centimeters. It is frequently necessary to convert centimeters to inches if people ask you their height measurement. To convert from centimeters to inches, divide the number of centimeters by 2.5 (there are 2.5 cm to each inch). Blood pressure is an example of a measurement that is made in millimeters (of mercury).

The *liter* (l) is the amount of water contained in a cube 10 cm on each side; it contains 1000 cubic centimeters (cc), 10 cubic m. A liter can be divided into smaller divisions like the meter. The most commonly used division is a *milliliter* (ml), 0.001 L. This measurement is identical to the cubic centimeter so ml and cc are interchangeable terms. Interestingly enough, medication is usually ordered in mls, but syringes for measuring medication are scored in cc.

The *gram* (gm) is the basic dry measurement. It is comparable to a ml in liquid weight. Drugs may be ordered as grams or fractions of grams, usually milligrams (mg), 0.001 gm. People are weighed in kilograms (kg), 1000 gm.

It is often necessary to convert kg to pounds for patients who ask how much they weigh. To do this, multiply the number of kg by 2.2 (there are 2.2 pounds to a kg). The number of grams is written before the unit in

Arabic numerals (5 gm). The number of grains being ordered is written in Roman numerals after the unit (gr IV).

APOTHECARY SYSTEM. The apothecary system of measurement was inherited from the system of measurement in practice in England at the time the United States was colonized. The basic unit of weight in this system is the *grain* (g or gr), originally the weight of a grain of wheat. Heavier quantities are expressed in *drams*, *ounces*, or *pounds*. Pound (lb) is abbreviated for *libra*, the Latin word for "pound." Other divisions besides the grain or pound are not commonly used today because of the great danger that their symbols may be easily confused, resulting in drug error.

In the apothecary system, the basic fluid measurement is a *minim* (m), the quantity of water that would weigh a grain. Larger quantities are fluid *drams*, *pints*, *quarts*, and *gallons*.

Theoretically, a minim also equals a *drop* (gtt), abbreviated for the Latin *gutta*. However, in actual practice, because the viscosity of the fluid and the size of the dropper from which the liquid falls may vary the size of the drop, these measurements cannot be interchanged in medicine administration.

A summary of apothecary values are shown in Table 29-6.

HOUSEHOLD MEASUREMENTS. Household measurements are not accurate because manufacturers of items such as teaspoons, tablespoons, and cups are not required to meet strict measurements unless the tool is specifically designed as a measuring device. (A spoon called a dinner teaspoon may vary from as much as 5—20 ml.) In discussing household measurements, you must stress that you are talking about a measuring teaspoon or a measuring tablespoon, not just any teaspoon or tablespoon.

Comparison of household measurements to the metric system and apothecary system are shown in Table 29-7.

TABLE 29-6. COMMON WEIGHTS AND MEASUREMENTS

Metric System
Length
1 meter (m) = 1000 millimeters (mm)
1 meter (m) = 100 centimeters (cm)
1 centimeter (cm) = 10 millimeters (mm)
Liquid volume
1 liter (l) = 1000 milliliters (ml)
1 cubic centimeter (cc) = 1 milliliter (ml)
Weight
1 gram (gm) = 1000 milligrams (mg)
1000 grams (gm) = 1 kilogram (kg)

Apothecary system
Weight
1 dram (ʒ) = 60 grains (gr)
1 ounce (℥) = 8 drams (ʒ)
1 pound (lb) = 12 ounces (℥)
Liquid volume
1 fluid dram (fʒ) = 60 minims (m)
1 fluid ounce (f℥) = 8 fluid drams (f ʒ)
1 pint (pt) = 16 fluid ounces (f ℥)
1 quart (qt) = 2 pints (pt)
1 gallon (gal) = 4 quarts (qt)
1 minim (m) = 1 grain (gr)

Household measures
1 teaspoon = 5 milliliters (ml)
3 teaspoons (tsp) = 1 tablespoon (tbl)
6 fluid ounces (180 ml) = 1 cupful
8 fluid ounces (240 ml) = 1 glassful

DRUG DOSAGE COMPUTATION FOR DRUGS IN LIQUID FORM

One mathematical formula (equation) will enable you to calculate the correct drug dosage for an oral or parenteral drug. A traditional formula used to determine drug dosage is:

$$\frac{\text{strength desired (the quantity you want to administer)}}{\text{strength you have (the strength on the bottle label)}} \times \frac{\text{quantity desired}}{\text{quantity you have}} = \text{answer}$$

This formula is often abbreviated as:

$$\frac{D}{H} \times \frac{QD}{QH} = \text{answer}$$

A newer, quicker way to compute drug dosages is:

amount ordered × dose on hand = answer*

Suppose as an example, you have a medication prescription for Tylenol (acetaminophen) 90 mg. It is supplied 125 mg drug in 5 ml liquid. Calculate how much you would administer by the traditional formula.

$$\frac{\text{90 mg (strength you desire to give)}}{\text{125 mg (strength in which the drug is supplied or you have)}} \times \frac{\text{Y (unknown or what you are asking in ml)}}{\text{5 ml (the quantity that 125 mg is in)}}$$

TABLE 29-7. RELATIONSHIP OF METRIC TO APOTHECARY AND HOUSEHOLD SYSTEMS

Apothecary	Metric	Household
1 grain	60 mg	—
15—16 minims	1 ml = 1 gram	15 gtts
1 dram	5 ml	1 teaspoon
1/2 ounce	15 ml	1 tablespoon
1 ounce	30 ml	1 ounce
—	180 ml	1 cupful
—	240 ml	1 glassful
1 liter	1000 ml	1 quart

*Peery, H. E. Personal communication, 1983.

To solve this type of ratio or algebraic equation, you must cross multiply the top right number by the lower left, and the lower right number by the top left number.

125 × unknown Y = 450

The method for solving this type of algebraic equation is to divide the value of Y into the opposite half of the equation (450 ÷ 125). The answer to this equation is 3.6 ml; therefore, you would need to administer 3.6 ml of liquid to administer 90 mg of the drug.

To use the shorter formula, place the figures you have into their appropriate places in the formula.

amount ordered = 90 mg

dose on hand = 125 mg in 5 ml

Always put the number and unit of measurement representing the *amount ordered* in place first. When you place the *dose on hand* numbers, put them so the measurement unit on the bottom of the fraction matches the measurement unit of the *amount ordered* value (mg is on the top of the first fraction and on the bottom of the second fraction).

$$\frac{90\text{ mg}}{1} \times \frac{5\text{ ml}}{125\text{ mg}} = \text{answer}$$

Solve the problem by cancelling units and reducing to the lowest denominator.

$$\frac{\overset{18}{\cancel{90}}\text{ mg}}{1} \times \frac{\overset{1}{\cancel{5}}\text{ ml}}{\underset{\underset{5}{\cancel{25}}}{\cancel{125}}\text{ mg}} = \frac{18}{5} = 3.6\text{ ml}$$

The unit of measurement for the answer (ml) is always the unit of measurement stated on the top of the last fraction.

As mentioned previously, the same calculation process is used whether you are preparing a liquid medication to be given orally (as in the above example) or a liquid medication to be given with a syringe intramuscularly, subcutaneously, or intravenously.

For example, suppose you have a medication prescription for chloramphenicol 200 mg. The vial states there is 300 mg of drug to each 5 ml of fluid. Use the traditional formula to determine drug dosage.

$$\frac{200\text{ mg (strength you desire to give)}}{300\text{ mg (strength in which drug is supplied or you have)}} \times \frac{\text{Y (unknown or what you are asking in ml)}}{5\text{ ml (the quantity that 300 mg is in)}}$$

Cross multiply to clear the equation.

300 Y = 1000

Divide the value of Y into the opposite half of the equation.

1000 ÷ 300 = 3.3

You would inject 3.3 ml to administer 200 mg of the drug. The same problem may be solved using the shorter formula.

$$\frac{200\text{ mg (amount ordered)}}{1} \times \frac{5\text{ ml}}{300\text{ mg}}\ \text{(dose on hand)} = \text{answer}$$

Solve the equation.

$$\frac{\overset{2}{\cancel{200}}\text{ mg}}{1} \times \frac{5\text{ ml}}{\underset{3}{\cancel{300}}\text{ mg}} = \frac{10}{3} = 3.3\text{ ml}$$

Developing the ability to solve mathematical problems like these may take practice. Appendix H contains more medication problems and their solutions. If solving these problems is difficult for you, take some time to work through a number of problems. Learning mathematical computations in a step by step manner will enable you to administer medication dosages safely.

Drug Dosage Computation for Tablets and Capsules. Calculating the correct drug dosage for drugs in the form of tablets or capsules presents a slightly different problem. You must determine how many tablets or half tablets to administer rather than how much liquid you will pour.

Suppose, as an example, you have a prescription order for a medication for 120 mg. You have tablets available that contain 40 mg each. How many tablets would you need to administer to equal 120 mg? As with liquid measures, substitute the amounts you have into the standard or shortened formulas.

$$\frac{120\text{ mg (strength you desire to give)}}{40\text{ mg (the strength of tablet you have)}} \times \frac{\text{Y (unknown or what you are asking)}}{1\text{ tablet (the quantity that 40 mg is in)}}$$

Cross multiply and divide the value of Y into the opposite half of the equation.

40 Y = 120

Y = 120 ÷ 40

Y = 3

3 tablets of this particular medication equals 120 mg.

The same problem may be solved with the shorter formula.

$$\frac{120\text{ mg (amount ordered)}}{1} \times \frac{1\text{ tablet}}{40\text{ mg}}\ \text{(dose on hand)} = \text{answer}$$

$$\frac{\overset{3}{\cancel{120}}\text{ mg}}{1} \times \frac{1}{\underset{1}{\cancel{40}}\text{ mg}} = 3\text{ tablets}$$

CONVERTING FROM DIFFERENT MEASUREMENT SYSTEMS

Calculating correct medication dosages grows more complicated when a physician orders a drug in one system of measurement (apothecary) and the pharmacist dispenses it to you in another system (metric or household). For example, suppose you have a drug prescription to administer atropine sulfate gr 1/300 and the ampule that is supplied to you contains 1 mg of atropine sulfate in each 1 ml. You cannot calculate drug dosages until you convert the strengths into the same system. Memorize the two conversion factors that you will use 95% of the time: gr 1 = 60 mg and 1/60 gr = 1 mg.

To use a conversion factor with the traditional system, set up the standard formula: D/H × QD/QH.

$$\frac{\text{grain 1/300 (strength you desire)}}{\text{grain 1 (the strength you have or the conversion factor you know)}} \times \frac{\text{Y (unknown or what you are asking in mg)}}{\text{60 mg (the second half of the conversion factor you know)}}$$

To solve the equation, cross multiply and divide the value of Y into the opposite half of the equation.

$$1\text{Y} = \frac{1}{\underset{5}{\cancel{300}}} \times \frac{\overset{1}{\cancel{60}}}{1} = \frac{1}{5}$$

Milligrams are expressed as decimals, not fractions, so change this fraction to a decimal by dividing the denominator into the numerator (5 into 1). Y = 0.2 mg. Fitting this number back into your original equation gives you grain 1/300 = 0.2 mg. You now have drug desired and drug supplied dosages in the metric system. Now solve the problem using the standard formula:

$$\frac{\text{0.2 mg (strength you desire; formerly grain 1/300)}}{\text{1 mg (strength you have)}} \times \frac{\text{Y (unknown or what you are asking in mg)}}{\text{1 ml (the quantity that 1 mg is in)}}$$

Solve the equation by cross multiplying and dividing the value of Y into the opposite half of the equation or Y = 0.2. In order to administer grains 1/300 of atropine sulfate you would need to administer 0.2 ml of solution.

To convert from one system of measurement using the shorter formula, incorporate the conversion into the formula or state the formula as:

amount ordered × conversion factor × dose on hand = answer

As before, always place the amount ordered first. Place the conversion factor second, with the unit of measurement stated in the amount ordered on the bottom of the conversion factor (top to bottom); place the numbers of the dose on hand last.

Once again, you want to administer gr 1/300 of atropine sulfate. The ampule you have supplies 1 mg in 1 ml. The conversion factor you need is (gr i = 60 mg).

$$\underset{\text{amount ordered}}{\frac{\text{gr i}}{300}} \times \underset{\text{conversion factor}}{\frac{60\text{ mg}}{\text{gr i}}} \times \underset{\text{dose on hand}}{\frac{1\text{ ml}}{1\text{ mg}}} = \frac{1}{5} = 0.2\text{ ml}$$

Notice that in this formula, the grains quantity of the amount ordered is on top and the grains amount of the conversion factor is on the bottom. The mg measurement is on the top of the conversion factor; therefore it is on the bottom of the dose on hand factors. The unit of measurement at the top of the dose on hand fraction is the unit of measurement of the answer.

DRUGS PREPARED IN UNITS

Some parenteral medications, such as antibiotics, are ordered and dispensed in USP *(United States Pharmacopeia)* units rather than metric or apothecary measurements. Suppose, for example, you have a drug order for 200,000 units of penicillin. The vial states that each milliliter of solution contains 1,000,000 units. To solve this problem, use the standard formula:

$$\frac{\text{200,000 units (strength you desire)}}{\text{1,000,000 units (strength you have)}} \times \frac{\text{Y (unknown or what you are asking in ml)}}{\text{1 ml (the amount that 1,000,000 units is in)}}$$

To solve the equation, cross multiply and divide the value of Y into the opposite half of the equation.

$$1{,}000{,}000\text{ Y} = 200{,}000$$

$$\text{Y} = 200{,}000 \div 1{,}000{,}000$$

$$\text{Y} = 0.2\text{ ml}$$

In order to administer 200,000 units of penicillin, you would administer 0.2 ml of solution.

Using the shorter formula:

amount ordered × dose on hand

$$\frac{\overset{1}{\cancel{200{,}000}}\text{ units}}{1} \times \frac{1\text{ ml}}{\underset{5}{\cancel{1{,}000{,}000}}\text{ units}} = \frac{1}{5} = 0.2\text{ ml}$$

INSULIN DOSAGES

At one time, insulin was supplied in different strengths and some calculation for dosage was necessary. Now, insulin is supplied in a standard strength of 100 units per 1 ml. Insulin is always administered in an insulin syringe (the only type of syringe that offers enough accuracy for this extremely sensitive drug). With the use of a U-100 insulin syringe, no calculation of dosage is necessary. If the physician's order is for 10 units of insulin, you measure 10 units on the syringe; if the order is for 40 units, you measure 40 units, etc.

PARENTERAL SOLUTIONS FROM TABLETS

At one time, medicine for injection was supplied as a sterile tablet. This tablet had to be dissolved in sterile water before the amount of the dissolved solution that would comprise the correct dose could be determined. Such a system often led to contaminated injection solutions or, if medicine did not completely dissolve in the water, inaccurate dosages despite correct calculations. Dissolving tablets (called *titrated* tablets) are no longer used today, so it is unnecessary to learn this form of calculation. Dissolving tablets are interesting from a historical standpoint only.

STRENGTHS OF SOLUTIONS

At one time, solutions such as weak antibiotic solutions for wound irrigation, were furnished in stock strengths (perhaps 100%). In order to use them in the strength ordered (perhaps a 10% solution), you would need to calculate how much diluent is needed to dilute the solution to the required strength. Today pharmacists take responsibility for preparing and dispensing correct strength solutions for instillations and irrigations. There is one instance, however, in which you still need to use this form of calculation. It is used to calculate how many calories a person is receiving in intravenous fluid. This is particularly important when the person is receiving his entire nutritional intake by an intravenous route (total parenteral nutrition).

To solve this type of problem, you need to determine how many grams of carbohydrate are being administered. A 5% solution of glucose in water, for example, means that there are 5 ml of dissolved carbohydrate (glucose) for every 100 ml of solution. In a 1000 ml bottle of a 5% solution of glucose in water, there is 50 ml of dissolved carbohydrate (5% of 1000 ml).

A gram of carbohydrate yields 4 kilocalories (kcal) when it is metabolized in the body. One gram equals one milliliter (Table 29-7); therefore, 50 ml of carbohydrate are also 50 gm of carbohydrate (the difference between a wet and dry form). Use the standard formula to find the caloric value.

$$\frac{\text{Y (unknown or what you are asking in gm)}}{\text{4 kcal (strength you know)}} \times \frac{\text{50 gm (amount you desire to know about)}}{\text{1 gm (amount 4 kcal is in)}}$$

Y = 200 kcal. Therefore, each 1000 ml of 5% glucose/water solution a person receives supplies 200 kcal. Using the shorter formula:

amount ordered × dose on hand = answer

$$\frac{50\text{ gm}}{1} \times \frac{4\text{ kcal}}{1\text{ gm}} = 200\text{ kcal}$$

Converting Milliliters to Minims. Many times when you are preparing medication for intravenous or intramuscular injections, the amount of solution you will be drawing up is very small (for example, 0.2 ml). In some instances, it is easier to measure in minims than in ml to view your measurement more clearly on the syringe.

This type of conversion may be illustrated with the penicillin problem used earlier. The order is for 200,000 units of penicillin. It is supplied as 1,000,000 units per 1 ml. What is the equivalent measure in minims? In order to solve this problem you need a conversion factor (15 minims = 1 ml). It is important to remember that you must determine how many ml to administer before you convert to minims. The conversion factor is used at the end of the formula.

amount ordered × dose on hand × conversion factor = answer

$$\frac{\overset{1}{\cancel{200{,}000}}\text{ units}}{1} \times \frac{1\text{ ml}}{\underset{5}{\cancel{1{,}000{,}000}}\text{ units}} \times \frac{15\text{ minims}}{1\text{ ml}} = \frac{15}{5} = 3\text{ minims}$$

Notice that, as always, the unit of measurement at the top of the first fraction is at the bottom of the second; the unit of measurement at the top of the second fraction is at the bottom of the third fraction; the unit of measurement at the top of the last fraction is the unit of measurement of the answer.

General Rules For Calculations

Calculating drug dosages may be hard for you if you have difficulty with mathematics. Drug dosage calculations will become easier with practice. Using the shortened formula omits steps and simplifies the procedure.

Never be embarrassed to ask for help with a drug dosage calculation. Administering a wrong dosage could affect a patient's safety. Feel free to consult the hospital pharmacist for help in calculating dosages; he is as interested in patient safety as you are. Question all dosages that seem excessive after calculation (a person would have to swallow 10 tablets, for example, in order to take the correct dose) or so small that the dosage would be lost in a syringe (0.001 ml). Physicians may have calculated incorrectly when they wrote the drug prescription or they may have been unaware of the strength the health care agency would supply and so did not appreciate the difficulty of the calculation.

In most instances when a conversion is required, gr 1 = 60 mg or 1/60 gr = 1 mg is the conversion factor needed. In order to convert to household measurements, the two conversion factors usually needed are 1 teaspoon = 5 ml and 1 tablespoon = 15 ml. Drug calculation may not seem so frightening if you remember that, although there are over 25,000 substances listed as medication in the *United States Pharmacopeia*, there is only one formula and a minimum number of conversion factors that solve all dosage calculations for the 25,000 substances.

CHILDREN'S DOSAGES

At one time, various formulas that used an adjusted adult dose of a drug after taking into consideration the child's age or weight were used as the basis for prescribing children's medicine. These formulas often resulted in excessive or inadequate dosage of drugs for children because there is a big difference in the size of children at any one age, and it is not true that dosage for children is merely a proportion of adult dosages (children are more than just small adults). Because of a child's more rapid metabolism, a drug may be ordered in a greater dose per pound of body weight for a child than it would be for an adult.

Today these formulas have been replaced by the more accurate method of comparing the recommended drug manufacturer dose per pound of body weight or surface area of the child (obtained from height and weight) with the actual weight or surface area of the child. A nomogram is used for determining surface area. To determine surface area from a nomogram, find the child's height in column one and his weight in column three. Draw a line between these two points; the number that the line crosses in column two is the child's body surface area.

If, for example, the recommended dosage of a drug is 50 mg per pound of body weight every 24 hours and a child weighs 10 pounds, he should receive 500 mg (50 × 10) of the drug every 24 hours (probably given in 3 to 4 divided doses depending on the particular drug).

If a newborn is 21 inches tall and weighs 7 lbs, his body surface area would be 0.2 m^2. If the recommended dosage of a drug is 50 mg per 1 m^2, the newborn would receive 10 mg (0.2 × 50), probably given in 3 to 4 divided doses depending on the particular drug.

THE SEVEN "RIGHTS"

Basic rules for safe medication administration traditionally include five "rights," namely, "right drug, right dosage, right route of administration, right time, and right patient." All people should know the reason they are taking medication, and therefore, a sixth right should be added to this list. The right to refuse medication should be added as a seventh right in honor of a patient's right to decide.

To determine that you have the right drug, check the name of the medicine against the prescription for the drug. If the physician's order is unclear, have it clarified in order to avoid gross medication errors. If this is the first time the drug is to be administered, you should use the original physician's order. Otherwise, you may use the copied medication card or Kardex system. Read the label of the medicine three times: (1) when you select the drug, (2) when you pour the drug or remove a tablet from a container, and (3) when the bottle is returned to the shelf or before you throw away a disposable container.

To be certain that you have the right dosage, compare the dosage of the tablet or liquid with the dosage written on the prescription. Some medications may be toxic if given in wrong dosages. Thus, some health care facilities ask you to double check these dosages with another nurse before administration.

To ensure that you have the right route of administration, look one more time at the prescription source. Medications are available in a variety of forms and are not interchangeable.

To be certain that you have the correct time, recheck either the prescription or the nursing care plan. Medications are prescribed either to be given at specified times of the day or by the number of times they should be administered each day. When drugs are ordered by the number of times they are to be administered each day, the nurse establishes the times that medication will be given. She needs to be aware of specific drug actions in order to determine the best time of day to administer the drug (for example, before meals). Typical times for medication administration are shown in Table 29-8 (see App. E for further explanation).

Medicine must be given "on time" so that a therapeutic blood level is maintained. Given too early, excessive drug levels might be reached; given too late, low dosages and inadequate effects may result. Medication is considered "on time" if it is given within a half hour time period of the administration time (a 10:00 A.M. medication could be given as early as 9:30 A.M. and as late as 10:30 A.M.).

In order to determine that you have the right patient, check the name on the prescription source with the

TABLE 29-8. ROUTINE DRUG ADMINISTRATION TIMES

Abbreviation	Times
BID	9 A.M., 9 P.M.
TID	10 A.M., 2 P.M., 6 P.M.
QID	10 A.M., 2 P.M., 6 P.M., 10 P.M.
qd	10 A.M.
q12h	12 noon and 12 midnight or 8 A.M. and 8 P.M.
q6h	6 A.M., 12 noon, 6 P.M., 12 midnight
q2h	10 A.M., 12 noon, 2 P.M., 4 P.M., 6 P.M., 8 P.M., 10 P.M., 12 midnight, 2 A.M., 4 A.M., 6 A.M., 8 A.M.

patient's identification band prior to administering the drug (Fig. 29-9). Do not use the name tag on a bed or on the room door instead of the arm band. A person may be sitting on the wrong bed or have had his room transferred without your knowledge. Do not ask the patient his name by saying it (Are you Mr. Jones?). Under stress and strain, his perception may be distorted and he may answer incorrectly. If a person has no arm band, ask another nurse to verify his identification. Be extremely careful when there are two patients with the same name on a nursing unit.

Always watch a patient swallow his medicine. Do not leave medication at the bedside for a patient to take later. Some patients will forget to take it; some patients may discard it because they do not like the taste. Another patient coming into the room may take it believing it was meant for him. If a patient is not in his room when you bring the medicine, return it to the medicine preparation area and bring it to the patient at a later time. If you leave medication on a medicine preparation counter, be certain that you leave the medication's identity (the medicine card) with it. If necessary, write the patient's name, room number, drug name, and dosage on a piece of adhesive tape and anchor the medicine cup or syringe to the medication tray or counter (Fig. 29-10). Be certain that you keep medication only temporarily and always in a safe area where it will be out of the reach of other patients and not be contaminated.

Right to Know. Today it is widely recognized that patients have the right to know about any therapy prescribed for them. They are more apt to cooperate and comply with medical personnel if they understand the importance of their therapy and the actions of the drugs.

Right to Refuse. If a person refuses a medication, explore with him his reason for refusing it. In most instances, a patient refuses medicine because of a lack of information. Offering the reason for and the benefits of the medicine is generally all that is necessary for a person to change his mind about medicine administration.

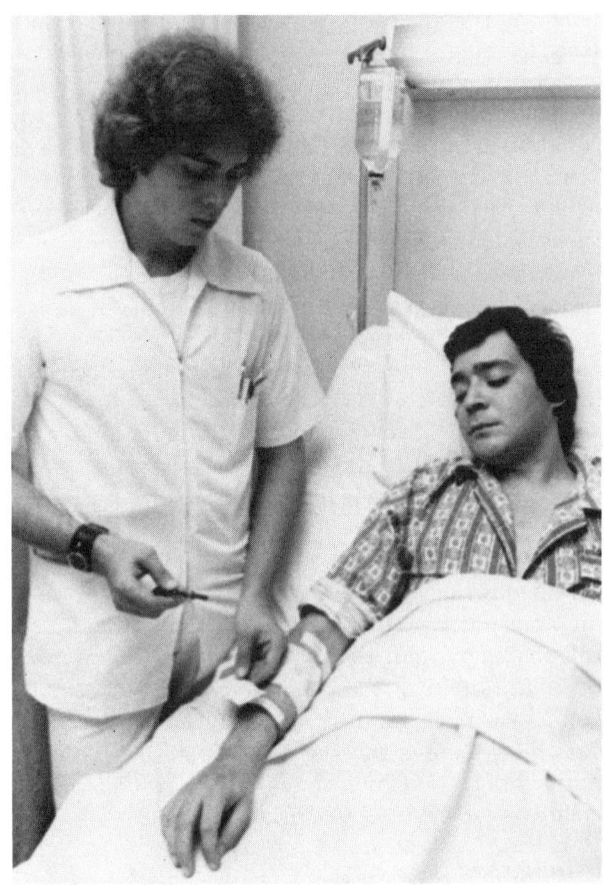

A

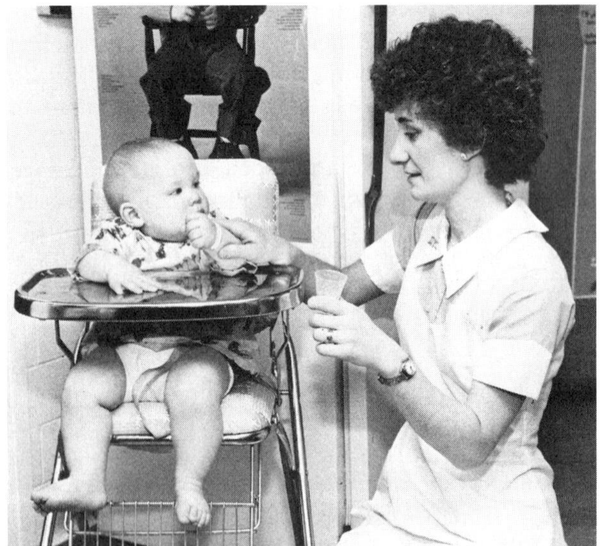

B

FIGURE 29-9. Always check the name on the prescription source with the identification band of the patient—adult (A) or child (B)—just prior to administering the drug.

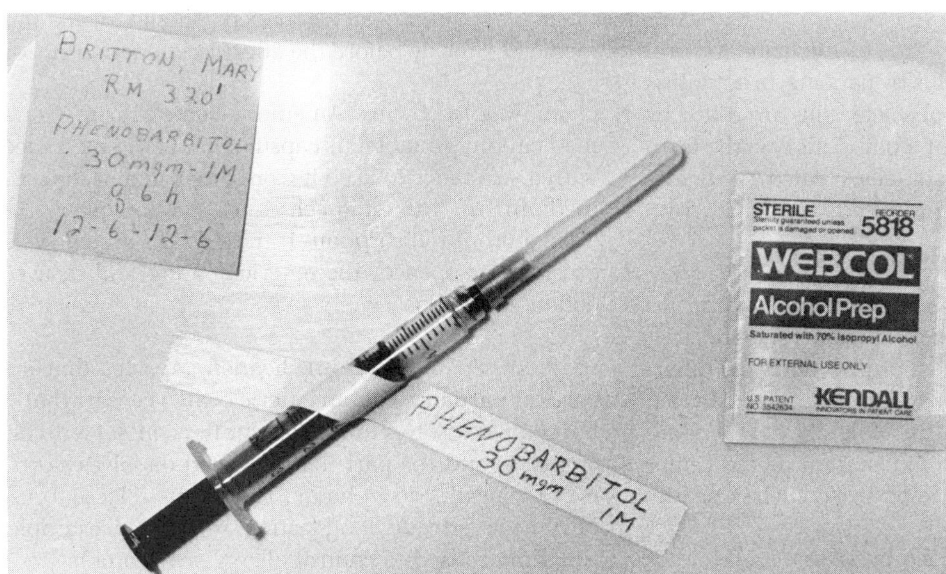

FIGURE 29-10. To save this injectable medicine, take a piece of adhesive tape (write the name of the drug and dosage), and tape the syringe to the medicine tray. Notice that the medicine card remains on the tray to identify the patient and his room number.

Sometimes a person refuses a medicine because an oral capsule or tablet is difficult to swallow, or a liquid medicine tastes bitter. Crushing tablets or offering "chasers" to go with the medicine may solve these problems. If the medicine cannot be modified into an acceptable form for administration, consult with the person's physician about an alternate form that is acceptable.

If a patient feels that his prognosis is poor, he may refuse medicine (I'm going to die anyway so what's the use?). If this is the reason for refusal, the patient should discuss his prognosis with his physician to be certain this is an accurate assessment.

Some people refuse medication because they are afraid that they may have an allergic or other untoward response to it. Listen carefully to statements about allergic responses. On admission to a health care facility, a person may be under stress and forget he once had an allergic reaction to a drug. When he hears the name of the drug or sees the capsule, he may remember a past response. Postpone the drug administration until it can be better determined if an allergic response was present.

Patients sometimes refuse medicine because they do not experience instant results from it and, thus, do not believe it is helping them. Tetracycline, for example, an antibiotic prescribed to help clear facial acne, must be taken for almost two weeks before improvement can be seen. (Many people stop taking it before this time and never see results.) Explaining the action and effect of the medicine helps to improve compliance.

If a medication is refused, record the reason for refusal. The patient's physician should be told immediately that a dose was omitted. A time delay in medication administration may lead to detrimental results.

EVALUATION OF MEDICINE EFFECTIVENESS

Because people may have idiosyncratic effects from medicine administration and because abnormal absorption, distribution, utilization, and excretion of drugs can occur, all people receiving medication need to be monitored to be certain that the drug's action is adequate and that no untoward reactions are occurring.

CHARTING MEDICATION

Medicine should be charted as being administered only after it actually has been administered. Do not chart it at the time of preparation because you have no assurance at that point that the person is going to take the medication. Also, when you assess a patient's condition just prior to administration, you may decide that some factor is present that makes medicine administration inappropriate.

Different health care agencies use different systems to record medicine administration. The information to be recorded, however, is basically the same in all agencies and includes the name of the drug, the dosage, route of administration, time of administration, and if it was injected, the site of injection. Some systems provide forms that only require you to fill in your initials in the appropriate space that lists the time of administration.

Oral Medication

Oral medication is the most common form of medicine administered because it is economic and convenient. Medicine for oral administration is available in either solid or liquid forms.

SOLID FORMS

Although almost all solid forms of medicine for oral administration are called pills by patients, in actuality, the use of the term *pills* is obsolete. Pills are rolled by hand and are in the shape of a ball. This was the form used when a pharmacist actually created medicines rather than using mass-produced medicine from pharmaceutical companies.

Tablets. Drugs are pressed into tablet forms and may be different shapes. They can be triangular, octagonal, or round. They typically are stamped with the pharmaceutical company initials or a code number that makes it possible to identify the tablet. Most tablets are scored or marked with an indentation at the center point that allows the tablet to be broken in half neatly.

Capsules. Capsules are formed by pressing a liquid or powder into a gelatin mold. Drugs prepared in this manner generally are those that are bitter tasting (the gelatin capsule conceals the taste). Because of this, capsules should never be chewed. If opened to ease administration, the powder or liquid usually must be mixed with something like applesauce to disguise its taste. Capsules are color-coded and often stamped with a code number that allows them, like tablets, to be identified easily. Figure 29-11 shows a capsule, a scored tablet, and a tablet.

Lozenges or Troches. Lozenges or troches are tablets designed to be held in the mouth until they dissolve. The medication is absorbed across the mucous membrane of the mouth. Medicine that would be destroyed by stomach acid or medicine that is designed to be absorbed slowly or have a local therapeutic effect are put into lozenge form.

Powder. A powder is a medication packaged in its loose, noncompressed form. In order for it to be administered, it must be mixed with a liquid or food. Calcium is often packaged this way.

Effervescent Powders and Tablets. These foam as they are mixed with liquid. Effervescent action can mask a medicine's bitter taste; a patient should drink this medicine quickly before the effervescent action stops.

FIGURE 29-11. Capsules, scored tablets, and tablets are forms of medicine for oral administration.

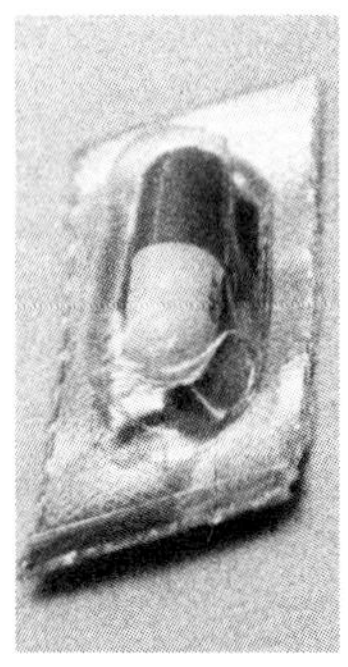
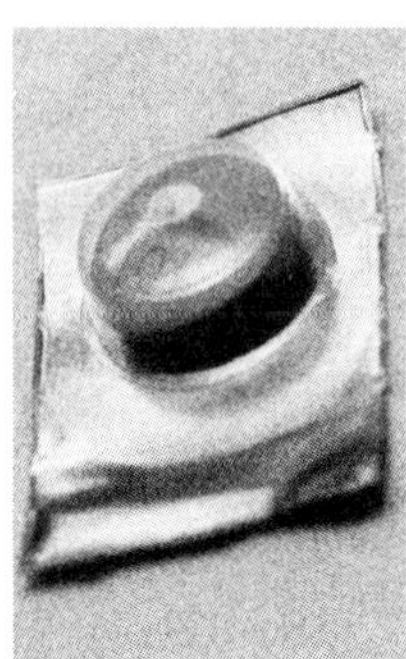
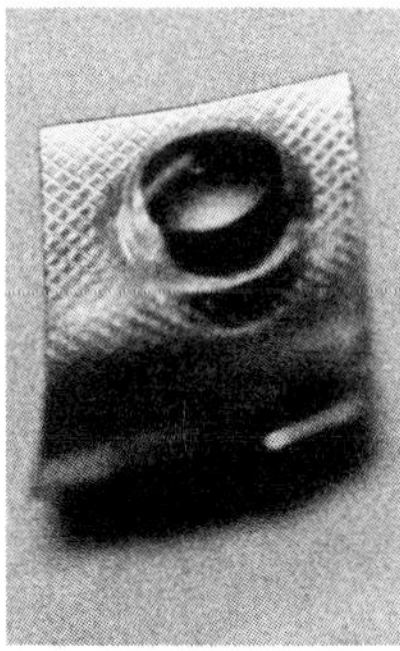

Enteric-Coated Forms. An enteric-coated form of oral medication is a tablet or capsule that has been coated with a substance to keep it from dissolving in the acid medium of the stomach and passing into the duodenum for absorption. If these forms are chewed, crushed, or opened, the enteric coating and delayed action will be lost.

Spanules. Spanules are medication capsules that are covered partially with an enteric coat. The part that is not coated dissolves immediately after contact with the stomach, and the part that is coated dissolves slowly over the next 12 to 24 hours. These time-release forms effectively provide long-lasting relief (for example, medication used to control allergy symptoms).

LIQUID FORMS

Liquid forms of oral medication are used when the person has difficulty swallowing solid forms or when a particular medication action is complemented by being administered in a liquid form. Medicine is often administered to children in this form but it is not unusual to find an adult who prefers liquid forms (Fig. 29-12). Liquid forms usually are flavored with a syrup (strawberry, raspberry) to give them a pleasant taste.

Solutions. Solutions are mixtures of medication dissolved in water. A solution may have a bitter aftertaste, so the person may want a "chaser" of something such as orange juice following the drinking of the solution.

Suspension. A suspension is a mixture of medicines in which the ingredients separate. A *magma* is a thick suspension with water as a base; an *emulsion* has an oil base. Suspensions must be shaken well before administration or improper drug dosages may result. Phenytoin (Dilantin), for example, is an anticonvulsant medication. if you do not shake the bottle well before pouring a dose, the person will receive a dilute dosage of medicine from the top of the bottle that will not control his convulsions. The dosage from the bottom of the bottle will be very strong and could produce toxic effects.

An *elixir,* a *spirit,* a *fluid extract,* and a *tincture* are medicines dissolved in an alcohol base. These mixtures are heavily concentrated and, therefore, usually are administered in very small dosages.

A *syrup* is a medicine dissolved in a sugar and water base. Syrups are used for a soothing local effect or to disguise the taste of a bitter-tasting medication. Because they taste so sweet and tend to be sticky, a person may desire a "chaser" of water or orange juice following administration. However, drinking water immediately after administration of cough syrup might destroy its soothing effect.

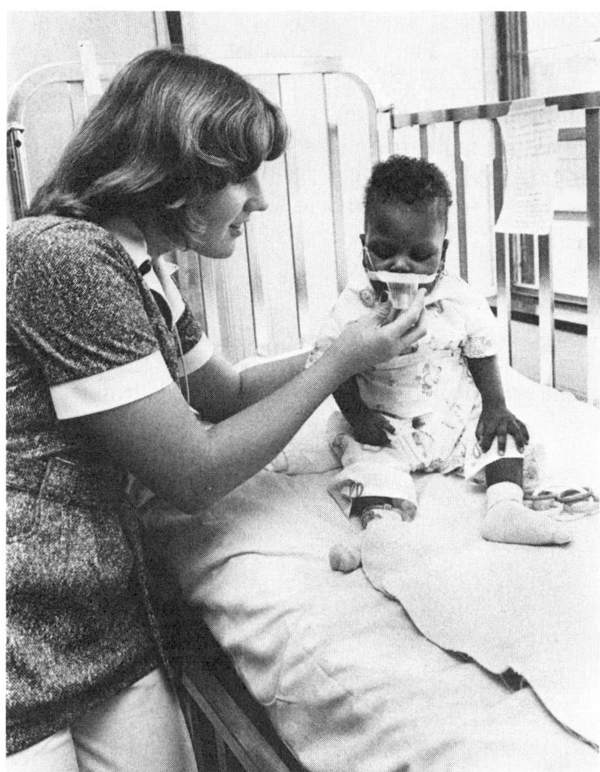

FIGURE 29-12. Administration of medicine in liquid form to a child. Adults (particularly older adults) may prefer or need a liquid form.

CONTRAINDICATIONS TO ORAL MEDICATIONS

Although oral medications are the most convenient form of medicine, they can also be dangerous. Oral medication cannot be used if a person's swallowing ability is impaired (for example, from unconsciousness). Giving an oral medication under such circumstances may cause aspiration (fluid entering the trachea), a potentially lethal state. Oral medicine administration may be contraindicated if mouth trauma is present because of the inability to swallow or irritation of the traumatized tissue. It is contraindicated if nausea or vomiting is present because it cannot be retained long enough to be absorbed. If a person is receiving no fluid or food by mouth, oral medications also are prohibited.

Administration of Oral Medication

Administration of oral medicine requires clean, not sterile technique. To follow a safe rule of medicine administration, choose the container of medicine from a stock collection or the patient's unit dose storage area and read the label for name, dose, and route of administration three times: (1) as you select the bottle or package, (2) just before you pour it or open the package, and (3) as you return the stock bottle to the shelf or dispose of the package.

To remove tablets or capsules from a stock bottle, use the lid of the vial to prevent the flow of too much medication so that only the number of tablets or capsules desired will enter the lid (Fig. 29-13).This tech-

FIGURE 29-13. Taking tablets from a stock bottle with the lid of the bottle prevents the removal of too many tablets.

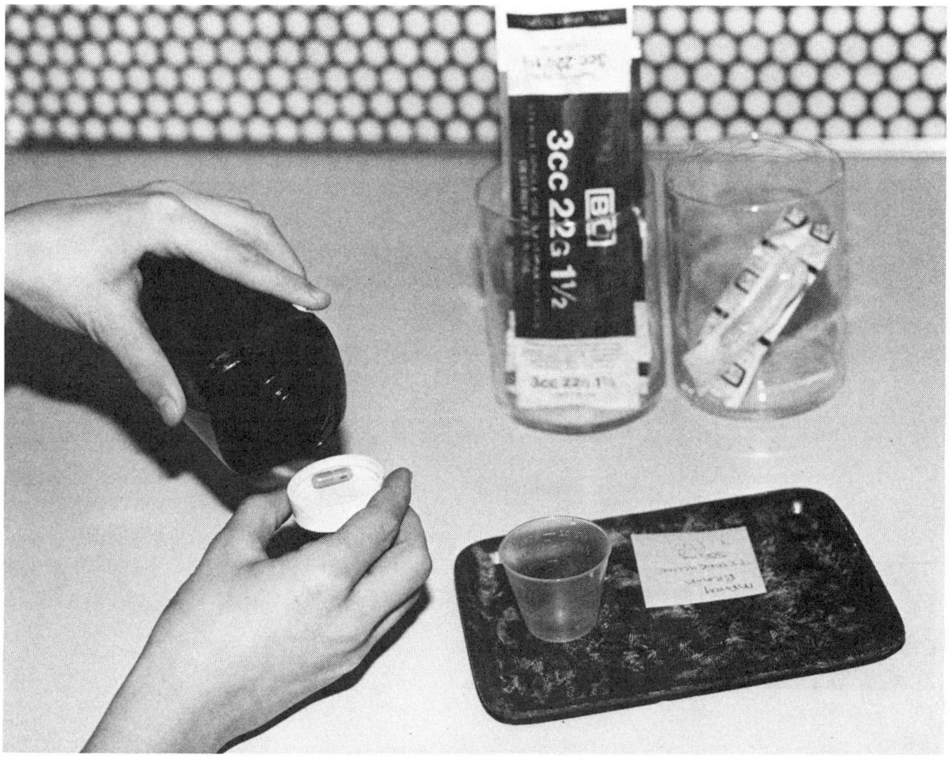

nique is better than allowing extra unwanted tablets or capsules to pour into the medicine cup because you should never return medicine to a stock bottle. Two reasons not to return medicine to a stock bottle are: (1) accidental return of the medicine to the wrong bottle and (2) possibility of contaminating the stock supply with bacteria (a medicine cup is clean, not sterile). Never pour tablets or capsules into your hand because your hand is very heavily contaminated with bacteria.

Assess whether the person will be able to swallow the medicine without it being modified in some way. Medicine stations should have a commercial tablet crusher or a mortar and pestle to crush tablets (Fig. 29-14A). If one is not available, you can crush tablets between two spoons (a technique you teach people to use at home). Placing a tablet between two medicine souffle cups and pressing down on the top cup with a solid object (for example, a spoon) is a method that prevents a tablet from splattering as it is crushed (Fig. 29-14B). Crushed tablets are often mixed with fruit flavors of baby food because most people enjoy the taste.

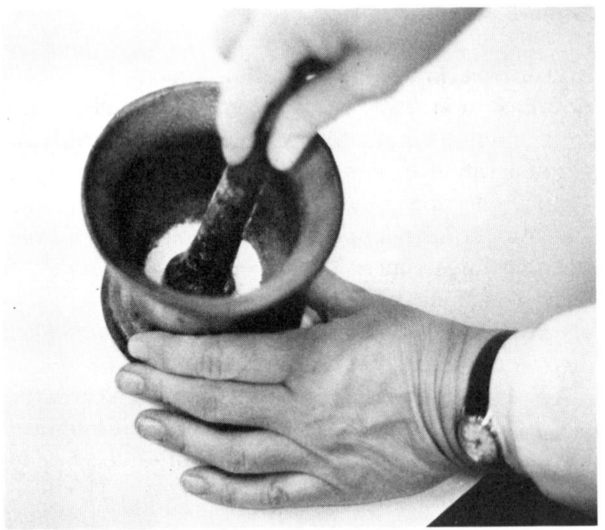

A

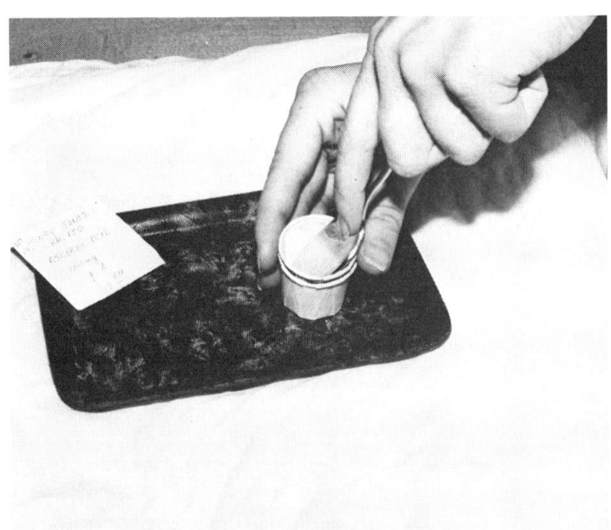

B

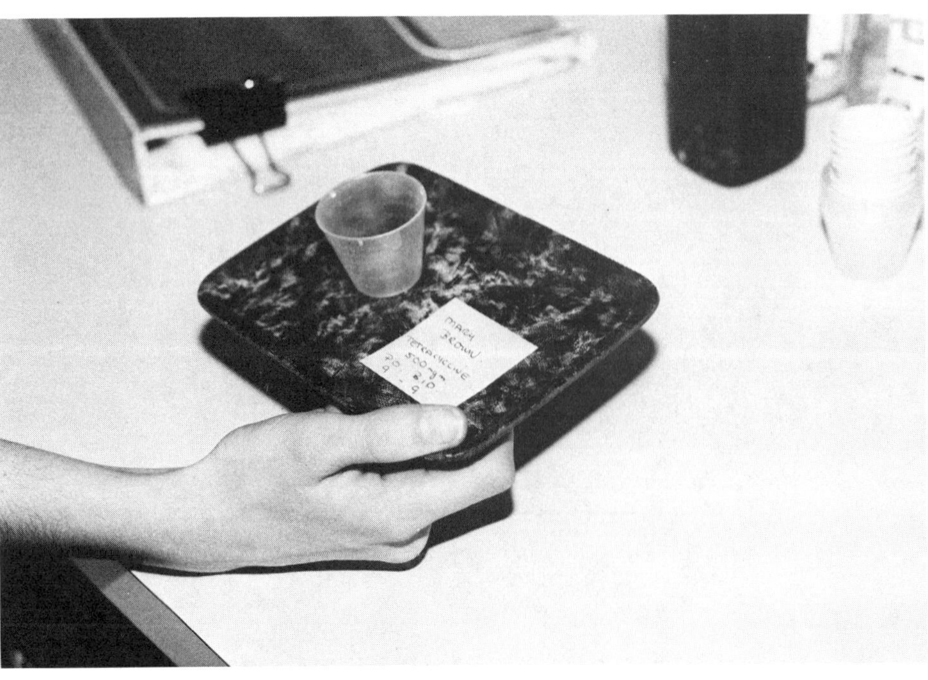

C

FIGURE 29-14. A. A tablet crusher or, as shown here, mortar and pestle may be used to crush tablets for easier administration. B. You can crush a tablet held between two souffle medicine cups. C. Carrying medicine on a medicine tray ensures you of a professional appearance.

Evaluate whether the tablet is one that can be crushed safely. If enteric-coated, crushing and releasing the medicine from its shell destroys the delayed action and probably changes the effect of the medicine. As a rule of thumb, capsules should not be opened. The substance in most capsules tastes bitter so its taste is not easily disguised; time release forms may lose their time release properties if separated from the capsule.

If enteric or time release capsules have been ordered and cannot be swallowed, notify the person's physician. She may want to change the medicine order to a nonenteric or nontime release form. Time release forms of medicine are ordered for long time intervals (12 to 24 hours); without a time release form, the medicine may need to be ordered at more frequent intervals in order to achieve optimal effects.

Scored tablets may be broken in half. Hold the tablet between your two thumbs and fingers (place a clean piece of gauze or paper towel between the tablet and your hands to keep the tablet clean), and put pressure on the tablet with both thumbs to snap it in two. It it does not snap readily, you can score it deeper with a sterile scalpel blade. Do not attempt to break tablets that are not scored. They do not break cleanly and your dosage will be only an approximation and not accurate. If you cannot prepare an accurate dose without breaking a nonbreakable tablet, consult the pharmacist or the person's physician (a workable drug prescription should be the responsibility of the prescribing or dispensing person).

There is sometimes a question as to how many different types of medicine you can place together in a patient's medicine cup. All of the tablets and capsules that will be taken together can be placed together in the same medicine cup. However, any medication that requires a special assessment check before administration (you must first count pulse or respirations, examine a laboratory report) must not be added to a medicine cup with other medicine. Once added, it would be easy to forget that some specific action before administration is necessary. Placing each type of tablet a person may be receiving in a separate cup is not cost efficient (a person on an acute therapy service might receive 5 or 6 different types of medication requiring 5 or 6 different medicine cups) and may be overwhelming to a person (12 tablets in one medicine cup seems less than 6 medicine cups with 2 tablets in each). Urge the person to swallow tablets or capsules one at a time so that if he should choke and cough and thereby destroy a medication, you know exactly what he has taken and which one to replace.

If the person will be able to chew or swallow the tablet whole, but it will leave a bitter aftertaste, provide a glass of iced or acid (fruit juice) liquid if desired to take immediately afterward. If you have no reason to believe the medication will taste badly, you will be able to use the water supply in the patient's room. Do not supply accompanying liquid for sublingual or buccal membrane tablets (lozenges or troches) because these must dissolve slowly under the tongue or against the cheek and should not be swallowed. You might want the person to take a swallow or two of water before sublingual or buccal membrane tablets are administered to stimulate saliva production and promote quicker absorbent action.

Place the prepared cups of medicine and the identification marker (the medicine card or Kardex system sheet) on a small tray to carry the medicine to the bedside (Fig. 29-14C). To ensure safe medication administration, do not be reluctant to add any specific assessment instructions on a separate sheet of paper as a reminder to yourself (take pulse, take respirations, ask about urinary output). Some nurses who administer medicine to many patients every day use colored strips of paper as "markers" (a red strip means take respirations, a yellow one means take pulse, and so on). It seems as if one would not need this type of instruction if she is going right from the medication preparation area to a patient's bedside but at the bedside, the patient can ask you a question that will distract you. "Cheat sheets" of this nature are not unprofessional; forgetting to make an assessment of this nature and thereby giving medicine unsafely is unprofessional.

At the patient's bedside, check the name on his identification band with the name on the working prescription form. Help the patient as necessary to take the tablet or capsule or hold his glass of water or other liquid. Be certain that people taking oral medication are sitting up. Attempting to swallow in a lying down position can lead to aspiration.

Unit Dose Tablets and Capsules. All unit dose administration systems provide oral medication forms in individual foil, cellophane, or plastic-wrapped packages. Some are supplied in enclosed plastic strips where you tear off the number of tablets or capsules that you need in the same way you remove scotch tape from a dispenser. Some health care agencies suggest that you do not unwrap the tablet or capsule from its package until you are at the patient's bedside.

Some patients enjoy opening their own medicine packages because it offers them a sense of independence. The patients may read the package and be aware of what they are taking. Others feel more impatience than reward. If the person's hand coordination is poor, he may drop the tablet on the floor and contaminate it. Use common sense to determine when it will be best to open the packets yourself or allow a patient to do so.

ADMINISTRATION OF ORAL LIQUID MEDICINE

To pour liquid medicine from a bottle, begin with the three identification checks to be certain that it is the

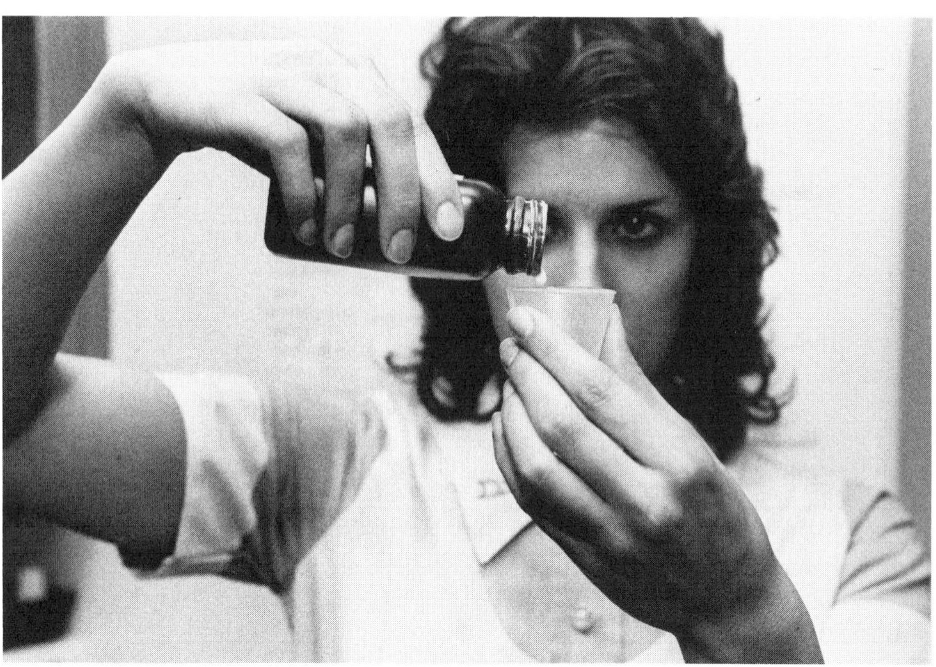

FIGURE 29-15. At eye level, pour all liquid medicine with the label against the palm of your hand; pour it in a direction away from the label to prevent medication from staining the label (label is partially obscured under student nurse's hand).

right medicine. Always hold all liquid medication with the label up against the palm of your hand so you pour *away* from the label (Fig. 29-15) to prevent any medicine from running down the side of the bottle and obscuring the label. Always place the cap of the bottle with its top side on the medicine preparation counter so the inside of the cap will remain clean. Hold the medicine glass you are using to measure the amount of medicine so that the meniscus of the medicine you pour is at eye level. Looking down or up at a liquid level distorts your vision and could give you an inaccurate reading. The medication level is read from the bottom of the meniscus.

Never use a medication if the label has been obscured by medication that has dripped over it. Never relabel a bottle with an obscured label. Return this bottle to the pharmacy to be relabeled. Relabeling is technically a dispensing step and is the pharmacist's responsibility.

If you do not have a medicine glass with small enough markings to determine a very small dose accurately, use a syringe marked in minims to measure the dose. If the patient is an infant, you might choose to leave the medicine in the syringe for administration (place the tip of the syringe without a needle at the side of the infant's tongue and inject small amounts slowly into his mouth). If medicine will be given by a nasogastric tube, you can also leave it in the syringe. If feeding is being done through a nasogastric tube, administer the medicine first so you can be certain it is flushed through the tubing completely and is not retained in the tubing.

Because many liquid medications taste sweet, a person often needs to drink something after them. It is better to urge a person to swallow the medicine dose first and then drink something rather than trying to dilute the medicine with a liquid because once you dilute it, the person must drink the entire solution in order to derive the benefit of the medicine, and a person may be unwilling to drink such a large amount.

Do not supply fluid to accompany cough syrups or medication that has topical application in the mouth (an antifungal drug or local anesthetic). These types of medicine should remain in contact with the oral mucosa and not be washed away for at least 15 minutes after administration.

Some liquid medicines are measured in drops. Medicine droppers vary in size. Never interchange a dropper that is supplied with one medicine with that from another because if the drop size differs from what the manufacturer recommends, the dose measured will be different.

Unit Dose Systems. In a unit dose medication system, liquid medicine may be supplied in small individual dose screw-top bottles or in vials similar to the vials that parenteral medicaton is supplied in (rubber-topped vials). If the medication is in powder form, you need to pour a designated amount of water into the bottle to activate it. You can use tap water for this because oral administration is not sterile. (Pour an amount from the faucet into a medicine glass before mixing with the powder. Pouring from the faucet directly into the powder can cause the powder to fly upward and spill from the container, causing the correct dose to be lost.)

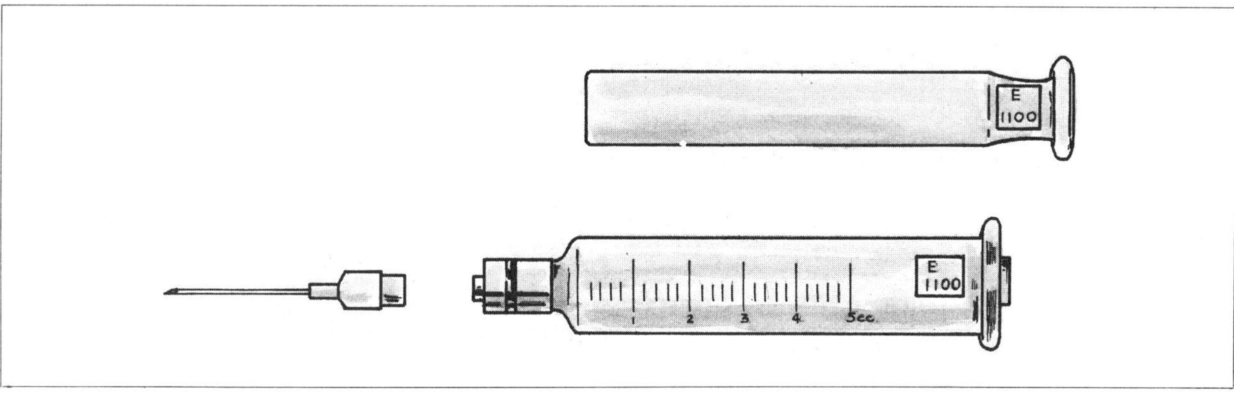

A

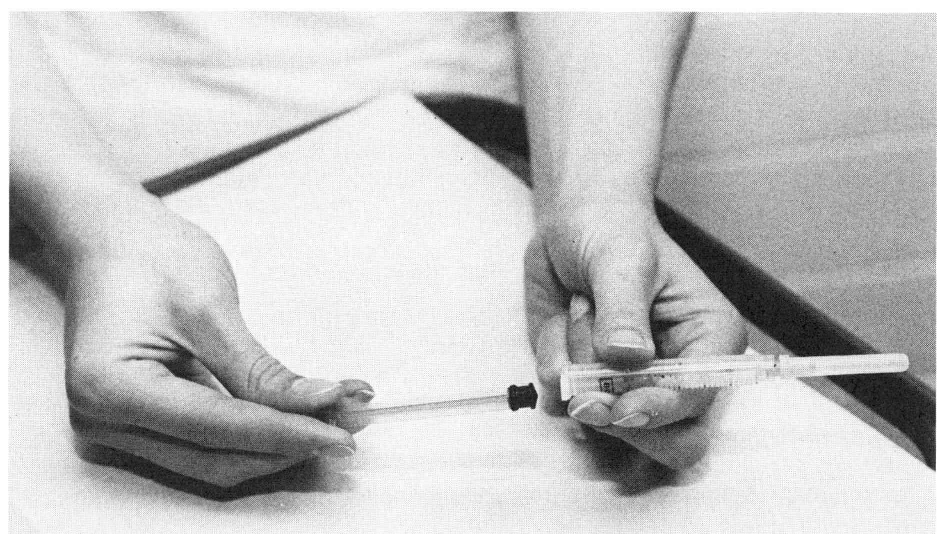

B

FIGURE 29-16. A. Syringes are composed of two parts: an outside barrel and an inside plunger. B. Avoid touching the inside plunger except by the base to maintain sterility.

Some health care agencies suggest that a person drink the medication directly from the vial in which it is supplied in order to avoid spillage or waste. Some people do not find swallowing from the bottle irregular; others find it uncomfortable or strange; children may be very suspicious of drinking from the bottle. Use common sense in deciding whether or not to pour medicine into a glass. If you are going to use the system of drinking directly from the vial, remember that your habit of three safety checks is compromised. Therefore, take the responsibility to check the name, dosage, and route of administration against your working prescription source three times in the medication preparation area. Do not mix oral liquid medications together because incompatible precipitates could occur.

ADMINISTRATION OF MEDICATIONS BY INJECTION

In common usage the term *parenteral* is used to mean the administration of medicine by injection. Although injection may be intradermally, subcutaneously, intramuscularly, intrathecally (into the spinal canal), intracardially, intra-articular (into a joint), or intravenously, the preparation for injection will be the same.

Preparation of medicine for injection must be done with *sterile* technique (any object that pierces the skin always must be sterile so that pathogenic [disease causing] microorganisms are not introduced).

SYRINGES

Both a syringe and needle are necessary for parenteral injection. Syringes are commonly available in 1 ml, 3 ml, 5 ml, 10 ml, and 20 ml sizes. For most administration, a 3 ml size is an adequate and easily manipulated syringe.

It is the ideal size for medicine administration because you rarely administer more than this amount and it is calibrated in both tenths of mls and minims for the easy measurement of medications. Extremely small doses of medicine are best and most accurately measured in a 1 ml syringe (often called a tuberculin syringe because small syringes originally were designed to administer tuberculin antigen for skin testing for tuberculosis).

Syringes are composed of two parts: an outside *barrel* and an inside *plunger* (Fig. 29-16). To assemble a syringe if it was not prepackaged assembled, you can touch the outside of the barrel at any point. However, the only portion of the plunger that you can touch is the wide flange. Hold this portion and slip the plunger down into the barrel. While you hold a syringe and fill it with medication, you must never let your fingers or your hand touch anything other than the outside flange. If you do touch anything beyond this point, microorganisms from your hand will be pushed into the syringe and the medication will be contaminated; you must reprepare the medication or you will be injecting an unsterile product that could cause a serious infection.

NEEDLES

Needles for injection have two separate portions: a *hub* and a *cannula*. The tip of the cannula is termed the *bevel*. When handling needles, touch only the hub to avoid contaminating the part that will pierce the skin. Needles are available in the common sizes of 18, 19, 20, 21, 22, and 25 gauge (diameter of the bore) and 5/8, 1, and 1 1/2 inch lengths (Fig. 29-17). The needle size chosen depends on the depth of the injection (intramuscular injections are placed deeper than subcutaneous injections) and the amount of adipose tissue present (a longer needle is needed for a person with large amounts of adipose [fatty tissue] than for an extremely slender person).

The size of the lumen (gauge) of the needle is selected depending on the viscosity of the medicine that will be injected through it. Blood is viscous so 18 and 19 gauge needles are generally used to withdraw blood; antibiotics are fairly thick substances usually injected through a 20 gauge needle; water-based medicine is injected successfully through a 22 or 25 gauge needle. Use the smallest needle gauge and the shortest needle length possible in order to reduce patient discomfort and increase the ease of administration. Do not be fooled into thinking that only small needles can be used on infants. If you are going to inject a newborn with a thick antibiotic, you might choose a fairly short needle (1 inch), but you would still have to use a fairly large gauge (a #20) in order for the thick fluid to be administered. Intradermal injections are very shallow and thus require a very short needle length (1/2 or 5/8 inch) and a fine needle gauge (25 or even 27).

INJECTION SITES

A suitable site for parenteral injection must be selected. The site depends on the type of injection (intradermal, subcutaneous, intramuscular, or intravenous) and the amount of medicine to be administered. Intra-articular, intrathecal, and intracardial injections are injections you will be assisting with but are primarily physician responsibility. As a result, you do not have the responsibility of selecting these injection sites.

Intradermal Injections

Intradermal injections (into the skin) are the most shallow injections. This type of injection is used not for medicine administration as such but for the injection of antigens to stimulate immunological reactions for allergy skin testing or for the administration of tuberculosis antigen to test for immunity to tuberculosis.

If the person is sensitive to the antigen administered, the site will show a "reaction" (a reddened, elevated area) within 24 to 48 hours after injection.

FIGURE 29-17. In choosing a needle for injection, you must choose the appropriate gauge (diameter of the bore) and length. Shown here are typical needles.

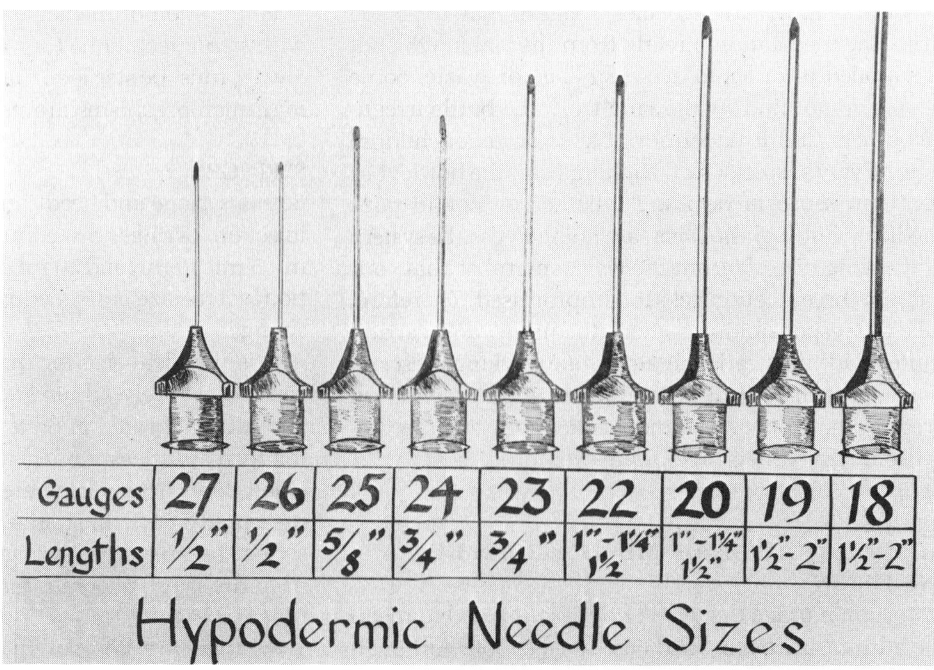

Sites chosen are areas of the body readily available for examination where the skin lifts easily and readily admits a small dose of fluid. If only one injection is to be administered, the inner aspect of the left forearm traditionally is selected. If many injections are planned, such as in extensive allergy testing, the outer aspect of the upper arms and the broad area of the back between the scapula are chosen. Although intradermal injections are almost painless, the thought of any injection creates a stressful situation, so give the patient adequate preparation and praise for cooperation.

Subcutaneous Injections

Subcutaneous injections are given into the layer of subcutaneous tissue between the skin layers and the muscle mass. Two commonly used sites for subcutaneous injections are over the deltoid and vastus lateralis muscles. The lower portion of the abdomen also may be used. In order to be certain that the needle tip comes to rest in this space, always "bunch" the skin over the injection site prior to injection.

Vastus Lateralis. The *vastus lateralis* is the muscle of the anterior thigh. This muscle is large and if the lateral aspect of it is used, it is a body area free of major interfering blood vessels and nerves. To locate a correct injection site, measure at least a hand's width from the knee upward; draw an imaginary line down the longitudinal center of the thigh; give the injection laterally to the line at that point (Fig. 29-18A). With an infant, measure about three fingers width from the knee upward. The thigh is less sensitive on the lateral surface than the inner surface, so injections on the lateral side are not apt to be painful.

Deltoid. The *deltoid* muscle is not as large a muscle as the vastus lateralis, but it marks the location of a subcutaneous injection site. To locate the bulk of the muscle, find the acromion process by palpation. In adults, the site for injection is a hand's width beneath the acromion process; in infants, it is at least 2 fingers' width below the acromion process (Fig. 29-18B). Palpate the muscle at this point; you should be able to sense by the bulk that you have located the heart of the muscle.

Deltoid area injections are convenient because the deltoid is an easy muscle to expose; it is a frequently used site for injection in ambulatory settings. This injection site can be used when a person is in a side-lying, prone, supine, sitting, or standing position.

FIGURE 29-18. A. Vastus lateralis injection site. B. Deltoid injection site. This site can be used in older children and adults. (Courtesy Department of Medical Illustration, State University of New York at Buffalo, Buffalo, New York.)

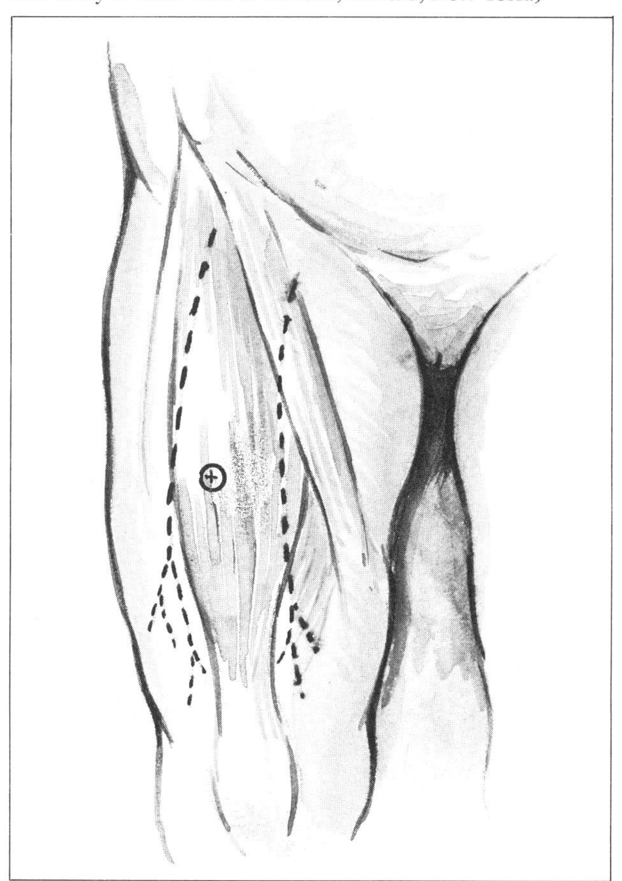

A

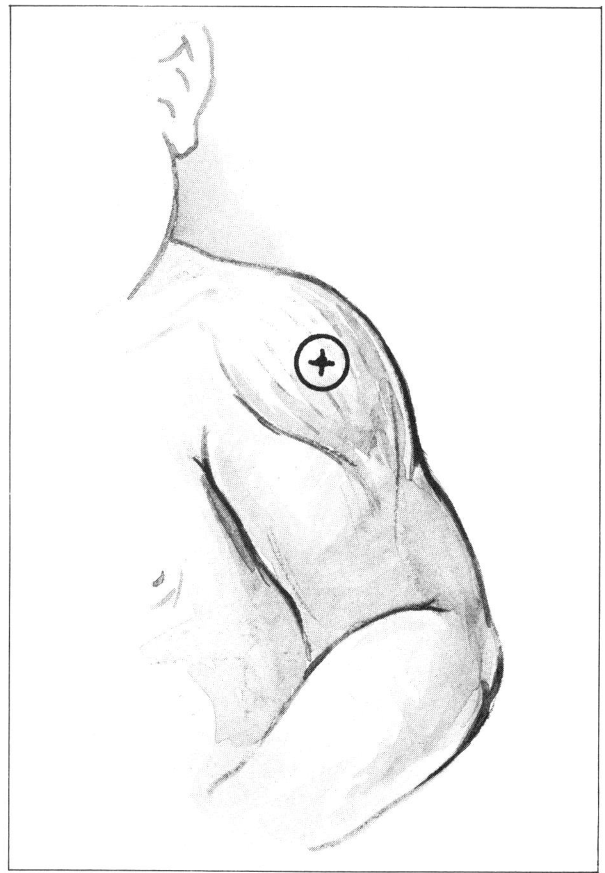

B

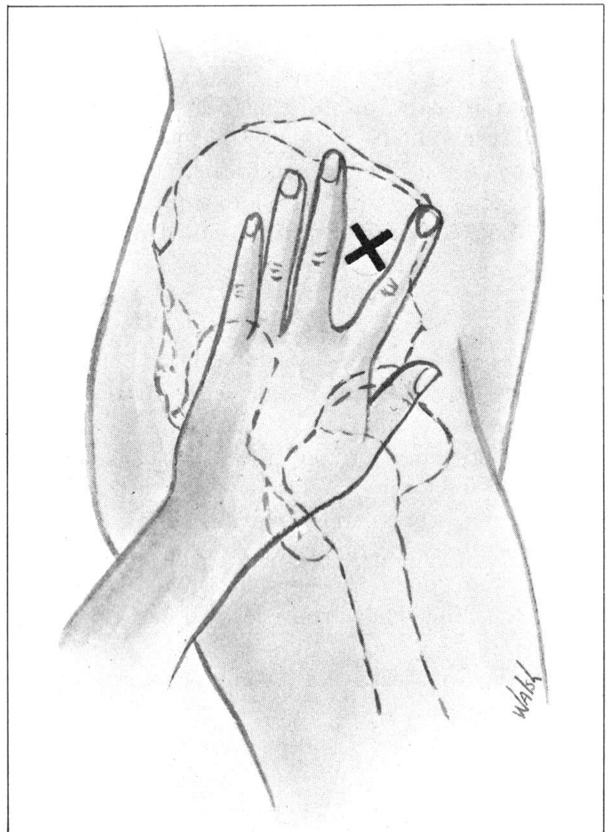

A

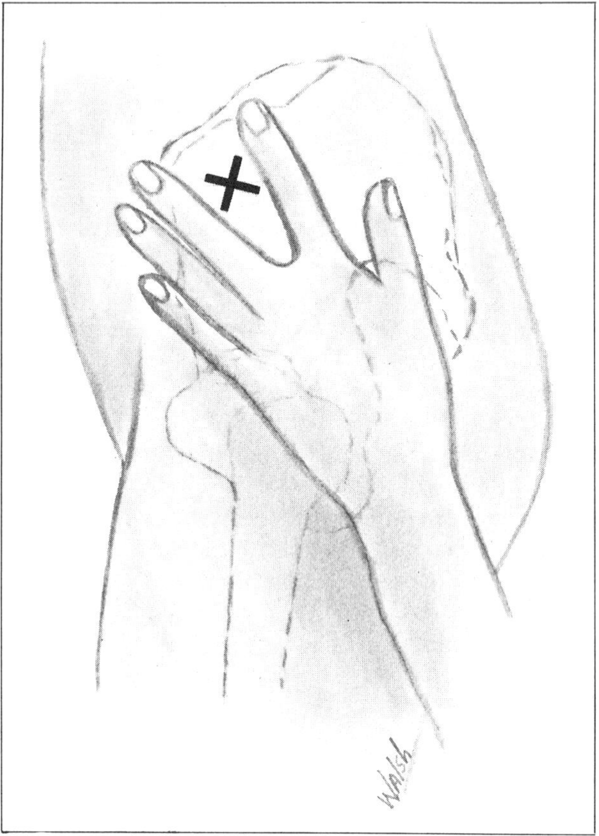

B

FIGURE 29-19. Ventrogluteal injection site. Mark the site by locating the greater trochanter and the anterior iliac crest, and spreading your fingers. A. Right side. B. Left side.

Lower Abdomen. A suitable *lower abdominal* injection site for subcutaneous injections is the area below the umbilicus, above the pubic hair, and medial to the iliac crests. This area is more sensitive in most people than the area over the deltoid and vastus lateralis, so it is never the site of choice for a single injection. It is the site chosen when many injections must be administered as in the case of heparin or insulin administration.

Intramuscular Injections

An *intramuscular* injection is placed deeply so that it enters a major muscle. The muscles acceptable for injection are the deltoid, vastus lateralis, ventrogluteal, and dorsogluteal. To be certain your needle will pierce deeply into the muscle, always "spread" skin over the muscle points to be injected.

Deltoid. The *deltoid* muscle site is chosen in the same way as described for subcutaneous injections.

Vastus Lateralis. The *vastus lateralis* site is chosen in the same way as described for subcutaneous injections. *This is the only acceptable intramuscular injection site for infants who have been walking less than one year.* It is a useful site for a person lying supine or sitting in a chair. Because it is easy to locate, it rapidly is becoming a common injection site for all ages.

Ventrogluteal. The *ventrogluteal* site is a good injection site to use with adults because subcutaneous fat at the site is fairly shallow, the muscle is comparably dense, and it is a site free of major blood vessels and nerves. It is an easy site to locate because the landmarks are identified easily in the average person (you may be unable to determine them accurately in the obese individual). It is best to use when the person is lying on his side, but it can be used with the person in a standing position, a supine position, or a prone position.

To determine the injection site on the patient's right hip, locate the protrusion of the greater trochanter of the femur and place the bottom edge of your left palm over it.* Locate the anterior iliac spine with your first finger; keep that finger in place and spread your first and second fingers apart; the injection site is in the center of the triangle formed by your fingers (Fig. 29-19). To locate the injection site on the left hip, place your left palm on the trochanter; place your second (middle) finger on the anterior iliac spine; spread your

*This book makes the assumption that all nurses are right-handed so that administration techniques may be explained in a more detailed way. If you are left-handed, simply use the opposite hands.

middle and index fingers; use the triangle formed by your fingers as the injection site. Always make a habit of using your left hand to locate the site because once you locate this site, you need to leave the locating hand in place to mark it. If you mark it with one hand and then lift that hand to pick up the syringe, you have lost the site.

Dorsogluteal. Once the intramuscular site of choice because the gluteus maximus is the largest muscle in the body, the *dorsogluteal* site is now used less often because of its close proximity to the sciatic nerve and the major blood vessels (the supragluteal artery) of the muscle. It is still an acceptable injection site, however, if the site is marked carefully.

To determine the injection site, locate the greater trochanter of the femur and the posterior superior iliac spine. Draw an imaginary line between them and give the injection in the area superior and lateral to the line (Fig. 29-20). These landmarks sometimes are difficult to locate in obese individuals.

A second method used to locate the injection site is to draw an imaginary line across the person's buttock both horizontally and vertically to divide it into four quadrants. The sciatic nerve crosses under both inner quadrants and then under the outer lower quadrant. *The only acceptable injection site, therefore, when imaginary lines are drawn on the buttock dividing it into 4 quadrants, is the upper outer quadrant.*

A person's buttock must be exposed fully in order to estimate quadrants or locate the trochanter and superior iliac spine. Always expose both buttocks fully and do not allow a feeling of modesty to interfere. A dorsogluteus site can be used with the person side-lying or prone. Lying prone with the toes "turned in" is the best position because this position relaxes the muscle, making the injection easy. This position also allows the best buttock exposure for marking the site.

FIGURE 29-20. Dorsogluteal injection site. Locate the greater trochanter of the femur and the posterior superior iliac spine; draw an imaginary line between them and give the injection in the area superior and lateral to the line; or envision the buttock as four quarters and inject in the upper outer quadrant as shown here.

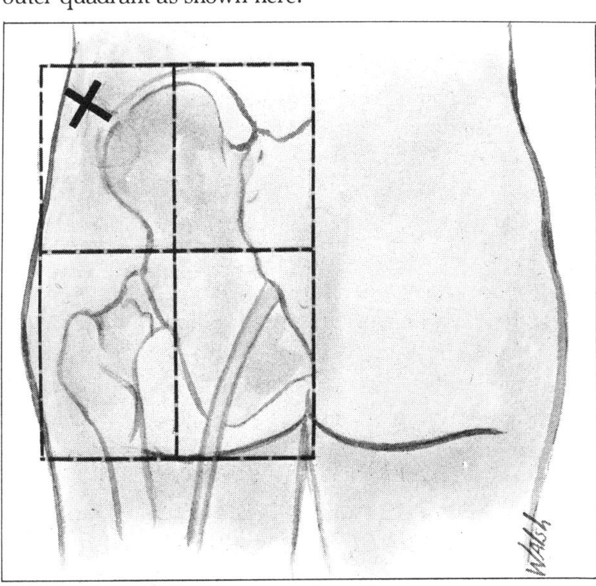

Forms of Parenteral Medication

Medicine for parenteral injection must be supplied as a sterile solution. You must use careful technique while preparing such medication to be certain that it remains sterile during preparation.

STERILE VIALS

Parenteral medication is commonly packaged in an airtight glass vial with a rubber stopper top. A metal cap covers the rubber top and must be removed to expose the top. Before you can introduce a needle into the vial to withdraw medication, you must remove surface bacteria contamination from the rubber top by wiping it with a suitable antiseptic such as 70% alcohol. Every time you remove your needle from the vial during preparation and then wish to pierce the top again for re-entrance, you must repeat this step of disinfection. Otherwise, you will push bacterial contaminants from the top of the vial into the medicine and you will be administering contaminated solution.

In order to remove liquid from the vial, you first must inject an amount of air equal to the amount of liquid medication you intend to withdraw into the vial. Attach your chosen needle to the syringe, being careful not to touch the plunger of the syringe anywhere but on the outside flange or the shaft of the needle. Withdraw the plunger of the syringe to fill the barrel of the syringe with an amount of air equal to the amount of medicine you wish to withdraw. With the vial inverted, and the rubber top cleaned with 70% alcohol, pierce the rubber top of the vial and inject this amount of air; pierce the needle into the vial so that the needle tip is above the surface of the liquid in the vial (Fig. 29-21). If the needle tip is below the liquid surface, the air will bubble through the liquid and these bubbles will make withdrawing an accurate amount of medicine more difficult.

As soon as all the air is injected from the syringe, withdraw the needle slightly so the liquid level covers the needle tip. Using the plunger of the syringe, withdraw the desired amount of solution into the syringe (Fig. 29-22). Make a habit of keeping the tip of the needle as close to the inner surface of the rubber stopper as possible so when you withdraw medication, even when the vial contains only a small amount of fluid, your needle tip will rest in the fluid and not above the level of fluid and air. An alternate technique of keeping the vial upright for air injection and inverted only for fluid withdrawal will also prevent air from being drawn back into your syringe.

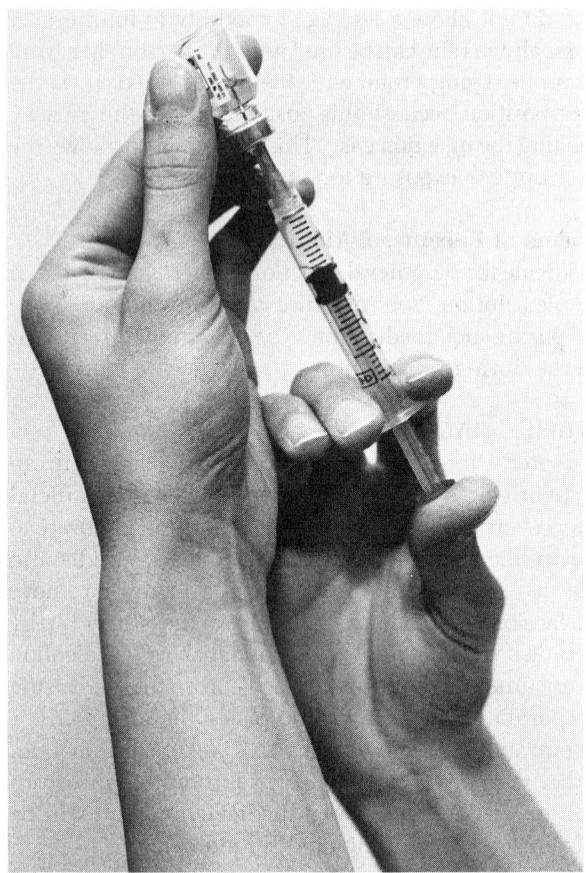

FIGURE 29-21. To remove liquid medication from a vial, inject an amount of air equal to the amount of liquid you intend to withdraw. Notice that the needle tip is above the level of the liquid to prevent bubbles.

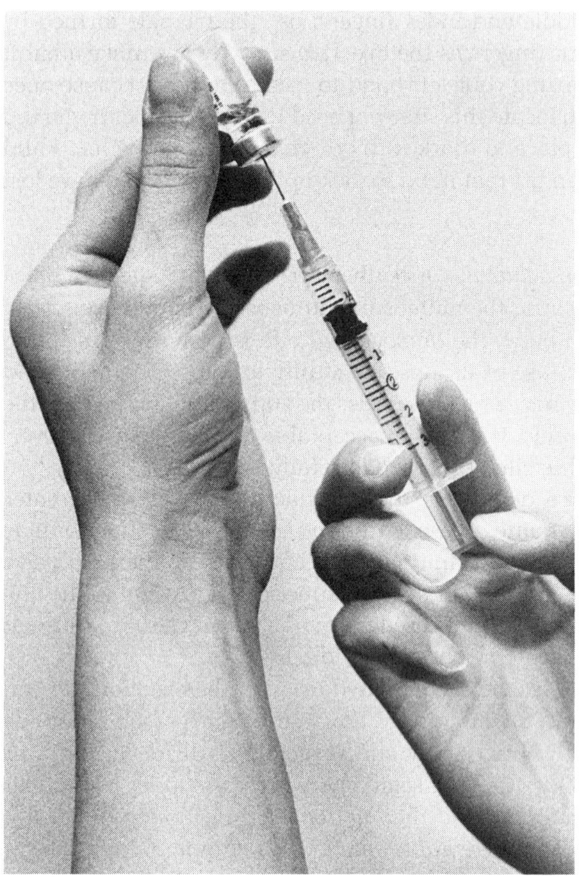

FIGURE 29-22. Withdraw the desired amount of solution into the syringe. The liquid level covers the needle tip to avoid introducing air.

Occasionally, despite your best effort, an air bubble will form at the top of the plunger as you withdraw the medicine. You must clear this bubble from the syringe or the measured amount of solution in the syringe will be inaccurate (you have only 0.8 ml medicine and 0.2 ml air, not 1 ml of medicine). To clear such a bubble, with the needle and syringe still in place in the inverted vial, tap the side of the syringe barrel sharply with your finger; this will cause the bubble to rise up the needle and return to the vial (for persistent bubbles, use a hard snapping motion; do not worry about breaking a syringe; you will hurt your finger long before you will break either a plastic or glass syringe with this motion). If the bubble does not clear even with sharp snapping, reinject the entire amount of fluid withdrawn back into the vial and withdraw again. Hopefully, the bubble will not reappear.

When you have the correct measurement of medicine in the syringe (hold the syringe at eye level), withdraw the needle from the vial and cap it with its plastic sheath to keep it sterile until you are ready to administer the medication. Be certain to make three safety checks for medicine identification during this process: (1) as you select the vial from its storage area, (2) just before you add the air to withdraw, and (3) just before you discard or return the vial to a storage area.

AMPULES

Many single dose injections of medicine are packaged in small glass ampules rather than in vials. Medicine in ampules tends to collect in the top section of an ampule. After your first safety check for correct medication, hold the ampule upright and tap the top of it sharply with your finger. This causes the liquid collected in the tip to flow down into the body of the ampule. Again, do not worry about breaking the medicine container with this motion. Ampules are not as fragile as they look.

When ampules were first manufactured, there was no ready way to remove the tip of the ampule from the body. At that time, the neck had to be scored with a small file to weaken it so that it could be snapped off. Today, the neck of ampules are prescored by the manufacturer to omit this filing step. A colored line on the neck of the ampule is the manufacturer's confirmation that the ampule is prescored and will break free readily. It is unlikely that you will work with medication not prescored in this way.

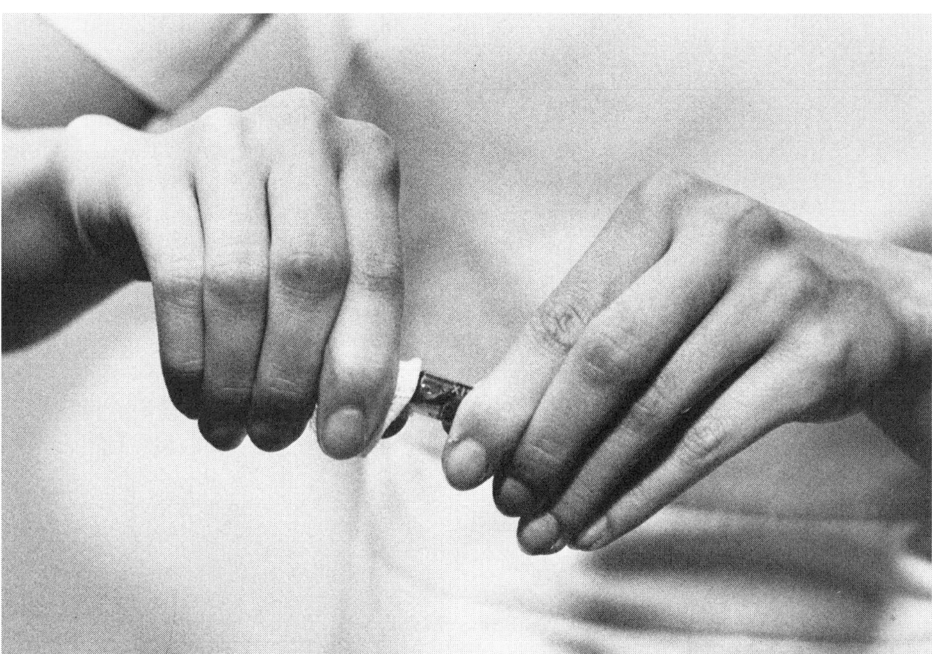

FIGURE 29-23. To open a glass ampule, flick fluid from the tip of the ampule; place a clean piece of gauze on the neck of the ampule and, by holding the body of the ampule in one hand and the tip between the thumb and finger of your other hand, snap off the tip.

To open the ampule, place a clean piece of gauze on its neck. While holding the body of the ampule in one hand and its tip between the thumb and finger of your other hand, snap off the tip (Fig. 29-23). The piece of gauze is necessary to prevent cutting your fingers with the sharp glass edge when the two portions break free. Do not use an alcohol-soaked pad to do this because you could squeeze some alcohol from the pad into the body of the ampule that could mix with the medicine (possibly changing its composition and forming a dangerous precipitate). Always inspect the medicine in the ampule after breakage to try and determine if any minute particles of glass fell into the solution. This rarely occurs, but if it does, you should discard the solution rather than risk withdrawing any glass particles into the syringe and injecting them into a patient. It is not necessary to wipe the sides of an ampule with alcohol similar to the way you wipe a vial before withdrawal of medicine because you are not going to pierce through any portion of the ampule. Also, a wet ampule is very difficult to grasp and break cleanly.

The solution in the broken ampule is not under pressure so you do not need to add an equal amount of air to the ampule prior to withdrawal of fluid from it (and adding any will cause the fluid level to overflow and be lost from the ampule). To withdraw fluid, simply place the tip of the needle and syringe into the ampule while it is in an upright position and, using the plunger of the syringe, withdraw fluid into the syringe. Due to surface tension of the fluid in the ampule, it is possible to invert an ampule and withdraw the medicine in the same position you use to withdraw fluid from a rubber-topped vial once the needle has been inserted into the ampule (Fig. 29-24). This is a desirable technique to practice because it is easier to see the calibrations on the syringe in this position and easier to bring the ampule and syringe to eye level for greater accuracy. Fluid will run from the ampule in this position if the side of the needle touches the side of the ampule, so you must keep the needle centered in the opening of the ampule. If you overdraw the amount of fluid needed, you cannot reinject or return it to the ampule in the inverted position, or this will break the surface tension and any medicine remaining in the ampule will flow out. Place the ampule upright to return the medication to it.

A bubble may form in the syringe during ampule withdrawal as well as during vial withdrawal. Remove it in the same way, either by tapping or returning the solution to the ampule (turned upright).

After you have the correct dosage in the syringe, recap the needle to keep the shaft sterile before injection. Be certain that you included three safety checks for medicine identification as you proceeded: (1) as you chose the ampule, (2) before you broke the tip, and (3) a final time as you discarded the ampule.

POWDERED MEDICATION IN VIALS

Some medications, particularly antibiotics, are provided in a fine dry, powder form that must be reconstituted into a solution before administration. Drugs packaged this way are accompanied by instructions (either on the bottle label or in the accompanying drug insert) that suggest which diluent (sterile water, isotonic sodium chloride, or a special diluent provided

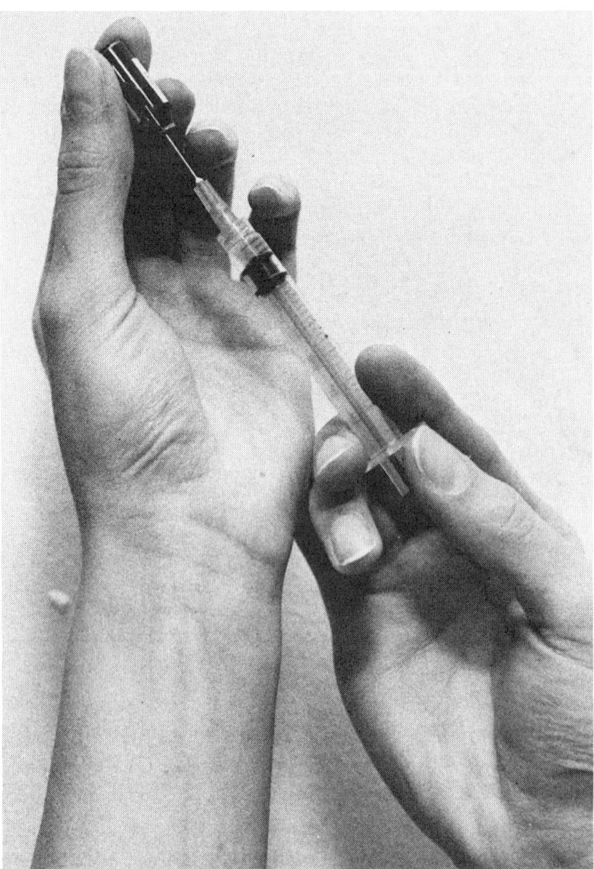

FIGURE 29-24. To withdraw fluid from an ampule, insert your needle into the ampule, invert the ampule, and withdraw the medicine in the same position that you use to withdraw fluid from a rubber-topped vial (or leave it right side up if you choose). Do not inject air into the ampule.

by the manufacturer) to use and how much of the diluent should be added to the vial to reconstitute the powder. If you do not follow these instructions, the powder will not dissolve well and will be impossible to inject.

Proceed with the preparation of the solution by wiping the top of the vial and adding the correct amount of the appropriate diluent. After adding this amount, remove the needle from the vial; recap the needle to keep it sterile and roll the bottle between your palms to mix the powder with the diluent. Do not shake the vial vigorously because this will cause bubbles to form; bubbles in the liquid will distort measurement in the syringe.

In some instances, as the powder dissolves in the diluent, it expands and creates bulk. In these instances, the directions accompanying the medication predict how much volume will be added by this expansion. It is important to note the fact that increased volume will occur because this increased volume will influence how you calculate the correct dosage. Suppose, for example, you wish to administer 250 mg of a drug from a vial containing a total of 500 mg of a powdered drug. The bottle label suggests that you add 2 ml of sterile water to the vial. Simple math tells you that if there is 500 mg in 2 ml of solution, 250 mg will be in 1 ml of solution. For the proper dose, it seems as if you would add 2 ml of water and withdraw 1 ml of solution. If the powder in the vial is a bulk-expansion type, however, the instructions will read, "Add 2 ml diluent to the vial; after reconstitution, total vial content will equal 3 ml." In other words, the powder will increase the volume of the vial by 1 ml. Now, the proportion of the drug to total solution is 500 mg to 3 ml, not 500 mg to 2 ml. In order to calculate the correct dosage, use the same calculation formula as with any problem. No conversion factor is necessary.

ordered amount × dose on hand = answer

or

$$\frac{\overset{1}{\cancel{250}}\text{ mg}}{1\text{ ml}} \times \frac{3\text{ ml}}{\underset{2}{\cancel{500}}\text{ mg}} = \frac{3\text{ ml}}{2\text{ ml}} = 1.5\text{ ml}$$

In other words, in order to administer 250 mg of the drug, you need to administer an increase of 0.5 ml over what you would have administered if you had not accounted for the expansion characteristic of the powder.

If the instructions accompanying a powdered vial do not specifically state that the powder will increase volume, you may assume safely that it will not. If in doubt, call the pharmacy to double-check.

Once a powdered vial has been reconstituted to a liquid form, proceed to prepare it the same as if it were a pre-liquidized form (inject air, withdraw solution). Be certain that when you re-enter the vial after mixing the powder into the diluent that you rewipe the top of the rubber stopper with an alcohol wipe.

READY-MIX VIALS

A number of medications must be reconstituted from a dry powder using *not* sterile water or sterile isotonic saline, but a diluent specific to that drug. Because solutions other than sterile water or sterile saline are not readily available at the average medication preparation area, these drugs are often packaged in vials containing the dry powder in the bottom chamber and the special solvent in the top. A sterile rubber stopper separates the two components (Fig. 29-25).

To reconstitute this type of powder, remove the protective metal cap of the vial and press down on the elevated rubber stopper. This action increases the pressure in the top diluent chamber and forces the separating rubber stopper down into the bottom powder-filled chamber accompanied by the diluent. Tip the vial as necessary to be certain that all diluent from the top chamber drains into the bottom chamber. Roll the vial

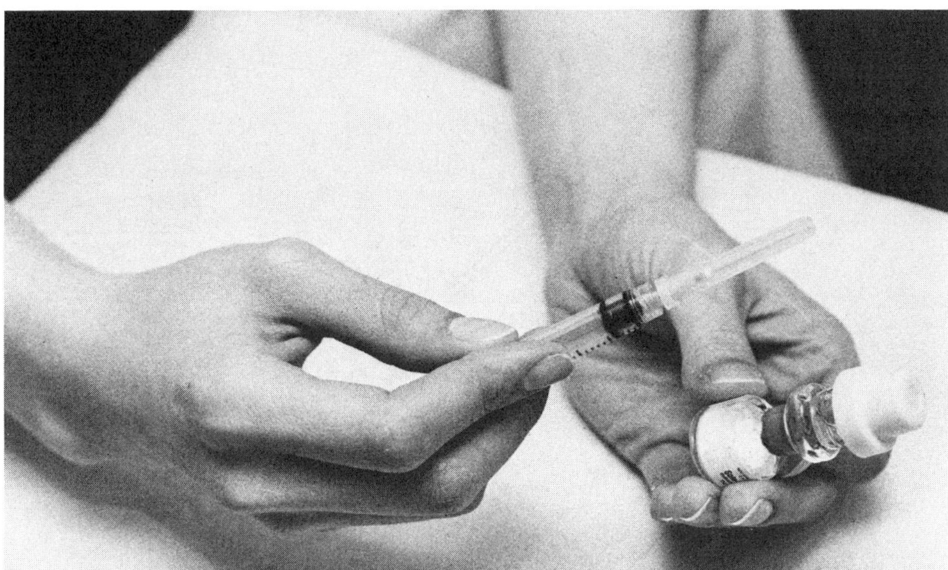

FIGURE 29-25. A ready-mix vial contains dry powder in the bottom chamber and a special liquid solvent in the top. A sterile rubber stopper separates the two compartments. To mix the two substances, press down on the rubber top of the vial.

between your palms to allow the diluent and powder to mix well. As soon as the powder is mixed, proceed to wipe the top stopper, inject air, and withdraw the required amount of medicine from the vial as if it was a regular vial (the center rubber stopper will remain in the bottom chamber of the solution, but this is no problem because it remains intact and is sterile).

PREFILLED SYRINGES

In a unit dose medication system, medicine for syringe injection comes from the pharmacy already premeasured and drawn into the syringe. To prepare such medication, all you need to do is add the needle to the syringe. A pharmacist's label is in place on the syringe stating its contents. Although this type of premeasurement economizes your time because you are not withdrawing the medicine from the vial or ampule, you lose the three safety checks that you ordinarily use to check to see if it is the right medicine. You must be certain when using this type of prefilled syringe that you establish three checkpoints: (1) perhaps as you choose the syringe from the patient's medication drawer, (2) before you place it on the tray you will use to carry it to the bedside, and (3) before you walk away from the preparation area. Prefilled syringes administered without these checks may cause medication errors.

TUBEX SYRINGES

Tubex syringes are syringes that are prefilled by the pharmaceutical company that manufactures this type of equipment (Wyeth Laboratories). The medication is contained in a glass or hard plastic cartridge with a needle for injection permanently attached. To prepare the medicine for injection, obtain a Tubex "barrel" (they are available in metal or plastic shapes), and "break" the barrel by separating the plunger of the unit from it (Fig. 29-26A). Insert the medicine cartridge into the hollow barrel and rotate it clockwise to set the top threads; bring the plunger back into place and screw it in until it locks sungly against the bottom of the medicine cartridge.

As with any prefilled syringe system, it is easy to assume that because 1 ml of medicine has been ordered, the pharmacist has sent you 1 ml of medicine. Do not assume. Check three times that the medication dose is correct: (1) perhaps as you select the cartridge from its drawer, (2) just before insertion into the barrel, and (3) when it is finally screwed into place. Remember that it is an amount standardized for the average dose; anytime you have an "unaverage" patient, you have a medication error waiting to happen unless you build in three safety checkpoints. (As a rule of thumb, "unaverage" patients may be every patient.)

If more dosage is present in the cartridge than is required, remove the needle sheath and gently expel the medicine that is not required. Be extremely careful not to touch the shaft of the needle against any object while doing this. With a regular syringe and detachable needle, if you should contaminate your needle, you can replace it; with a permanently attached needle, a contaminated needle means a contaminated cartridge. If the liquid you are expelling is a scheduled drug, you need someone to witness and sign a permanent record that the scheduled drug was truly discarded (specifying the amount that was discarded).

Once you have a Tubex syringe prepared and are certain that your type and dosage of medicine is correct, the actual administration of the medication will

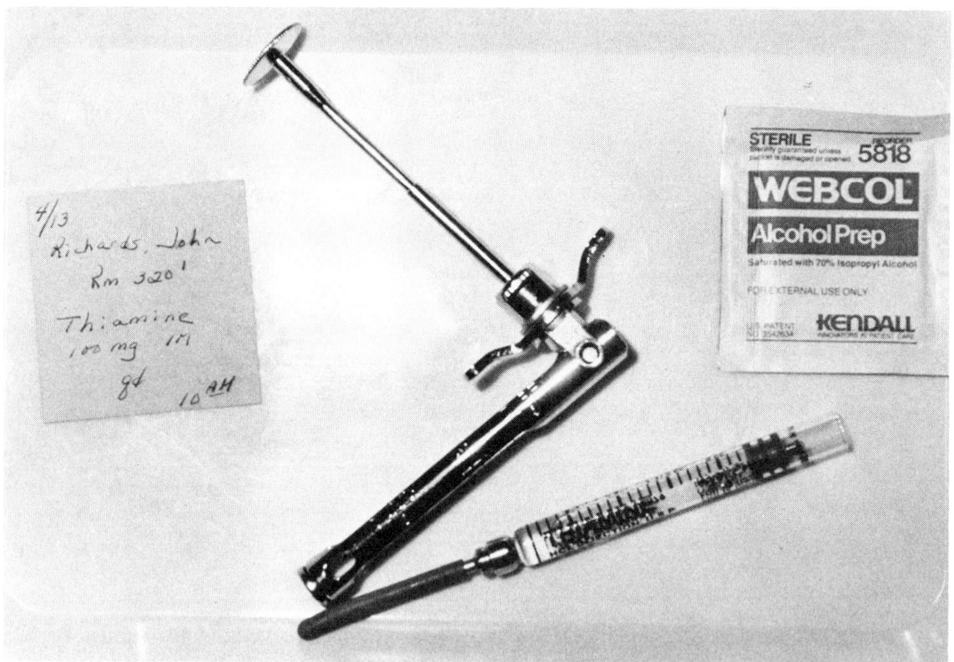

A

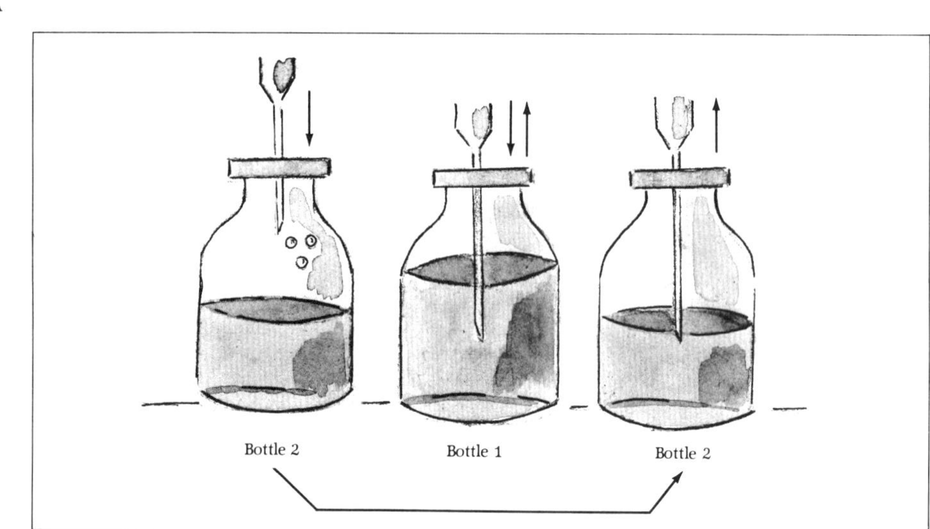

B

FIGURE 29-26. A. To use a Tubex barrel, "break" the barrel by separating it from the plunger of the unit; the container of medication will then "load." B. Double vial technique. Notice that the first step is to inject the measured amount of air into the *second* vial.

be no different than with a regular syringe and needle. However, because the syringe is heavier, you may need to use less thrust to give the injection.

Mixing Medication for Parenteral Administration

If at all possible, it is always preferable to administer one injection rather than two to reduce the amount of pain involved and to conserve injection sites. Using injection sites too close together can cause tissue atrophy with fibrotic scarring. This ultimately results in a "pitted" skin appearance as well as poor absorption of medication from the atrophied site. Mixing two parenteral medicines is contraindicated if the two medicines have synergistic or antagonistic properties or if the combined volume of medicine would make a single injection too great. Medicine may be mixed in a syringe from vials or ampules, however, always be sure to check for incompatibility before mixing medications this way.

DOUBLE VIAL TECHNIQUE

In order to withdraw medicine from two vials, prepare the two vials by identifying the contents against your working prescription source in the same way as if you had a single medicine; prepare both tops by opening them and wiping them with 70% alcohol. Prepare the syringe and needle as with a single medication injection.

To combine the medicine from the vials, draw up the amount of air equal to the amount of medicine you need for the *second* vial and inject it into the second vial. Do not withdraw any medicine; simply inject the air and remove the needle from the vial. Next, draw back the amount of air equal to the amount of volume you will withdraw from the *first* vial, inject it into the first vial, and draw back the needed amount of medicine. Expel bubbles as necessary. Withdraw the needle from the vial. Reclean the top of the second vial, insert the needle into the second vial, and withdraw the amount of medicine desired from the second vial. Do not inject air prior to withdrawing solution from the second vial because that was accomplished in the very first step (Fig. 29-26B).

The advantage of adding air to the second vial as your first step is that, once you have solution in the syringe from the first vial, adding air at that point might end with you also adding some of the solution in the syringe to the second vial. Mixing two types of medication this way may make it necessary to discard the second vial. If there is not enough air in the second vial when you insert the syringe with the first medicine into that vial, the negative pressure in the second vial will pull the medicine from the syringe, and again, you will contaminate the second vial. To prevent this from happening, always add a generous amount of air to the second vial.

A second danger is that you could confuse the two medicines in terms of dosage (you draw up 1 ml of the medicine you needed 2 ml of and 2 ml of the one you needed 1 ml of). The only way to prevent this is to concentrate and to use checks to verify medicine and dosage. You must also be careful not to overdraw the second amount of medicine added to the syringe. If you do, you must discard all the medicine in the syringe and begin preparation again because the proportion is now incorrect.

DOUBLE AMPULE TECHNIQUE

To mix medicine from two ampules, check the identification of both ampules against your working prescription source. Open both ampules by snapping their tops. Draw up one medicine and carefully expel any air or bubbles. Insert the needle into the second ampule and withdraw the amount needed of the second medicine.

Mixing medication from two ampules is the easiest type of mixing to accomplish. Again, be certain that you do not overdraw the second type of medicine needed. If you do this, you must discard everything in the syringe and begin again.

VIAL AND AMPULE TECHNIQUE

To mix medicine from an ampule and a vial, identify both medicines by your working prescription source. Clean the top of the vial with 70% alcohol; snap off the top of the ampule. Inject an amount of air into the vial equal to the amount of the volume desired and withdraw the dosage of medicine required. Insert the needle into the ampule and draw the amount of medication desired from the ampule into the syringe. Withdrawing the medicine from the vial first avoids the problems of having to add air to the vial after you have solution from the ampule in the syringe, thus avoiding contamination.

INSULIN TECHNIQUE

Preparing and administering insulin differs slightly from other medicines in that it is measured in USP units rather than mg or ml. As mentioned previously, never withdraw or administer insulin unless you are using an insulin syringe because this is the only accurate way to measure insulin units. Insulin strength is U-100, or there are 100 USP units to each 1 ml; to measure this strength accurately, your syringe must also be marked U-100.

Insulin is supplied in long-acting (has an effect of about 24 hours), intermediate-acting (has an effect of 8 to 18 hours), and short-acting (begins to have effect immediately but only lasts 2 to 4 hours) forms. The short-acting form of insulin is also termed *regular* insulin. Check the type of insulin closely against your working prescription source because vials look similar.

Insulin regulates blood glucose levels in the body. If too little insulin is present, the blood glucose level rises beyond normal limits; if too much insulin is present, the blood glucose level is decreased below normal limits. Because cells need glucose to function (particularly brain cells), it is extremely important that regular (short-acting) insulin is always available for emergency injection. This form must never be contaminated by another form of insulin. If another form of insulin was added to this vial, the action of the regular insulin would be slowed and it would no longer be effective in an emergency situation.

Ordinarily, when you are mixing medicine for injection from two vials, it is immaterial which one you designate as the first vial to withdraw from and which one you designate as the second vial. However, *when mixing insulins, protect the regular (short-acting) insulin.* In other words, always use the regular insulin as the first vial. Inject an amount of air into the second vial equal to the volume you intend to withdraw; remove the needle without removing any fluid from the vial. Inject air into the first vial (the regular insulin) and remove the required amount. Insert the needle into the second vial and withdraw the needed amount (Fig. 29-26B). Never place the needle into the regular insulin after it has entered a long-acting or intermediate-acting insulin so there is never a possibility that the other insulins will contaminate the regular insulin.

Administration of Parenteral Medicine

Giving an injection without a person's consent is a violation of his legal right (it is assault and battery). A person does not have to allow another person to touch his body unless he so desires. When you approach a patient with an injection, therefore, you must inform him of how the medicine will be administered ("I have your medicine, Mr. Jones. It's an injection." or "I have your injection for you, Mr. Jones").

Never give injections to patients who are asleep. Not only is this a violation of their rights, but it may be dangerous. If they wake suddenly as the medicine begins to enter body tissue (the point at which pain is felt), they may turn quickly and brush your hand, causing the needle to break.

Never call injections "shots." Approaching a dozing army veteran and saying, "I have a shot for you" may revive battlefield scenes and elicit extreme fear. In any event, it is an unprofessional term and the only time it should be used is with health histories when you are asking about childhood immunizations. Mothers refer to a basic infant immunization series (diphtheria, tetanus, and pertussis vaccines) as "baby shots" and may not understand your question otherwise.

Always place injection syringes on a medicine tray with your working prescription source for identification. Carrying a syringe without a tray is unprofessional. Be certain to make accurate patient identification. An injected medication is absorbed into the bloodstream very quickly. If injected into the wrong individual, it could have immediate, fatal results.

Once you have announced to a person what you are going to do, proceed with a degree of speed (but never so much that safety is impaired) because from that point on, the threat of the injection is often as frightening and traumatic as the injection itself.

Technique for Intramuscular Injection

The medicine is placed deeply into a major muscle with an intramuscular injection. Although correct needle gauge and length is determined according to the person's build and amount of adipose tissue present, medicines administered intramuscularly are generally thick in consistency and require a fairly large gauge (#20, #22); in order to reach a muscle beneath subcutaneous tissue, you need a needle 1 inch in length or longer. The volume of solution injected should not exceed 2 ml. if the preparation exceeds this volume, you need to prepare two injections.

It is common practice to "seal" the medication into the muscle so that none retreats as the needle is withdrawn. In order to accomplish this, as soon as you have the accurate dose of medicine in your syringe, pull the plunger back approximately two minims so that you add two minims of air to the syringe. This air is added at the needle end of the syringe. When administering an injection, it is very important that you do not inject air into body tissue because, if the needle has accidentally been placed in a blood vessel, the air would become an embolus (a possible lethal complication). As you tip the syringe to inject the medication into a muscle, the air from the needle end of the syringe will rise in the syringe to the plunger end and will follow the medication as it is being injected. This is safe because you already have checked to see that you are not entering a blood vessel (see p. 697) and so a safe "seal" has been created to prevent medication from following the route of the needle out of the muscle back into the subcutaneous tissue.

With any injection, be certain to take time to expose adequately the site you have selected. If a person is wearing a sleeveless blouse or a loose-sleeved gown, the deltoid area can be exposed adequately by pushing up the cloth. If the person is wearing a long-sleeved blouse or shirt, he may have to remove his arm from that sleeve. Pushing up a long sleeve often puts pressure on the deltoid so that it cannot retain the medication well; after you withdraw your needle, medicine under pressure flows back through the needle track and is expelled.

For ventrogluteal, vastus lateralis, and dorsogluteal injection sites, the full site also must be exposed. Attempting to administer an injection without adequate exposure leads to misjudgment of the safe site and possible severe patient injury.

Clean the injection site with an alcohol wipe, moving in a circular motion, inside to outside (a principle of asepsis so that you are moving bacteria away from the injection site, not merely streaking them side to side). Hold the wipe between the fingers of your left hand for safe and convenient keeping during the rest of the procedure. Do not place it back on your medicine tray because you want it within reach if you need it quickly. Uncap the needle sheath that is protecting the sterility of the needle shaft and return it to the medicine tray (you will need this again, too, but not quickly).

Place your left hand over the site you have selected, spreading the skin with your index finger and thumb so it is flat over the site. Flattening the surface skin ensures that the needle tip will reach far down into muscle. Injecting the medicine at a sharp angle is another technique used to guarantee that the needle has pierced deeply (Fig. 29-27).

Hold a syringe for injection in the same manner you would hold a dart. Use a quick thrust technique for injection (it is surprising how strong and resistant skin is to a very sharp needle). Do not be concerned that the needle will pierce too deeply. If you have chosen the appropriate site and needle length, this will not occur. A larger concern should be that too soft an injection technique will not pierce the skin and you will have to attempt the procedure again. Inject the needle as rapidly as possible. A needle passing rapidly through tissue causes no pain; a needle pushed slowly through tissue can cause intense pain.

One of the greatest dangers of intramuscular injections is that the needle may enter a blood vessel accidentally. Therefore, when you inject the medicine, you may inject it into a blood vessel rather than muscle tissue. This is always a serious complication because the medication could become an embolus in the bloodstream if it precipitates into particles. To determine that the tip of the needle is not resting in a blood vessel, steady the syringe with the thumb and fingers of your left hand (Fig. 29-28), and with your right hand, pull back slightly on the plunger. If the tip of the needle is resting in a blood vessel, this action will cause blood to be pulled back into the syringe.

If you obtain blood on aspiration (pulling back on the plunger), do not inject the drug because you will be injecting it intravenously rather than intramuscularly. Withdraw the needle and syringe and apply pressure to the site to promote coagulation of the pierced blood vessel. Draw up new medication in a new syringe; reselect an injection site at least one-half inch away from the original one; reinject and reaspirate. Changing the needle after entering a blood vessel prevents you from depositing clotted blood held in the needle into the muscle. Accidentally entering a blood vessel is a rare occurrence. Because it is a danger, however, with each injection, you must test for the possibility that your needle tip has entered a blood vessel.

If you do not obtain blood on aspiration, the needle is in the proper place and you may administer the drug safely. Push the plunger with firm, steady pressure in order to force the medication through the needle. When the syringe is empty, place the alcohol wipe from your left hand at the base of the needle, and apply gentle pressure with your left hand as you withdraw the needle with your right hand. This action prevents medication from following the needle back through the track and thus, no medication is lost. As a last step, gently rub the area for a few seconds to increase blood supply and aid in the absorption from the site.

FIGURE 29-27. A. An intramuscular injection is administered at a 90-degree angle to ensure that it reaches the muscle layer. B. Giving an intramuscular injection.

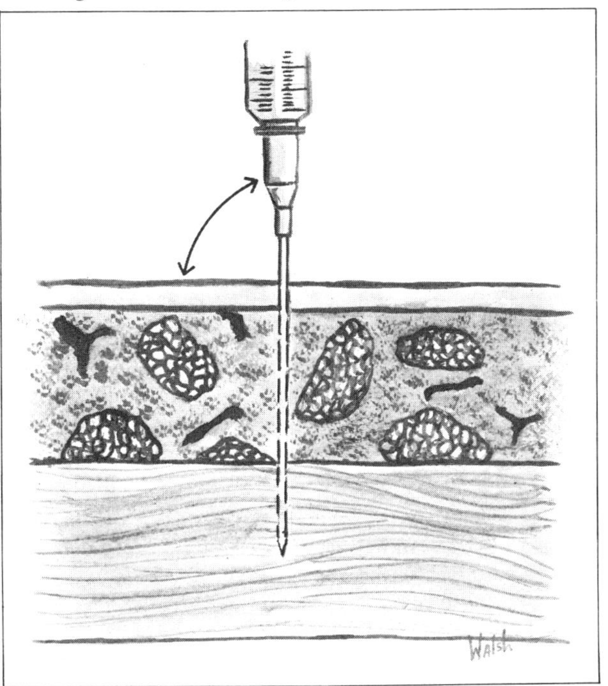

A

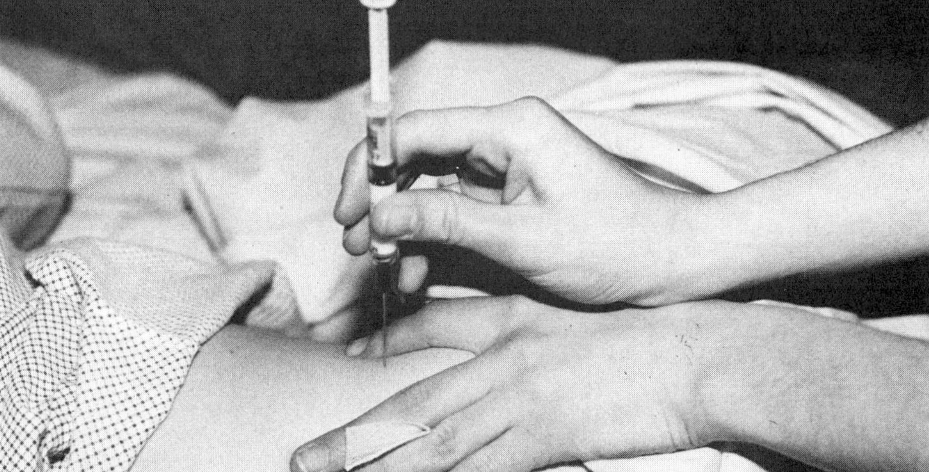

B

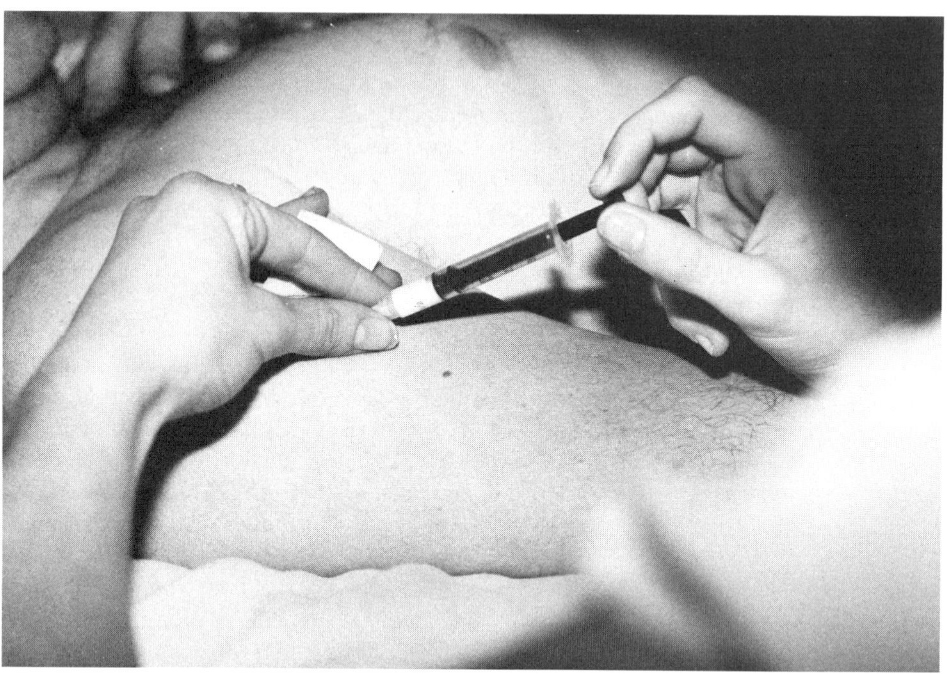

FIGURE 29-28. To determine that the tip of the needle is not resting in a blood vessel, steady the syringe with the thumb and fingers of your left hand and, with your right hand, pull back slightly on the plunger of the syringe to assess if air appears in the syringe (aspiration). A blood return means that you are in a blood vessel. Do not inject medicine, and immediately withdraw needle.

In some instances, after you withdraw the needle following an injection, you may notice a small amount of blood oozing from the injection site. This is caused by the needle passing through a broken capillary. It is always a small amount of blood and is not worrisome. Apply pressure at the site with a dry, sterile compress to halt the bleeding rather than the alcohol soaked one because alcohol prevents the formation of a clot at the surface. Applying a Band-Aid snugly to the site will prevent the clot from being dislodged until the coagulation at the site is complete. This is important because

FIGURE 29-29. A. A subcutaneous injection is administered at a 45-degree angle. B. Giving a subcutaneous injection. C. Removing the needle; notice the placement of the alcohol swab.

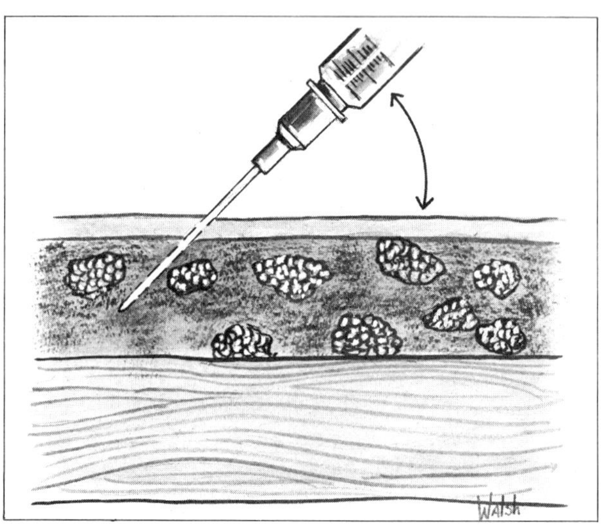

A

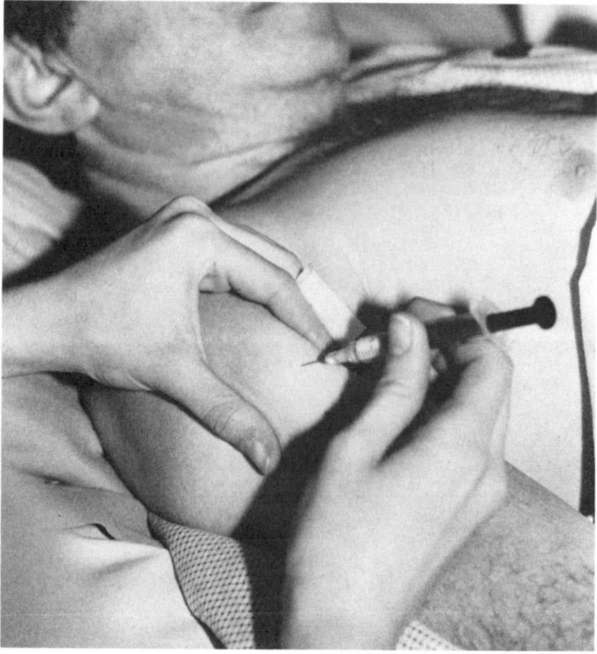

B

bleeding from an injection site is always frightening to a patient; assure the patient that this is minimal bleeding.

Technique for Subcutaneous Injection

In order to ensure that the drug is placed in the subcutaneous tissue rather than the intramuscular tissue, bunch the tissue between your left thumb and index finger. To ensure that the needle does not pierce beneath the subcutaneous tissue, use an injection angle of 45 degrees (Fig. 29-29).

Drugs that are administered subcutaneously are thin and readily absorbed so you can use a needle with a fine gauge (#22, #25). Because you are injecting into shallow tissue, you should use a relatively short needle (1 inch or 5/8 inch). Subcutaneous tissue will not hold as much volume as a large muscle space. The volume of a subcutaneous injection should not exceed 1 ml.

Because subcutaneous injections are not administered at a 90-degree angle, the air does not rise to the plunger end of the syringe with the injection. Therefore, you do not need to add an extra 2 minims of air to a subcutaneous injection like you do with an intramuscular injection.

A needle slides in best if the bevel of the needle (Fig. 29-30) is up, but it really does not matter which way the bevel faces. If the needle length used is extremely short (1/2 inch), a 90° angle can be used for injection. Because the needle length is so short, the medicine is deposited in shallow tissue although the angle used is the type used in an intramuscular injection. People with diabetes who inject their own insulin daily use short needles and inject with a 90-degree angle. Injection at a 90-degree angle is easier to learn and feel confident about more quickly.

INTRADERMAL INJECTIONS

An intradermal injection requires a very short needle (3/8 inch) and a very narrow gauge (#25 or #26). Intradermal injections are always small (0.01 to 0.1 ml) so a 1 ml syringe may be necessary for accurate preparation. The injection angle is shallow (10 to 15 degrees) so that the needle just pierces into the dermal layer of skin and not farther down into the subcutaneous tissue. Pull the skin taut when you inject to ensure shallow penetration. The injection of a solution into this layer will cause a wheal (welt) to form at the site.

Do not rub intradermal injections following administration; merely blot away any extra solution that is left at the site. If a skin reaction is expected to form at the site, take a ball-point pen and draw a circle around the site of administration so the area to be observed is well-marked.

Z-TRACK INJECTION TECHNIQUE

Some medicine is so irritating to subcutaneous tissue that it must not be allowed to escape back into the tissue as the injection needle is withdrawn from the muscle. A technique to trap medicine in intramuscular tissue this way is termed a *Z-track* technique.

After the medicine has been prepared in the syringe, the needle should be changed so that medicine clinging to the sides of the needle will not be left in subcutaneous tissue as the needle is inserted. Be certain to add the two minims of air as with all intramuscular injections to create a "seal."

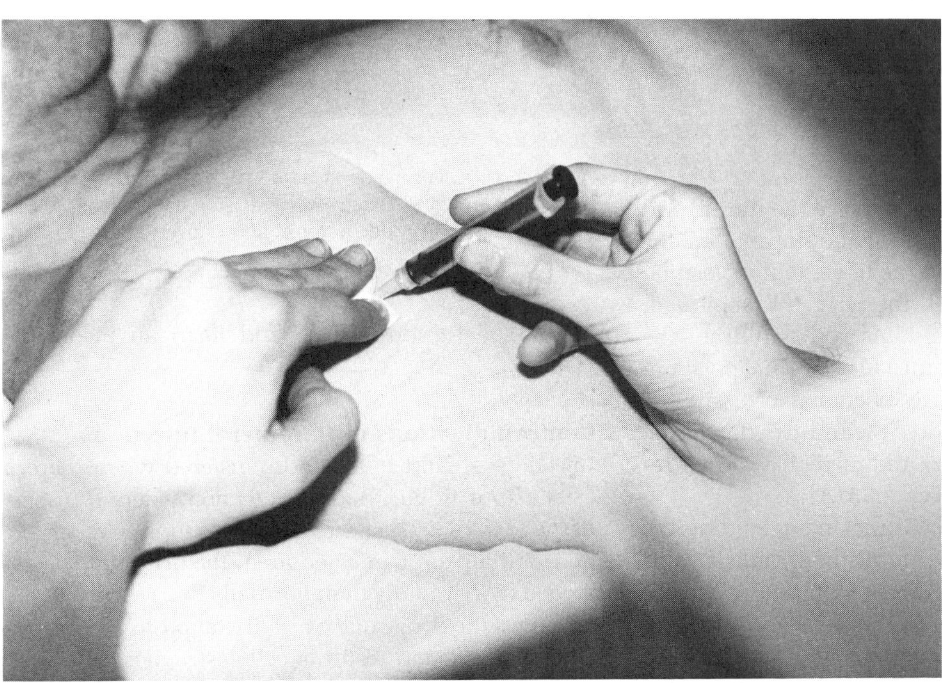

C

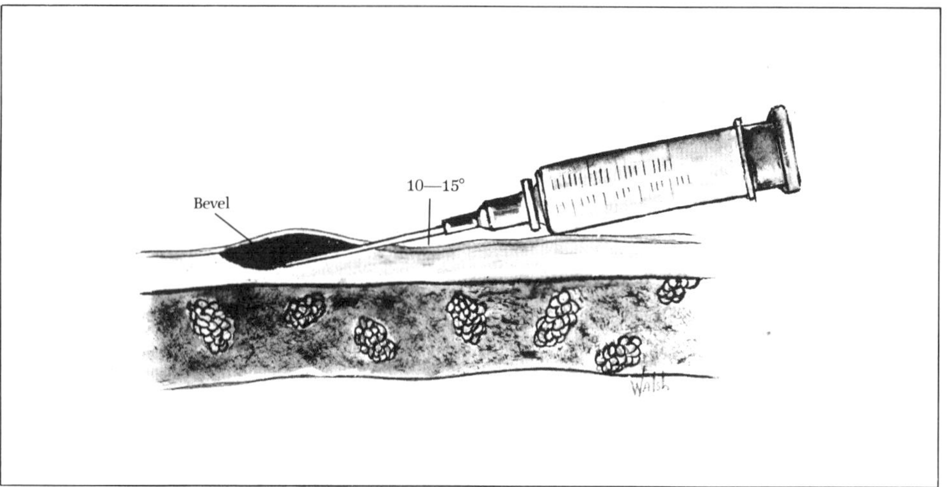

A

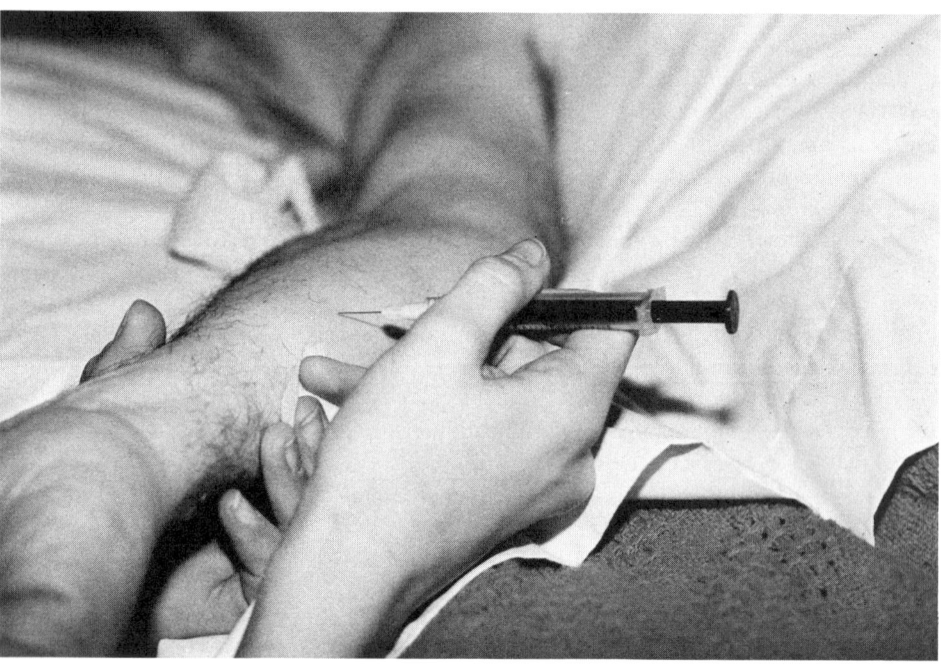

B

FIGURE 29-30. A. For injections, a needle slides in best if the bevel faces upward. Illustrated here is an intradermal injection. B. An intradermal injection is given at a 10 to 15-degree angle.

To inject by a Z-track method, place the thumb and finger of your left hand on the injection site and pull the tissue firmly to the left. Hold the tissue in this position while the needle is inserted, the syringe is aspirated, and the medicine is injected. As you withdraw the needle, allow the tissue to return to its normal position. Because the needle pierced the subcutaneous tissue at a different path than is now over the muscle, the needle track is "broken" (irregular) and medicine cannot return by way of the track (Fig. 29-31A).

The major difficulty with Z-tracking is holding the tissue to one side while you aspirate the syringe. Do this by applying pressure with the side of your left hand while you stretch your index finger and thumb to steady the syringe tip. Do not avoid aspirating because you find it awkward. Injecting an irritating medicine intravenously might be far more dangerous than allowing tissue to slip a little and form an incomplete Z-track.

Contraindications to Parenteral Injections

Injections should not be administered when there is evidence of inflammation, infection, edema, or scar tissue at the site. Because the blood supply is very rapid in an inflamed or infected area, the drug may be absorbed more rapidly than normally from these sites. In addition, the drug may cause irritation to already abnormal tissue and result in cell destruction and death (necrosis) at the site. Blood supply to edematous or scar tissue is limited, so the absorption of a drug will be

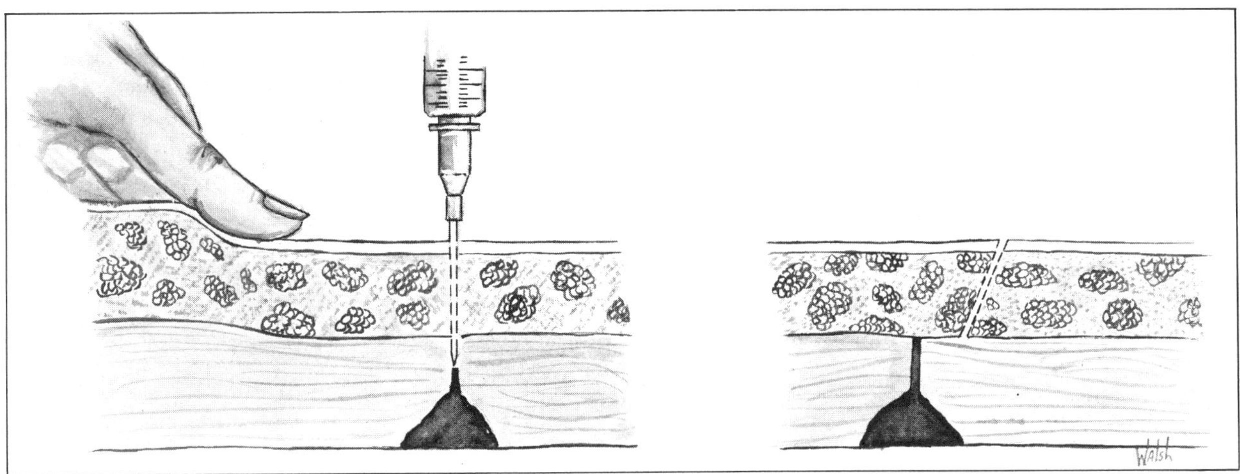

A

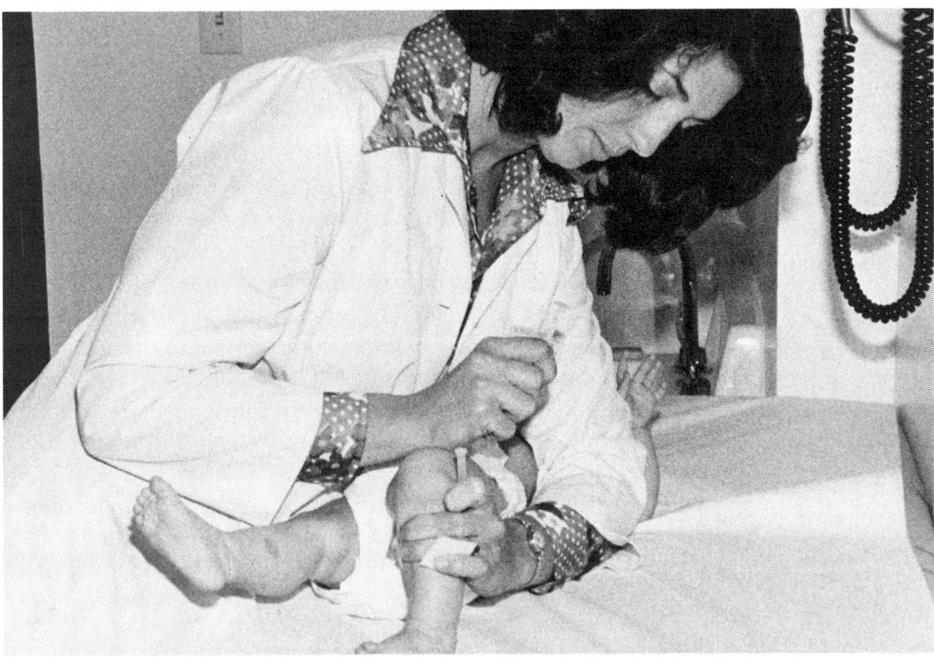

B

FIGURE 29-31. A. Z-tracking, a technique used to avoid a medicine that is irritating to subcutaneous tissue returning by needle track. Retract skin during injection (left); tissue returns to normal position following injection (right). B. To restrain a child for an anterior thigh site (vastus lateralis), secure the knee of the selected leg with your left hand; lean your body weight over the child's body to prevent his torso from moving. Use your right hand to administer the injection.

delayed or negligible if these conditions are present. Edema tends to occur in the lowest body parts. This means that the gluteus maximus and vastus lateralis sites in the person confined to bed rest may be poor injection sites if he has accompanying edema. The deltoid site usually is not affected by systemic edema because it tends to be a body part that always is elevated and, thus, may by the injection site of choice in persons with dependent edema. The difficulty with using a deltoid site is that you must have a small volume to inject (not over 1 ml) and you must use the heart of the muscle.

Many people have vaccination scars over the body of their deltoid muscle. Never inject a drug into a vaccination scar because the scar is often too tense to allow needle entrance and consists of such firm scar tissue that no absorption from the site will occur.

REDUCING THE PAIN OF PARENTERAL INJECTIONS

Contrary to popular belief, the penetration of the skin, subcutaneous tissue, and muscle by a needle does not hurt if the needle is sharp (new) and is administered swiftly. Practice injection technique, therefore, until you feel confident with a quick and sure motion. If pain is felt with the injection, it will be at the moment the medicine is injected because this action causes the stretching of tissue. After aspirating to check that the needle is in a safe location, inject the medicine fairly rapidly to minimize this moment of pain. No pain is felt when the needle is removed if the movement is, once again, quick and steady.

Pain can be relieved by massaging the area for a few seconds immediately following an injection. Counterirritation of this nature (rubbing your elbow after you bump it is the same phenomenon) decreases pain because the nerve endings at the site then transmit the feeling of rubbing rather than the stretched or painful sensation.

Parenteral injections are less painful if a person is relaxed because there will be less tension on the tissue. Relaxation can be accomplished by proper positioning (toes turned in for a dorsogluteal injection). It can also be accomplished psychologically by distracting the patient (for example, ask him to count to ten or hold his breath). In most instances, however, a nurse's confident manner is able to allay an adult's fear of an injection and help him to relax.

INFANTS AND PARENTERAL INJECTIONS

Infants and children up to about 5 years of age must be restrained for parenteral injections. Even though they say they will not move, they may be unable to hold still once you begin to inject the medicine. Quick movement by children once the needle has been injected could break the needle shaft.

The only acceptable injection site for intramuscular injection in infants is the anterior thigh (vastus lateralis); the only acceptable subcutaneous sites for injection in infants are the anterior thigh and the deltoid area. To prepare an infant for an injection in the anterior thigh site, clean the site with 70% alcohol. Restrain the knee of the selected leg with your left hand; lean your body weight over the child's body to prevent his torso from moving. Use your right hand to administer the injection (Fig. 29-31B). If the infant is very strong (the strength of a newborn when he is angry may be deceptive), ask for assistance to help restrain him. With an older child, you must have assistance because the child is far too strong to restrain by yourself. When assisting in this type of restraint, use a "Let me help you hold still" approach so the child will realize that you are asking for his cooperation rather than forcing him to do something unwillingly.

Do not ask parents to help restrain their child for injections because there is some pain associated with injections. Parents must be regarded as protectors rather than people who cause pain. Hand the child to the parents immediately after the injection to be comforted. Praise and comfort the child.

Aftercare of Injection Equipment

Syringes and needles must be discarded in safe receptacles so people cannot use them for illegal drug administration. Disposable needles must be broken at the hub and disposable syringes must be crushed at the tip (Fig. 29-32) and then discarded in predetermined places for removal from the nursing care unit. Glass syringes and reusable needles must be rinsed with tap water and placed in a suitable container for safe return to central supply for resterilization.

A syringe used for oral medication measurement or administration must be discarded with the same thorough actions described above. Safe disposal of needles and syringes is as much a responsibility of drug administration as any other step; do not regard it lightly just because the step occurs late in the procedure.

INTRAVENOUS MEDICATION

In many health care agencies, student nurses are not allowed to administer intravenous medication. You should learn the administration technique, however, because as a graduate, you will be administering many drugs by this route.

Intravenous administration (injection directly into the venous bloodstream) is the most rapid way to administer a drug because it bypasses the step of drug absorption completely. This also makes it the most dangerous form of medicine administration. If the wrong medicine is administered accidentally, it will begin to take action before you have the chance to counteract the error.

The steps of beginning an intravenous infusion are discussed in Chap. 30 because the intravenous route is used to stabilize body fluids as well as to administer medicine. Medicine can be injected by this technique (piercing the skin and sliding the needle of the syringe into an evident, available vein), but this form of medication therapy is used only in emergencies because it requires a puncture of the vein that is accompanied by pain; it is generally reserved as a physician's responsibility. Because veins cannot be entered too many times at the same site before inflammation results and some oozing of blood into subcutaneous tissue (hematoma) occurs and obliterates the site, this technique is not an ideal one for medicine administration. As a rule then, medicine for intravenous administration is added, not directly at the vein site, but to an already existing intravenous line. This can be done in four ways: (1) directly into the bottle or bag of intravenous fluid, (2) into a volume-controlled chamber in the intravenous tubing, (3) directly into the lower tubing at a bolus injection site on the tubing, or (4) directly into a heparin lock.

These techniques of medication administration are discussed in Chap. 30 with other techniques concerned with intravenous fluid therapy. Quick Reference Stop 29-4 presents some interesting findings about the safe administration of injections and intravenous medications.

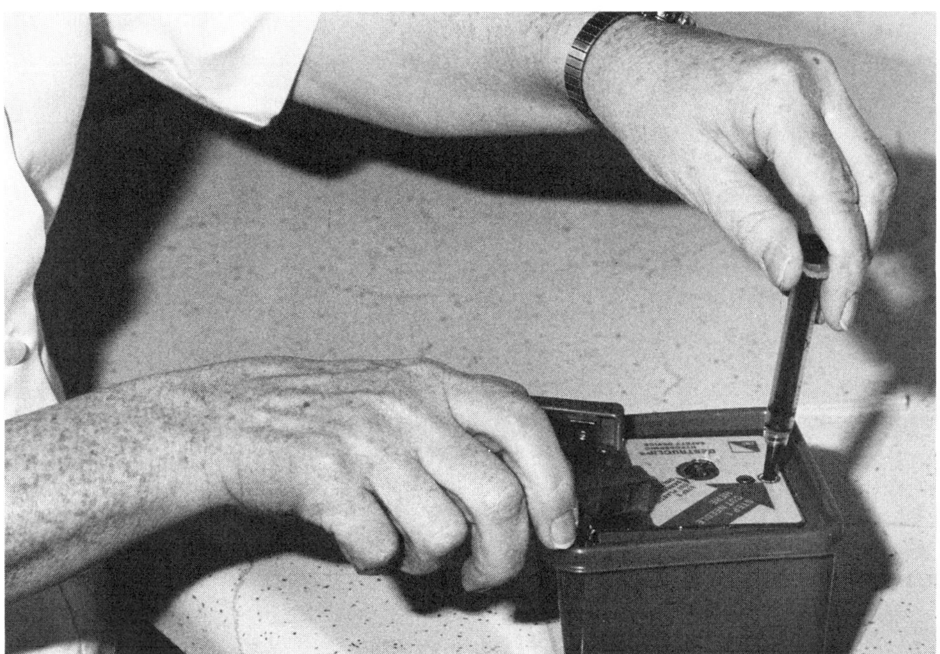

A

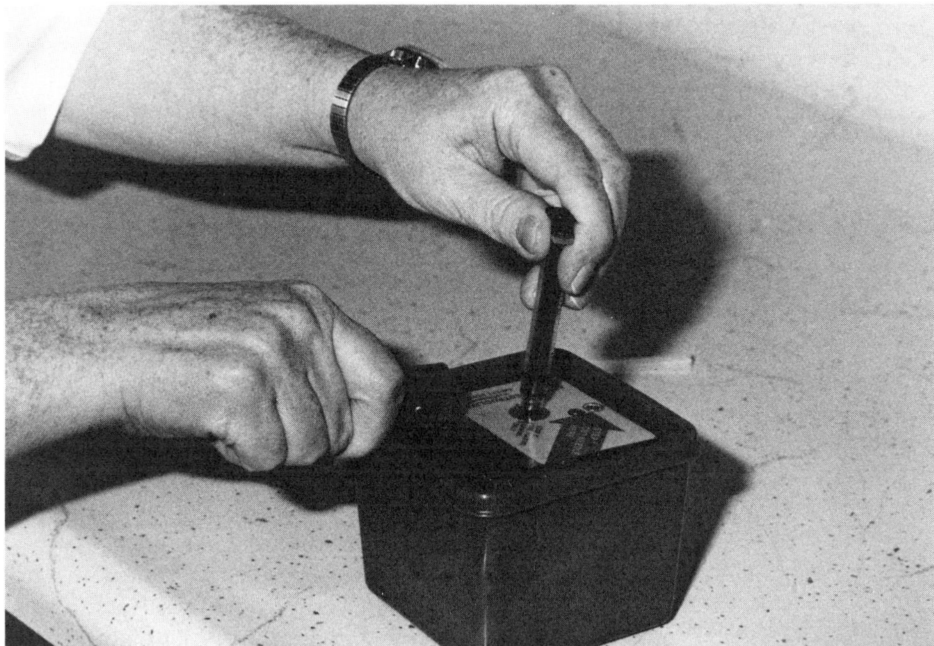

B

FIGURE 29-32. After use, break disposable needles at the hub (A) and crush disposable syringes at the tip (B).

TOPICAL ADMINISTRATION OF MEDICINE

Topical administration of drugs is the application of medicine to the skin by rubbing (inunction) or instillation (flushing a body cavity such as the conjunctiva of the eye with medication).

Types of Medicine

Topical preparations of medicine vary in concentration and consistency depending on the effect intended by the medicine. They differ from oral or parenteral administration preparations because they are designed to be used only for external use. *Lotions* are water-based suspensions. They are patted onto the skin to soothe and reduce irritation at a local site. A *liniment* is a liquid suspension that is applied to the skin by rubbing to relieve pain and redden the skin. It relieves pain and swelling at the site by counterirritation and improves blood supply to the body part. *Plaster* is the older term used for a counterirritant medication.

An *ointment*, in contrast, has an oil base such as petrolatum or lanolin. Ointments tend to cling to skin more firmly than lotions and, thus, do not wash off as easily as lotions. Ointments may be prepared in sterile forms as in the case of eye applications (ophthalmic ointments).

☐ **QUICK REFERENCE STOP 29-4: RESEARCH**

One of the nurse's major responsibilities is to insure that medications are administered safely and that they will be effective in the treatment of patients. The research presented below provides some data that nurses can utilize to assist them in administering medications safely and effectively to patients.

Hypodermoclysis—outdated and ineffective?
Hypodermoclysis, commonly known as clysis, is administration of fluids into subcutaneous tissue. Many nurses have felt this procedure to be unsafe and ineffective. According to Shen and Singer-Edelstein (1981), however, clysis can be a safe and effective way to administer fluids to confused, dysphagic, or comatose elderly patients and can provide a useful alternative to intravenous (IV) therapy. In their study, a sample of 270 elderly patients received a total of 1,850 infusions of isotonic fluids via the clysis method. Effective administration of 1 to 2.5 liters over a 2 to 4 hour period was achieved with only a small percentage of complications noted. The authors caution, however, that clysis should not be considered an alternative to IV therapy in life-threatening conditions.

Which position is best for dorsogluteal injection?
An experimental study by Rettig and Southby (1982) sought to determine whether patient position (prone or side-lying) affects the discomfort a patient experiences when receiving an intramuscular (IM) injection in the dorsogluteal region. The findings of this study suggest that, "an injection into a relaxed muscle reduces discomfort; that relaxation of the dorsogluteal muscle is insured when the femur is internally rotated" (p. 221).

It was concluded by the researchers that either the prone or the side-lying position can be used when the patient is receiving an IM injection into the dorsogluteal region, provided muscle relaxation is insured by internal rotation of the femur.

Are students adequately prepared to administer IM injections safely to patients?
According to Mitchell (1982), the answer may be *no*! In a study of nursing students who had previously been taught and apparently had learned the skill of administering an intramuscular injection, overwhelming failure was demonstrated when students attempted to administer IM injections. The greatest number of failures was due to student inability to accurately identify boundaries and/or palpate bony landmarks. The author identifies the need for more adequate teaching by faculty and greater learning by students in order to insure safe administration of medication by IM injection.

SUGGESTED READINGS

Mitchell, C. A. Development of an instrument to measure process components of the skill, intramuscular injection. *PRN: The Adelphi Report 1981—82*, Project for Research in Nursing, School of Nursing, Adelphi University, Garden City, N.Y.

Rettig, F. M., and Southby, J. R. Using different body positions to reduce discomfort from dorsogluteal injection. *Nursing Research* 31(4):219, 1982.

Shen, R. J., and Singer-Edelstein, M. Subcutaneous infusions in the elderly. *Journal of the American Geriatric Society* 29(12):583, 1981. As reported in: Hypodermoclysis revisited. Medical Highlights. *Am. J. Nurs.* 82(3):466, 1982.

Pastes are thick, stiff ointments. They are used to protect skin from things such as drainage from a wound that would otherwise quickly excoriate the skin because of the presence of constant moisture.

Skin Application

Many preparations of topical applications are supplied in jars with screw-top lids. Others are supplied in toothpaste-like squeeze tubes. Skin applications require clean (not sterile) technique. However, if there is a break in the skin, topical application requires sterile technique in order to prevent the spread of microorganisms internally.

To remove a medication from a jar, use a clean tongue blade and remove the amount of medication that you judge necessary for application (Fig. 29-33). Place the tongue blade on a clean piece of gauze and carry it to the patient's bedside on a tray. In many instances, a layer of old lotion or ointment needs to be washed away from the administration site before a new one is applied. To apply the new ointment, use the tongue blade or the gauze to spread the substance on the skin. If the area of application is tender, use softer gauze for application to reduce the possibility of causing discomfort. It is important that you do not spread topical medicine with your fingers; some absorption always take place from the skin, so over a period of time, you would absorb some of the medicine through the skin of your fingers.

Following application of a topical substance, the person's physician may or may not want the site covered with a dressing. A dressing keeps the substance from rubbing off against the bedclothes but it also holds in moisture and may cause the site to become macerated.

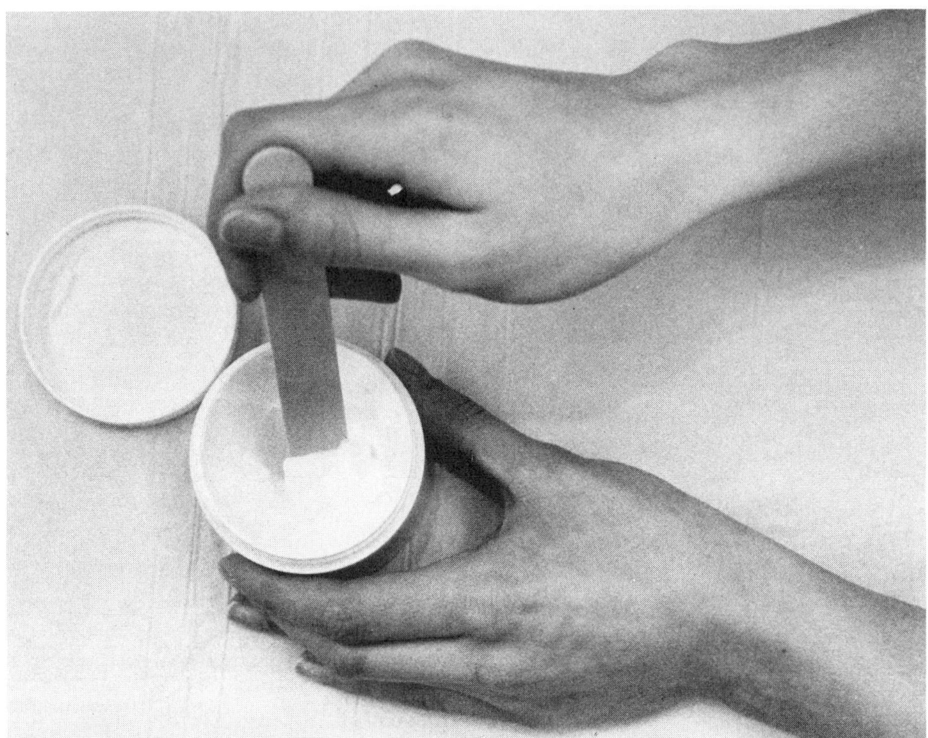

FIGURE 29-33. To remove medication from a jar, use a clean tongue blade.

Instillations

An *instillation* is the placement of a solution or medication in a body cavity in order to obtain a therapeutic effect.

EYE INSTILLATION

Medication is applied to the eye either in the form of drops or ointment. All medication for use in the eye must be labeled "ophthalmic preparation" (safe for use in contact with the eye). The medication must be kept sterile and applied sterilely to prevent the development of eye infection.

Eye Drops. For comfort, eye drops should be at room temperature when administered. To instill eye drops, position the patient so his head is held back if he is sitting; his head is flat if he is supine (Fig. 29-34). Expose the conjuctiva of the lower eyelid by placing a finger on the skin beneath the eye and gently retract the eyelid downward. If the person is an adult, ask him to look up so that his cornea will move as far away from the bottom of the eye globe as possible.

Using a sterile eye dropper that is supplied with the medication, let the required number of drops of medication fall onto the pocket of the lower conjunctival sac. Be certain that the drops do not fall on the cornea because this will be painful (a corneal reflex). Also be certain that the drops do not fall on the inner canthus or they will be immediately lost through the nasolacrimal duct. Allow the person to close his eye and blink immediately afterward to wash the medication across the entire surface of the eye.

Use a degree of speed when administering eye drops (but not to the point that you compromise safety) because having eye drops placed is not a pleasant sensation. Remember that once you have explained what you are going to do, the anticipation of the administration of eye drops may be unnerving. Be certain that the tip of the eye dropper does not touch the eye or it will become contaminated. If this does occur, you cannot return it to the bottle of medication because it would contaminate the entire bottle. In addition, the tip of the dropper could actually scar the cornea.

It is general practice to discard any unused medication drawn up into the medicine dropper rather than return it to the bottle. (As a general principle, never return medication to bottles in order to avoid the possibility of returning it to the wrong bottle.) Be certain that you include three safety checks to identify the medicine with eye instillations: (1) when you select the medication, (2) when you leave the medication area, and (3) when you draw the medicine into the dropper.

Ointment Application. To apply ointment to the eye, take the tube of ophthalmic ointment and a piece of sterile gauze to the bedside. Unscrew and place the cap of the tube right-side up on the bedside table to keep it clean. Squeeze a drop of ointment out onto the gauze. This is a precautionary step in case the drop was contaminated when this tube of ointment was used previously. After the first drop has been dispelled, open the lower conjunctival sac in the same manner as if instilling eye drops; place a rim of ointment along the con-

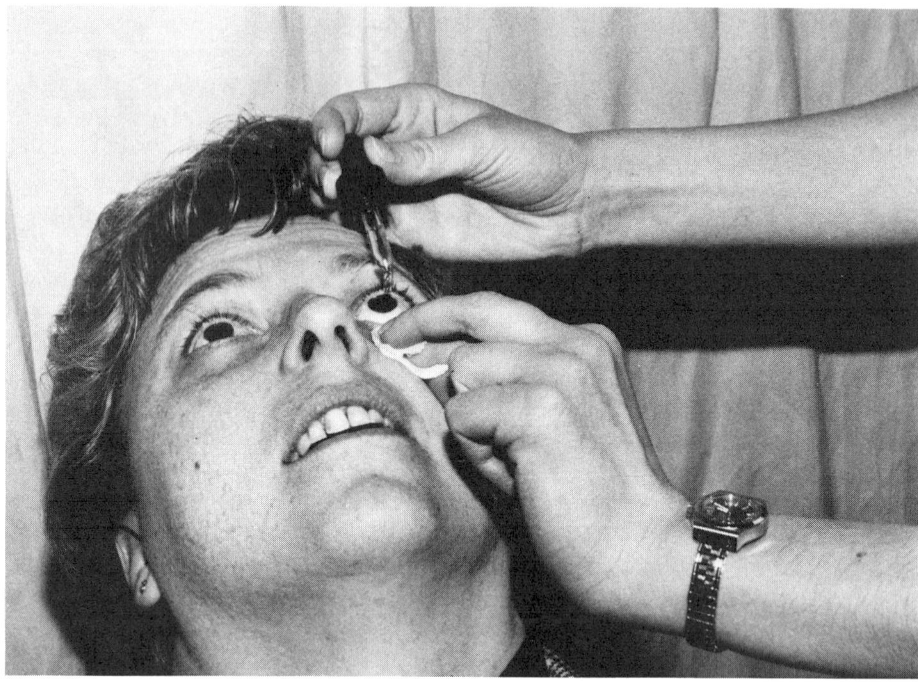

FIGURE 29-34. Installation of eye drops. The medication is dropped into the lower conjunctiva.

junctival sac from the inner canthus to the outer canthus. Always begin at the inner canthus and move to the other so that if any infection is present, it will not be carried into the nasolacrimal duct and possibly into the second eye. Allow the person to close his eye and blink in order to spread the ointment over the eye globe.

Before replacing the cap on the ointment tube, squeeze out and discard a drop. This will protect the ointment in the tube from being contaminated in case it made contact with the eye during administration.

Be certain to include three safety checks to properly identify eye ointment. Sometimes medications such as ointments do not seem as serious as other medications. No medication administration should be taken lightly.

NOSE DROPS

Nose drops should be at room temperature when administered for greatest comfort. Be certain to maintain three identification safety checks with nose drops and sprays. To instill nose drops, position the person with his head held back if he is sitting in a chair; if lying supine, place a pillow under his neck so his head is tipped slightly backward (hyperextended) (Fig. 29-35).

Instill the drops by letting them fall gently into each nostril from the medicine dropper provided with the medicine. Be careful not to touch the nasal mucosa with the dropper tip or you will be unable to return the dropper to the bottle again because it will be contaminated with bacteria. Ask the person to hold his head in this extended position for 3 to 5 minutes.

If the medication is being administered for sinus congestion, its purpose is to shrink nasal mucous membrane and allow drainage of secretions from the sinuses. The most effective way to administer this type of drop is to position the person with his head to the right side (still hyperextended) while you administer drops to the right nostril; turn his head to the left side to administer drops in the left nostril. After administration to the right side, pause at least a minute to allow penetration on that side; have the patient also hold his head in the left-sided position for a minute after administration to allow penetration. After the drops are instilled, ask him to "sniff" or attempt to move the medication back into the deep recesses of his nasal cavity.

If nose medication is furnished in a squeeze-type tube, the best position for administration is to have the person sit upright so the position of the squeeze bottle is also upright. Most people prefer to administer this type of medication to themselves and certainly can do so. They merely squeeze the plastic soft-sided bottle the number of times prescribed and "sniff" each time to draw the medication well into the nasal folds. Do not tip this type of dispenser up to squeeze it or, instead of a spray of medication, a stream of medication will pour out. This is a larger dose of medication than was prescribed (a single spray holds no more than a drop; a stream of medication could hold a hundred drops) and may be frightening because it will run to the back of the throat (a smothering feeling). It could lead to aspiration.

EAR DROPS

It is important that ear drops be at room temperature when administered. If a cold substance is placed in the ear, it can affect the equilibrium of the body so drastically that the person may vomit from the sudden spinning sensation he experiences; it can cause acute pain

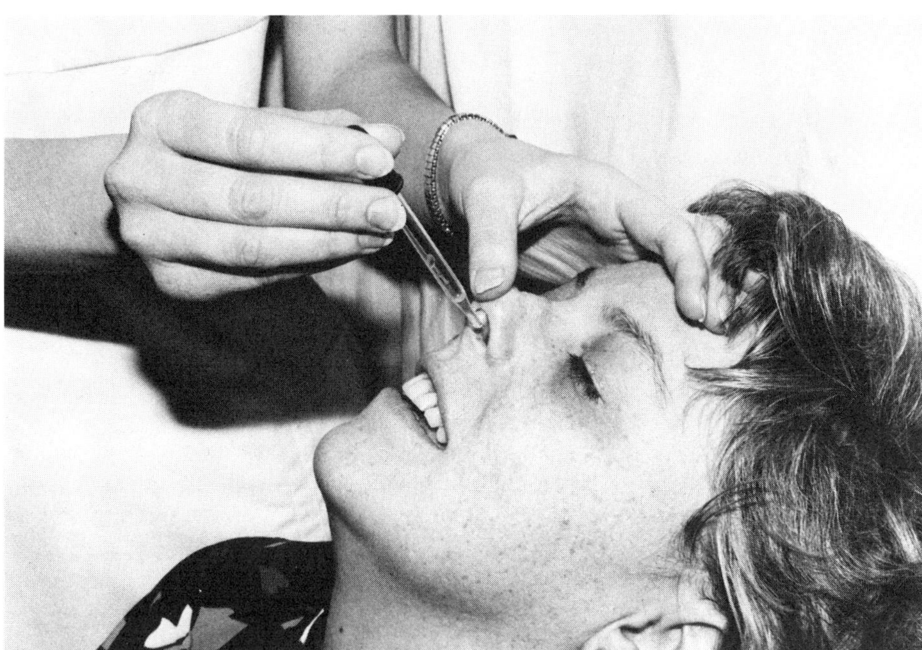

FIGURE 29-35. Installation of nose drops. Be careful that the tip of the dropper does not touch the nose; if it does, you should not return it to the medicine vial.

from the membrane contraction. All ear medication will be marked *otic* solution. Remember to include three safety checks for medicine identification.

Ear drops are instilled for bacterial or fungal infections, to reduce local inflammation, or to soften cerumen (earwax). To instill drops, position the person with his head to the side if he is sitting; turn him on his side if he is in bed. To be certain that the drops of medicine penetrate deeply into the external canal, you must straighten the track of the external ear canal. To do this in a child under the age of two years, pull the pinna of the ear down and back; in an adult, pull the pinna up and back. Allow the number of prescribed drops of medicine to fall into the ear canal using the medicine dropper supplied with the medicine. To prevent contamination, be careful not to touch the dropper against the ear (Fig. 29-36). Have the person hold his position for 3 to 5 minutes following the instillation so that the medicine can travel the length of the external ear canal. There is controversy concerning whether or not placing a cotton pledget in the external ear following ear drop placement helps to hold the medicine in place. In some instances, this may be helpful; in others, the cotton actually may act as a wick and draw medication out of the inner part of the external canal.

Having ear drops placed may be uncomfortable. Give support for cooperation, especially in children who may be frightened.

BLADDER INSTILLATION

Bladder instillations are not common procedures. They may be used to instill an antibiotic solution into the bladder but are used mostly in combination with diagnostic testing (the bladder is filled with a radio opaque solution that shows on x-ray; the person voids and the function of the bladder and the urethra can be demonstrated on x-ray).

The bladder first is catheterized to remove the urine in the bladder (see Chap. 38 for bladder catheterization technique). The solution is allowed to infuse into the bladder by gravity drainage or gentle syringe pressure.

Following the instillation, it may be necessary to press a sterile gauze square against the external urinary meatus for a few minutes. This will minimize the sensation of having to void so that the medication can be retained in the bladder for the designated or desired length of time.

The bladder is a sterile, internal cavity prone to infection. Therefore, intrusive bladder procedure must utilize a totally sterile technique to avoid introducing microorganisms into the bladder. With diagnostic testing, you often are assisting with the catheterization and instillation rather than being the primary caregiver. Remember that if you hand a caregiver the wrong solution or strength of solution to instill, you are as legally responsible for the error as the person who actually instills it. Include three medicine identification checks for yourself in the procedure; show the person to whom you are handing the solution the label of the medicine.

RECTAL INSTILLATION

Rectal instillations are of two types: (1) fluid instillation and (2) suppository insertion.

Suppository Insertion. Rectal suppositories are medicines combined with a glycerin or cocoa butter base. They are kept refrigerated prior to insertion. After

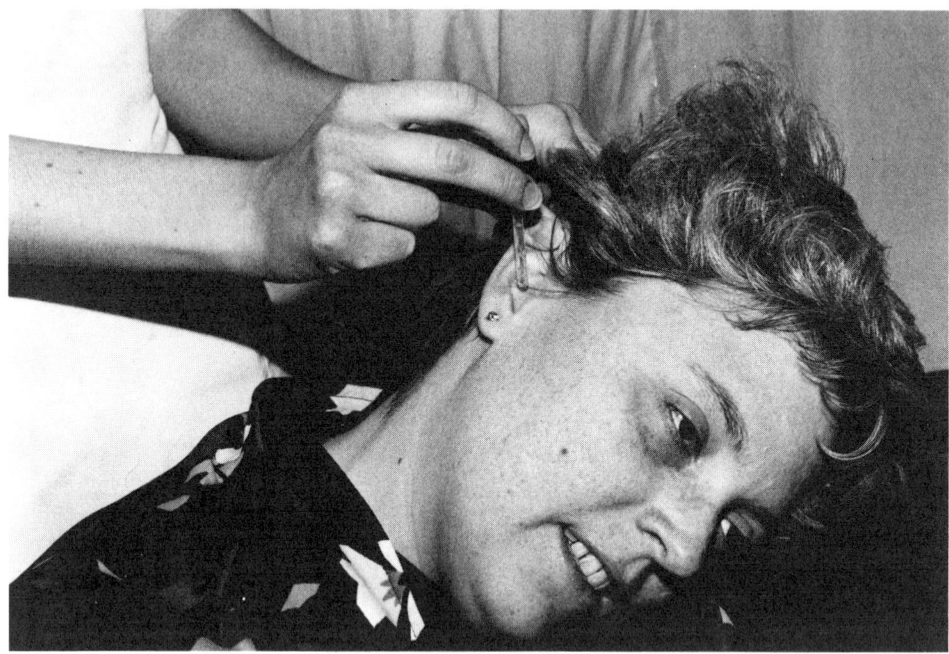

FIGURE 29-36. Installation of ear drops. In an adult, the ear is pulled up and back.

FIGURE 29-37. Insertion of a rectal suppository. To correspond with the slant of the rectum, the angle of insertion should be toward the umbilicus. Protect your hand with a clean glove or finger cot.

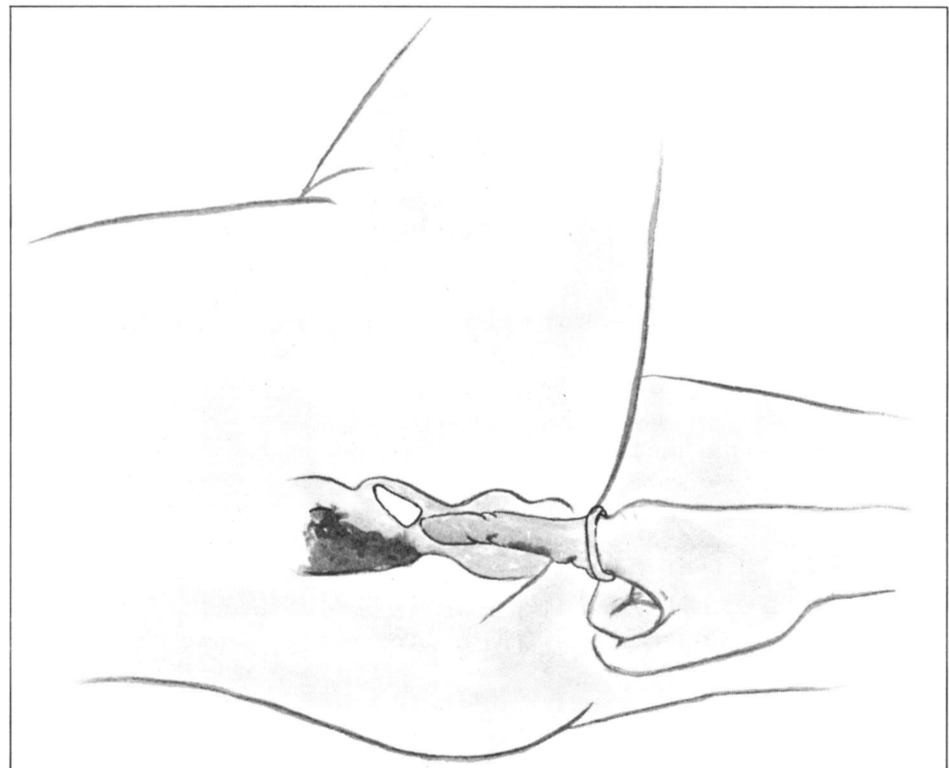

insertion, as the base substance reaches body temperature, it melts and releases the drug to be absorbed across the mucous membrane of the rectum.

To insert a suppository, ask the person to turn on his side in a Sim's position. Cover your index finger with a rubber finger cot or a clean rubber glove (use your smallest finger with infants). Lubricate the tip of the suppository with a water-based lubricant. Place the lubricated end of the suppository at the anal meatus and, using your covered finger, gently insert it the full length of your finger. It is necessary to place a suppository this deep because you must place it beyond both the first and second rectal sphincters. Otherwise, it will initiate rectal contractions and the medicine will be expelled. The angle of insertion should be toward the umbilicus because that is the slant of the rectum (Fig. 29-37).

Withdraw your finger gently and press the person's buttocks together for a full minute. This relieves any feeling of having to defecate caused by rectal intrusion and, therefore, prevents the suppository from being expelled. At the end of the minute of compression, wipe away any excess lubricant; help the person to a comfortable position.

Always use extremely gentle pressure for rectal insertion to relieve the sensation of having to defecate. Gentle pressure is also important if a person has hemorrhoidal tissue present (distended rectal veins) because hemorrhoids may make rectal insertion very painful; extremely distended rectal veins could actually rupture with rough handling. Appreciate the fact that many people are embarrassed by having rectal medications administered. Offer support as necessary.

Fluid Instillation. Small amounts of liquid medicines can be inserted rectally for absorption across the membrane. These are instilled using the enema administration technique that is discussed in Chap. 37.

Any medication administered rectally is administered using clean (not sterile) technique. Do not discount the importance of the medicine you are administering by this method; carefully identify the medicine and strength before administration.

VAGINAL INSTILLATIONS

Vaginal medication generally is administered to combat local fungal or bacterial infections. Vaginal medication may be in suppository, foam, or fluid forms.

Vaginal Suppositories. Vaginal suppositories are medications combined with a base such as cocoa butter. At body temperature, the suppository melts and allows the drug to contact the vaginal membrane. Most vaginal medications are supplied with an applicator to facilitate effective insertion.

Vaginal administration is always accomplished with sterile technique to avoid introducing microorganisms into the vagina that could spread to the uterus and cause a lethal infection. For administration, insert the suppository into its accompanying applicator, being careful not to touch any portion of the applicator except the distal tip that will not enter the vagina. If it is not prelubricated, lubricate the tip of the applicator with sterile petroleum jelly or a similar water-based lubricant (discard the first drop of lubricant onto a sterile gauze to ensure that the drop you use is sterile). Help the woman position herself supine with her knees elevated (a dorsal recumbent position). Place a draw sheet or bath blanket over her abdomen and upper torso to prevent embarrassment. Expose the vaginal opening by gently spreading the vulva with one hand; insert the applicator and direct it downward toward the patient's back because that is the anatomical slant of the vagina (Fig. 29-38).

If excessive vaginal discharge is present, wipe away the accumulated discharge on the vulva before insertion (a washcloth with soap and water will serve this purpose) so accumulated vulvar secretions will not be introduced when the applicator is inserted. If an infectious process is present, you might want to wear a clean glove to protect your hand that touches the infected vulvar tissue. Following the deposition of the suppository, gently remove the applicator. Wipe away any excess lubricant from the vaginal opening with a sterile gauze square. Urge the patient to lay flat on her back for about 15 minutes because standing upright might cause expulsion of the suppository before the medicine can be released.

Be aware that many women are embarrassed by vaginal medication insertion. The average, responsible woman can be depended on to administer this type of

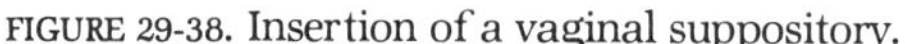
FIGURE 29-38. Insertion of a vaginal suppository.

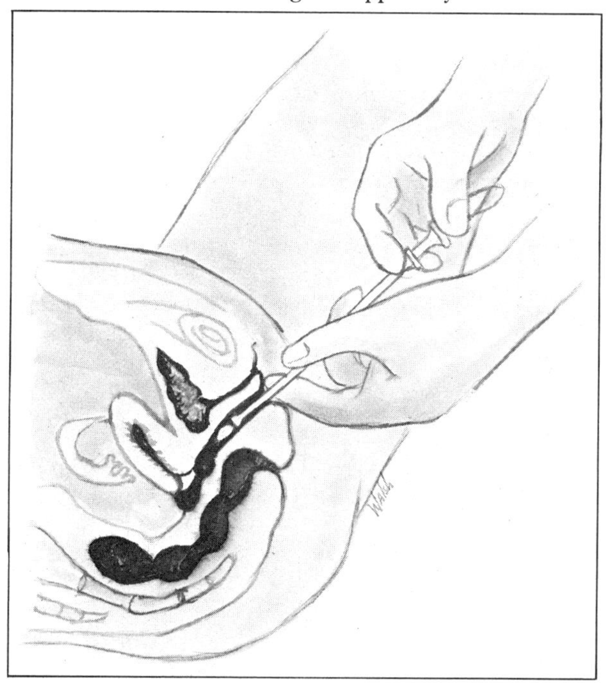

medication to herself after you have reviewed the procedure with her. Emphasize the fact that she must be careful not to touch the tip of the applicator prior to insertion. Make sure she understands the anatomical position of the vagina and the necessity for remaining flat for 15 minutes after medication insertion.

Remember that legally, whether you administer a medicine or give it to a woman to administer to herself, your responsibility concerning medicine administration is the same. Include three checks to identify the type and strength of medicine in your preparation, whether or not you will perform the actual administration.

Douching. Technically, the instillation of medicine vaginally by fluid administration is not really an instillation. Because the vagina has no external sphincter, the fluid is not retained. Therefore, this form of administration actually is an *irrigation* (douching). Allowing fluid to flow across the membrane surface is an effective method of cleaning the vaginal mucosa or exposing it to a drug.

As with all medication, be certain to check the type and strength of medication you are using three times. Solutions for vaginal insertion should be room temperature or feel pleasantly warm on the inner wrist; cold solutions may cause uterine cramping and discomfort. Prepare the solution in an irrigating container with the appropriate tubing and douche tip as specified. Douche tips are plastic or glass and are curved to conform to the shape of the vagina. Inspect such tips carefully for sharp edges or cracks because vaginal membrane is fragile, and an accidental laceration may be very painful. Help the woman to lie in a dorsal recumbent position. Position a bedpan comfortably under her buttocks; use appropriate draping for modesty. Lubricate the tip of the tubing with a water-based lubricant (discard the first drop to avoid the possibility of contaminated lubricant) and gently insert the douche tip into the vagina.

It is good practice to allow a small amount of the solution to flow over the woman's vulva to cleanse the area of the vagina before inserting the douche tip so you do not introduce accumulated vulvar secretions into the vagina. If this simple cleansing procedure is not adequate, clean the vulva thoroughly (with a washcloth and soap and water) before beginning. Following cleansing or rinsing, allow the solution to flow from a height of no more than 18 inches (Fig. 29-39).

FIGURE 29-39. Installation of a vaginal douche.

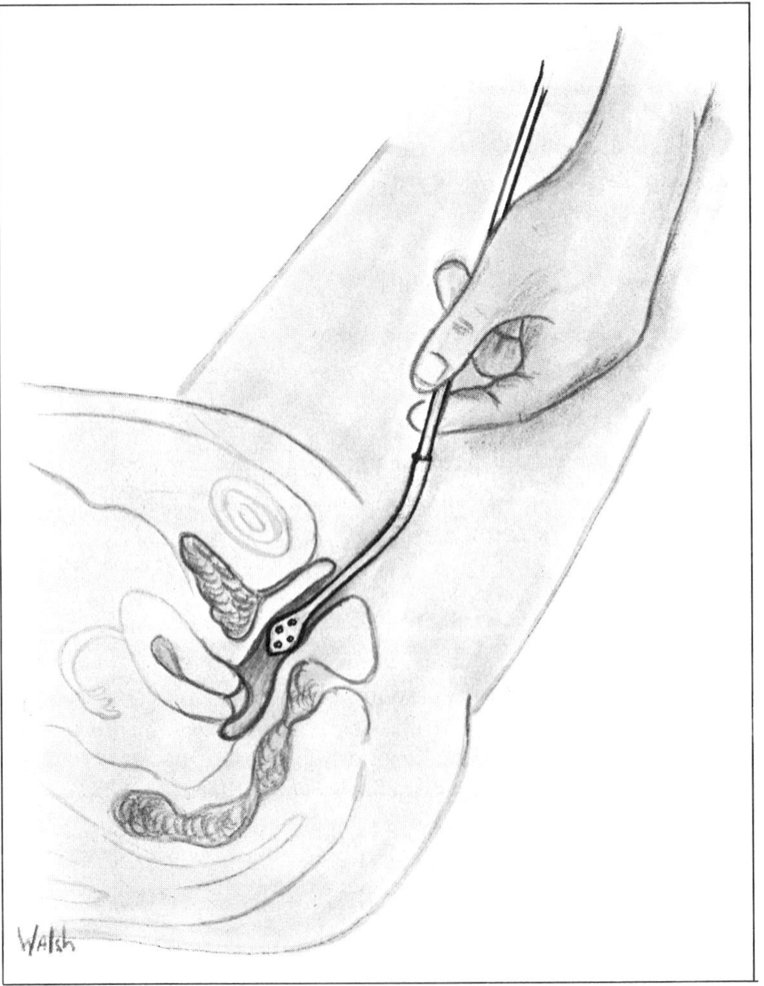

Many women are asked to continue to administer douches to themselves at home. Sitting in a bathtub is the recommended position for them to use at home. When reviewing instructions with them, be certain to emphasize that the solution should be at a sensible temperature (some people think that "burning out" an infection is desirable; this will burn vaginal membrane before it will be effective against microorganisms) and also explain the importance of regulating the height of the solution container (too high a position could cause pressure that could conceivably force solution into the cervix and uterus, causing a uterine infection).

There are commercial douche sets that women can buy over-the-counter that consist of a bulb-type syringe; many women ask if they can use these instead. They are not recommended as being as effective for general use as the other type. In fact, these types of administration sets are dangerous if the woman is pregnant because if any cervical dilatation is occurring, solution surely would enter the uterus and may cause fetal damage if administered under pressure this way.

Inhalation Administration

Drugs may be administered by inhalation for local effect on respiratory membranes. Such administration is by nebulizer (a fine-mist spray) or by a pressurized device that sprays medicine. Oxygen given by inhalation may be considered a medicine. All these forms of therapy are discussed in Chap. 32 with other aspects of respiratory therapy.

TEACHING SAFE MEDICINE ADMINISTRATION

Although you may administer the initial or first few dosages of medicine to a person, you very often will need to give him instructions to continue to take the medication by himself at home. The following box lists guidelines for the patient to follow when self-administering medicine.

Before a person can self-administer a drug safely, he needs the same information that you require before you can administer a drug safely: name of the drug, purpose or expected action, correct dosage and route, what to do if a dose is missed (just skip a dose or double up the next time?), any foods or other medicine that cannot be taken with this drug, expected side effects, and any special instructions (how to administer an injection, etc.) (Fig. 29-40).

Usually, a person does not ask enough questions about the medicine he will be taking at home to know the answers to the above questions. If something happens that he does not expect because he was not forewarned about it, his first solution to the problem will probably be to stop taking the drug. Every patient must understand clearly the importance of his drug therapy so that he will continue to administer the medicine.

Do not wait for people to ask questions about the medication they are taking. Do not just hand people their prescriptions. Always explain to them what the medicine is and why they will be taking it.

Guidelines for Self-Administration of Medicine

1. Take drugs only when necessary. Use a minimum of over-the-counter medications to prevent inadvertent drug interactions.
2. Never take a medication unless you understand the action, dosage, untoward or side effects, and rules for safe storage of the drug.
3. Store medicine in its original labeled container; the label is a safeguard against medicine error.
4. Do not store unused portions of drugs because their composition may change after a period of time. Do not discard them in the garbage because there is a possibility that children might find and ingest them. Discard them by flushing them down a toilet.
5. Keep all medicine out of the reach of children. Try not to take medicine in the presence of children or refer to medicine as candy because children mimic adult behavior and accidentally may poison themselves.
6. Keep oral medication in a different storage area than medication to be used externally so external medicine will not be ingested accidentally.
7. Examine medication for expiration dates; do not use after these dates because the composition of drugs changes with time.
8. Refrigerate all drugs that require refrigeration.
9. Insist that the pharmacist put the name of the drug on the label of the medication. Having the name of the drug on the label helps prevent medicine errors and, in case of accidental poisoning or an untoward effect, it allows proper interventions to be started quickly.
10. Do not take drugs in the dark because you will not be able to read and identify the label. If vision is a problem, have a support person set up the medicine in a prefilled dispenser kit or mark the bottle of medicine with a form of identification that you can feel with your fingertips (a 1/2 inch square of sandpaper, for example).
11. If remembering to take medicine is a problem, make out a reminder chart so that doses are checked off as they are taken.
12. If you experience effects with drug administration that your physician had not warned you about, consult your physician before you continue to take the medicine.

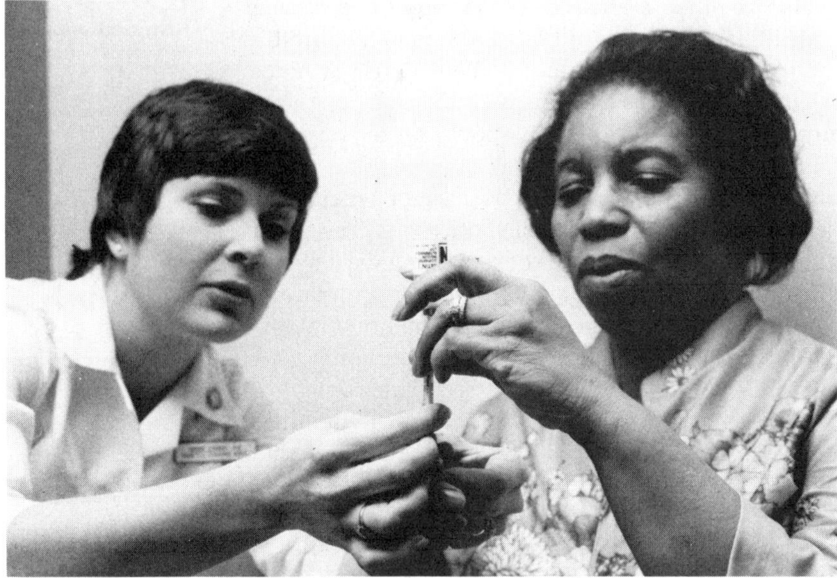

A

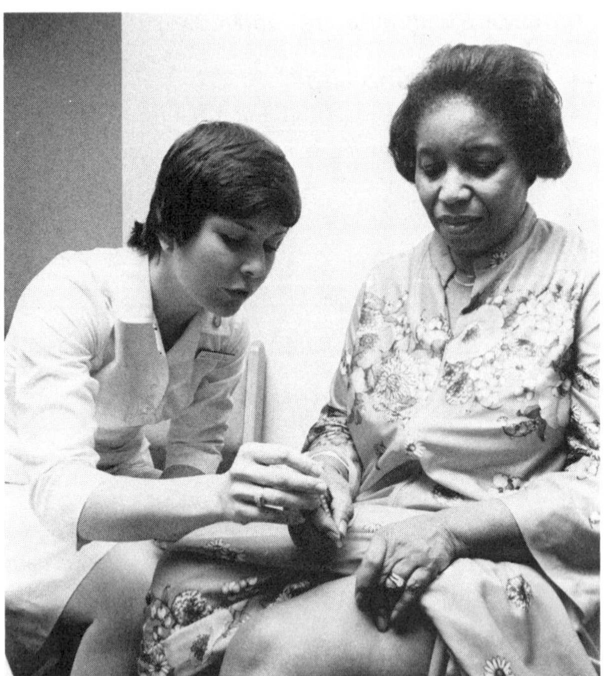

B

FIGURE 29-40. Teaching how to administer medicine is a major nursing role. Here a woman learns how to withdraw a correct dose of insulin (A) and administer her own injection (B).

UTILIZING NURSING PROCESS

To be certain that the administration of medications is done thoroughly, utilize nursing process.

ASSESSMENT

Always assess whether a medicine is currently needed before you administer it. When a patient's condition changes, the need for medicine changes. Because you spend so much time with a patient, your judgment as a caregiver as to whether a person's condition is changing is often the most accurate of all his caregivers, especially when estimations of mood or patterns of behavior are considered. Use findings from patient history, physical assessment, and laboratory reports to assess thoroughly.

ANALYSIS

Although medication administration begins as a dependent nursing function (you follow the instructions of someone else), there is a need for independent action. Assessment often leads you to conclude that a person who was prescribed a potent pain medication on Monday for his severe pain no longer needs such a strong pain medication; your independent action is to ask for a change in order. In other instances, a person's physician may underestimate the degree of pain a person will have and prescribe a pain medication that is not strong enough. Once again, you would ask for a change in order. Sometimes, prior to administration of an antibiotic (a classification of drugs with high allergy potential), you notice that the person has a widespread body rash. Analysis tells you not to administer the medication until the rash can be evaluated. Another example might be realizing that a laboratory report you have just received shows that a person has a strain of bacteria that is resistant to the type of antibiotic that has been prescribed for him. He needs a change of prescription because administering this antibiotic to him will provide no effect at all. The recognition of ineffective or excessive drug administration is an important part of your duty; you must pull your assessments together and, based on their meaning and importance, make a conclusion concerning the administration of a particular medicine (see QRS 29-5 to 29-7).

☐ **QUICK REFERENCE STOP 29-5: SAFETY**
General Rules for Safe Medication Administration

1. Be certain that you have a clear written order for each medication administered unless a true emergency situation exists.
2. Concentrate on the act of preparing and administering medicine; do not let yourself be distracted during this potentially dangerous time.
3. Never take a medicine from an unlabeled or illegibly labeled container.
4. Check a medicine Kardex or card with the original physician's order the first time a medicine is to be administered to be certain that a transcription error did not occur.
5. Always check the patient's identification band before administering medicine. The advantage of this identification check is that it allows you to care for responsible adults (who could tell you their name correctly) and persons who cannot do this reliably (children, people with mental illness) without changing your preparation habits.
6. Do not leave medicine by a bedside; if it is not taken immediately, return it to the medication area.
7. Never return an unused portion of medicine to a stock medicine bottle because of the potential danger of returning it to the wrong bottle and contaminating the medication.
8. Do not administer medication prepared by someone else (except for unit dose forms prepared by a pharmacist). If an error was made in preparation, you would be equally responsible for this error.
9. Do not prepare medication for another person to administer (encouraging them to break rule 8).
10. Question any drug order that is not clear or, in your opinion, would cause harm if administered.
11. Refuse to administer any medication that, in your opinion, would cause harm to the patient.
12. Chart all medicine administration as soon as administration has been completed so a dose will not be repeated accidentally by another caregiver.

PLANNING

Planning medicine administration often means planning appropriate times to administer medicine in conjunction with other therapies the person is receiving (not offering a sedative just before physical therapy, for example) or in conjunction with meals or not. The method of administration (crushed tablets, for example) requires planning so the method that will ensure compliance is used.

☐ **QUICK REFERENCE STOP 29-6: PSYCHOLOGICAL CONSIDERATIONS**

People may have unrealistic expectations about the medicine prescribed for them, expecting it to work immediately in controlling or eliminating their symptoms, and are disappointed when less than total relief occurs. Educate people that few medications are "miracle" drugs; often times, people must do more than just take a medicine (do breathing exercises, return for frequent blood work, learn to cope with stress better) in order to feel well again. On the other hand, inform people that if a medicine does not seem to be effective, they should notify their physician. An idiosyncratic or other effect may be occurring that is making the medication less effective than their physician anticipated.

☐ **QUICK REFERENCE STOP 29-7: COMMUNITY CONSIDERATIONS**

Many people are given a prescription on discharge from a health care agency. It is their responsibility to have it filled and take it as prescribed.

Always review prescriptions with people to be certain they understand the purpose of the medication they will be taking and the correct dosage and time. A person probably will be more conscientious about taking a medicine if he understands its purpose.

Ask if people foresee any problems with buying or taking a medication. This may expose problems such as not being able to afford a medication, concern they will not be able to remember which medication to take in the morning and which one to take at night, or difficulty with swallowing.

If the measurement of a medication will be difficult for a person to make such as 3/4 of a teaspoon, you might want to mark the corresponding number of mls with a ball-point pen on a plastic medicine cup for a patient to take home with him to ensure accuracy of dosage.

IMPLEMENTATION

The same steps prior to medicine administration should be used with every patient each time a medicine needs to be administered. The administration of any kind of medicine must be viewed as a large responsibility. Learn medication administration habits thoroughly so that your technique is flawless in any situation (in either a busy emergency unit or in a private home with only one patient). A practicing nurse must have the ingrained habit of reading all medication labels three times.

EVALUATION

Always include evaluation as the final step in the administration of medication. You never can be certain that a medication is having therapeutic effects until you reassess the situation and see that therapeutic effects actually are occurring.

NURSING CARE PLAN

Billy is a 2-year-old who is admitted to the hospital for otitis media (middle ear infection). He will be hospitalized for 2 days and then will be discharged. He will continue to take an antibiotic (ampicillin 250 mg QID) for an additional 8 days at home.

NURSING DIAGNOSIS

Potential for poor compliance with medication administration related to age.

Locus of Decision-Making: Shared by nurse and parent.

Goal: Billy will take medicine as prescribed.

Criteria: Billy will take ampicillin 250 mg qid for 10 days.

NURSING ORDERS

1. Ask pharmacy for liquid form; child is too young to swallow capsules.
2. Administer medicine from medicine cup following by grape juice or cherry Koolaid (his favorite).
3. Do not give medicine with syringe because he is very frightened at the sight of syringe.
4. Do not give medicine followed by orange juice; mother is worried he will associate taste of medicine with orange juice and not drink it in the future.
5. Explain action of drug to parent and importance of continuing it for the full 10 days.
6. Help mother to make a reminder sheet for refrigerator door. (Difficult for busy moms to remember meds.)
7. Praise lavishly for good compliance; needs positive association with medicine administration in order to continue to take it for the full 8 days at home.

SUGGESTED READINGS

Boyles, V. Injection aids for blind diabetic patients. *Am. J. Nurs.* 77:1456, 1977.

Clarke, T. R. Pharmacy prepared drug history: A tool to medication. *Nurs. Homes* 29:2, 1980.

Cohen, M. R. Medication errors: If a drug doesn't look right, check with the pharmacist. *Nursing* (Horsham) 11(10):81, 1981.

Cohen, M. R. Medication errors: Report errors caused by misleading package labels. *Nursing* (Horsham) 12(4):114, 1982.

Cohen, M. R. Always clean the mortar and pestle after crushing tablets. *Nursing* (Horsham) 12(12):25, 1982.

Cohen, M. R. Medication errors. Watch out for look-alike drugs. *Nursing* (Horsham) 13(1):29, 1983.

Cohen, M. R. Don't forget to check the administration route. *Nursing* (Horsham) 13(2):116, 1983.

Cohen, M. R. Look up unfamiliar drug before administering it. *Nursing* (Horsham) 13(3):74, 1983.

Creighton, H. Law for the nurse manager: Liability of nurse floated to another unit. *Nurs. Manage.* 13(3):54, 1982.

Cushing, M. Fears of a floating nurse . . . the legal side. *Am. J. Nurs.* 83(2):297, 1983.

Davis, N. M., et al. Learning from mistakes: 20 tips for avoiding medication areas. *Nursing* (Horsham) 12:65, 1982.

Dorsett, T. Administration of medications during school hours. *J. Sch. Health* 52(7):444, 1982.

Goldberg, P. B. How risky is self-care with over the counter medicines? *Geriat. Nurs.* 1:279, 1980.

Gotz, B., and Taylor, A. Drugs and the elderly. *Am. J. Nurs.* 78:1347, 1978.

Gringuaz, A. *Drugs: How They Act and Why*. St. Louis: Mosby, 1978.

Hickman, R. A. When you have to reconstitute meds . . . guide to diluents and storage times for commonly ordered drugs. *RN* 44:40, 1981.

Hopkins, S. J. Drug dosage and the elderly. *Nurs. Mirror* 152:41, 1981.

Johnston-Early, A., et al. Venipuncture and problem veins. *Am. J. Nurs.* 81:1636, 1981.

Kennedy, B. Self-medication. *Can. Nurse* 77:36, 1981.

Long, G. The effect of medication distribution systems on medication errors. *Nurs. Manage.* 13(3):182, 1982.

Markowitz, J. S., et al. Nurses, physicians, and pharmacists: Their knowledge of hazards of medications. *Nurs. Res.* 30(6):366, 1981.

Meguerdichian, D. Improving self-medication in an HRF. *Geriatr. Nurs.* (New York) 4(1):30, 1983.

Mullen, E. M., et al. Drugs and the elderly patient. *J. Gerontol. Nurs.* 7:108, 1981.

Newton, M. Guidelines for handling drug errors. *Nursing 77* 7:62, 1977.

Newton, D., and Newton, M. Route, site and technique: Three key decisions in giving parenteral medications. *Nursing 79* 9:18, 1979.

Nynick, A. Instituting a post partum self-medication program. *M.C.N.* 6(6):422, 1981.

Palmer, D. A. Unit dose. *Am. J. Nurs.* 80:2062, 1980.

Pavkou, J., et al. The older adult and drug therapy: Part one. Special considerations for the community-based elderly. *Geriatr. Nurs.* (N.Y.) 2(6):422, 1981.

Pogrund, R., et al. The aggregate approach: A student experience . . . medication errors among homebound elderly patients. *J. Gerentol. Nurs.* 8(12):696, 1982.

Ptaszynski, E. M., et al. Experience in posology. *J.N.E.* 20(8):41, 1981.

Rodman, M. J. The drug interaction we all overlook—Antacids. *RN* 43:46, 1980.

Romankiewicz, J., et al. To improve patient adherence to drug regimens: An interdisciplinary approach. *Am. J. Nurs.* 78:1211, 1978.

Royle, J., et al. Implementation of a unit dose medication system: Making change strategy relevant throughout a hospital. *Can. Nurse* 78(9):36, 1982.

Sklar, C. What constitutes nursing negligence in the administration of medications? *Can. Nurse* 77:48, 1981.

Smith, L. L. Fun and frolic with unit dose. *RN* 44:99, 1981.

Todd, B. Could your patient's confusion be caused by drugs? *Geriatr. Nurs.* 2:219, 1981.

Todd, B. What does a good drug history include? *Geriatr. Nurs.* 2:63, 1981.

Topical Therapy: Choosing and using the proper vehicle. *Nursing 77* 7:8, 1977.

QUESTIONS FOR REVIEW

A1. The patient you are assigned to care for has regular insulin (short-acting insulin) 4 units and NPH (long-acting insulin) ordered to be given at 7:30 A.M. every morning before breakfast. The night nurse tells you that she prepared it in the syringe to save time for you; she hands you the syringe of medicine. Your best action in this situation would be:

1. Place the syringe and the two vials she used to prepare the medicine in the refrigerator until 7:30 A.M.
2. Recheck the medication card against the physician's order before administering the medication.
3. Check a drug reference before giving the injection to see if regular insulin and NPH insulin are compatible when mixed.
4. Refuse to give an injection that another person has prepared.

If you chose answer 1, proceed to A2.
If you chose answer 2, proceed to A3.
If you chose answer 3, proceed to A4.
If you chose answer 4, proceed to A5.

A2. This is not the best answer because insulin should be administered at room temperature to prevent atrophy of subcutaneous tissue. Also, because you are legally responsible for your own actions, if you administered a wrong dose of insulin, even though you did not prepare it, you would be liable for the consequences. The correct answer is option 4: refuse to administer any medication you did not prepare. Go to B1 for the next problem.

A3. Although this is a procedure used to ensure that no error was made in transferring the information to the medicine card, it is not the best answer. The correct answer is option 4: refuse to administer any medication you did not prepare, because you would be liable if a mistake was made in the preparation that could be harmful to the patient. Go to B1 for the next problem.

A4. Although this is an important practice before mixing any medications in a syringe to be certain that a drug interaction will not occur, it is not the best answer. The correct answer is option 4: refuse to administer any medication you did not prepare, because you would be liable if a mistake was made in preparation that could be harmful to the patient. Go to B1 for the next problem.

A5. Right. You are legally responsible for your actions. Thus, if the nurse had made a mistake in calculating the dosage, and caused you to administer a wrong dosage, you would be liable for the consequences. As a student, refusing to administer any medication that you did not prepare is not always an easy thing to do; however, refusing is your only safe action. Most nurses will recognize the significance of your action and commend you for not breaking this important rule. Go to B1 for the next problem.

B1. Billy, 6 months old, has ampicillin 250 mg IM every 6 hr prescribed. The vial states there is 1000 mg in 1 ml of solution. How many *minims* would you administer?

1. 0.25
2. 2.5
3. 4
4. 6

If you chose answer 1, proceed to B2.
If you chose answer 2, proceed to B3.
If you chose answer 3, proceed to B4.
If you chose answer 4, proceed to B5.

B2. If you arrived at this answer, you probably misread the question. Your answer is the number of ml needed, not the number of *minims* needed. Add a conversion factor to the formula and select a new option from those in B1.

B3. If you arrived at this answer, you must have computed wrong. Look at B5 for the correct solution to the problem.

B4. Right. If you want to verify the formula and the steps needed to solve this problem see B5. Proceed to C1 for the next problem.

B5. If you arrived at this answer, you computed wrong or used a wrong formula. To solve this type of problem, you need to determine the number of ml needed and convert that number to minims. Therefore, you need to set up the formula as:

ordered amount × dose on hand

× conversion factor = answer

The conversion factor you need is 16 minims = 1 ml, so:

$$\frac{\overset{1}{\cancel{250}}\text{ mg}}{1\text{ ml}} \times \frac{1\text{ ml}}{\underset{\underset{1}{\cancel{4}}}{\cancel{1000}}\text{ mg}} \times \frac{\overset{4}{\cancel{16}}\text{ minims}}{1\text{ ml}} = 4\text{ minims}$$

C1. The best injection site to choose for 6-month-old Billy would be:

1. vastus lateralis (see C2)
2. dorsogluteal (see C3)
3. deltoid (see C4)
4. ventrogluteal (see C5)

C2. Right. The only acceptable site for an intramuscular injection in an infant who does not walk yet is the vastus lateralis muscle. Proceed to D1 for the next problem.

C3. No. This is an extremely dangerous site for an injection in an infant who does not walk yet because until this muscle strengthens with walking, the sciatic nerve occupies almost the entire muscle area. In an infant who does not walk yet, never use any intramuscular injection site except the vastus lateralis. Proceed to D1 for the next problem.

C4. Although you know that the dosage you are going to administer is small (only 4 minims), a deltoid muscle is not the best choice for an intramuscular injection site in an infant (subcutaneous injections can be given in this site to infants). In an infant who does not walk yet, never use any intramuscular injection site except the vastus lateralis. Proceed to D1 for the next problem.

C5. No. This muscle is not well-developed in infants until they walk. In an infant who does not walk yet, never use any intramuscular injection site except the vastus lateralis. Proceed to D1 for the next problem.

D1. You bring 2 tablets of Tylenol (acetaminophen) into Mr. Jones's hospital room. He is not there but his roommate tells you he is having an x-ray done in another department and will return in 15 minutes. Your best action would be:

1. Leave the medicine on Mr. Jones's bedside stand and ask his roommate to remind him to take it when he returns (see D2).
2. Place the medicine inside the top drawer of Mr. Jones's bedside stand and place a note on top of the stand telling him to take it (see D3).
3. Remove the medicine from the room and return with it when Mr. Jones returns (see D4).
4. Telephone the x-ray department and ask the nurse there to give Mr. Jones the medicine (you know they have Tylenol available) (see D5).

D2. Do not give a roommate the responsibility for reminding a patient to take his medication. Never leave medicine on a bedside stand where another patient could swallow it accidentally, thinking it was meant for him. Also Mr. Jones may decide not to take the pills and receive inadequate therapy or hoard them day by day until he has accumulated a lethal dose (stress may be the cause of suicide). Return to D1 and choose another option.

D3. This is not a responsible practice because the note might blow away before Mr. Jones returns. Remember, also, that when you are accounting for the administration of medicine, you must sign a sheet stating that you witnessed the ingestion of the medicine. Return to D1 and select another option.

D4. Right. This is the only safe procedure because it will prevent Mr. Jones from forgetting to take the medicine and prevent him from hoarding the medicine. It is important that you witness the ingestion of the medicine. Proceed to E1 for the next problem.

D5. This is not advisable. The nurse in the x-ray department will not be able to administer medicine based on your telephone order (she has no written prescription to work from). If it were imperative that Mr. Jones receive the medicine exactly at the moment you have it prepared, you could take the tray of medicine with its identifying card to the x-ray department and, providing it does not interfere with the x-ray currently being done, administer it in the x-ray department. As a rule, if a patient is not available to take a medcine when you enter his room, simply remove the medicine from the room and bring it back when the patient returns. Proceed to E1 for the next problem.

E1. You are going to apply an ophthalmic antibacterial ointment to Mrs. Smith's eye. Your best procedure would be:

1. Line the lower conjunctival rim of the eye with the ointment from the outer canthus to the inner canthus (see E2).
2. Squeeze a drop of the ointment on a sterile pad and pat the eye globe gently (see E3).
3. Drop the ointment directly onto the cornea, being careful not to contaminate the tip of the tube (see E4).
4. Line the lower conjunctival rim of the eye with the ointment from the inner canthus to the outer canthus (see E5).

E2. No. Lining the lower conjunctival rim is correct, but your motion should be from the inner canthus toward the outer canthus. This motion prevents any secretions from being pushed into the nasolacrimal duct and into the other eye. Proceed to F1 for the next problem.

E3. No. Eye ointments or drops are applied to the lower conjuctival sac, not to the eye globe, to avoid touching the cornea. Touching the cornea causes sharp pain and tearing. Select another option.

E4. No. It is important not to contaminate the tip of the ointment tube, but never place eye medicine directly on the cornea. Touching the cornea causes extreme pain and tearing. Select another option.

E5. Right. Both eye drops and eye ointment are placed in the lower conjunctival rim. Never place them on the eye globe so that you will avoid touching the cornea because touching the cornea causes extreme pain and tearing. Placing the ointment from the inner canthus to the outer canthus prevents secretions from being forced into the nasolacrimal duct and pushed into the other eye. Proceed to F1 for the next problem.

F1. When preparing an oral medication, which option is not good technique?
1. Pour liquid medicine at eye level (see F2).
2. Crush enteric-coated tablets (see F3).
3. Check the medicine label three times (see F4).
4. Use clean, not sterile, technique (see F5).

F2. In order to determine a liquid level accurately, you must look straight across at the top of the fluid. Always pour liquid medicine at eye level. Select another option.

F3. Right. Tablets should not be crushed when they are enteric-coated because crushing destroys the coating and may change or alter the drug's action. If a person cannot swallow an enteric-coated tablet, his physician should be notified so that he can change the therapy accordingly. Proceed to G1 for the next problem.

F4. You should always check the medicine label three times. Select another option.

F5. Clean, not sterile, technique is appropriate for oral medication preparation. Select another option.

G1. When preparing a subcutaneous injection of 1 ml from an ampule, which option reflects good technique?
1. Inject 1 ml of air into the ampule prior to withdrawal of 1 ml of drug. (see G2).
2. Wipe the neck of the ampule with 70% alcohol prior to opening it (see G3).
3. Use a 20 gauge, 1-1/2 inch needle for injection (see G4).
4. Hold the ampule upside down while withdrawing the medicine (see G5).

G2. No. Because ampules do not have negative pressure in them, it is unnecessary (and causes the drug level to overflow) to inject air into the ampule. Select another option.

G3. No. This is not necessary because your needle does not penetrate through the outside of the ampule as it does through the outside of a vial. Leaving alcohol on the neck of the ampule when it is broken may cause alcohol to mix with the drug, distorting or inhibiting its effect. Select another option.

G4. No. A needle of this length is too long for a subcutaneous tissue injection. It is also a very heavy gauge. A 22 gauge, 1 inch needle would be better to use to place medicine into subcutaneous tissue unless the patient is obese (with thick adipose tissue). Select another option.

G5. Right. Although at first this seems impossible, the surface tension of the liquid will hold the liquid in the ampule while you withdraw it, as long as your needle remains in the center of the ampule (touching the side of the ampule will break the surface tension and cause the liquid to flow down the needle). It is not necessary to invert an ampule to withdraw the medicine from it if positioning the ampule upside down makes you uncomfortable. Proceed to H1 for the next problem.

H1. A medication you are going to administer is ordered to be given QID. This means you would administer it:
1. 4 times a day (see H2).
2. every 4 hours (see H3).
3. twice before noon and twice after noon (see H4)
4. 2 times a day (see H5).

H2. Right. QID is the abbreviation for *quatis in die* or "4 times a day." Doses, as a rule, are spaced throughout the waking hours: 10 A.M., 2 P.M., 6 P.M., and 10 P.M. At home, people usually take QID medications with each of 3 meals and a bedtime dose. People are less apt to forget to take medication if they do it this way. Proceed to I1 for the last problem.

H3. No. Administering a drug every 4 hours would mean that it would be administered 6 times every 24 hours. QID stands for *quatis in die* or "4 times a day." Proceed to I1 for the last problem.

H4. Not necessarily. QID stands for *quatis in die* or "4 times a day," but depending on the drug, these time intervals might be spaced to cover long time spans (for example, 8 A.M., 2 P.M., 8 P.M., 2 A.M.). Spacing throughout the waking hours (10A.M., 2 P.M., 6 P.M., 10 P.M.) is the way that health care facilities usually administer QID medications. Proceed to I1.

H5. No. Two times a day is abbreviated BID. QID is the abbreviation for *quatis in die* or "4 times a day." Proceed to I1 for the next problem.

I1. When administering ear drops to 22-year-old Mr. Oswald, which option reflects good technique?
1. Pull the pinna of the ear up and back (see I2).
2. Chill the drops to reduce pain sensation (see I3).
3. Do not return the dropper to the bottle after use. (see I4).
4. Hold a warm compress to the ear following instillation (see I5).

I2. Right. This action straightens the adult's outer ear canal and allows ear drops to reach the tympanic membrane. If the patient is a child under the age of 2 years, you would pull the pinna down and back.

I3. No. Administering chilled ear drops can provoke an inner ear response that causes pain and vomiting from vertigo. Select another option.

I4. No. As long as you do not touch the ear lobe or canal with the tip of the dropper, there is no fear of contamination, and you may return the dropper to the bottle. Select another option.

I5. No. This would not be done unless specifically ordered because it might be dangerous, causing rupture of the tympanic membrane from the increased collection of fluid in the area due to the warmth. Select another option.

IX. NURSING PROCESS IN ACTION: BODY MAINTENANCE NEEDS

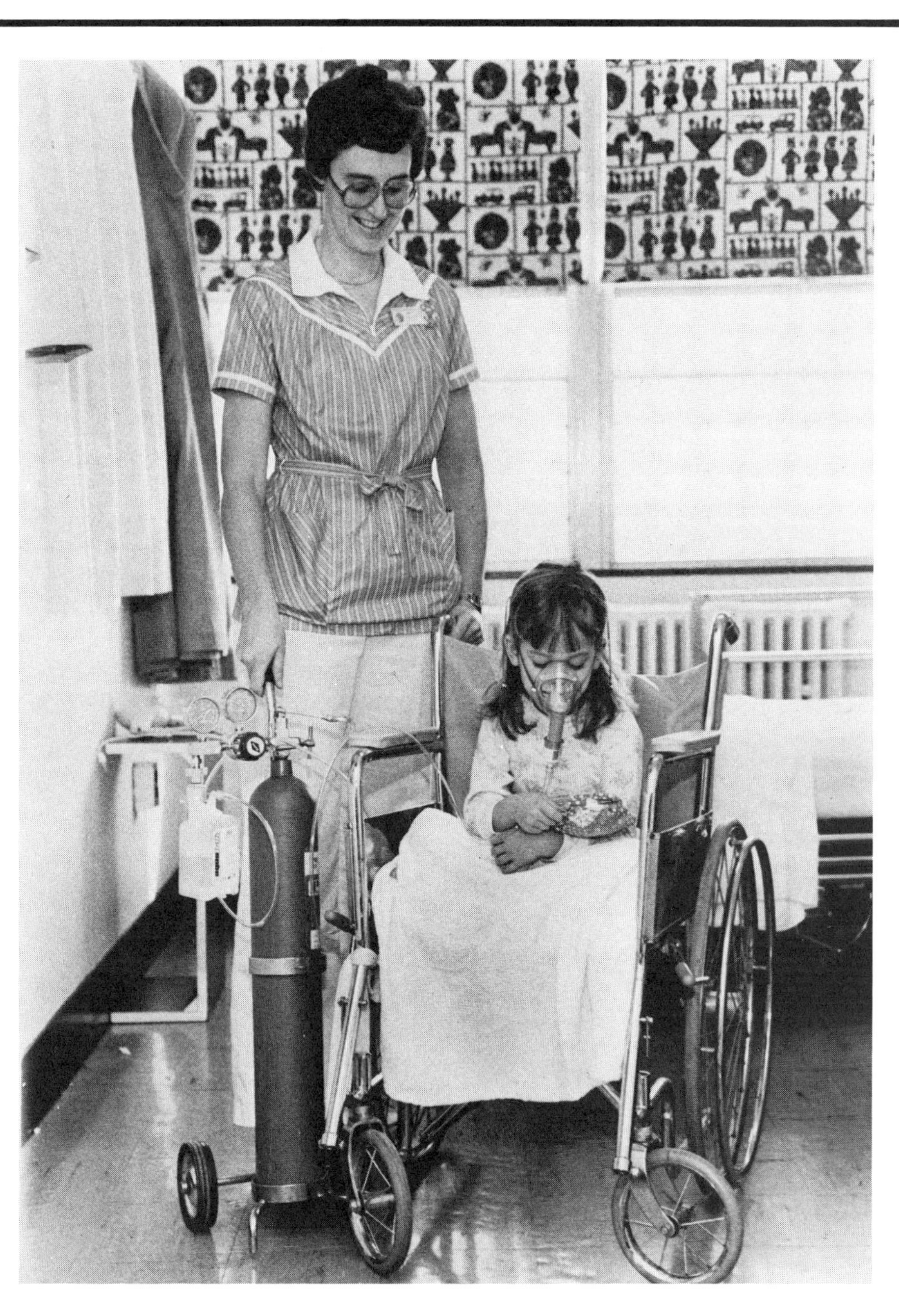

30. FLUID AND ELECTROLYTE BALANCE

OBJECTIVES
Upon mastery of the material in this chapter, you should be able to:

1. Describe water and electrolyte distributions in the human body.
2. Describe the role of a semipermeable membrane in the movement of fluid.
3. Describe the body regulatory mechanism for fluid and electrolyte balance.
4. Assess patients to detect those at risk for electrolyte or fluid imbalance.
5. Describe primary, secondary, and teritiary prevention measures for correcting fluid and electrolyte imbalance.
6. Describe nursing responsibilities for replacing fluid and electrolytes by oral and intravenous routes.
7. Describe the use and importance of intake and output records.
8. Describe nursing responsibility for replacement of fluid by blood or blood product transfusion.

TERMS
The terms important for an understanding of this chapter are shown below and defined in the glossary:

edema
electrolytes
extracellular fluid compartment
hydrostatic pressure
hypertonic
hypervolemia
hypotonic
hypovolemia
infiltration
infusion pump
intracellular fluid compartment
intravenous fluid
intravenous medication
isotonic
osmolarity
osmotic pressure
venipuncture
volume control set

Maintaining fluid and electrolyte balance is a body need of the highest priority; if an actual imbalance of either factor is threatened, the body will very quickly effect a change to bring these levels back into balance, or to a state of *homeostasis*. Because all illnesses affect fluid and electrolyte balance in some way, and because fluid and electrolytes must be in balance for health, monitoring this balance and initiating measures to achieve it are part of all patient contact and of all nursing care.

BODY FLUID

Sixty to seventy percent of the body weight of an adult is composed of water (Fig. 30-1). A thin person has proportionally more water in his body than an obese one because fat is almost water-free. Women's bodies contain proportionally less water than men's because a woman's body is composed of more fat than a man's body.

Infants have a greater proportion of water than adults (about 77 percent in a newborn; 60 percent by 2 years of age—Fig. 30-1). It would seem that fluid loss in infants is less serious than it is in adults because of the greater proportion of water. Actually, just the opposite is true. Because body content has a higher proportion of water in the young child, a change in the water level influences more of the infant's systems and so is more serious. Older adults tend to have reduced interstitial fluid, which accounts for the dry skin seen in this age group. Because the older person may also have more difficulty shifting or regulating fluid as necessary, water and electrolyte imbalance is particularly important in these adults.

Fluid Distribution

Fluid is distributed in the body between two major compartments: the extracellular compartment (fluid in spaces outside cells) and the intracellular compartment (fluid in cells). Extracellular fluid can be divided still further into intravascular fluid (fluid within blood vessels) and interstitial fluid (fluid surrounding cells and including cerebral spinal fluid, pleural and abdominal fluid, gastrointestinal fluid, and lymph).

In an adult, 45 percent of body weight is water in cells, leaving only 15 percent in extracellular spaces. Of this extracellular fluid, 4.5 percent is found as plasma in blood vessels, and 11 percent is found in the interstitial space. In infants, about 35 percent is intracellular, 4.3 percent is intravascular, and 38 percent is interstitial. These proportions are shown diagrammatically in Fig. 30-2.

Fluid is important to the body because it transports cells by way of the bloodstream and therefore is indirectly responsible for nutrient and oxygen supplies and

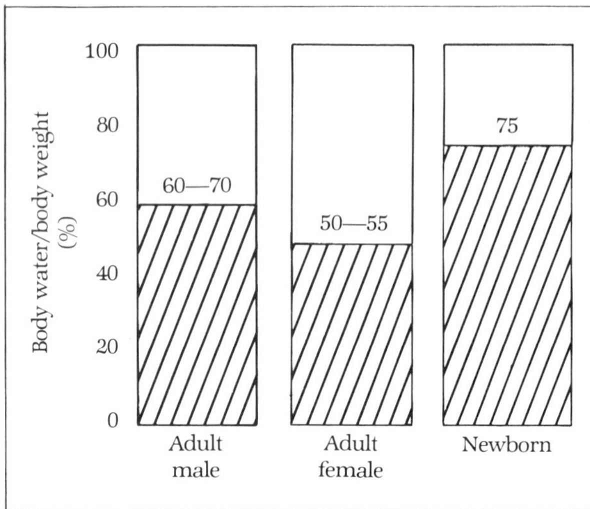

FIGURE 30-1. The relationship of body water to body weight. In an adult, 60 to 70% of body weight is composed of water. Infants have a greater proportion of water than adults; about 77% in newborn, 60% by 2 years of age.

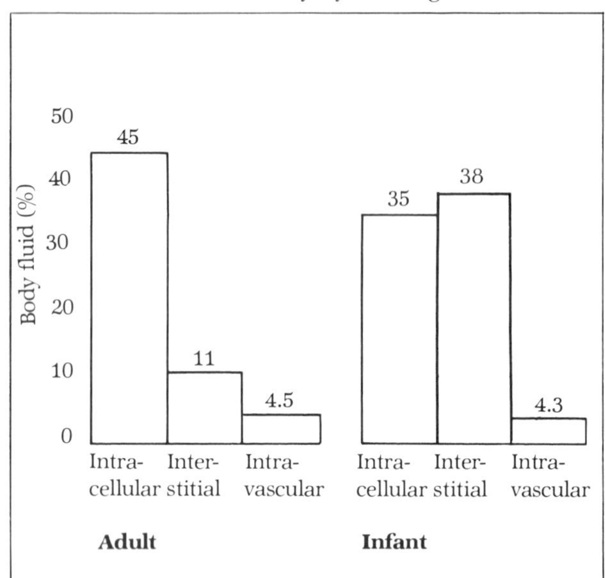

FIGURE 30-2. Percent of body fluid distributed in different body compartments.

the availability of protective white blood cells. It maintains the volume and patency of blood vessels, is necessary for the chemical synthesis of cell metabolism and growth, is important for body temperature regulation, and serves as the medium for removing waste materials from the cells and excreting them from the body.

Homeostasis

Water balance in the body depends on the body's ability to maintain a balance in the face of disturbances in intake or output. In health, water is ingested orally. It is derived not only from obvious fluid intake but also from solid foods and from the metabolism of food, which releases water. Both fat and carbohydrate metabolism release 100 ml of water for each 1100 g of fat or carbohydrate; protein produces 40 ml of fluid for each 100 g of protein.

Water is lost from the body mainly by urine output; subtle amounts are excreted in feces, sweat, and water vapor from the lungs. Water loss from sweat and lungs is termed *insensible* water loss; it is a constant source of water loss but is difficult to measure. In extreme dehydration, even though a person seems to be losing no more body water, he will continue to lose some through insensible loss. Profuse sweating (diaphoresis) or heavy breathing indicates that more fluid than usual is being lost through insensible loss, and fluid replacement will have to be greater to compensate for it.

All means of fluid intake and output are summarized in Table 30-1. Because oral intake of fluid is the chief means of water intake and urine elimination is the chief means of water output, measuring and comparing these is the main method of estimating fluid balance. As a rule, the average adult must take in 2000 ml of fluid daily to balance his fluid output.

Disturbances in Water Balance

Disturbances in water balance occur if water intake exceeds or is less than water output or if water output exceeds or is less than water intake. Circumstances that can cause any of these four situations are shown in Table 30-2. Table 30-3 lists the symptoms or signs that accompany dehydration (a state of less than normal body water) and overhydration (a state of more than normal body water).

TABLE 30-1. WATER BALANCE IN THE HUMAN BODY FOR 24 HOURS

Intake		Output	
Oral fluid	1200 ml	Urine	1500 ml
Solid food	1100 ml	Water lost from lungs	400 ml
Water of oxidation	300 ml	Sweat	600 ml
		Feces	100 ml
Total	2600 ml		2600 ml

TABLE 30-2. FACTORS THAT INFLUENCE FLUID INTAKE AND OUTPUT

Increased fluid intake	Caused by too vigorous intravenous fluid administration; "crash" water intake programs as fad diets
Decreased fluid intake	Caused by nausea, vomiting, refusal to eat or drink, depression (which limits appetite and fluid intake)
Increased fluid output	Caused by decreased production of antidiuretic hormone or aldosterone, nasogastric drainage, diaphoresis, diarrhea, increased respiratory rate and depth
Decreased fluid output	Caused by increased antidiuretic hormone production, kidney failure

TABLE 30-3. COMMON SYMPTOMS OF DEHYDRATION AND OVERHYDRATION

Percent of Water Loss	Symptoms
Dehydration	
1%	Thirst
5—8%	Lethargy, increased pulse rate, increased temperature, decreased mental functioning, decreased body weight, concentrated urine
11—15%	Delirium, kidney failure
Over 20%	Death
Overhydration	Weight gain, mental confusion, dyspnea (difficulty breathing from fluid accumulation in lung spaces), increased blood pressure, edema, distention of neck veins

Electrolytes

An electrolyte is a substance that when dissolved in water dissociates into component particles termed *ions*. If these ions are positively charged, they are cations, if negatively charged, they are anions. In the human body, important cations are sodium (Na^+), potassium (K^+), calcium (Ca^{++}), and magnesium (Mg^{++}). Important anions are chloride (Cl^-), phosphate ($HPO_4^=$), sulfate ($SO_4^=$) and bicarbonate (HCO_3^-).

For body fluid to be balanced, the number of positively charged cations present must equal the number of negatively charged anions present. The body is capable of making many quick changes because if the number of cations increases, the number of anions must also increase if the electrolyte composition is to remain balanced; if the number of cations decreases, the number of anions must also decrease.

SODIUM

Sodium (Na^+) is instrumental in the body for regulating the amount of body water and therefore for blood viscosity and volume because it "holds" or draws water to it. A person with a low sodium level is in danger of dehydration; a high sodium level presents a danger of overhydration. Dehydration of body tissue may also occur when the blood sodium level is high, drawing body fluid away from body cells into the bloodstream. In the blood, sodium combines with bicarbonate to form an important buffer (sodium bicarbonate), and in this way is also instrumental in regulating the pH or acid-base balance in the body. The amount of sodium retained or lost from the body is regulated by aldosterone, an adrenal hormone.

CALCIUM

Calcium (Ca^{++}) is instrumental for the health of bone and teeth enamel, serves as an intrinsic factor in blood coagulation, and is necessary for normal conduction of nerve impulses and cell growth as well as for absorption and utilization of vitamin B_{12}. With calcium deficiency and resultant decreased nerve conduction ability, generalized irritability of nerve tissue occurs, resulting in convulsions (tetany) at its extreme point. Calcium levels in the body are regulated by activity of the parathyroid glands. Calcium is utilized for bone growth only in the presence of vitamin D. Calcium level is also influenced by the level of phosphorus present because these two electrolytes exist in inverse proportion to each other (if the calcium level rises, the phosphorus level decreases; if the calcium level decreases, the phosphorus level will increase).

POTASSIUM

Potassium (K^+), the chief cation in the cells, is instrumental in nerve impulse conduction, particularly in the heart and skeletal muscles. It is important in acid-base (pH) regulation. The kidneys play a strong role in the regulation of potassium, conserving it when the potassium level begins to fall. Too much or too little potassium in the body can cause severe arrhythmias of heart muscle (enough to actually stop the heart). Never administer potassium in intravenous fluid unless you are certain that the person's kidneys are functioning so that if this potassium represents an excess, it can safely be excreted before dangerous levels are reached.

MAGNESIUM

Magnesium (Mg^{++}) is important for neuromuscular regulation within the body and aids protein and vitamin B metabolism. Magnesium, like calcium, is regulated by the parathyroid gland.

ANIONS

Anions in body fluid (chloride, phosphate, sulfate, and bicarbonate) are important in regulating the pH balance of the body. Chloride is lost readily with vomiting because it is a constituent of hydrochloric acid from the stomach; bicarbonate is the form that is administered intravenously if it is necessary to change the proportion of anions as therapy.

MEASUREMENT OF ELECTROLYTES

Electrolytes are measured not according to their weight but according to milliequivalents (mEq), or the chemical combining power of each. One milliequivalent of any electrolyte equals one milliequivalent of any other even though one might weigh twice as much as the other in milligrams.

Osmotic and Hydrostatic Pressure

Fluid shifts easily between the blood vessels (intravascular compartment) and the interstitial space because fluid in these spaces is very similar in content (they differ primarily in that blood plasma contains protein and interstitial fluid does not). The flow of fluid be-

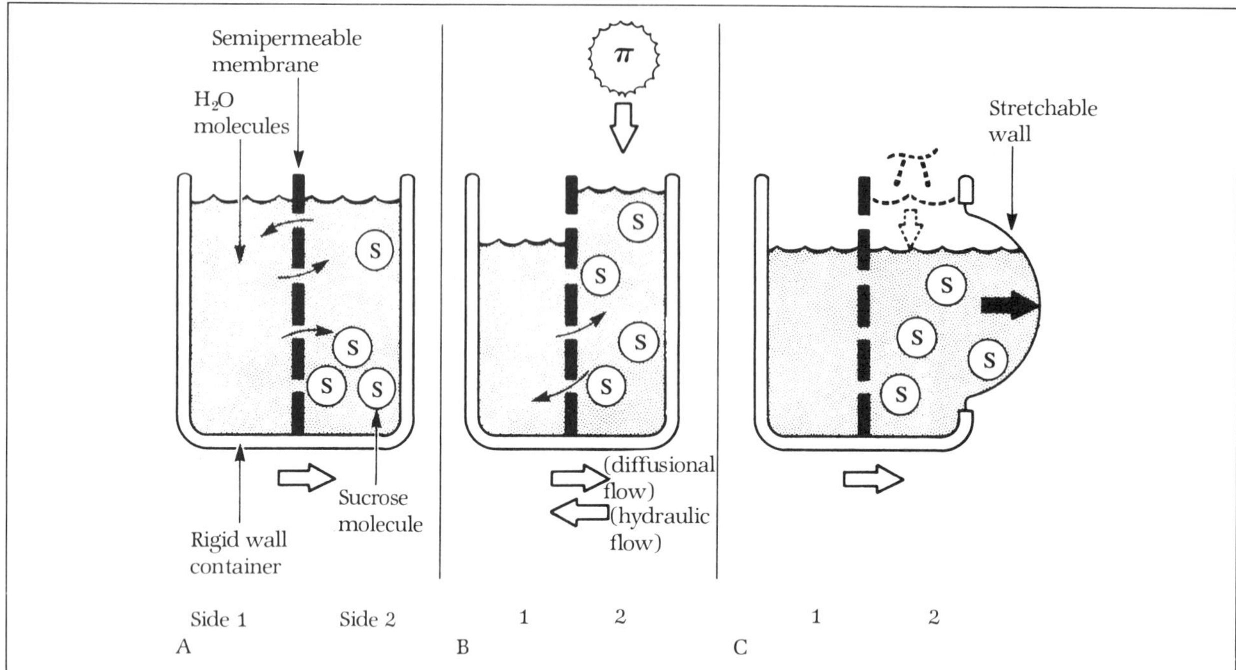

FIGURE 30-3. Osmotic pressure. Fluid diffuses from an area of lesser osmotic strength to one of more pressure to dilute the stronger solution; for example, if the bloodstream contains a heavy proportion of sucrose particles, fluid will shift from the interstitial space onto the bloodstream to dilute it. This figure illustrates water movements across semipermeable membranes. A. Water tends to move by diffusion down its concentration gradient from side 1 to side 2 of a rigid-walled container. B. The net flow of water causes the column of fluid on side 2 to rise. A hydrostatic pressure (π) is thus built up across the membrane between side 1 and 2. C. If the wall of side 2 is stretchable, the hydrostatic pressure pushes outward, causing an increase in volume. (From E. Selkurt [Ed.], *Basic Physiology for the Health Sciences* [2nd ed.]. Boston: Little, Brown, 1982.)

tween these two compartments depends on osmotic pressure: Fluid flow always occurs from the area of lesser concentration to the area of greater concentration.

The osmolarity of a solution refers to the proportion of dissolved particles present (solute) to that of solvent. Fluid diffuses from an area of lesser osmotic strength (less solute) to one of more pressure (more solute) to dilute the stronger solution and even the pressure as shown in Fig. 30-3. If the bloodstream contains a heavy proportion of protein particles, fluid will flow from the interstitial space into the bloodstream. If many protein molecules have been excreted by a damaged kidney, making the blood deficient in protein molecules, fluid will shift from the blood (which now has less osmotic pressure) into the interstitial tissue. This is the reason why persons with kidney disease invariably have at least some degree of edema (fluid in subcutaneous tissue), because protein tends to be excreted in this way with kidney disease. This type of edema can be relieved by intravenous administration of a strong solution of protein (albumin), which will "call" the fluid back into the circulatory system. Such regulation of fluid balance requires close observation of the person's circulatory status to prevent fluid overload (a strain on the heart).

Fluid shift is also influenced by hydrostatic (oncotic) pressure. Hydrostatic pressure is the pressure exerted on the blood cells and plasma due to the size of the lumen of the blood vessels, blood volume, and heart action. Hydrostatic pressure causes fluid to move by filtration rather than by diffusion as with osmotic pressure. If hydrostatic pressure in the blood rises owing to the presence of a large amount of fluid in the circulatory system (as could occur with intravenous fluid administration or arteriosclerosis), fluid will shift from the vascular system to the interstitial space (or from an area of greater pressure to one of lower pressure). Oncotic and osmotic pressures are compared in Table 30-4.

Hormone Control of Water Balance

ANTIDIURETIC HORMONE

Antidiuretic hormone (ADH) is regulated by the hypothalamus but distributed by the posterior pituitary gland. *Diuresis* means increased urine volume and consequent fluid loss; antidiuretic hormone, therefore, prevents fluid loss by decreasing urine output. When blood osmolarity (concentration) increases, additional ADH will be secreted; there will be increased renal retention of water due to its effect on the kidney, and urine output will be decreased. If blood osmolarity falls, the level of ADH produced will be decreased; there will be increased renal excretion of water and increased urinary output.

The body's ability to interpret blood osmolarity (and consequently respond to correct it) is threatened in the

TABLE 30-4. COMPARISON OF ONCOTIC AND OSMOTIC PRESSURE

Comparison Factor	Osmotic Pressure	Oncotic (Hydrostatic) Pressure
Source of pressure	Pressure determined by concentration of molecules in fluid	Pressure determined by volume of blood, action of heart, and size and tension of blood vessels
Direction of movement	Fluid moves from area of lesser concentration to one of greater concentration	Fluid moves from area of greater to lesser concentration
Method of fluid movement	Diffusion	Filtration
Relation to illness	Decreased protein molecule level in blood vessels leads to edema	Increased pressure in circulatory system will lead to edema
	Increased molecule concentration in blood vessels moves fluid from interstitial spaces into bloodstream	Rarely, enough pressure in interstitial tissue is created to cause a reverse fluid shift of this nature

presence of physical or psychological stress. Frequently a great increase in the amount of ADH secretion occurs following trauma, decreasing urinary output markedly. Always measure urine output and specific gravity in patients following any form of stress to ascertain that ADH secretion is not excessive. Be extremely careful in administering intravenous fluid to such people because a "normal" amount of fluid at this time may cause fluid overload due to the small amount of urine being excreted.

Exposure to cold or acute alcohol ingestion will decrease ADH secretion, causing larger than normal amounts of urine to be excreted. Diabetes insipidus is a disease state in which ADH is constantly undersecreted and diuresis constantly occurs. This disease can occur either as a congenital syndrome or following a head injury or infection with consequent damage to the hypothalamus or pituitary gland.

ALDOSTERONE

Aldosterone is manufactured and released by the adrenal glands. Unlike antidiuretic hormone, it acts not by controlling water absorbed or not absorbed in the kidney but by regulating sodium ion concentration. Because sodium "holds" water, if a high concentration of sodium is present, little fluid will be excreted by the kidneys; if sodium ion concentration is low, a great deal of water will be excreted by the renal tubules.

The most important stimulus for aldosterone secretion is a low sodium concentration. A low sodium level can occur if salt intake is low or if perspiration is excessive, causing sodium chloride to be lost in sweat. Lesser factors that can lead to increased aldosterone secretion are constriction of major arteries, the presence of stress (physical or psychological), and a decreased intravascular volume (as could occur with hemorrhage).

Aldosterone production will be decreased if the intravascular volume is increased. Hypoaldosteronism may occur as a congenital defect. To maintain a balance of cations and ions in body fluid if a great deal of sodium is being retained, large proportions of potassium may be excreted. Under severe stress, therefore, because of the interplay of aldosterone and sodium, potassium deficiency may occur secondary to the primary problem of fluid regulation.

THYROID AND PARATHYROID HORMONES

The thyroid hormones tetraiodothyronine (thyroxine, T_4) and triiodothyronine (T_3) increase cardiac output by increasing heart rate. Increased heart rate causes more effective perfusion of the kidney glomeruli; more water is cleared from the body by this action.

Kidney Regulation

Because urine output is the chief method by which water is lost from the body, the amount of urine formed by the kidney greatly influences water balance. The functional unit of the kidney is the nephron. Blood flows into the kidney nephron from the arterial circulation by way of the renal artery; this artery divides into thousands of afferent capillaries, each of which carries arterial blood to a glomerulus. The hydrostatic pressure of the blood in the artery is higher than that of the filtrate in the proximal tubule, causing water and electrolytes to pass from the artery into the proximal tubule. In the proximal tubule, all of the glucose and amino acids are reabsorbed, and almost all of the sodium, vitamins, and chloride ions are reabsorbed. As the sodium is reabsorbed, an equal balance of water is reabsorbed also. This is passive reabsorption—it occurs because of the sodium reabsorption, not because of body need or usefulness. In the distal tubule, additional water is reabsorbed, this time in response to aldosterone and antidiuretic hormone levels; this reabsorption reflects an active process or response to body need. In health, so much water is reabsorbed between the two reabsorption sites that of every 100 ml of water that originally crossed to the tubule in the glomerulus, only 2 ml remains to be excreted as urine.

Kidney regulation of water balance will be faulty if the arterial blood pressure falls below the pressure in the proximal tubule. People who have had hemorrhage or reduced cardiac output may have difficulty with inadequate water balance in addition to their initial problem.

Primary kidney disease such as kidney infection (glomerulonephritis) impairs the function of the glomeruli and allows products it would normally exclude such as protein to pass into the filtrate. This loss of protein from the blood circulation may reduce the osmotic pressure in the blood so greatly that fluid shifts from the bloodstream to the interstitial space, not only causing edema, as mentioned previously, but also lowering blood pressure because of the decreased blood volume.

The presence and absence of aldosterone and antidiuretic hormone influence the amount of sodium reabsorbed (and therefore the amount of water reabsorbed). Kidneys lose some of their ability to function effectively under extreme physical or psychological stress. Any acute illness, therefore, may cause a water balance problem superimposed on existing difficulties.

Thirst as a Regulator of Water Balance

Thirst is a sensation to which the brain responds (by way of the hypothalamus) in much the same way that it responds to pain or increased or decreased carbon dioxide levels. The sensation of thirst arises from decreased water intake, increased water loss, or increased sodium intake (the abnormal sodium level "demands" more water to balance it). The hypothalamus recognizes that the blood osmolarity is high or the blood volume is low and that cells are experiencing difficulty with metabolism due to lack of water. Nerve impulses initiate a thirst reaction; under ordinary circumstances, a person drinks water or other fluid as soon as possible and continues to drink until the thirst sensation passes.

In disease, the presence of thirst may or may not be helpful; in some instances drinking to relieve thirst would actually compound the disease state (with a gastrointestinal infection, for example, drinking might cause vomiting, which would cause loss of electrolytes, and the person would be short of both fluid and electrolytes). A person who has lost a great deal of water (severe dehydration) is often not thirsty because after a certain point this warning system is no longer responsive. Excessive thirst is termed *polydipsia.*

Acid-Base Balance

The term pH is an abbreviation for two French words that mean the "power of hydrogen"; it denotes whether a fluid is acid or alkaline. Water (H_2O) can be dissociated into H^+ and OH^- ions. A solution is acid (pH under 7) if it contains more H^+ ions than OH^- ions. It is alkaline (pH over 7) if the number of OH^- ions exceeds the number of H^+ ions. The pH of blood is normally 7.4, or slightly alkaline. In health, when the number of cations in the blood equals the number of anions, the number of H^+ ions balances the number of OH^- ions for all practical purposes. If the number of anions (Cl^-, for example) should fall by, say, 10, however (as would occur when hydrochloric acid is lost in vomiting), the number of H^+ ions must also be decreased by 10 to keep the number of positive and negative charges equal. Because this would make the OH^- concentration in the blood greater than the H^+ concentration, the plasma would become alkaline, which is the typical picture in vomiting. Conversely, if the number of Na^+ ions were decreased by 10, the number of H^+ ions would increase by 10, and the blood would become acidotic because more H^+ ions would then be present than OH^- ions. A low pH of this nature leads to vascular constriction, particularly of the pulmonary vessels; hemoglobin is unable to carry as much oxygen in an acidic state as in a normal pH state. Thus, overall circulatory and oxygenation function and ultimately cell function are affected by pH.

There are three buffer systems in the body that work to keep the number of H^+ and OH^- ions as nearly equal as possible so that pH remains at the usual point of near neutrality (7.35 to 7.45). A pH of under 7.0 or over 7.8 is too extreme to be compatible with life.

Buffer Salts. Buffer salts are basic or acidic substances that convert strong acids or bases into weaker ones. After being buffered, an acid that normally would yield many H^+ ions is changed into one that ionizes only slightly, yielding only a few H^+ ions. A strong base is converted to a substance that yields only a few OH^- ions. By this mechanism, dramatic changes in blood pH are avoided because fewer H^+ ions or OH^- ions are added to the blood at one time.

Respiratory Excretion. The lungs are capable of both removing excess H^+ ions from the blood and conserving them. Hydrogen ions (H^+) combine with bicarbonate ions (HCO_3^-) in the blood to form carbonic acid (H_2CO_3). In the lungs, carbonic acid is converted to CO_2 and H_2O. The CO_2 is excreted from the lungs; the hydrogen ion is tied up in the production of H_2O and no longer affects the acidity of the blood. Conversely, with a rising pH, the lungs will retain CO_2 and the reverse equation results: CO_2 and H_2O combine to form carbonic acid, which is then converted into H^+ and HCO_3^-. This adds additional H^+ ions to the bloodstream, decreasing pH.

Kidney Excretion. H^+ by itself or as NH_4 (ammonia) can be excreted in the urine in exchange for sodium and potassium. Conversely, when the serum HCO_3^- and serum pH rise, H^+ ion secretion stops, and potassium excretion may be excessive.

BLOOD CO_2 AS AN INDICATOR OF BLOOD PH

Disturbances in acid-base balance lead to acidosis or alkalosis (low or high pH, respectively). The amount of

TABLE 30-5. COMPARISON OF COMPENSATED METABOLIC ALKALOSIS AND ACIDOSIS

Comparison Factor	Metabolic Alkalosis	Metabolic Acidosis
pH	Increased (above 7.45)	Decreased (below 7.35)
HCO_3	Elevated (above 29 mEq/L)	Decreased (below 25 mEq/L)
CO_2	Increased (above 32 mEq/L)	Decreased (below 22 mEq/L)
Potassium	Decreased (below 4 mEq/L)	Increased (above 6 mEq/L)
Signs and symptoms	Confusion, numbness, and tingling in extremities, muscle twitching, convulsions Shallow breathing	Headache, confusion, coma Deep respirations
Possible causes	Vomiting, excess intake of bicarbonate by antacid medication, nasogastric tube secretions, diuretic therapy with loss of potassium	Diarrhea, excess acid ingestion such as aspirin poisoning, renal failure, starvation leading to fat breakdown, metabolic illness such as diabetes mellitus

each of these is reflected in the measured blood CO_2 level.

Blood CO_2 represents all the CO_2 present in the plasma. Most of this is in the form of bicarbonate; a small amount is held at the intermediary stage as carbonic acid, which is actually dissolved CO_2. The carbon dioxide concentration is expressed as milliequivalents per liter. The normal value is 22 to 28 mEq per liter.

When, as in diarrhea, excessive Na^+ ion is lost, the body conserves H^+ ions to keep the positive and negative charges equal in number. The blood begins to become acidotic as the number of H^+ ions in the blood increases in relation to the number of OH^- ions present. To correct (compensate for) the blood pH, the body can excrete H^+ ions through the kidney; the most rapid way, however, is by combining H^+ ions with HCO_3^- ions in the blood to form carbonic acid and then CO_2 and H_2O for lung excretion. When this has continued for a time, the CO_2 level will fall lower and lower as the body uses up its store of bicarbonate. Acidosis occurring from other than a respiratory cause is termed *metabolic acidosis.* In compensated metabolic acidosis, the blood CO_2 is invariably low. The lower the blood CO_2 value, presumably, the larger the number of Na^+ ions that have been lost, and the greater the severity or duration of diarrhea that was present.

When Cl^- ions are lost, as with vomiting, the body decreases the number of H^+ ions present to keep the number of positive and negative charges equal. The blood will now become alkalotic because the number of H^+ ions is smaller than the number of OH^- ions present. To correct this state, the kidneys can conserve H^+ ions; a more immediate solution, however, is for the lungs to conserve CO_2. The person's respirations slow and become shallow (hypopnea) with this compensation effort. The excessive CO_2 accumulated is dissolved in the blood as carbonic acid and then converted into H^+ and HCO_3^-. The total blood CO_2 content (HCO_3^- and carbonic acid) will rise. In compensated metabolic alkalosis, therefore, the blood CO_2 level will invariably be high. The higher it is, presumably the larger the number of Cl^- ions that have been lost. Table 30-5 summarizes comparative findings of metabolic alkalosis and acidosis. If excessive or deep breathing is the primary cause of an acid-base dysfunction, this is termed *respiratory* alkalosis or acidosis. These conditions are discussed in Chap. 32 with other respiratory effects.

Patients at Risk of Fluid and Electrolyte Imbalance

VOMITING

Vomiting depletes the body of both hydrogen and chloride ions because they are lost in hydrochloric acid. As mentioned previously, this leads to alkalosis from the shift of hydrogen ions. In addition to the electrolyte disruption, vomiting will lead to decreased fluid volume; prolonged vomiting will force the body to break down fat cells for cell energy because glucose and protein are no longer being supplied. The fatty acids released by fat breakdown will lead to eventual acidosis. Vomiting may occur as an accompaniment to any illness; in any case it immediately complicates any illness.

DIARRHEA

Diarrhea, or frequent and loose watery stools, leads to decreased fluid volume and loss of sodium, evoking H^+ shifts and eventual acidosis. Diarrhea leads to volume depletion very quickly in infants. As a rule, there is no innocent diarrhea in infants; every case needs medical investigation to permit prompt treatment before dehydration occurs.

GASTRIC SUCTION

A nasogastric tube is inserted through the nostrils to the stomach in a person with a gastrointestinal obstruction; gentle suction attached to the distal end of the tube will remove fluid and air from the stomach to keep him from vomiting and possibly aspirating. If a person is being fed by a nasogastric tube, gastric secretions are often aspirated from the stomach prior to a feeding to check that the tube is in the stomach and that the feedings are not so large that the stomach cannot digest them and empty before another feeding.

The few milliliters of gastric contents should always be returned prior to feeding so that electrolyte depletion does not occur. When computing intake and output in a person with gastrointestinal suction, be sure to keep track of any amount removed and discarded. Although this amount is invariably small, the total during 24 hours can be excessive.

INTESTINAL SUCTION

A person who has an obstruction in the lower gastrointestinal tract may have a nasoduodenal tube inserted through the nostril to the intestine; gentle suction will remove fluid and air from the intestine. The constant removal of secretions from this portion of the gastrointestinal tract will lead to the same problems associated with diarrhea (acidosis and fluid volume deficit). When computing intake and output in such a patient, be sure to account for all secretions removed so that this amount is not underestimated.

HIGH FEVER

Severe diaphoresis (profuse sweating) occurs with all fever; the higher the fever, the more fluid is lost by this route. Besides fluid volume deficit, fever also causes the person to breathe rapidly and deeply to increase the cooling effect of this adaptation. Respiratory alkalosis from increased carbon dioxide loss may occur. Such high fevers can occur in the person with an acute infection or with a central nervous system injury in which the hypothalamus (the temperature regulating center) is temporarily dysfunctional.

HEMORRHAGE

Hemorrhage (profuse bleeding) depletes fluid volume in the body. It can occur suddenly and in large amounts whenever there is interference with skin integrity (surgery, burns, accidents). Hemorrhage is the most frequent cause of death from childbirth. It may be slow but continuous in such conditions as peptic ulcer or blood-clotting defects.

DRAINING WOUNDS

A draining wound leads to fluid volume deficit and often protein deficit because the exudate from this type of wound contains protein. This is a paradoxical situation because without a high level of protein, healing of the wound cannot occur; it is the wound drainage that leads to a low protein blood level and interference with healing. Wounds such as burns and decubiti (pressure sores) and "dirty" wounds such as grease-smeared ones are most prone to become draining wounds.

EDEMA

Edema is excess fluid in the interstitial space. It occurs when the hydrostatic pressure is greater or the osmotic pressure is lesser in blood vessels than in the interstitial space or as a primary response to inflammation (fluid flowing from the vascular system to an injured area brings with it platelets for clotting potential, white blood cells, and antibodies to fight infection). A rare cause is lymphatic obstruction. Edema in all instances is a symptom of an underlying disease, not a disease in itself. Edema will not subside until the original problem is corrected.

Generalized edema is termed *anasacra*. Edema is always serious because as fluid fills the spaces between cells, it pushes the cells further away from the surrounding capillaries than is normal. This limits the availability of nutrients and oxygen to cells. A great deal of edema can be present before it becomes obvious. In an adult, for example, as much as 10 pounds of fluid can accumulate before the typical look and puffiness of edema is evident. Edema is classified by extent according to a 4^+ scale (see Chap. 25, Fig. 25-2).

Pulmonary and cerebral edema are particularly serious. Edema collecting in the lungs and head puts pressure on critical centers and interferes with function of the lungs and brain cells. Signs that pulmonary edema are present are cough, dyspnea, and tachypnea (fluid diffuses across the alveolar membrane into the alveolar spaces, blocking out oxygen—carbon dioxide exchange space). Symptoms of cerebral edema are disorientation and confusion.

ASCITES

Ascites is a special type of edema or accumulation of fluid in the abdominal cavity (Fig. 30-4). Ascites fluid is very similar in composition to blood plasma; a person with severe ascites can develop a fluid volume deficit and a protein deficit. Ascites tends to occur in kidney disease, liver disease, and congestive heart disease. Ascites fluid is removed either by insertion of a cannula into the abdominal cavity to drain the fluid or by causing it to diffuse into the bloodstream by administration of albumin, which increases the protein content of the blood.

DIURETIC THERAPY

A diuretic is a drug that increases urine output. Many diuretics act by preventing sodium reabsorption in the distal kidney tubule; if sodium is not reabsorbed there, water is not reabsorbed either, causing a greater urine output. Because many diuretics also prevent reabsorption of potassium, a side effect of these drugs is hypokalemia (lowered potassium blood level). To counteract this difficulty, many people taking daily diuretics also must take a daily potassium supplement; everyone who takes a diuretic needs to have the potassium level monitored.

SPECIAL DIET THERAPY

Special diets may lead to fluid or electrolyte imbalance. A low sodium diet, for example, may prevent reabsorption of water in the distal tubules. Low sodium diets are often ordered for people with heart disease to cause this loss of water and lower the circulating blood volume,

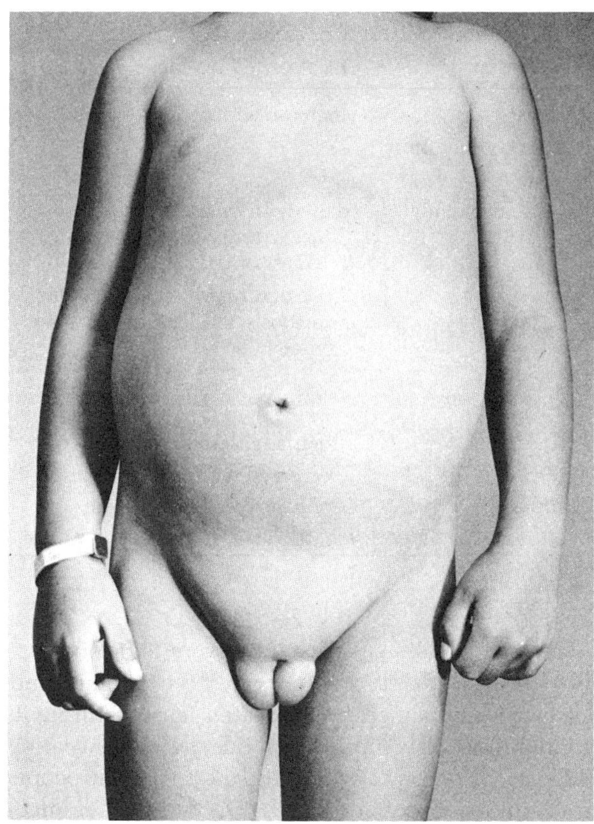

FIGURE 30-4. This child has ascites. The abdomen is distended with fluid.

thus decreasing the work load on the heart. With such a diet there is a possibility that a person may develop hyponatremia (lowered sodium blood level) and excessive fluid loss.

A person on a high-protein, low-carbohydrate diet may develop severe acidosis if there is so little carbohydrate that the person has to break down fat for body fuel.

PSYCHOLOGICAL MANIFESTATIONS

Stress of any kind affects appetite (nausea or heartburn before a test). People with severe depression are usually not interested in food and consequently may eat so little that they can develop a fluid or electrolyte imbalance.

Anorexia nervosa is a specific psychological illness in which the person views food as repugnant; if he can be coaxed into eating, he will generally vomit the food immediately afterward (behavior termed *bulemia*). In other psychological illnesses, a person may believe that eating or drinking will harm him (believing that all his food is poisoned, for example).

Assessment of the Person with a Fluid and Electrolyte Imbalance

Because fluid and electrolyte imbalance is a secondary complication of any illness, every patient must be assessed for the possibility of its occurrence.

HEALTH HISTORY

The signs and symptoms of fluid and electrolyte imbalance usually begin in subtle ways. A sudden gain in weight, for example, may be the first indication of edema. Other signs that may be reported are hands so swollen that a wedding ring will no longer fit or feet so swollen that the person cannot put on bedroom slippers.

In people reporting vomiting and diarrhea, ask about the duration, intensity, frequency, description, associated symptoms, and actions that have been taken to relieve the condition. In a young child the fluid volume is so small that there is no such thing as "a little" diarrhea or "a little" vomiting. All diarrhea and vomiting are serious in young children and need further investigation.

Ask about recent dieting for weight loss, special diets such as liquid protein diets, diuretic use, and kidney, heart, and gastrointestinal illnesses because all of these may lead to fluid or electrolyte imbalance. Dieting for weight loss may lead to dehydration if fluid intake as well as caloric intake is reduced; a high-protein liquid diet can lead to such a high plasma protein level that water is drawn into the bloodstream from the surrounding tissue by osmotic pressure; the kidneys, unable to handle the high level of urea (a breakdown product of protein), may fail. Diuretics are drugs that increase urine output; excessive use of these can lead to dehydration. Gastrointestinal illnesses prevent ready intake of fluid, cardiac illness can impair the circulation of fluid, and kidney illness can compromise the excretion of fluid.

The symptoms of electrolyte deficits are specific for the electrolyte lost. Calcium deficit leads to tingling or numbness of fingers and toes or muscle cramping. Potassium deficiency leads to cardiac arrhythmias (reported as fluttering or skipped heartbeats).

PHYSICAL EXAMINATION

Physical examination often reveals signs of fluid imbalance (Table 30-6). Weight is an important determinant of fluid loss or gain. The weight of all patients admitted to a health care facility is recorded on admission. In patients scheduled for surgery such as cardiac surgery, in which a change in the amount of circulating blood after surgery would have a serious effect on heart function if it were suddenly either less or more, weight is recorded immediately after surgery. As a rule, a sudden weight gain of more than 0.5 kg in 24 hours is probably caused by edematous fluid collection. A weight loss of over 10 percent of total weight reflects extreme fluid loss and a situation that needs immediate medical intervention. Chronic weight loss may reflect protein deficiency or a poor nutritional intake. It is also a preliminary sign of cancer.

Peripheral vein assessment is a method of judging the amount of fluid in a person's vascular system. To assess peripheral vein filling, raise the person's hand

TABLE 30-6. SIGNS AND SYMPTOMS OF FLUID AND ELECTROLYTE IMBALANCE

Assessment Factor	Overhydration	Dehydration	Electrolyte Imbalance
Weight	Increased	Decreased	Increase with sodium excess
Peripheral vein filling time	Increased emptying time	Increased filling time	—
Neck vein distention	Present	Not present	—
Pulse	Rapid and bounding	Rapid and thready	Slow with magnesium excess; arrhythmias with potassium excess or deficit
Respiratory pattern	Shallow if ascites is present; rales present in lungs	—	Deep and rapid with metabolic acidosis; shallow and slow with metabolic alkalosis
Temperature	Normal	Increased	—
Blood pressure	Increased	Decreased	—
Skin	Edema	Poor turgor	Edema with sodium excess
Urinary output	Increased	Decreased	Decreased with sodium excess
Level of consciousness	Confusion	Confusion	Confusion with magnesium deficit

and hold it in an elevated position above heart level. Count the number of seconds that it takes for blood to empty from the veins on the back of the hand (veins become flat and barely noticeable). Next, lower the person's hand below heart level and count how many seconds it takes for blood to fill the veins (they become distended and prominent). Normally, peripheral vein emptying or refilling time is under 3 seconds. If vascular volume is excessive, it will take longer than normal for the veins to empty; if vascular volume is less, it will take longer for the veins to fill.

Observation of neck veins can offer the same information. If the person's head is elevated more than 45 degrees, neck vein distention should not be noticeable. If it is present, it suggests circulating fluid overload.

Pulse rate suggests vascular volume. With an increased circulatory volume, the pulse rate is bounding (strong) and rapid (the heart is trying to move the excess blood as rapidly as possible to keep itself from being overloaded); with decreased vascular volume, the pulse will be thready and rapid (the heart is pumping faster than normal in an attempt to circulate oxygen faster than normal). Electrolyte disturbances such as potassium deficiency or excess will cause cardiac arrhythmias; magnesium deficit can cause bradycardia (slowed heart rate).

Respiratory rate also suggests fluid and electrolyte status. Deep rapid breathing (termed *Kussmaul respirations*) occurs with respiratory alkalosis or as compensation in metabolic acidosis. Shallow respirations may be caused by potassium deficits or excess if the cardiac muscle weakens. An abdominal cavity filled with ascites fluid prevents full expansion of the diaphragm and therefore causes shallow respirations. If there is circulatory overload, leading to effusion of fluid into the lungs, the sound of rales or a crackling sound can be heard on auscultation of lung tissue.

The other vital signs, blood pressure and temperature, are also changed in the presence of fluid and electrolyte imbalances. An elevated temperature will occur with blood volume deficit due to loss of sweating and local irritation of cells. After surgery many people develop a low-grade fever (101°F), not from an infection (the complication that is always feared after surgery) or inflammation but from lack of fluid for 8 hours before surgery and during the procedure itself. As soon as intravenous fluid is begun or they begin to drink, this mild temperature increase will fade. Blood pressure is the measurement of tension within the arterial circulation; this will increase with fluid overload and decrease with fluid deficit.

The skin reveals a number of findings that suggest fluid deficit or excess. To assess skin turgor (the degree of fluid in subcutaneous tissue), pinch a ridge of skin on the abdomen or an extremity (any spot where it lifts readily). Normally, if you lift a ridge of tissue this way, the skin returns immediately to its normal position as soon as you take your hand away. If subcutaneous fluid is decreased, the ridge of skin will not return to normal but will stay in this raised position. Poor skin turgor is a late severe sign of dehydration. When it is discernible, a severe fluid deficit is already present.

When there is excess body fluid, edema will be present. Edema always tends to be dependent or collect in the lowest body parts. In the person who has been standing, the feet and lower legs will become edematous; in a person lying in bed, the buttocks and the back surface of the legs will show signs of edema. If the person has been sleeping with a flat pillow or no pillow, his eyelids may be so edematous that he has difficulty opening his eyes or speaking because his tongue is so swollen.

With dehydration, the eyeballs appear sunken and there are deep dark lines under the eyes. The person's lips may be dried and cracking; sweating is not apparent even in the person with a high temperature.

Assessment for electrolyte imbalance includes listening for cardiac irregularities (increased or decreased heart rate or uneven rate). Assessment of muscle contraction will reveal calcium deficiency. A test that is helpful for revealing this is a test for *clonus*. Hold the person's foot and ankle in your hand and dorsiflex the foot three times in rapid succession. If calcium is at normal levels, when you remove your hand, the foot will remain still; in persons with a low circulating calcium level, however, the foot will continue to dorsiflex for 10 to 12 more times (clonus).

LABORATORY ANALYSIS

Laboratory analysis, the third prong of nursing assessment, is also important in revealing fluid and electrolyte imbalances. Hematocrit level (the proportion of red blood cells to plasma present) will reflect fluid deficit or excess. If little fluid is present, the hematocrit level will be abnormally high; it will be abnormally low in the presence of excess fluid. The amount of urine output and the specific gravity of urine are prime indicators of fluid excess or deficit. With excess, urine output will be increased and specific gravity will be low; with a deficit, urine output will be decreased and specific gravity will be elevated.

Electrolyte excesses or deficits are determined by measurement of the specific electrolyte in the blood plasma. Normal values of the chief body electrolytes are shown in Appendix G. Each laboratory determines a normal level for these electrolytes depending somewhat on the equipment used and the method of analysis. In any health care agency, therefore, always use the exact levels determined by that agency as normal for their analysis.

Urine tests are a less accurate but still useful method of determining some levels of electrolytes in the body. With alkalosis, for example, the urine is alkaline also; if protein is present in urine, it suggests that hypoproteinemia (low protein blood level) may occur (this will eventually lead to water leaving the bloodstream for interstitial spaces).

NURSING DIAGNOSIS

The Fourth National Conference on Nursing Diagnoses accepted two diagnoses in reference to fluid balance: Fluid volume deficit, actual, and Fluid volume deficit, potential. These diagnoses with their defining characteristics are shown in Appendix C.

Planning Care for People with Fluid and Electrolyte Imbalances

The goal of care for people with fluid and electrolyte disturbances from a medical standpoint is either to limit the loss of water and electrolytes or to institute fluid and electrolyte administration to bring these levels back to normal as quickly as possible. If the person has a fluid and electrolyte deficit resulting from an acute condition such as vomiting or diarrhea and the acute symptoms have now stopped, regulation of fluid or electrolyte levels is generally accomplished without difficulty. If the loss of fluid or electrolytes is still continuing, however, not only must the deficient level be replaced but the amount of concurrent losses must be anticipated and replaced as well. To accomplish this, medical and nursing care must cooperate closely.

If fluids and electrolytes will be regulated orally, the person's cooperation will be necessary because he must swallow the needed quantity. If restriction of oral fluid is necessary, he must agree not to drink or eat. If intravenous therapy is part of the plan of care, he must agree to lie still to prevent the fluid from infiltrating (infusing into subcutaneous tissue rather than into a vein). If he cannot cooperate in this way (in the case of an infant or small child, for example), your planning must involve the use of restraints to limit movement for safe administration of intravenous fluids.

People with edema or poor skin turgor need frequent turning and skin care (at least every 2 hours) to prevent skin breakdown because in these conditions cells are not receiving the normal oxygen and nutrient supply and are therefore already threatened. Sustained pressure quickly compromises them to a point of dysfunction. If edema is localized, elevating the body part generally helps to relieve it (it lowers hydrostatic pressure in the involved part). Anti-embolic stockings may have been ordered before ambulation to prevent edema in the lower extremities. When the patient sits in a chair he should elevate his feet and legs on a footstool to prevent excess accumulation in his feet. He may need two pillows to sleep with at night to keep edema from accumulating in his face.

Implementation of Fluid and Electrolyte Replacement

ORAL FLUID ADMINISTRATION

Always be aware of how much a person is drinking during each 24-hour period. When the person has a fluid deficit, he must be encouraged to drink more fluid than normal. Increasing oral fluid intake in this way has traditionally been called forcing fluids; this is an obsolete term because it implies that you would actually force someone to drink. A better term is "encouraging" fluid. A physician's order for encouraging fluid should state in detail the amount of fluid the person should receive during 24 hours. This specified amount can then be divided into the amounts to be given by each nursing shift. The major amount of fluid (two-thirds) is generally administered during the day because this shift includes the breakfast and lunch periods; another third is administered during the evening and night shifts. People drink fluid most readily if they like the fluid given. You often have to ask the dietary department to supply a special type of fluid. Be creative with suggestions. When a person tires of drinking cold fluids, a hot liquid such as a clear soup or hot cocoa might be acceptable. Jello and Popsicles are considered fluids.

People can usually drink more clear fluids (ginger ale, water, tea) than thicker fluids such as milkshakes or cream soups because the thicker fluids are absorbed from the stomach more slowly. Be cautious in offering fluids with caffeine content because a person may become nervous or jittery from the effect of the caffeine. Broth provides a change of taste but tends to have a relatively high salt content so is contraindicated for people who need a low sodium intake. People with mouth lesions (caused by cracking of the mucous membrane due to dehydration) may not be able to drink fruit juices because the acid content stings their mouths; carbonated beverages may also be uncomfortable for people with mouth lesions unless they are allowed to stand for a few minutes to become flat.

Fruit juices, especially cranberry juice, will increase the acidity of urine. Remember this when testing urine for pH in a person who is receiving a great deal of fluid. Ice chips are another form of fluid that makes a nice change from drinking fluid. Because ice melts to half its volume, a glass of ice chips is counted as half a glass of fluid for the intake record. Most people drink more fluid if it is offered in small amounts rather than as larger amounts spaced further apart.

Sometimes, particularly in people with heart or kidney diseases, it may be necessary to restrict the amount of fluid ingested to keep the circulatory system from becoming overloaded. Some people on restricted fluid intake like to have the fluid given in small amounts carefully spaced during the day; others like it given in less frequent but larger amounts. Avoid foods that have a high salt content such as potato chips or luncheon meat because these tend to increase thirst; sweet foods and milk products tend to have the same effect. Keep beverages out of sight, and try to arrange to keep the smell of coffee from a service cart away from the patient's room. Adults on restricted fluid may enjoy rinsing their mouth with water or mouthwash to keep the mucous membranes from drying. Do not allow children to do this because they invariably swallow the rinse solution (no water for rinsing after teethbrushing is allowed for the same reason).

ORAL CARE

People who are receiving either added fluid or restricted fluid need frequent oral care. People who are receiving increased fluid are receiving it because their body is deficient in fluid; this is manifested by dry mucous membranes. People on restricted fluid develop dry mucous membrane from the fluid restriction. Apply petroleum jelly (Vaseline) as necessary to keep the lips from drying. Coating the mucous membrane with glycerine and lemon juice is sometimes effective in preventing drying, but for other people, the compound may actually cause additional drying.

THERAPEUTIC DIETS

Fluid and electrolyte imbalances can be modified to some extent by special diets. Although some diuretics spare the excretion of potassium, people taking diuretics should as a rule be urged to eat foods high in potassium to minimize the amount of potassium lost with water in the urine. Orange juice and bananas are two foods high in potassium; such administration might be contraindicated in people with cardiac disorders that make the heart especially sensitive to potassium regulation. People with calcium deficiency can increase their calcium intake by drinking milk or eating milk products and green leafy vegetables. People with low protein levels can increase their blood protein level by eating protein-rich foods such as meat, fish, and eggs. Unfortunately, a side effect of protein deficiency is anorexia or loss of appetite, so eating large quantities of these rich foods may be very unappealing and very difficult to accomplish.

Infants with electrolyte imbalances may be given additional electrolyte solutions (Pediolyte, for example). Because these solutions look like water, a mother may not realize their importance.

To reduce fluid load in the body, a salt-restricted (low-sodium) diet may be ordered. These diets may be very strict, or they may involve restricting only obviously salty foods and added salt in cooking or before eating. In either instance, a low-sodium diet tends to become tasteless and unappealing after awhile. Remember that companionship and conversation are part of mealtime; supplying these will often allow a person to eat a diet that would otherwise be too unappetizing to be touched.

RECORDING INTAKE AND OUTPUT

Be aware of fluid intake and output in all patients because fluid balance is compromised to some extent in all illnesses. In some patients, intake and output are so critical that it is necessary to measure them. To measure intake and output accurately you must actually measure, not estimate, the amount of fluid taken in or excreted, because estimated amounts are often very inaccurate. Consider all output (gastric drainage, liquid stool, wound drainage) in your total. In some instances you must administer fluid of one type to equalize the urine output and fluid of another type to replace wound drainage or liquid stool, so these amounts should be kept separate except as a final total (urine output might be replaced with a balanced electrolyte solution, liquid stool with a solution higher in sodium because sodium is lost in stool, and drainage from a nasogastric tube with normal saline).

In infants it is difficult to separate liquid stool from urine because these blend together in a diaper. Separate urine from stool by applying a urine collector (see

Chap. 38); check it frequently. In women, to prevent a loss of urine that cannot be measured, ask the woman to void first before trying to move her bowels. If a person is incontinent, output can only be estimated because it is impossible to measure accurately the amount of urine contained in sheets. To establish a more accurate measure of urine output, offer a bedpan frequently (every 2 hours) to such people.

Diapers can be readily used as a method of measuring urine output. Weigh the diaper before it is placed on the infant and record this weight conspicuously in case you are not the person who removes it from the baby (commercial or disposable diapers can be marked with a ballpoint pen on the plastic surface). Reweigh the diaper after it is wet and subtract the difference to determine the amount of urine present. This difference will be a number of grams. Because a gram equals a milliliter, the total can be recorded in milliliters.

If urine will be not only measured for amount but tested for blood, protein, or specific gravity, it is important that menstrual blood not be mixed with the specimen. A woman who is having her menstrual period should wash her vulva with clear water and place a clean cotton ball in her vagina before voiding to prevent menstrual blood from contaminating the urine. Even if no blood is apparent in the urine on gross inspection, mark such specimens "possible menstrual blood contamination" if you are sending the sample to a laboratory because microscopic examination may well reveal the presence of red blood cells. If you are testing the urine yourself, indicate in the record that menstrual blood may have been present.

Many adults will take full responsibility for recording the amount of their liquid intake if they are supplied with the necessary form and instructions. If you want the amount of fluid recorded in milliliters, supply the person with whatever conversion factors he will need (a cupful is 150 ml; a glassful is 180 ml) or ask him to record in cupfuls, which you will convert to metric numbers. If you intend to observe the amount taken with a meal and record this yourself, be present when the meal tray is removed from the room. Do not ask the patient to remember later what he drank (see Quick Reference Stop 30-1).

Many ancillary personnel in health care settings do not realize the importance of measuring intake and output because they do not know how lethal fluid and electrolyte imbalances can become. Be certain that everyone on a nursing unit is informed about who needs to have intake and output measured; post signs as necessary on room doors, room bathrooms, and utility rooms as necessary to alert all personnel and family members who will be helping with care.

☐ QUICK REFERENCE STOP 30-1: RESEARCH
Intake/Output Measurements

Many nursing skills are involved in maintaining adequate fluid and electrolyte needs of patients. Intake and output measurements are frequently performed by nurses, yet questions have been raised about the accuracy of these measurements. The research below tests the accuracy of this technique empirically.

Intake and Output Measurements—Accurate?
Pflaum (1979) studied 30 patients and compared their intake and output measurements with true fluid changes as indicated by weight measurements. "This study had demonstrated a mean error in I-O figures of 799.5 cc per day when compared with daily weight calculations. There was no statistically different correlation between the two values. It is suggested that a change be made in nursing practice. If recording of intake and output is to continue as a nursing practice, then it must be coupled with daily weighings and used only in cases where intake must be limited and/or output carefully monitored" (p. 498).

SUGGESTED READING

Pflaum, S. S. Investigation of intake-output as a means of assessing body fluid balance. *Heart and Lung* 8(3):495, 1979.

WEIGHT

Weight measurement on a daily basis (or even more frequently) may be ordered for certain patients to document weight gain or loss. This type of measurement is important for estimating increase or loss of body fluid. Weight should be recorded at the same time daily on the same scale with the person wearing the same clothing or amount of clothing each time. Infants are weighed nude to discount the influence of clothing on their weight. A daily weight is most accurate if it is done before breakfast after the person voids.

MEDICATION ADMINISTRATION

Some electrolytes such as potassium and calcium may be increased by oral or intravenous supplementation. Before administering potassium as a supplement, ascertain that the person still needs the supplement by a recent laboratory report (preferably no longer than the day before for oral administration, that morning for intravenous administration). Both deficits and excesses of potassium can cause cardiac arrhythmias.

Sodium bicarbonate to correct acidosis may be administered intravenously. Intravenous fluid containing any electrolyte supplement should run at a constant rate so that the person does not receive a great deal of the supplement during one hour and then a small amount the next. "Rebound" effects of such erratic electrolyte administration may precipitate greater deficits or excesses than were originally present. These strong solutions also have a potential for causing extreme irritation if they infuse into subcutaneous tissue and need to be observed carefully. Magnesium or ammonium chloride may be administered intravenously, but these are not seen as frequently as potassium, calcium, and sodium bicarbonate supplements.

INTRAVENOUS THERAPY

The intravenous route is the fastest method of replacing fluid and electrolytes because the fluid enters the circulatory system immediately and does not need to be absorbed from the gastrointestinal tract. It is the method of choice in emergencies; it is an effective method for administering fluid and electrolytes to people who are unable to drink oral fluids due to conditions such as vomiting and nausea, gastrointestinal obstruction, mouth or throat surgery, or unconsciousness (see QRS 30-2). The intravenous route may also be used as a primary method for administering medication.

Common Intravenous Sites. Common sites utilized for intravenous therapy are the dorsal veins of the hands, forearm veins (basilic and cephalic), and veins in the antecubital space (inner elbow). Lesser used but acceptable sites are veins in the foot or scalp (see Chap. 20, Fig. 20-2). Because intravenous fluid will infuse during a period of time, the site selected must be one that can be preserved despite body movement and that will not greatly inconvenience the person in everyday activities if possible. In a right-handed person, for example, an intravenous infusion is usually begun in the left hand so that the dominant hand is free for eating. Veins in the lower extremities of adults are little used, partly because such veins may be more prone to thrombus (clot) formation than those in the upper extremities but also because maximum ambulatory ability should be maintained. The antecubital space, formerly frequently used, is little used today because although the veins there are large and accept fluid well, elbow flexion tends to cause a needle placed there to infiltrate, necessitating termination of the infusion.

Although many people do not like intravenous fluid in the back of their hand (they are worried it will leave a scar there), this is an optimal site because if infiltration does occur there, it can be easily seen as soon as it occurs, and the infusion site can then be advanced further up the arm. If a more proximal site is chosen first and the infusion is then moved to a more distal site, there is often "leaking" from the point where the vein was pierced initially due to the increased pressure of the intravenous fluid in the vein and continuing infiltration at that point. People can be assured that an intravenous infusion will leave no mark on their skin other than a pinpoint scab that forms when the needle is removed; this disappears without any mark within three days.

The actual site chosen depends on the availability of veins (a cut on an arm cancels a usually available site) and on the type, volume, and rate of fluid to be infused. Small hand veins, for example, are generally not used if the fluid to be infused is irritating or causes pain. Infusing such a fluid into a larger vein causes it to be diluted more quickly and reduces discomfort. Fluid cannot be infused as quickly in a small vein as in a larger one, so if the fluid will have to be administered during a short time span in large amounts, a larger vein that will better handle this volume is chosen. Blood, because it is viscous, is often administered in larger veins.

Intravenous Needles. Intravenous fluid is most commonly administered through a large metal needle (No. 22, 20, or 18). Infants and some older adults have such narrow veins that a No. 22 or even a No. 25 needle must be used.

"Butterflies" are metal needles with an extra flange of plastic added on both sides of the needle hub to give the person beginning the infusion a wider surface to grasp, thereby guiding needle placement better. Butterflies are also termed *scalp vein needles* because they were designed originally for entrance into small infant scalp veins. A length of very narrow tubing leads from the needle to the fluid administration tubing. Today,

☐ QUICK REFERENCE STOP 30-2: NUTRITION
Limitations of Intravenous Therapy

1. Regular intravenous therapy supplies electrolytes, glucose, and fluid and, if specifically added, vitamins, but not protein and fat. It is only a temporary means of sustenance; therefore, when ingestion of oral substances is prohibited, it is not a long-term method for nutrition. Hyperalimentation solutions (total parenteral nutrition [TPN]) do provide total nutrition. These solutions are generally administered into the central veins rather than into peripheral veins because of their high molecular weight. They are discussed further in Chap. 35.
2. To calculate the number of calories a person is receiving in intravenous fluid, determine the number of grams of carbohydrate in the solution. A 5 percent glucose solution means that 5 ml of every 100 is sugar (in a 1000-ml bottle there are 50 g of sugar; 1 ml equals 1 g). One gram of carbohydrate (sugar) yields four calories.
3. Be aware that mealtime for most people means more than eating. It is also a time for conversation and social interaction. For the person receiving intravenous therapy who is not eating any meals, provide these experiences for him at set visiting times. Otherwise he may become depressed.

scalp vein needles are used at any site that is difficult to enter.

Intracaths are plastic needles with a metal guide inserted in the lumen to give the plastic rigidity. As soon as the intracath is placed in the vein, the metal guide is withdrawn, and only the hollow plastic needle remains. Because such a needle is more flexible than a metal needle, theoretically it will not infiltrate or pierce the vein wall to infiltrate as much. Intracaths may be no longer than a regular needle (1 1/2 inches), or they may be as long as 12 to 18 inches. These longer intracaths are "through the needle" insertions—structured so that a metal needle is inserted into the vein; the thinner intracath is then threaded through the hollow metal needle into the vein. A long intracath can be inserted into a vein at the forearm, yet actually deliver the intravenous fluid into the antecubital space or into a very large vein for quick distribution of an irritating fluid (thereby achieving the benefits of administering fluid at the antecubital space without risking infiltration due to elbow bending).

If there is a disadvantage to intracaths it is that they are made of plastic and could conceivably break while being placed or removed. The tips of intracaths are beveled or slanted to make the tip easily recognizable. After removal of an intracath, always check the tip to be certain that the entire intracath has been removed and that a portion did not break off inside the vein (you can identify the tip if it is present). If you do remove an intracath and suspect that it did break, immediately place a constricting tourniquet above the level of the intravenous site (between the site and the heart) to keep the broken piece from moving with venous bloodflow, and immediately notify the person's physician. Intracaths are radiopaque (visualizeable on x-ray film) so that the missing piece can be located by a radiograph; sometimes gentle palpation of the vein will reveal the presence of the piece. It must be removed by a cut-down or surgical incision into the vein at that point. A broken intracath is a rare occurrence but is an emergency when it does occur. An unrecognized tip would move through the venous circulation and cause obstruction in the lung or the heart.

Venipuncture. Venipuncture is, as the name implies, a puncture into a vein to initiate intravenous therapy. Sterile techniques must be used for venipuncture to prevent microorganisms from being introduced by the needle or from the skin during the puncture. Whether nurses perform venipuncture or not depends on health care agency policy. In many agencies, intravenous fluid is begun by special intravenous teams or physicians. All nurses need to know how to perform a venipuncture so that in an emergency they can draw blood or establish an intravenous route. They also need to be familiar with the technique to assist a physician with the procedure. See Procedures 30-1 and 30-2.

To do a venipuncture, a tourniquet is placed about 2 inches above the chosen venipuncture site (Procedure 30-1, Fig. 1). The purpose of the tourniquet is to cause buildup of blood behind it that will distend the vein; distending the vein will make it easier to penetrate because it is wider and fatter than normal and will minimize the danger of the needle piercing the back wall of the vein as it is inserted (ineffective placement that must then be removed). The tourniquet should be snug but not tight enough to pinch and be uncomfortable. A pinching tourniquet is probably cutting off arterial flow as well, and that is an unnecessary fluid restriction to the body part distal to the tourniquet. Lowering the extremity below heart level will cause even greater vein distention. Asking the person to open and close his fist several times and lightly tapping the vein over the chosen site are other techniques that cause the veins to fill fully and allow for easiest needle insertion.

The skin surface over the chosen site must be washed thoroughly with a suitable antiseptic such as 70 percent alcohol; washing should be done in a circular motion from the site outward (moving surface microorganisms away from the site). Povidone-iodine solution (Betadine) is a better bactericidal, sporicidal, and fungicidal solution than alcohol, but occasionally people are allergic to it, so it is not used routinely. If using povidone-iodine to wash, ask the person about a possible allergy to iodine first. Shaving of intravenous sites, except for scalp sites, is unnecessary even if considerable hair is present. Shaving hair makes removal of the tape used to secure the needle easier, but nicks caused by shaving may predispose the patient to infection dangerously near the venipuncture site.

To insert the needle, hold the skin taut against the vein by placing your left hand near the site and stretching the skin over it with your index finger and thumb. Holding the needle in your right hand with the bevel up, pierce the skin just to the side of and about half an inch below the point where the needle will pierce the vein. Enter the skin with the needle held at a 45-degree angle; immediately decrease this angle to 30 degrees, pierce the vein from the side, and thread the needle gently one-half to three-quarters of an inch into the vein (Procedure 30-1, Fig. 2). You can tell that the needle has entered the vein because the pressure or resistance you feel will immediately decrease as you enter the vein; a thin stream of blood will enter the needle owing to the increased pressure in the vein, appearing in the intravenous tubing (or if you are performing a venipuncture to withdraw blood in the syringe you would attach to your needle), proof that you have entered the vein.

Remove the tourniquet as soon as the needle is in place; open the clamp on the intravenous tubing to allow fluid to flow. Observe the site for swelling (a sure sign that the needle has punctured the posterior wall

PROCEDURE 30-1
Venipuncture for Intravenous Therapy

Purpose: Entrance into a vein by a needle using sterile technique to initiate intravenous therapy.

Plan	*Principle*
1. Wash your hands, identify patient, explain procedure.	1. Prevent spread of microorganisms; provide for patient safety and cooperation.
2. Assess appropriateness of procedure; analyze and plan modifications depending on specific patient need.	2. People vary greatly in ease and accessibility of veins. Consider age of patient, type and length of infusion.
3. Implement procedure by organizing equipment: scalp vein needle, alcohol pledgelet, tourniquet, sterile syringe if a blood sample is needed.	3. Scalp vein needles are easiest to place because of the "butterfly" flange.
4. Place a tourniquet 2 inches above chosen venipuncture site; ask the person to open and close his hand. Tap chosen site lightly to cause vein distention (Fig. 1).	4. Do not use a person's dominant arm if at all possible. Use the most distal site possible to allow further administration.

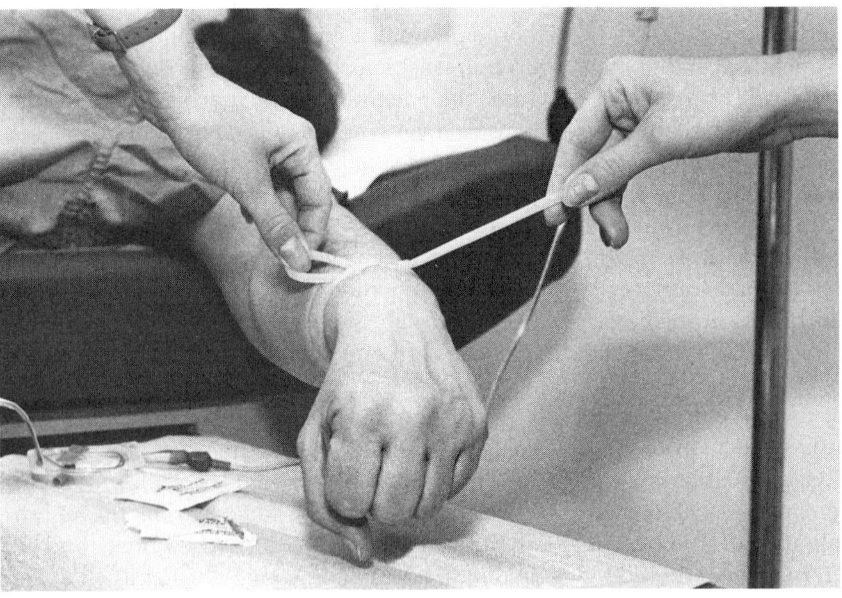

FIGURE 1. To apply a tourniquet, place it about 2 inches above the chosen venipuncture site; to remove it with one hand, grasp the free end and pull.

5. Cleanse the skin at the site with alcohol in a circular manner. Do not palpate or tap the site after cleansing it or you will contaminate it again.	5. Skin always contains surface bacteria. A circular motion (inside to outside) wipes bacteria away from the site.
6. Place a thumb on the vein just distal to the venipuncture site to stabilize it; insert the needle of the scalp vein bevel up at a 45-degree angle just to the side of the vein and 1/2 inch distal to the point where you want to enter the vein.	6. Piercing the skin takes pressure; this pressure could be enough to pierce completely through the vein if you are on top of it. Entering from the side gives more control.

7. When the needle has pierced the skin, lower the angle of the needle until it is about parallel with the skin surface; thread it into the vein 1/2 to 3/4 inch (Fig. 2).

7. A flat angle prevents piercing the vein.

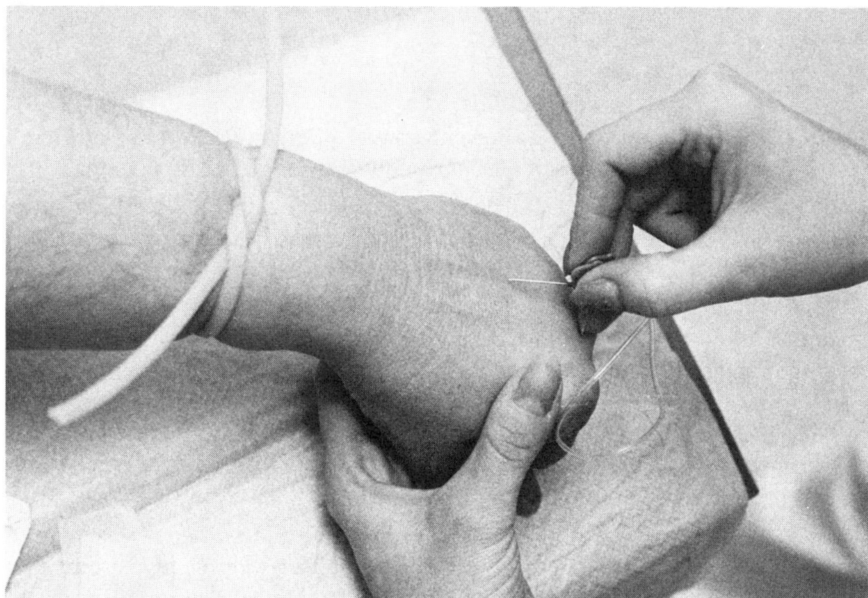

FIGURE 2. For a venipuncture, hold the needle in your hand, bevel up, and pierce the skin just to side of and about 1/2 inch below the point where the needle will pierce the vein. Keep needle at a 45-degree angle to puncture.

8. Allow blood from the vein to flow back to completely fill the scalp vein tubing (to take a blood sample, attach the syringe to tubing and gently aspirate blood back into the syringe).

8. Pressure in the vein is greater than in the empty tubing. Unless you completely fill the tubing with blood, you will administer air when you administer intravenous fluid. Aspirate gently to avoid collapsing the vein.

9. If blood drawing was the goal of venipuncture, press alcohol pledgelet over needle tip and withdraw needle flat with skin surface. Hold for at least 10 seconds to stop blood flow. Apply band-aid to site as necessary. Prepare specimen for laboratory.

9. If there is oozing at a venipuncture site from improper compression afterward, the site will be obscured for further venipuncture.

10. If purpose of venipuncture was to initiate intravenous fluid, follow with steps outlined in Procedure 30-2.

MODIFICATIONS FOR CARE OF CHILD

Children under about age 10 are not able to hold still long enough for a venipuncture without a second person present to restrain them as necessary.

The femoral or jugular vein can be used for venipuncture for drawing blood, but if everyone has been careful with compression afterward and has preserved venipuncture sites, it is rarely necessary to use them.

MODIFICATIONS FOR CARE OF OLDER ADULT

Older adults with arteriosclerotic vessel changes have veins that are very difficult to penetrate (they are narrow and hard). Compress adequately to preserve venipuncture sites because they may be few in number.

PROCEDURE 30-2
Assisting with Venipuncture and Beginning Intravenous Administration

Purpose: To provide assistance in administering fluid when the oral route is not accessible; to provide assistance in administering replacement fluid, electrolytes, or nutrients. To provide assistance in offering a vehicle for intravenous medication administration.

Plan	*Principle*
1. Wash hands, identify patient, explain procedure to patient.	1. Prevent spread of microorganisms; provide for patient safety and cooperation.
2. Assess appropriateness of procedure based on patient condition and circumstances.	2. People who would benefit from mobility and are having intermittent administration might benefit from a heparin lock.
3. Implement procedure by assembling equipment: appropriate intravenous solution (label checked three times); tubing that will supply desired drip rate; appropriate needle; three strips of 1/2-inch tape; two strips of 1-inch tape; two 4 × 4 gauze squares, one sterile 2 × 2 gauze square, alcohol for skin preparation; armboard; tourniquet.	3. Adhesive tape will be used to secure needle in place and arm to armboard. Backing the wide adhesive strips with gauze prevents them from pulling hair when they are removed at end of infusion.
4. To prepare solution, open bottle or bag and attach tubing; flush tubing with solution to evacuate all air from the tubing. Reclose the tubing clamp and recap end of tubing to keep them sterile. Label bottle and tubing with date, time, any additives, and your initials.	4. Be certain that all air is evacuated from tubing to prevent an air embolus. Tap small air bubbles to cause them to rise in fluid and evacuate into solution container.
5. Restrain patient appropriately; effective venipuncture requires a nonmoving patient.	5. Restrain adults by resting your hand on their arm with a comment such as, "Let me help you hold this still."
6. Assist as necessary as the physician beginning the venipuncture applies the tourniquet, swabs the chosen site, and inserts the needle; release the tourniquet and open the clamp on the infusion tubing to allow solution to flow into the needle.	6. If a regular needle is used, it is attached to the intravenous tubing just prior to insertion. If a scalp vein needle is used, blood must flow the length of the attached tubing before the infusion tubing can be attached.

7. When the infusion is infusing well, the needle is stabilized by one criss-crossed piece of tape; one piece of tape directly over the hub may tip it slightly downward, helping the position (Fig. 1).

7. Stabilizing the needle well prevents irritation of the vein.

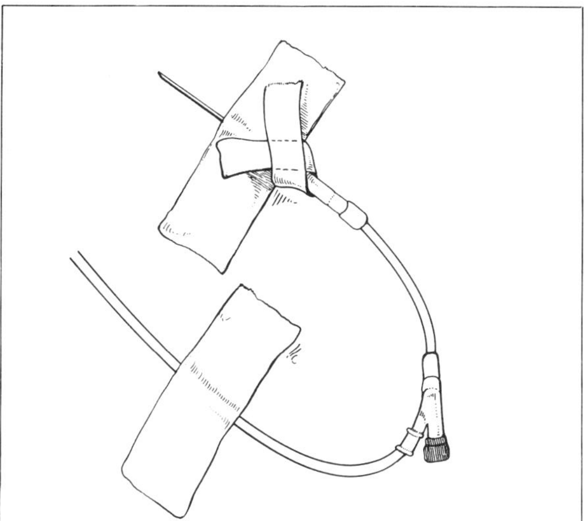

FIGURE 1. Securing the needle. Note that the tape securing the tubing is independent of the needle; an accidental pull will not dislodge the needle. (From A. Plumer, *Principles and Practice on Intravenous Therapy* [3rd ed.]. Boston: Little, Brown, 1982.)

8. Loop the tubing once and attach it with a third strip of narrow tape. Attach armboard with wide strips of tape above and below the venipuncture site (Fig. 2). An armboard in adults is a "reminder," not a restraint.

8. Looping the tubing prevents the needle from being dislodged if the tubing is tugged because it causes the pull to stop at the loop rather than the needle.

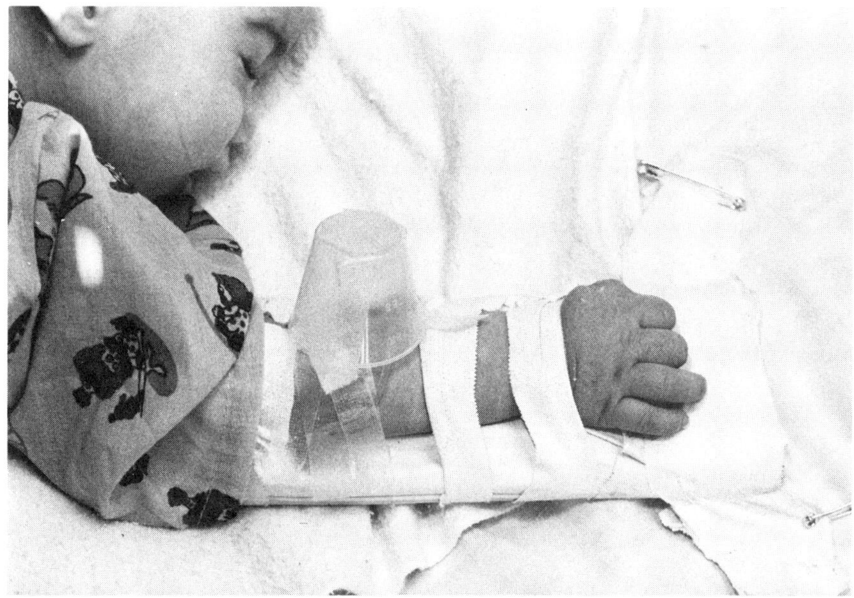

FIGURE 2. In infants and young children, attach "wings" to the armboard and pin the board to the mattress to stabilize the board. The medicine cup over the insertion site protects the site.

9. Regulate infusion flow rate by clamping the tubing or attaching an infusion regulation pump.	9. Never walk away from a new infusion without checking twice that the flow rate is correct. The rate of infusion may increase in the first few minutes as vein spasm from the venipuncture subsides.
10. Attach tape to bottle or bag, anticipating emptying times. Position patient comfortably. Provide diversion as necessary.	10. People at first are very aware of an infusion, but if it is taped comfortably they soon forget it and begin to resume regular activities.
11. Assess efficiency, effectiveness, cost, safety, and comfort aspects of procedure. Chart the venipuncture site used, type and rate of infusion and patient's response to procedure.	11. Documentation of patient status and nursing care.
12. Plan health teaching as necessary such as necessity to guard intravenous site; keep it dry and so on.	12. Health teaching is an independent nursing action always included as part of care.

MODIFICATIONS FOR CARE OF CHILD

In infants it is helpful to tape the armboard in place before the venipuncture is done so that struggling between the time the needle is placed and the infusion is attached does not dislodge the needle.

The dorsal surface of the foot and the scalp veins are additional sites that may be used in infants because they do not have the same problems of circulatory stasis in the lower extremities as adults. Using such a site may leave the child's arms free to play and eat by himself.

A child up to about 3 or 4 years of age needs restraints with an intravenous line when an adult is not with him. Attaching "wings" to the armboard and pinning the board to the mattress (Fig. 3) stabilizes the board.

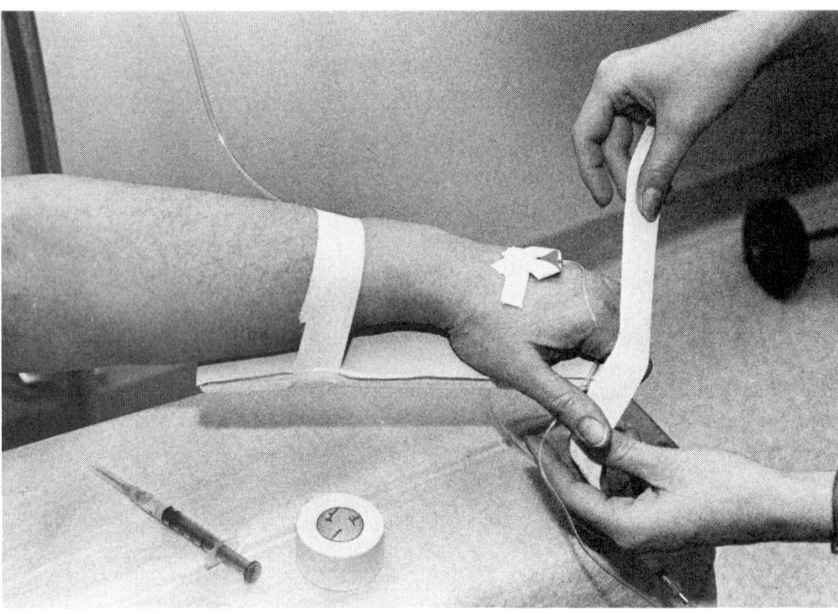

FIGURE 3. Securing an arm to an armboard. Be certain that the body part is in good anatomical alignment first.

Always provide an activity to occupy a child while an infusion is running. If the infusion is the most interesting thing in his environment, he is tempted to change the flow rate or perform other hazardous acts out of boredom.

In all children under 2 years of age a volume control chamber should be an intrinsic part of the fluid line for safety. If a crib is being used, attach an extension tubing to allow the crib rail to rise freely.

Remaining on bed rest because an intravenous infusion is running is very difficult for children. Suggest heparin locks when appropriate to allow greater mobility.

MODIFICATIONS FOR CARE OF OLDER ADULT

Be very careful to prevent circulatory overload in older adults by careful regulation of fluid flow. Older adults with heart disease should have volume control chambers for safety.

Many older adults need stimulation to receive enough sensory input. Provide ambulation by assisting them to walk or move to a wheelchair despite the presence of the infusion. A person with a hearing deficit may be bothered by the tone of an infusion pump. Explain the sound and locate it either close enough to the bed so that he can hear it well or far enough that he cannot hear it, whichever position suits him best.

Release armboard restraints and do passive range-of-motion exercises every 2 hours (unless this would lead to venipuncture infiltration) to ensure good circulation in older adults, particularly those with arteriosclerotic vessel changes.

and fluid is infiltrating into the subcutaneous tissue rather than the vein). Remove the needle and apply pressure to the site if swelling occurs in order to halt any bleeding from the punctured vein. Choose another site for a second attempt, preferably on the opposite extremity since applying a tourniquet above the site will cause at least minimal oozing under the skin (a hematoma) at that site as the pressure rises in the vein again.

If no swelling occurs, the needle is undoubtedly well positioned. Anchor the needle by a narrow piece of tape pulled beneath the needle and crossed on top; further stabilize the needle hub by a second piece of tape directly over the hub (Procedure 30-2, Fig. 1). Securely anchoring the needle prevents it from moving in the vein; such movement is painful and the irritation of the motion can lead to phlebitis (vein inflammation).

To further protect the site, place a sterile piece of gauze (a 2 × 2) or an occlusive dressing such as Op-site directly over the puncture site and secure it in place with added tape. A health care agency policy may require an application of povidone-iodine or a bacterial ointment at the site under the dressing. Use a single-use packet ointment for this purpose so there is no danger of cross contamination between patients. Loop the intravenous tubing and secure it as necessary as a final step to prevent it from snagging on bedclothes and dislodging the needle (tape it so an accidental tug on the tubing will pull at the tape, not the needle site). Use no more tape than necessary since the tubing will need to be changed every 24 hours to prevent bacterial contamination.

Write the date and time of insertion and your name on a separate piece of tape and apply it to the dressing so there is no question as to when the intravenous fluid was begun (do not apply the tape first and then write time and date, or the pressure of your pen may push the needle through the posterior vein wall, destroying the site).

Most people want an armboard attached to remind them to hold their extremity still (and actually need a board attached to remind them to hold it still). Be certain that an extremity taped to an armboard is in good anatomical position (Procedure 30-2, Fig. 2). Padding strips of adhesive tape with gauze squares allows this tape to hold the board in place yet removes easily without pulling hairs.

Intravenous Fluid. Intravenous fluid is considered a medicine and is ordered with the same precise specifications as oral or injectable medication. The physician's order should specify the type and amount of fluid to be administered and the rate at which it should be administered. If additives such as vitamins or additional electrolytes are to be added, the amount and type of these should be specified exactly. If more than one bottle of intravenous fluid is to be administered, the order of administration should be specified. Calculating the rate of administration (how many drops per minute) may or may not be determined by the physician. If it is not, it is calculated by you (see below).

TYPES OF INTRAVENOUS FLUID. The type of intravenous fluid ordered depends on the exact fluid and electrolyte imbalance present. A fluid that exactly resembles blood plasma is an *isotonic* solution; a solution that has more molecular weight than blood plasma is *hypertonic*, less molecular weight, *hypotonic*. If hypotonic fluid is administered, fluid will leave the vascular compartment and enter the interstitial tissue (fluid will flow from an area of lesser osmotic concentration to one of higher concentration). It may enter the red blood cells to such an extent that they will rupture. If a solution is hypertonic, fluid in the red blood cells will leave them and enter the plasma, shrinking and disintegrating the cells; additional fluid will be drawn from the interstitial tissue into the bloodstream. The least traumatic solution used for intravenous therapy, therefore, is an isotonic one—one that is the same molecular weight as the blood. Normal saline (0.9 sodium chloride in water), 5 percent dextrose in water, and lactated Ringer's solution are the three solutions considered to be isotonic.

When brain edema is present, a hypertonic solution (10% dextrose in water) is administered intravenously for its osmotic effect (fluid in the subcutaneous tissue will move into the suddenly more concentrated bloodstream). This evacuates edematous fluid and prevents pressure on brain cells from edema. It is important to monitor urine output in all patients receiving intravenous fluid to be certain that it is maintained at an adequate rate. For people receiving hypertonic solutions this is doubly important; if urinary output is compromised in some way, the person's circulatory system can be easily overloaded because of all the fluid being drawn from subcutaneous spaces. Table 30-7 summarizes the commonly used intravenous fluids and situations in which they are used.

CONTAINERS FOR INTRAVENOUS FLUID. Intravenous fluid has traditionally been furnished in glass bottles. The inside of the bottle and the fluid are sterilized at the manufacturing plant; the bottle has a rubber stopper top and negative pressure or a vacuum inside. Glass bottles must be vented either by an opening in the rubber stopper separate from the place where the infusion tubing inserts or by an indirect vent in the administration tubing. The advantage of glass bottles is the ease of determining the fluid level left in the bottle; the disadvantage is that they require more shelf space than plastic containers and are potentially more dangerous if they break.

Plastic bags for intravenous therapy have been available for about 10 years but have taken a long time to be accepted (Fig. 30-5). Because a plastic bag collapses as it empties, it needs no air vent. Plastic bags are difficult to manipulate at first but are no more difficult to work with when you are accustomed to them. Some medications (such as insulin) cannot be added to plastic bags because the bag absorbs the medication. They cannot be used in a series (one bag connected directly to another, a system used when large amounts of fluid are being administered rapidly) because as the first bag empties, air in the bag can be drawn into the intravenous line, possibly causing an air embolus if it enters the person's bloodstream. Plastic bags have the advantage of taking little storage space. The bag should be stored in the additional plastic wrap furnished with it by the manufacturer to keep fluid inside the bag from gradually seeping through the bag, causing the amount of fluid inside to decrease in amount and increase in strength. Both plastic and glass systems supply fluid in 250-, 500-, and 1000-ml containers.

TABLE 30-7. COMMONLY USED INTRAVENOUS SOLUTIONS

Solution	Tonicity	Common Purposes
0.9% sodium chloride (normal saline)	Isotonic	Replacement of fluid loss
5% dextrose and water	Isotonic	Replacement of fluid loss and to supply minimal calories
Lactated Ringer's	Isotonic	Replacement of fluid loss and electrolytes
0.45% sodium chloride	Hypotonic	Rapid hydration (fluid moves from vascular space to interstitial spaces, quickly hydrating tissue)
5% dextrose in 0.9% sodium chloride	Hypertonic	Replacement of body fluid loss and minimal calories

PREPARATION OF INTRAVENOUS FLUID. All intravenous fluid, whether in plastic bags or glass bottles, appears much the same at first glance. In selecting fluid, follow the basic rules of medicine administration: Read the label three times before you remove it from the shelf, before you insert the tubing, once more before you hang the bottle over a patient's head or leave the medi-

FIGURE 30-5. A. A plastic bag of intravenous fluid. B. A glass bottle of intravenous fluid has a rubber stopper to protect the negative pressure, or vacuum, inside. Here a student nurse carefully selects the correct solution from a supply cart.

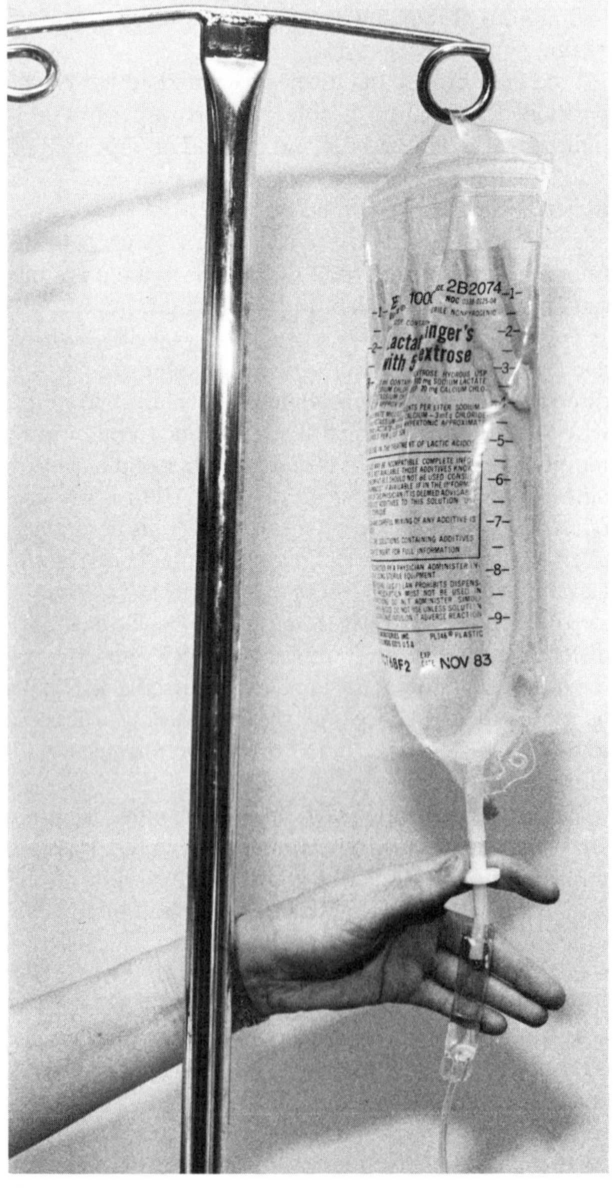

A

cation preparation area; see Fig. 30-5 and Quick Reference Stop 30-3.

Always check the expiration date on intravenous fluid as you do on drug bottles. Expiration dates are marked to establish the point at which bacterial contamination or disintegration of contents could have occurred.

With plastic bags, gently squeeze the bag to detect any leaks; inspect glass bottles for cracks where contamination could enter. Discard or return to the pharmacy any fluid that is discolored or cloudy even if the expiration date has not been reached. Sometimes discoloration is the result of the sterilization of the fluid, but you cannot tell this from observation.

Intravenous Tubing. The choice of intravenous tubing depends on the amount and number of solutions that will be infused, the rate of infusion desired, and whether special safety measures to prevent a larger amount of fluid accidentally infusing at once or not is desired.

Figure 30-6 illustrates the opening of a glass bottle of fluid. After the metal ring and rubber disk that seal the top of the bottle have been removed, the tubing is inserted into the bottle by puncturing the rubber top with the point of the tubing. It is not necessary to wipe the top of the bottle with alcohol before puncturing it

☐ QUICK REFERENCE STOP 30-3: SAFETY
Intravenous Fluid Administration

1. Use strict sterile technique with intravenous equipment. Any bacterial contamination from careless handling enters the bloodstream immediately.
2. Check the rate of intravenous fluid infusion at least hourly. Check more frequently if the patient is a child or an adult who cannot be responsible for monitoring his own care or if medication is added to the infusion.
3. All intravenous fluid is considered medication. Check all labels as carefully (three times) as you would a drug.
4. Mark with a piece of adhesive tape or a label the time and date when intravenous solutions and tubing were opened. The bacterial count begins to increase when they are opened, not when they are actually used.
5. When irrigating an intravenous needle, withdraw the syringe plunger, do not inject it, to avoid pushing a blood clot into the person's circulation.
6. Be certain that intravenous fluid tubing is changed every 24 to 48 hours to reduce the risk of bacterial contamination.

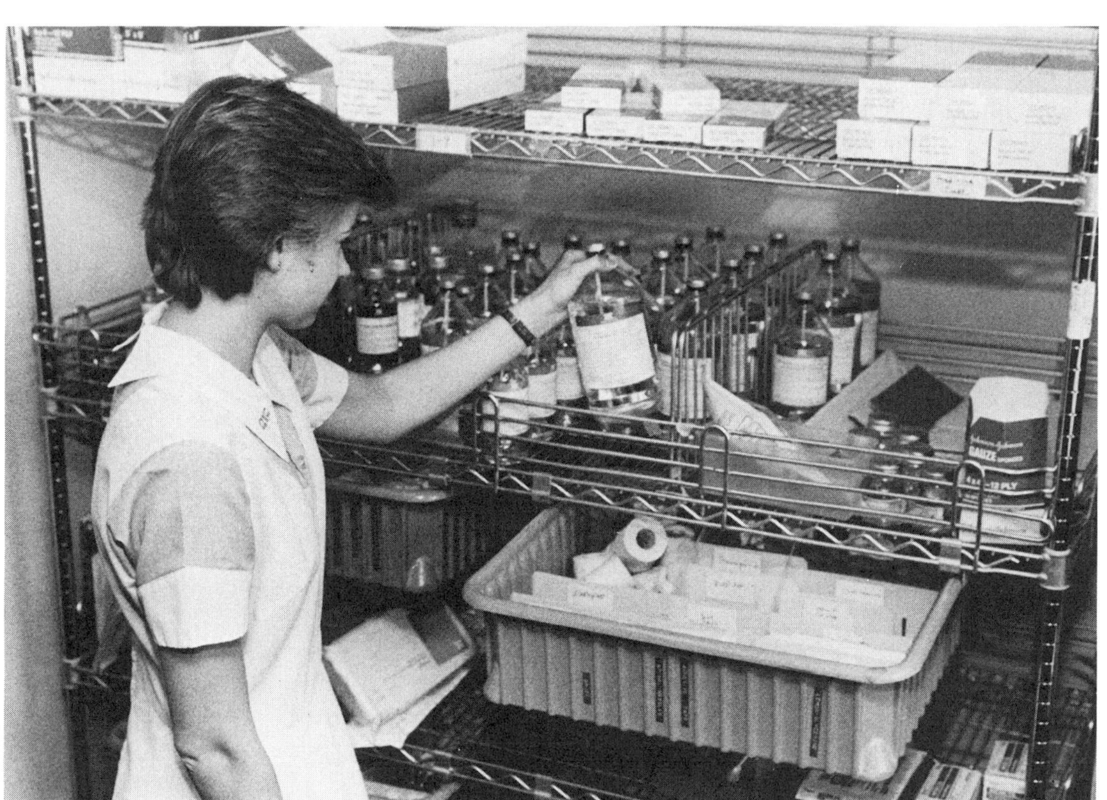

B

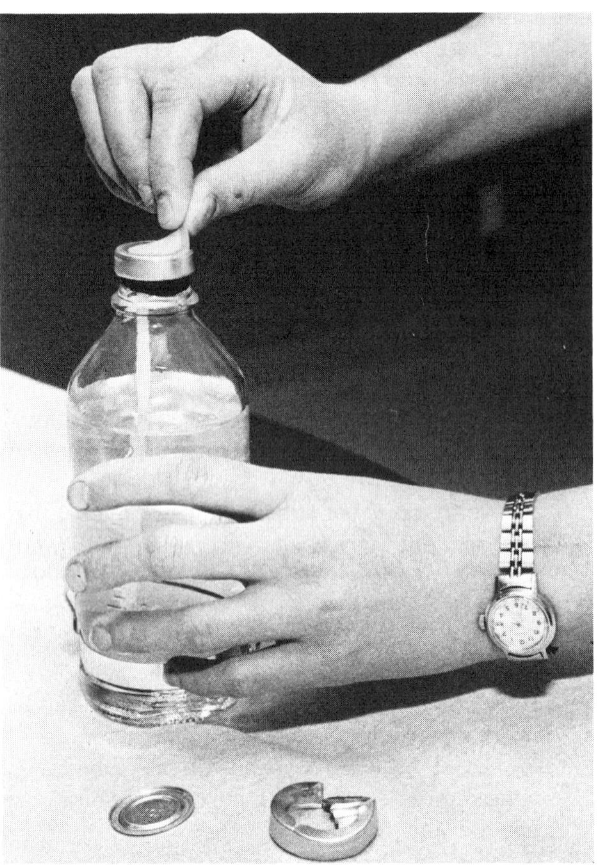

A

as is done with vials of medication because the rubber top is sterile under the rubber disk and wiping with alcohol might allow alcohol to drop into the solution, changing its composition. Fluid flows from the bottle (Fig. 30-7) through the tubing to a drop chamber, where drops of fluid can be observed as they fall, and then on down the tubing into the patient. The size of drop that a drop chamber creates differs according to the brand of intravenous equipment. Equipment from different manufacturers will deliver either 10, 15, or 20 drops per milliliter of fluid. If you have memorized a conversion factor such as 15 drops to a milliliter, forget it when working with intravenous fluid. Consult the tubing package for the manufacturer's statement of the number of drops in a milliliter of fluid dripping from that chamber and use that conversion factor only.

Figure 30-8 shows a different type of drop chamber, or a *minidrip* chamber. The thin silver tubing through which the drops must fall in this set-up limits the size of the drops considerably. Depending on the brand of equipment, the drop size for a minidrip apparatus will supply either 50 or 60 drops per milliliter.

Figure 30-8 also illustrates a volume control set that can be added to the plain tubing. This is a calibrated chamber (Buretrol, Metriset, and Soluset are various

FIGURE 30-6. Connecting intravenous tubing to the bottle. A. Remove the metal and rubber disk from the IV bottle. B. Puncture the rubber top of the bottle with the point of the tubing.

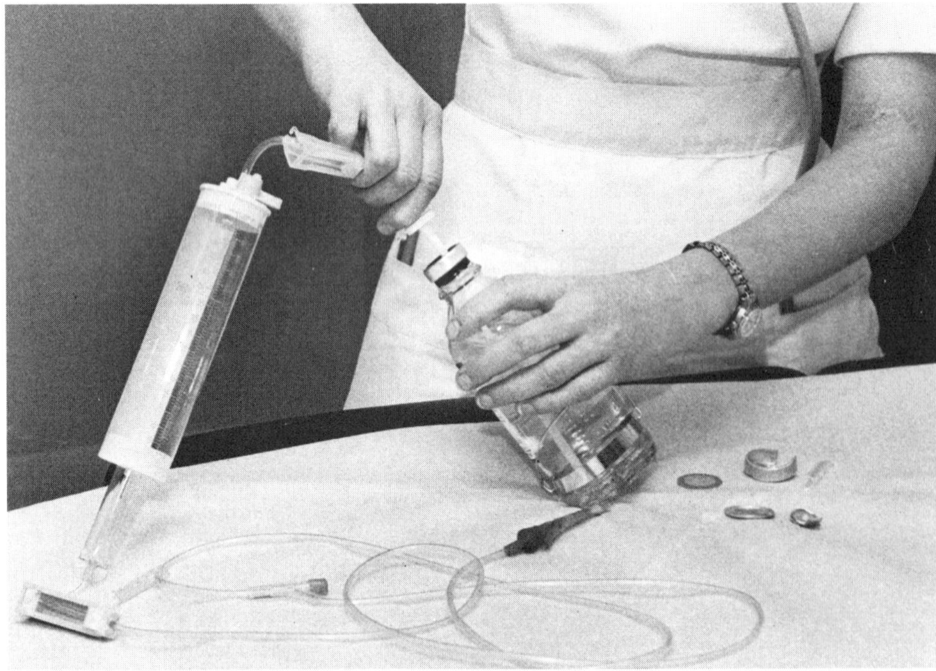

B

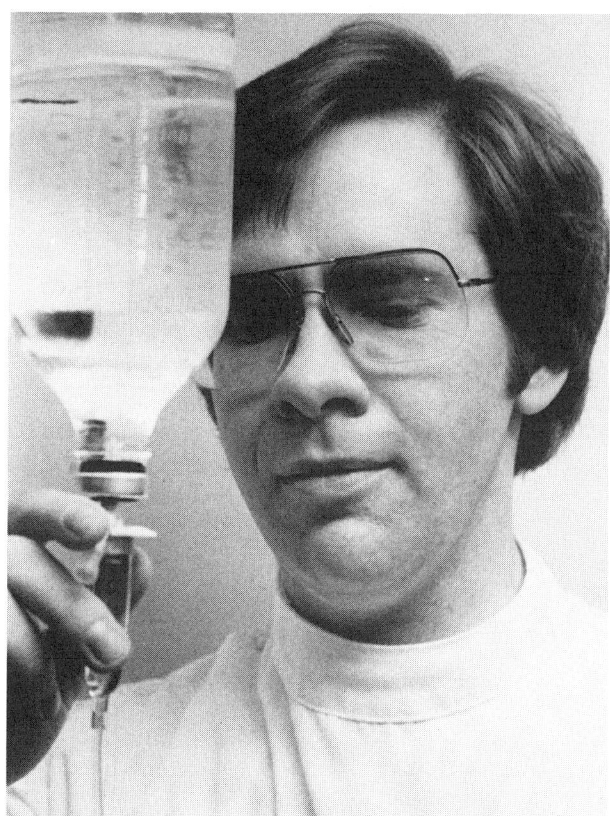

FIGURE 30-7. Fluid flows from the bottle through the tubing into a drip chamber and then into the patient. You can observe the drops of fluid as they fall into the drip chamber to count the rate of flow.

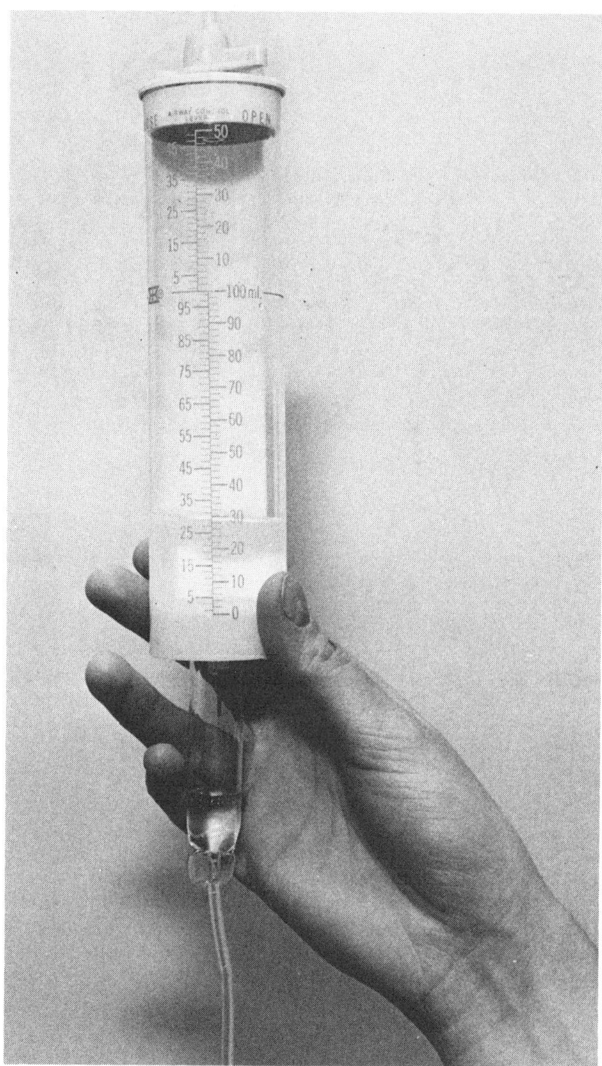

FIGURE 30-8. A mini-drip chamber limits the size of the drops and allows small amounts to be administered safely. Here a mini-drip and volume control chamber are combined into a single unit.

brand names), 100 to 250 ml in size, which is filled with intravenous fluid from the solution bag overhead. The clamp above the volume control chamber is closed after a set amount of fluid has filled the chamber so that no more fluid from the bag can enter the drip chamber. Such a device is a safety measure in that if the tubing clamp should be accidentally released (or deliberately released by a child), the person could receive no more fluid than that contained in the volume control chamber. Intravenous therapy is not administered to children under 2 years of age without such a safety feature in place to eliminate the danger of circulatory overload. For such children, fill the volume control chamber with no more fluid than the child is to receive in an hour's time (a safe amount no matter how unstable the tubing clamp). Volume control chambers are also useful if the solution contains a medication such as potassium or heparin to ensure that a large volume of potentially lethal medication cannot accidentally be administered too rapidly (Fig. 30-9).

Volume control sets are designed to deliver a variety of different-sized drops (10, 15, 50, or 60 drops per milliliter). Allow volume control chambers to fill according to manufacturers' directions. As a rule, pinching such chambers to help them fill distorts the pressure inside and results in poor flow thereafter.

If a person is to receive a great deal of fluid during a day's time, two bottles of fluid may be hung in a series (Fig. 30-10). The two bottles are connected by plastic tubing; keep the air vent closed on the primary or first bottle to be infused; open the air vent on the second bottle. With a series connection, the second bottle will empty first; when it is empty, the primary bottle will begin to empty. A series arrangement is best used if the two solutions are the same type. If the primary bottle contains a solution that is hypotonic to the second one, there will be minimal mixing of the solutions. If the primary bottle is hypertonic to the second one, osmotic pressure will cause extensive mixing of the solutions. If a person is to receive 1000 ml of 0.9 percent sodium chloride (isotonic solution) and following that, 1000 ml of 10 percent dextrose and water (hypertonic solution), for example, you could not use a series connection. The two solutions will mix, and the person would receive a

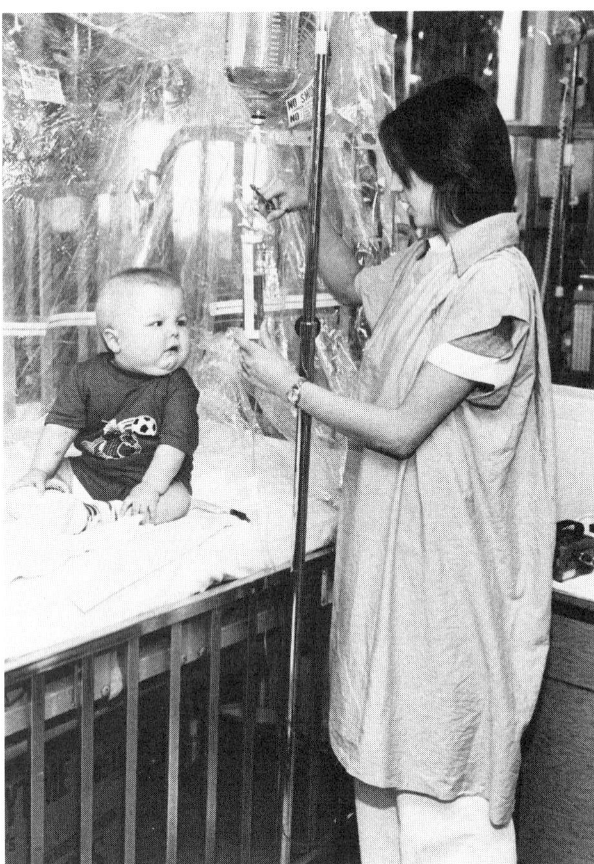

FIGURE 30-9. A volume control set that can be added to plain tubing is a calibrated chamber, 100 to 250 ml in size. It is both a safety control and a convenient port for adding medication.

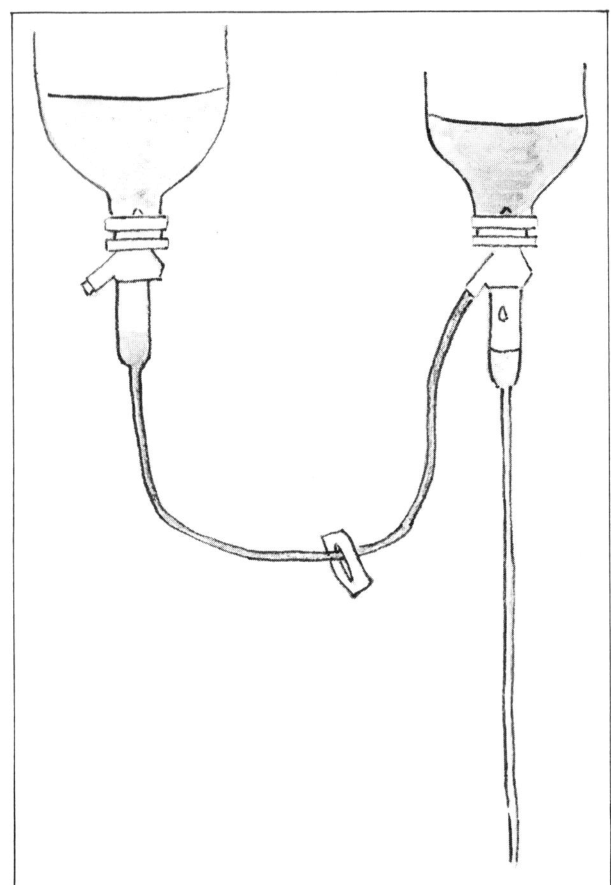

FIGURE 30-10. Two bottles may be hung in a series connected by plastic tubing. The second bottle (the one with the open air vent on the left) will empty first. When this second bottle is empty, the primary bottle will begin to empty.

combination of both solutions, not one first and then the other.

The rate of infusion of the two solutions may make a series connection not practical because of the possibility of infection. If it is to take 8 hours, for example, for the second bottle to empty, the primary bottle will have been open for 8 hours before it ever begins to empty. The possibility of bacterial contamination is minimized by simply infusing the second bottle by a single tubing arrangement and then, 8 hours later, infusing the primary bottle.

Figure 30-11A shows a Y-type or parallel arrangement, which allows two solutions to be administered either alternately (by opening first one clamp and then the other) or simultaneously (by opening both clamps). Such a setup might be used to administer a hypotensive drug (a drug to reduce blood pressure). In this instance, one solution bottle is filled with an isotonic solution such as 5 percent dextrose and water, and the drug is added to the other bottle. The clamp to the plain bottle is opened, and the drug-added bottle clamp is closed so that the plain solution will infuse most of the time. If, after taking vital signs, the person's blood pressure is found to be elevated, the plain solution bottle clamp is closed, the drug-added solution bottle clamp is opened, and the person is administered enough of the hypotensive solution to raise and stabilize the blood pressure. At that point, the clamps will be reversed and the plain solution infused again.

Blood is typically administered with a Y-type connection (blood on one side, normal saline on the other) because the normal saline infusion can be used to "thin" the blood infusion as needed. With a Y-type setup, whenever one bottle empties completely, air can enter the tubing from the empty bottle and cause an air embolus if the clamp to the empty bottle is not securely closed. To prevent this, make a habit of not allowing solution bottles to empty completely (leave a rim of fluid in the bottle).

Figure 30-11B shows yet another tandem arrangement—a "piggyback" setup. This arrangement is used to infuse a primary solution continually and a second solution (the piggyback) intermittently. It is often used to infuse a medication contained in the piggyback solution. To attach a piggyback tubing, the needle used should be no longer than 1 inch so that it will not puncture the side of the primary tubing as it is inserted. Lower the height of the primary bottle so it

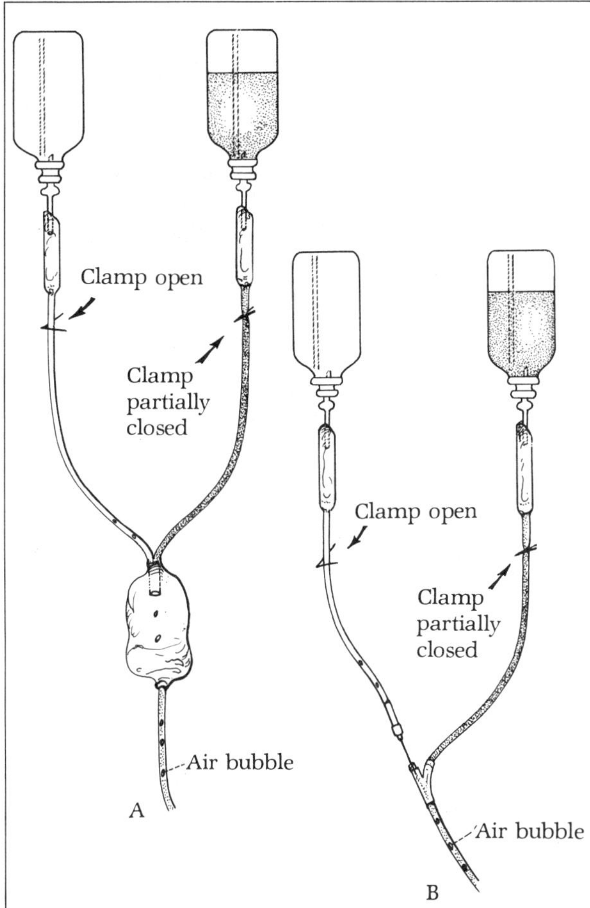

FIGURE 30-11. A Y-type tubing allows two solutions to be administered either alternately or simultaneously. A tandem or "piggyback" setup is used to infuse a primary solution continually and a second solution (piggyback) intermittently. Medication is often administered by this system. A. Bottle runs dry during simultaneous infusion of fluids through Y-type administration set. Pressure below the partially constricted clamp is less than atmospheric, allowing air from the empty bottle (atmospheric) to enter infusion. B. Secondary infusion piggybacked through injection site of a primary intravenous set. Lacking an automatic shut-off valve, air from the empty container will enter the circulation. The same principle is involved as in the Y-type set. (From A. Plumer, *Principles and Practice of Intravenous Therapy* [3rd ed.]. Boston: Little, Brown, 1982.)

hangs lower than the piggyback; open the clamp on the piggyback line. The greater hydrostatic pressure in the piggyback bottle will cause that fluid to infuse. A valve in the primary tubing connection automatically closes to stop the primary infusion while the piggyback solution flows past it if the tube is specifically designed for this type of setup; as the piggyback solution finishes, the valve allows the primary solution to infuse once more. If the tubing is merely plain intravenous tubing with a piggyback attached to it, no such valve is present, and the primary clamp must be closed to allow the piggyback solution to infuse and opened again to allow the primary infusion to be restarted. Know your equipment.

In a piggyback arrangement, if a glass bottle empties completely, air can enter the tubing and cause an air embolus (it is basically a Y-type arrangement). Not allowing a bottle to empty completely prevents this.

Filters. Filters are screens that trap any particles in intravenous fluid and prevent them from entering the patient's bloodstream. A filter must be used with blood or its products because of the danger of clots or agglutinated cells that might be present, or with intravenous fluid that contains a high proportion of additives (the possibility that mineral precipitate or undissolved particulate matter will be present increases with the number of additives). A filter is always used for total parenteral nutrition solutions because these contain so many additives. Careful taping and support of the filter with a strong backing such as a tongue blade helps to minimize snagging on bedclothes.

Determining Fluid Flow Rate. The type and amount of intravenous fluid and the rate of infusion is ordered by the physician. From this information you must calculate the number of drops per minute of the infusion to administer the total amount within the specified time span.

As mentioned in the discussion of intravenous tubing, the drop chamber of the apparatus forms drops of fluid of different sizes—10, 15, 20, 50, or 60 drops to a milliliter. This drop size is termed the *drop factor.* To calculate the correct rate for the infusion you need to examine the equipment and determine the drop factor. To calculate the flow rate, use the following formula:

$$\frac{\text{total volume to be infused (ml)} \times \text{drop factor}}{\text{total time of infusion in minutes}}$$

In this example, the total volume to be infused is 1000 ml; the drop factor will be 15; time of the infusion is 8 hours (480 minutes). Solved, the equation looks like this:

$$\frac{1000 \times 15}{480} = \frac{15{,}000}{480} = 31 \text{ gtt/minute}$$

Suppose the drop factor of the equipment used is 60 gt per milliliter; the equation would then be:

$$\frac{1000 \times 60}{480} = \frac{60{,}000}{480} = 125 \text{ gtt/minute}$$

Place a strip of adhesive tape on the infusion bottle (Fig. 30-12) and mark on it how much fluid should be infused at each successive 1-hour interval so that you will know that the fluid is infusing properly. The calculated drip rate is only a means to the end; the hourly totals are really the goal to strive for to reach the total

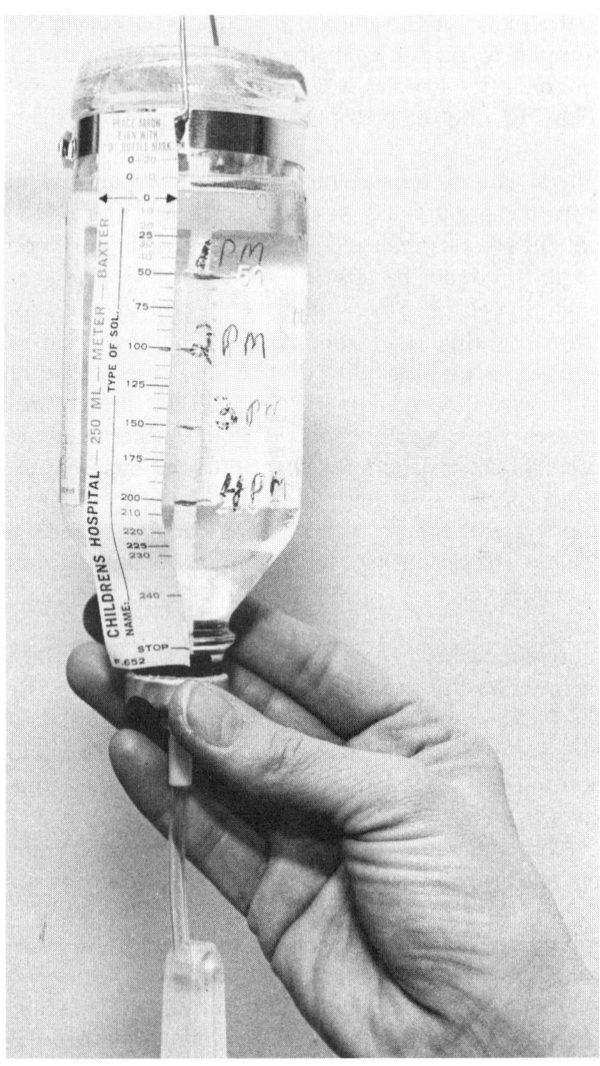

FIGURE 30-12. Placing a strip of adhesive tape (commercially prepared strips are also available) on the infusion bottle and marking how much fluid should be infused at successive 1-hour intervals allows you to assess if fluid is infusing at the proper rate.

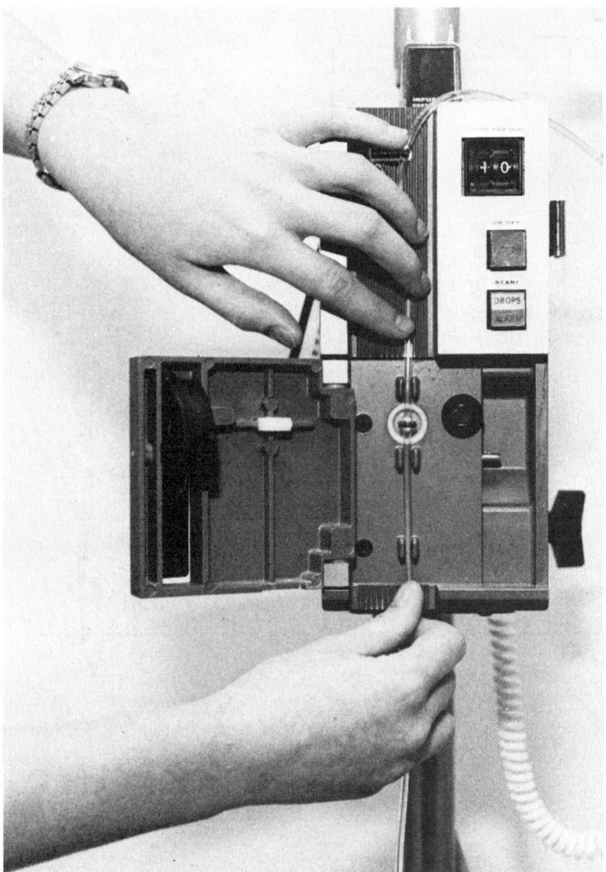

FIGURE 30-13. An automatic infusion pump. With this brand pump, the intravenous tubing is threaded through the pumping mechanism.

fluid intake. If at the end of an hour, more or less fluid than the predetermined hourly amount has been infused, slow or increase the drip rate accordingly (within reason). Adjusting a drip rate 10 drops faster or slower is a reasonable rate adjustment; more than this would probably cause a fluid overload. In people with cardiovascular conditions the physician may not wish you to advance the rate but allow the fluid to run behind to prevent any threat to an already overworked heart. This is true if medications have been added to the fluid. Fluid used in total parenteral nutrition, because it is so heavy in molecular weight, is never allowed to run faster because of the problem of overload on cardiac circulation. Adjusting the drip rate always calls for judgment, depending on the solution being infused and the patient's condition. Checking the amount of fluid infused during each half hour and making a smaller adjustment at that time often corrects the problem without the necessity for a major adjustment.

Infusion Administration Pumps. A number of infusion pumps that automatically push intravenous fluid into a vein rather than letting it merely drop by gravity pressure are available. Such pumps provide a stricter regulation of flow rate than gravity flow alone because they compensate to some extent for positional resistance caused by the needle touching the side of the vein (or at least warn that such resistance is present). They are used routinely with children under 2 years of age, to administer potent medications such as heparin, and with total parenteral nutrition solutions (TPN).

Figure 30-13 shows an IVAC pump, which is typical of those available. The intravenous tubing is threaded through the pumping mechanism at the front of the pump and from there to the patient. It moves fluid, periodically compressing the tubing. An alarm will sound if the pump is unable to administer the amount of fluid (milliliters per hour) it has been set to deliver due to increased venous pressure, for example, or a clotted needle. Pumping will halt when the solution bottle empties so that air cannot accidentally be pumped into the vein, creating an air embolus. It will

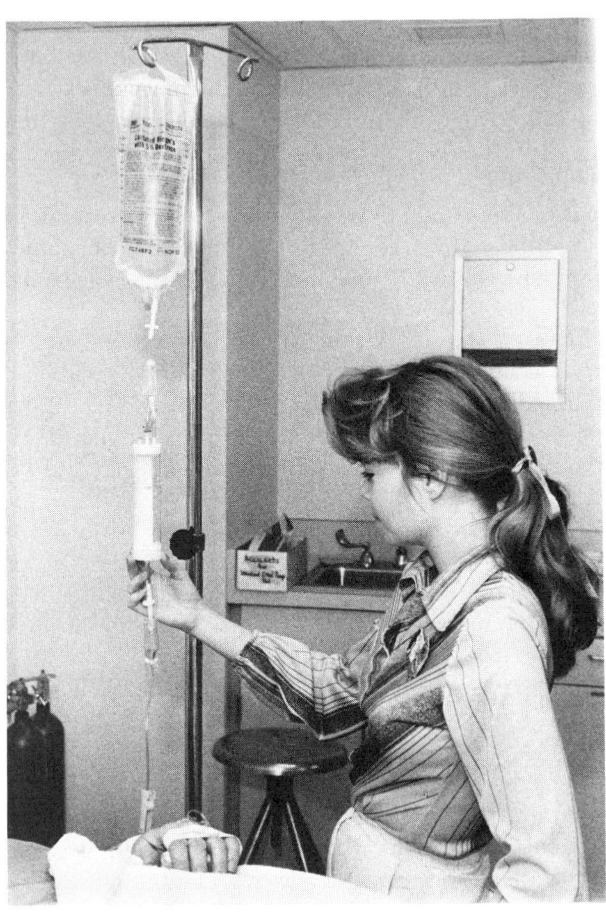

A

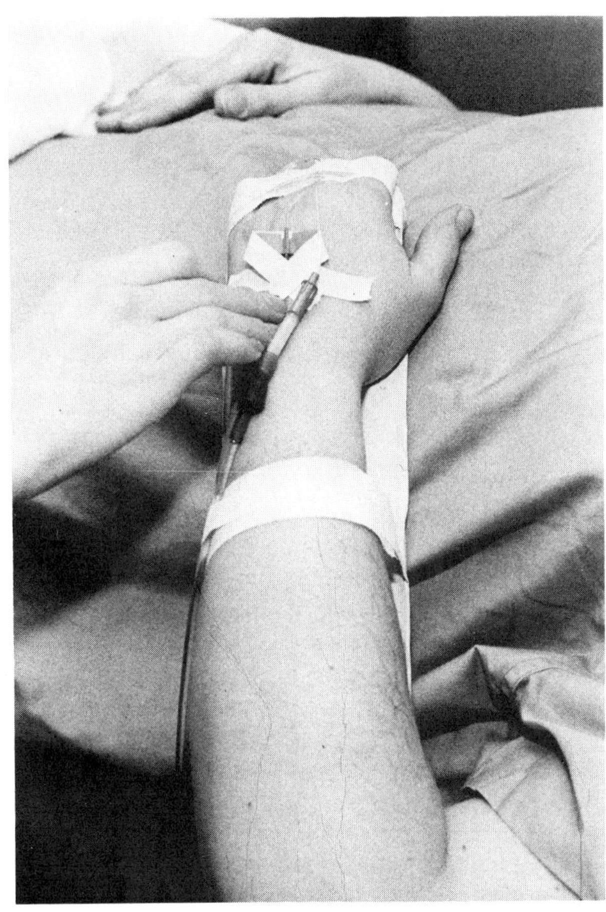

B

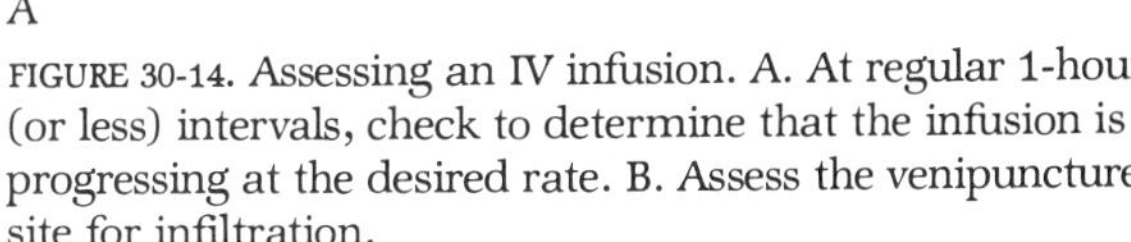

FIGURE 30-14. Assessing an IV infusion. A. At regular 1-hour (or less) intervals, check to determine that the infusion is progressing at the desired rate. B. Assess the venipuncture site for infiltration.

run as a portable unit on rechargeable batteries to allow for patient mobility.

Charts are printed on infusion pumps that name the types of tubing and consequent flow rates to be used to infuse hourly totals. Read the instructions for all infusion pumps carefully because different brands and models vary in capability. Some manufacturers suggest that their models not be used for blood administration because the specific pumping action will destroy red blood cells. Some in-line filters cause such resistance that they cannot be used with infusion pumps because the pump interprets the filter's resistance as venous pressure buildup and sets off an alarm.

The presence of an infusion pump does not relieve you of the responsibility to check the venipuncture site frequently for infiltration and for flow rate (Fig. 30-14). All infusion pumps have some degree of inaccuracy and some limits to the amount they can adjust if a patient moves and constricts venous blood flow. If a needle should infiltrate, the pump may push more fluid into the subcutaneous tissue than would occur by simple gravity flow.

Keep Vein Open (KVO) Infusions. Keep vein open infusions are infusions of intravenous fluid that are run at a rate that is just fast enough to keep the needle from plugging, thereby keeping the fluid line open for periodic or emergency medicine administration but not fast enough to supply an appreciable amount of fluid to the circulatory system. The type of solution to be infused is specified, but the total amount and rate other than KVO is not. In common practice, the rate of a KVO infusion is set at 10 to 20 ml per hour.

Factors that Influence Flow Rate. Flow rate is influenced by other factors than the drop factor, so even after the flow rate is established it must be observed frequently to be certain that other factors are not interfering with the actual flow rate. Possible solutions to common problems with intravenous fluid administration are shown in the following box.

Trouble-Shooting with Intravenous Fluid Administration

Problem	*Possible Solution*
Fluid has halted flow in tubing	Check for infiltration of needle Check for positional change or kink or compression of tubing Elevate fluid solution higher for greater gravitational effect "Prime" needle with compression of rubber connector in tubing
Drip chamber is so full that no drops can be observed	Clamp tubing; turn solution bag or bottle upside down and squeeze drip chamber to empty drip chamber back into solution bottle; rehang bottle; reopen clamp
Air bubbles are present in tubing	Tap side of tubing to allow bubbles to rise
Amount of fluid is not infusing as expected according to calculated drip rate	Reexamine drop factor expected for that equipment; recalculate drip rate. Increase rate up to 10 drops faster to achieve hourly goal (calculated rate is only theoretical rate)
Patient states that arm is stiff after infusion is removed	Urge patient to exercise arm; do active or passive range of motion exercises; give reassurance that this is normal (similar to stiffness in a leg after elevating it on a footstool)

POSITIONAL CHANGES. Elevating an extremity will slow the infusion rate because the fluid has to run "uphill" in this position. A person often is not aware of the importance of position and rests his hand on his overbed table while he reads or watches television. Bending the elbow sharply will have the same effect. Reminding the person to keep the infusion site level and the arm straight will increase the flow again. If a person raises his arm so high that the venous pressure equals the gravity pressure of the solution, blood will flow from the infusion site into the tubing. This is frightening for patients, and if an infusion pump is being used it will cause the pump to alarm. Lowering the extremity will quickly sweep this blood back into the vein (with a KVO apparatus you might increase the rate for a few seconds to accomplish this). You may often notice this phenomenon when you help people to sit up on the side of the bed or to walk.

CHANGE IN NEEDLE POSITION. If the needle bevel is resting against the vein wall, the infusion rate will slow markedly. A needle can change position this way if the person forgets to guard the site and accidentally allows the needle to be tugged as the tubing is snagged on bedding. A positional change can also cause this. Adjusting the needle by realigning the stabilizing tape will free the bevel and again allow free flow of fluid. Do not push the needle farther into the vein because this will cause the bevel to puncture the side of the vein and could introduce microorganisms; pulling it back a barely perceptible amount is another acceptable solution.

CONSTRICTING TAPE. Tape applied tightly to anchor the needle or the armboard will interfere with venous return and slow the flow of fluid. Releasing the tape will solve the problem. The tape may be tight because infiltration is occurring at the site, causing swelling of subcutaneous tissues.

HEIGHT OF SOLUTION BOTTLE. Intravenous solutions flow by gravity and therefore flow only when the external pressure of the fluid is greater than the internal venous pressure. The greater the height, the greater the external pressure and the more rapid the flow. Even with an automatic infusion pump in place, the height of fluid influences the ease of flow.

INCREASED VENOUS PRESSURE. If the person's venous pressure increases, the solution will not infuse because the increased venous pressure then makes the internal pressure equal to the external pressure. Venous pressure can increase because of cardiac overload (the heart cannot handle all the fluid arriving there, so blood is pushed back, pooling in the venous circulation). It can be caused by such simple factors as the person turning or lying on his arm (constriction causes local venous pooling) or by an infant's crying, which increases systemic blood pressure.

NONPATENT AIR VENT. If the air vent on the volume control chamber or a solution bottle should become plugged, fluid cannot leave the volume control chamber or the solution bottle because air cannot enter and replace it. If this is the problem, the solution bottle may need to be replaced.

NONPATENT NEEDLE. Blood has an intrinsic tendency to clot. Whenever there is stasis of blood, as in a vein that is partially obstructed by a needle, clot formation at the needle tip may occur. This will slow or halt the

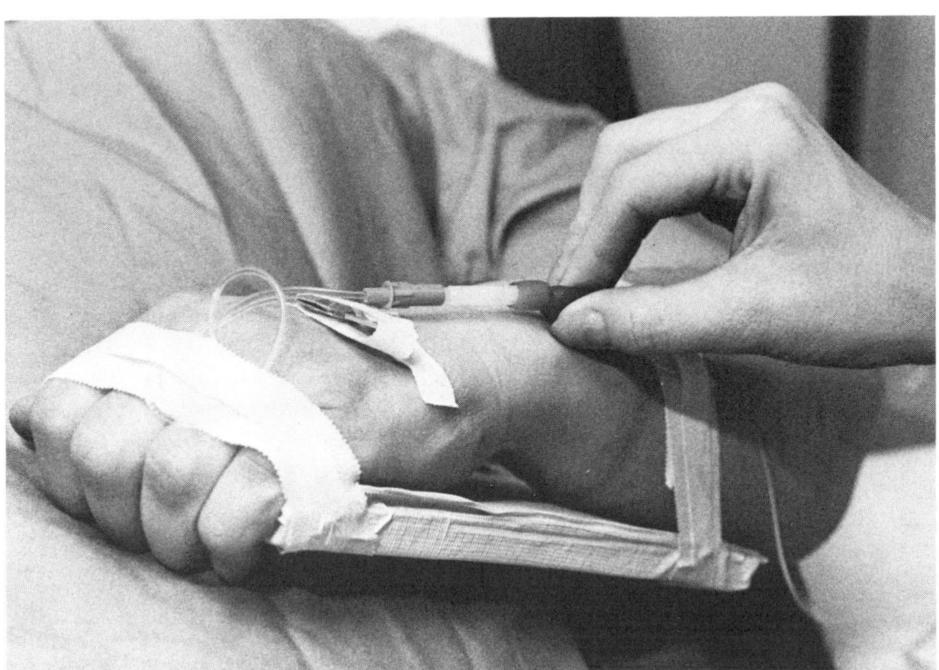

FIGURE 30-15. To prevent blood clot formation at the needle tip, pinch the rubber connection of the tubing to force a small spurt of fluid rapidly through the needle and "stir up" blood around the needle tip.

flow of fluid. To prevent clot formation, at least every 8 hours pinch the rubber connection of the tubing to force a small spurt of fluid rapidly through the needle and stir up the blood around the needle (Fig. 30-15). To test whether a needle has been plugged by a clot, pinch the rubber connector or the tubing just above the needle and quickly release it. If the needle is patent, a flashback of blood will appear in the tubing just above the needle. Another check is to lower the solution bottle below the level of the venipuncture site. If the needle is patent, blood will flow back into the tubing. Following these checks for patency, be sure that all blood flashbacks are immediately washed back into the patient by the force of the solution flow (for KVO infusions you may need to increase the rate of flow momentarily to achieve this). If you leave the blood in the tubing or needle, it will clot, and your check for patency has actually caused clotting and nonpatency.

If no blood returns by these methods, one of three reasons exists: Either the needle bevel is out of the vein or it is plugged or positioned so tightly against the vein wall that blood cannot flow into it. Move the needle away from the vein wall by manipulating its hub and test it again.

You can attempt to remove a clot from a needle by disconnecting the tubing from the needle, attaching a syringe to the needle, and aspirating it to see if the clot will return to the syringe (or insert the needle into the flashback bulb because this will reseal). Do not inject a solution into the needle to free a clot; this could cause the clot to break free into the bloodstream and become an embolus. Aspiration pressure must be gentle to prevent collapsing the vein (which will invariably cause the needle bevel to pierce the vein wall and leave the vein). If aspiration is not effective, the needle will have to be removed and another needle inserted at a different site.

Clots should not be allowed to form at needle tips. Checking frequently to make sure that the fluid is infusing constantly and that the patient has not interfered with flow in some way by bending his elbow or elevating his arm and "priming" by injecting a small burst of fluid every 8 hours are important prevention measures.

Changing Solution Bottles. Whenever a new and different solution is ordered or just before a solution bottle empties, a new solution is attached to the existing tubing and needle. To do this, carefully select a new solution, label the bottle with the date, time, and your initials or name, and attach a tape with the anticipated hourly emptying times. At the bedside, remove the metal and rubber disks from a glass bottle top or the tear tab from a plastic bag, being careful not to touch the top of the glass bottle or the insertion site of the plastic bag to keep this site sterile. Set the bag or bottle on the bedside stand with the insertion site up. Clamp the tubing of the existing fluid line; take down the empty bottle and turn it right side up; pull out the tubing tip. Do not touch the tip to the side of the bottle because it must be kept sterile for the new insertion. Push the still sterile tip into the new bottle or bag until it fits snugly, turn the new bottle or bag upside down, hang it, and reopen the clamp to the proper drip rate.

A few drops may fall when a bottle of fluid is first turned upside down if the bottle has an air vent incorporated in the rubber stopper top. This is annoying because its glucose content makes most intravenous fluid very sticky as it dries, but not important to the functioning of the system.

Changing Solution and Tubing. Intravenous solution and tubing should not be used longer that 48 hours or the bacterial count (particularly if a solution with a high sugar count is being used) grows very high. Many health care agencies do not allow intravenous tubing or solutions to be used longer than 24 hours. To change a bottle or bag and tubing, select a new solution as if it were the first time the infusion was being started. Flush the tubing to be certain that all air is removed; label time, date, your initials, and anticipated emptying times on the bottle. At the bedside, hang the new infusion setup on the intravenous pole next to the existing setup; pull enough tape away from the venipuncture site to reveal the needle hub. Close the clamp on the existing tubing to halt the flow of fluid; grasp the needle hub firmly with one hand; twist and gently remove the existing tubing. Immediately uncap and plug the new tubing into the needle hub. Open the clamp on the new tubing to allow for fluid flow. Once the new fluid is flowing well, replace tape as necessary to restabilize the needle. It is important to remember when changing tubing to grasp the needle hub firmly so that the needle tip does not move more than necessary (and so will not pierce the vein wall by movement) and to make the interval during which fluid is not infusing as short as possible (a matter of seconds). This prevents clotting at the needle tip during the change of tubing and fluid.

Do not use scissors to cut tape or you may accidentally cut the tubing. This is particularly true if a scalp vein is in place because the tubing involved is so fine that it is difficult to see; if the tubing, which is actually an extension of the needle, is cut, the needle will have to be replaced. As you remove the existing tubing from the hub of the needle, you may notice a small amount of blood ooze from the needle. Do not be alarmed; this is proof of the patency of the needle and correct location in a blood vessel. Merely wipe this blood away after the new tubing is connected and infusing; leaving moisture from the bleeding under the tape or dressing could lead to macerated skin.

COMPLICATIONS OF INTRAVENOUS THERAPY

Although intravenous therapy is life-saving for many patients who cannot take oral fluid, it is not a therapy without risk and some danger. Whenever you are administering intravenous fluid, you must be alert to signs of complications.

Local Infiltration. Local infiltration is the most frequent complication of intravenous therapy. As fluid enters the subcutaneous tissue from the needle that has pierced the vein wall, the site becomes edematous (puffy or swollen); it generally feels cooler to the back of your hand than the surrounding tissue because of the fluid content. The best way to assess whether edema is occurring is to compare the site with the same area on the opposite extremity. This prevents you from confusing the normal puffiness of "baby fat" at wrists with true edema.

As edema becomes extensive, the area begins to feel painful to the person, and inflammation with erythema (redness) occurs. At this point of inflammation, the area feels warm to the back of your hand (vasodilation has occurred, calling plasma and white blood cells to the area). The rate of flow of an infusion will slow or halt with infiltration; you are unable to obtain flashback blood when you squeeze the rubber connection in the tubing or lower the bottle level.

Infiltration is a harmful event because the accumulated fluid in tissue pushes cells farther away from capillaries than normally, depleting them of oxygen and nutrients. If the infiltrated solution is hypertonic, fluid will leave nearby cells by osmotic pressure (flow is from a lesser to a greater osmotic pressure), further destroying local cells. If the process continues unchecked, cell death and actual sloughing of tissue can occur. This leaves an area susceptible to secondary infection or superimposes a second illness on a person who already has an illness for which the fluid is being administered to correct. In addition, infiltrated fluid is poorly absorbed from subcutaneous tissue so the person no longer has the benefit of the fluid administration. The site is not available for further administration until it has time to heal and stabilize again.

Discontinue fluid flow immediately when you recognize that infiltration has occurred. Assess that a pulse is present in the distal extremity or that nailbed blanching occurs to be assured that the edema is not obstructing arterial circulation. Placing a warm wet compress for about 20 minutes on the site hastens absorption of edematous fluid and improvement in cell function.

Thrombophlebitis. Phlebitis is inflammation of a vein. Thrombophlebitis is inflammation of a vein with clot formation. This complication occurs most often when the intravenous fluid has been infusing into a venipuncture site for an extended period of time (24 to 48 hours) or an irritating solution (nonisotonic) is being infused. There is erythema and pain at the venipuncture site (hydrostatic pressure in the vein increases distal to the clot and causes fluid to leave the vein and enter the subcutaneous tissue). Red streaks and pain may be apparent along the course of the vein.

If you suspect thrombophlebitis, discontinue the infusion and remove the needle. Apply a cold wet compress to the site for about 20 minutes to reduce further inflammation. Assess that a pulse is present distal to the venipuncture site or that blanching and filling of nailbeds occurs to be assured that the edema is not obstructing arterial circulation. If the site is still inflammed and tender after an hour, apply a warm compress to the site for comfort.

Do not rub or massage the area; rubbing a thrombus may cause it to move and become a systemic embolus. Notify the person's physician of the complication. A thrombus will gradually dissolve and vein patency will be restored again; until that time, the risk of emboli is present and a potential lethal situation exists. Many health care agencies have policies that the sites of intravenous infusions must be changed every 48 hours to reduce the possibility of thrombus formation.

Air Embolus. The symptoms of air embolus are weak rapid pulse, cyanosis, and loss of consciousness. Blood pressure will be low (hypotensive). Theoretically, the amount of air necessary to cause an embolus is 5 to 15 ml per kg tf body weight; in an adult, this is 200 ml. This is a stretch of air that is much longer than the length of a normal infusion tubing. This is a theoretical amount, however, and in a seriously ill person (or in a 7-pound infant), it may be as little as 10 ml (easily the length of a stretch of tubing). Never allow any air to enter a venipuncture site to be certain that you do not reach this limit. If air does enter the tubing, clamp the tubing, unconnect it from the needle, and flush out the air by allowing the solution to flow briefly into an emesis basin or other container until the column has been discharged; then reconnect the tubing. Cause small bubbles in a tubing to rise by flicking them with your thumb and finger the same way you flick bubbles from a medication syringe.

Circulatory Overload. The infusion of too much fluid or fluid infused too rapidly can lead to circulatory overload. This is a particular danger in people with cardiac or kidney disease. Signs of circulatory overload are venous distention (marked neck vein engorgement) and increased blood pressure. If pulmonary edema is developing from increased hydrostatic pressure in the venous circulation, cough, dyspnea, and shortness of breath will occur.

If you suspect circulatory overload, slow the infusion rate until it is barely dripping but do not stop it (a person with pulmonary edema is in critical respiratory distress and needs an emergency line for medication). Raise the head of the bed to increase ease of respiration, and notify the person's physician. The person may need a diuretic administered to help evacuate the excess fluid. Until the overload is evacuated he is in danger of heart and respiratory failure.

Nursing Care During Fluid Administration. Most people expect to feel intravenous fluid entering the vein and are surprised to discover that after the initial painful puncture, they feel no pain and no sensation associated with the line at all. Intravenous fluid administration is, in fact, so unnoticeable that the person may easily forget that fluid is infusing. That is why it is important to add an armboard to stabilize the arm and remind the patient as soon as he moves that he must not tug at the needle or the tubing with the movement.

Because people tend to forget that an intravenous infusion is in place, you must be extremely aware that it is. Check the venipuncture site at least hourly for signs of local infiltration and phlebitis. There is some disagreement about whether the dressing over the venipuncture site should be disturbed. In some health care agencies, the dressing is removed daily, new antibiotic ointment is applied to the site, and a new sterile dressing is applied. In other agencies, the initial dressing stays in place undisturbed unless it is obviously soiled or must be removed to renew the venipuncture site or to view it adequately to assess infiltration. This is particularly true in caring for children. Follow health care agency policy as to dressing site care.

At least every 2 hours ask the person to move (or move for him) his wrist, elbow, and fingers through range-of-motion exercises (providing this will not disrupt the needle) to ensure adequate circulation to the distal extremity. Do not exercise the elbow if the needle is inserted in the antecubital space because this would cause the needle to infiltrate as the elbow flexes. Loosen any restraints used every 2 hours, and assess the condition of the skin under the restraint and the distal extremity to be certain that the restraint is not impairing circulation due to pressure or causing local irritation.

An intravenous infusion means that the person must guard the venipuncture site; it does not mean that he has to lie frozen, unable to move. He certainly can move from his bed to a wheelchair or bedside chair. He can be ambulatory with the use of a movable intravenous infusion pole.

To change pajama tops or a hospital gown with an intravenous infusion in place, simply consider the tubing and the solution as part of a very long arm. To remove the gown or pajama top, slide it all the way along the tubing and up over the bottle or bag, being careful not to snag the material on a connection. Replace a gown by placing one armhole over the bottle or bag as if that were the fingers of the person's arm and slide it gently down and over the armboard as necessary. If an automatic infusion pump is in place, temporarily disconnect it during this time (set the infusion rate by the tubing clamp to a "ballpark" drip rate); reconnect it to the infusion pump when the new piece of clothing is in place. Infant gowns or tops do not slide over a solution bottle or bag because the arm opening is too small. The average child who has this small a gown, however, is in a crib and therefore has an additional crib rail extension piece of tubing (to allow the crib rail to be raised or lowered without pulling on the tubing). You can temporarily clamp shut the infusion flow, disconnect the tubing at that point, and slide the gown over just the extension tubing and arm to change it, being careful not to touch the ends of the tubing connection to the material as you work to keep it sterile.

Although intravenous fluid treatment was first attempted as early as 1662, it was not possible safely until the 1930s, when a method of sterilizing bottle fluid was developed. Administration of intravenous fluid has been considered until recently a "last resort" measure. The person who is told that he will receive intravenous fluid, therefore, may worry that he is extremely ill when he thought that he was only moderately ill. This sudden worry about illness can precipitate a grief reaction, just as if the person were told that he was really seriously ill. As the person passes through the different stages of grief (denial, anger, bargaining, depression, acceptance), he may resist intravenous fluid administration in various ways. With the acceptance phase of grief, a person again becomes accepting of fluid therapy. Careful explanation of why intravenous fluid is necessary helps to prevent this type of reaction. In many instances, for example, fluid is administered intravenously as a vehicle of medication; it is not a last resort at all but a routine first resort.

Because preschool children fear any intrusive procedures, they fear intravenous fluid administration greatly. Guarding an administration site so that the needle does not infiltrate is vitally important in such children to keep the hospital experience within an acceptable level of stress.

Be honest with people about the degree of pain they can expect from intravenous needle insertion. Some medications, particularly penicillin, sting when they are administered intravenously. Being honest about when a person will feel pain helps him to accept procedures that are both painful and nonpainful because he knows he can trust you.

Removing an Intravenous Needle. Removal of an intravenous needle, unlike insertion, is not painful. To remove the needle, clamp off the tubing so that no more fluid can infuse; remove the dressing and tape to reveal the venipuncture site. Press an alcohol compress against the point where the needle enters the skin and pull the needle back flat with the surface of the skin. Apply pressure to the site until any bleeding halts. If the person wishes, a bandaid can be applied. Check the needle to be certain that it is intact (this is particularly important if a plastic intracath, not a metal needle was used).

Most people expect needle removal to be painful. It will be painful only if, because of fear, they pull their hand away as you begin to withdraw the needle, causing the needle to repuncture them. Reassure the patient that removal does not hurt. Be honest about the pain involved in removing the adhesive tape that held the needle and armboard in place (adhesive strips that remove hair with them *do* hurt).

Venous Cut-Down. If a person has very narrow, hardened veins (arteriosclerosis) or such low blood pressure (hypotension) that the veins will not distend enough to be penetrated with a needle, a cut-down may be necessary to begin intravenous fluid. Because a cut-down is a minor surgical procedure, in most health care facilities a separate permission signature is required. Most health care agencies have cut-down trays supplied from a central source that supply all equipment needed for the procedure but the antiseptic needed to wash the skin and a local anesthetic (Xylocaine). In addition, the bottle of intravenous solution and the proper tubing must be prepared.

The physician performing the cut-down needs a good light because she must see to dissect a very small vein. Secure a gooseneck light if the patient's overhead or a treatment room light is not adequate for close visualization. She needs a place to prepare a sterile field and room to put on sterile gloves (a clean flat surface above waist level). The skin over the selected vein is washed with an antiseptic solution (usually povidone-iodine); local anesthetic is injected into the site. After a few minutes, a small 1-inch incision is made horizontally over the vein; the incision is spread apart by a hemostat (clamp) and the vein located. It is isolated by slipping the hemostat underneath it to bring it into clear view. Next, the vein is ligated (tied shut). It is cut just proximal to the tie with a scalpel, and a thin, sterile polyethylene tube is threaded into the lumen. The intravenous tubing is attached to this threaded catheter as it exits through the small incision and the infusion begun. A few stitches are generally needed to close the sides of the incision and secure the polyethylene tube in place, ensuring that the incision will heal with only a thin pencil-line scar.

An antibiotic ointment is generally added to the closed incision and a small, dry sterile dressing secured on top of that. Cut-downs do not infiltrate as easily as regular venipuncture sites because they have no sharp needle tip to pierce the vein wall. They allow the person to have more mobility because there is not so much danger of infiltration. They are left in place as a rule for about a week. Although the initial procedure is more serious than a regular venipuncture, the person may have to experience only one procedure rather than several due to constantly infiltrating venipunctures. Most cut-down skin sutures must be removed after 7 days to prevent the sutures (usually silk, which is not absorbed) from causing irritation and inflammation. Check daily for inflammation or any purulent exudate at the site that would indicate an infection from skin surface bacteria.

In newborns who are to receive fluid therapy or frequent blood gas determinations, an umbilical vessel catheterization may be done using a basic cut-down technique for infusion of intravenous fluid into an umbilical vessel.

Scalp Vein Insertion. The scalp veins (especially the superficial temporal vein) are good sites for intravenous infusion in infants when other sites are inaccessible

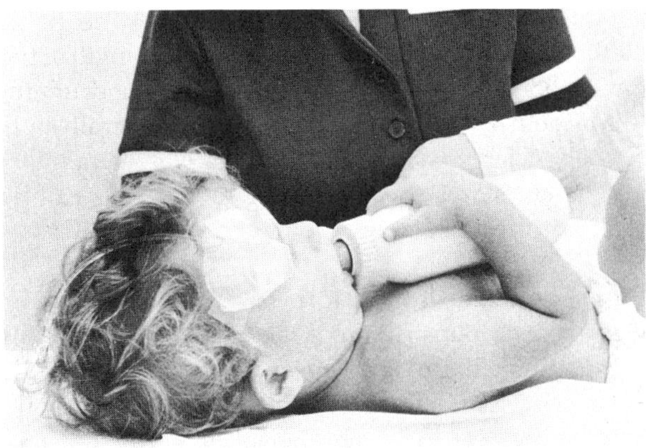

FIGURE 30-16. A scalp vein used for intravenous administration. The inverted medicine cup over the insertion site protects the site if the child turns.

(Fig. 30-16). Parents may find the use of such veins very frightening but they can be assured that a scalp vein is basically just another infusion site and has some advantages because it infiltrates very infrequently, therefore allowing the infant more movement than he could possibly have if an arm or hand site were used.

For scalp vein venipuncture, a rubber band stretched snugly across the forehead and over the occiput is used for a tourniquet; to remove it after the needle is in place simply snip it with your bandage scissors.

If infiltration occurs when a scalp infusion is in place, gravity tends to cause the swelling to appear behind the ear or toward the back of the head. To inspect the site, always palpate the posterior scalp surface to assess for such infiltration.

Bone Marrow Transfusion. An alternative route for administering intravenous fluid is by way of the bone marrow. The technique appears to have little advantage over regular intravenous therapy and carries with it the potential danger of causing osteomyelitis, a severe bone infection. It is not, therefore, a method of fluid replacement except in experimental programs.

INTRAVENOUS SOLUTION AS A VEHICLE FOR MEDICATION ADMINISTRATION

Intravenous therapy may be used as an efficient vehicle for medication administration. Medicine given by this route may be added to the solution bottle, to a volume control chamber, or directly into the venipuncture site (a bolus or heparin lock technique) (see QRS 30-4).

Fluid Bottle Administration

Medications to be added to a solution bottle are ordered according to the type and amount of medication needed and the amount of fluid to which the medication is to be added (20 mEq of potassium in 1000 ml of 5 percent dextrose in water, for example). When adding medicine to a solution bottle or bag, the medicine

☐ QUICK REFERENCE STOP 30-4: PHARMACOLOGY
Administering Medication Intravenously

1. Before mixing any medication in a bottle of intravenous fluid or a volume control chamber check with an approved list or a pharmacist to be sure that the drugs are compatible. Otherwise, a precipitate may form that could cause an embolus, or the drugs could be inactivated in the tubing.
2. Medication administered intravenously bypasses the step of absorption and begins to act immediately. Always remain with a person for a few minutes after such medication administration to assess for untoward effects.
3. Always check to be sure that the intravenous needle is in the vein (you can detect flashback blood) before adding medication to a fluid line. Medication infused into subcutaneous tissue because of needle infiltration can cause extensive tissue damage.
4. Always check that medication administered intravenously is clearly labeled that it is intended for intravenous injection. The word *parenteral* alone does not imply this.

should be added before the tubing is flushed. If you flush the tubing first, you will add the medicine only to the fluid remaining in the bottle or bag, not the total amount of fluid (900 ml, not 1000 ml). This concentrates the medicine (administers a stronger dosage of medicine) more than the ordering physician intended. This can lead to a serious medication error, especially when involving intravenous fluid. Attach a label to the bottle designating the additives so that anyone can easily identify the medicine added to the fluid.

Volume Control Chamber

If the medicine is to be added to a volume control chamber, fill the chamber with the designated amount of fluid to dilute the medicine properly. If the physician did not order a set amount of fluid, read the drug literature or ask the agency pharmacist for the correct dilution for that particular medication, or ask the physician to specify the amount she desires. Diluting medicine in this way allows it to enter the circulation without irritating the vein walls. Allow the volume control chamber to fill with the determined amount of dilution fluid (usually about 30 ml); then clean the medication injection port with 70 percent alcohol and inject the correct dose of medication with a syringe and needle into the chamber. Attach a label to the chamber that specifies the drug and amount (Fig. 30-17). Careful labeling is a safeguard for correct drug and dosage; also, if the person should develop symptoms from the administration of medication, anyone can quickly

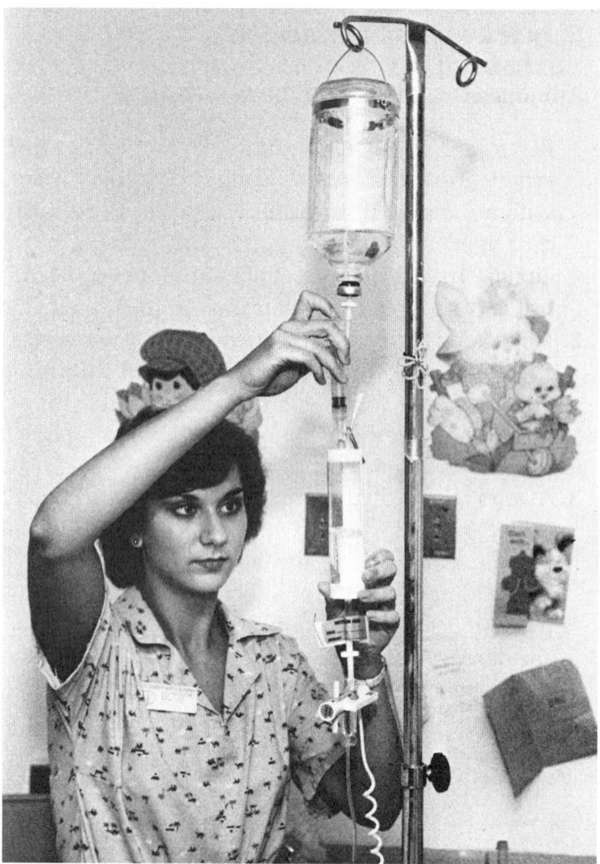

FIGURE 30-17. Adding medicine to a volume control chamber. After cleaning the medication injection port with an antiseptic, inject the correct dosage of medication with a syringe into the chamber. Notice the medicine label attached just below the chamber, which signals that medication will be infusing.

evaluate them based on the information in the label. Medication from a volume control chamber is generally administered at a fairly rapid rate, allowing the medicine to reach high blood levels quickly. After the medicine and its dilution fluid have infused, you will refill the chamber for an hourly rate if the intravenous fluid is going to continue to flow at a fairly rapid rate. Regulate the flow rate at its designated speed, and proceed with regular intravenous fluid administration. If the intravenous fluid is being used only to maintain an open line, however (set at a KVO rate), you will refill the chamber with 10 to 20 ml of additional fluid and let this also flow through the tubing at a fairly rapid rate as a "flush" to the tubing. If this is not done, the last portion of the medication will remain in the tubing for a long time, and without this additional amount, the blood level may not rise to the therapeutic level desired. Flushing may be contraindicated in very small infants or in anyone with a threat of cardiac overload.

Bolus Injections

In the bolus injection method intravenous medicine is delivered directly into the medication injection port of the tubing using a syringe and needle. The bolus method of administration places the full strength of the medication almost immediately into the bloodstream. It is a method used in emergencies and generally only by a physician or when a physician is closely monitoring patient status so that side or toxic effects can be dealt with immediately.

Piggyback Administration

Piggyback administration of medication is convenient because in health care agencies using this system, the medication is added to a separate small bag of diluent fluid (a piggyback) in the pharmacy and is therefore supplied already prepared (in a unit dose system) and ready to hang. Be extremely careful to check the label three times for the correct drug and dose on these prepared administration units because medicine administered by such a route is present in the bloodstream immediately and operating; there is no way to reverse a drug error. Some medicine prepared in such a way must be administered immediately, so you must coordinate your care with a pharmacy delivery to accomplish this.

Heparin Lock

Heparin locks are a method of administering intravenous medications intermittently without the necessity of maintaining a constantly infusing intravenous solution. This allows the patient greater mobility and reduces the possibility of fluid overload. The "lock" is a scalp vein and its short connected tubing used with an injection adaptor or a commercial lock (Fig. 30-18A). The needle is inserted into a vein at any venipuncture site, but generally the dorsal surface of the hand is used. The site is guarded in the usual way. To keep the needle patent and prevent a blood clot from forming at the tip and blocking the lumen, the short attached tubing and the needle and tubing are filled with a dilute solution of heparin and sterile water (heparin is a drug that prevents blood coagulation; see Fig. 30-18B).

Medication may be injected into a heparin lock by reattaching intravenous fluid or by a direct "push." To inject medicine into a heparin lock, you need a syringe and needle (as small a needle as possible, preferably a 25-gauge) filled with the medication, an empty syringe, and a syringe with at least 1 ml of dilute heparin solution. Wipe off the injection adaptor with alcohol, insert the needle of the empty syringe, and aspirate the dilute heparin solution from the tubing (use about 1 ml to fill the tubing). As you aspirate, first the heparin solution will return and then the tubing will fill with blood, letting you know you have removed all of the flush solution. Change syringes, and inject the specified medicine; then change syringes once more to the dilute heparin-filled one. Inject enough diluted heparin solution to fill the tubing and needle completely to maintain patency until the medication port is needed again. It is important to aspirate the heparin solution from the tubing before injecting each time rather than injecting it with the medication because this action not only proves that the needle is inserted into a vein (you aspirate blood) but avoids injecting heparin into the person's system each time. The addition of even dilute heparin over a long period of time might have systemic anticlotting effects.

If there are long periods between medication injections, a heparin lock may need to be flushed by aspirating the heparin solution and placing the new solution in the lock between medication injections (about every 2 hours). Heparin locks are also used for withdrawal of blood and with patients who will be having blood aspirated frequently for diagnostic tests such as blood glucose levels in newly diagnosed diabetes. As with intravenous fluid administration, the site should be changed every 48 hours to prevent irritation and inflammation at the site, which could lead to infection or thrombophlebitis.

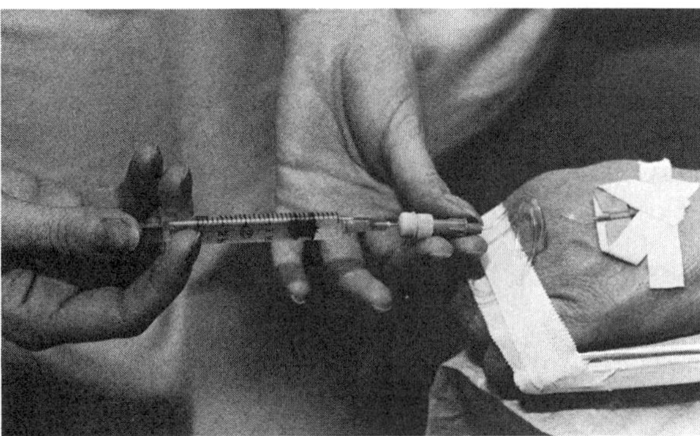

A

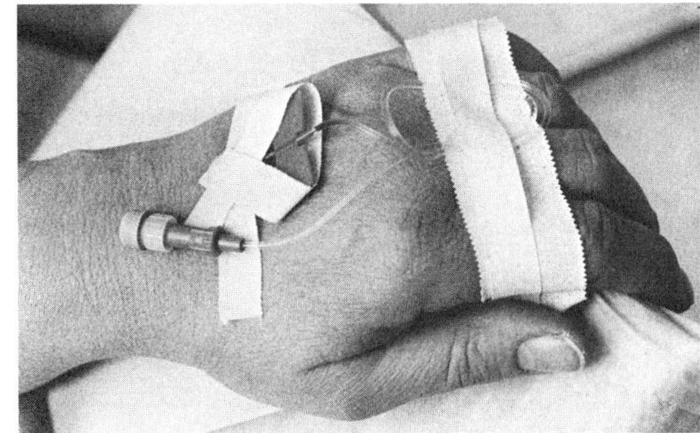

B

FIGURE 30-18. A heparin lock. A. A heparin lock is an injection adaptor that fits into the distal end of scalp vein tubing; it is used to administer intermittent intravenous medications. B. When not in use, it is kept patent by periodically injecting a dilute heparin solution through the tubing.

BLOOD TRANSFUSION

Although a blood transfusion is a form of intravenous therapy, it requires important considerations in addition to those involving regular intravenous therapy. The word *transfusion* is used with blood administration rather than *infusion* because originally, before blood or its products could be stored safely for administration, it was given immediately, or transfused, from the donor to the recipient.

Types of Blood Transfusions

Blood transfusions may consist of either whole blood (plasma and all its constituents) or a single constituent, depending on the need of the person receiving the transfusion.

WHOLE BLOOD

Whole blood (plasma, blood cells, and all other constituents such as platelets, antibodies, and protein) is transfused to people who need both blood cells and volume replacement; a unit is about 500 ml in volume. Whole blood is given following hemorrhage or burns. If the person's primary need is additional blood cells but not volume, whole blood may not be the transfusion of choice because the amount of volume needed to administer the necessary number of replacement blood cells could overload the circulatory system.

PACKED RED BLOOD CELLS

Packed red blood cells are what the name implies—a concentration of red cells (the plasma has been removed); a unit is about 250 ml in volume. Packed cells are administered when cell replacement but not volume replacement is required.

WASHED PACKED RED BLOOD CELLS

Most antibodies are removed from cells that are "washed." Such cells are less apt to initiate an allergic reaction in people who are prone to allergic manifestations.

WHITE BLOOD CELLS

Leukocytes may be administered separately from red blood cells and plasma to people who have an abnormally low white cell count but do not need red blood cells or volume replacement. Patients who receive white blood cells are generally people who have received anticancer (chemotherapy) drugs because these drugs act by killing fast-growing cells in the body (cancer cells). Because white blood cells also grow quickly, they are also usually destroyed by chemotherapy.

PLASMA

Plasma may be used as a quick volume expander, but recent experience has shown that plasma administration carries a high risk of hepatitis contamination. In most instances, today, therefore, the protein of plasma (albumin) may be administered instead of the actual full plasma. Synthetic volume expanders are being developed that simulate plasma in their effective volume expansion properties but carry no risk of hepatitis contamination.

CRYOPRECIPITATE

Cryoprecipitate is a plasma fraction high in fibrinogen and blood clotting Factor VIII. Cryoprecipitate is administered to people with bleeding disorders (hemophiliacs). Isolating a factor in this way allows a great deal of it to be administered without risk of volume overload.

PLATELETS

People who receive chemotherapy for cancer may also develop a deficiency in platelet level. Platelets administered intravenously can correct this potential blood clotting deficiency.

RHOGAM

Whenever a person's body is invaded by a foreign protein (an antigen), the lymphatic system produces antibodies or defense structures against the invading protein. RhoGam is the commercial name for antibodies directed against the Rh factor in blood. Such antibodies are removed from donor blood and injected intramuscularly into an Rh-negative woman following the birth of an Rh-positive child or abortion of a fetus. With these foreign antibodies in her system, she does not develop her own antibodies against the Rh factor. After about three months the foreign antibodies are destroyed, so with any future pregnancy, no antibodies against the Rh factor will be present. If such antibodies were present, they could act to destroy the red blood cells of a new Rh-positive fetus (erythroblastosis fetalis).

Blood Groups

Blood type in persons is inherited. Types are grouped into ABO and Rh systems.

ABO BLOOD GROUPS

A person has either A, B, AB, or O type blood. In A type blood there is an A antigen on each red blood cell; in B type a B antigen is present; in AB type both the A and B antigens are present; and in O type neither A nor B antigen is present.

In addition to these antigens, naturally occurring antibodies (antibodies present without any stimulation) are also present. A person with A type blood has anti-B antibodies; a person with B type blood has anti-A antibodies; a person with AB type blood has neither anti-A nor anti-B antibodies; a person with O type blood has both anti-A and anti-B antibodies. Anti-A antibodies destroy A antigens that come in contact with them; anti-B antibodies destroy B antigens. This is the basis for the often-heard statement that O type blood is a universal donor. A person with O type blood can donate blood to anyone because O blood, with no A or B antigens present, will not be destroyed by the recipient's anti-A or anti-B antibodies. People with AB blood are viewed as universal recipients because their blood has no antibodies and will not destroy any type of blood administered to them. These statements are only true within limits, however, because Rh blood status also affects blood compatibility, and in many instances a difference in subgroup of blood types can cause a reaction. Destruction of red blood cells by anti-A or anti-B antibodies is termed *hemolysis.* A blood transfusion reaction occurring from improperly typed or matched blood between donor and recipient is termed a *hemolytic* reaction.

RH BLOOD GROUPS (D ANTIGENS)

The term *Rh* stems from Rhesus monkey, the animals used in the original experiments in which an additional blood antigen was discovered. Today this blood antigen is classified more accurately as the D antigen. In about 85 percent of Caucasian persons a D antigen is present in the blood; they are said to be Rh (D antigen)-positive. The other 15 percent of Caucasian persons lack the antigen or are Rh-negative. These proportions differ according to nationality and race. Almost the total population of Japan and China, for example, are Rh (D antigen)-positive.

The person with a D antigen does not have an anti-D antibody. If a person who is D antigen-negative is administered D antigen (Rh)-positive blood, he will develop anti-D antibodies, which will hemolyze D antigen red blood cells in the same way that anti-A or anti-B antibodies do. In contrast to anti-A or anti-B antibodies, however, which occur naturally, anti-D antibodies do not form until the blood system has been invaded by the D antigen. This occurs in two ways—either by an improperly matched blood transfusion or by exchange across the placenta when a fetus has the D antigen and the mother does not as the placenta (afterbirth) is freed from the uterus at birth. With an anti-A or anti-B hemolytic reaction, this will occur the very first time that the offending antigen is introduced. The first time the D antigen is introduced to the person with Rh-negative blood, a hemolytic reaction will not occur because the anti-D antibodies must first be stimulated.

A hemolytic reaction will occur a second time, however. In the Rh (D antigen)-negative mother, carrying a D (Rh)-positive fetus, no hemolytic reaction occurs if this is the first pregnancy; because antibody formation against the D antigen is provoked, however, in a second pregnancy, if the fetus is again D-positive, anti-D antibodies in the mother will cross the placenta and begin red cell destruction in the fetus while it is still in utero. This problem can be prevented by administering anti-D (RhoGam) antibodies to the woman within 72 hours after delivery of a D-positive fetus. The woman's body does not continue to form anti-D antibodies because the injection has made them instantly present. These foreign antibodies are destroyed by the woman's body in about three months (as in all passive immunizations). Therefore, because the woman did not form anti-D antibodies she has no anti-D antibodies (or very few) present. This process makes each pregnancy she undertakes the same as a first pregnancy in terms of D antigen incompatibility risk. If the fetal blood type was not determined at birth, as in an abortion or a tubal pregnancy, RhoGam is also given on the chance that the fetal blood type was D-positive.

Blood Donor Storage Regulations

At one time donors were not carefully screened for possible diseases that could be carried in blood, so the recipient of a blood transfusion was very susceptible to developing a secondary disease such as hepatitis. Today, blood donors are carefully screened to be certain that they have no form of heart, kidney, lung, or liver disease, are not taking any medication (birth control pills are an exception), have not had recent surgery, or are not drug abusers. They should not have donated blood in the last 90 days to be certain that they can withstand the systemic shock of losing 250 ml of blood. They are also screened for a history of cancer, allergies, jaundice, and hepatitis to be certain that no disease will be transmitted to the recipient.

The donor's blood pressure and pulse are taken; his blood is tested for hematocrit level to be certain that he is not anemic (anemia would make it hazardous for him to donate blood, and his blood would not contain the high level of red blood cells or hemoglobin needed by the recipient). Donor blood is marked immediately with the donor's name, number, ABO and Rh type, results of tests for syphilis and hepatitis, name and address of the blood bank, and anticipated expiration date. Donor blood has an anticoagulant added to it, either ACD (acid-citrate-dextrose), CPD (citrate-phosphate-dextrose), or ATP (adenosine triphosphate). These additives prolong the length of time the blood can be used. When ATP is added, shelf life can be as long as 35 days.

Donor blood is stored in heavy plastic bags. It must be stored separately from other products in health care agencies in a registered blood bank. It must not be removed from refrigeration longer than 30 minutes before administration to prevent spoilage of blood cells. If brought to a hospital unit in anticipation of administration, it should be placed in the medicine refrigerator for safe-keeping until just prior to administration.

Blood Typing and Cross Matching

The person who is to receive a blood transfusion must first have blood drawn; this is sent to the blood bank for determination of blood type and to allow a portion to be mixed with a sample of the proposed donor blood to check for hemolytic reaction. Marked on the unit of blood when it leaves the blood bank after this careful typing and cross matching will be the donor's and recipient's names, hospital name of recipient, blood type of donor and recipient, and results of cross matching (compatible).

Blood Transfusion

The first step in safe administration of blood is identification of the proper blood for the proper patient. Most health care agencies require that two responsible people (nurse and physician or two nurses) check the blood received on the unit to make sure that the blood is properly cross-matched for the recipient and to sign that they have verified this information. Never administer any blood that you have even the slightest doubt is not compatible with the recipient because, if it is not, the hemolyzed red blood cells that will result will cause blockage and interference with kidney and heart function (the red cells become emboli) with possible fatal consequences.

The second step in blood transfusion is to establish a baseline temperature, pulse, and blood pressure rate for the patient. These measures will be taken throughout the transfusion and assessed against the baseline values to detect a transfusion reaction at the earliest possible point.

Blood must be administered through a special transfusion set that contains a blood filter (Fig. 30-19). A filter is necessary to remove any clots or clumped blood cells, which, if they entered the bloodstream, might lead to a pulmonary embolus. A large gauge needle (No. 18 in adults, No. 20 in infants) is used so that red blood cells will not be crushed and the heavy viscosity of blood (blood is four to five times thicker than water) will not slow the flow so much that clotting occurs in the tubing.

To begin the transfusion, normal saline is first begun from a Y-type infusion setup. It is difficult to tell if the intravenous needle is inserted properly if the transfusion is not begun with normal saline because you cannot easily see the blood return in the needle due to the flowing blood. Normal saline is also available for use at any point during the transfusion if the blood flow slows due to viscosity. This is particularly important in the administration of packed red blood cells, which are very thick in consistency.

Never use any other intravenous fluid with blood or blood products than normal saline, the most isotonic of intravenous fluids, to prevent hemolysis of red blood cells in the tubing. Ringer's lactate, considered isotonic for intravenous therapy, cannot be used because the calcium content may cause clotting in blood; a 5 percent dextrose and water solution will cause hemolysis because it is not exactly isotonic. Never add any medication to a blood transfusion for the same reason.

Blood should be administered within 4 hours time because after this time the temperature of the blood left in the bag has probably reached room temperature and spoilage of cells may begin. The initial rate of administration should be slow (1 ml per kg body weight per

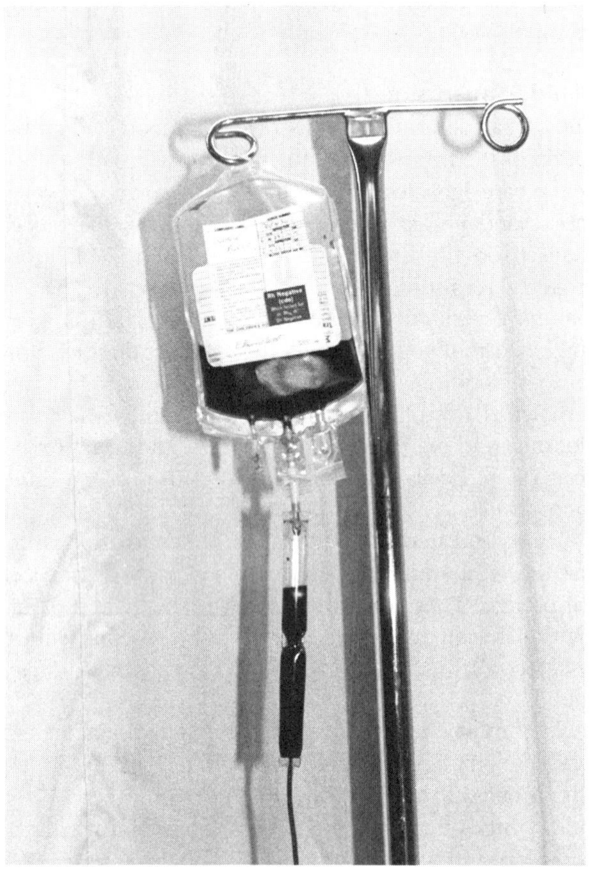
A

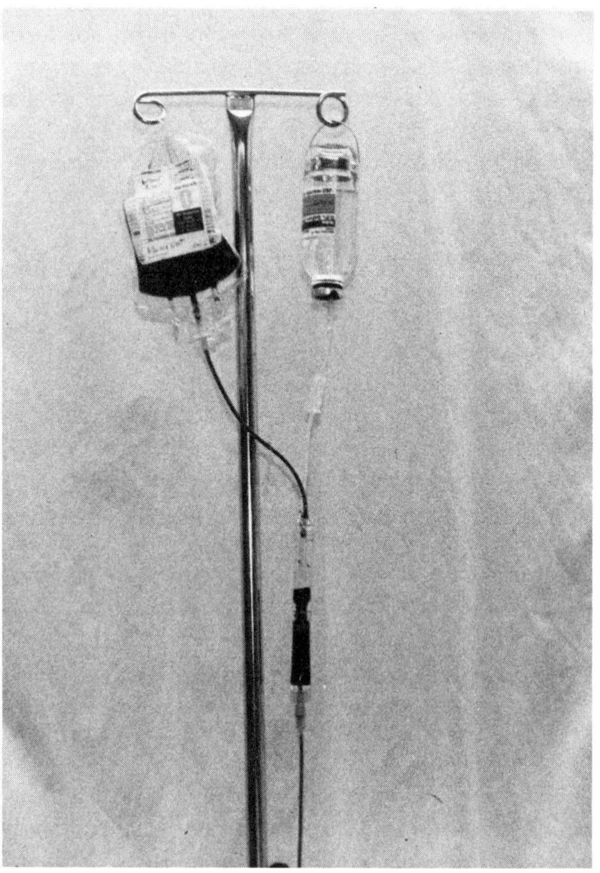
B

FIGURE 30-19. A. To administer blood, a special transfusion set that contains a blood filter to remove any clots or clumping of blood cells must be used. B. Normal saline is hung with transfusion in a Y setup.

hour) because if a transfusion reaction is going to occur, it generally occurs in the early minutes of the transfusion, and the less blood that has been transfused at this time the better. This rate means that the average adult of 150 pounds (68 kg) would receive 68 ml per hour, or, with a drop factor of 10 drops per milliliter, a rate of 10 drops per minute. Do not add a minidrop apparatus to a blood transfusion even though the rate would be easier to calculate with a higher drop factor because the smaller lumen of the minidrop tubing will crush cells just as much as a small needle lumen at the venipuncture site might.

Remember that blood is a viscous fluid; it should never be given extremely rapidly even after the initial cautious time period because it can cause circulatory overload very readily. The exception is in extreme hypovolemia emergencies, when blood may actually be "pumped" into the recipient by squeezing the plastic donor bag by hand or attaching an inflated blood pressure cuff to it. It is very important to prevent infiltration during a blood transfusion because blood is absorbed poorly from the subcutaneous tissue. It may remain there for such a long time that infection occurs at the site. Observe the venipuncture site at half-hour intervals for signs of infiltration (swelling, pain, and a sensation of coolness at the site). Take vital signs (temperature, pulse, respiration, and blood pressure) according to health care agency policy during the transfusion and for 1 hour afterward. The time interval for these measurements will vary in different agencies, but the maximum time span is once every hour.

Transfusion Reactions

Transfusion reactions can have a number of causes. The time of the reaction's occurrence and the actions to be taken depend on the cause and extent of the reaction.

HEMOLYTIC REACTIONS

Hemolytic reactions involve the rupture of red blood cells with release of hemoglobin. They are caused by administration of incompatible blood or blood that was accidentally frozen or warmed beyond safe limits. Because there are about 300 subgroups of blood antigens in addition to those cross-matched for A and B, a hemolytic reaction from one of these untested antigens is always a possibility with any transfusion. Fortunately, most of these other antigens produce little red cell destruction, and the reaction, if present, will be mild. Symptoms of a hemolytic reaction are tachypnea, tachycardia, decreased blood pressure, chills and fever, cyanosis, anxiety, and hemoglobinuria (blood in urine). If the blood pressure falls too low, shock and renal failure will result.

Take immediate action by halting the blood transfusion, open the normal saline attached to the Y-tubing, and allow it to infuse slowly to keep the vein open so that if emergency drugs must be administered, an immediate route will be available. As soon as possible, change the tubing to prevent any blood cells left in the tubing from infusing. Notify the person's physician immediately so interventions to combat shock can be begun. Administer oxyen as necessary for cyanosis.

ALLERGIC REACTIONS

Manifestations of an allergic reaction are urticaria (hives) with pruritus (itching) and a rash. Stop the transfusion at the first sign of such a reaction because in an extremely sensitive individual, the beginning symptoms (annoying but not harmful) may progress rapidly to laryngeal edema and anaphylactic shock (halting of respiratory and cardiac function). Notify the physician immediately. In most instances an intramuscular injection of an antihistamine such as Benadryl will halt the reaction.

PYROGENIC REACTIONS

A pyrogenic reaction is a reaction to contaminates in the donor blood. *Pseudomonas* is the chief bacterial offender in contaminated blood; it usually enters the donor blood because of improper site preparation at the time of blood donation. Symptoms of a pyrogenic reaction are abdominal pain, vomiting, and severe hypotension leading to renal failure. Discontinue the infusion, keeping the vein open, and alert the physician so that interventions to combat shock can be initiated.

CIRCULATORY OVERLOAD

Circulatory overload is most apt to occur in persons with cardiac or kidney disorders. As the circulatory system becomes overloaded, edema, particularly pulmonary edema, may develop. The patient will develop a cough, chest pain, shortness of breath (dyspnea), and cyanosis. Discontinue the infusion, leaving the vein open, by slowly infusing normal saline; notify the physician of the occurrence, and administer oxygen as necessary for cyanosis. Circulatory overload is treated by administering a diuretic to remove the excessive fluid quickly by way of the kidneys. A person who has a circulatory overload reaction is generally a candidate for packed red cells rather than whole blood if a second transfusion should be necessary.

POTASSIUM EXCESS

Blood cells begin to deteriorate the moment they are withdrawn from the donor. The longer the blood is stored, the more breakdown occurs. As cells deteriorate, potassium is released. Always double-check expiration dates on blood to be certain that no blood past the expiration date (that is, blood with a dangerously high potassium level) is infused. In people with calcium or kidney disorders, blood that is not more than 24 hours old is generally administered to keep potassium level to a minimum.

CITRATE REACTION

Acid-citrate-dextrose (ACD), the preservative in blood, can combine with calcium in the bloodstream to form calcium citrate. This binding of calcium lowers the level of usable calcium, causing the same effect as if calcium were suddenly lost from the bloodstream. The body compensates for this by releasing additional calcium from bones and by quickly removing citrate by way of the liver before any more calcium-binding can occur. The person with a liver disorder is particularly prone to calcium deficit from a transfusion. Symptoms of a low calcium level are tetany (tingling and numbness of fingers and toes), increased irritability, laryngeal spasm, and convulsions. Infusing blood slowly is the best method of preventing such a reaction because it gives the body time to compensate for calcium loss.

HEMOSIDEROSIS

Hemosiderosis is the infiltration of iron into body tissues. A person who receives a great many blood transfusions over a period of time will develop hemosiderosis from the large amount of iron transfused to him in red blood cells. Hemosiderosis causes skin discoloration (a bronze color) and can be so severe that the heart, lungs, and kidneys are invaded, causing lack of function in these organs. Iron stores of this nature can be chelated (excreted) from the body by administration of specific iron-chelating agents; future blood transfusions should be kept to a minimum.

POSTREACTION PROCEDURES

Following a blood reaction, a blood sample must be drawn and returned to the blood bank along with the unused blood so that the cross match can be rechecked and the exact cause of the reaction established. A urine sample must be obtained and sent for urinalysis to determine whether blood is present. Describe the exact nature of the reaction as you observed it and the therapy initiated. A reaction with one blood transfusion does not mean that the person will have a reaction with another.

Special Blood Transfusion Situations

Exchange blood transfusion is a technique in which a small amount of blood is withdrawn by syringe from a person's venous circulation and discarded. The same amount of donor blood is injected; a second sample of blood is withdrawn, more blood is introduced, and so on until about 80 percent of blood volume has been replaced with new blood. This technique washes out substances such as bilirubin and toxic drug levels from the bloodstream. It is used particularly in infants with blood incompatibility reactions from Rh factor. It is not a procedure without risk due to the frequent adjustments the cardiac system must make to changes in volume load.

Blood may be given to a fetus by an intrauterine transfusion. Because it is impossible to locate a fetal vein for such a transfusion, blood is injected into the fetal abdomen (located by sonogram). The blood is gradually absorbed across the peritoneal membrane and into the fetal bloodstream.

Autotransfusion is the transfusion of one's own blood. If a person who is anticipating surgery chooses to do so, he may donate a unit of his own blood a month in advance. At the time of surgery his own blood is transfused to him if needed rather than donor blood. Such a procedure is often suggested for a person who has multiple allergies and may in the future become a common procedure in all elective surgery.

SHOCK AND ITS RELATION TO FLUID AND ELECTROLYTE BALANCE

Shock is a condition in which the blood volume has been reduced to such an extent that cell perfusion is no longer adequate. A person in shock will have signs of hypotension due to the small circulating volume: cold and pale skin (due to vasoconstriction, which is the body's attempt to hold blood in the central core); poor or no kidney output (blood pressure is too low for fluid to pass into the tubule filtrate); apprehension (epinephrine and norepinephrine are released in response to stress); increased pulse rate (as the circulatory system tries to push the remaining blood as quickly as possible); increased respiratory rate (more oxygen is needed for tissue that is becoming short of adequate oxygen); and possibly mental changes (brain cells are not receiving enough oxygen due to lowered perfusion levels).

Physiological shock of this nature can occur rapidly from hemorrhage. Shock must be considered a possibility in all patients with any degree of blood loss because the amount of blood that is visibly lost may not be indicative of the total loss. Also, in many accident victims, blood is being lost internally into the abdominal cavity from a ruptured spleen or liver. These people develop severe physiologic shock, yet no blood loss is evident.

Because most people know that blood volume is important for life, they seek health care after losing blood or after a traumatic accident on the chance that shock may develop. Most people are not aware, however, that shock can also develop from fluid loss. The person with vomiting or diarrhea can lose so much blood volume in the body's attempt to replace lost interstitial fluid that he can develop shock as deep and serious as the person actively hemorrhaging. In a person with kidney damage who is losing large amounts of protein, blood will leave the circulatory system to enter the interstitial space by osmotic pressure. This will result in massive generalized edema and ascites. Although no fluid has left the body, the person's blood volume may be as low as if he were hemorrhaging, and shock can result.

Other reasons for shock are poor heart output (blood pressure is maintained by a combination of heart rate and cardiac output) such as can occur following a heart attack. Blood volume is not actually decreased but the effect is the same because it is not being circulated. This is termed *cardiogenic* shock.

In *neurogenic* shock, the peripheral circulation dilates so much that a large proportion of blood pools in the body periphery; this lowers blood pressure to vital organs and produces the same symptoms as if volume were actually decreased. This type of shock occurs following spinal cord injury as the normal nerve impulses are cut off.

Septic shock occurs in the person with an overwhelming infection. The blood vessels appear to respond to the high level of toxins present by failing to constrict; blood then pools in the peripheral circulation as it does in neurogenic shock.

Obstructive shock occurs when a major circulatory route is blocked. Pulmonary embolism (a blood clot in the pulmonary artery) blocking flow of blood to the lungs and left side of the heart may cause this type of shock. Blood volume is not actually decreased, but because of the blockage it is decreased to the vital organs and has the same effect as if total volume were decreased.

Volume Loss. In an adult blood volume loss (or volume pooling) is extensive (perhaps as much as 1500 ml) before shock becomes severe because of the body's ability to compensate for volume loss in a number of ways. Peripheral vasoconstriction pushes blood into the central circulation and helps to maintain pressure. A person experiencing low blood volume automatically sits or lies down because he feels weak; this circulates blood to the brain cells and provides more readily for function of vital centers. If psychological shock (inability to think or solve problems) is also present, the person may not do this, compounding the problem. This stage of shock (when vasoconstriction is present) is termed *compensated* shock.

If fluid loss continues, compensation mechanisms will eventually fail. Cells are not supplied with enough oxygen and begin to die. Anaerobic metabolism (metabolism without oxygen) begins. This results in severe acidosis, which further compromises cell function. Unless blood volume can be restored, the ultimate consequence of uncompensated physiological shock will be death.

Assessment of Shock

Blood pressure recordings are the most dramatic evidence of beginning symptoms of shock. The point at which the blood pressure suddenly falls is the point at which compensation measures have failed and the person is extremely ill. Subtle blood pressure and pulse changes must be recognized before this; a slowly increasing pulse rate and a slow but steadily decreasing blood pressure reading are such changes. A decreasing pulse pressure (the difference between systolic and diastolic readings) may be helpful. If fluid loss is ongoing, however, the diastolic level decreases with the systolic level, so the measurement is not helpful in itself.

Decreased urine output is an important measure. The kidneys filter urine because the blood pressure in the arterial system is greater than that in the kidney glomeruli; poor filtration in a person without known kidney disease generally suggests that arterial pressure is so low that filtration cannot occur. The normal urine output of an adult is 30 ml per hour. A urinary output below this suggests shock.

Restlessness and increasing anxiety are signs of oxygen hunger (hypoxia). If you are observing a person following a traumatic accident it is sometimes difficult to determine whether these signs are related to psychological stress or shock. If you have made every effort, however, to allow the person to talk about the accident and have given adequate assurance that the danger is past, consider shock if restlessness and anxiety continue. Such mental changes as increased sleepiness and difficulty with orientation are severe and suggest that shock is uncompensated.

Specific Nursing Interventions

If shock is recognized in time, therapy to correct it can be initiated and the situation corrected. Uncompensated shock is always an emergency because the person is very close to total dysfunction of the body system. Place the person in a supine position to allow as much fluid as possible to flow to the cerebral vessels. At one time people in shock were placed in a Trendelenburg position (head lower than chest) in an attempt to fully oxygenate brain tissue. This is no longer done, however, because it may force so much blood to the cerebral arteries that rupture of arteries can occur and blood flow to the heart and kidneys may be compromised. Depriving the coronary arteries of blood produces the same effect as a heart attack.

The person in uncompensated shock has hypoxia in all body cells. Oxygen administration by face mask is the best emergency source of oxygen. Further oxygen aids such as an endotracheal tube or a ventilator mask may be necessary if the respiratory system is so depressed that effective breathing is difficult to reestablish. Circulating blood volume needs to be increased as quickly as possible. When bleeding occurs, blood transfusion is the ideal method to accomplish this. In most emergency situations, however, blood is not available for transfusion because it must be carefully matched to the person's blood type before it can be administered. Intravenous fluid (Ringer's lactate or normal saline) is usually the first choice, therefore. It may be very difficult for a physician to locate an acceptable vein for fluid administration because the veins are collapsed due to the depleted circulatory load. The physician may need to do a cut-down to insert an intravenous fluid line. Plasma may be administered without cross matching and may be administered as a second fluid. Plasma expanders (albumin and dextran), which do not need to be cross matched for blood type, may also be used in this way.

Keep the person warm by not allowing him to be unnecessarily exposed during procedures but avoid increasing his temperature rapidly. Increased temperature causes vasodilatation; the small amount of vasoconstriction that the person is able to maintain may be the difference between heart function and heart failure until he has received enough intravenous fluid to increase his blood volume.

Intravenous fluid is administered rapidly at first and then slowed and continued at the slower rate for a period of hours. The additional fluid is as important as the initial fluid in restoring fluid volume. Be certain that the intravenous line does not infiltrate and block the supply of this vital fluid. Measure intake and output and specific gravity of urine to be certain that too much fluid is not administered, causing overhydration. Sitting up with lowered blood pressure can cause dizziness and shortness of breath; maintain a supine or only a slightly raised head position until fluid volume is completely corrected.

Be aware that shock is a symptom of an underlying process. Measures to correct the underlying condition must be started as soon as the emergency phase of care is complete or both hypovolemia and shock will recur. If the shock resulted from fluid loss into the interstitial tissue as edema, careful observation is needed as fluid is "called back" into the circulatory system to prevent circulatory overload. A diuretic is generally administered in such cases to ensure that the fluid that returns to the circulatory system will be quickly removed from the body.

LIFE SPAN CONCEPTS AND FLUID AND ELECTROLYTE BALANCE

The Infant

When an infant is ill, his food and fluid intake often drops dramatically. Sucking to obtain fluid requires muscle strength, and he tires before he drinks his normal amount of breast milk or formula. In an illness involving the throat or ear, sucking causes pain and he drinks less. In addition, vomiting often occurs as a systemic symptom in infants and can be superimposed on any illness. Diarrhea is a grave danger in infants because the amount of fluid lost is extreme compared with total fluid volume. The ability to concentrate urine and thus conserve body fluid is not fully developed until 1 year of age. Because of these factors, extremely simple illnesses in infants may be quickly complicated by a fluid or electrolyte imbalance.

It is difficult to encourage infants to drink more than they want. Try cool fluids if fever is present; try different flavored juices for a change of pace. Use apple juice sparingly because it tends to cause diarrhea. Infants accept fluid best from their mother (or primary caregiver); encourage parents to visit and hold the infant for feeding to achieve the best fluid volume intake.

The Toddler and Preschooler

It is also difficult to persuade toddlers to drink extra fluid. Popsicles, ice cream bars, ice cream, sherbet, and jello are good solutions.

Preschoolers tend to be fussy eaters and may have difficulty finding any food they like. Offer small amounts frequently for best results. A game such as Simon Says may be helpful in getting a child to take small amounts of fluid, but do not bribe children to drink. Preschoolers dislike intravenous therapy and need a great deal of support and praise for cooperation during a venipuncture. Children up to at least 3 years of age need restraints for safe administration of intravenous therapy when an adult is not with them.

The Schoolager and Adolescent

Schoolagers and adolescents like to feel in control of their bodies and their situations. They cooperate best in a program of increased fluid administration if they are allowed to select the fluid they will drink and help keep a record of their intake. Children this age choose drinks such as Kool-Aid or carbonated beverages over more nutritious fluids such as milk if given a free choice.

Some adolescents can become dehydrated while trying to reduce weight for competitive sports such as wrestling or from quick-loss fad reducing diets. They need diet counseling on how to lose weight by other means than totally halting fluid input.

The Young and Middle-Aged Adult

Young and middle-aged adults are cooperative about fluid regulation programs because they fully understand the importance of the actions being taken. They will cooperate to drink any fluid you offer (within reason). Plain water is often the most refreshing drink for relieving thirst and is often overlooked in favor of something more creative.

The Older Adult

Because the older adult may have some loss of kidney function, he may be less able to concentrate urine than previously, leading to dehydration. The older adult living alone may become dehydrated if his food budget does not allow him a choice of beverages, especially in summer.

Guard intravenous sites carefully in older adults if there are arteriosclerotic changes in blood vessels. Many older adults are passive in their acceptance of therapy; assess fluid intake carefully because they may not ask for as many things as younger people. Many older adults with arteriosclerosis are taking a daily diuretic to help them excrete body fluid for better heart function; encourage foods high in potassium (orange juice and bananas, for example) for such people.

NURSING CARE PLAN

John is a 6-month-old infant patient of yours. He is hospitalized for diarrhea and dehydration. His physician's orders are NPO; intravenous fluid: 500 ml 5 percent dextrose and normal saline to infuse at 50 ml per hour. Temperature, respiration, and pulse taken every 4 hours; intake and output to be measured.

The nursing care plan you might write for him is as follows:

NURSING DIAGNOSIS

Fluid volume deficit, actual related to diarrhea.

Assessment: Lips and mucous membrane dry; eye globes slightly sunken; crying without tears. Skin turgor moderately poor, ridge of skin returns to place, but slowly. Diaper area reddened and excoriated. Has had two liquid green stools (70 ml and 120 ml) since admission 30 minutes ago. Voided 20 ml concentrated urine; specific gravity: 1.035. Temperature 102.4°F. Pulse: 100; R:20.

Locus of Decision-Making: Shared with parent and nurse.

Goal: Patient to have improved hydration by 4 hours time.

Criteria: Skin turgor will be improved; urine specific gravity will be under 1.030.

NURSING ORDERS

1. Intravenous therapy to be begun on dorsal surface of left hand (5 percent dextrose and normal saline) at 50 ml per hour.
2. Use Buretral, minidrip apparatus, and IVAC pump in intravenous line for safety. Fill Buretral to 30 ml + 10 every hour.
3. Drop factor is 60 gtt per milliliter. Infuse at 50 gtt per minute to achieve infusion of 50 ml per hour.
4. Keep NPO. Use Vaseline to lips for comfort.
5. Apply urine collector to separate urine from liquid stool. Test specific gravity of all urine.
6. Weigh diapers for stool quantity; test all stool for occult blood, reducing substances (sugar), and pH.
7. Apply A & D ointment to diaper area following diaper change to protect skin from acid stool.
8. Encourage mother to touch and stroke child to reduce fear of strange surroundings and hurtful procedures.
9. Apply clove-hitch wrist restraints to safeguard IV. Loosen and assess pulse and skin every 2 hours.

SUGGESTED READINGS

Amonsen, S., and J. Gren. Relationship between length of time and contamination in open intravenous solutions. *Nurs. Res.* 27:372, 1978.

Anderson, M. A., et al. The double-lumen Hickman catheter. *Am. J. Nurs.* 82:272, 1982.

Beaumont, E. The new I.V. infusion pumps. *Nursing 77* 7:31, 1977.

Burgess, A. *The Nurse's Guide to Fluid and Electrolyte Balance* (2nd ed.). New York: McGraw-Hill, 1979.

Coco, C. D. *Intravenous Therapy: A Handbook for Practice.* St. Louis: Mosby, 1980.

Correcting fluid and electrolyte problems . . . managing IVs. *Nursing* (Horsham) 13(1):79, 1983.

Cunningham, S. G. Fluid and electrolyte disturbances associated with cancer and its treatment. *Nurs. Clin. North Am.* 17(4):579, 1982.

Felver, L. Understanding the electrolyte maze. *Am. J. Nurs.* 80(9):1591, 1980.

Fineman, V., et al. Toward impeccable I.V. technique. The right things to say about I.V.s. *RN* 44(8):29, 1981.

Gruber, D. L. Helping the child accept I.V. therapy. *Am. J. I.V. Ther.* 4:50, 1977.

Habel, M. What you need to know about infusing plasma expanders. *RN* 43:30, 1980.

Juliani, L. M. Keep this quick flow-rate calculator handy and hold onto this glossary of IV fluid terms, too. *RN* 44(10):64, 1981.

Keithley, J. K., et al. What's behind that I.V. line? *Nursing* (Horsham) 12:32, 1982.

Lane, G., et al. When persistence pays off: Resolving the mystery of an unexplained electrolyte imbalance. *Nursing* (Horsham) 12:44, 1982.

Lawson, M., et al. Long-term I.V. therapy: A new approach. *Am. J. Nurs.* 79:1100, 1979.

Masoorlie, S. T. Trouble-free I.V. starters. *RN* 44:20, 1981.

Metabolic acid-base disorders: Chemistry and physiology (programmed instruction, part I). *Am. J. Nurs.* 77:1619, 1977.

Metabolic acid-base disorders: Physiological abnormalities and nursing actions (programmed instruction, part II). *Am. J. Nurs.* 78:87, 1978.

Metheny, N. Preoperative fluid balance assessment. *A.O.R.N. J.* 33(1):51, 1981.

Metheny, N. M., and W. D. Snively. Perioperative fluids and electrolytes. *Am. J. Nurs.* 78:840, 1978.

Metheny, N. M., and W. D. Snively. *Nurses' Handbook of Fluid Balance.* Philadelphia: Lippincott, 1979.

Michael, S. Home I.V. therapy. *Am. J. Nurs.* 78:1223, 1978.

Millan, D. A., et al. Intravenous therapy: A special feature. *Am. J. Nurs.* 79:1268, 1979.

Oelerich, W. J., et al. Mini I.V. patients . . . maximum precautions . . . infant I.V. insertion: Step by step. *RN* 44:43, 1981.

Quinlan, M. Would you spot this dangerous electrolyte imbalance? *RN* 46(3):50, 1983.

Rando, J. T. Fluid and electrolyte management of the adult surgical patient. *A.A.N.A. J.* 50(1):49, 1982.

Rando, J. T. A review of past and current thinking in pediatric fluid therapy. *A.A.N.A. J.* 48(5):437, 1980.

Reed, G., and V. Sheppard. *Regulation of Fluid and Electrolyte Balance* (2nd ed.). Philadelphia: Saunders, 1977.

Robinson, L. A., and N. F. Whitacre. Intravenous administration of antibiotics in children. *Pediatr. Nurs.* 3:21, 1977.

Rosenthal, K. A. Converting micrograms/kilograms/minute to microdrops . . . chart vs. formula method. Part I. *D.C.C.N.* 1(6):326, 1982.

Rutman, R., et al. Blood therapy. *Am. J. Nurs.* 79:925, 1979.

Sager, D. P., and S. K. Bomar. *Intravenous Medications.* Philadelphia: Lippincott, 1980.

Samson, L. F. Use of a preemie needle . . . a 27 gauge IV needle designed for use with small infants. *Crit. Care Nurse* 2(5):6, 1982.

Scarlato, M. Blood transfusions today: What you should know and do. *Nursing 78* 8:68, 1978.

Scott, M. A. *Calculations of Medications.* Norwalk, Conn.: Appleton-Century-Ceofts, 1982.

Selye, H. *Stress in Health and Disease.* Boston: Butterworths, 1976.

Symposium on fluid, electrolyte, and acid-base balance. *Nurs. Clin. North Am.* 15(3):535, 1980.

Twombly, M. The shift into third space. *Nursing 78* 8:38, 1978.

Vogel, T. C., et al. Teaching parents to give indwelling C. V. catheter care . . . a child going home with an indwelling central venous catheter. *Nursing* (Horsham) 13(1):54, 1983.

Weinstein, S. M. The I.V. nurse: Recognizing a growing specialty. *Nurs. Manage.* 13:22, 1982.

Weldy, N. J. *Body Fluids and Electrolytes.* St. Louis: Mosby, 1980.

Woodland, C. How to make infusion control devices work for you. *R.N.* 44:58, 1981.

QUESTIONS FOR REVIEW

1. Mrs. Fox is a patient of yours. She is to have intravenous fluid administration. In planning care, it is important for you to know that which electrolyte is the most common cation of extracellular fluid?
   a. Sodium.
   b. Potassium.
   c. Magnesium.
   d. Sulfate.

2. Fluid in the body often moves by osmotic pressure. As part of health teaching, you could explain this to Mrs. Fox as:
   a. Movement of solvent through a semi-permeable membrane from a lesser to a greater concentration.
   b. Movement of molecules through a semi-permeable membrane from a lesser to a greater concentration.
   c. Movement of solvent through a semi-permeable membrane from a greater to a lesser concentration.
   d. Movement of molecules through a semi-permeable membrane from a greater to a lesser concentration.

3. Mrs. Fox's physician asks you to assess whether Mrs. Fox's aldosterone level is adequate. To do this you need to know that aldosterone acts to regulate fluid balance by:
   a. Excreting excess body fluid.
   b. Increasing sodium reabsorption.
   c. Decreasing potassium absorption.
   d. Increasing sodium excretion.

4. Mrs. Fox's physician is also concerned about her becoming acidotic. A body fluid is acid if it has:
   a. More OH^- ions than H^+ ions.
   b. A pH over 7.00.
   c. More H^+ ions than OH^- ions.
   d. Nearly equal H^+ and OH^- ions.

5. To implement care, you will be administering an isotonic fluid. Which of the following solutions is considered isotonic?
   a. 0.45% sodium chloride.
   b. Whole saline.
   c. 5% dextrose and water.
   d. Potassium in saline.

6. If an infusion is to run at 50 ml per hour and the equipment furnishes a drop factor of 15, at what rate will you set the flow?
   a. 5 gtt per minute.
   b. 12 gtt per minute.
   c. 25 gtt per minute.
   d. 50 gtt per minute.

7. If whole blood is ordered for Mrs. Fox, which intravenous fluid would you choose to begin the transfusion?
   a. 5% dextrose and saline.
   b. Lactated Ringer's solution.
   c. 5% dextrose and water.
   d. 0.9% sodium chloride.

8. If the blood infusion should infiltrate, the symptoms you would assess for would be:
   a. Cyanosis at the venipuncture site.
   b. Edema at the venipuncture site.
   c. Red streaking of veins distal to the site.
   d. Pain proximal to the site.

31. CARDIOVASCULAR RESPONSES

OBJECTIVES
Upon mastery of the material in this chapter, you should be able to:

1. Describe the physiological principles of normal heart action that influence pulse and blood pressure readings.
2. Describe the techniques for determining pulse and blood pressure.
3. List the common sites used to assess pulse.
4. List the normal values for pulse and blood pressure according to age.
5. Describe the conditions that cause deviations in pulse and blood pressure readings.
6. Describe the role of pressure bandages in maintaining cardiovascular function.
7. Apply the nursing process to give safe and planned care to a patient whose care involves principles of cardiovascular regulation.

TERMS
The terms important for an understanding of this chapter are shown below and defined in the glossary:

apical heart rate
blood pressure
bradycardia
diastole
diastolic blood pressure
heart rate
hypertension
hypotension
Korotkoff's sounds
murmur
premature beat
pulse
pulse deficit
pulse pressure
sinus arrhythmia
systole
tachycardia

Maintaining cardiovascular function is important because such function is instrumental in transporting oxygen and nutrients to body cells and removing waste products from cells; when cardiovascular function fails, all cells of the body are to some degree affected.

CARDIOVASCULAR FUNCTIONING

The efficiency of cardiovascular function depends on the function of the heart, blood vessels, and fluid within the vessels (the blood).

THE HEART

Take a minute to review normal blood circulation through the heart because the sounds you hear when listening to a heart beat are direct consequences of blood flow through the heart. As illustrated in Fig. 31-1, venous or nonoxygenated blood returning from the body enters the right atrium from the vena cava. Both atria contract; blood is forced through the tricuspid valve into the right ventricle. As the ventricles contract, blood is forced through the pulmonary valve into the pulmonary artery. From the pulmonary artery, it circulates through the lungs; oxygen is diffused into it from lung alveoli; the oxygenated blood returns to the heart by way of the pulmonary veins and empties into the left atrium. With atrial contraction, it crosses the mitral valve to the left ventricle. With ventricle contraction, it is forced through the aortic valve to the aorta and out to the aorta and the body.

The sound of the mitral and tricuspid valves closing as ventricles contract is the first heart sound heard (the *lub* of "lub-dub"). This phase of heart action is termed *systole.* The sound of the pulmonary and aortic valves closing is the second heart sound heard (the *dub* of "lub-dub"). Atrial contraction and closure of these valves is termed *diastole.* The heart beat originates in the sinoatrial (SA) node located on the back wall of the right atrium. An electrical impulse that arises from this point spreads 60 to 100 times a minute across the atrium to cause contraction (diastole). When the impulse reaches the atrioventricular (AV) node, it continues to spread across the ventricles, causing them to contract (systole).

Cardiac Output. Cardiac output is the product of the volume of blood that is pumped from the left ventricle times the heart rate per minute. In order to keep cells oxygenated, the heart attempts under normal conditions to maintain its cardiac output by varying either the heart rate or filling of the ventricles.

BLOOD VESSELS

The ability of blood vessels to function effectively depends on how they respond to autonomic nervous system stimulation and combat effects of gravity or body environmental changes. The wider (more dilated) a blood vessel, the less resistance it offers to blood flow

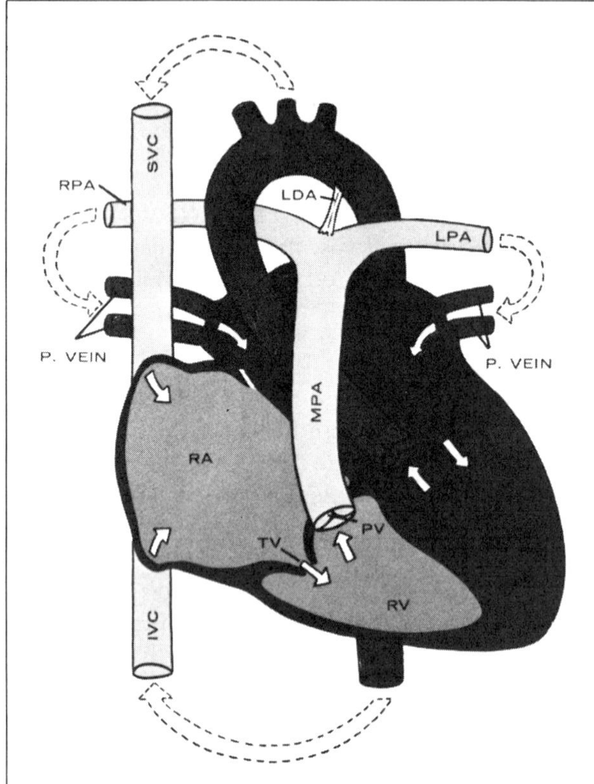

FIGURE 31-1. Normal blood circulation through the heart. AO=aorta; AV=aortic valve; IVC=inferior vena cava; LA=left atrium; LPA=left pulmonary artery; LV=left ventricle; MPA=main pulmonary artery; MV=mitral valve; LDA=ligamentum ductus arteriosus; PV=pulmonary valve; p. vein=pulmonary vein; RA=right atrium; RPA=right pulmonary artery; RV=right ventricle; SVC=superior vena cava; TV=tricuspid valve.

and the less strength it needs to move blood through it; hence the lower the blood pressure. Blood vessels constrict in response to cold; they dilate in response to warmth.

Valves in the venous circulation are instrumental in moving blood through the venous system. Such valves are necessary because, when a person is standing, blood in the venous system is flowing against gravity. Inadequate venous valve function will lead to edema in lower extremities (fluid pools in these vessels and then diffuses into subcutaneous tissue because of the increased hydrostatic pressure) and to varicose veins (veins distended and visible on the skin surface).

THE BLOOD

The efficiency of blood depends on the amount of plasma and the number of platelets, and red and white blood cells present. The plasma level will decline if a person is dehydrated; cellular totals to a large extent depend on nutrition. All blood factors may be decreased if blood loss from a break in the circulatory system (hemorrhage) has occurred.

ASSESSMENT OF CIRCULATORY STATUS

Because cardiovascular function is so important for cell function, assessment of cardiovascular function must be a continuous, ongoing process with any patient interaction.

Health Interview

A patient with a fault in cardiovascular function typically reports feeling "tired" as a major symptom. It is easy to ignore such a statement as not important since fatigue is much vaguer than most reported symptoms and, for students, a common condition. Always listen carefully to a report of fatigue, however, and ask the person to describe specifically what he means by the symptom. Everyone should be able to walk up one flight of stairs, for example, without feeling short of breath. Be sure to evaluate when listening to parents describe a child's behavior whether they are describing sedentary activities or fatigue. A child who comes home from school and lays down to read is probably only a child more interested in reading than in playing baseball; a child, on the other hand, who comes home from school and sleeps is abnormally fatigued. Children with congenital heart disease typically stop active games and assume a knee chest or squatting position, a position that traps blood in lower extremities and reduces the amount that the heart must oxygenate. Listen for reports of "heart skipping beats" or "heart knocking against chest," which describe the common symptom of arrhythmia or irregular heart action.

If a person's heart action is weak, blood does not circulate well to distal parts (or blood vessels are constricted so much that even a very strong heart action cannot pump blood through them effectively). People report symptoms of cold, tingling, or numb hands and feet. Inadequate circulation to hands can cause "clubbing" of fingers or "spoon-shaped" fingertips from increased capillary growth at the fingertips. There is less growth of hair, especially on the legs; nails become brittle and yellow.

Inadequate oxygen perfusion of tissue is always accompanied by an increase in respiratory rate (the body tries to compensate for slow circulation by "overloading" the blood with oxygen). As a result, some people may not be as aware of irregular heart action as they are of a change in respiratory rate. Increased blood pressure gives symptoms of headache, "buzzing in the ears," and vertigo (dizziness) on arising. Lower blood pressure also gives symptoms of vertigo on arising until blood pressure in cerebral arteries is readjusted.

Physical Assessment

Physical assessment for cardiovascular function includes assessment of the heart rate and quality (reflected by the pulse rate and quality), skin color, urine output, blood pressure, and lower extremities.

HEART RATE

Heart rate is the speed of the heart beat; it is referred to as the number of times the heart beats in the span of 1 minute. In fetuses and newborns, this rate is as high as 120 to 160 beats per minute; in adults the usual heart rate is 70 to 80 beats per minute. Usual rates for different age children are shown in Table 31-1. To count a heart rate, place your stethoscope against the chest over the heart apex or the place where the mitral valve sound is heard best. This is the fifth intercostal space just medial to the midclavicular line in the adult (see Fig. 19-3); the fourth or fifth space in the infant. The heart beat can often be palpated at this point with the palm of your hand but the rate cannot be accurately assessed by palpation. Listen with a stethoscope for the rate (called an *apical pulse rate*).

An apical pulse rate is generally measured in infants because their peripheral pulses tend to be too faint to be accurate; an apical rate should be obtained before the administration of cardiac medicine and whenever peripheral pulse points are obscured or too weak to evaluate accurately. Because it is difficult to hear a heart beat over the sound of loud crying, try to listen to an apical beat in an infant before you attempt any type of care that would frighten him (take heart rate before temperature, for example).

As blood is pumped into the aorta with systole, it initiates a wave throughout the circulatory system. This wave represents ventricular contraction. It can be felt at any point where an artery passes close to the skin surface as a pulse.

PULSE RATE

Common arteries and the sites that can be used to measure pulse rate are shown in Table 31-2. A peripheral pulse rate is recorded more often than an apical heart rate because determination does not require a stethoscope, only your fingertips. Pulse rate is an indirect measurement of heart rate, however, so it does not reveal as much information about the heart as an apical assessment. In the person with narrowed arteries, for example, the pulse rate may be distorted because it is difficult for the blood to reach a distal pulse site. The measurement of apical and peripheral pulse rates are described in Procedures 31-1 and 31-2.

Abnormalities with Rate. Tachycardia is an increased heart rate, measuring in adults over 100 beats per minute. The heart rate increases with exercise, fever, hypoxemia (low oxygen level in blood), or lowered blood pressure in order to better supply body cells with oxygen. Stress caused by worry, fear, or pain can increase heart rate. It is difficult to count a rapid pulse because the sensations against your fingertips are light and barely felt before they disappear. The best assurance that you will be able to count these rapid rates is to remain

TABLE 31-1. AVERAGE PULSE RATE FOR DIFFERENT AGE GROUPS

	Pulse Rate (per min)	
Age Group	Average	Range
Newborn	125	70—190
1 year	120	80—160
2 years	110	80—130
4 years	100	80—120
6 years	100	75—115
8 years	90	70—110
10 years	90	70—110
12 years		
Females	90	70—110
Males	85	65—105
14 years		
Females	85	65—105
Males	80	60—100
16 years		
Females	80	60—100
Males	75	55—95
18+ adult		
Females	75	55—95
Males	70	50—90

Source: From V. C. Vaughan III and R. J. McKay, Jr. (Eds.), *Textbook of Pediatrics* (11th ed.). Philadelphia: Saunders, 1979.

TABLE 31-2. COMMON SITES FOR ASSESSMENT OF ARTERIAL PULSE

Pulse	Location
Carotid	To the right or left of the trachea, anterior to sternocleidomastoid muscle.
Brachial	Antecubital fossa at point where brachial artery passes over ulna.
Dorsalis pedis	Dorsum of foot at point where dorsalis pedis artery passes over proximal phalanges (in line between first and second toe).
Apical	Auscultated at 5th intercostal interspace at the left midclavicular line.
Femoral	At the left or right groin at point where femoral artery passes over the body of the ischium.
Popliteal	At the popliteal fossa (posterior surface of the knee) at the point where popliteal artery passes over the articular surface of the femur.
Posterior tibialis	Lateral surface of ankle at point where posterior tibialis artery passes over lateral malleolus.
Radial	Inner surface of the wrist at point where radial artery passes over radius.
Temporal	At the temple at point where temporal artery passes over temporal bone.

PROCEDURE 31-1
Obtaining an Apical Pulse

Purpose: To assess circulatory function by evaluating the rate, rhythm, and quality of the pulse at an easily accessible central site.

Plan	*Principle*
1. Wash your hands; identify patient; explain the procedure.	1. Prevent the spread of microorganisms; ensure patient safety and cooperation.
2. Assess patient status; analyze appropriateness of procedure. Plan modifications as necessary. Implement procedure by obtaining equipment: stethoscope, notepad and pencil for recording reading.	2. Pulse rate is an easy-to-forget item. Determining apical rate necessitates the use of a stethoscope in contrast to other pulse points.
3. Position the patient comfortably; preferably lying or sitting.	3. Pulse rate changes with exercise. A resting position helps to make comparison between readings at different times more meaningful.
4. Warm the diaphragm of the stethoscope by holding it in your palm for a few seconds. Expose patient's chest as neccessary so you can palpate point of maximum impulse (PMI) on chest. Place stethoscope diaphragm over this point.	4. The point of maximum impulse in most people is the 5th intercostal space at the left midclavicular line. Avoid exposing the person unnecessarily for the sake of modesty.
5. Looking at your watch, count the number of apical beats heard for 30 seconds; multiply by 2. Sinus arrhythmia (slowing and increasing with respirations) makes 15 seconds too short a time to count an apical rate.	5. If rhythm is irregular or very fast you need to count for a full minute for accuracy. When counting heart beats, count both systole and diastole (lub-dub) as one beat.
6. Leave your stethoscope in place and evaluate the rhythm (irregular, regular) and strength (forceful, weak, soft).	6. An irregularity in beat may be as important in determining ineffective heart action as the rate of the beat.
7. Remove stethoscope, reinstate clothing as necessary; position patient comfortably; provide for activity or stimulation as necessary.	
8. Evaluate effectiveness, efficiency, cost, comfort, and safety of procedure. Record rate, rhythm, and quality immediately. Plan health teaching as necessary; indicate, for example, the importance of checking pulse rate before cardiac medication administration (many people will be doing so independently at home and need to understand its importance to continue to check pulse rate conscientiously).	8. Document patient status and nursing care. Health teaching is an independent nursing action always included with care.

MODIFICATIONS FOR CARE OF CHILD

Infants and young children are very wary of stethoscopes, afraid that stethoscopes will hurt when pressed against their skin. Be certain that the stethoscope diaphragm is warm to avoid frightening a child with a cold disk. Letting an infant be held by his mother while you assess heart rate is often helpful. Showing the child that a stethoscope does not hurt by placing the diaphragm on the back of his hand first is often helpful. Be cautious about letting children handle your stethoscope to listen through it (they tend to stretch it so that it does not fit your ears well afterward).

MODIFICATIONS FOR CARE OF OLDER ADULT

Older men tend to develop some degree of air retention in alveoli after expiration (emphysema) which may increase sinus arrhythmia effects. Emphysema often causes accessory chest sounds such as rhonchi; learn to "tune out" lung sounds while you listen to the heart beat.

PROCEDURE 31-2
Obtaining a Radial Pulse

Purpose: To assess circulatory function by evaluating the rate, strength, and quality of the pulse of a readily available peripheral artery.

Plan	*Principal*
1. Wash your hands; identify the patient; explain the procedure.	1. Prevent the spread of microorganisms; ensure patient safety and cooperation.
2. Assess patient status; analyze appropriateness of procedure. Plan modifications as necessary. Position patient comfortably; preferably supine or sitting with arm across chest or at side.	2. Pulse increases with exercise; a resting position gives an accurate comparison with the previous pulse recording.
3. Obtain equipment: notepad and pencil to record information obtained.	3. Pulse rate is an easily forgotten factor unless written down immediately.
4. Place two or three fingertips on the radial artery on the inside of the patient's wrist.	4. Your fingertips are sensitive to the vibration of the artery. Never use your thumb or you may feel your own pulse, not that of the patient.
5. Look at your watch and count the pulsations that you detect for 15 seconds.	5. A 15-second interval allows an accurate measurement unless the pulse is irregular or very rapid.
6. Continue to hold your fingertips against the artery while you evaluate the strength (full, bounding, weak, thready) and rhythm (regular, irregular) of the pulse.	6. Observations of rhythm and strength are as indicative of cardiovascular illness as abnormal rate.
7. Remove your hand; position patient comfortably and provide adequate stimulation activity.	
8. Record rate, strength, and rhythm. Evaluate effectiveness, efficiency, cost, comfort, and safety of procedure. Plan any patient teaching necessary; describe, for example, how to assess one's own pulse for the person who will be doing so at home prior to cardiac medicine administration.	8. Document patient status and nursing care. Health teaching is an independent nursing action always included in care.

MODIFICATIONS FOR CARE OF CHILD

Pulse rate increases greatly with crying. To decrease crying, take a minute to allow the child to be comfortable with you before touching him. As a rule, do not use radial pulse sites with infants. Take an apical assessment for highest accuracy.

MODIFICATIONS FOR CARE OF OLDER ADULT

Since many older adults have a weak radial pulse, you may need to take the pulse, using the same technique, at the brachial artery in the antecubital space instead. If arteriosclerosis is present, a person's blood vessels feel hard and unyielding under your fingertips.

undistracted while you count. You may have to say to a patient, "I'll answer your question in just a second," to prevent him from interrupting while you count the pulse rate.

Bradycardia is a slow heart rate, measuring below 60 beats per minute in adults. It is a response to parasympathetic nerve stimulation and is seen in people with heart block (poor conduction between atria and ventricles) or increased intracranial pressure; it can also be momentarily caused by vagal nerve stimulation, the result of bronchial suctioning, forceful vomiting, and so on. Some well-conditiond athletes have a mild bradycardia because their hearts' stroke volume is so great that their hearts can beat more slowly than normally and still adequately perfuse their tissues.

A person with bradycardia may have a cardiac pacemaker, an electrode implanted into the heart that initiates a faster cardiac rate. Pacemakers can be activated either constantly or only when the heart fails to beat. A cardiac pacemaker always functions at a beat specifically set for that person. A patient with a pacemaker will show you its location (under the skin on the chest) and know his normal heart rate; ask what his normal rate is on hospital admission or when beginning care in his home. If you take the pulse of someone with a pacemaker in place and discover it is less than normal, it generally means that the pacemaker's batteries are beginning to fail (batteries in pacemakers lose their strength slowly with ample time for the person to see his physician and have the pacemaker changed before it fails). People with pacemakers should not have electric cautery, diathermy, or microwaves used around them as these sources of electricity may interfere with pacemaker performance. Double-check that all electrical plugs used near the person are three-pronged (not just adapted to be three-pronged), so no possible shock could occur around the person (and possibly interfere with pacemaker ability). Men are cautioned at home not to use electrical drills or work on a car engine by leaning directly over it. No electrical razor should be used directly over the pacemaker when preparing for surgery or performing other procedures.

RHYTHM

Heart rhythm (the time interval between beats) is as important as heart rate in detecting normal function. This assessment is done best by listening directly to the heart rate, but it can also be evaluated by pulse palpation.

Abnormalities with Rhythm. Usually a pulse rhythm is evenly spaced (regular). Two irregularities that are normal, however, may be noticed on occasion. *Sinus arrhythmia* is a variation in heart rate due to the pressure changes that occur in the chest during respiration. You may notice it in adults, schoolagers, and adolescents. With sinus arrhythmia, the heart rate increases on inspiration as pressure in the lungs traps a maximum amount of blood in the lungs and allows a reduced amount to return to the heart. To counteract the reduced amount of blood returning to it, the heart increases its rate slightly to maintain the cardiac output level. As the lungs empty with expiration, the backlogged blood returns to the heart; as stroke volume is increased, the rate slows. If you have any doubt whether or not you are listening to sinus arrhythmia, observe the respiratory pattern while you simultaneously count the apical beat; ask the person to hold his breath (the heart rate remains constant with the breath held).

A second variation in rhythm which you may occasionally hear is the presence of a premature beat. You can feel this by palpating a peripheral pulse or listening for an apical pulse. The sensation is simply an extra beat suddenly interspaced in a normal rhythm (beat . . . beat . . . beat beat . . . beat). It means that a point in the heart other than the SA node initiated a heart beat. This happens with emotional stress (brought on by a physical examination, hospitalization, worry over surgery). It happens in early pregnancy due to the increased blood volume. The person can usually describe the abnormal sensation, often with the phrase "my heart skipped a beat"). By itself, such a one-time situation is normal. If you feel or hear a premature beat, listen for a full minute to be certain that you cannot hear others. Serious heart pathology may be suggested if you hear more than one during that time (or every time you take the pulse, you hear or feel one), and the finding should be reported to the patient's physician for additional assessment.

Abnormal pulse patterns that do reflect cardiac or vessel pathology are shown in Table 31-3.

QUALITY

The quality of heart rate refers to the strength (forceful or faint) and whether or not murmurs are present. Murmurs are the result of an interference of blood flow through the heart (blood moving at an abnormally fast pace through a poorly operating valve or stopped in some way by a nonfunctioning valve; in children they can result from congenital heart defects such as septal

TABLE 31-3. ABNORMAL PULSE FINDINGS

Finding	Description	Possible Cause
Bigeminal pulse	Irregular rhythm in which every other beat is premature (early) and weak; an irregularly regular beat.	Ventricles contract early so that stroke volume is weak; occurs following heart attacks (myocardial infarction) or certain drug intoxifications.
Pulsus alternans	Rhythm is regular but the strength is alternately strong or weak.	Occurs with left side heart failure or heart block.
Paradoxical pulse	Rhythm is regular but the strength of the beat weakens when the person inhales.	Blood is accumulating in the heart, or edema is compressing major blood vessels near the heart.
Corrigan's (water-hammer) pulse	Pulse "slaps" against your palpating fingers, then collapses; an extreme "bounding" feeling.	Aortic valve is failing to close properly.
Dicrotic pulse	Two pulse waves for each heartbeat are present.	Reflects nervous system depression.

defects). Murmurs may be "innocent," merely reflecting disturbed but not serious flow problems, or "pathologic," reflecting serious heart pathology. Murmurs can be assessed only by listening to the heart directly with a stethoscope; they are discussed in Chap. 19 with aspects of physical assessment.

The strength of the heartbeat can be assessed by palpating the pulse not just for the rate but for the force of the wave that the heartbeat originated. The elasticity of the blood vessel can also be evaluated by estimating the vessel's "spring" under your fingertips when palpating.

Abnormalities of Pulse Quality. Two measures of pulse quality that you want to assess are the strength of the vibration and the elasticity of the vessel wall. If the stroke volume of the heart increases, the wave of pressure through the vessel can be felt strongly; if the amount of blood pumped with each heart contraction is decreased, the pulse wave at a peripheral point becomes less easy to feel. The quality of pulse may be described as 4+ (abnormally strong and bounding); 3+ (strong but not abnormal, as might be felt following strong exercise); 2+ (normal); 1+ (weak or thready); or 0 (absent).

Elasticity of the arterial walls is assessed by pressing against them with your fingertips and judging their degree of resiliency. Normal arteries compress easily, and you are aware only of the sensation of the pulse beat, not of the artery itself. In people with arteriosclerosis, however, the artery feels hardened and inflexible. If the blood pressure is very high, the tension in the artery will make it less easy to compress. It takes much practice before you can claim with confidence the ability to assess the elasticity of arterial walls.

PULSE DEFICIT

Pulse deficit is the difference between a radial pulse rate and an apical pulse rate. If ventricular contractions are not strong or regular, some of them may be so weak that the wave caused by the contractions does not reach the peripheral pulse site. In these instances, the peripheral pulse reading is inaccurate (the peripheral pulse count is 60; the apical rate is 80).

To assess if a pulse deficit is present, you need two examiners. Place a watch in a conspicuous place where you both can observe it. Have one person count the apical heart rate with a sthethoscope while the other palpates the radial pulse rate, beginning the counts when one of you say "Now" or "Start" (see Procedure 31-3). Because pulse deficits do exist is why the apical rate should be used for medication that must be administered based on heart rate, such as digitalis.

PROCEDURE 31-3
Obtaining a Pulse Deficit

Purpose: To assess the difference between the apical and radial pulse rates by comparing the number of ventricle beats to the number of pulse beats at a peripheral vessel site.

Plan	*Principle*
1. Wash your hands; identify the patient; explain the procedure. Ask another nurse for assistance.	1. Prevent spread of microorganisms; ensure patient safety and cooperation. Two people are necessary since one must count the apical rate while the other will count the radial rate.
2. Assess patient status. Analyze appropriateness of procedure. Plan any necessary care modifications. Implement procedure by assembling equipment: stethoscope, notepad and pencil, and watch with second hand.	
3. Position patient comfortably. Remove clothing as necessary to palpate and locate point of maximum impulse (PMI) on chest; place stethoscope over PMI.	3. The point of maximum impulse is located at the 5th intercostal space at the left midclavicular line in adults; slightly lower and outside in infants.
4. Position a watch so that both examiners can readily observe it.	4. Having both examiners use the same watch ensures accuracy.
5. Agree to begin counting when the second hand of the watch reaches a certain number or when you say "start."	5. A pulse deficit will be accurate only if the apical and radial beats are counted simultaneously.
6. Count the number of beats heard or sensed for a full 60 seconds.	6. A 60-second time frame ensures best accuracy.

7. Leave patient positioned comfortably; reposition clothing as necessary; provide diversion or stimulation as necessary.
8. Evaluate effectiveness, efficiency, cost, comfort, and safety of procedure. Record the apical and peripheral rates immediately. Plan health teaching as indicated; describe, for example, the importance of the procedure.

8. Document patient status and nursing care; health teaching is an independent nursing action always included in nursing care.

MODIFICATIONS FOR CARE OF CHILD

It is difficult for a small child to hold still for a full minute. Fortunately, pulse deficits, which tend to be a problem of the older age group, are not evaluated often in children.

MODIFICATIONS FOR CARE OF OLDER ADULT

The radial pulse in some older adults is very faint and difficult to count accurately. You may have to repeat the procedure for another minute to be sure that the radial pulse count is accurate (otherwise you would mistakenly record the deficit as very extreme).

PROCEDURE 31-4
Obtaining a Blood Pressure

Purpose: To assess the force of blood ejected against vessel walls by use of a sphygomomanometer and stethoscope.

Plan

1. Wash your hands; identify the patient; explain the procedure.
2. Assess patient status; analyze appropriateness of procedure; plan care modifications. Implement procedure by assembling equipment: stethoscope, sphygomomanometer, notepad, and pencil. Check that sphygomomanometer is calibrated at zero.
3. Position patient comfortably in a lying or sitting position. Remove clothing as necessary to expose left arm.
4. Place the cuff around the patient's bare arm just above the antecubital space. Position the sphygomomanometer gauge so that it is easily read.
5. Warm the diaphragm of the stethoscope by holding it in your palm for a few seconds; place eartips in your ears pointing forward; palpate brachial artery at antecubital space; and fit diaphragm over the pulse point.
6. Close the valve on the bulb of the sphygomomanometer; pump the bulb until the gauge or mercury column rises to 40 mm Hg over anticipated systolic pressure.
7. Turn the valve to allow air to leave the cuff at a rate of about 2 mm Hg per minute; listen for Korotkoff's sounds.

Principle

1. Prevent spread of microorganisms; ensure patient safety and cooperation.
2. Choose a cuff size that is no wider than two-thirds of the upper arm width. A cuff size wider than this gives a false low reading; narrower than this, a false high reading.
3. Always using the patient's left arm makes blood pressure readings more consistent over time. Cuff must be applied to bare arm, not over clothing.
4. A mercury column should be read at eye level for greatest accuracy.
5. The brachial pulse point (located on the medial aspect of antecubital space) is an easy place to palpate as a whole.
6. Inflating the cuff to 40 mm Hg over anticipated systolic pressure allows you to hear systolic pressure clearly.
7. Using a very slow deflating rate allows you to determine the point on the gauge or scale at which you heard a sound.

8. Note the number on the gauge or scale at which you first hear sound.	8. This point represents the systolic pressure.
9. Continue to deflate cuff until you note the point at which the sound muffles.	9. This point represents the diastolic pressure.
10. Remove the cuff from the patient's arm. Position patient comfortably; supply stimulation activity as necessary.	10. If you want to repeat the reading, wait at least a full minute after cuff is deflated before reinflating it to allow for unrestricted circulation to arm.
11. Evaluate the effectiveness, efficiency, cost, comfort, and safety of procedure. Record the readings obtained; plan health teaching as necessary (for example, inform patient about the importance of knowing his blood pressure).	11. Document patient status and nursing care; health teaching is an independent nursing action always included in care.

MODIFICATIONS FOR CARE OF CHILD

Blood pressures are rarely taken in a child under 3 because the sight of equipment often makes him cry, which causes blood pressure to rise and therefore be inaccurate. With preschoolers and early schoolage children, take a minute to explain that the cuff will not hurt (it "hugs" their arm) so that they will not be unnecessarily frightened by a painless procedure.

MODIFICATIONS FOR CARE OF OLDER ADULT

People with arteriosclerosis tend to have auscultatory gaps in blood pressure. To be certain that you have inflated the cuff above this point, palpate the brachial artery as you inflate the cuff; inflate to a point above which you can no longer feel the pulse sensation.

OBSERVATION OF PULSE POINTS

Ordinarily the only points where you can actually observe a pulse are the carotid artery (in the groove between the trachea and sternocleidomastoid muscle) and the jugular vein (lateral to the sternal notch). There are noticeable fluctuations in many people when they are lying supine at these points. As you elevate the person's head to about 45 degrees, the venous pulsations should disappear; if still present, they suggest extremely strong central venous pressure, which occurs when the heart cannot handle all the blood returning to it.

As mentioned, the heart beat can be palpated at the fifth intercostal chest space in most patients (in slim people and infants, the beat can be observed here as well). This space is referred to as the *point of maximum impulse* (PMI); it represents ventricular contraction, or systole. A heart beat apparent elsewhere in the chest suggests that the heart is beating very forcefully as the result of blood overload.

PULSE SITES

Common arterial pulse sites are shown in Fig. 31-2. Table 31-2 describes common arterial sites used to measure pulse rate. A pulse can be palpated wherever an artery courses near the skin surface and has a bone or other firm structure immediately below it to provide a point of pressure. The most common site used in adults and children is the radial artery; in infants peripheral pulses may be difficult to palpate, so the apical heart rate is more often routinely assessed. The best point at which to palpate the radial artery is by the radius (below the thumb on the inner surface of the wrist). The brachial artery courses in the groove between the biceps and triceps muscles just at the inner surface of the elbow (antecubital fossa). This is the artery you palpate to determine proper placement of your stethoscope for a blood pressure reading also.

The temporal artery is a good pulse site to use with people who have large dressings, bruises, or other obstructions to usual sites. The best site to palpate this pulse is the temple area between the eye and hairline. The bone that you press against is the temporal.

The carotid artery is the major artery supplying the head; it is a pulse site used in cardiopulmonary resuscitation because it is the pulse closest to you when you are doing external cardiac massage or mouth-to-mouth ventilation. The best place to locate this pulse is lateral to the trachea at the level of the larynx. Remember that the blood supply to the head is carried by this artery; never palpate for over a minute at this site so as not to obscure blood flow to the head for too long (the person will feel faint from lack of cerebral blood supply). Never palpate both carotid arteries at the same time, which would totally obstruct blood flow to the head. Because palpating carotid arteries can slow heart rate due to special receptors present, never use a carotid artery as a routine pulse site.

The femoral artery crosses the groin just slightly on the medial side of the thigh. It is bordered by muscles on the sides and the inguinal ligament just superior to it.

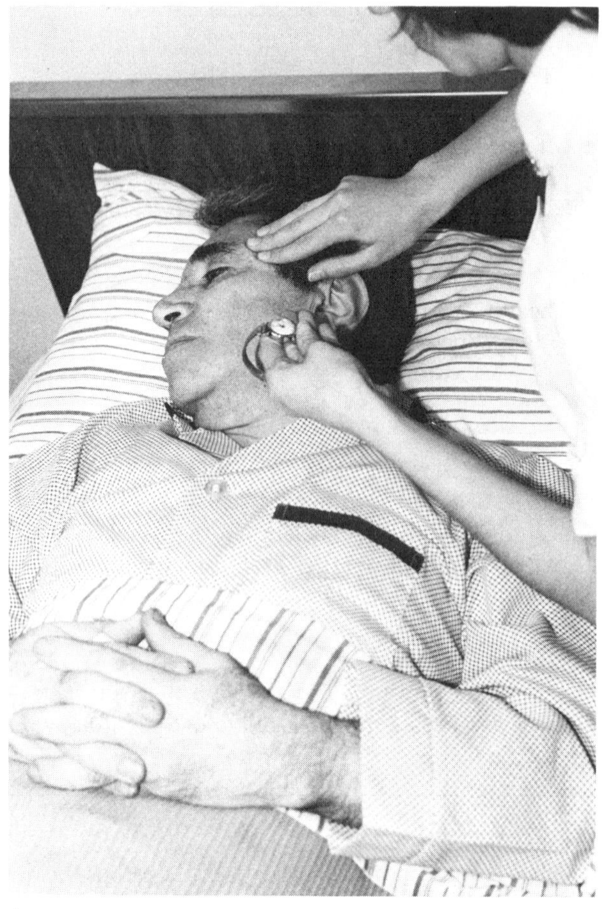
A

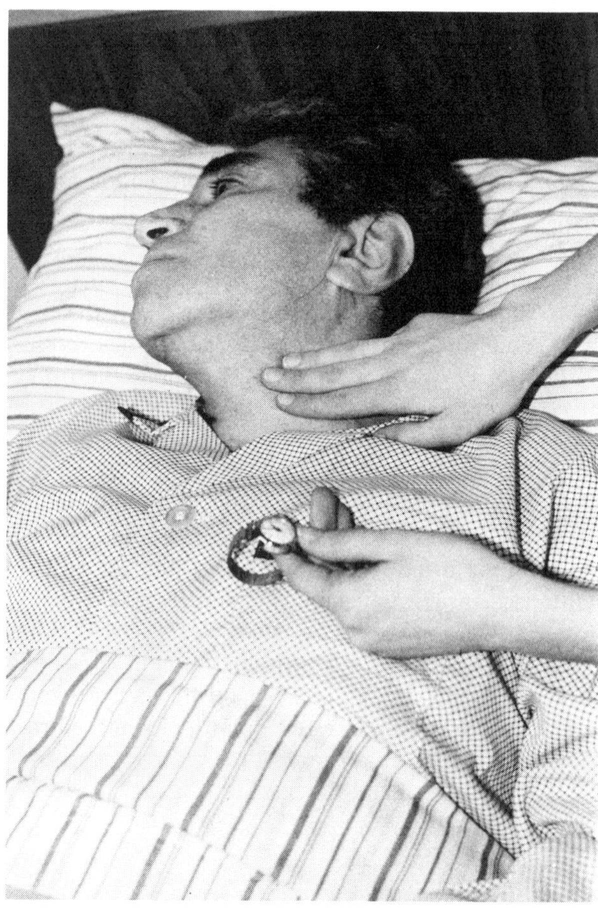
B

FIGURE 31-2. Common sites for taking pulses. A. Temporal. B. Carotid. C. Brachial. D. Radial. E. Apical. F. Femoral. G. Popliteal. H. Posterior tibial. I. Dorsalis pedis.

That femoral artery pulsations are present in newborns is important as it rules out a common cardiac defect (stenosis of the aorta); with aortic stenosis, not enough blood reaches the lower extremities to make femoral pulses palpable.

The popliteal is a possible, but not common, site for pulse assessment because it is only a continuation of the femoral artery and is difficult to locate in many people. The best place to palpate it is at the popliteal fossa (the back of the knee) along the outer surface of the medial tendon. The pulse is apparent if you bend the person's knee 45 degrees before beginning palpation. It is often easier to obtain with the person in a prone position.

The dorsalis pedis (pedal) pulse is helpful in showing that circulation to distal lower extremities is present. The pulse is located on the top surface of the foot (dorsum) just lateral to the extensor tendon of the large toe. A lesser used site that evaluates the efficiency of lower extremity circulation is the posterior tibial pulse (located just behind the medial malleolus). These pulses are assessed following leg surgery or if a cast, splint, or other possibly constricting apparatus is in place to determine whether good circulation to the leg is present. Popliteal, posterior tibial, and pedal pulses are not assessed for rate as much as for presence and quality. They are often compared bilaterally.

TECHNIQUE FOR EVALUATING PULSES

If the pattern of a pulse rate is regular, you can count it for 15 seconds and multiply by 4 to determine the person's pulse rate per minute. If it is not regular, you must count the rate for a full minute. Before you begin to take a pulse, be certain that the person is in a comfortable position since you do not know how long you will need to count. If he is lying supine, place his forearm across his chest and his palm downward; if he is sitting, bend his elbow 90 degrees and rest the elbow on the chair armrest. Gently place three of your fingertips on the designated pulse point with very light pressure. If you press on the artery too strongly, you will obscure blood flow and so not be able to feel a pulse any longer. Never palpate for a pulse with your thumb, which has such a strong pulse that it is possible to feel your own pulse when you press with it. Table 31-4 summarizes factors that influence pulse rate.

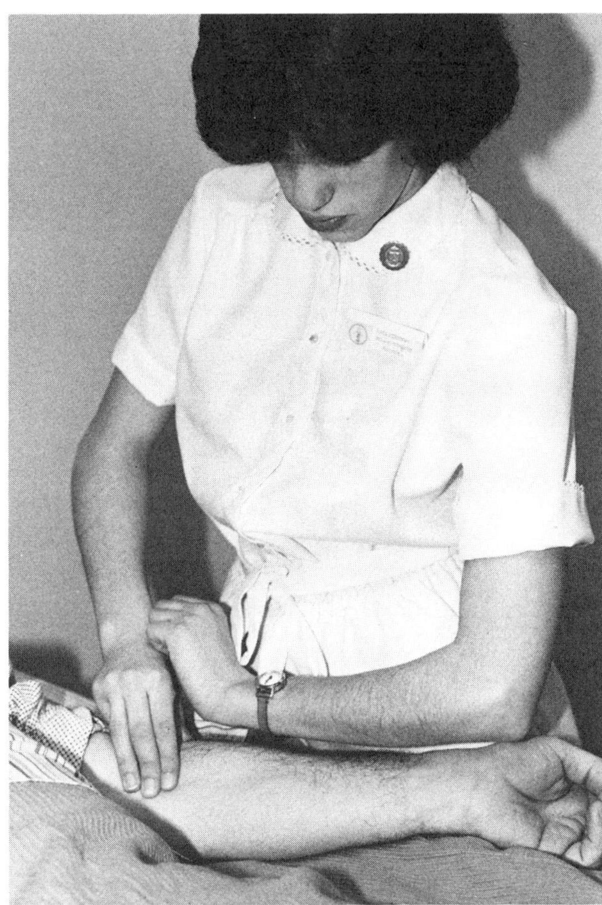

C

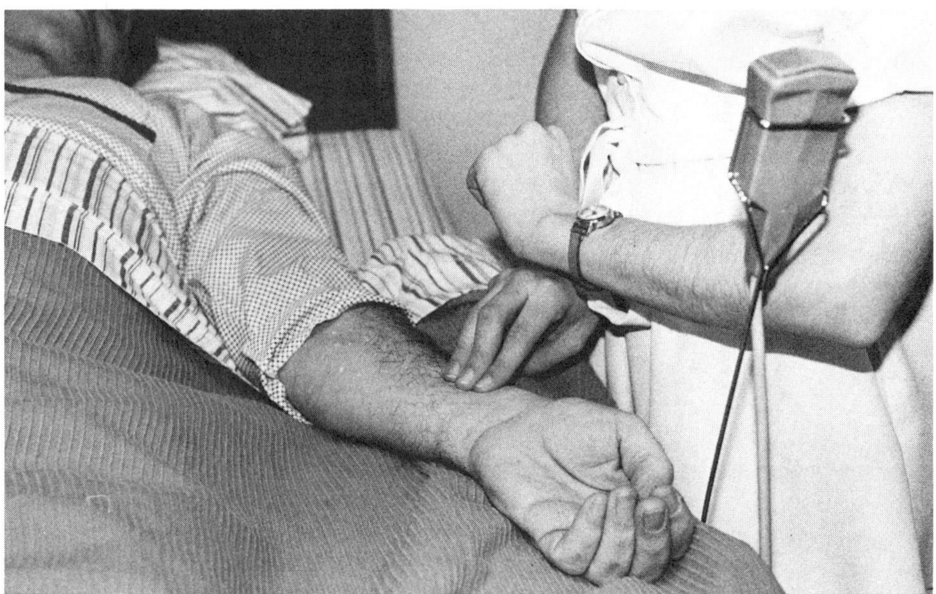

D

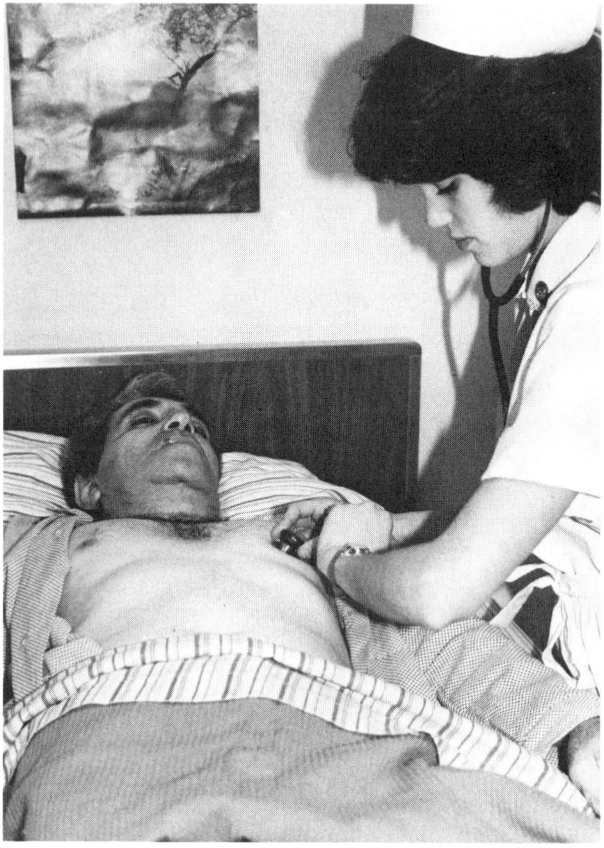

E

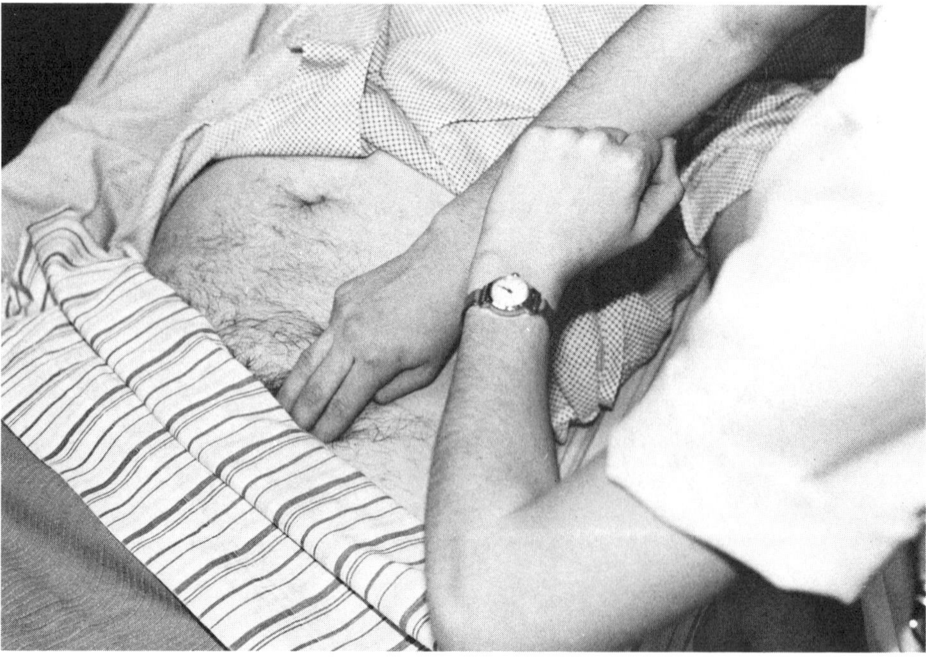

F

FIGURE 31-2 (CONTINUED)

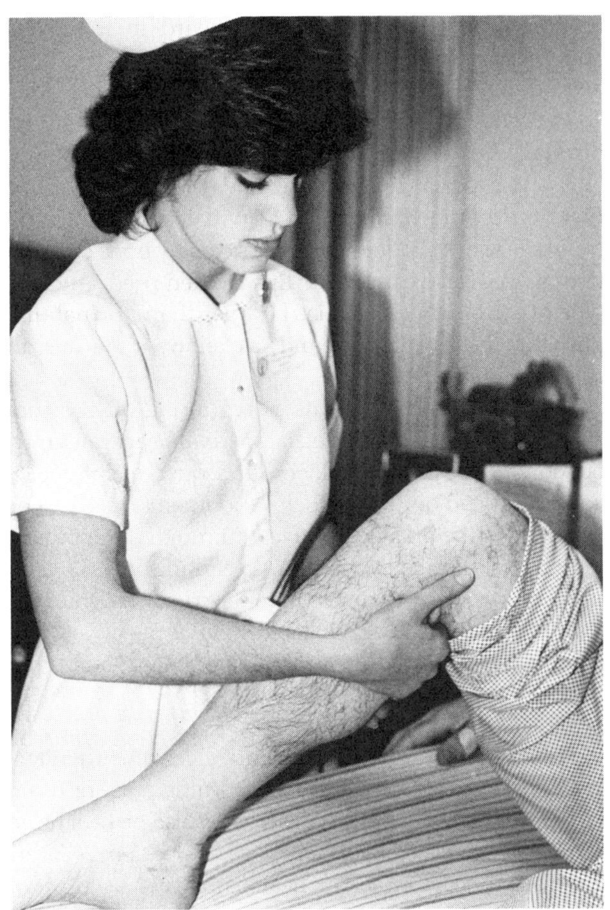

G

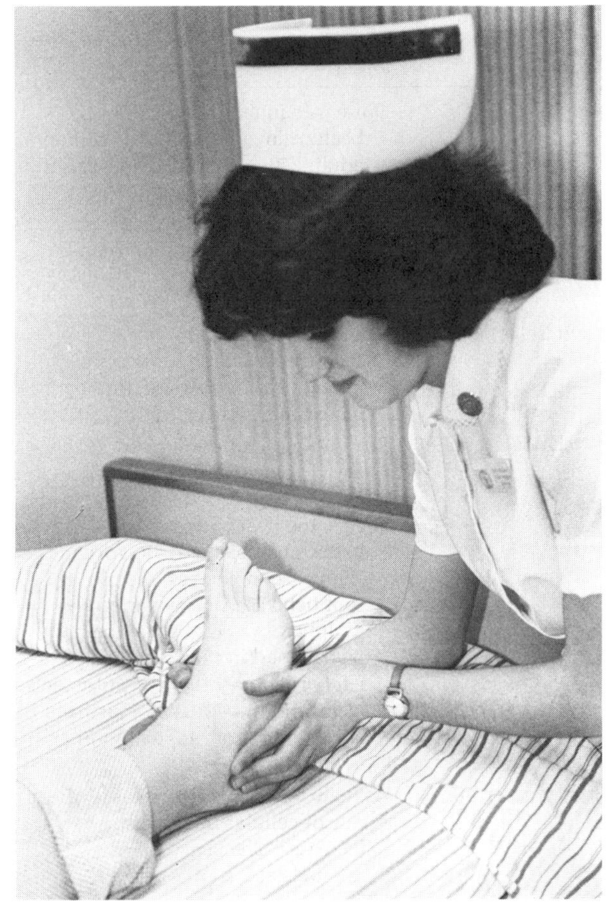

H

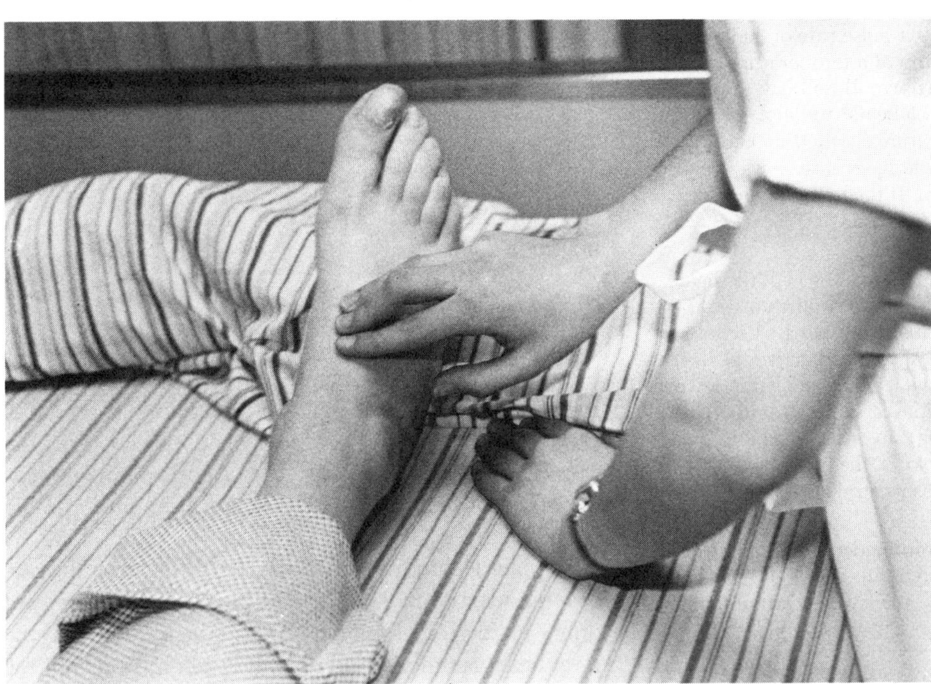

I

TABLE 31-4. FACTORS THAT INFLUENCE PULSE RATE

Factor	Influence
Age	Pulse rate in fetal life is 120—160 beats/min; at birth, 120—160; in adults, 70—80; it increases slightly again in the older adult.
Sex	Women tend to have a pulse rate slightly more rapid than men but still within the normal 70—80 beats/min.
Exercise	The heart increases its rate to supply the increased amount of oxygen needed during exercise, thus increasing pulse rate.
Psychological state	Stress of either a physical or psychological nature initiates a general adaptation response. With this, the heart rate increases to better push blood to vital organs. With excessive stress, there may be so much vasoconstriction to the peripheral vessels (while the body holds blood in the central core for vital organ use) that the pulse feels weak and thready. You may need to assess an apical rate to obtain an accurate rate.
Body temperature	As body temperature increases, the rate of cellular metabolism increases. The heart increases its rate to better supply oxygen to cells. The pulse rate rises about 5 beats/min for each degree of temperature elevation (a person who has a pulse rate of 80 beats/min at a temperature of 98.6°F (normal) will have a pulse rate of 85 beats/min at a temperature elevated to 99.6°F). Low body temperature slows heart function. If the body should be cooled as low as 84°F, heart function halts.
Body position	For blood to move through the heart of a person in a supine position, the heart must work harder because a great deal of blood arrives at the vena cava (none is pooled in lower extremities as happens with standing). In order to handle this excess blood, the heart both increases its stroke volume and rate.
Blood volume	If blood volume decreases, the heart will increase its rate to try to circulate the lowered amount of blood present more rapidly.

FETAL HEART SOUNDS

Fetal heart rate is used to diagnose pregnancy and to assess the health of the growing fetus.

Fetal heart sounds may be heard through the abdomen when the mother is about four and one-half months pregnant. They are best heard in the lower abdomen (right or left) if the fetus is positioned with his head down (vertex position) or upper abdomen if his head is superior (breech position), and are best heard through the fetal back.

In order to hear fetal heart sounds best, a stethoscope that fits over the examiner's head with a metal band and conducts sounds to the examiner's ears by bone conduction as well as the usual ear tips is often used. Another type of stethoscope used has a larger than normal diaphragm (the extra weight and size allows it to transmit sound better).

Fetal heart sounds are assessed during all prenatal visits as well as labor. During labor, fetal heart rates may be monitored by the Doppler or ultrasound technique by a monitor lead on the mother's abdomen (Fig. 31-3) or detected by the insertion of a lead through the mother's vagina and uterine cervix that is then fixed to the fetal scalp. It is very reassuring to parents to hear the sound of their baby's heart beat while he is in utero: Always give parents the opportunity. Normal fetal heart sounds are 120 to 160 beats per minute.

Electronic Monitoring. A number of electronic monitoring techniques are available for recording pulse or heart rate. These are generally used when pulse or heart rate needs to be assessed continually, as in a patient recovering from a heart attack or heart surgery.

Photocells. Photocells are small fingertip-sized leads that can be attached to peripheral body parts such as the ear and, by bouncing light off moving red blood cells, project a pulse pattern on a monitor screen. By comparing such a readout with an electrocardiogram done at the same time, it can be demonstrated that each ventricular contraction of the person does carry a discernible wave into the peripheral circulation or that heart action is adequate.

Doppler Technique. With the Doppler technique, high frequency sound waves are "bounced off" body tissue; the rate and pitch at which they return demonstrate the movement and density of the underlying tissue. If a Doppler transducer is placed over a pulse point, the pulse can be converted either into a pattern on an oscilloscope that can be read like a graph or into audible sound (Fig. 31-3).

Doppler technique is used frequently to count the rate of fetal heart sounds as the audible beating assures not only you and the physician but also the mother that the fetal heart is functioning well. It is a helpful technique for evaluating lower extremity pulsations.

Skin Color

If blood vessels are constricted, the color of the overlying skin is pale compared to normal skin. The skin may also feel cool rather than warm, a phenomenon caused by

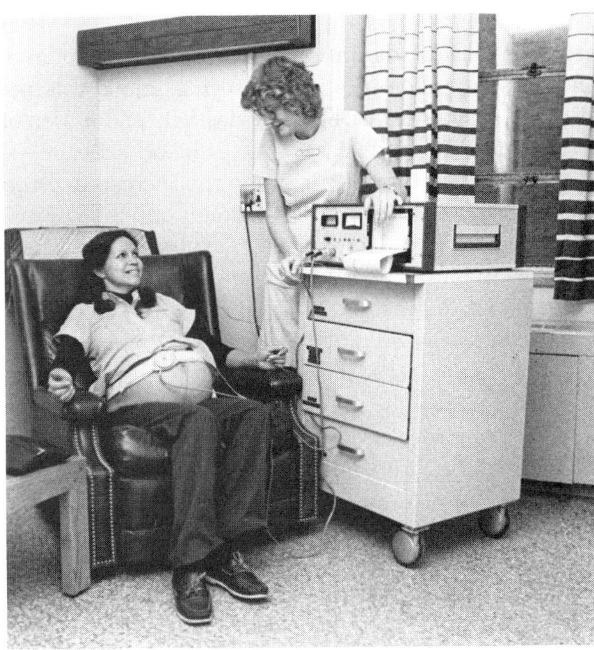

FIGURE 31-3. External monitoring of fetal heart sounds by ultrasonic technique, shown here in an ambulatory setting. Notice the lead on the mother's abdomen attached to the monitor that records the fetal heart rate.

arteriosclerosis, which lessens the lumen of a blood vessel and thus reduces the amount of blood circulating through it. Vasoconstriction occurs in response to cold, stress, vasoconstricting agents (including cigarettes), and a number of peripheral vessel diseases.

With vasodilatation, the area appears reddened and will feel warm to touch. Vasodilatation occurs in response to warmth, inflammation, increased metabolic rate, fever, and infection. Mottling (blue-gray patches on the skin) suggests generalized but irregular peripheral vascular constriction due either to exposure to cold or vascular disease.

People with fewer than normal red blood cells (anemia) often appear pale; people with lower than normal blood pressure, or constriction to a body part, have poor capillary filling—if you press on a body part (for instance, a fingernail), it blanches white immediately, but the color takes longer than usual to return (normal filling time is under 3 seconds). Mucous membrane, such as the oral mucosa, or the conjunctiva of the eyelid may appear very pale. It is more difficult to assess changes in skin color in black patients. Buccal membrane is most indicative of color changes.

Edema

Edema is the collection of fluid in subcutaneous tissue. It occurs in circulatory disease when the heart is unable to handle the blood load returning to it. This backlog of blood leads to increased pressure in the venous circulation, which causes fluid to shift from the bloodstream into the subcutaneous tissue (fluid shifts from an area of higher hydrostatic pressure to one of lower hydrostatic pressure). Edema tends to be dependent (will occur in the lowest body parts). In an ambulatory person, feet and lower legs will be most edematous. For a person on bedrest, his buttocks and posterior lower legs will be edematous; if he sleeps supine without a pillow, his face may be so edematous in the morning that he may be unable to open his eyes or move his tongue.

The degree of edema present is rated on a 4+ scale (see Fig. 25-2), ranging from 4+ (the greatest degree of edema) to 0 (no edema). When edema is most extensive or intense, it is termed *pitting edema:* When your finger is pressed against the skin, it sinks in and actually leaves an indentation (pit) once it is removed.

Urine Output

The kidney filters the blood that passes through it to extract fluid for excretion. Kidney output depends, therefore, on the amount of blood passing through the kidney (reduced blood flow will cause reduced urine output). The main reason why fluid filters from the bloodstream to the kidney glomeruli is that hydrostatic pressure in the bloodstream is greater than that in the kidney. Consequently, whenever blood pressure decreases, not enough pressure in the blood vessel side will be present to effect adequate filtration, and urine output will be decreased.

It is easy to think of urine output as measuring mainly kidney function and overlook the importance of urine output as a major means of circulatory assessment as well.

Varicosities

Varicosities or varicose veins are tortuous, bulging veins. Varicosities tend to occur as a complication of pregnancy or an abdominal tumor causing increased intraabdominal pressure. In most instances, the collection of blood in lower extremity veins has become so great that the vein valves can no longer move the blood appropriately; the vein becomes so distended that actual destruction occurs to its wall, causing it never to return to its former shape (Fig. 31-4).

People with varicosities often experience an aching feeling in their legs on standing over a period of time. They are at risk following surgery or any period of immobility because blood cannot flow normally through such distended veins and, as a result, the chance of venous thrombus (blood clot) is greater than in the person with better circulatory function.

Arteriosclerosis and Atherosclerosis

Arteriosclerosis is the hardening and narrowing of arteries due to the effects of aging. Atherosclerosis is the deposition of fatty plaques in the lumen of arteries (which narrows the lumens). Atherosclerosis tends to be

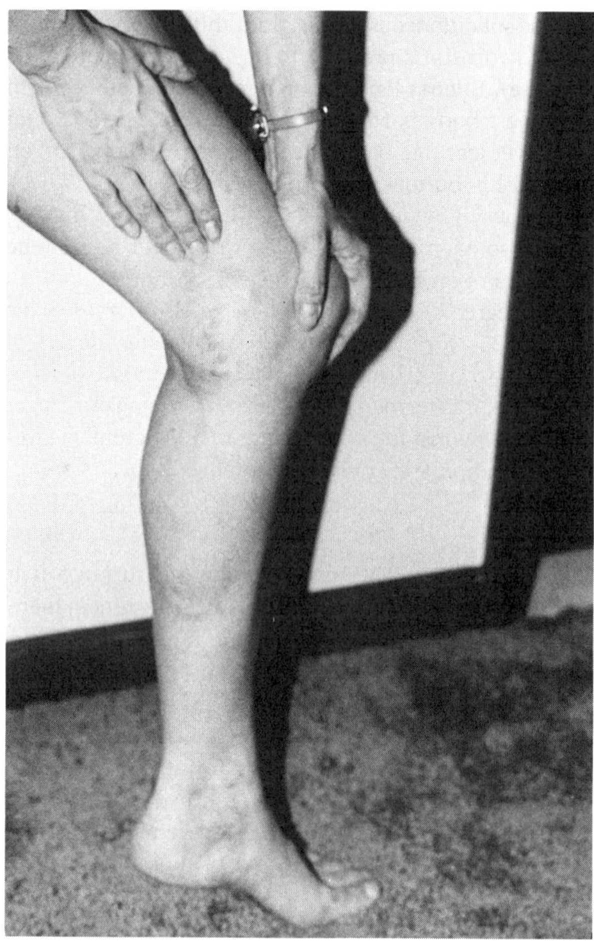

FIGURE 31-4. Varicosities are tortuous distended veins; thrombophlebitis develops readily in them.

familial and increase with age. That either arteriosclerosis or atherosclerosis is present can best be detected by estimating the quality of blood vessels when you take a pulse (does the vessel feel springy or hard under your touch?) and by testing for capillary filling (blanching of fingerbeds) and venous filling (hold an extremity below heart level and watch for filling of the veins; normal time is 5 seconds).

Blood Pressure

Blood pressure (the force exerted by arterial blood against vessel walls) is a common health assessment measure today; it is not an old assessment measure. It was not until 1855 that a technique of using counterpressure to record the finding was discovered. Up until the 1940s, the technique was considered so complicated that it was a physician's, not a nurse's, responsibility.

THE BASIS OF BLOOD PRESSURE

The force or pressure of blood against arterial walls is a product of heart rate plus stroke volume (the cardiac output) times the resistance to blood flow in the vessels (peripheral vascular resistance). Any change in heart rate, volume, or vessel resistance will influence blood pressure. Because they affect heart rate, stroke volume, and resistance to vessels factors such as blood volume, viscosity, response to stress, and elasticity and lumen of vessels are indirect determinants of blood pressure.

When cardiac output or resistance is increased, blood pressure will increase. When cardiac output or resistance is decreased, blood pressure will decrease. There are receptors in the aortic arch and carotid artery that are sensitive to blood pressure; if they detect a high or low pressure, the circulatory system can adjust by altering heart rate. The presence of these receptors is another reason why carotid arteries are not routine sites for pulse pressure measurements. Pressure on the carotid arteries from an external force such as your fingertips may be interpreted by these receptors as elevated blood pressure, and the person's heart rate may reflexly slow.

An elevated blood pressure (over 140/90 in adults) is termed *hypertension;* a decreased one (under 95/60 in adults) is *hypotension.* Table 31-5 summarizes factors that influence blood pressure.

AVERAGE BLOOD PRESSURE

Like average pulse rate, average blood pressure varies greatly. An average blood pressure in newborns is difficult to measure accurately but is about 80/45. This pressure gradually increases in life until it reaches an adult average of 140/90; 170/95 for the older adult. Blood pressure for all age groups is listed in Table 31-6.

Notice that there is no difference in blood pressure between girls and boys until puberty. After puberty, women tend to have a slightly lower blood pressure than men. Blood pressure is generally lowest in the early morning when basal metabolism rate is slowest due to sleep; the level rises slightly during the day to correspond with the increase in basal metabolism rate until it reaches a peak at late afternoon or early evening; it then declines again. This circadian rhythm explains why a blood pressure recording ordered once daily should be taken approximately the same time each day, not in the morning one day and the afternoon the next.

Sodium (table salt) can lead to elevated blood pressure because it tends to hold fluid in the body, thereby increasing the total circulatory load and the peripheral resistance. It is important to remember when recording blood pressure that exercise also affects the level. Blood pressure is most accurate when a person has been resting for 5 minutes prior to the recording. Some people have a noticeable difference (up to 20 mm Hg) in blood pressure between their right and left arm. To avoid having this finding interfere with blood pressure recording, as well as causing other health providers to check continually which site was used last, always take a person's blood pressure in his left arm unless contraindicated by reasons such as bulky dressings or intravenous therapy in that arm (see QRS 31-1).

TABLE 31-5. FACTORS THAT INFLUENCE BLOOD PRESSURE

Factor	Influence	Blood Pressure Effect
Age	Blood pressure increases with age since the larger the circulatory space, the more force is necessary.	↑
Exercise	Increases stroke volume of heart.	↑
Fever	Increases metabolic rate, which increases stroke volume and rate.	↑
Exposure to cold	Causes vasoconstriction with increased vessel resistance.	↑
Psychological stress	Increases heart rate.	↑
Polycythemia (increased number of red blood cells)	Increases viscosity of blood and peripheral resistance.	↑
Vascular fluid overload	Increases amount of blood to be moved, which increases heart rate.	↑
Arteriosclerosis or atherosclerosis	Decreases elasticity of vessel walls and increases peripheral resistance.	↑
Obesity	More force is needed to pump blood through bigger system.	↑
Exposure to warmth	Causes vasodilation with decreased vessel resistance.	↓
Hemmorrhage	Decreases blood volume and vascular resistance.	↓
Anemia (less than average number of red blood cells)	Decreases blood viscosity and vascular resistance.	↓
Decreased heart action	Decreases cardiac output.	↓

TABLE 31-6. BLOOD PRESSURE FOR DIFFERENT AGE GROUPS

Age	Blood Pressure (mm Hg)
Newborn	80/45
Infant	90/60
3—6 years	110/70
7—10 years	120/80
11—15 years	130/80
15—20 years	130/85
20—40 years	140/90
40—60 years	160/95
60—75 years	170/95
Over 75 years	180/100

Source: From the American Heart Association.

☐ QUICK REFERENCE STOP 31-1: NUTRITION

Nutrition influences blood pressure levels in the form of obesity (a condition generally attributed to poor nutrition), which increases blood pressure. A high salt level (salt retains fluid) increases the blood volume and also increases blood pressure. A high intake of triglycerides and sterols may be responsible for atherosclerotic plaques in susceptible individuals; atherosclerosis increases blood pressure because it narrows the lumen of arteries.

A diet too low in iron may lead to anemia (reduced number of red blood cells); the heart beats faster to try to better oxygenate body cells. Low blood viscosity from anemia may lower blood pressure; the faster heart rate may increase blood pressure.

ORTHOSTATIC HYPOTENSION

Normally blood pressure increases slightly on standing (the heart has to work harder to push against gravity). Orthostatic hypotension is a low blood pressure caused by the effect of standing. Some people have such a noticeable orthostatic hypotension change that they typically experience vertigo (dizziness) on rising rapidly. Such a person has to learn to rise slowly from a lying to sitting or a sitting to standing position. If he does experience acute vertigo, sitting down and lowering his head or lying down again will immediately restore adequate pressure.

If a person has been immobile for a long period of time (days to weeks), orthostatic hypotension is very apparent the first time he is helped out of bed. For this reason, help a patient who has had surgery or been on bedrest to sit up for the first time in set stages (sitting on the side of the bed first [dangling], standing before attempting to walk, etc.).

SUPINE HYPOTENSION

When a pregnant woman lies on her back (supine), the weight of the filled uterus presses against the vena cava and blocks return of blood from the lower extremities. The woman is suddenly hypotensive, just as if she had lost this amount of blood from her circulatory system. She develops symptoms of vertigo, shortness of breath, and heart palpations. To restore her blood pressure quickly, turn her to her left side (which removes the uterine pressure from the vena cava and restores blood volume). The same phenomena can occur in a patient with an abdominal obstruction or tumor that causes the same sort of pressure disturbance.

RECORDING BLOOD PRESSURE

Blood pressure can be recorded by direct or indirect methods. Indirect methods are commonly used because they are nonintrusive. The most frequently used indirect method is to apply counterpressure against an artery wall until the external pressure applied is greater than the internal pressure present. This collapses (or nearly collapses) the artery walls. When you gradually lessen the external pressure, a number of phenomena occur.

Systolic Pressure. When an artery blood flow is completely occluded due to high external pressure, you can hear no sound of blood flowing when listening to the artery with a stethoscope. As you gradually reduce the amount of external pressure present to the point at which the external pressure is less than the pressure in the artery, you will hear the sound of this initial blood flow (a sharp tapping sound). This sound is termed the *systolic pressure,* and reflects the maximum force of blood in the system during ventricular contraction (systole).

Diastolic Pressure. As you continue to decrease your external pressure, the blood in the artery continues to flow easier and faster. At the point at which the external pressure equals that of the blood flow, the sound you hear "damps" or muffles to a sound described as blowing rather than sharp or tapping. This point of muffling is the *diastolic pressure,* and reflects the lowest level of pressure in the circulatory system (relaxation of the ventricles or diastole). Diastolic pressure will be abnormally high in people who have increased resistance in artery walls (hardened arteries); it will be abnormally low in people who have shunts between blood vessels or active bleeding.

Korotkoff's Sounds. Korotkoff was a Russian surgeon who first appreciated the significance of the sounds heard with blood pressure determination. Table 31-7 summarizes the four distinct sounds (or lack of sound) that you hear on blood pressure assessment as you deflate the external pressure.

Pulse Pressure. The difference between systolic and diastolic readings is the pulse pressure, the value of which normally ranges from 40 to 60 mm Hg. It will be reduced if there is little arterial compliance (diastolic pressure is increased because there is never a totally low point of pressure); it may be wide if a shunt for blood is present (diastolic pressure is greatly reduced) or cardiac stroke volume is great (systolic pressure is great).

TABLE 31-7. KOROTKOFF'S SOUNDS

Phase	Sound Heard	Importance
I	Sound is first heard as a sharp tapping sound.	Systolic pressure
II	Sound changes and has a murmuring quality.	
III	Sound is crisper, more intense.	
IV	Sound is muffled or damped.	Diastolic pressure
V	Sound disappears (can no longer be heard).	

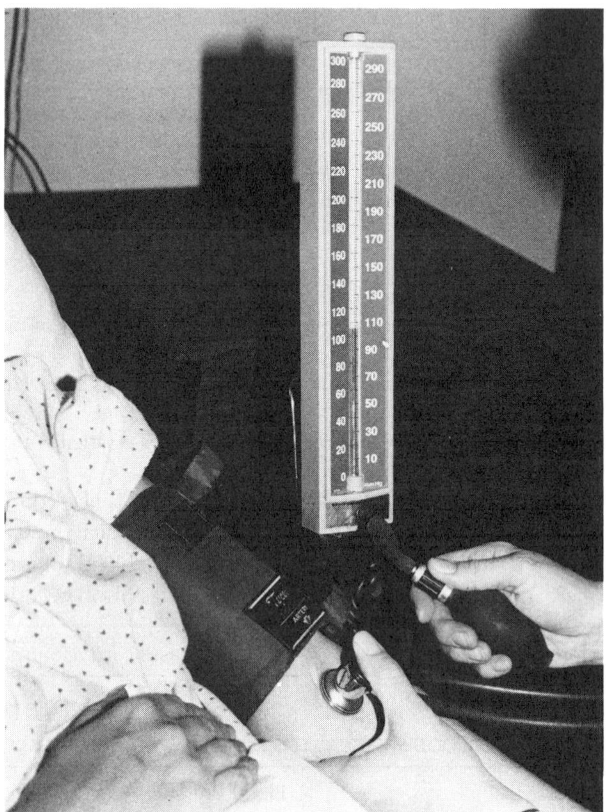

FIGURE 31-5. Blood pressure taken by a mercury sphygomomanometer. Notice how the left hand supports both the elbow and the stethoscope.

Blood Pressure Recording Equipment. The instrument used to measure blood pressure is a sphygomomanometer. Two types are available: one works by measuring resistance to mercury and the other by measuring resistance to air (an aneroid model). Both are accurate and consist of three main parts—a pressure manometer, an inflatable rubber bladder cuff (covered with a cloth sleeve), and a pressure bulb to inflate and deflate the cuff.

A mercury sphygomomanometer (Fig. 31-5) has a large glass cylinder filled with mercury, similar to a glass thermometer. As you inflate the pressure cuff, the mercury level in the cylinder rises; as you release the pressure cuff, the mercury level falls. By reading the number on the cylinder at the point when you hear the first Korotkoff's sound and the damping of sound, you establish your blood pressure reading. The measure used is millimeters of mercury (mm Hg).

An aneroid manometer (Fig. 31-6) contains a small bellows with a round pressure gauge. As the bellows

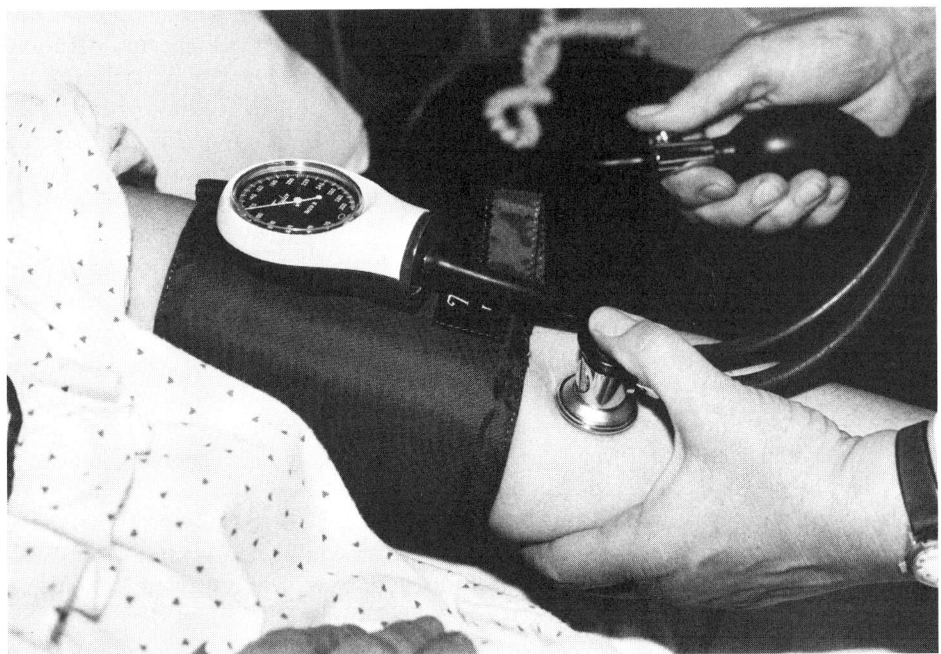

FIGURE 31-6. Aneroid sphygomomanometer used in blood pressure reading.

expands with pressure, the needle in the circular gauge registers a high number; as the bellows deflates, the needle indicator falls. Although such a meter uses air, it is also read in millimeters of mercury.

Mercury sphygomomanometers need never be recalibrated (realigned to be accurate); disadvantages of using them are their bulk and the need to maintain the mercury column in an upright position during use. An aneroid system needs to be recalibrated at least once yearly to ensure its accuracy; it has the advantage of being smaller and more easily portable and so more useful in confined patient care spaces. Be certain that the gauge registers zero before beginning or has been recalibrated accurately.

The usual problem in taking blood pressure does not concern, however, the manometer but the selection of proper cuff size. This proper size is two-thirds the length of the patient's upper arm, or 20 percent greater than the diameter of the upper arm (comparable measurements are used for a lower extremity). If a cuff is too narrow, the blood pressure reading will be abnormally high because so much extra pressure is necessary to compress the artery; a too wide cuff will give a false low reading as the artery is too easily compressed. Table 31-8 lists normal blood pressure cuff sizes.

If a person is going to have several blood pressures recorded (once every day, 4 times daily, every 15 minutes, etc.), mark on the person's care plan the size cuff and type of sphygomomanometer you used for the baseline measurement so that any differences in subsequent readings truly reflect a change in blood pressure and not merely a difference in equipment.

TABLE 31-8. NORMAL BLOOD PRESSURE CUFF SIZE

Age Group	Size (cm)
Newborn	2.5—3
Infant	3—5
Child	5—8
Adult	12—14
Obese adult	18—20

The other piece of equipment necessary for blood pressure recording is a functioning stethoscope. (Blood pressure can be determined by palpation and observation, but only the systolic reading can be recorded by these methods, which are not as trustworthy as an auscultatory technique.) Be sure that the diaphragm of the chosen stethoscope is small enough to fit comfortably over the brachial artery in the antecubital space. Too large a diaphragm does not fit snugly enough for you to discern the muffling of sound that indicates the diastolic pressure.

Technique of Blood Pressure Recording. Blood pressure readings are affected by exercise, psychological stress, and body position. Be certain that the person has been resting (or at least engaged in a sedentary activity) for 5 to 10 minutes before a recording. For best accuracy, take blood pressure on the left arm with the person either sitting or lying down (see Procedure 31-4). The room must be quiet for you to hear sounds accurately; you may have to ask visitors or the patient himself to restrain from talking while you listen to the sounds.

The best artery to compress and listen to is the brachial artery in the medial side of the antecubital fossa (inner surface of the elbow). Be certain that the cuff size you have chosen is correct (two-thirds the distance of the upper arm) and that the rubber inflatable bladder of the cuff is completely deflated. Because rubber can be irritating to skin, cuffs have removable and washable cloth covers. Wrap the deflated cuff around the person's upper bare arm and fasten it securely (most brands have velcro or hook and eye fasteners). Attempting to place a cuff over clothing will lead to an abnormal pressure reading since the cuff then has to compress the cloth as well. Locate the brachial artery by the antecubital fossa by palpating it with your fingertip (the cuff must be above this spot before you can palpate accurately). Place the diaphragm of your stethoscope firmly over the brachial artery at the spot where you palpated it; fit the stethoscope tips into your ears. Inflate the pressure cuff of the apparatus by pumping the pressure bulb until the mercury column or aneroid gauge reads a pressure approximately 40 mm Hg over the person's systolic measurement. (An adult's pressure is normally 140/90, so inflate to about 180 mm Hg; a newborn's normal pressure is 80/45, so inflate to 120 mm Hg.)

If you are unaware of the person's previous blood pressure reading or have reason to think his pressure is higher or lower than normal, you can palpate the brachial artery while you inflate the cuff. Inflate until the pulse disappears and then continue until the reading has increased about 40 mm Hg. Now position your stethoscope for listening.

Before deflating the cuff, you should hear no Korotkoff's sounds through the stethoscope. Release the pressure bulb slowly and regularly while you listen. Note the point at which you first hear sound (systolic reading) and the point at which the sound muffles (diastolic reading).

At one time, the fifth Korotkoff's sound (the point at which the sounds disappeared) was considered the diastolic pressure. Although the American Heart Association has determined that the muffling of the sounds is a more accurate point for a diastolic reading than the disappearance of the sounds, there is still some controversy. In cases where medication administration is based on blood pressure measurements, you may be asked to record both these points or to record a blood pressure with three instead of two numbers (120/70/40, not 120/70).

If you are distracted while recording a blood pressure, completely deflate the cuff and allow at least a minute to pass before reinflating the cuff (compressing the artery) and repeating the reading to allow a surge of blood to enter the arm and supply nutrients to cells.

Auscultatory Gaps. In some individuals, particularly those with hypertension, immediately after you hear the first Korotkoff's sound, you suddenly hear nothing; at a point 30 to 40 mm Hg below this, sounds are recognizable again and continue to be present normally until they muffle and disappear. This gap in sound is termed an *auscultatory gap*. It can lead to an inaccurate reading if the point between the gap is interpreted as the systolic pressure rather than the first sound heard. An auscultatory gap should be suspected if you have an unreasonably low systolic blood pressure reading (a young healthy male has a blood pressure of 90/70).

Paradoxical Blood Pressure. With a paradoxical blood pressure, Korotkoff's sounds are clear and sharp on expiration, but become faint and difficult to auscultate on inspiration. Although rare, this can occur if the person is breathing very deeply or has an abnormal amount of pressure on the heart (for instance, from accumulated blood in the chest). With a paradoxical blood pressure, be careful not to confuse a hard-to-hear point of sounds with the muffling of sound (the diastolic pressure). If the person holds his breath while you auscultate, this variation in the strength of beats will not occur (but such a request is unreasonable if he is breathing deeply because short of breath). Palpating to determine the systolic pressure may be helpful.

Palpating Blood Pressure. It is possible to palpate a systolic blood pressure and, in some instances of very low blood pressure, necessary because you cannot auscultate one. To record this, merely rest a fingertip on the brachial artery in the antecubital space while you inflate the cuff. The point at which you can first palpate a pulse as you deflate the cuff is the systolic pressure.

You cannot obtain a diastolic reading by this method, and the systolic pressure you record is probably 5 to 10 mm Hg lower than the reading you would obtain by auscultation. The method is not used as a routine method of blood pressure reading but is a useful emergency technique. When charting a blood pressure taken by this method, note only the systolic number; then write "P" or "Palpated" to account for the single number.

You can also determine a systolic pressure by inflating a cuff and observing the mercury column or aneroid needle as the cuff is decreased. The mercury column or needle will begin to jiggle at the level of the systolic pressure. This method is very inaccurate; it is helpful if you are teaching a person to take his own blood pressure since you can determine whether his systolic reading value is accurate (your instructor uses this method to assess your systolic readings).

Flush Blood Pressure. It is often difficult to locate a blood pressure cuff small enough to record an infant's blood pressure accurately. In these instances you can take blood pressure by a flush method. To do this, apply a blood pressure cuff (size is unimportant) to the child's upper arm. Wrap the extremity from the fingers up to the cuff with an elastic bandage. Inflate the blood pressure cuff to a point about 40 mm Hg over the anticipated blood pressure. Unwrap the bandage. The arm will

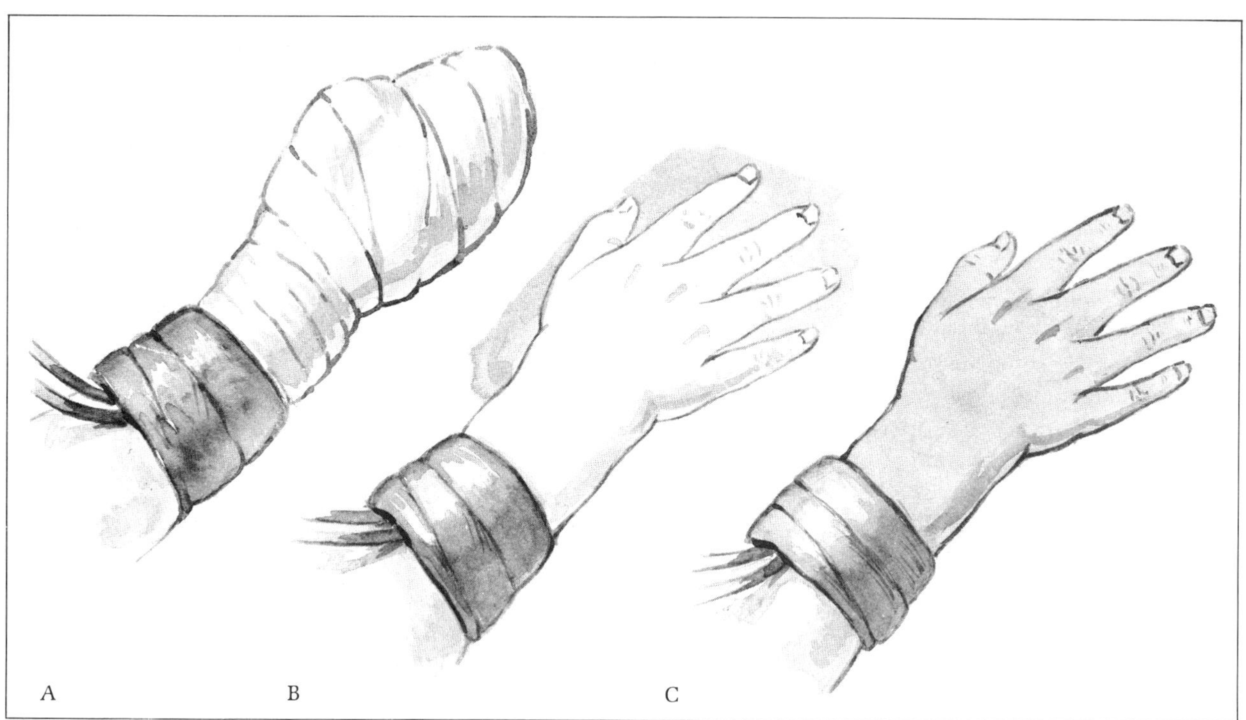

FIGURE 31-7. Flush blood pressure measurement. A. A blood pressure cuff is applied and the distal extremity is wrapped snugly with an Ace bandage. B. The cuff is inflated; the Ace bandage is removed. C. The point at which the distal extremity "flushes" or pinkens as the pressure in the cuff is released is the flush blood pressure. (Courtesy Department of Medical Illustration, State University of New York at Buffalo, Buffalo, New York.)

appear pale because the pressure of the bandage and cuff has caused a great deal of blood to leave the extremity.

To obtain the blood pressure, reduce the cuff pressure gradually, watching the arm for a color change as you do. Read the level at the point that the extremity flushes pink. At this point, blood flows through the extremity again and inner arterial pressure equals your external pressure (Fig. 31-7).

This technique gives you only one reading; record it as "Flush" pressure. A flush pressure is about halfway between the child's systolic and diastolic pressure (if the child's blood pressure is 80/40, his flush pressure will be about 60). Normal flush pressures are shown in Table 31-9.

TABLE 31-9. FLUSH BLOOD PRESSURE IN INFANT ARM

	Blood Pressure (mm Hg)	
Age	Average	Range
1—7 days	41	22—66
1—3 months	67	48—90
4—6 months	73	42—100
7—9 months	76	52—96
10—12 months	57	62—94

Source: From Mass, A. J. Indirect methods of blood pressure measurement. *Pediatr. Clin. North Am.* 25:3, 1978.

Orthostatis Blood Pressure. In some instances an orthostatic blood pressure—an estimation of the difference between a person's blood pressure when supine and that when standing—may be needed. To obtain such a pressure, the person must have been lying flat in bed for at least 5 minutes. Take his blood pressure in this position. Help or ask him to stand and immediately retake his blood pressure in this position.

You may want a second person to help you because a person with orthostatic hypotension grows very dizzy and may actually faint on standing. If you do determine a systolic pressure difference over 10 mm Hg between lying and standing positions, note on the person's nursing care plan that he should always be assisted gradually to a standing or sitting position in order to prevent fainting or extreme vertigo.

The most practical way to obtain an orthostatic blood pressure is to take it first thing in the morning because you can be assured that the person has been lying quietly for an extended time.

Lower Extremity Blood Pressure. Like systolic blood pressure, diastolic pressure is normally 10 to 40 mm Hg higher in the lower extremities than in the upper extremities. If you are unable to obtain upper extremity blood pressure due to the presence of a surgical dressing or intravenous therapy, you can record lower extremity pressure, wrapping the cuff around the thigh and auscultating the popliteal artery at the posterior knee. Lower extremity blood pressure may be asked for in patients with heart disease to establish the person's ability to perfuse lower extremities adequately despite lessened heart action.

Lower extremity blood pressures are more difficult to obtain than upper extremity pressures because many cuffs are not large enough to circle the thigh adequately and the popliteal artery is more difficult to locate and auscultate than the brachial.

Contraindications to Blood Pressure Recording. Because blood vessels are temporarily occluded during a blood pressure reading, it is not good technique to measure blood pressure in an arm or leg if an intravenous infusion is flowing into that extremity. The occlusion may raise the pressure so greatly in the vein that the needle will be dislodged. If the person has had surgery on an extremity (or chest muscle or breast surgery), the resulting edema will distort a blood pressure reading. If the antecubital fossa is not accessible due to constrictive clothing or dressings, you cannot read a blood pressure on that arm. Some solutions to blood pressure assessment problems are provided in the following box.

Trouble-Shooting With Blood Pressure Assessment

Problem	*Possible Solution*
Cuff does not inflate.	Check that tubing connection to manometer is tight. Turn valve on bulb in the opposite direction.
Unable to hear Korotkoff's sounds.	Test whether stethoscope is conducting sound by tapping on diaphragm. Check that stethoscope tips are pointing forward in your ears. Palpate a pressure to locate the systolic point; be certain you inflate cuff over this point.
Person's arm is too contracted for stethoscope to fit snugly against brachial artery.	Use the bell of the stethoscope as it fits better into a smaller space. Ask a second person to help you to position arm better. Consider possibility of a lower extremity blood pressure or a flush pressure.
Reading obtained is probably inaccurate because proper size cuff was not available.	Chart pressure obtained as questionable due to improper size cuff. Question antihypertensive medication administration orders based on inaccurate blood pressure values. Mark the cuff that was used; if the same cuff is used consistently, it will demonstrate *changes* in blood pressure. Report your problem of inadequate equipment to nursing supervisor; saving pennies on equipment can cost a health care facility patient safety.

Electronic Monitoring. With space exploration, it became necessary to monitor pulse and blood pressure readings of astronauts constantly while in space yet leave them freedom of movement. This problem led to the use of electronic monitoring equipment.

ULTRASONIC DOPPLERS. As noted earlier, Doppler technique bounces high frequency sound waves off body parts; the rate and pitch at which they return depend on the density of the body part that is struck. If a Doppler lead is placed over an artery, either the movement of the blood (pulse wave) or the tension of the blood (blood pressure) can be interpreted as a digital readout or a monitor print; Dopplers can be adapted to emit the sound of the pulse waves for auscultatory assessment.

Electronic blood pressure recording is used when an almost continuous assessment is necessary; it is helpful in infants whose blood pressure is difficult to obtain by usual methods and in patients too obese to be fitted with a regular size cuff.

Direct Blood Pressure Measurement. In critical care situations or in diagnoses of heart and blood vessel diseases, blood pressure can be measured directly by insertion of a catheter into an artery. Such a catheter, termed an *indwelling catheter*, is most frequently placed into the radial or femoral artery (under strict aseptic conditions). The catheter is first flushed with dilute heparin to keep blood from clotting in it and then attached by tubing to a pressure sensor or transducer at the patient's bedside. A transducer converts the pressure sensed into electrical energy. The blood pressure reading can be displaced on a monitor as a flickering light, graph, or digital number.

Such equipment works by measuring the internal arterial tension against external air pressure. Never attempt to use this type of equipment until you have been well oriented to it; if you are unfamiliar with the equipment, you may inject the air not into the transducer receptor but into the person's artery. This creates an air embolus, which, because the air blocks the blood supply to the coronary blood vessels, could be lethal.

Direct pressure measurements are used in patients following heart surgery, severe burns, severe heart failure, or cerebrovascular accidents. Cardiac catheterization (insertion of a catheter through the radial or femoral vein into the heart to measure blood pressure levels in the heart chambers) is another form of direct blood pressure measurement. It is a diagnostic technique used to establish the degree of cardiac involvement present prior to cardiac surgery.

The person with an arterial catheter in place must have the extremity distal to the catheter insertion assessed every hour for good circulation (palpate a distal pulse or test for capillary filling) to be certain that the catheter or a hematoma at the insertion site is not obstructing the major circulatory route to the distal extremity.

Hypertension. Although it depends on the individual, hypertension in adults is usually defined as a persistent systolic blood pressure over 140 mm Hg and a diastolic pressure over 90 mm Hg. There is a familial tendency for elevated blood pressure; it also occurs in combination with kidney disease, adrenal tumors, hyperthyroidism, coarctation (stenosis) of the aorta, and increased intracranial pressure.

Hypotension. Hypotension in adults is defined as a blood pressure below 95/60 mm Hg. This value, however, may reflect a normal reading in the very light weight adult (whose body build is still more adolescent than adult).

ANTIHYPOTENSIVE AND ANTIHYPERTENSIVE MEDICATION. Many different medications are available for stabilizing blood pressure within normal limits. These medications are always potentially dangerous because the point at which they are therapeutic (raise or decrease blood pressure appropriately) is extremely close to the point at which they are toxic (increase or decrease blood pressure into hypotensive or hypertensive limits). When administering such medication, be certain that the spacing between administrations is correct (neither too long nor too short) and that the medication is still indicated based on a recent assessment of blood pressure (see QRS 31-2).

CENTRAL VENOUS PRESSURE

Central venous pressure (CVP) is a measurement of venous blood pressure rather than the usual arterial blood pressure. For this measurement, a thin catheter is inserted into a distal vein (usually the brachial) and advanced to rest in the superior or inferior vena cava just outside the heart (Fig. 31-8A). It is measured in patients receiving a great deal of intravenous fluid (to be certain that fluid overload does not occur) and in those with heart failure. Central venous pressure increases when blood begins to pool in the vena cava because the heart cannot handle the amount returning to it; it decreases following hemorrhage or severe vasodilatation.

Unlike arterial blood pressure, which is measured in millimeters mercury, CVP is measured in centimeters water. In order to record a CVP level, the patient's bed must be flat (or always elevated to the exact same point) at the time of the reading. The CVP catheter is attached to intravenous tubing as it leaves the patient's vein; the tubing is always kept patent by a slowly infusing intravenous fluid. A stopcock inserted in the tubing allows the fluid to be diverted from the intravenous fluid bottle into either the tubing, catheter, and patient, or into a manometer (the gauge where the level will be read). The manometer is taped to an intravenous pole beside the bed; the zero mark on the gauge should be level with the patient's midaxillary line at the third or fourth interspace as he lies supine. This point is even with the atria of the heart (Fig. 31-8B).

To do an actual reading, turn the stopcock so that fluid from the intravenous bottle flows into the manometer until the fluid column measures about 30 cm H_2O; turn the stopcock to end the flow from the bottle to the manometer. The fluid in the fluid column will then fall until its pressure equals the person's CVP. The fluid level will fluctuate by 1 to 2 cm H_2O at the bottom point as the person breathes; at the highest point of oscillation, read the level (normally 5 to 15 cm H_2O).

Following a reading, it is important to reverse the stopcock and reopen the fluid flow between the bottle and the catheter. If this is not done, blood will clot at the tip of the catheter, not only making the catheter inoperative but possibly causing a thrombus or emboli in the vessel.

Do not attempt to take CVP readings until you are familiar with the exact equipment used. Incorrect technique may cause an air embolus (air in the vein), a potentially fatal condition.

LIFE SPAN CONCEPTS

THE INFANT

An infant's blood pressure is not recorded routinely until he is 3 years of age because his arm is too small to fit with a stethoscope diaphragm and, if he cries, blood pressure rises inaccurately. Infants generally cry whenever faced with manipulative procedures such as blood pressure recording.

If you are taking all vital signs (temperature, pulse, respirations and blood pressure), always take respirations first (you do not need to disturb the infant in any way); pulse next (you disturb only to the extent of fingertip touch); blood pressure next (a cuff feels snug but does not really cause discomfort); and temperature last (a rectal temperature is intrusive; an axillary one requires you to restrain the arm). Never take temperature before other vital signs, or other vital signs will be distorted.

☐ QUICK REFERENCE STOP 31-2: PHARMACOLOGY
Antihypertensive Medications

Antihypertensives act by one of three methods: (1) slowing the heart rate, (2) dilating blood vessels, or (3) reducing the amount of fluid in the circulatory system through use of a diuretic. A major problem with antihypertensive medication is that the number and quality of side effects cause people to stop taking them and allow their condition to grow worse.

Medication	*Action and Precautions*
Vasodilators (widen lumen of vessels to reduce peripheral resistance)	
Papaverine (papaverine hydrochloride)	Side effects include flushing of face and mild sedation.
Unitensin (unitensin acetate)	Very narrow range between therapeutic and toxic doses; used in emergencies for its rapid action.
Apresoline (hydralazine hydrochloride)	Heart arrhythmias may occur with high dosages.
Nitroglycerin (glyceryl trinitrate)	Administer sublingually; has specific vasodilation effect on coronary vessels.
Diuretics (block sodium reabsorption in ascending tubules, allowing additional excretion of water from body)	May cause hypovolemia. Excessive potassium may be lost in urine.
Edecrin (ethacrynic acid)	
Hydodiuril (hydrochlorothiazide)	
Lasix (furosemide)	
Drugs acting on central nervous system	
Aldomet (methyldopa)	Orthostatic hypertension may occur.
Inderal (propranolol)	Gastrointestinal tract disturbance and aggravation of asthma may occur.
Serpasil (reserpine)	Drowsiness, lethargy may occur.

Take apical pulse rate in infants rather than peripheral pulse rate for best accuracy.

THE TODDLER AND PRESCHOOLER

Beginning at age 3, blood pressure is incorporated as a routine technique of health assessment. This new equipment is frightening for children; give them time to handle it first and explain that the cuff "hugs" but does not really hurt the arm.

THE SCHOOLAGER AND ADOLESCENT

Because schoolage children and adolescents tend to be very active, you need to know their level of activity prior to pulse and blood pressure recordings. If a child races to a treatment room to meet you, his reading will surely be higher than one obtained while he was quietly sitting in bed.

Assess carefully the size of blood pressure cuff used with children of all ages. A cuff appropriate in size for one 12-year-old may not be appropriate for another 12-year-old because children grow at such different rates during this time.

THE ADULT

Most people are aware that elevated blood pressure is a major health problem. Some people place more importance on blood pressure determination than is warranted (feeling that if their blood pressure is normal, they are totally well). Many adults, therefore, want to know their blood pressure after you take it; indeed, it is

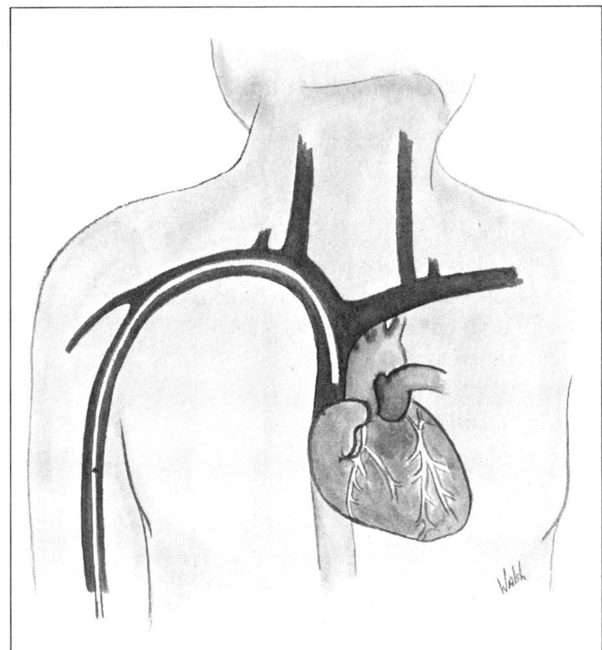

A

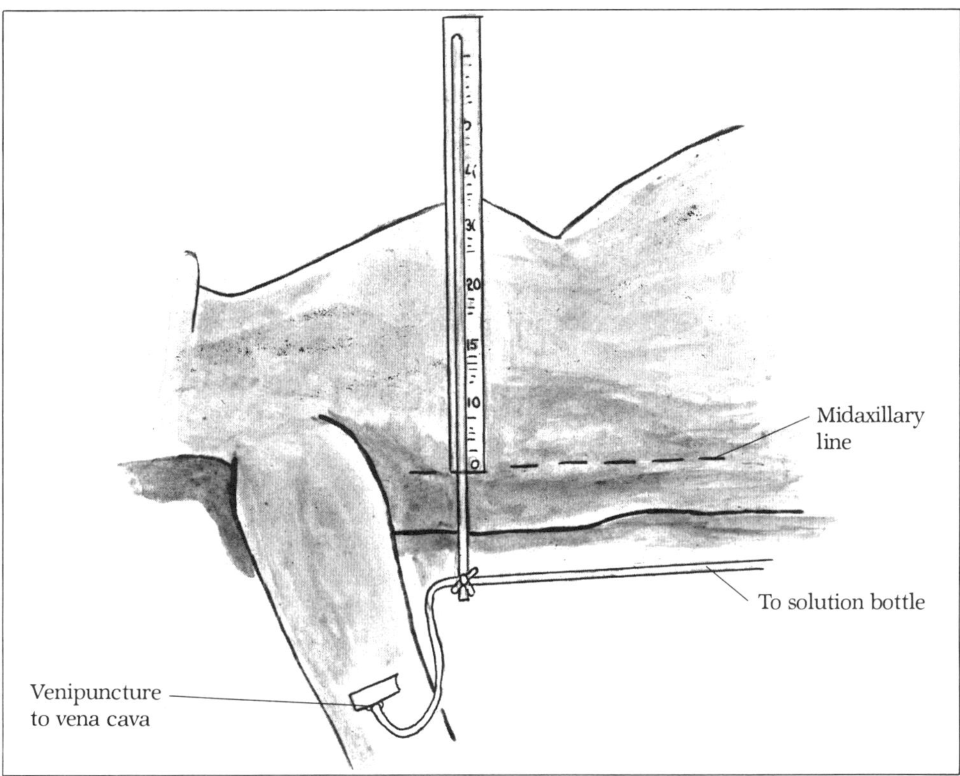

B

FIGURE 31-8. A. Placement of catheter. B. Measurement of central venous pressure.

important that people know their vital signs in order to offer this information at future health assessments as baseline data. There is a well-known rule of thumb that a normal systolic blood pressure reading is your age in years plus 100 (a person of 40 would have a systolic blood pressure of 140). Be aware that people are probably using this guideline, which is not really accurate, to evaluate the information you give them. When you tell a patient his reading, remember also to prefix it with a statement such as "It's normal for your age" or "Blood pressure increases when a person is worried, so I'm not surprised that yours is slightly high right now" (see QRS 31-3).

Pregnant women have their blood pressure checked at each prenatal visit to detect the possible complication of pregnancy-induced hypertension, which can be fatal to both mother and fetus if left untreated. Why this response occurs is unknown, but all blood vessels in the woman's body appear to spasm or contract, and the narrowed vessel lumens cause blood pressure to increase greatly. A blood pressure reading 30 mm Hg above the woman's prepregnancy level suggests that hypertension may be developing. She needs to be referred to her physician immediately for further evaluation of her condition before circulation to her cerebral arteries and the fetal circulation is any further affected.

Hypertension begins to become a general health problem as people enter middle age (see QRS 31-4). Most people with this involvement are placed on an antihypertensive to reduce blood pressure. It is important that this type of medication be taken consistently (four times a day every day, for example) not sporadically (four times one day, none the next, twice the next). With sporadic administration, the blood pressure is sometimes elevated, sometimes not, a situation that may give more symptoms, such as buzzing in the ears, headache, and vertigo, than untreated hypertension (and may lead just as dangerously to cerebral vessel or cardiac damage). On the other hand, if a person forgets his medication one day, he should not double his dosage the next day, and thereby possibly lower blood pressure to below cerebral perfusion effectiveness.

Side effects of antihypertensives are so common that many people quickly discontinue taking them; also, unlike symptoms such as pain or shortness of breath, hypertension symptoms are not acute (a dull headache, vertigo), and the threat of future disability is so vague that people do not continue to take this type of medication well. Teach both the importance of taking hypertensive medication and the necessity of rechecking dosage or type of medication with a physician in order to reduce side effects. A reminder chart, taped to the kitchen cupboard or medicine cabinet, may be necessary in order for them to remember to take this type of medicine everyday (see QRS 31-5).

☐ QUICK REFERENCE STOP 31-3: PSYCHOLOGICAL CONSIDERATIONS

Even very young children appreciate that heart function is necessary for health and life. Taking vital signs is done so commonly by nurses that it is easy to forget the procedure is not "common" and may be very stressful for the person you are assessing.

Remember that raising your eyebrows or murmuring "Hmm" as you discover an elevated blood pressure means as much to the patient as saying that you are surprised at the reading.

☐ QUICK REFERENCE STOP 31-4: HEALTH TEACHING
Risk Factors Associated With the Development of Hypertension

Age (over 50 years)
Sex (male)
Race (black)
Obesity (10% over normal weight)
Stress caused by type A personality (characterized by a high achievement drive)
Cigarette smoking
Alcohol consumption
Caffeine consumption
Presence of hyperlipidemia (increased cholesterol blood level)
Use of oral contraceptives

THE OLDER ADULT

Blood pressure is typically elevated slightly in older adults because peripheral resistance is increased in the presence of arteriosclerosis or atherosclerosis. Elevated blood pressure in older adults combined with some decrease in the integrity of blood vessel walls cause cerebrovascular accidents (stroke) to be a major health problem in this age group.

IMPROVING CARDIOVASCULAR FUNCTION

Assessment of cardiovascular function is always an independent nursing action with each patient contact; in addition, independent nursing interventions to promote cardiovascular function should always be considered in planning care.

BODY POSITION

A continuous supine position causes the heart to beat faster and harder in order to handle the large amount of

□ QUICK REFERENCE STOP 31-5: COMMUNITY CONSIDERATIONS

Hypertension affects 15 to 20 percent of the United States population. In the majority of people, hypertension is a chronic illness that can be controlled by proper medication, diet, and exercise but will never be cured. Help people to understand that any chronic illness of this nature requires them to follow their physician's instructions consistently.

People who are discharged from a health care agency and will be taking antihypertension medications at home need to observe certain precautions.

1. Always rise gradually from lying to sitting, and sitting to standing positions to prevent orthostatic hypotension and a sense of dizziness, faintness, or flashing lights.
2. Standing in one position for any length of time should be avoided as this allows blood to pool in the venous circulation and add to or cause orthostatic hypotension. People who work on production lines, have filing jobs, or teach are apt to do this.
3. When lying down for over an hour, exercise legs by wiggling toes and flexing knees to promote blood movement from lower extremities. People who watch television can learn to do this routinely at the end of every program.
4. A hot bath or steam bath may cause extreme vasodilation of lower extremities and cause severe hypotension. Have the person shower or modify bathtub water temperature. Caution him not to take baths when alone in the house until he is sure that doing so is not a problem.
5. Medication must be taken conscientiously. Teach people not to be reluctant to use a memory aid such as a marked pill container or a sign on the refrigerator. These are not "babyish" or "poor memory" aids. Everyone needs this type of aid to remember to take medication over a long time period.
6. The patient should not discontinue medication abruptly since extreme rebound hypertension could result. Plan ahead to have a supply of medicine for vacations or holidays.
7. Dizziness is most apt to occur during the first 2 hours following medicine administration, so the patient should use caution when driving or working with machinery.
8. If side effects are bothersome, the person should consult his physician for a change of medication or dosage. There are many types of such medication and he may need to try several before he finds one that is compatible.
9. The patient should not experiment with a change of dosage himself. He could cause hypotension or rebound hypertension with only a small dosage adjustment.

blood supplied to it by the vena cava. Nurses often place people on bedrest in a supine position and conscientiously turn them side to side, but do not consider the possibility of a semi-Fowler's position. Proper position is especially important for patients who are immobilized due to a bulky cast or orthopedic traction. Ask for clear orders on whether or not a semi-Fowler's position can be used (if so, use it in preference to a supine position for at least a portion of the day to reduce heart action, allow a better view of surroundings, and promote better self-care ability). Do not use a knee gatch on a bed to maintain a semi-Fowler's position as a continually bent knee causes lower leg vessel constriction and possible thrombophlebitis. With the patient's head elevated, assess the skin area of the buttocks and base of the spine well: Weight is shifted to this area and a decubitus ulcer (pressure ulcer) may form.

Always make sure that a patient is not lying with one arm underneath him or is lying or sitting with knees crossed as lower extremity vessel constriction may result and interfere with venous return.

CONSTRICTING OBJECTS

Whenever an object that causes possible circulatory constriction, such as a cast or a dressing, is in place, you must carefully assess the circulation to the distal body part. Check circulation by blanching fingernails or toenails and watching them refill, palpating for normal warmth in the distal part, and asking the person if he feels any sensation such as tingling or numbness.

ELEVATION OF BODY PARTS

Edema tends to occur secondary to an injury to a body part because the body allows excess blood to enter the area of injury, bringing a ready supply of platelets for blood clotting and white blood cells and antibodies for infection control. The additional pressure of the distended blood causes loss of plasma to subcutaneous tissue by hydrostatic pressure. In some injuries, the pressure is so acute that it can cause pain and constriction of blood vessels in the area. Elevating the body part decreases the amount of blood flow to the part and so reduces the edema present.

Be careful when elevating body parts to reduce edema that you do not elevate so far that you cause a sharp bend at the groin, elbow, or shoulder, which will actually increase constriction to the extremity, not improve circulatory flow.

EXERCISE
Muscle contraction against veins aids in pumping blood. Medical condition permitting, active leg contraction (wiggling the toes, flexing and extending the knee) is effective in helping patients on bedrest to move venous blood. Encouraging active range-of-motion exercise three times a day is helpful (passive range-of-motion exercise is less effective but still helpful). People who work at jobs that require long periods of standing are well advised to bend their knees deliberately and shift their weight from foot to foot about every 15 minutes to reduce venous stasis. You need a physician's order for exercise for a patient with cardiac limitations.

ANTIEMBOLIC (ELASTIC) STOCKINGS
Stockings that apply gentle compression to lower extremities supplement the action of muscle contraction or aid venous return. Like exercises, they should be used with a physician's order. Such stockings extend from the foot to below the knee or all the way over the knee to the groin. Always apply antiembolic stockings with the patient in a supine position so veins are empty at the time they are positioned. To apply such a stocking, pull the foot and heel into place and then gently pull the stocking over the leg (Fig. 31-9). Check to be certain that the heel fits snugly and no wrinkles are present along the stocking that could cause pressure.

After an antiembolic stocking has been in place for about an hour, check the area at the top of the stocking carefully to be certain that the top is not binding and causing obstruction at that point. Antiembolic stockings should be removed at least twice a day so the underlying skin can be inspected for irritation or edema. Check the toes for circulation and warmth.

If a person is going to be discharged from a health care agency with instructions to purchase elastic stockings or continue to wear them at home, be sure they understand that the prescription for stockings is referring to *medical*, not commercial, support stockings.

ELASTIC BANDAGES
Elastic bandages are elasticized roller bandages wound around an extremity to offer the same encouragement to venous return as fitted elastic stockings. Elastic bandages are frequently referred to as *Ace bandages* (a common brand name). As with elastic stockings, such a bandage should be put in place when the person is lying down so veins are not distended at the time of application. You must be certain that it is applied smoothly and with even pressure. Begin such an application by holding the roll of bandage over the middle of the foot and making two circular turns to anchor the bottom edge of the bandage. Continue to apply it by making spiral turns (each turn overlaps the previous turn by about one-half the bandage width) to just below the knee (Fig. 31-10). If the bandage is to cover the knee or any other joint, you must wrap the joint with a figure eight technique to allow for joint mobility (Fig. 31-11). You would proceed to wrap the leg above the knee with spiral turns again. Anchor the last turn in place with a metal clip, safety pin, or piece of tape.

FIGURE 31-9. To apply elastic stockings, position the foot and heel in place and then pull the stocking up over the leg.

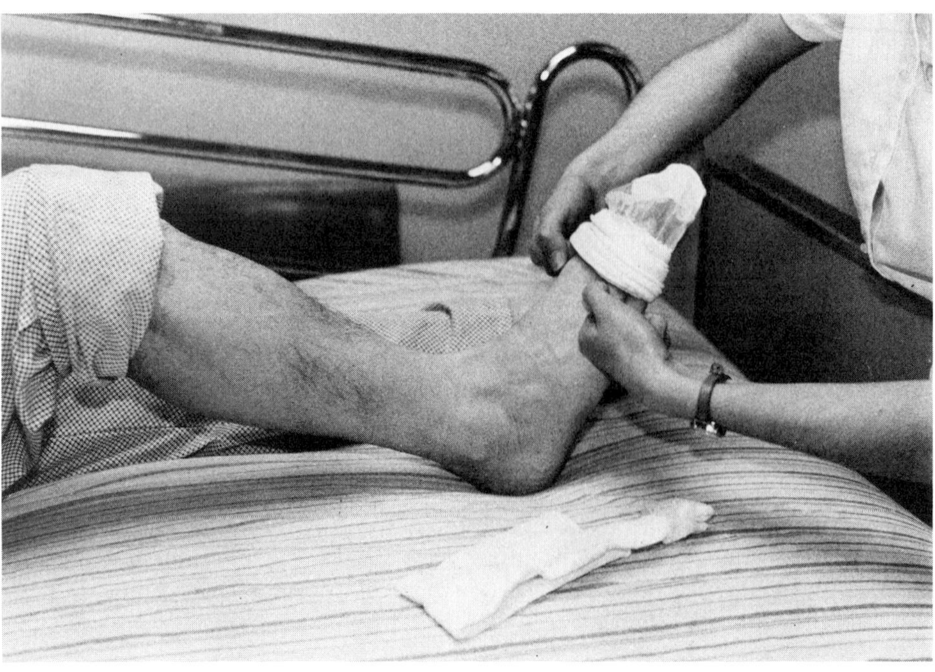

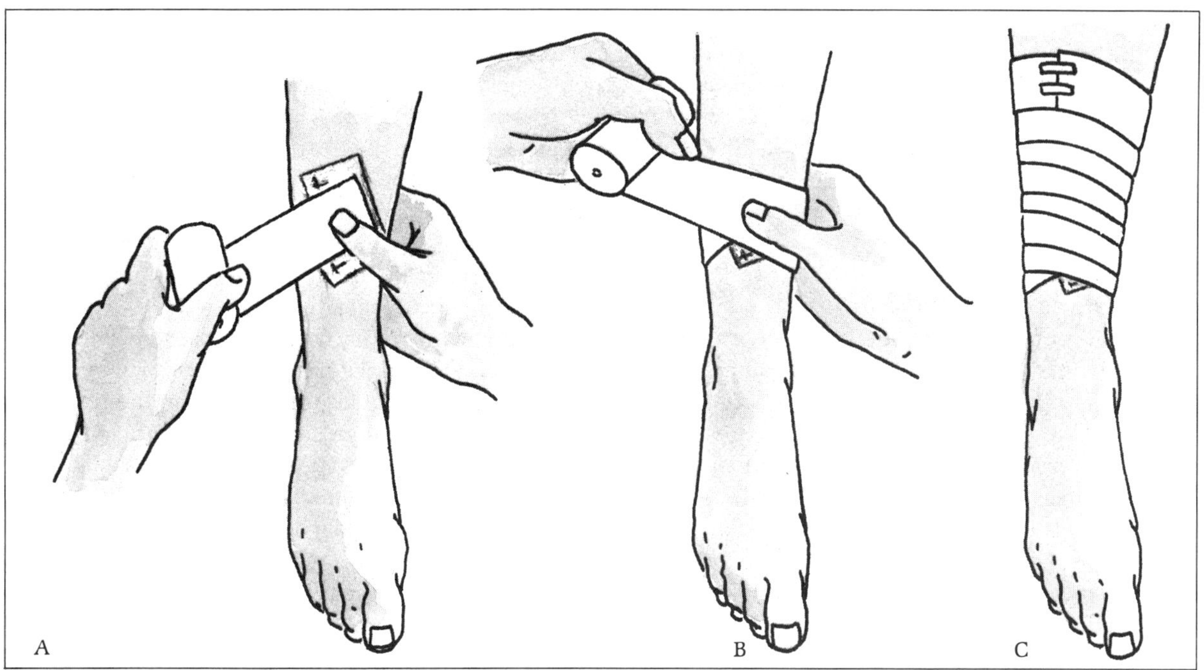

FIGURE 31-10. To apply an ace bandage, start at the dressing site (A), make spiral turns up the leg (B), and secure (C).

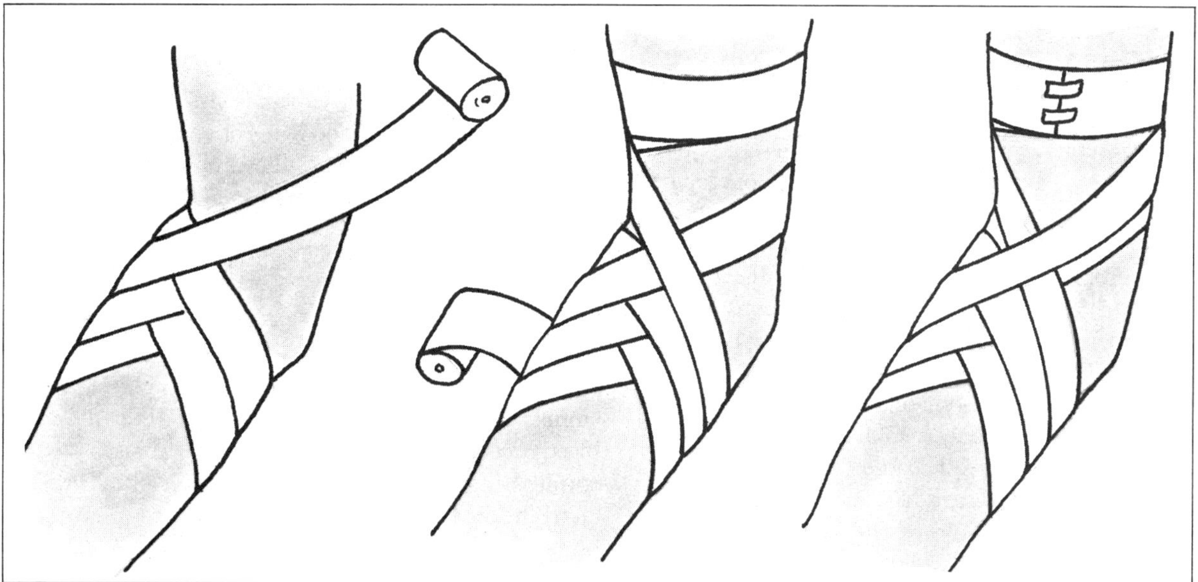

FIGURE 31-11. If an ace bandage is to cover a joint (here, the elbow) use a figure eight technique when wrapping; this allows for joint mobility.

Elastic bandages should be applied snugly but not tightly. The elastic thread used in their construction draws taut after application; if you apply the bandage with undue pressure, the additional elastic tightening will, after a few minutes, impair rather than aid circulation. Always assess an extremity for circulation within the first hour after application unless such stockings have been applied following vascular surgery; as with elastic stockings, the bandage should be removed at least twice daily so the skin underneath can be assessed and the body part cleansed. Following vascular surgery they are not removed until specifically ordered by the person's physician.

HEAT AND COLD APPLICATION

Application of heat to an area causes vasodilation, or "pulls" blood into the area. Applying cold causes the opposite effect of venous constriction, or reduces blood flow to the area. Following a traumatic injury such as an ankle sprain, applying ice intermittently (20 minutes on, 20 minutes off) to the injured area for the first 24 hours will keep edema in the area to a minimum. Applying heat after that time will aid the absorption of any blood and reduce edema at the site. Application of heat and cold always calls for diligent observation to prevent burns. The full effect of heat and cold application and responsibilities for nursing care are discussed in Chap. 33.

EDUCATION AND MOTIVATION

Most people are not aware of the importance of venous circulation; they do not appreciate that an exercise as simple as flexing and extending their knee can be helpful. If left with instructions such as, "every hour, bend your knee a few times," they will remember to do this no more than once or twice a day. Explain the importance of such an exercise; be available to observe and either remind a patient to exercise or help him construct a reminder chart of some kind to hang by his bed. Quick Reference Stop 31-5 lists important rules for the self-administration of antihypertensive medication.

BLOOD LOSS

One of the most hazardous problems for a human body is blood loss. In many instances the basic problem of a patient is either chronic blood loss (a stomach ulcer) or acute blood loss (hemorrhage from a large cut). Blood loss lowers blood volume, so the person typically appears pale (vasoconstriction of peripheral vessels pushes blood to the central core for vital organ use); has a rapid pulse rate (the heart is beating rapidly, trying to oxygenate cells with a decreased volume of blood); breathing rapidly (trying to supply oxygen to cells despite the transport problem); has a low blood pressure (blood pressure depends on blood volume); and anxious (either from the knowledge that he has a blood loss or as an alerting body response to the increased heart rate).

The best position for someone with lowered blood volume is supine (with only a small flat pillow or legs elevated about 20 degrees) because this better helps to supply blood to cerebral arteries. At one time, people with blood loss were placed in a Trendelenburg (head-dependent) position. This is no longer done except in special circumstances as it may decrease blood to kidney arteries and cause excess blood in the cerebrum. Remaining quiet is helpful because movement requires increased cellular metabolism and places a greater strain on the heart. For a body to keep itself warm requires an increased metabolism level and more oxygen, so prevent the person from becoming chilled.

Blood volume is replaced by the infusion of intravenous fluid or blood products. Blood pressure can be maintained by the addition of a medication to cause vasoconstriction and elevate the pressure of blood in the body's central core.

HALTING BLEEDING

An extremely helpful emergency measure is the halting of bleeding. The most effective way to halt active bleeding is generally to apply firm compression to the site. Always be aware when caring for people with recent surgical incisions or other wounds that bleeding from the site is a possibility. Assess not only the site itself for active bleeding but turn the person to be certain that blood has not oozed from the edge of a covering dressing and is pooling underneath the person.

Tourniquets are rarely used today because, while their application does reduce bleeding at the injured area, it also decreases the blood supply to the entire body part and thus can cause more harm than the original injury. Pressure on pulse points (pressure to the brachial artery to halt bleeding in a hand, for example) is another technique little used today for the same reason.

Nosebleeds. Nosebleeds are a common source of blood loss that can occur during the course of normal patient care. Dry heat in health care agencies tends to dry and crack the mucous membrane of the nose and lead to bleeding; children tend to rub or pick their noses, which causes bleeding. To best halt a nosebleed, sit the person up (to take pressure off the small capillaries in the nose) and press your fingers against the sides of the nose (Fig. 31-12). You must maintain pressure for about 5 minutes for effective results. Most people are frightened by a nosebleed because the blood is so obvious; if blood flows to the back of the throat, they may choke and feel suffocated by it. You can be assured that unless the person has a blood coagulation problem, the amount of blood lost by a nosebleed is really very small and will not cause systemic effects.

Many children with nosebleeds swallow some blood, which may lead them to vomit about an hour later (the vomitus is black or dark brown from the action of stomach enzymes on it). Remembering that the nosebleed occurred helps you to assess the seriousness of the vomited blood (not serious if blood is "old"). Always chart the occurrence of the nosebleed since you may not be present when the patient vomits.

Following any blood loss, remove signs of bleeding from the person's environment (soiled linen, dressings, etc.). It is easy for a nurse to become accustomed to the sight of blood but the person himself is not apt to witness it as casually and can be unnecessarily frightened by the sight of soiled linen or carelessly disposed care articles.

PHLEBITIS AND THROMBOPHLEBITIS

Phlebitis is inflammation of a vein. Although it tends to occur when a vein has been intubated as part of an intravenous fluid or diagnostic procedure, it can result from prolonged inactivity (for example, bedrest) or the

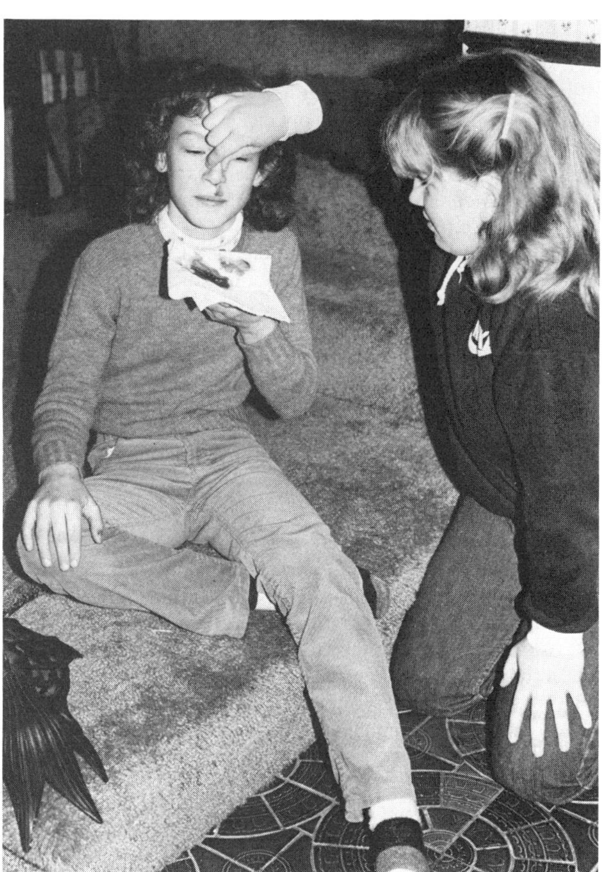

FIGURE 31-12. To stop a nosebleed, sit the person upright and press your fingers against the sides of the person's nose; maintain pressure for about 5 minutes.

pressing on a body part of a constricting object (such as a cast). The skin over the area becomes warm to touch and appears reddened (erythematous). The person reports pain at the site.

Thrombophlebitis is inflammation of the vein with an accompanying blood clot formed at the inflammation site. The symptoms of thrombophlebitis are more intense manifestations than those of phlebitis. A thrombophlebitis is always a serious problem because, if the blood clot moves from the original site, it may either occlude the pulmonary artery, blocking blood flow to the lungs and preventing oxygen exchange, or obstruct the coronary arteries, blocking blood supply to the heart (a heart attack).

Never massage a body area where you suspect phlebitis or thrombophlebitis since massage could cause this type of movement. In order to reduce the inflammation and clot formation, the person's physician will order any irritating intubation removed from the site, immobilization of the body part, application of heat, and possibly the administration of an anticoagulant to prevent further clot formation. Under these conditions, the clot found will gradually dissolve.

HOMANS' SIGN

Homans' sign indicates the presence of a thrombophlebitis in a leg vein. Flex the person's knee and dorsiflex his foot. If the person has pain, a thrombophlebitis in the leg calf is suggested (see Procedure 25-3, Fig. 5). Check for Homans' sign at least every 8 hours in patients who have lower extremity intubation or are on bedrest. Including this assessment as a routine part of patient bathing is an easy way to include it in routine care.

Luke's sign is a similar finding used in assessment. It is pain in the calf on standing (a position that partially dorsiflexes the foot).

PREVENTING THROMBOPHLEBITIS

Thrombophlebitis can be prevented by implementations to encourage venous return (range-of-motion exercises, elevation of body parts, etc.). Being certain that intravenous sites are changed every 48 hours in adults helps to limit their formation. Intravenous lines are left for a longer period of time in children as they have a much lower incidence of thrombus formation than adults.

UTILIZING NURSING PROCESS

Because cardiovascular function is so important, careful assessment, planning, and care interventions must be considered with all patients.

ASSESSMENT

The usual assessment measures for cardiovascular status (pulse and blood pressure) are so common that their importance is easily discounted. Since these techniques are easily learned, nursing aides take and record these measurements in many health care agencies. Always ask what measurements were done on people you care for, even if you do not actually take them yourself. Do not confuse the fact that, although these measures are easy to record, they are not "simple" (see QRS 31-6).

☐ QUICK REFERENCE STOP 31-6: ADVOCACY

Vital sign assessment is ordered every 8 hours or every 4 hours around the clock in many health care agency settings. When a person is very ill these frequent assessments are necessary; as a person's health improves, such frequent recording of vital signs is no longer necessary and, in addition to spending a large amount of nursing time ineffectively, results in much loss of sleep for the patient.

You may need to advocate that the number of times a patient is awakened during the night or interrupted during the day be reduced.

Remember as well to record these readings immediately: They are as easy to forget as to take.

ANALYSIS

Use common sense to determine the significance of vital sign readings. A person with a high temperature, for example, can be expected to have an elevated pulse rate. Ordinarily, this is not important; the fever is the chief problem. In a person with cardiovascular illness, however, the increased pulse rate might be the chief danger to the person, not the fever. Do not be reluctant to recheck vital signs taken by a nursing aide if your observation of a person's condition leads you to question the reading's accuracy. If an aide tells you that the blood pressure of a patient whom you know has ringing in his ears and an occipital headache is normal, you might suspect that the aide missed an auscultatory gap and has recorded a falsely low reading.

The Fourth Annual Conference on Nursing Diagnosis accepted two diagnoses in reference to cardiovascular functioning: "cardiac output, alteration in: decreased," and "tissue perfusion, alteration in: cerebral, cardiopulmonary, renal, or peripheral." The defining characteristics of these diagnoses are shown in Appendix C.

EVALUATION

Always compare pulse and blood pressure readings to a person's last reading. Average levels vary so much among people that, unless you do so, you can miss the fact that a person's vital signs, while still within normal limits, have moved during the last 4 hours from a pulse rate of 68 at 10:00, to 72 at 11:00, to 76 at 12:00, and to 80 at 2:00. This slow increase or decrease in pulse or blood pressure may be as serious as a sudden increase or decrease. Evaluation is the step that best lets you detect these subtle changes before they become apparently drastic increases or decreases.

NURSING CARE PLAN

Andrea O'Malley is a 68-year-old woman admitted to the hospital for a persistent urinary tract infection. In addition, she has mild hypertension (150/90). Although she has been taking an antihypertensive at home for a year, her physician suspects that she does not take it regularly. In the hospital, she tends to spend a high proportion of her time lying in bed and knitting a sweater for her grandson, although she has been told to be as ambulatory as possible. She states that bedrest is comfortable for her because she feels dizzy when walking alone. Her physician ordered blood pressure readings TID and orthostatic reading qd, and antiembolic stockings. In addition, she wrote on the chart, "Prevent thrombophlebitis."

The following is a nursing care plan you might write for Mrs. O'Malley in reference to cardiovascular function.

NURSING DIAGNOSIS

Knowledge deficit related to use of antihypertensive and antithrombophlebitic prescriptions.

Goal: Patient will remain free of cardiovascular complications during period of hospitalization.

Criteria: Pulse, blood pressure, and venous return will remain within normal limits during hospitalization.

NURSING ORDERS

1. Patient has auscultatory gap on blood pressure reading. Palpate brachial pulse as you inflate cuff, and inflate cuff to above auscultatory gap.
2. Consistently use left arm for measurement; use aneroid manometer with #2 cuff.
3. Take orthostatic blood pressure one time daily before she arises in A.M. Chart whether sleep was restful or troubled (a true resting supine pressure or not).
4. Always help and teach patient to rise to standing or sitting position gradually from supine position to prevent orthostatic hypotension.
5. Remove TED antiembolic stockings BID to assess skin. Reapply with patient in supine position.
6. Encourage patient to ambulate at least three times daily by walking with her the length of hallway and back.
7. Ask patient to knee flex and push against foot board q4h. Remain with her to emphasize importance of exercise.
8. Caution patient not to lie with knees crossed while in bed; do not use knee gatch on bed or pillows under knees.
9. Explore reason for poor compliance with antihypertensive medicine (lack of understanding of importance? poor memory? inability to refill prescription?).
10. Teach effect of medication and ways to increase compliance of self-administration (medication chart? association with mealtime?).

SUGGESTED READINGS

Abelmann, W. H. Effects of alcohol on the cardio-vascular system. *Hosp. Pract.* 16(11):80A, 1981.

Bahr, R. T., et al. Blood pressure readings and selected parameter relationships on an elderly ambulatory population. *J. Gerontol. Nurs.* 8(3):159, 1982.

Baldini, J. Knowledge about hypertension in affected elderly persons. *J. Gerontol. Nurs.* 7:542, 1981.

Brown, A. L., et al. Elevated blood pressure among Harlem residents. *Nurse Pract.* 7(3):26, 1982.

Evans, M. J. Tips for taking a child's blood pressure quickly. *Nursing* (Horsham) 13(3):61, 1983.

Foster, S., and Kousch, D. C. Promoting patient adherence to blood pressure regime. *Am. J. Nurs.* 78:829, 1978.

Giblin, E. Controlling high blood pressure. *Am. J. Nurs.* 78:824, 1978.

Grim, C. M. Nursing assessment of the patient with high blood pressure. *Nurs. Clin. North Am.* 16:349, 1981.

Hall, D. Teaching ideas: Cardiovascular health. The assessment of type A behavior in children. *Health Educ.* (Washington) 13(1):55, 1982.

Harrison, D. C., et al. Cardiovascular risk reduction: The problems facing our society. *Health Educ.* 13:9, 1982.

Hazinski, M. F. Critical care of the pediatric cardiovascular patient. *Nurs. Clin. North Am.* 16(4):671, 1981.

Hill, M. N., et al. Seeking and finding all those patients with high blood pressure. *Nursing* (Horsham) 12(2):72, 1982.

Hill, M. W. What can go wrong when you measure blood pressure. *Am. J. Nurs.* 80:942, 1980.

Hill, M., et al. In hypertensive emergencies, act quickly but also act cautiously. *Nursing* (Horsham) 13(2):34, 1983.

Hinds, C. A hypertensive survey: Respondents' knowledge of high blood pressure. *Int. Nurs. Rev.* 30(1):12, 1983.

Huebsch, J. A. Health assessment of the cardiovascular patient. *Occup. Health Nurs.* 29:11, 1981.

Ivenson-Ivenson, J. Pulse taking . . . students' forum. *Nurs. Mirror* 154:28, 1982.

Ivenson-Iveson, J. Blood pressure: How to measure it and what the readings mean. *Nurs. Mirror* 154:41, 1982.

King, D. E. Assessment and evaluation of the paradoxical pulse. *D.C.C.N.* 1(5):266, 1982.

McConnell, E. Fitting antiembolism stockings. *Nursing 78* 8:67, 1978.

Miller, K. Assessing peripheral perfusion. *Am. J. Nurs.* 78:1673, 1978.

Moller, J. H. Cardiovascular risk reduction: The problem facing the school age population. *Health Educ.* 13:13, 1982.

Norris, D. L., et al. What all those pressure readings mean—and why. *RN* 44:34, 1981.

Peitzman, S. J., et al. Care of elderly patients in a special hypertension clinic. *J. Am. Geriatr. Soc.* 30(1):2, 1982.

Pepler, C. J. Your fingers on the pulse: Evaluating what you feel. *Nursing* (Horsham) 10:32, 1980.

Powers, M. J., et al. Factors influencing knowledge, attitudes, and compliance of hypertensive patients . . . four aspects of an educational program. *Res. Nurs. Health* 5(4):171, 1982.

Reed, W. L. Racial differences in blood pressure levels of adolescents. *Am. J. Public Health* 71:1165, 1981.

Scharping, E. M. Physiological measurements of the neonate . . . methods for accurately measuring vital signs are constantly being refined. *M.C.N.* 8(1):70, 1983.

Shanker, B. S., et al. Patterns of care for hypertension among hospitalized patients. *Public Health Rep.* 97(6):521, 1982.

Sparacino, J. Blood pressure, stress and mental health. *Nurs. Res.* 31:89, 1982.

Stright, P. A., and Soukup, S. M. How to hear it right: Evaluating and choosing a stethoscope. *Am. J. Nurs.* 77:1477, 1977.

Ward, G. W., et al. Treating and counseling the hypertensive patient. *Am. J. Nurs.* 78:824, 1978.

Willis, S. E. Hypertension in pregnancy: Pathophysiology. *Am. J. Nurs.* 82(5):792, 1982.

Willis, S. E., et al. Hypertension in pregnancy: Prenatal detection and management. *Am. J. Nurs.* 82(5):798, 1982.

Wolfgang, J., et al. An investigation of cardiovascular disease risk factors in an adolescent population. *J. Sch. Health* 52:218, 1982.

QUESTIONS FOR REVIEW

Mrs. Smith is a patient for whom you provide care. Frequent pulse and blood pressure readings have been ordered to be taken on her during a hospitalization.

1. Which of the following would be a normal pulse pressure for Mrs. Smith?
   a. 0—10 mm Hg
   b. 20—30 mm Hg
   c. 40—50 mm Hg
   d. 70—80 mm Hg

2. Which of the following would *not* increase her blood pressure?
   a. Exercise.
   b. Psychological stress.
   c. Exposure to warmth.
   d. Obesity.

3. To avoid missing an auscultatory gap when inflating her blood pressure, which technique would you use?
   a. Inflate the cuff to above 200 mm Hg.
   b. Palpate the brachial artery as you inflate the cuff.
   c. Inflate the cuff before you apply it.
   d. Do not inflate the cuff over 160 mm Hg.

4. Pulse deficit is defined as the difference between:
   a. The radial and apical pulse rates.
   b. Radial determinations 4 hours apart.
   c. The systolic and diastolic blood pressures.
   d. The first and second Korotkoff sounds.

5. Blood pressure, as commonly used, is a measure of:
   a. Arterial pressure.
   b. Venous pressure.
   c. Capillary pressure.
   d. Left ventricular pressure.

6. If Mrs. Smith's blood pressure is 122/70, her diastolic pressure is:
   a. 122
   b. 70
   c. 52
   d. 192

7. If Mrs. Smith has orthostatic hypotension, which measure would you want to use with her?
   a. Never place her in a supine position.
   b. Never allow her to sit up suddenly.
   c. Never allow her to drink fluid rapidly.
   d. Never allow her to stand.

8. An aid to venous return from Mrs. Smith's right leg would be to:
   a. Elevate the knee gatch of her bed.
   b. Apply cold packs to the leg.
   c. Elevate the head of the bed.
   d. Elevate the leg and foot on two pillows.

9. Antiembolic stockings are ordered for Mrs. Smith. When putting these on her:
   a. Be certain that she walks 10 feet first.
   b. Be certain that her toes are fully covered.
   c. Do range-of-motion exercises first.
   d. Put them on her before she rises in the morning.

10. Which of the following descriptions reflects the best technique for assessing the radial pulse?
    a. Place your fingertips lightly on the lateral side of the inner surface of the wrist.
    b. Place two fingertips snugly on the midline of the inner surface of the wrist.
    c. Rest your fingertips lightly on the medial side of the antecubital space.
    d. Press your fingertips against the lateral side of the inner surface of the wrist.

32. OXYGEN REGULATION

Oxygen regulation is the most critical of all life functions because without it other life processes halt. To understand the assessment and therapy of patients with respiratory dysfunction, it is important to understand the full extent of the respiratory process.

OBJECTIVES

Upon mastery of the material in this chapter, you should be able to:

1. Describe the process and role of respiration in maintaining wellness.
2. Describe common interferences with proper respiration.
3. List the signs of hypoxemia and hypoxia.
4. List the common reasons for administering oxygen.
5. Describe safe techniques of oxygen administration.
6. Describe proper suctioning, coughing, and breathing techniques.
7. Describe the important role of psychological support for persons with respiratory distress.

TERMS

The terms important for an understanding of this chapter are shown below and defined in the glossary:

apnea
bradypnea
Cheyne-Stokes respirations
cyanosis
dyspnea
hypercapnea
hyperpnea
hyperventilation
hypoventilation
hypoxemia
Kussmaul respirations
orthopnea
phlegm
sputum
tachypnea

RESPIRATION

Respiration can be divided into two major phases—external and internal. External respiration is the process of moving oxygen into the alveoli of the lungs and its diffusion across the alveolar membrane to the blood capillaries while carbon dioxide diffuses from the capillaries back to the alveoli and then outside to the atmosphere. Other terms for this phase are *ventilation* and *diffusion*. Internal respiration is the transport and utilization of oxygen by cells and the exchange of carbon dioxide for oxygen in the blood capillaries.

Respiratory dysfunction may develop at the level of the upper or lower respiratory tract, the blood, or the cells. To assess the adequacy of the respiratory status, therefore, it is necessary to assess not only the pulmonary system function but also indications of blood and cell function.

Ventilation

Air always flows from an area of greater pressure or concentration to an area of lower pressure. When the diaphragm descends on inspiration, the chest cavity enlarges and the lung space expands. This increase in space causes the pressure in the lungs to decrease to a point just below the pressure of the atmosphere, and therefore air (which has an oxygen content of 21 percent) is sucked in through the nostrils to flow through the pharynx, the trachea, the bronchi, and the bronchioles and finally into the alveoli. Normal inspiration lasts 2 to 3 seconds. Following inspiration, the lung tissue is stretched taut; it then recoils to empty the air from the lungs (this takes about 2 seconds).

Inspiration is initiated by stimulation of the respiratory center in the medulla oblongata and, to a lesser extent, by stretch receptors in the lungs (the Hering-Breuer reflex). The medulla responds to cues based on the level of oxygen, carbon dioxide, and pH (acid-base) of the blood. Of these three factors, the carbon dioxide level is the most important. If the carbon dioxide level in the blood (PCO_2) rises, both the rate and depth of ventilation will increase to clear the body of the excess; when PCO_2 falls, ventilation will decrease in rate and depth to conserve carbon dioxide (to prevent excessive "blow off"). When a decrease in the blood oxygen level (PO_2) or a decrease in pH occurs (as the body becomes more acidotic), ventilation will also increase to pull in more oxygen and blow off carbon dioxide (carbon dioxide will then not be able to combine with water (H_2O) to form carbonic acid (H_2CO_3) and then bicarbonate (HCO_3^-) and H^+ ions. The absence of H^+ ions increases the pH of blood (acidity occurs when more H^+ ions are present than OH^- ions).

Small cilia and mucus in the nose serve the important function of moistening the air and filtering and trapping small particles of dirt to keep the lower respiratory tract continually moist and free of foreign organisms. If for any reason the nose and upper pharynx are bypassed during respiration (for instance, when the patient has a tracheotomy or when a tube [a nasotracheal or oral tracheal tube] is passed through the nose or mouth into the trachea to ensure an open larynx), these important functions of moistening and filtering are lost. Patients with these bypass techniques need special precautions (such as sterile technique to limit the introduction of microorganisms and administration of premoistened air; otherwise they are likely to develop pneumonia (lung infection) from the invasion of microorganisms into the drying mucous membranes.

When caring for persons with respiratory illness, it is important to remember that when the trachea divides into the two main stem bronchi, the right main bronchi is a little wider and straighter than the left (Fig. 32-1). This means that when you pass a suction catheter to remove accumulating mucus in the bronchi, it will invariably enter the right bronchi unless special measures are taken to make it turn to the left (twist it as you insert it).

Factors that may interfere with ventilation are basically physical or obstructive problems such as edema, spasm, or a contraction that narrows the upper airway passages, or the presence of tumors or a collection of fluid that obstructs the airway. A muscle or bone disease that does not allow expansion of the chest muscles such as scoliosis (sideways curvature of the spine) can also interfere with adequate ventilation. Inspiration is a more forceful action than expiration; in most instances, expiration is more affected than inspiration with muscular diseases.

FIGURE 32-1. Normal lung anatomy. Notice the straighter, wider right bronchus.

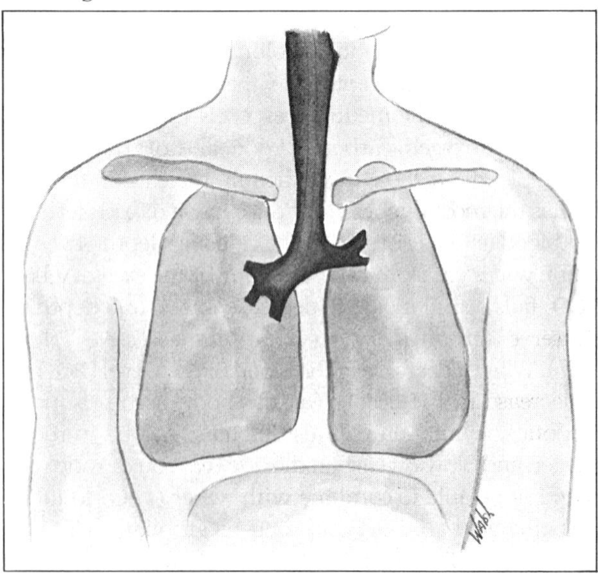

Diffusion

The alevoli of the lungs are normally only one cell deep in thickness, allowing gases to be exchanged (diffused) across them with ease. The atmospheric pressure of air is about 759 mm Hg. Oxygen comprises about 21% of room air, and the pressure of oxygen is therefore about 159 mm Hg (21% of 759 mm Hg). Because the alveoli are never fully emptied (to prevent the space from fully collapsing at the end of expiration), a small amount of CO_2 is always retained in the lungs. As atmospheric air is pulled into the lungs on inspiration, it mixes with this CO_2; the partial pressure of O_2 at the alveolar level is less than the atmospheric pressure, therefore, or 100 to 110 mm Hg. The pressure of oxygen in unoxygenated (venous) blood is only about 40 mm Hg. Under normal circumstances, therefore, O_2 will diffuse readily across the alveoli into the unoxygenated venous system because of such a sharp pressure gradient. Not all O_2 in the alveoli diffuses into the bloodstream even with this pressure gradient, so the partial pressure of O_2 in heavily oxygenated blood (now arterial blood) is slightly less than this, or about 95 mm Hg.

In addition, for respiration to be effective CO_2 must leave the venous blood. The pressure of carbon dioxide in the venous circulation is about 46 mm Hg; in the alveoli it is about 40 mm Hg, and in atmospheric air it is negligible, or 0 mm Hg. This difference allows CO_2 to cross from the venous capillaries to the alveoli at the beginning of expiration. Note that the difference in gradient of CO_2 is not as great as that of oxygen. This means that in many diseases it may be more difficult for a person to breathe off CO_2 than to breathe in oxygen. Assessment of a person with a respiratory illness must involve both considerations; not only must the person's intake of O_2 be adequate but his output of CO_2 must be adequate as well.

Difficulty with diffusion will occur if the alveolar membrane is thicker than usual, is coated by a fibrous secretion or has deteriorated in some way. The presence of blood or secretions coating the alveoli, as in pneumonia, reduces the amount of the exchange surface. The pressure of gases that are present also affects the exchange (the oxygen pressure in the lungs must be higher than that in pulmonary capillaries for exchange to take place, and the CO_2 pressure in the capillaries must be higher than that in the alveoli). If the lung alveoli collapse (atelectasis), the exchange surface is no longer present, so no exchange can take place. If a puncture in the lung occurs, allowing alveolar air to enter the pleural space, this will collapse the lung tissue (pneumothorax); pneumothorax may also be caused by a puncture in the chest wall as in a traumatic injury. Such a situation is always an emergency because the person's ability to diffuse gases is compromised so suddenly.

Transport

In the next step in respiration, oxygen is carried by the blood to cells. This is accomplished mainly by oxygen combining with hemoglobin in the red blood cells; some oxygen is carried freely (dissociated) in the bloodstream. Poor transport of oxygen will occur if a less than normal number of red blood cells are present (anemia), if the red blood cells are defective (sickle cell anemia), if blood flow is sluggish (blood pressure is decreased), or if there is a stricture or blockage of the blood flow (arteriosclerosis, for example). Because blood pressure may be decreased owing to loss of blood or inadequate heart action, all patients with trauma involving blood loss or cardiac illness must be assessed carefully not only for the direct effects of their illness but for internal respiratory efficiency as well.

Cellular Perfusion

Oxygen passes from the bloodstream into the cells because of a positive gradient between the pressure of oxygen in the small arterioles that contact the cells and the oxygen pressure within the cells. Although the pressure of oxygen in the lung alveoli is 159 mm Hg, the alveolar system does not allow all oxygen to cross, so the oxygen pressure in the arterial system is about 95 mm Hg, and in cells it is about 40 mm Hg. The pressure of carbon dioxide in cells is about 46 mm Hg; the pressure in the blood capillaries near cells is about 40 mm Hg, so carbon dioxide diffuses from cells to vessels equally well.

Exchange at the cellular level is inhibited if there is thickening of the blood vessel walls (arteriosclerosis); if blood pressure is decreased (with blood loss or inadequate pump capacity of the heart); if there is an obstruction to the flow of blood (a thrombus), preventing the blood from contacting the cells; or if the cells are unable to receive the oxygen owing to a disturbed metabolic process such as acid-base imbalance. This is the difficulty in a metabolic disease such as diabetes mellitus. Adequate oxygen reaches the cells; cells are then unable to use it because of poor functioning. Assessment of respiratory function is necessary in metabolic disease, therefore, as well as in cardiac and respiratory-based illnesses.

Blood Gases

The term *blood gases* refers to the amount of oxygen and carbon dioxide in the arterial bloodstream. They are reported as PO_2 and PCO_2, referring to the partial pressure of these gases. To make it clear that the analysis is of arterial blood, some institutions report blood gases as PaO_2 and $PaCO_2$.

PO_2

As mentioned earlier, oxygen comprises 21 percent of atmospheric air, so its partial pressure is 21 percent of 759 mm Hg, or 159 mm Hg. In arterial blood its partial pressure is 80 to 100 mm Hg.

The partial pressure of carbon dioxide in atmospheric air is negligible and is considered to be 0 mm Hg. In arterial blood it is 38 to 42 mm Hg.

Arterial levels of PO_2 will fall if adequate oxygen cannot perfuse the alveoli (when the level is below 60 mm Hg oxygen is generally administered); rising PCO_2 levels indicate the presence of poor respiratory function or an inability of the person to expire adequately.

OXYGEN SATURATION

Blood gas reports also include the proportion of hemoglobin in red blood cells that is saturated (that is, hemoglobin that has picked up all the oxygen it can carry). The oxygen saturation level helps to isolate the level of the respiratory problem. If hemoglobin is 100 percent saturated and yet the cells are not receiving enough oxygen, either there is not enough hemoglobin present to carry the total amount of oxygen needed or the cells cannot pick up the oxygen from the hemoglobin. If hemoglobin is very unsaturated, either the hemoglobin is defective and thus cannot carry adequate oxygen or adequate oxygen to saturate it has not diffused to the blood system from the alveoli. The normal saturation level of hemoglobin is 95 to 98 percent.

ACID-BASE BALANCE

The body's acid-base balance affects the blood gas balance because hemoglobin does not become as well saturated with oxygen if the bloodstream is acidotic; body cells do not allow oxygen to diffuse into them if they are suffering acidosis.

Hydrogen Ion Concentration. In the bloodstream water (H_2O) dissociates into its two components, hydrogen (H^+) and hydroxide ions (OH^-). If a solution has more hydrogen ions present than hydroxide ions, it is an *acid* solution; if fewer hydrogen ions are present than hydroxide ions, it is *alkalotic*. The presence of H^+ ions (pH) is expressed as a numerical value. A value of 7.0 is neutral; a value below 7.0 reflects a solution that has an excess of hydrogen ions (acid); a value above 7.0 reflects a solution with a deficit of hydrogen ions (alkaline). The pH of blood is always slightly alkaline and normally has a very narrow range—7.35 to 7.44. A level as low as 7.0 or as high as 7.8 is incompatible with life.

The lungs play a vital role in regulating the acid-base level of the blood because they are an important means of either conserving or blowing off hydrogen ions, whichever mechanism is needed to stabilize blood pH. For example, if the blood pH is becoming alkalotic (nearing 7.44), the person begins to breathe shallowly (hypoventilation), allowing less CO_2 to be expired than normal. This retained CO_2 combines with water to form carbonic acid (H_2CO_3) in the bloodstream. It then dissolves as needed into H^+ and HCO_3 (bicarbonate), increasing the number of hydrogen ions present and decreasing the pH. If the blood pH approaches its low normal level (near 7.35), the body combines free H^+ ions with bicarbonate to form carbonic acid and then dissociates these into H_2O and CO_2. The CO_2 is blown off from the body by deep rapid respirations (hyperventilation) to lower the total H^+ level and restore the acid-base balance.

In lung disease, hypoventilation often occurs as part of the disease (fluid blocks the airways, constricting and not allowing air to pass). Table 32-1 summarizes the blood patterns in which respiratory alkalosis or acidosis is present.

Base Excess. Base excess is a report of the amount of bicarbonate that is free to be utilized by the body to counteract acidosis (by combining with H^+ ions to form carbonic acid). A positive base excess (a plus value) shows that excess bicarbonate is present; a negative (or minus) value shows that no bicarbonate is available.

Bicarbonate. In some laboratories not only the base excess but also the actual bicarbonate level is reported. The normal bicarbonate level is 22 to 28 mEq per liter.

Potassium can be shifted easily from the bloodstream into cells or vice versa. If the blood is becoming acidotic, the body can shift potassium ions (K^+) in exchange for H^+ into the bloodstream from the cells, increasing the number of positively charged ions present and maintaining a balance between the positively and negatively charged ions in the blood. If the blood is becoming more alkalotic than normal, the body can secrete potassium in urine in added quantities, reducing the amount of potassium ions present in the blood and keeping the number of positively and negatively charged ions equal.

With long-term respiratory illness or alterations, therefore, potassium levels are affected at least to some extent. The blood potassium level will be decreased with respiratory alkalosis. Levels of potassium both above and below normal can cause severe cardiac arrhythmias; in extremely abnormal concentrations, they can cause complete heart block. The potassium level is not a part of blood gas reports per se but is usually ordered at the same time because it tends to show the duration or acute extent of the respiratory problem.

RESPIRATION AND LIFE SPAN CONCEPTS

The efficiency of external and internal respiratory function is affected by age.

The Fetus

The exchange site for oxygen in a fetus is not the alveolar-capillary interface but the placenta-uterine interface. Early in intrauterine life, villi, the two-cell-thick "fingers" from the growing zygote, dip down into the uterine sinuses or systems of maternal blood. Oxygen diffuses across from the maternal blood by osmosis into the villi and back through the umbilical cord to the fetus. Carbon dioxide returning from the fetus diffuses by the same process back to the maternal blood. A fetus exists at about 90 percent of his mother's oxygen level. A pregnant woman who develops an illness such as pneumonia that can interfere with the alveolar exchange of oxygen, thus decreasing the oxygen level in her arteries, is often administered oxygen because she must maintain an adequate oxygen level in the blood to keep the fetal oxygen level high; another patient who is not pregnant might not be administered oxygen in the same situation. Pregnant women are advised not to fly in aircraft with unpressurized cabins that lack oxygen administration capability because if the oxygen level in the airplane failed at a high altitude, the woman's blood oxygen level might be severely compromised.

TABLE 32-1. RESPIRATORY AND METABOLIC ACIDOSIS AND ALKALOSIS

Condition	Definition	Possible Causes	Symptoms	Typical Values
Respiratory acidosis (acidemia)	Increased number of H^+ ions present	Hypoventilation causing retention of CO_2	Shallow respirations, lethargy, coma	pH, ↓ 7.35; HCO_3, ↑ 27 mEq/L PCO_2, ↑ 40 mm Hg PO_2, normal Potassium, ↑
Respiratory alkalosis (alkalemia)	Decreased number of H^+ ions present	Hyperventilation with excess blowing off of CO_2	Deep respirations, numbing, tingling in hands	pH, ↑ 7.45; HCO_3, ↓ 22 mEq/L PCO_2, ↓ 40 mm Hg PO_2, normal Potassium, ↓
Metabolic acidosis (acidemia)	Abnormal accumulation of fixed acids	Excess keto acid production	Increased respiration	pH, ↓ 7.35; HCO_3, ↓ 22 mEq/L PCO_2, ↓ 40 mm Hg
Metabolic alkalosis (alkalemia)	Loss of H^+ ions or addition of fixed base to body fluids	Loss of acid gastric juice	Decreased respiration	pH, ↑ 7.45; HCO_3, ↑ 28 mEq/L PCO_2, ↑ 40 mm Hg

Fetal lungs are coated with a serous fluid that keeps the alveolar surfaces from adhering to each other while they are unused in uterine life. This fluid is absorbed across the alveoli into the pulmonary capillaries in the first few moments of extrauterine life.

The Newborn

Because the alveoli have not been used in utero, at birth, although they are not adherent to each other due to the presence of lung fluid, neither have they ever been expanded before. A first inspiration occurs because when the infant's umbilical cord is clamped following birth, he begins to experience anoxia (a low level of oxygen in cells). This, coupled with thermal stimulation (the temperature of the outside air on wet skin) and accumulating carbon dioxide in the blood, stimulates the respiratory center in the medulla to initiate an inspiration. The first inspiration takes a great deal of strength to accomplish (a pressure of about 40 mg Hg is needed). A baby's cry at birth is an announcement that he has taken this first important breath because crying is only possible if air is being pulled past the larynx. Newer techniques of childbirth that encourage immediate warming of the baby at birth and delivery in a room devoid of bright lights tend to prevent crying. The lack of crying, however, may not allow such babies to aerate their lungs as well at birth.

Newborns have a more rapid respiratory rate than adults—between 30 and 50 breaths per minute. The pattern is often slightly irregular; there may be an occasional sigh or two or three rapid inspirations followed by a longer than normal pause. There may be a quick "snoring" noise due to mucus collected in the nose. These are normal patterns for newborns; all new mothers need time to become familiar with this irregular pattern so that they will not worry about it.

Newborn infants are nose breathers. They do not have the coordination necessary to open their mouths to breathe if their nasal passages should become blocked. All newborns should be carefully assessed for respiratory function. A newborn with an obstruction of the nostrils or the posterior aspect of the nostrils (the choanae) needs to have an oral airway inserted to help him breathe through his mouth until the obstruction can be relieved. Mucus collected in the nose from an upper respiratory infection (a common cold) will cause the baby extreme distress and may need to be suctioned away to offer him breathing space.

The Infant

Because the infant continues to be a nose breather for the first year, his problems generally center around nasal obstruction. Infants begin to contract upper respiratory infections as soon as they are exposed to visiting friends and relatives, and most infants have at least one cold during their first year. Although it is a simple illness, the infant often has a high fever with it, and he may need nose drops to keep the nasal secretions liquid and flowing. Nasal secretions may have to be removed, especially before feeding, because the baby cannot breathe through his nose if his nostrils are blocked while he sucks on a bottle or his mother's breast.

The skin under the nose may become easily excoriated from nasal drainage with an upper respiratory infection because an infant cannot wipe this away as does an adult. Coating the skin with a water-based ointment will protect it. Caution the parents never to use an oil-based ointment for this purpose because if the baby should aspirate such a product, it could lead to inflammation of the alveoli (lipid pneumonia) and interfere with oxygen exchange at the alveolar level.

Upper respiratory tract infections in infants can spread quickly to become middle ear infections (otitis media) because of the short horizontal slant of the eustachian tube from the posterior pharynx in infants. This is another reason why a cold in an infant is rarely "just a cold."

The Toddler and Preschooler

Toddlers and preschoolers begin to have many new contacts outside their homes and are therefore exposed to many more people with upper respiratory tract infections. Because of such exposure they contract many of these infections (as many as 12 a year).

A preschool child who "keeps a cold" or "goes from one cold to another," may be developing an allergy to respiratory inhalants. In such children one criterion of assessment is the mucous membrane of the nose. A child with a cold has a reddened membrane; a child with an allergy often has a pale, edematous nasal membrane. The exudate with an upper respiratory infection may become thick and yellow (purulent); the exudate with an allergy is usually thin and watery. A history of frequent colds may also describe a child who has a chronic illness of some type and therefore has less resistance to disease than other children.

Many preschoolers contact "strep" throats—infection with beta hemolytic streptococcus, group A organisms. These are serious infections, not only because they are extremely painful (the throat appears beet red and pus is evident on the crypts of the tonsils) but also because beta hemolytic streptococci, group A, distribute toxins to body tissues as they grow. These toxins cause an extremely high fever and lassitude during the infection. This type of infection may result in permanent heart disease (rheumatic fever) or permanent kidney disease (glomerulonephritis). All children with sore throats should be seen by a health care provider because the only means of preventing the toxin outlay of the organism is antibiotic therapy. An important nursing role is teaching parents that not every sore throat is caused by streptococci (many are viral in origin), and therefore not every sore throat needs antibiotics; when an antibiotic is prescribed for a sore throat it means that a streptococcal infection was suspected, and the medicine should be taken for the full 10 days prescribed to be maximally effective. Often a medicine chart for this age child needs to be made to hang on the refrigerator door as a reminder of what times and for how long the medicine needs to be taken.

The Schoolager and Adolescent

Schoolagers and adolescents, as a rule, continue to have many upper respiratory infections that are passed back and forth in school. A disease with respiratory symptoms that tends to become manifest during the school-age period is asthma. Asthma is an allergic response that causes inflammation and narrowing of the bronchi. As a rule, a child with asthma can breathe in normally, but his bronchi are so narrowed and so much mucus collects from the inflammatory process that it is almost impossible for him to breathe out again. Children with asthma are always frightened by the sudden inability to breathe; a nurse needs not only to supply oxygen quickly but also to provide interventions to help the child feel secure and less frightened, thereby slowing his respiratory rate and making each breath more efficient (Fig. 32-2).

Nurses have a major role in educating school-age and adolescent children not to begin smoking cigarettes to reduce their risk of developing lung cancer or cardiovascular problems. This responsibility begins with a good role model of not smoking themselves.

The Young and Middle-Aged Adult

Respiratory difficulties in young adults tend to occur to some extent from infections such as pneumonia but more often are due to accidents that cause a broken rib or an injury to the lung itself. Adults who are placed on bed rest due to automobile or motorcycle accidents must be assessed thoroughly for respiratory function because immobility decreases lung function (the chest must expand against gravity) and predisposes the lungs to stasis of secretion and bacterial growth.

The middle-aged adult begins to be prone to lung diseases such as lung cancer (which is strongly associated with cigarette smoking) and emphysema (overdistention of the alveoli so that they never effectively empty, leaving a high residual amount of unexpired CO_2), as well as to cardiovascular diseases such as arteriosclerosis and myocardial infarction.

Certain occupations such as coal mining and working in cotton mills expose workers to irritating substances that eventually lead to deterioration of the alveoli. Pollution from motor vehicle emissions or other industrial wastes may cause the same phenomenon. Many people in this age group ask if taking supplementary vitamin C daily will keep them from developing respiratory infections or illnesses. There is little documented proof that intake of vitamin C prevents respiratory infections. The large amount of vitamin C recommended by those who advocate its use may actually be toxic.

The Older Adult

Because the older adult may not be as active during the day as he was formerly he may not take as many deep breaths as he used to. This, combined with decreased muscle movement of the rib cage may cause him to "pocket" or increase his residual lung volume. This "dead air" tends to invite infection.

FIGURE 32-2. Many people experience a suffocating feeling with oxygen administration equipment. Here a girl manages a smile for a camera despite her shortness of breath.

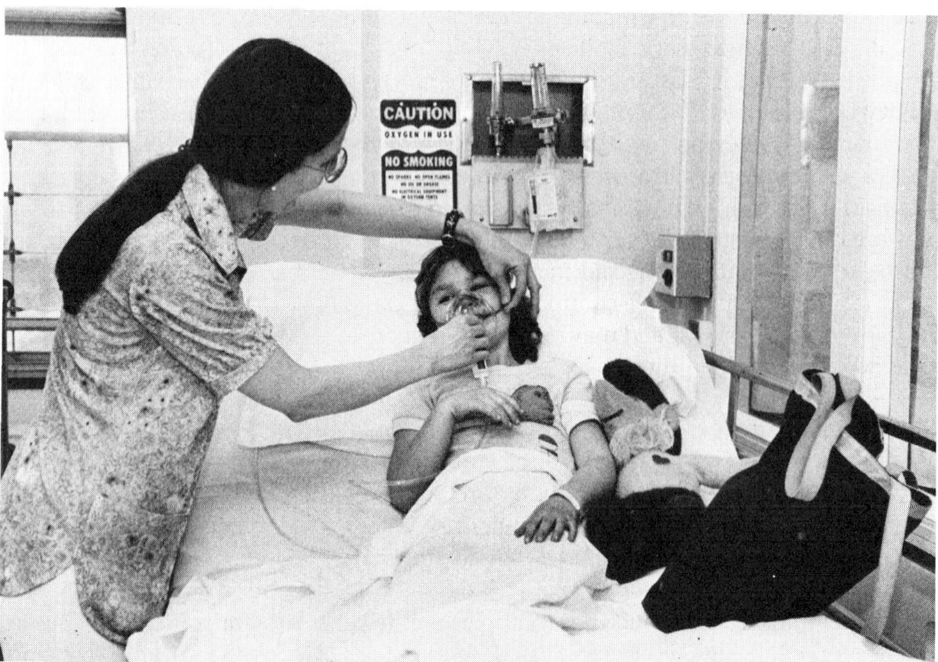

Older people often have some degree of arteriosclerosis, which narrows the arteries and makes them less pliable, making transport of oxygen less reliable than formerly. If the person has difficulty in buying iron-rich foods owing to a fixed income, his red blood cell count may also be decreased, which further decreases transport of oxygen.

Whenever an older adult is placed on sedentary activity or on bed rest, his respiratory function should be assessed thoroughly every day, and some preventive measures such as taking several good deep breaths several times a day should be instituted. Without these preventive measures his chances of developing a respiratory infection as a secondary problem are high.

ASSESSMENT OF RESPIRATORY FUNCTION

The assessment step of the nursing process typically has three parts—health interview, physical examination, and allied laboratory studies.

Interviewing

Despite the fact that everyone knows that breathing is essential to life, many adults at a health interview regard symptoms such as shortness of breath on walking upstairs, chronic cough, or fatigue as unimportant and therefore mention them in an almost off hand manner. A nurse must listen carefully when interviewing a patient for respiratory function to avoid missing the importance of these symptoms. Shortness of breath or fatigue may reflect a transport problem, whereas a chronic cough may be caused only by an irritated throat due to a mild allergy, or it may be the beginning sign of something as serious as lung cancer. Asking how many pillows a person uses to sleep on often reveals respiratory distress (an elevated chest position lowers the position of the abdominal contents and offers more potential for chest expansion). Asking if a person sleeps soundly often reveals the presence of a chronic cough that wakes the patient periodically during the night. Be certain to ask about occupation and smoking history (marijuana as well as cigarettes) to establish possible risk.

A mother of a small infant may not report that the infant's respirations are distressed (for instance, they may be rapid, but she knows that an infant's respiratory rate is more rapid than that of adults so she thinks they are all right), but she may report that the infant has difficulty in drinking or never sucks for long periods at the breast or finish an entire bottle. This is because the baby cannot swallow and breathe at the same time; he has to stop sucking to maintain his rapid respiratory rate because of some form of distress. Listening for reports of feeding problems in infants, then, is a vital part not only of nutrition assessment but of respiratory assessment as well.

A history of frequent upper respiratory tract disease needs to be investigated because it may be a sign of an allergy, an unsafe environment (high in pollutants), or an altered immunosuppressive activity in the body. See the following box for pertinent questions to include in the interview for respiratory function.

Physical Examination

The first step in physical assessment is observation. Important signs to note are the general appearance, skin color, rate and quality of respirations, chest contour, fingertip clubbing, the quality of speech, and breath odor.

GENERAL APPEARANCE

A person who has difficulty with breathing feels uncomfortable and may be in acute distress or pain. If he is covered by many clothes or bedcovers so that his chest cannot be readily observed for respiratory movement, these forms of distress may be evident first by noticing facial expression. Distress may also be evident by an attempt to find a position of comfort (sitting up in an emergency room even though the patient appears otherwise exhausted). Infants with respiratory distress typically struggle and do not comfort readily when held. Nasal flaring and use of accessory respiratory muscles (pectorals or sternocleidomastoid muscles) may be observed. Many people with respiratory distress are comfortable while they are at rest, but grow uncomfortable when they exercise. Note carefully the degree of exercise that causes this. If discomfort is noticeable on simply turning in bed or walking a few steps, the degree of respiratory impairment is obviously greater than it is if the person experiences no distress until he has walked the length of the hallway or a flight of stairs.

Interviewing Questions for Assessing Health of Respiratory System

Has the person ever had: Chest pain? Shortness of breath? Frequent respiratory tract infections?
Can he breathe equally well lying down and sitting up?
Does he have a cough?
Does he produce sputum?
Does he have a nasal discharge?
Is he exposed to environmental contaminants at home or work?
Does he ever notice cyanosis?
Is he constantly fatigued?
When was his last chest x-ray?
Is he a smoker (cigars, pipes, cigarettes, or marijuana)?
Does he use cocaine?

ORTHOPNEA

Orthopnea is difficulty in breathing except in an upright position. It is a subjective finding—that is, it can be reported by the person although it may not be observed by you. Always observe a person's respiratory activity not only while he is standing or sitting but also when he is lying down. Orthopnea generally results from excessive pulmonary congestion due to poor circulation.

DYSPNEA

Dyspnea is a broad term that denotes difficulty in breathing in any form. The term is used for both a purely subjective finding (the person experiences difficulty in breathing even though you do not notice any evidence of distress) and for an objective finding (you notice distress). It may be caused by cardiac, respiratory, or psychological factors. The person with dyspnea generally struggles to sit upright; he is very frightened as his increasing oxygen hunger grows stronger. He needs immediate intervention (probably including oxygen therapy) to relieve his difficulty. Dyspnea is always serious because it may precede *apnea*, or cessation of breathing.

SKIN COLOR

The skin color of a person who is transporting an adequate level of oxygenated hemoglobin (which is red) through his arteries appears pink (in deeply pigmented skin a pink hue appears when it is pressed and blanched). If the arterial blood contains a larger than normal portion of unoxygenated hemoglobin (blue to purple in appearance) the skin color becomes pale and then dusky blue. In people with deeply pigmented skin, this blue tinge is most perceptible in the mucous membranes such as the lips or the conjunctival sac of the eye. Such blue discoloration is termed *cyanosis*. Cyanosis may be first apparent in the skin around the mouth (circumoral cyanosis); in all people it is often more noticeable in mucous membranes or the nail beds than in the skin itself. The buccal membrane of the mouth (inner surface of the cheek) is considered by many the best place to assess for cyanosis in deeply pigmented individuals.

Because cyanosis does not appear until 80 percent of hemoglobin is unoxygenated, it is a late sign of oxygen lack (normal hemoglobin is 95 to 98 percent saturated). It will not be apparent if less than 5 gm of hemoglobin is present because in such cases so little hemoglobin is present that all of it is saturated despite the fact the cells are very short in oxygen. People with severe anemia, therefore, lack this important finding of cyanotic appearance.

RESPIRATIONS

Observe not only the rate of respirations (see Procedure 32-1) but their depth and rhythm as well. Average respiratory rates for different age groups are shown in Table 32-2. If the respiratory rate is above this norm, the person has *tachypnea;* if below it, he has *bradypnea.* Tachypnea generally occurs because of lack of oxygen or increased blood carbon dioxide levels (the respiratory rate increases spontaneously to take in or blow off needed gases). Bradypnea generally occurs either because of lowered blood carbon dioxide levels (the person breathes slowly to conserve carbon dioxide) or because the respiratory center is directly affected by trauma such as increased intracranial pressure.

Breathing should be quiet and without effort. Note the time of both respiratory phases (inspiratory and expiratory). If the inspiratory phase is unusually long (more than 3 seconds), it generally denotes at least a partial obstruction of the airway. If expiration is unusually prolonged (more than 2 seconds), either there is an obstruction or the alveoli are so hyperdistended that it takes longer than usual to empty them.

Metabolic disease may cause abnormal breathing patterns because the person attempts to adjust the acid-base balance by using respiratory compensatory mechanisms. Typical breathing patterns in these diseases and their causes are shown in Table 32-1.

CHEST CONTOUR

Observe the chest contour for anteroposterior diameter in contrast to lateral diameter. An increased anteroposterior diameter suggests chronic lung disease (a barrel or pouting pigeon chest). A decreased anteroposterior diameter may suggest a congenital bone defect (pectus excavatum), a condition that may limit lung expansion. Observe the spinal column. Kyphosis (posterior curvature of the spine) and scoliosis (lateral curvature of the spine) may both distort the chest cavity and limit lung expansion.

Observe also the accessory muscles of respiration (the sternocleidomastoids, intercostals, and trapezius). Normally these are barely noticeable with respiratory movement. If the person has difficulty inhaling, however, he must use these muscles to accomplish adequate rib expansion. If inhalation is extremely difficult, the supracostal, intracostal, and subcostal spaces are actually sucked inward. This is termed *retraction* and is described by the muscle involved (supracostal retraction, subcostal retraction, or intracostal retraction).

Many infants normally use their abdominal muscles to assist in respiration. This is abnormal in older children and adults, however, and again reveals that the person is using accessory muscles because inspiration is difficult.

Notice whether chest contour is symmetrical right to left and whether there is a midline trachea on the anterior throat. A collapsed lung (atelectasis) may be revealed by a smaller appearing chest cavity on that side or a deviated trachea.

PROCEDURE 32-1
Obtaining the Rate of Respirations

Purpose: To assess respiratory function by counting and evaluating respiratory rate and quality.

Plan	*Principle*
1. Wash hands; identify patient. Analyze appropriateness of procedure.	1. Omit explaining the procedure; if a person is aware that his respirations are being assessed, self-consciousness causes the rate to change. Delay counting if the person has been exercising strenuously because this will increase the rate disproportionately.
2. Implement procedure by obtaining necessary equipment; only a note pad or chart to record findings is needed.	2. Make a habit of recording vital sign assessments immediately; important as they are, they are also easily forgotten.
3. Following pulse assessment, with your fingers still resting on the patient's wrist or with your stethoscope still in place on his chest, observe the rising and falling of the chest.	3. By pretending to continue pulse assessment you will not alert the patient to the fact that you are now counting and evaluating respirations.
4. Count respirations for at least 30 seconds for accuracy.	4. If the respiratory rate is very rapid or irregular, you need to count for a full minute for accuracy.
5. Assess additional qualities of respiration—rhythm (regular, irregular, depth); any accessory sounds heard (wheezing, stridor).	5. Abnormal depth or rhythm or accessory sounds of respirations may be as important as the rate.
6. Evaluate effectiveness, efficiency, cost, safety and comfort aspects of procedure. Record rate, depth, rhythm, and accessory sounds immediately on the note pad or chart. Plan health teaching as needed such as the importance of not resting the arms on the chest to allow for greater lung expansion.	6. Document patient status and nursing care. Health teaching is an independent nursing action always included as part of nursing care.

MODIFICATIONS FOR CARE OF CHILD

An infant's respiratory rate changes markedly if the infant cries. Make a point of counting an infant's respiratory rate when you first approach his crib, before you lower the crib rail (which will wake him and possibly provoke crying). Always try to quiet a crying infant by sitting and rocking him or walking with him momentarily before counting the respiratory rate. If the infant is crying when the rate is counted, mark the word *crying* on the record or graph so that it can be evaluated in its proper perspective.

MODIFICATIONS FOR CARE OF OLDER ADULT

Many older adults have a very shallow rib cage movement with respiration. It may be necessary to auscultate breath sounds with a stethoscope to be accurate in such people. Make a point of saying you are listening to the heart, not the lungs so that the pattern of respiratory movements remains unchanged.

TABLE 32-2. NORMAL RESPIRATORY RATES IN DIFFERENT AGE GROUPS

Age	Normal Rate per Minute
Newborn	30—50 breaths per minute
Infant	Up to 45 breaths per minute
Toddler	Up to 40 breaths per minute
Schoolager and adolescent	16—20 breaths per minute
Adult	14—20 breaths per minute

FINGERTIP ASSESSMENT

People who are chronically unable to supply oxygen to the body cells develop "clubbing" or lateral expansion of the fingertips (Fig. 32-3). This occurs because the capillary endings in the fingertips proliferate in an attempt to bring more oxygen to the oxygen-starved cells there. Clubbing can occur either in people with severe cardiac disease (oxygen is not reaching the distal cells owing to poor transport) or in people with chronic obstructive pulmonary disease (oxygen is not reaching the

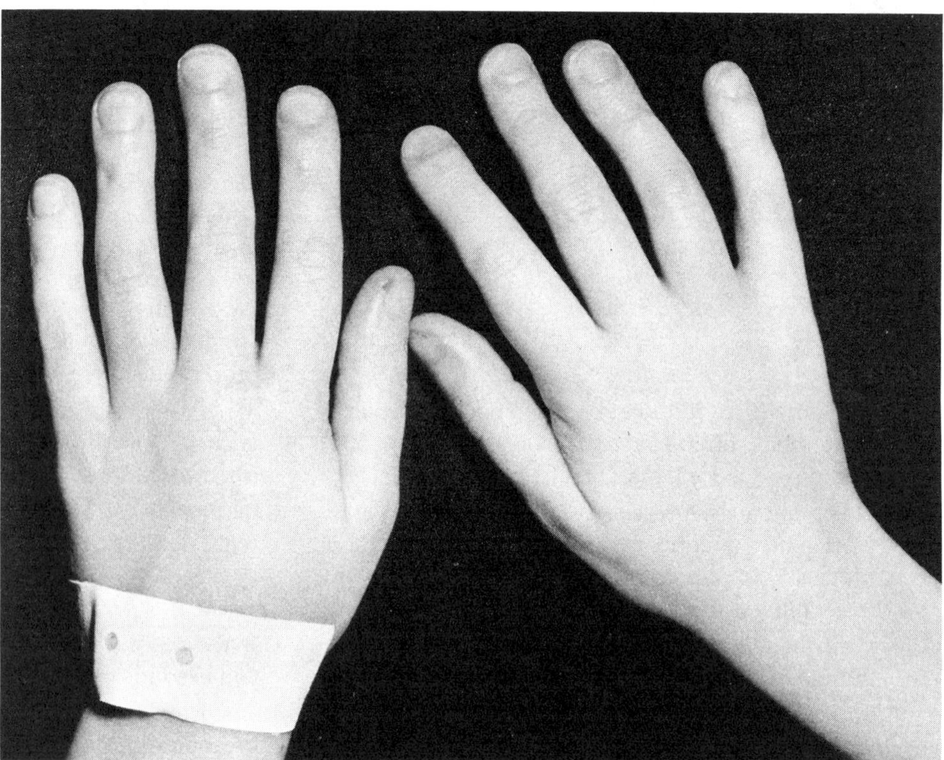

FIGURE 32-3. "Clubbing" of fingertips occurs in people chronically unable to oxygenate body cells.

bloodstream for transport because it is not crossing the alveolar-blood interface).

SPEECH PATTERN

People with normal respiratory function are able to finish long sentences without pausing for breath; they speak with an adequate volume of air to make their voice well heard. In contrast, people who cannot move a sufficient volume of air through the larynx may not be able to speak above a whisper; the tone of voice may be high pitched rather than resonant. They may need to pause every few words to take a breath. When observing a person for respiratory function, assess not only what the person is saying but how he is speaking for extra clues to breathing difficulty.

BREATH ODOR

Breath odor generally denotes poor oral hygiene rather than a respiratory difficulty, but there are exceptions. An inhaled foreign body such as a peanut that has been lodged in a bronchus for a period of time and has produced a local infection may produce a breath odor. Other breath odors, such as a sweet odor, may indicate a metabolic process that has resulted in acidosis; the odor of alcohol often gives a clue to the reason for an accompanying bradypnea.

Palpation

Palpation is a useful technique for discovering abnormalities in respiration. By palpating the chest you may be able to discover that fluid is present in the alveoli (air passing through the bronchi normally causes "fremitus," or small vibrations that can be felt by placing the palms of your hands on the person's chest). When fluid is present this vibration may be increased. If so much fluid is present that no air enters the bronchus, no fremitus will be present. The technique of palpation is discussed more fully in Chap. 19.

Auscultation

Always make a point of listening to the sounds of respiration at the same time you are counting the rate and assessing the depth and rhythm. Normally, respirations should make only very quiet sounds. Adventitious sounds and their likely causes and seriousness are summarized in Table 32-3.

People whose lungs are collapsed (pneumothorax) or who are unable to move any air at all through their airways have "silent lungs"—breath sounds are inaudible on auscultation of the chest. This is obviously serious because it indicates either lungs that are so filled with fluid that air can no longer pass through them or lungs or chest muscles that are so diseased that they are unable to maintain normal chest pressure.

Cough

Listen for coughing and evaluate whether it is a "dry" cough or a "moist" one (rasping and has the sound of

TABLE 32-3. ADVENTIOUS SOUNDS HEARD ON LUNG AUSCULTATION

Sound	Description	Importance
Rales	Crackling	The sound of air moving through moisture in the alveoli; pathologic
Rhonchi	Coarse, snoring	The sound of air moving through moisture in large bronchi; normal
Stridor	Shrill, "crowing"	The sound of air being pulled past a constricted larynx; pathologic
Wheezing	High, whistling	The sound of air being pushed through constricted bronchioles; pathologic

mucus being moved by the flow of air). Evaluate whether the sound indicates merely a clearing of the throat or is initiated from deep in the chest and whether it is productive (raises mucus that can then be expectorated) or nonproductive (raises no mucus). Evaluate the quality (small, moderate, or large) of mucus raised and its appearance (for example, yellow, purulent, or blood tinged). Children under 3 years of age, as a rule, are unable to coordinate coughing and expectorating and so always have nonproductive coughs (they swallow mucus).

The pattern or sound of coughing is often diagnostic of its cause. Children with croup (tracheolaryngobronchitis) have such severe spasms of the larynx and trachea due to inflammation that they have a "seallike" or barking cough. Children with pertussis (whooping cough) have a paroxysmal cough followed by a high crowing sound (a pattern of cough, cough, cough, whoop, cough, cough, cough, whoop, and so on).

Coughing may have psychological causes (a nervous response similar to biting fingernails). Evaluating the surrounding circumstances may highlight the reason for a cough. It also helps to determine the reason for coughs caused by physical illness (for instance, coughing that occurs only when the person lies on his right side or only in the presence of cigarette smoke).

Laboratory Analysis

A number of laboratory tests are helpful in assessing lung function. Sputum culture or analysis of nose and throat cultures may be ordered. Techniques for obtaining these specimens are discussed in Chap. 20 with other culture techniques. A radiograph of the chest or specific radiographic studies such as a bronchogram may be ordered. Be certain that people having a chest radiograph are not wearing necklaces or gold neckchains because these will block out a portion of the x-ray film. Many people are not aware that lung tissue extends above the level of the clavicle and therefore don't know that such jewelry will interfere with the radiograph. Thoracocentesis (aspiration of fluid from the pleural space by a puncture through the chest wall) and bronchoscopy (insertion of a thin hollow tube into the bronchus through the mouth for visual inspection) may be ordered. A biopsy (removal of a piece of tissue) may be done at the same time as bronchoscopy. Blood gas analysis (analysis of PO_2 and PCO_2) is another useful procedure. These diagnostic studies are discussed in Chap. 20; blood gases are shown in App. G.

Pulmonary Function Studies

Pulmonary function studies are studies that evaluate ventilation function. For these procedures, the person is seated by a spirometer, an apparatus that consists of a revolving drum with graph paper attached to its outside surface. The person breathes into the spirometer through a tube and mouthpiece (Fig. 32-4). Common measurements made are vital capacity, maximal breathing capacity, and forced expiratory volume. Table 32-4 summarizes these studies.

RELIEVING RESPIRATORY DISTRESS

Techniques for relieving respiratory distress are specific for the cause of the distress, but some common nursing interventions are psychological interventions, oxygen administration, and mobilization of mucous secretions from the chest by such means as postural drainage and administration of medication.

Psychological Considerations

All respiratory distress almost automatically brings with it some psychological distress (worry or fright because even preschoolers appreciate the importance of breathing for life). Providing an environment as stress-free as possible, therefore, generally aids a person's respiratory response greatly. Most people with respiratory illness are relieved at being placed in an intensive care unit because there they know that someone is constantly watching them or that the monitor leads attached to their chest will raise an alarm and call for help if their respiratory condition deteriorates.

These people are very fearful the first day they are moved from such a unit to a regular patient care unit because the bed is no longer instantly visible from the nursing station desk. In planning patient room placement, try to place a person with respiratory illness as close to the nursing station as possible. Make sure that the room has functioning oxygen wall outlets. In an emergency room be certain that the patient is examined near an oxygen source.

Be certain to include a system of "careful watch" techniques in your plan of nursing care, not only because frequent observations of a person with any degree of respiratory illness are necessary, but also because the person needs the reassurance that he is being frequently checked as much as he needs the check. Make a habit of

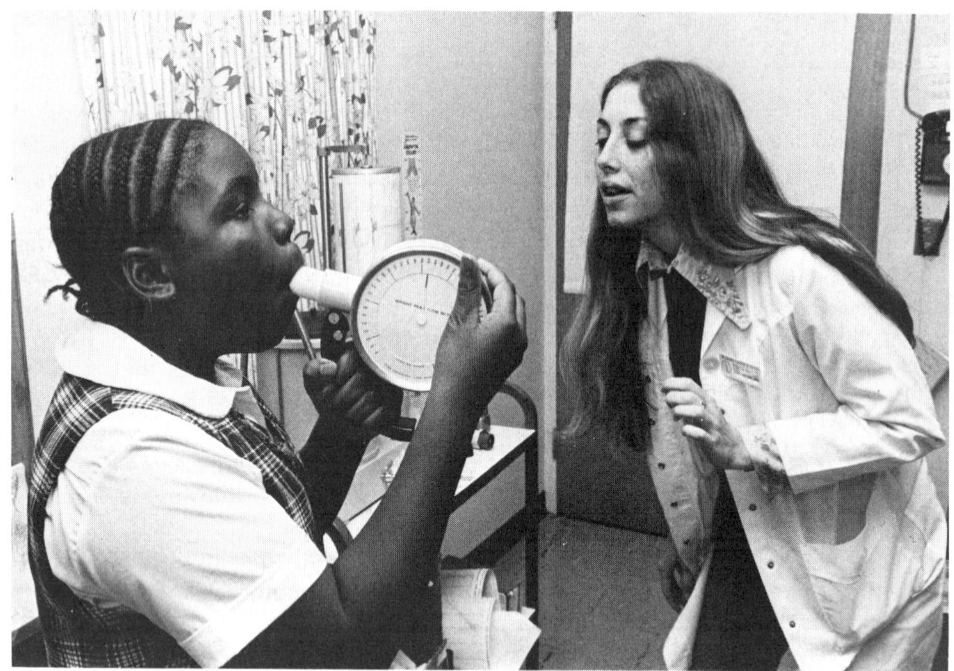

A

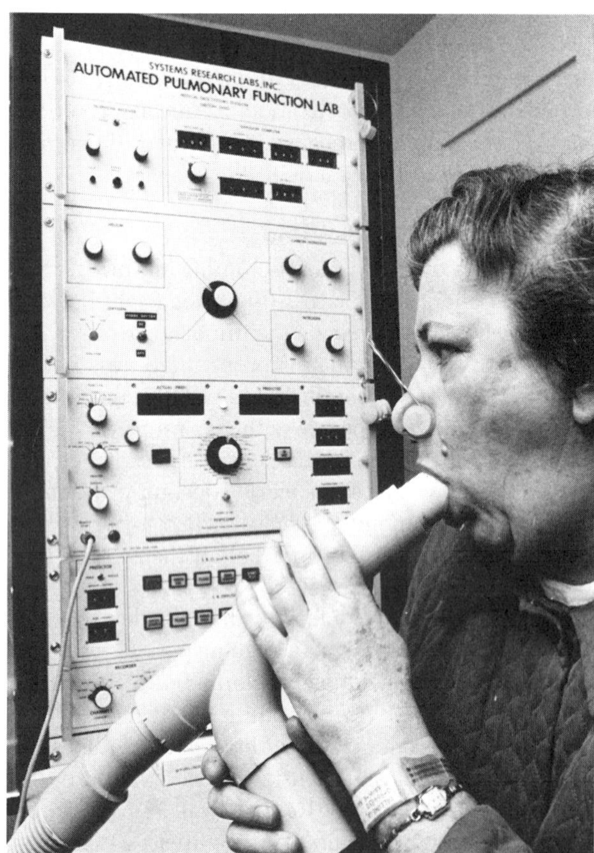

B

FIGURE 32-4. Equipment utilized in pulmonary function studies of child (A) and adult (B).

TABLE 32-4. PULMONARY FUNCTION STUDIES

Study	Definition
Vital capacity	The maximum amount of air that can be exhaled after a maximum inhalation.
Forced expiratory volume	Volume of a forcefully expired breath after a deep inhalation.
Maximal breathing capacity	Maximum amount of air a person can breathe in and out in 1 minute.
Residual volume	Volume of air that remains in lungs after a normal expiration.
Expiratory reserve volume	Volume of air that can be expired after a normal expiration.
Tidal volume	Amount of air normally inhaled and exhaled.
Inspiratory reserve volume	Amount of air that can be inspired over and above a normal inhalation.

going into the room at times other than to carry out a specific procedure.

Many people with respiratory illness are afraid to fall asleep for fear they will stop breathing while asleep. You may need to sit by the side of the bed to allow them to rest comfortably and prevent a secondary problem of physical exhaustion. This is particularly true of people who have had some form of ventilatory assistance (such as a respirator) or respiratory monitor for the first few nights they are without this equipment. People who become extremely anxious about their ability to breathe normally often hyperventilate because of anxiety, thus realizing their worst fears.

People who are using an oxygen tent (children) or face mask often feel shut off from you and may worry that if they need immediate help you will not be able to reach them quickly. When caring for people using such equipment, make a habit of showing them how the tent or mask lifts away easily so that they know they can be reached easily and can begin to appreciate the equipment as helpful rather than as a form of interference.

Do not try to relieve a patient's altered respiratory pattern by such statements as "Breathe normally" or "Don't think about your breathing." Such statements actually call attention to the problem rather than relieving it. Instead, give specific instructions that distract the person such as "Count to twenty for me" or "Take a really deep breath and then blow it all out." Remember that people who are short of breath often have difficulty speaking. Make a habit of carrying the responsibility for conversation by making reassuring statements.

People with respiratory illness who are being transported to another area of a health care facility such as the x-ray department often need a strong support person to accompany them; otherwise, their worry that they will not be safe outside the careful watch care causes them to hyperventilate, again realizing their worst fears. Never underestimate how frightening it is to be unable to breathe, and always accompany intervention for respiratory distress with assurance and comfort to decrease apprehension and anxiety.

Mobilizing Secretions

Raising mucus from the respiratory tract is called *expectoration.* The mucus raised is termed *sputum.* Various techniques are helpful in stimulating expectoration.

COUGHING

Coughing is a reflex generated by irritation of the pharynx, trachea, or bronchi (neurological impulses pass through the vagus nerve to the medulla oblongata and from there to the cough center). Coughing is an important procedure for raising mucus from the respiratory tract unless it is so excessive that it becomes exhausting or so forceful that it irritates the mucous lining of the respiratory tree. If the mucus is liquid and mobile, the cough will raise the secretions, and when the tract is clear coughing will halt. Medications generally given for cough, therefore, are expectorants (medications that loosen and aid the removal of sputum) rather than antitussives (medications that halt coughing). If the cough is caused by nasal secretions dripping into the pharynx, as happens with upper respiratory tract infections, an antihistamine medication to dry the upper airway secretions will halt the cough. Common expectorants, antihistamines, and antitussives are shown in Quick Reference Stop 32-1.

The coughing mechanism begins with a rapid inhalation that distends the lungs bilaterally. The glottis closes as the inhalation ends, and high intrathoracic pressure is momentarily present; because the diaphragm is in a descended position, intra-abdominal pressure is also high. After this initial second, the glottis reopens, the increased abdominal pressure pushes up violently against the diaphragm and the person exhales rapidly. The sound of coughing is the sound of mucus being mobilized and the forceful rush of air out of the larynx.

If a person has alveolar disease that has weakened the alveoli, the intrathoracic pressure attained by coughing may be enough to burst the alveoli at a weak point. This causes a pneumothorax (air from the alveolar space rushes into the pleural space and collapses the lung or lobe on that side, causing atelectasis). Pneumothorax is more often a problem of forceful ventilation, however, than of coughing (ventilators operate by pushing oxygen into the alveoli under pressure).

People with surgical incisions of the chest or abdomen generally need splinting of the incision area while they cough (hold a pillow or your hand snugly against the area or teach the person to do this for himself). This limits pain at the incision site and possibly prevents tearing of the healing tissue. It also is very reassuring because most people are concerned about the possibility of sutures tearing after surgery. Postoperative patients, particularly those who have had a general anesthesia, who do not cough and breathe deeply following surgery to aerate their lungs tend to collect many secretions in the bronchial tree and may develop pneumonia (alveolar infection) as a secondary complication of surgery. Methods of teaching coughing and deep breathing in the preoperative period are discussed in Chap. 40.

Provide a paper bag or other container for proper disposal of tissues used for coughing. The person who is coughing needs to wash his hands well before eating because even with the proper use of tissues, his hands will become contaminated with microorganisms that grow readily in any pooled body fluid.

Teach people that coughing as a rule is a helpful, not a harmful phenomenon that does not need to be halted because when the underlying reason for the coughing improves, the coughing will stop.

TURNING

All patients on bed rest should be turned or asked to turn every 2 hours to help keep respiratory tract secretions mobile. They should get out of bed and sit in a bedside chair or wheelchair or should be ambulatory as soon as possible. This is particularly important for people with respiratory illness, yet people who have experienced an episode of acute respiratory distress may be most reluctant to leave their hospital room and their source of oxygen. If a person is reluctant to leave his room when he is ambulatory, walking back and forth in the room for 15 minutes will provide the same

□ **QUICK REFERENCE STOP 32-1: PHARMACOLOGY**
Commonly Used Drugs to Reduce Cough

Classification	*Action*	*Example*	*Precautions*
Expectorants	Aid in removal of viscid mucus	Potassium iodide	Use interferes with thyroid tests. Continual use may cause hyperthyroidism.
Nasal decongestants (antihistamines)	Relieve congestion in nose by constriction of arterioles	Ephedrine	Topical application produces few adverse effects, although transient hypertension can occur from vasoconstriction. Has a rebound effect; after more than three days of therapy, great vasodilatation and increased congestion occurs.
Demulcents	Soothes mucous membrane with glycerin	Many commercial brands (cough drops)	Continuous use can add to dental caries if type chosen contains sweetened flavorers. Remind patient to suck slowly to offer sustained effect.
Antitussives	Suppresses cough	Tessalon (benzonatate)	Non-narcotic; temporary local anesthesia of oral mucosa may result.
		Romilar (dextromethorphan hydrobromide)	Non-narcotic; increases threshold of medullary cough center. Has no depressant effect on respirations.
		Codiene phosphate	Narcotic; inhibits medullary cough center. Causes drying of mucous membrane. Respiratory depression may result.

amount of activity as walking in the hallway for 15 minutes.

A few people with specific lung disorders should not be turned to the affected side. If the diseased lung is not ventilating well, lying on that side causes a great deal of blood to flow into the poorly functioning lung, leaving less blood to circulate through the functioning lung. Hypoxemia or poorly saturated hemoglobin levels may result. The person can generally be turned in every other way, however (supine, prone, and on the unaffected side).

A change in position from side to side or from a flat position to a sitting or standing position often promotes coughing as respiratory secretions move, stimulating the cough reflex. Some people are reluctant to sit up in bed or walk because coughing does occur at these times. Teach them that they should not stop activity because it provokes coughing, but should, in fact, welcome it.

Some patients need to have oxygen administered while they ambulate. They may be reluctant to change from a wall outlet source (which seems so secure) to a

☐ **QUICK REFERENCE STOP 32-2: PHARMACOLOGY**
Drugs Commonly Administered by Aerosol Route

Classification	*Action*	*Example*	*Precautions*
Bronchodilators	Relax smooth muscles to dilate bronchi	Bronkosol (isoetharine) Isuprel (isoproterenol hydrochloride)	Most bronchial dilators have the side effect of increasing heart rate and blood pressure. Check the pulse rate before and after administration.
Mucolytics (detergents)	Mobilize respiratory secretions by liquefying and changing the surface tension of mucus	Mucomyst (mucolytic) Alevaire (detergent) Dornavac (mucolytic plus proteolytic)	Bronchospasm may occur as an idiosyncratic reaction to any aerosol medication. If large amounts of mucus are mobilized, mucus may cause obstruction if not expectorated or suctioned.
Immunosuppressants	Prevent allergic response to antigens	Cromolyn sodium (Aarane)	Is not effective after bronchospasm has already begun; it has a preventive action.
Corticosteroids	Anti-flammatory	Decadron (dexamethasone sodium phosphate) Vanceril (beclomethasone dipropropionate)	Localized fungus infection in mouth or larynx may occur.
Antibiotics	Reduce bacteria count in respiratory tract (largely local action rather than systemic)	Polymyxin B	Bronchospasm may occur with any aerosol therapy as a response to foreign particles in the airway.

portable tank (which seems temporary and undependable). Make a point of assuring them that you have checked the tank's supply and you know it will be adequate for the time they will be using it.

NEBULIZATION

Nebulizers are devices that provide a stream of moistened air into the respiratory tract. Ultrasonic nebulization delivers such miniscule droplets into the respiratory tract that even the finest bronchioles can be moistened. Drugs such as detergents can be combined with the nebulized mist (this is termed aerosol therapy) to loosen secretions and help move them out of the respiratory tract; antibiotics may also be administered for local action by this route. Common aerosol medications are summarized in Quick Reference Stop 32-2. If a drug is being administered by aerosol to loosen and move secretions it will cause coughing. If the medication is an antibiotic that is meant to remain in the lungs, caution the person to try not to cough (not always possible because the moistened air of the treatment may cause tracheal irritation and a cough reflex).

Many people find nebulizer treatments uncomfortable (because they are frightened or feel as if they are drowning). Many people do not realize that aerosol administration is the most effective route for medications that loosen respiratory secretions, and they need support to continue such treatments.

Administration of aerosol medication carries the same responsibility as does administration of other forms of medication. It is prescribed according to dose, route, and times of administration like any other drug, and the particular vehicle that will be added to the nebulizer to create the mist is specified (usually distilled water so that impurities in water do not clog the

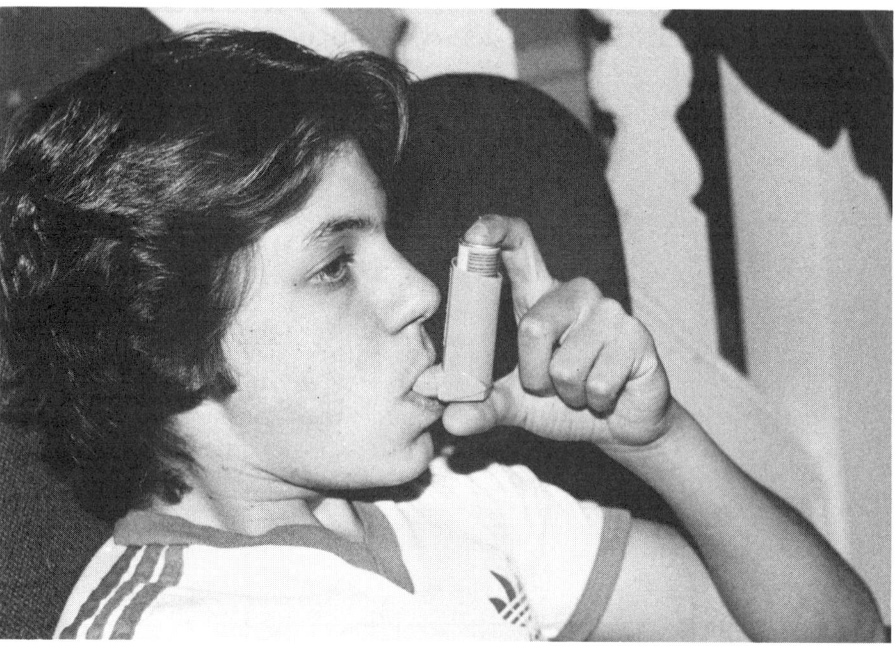

FIGURE 32-5. This teenage boy uses a hand-held nebulizer to relieve bronchial spasm.

nebulizer tip, or normal saline, which is isotonic with respiratory tract tissue). Do not be careless with this form of drug administration; check labels of drugs three times as in any other medication preparation.

The nebulizer used may be simple hand-held apparatus, or it may be connected to an electrical pump as a power source. Be familiar with the type of nebulizer you will be using before attempting to assist a patient with aerosol therapy. Small hand-held nebulizers may be used by some people, particularly those who have bronchial spasm (Fig. 32-5). They need good instructions in the use of such nebulizers and should be cautioned that although a little medication is good for them, a lot is not necessarily better so that they will use the device responsibly and not continually.

HUMIDIFIERS

A humidifier is a device that delivers water vapor to the air. It differs from a nebulizer in that it moistens the air in the entire room; the person then breathes in this moistened air. As a rule, humidifiers use water heated to the boiling point to provide warm, moistened air. Newer cool air humidifiers are available. Aerosol medications can be added to humidifiers so that the medication is delivered to the room at large. Because the particles of water produced by humidifiers are rarely as small as those produced by nebulizers, they do not penetrate the small bronchioles as well as nebulized air. They have other disadvantages in that they change not only the patient's immediate environment but the health care provider's environment as well. If they use a hot water source, they are potentially dangerous because they can cause severe scalding if tipped over near the patient. Mothers frequently use humidifiers in their infant's room at home when the infant has an upper respiratory infection. They can be assured that a cold air nebulizer used in a care setting will provide the same effect without the risk of having scalding water nearby.

Safety with Nebulizers and Humidifiers. Both nebulizers and humidifiers can become potential reservoirs for infection unless all medications and solutions used in them are sterile. They need to be thoroughly cleaned between uses for different patients so that they do not become the cause of nosocomial (hospital-based) infections. Observe patients carefully while they are receiving nebulizer therapy to be certain that they do not receive so much moisture that the moisture begins to add to the fluid load in the lungs instead of loosening and liquefying secretions. Respiratory membranes absorb solutions well, and children particularly may develop water intoxication from absorption of fluid across the respiratory tract membrane.

During administration of aerosol medications, watch carefully for signs of tracheal or bronchial irritation (bronchial spasm or bronchial edema) or systemic symptoms which may result from absorption by the membrane. It is easy for patients to discount aerosol drugs as unimportant and therefore take too much or not enough; be careful not to make the same error.

Intermittent Positive Pressure Breathing (IPPB)

An IPPB machine delivers oxygen or room air under pressure to the respiratory system to aerate the alveoli fully and prevent pooling of respiratory secretions. The person puts the mouthpiece of the attached tubing

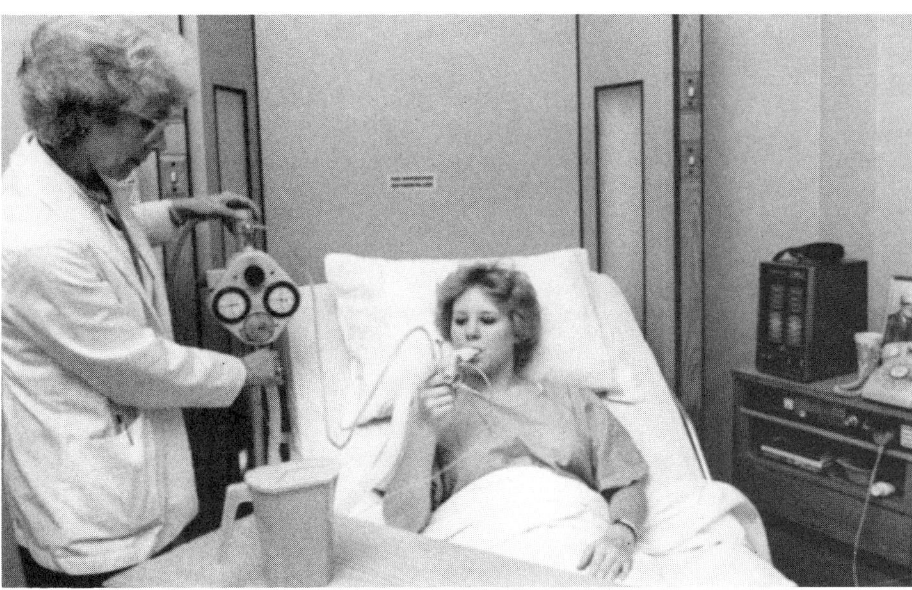

FIGURE 32-6. An IIPB treatment.

securely into his mouth and breathes in. This "triggers" the machine to produce the prescribed flow of oxygen or atmospheric air into his lungs (Fig. 32-6). IPPB machines are pressure-sensitive; when the person begins to expire, the machine clicks off and the person can expire easily. People need a good explanation of how the machine works, emphasizing that it will shut off as they begin to expire; otherwise, they will be very reluctant to use it because they are afraid that their lungs will burst from the continual pressure. IPPB machines make sighing, clicking, and hissing noises that are disturbing to some people; familiarize them with the equipment to make them comfortable. Aerosol medication mist can be delivered by IPPB machines as well as by nebulizers and humidifiers.

Observe a person carefully during an IPPB treatment for signs of dizziness or tremors (signs that overventilation is occurring or that too much carbon dioxide is being expired due to such deep breathing); increased pulse (venous blood returning to the heart is being impaired owing to the intermittently increased pressure in the chest); sharp headache (increased chest pressure is preventing good cerebral venous return and cerebral pressure is increasing); nausea or burping (the person's stomach is filling with air; he needs to breathe in with the machine so that the air enters his respiratory tract instead of fighting it, which allows at least a portion of it to enter the esophogus and stomach); and sudden dyspnea or shortness of breath (the pressure may have ruptured a weakened aveolus, leading to pneumothorax and collapse of a lung lobe).

If these complications should occur, halt the IPPB treatment and consult about what further care is necessary. These complications generally do not occur and, although IPPB therapy is not used as frequently as other forms of therapy, its benefits in administering aerosol medications and in helping to fully aerate and liquefy secretions can be considerable.

Postural Drainage

Postural drainage in its simplest form means moving secretions from the respiratory tract by means of the flow of gravity (a change in position). Additional techniques of clapping, vibrating, and percussion assist the flow of secretions. Postural drainage may be done by a respiratory therapist who comes periodically during the day, or it may be a nursing activity (particularly with infants). It may be a combined procedure (the respiratory therapist does it one of the four times ordered each day; a nurse does it the other three times).

Postural drainage causes coughing because it loosens and moves secretions. Sometimes the cough is so forceful that it causes vomiting. As a rule, therefore, postural drainage should never be done just after a meal when the stomach is full and the danger of aspiration from vomiting is most acute. If all sections of the lungs are to be drained, it is a long, exhausting procedure. Therefore, it should not follow immediately another procedure such as bathing or bed making that may drain energy. If the person is taking an expectorant, postural drainage should be scheduled when the expectorant will be operating at its peak level. If the person is having aerosol medication therapy to loosen secretions, postural drainage should follow this treatment immediately. Therefore, no matter who is actually doing the postural drainage, you will need to coordinate the timing.

Table 32-5 shows positions used to drain various lung lobes. The technique of clapping (Fig. 32-7) is done by striking the area over a particular lung lobe with the palm of the cupped hand (in infants, a soft nipple may be held in the palm to reduce the size of the

TABLE 32-5. COMMON POSITIONS FOR POSTURAL DRAINAGE

Lung Area	Patient Position	Area To Be Clapped and Vibrated
Upper lobes		
Apical segment	Sit upright, leaning forward slightly	Upper back and shoulders above shoulder blades
Right posterior segment	Sims's position on left side, bed flat	Area surrounding right scapula
Left posterior segment	Bed flat, Sims's position on right side	Area surrounding left scapula
Anterior portion	Bed flat, supine position	Upper anterior chest below clavicle
Lingula (middle segment of left lung)	Raise foot of bed 15—30 degrees. Position patient turned partially to back and partially to right side with pillow under back.	Left lateral chest at nipple line
Middle lobe of right lung	Raise foot of bed 15—30 degrees. Position patient turned partially to back and partially to left side with pillow under back.	Right lateral chest at nipple line
Lower lobes		
Superior segments	Bed flat; supine position	Area over lower third of anterior rib cage
Posterior segments	Raise foot of bed 30 degrees; prone position	Lower third of posterior rib cage
Anterior segments	Raise foot of bed 30 degrees; supine position	Lower anterior ribs
Left lateral segment	Raise foot of bed 30 degrees; right side position	Lower third of left lateral rib cage
Right lateral segment	Raise foot of bed 30 degrees; left side position	Lower third of right lateral rib cage

FIGURE 32-7. Clapping technique. Striking the area over a lung lobe with a cupped hand produces a large cracking noise from the force of the compressed air.

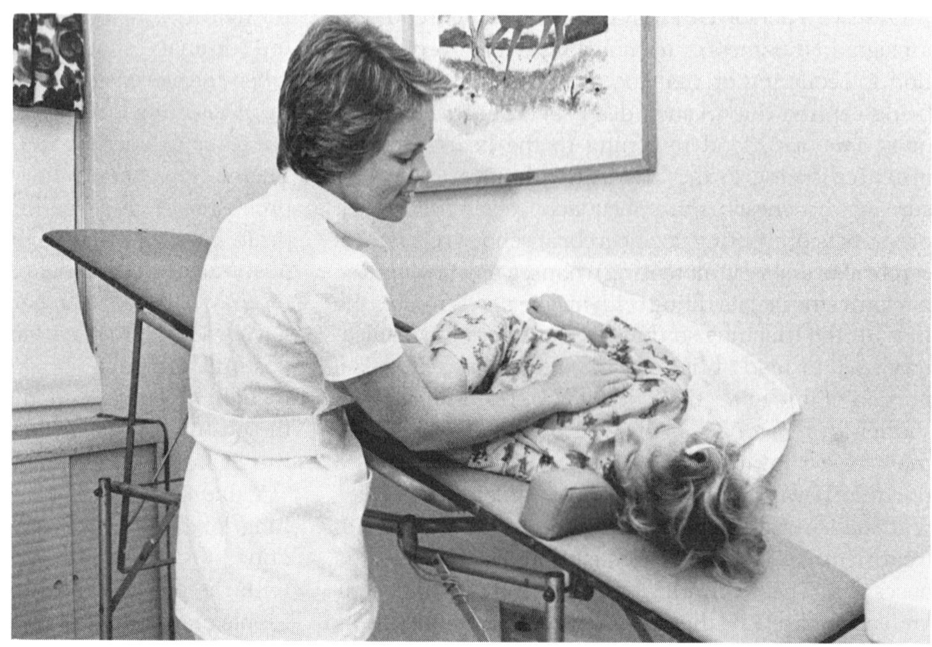

area struck). Clapping sounds as if the striking is much harder than it actually is. Parents and other support people need to be assured that the process is not painful. Vibrating is done by placing the cupped palm on the skin over the chosen area and literally vibrating it in that position for a minute at a time.

Many people with chronic lung disease will need postural drainage after they return home, so someone in the family (wife, husband, or parent) will need to learn the technique. Most people do not understand the value of postural drainage and therefore will not continue to do it well at home. Educate them about its value (it is the most inexpensive and effective means of raising tenacious mucus available).

Suctioning

Suctioning is the removal of respiratory tract secretions by means of a catheter. This is necessary whenever a person cannot cough adequately to clear secretions from the tract. Deep suctioning (endotracheal suctioning) is used when the patient has been intubated (an endotracheal tube has been passed through the nose or mouth into the trachea to maintain an open upper airway) or when a tracheostomy has been done (a tube has been passed through an incision on the anterior trachea). Oral and nasal suctioning is a simpler procedure and is used when excess secretions in the upper respiratory tract are interfering with the exchange of air to the lower tract.

ORAL OR NASAL SUCTION BY BULB SYRINGE

A bulb syringe initiates very gentle suction and is the method used for clearing secretions from the nasal passage and the mouth of a newborn or infant. Such suctioning is often done just before feeding because the infant cannot breathe through his mouth and suck at the same time; he must have his nose free of secretions to feed comfortably.

To use a bulb syringe, first compress the bulb of the syringe, insert the tip gently about half an inch into a nostril, and allow the bulb to re-expand gently. This sucks nasal secretions into the bulb. Remove the syringe from the nostril, press the bulb again, and expel the contents into a paper tissue or other container for disposal. Repeat the process as many times as needed with both nostrils. When teaching parents how to use a nasal syringe, be certain they understand the importance of compressing the bulb *before* inserting it into the nostril. Inserting the syringe and then compressing the bulb would force the secretions further back into the nose, compounding the blockage rather than relieving it. When suctioning both the oral and nasal passages, clear the oral cavity first and then the nostrils or use separate syringes to avoid spreading microorganisms in nasal secretions to the oral cavity.

NASAL OR ORAL SUCTION BY CATHETER

Procedures 32-2, 32-3, and 32-4 describe the process of nasal and oral suctioning using a catheter. Such suctioning may consist of nasopharyngeal (nose and

PROCEDURE 32-2
Nasopharyngeal Suctioning

Purpose: To remove secretions from the nose and pharynx by introducing a sterile catheter and applying vacuum suction; to prevent obstruction or infection of the upper airway caused by retained secretions; to obtain a nasopharyngeal secretion specimen for laboratory analysis.

Plan	*Principle*
1. Wash your hands, identify patient; explain procedure to patient.	1. Prevent spread of microorganisms; ensure patient safety and compliance.
2. Assess respiratory rate and dyspnea; analyze appropriateness of procedure; modify plan as necessary.	2. Need for suction is evident by noisy respirations, increased respiratory rate, subjective feeling of dyspnea.
3. Implement procedure by assembling equipment: suction source (wall or portable), connecting tubing, sterile catheter, sterile glove, sterile rinsing solution (0.9% normal saline or sterile distilled water), sputum trap if specimen is desired.	3. Use of sterile equipment prevents the introduction of microorganisms into the respiratory tract, thus initiating a secondary infection; the glove serves the secondary purpose of protecting your hand from possibly infected respiratory secretions.
4. Position patient comfortably; provide privacy.	4. Most people with respiratory distress feel most comfortable in a Fowler's or semi-Fowler's position; for ease in suctioning, place a small pillow or rolled towel behind the neck so that the head tips slilghtly backward (hyperextends).

5. Open bottle of sterile rinsing solution; open sterile catheter; put on sterile glove and attach catheter to connecting tubing from suction source. Test whether catheter is patent and suction apparatus is operating by dipping the catheter in sterile rinse solution (with gloved hand) and suctioning small amount of solution through catheter.	5. Suction is transmitted to the inner core of the catheter by pressing your thumb against the suction vent in the connecting tubing with your unsterile hand. Dipping the tip of the catheter also moistens it, making nontraumatic insertion easier.
6. Remove your thumb from the suction vent so that suction pressure is not operating; measure the length of the distance between the person's nose and earlobe. Insert catheter gently into nostril. Do not force the catheter if you meet resistance.	6. Use no suction as the catheter is inserted so that it will slide easily against the mucous membrane. Always use a gentle technique to avoid trauma to the sensitive mucosa. In many people one nostril is smaller than the other and does not allow a catheter to pass easily. Be careful as you hold the catheter to measure the distance between the nose and earlobe that you do not touch the catheter against the face and contaminate it.
7. Press your thumb against the suction vent intermittently and withdraw the catheter gently, rotating it as you withdraw it. Be certain that the catheter remains in the nasopharyngeal cavity no longer than 10—15 seconds. Contain the catheter in the gloved hand as it is removed so that it does not touch any nearby object.	7. Rotating the catheter allows it to reach more pockets of secretions; intermittent suction prevents the mucous membrane from being pulled into the catheter and injured. Limiting the time of insertion ensures that excessive oxygen is not removed from the airway. Holding the catheter contained prevents it from striking objects.
8. If an aspiration trap or specimen trap is used, it should be inserted between the catheter and suction tubing before they are inserted. Secretions obtained will be deposited in the "trap." If a trap was used, remove it at this point from the tubing.	8. When obtaining a specimen, always connect the trap before the first suctioning attempt because this attempt will undoubtedly remove most of the secretions. Remove the trap from the system before rinse solution is added in the next step.
9. Dip the catheter tip in rinsing solution; rinse the inner core by suction pressure.	9. If secretions are thick and tenacious they can easily plug the lumen of the catheter if they are not rinsed away after each suctioning attempt.
10. Assess effectiveness of the procedure; take respiratory rate. If the airway still appears obstructed, repeat catheter insertion and suction.	10. Suction as few times as necessary to prevent mucosal irritation, but be certain to perform adequate suction to clear the airway. Unless the patient is in acute distress allow a number of inhalations before a second suction attempt to allow lung aeration.
11. Turn off suction source; discard catheter and sterile glove and used rinsing solution.	11. Do not place the catheter in rinsing solution for reuse. A rinsing solution supports the growth of microorganisms, so reuse of either the catheter or the solution would insert a high proportion of microorganisms into the respiratory tract.
12. Cover end of connecting tubing with gauze to keep it clean; empty and rinse to clean collecting bottle of suctioned material as necessary; leave patient comfortable.	12. Connecting tubing and bottle are reused and are clean but not sterile.
13. Offer support for patient cooperation; plan health teaching as necessary, such as need for suctioning, helpfulness of good hydration to keep secretions moist.	13. Nasopharyngeal suctioning is not comfortable. Any degree of cooperation, then, is good cooperation and deserves praise. Health teaching is an independent nursing function that is always included in nursing care.

14. Evaluate effectiveness, efficiency, cost, comfort, and safety of procedure. Record procedure, appearance of secretions obtained, and patient tolerance, as well as patient status after the procedure.

14. Document patient status and nursing care.

MODIFICATIONS FOR CARE OF CHILDREN

Small children respond poorly to intrusive procedures. They also have been told many times not to push anything into their noses. Give a careful explanation that includes a statement that it is all right to insert this catheter; caution that the catheter will "tickle" when they feel it in the nose.

Small children generally need their hands held by a second person to keep them from pushing the catheter away. Urge the restraining person to use an explanation such as "Let me help you keep your hands down" rather than a punitive attitude. Infants can be effectively restrained by a mummy restraint for nasopharyngeal suctioning.

Praise lavishly. Any degree of cooperation short of hysterical screaming is good for an intrusive procedure with a small child.

MODIFICATIONS FOR CARE OF OLDER ADULT

Mucous membranes in the older adult are traumatized easily. Be extremely gentle with catheter insertion. Many older men have partially deviated nasal septa (they have struck it or fallen on it by that time of life), so one side of the nose receives a catheter more easily than the other. You may need to use a catheter with a smaller lumen than you anticipated in many older adults to compensate for septal deviations. If one side of the nose is much smaller than the other, the person uses the larger side almost entirely for air exchange. Keeping it free of accumulated secretions is that much more important because it is the patient's chief route for oxygen.

PROCEDURE 32-3
Oral Suctioning

Purpose: To remove accumulating secretions in the oral cavity by means of a sterile suction catheter and a vacuum suction source.

Proceed in the same manner as for nasopharyngeal suction. Positioning the patient on his side is advantageous because it allows secretions to pocket against the buccal membrane where they can be easily reached by the catheter. Never position a person supine for oral suction because he could aspirate oral secretions from this position.

Slide the catheter along the side of the tongue to the rear of the mouth before initiating suction pressure; rotate and use intermittent suction as you remove the catheter. Be careful not to touch the uvula at the posterior end of the mouth with the catheter tip or you will initiate a vomiting reflex.

If you are suctioning both oral and nasal secretions, change catheters, gloves, and rinsing solution before beginning the new route of suction. If the patient is unconscious or uncooperative, never place your fingers in his mouth to assist with the catheter entry or to keep his jaws apart. A muscle spasm in an unconscious patient or resistance from an uncooperative one could result in a severe laceration to your fingers. Use a tongue blade padded with wrapped gauze if it is necessary to move the tongue away from the catheter.

MODIFICATIONS FOR CARE OF CHILD

Remember that children often have loose teeth between the ages of 5 and 8. Tap teeth with a tongue blade in the unconscious child to determine if any are loose prior to suctioning. Use caution while suctioning to avoid striking an extremely loose tooth. If you find a loose tooth before undertaking suctioning, mark this on the nursing care plan; inform the physician of the tooth's condition (she will either allow it to be worked loose by the nursing staff or refer it to a dentist for removal). Do not ignore the problem because a loose tooth can be aspirated by an unconscious child.

MODIFICATIONS FOR CARE OF OLDER ADULT

Many older adults have some periodontal disease (infection of gum tissue surrounding the teeth, causing them to be loose). Use the same precautions as with children to determine whether teeth are loose or not. Touching gum tissue affected by periodontal disease causes it to bleed readily. Try to avoid touching the gum line just at the base of the teeth to avoid this problem.

PROCEDURE 32-4
Tracheobronchial Suctioning by Intubation Routes

Purpose: To remove accumulated respiratory secretions by introducing a catheter and a vacuum suction source; to prevent obstruction or infection of the upper respiratory tract caused by retained secretions; to obtain a tracheal secretion specimen for laboratory analysis.

The suctioning procedure by this deep route is basically the same as that used for nasopharyngeal suctioning. It can be done through the nasal or oral route. If the nasal route is used, insert the catheter during inhalation so that the epiglottis is raised, freeing the route to the trachea. The oral route is very ineffective because the gag reflex interferes.

Suctioning may be ordered as "only length of tube" or "deep suction." To estimate the length of a tube you must obviously be familiar with the equipment used, but as a rule, a tracheostomy tube is about 3 to 5 cm in length. An endotracheal tube rests just proximal to the bifurcation of the major bronchi, so estimating a length of catheter from the distal end of the tube to the sternal tip will provide estimation of the depth of suction required.

To direct a catheter into the left bronchus, rotate the catheter clockwise as you insert it; to direct it toward the right bronchus, rotate it counter clockwise (Fig. 1). A Coudé tip catheter is a better way of ensuring that a catheter enters the left or less straight bronchus. Be certain to use strict sterile technique with deep suction. Microorganisms introduced into the trachea this way will surely cause a secondary infection (Fig. 2). Oxygen administration may be prescribed immediately before and after suctioning because a high percentage of oxygen is removed from the lungs by suction at this depth.

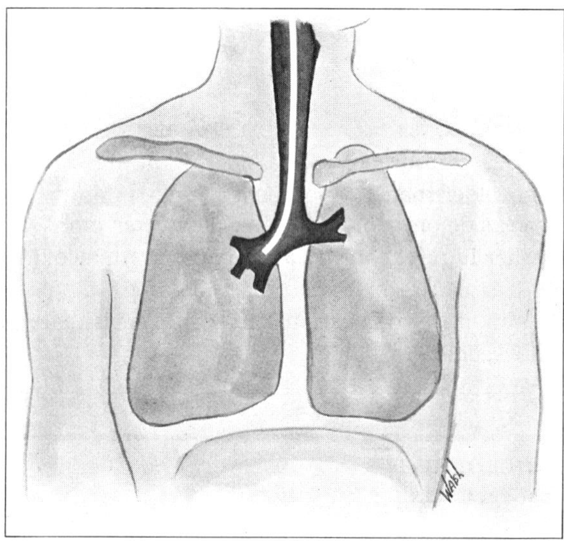

FIGURE 1. A suction catheter anatomically enters the right bronchus because of the straighter and wider angle.

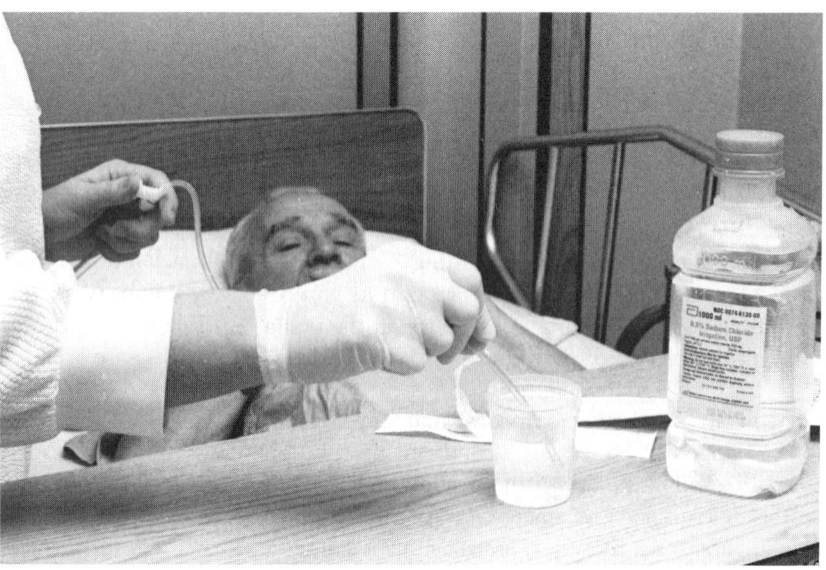

FIGURE 2. Rinse suction catheters between suctionings in sterile water or normal saline.

throat) suction or oral suction if the mucus present is mainly a collection of oral secretions. Suctioning can be a life-saving process that prevents mucus secretions from plugging the respiratory tract and blocking air exchange. It is, unfortunately, also a procedure that is not without risks, so it should be done only as needed and should be carried out with good technique and continuous observation of the patient's condition.

The need for suction can be evaluated from subjective and objective observations. The patient who is awake and aware feels apprehensive as he begins to experience oxygen hunger as the first respiratory secretions clog and obstruct his airway. People who are intubated cannot speak to call your attention to their distress, so you must check frequently on such people to recognize the feeling of distress and act quickly to relieve it.

Objective signs are rasping and gurgling respirations or an observable rapid or distressed breathing pattern; if you palpate the chest you can often feel the vibration of air moving through pooled secretions (tactile fremitus). If you listen to the person's chest with a stethoscope you can usually hear the sound of air passing through secretions in the upper airway (rhonchi) if suctioning is needed (the sound is a loud, harsh snoring or rattling sound). You may also hear moist rales (the sound of air passing over fluid; as very narrow bronchioles are reopened on inspiration, they make a crackling sound similar to crinkling tissue paper). Following suction, listen to the person's chest again. Suctioning should clear (or reduce) the sound of rhonchi. It will not clear the sound of small bronchiolar or alveolar rales because the catheter, even with deep suctioning, does not pass much beyond the point of the bifurcation of the bronchi, so it cannot clear secretions at this level.

Suctioning is accomplished by first passing a thin, pliable catheter to the depth of the respiratory tract desired and then initiating an intermittent suction power source, gently removing the catheter while the suction removes the secretions as the tip of the catheter passes them. The source of suction is negative pressure or vacuum extraction (secretions will be pulled from their location at the level of higher pressure into the vacuum or the place of lower pressure). Most health care agencies have built-in wall suction units close to the built-in oxygen outlets (Fig. 32-8) because many people who need oxygen also need suctioning. If there is no wall suction unit available, a portable suction unit (a Gomco apparatus) can be used (Fig. 32-9). The amount of pressure used should be the least amount necessary to remove the secretions so that trauma to the respiratory tract is minimal. A safe pressure to use with adults is between 80 and 140 mm Hg; pressure for infants and small children should be ordered specifically. Portable suction units have controls that allow suction pressure to be regulated only as high or low (strong or gentle pressure). Always use the low suction

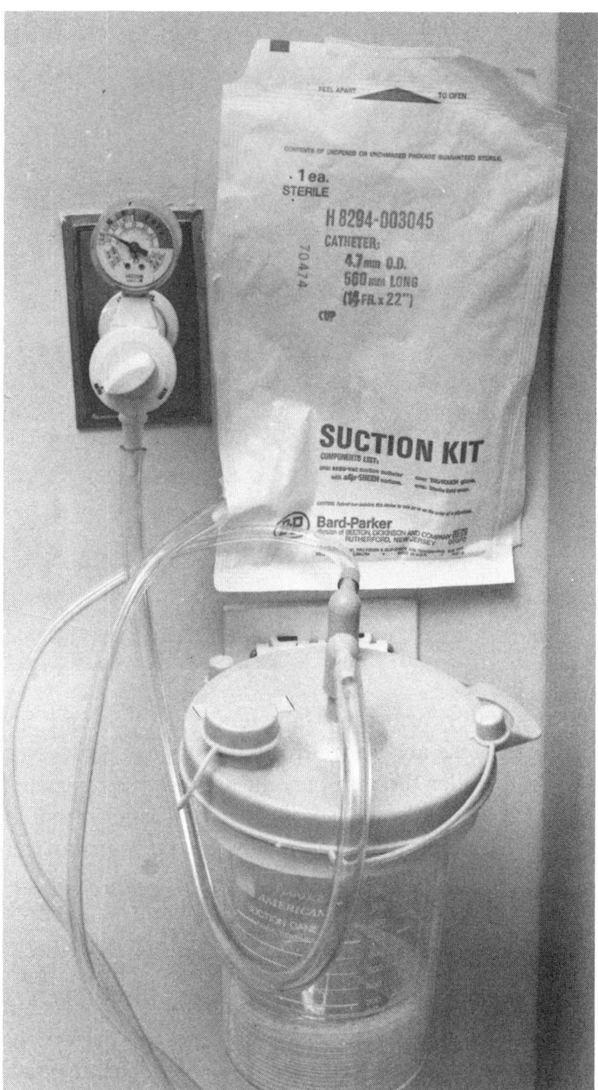

FIGURE 32-8. A wall suction unit. Pressure is regulated by the gauge attached to the suction source.

level on portable units. If this pressure setting is not strong enough to remove the mucus, the problem is probably not the strength of the vacuum pressure but the thickness of the mucus, which must be liquefied first. The problem will probably best be managed by securing an order for a liquefying agent (adding a drop or two of normal saline just prior to suction of the nostrils or the intubation tube, or administering an aerosol detergent several times a day, for instance) rather than by increasing the pressure of suctioning. Too forceful suctioning can cause severe damage and bleeding to the respiratory mucosa.

Suction catheters have several openings along the sides rather than a single one at the tip (as in a French style catheter) or one or two openings near the tip (as in the whistle-tip style). The presence of several openings prevents easy occlusion of the catheter, and less pressure is exerted at each opening, preventing damage to

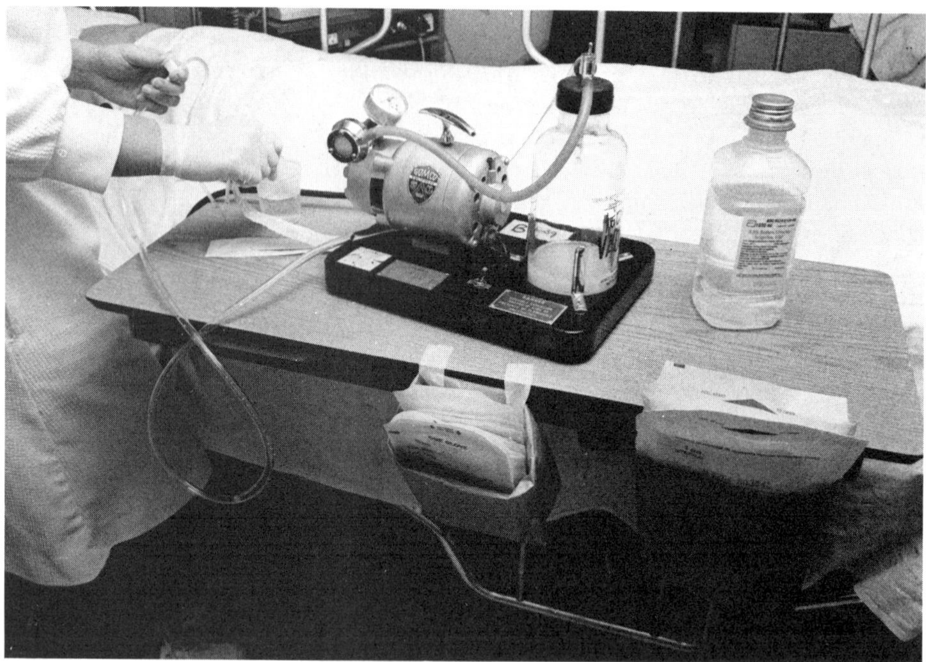

FIGURE 32-9. A portable suction unit. Always use low pressure with portable suction units to avoid injury to mucous membrane.

the respiratory mucosa. Catheters are numbered according to size and range from about a No. 5 to a No. 18. The smaller the number, the smaller the diameter of the catheter. Use the smallest size catheter possible so that the respiratory tract walls will be traumatized as little as possible by the catheter insertion. A small catheter also has the advantage of allowing air to enter the respiratory tract beside it; a large catheter obstructs any free entry of air. Secretions are removed by suction, which also removes oxygen from the lungs. The larger the catheter, the more air is removed (an extremely large amount of air removed could lead to alveolar collapse).

RISKS OF SUCTIONING

Trauma to Airway. Friction of the catheter against the respiratory mucosa combined with the suction applied to the mucous membranes can be very irritating to the respiratory mucosa. It is not uncommon after a long period of suctioning to see the secretions begin to become blood-tinged as active miniature bleeding sites result from mucous membrane irritation. To reduce trauma to the airway, never force a suction catheter. If it will not pass freely through the posterior nares, use the oral route for suction. Lubricate the tip with sterile water or normal saline before insertion. Never apply suction pressure as the catheter is advanced, only when it is being removed. Rotating the catheter as you remove it also helps to prevent the membranes from being "grabbed" by the suction pressure and injured.

Alveolar Collapse. The suction pressure that is applied to remove secretions also removes air from the bronchi and alveoli. If a great deal of air is removed (during prolonged suction or high-pressure suctioning), so little may remain that the alveoli collapse. Administering oxygen just prior to suctioning helps to "load" the airway with oxygen and minimize the problem. To avoid this it is a helpful practice to avoid applying suction for a longer period of time than you can comfortably hold your own breath.

Vagal Stimulation. Stimulation of the vagal nerve may result in bradycardia. The irritation of a catheter against the respiratory tract walls may be enough to cause severe bradycardia from this source. If bradycardia should occur during suctioning, stop the suction immediately and offer oxygen. The effect of bradycardia is transitory as a rule if oxygen therapy is begun. Oxygen therapy is necessary to aid oxygen transport during the period of reduced heart rate.

Paroxysmal Cough. The respiratory mucosa may be so irritated by the passage of a catheter that violent, spasmlike coughing is induced. This type of coughing expends a great deal of energy and can lead to hypoxemia (low blood PO_2 level) because no air can enter the airway during such violent coughing. To prevent this complication, always suction gently.

Hypotension. Hypotension may occur if there is severe bradycardia from vagal stimulation. Unless respiratory distress dictates otherwise, place the person in the supine position; as the bradycardia improves with oxygen administration, the hypotension will also be relieved.

Hypoxemia. When the suction source is turned on and air is removed from the respiratory tract, the amount of air removed may not be enough to cause atelectasis or collapse of the lung tissue, but it may remove so much oxygen that an inadequate supply diffuses across the alveoli, resulting in hypoxemia. To reduce this problem it may be necessary to administer oxygen just prior to and immediately after suctioning, limiting suctioning time to 10 to 15 seconds. If more suction is needed after the catheter is removed, allow the person to take at least five good deep breaths (or administer oxygen for five breaths as appropriate) before you reintroduce the catheter. The symptom that reveals the presence of hypoxemia is tachypnea that occurs each time following suction.

Moistening Secretions

One important way of keeping respiratory secretions moist and readily moveable is by making sure that the patient remains well hydrated. Offer fluid frequently (unless it is otherwise contraindicated); if intravenous fluid is being administered, check frequently to be certain that it is flowing at the desired rate.

People who cough vigorously may vomit from the force of coughing. Ordinarily, when people are vomiting they should stop intake of all fluid or food for about 4 hours to rest the gastrointestinal tract. Be certain that the person who has vomited in this way understands that it is caused by the coughing. Urge him to drink fluid to help keep the respiratory secretions moist and easy to expectorate.

Mouth Care

People with any degree of respiratory distress (except infants, who are total nose breathers) begin to breathe through their mouths. The nasal filtering of air by the nasal cilia is then lost, and the oral mucous membrane will begin to become dry. If the person continues to breathe through his mouth for any length of time, the oral mucous membrane and lips will actually form crusts or crack with small fissures. These are extremely painful when the person speaks or swallows and invite invasion of microorganisms and a secondary infection.

Frequent sips of fluid (which also liquefies and helps raise respiratory secretions) help to keep the oral mucous membrane moist. Rinsing the mouth with mouthwash at least every hour is helpful. Swabbing the patient's lips with a water-soluble lubricant as needed reduces lip trauma. "Bad breath" is caused by the growth of microorganisms on the gums and tongue. Brushing the teeth (including the tongue) about every 4 hours will effectively reduce mouth odor caused by mouth breathing.

☐ QUICK REFERENCE STOP 32-3: NUTRITION
Need for Additional Fluids

As a rule of thumb, people with respiratory distress need additional fluid to compensate for the drying effect of mouth breathing and to keep respiratory secretions moist and movable. Unless otherwise contraindicated, offer such patients additional fluids. Keep an estimated intake and output record to be certain they are receiving adequate fluid.

These measures should be included in the initial planning of nursing care so that they are begun before mouth drying begins. You can anticipate that with respiratory distress some degree of drying will occur; it is best to prevent it as much as possible rather than having to initiate action to restore oral health after fissuring or other damage has occurred (see QRS 32-3).

Techniques for Better Aeration of the Lungs

Aerating the alveoli not only helps to move respiratory secretions but also ensures that adequate alveolar space is kept open for sufficient air exchange.

INCENTIVE RESPIRATORY DEVICES

Incentive respiratory devices are devices that encourage a person to inhale deeply to aerate the lungs fully, thereby helping to diffuse oxygen and prevent atelectasis. They are plastic, brightly colored devices that usually have colored balls floating in cylinder chambers or boxlike structures that flash colored lights when a set pressure is applied to them. The person places his mouth on the mouthpiece and tubing of the apparatus. He then breathes in strongly or exhales forcefully, depending on the type of device. Those that depend on inspiration are thought to be more effective. The patient needs to use not only a strong inhalation or exhalation but a sustained one for best results (Fig. 32-10).

A person must be well motivated to do this type of exercise and must understand the importance of keeping air moving through the lungs (to avoid stasis of secretions, which can lead to infection, and to better diffuse oxygen into his bloodstream) before he can use an incentive respiratory device properly. Use of such devices is prescribed by a physician; the actual number of breaths to be taken (5 to 20 deep breaths an hour, for example) may actually be determined by a respiratory therapist. Observe the patient while he uses such a device because some people cannot carry out the instructions as prescribed (taking 20 very deep inhalations in a row could lead to hyperventilation and dizziness in many people). You may need to break the prescription down into smaller units (10 breaths every 30 minutes) until the patient grows more used to full lung expansion. Incentive spirometry devices are, as a

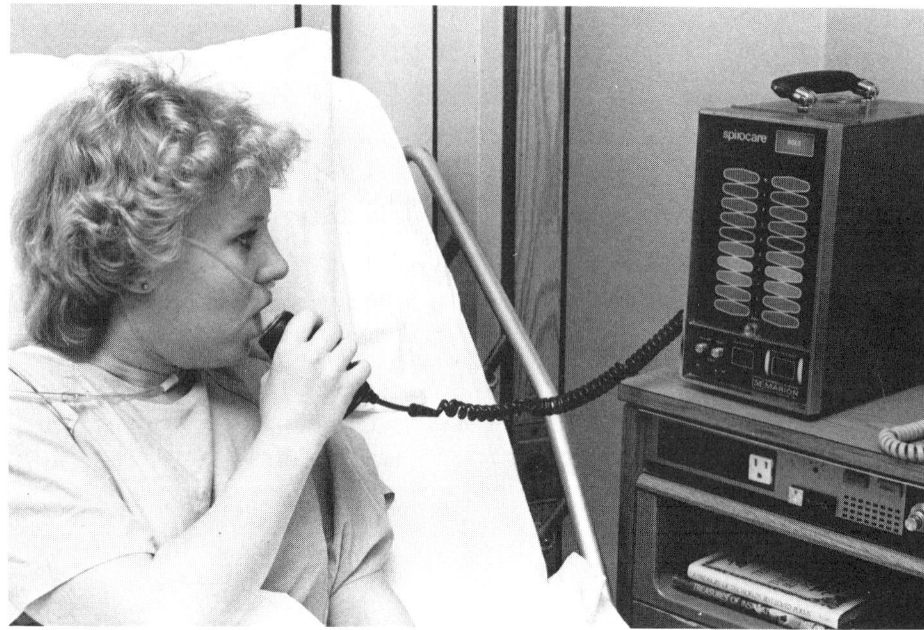

FIGURE 32-10. An incentive spirometer. Adequate respiratory movements light up colors on machine.

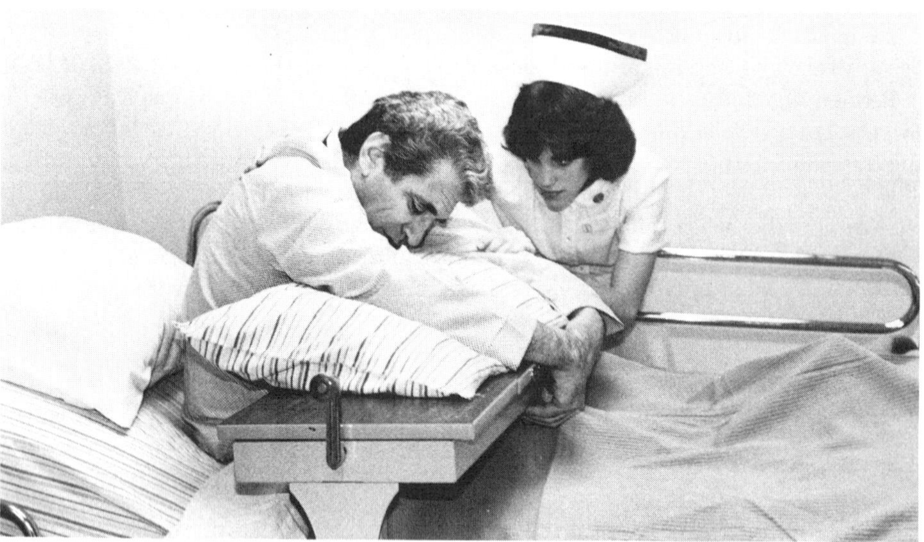

FIGURE 32-11. Patients with orthopnea may not be able to breathe comfortably unless they are sitting upright. Leaning forward over a bedside table is often an effective position for them.

rule, fun to use if they do not cause discomfort because the person is rewarded for his effort, but they also are serious exercises that should be continued conscientiously.

POSITIONING AND COMFORT

Most people with respiratory distress or orthopnea are most comfortable in a Fowler's or semi-Fowler's position. You may need to administer a bedbath to such a person and to make the bed with the head of the bed continually elevated. Infants are most comfortable if placed in an infant seat to maintain a head-elevated position. Make certain that the person's arms do not rest across his chest; the weight of them reduces chest movement and lung aeration. Some people are most comfortable sitting far forward and leaning against an overbed table (Fig. 32-11). Be certain that this position does not occlude chest movement by pressure of the table against the rib cage.

If a person has abdominal pain or a surgical incision that limits chest expansion, he cannot inspire deeply because of the increased pain. Administer adequate analgesic to limit the degree of pain to a level that does not interfere with good chest expansion. On the other hand, analgesics or sedatives should never be administered to people with respiratory distress without first

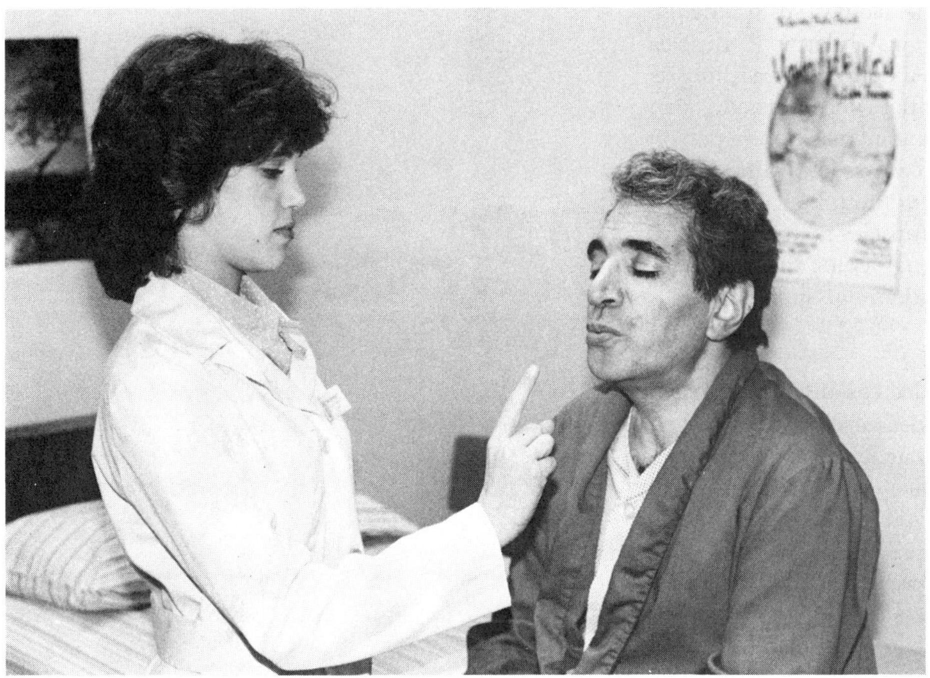

FIGURE 32-12. To teach pursed lip breathing, hold your finger about 10 inches in front of the patient's mouth. Instruct him to "blow out the candle."

assessing the effect of the drug on respiratory function because most drugs in these categories cause at least some decrease in respiratory function. Use judgment to find the point of pain relief or sedative effect that best offers comfort but still allows good lung expansion.

□ QUICK REFERENCE STOP 32-4: HEALTH TEACHING
Pursed Lip Breathing

Chronic obstructive pulmonary disease (COPD)—sometimes abbreviated COLD for chronic obstructive lung disease—is a major health problem for middle-aged and older adults. They tend to "pocket" air in overexpanded alveoli. To evacuate more of this air, they need to learn pursed lip breathing, or breathing out against pressure. This sustains the length of the expiration, increases pressure in the bronchi, and keeps them from collapsing with exhalation until more air can be evacuated. To teach pursed lip breathing:

1. Ask the patient to inhale comfortably but to aerate the alveoli fully. Time the inhalation.
2. Teach the patient to purse his lips and expire slowly against the pressure this causes as if he were gently blowing out a candle. Press on the upper abdomen with your hand during the exhalation to help the diaphragm rise and to empty the alveoli more fully. Time the exhalation.
3. Urge the patient to practice until he achieves an exhalation against pressure that is twice as long as an inhalation.

BREATHING TECHNIQUES

People with chronic obstructive lung disease (COLD) tend to "pocket" air in the alveoli and never empty the alveoli at the end of expiration as fully as is normal. This leads to poor oxygenation (little oxygen can enter because so much carbon dioxide is present) and infection (stasis in any body compartment invites the growth of microorganisms).

Learning a breathing technique that helps to empty the alveoli more fully is important in improving air exchange. Normally, at the end of expiration, the bronchi collapse, allowing no more air to be expired through them (a system designed to prevent the alveoli from fully emptying with each expiration so that they have to be opened each time). The secret of better emptying of distended and pocketed alveoli is to breathe out against pressure, which delays the collapse of the bronchi for a longer space of time and allows more air to be emptied from the alveoli (Fig. 32-12 and QRS 32-4).

Abdominal Muscle Breathing. Using the abdominal muscles in breathing is also a means of prolonging exhalation and promoting greater alveoli emptying. The person breathes in, concentrating on using his abdominal muscles with the effort. If he is truly using the abdominal muscles, the abdomen will rise as he inhales. The person then exhales slowly (sustaining the effort for at least 7 seconds); his abdominal muscles will flatten as he exhales. Abdominal breathing is easier to learn in a supine position; once learned, it can be done well in a sitting or standing position (a person sitting at a desk or standing at an assembly line can do it many times during the day without interfering with work). Using the abdominal muscles to breathe serves the secondary purpose of strengthening these muscles and presenting a slimmer abdominal appearance.

OXYGEN ADMINISTRATION

Hypoxemia. Hypoxemia is a decreased level of oxygen (PO_2) in blood. *Hypoxia* is a decreased level of oxygen in body cells. It is possible to analyze the presence of hypoxemia by both objective and subjective assessments; the presence of hypoxia can only be measured subjectively.

Objective measures of hypoxemia are blood gases, tachypnea, tachycardia, restlessness, and mental confusion. Tachypnea and tachycardia occur as the body tries to pull in more oxygen and distribute it more quickly to body cells. The symptoms of mental confusion and restlessness result from brain cells that are beginning to function with less than the desired amount of oxygen.

If hypoxemia becomes severe (in such a case some hypoxia is undoubtedly present), symptoms of bradycardia, bradypnea, cyanosis, lethargy, or somnolence occur. If hypoxemia continues uncorrected it will ultimately lead to coma and death.

Cyanosis is only one symptom of hypoxemia and is not always reliable. Its presence is influenced by the presence of subcutaneous fat, skin pigment, hemoglobin concentration, and environment (such as the amount of light in the room and the color of the walls).

Oxygen administration almost immediately increases the proportion of oxygen at the alveoli-blood interface. It does not immediately increase the PO_2 level in those conditions in which diffusion across the alveoli is the basic difficulty. It is important to determine blood gas levels before oxygen is administered to be certain that oxygen is truly needed (the PO_2 level is low) and to measure the PCO_2 level. A PCO_2 level that has been high for some time (more than 45 mm Hg) causes numbness of the respiratory center so that the person is no longer stimulated to respiration from a rising carbon dioxide level. In these instances, the main stimulation to breathing is oxygen want. If people with this clinical picture are flooded with oxygen, their stimulation for breathing is lost.

In an emergency (if the person is cyanotic and gasping for breath), oxygen should be administered immediately at about 10 liters per minute and blood gases are determined within the next few minutes.

If oxygen administration is effective, the person's respiratory rate will begin to approach normal, the effort expended for breathing is reduced (use of accessory chest or abdominal muscles lessens), and tachycardia, cyanosis, and mental confusion are also reduced. These symptoms must be accompanied by blood gas assessment to prevent overdosing (toxicity) of oxygen when it is no longer necessary. Oxygen administration is palliative therapy—it merely relieves the symptoms and signs of distress. It must be continued until the underlying cause of the distress is relieved.

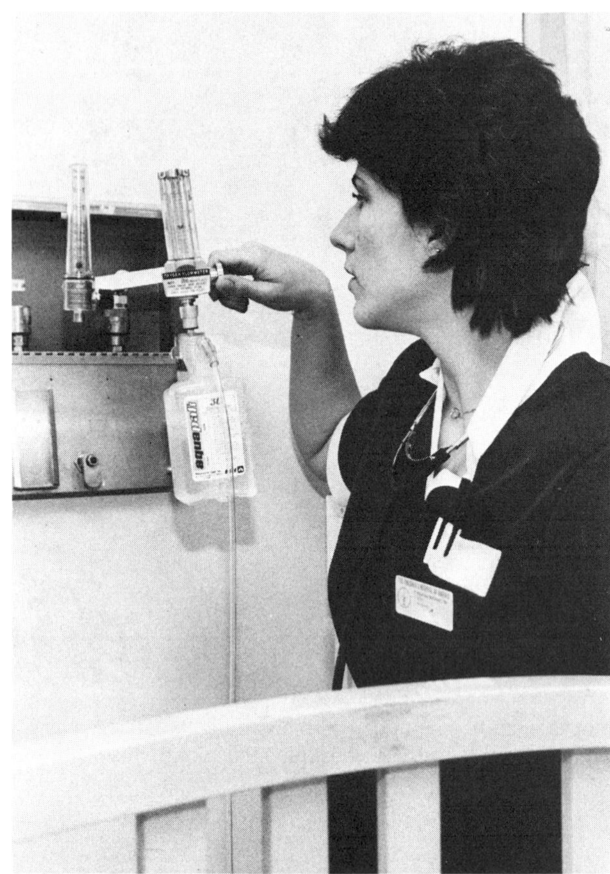

FIGURE 32-13. Wall outlet oxygen unit. The height of the metal ball in the flow meter reveals the number of liters of oxygen being administered. Oxygen bubbles through a humidifier to moisten it.

Oxygen Administration Techniques. Oxygen in most health care agencies is supplied by wall outlets; in some older institutions or in emergency rooms it may be supplied by portable tanks. People who are being transported from one area of an agency to another (or from home to an agency) receive oxygen from small portable tanks.

To measure the amount of oxygen being administered by a wall outlet, an oxygen flow meter is attached to the outlet (Fig. 32-13). These typically screw into the wall outlet with a twisting motion. To turn on the oxygen, open the valve; a mercury ball will rise in the flow meter cylinder liter gauge to indicate how much

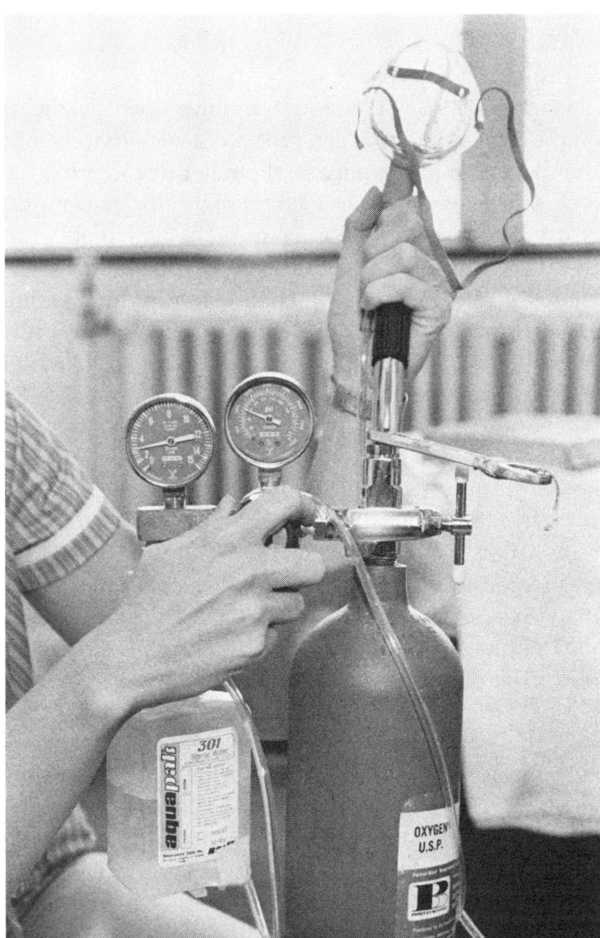

FIGURE 32-14. Portable oxygen tank. The gauge on the left shows the liters of oxygen being administered; the gauge on the right the amount of oxygen remaining in the tank.

oxygen is flowing. Like all drugs, oxygen is ordered by prescription (4 liters per minute or 8 liters per minute, for example). The percentage of oxygen delivered varies with the amount used, but as a rule, flow of 4 to 6 liters per minute will provide 30 to 40 percent of oxygen; 10 to 12 liters per minute will provide about 70 to 80 percent. Oxygen tanks have a similar valve and liter flow meter attached to them. They have a second valve that shows the amount of oxygen left in the tank (actually, it shows the pressure in the tank, which is an indirect measure of the amount of oxygen).

Oxygen must be bubbled through distilled water to be moistened so that it does not dry the respiratory tract excessively. A glass or plastic jar attached to the oxygen flow meter in Figure 32-14 is the moistening source. In most institutions oxygen equipment is maintained by the respiratory therapy department; the nurse's role involves being sure that sterile distilled water is present in the moistening source. Filling the jar is simply a matter of temporarily turning off the oxygen flow, unscrewing the jar, filling it half full with distilled water, reattaching it, and reestablishing the oxygen flow.

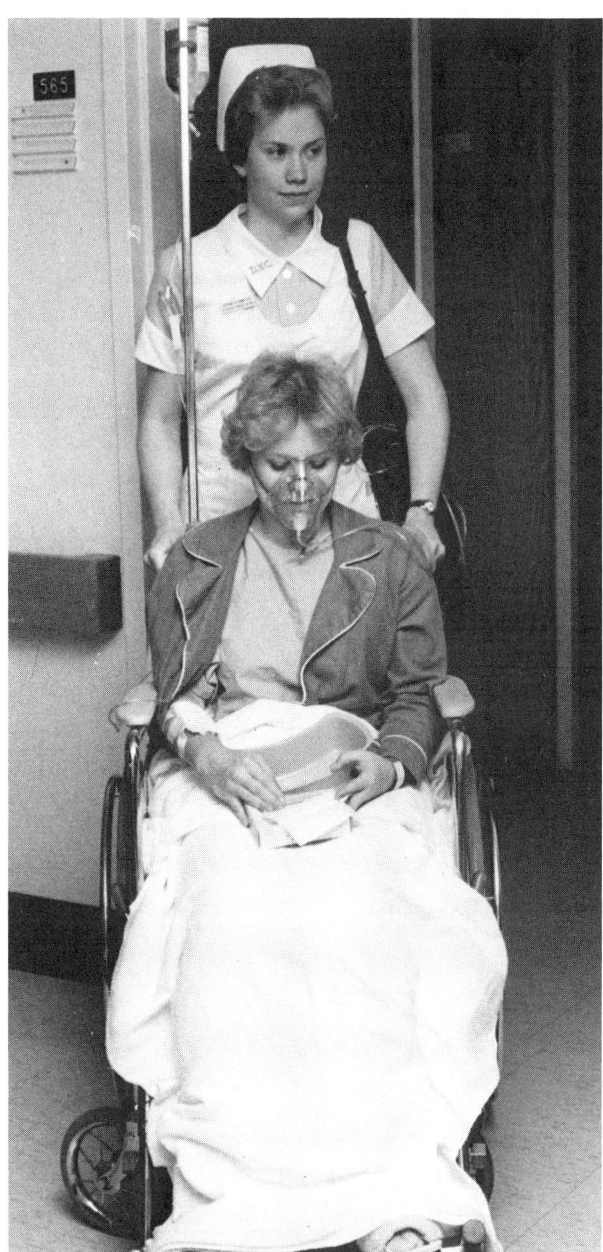

FIGURE 32-15. The advantage of a portable oxygen source is that it allows a person greater mobility. This adult is being transported for diagnostic testing. The newer portable oxygen equipment is contained in the student nurse's over-the-shoulder bag.

The method by which oxygen is actually delivered to the patient depends on the concentration prescribed and the advantages and disadvantages of different types of equipment. Portable oxygen equipment allows greater mobility for the patient (Fig. 32-15 and QRS 32-5).

OXYGEN MASKS. An oxygen mask is the easiest method for administering oxygen (Fig. 32-16). A properly fitting mask covers both the nose and the mouth and is therefore effective with people in acute distress (who tend to breathe through the mouth). Masks used today

☐ QUICK REFERENCE STOP 32-5: ADVOCACY
Oxygen Administration

Oxygen may be administered by different methods depending on the amount needed and the disease. Individual preference is important also. You may need to intercede for a patient who wants a mask instead of nasal prongs, or nasal prongs in place of a mask. Oxygen administration is not effective if a person is breathing rapidly from anxiety. Reducing anxiety by suiting the type of equipment to the patient can improve the success of therapy.

are made of clear plastic so that you can continue to assess skin color under them; they are lightweight so that they do not feel heavy and confining to the patient, and they are disposable after use to prevent the spread of microorganisms from person to person.

It is important that a mask fit snugly to prevent oxygen from escaping around it. With flow rates of 6 to 8 liters per minute, a mask can supply an oxygen concentration of between 35 and 55 percent. The advantages of oxygen administration by mask are that it can be applied quickly in an emergency and it supplies high concentrations of oxygen. Some people may have difficulty in adjusting to an oxygen mask because they feel confined by it; they cannot expectorate or eat or drink with the mask in place.

FIGURE 32-16. Oxygen mask. The mask should cover both mouth and nose.

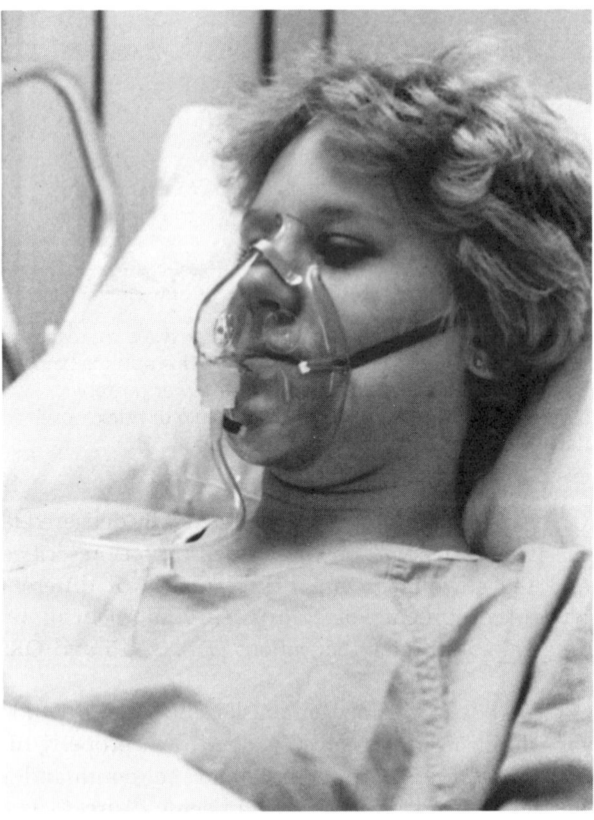

VENTURI MASKS. Venturi masks have open portholes on the side, and the oxygen tube has a wide diameter at the distal end and a narrow diameter at the proximal end. As oxygen pours through these different openings, a drop in pressure occurs, creating a suction effect in the mask. The holes at the sides of the mask allow room air to entrain (enter) with each inspiration, ensuring enough air to provide full lung expansion. Venturi masks, unlike regular masks, can be set to deliver a selected percentage of oxygen flow—30 percent, 35 percent, or 40 percent. They are ideal for use with the person who must not be given excessive oxygen because his respiratory stimulation operates on oxygen want.

Oxygen administered by a Venturi mask need not be humidified. Water vapor restricts the flow of oxygen and increases the suction effect (delivers more oxygen than specified, thus destroying one of the features of the Venturi mask). A Venturi mask employs the principle of High Air Flow Oxygen Enrichment; or it may be referred to as a HAFOE mask by the oxygen therapy department.

NONREBREATHING BAGS. A rubber or plastic bag may be attached to an oxygen mask to increase the percentage of oxygen administered. With a nonrebreathing bag, a one-way valve between the bag and the mask allows oxygen to enter both the bag and the mask. When the person breathes in, air is entrained from both the mask and the bag. This air is richer in oxygen than that offered by a regular mask alone because the oxygen source is not only the mask but the oxygen pool accumulated in the breathing bag as well. It is called a nonrebreathing bag because the one-way valve between the mask and the bag prevents exhaled carbon dioxide from being rebreathed into the attached bag (i.e., the person does not rebreathe his expired air). A nonrebreathing bag can increase the oxygen administered up to 90 percent. A high liter flow of 6 to 15 liters per minute is necessary to accomplish this. The liter flow should be strong enough to prevent the bag from fully collapsing with each inspiration but allow it to remain about one-third full.

REBREATHING BAGS. Masks may have a rubber or plastic bag attached to them with a two-way valve insert. The person breathes in a mixture of oxygen from the mask and accumulated expired air from the bag. Air from the bag is high in carbon dioxide. People who are hyperventilating (blowing off excess carbon dioxide) may benefit from rebreathing bags to increase their carbon dioxide level as well as their oxygen level.

NASAL PRONGS. Nasal prongs are also a rapid and convenient method of the administration of oxygen. They consist of a rubber or plastic appliance with prongs one-quarter to one-half inch long that insert

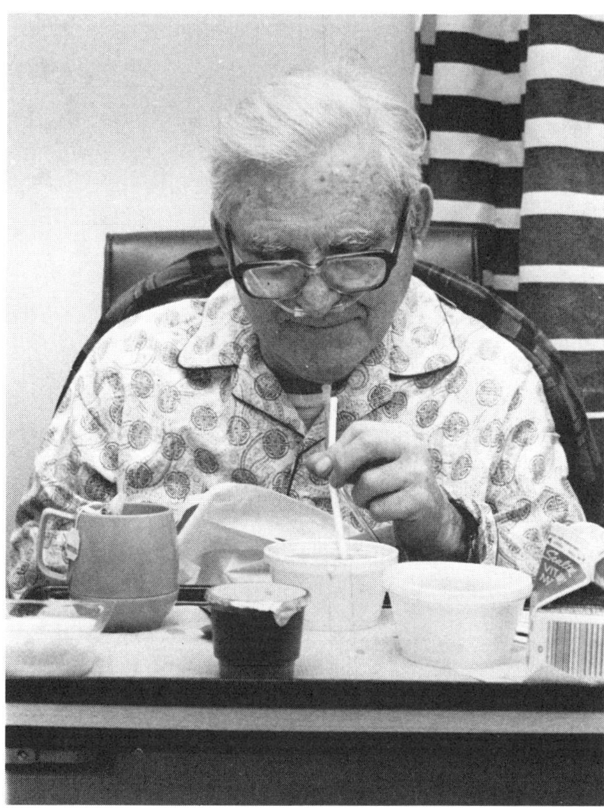

FIGURE 32-17. Oxygenation by nasal prongs. An advantage of oxygen prongs is that the person can eat with them in place.

into both nostrils (Fig. 32-17). Nasal prongs must be checked frequently because they tend to become dislodged when a person turns his head; some people report sinus pain from the presence of the oxygen so close to the maxillary sinuses. They provide an ineffective route of oxygen administration for a person with nasal congestion because the flow of oxygen is blocked in the nasal cavity. Oxygen administered at about 6 liters per minute will provide up to 40 percent oxygen by this source.

Nasal prongs cause extreme drying of the nasal mucosa and may cause local irritation and a pressure sore at the nostril. Coating the mucous membrane of the nose with a water-soluble lubricant may offer comfort (but the nasal prongs will then not stay in place well). Remove the prongs at least every 4 hours to check for excessive dryness and irritation from compression; if these problems are occurring, oxygen should probably be administered by a mask until the problem clears.

Because small children of preschool age dislike intrusive procedures, they generally do not tolerate nasal prongs. In infants prongs tend to cause extreme pressure on the nasal septum and must be checked at least hourly. Nasal prongs are effective even if the person is mouth breathing because the pressure of the oxygen flow forces the oxygen back to the pharynx, where it is then further inhaled. A person does not have to struggle to breathe through his nose when nasal prongs are in place, therefore, but can continue mouth breathing if that is more comfortable for him.

NASOPHARYNGEAL CATHETERS. Oxygen may also be administered through a pliable plastic catheter inserted through the nostril, back to the upper pharynx. Prior to insertion, the catheter should be coated lightly with a water-soluble lubricant (as mentioned earlier, never use an oil-based lubricant; aspirated oil can cause severe lung inflammation and lipid pneumonia). The proper distance for insertion is the measurement of the distance between the person's nose and the earlobe (Fig. 32-18). The catheter is inserted this distance. If it is inserted too far, it will cause vomiting (by initiating the gag reflex at the back of the throat). If it is inserted so far that it enters the esophagus rather than the trachea (a catheter passed to the back of the throat normally enters the esophagus rather than the trachea, a reassuring fact when administering tube feedings), the stomach will fill with oxygen, and vomiting will ensue.

The insertion of a nasal catheter causes temporary discomfort (a tickling or sneezing feeling) but should not be painful (Fig. 32-19). Once it is in place it should no longer be felt. If it is properly placed, the tip should be visible just behind the uvula but should not be readily visible in the back of the throat (Fig. 32-20).

Most people do not have a truly symmetrical nose—one side of the nose is slightly larger on the inside than the other. Never force a catheter when inserting it. If resistance is felt in one nostril, invariably the catheter will insert smoothly and without resistance on the other nostril (the larger side). Oxygen catheters range in size from about 10 to 14 (the larger the number, the larger the lumen). They are French catheters with openings on the sides that prevent them from becoming easily occluded by nasal mucus. Feeding tubes, which come in very small sizes—6 French, for example, can be used in infants for the administration of oxygen.

A nasopharyngeal catheter must be taped in place after insertion, or it will quickly become dislodged with any change in position. Never bring a catheter up and tape it to the forehead. This puts excessive pressure on the anterior surface of the nostril and can actually cause necrosis of the area (or at least painful ulceration). Bring it instead to the side and tape it to the cheek (Fig. 32-21). If the person is perspiring freely, tapes other than adhesive tape do not adhere well; on the other hand, adhesive tape is irritating if it is changed frequently. You can solve this problem by first taping a piece of eye tape (clear or nonallergenic tape) to the cheek and then taping the catheter to this with adhesive tape. This holds well and does not irritate sensitive facial skin.

A nasopharyngeal catheter should be removed about every 8 hours and replaced with a fresh one (in the

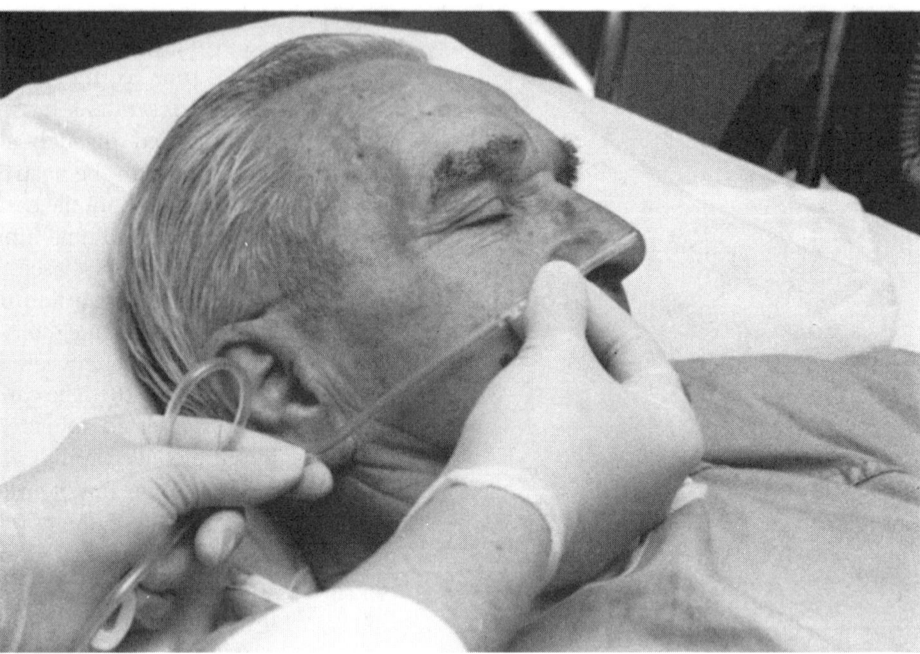

FIGURE 32-18. Measure the proper distance for inserting a nasopharyngeal catheter by measuring the distance between the patient's nose and earlobe.

opposite nostril if both nostrils can be intubated). Catheters left in place for longer periods collect a coating of secretions that may plug the cannula and disrupt the oxygen flow, and stasis of moist secretions invites local infection.

Nasopharyngeal catheters supply a concentration of 40 to 50 percent oxygen at a flow rate of 6 to 8 liters per minute. This is not as convenient a method of oxygen administration as nasal prongs or an oxygen mask because the patient cannot remove and then replace the oxygen source, but if introduced initially as a dependable method of oxygen administration it will be well accepted by most people.

OXYGEN TENTS. An oxygen tent has the advantage of being a nonintrusive method of supplying oxygen; it also can be flooded with moisture as well as oxygen to offer a high-humidity environment as well as an oxygen-rich one. The disadvantages of tents are that they are not able to deliver high concentrations of oxygen and cause many people to feel "boxed in" or claustrophobic. Oxygen in concentrations of over 21 percent is heavier than room air, so oxygen easily escapes through the bottom of a poorly tucked-in tent. The highest concentration that can be achieved in a tent is about 50 percent, and this can be achieved only at very high flow rates of 12 to 15 liters per minute.

When caring for people in oxygen tents, be certain that the bottom of the tent is securely tucked under the edges of the mattress. The bottom edge should be brought out as far away from the person as possible to give adequate space in the tent. Cover the bottom edge by laying a cotton blanket or folded sheet across it and tucking the blanket or sheet under the mattress on both sides. Some brands of tents tend to build up a high

FIGURE 32-19. Insertion of nasopharyngeal catheter. Use gentle technique; inform the patient about what you are doing.

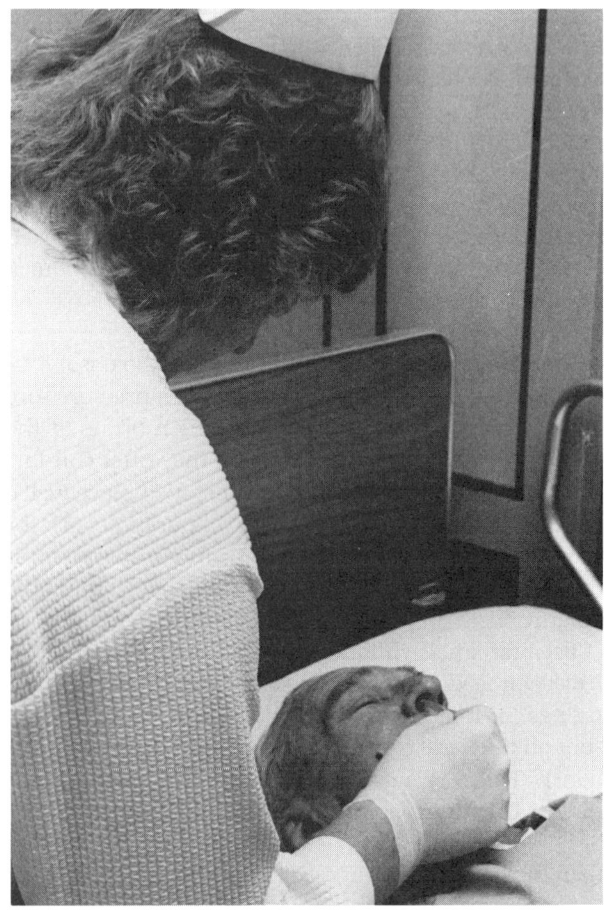

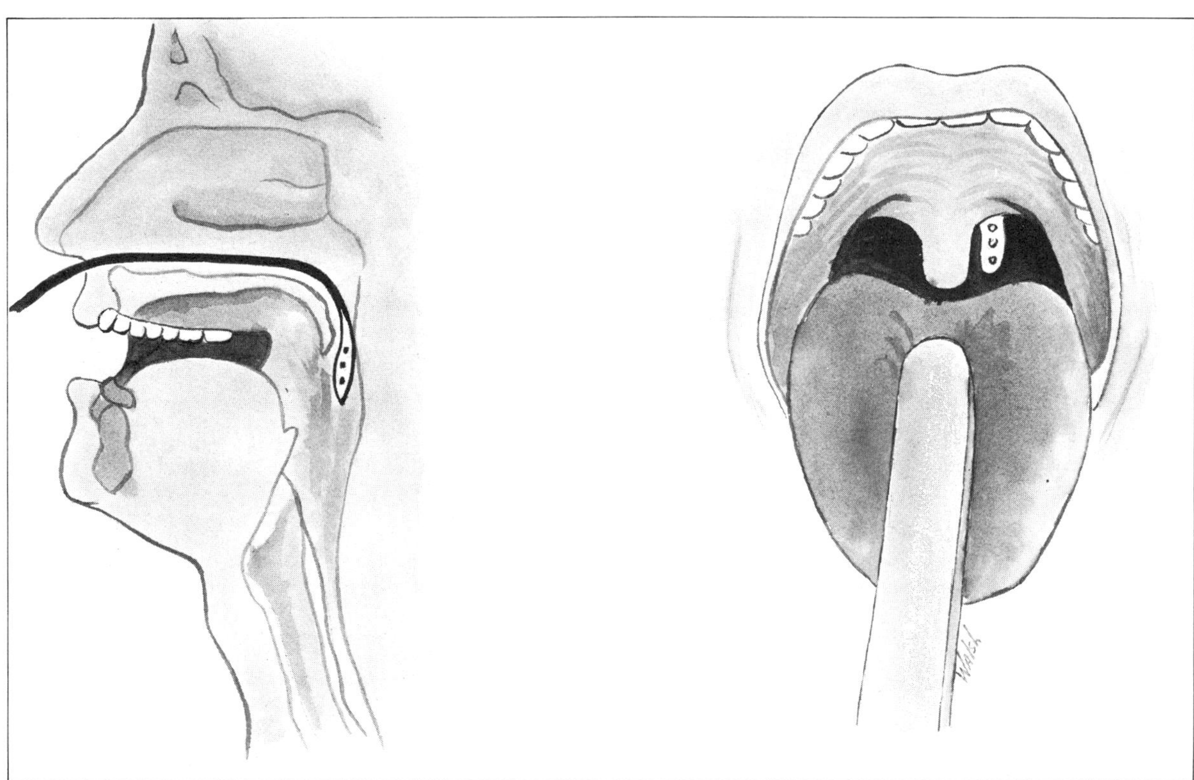

FIGURE 32-20. An oxygen cannula in place; it should be just visible in the back of the throat.

FIGURE 32-21. Nasopharyngeal catheter taped in place. Notice that it crosses the cheek; to avoid irritation to nare, it does not pull upward across the forehead.

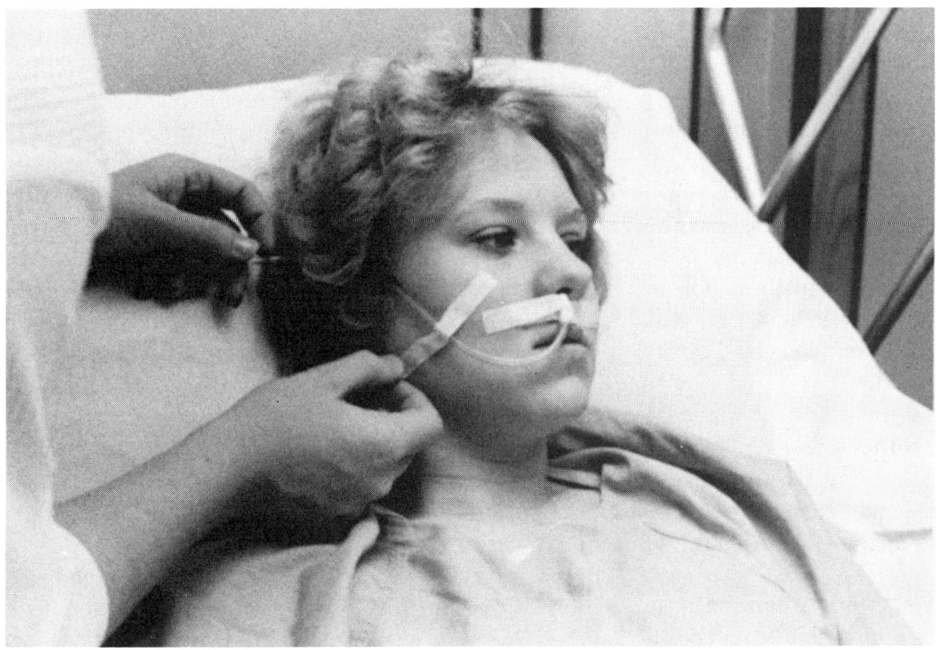

carbon dioxide level when the bottom edge is tucked in, so in some instances this should be left untucked to allow expired carbon dioxide to be removed from the tent. If the tent size is properly chosen, however, the problem of expired carbon dioxide retention should be minimal.

Plan nursing care carefully so that the tent needs to be opened as seldom as possible. Tents have zippered side openings that may be used for access, or you may lift the bottom edge of the tent. Try to make use of the zippered openings when possible (because they are high in the tent less oxygen is lost than when the bottom is lifted). When carrying out a procedure such as a bedbath in which you need access to the person's whole body, untuck the bottom of the tent and retuck it only under the pillow. Do not use a tent in this manner for a long period of time because carbon dioxide levels can build up in such a small enclosed space.

A person in an oxygen tent may feel cold, especially if the oxygen is blowing directly on him. Try to position the oxygen flow so it strikes the side of the tent, not the patient. Cover the shoulders and chest with a bath blanket or cotton robe as necessary for warmth. If the tent is being used to supply humidity as well as oxygen, the bedding may grow very damp and feel chilly. In these instances, you need to change the bedding frequently to keep the person from feeling chilled. If there is high humidity in the tent, it will be manifest as "fog" in the tent. Such a moist environment loosens or keeps the respiratory secretions loose, so the person tends to cough frequently. Be certain that adequate disposable tissues and a disposal bag are available. People with a respiratory illness that has necessitated the use of an oxygen tent frequently have an infectious process that causes a high temperature. The coolness of the tent may keep their temperature at a normal level, but when they are removed from the tent for any period, their temperature may rise. As a rule, people who have elevated temperatures should never be dressed or be allowed to use blankets because this additional heat adds to the temperature elevation. Caring for people in oxygen tents is an exception to this rule. To prevent chilling, provide blankets as necessary to keep the person from feeling damp and cold.

People in tents with very high humidity levels often feel very isolated (they have difficulty seeing you and know that you have difficulty seeing them). Make a special effort to show such people that you are frequently checking on them to increase their feeling of security.

Oxygen tents are used rarely with adults because they do not supply high levels of oxygen and can complicate nursing care because of their bulk. They are the method of choice for supplying oxygen to children in the preschool-age group because children in this age group dislike intrusive procedures and prefer a tent to nasal prongs or a cannula (Fig. 32-22). Some children are afraid of oxygen tents at first because they have been told many times by their parents not to put their heads in plastic bags. It often helps to reassure them by asking their mother to tuck her head into the tent with them or putting the tent over both you and the child initially. Always speak to a person immediately after putting an oxygen tent in place to reassure them that they can hear within the tent and you can hear them.

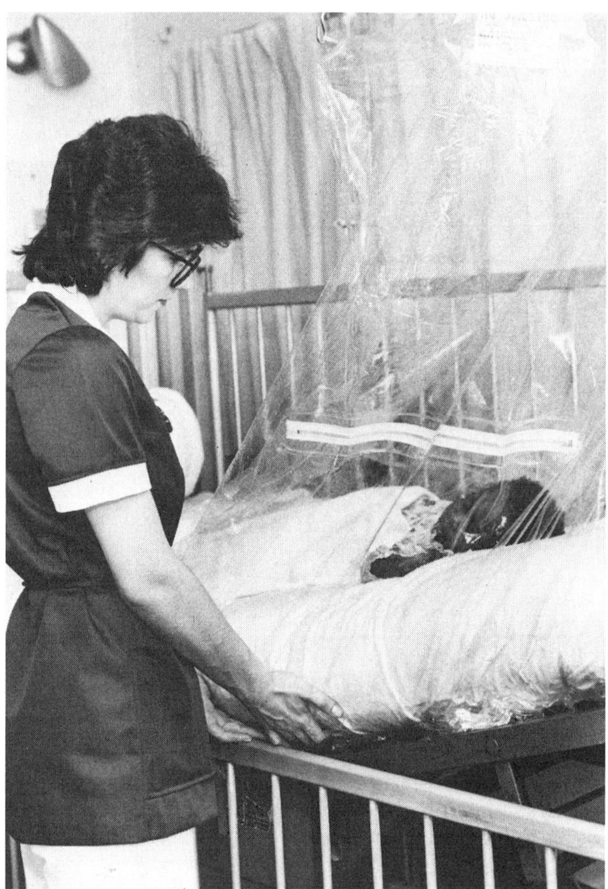

FIGURE 32-22. An oxygen tent. Oxygen is heavier than room air; tuck the bottom of tents well to prevent oxygen loss.

MIST TENTS. Oxygen tents can be used solely for their ability to provide mist or moisture. Although still an "oxygen tent," it is filled with room air or compressed air plus mist made by a nebulizer that floods the internal space with droplets of moisture created by blowing the air over distilled water or a bronchial detergent such as Mucomyst.

ISOLETTES. Isolettes (incubators) (Fig. 32-23) are frequently used to administer oxygen to infants and newborns. The Isolette can be flooded with oxygen and moisture in much the same way as an oxygen tent. When working with Isolettes that are being used to supply oxygen, organize care so that you open the top of the Isolette or the portholes as little as possible to prevent escape of the oxygen. It is difficult to maintain high levels of oxygen in Isolettes as in tents, but they have the advantage of being nonintrusive and not in-

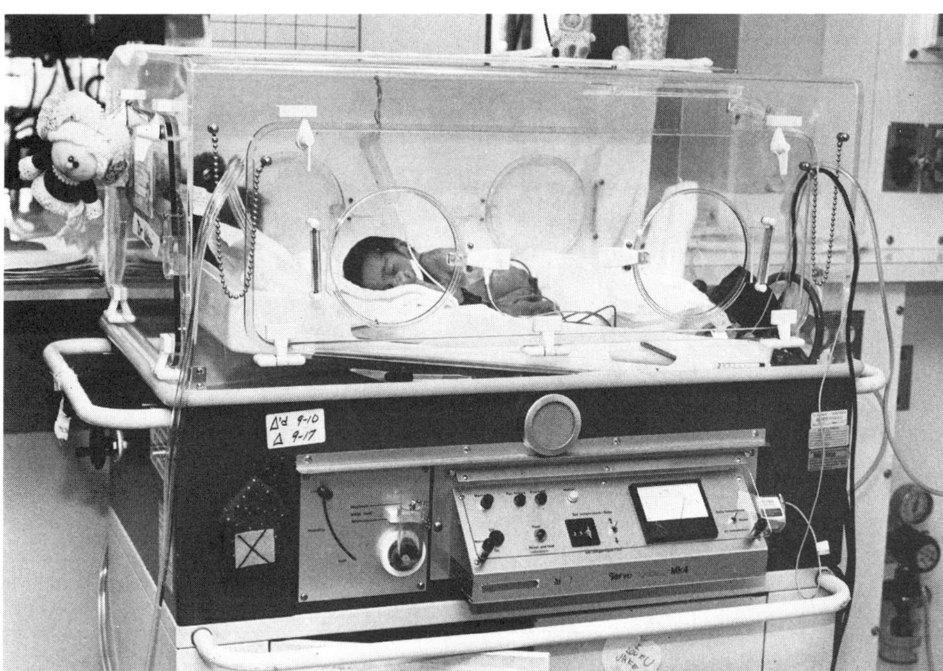

FIGURE 32-23. An Isolette is a means of oxygen administration for this newborn.

itiating nasal irritation as do nasal prongs and catheters.

OXYGEN HOODS. Oxygen hoods are clear plastic hoods that fit over an infant's head to supply oxygen. A hood has the advantage of supplying high levels of oxygen without being intrusive; it allows procedures with the remainder of the infant's body to be carried out without interference by the oxygen apparatus. A disadvantage of a hood is that it can be used only by a small infant or the amount of carbon dioxide buildup will be excessive. Older infants tend to find hoods constricting or "suffocating" and dislike them.

VENTILATORS. Ventilators (respirators) are another means of delivering oxygen under pressure. There are two main types of ventilators—the pressure-sensitive type, which delivers oxygen until a set pressure in the respiratory tract is reached, and the volume-sensitive type, which delivers oxygen until a certain volume has been delivered. At this point, the ventilator clicks off and the person expires air by the automatic recoil action of his lungs. Ventilators may be set to deliver an extra volume of air just at the end of exhalation (positive end expiratory pressure, or PEEP) to increase the intrapulmonary pressure and help keep the alveoli from collapsing, or continuous positive airway pressure (CPAP), which maintains increased pressure all during exhalation. Excessive pressure can cause rupture of the alveoli, resulting in air entering the chest cavity. This results in a collapsed lung and is called a pneumothorax (Fig. 32-24).

Ventilators may be used to assist respiration (when the person inhales spontaneously, the ventilator adds to his effort) or for total initiation of inhalation at a set timed rate.

Safety and Oxygen Administration. Oxygen does not burn but it supports combustion. This means that if a flame or electrical spark comes in contact with oxygen, a rapid explosion will occur. All rooms in which oxygen is being administered must be well marked and should be well ventilated so that excess oxygen does not "pocket" in the room. Caution visitors and patients that they must not smoke near oxygen sources. All electrical equipment used in the room must be well grounded (have a three-prong plug) so no sparks are generated from this source. Be extra cautious that cords of electrical appliances are not frayed to avoid sparks. Do not use wool sweaters or blankets with oxygen tents because they tend to cause static electrical sparks, and be careful of metal wind-up toys for children in oxygen tents for the same reason. Do not use electrical call bells with oxygen tents; supply a metal hand bell such as that used on registration desks instead.

Determining Safe Oxygen Concentrations. The oxygen concentration actually achieved in the oxygen apparatus should be tested by an oxygen analyzer every 4 hours to be certain that an adequate level of oxygen is being maintained. Blood gas levels should be determined before oxygen therapy is begun; blood gases should be assessed frequently during the course of oxygen administration to determine that the amount of oxygen being administered is neither excessive nor inadequate. In an emergency, blood gas levels will not always be available, and you can feel free to administer oxygen until cyanosis decreases. At that point, decrease the oxygen liter flow 5 liters per minute and observe the

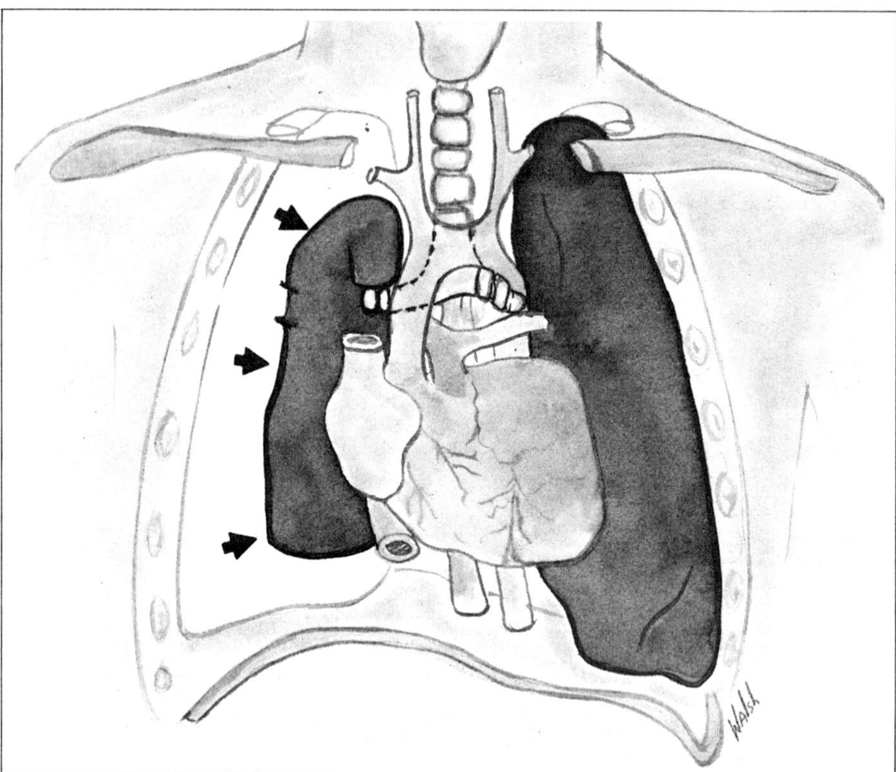

FIGURE 32-24. A complication of ventilator therapy can be rupture of alveoli which causes air to enter the chest cavity and possibly collapse the lung (pneumothorax).

patient again. Keep reducing the liter flow rate by 5-liter decrements until cyanosis reappears. Then increase the liter flow rate 5 liters per minute above this level.

RETROLENTAL FIBROPLASIA. The capillaries of the retina do not mature until late in intrauterine life. In an infant who has been born prematurely, the retina is very susceptible to the effects of oxygen administration. Whenever the PO_2 level rises over 100 mm Hg, there is danger that vasoconstriction of the susceptible capillaries may occur; this decreases the supply of blood to the retina. The retina then dies and is replaced by fibrous tissue and sloughs forward. No vision is possible in the damaged segment. If the entire retina is involved, total blindness results (retrolental fibroplasia). Blood gas levels must be determined frequently with administration of oxygen to immature infants to ensure that the PO_2 does not rise above 100 mm Hg. Recent studies document that even in adults, if the arterial oxygen tension is allowed to rise as high as 250 mm Hg, the same phenomenon can occur.

OXYGEN TOXICITY. Long-term use (at least 24 hours) of high concentrations (more than 50 percent) of oxygen appears to cause a thickening of the lung alveolar walls. When this occurs, the diffusion of gases across the alveoli is no longer easy to accomplish. Symptoms that the person may be developing oxygen toxicity are restlessness and increasing respiratory distress despite the high concentration of oxygen being administered. Some people develop a nonproductive cough; some report a burning or aching sensation in the midchest area (below the sternum). The PO_2 level begins to decrease. Oxygen toxicity may become, unfortunately, a "catch-22" situation. The person needs high concentrations of oxygen so that enough oxygen can diffuse across the alveoli to be effective; high concentrations of oxygen actually harm the alveoli and make it more difficult for diffusion to occur.

Oxygen toxicity cannot be totally prevented but can be minimized if the lowest dose of oxygen needed to maintain blood arterial levels is administered. Think of oxygen as a drug (which it is), not as "just oxygen."

ATELECTASIS. Normally, oxygen comprises only 21 percent of room air; nitrogen comprises almost all the remaining 79 percent. Nitrogen is inhaled with each inhalation of room air along with oxygen; it does not cross into the bloodstream but remains in the lungs as "filler," maintaining tension in the alveoli that keeps them from collapsing and aids in diffusing oxygen.

If high concentrations of oxygen are being administered (over 80 percent), little nitrogen is present in the lungs (20 percent compared to the usual 79 percent). Because almost all the oxygen delivered diffuses into the pulmonary capillaries, the alveoli are left almost empty (no free nitrogen is present any longer) at the end of inhalation. Empty alveoli may collapse (atelectasis). Collapsed alveoli require a great deal of inspiratory effort to reopen; the person with a respiratory illness may be unable to accomplish this. When the alveoli are unopened, there is no exchange surface on which oxygen diffusion can take place.

Periodic deep breaths aid in pulling in room air or adding "filler" to the alveoli; moving and changing position automatically causes a person to inspire more deeply and thus aids in filling the alveoli also. Most ventilators have a "sigh" capacity that periodically forces an additional amount of air into the lungs to provide filler air and in an attempt to prevent atelectasis.

AIRWAY OBSTRUCTION

Airway obstruction generally results from the gradual accumulation of respiratory secretions. It can occur abruptly due to aspiration (taking in) of fluid, pieces of meat (unchewed meat is a frequent offender), or any other object such as a safety pin, paper clip, or deflated balloon. Aspiration results from laughing or talking while swallowing (air passing out of the trachea opens the epiglottis), from eating rapidly (swallowing and breathing become uncoordinated), and from a decreased gag reflex due to alcohol or other drug use or cerebral illness. The initial response to aspiration is abrupt coughing, tearing, gasping, noisy respirations, or struggling to achieve an inhalation. Bronchospasm (closing off the bronchi to prevent any further foreign invasion) occurs in response to the foreign material present, totally occluding the airway in many instances.

Aspiration is always an emergency situation. If the foreign material is a liquid, violent coughing often removes it. This does not necessarily correct the problem, however, because bronchospasm and accompanying inflammation may continue to make breathing difficult. The foreign material may provoke irritation and "chemical" pneumonia during the next 24 hours.

If the swallowed object is not removed by violent coughing, slapping the person sharply on the back with the heel of the hand between the shoulder blades may dislodge it. An even more effective method is a thrust inward and upward on the abdomen just under the sternum (the Heimlich maneuver, described in Procedure 32-5). This maneuver forces the diaphragm up abruptly, creating sudden pressure in the respiratory tract and forcing the aspirated object upward. The person coughs violently as the object moves, and this additional force fully dislodges the object.

If the aspirated object is a safety pin or paper clip, for example, it may need to be removed by a bronchoscopy (a flexible tube inserted into the bronchus through the mouth). Although such foreign objects are potentially very serious because of sharp points, they rarely cause complete obstruction of the airway, so there is time for transport to the hospital and removal of the object.

CARDIOPULMONARY ARREST

The most serious threat to life at all times is cardiopulmonary arrest or a sudden halt in respirations

PROCEDURE 32-5
Abdominal Thrust (Heimlich Manuever)

Purpose: To re-establish a patent airway by emergency removal of a foreign object from the trachea by an inward and upward abdominal thrust.

Plan	*Principle*
If the person is standing or sitting: Stand behind the person, make a fist with one hand, and clasp it with your other hand. Pull it sharply inward and upward between the umbilicus and the sternum of the person in front of you. Repeat procedure until the foreign object is expectorated.	Technique ensures maximum thrusting ability. An abdominal thrust puts increased abdominal pressure on the diaphragm, which increases the intrathoracic pressure and dislodges the object from the trachea.
If person is supine: Kneel over person, and place the heel of one hand on his abdomen between the umbilicus and the sternum. Press inward and toward the sternum with a quick hard motion. Turn the person's head to the side to prevent reaspiration of the object as it is expectorated.	Use this technique also if the person is so obese that you cannot effectively reach around him.
If the person is an infant: Turn the infant upside down and support him by your forearm. Administer several quick sharp thrusts to the back between the scapulae. Inspect the back of the throat for the object and remove it immediately.	An abdominal thrust is not used in infants because they do not have space in their abdomen; the abdominal contents (particularly the spleen and the liver) can be injured.

and heart failure. This is always an emergency because brain tissue, the most sensitive tissue in the body to oxygen want, can survive only 4 to 5 minutes with total respiratory and cardiac arrest.

Such an arrest may result from an allergic response (anaphylactic shock) after food ingestion or inhalation or vaccine administration, from drowning, from choking on a foreign object such as a piece of meat, or from blockage of the respiratory tree by mucus or edema, or it may occur in a person with heart disease if his heart fails or becomes short of oxygen (a heart attack).

Death from cardiopulmonary arrest is preventable if care is initiated promptly within a minute or two after the arrest is recognized. Two cardinal rules apply: (1) speed is necessary, and (2) organization of interventions is necessary to avoid wasting time on unimportant details. All nurses should be certified as proficient in CPR (cardiopulmonary resuscitation) so they can assist effectively in such emergencies.

Cardiopulmonary Resuscitation in a Structured Setting

The first step in initiating cardiopulmonary resuscitation is assessment of respiratory function. Inspect the person's chest and abdominal muscles for respiratory movement. Place your ear close to his mouth and nose and listen for any sound of respiratory air exchange.

If you hear no sound or can detect no chest movement, respiratory arrest is present. Summon help by shouting if you are alone or pressing the person's call button if it is readily available with a persistent motion. Proceed to begin resuscitation based on A, B, C, and D steps—airway, breathing, circulation, and drugs.

AIRWAY

Position the person on his back (supine), open his mouth, and inspect it quickly for any object that could be causing obstruction. Sweep the person's mouth from side to side with your finger, bringing any object in the mouth forward and out. Hyperextend the person's head a small amount by placing an object such as a pillow, a purse, or a hand towel under the neck. This position opens the airway and in some instances will be enough in itself to initiate respirations. Be careful not to *over*extend the head because this will actually close the airway due to the sharp bend at the neck. This is most true in infants and newborns. If the person has a cervical injury or a suspected cervical injury, merely bring the lower jaw forward to effect airway opening.

BREATHING

If breathing does not begin spontaneously with the person's head in a hyperextended position, true pulmonary arrest is present, and ventilation by mouth-to-mouth breathing must be begun. Fit your mouth firmly on the open mouth of the person to be resuscitated, close his nostrils with the fingers of a free hand, and breathe into his mouth with a short but forceful expiration (Fig. 32-25). Lift your mouth away, turn your head to the side and inhale; repeat for four ventilations. Turn so your ear is over his mouth and you can see his chest. The chest will have risen during your exhalations if your action was forceful enough; it should fall during your inhalation. You should be able to hear the sound of air being exhaled by him (normal

FIGURE 32-25. In cardiopulmonary resuscitation, hyperextend the patient's head by placing an object under his neck. Pinch his nostrils closed. Ventilate by mouth-to-mouth breathing, using short, forceful expirations.

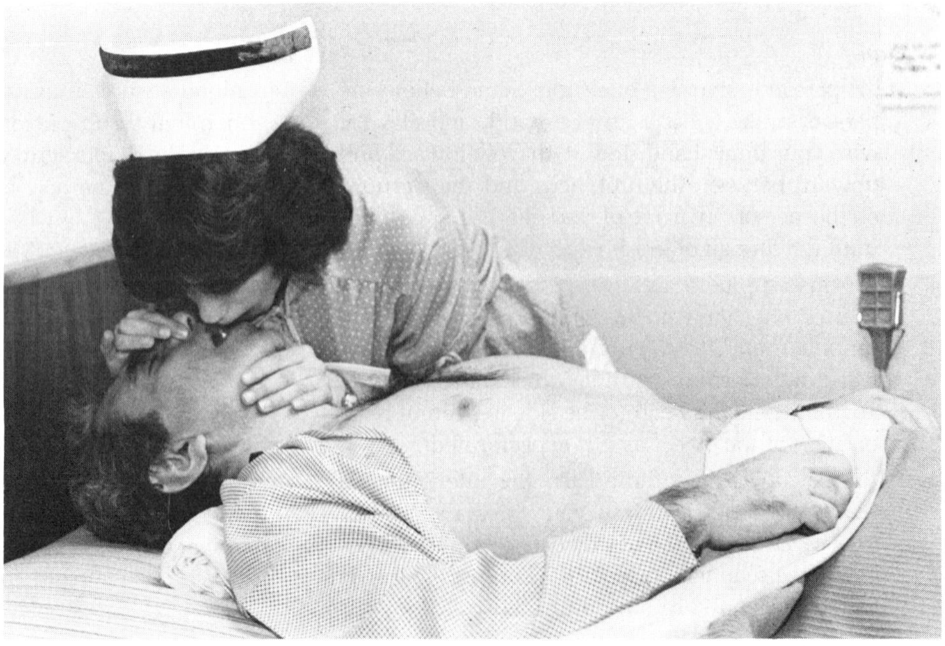

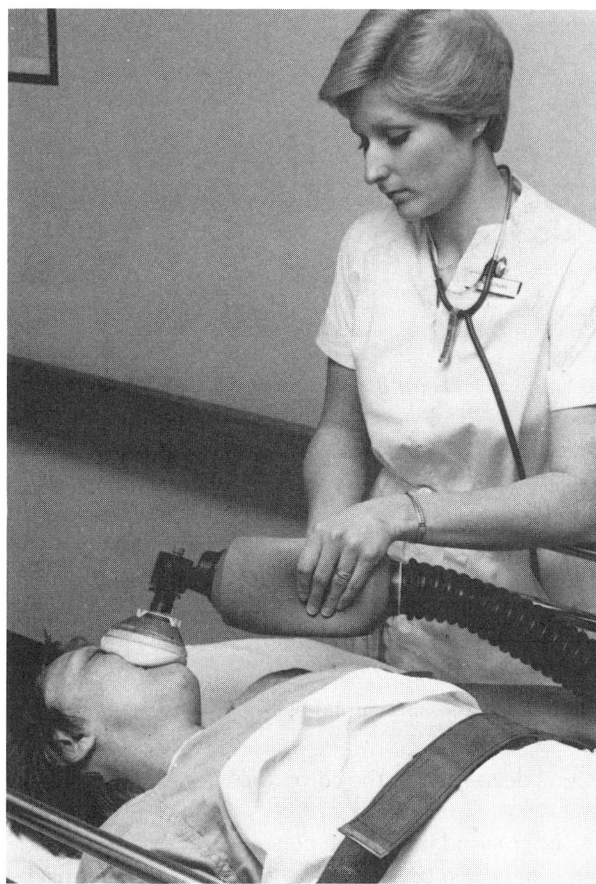

FIGURE 32-26. A resuscitation bag. Compression of the bag forces oxygen into the person's lungs.

lung recoil will empty the lungs). Many people worry that mouth-to-mouth resuscitation does not deliver enough oxygen or that you are not breathing anything but carbon dioxide into the person. Expired air, however, contains about 16 percent oxygen, or not that much less than the content of atmospheric air (21 percent).

If a resuscitation bag (an Ambu bag) is available, fit the mask of the bag firmly over the person's mouth and nose and press on the bag instead of using your own breaths (Fig. 32-26). Watch for chest expansion during inhalation and a falling chest during exhalation for proof that the lungs are expanding. Resuscitation bags of this type have the advantage of delivering standard amounts of air for ventilation; because they deliver room air unless attached to oxygen sources, for practical purposes they deliver air that has no advantage over expired breaths.

If a person has an endotracheal or tracheotomy tube in place, obviously you must either breathe into the tube or position the bag into it rather than the mouth because there is some type of obstruction to the airway that the tube is bypassing or correcting.

If on breathing or bagging, you feel resistance, it means that there is an obstruction of some type in the

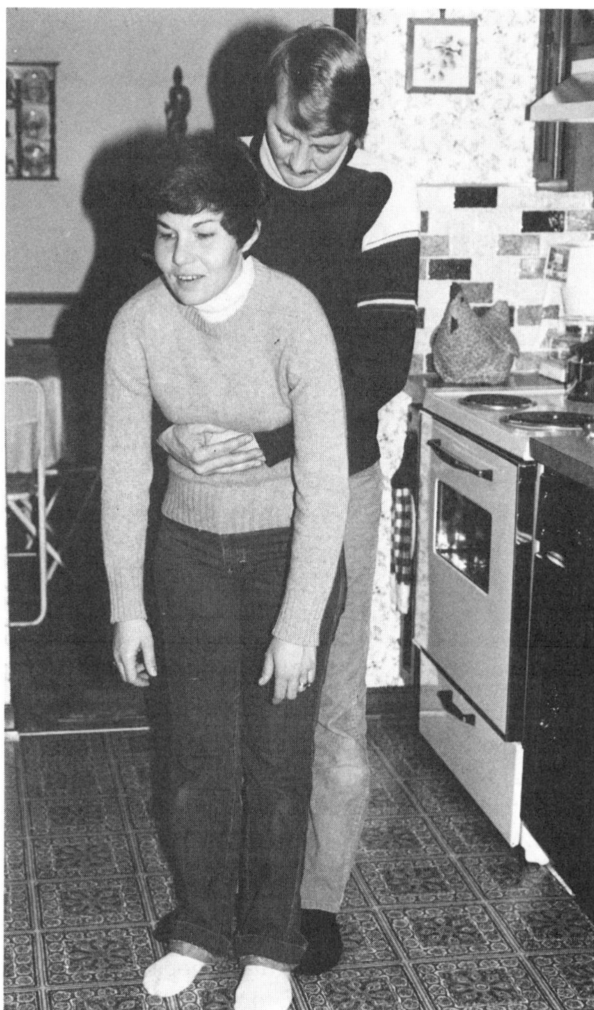

FIGURE 32-27. A Heimlich maneuver can be used in any setting; in this instance, the home.

airway. Assess the angle of the neck to be certain that it is extended but not overextended. Turn the person to his side and strike the space between the scapulae sharply three or four times with the heel of your hand; turn the person supine and press inward and upward on the abdomen just below the diaphragm (Heimlich maneuver or abdominal thrust [Fig. 32-27]) to dislodge any obstructing object. Sweep your hand through the person's mouth for any foreign object that was dislodged. In many instances, ventilation will begin spontaneously if an object was dislodged by one of these two actions.

If no object was dislodged, or if respirations do not start spontaneously, begin mouth-to-mouth breathing again for four more ventilations. Even if an object is present in the trachea, in many instances some air will pass around it, and your ventilation efforts will still be successful.

When help arrives (in a health care setting, if your first call for help was heard, persons experienced in resuscitation will begin arriving at this point) a person

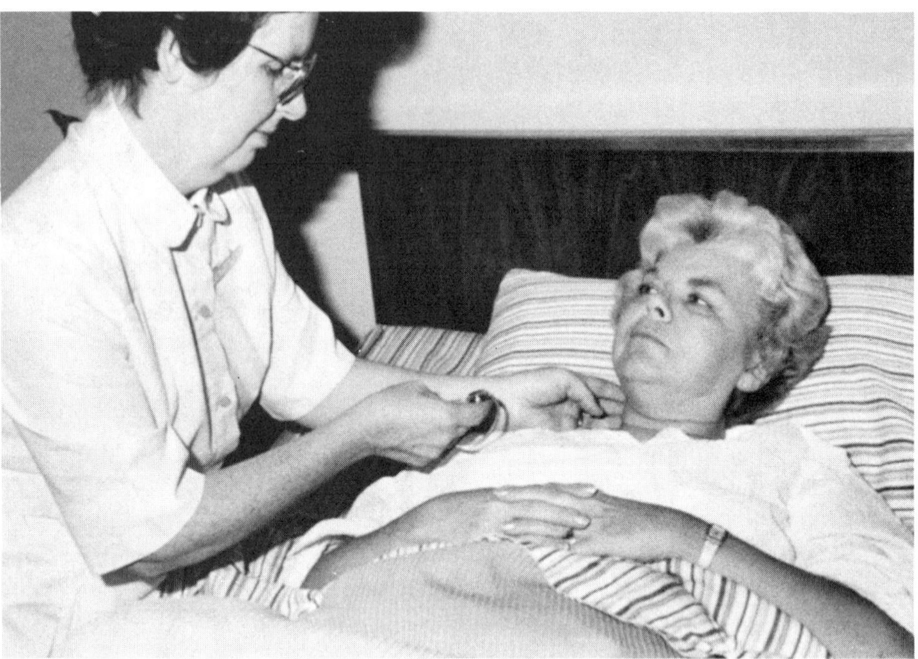

FIGURE 32-28. Assessing carotid pulse.

able to perform a tracheotomy (an opening into the trachea just below the cricoid cartilage to relieve upper respiratory obstruction) will be able to relieve the persistent obstruction to ventilation.

CIRCULATION

Ventilation by itself will be unsuccessful in resuscitation if the person's heart has also stopped functioning because the oxygen delivered to the lungs cannot leave the lungs and reach the cells. After administering the initial four ventilations, place a hand on the person's carotid pulse (on the anterior neck just lateral to the larynx, Fig. 32-28) and assess the heartbeat. If you feel none, open the person's eyes and assess pupil size. Constriction of pupils is controlled by the third cranial (oculomotor) nerve. Normally, if you allow bright light to strike the iris, it constricts, but if the oculomotor nerve is compromised by a low oxygen level, it will not initiate the reflex and the iris will remain widely dilated. Widely dilated pupils, therefore, indicate a circulation that is not functioning adequately (the person has heart arrest as well as respiratory arrest).

After as little as 1 to 2 minutes of hypoxia, the pupils will be widely dilated; after 4 to 6 minutes of severe hypoxia, they remain fixed or nonreactive to light, an indication that probably severe brain damage from hypoxia has occurred.

If there is no carotid pulse (if there are dressings or other conditions that obscure the carotid artery, use the femoral or radial pulse site) and the pupils are dilated, the person needs cardiac resuscitation as well as pulmonary resuscitation. This is accomplished by external cardiac compression. Cardiac arrest occurs fairly quickly following pulmonary arrest because when the PO_2 is decreased in the coronary arteries, heart action halts.

Either stand beside the person's bed or kneel beside him on the bed depending on your height (you must be above the person to initiate enough pressure to begin heart action) and place the heel of your hand on the bottom of the sternum (1 inch above the xyphoid process). Use the heel of your hand rather than your fingers for this action to increase the amount of pressure you will be able to apply; keep your elbow straight so you will be able to apply adequate pressure (Fig. 32-29). Be certain that your hand is not resting on the rib cage (ribs can break under this much pressure, lacerating a lung) or on the xyphoid process (it can break off and lacerate a lung or the liver).

Press and release the sternum at a rate of about 80 compressions a minute. Do not remove your hands from the chest at the end of a compression; merely let them rise so you do not waste time repositioning them with each compression. If you are by yourself, compress the person's heart 15 times, then ventilate his lungs with two exhalations, repeat with 15 compressions, two ventilations, and so on. Do not hurry the ventilations so much that the person does not exhale during the effort; however, try to limit the time of the ventilation attempts to about 6 seconds.

If someone else is with you, one of you should perform cardiac compression while the other is responsible for lung ventilation. *You cannot ventilate while someone compresses at the same time* or the ventilation will not be effective because air cannot enter the lungs when the chest is compressed. Establish a rhythm of five cardiac compressions by one person, one lung ven-

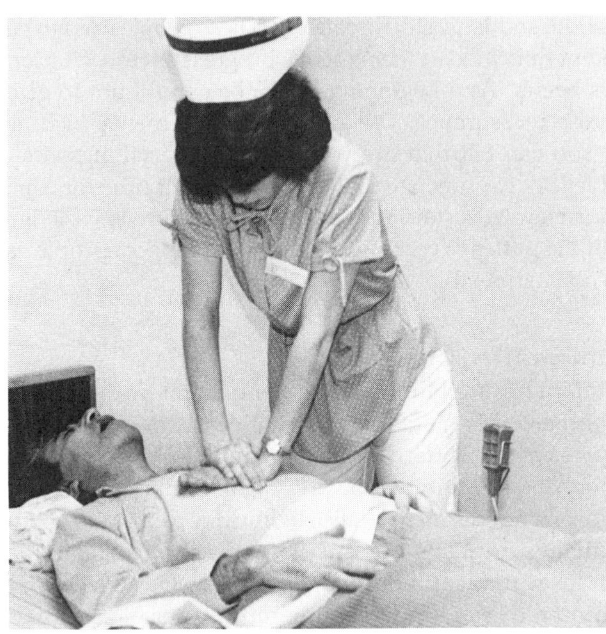

FIGURE 32-29. To perform external cardiac compression, place the heel of one hand on the bottom of the person's sternum. Place the heel of the other hand on top of the first. Keep elbows straight.

tilation by the second person, then five cardiac compressions and one lung ventilation and so forth. Ventilation should be done without interrupting the cardiac compression. This is best coordinated if the person doing cardiac compression counts "one and two and three and four and five and" as she works, saying the number as she compresses and the "and" as her hand rises; the person responsible for lung ventilation begins the breath or bag compression on the "and" after five. Counting this way also allows two people to change places because the new person knows when to enter the cycle.

After the first full minute of cardiac compression, check the carotid pulse and the person's pupils to see whether the pulse is present with cardiac compression and the pupils have begun to constrict once more (proof that cardiac compression is adequate to circulate blood).

DRUGS

The next step in cardiopulmonary resuscitation is the administration of drugs to improve respiratory response or help initiate cardiac function. Every health care agency has a "crash" or emergency cart provided with drugs necessary for cardiac pulmonary arrest procedures. The first physician to arrive on the scene will determine what medication, if any, is needed in the particular resuscitation attempt and the needed dosage. During the time that lung ventilation is compromised, considerable carbon dioxide builds up in the blood because it is not blowing off well. This can quickly lead to severe acidosis. Generally sodium bicarbonate is administered intravenously to counteract this. If the heart is not functioning, a stimulant drug such as epinephrine (injected directly into the heart with a long cardiac needle) may be necessary. Other frequently used drugs are isoproterenol (Isuprel), a drug that increases the contractability of the heart muscle, and calcium gluconate, which strengthens cardiac contractions.

An intravenous fluid line is begun to administer these and other specific medications quickly, depending on the person's medical condition (as a rule, medication cannot be administered intramuscularly when cardiac action is in doubt because muscle perfusion will not be adequate to pick up and absorb the medicine from the site, and oral administration is impossible because the person is unconscious).

Cardiopulmonary resuscitation is continued until it is apparent that the person is capable of spontaneous heart and lung function or until it is determined by the physician coordinating the resuscitation attempt that the effort is ineffective. An attempt may be carried out for as short a time as 5 or 10 minutes or for an hour or more. Following successful resuscitation, the underlying reason for the pulmonary cardiac arrest must be determined and therapy begun to improve it or arrest will very quickly occur again.

Roles in Life-Saving Attempts

To coordinate care during cardiopulmonary arrest, all health care agencies follow set procedures. You need to familiarize yourself with the procedures used in each health care agency in which you practice. The first person present at an arrest should assess whether an arrest has truly occurred and then begin ventilation; the second person to arrive should assume responsibility for circulation, and the third should help with the intravenous administration of drugs (inserting the line, drawing up and possibly administering the drug). The fourth person is generally most helpful as a relief person for compression or ventilation (compression of an adult chest is fatiguing because a great deal of effort is required to compress a large man's sternum effectively), as a family advocate, or as a helper to bring extra supplies not included on the emergency cart. The roles assumed also differ according to each person's experience and expertise.

When helping with administration of medication, you will be following verbal orders. Always repeat a verbal order so that the physician giving it to you can verify that you have heard it correctly and has an opportunity to hear and review the order herself before it is acted on. Record immediately on a flow sheet any medication you have administered and the dosage and time of administration. By the same token, if you draw up medication in anticipation that it will be needed, label the filled syringe immediately with the drug and dosage or you may forget what medication you drew up

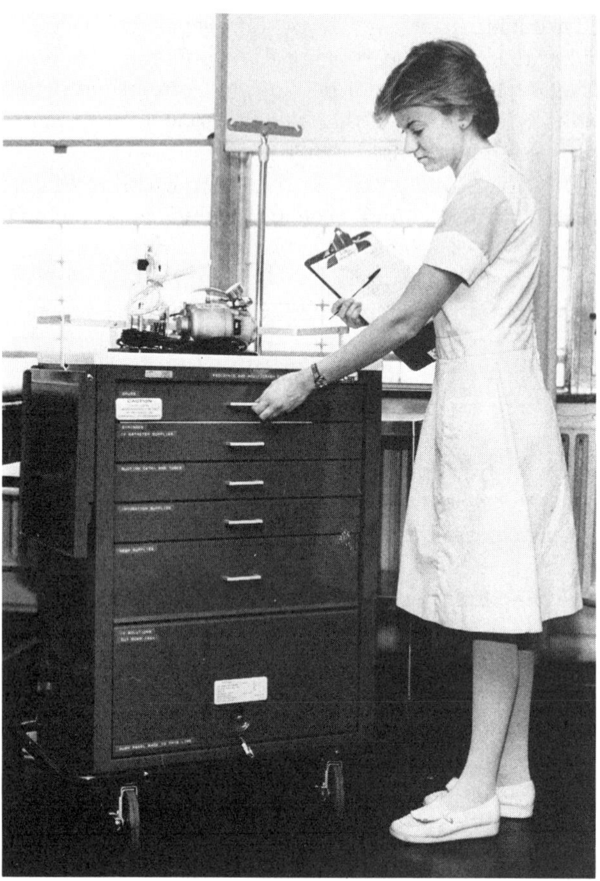

FIGURE 32-30. An emergency cart should be checked daily to see that all supplies are in place and in good repair.

when the drug is needed. Do not hesitate to ask people to repeat drug names or dosages for you.

Theoretically, an emergency cart has everything on it that will be necessary for a resuscitation attempt (a resuscitation bag, airways, oxygen administration equipment, suction equipment, a chest board, intravenous infusion equipment, and emergency drugs). As part of the routine management of a nursing unit, such a cart should be checked daily (Fig. 32-30) to see that all supplies listed as belonging on the cart are there, drugs are not outdated, and all equipment is functioning.

Never remove anything from an emergency cart except for use in an emergency situation. To reach for a lifesaving drug or piece of equipment on an emergency cart and realize that it is missing because it was used for routine care produces a most helpless feeling. Never change the usual storage place of an emergency cart unless all unit personnel agree that the new position is advantageous and are aware of it. Important seconds can be lost in an emergency situation if the cart has been moved from its usual location.

Family advocacy or concern for the patient's roommate is an important role that should not be taken lightly in an emergency situation. It is terrifying for a family member or a roommate to see someone he cares about suddenly stop breathing. These people need to be kept informed of the patient's progress as resuscitation is begun. As a beginning nurse, be careful not to give false reassurance. Use supportive statements such as "You can tell that everyone is doing everything possible" or "I appreciate that this is a difficult time for you" instead. Be certain that a person with sure knowledge of the patient's condition does talk to support people as soon as possible.

Infant Resuscitation

Infant resuscitation differs from adult resuscitation because the rate and rhythm of ventilation and compression are different due to an infant's small circulatory and ventilatory capacity. With an infant, be certain to extend the neck only slightly for ventilation. An infant's trachea is very supple, and a sharp bend in the trachea may compress, not open the airway. Place your mouth over both the mouth and the nose for ventilation. Use only a mouthful of air for exhalation or the alveoli may burst from undue volume and pressure.

For cardiac compression, use the fingers, not the heel, of your hand (only two for a newborn) and place them *midway* on the sternum (the liver is high in infants, under the bottom of the sternum). Compress at a rate of 80 to 100 compressions per minute. Use the same proportion of five compressions to one exhalation for cardiac and ventilation support as used in adults. You need to compress only one-half to three-quarters of an inch to initiate cardiac compression effectively. Alternatively, cardiac compression in infants can be done by placing the palms of the hands under the infant's back and extending the thumbs across the chest to perform sternal compression.

In many cases, with nose and mouth ventilation the infant's stomach becomes distended with air after a few minutes. This is potentially dangerous because it interferes with diaphragm expansion, and sternal compression may cause vomiting with accompanying aspiration of stomach contents. To relieve this stomach distention, a nasogastric tube can be quickly inserted and left in the side of the infant's mouth to be a release for this volume of air. Passing a nasogastric tube in an unconscious infant takes only a few seconds because there is no resistance to the tube.

Tracheostomy

A tracheotomy is a permanent incision into the anterior trachea; a tracheostomy is a temporary incision into the anterior trachea (Fig. 32-31). In most instances such an incision is temporary to allow suctioning of respiratory secretions or to bypass a temporary obstruction of some type in the upper airway. People with tracheostomies or tracheotomies cannot speak because voice sounds are made by air passing over the vocal cords, and after such an opening in the trachea,

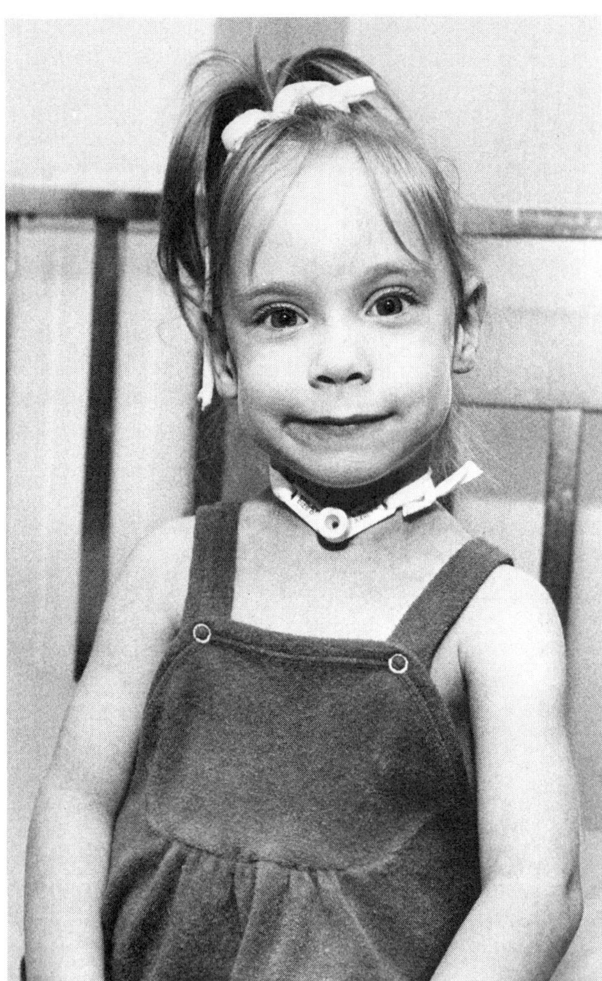

FIGURE 32-31. Child with a tracheotomy tube in place; notice the tape, which holds it securely.

air enters the lungs below the level of the vocal cords. Because most tracheostomies are done as emergency procedures (when the person suddenly becomes cyanotic due to upper respiratory tract obstruction), the person is at first extremely frightened, not only because of what has happened (a suffocating feeling of not being able to breathe and someone cutting his throat) but because he thinks of what could have happened if emergency help had not been immediately available. Almost as frightening is the realization that he now can no longer talk (if he becomes obstructed again, he cannot call for help, and he worries that this time he will die). He can talk, however, if he places a hand over the opening of the tracheostomy tube that is inserted in the tracheal incision and air is again drawn up over the vocal cords. He needs to be shown how to do this early following the tracheostomy so he can communicate effectively with it in place.

A tracheostomy tube is usually inserted because excess respiratory secretions are present; frequent suctioning through the tracheostomy tube is usually necessary to keep the secretions from obstructing the tube and occluding the airway. With a tracheostomy tube in place, the normal filtering and moistening action of inhaled air is lost, and the person is more prone to respiratory tract infections than most people. All suctioning must be done with strict sterile technique to limit the introduction of infection as much as possible.

Tracheostomy tubes are made of either silver or plastic. Those made of silver consist of three parts—an outer cannula, an inner cannula, and an obturator (Fig. 32-32A). The obturator is inserted into the outer cannula when the tube is initially inserted (the tube has a flat tip; the obturator fits into it to make a smooth rounded tip for easy and untraumatic insertion). It is removed immediately after insertion because it is not hollow and would obstruct the tube if left in place. It is replaced by the inner cannula, which is hollow; with the inner cannula in place there is no possibility that the tube can become seriously obstructed because the inner cannula containing the obstruction can be quickly removed, freeing the airway. Plastic tubes do not have inner cannulas, but they are not as easily coated with obstructive mucus.

In addition to frequent suctioning, the inner cannula must be removed at least every 8 hours and cleaned (soaking it in a solution of half hydrogen peroxide and half distilled water effectively removes mucus) and replaced or crusted mucus will adhere so tightly that the cannula can no longer be removed, and its safety feature is lost. The area around the tracheostomy must be kept from becoming moist from secretions because it will become excoriated by having a piece of gauze fitted around it. The strings that hold the tube in place may be replaced as they become soiled. When the strings are untied a second person must be present to hold the tube in place so that if the person should cough at that moment, the tube will not be dislodged. If the tube should be dislodged, the incision in most instances remains open, and although respirations are threatened, they are rarely seriously impaired. Remain with the patient and place your fingers on both sides of the tracheal incision to separate it and keep it patent (if a hemostat is at the bedside, gently insert the clamp and spread the incision). Summon experienced help to replace the tube.

Intubation with an Endotracheal Tube

An endotracheal tube serves the same purpose as a tracheostomy tube—to provide a patent airway for the person with a temporary upper airway obstruction. This is a thin, pliable tube that can be inserted as a nasotracheal tube but is generally inserted by the oral-tracheal route (Fig. 32-32B). Endotracheal tubes are taped in place rather than tied. Because they tend to cause tissue irritation by pressure against the pharynx, they are left in place only three to four days. They are then replaced by a tracheostomy tube if an alternate airway is still necessary.

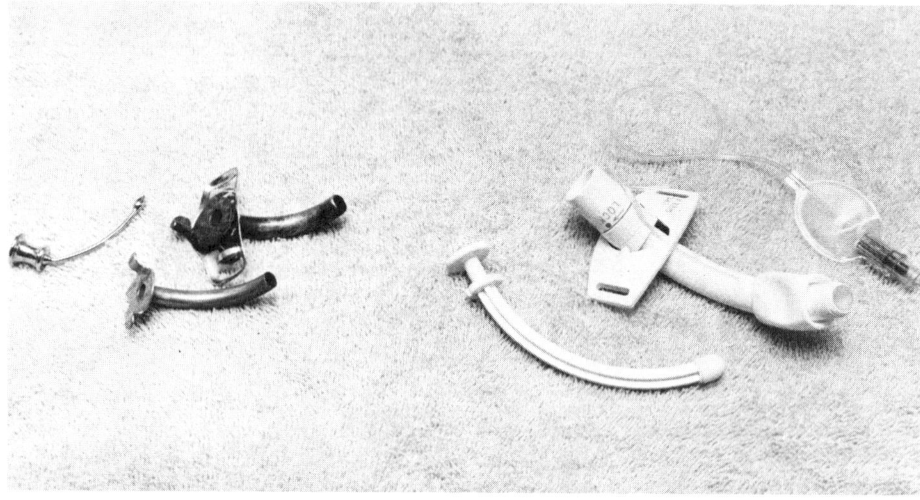

A

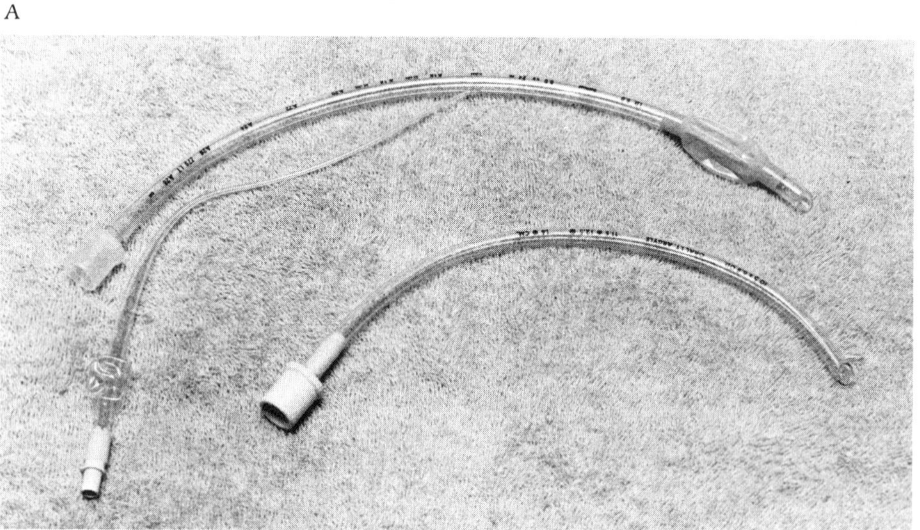

B

FIGURE 32-32. A. Tracheotomy tubes. On the left is a metal one; on the right a plastic one. The plastic one is "cuffed." B. Endotrachial tubes. The one on the left is "cuffed." The cuff seals the airway against aspiration.

Endotracheal airways have the advantages of being easily inserted without a surgical procedure (no incision is made) and leaving no neck scar (Fig. 32-33). They also allow air to enter the lungs from the mouth or nose rather than directly into the trachea, and therefore possibly carry less risk of a lung infection.

Respiratory Monitors

The respiratory rate can be monitored by means of "leads" placed on the chest (Fig. 32-34) or, in some instances with infants, by a special mattress that senses changes in chest movements. With such monitors, if there is no chest movement for a predetermined period of time (30 seconds to 1 minute, as a rule) the attached monitor will sound an alarm.

When caring for a person with an apnea monitor, be certain that you do not go so far away from the patient that you cannot hear the alarm. In a hospital equipped with an intercom system of two-way communication, the device can be left turned on. The sound of the alarm will then be heard in the nursing station. Be aware that

FIGURE 32-33. Inserting an endotrachial tube through a laryngoscope.

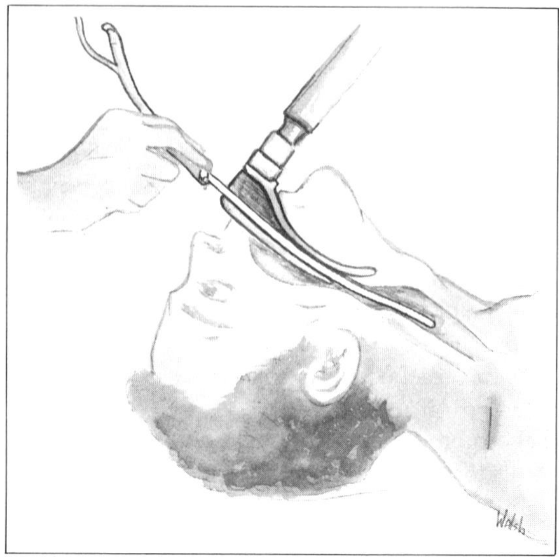

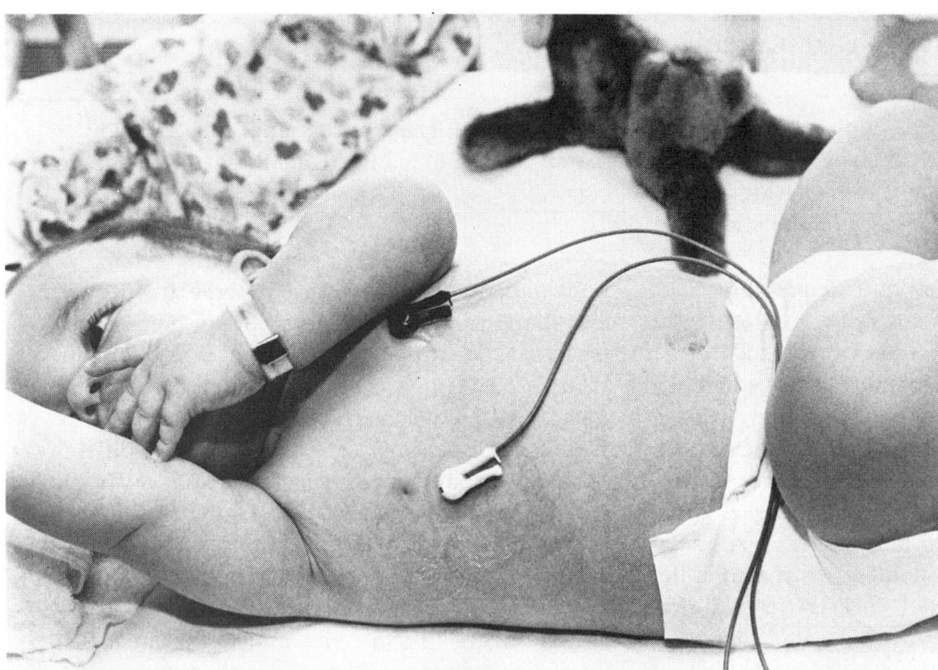

FIGURE 32-34. Apnea monitor leads. Cessation of breathing triggers an alarm to sound.

such leads often become disconnected if the person turns suddenly, sounding a false alarm. Some people are afraid to fall asleep with a monitor in place because they are concerned that it will malfunction and not alarm you of their distress. With such people you might want to make a point of testing the alarm either by temporarily removing a lead or by asking the patient to hold his breath. If a person has frequent false alarms, you might want to assess whether he is frequently testing the monitor by holding his breath.

Some infants return home with apnea monitors in place. Help a mother to plan her day carefully. She may have to omit showering, vacuum cleaning, or playing a radio or television if these sounds would obscure the sound of the alarm from an upstairs bedroom.

UTILIZING NURSING PROCESS

People who have any degree of respiratory illness are worried about their condition. They appreciate having caregivers around them who have planned their care in a logical and sound manner. Quick Reference Stop 32-6 presents some recent findings related to research in the care of patients with respiratory dysfunction.

Assessment

Respiratory function is a vital life function. Make a point of always observing respiratory function in every patient. Do not discount the importance of counting respiratory rate just because it is the easiest vital sign measurement to take. When respiratory distress occurs, an increase in respiratory rate or a deviation in its character will be one of the first apparent signs, and it will be present much before more obvious signs such as cyanosis.

Analysis

The number of problems related to respiratory dysfunction is high because there are many types of respiratory illnesses. Three common nursing diagnoses accepted by the Fourth National Conference on Nursing Diagnoses are airway clearance, ineffective; breathing pattern, ineffective; and gas exchange, impaired. These are shown in Appendix C with their defining characteristics.

A nursing diagnosis for the person with respiratory difficulty is established following careful assessment. Because any difficulty with respiration leads to distress, the main problem may not actually be the respiratory difficulty itself but the person's anxiety about the difficulty. A nursing diagnosis in relation to respiratory function, therefore is often listed not as "inadequate air exchange related to chronic lung pathology changes" but rather as "anxiety related to difficulty with respiration." You may be able to accomplish very little change in a person's ability to exchange air, but you can accomplish a great deal of change in his ability to deal with the problem (see QRS 32-7).

Planning

Because all respiratory difficulty is accompanied by psychological distress, planning for the patient with any kind of respiratory illness must include input from the patient. Many people with respiratory distress lie very still (instinctively conserving energy for this vital function, which suddenly requires energy to accomplish). This means that you must consider them immobilized and plan to combat the effects of immobility

☐ **QUICK REFERENCE STOP 32-6: RESEARCH**
Oxygen Regulation

Meeting the respiratory needs of patients is a major nursing responsibility. Many nursing skills are associated with the care of patients receiving oxygen therapy, those with altered respiratory function, and those prone to respiratory infection. Nursing research has begun to investigate these topics, as noted below.

Does oxygen inhalation affect oral temperature readings?
Assessing temperature by the oral method rather than the rectal or axillary method has traditionally been avoided when the patient is receiving oxygen therapy. It has been thought that such therapy resulted in oral temperature readings that were inconsistent with the overall body temperature. A study by Lim-Levy (1982) empirically tested this assumption. One hundred healthy adults participated in the study, which was conducted to ascertain how oral temperature was affected by oxygen inhalation through a nasal cannula. Subjects were tested before and after oxygen inhalation, under three different liter flow conditions. The results showed no significant alterations in temperature because of oxygen inhalation.

Early assessment of respiratory infection in elderly patients.
Early identification of respiratory tract infection is beneficial, especially in elderly patients. A retrospective study of 60 elderly patients showed that those who developed lower respiratory tract infections had a respiratory rate of greater than 25 breaths per minute for three to four days prior to the onset of clinical signs and symptoms. A normal respiratory rate was considered 16 to 25 breaths per minute (Increased respiratory rate is a tip-off to infection in the elderly, *Nursing* 1983).

Tracheotomy care—clean versus sterile.
Harris (1980, 1981) questions the need for maintaining sterility in tracheotomy care management. Sterile technique has traditionally been used for this procedure, although recently clean and modified sterile techniques have been introduced. In this investigation, patients who were given sterile tracheotomy care demonstrated higher levels of pulmonary infection than those undergoing clean care techniques (Harris, 1981). It was also found that 50 percent of nurses and physicians responsible for caring for patients with tracheotomies were unable to differentiate satisfactorily between sterile and clean care techniques in terms of gloving, equipment, and solutions used (Harris, 1980); no two hospitals, nursing texts, or other nursing references were alike in tracheotomy care procedures (Harris, 1980). The author suggests further research to be directed toward differences in cost to the patient and the hospital in terms of nursing time and equipment, patient anxiety, and patient self-care possibilities. This research certainly raises serious questions about current nursing practice in this area.

SUGGESTED READINGS

Increased respiratory rate is a tip-off to infection in the elderly. *Nursing* 13(2):22, 1983. Report of research study previously reported in *Geriatric Medicine Currents* and conducted at Southhamptom General Hospital, Southhamptom, England.

Harris, R. B. National survey: Current status of aseptic tracheotomy care techniques and approximate rate of infection in hospitals with Head and Neck/ENT surgical departments. *PRN: The Adelphi Report 1979—1980*, Project for Research in Nursing, School of Nursing, Adelphi University, Garden City, N.Y., 1980.

Harris, R. B. Clean vs. sterile tracheotomy care on level of infection on first-week postoperative head and neck/ENT surgical patients—A retrospective pilot study. *PRN: The Adelphi Report 1980—1981*, Project for Research in Nursing, School of Nursing, Adelphi University, Garden City, N.Y., 1981.

Lim-Levy, F. The effect of oxygen inhalation on oral temperature. *Nurs. Res.* 31(3):150, 1982.

just as if their basic problem was a musculoskeletal one (turning, deep breathing, ambulation, and stimulation). One of the effects of immobility is the formation of decubitus ulcers, which tend to develop quickly in people with impaired respiratory function because the skin cells are deprived of oxygen owing to the basic disease as well as to pressure points resulting from the "frozen" body posture.

Implementation

Implementation of care in people with respiratory illness is always two-pronged: Physical care measures are important, but teaching or psychological measures to help patients accept or adjust to this change in a vital life function is extremely important also. Persons with any chronic disease should be encouraged to maintain as active a life as possible within the limitations of their

☐ **QUICK REFERENCE STOP 32-7: PSYCHOLOGICAL CONSIDERATIONS**
Overcoming Anxiety

The rate and depth of respiration are strongly influenced by emotions. In many instances the most effective way to help a person stabilize his breathing pattern is by giving reassuring support. Many people are afraid that oxygen equipment will force too much oxygen into their lungs and rupture them. Pay careful attention to the equipment you are using. With time it will become very familiar to you; it is rarely familiar or comfortable for a person in respiratory distress.

disease process. Some adults with lung disease may have to change occupations to a position that removes them from a source of lung pollution; they may not be able to continue to work outside in the cold or rain if this would increase the likelihood of upper respiratory tract infections for them. Children should be encouraged to attend school and participate in extracurricular activities to maintain social interaction. Swimming is an activity that is generally suggested for people with lung illnesses because it exercises the chest muscles and keeps them strong; it also encourages deep inhalations that fully expand the lung tissue.

In addition to such activities as swimming, breathing exercises are often prescribed for many people with chronic respiratory involvement. They should be done three or more times a day, and these times need to be planned definitely each day so that this type of therapy is reliably followed (see QRS 32-8).

Evaluation

Evaluation of a person with respiratory illness should involve not only an improvement in his physical ability to breathe, but also to his life-style and whether he has returned to thinking of himself as a person now well after an illness and able to function fully, or as someone who will never again be wholly able to take care of himself. Ask about work performance or school performance and whether the person initiates activities that are independent of his support people. Many people with respiratory illness want to live alone and be independent but also feel a strong need to have dependable people around them who do check on them frequently. You may need to help a person establish a network of support people among family members or friends who serve this function for him (see QRS 32-9).

Nursing Care Plan

Mr. Summers is a 50-year-old man who has been admitted to the hospital following an episode of chest pain and shortness of breath while at work. The following is a problem-oriented record note written in the emergency room on him:

Problem: Shortness of Breath
Subjective: Patient states that he became short of breath following the news that the plant where he has worked for 14 years is going to close. Chest pain was momentary, but shortness of breath has persisted. Feels "light-headed" and "unable to get enough air."
Objective: Respiratory rate is 50 per minute. Minimal subcostal retraction. Oxygen being administered by mask at 6 liters per minute; respiratory rate slowed to 30 per minute.
Analysis: Shortness of breath and rapid respiratory rate improved by oxygen administration.
Planning Goal: Patient will have normal breathing pattern within 30 minutes.
Criteria: Patient's respiratory rate to be below 20 per minute within 30 minutes.

☐ **QUICK REFERENCE STOP 32-8: HEALTH TEACHING**
Lung Function Exercises

Exercises to increase lung function such as incentive spirometry, pursed lip breathing, or swimming seem so simple that people tend to discount them as unimportant. You may need to help people make a chart to hang on their refrigerator or bathroom mirror to remind them to do these exercises. They need careful instruction in the importance and purpose of these exercises or they will not continue to do them long enough to be effective.

☐ **QUICK REFERENCE STOP 32-9: COMMUNITY CONSIDERATIONS**
Respiratory Emergencies At Home

Many people return to their homes following hospitalization for a respiratory illness with chronic symptoms of illness. Because respiratory illnesses are always frightening, be certain that the person has a clear understanding of what he should do if his symptoms should suddenly grow acute. Should he call the hospital for an ambulance? Call his physician? Call a local paramedic number? Inject epinephrine? Help him think through what he would do if an emergency arose while his wife was at work, or if he were on vacation in a strange city; if eyesight is a problem, how would he see to telephone for help? (A push button phone or a community 911 number are possible solutions to this problem.)

When acute respiratory symptoms occur, they can be incapacitating. Preplanning helps to avoid this problem for the patient at home.

NURSING ORDERS

1. Keep patient in semi-Fowler's position for comfort.
2. Continue oxygen administration until blood gas results are returned.
3. Reassure patient that he is being watched closely. Encourage him to remain quiet to save energy for breathing (unless he feels that discussing the news that began the discomfort would be helpful to him).

SUGGESTED READINGS

Albanese, A., and Riley, J. Caring for the intubated patient. *RN* 43:38, 1980.

Belman, M., et al. Incentive spirometry. *Chest* 79:254, 1981.

Budassi, S. A. Management of cardiopulmonary arrest. *Nurs. Clin. North Am.* 16:37, 1981.

Cannon, C. Palpation and auscultation. *RN* 43:20, 1980.

Cline, B. A., et al. A.R.D.S. means emergency. *Nursing* (Horsham) 12(2):62, 1982.

Conine, T. A., et al. Sexual adjustment in chronic obstructive pulmonary disease. *Resp. Care* 26:871, 1981.

Cugell, D. W. Guide to modern lung function tests. *Hosp. Med.* 14:57, 1978.

Del Bueno, D. J. A quick review on using blood-gas determinations. *RN* 41:68, 1978.

Detoledo, L. W. Caring for the patient, instead of the ventilator. *RN* 43:20, 1980.

Egan, D. F. *Fundamentals of Respiratory Therapy* (2nd ed.). St. Louis: Mosby, 1973.

Ellmyer, P., et al. Ambulatory nursing. A guide to your patient's safe home use of oxygen. *Nursing* (Horsham) 12(1):56, 1982.

Fuchs, P. L. Getting the best out of oxygen delivery systems. *Nursing (Horsham)* 10:34, 1980.

Glass, L. B. Exercise therapy for the patient with pulmonary dysfunction. *Top. Clin. Nurs.* 3:87, 1981.

Hasler, M. E., et al. The effect of oxygen administration on oral temperature assessment. *Nurs. Res.* 31(5):265, 1982.

Hoops, E. J. Cardiopulmonary resuscitation of children. *Nurs. Clin. North Am.* 16:623, 1981.

Hotter, A. N. Adult respiratory distress syndrome. *Crit. Care Update* 8(8):26, 1981.

Hunter, P. N. Bedside monitoring of respiratory function. *Nurs. Clin. North Am.* 16:211, 1981.

Jennings, C. An alternative: Nasal cannula oxygen therapy for infants who are oxygen dependent. *M.C.N.* 7(2):89, 1982.

Kanto, W. P., Jr. Dealing with respiratory distress. *Emerg. Med.* 9:67, 1977.

Kaufman, J. S., and Woody, J. W. For patients with COPD: Better living . . . through teaching. *Nursing 80* 10:57, 1980.

Keogh, B. A., et al. Clinical significance of pulmonary function tests. *Chest* 78:856, 1980.

McFadden, R. Decreasing respiratory compromise during infant suctioning. *Am. J. Nurs.* 81(12):2158, 1981.

Monitors that need nursing . . . trancutaneous oxygen monitors. *Health Soc. Serv. J.* 92(4809):970, 1982.

Morrison, M. L. (Ed.). *Respiratory Intensive Care Nursing.* Boston: Little, Brown, 1979.

Nielson, L. Mechanical ventilation: Patient assessment and nursing care. *Am. J. Nurs.* 80:2191, 1980.

O'Malley, P., and Zankofski, M. A. Disposable suction catheters. *Nursing 79* 9:70, 1979.

Peterson, G. M. Application and assessment of oxygen therapy devices. *Nurs. Clin. North Am.* 16:241, 1981.

Rau, J., and Rau, M. To breathe or to be breathed: Understanding IPPB. *Am. J. Nurs.* 77:613, 1977.

Rifas, E. M. How you . . . and your patient . . . can manage dyspnea. *Nursing 80* 10:34, 1980.

Rokosky, J. S. Assessment of the individual with altered respiratory function. *Nurs. Clin. North Am.* 16:195, 1981.

Sandham, G., and Reid, B. Some Q's and A's about suctioning. *Nursing 77* 7:60, 1977.

Shake, K. The ABC's of ABC's. *Nursing 79* 9:26, 1979.

Stanley, L. You really can teach COPD patients to breathe better. *RN* 41:43, 1978.

Sumner, S. N. Refining your technique for drawing blood gases. *Nursing 80* 10:65, 1980.

Waldron, M. W. Oxygen transport. *Am. J. Nurs.* 79:272, 1979.

Waterson, M. Teaching your patients postural drainage. *Nursing 78* 8:51, 1978.

Weaver, T. E. New Life for lungs . . . through incentive spirometers. *Nursing 81* 11:54, 1981.

Weaver, T. E. ABGs: Taking the sample, interpreting the results. *RN* 46(3):64, 1983.

QUESTIONS FOR REVIEW

1. Mr. Jones is a black, 45-year-old patient of yours. He has dyspnea. This means that:
   a. His respirations are deep.
   b. He feels he has difficulty breathing.
   c. His respiratory rate is more than 30 breaths per minute.
   d. He feels dizzy with inspiration.

2. If he has orthopnea, this would mean that:
   a. He cannot breathe except lying down.
   b. He needs to raise his arms to breathe.
   c. He has difficulty breathing unless he is sitting up.
   d. He breathes rapidly unless sitting upright.

3. To assess whether Mr. Jones has cyanosis, the best body part would be:
   a. The skin area around his mouth.
   b. The back of the hands.
   c. The buccal membrane.
   d. The nail beds.

4. Oxygen by nasal prongs is ordered for Mr. Jones. To analyze whether this form of therapy is suitable for him, which factor would *not* be a contraindication to its use?
   a. Mr. Jones has a nasal obstruction.
   b. Mr. Jones moves in bed a great deal.
   c. Mr. Jones needs an oxygen concentration of 100 percent.
   d. Mr. Jones has a slightly elevated PCO_2.

5. In planning care for Mr. Jones, which factor can you anticipate will *not* be included in your care?
   a. Periodic blood gas analysis.
   b. Periods of alternating humidification and dry oxygen administration.
   c. Continuous restriction on no smoking.
   d. Increasing fluid intake.

6. If you saw Mr. Jones choking on a piece of meat, your best action would be to:
   a. Reach into his mouth to try and remove it.
   b. Strike his anterior chest three times.
   c. Apply inward and upward abdominal pressure.
   d. Increase his oxygen supply to above 10 liters per minute.

7. If Mr. Jones has a chronic lung disease and his carbon dioxide level is constantly high, the effect of administering oxygen to him could be to:
   a. Increase the blood pressure in the distal capillaries.
   b. Decrease the pulse rate.
   c. Decrease the alveolar diffusion of carbon dioxide.
   d. Halt respirations.

8. In evaluating Mr. Jones's blood gases, which of the following would you accept as a normal value?
   a. PCO_2 = 40 mm Hg; PO_2 = 80 mm Hg; saturation = 97%.
   b. PCO_2 = 90 mm Hg; PO_2 = 30 mm Hg; saturation = 40%.
   c. PCO_2 = 30 mm Hg; PO_2 = 90 mm Hg; saturation = 60%.
   d. PCO_2 = 60 mm Hg; PO_2 = 40 mm Hg; saturation = 90%.

9. To suction Mr. Jones with a nasopharyngeal catheter, what would be the longest period you would suction at one time?
   a. 1 to 5 seconds.
   b. 10 to 15 seconds.
   c. 30 to 35 seconds.
   d. 45 to 50 seconds.

10. You administer Mr. Jones an antitussive. This is a medication that:
    a. Liquefies secretions.
    b. Raises secretions.
    c. Dilates the bronchi.
    d. Halts coughing.

11. In cardiopulmonary resuscitation by two people, the proportion of heart compressions to lung ventilations should be:
    a. 1 to 4.
    b. 1 to 10.
    c. 10 to 5.
    d. 5 to 1.

33. THERMAL REGULATION

OBJECTIVES

Upon mastery of the material in this chapter, you should be able to:

1. Describe the body regulatory systems for conserving and dissipating heat.
2. Describe the techniques used for determining body temperature.
3. Describe common nursing procedures used to reduce an elevated temperature.
4. Describe the principles that govern the safe application of heat and cold.
5. List the safety measures that should be followed when using heat and cold applications.
6. Explain the body alterations that can occur following applications of heat and cold.
7. Apply the nursing process to give safe and planned care to a patient whose care involves principles of thermal regulation.

TERMS

The terms important for an understanding of this chapter are shown below and defined in the glossary:

antipyretic
conduction
convection
evaporation
fever
hyperthermia
hypothermia
pyrexia
pyrogen
radiation

Heat is constantly produced in the body and constantly lost from it. Unless the external environment is extremely warm or cold for an extended period, the average person is able to regulate the body temperature between a very narrow range of 96.8° to 100.4°F (36°—38°C). This is characteristic of a homeothermic or warm-blooded animal (in contrast to a poikilothermic or cold-blooded animal). Body heat is maintained within this narrow margin by keeping a careful balance between heat produced by the body and heat lost to the environment.

BODY HEAT PRODUCTION

Heat produced by the body is the result of body metabolism; the amount of heat produced is regulated, therefore, by the rate of metabolism. The metabolic rate is increased by muscular activity, the presence of fever or increased body temperature, increased secretion of thyroxine from the thyroid gland, increased oxidation of food, and increased sympathetic nerve stimulation. Shivering is a subtle type of muscular activity or form of exercise for raising body temperature that is effective in everyone but newborns, whose shivering mechanism is immature. To compensate for the lack of shivering response newborns have a special type of fat called brown fat, which is located mainly behind the sternum, in the neck and between the shoulder blades, and surrounding the kidneys and adrenal glands. This special form of fat produces heat or sustains body heat in much the same way as heat is maintained in hybernating bears.

Piloerection (goose bumps) is another mechanism used by animals with fur to maintain body heat. When hair shafts stand on end in animals with thick fur, a layer of air is trapped under the layer of fur, producing a layer of insulating air much as several layers of clothing or stitched and padded *(quilted)* clothing provides insulation for skiers. In humans, piloerection occurs but does not afford any protection against heat loss because body hair is not thick enough to trap air.

Maintaining body temperature is such a strong physiological need that even under stress conditions the body attempts to maintain heat so incessantly that it quickly burns up nutrients for warmth that might better be conserved for sustained cell nutrition. The same phenomenon occurs when the body has excess heat; a person will continue to perspire to cool body temperature to the point of dehydration.

METHODS OF HEAT LOSS

Four different principles govern heat lost from the body.

Conduction

Conduction is the loss of heat from a warmer to a colder object that is in direct contact with it. Heat from the body's central core is lost to peripheral body areas by conduction through tissue layers. If you touch an object colder than your skin, heat passes from your skin to the object. If you are trying to keep a patient warm, don't lay him on a cool bed surface, and don't place a newborn in a cool Isolette and then turn on the heat; warm the bedding first to prevent conduction loss. Subcutaneous fat is a good insulator because it is a poor conductor of heat and gives off heat poorly to contiguous colder objects. Vasoconstriction impairs heat losses by conduction because it pushes the blood back under subcutaneous fat. Dilatation of blood vessels improves conduction loss by pushing blood away from its insulating fat layer.

Convection

Convection is the loss of heat to moving air or liquid currents. Heat passes from the skin to the cooler air around it; the layer of air next to the skin becomes warmed, and although it rises slowly away from the body (hot air rises), it serves as a protective layer that limits more heat loss to the air. If this insulating air layer is moved away, however (by an air conditioner, the wind, or a fan, causing a convection current), additional heat loss will take place.

Radiation

Radiation is heat loss to a distant colder object. Body heat is radiated toward an object such as a cold window or an air conditioner unit; heat is radiated from a warm radiator toward the skin. The closer the two objects are, the quicker and more intense the radiation potential. Thus, when trying to keep someone warm, moving the bed further away from a large window on a cold day may be necessary. If the person has a fever that should be reduced, move the bed closer to a cold window or away from the room's heating source.

Evaporation

When a liquid changes to a gas, heat is released (because it is used as energy in the exchange). There are two forms of water loss from the body that are important in evaporation. One is insensible loss, or the water lost by way of the lungs and skin that one is unaware of, and the other is active perspiration (sweating). Sweat is basically a product of the exocrine glands. These glands are present almost everywhere in the body; large numbers of them are located in the forehead and the lower extremities. Sweating is limited when the body temperature falls below 37°C (98.6°F), but insensible water loss and evaporation from the lungs continue. In a person with a subnormal temperature, humidifying the room limits insensible water loss from this source.

If the humidity of the room air is high (e.g., there is a high proportion of water vapor in the air), less evaporation takes place (because the air is already loaded with as much water as it can carry), and sweating will decrease. This is the reason that just before a summer rainstorm you often feel so warm; after the storm, although the temperature is the same, you feel much more comfortable. Because the air contains less water, more evaporation from your skin can take place, and better body cooling results.

BODY TEMPERATURE

Body temperature refers to the core or internal temperature of the body (the temperature in the thoracic and abdominal cavities and the central nervous system). Because the skin is peripheral it invariably has a temperature lower than the core temperature. When taking a person's temperature, you should place the thermometer so that you are monitoring the internal body temperature, not merely the skin or mucous membrane temperature.

Factors Affecting Body Temperature

Although 98.6°F (37°C) is accepted as the average normal body temperature, you will discover that a person's temperature varies from this depending on environmental stimuli and individual differences. The ways in which a person regulates body temperature are shown in Fig. 33-1.

AGE

At the moment of birth, a newborn's temperature is slightly elevated (99.6°F or 37.6°C) because he has been living for nine months in a central or core organ in his mother. Almost immediately, however, his temperature falls to 98.6°F. He has little subcutaneous fat to conserve heat, relatively little muscle mass to produce heat, and a large surface area that invites excessive conduction loss. Because he cannot shiver, he has difficulty maintaining body temperature, particularly in a chilled delivery or birthing room (which is kept slightly cool to minimize the danger of exploding anesthesia gases). The only way he can maintain body temperature is by increasing the metabolic rate, which calls for increased oxygen. If the newborn has any difficulty with oxygenation (part of the alveoli-exchange space may be covered by lung fluid, or the alveoli may not yet be performing at their peak level), anaerobic (unoxygenated) metabolism may begin, a process that leads to acidosis because it involves the breakdown of body fat. Allowing a newborn to become chilled, therefore, is not a small error; it can severely compromise the newborn's entire metabolic function. Cooling should be prevented in a newborn by drying the skin well, wrapping the infant snugly to prevent evapora-

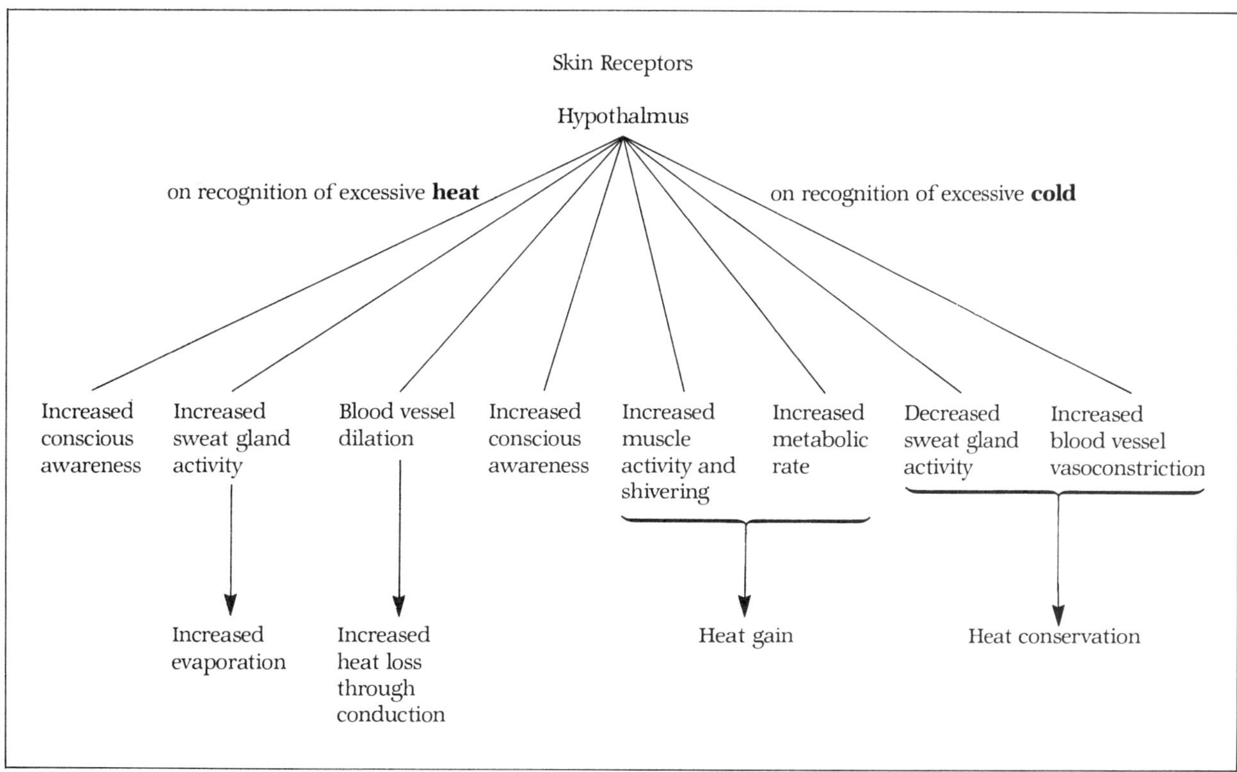

FIGURE 33-1. Responses of the body to heat and cold; balance of body temperature.

tion, and placing him in a heated bassinet or under a radiant heat warmer to prevent heat loss from conduction and convection.

Older adults tend to have a lower than average body temperature. As a group, they have less subcutaneous fat for body insulation, so they tend to lose more heat; if the level of activity is reduced, they do not initiate as much heat production as young persons. In a room where a young nurse is comfortable, therefore, an older adult may feel chilly. When transporting older adults through hospital corridors be particularly careful to provide a sweater or shawl or blanket to protect body warmth. Because surgical suites are kept slightly cool, the stretcher of an older adult being transported to surgery should always be covered to prevent chilling between the time of arrival in the surgical suite and the time anesthesia is actually administered.

EXTERNAL TEMPERATURE

The term *ambient* means "surrounding." Ambient air, therefore, is the surrounding external air (room air). The temperature of ambient air does not greatly affect internal body temperature until the difference between the two is extreme. Under normal circumstances, internal body temperature varies only 1°C (1.8°F) whether it is uncomfortably warm or uncomfortably cold in a room (this is why it is important to be certain that you are measuring the internal body temperature rather than the peripheral temperature).

CIRCADIAN RHYTHM

Circadian rhythm refers to the sleep-wake rhythm of the body, a pattern that varies slightly from person to person. For most people the period of deepest sleep is between midnight and 6 A.M.; basal metabolism is at its lowest point during this time, so body temperature is also at its lowest point. This period corresponds with the period of least body action and lowest hormone production. The average person's highest body temperature occurs between 4 and 8 P.M. These temperature variations are slight, ranging from 0.5° to 1.5°C (0.9°—2.7°F). Such low and high points tend to be reversed in the person who works at night; even when the worker changes to a night sleeping pattern, it takes one to three weeks for the temperature rhythm to change. The initial admission history to a health care facility should document a person's sleep-wake pattern so that high and low temperature points can be predicted.

Temperature rhythms are not present in newborns. A child is about three weeks old before such a pattern becomes apparent.

EXERCISE

Exercise increases the metabolic rate and therefore body temperature. Shivering, as mentioned earlier, is a series of rapid, involuntary muscle contractions and is therefore a subtle form of exercise that increases body temperature. As long as a person with a fever is shivering from an accompanying chill, the fever will be very difficult to reduce because the person is actively producing body heat.

HORMONE SECRETIONS

In women, just prior to ovulation, there is a fall in body temperature of 0.5°C (0.9°F) for one day and then a sudden increase of about 0.5° to 1.0°C (0.9°—1.8°F) that occurs with ovulation. The rise is caused by the high level of progesterone produced at the time of ovulation. The increased temperature will be sustained for the life of the ovum or until just before the next menstrual period. At this time progesterone levels fall, and so does body temperature. If a woman becomes pregnant, the temperature remains at the elevated stage for the first 3 months of pregnancy.

These changes in temperature can be used by women to locate their day of ovulation and so are helpful in family planning. The changes are so subtle that they do not need to be considered in normal temperature-recording.

Increases in levels of thyroxine and growth hormone increase body metabolism and may therefore elevate body temperature. This increase may be important in detecting whether adequate levels of these hormones are being produced.

PSYCHOLOGICAL INFLUENCES

The presence of a stressor increases the secretion of epinephrine and norepinephrine, which in turn increases the metabolic rate (to prepare the body for "flight or fight"). For such an increase to be considered in normal temperature-taking, however, the stress would have to be extremely intense and prolonged.

HYPOTHALAMIC REGULATION

The temperature of the blood passing through the hypothalamus regulates compensating mechanisms. The average person has a set-point or reference point for body temperature (37°C, 98.6°F). When the temperature of the blood arriving at the hypothalamus is above or below this point, the hypothalamus initiates a stimulation for heat loss or heat production as necessary through such measures as vasoconstriction or shivering. In hypothalamic regulation peripheral sensors in the skin relay heat and cold sensations to the hypothalamus. If the environment is cold, sympathetic nerve innervation causes vasoconstriction in peripheral vessels (causing the blood to pool in the body's central core, where its heat can be better maintained because of insulation by body fat and muscle). With vasoconstriction, the skin appears pale or mottled and is cool to the touch; finger and toe nailbeds and lips are blue or purple.

If the environment is warmer than body temperature vasodilatation occurs to promote blood pooling in the periphery of the body, where it is more readily cooled because it is spread thinner. With vasodilatation, the skin appears pink or red and feels warm to the touch. The anterior hypothalamus appears to control temperature-reducing measures (protecting against hyperthermia); the posterior portion appears to control heat-increasing measures (protecting against hypothermia). A brain injury is serious if it causes enough edema to produce pressure on the hypothalamus. When this occurs, the body appears to be unable to regulate its temperature; it is not unusual to see a body temperature of 106° to 107°F (41.1°—41.7°C) in a patient with severe brain compression and heat regulatory loss.

A too-high body temperature, or hyperthermia (over 107°F, 41°C), is dangerous because the protein in body cells becomes inactivated, and enzyme function appears to be impaired. A low body temperature, or hypothermia (80.6°F, 27°C), is also dangerous because the cell membranes are damaged. Hypothermia can be medically induced to slow body function deliberately to allow heart surgery, in which a quiet and nonbeating heart is necessary.

NEUROLOGICAL REGULATION

Nerve innervation not only helps to stimulate body actions such as shivering and vasoconstriction but also alerts the conscious mind to the sensation of warmth or cold. This conscious awareness causes a person to take actions to warm himself (by stomping the feet, clapping the hands, rubbing the arms, or putting on a sweater) or to become cooler (by taking off an article of clothing, stepping into the shade, and so forth). People who are unconscious lose this important awareness of discomfort, so a nurse must be very aware of body temperature in such individuals. People who are handicapped in a way that makes them less mobile must be guarded also, because even though they register the sensation of heat or cold, they may be unable to move independently to do something to adjust their body temperature.

Pain from heat occurs at about 45°C (113°F) and from cold at about 17°C (62.6°F). Pain from heat is sharp and localized at the point of contact; pain from cold is duller and often radiates to surrounding areas. The radiating pain probably is caused by spasm in the constricted blood vessels. Because cold pain is a dull sensation and is poorly localized, frostbite may occur before a person is aware that his fingertips or toes are really that cold.

FEVER

Fever (pyrexia) is an elevation in body temperature over the normal limits (36°—37°C; 96.8°—98.6°F). Fever results from an elevated temperature set-point in the hypothalamus. If body temperature is slightly elevated (37.1°—38.2°C; 98.8°—100.6°F) a low-grade fever is present. A temperature over 38.2°C (100.6°F) is a high-grade fever. An elevation over 40.5°C (104.9°F) is often referred to as hyperthermia or hyperpyrexia.

Fever reflects a disease process—infection, inflammation, allergy or drug reaction, or cerebral or neurological injury causing brain edema. Different disease processes can cause different patterns of fever. Note, therefore, not only a person's body temperature but also whether it is consistently or only intermittently high. Different types of fever are summarized in Table 33-1.

A pyrogen is any agent that causes an increase in body temperature. When white blood cells (polymorphonuclear leukocytes) are damaged, an endogenous pyrogen factor is released; this factor appears to elevate the hypothalamic temperature set-point. Substances such as bacteria, bacterial toxins, and antigens injure the leukocytes and cause release of the endogenous pyrogen factor. Prostaglandins (specific substances that influence enzyme function) may influence elevation of the hypothalamic temperature set-point. With an elevated set-point, the body simply does not respond to the fact that its temperature is above normal until that new set-point is reached, so its temperature reduction mechanisms are not activated as soon.

There are three stages in fever (Table 33-2). In actual practice, fever is dealt with so promptly by the use of antipyretics and other therapeutic measures that the three stages may not be readily apparent.

In itself, fever is a helpful body response. For example, bacteria that are pathogenic to humans survive only within a narrow temperature range. If the body temperature rises above this limit, bacteria are destroyed. At one time diseases such as pneumonia (caused by invasion of *Pneumococcus* bacteria) were treated by allowing the person's temperature to rise as high as it would. If the temperature was high enough, the bacteria were destroyed, the fever then dropped abruptly, and the person was cured. Unfortunately, in some instances the fever became so high for such an extended period that cell function was destroyed, and the patient died as a result of the fever. Curing infection by such a technique was termed a *crisis*. Today, infections are treated with antibacterial drugs that cause the gradual destruction of bacteria and a corresponding gradual reduction in fever (termed *lysis*).

TABLE 33-1. TYPES OF FEVER

Type	Description
Intermittent	Temperature alternates between elevated and normal levels on a day-to-day basis.
Remittent	Temperature is always elevated, but the daily highs vary widely.
Relapsing	Febrile periods are interspaced with periods of normal temperature; the febrile periods last several consecutive days.

TABLE 33-2. STAGES OF FEVER

Stage	Description
Onset	Period of time during which the temperature level is rising; this may be abrupt or gradual.
Stadium or fastigium	Period of time during which temperature remains high (*stadium* [Greek] meaning "distance"; *fastigium* [Latin] meaning "roof").
Subsiding or decline	Period during which fever returns to normal. If the period is abrupt, it is termed *crisis*; if gradual, *lysis*.

SYMPTOMS OF FEVER

When the body temperature begins to rise above normal, a person may begin to feel cold (because there is a marked difference between the body temperature and ambient air). He rubs his arms and puts on additional clothing; his skin feels cool to the touch owing to temporary vasoconstriction. His body responds to the sensation of cold by piloerection and shivering (a shaking chill) to produce heat. This reaction generally occurs when the onset of fever is rapid, as in acute infections.

The temperature rises during this chill reaction, which lasts 10 to 30 minutes, due to the heat produced by muscle activity. Always take a person's temperature following a chill of this kind to determine its upper level even if you took it just prior to the episode because it increases so much during this active time.

In addition to feeling cold, a person with a fever may develop a headache (from vasodilatation of the cerebral blood vessels) and general malaise. He appears flushed (reddened); he may be diaphoretic (have extreme perspiration) as he loses body water; his lips and mouth may be very dry; and he may be thirsty. For each 1°C (1.8°F) rise in temperature, the pulse increases 5 to 15 beats per minute. This means that a person who has a normal pulse of 80 may have a pulse rate of 100 if his temperature is 39°C (102.2°F). In addition to being rapid, the pulse is often thready or weak. As the pulse rate increases, the respiratory rate increases with it to supply enough oxygen for the increased metabolic rate.

Some people develop delirium (confusion) if the fever is high (usually more than 39°C [102°F]) owing to irritation of cerebral cells. If the fever occurs rapidly, children under 5 years of age are prone to convulsions owing to the sudden insult to the body cells.

Care of the Person with Fever

Measures that aid the body in achieving its own physiological responses to fever are most effective. At first it would seem that immediately making the person as cold as possible would be the most helpful measure. If a person is cooled too abruptly, however, so that he begins to shiver, this will be exactly the wrong action. Interventions for fever require judgment in deciding what is the most effective action at the right moment.

PROMOTE A COOL ENVIRONMENT

If a person is having a chill and is actively shivering, promote warmth by an extra blanket or a sweater until the shivering stops; as soon as the chill passes, remove the blanket or sweater but do not allow the shivering to begin again. Placing a cool cloth on the person's forehead feels soothing, especially if headache is present, and has a cooling effect as well. Sponging the face with cool (not cold) water often feels soothing.

To reduce a temperature quickly, the patient can be placed in a tepid (just slightly cool) bath of water. Never use cold water because this is shocking to the nervous system and may cause a convulsion, especially in young children. An older method of reducing fever quickly consisted of sponging the patient with alcohol, which evaporates so quickly from the skin that it causes almost immediate cooling. Such a practice can be extremely dangerous, however, because such rapid cooling can cause convulsions from the shock, and some children may inhale so many alcohol fumes that they actually become comatose from alcohol intoxication and suffer liver damage. *Never, therefore, use alcohol to reduce a child's temperature.* The procedure for a tepid bath is discussed later in this chapter under Heat and Cold Applications.

Change the person's bedclothes and clothing as often as necessary to keep them from becoming wet and cold from diaphoresis. Wet clothing not only is uncomfortable but also interferes with evaporation from the skin surface and therefore with the body's effort at cooling. Many people develop herpes simplex type 1 virus infections (pinpoint-sized, clustered vesicles called fever blisters or cold sores) on their lips when they have a high fever. These are painful each time the person moves his lips; because they are mildly contagious the person should not exchange drinking glasses or straws while the lesions are present. Keeping the blisters covered with petroleum jelly (Vaseline) or some other soothing ointment prevents cracking and pain. Healing takes place in five to seven days.

PROMOTE FLUID INTAKE

Perspiration rapidly depletes the body's fluid, so fluid intake should be encouraged (unless accompanying vomiting from a gastrointestinal illness is present). An older term for encouraging fluid intake is *forced fluids.* Such a term is misleading if it implies that actual force should be used. If the patient has a general feeling of not being well (malaise), there may not be many fluids that appeal to him. Try to determine his preferences so that he will drink more. Remember that Jello and Popsicles count as fluid; these may be acceptable if drinking liquid does not appeal to the person. Encourage cool fluids (soft drinks, fruit juices) before hot liquids (tea, coffee), but hot liquids may be more acceptable than cold ones (hot fluids may be more soothing to a person with a sore throat) and do not make an appreciable difference in terms of cooling, whereas the amount of fluid taken in does make a difference. Use good judgment in encouraging fruit juices, especially apple juice, because these may cause diarrhea (which will lead to fluid loss). A juice such as orange juice may be irritating if the person has a herpes infection. In adults, try to encourage an intake of 2500 to 3000 ml of fluid every 24 hours. Table 33-3 shows different average fluid requirements for other age groups.

Keep a careful record of fluid intake and output to document maintenance of a positive fluid balance; test the urine for specific gravity to show that the person is well hydrated. A person who needs more fluid concentrates urine above the normal limits to conserve fluid. A normal specific gravity of urine, therefore, demonstrates that the person is receiving enough fluid to offset that lost by diaphoresis. Normal specific gravity is 1.003 to 1.030. (See Chap. 20 for a complete discussion of the specific gravity of urine.)

If the mucous membranes of the patient's mouth are dry, they can easily crack, causing extreme tenderness and inviting infection from secondary bacteria. Rinsing the mouth with mouthwash about every hour or applying a soothing ointment such as petroleum jelly (Vaseline) to dry lips helps prevent this complication.

REDUCE ACTIVITY

A person with an elevated temperature should have rest. Because muscle activity increases heat production, activities such as running increase body temperature. In many instances it is necessary to reduce anxiety in order to reduce activity. A person lying in bed who is anxious and constantly moving will have an elevated temperature that will stay elevated longer than a person who is truly resting. This is particularly true of children. A child at home who is constantly calling for a parent from a bedroom may actually rest better on the living room couch or on a sleeping bag in the kitchen, where he does not have to seek out so many activities to entertain himself.

ADMINISTER ANTIPYRETICS

An antipyretic is a medication that reduces temperature. Acetylsalicylic acid (aspirin) is the antipyretic

TABLE 33-3. FLUID REQUIREMENTS PER AGE GROUP

Age	Average body weight (kg)	Fluid requirement per kg/24 hours (ml)	Fluid requirement per 24 hours (ml)
Newborn	3.0	80—100	250—300
3 months	5.4	140—160	750—850
6 months	7.3	130—155	950—1100
9 months	8.6	125—145	1100—1250
1 year	9.5	120—135	1150—1300
2 years	11.8	115—125	1350—1500
4 years	16.2	100—110	1600—1800
6 years	20.0	90—100	1800—2000
10 years	28.7	70—85	2000—2500
14 years	45.0	50—60	2200—2700
18 years and adult	54.0	40—50	2200—2700

Source: From V. C. Vaughan and R. J. McKay, *Nelson's Textbook of Pediatrics* (11th ed.). Philadelphia: Saunders, 1979.

that most people use first to reduce fever; it apparently works by interfering with prostaglandin synthesis (prostaglandin action increases body temperature). The action of acetaminophen (Tylenol), another commonly used antipyretic, is less well understood but acts to reduce the body temperature set-point. Acetaminophen causes less stomach irritation than aspirin if accompanying gastrointestinal symptoms are present. Physicians' orders for antipyretics as a rule specify not only drug, dose, and frequency but also the exact degree of temperature that should be reached before it is administered. If a physician writes an order such as, "Administer 10 grains aspirin for fever," ask for clarification. You need to be certain that you and she have the same concept of fever. If the patient is a child, ask if a rectal, axillary, or oral temperature reading is meant. A rectal temperature may be one degree higher than an oral one; an axillary temperature may be one degree lower than an oral one. If the order states, "Administer aspirin when fever reaches 101°F," referring to an oral temperature reading, you would administer the drug with a rectal reading of only 100°F. An axillary temperature reading would have to be 102°F to administer the medication.

Never "just" administer an antipyretic. Be certain that other measures such as the removal of blankets or flannel pajamas and an increase in fluid intake are undertaken at the same time so that the full effect of the medication can be realized. Acetysalicylic acid and acetaminophen are compared in Quick Reference Stop 33-1.

ADMINISTER MEASURES TO RELIEVE THE UNDERLYING DISEASE PROCESS

Fever is a symptom of a disease process, not a disease process itself. In most instances the patient's physician will order measures to be instituted to combat the underlying disease process (cure the infection, reduce the inflammation, and so on). Be conscientious in carrying out whatever actions are prescribed, because without control of the underlying disease process, the fever will return when the effect of the antipyretic has worn off. Remember, fever is only a symptom of disease.

The exception to this rule is a fever of unknown origin (FUO). The person appears to have no symptoms but fever; unless the fever is excessively high, the physician may ask that no medication be given to reduce the fever and for close observation for any symptoms or signs that will be a clue to the underlying disease process. Often FUOs are caused by mild urinary tract infections that produce urinary symptoms (pain and frequency of urination) within 48 hours. Parents need support to appreciate that a mild fever is not harmful to their child for a limited amount of time (again, the fever is not the illness).

HEAT STROKE

Heat stroke occurs in individuals who have been exposed to extreme heat for a prolonged period. It usually results from outdoor summertime activities but can occur in some workers, such as those who work in steel mills near open-hearth furnaces.

Owing to the excessive heat in the environment, the person's internal temperature rises well above normal. Apparently because of the excessive heat, however, the body's thermoregulatory mechanisms fail; sweating to cool the body does not occur. The person feels weak; delirium or coma develops, and the blood pressure falls too low to support body functions. If cooling cannot be effected, heat stroke is fatal due to ineffective circulation (such extensive vasodilatation occurs that the cen-

☐ QUICK REFERENCE STOP 33-1: PHARMACOLOGY
Commonly Used Antipyretics*

Drug	*Precautions*
Acetaminophen (Datril, Tylenol, Tempra)	Children's preparations are pleasantly flavored and therefore need to be stored carefully out of their reach to prevent poisoning. The drug is also an analgesic; be cautious when applying cold or heat because these sensations are decreased. Hepatic (liver) damage can occur with prolonged use or toxic dose.
Acetylsalicylic acid (aspirin)	Children's preparations are pleasantly flavored and need to be stored carefully out of their reach to prevent poisoning. The drug is also an anti-inflammatory and an analgesic. It inhibits prothrombin formation and thus may interfere with blood coagulation. It may cause gastrointestinal irritation with prolonged use. Not recommended for use if child has symptoms of flu or chickenpox. Reye's syndrome or encephalitis (inflammation of brain cells) may occur under these circumstances.

*An antipyretic is a drug that lowers body temperature.

tral core does not have adequate blood to oxygenate the vital organs).

Heat stroke tends to occur more frequently when humidity is high than when it is low; it occurs more frequently in people who are in poor physical condition than in those who exercise regularly in heat (e.g., the first day of football practice rather than during the football season). People who are taking atropine (a vasodilator) are more susceptible than others.

Therapy for heat stroke is aimed at reducing body temperature rapidly by sponging the body with cool water and supporting blood pressure by a measure such as intravenous fluid until the person can again utilize his thermoregulatory mechanism to adjust body temperature.

Heat Prostration or Heat Exhaustion

Heat prostration is a second condition that results from exercising in heat. It is not so much an effect of the heat, however, as it is a failure of the circulatory system due to the extreme exercise and diaphoresis without enough fluid replacement. A person with heat prostration is dyspneic (has difficulty in breathing), his skin feels cool, and he appears pale. He may be confused and have muscle cramps (due to sodium depletion in sweat). His body temperature is not greatly elevated. A person with heat prostration needs to be immediately placed in a supine position to provide blood flow to the cerebral vessels, and he needs medical support for his failing circulation such as intravenous fluid replacement. Taking a sufficient supply of sodium (salt tablets) on very warm days is advised for people who are prone to heat prostration (sodium holds body fluid and prevents excessive fluid loss).

Hyperthermia with Anesthesia

One of the dangers of a general anesthetic is that during administration, the thermoregulatory mechanisms of the hypothalamus are suppressed. Rarely, the body temperature may begin to rise unchecked, and extreme tachycardia (increased heart rate), possibly leading to a fatal cardiac arrhythmia, may occur. If the condition is not recognized, the temperature will rise so high that irreversible cell injury, particularly to brain cells, may occur during surgery.

Halting the administration of anesthesia alone will not reverse the condition. If the temperature can be brought down to normal, however (by cooling with a hypothermia blanket, for example), it does not tend to recur. The patient must be informed that a second administration of general anesthesia might carry the same risk so that he can make judgments about elective surgery from an informed standpoint.

HYPOTHERMIA

Hypothermia is a body temperature below normal. Most episodes of hypothermia occur because of accidental exposure to sustained cold; it can be medically induced as an adjunct to surgery or to halt bleeding.

Accidental Hypothermia

Accidental hypothermia occurs in such people as skiers or mountain climbers who do not protect themselves well enough before exposure to a cold environment, older adults who have decreased ability to sense cold, and chronic alcoholics as alcohol dilates the blood vessels, initiating excessive conductive heat loss.

Hypothermia in children should always be viewed as child neglect or abuse unless a reasonable circumstance for the cold exposure can be documented.

With hypothermia cell function in all body cells declines. This is reflected in a decreased respiratory rate and decreased cardiac rate. As the cardiac rate decreases, the pulse becomes slow and weak, and the blood pressure falls (blood pressure depends on a normal heart rate). The person's ability to think declines as cerebral cell function is affected; insulin production and other body processes such as kidney function fail. At a low temperature of 82.4°F (28°C) respirations cease. At 75.2°F (24°C) reflexes disappear, and ventricular fibrillation and cardiac arrest occur.

People with hypothermia must be warmed gradually or vasodilatation from the warming effect will draw so much blood away from the central circulation that cardiac failure will result. Gradual warming is generally achieved by covering the person with warm blankets or a hyperthermia blanket.

Frostbite

Frostbite results from extreme or prolonged cold exposure that is so intense that the toes, nose, or fingers are deprived of oxygen and nutrients owing to vasoconstriction; vasoconstriction, which keeps the blood in the body's central core, causes cells to die. A frostbitten area appears white and feels numb. To warm frostbitten extremities, cover the area with soft towels or blankets or submerge it in pleasantly warm water (100°F, 43.3°C) for about 20 minutes. Do not rub frostbitten areas to help bring back circulation. Rubbing may be harmful to cells already damaged by lack of oxygen. As feeling returns in frostbitten extremities, there is acute pain, and the person will need an analgesic to be comfortable. If there is extensive cell damage, a portion of the extremity may have to be amputated to prevent extensive infection from invading the area of necrosing cells.

Induced Hypothermia

Local hypothermic measures (such as an ice pack) may be used to reduce swelling following injury to the muscles or cartilage; ice water is used to reduce the pain of burns, and an ice saline lavage (saline injected and removed) from the stomach is used to halt stomach bleeding by causing local vessel vasoconstriction. General hypothermia reduces a person's metabolic rate and cell need for oxygen so dramatically during heart surgery that during surgery the heart can actually be stopped and repaired.

General hypothermia must be induced only under very strict conditions. The person is either immersed in a cool bath or wrapped in a hypothermia blanket. To prevent shivering as the process begins chlorpromazine (Thorazine) is often administered for both its antishivering and its sedative effects. Temperature and cardiac function must be constantly monitored, and equipment and personnel must be available to reverse the effects on the circulatory system. If hypothermia is being initiated for surgery, it is begun after the patient is anesthetized for comfort and because the reduction in body activity aids in cooling.

TEMPERATURE-TAKING

Temperature is a vital body sign because abnormal temperature reflects a disease process (it is never normal) and, if present for any length of time, can lead to fluid and electrolyte imbalance, which is always a serious health complication. Because temperature-taking is a common process (mothers appear to take temperatures with no difficulty), it is easy to discount the importance of the measure or the judgment needed to assess it accurately (mothers take temperatures easily at home because they have had good instructions; it requires a different level of responsibility to be the person giving the instructions).

Thermometers

Two types of thermometers are popularly used to record body temperature. The first is a mercury-in-glass type; the second is an electronic type.

GLASS THERMOMETERS

A mercury-in-glass thermometer (Fig. 33-2) is exactly that—a cylinder of mercury encased in a glass tube. When mercury is heated, it expands. The higher a person's temperature, the higher the column of mercury will rise in the glass tube as it expands. The advantage of mercury-in-glass thermometers is that they are economical. The disadvantages are that they can break, releasing mercury, which is a poison, and sharp glass edges that can cut; they register slowly and must be disinfected between patients or discarded after use.

These thermometers are shaped differently for oral and rectal use and are easily distinguishable by their shape. An oral thermometer has a long thin bulb (Fig. 33-3). This thin tip reaches well under the tongue, where it should be placed. A rectal tip is short and thick, allowing it to be inserted into the rectum without danger of breakage. Some health care agencies buy only the thick-tipped type of thermometer and then mark them for oral or rectal use by painting the tips blue for oral use and red for rectal use. The method of obtaining oral and rectal temperatures using a glass thermometer is shown in Procedures 33-1 and 33-2.

ELECTRONIC THERMOMETERS

Electronic thermometers are based on the principle that heat alters the voltage, or resistance, to a conduc-

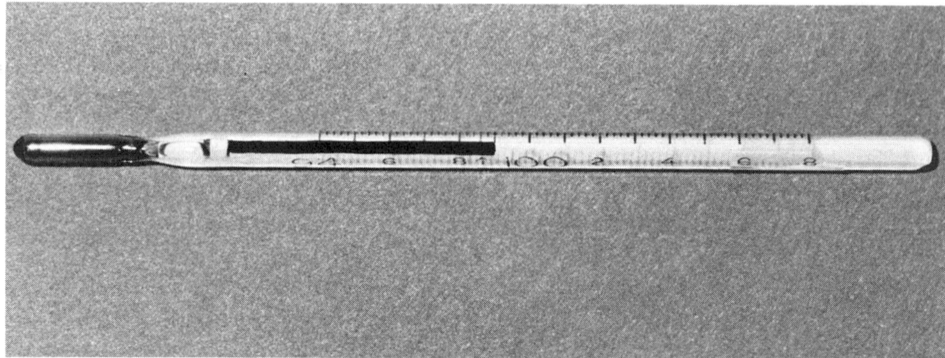

FIGURE 33-2. A glass-mercury thermometer. Temperature is read at the highest point to which the dark column of mercury rises in the center core.

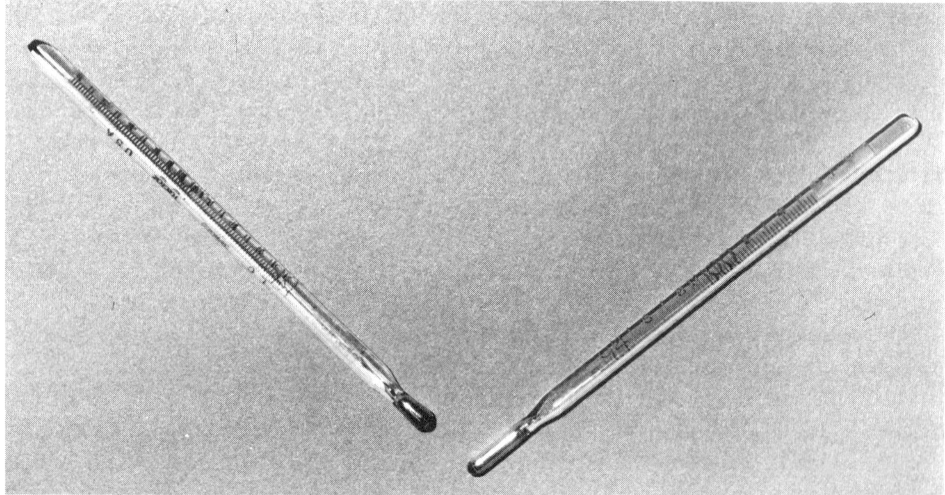

FIGURE 33-3. Comparison of rectal (left) and oral (right) thermometers.

PROCEDURE 33-1
Obtaining a Measurement of Oral Temperature Using a Glass Thermometer

Purpose: To assess the balance of body heat loss and production by means of a convenient indirect method.

Procedure	*Principle*
1. Wash your hands, identify the patient, explain the procedure.	1. Prevent the spread of microorganisms; ensure patient safety and cooperation.
2. Assess patient's condition. Analyze whether the patient's condition is correct for oral temperature-taking. Plan modifications as necessary.	2. Patients who are unconscious, cannot hold their mouths closed, breathe through their mouths, or are too immature (under 5 years of age) should not have a temperature taken orally. If the person has just taken a drink of ice water, wait at least 5 minutes.
3. Implement procedure by assembling equipment: clean glass oral thermometer, clean paper tissue, notepad and pencil to use to record reading.	

4. Hold the thermometer at eye level. Rotate it until the height of the column of mercury is discernible. Assess the highest calibrated number touched by the level of mercury in the thermometer.

4. The mercury should be below 96°F (35.5°C) to register accurately.

5. If the mercury column is not below 96°F (35.5°C), shake the thermometer with a quick downward flip to cause the mercury column to descend below 96°F.

6. Ask the patient to open his mouth; place the thermometer slightly to one side of the mouth under the tongue. Ask the person to close his lips to hold the thermometer securely in place and prevent air flow over it.

6. The thermometer tip must be in close contact with the sublingual blood vessels to record a body temperature not a mouth or peripheral temperature.

7. Leave the thermometer in place for 8 minutes.

7. This time interval is necessary to ensure a sufficient rise of the mercury column. Do not leave the person unattended during this time or he may fall asleep or become distracted and allow the thermometer to fall from his mouth or away from the sublingual blood vessels.

8. Remove the thermometer and wipe it with a tissue from your fingertips to the thermometer tip to remove oral secretions.

8. Oral secretions may obscure your view of the calibrations; wiping the thermometer from fingertips to thermometer tip prevents spread of microorganisms from the oral cavity to your fingertips.

9. Observe the new level of mercury in the thermometer.

9. Oral temperature is normally 98.6°F (37°C). If the column of mercury is below 97°F (36.1°C), the thermometer probably did not register.

10. Record the temperature obtained immediately. Shake the thermometer down below 96°F (35.5°C); return thermometer to proper place for disinfection. If you need to wash off a thermometer to remove excessive oral secretions, use room temperature water; hot water will cause the mercury to rise so high in the column it will break the thermometer.

10. This is an easy assessment number to forget. Having to repeat a temperature recording because you forgot the number causes a patient unnecessary inconvenience. Thermometers should be used once and disinfected before a second use to prevent spread of microorganisms.

11. Evaluate the effectiveness, efficiency, cost, comfort, and safety aspects of the procedure. Plan health teaching as necessary, such as what a normal temperature is and how to record one accurately.

11. Health teaching is an independent nursing action that is always included as a part of care.

MODIFICATIONS FOR CARE OF CHILD

Children under age 5 are, as a group, not responsible enough for oral temperature-taking. Be sure to stay with school-age children during temperature-taking because they are unaware of the danger of mercury (which is poisonous) should a thermometer break. Children sometimes ask if they can have the mercury from a broken thermometer to play with (it molds into balls and then repells itself in interesting patterns). Do not allow this; mercury can be absorbed through the skin in sufficient amounts to cause permanent extensive brain and neurological damage.

MODIFICATIONS FOR CARE OF OLDER ADULT

Many older adults develop a habit of "cat napping" during the day or fall very quickly asleep when they are comfortably sitting in a chair or lying in bed. Be certain to stay with the older adult during oral temperature-taking because cat napping will not allow the person to keep the thermometer firmly sealed in his mouth.

PROCEDURE 33-2
Obtaining a Rectal Temperature Using a Glass Thermometer

Purpose: To assess the balance between heat loss and heat production by measuring body temperature using a safe though intrusive procedure.

Procedure	*Principle*
1. Wash your hands; identify the patient; explain the procedure.	1. Prevent the spread of microorganisms; ensure patient safety and cooperation.
2. Assess patient condition. Analyze appropriateness of procedure. Plan necessary modifications.	2. Rectal temperature-taking is contraindicated in people who have had rectal surgery or rectal obstruction; it should be kept to a minimum in preschoolers because it is intrusive.
3. Implement procedure by assembling equipment: rectal glass thermometer, a lubricant of choice, a clean paper tissue, notepad and pencil for recording temperature obtained.	3. Rectal glass thermometers have rounded short bulbs in contrast to the long slender tips of oral thermometers. Never use an oral thermometer to take a rectal temperature. The longer bulb could break, causing laceration and deposition of mercury in the rectum.
4. Hold the thermometer at eye level. Rotate it until the height of the column of mercury is visible. Assess whether the level of the mercury is below 96°F (35.5°C). If not, shake the thermometer with a quick downward flip of your wrist to cause the mercury column to descend below 96°F.	4. The mercury should be below 96°F (35.5°C) to register accurately.
5. Lubricate the tip of the thermometer with mineral oil, water-soluble jelly, or clear tap water.	5. A lubricant is helpful in allowing the thermometer to pass freely through the anal sphincter. Never use hot water because the mercury will expand so much the glass will break.
6. Place adult patient in Sims's position. Drape appropriately to preserve modesty.	6. This position allows a clear view of the rectal area. Never attempt to place a rectal thermometer without good visibility of the anal area to avoid injury to rectal mucosa or, in women, insertion into the vagina by error.
7. With your left hand, raise the person's upper buttock slightly to fully expose the anal area; insert the thermometer about 1-1/2 to 2 inches. If the anal sphincter is very tense, ask the patient to take a deep breath. This distracting maneuver causes the sphincter to relax. Slant the thermometer toward the umbilicus because this is the slant of rectum.	7. The thermometer must be inserted far enough to rest against the mucosal wall so that body temperature, not anal or skin temperature, is recorded. Inserting the thermometer too far may cause rupture of the mucosa. Use a gentle touch with a patient who has hemorrhoidal tissue because this is very painful.
8. Leave the thermometer in place for 2 to 4 minutes, holding it securely in place with your hand.	8. Never leave a rectal thermometer in place without remaining with the patient; he might turn and break the thermometer. This time interval is necessary for the mercury column to expand to its greatest potential.
9. Remove the thermometer, wipe it with the tissue from your fingertips to the thermometer bulb to remove any feces present.	9. Feces will obscure your view of the height of the mercury column. Wiping from fingertips to bulb prevents spread of microorganisms to your fingertips.

10. Assess the height of the column of mercury; wipe away any lubricant left at the anus, and position the patient comfortably.

10. A normal rectal temperature is 99.6°F (37.6°C). If the thermometer remains at 96°F, repeat the procedure because for some reason the thermometer did not register. This can happen if there is a great deal of feces in the rectum and the thermometer entered the center of a fecal mass and so was not positioned against the mucosal wall.

11. Wash your hands. Record the reading immediately. Mark the recording as a rectal temperature.

11. Prevent spread of microorganisms. Document patient status and nursing care. A rectal temperature is one degree higher than an oral temperature.

12. Dispose of tissue; return thermometer to proper place for disinfection. Evaluate effectiveness, efficiency, cost, comfort, and safety of procedure. Plan health teaching as necessary, such as temperature-taking technique for self-care.

12. Thermometers should be disinfected after use to prevent spread of microorganisms. Health teaching is an independent nursing measure that is always included in nursing care.

MODIFICATIONS FOR CARE OF CHILD

In infants a thermometer is inserted only the length of the bulb and in children only an inch to avoid possible perforation of the rectal mucosa. Appreciate that this is an intrusive procedure and is disliked very much by the preschool-age child.

MODIFICATIONS FOR CARE OF OLDER ADULT

The average older adult has some formation of hemorrhoidal tissue (distended rectal veins). Use very gentle technique to avoid injury or pain as you insert a thermometer past this distended tissue.

tor of electric current. Such a thermometer system requires an initial high cost but has the advantage of registering quickly (under 30 seconds compared to 3 to 7 minutes for an oral temperature and 10 minutes for an axillary temperature with a glass thermometer); and furthermore, they do not contain mercury or glass, so these dangers are eliminated. Disposable covers are used to eliminate disinfection costs and time. Electronic thermometers have two probes, one coded red for rectal use and one coded blue for oral use. Because the probe is always covered by a plastic cover before use, however, these can be used interchangeably without worry of contamination from patient to patient (see Procedure 33-3, Fig. 1).

Electronic thermometers include a base unit, which contains rechargeable batteries, a probe, which is the sensor unit, and individual disposable probe covers to keep the thermic probe clean from one use to the next (see procedure 33-3, Fig. 2). To use such a thermometer, remove the probe from the power base and insert it into a disposable cover. Place the covered probe either orally, rectally, or in an axillary position following glass thermometer temperature-taking technique. Electronic thermometers begin to register immediately, and a read-out window on the base unit will show the temperature being recorded by flashing. Most units have a light or tone that indicates that the final temperature has been reached. Remember to read the temperature and record it before you eject the probe cover and return it to the unit. Returning the probe to the central base unit turns off the unit and causes the read-out window to register zero again.

If an electronic thermometer fails to register, the chances are high that uncharged batteries and not the patient's body temperature is at fault. Always return electronic thermometers to their designated storage place and know whether or not they should remain plugged into the wall unit when not in use. Procedure 33-3 shows how to obtain an oral temperature using an electronic thermometer.

CALIBRATION OF THERMOMETERS

Thermometers are calibrated according to a Fahrenheit or Celsius (centigrade) scale. On a glass thermometer, the scale is etched into the glass; with an electronic thermometer, the computerized number is read on the thermometer base. Comparison of Fahrenheit and Celsius scales is shown in Appendix F. The mathematical formula for converting Celsius to Fahrenheit and vice versa, is shown in Quick Reference Stop 33-2.

☐ PROCEDURE 33-3
Obtaining an Oral Temperature Using an Electric Thermometer

Purpose: To assess the balance between body heat loss and production by means of a convenient and rapid indirect procedure.

Procedure	*Principle*
1. Wash your hands, identify the patient, explain the procedure.	1. Prevent spread of microorganisms; ensure patient safety and cooperation.
2. Assess patient's condition; analyze appropriateness of procedure; plan modifications as necessary.	2. Never take an oral temperature in a person who is unable to cooperate. People who are unconscious, not mentally alert, are unable to hold their lips closed, or are under 3 years of age should not have their temperature taken by this method. Electronic thermometers can be used with younger children than glass thermometers because there is no danger of glass breakage.
3. Implement procedure by assembling equipment: designated oral electronic thermometer, sheath to cover thermometer probe, clean paper tissue, notepad and pencil to record reading obtained (Fig. 1).	3. Electronic thermometer probes must be covered by a disposable plastic sheath prior to use, not only to prevent spread of microorganisms but to activate sensation of temperature properly.

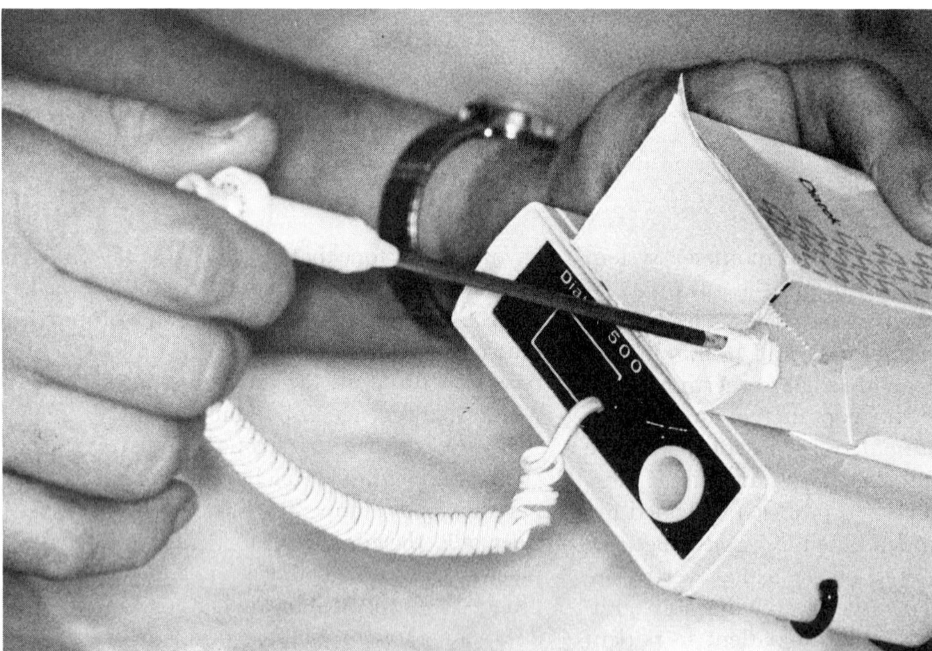

FIGURE 1. Electronic thermometers are covered with disposable shealths to keep them clean between patient encounters.

4. Remove the thermometer probe from its stored site in the thermometer base; this automatically turns on unit. A digital display of 94°F (34°C) appears on the read-out screen.	4. If base unit does not activate, it may be that the batteries need to be recharged before the unit can be used.

5. Insert the thermometer probe into a probe sheath. Ask the patient to open his mouth; insert the probe with sheath in place under the patient's tongue (Fig. 2).

5. An individual sheath for each patient prevents spread of microorganisms; tip of probe must be placed close to the major blood vessels so that the temperature recorded reflects the internal body temperature, not the mouth or peripheral temperature.

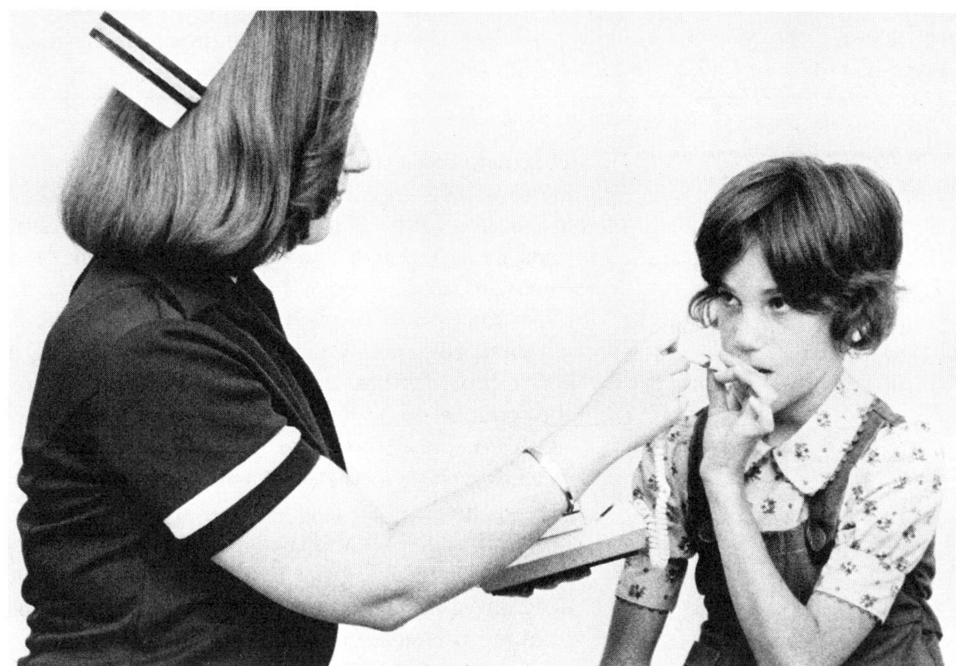

FIGURE 2. Recording an oral temperature with an electronic thermometer.

6. Hold the thermometer in place or allow the patient to do this (with his lips closed); observe the read-out screen as it records the body temperature. Depending on the model, a light will flash or the numbers change in some manner to indicate that the final number has been reached.

6. Electronic thermometers record in about 45 seconds.

7. Remove the probe and sheath; discard the sheath by ejecting it from the probe into a waste container.

7. Discarding the sheath immediately prevents it from being confused with a clean one. Do not be careless about disposing of sheaths; the average person has streptococcal bacteria in his mouth. Sheaths must be placed in waste containers, not on the bedside stand or other similar place.

8. Record the read-out number obtained; return the probe to the unit base. This action resets the read-out screen to 94°F (34°C) and turns off power in the unit.

8. Make a point of recording the read-out before you cause it to disappear. Be certain the unit does turn off to preserve battery life.

9. Evaluate effectiveness, efficiency, cost, comfort, and safety of procedure. Plan health teaching as necessary, such as what a normal temperature is and how to record one accurately. Return the thermometer base to its rechargeable storage space.

9. Health teaching is an independent nursing function that is always included as a part of care. Being conscientious about keeping the base unit charged makes the equipment available for emergencies when there is no time for recharging prior to use.

MODIFICATIONS FOR CARE OF CHILD

Because electronic thermometers are not breakable if they are bitten, they can be used with children as young as about 3 years old. Under this age, children do not understand the importance of keeping their mouths closed, so oral temperature-taking, even if safe, is not accurate.

MODIFICATIONS FOR CARE OF OLDER ADULT

Oral cancer, if present, tends to occur under the tongue. Always observe the mucous membrane under the tongue when you place an oral thermometer for an area of ulceration or discoloration, especially in people who smoke cigars or pipes (conditions of high risk for oral cancer).

☐ QUICK REFERENCE STOP 33-2: HEALTH TEACHING
Celsius and Fahrenheit Measurements

Temperature may be recorded either on a Fahrenheit scale, on which 32° marks the freezing point of water, 212° marks the boiling point of water, and a typical oral body temperature is 98.6°, or on a Celsius or centigrade scale, on which 0 and 100° are the freezing and boiling points of water and 37° is the oral body temperature.

A detailed comparison of Fahrenheit and Celsius scales is shown in Appendix F. To convert from a Fahrenheit to a Celsius measurement, subtract 32 and multiply by 5/9. To convert from Celsius to Fahrenheit, multiply by 9/5 and add 32.

Sites for Temperature-Taking

Three body sites for temperature-taking are commonly used—oral, rectal, and axillary. Skin temperature may be used when continuous monitoring is desirable, such as with small infants in Isolettes (incubators) when opening and closing the Isolette to repeat temperature readings would lower the oxygen or temperature level in the Isolette.

ORAL TEMPERATURE

To take an oral temperature, the tip of the thermometer must be placed under the tongue so that it rests against the major blood vessels there; ask the person to close his mouth to keep the thermometer in place and prevent air currents from being drawn across it. It is important that the thermometer tip (the point where both glass and electronic thermometers record the temperature) is in close contact with blood vessels so that the temperature assessed reflects that of the bloodstream (the internal body temperature) rather than the temperature of the mouth (which has a peripheral, or lower, temperature).

Never take an oral temperature of anyone who is not fully awake and alert and cooperative. This is extremely important when using a glass thermometer to prevent accidental breakage and to ensure that the temperature assessed is truly the bloodstream temperature. This means that oral temperatures should not be taken in people who are comatose or in any way confused and in children under 5 years of age. Other contraindications include people who cannot close their mouths (owing to jaw surgery or injury), mouth breathers (almost any person in respiratory distress), patients in whom nasal oxygen is being administered (cooled oxygen and mouth breathing in combination may lower the oral temperature readings), and people with localized mouth infection (the temperature may be elevated owing to the local heat produced). An oral temperature should not be taken immediately after a person drinks ice water (wait 5 minutes); the effect of smoking or drinking hot beverages may also make a difference, so it is usually recommended to wait 5 minutes after these activities as well.

The average oral temperature is 98.6°F (37°C). The range of normal is 97.6° to 99.4°F (36.5°—37.5°C). The time needed for a thermometer to record an oral temperature varies according to different research studies; 8 to 10 minutes for a glass thermometer is an accepted time interval. After the full time interval has passed, remove the thermometer, wipe the cylinder with a paper tissue to remove oral secretions that might obscure the calibrations on the glass, and read it immediately. Record the number immediately; it is easy to forget as you proceed to perform other aspects of care.

RECTAL TEMPERATURE

A rectal thermometer is inserted into the rectum about 2 to 3 inches in adults, 1 inch in children, and only the length of the glass bulb in infants. With electronic thermometers comparable lengths apply. The thermometer should rest against the side of the rectal mucosa and should not be embedded in a fecal mass. You must use a short-tipped glass thermometer, never a long-tipped one to avoid breakage of the tip (Fig. 33-4).

Rectal thermometers should be lubricated with water or a water-based jelly for easiest insertion; they must be held in place constantly. Rectal temperature-taking is contraindicated in patients who have had rectal surgery or injury or have rectal pathology (such as obstructive hemorrhoids), in newborns (the danger of mucosal perforation is great), and in patients who

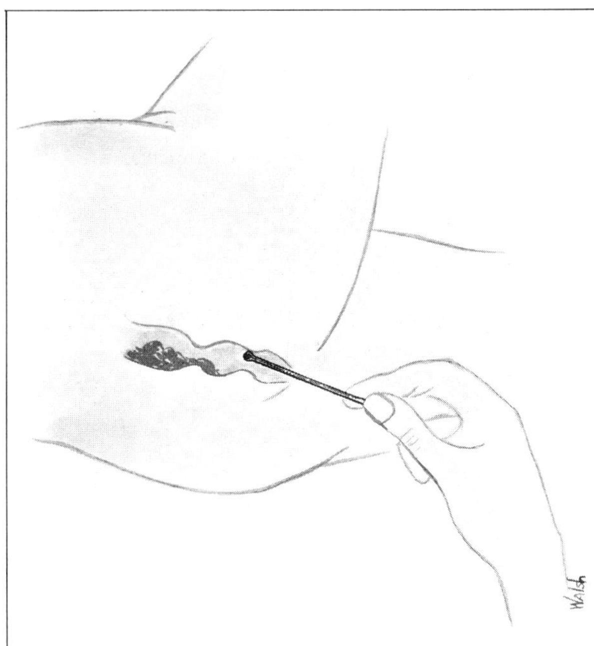

FIGURE 33-4. A rectal thermometer in place.

have had heart attacks (anal stimulation may cause bradycardia) or whose heart rates have been increased due to vagal stimulation. Intrusive procedures are very frightening to the preschool child and so should be kept to a minimum.

A normal rectal temperature is 99.6°F (37.6°C). The range is 98.6° to 100.4°F (37.0°—38°C). The time interval needed for a glass thermometer to register for a rectal temperature is also controversial but for an accurate reading it should remain in place about 2 to 4 minutes. After this time interval, remove the thermometer gently, wipe any fecal material away with a paper tissue, and read the height of the mercury immediately. Record the reading immediately with an R before it to indicate that it is a rectal reading. See Quick Reference Stops 33-3 and 33-4 for more information about oral and rectal temperature-taking. Quick Reference Stop 33-5 presents some of the research done by nurses on the accuracy and safety of rectal and oral routes.

AXILLARY TEMPERATURE

An axillary route of temperature measurement is helpful in people who cannot have an oral temperature recorded and are difficult to position for a rectal route or who are too young for an oral recording and have a contraindication for a rectal route. The normal axillary temperature is 97.6°F (36.4°C). The normal range is 96.6° to 98.4°F (36.0°—37.0°C). Always use a short-tipped thermometer to prevent breaking of the long thin bulb of a glass thermometer. Place the bulb of the thermometer well within the axilla, hold it in place by pressing the person's arm next to his side (Fig. 33-5). A glass thermometer should remain in place for about 10 minutes to register accurately. When recording the reading place an A in front of the number recorded to indicate that it is an axillary reading (about one degree lower than an oral reading).

☐ QUICK REFERENCE STOP 33-3: SAFETY
Temperature-Taking

1. Never use oral temperature-taking with people who are not fully conscious, mentally alert, and over age 5.
2. Never use rectal temperature-taking with people who have undergone rectal surgery or rectal obstruction.

☐ QUICK REFERENCE STOP 33-4: COMMUNITY CONSIDERATIONS
Self-Care and Temperature-Taking

Everyone should know how to take an oral temperature so he can care for himself. Every mother (or child's primary caregiver) needs to know how to take a rectal temperature so she can care for the child. A person who is able to tell his physician hat he has a temperature of 102°F will automatically receive more of his physician's attention than if he is able to say only that he feels warm and feverish. Help people to be better health care consumers by teaching them better methods of self-care.

CHEMICAL THERMOMETERS

A newer type of temperature-recording device now in use is a chemical thermometer strip (Fig. 33-6). These strips may be used either as oral thermometers or placed against the forehead, depending on the brand. These devices register quickly (about 45 seconds) and are therefore helpful with people who cannot keep an oral thermometer in place for 10 minutes. They are nonintrusive and can be used with small children. They are disposable after use and so do not need cleaning. Because their accuracy is still not well documented, many health care agencies have still not adopted them as their major temperature-taking system.

Continuous Temperature Monitoring

Patients with cerebral edema that is interfering with the temperature-regulating center, those who are immature, and those whose temperature regulation might not yet be functioning effectively or who have hypothermic or hyperthermic blankets in place may need continuous temperature monitoring. For this, a rectal thermic probe is inserted or thermic leads are taped in place on a central body location such as the

☐ **QUICK REFERENCE STOP 33-5: RESEARCH**
Temperature-Taking

Most nurses have been taught and continue to believe that rectal temperatures are the most accurate. Yet the rectal route is the least safe and the most inconvenient. It continues to remain the most preferred route, however. Is it *really* the best choice? Nurse and other health professional researchers have begun to question and investigate the various temperature-taking techniques (rectal, oral, axillary) for aspects of safety, accuracy, and convenience. Although research in this area still shows conflicting findings, the sample of research studies presented below gives nurses something to think about.

Is rectal most accurate?
In a small experimental study by Eoff and Joyce (1981), hospitalized toddlers and preschoolers were studied to determine whether a significant difference existed between readings obtained by the rectal and axillary routes. The authors knew the axillary route to be the safest and least disturbing to children of this age. They found no difference between the two routes. The authors strongly recommend axillary temperatures over rectal temperatures for this age group because both routes appear to be equally accurate.

How dangerous is rectal?
A survey by Lau and Ong (1981) demonstrated the dangers inherent in taking rectal temperatures. During a 10-year period, 16 infants and young children required hospitalization for injuries due to broken or retained rectal thermometers. Among those surveyed, neither rectal perforation nor peritonitis, the major complications associated with rectal thermometer insertion, occurred. With such complications mortality is reported as high as 70 percent. Readers are urged to provide careful parental instruction in taking rectal temperatures and to make sure that rectal thermometers are well lubricated. The authors believe that the axillary route is safer, although perhaps slightly less accurate.

Plastic-sheathed oral thermometers—Accurate?
To discourage transmission of bacteria from patient to patient when glass oral thermometers are used, disposable plastic sheaths have been introduced. Is the temperature reading still accurate with the use of the sheath on the thermometer? Findings of a large empirical study by Graves and Markarian (1979) revealed that plastic-sheathed thermometer recordings were consistent with those recorded from unsheathed thermometers.

SUGGESTED READINGS

Eoff, M. J., and Joyce, B. Temperature measurements in children. *Am. J. Nurs.* 81(5):1010, 1981.

Graves, R., and Markarian. Oral temperatures and plastic-sheathed thermometers. Presented in: For the Research Record, *Am. J. Nurs.* 79(3):465, 1979.

Lau, J., and Ong, G. Broken and retained rectal thermometers in infants and small children. *Aust. Paedriatr. J.* 17(2):93, 1981. Cited in: What happens when a rectal thermometer breaks in situ? *Nurses Drug Alert* 6(4):31, 1982.

abdomen. The coupling from the probe or lead is attached to a control system that registers the body temperature. Infants in special incubators (Servo-Control Isolettes) may be monitored by leads attached to the abdomen. When the thermostatic regulatory sensor of the Isolette registers a body temperature that is lower than normal, the control automatically switches on and begins warming the internal air of the Isolette; when the temperature probe again reflects a normal infant temperature, the heat turns off.

With people covered with hypothermia or hyperthermia blankets, the read-out on the temperature-recording device will indicate a body temperature above or below normal, and a change in the blanket controls can then be made to increase heating or cooling. When caring for people with continuous temperature probes or leads in place, always check that the probe or lead is secure after an activity such as turning the person. If the monitoring system records a subnormal temperature, always consider *first* that the lead or probe has become dislodged. Any mechanical monitor can malfunction; use common sense based on the patient's appearance as well as on the read-out on the recording device for best assessment.

Judgment and Temperature-Taking

Because thermometers must remain in place for a fairly long period of time to register accurately and are at best only mechanical devices, at times the reading may not correlate with other observed signs—for example, the person may be diaphoretic and flushed and his mucous membrane is dry and parched, yet the thermometer you have used shows a subnormal temperature. Use common sense. Secure another thermometer and retake the temperature. A person who looks as if he has a fever probably has a fever, despite what the piece of equipment you hold in your hand tells you.

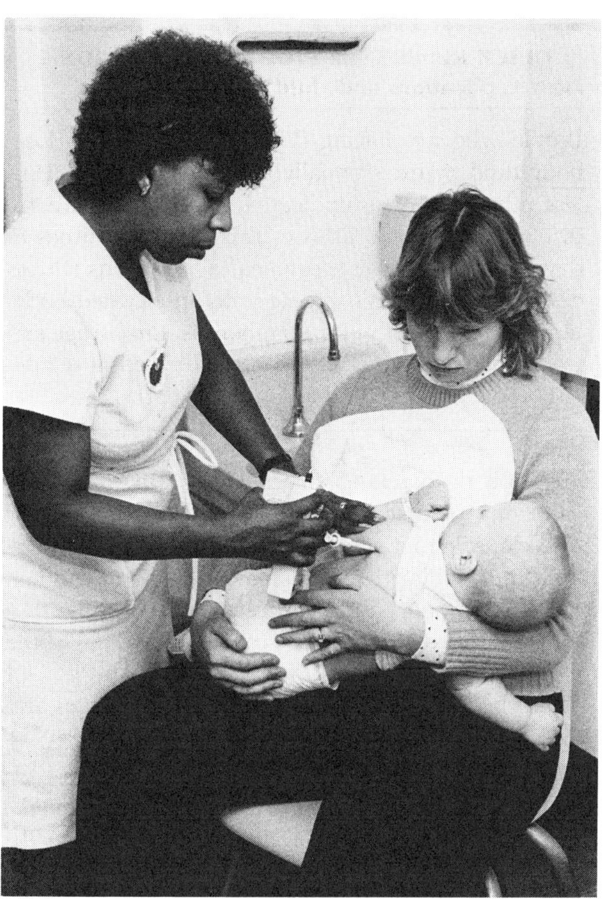

FIGURE 33-5. Recording an infant's axillary temperature. Notice how the baby's arm is held against his body to occlude air.

FIGURE 33-6. Use of a chemical strip thermometer. Such a nonintrusive method is rapid and convenient in an ambulatory department.

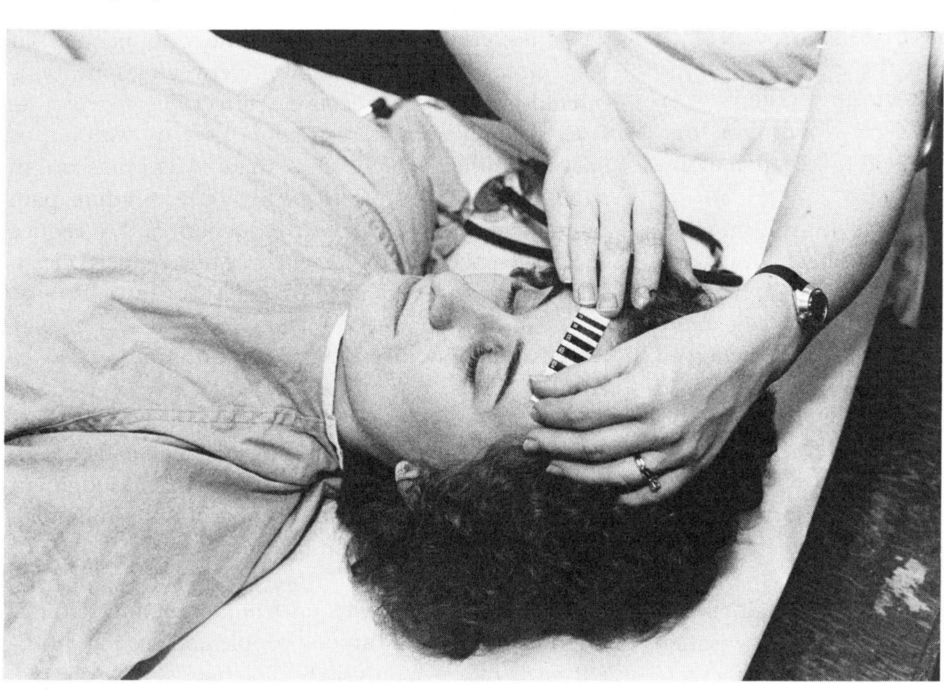

After Care of Thermometers

Following use, a glass thermometer needs to be wiped clean for the calibrations to be read clearly and for reuse after storage. Some health care agencies use a plastic slipcover for glass thermometers similar to the probe cover of an electronic thermometer; the cover is simply removed and discarded after use, eliminating the need to wipe the thermometer clean.

Thermometers should be stored dry. Standing them in a mild antiseptic solution is not advocated because unless the container and solution are both replaced every day, such a medium encourages growth of high levels of bacteria within a few hours.

HEAT AND COLD APPLICATIONS

The effects of heat and cold on the body are important not only in taking temperatures accurately but also in understanding how heat and cold applications can be used as therapeutic measures.

Sensory Receptors

The skin contains about twice as many receptors for cold as it does for heat, and, in addition, the cold receptors are located more superficially in the skin. A slight decrease in external temperature or a slight increase in external temperature will be registered as either cold or hot by these receptors; if the increase is great in either direction, the sensation is sensed not only by the hot and cold receptors but by pain receptors as well.

Sensation travels in two ways from the cutaneous receptors. An instant relay pattern by afferent (sensory) fibers carries the sensation back to the spinal cord; at the cord level, the message jumps to a motor tract, and efferent (motor) impulses cause the body part registering the sensation to contract or jerk away instantly from the source of discomfort. Sensations continue to travel up the spinal cord to the hypothalmus and then to the cerebral cortex, where the cause of the discomfort is analyzed and identified. Note that the first response is movement away from the object; the second response, which follows moments later, is, "The stove is hot and I shouldn't touch it."

As efficient as hot and cold receptors are at registering and relaying sensations, they have one drawback—they can become conditioned to a hot or cold stimulus. If you step into a bathtub of water that is at first uncomfortably hot, after a few minutes it feels comfortable. This mechanism is a defense against pain; unfortunately, it also allows people to become burned from heating pads or to develop frostbite.

Effects of Heat Application

Local heat application has a direct effect on cutaneous tissue. The most noticeable of these effects is vasodilation of the cutaneous blood arterioles by inhibition of sympathetic vasoconstricting nerves. Peripheral vasodilation due to local heat application increases blood flow through the surface capillaries, causing leukocytes to pour into the area. The pooling of the blood in capillaries causes plasma to leave the capillaries by osmosis, diffusing into the subcutaneous tissue (edema). The excess blood flow to local tissue supplies added oxygen to local cells; this increases the cells' metabolism rate (increased metabolism requires more oxygen). This fact should be remembered when applying heat to a hand or foot. Within minutes, the cells in the hand (or foot) need more oxygen than usual; if blood cannot reach them easily (for instance, if atherosclerosis or arteriosclerosis has caused narrowed blood vessels in the extremity, or if the elbow or knee is sharply bent), the cells will begin to register oxygen want and may be damaged. Heat application may actually interfere with cell function rather than aiding it.

The application of heat reaches its maximum effect in 20 to 30 minutes. After an hour of heat application capillary vasoconstriction occurs as a secondary effect. This means that after this time, heat will be more destructive than beneficial. Following application of heat, about an hour should elapse before it is applied again to avoid generating a secondary effect.

Extreme heat (hot enough to burn) causes extreme vasoconstriction. This principle needs to be remembered when working with persons with burns because the constrictive reaction may seriously interfere with circulation in the area of the burn.

Exactly why heat application relieves pain is not clearly understood. It may be that when the sensation of heat is relayed to the cerebral cortex pain receptors do not effectively relay pain sensations. Heat is helpful in relieving pain from muscle stiffness or spasm (it relaxes muscle tone and rejuvenates muscle strength), in dilating capillaries and increasing blood flow when circulation is poor, and in increasing blood flow in a blood-congested area, thereby moving blood out of the area.

Heat encourages healing by drawing leukocytes and lymph into the area and diffusing plasma with leukocytes and antibodies into subcutaneous tissue. Increased metabolism at the site may encourage wound healing; pus formation (suppuration) is increased with heat due to leukocyte invasion (see QRS 33-6).

> ☐ **QUICK REFERENCE STOP 33-6: NUTRITION**
> **Heat Applications and Fluid Loss**
>
> People who are having dry heat applications lose body fluid by exceptionally heavy perspiration. Unless otherwise contraindicated, encourage them to drink an additional glass of fluid as many times a day as they are having dry heat applications (three or four times a day). People with an elevated body temperature lose fluid by diaphoresis. Encourage extra fluid unless otherwise contraindicated at a rate of 6 to 8 glasses of fluid a day (2,000 ml).

Effects of Cold Application

The response of the body to cold application is opposite that to heat. Cold supports sympathetic vasoconstricting nerve endings, causing narrowed surface capillaries. This reduces cutaneous blood flow, reducing cell perfusion at the site and slowing metabolic function. Cold application reaches its maximum therapeutic effect in 30 to 60 minutes; after this time a secondary vasodilation will occur. As with heat application, at least an hour should be allowed between applications of cold to avoid this secondary effect.

Cold applications are used to prevent swelling or edema (with less blood flow there is less pressure in capillaries and less plasma diffusion), to reduce pain by reducing nerve impulse conduction, and to reduce the oxygen needs of tissue when there is reduced circulation to the area to avoid oxygen want by cells.

Assessment Factors Before Heat or Cold Application

Application of heat and cold is a major responsibility because extreme heat or extreme cold can cause damage if the application is not done with good judgment and caution. Always assess people for the following factors before application of heat or cold:

1. *Individual temperature tolerance.* Heat and cold tolerance varies greatly among people and among different parts of a person's body. The hands, for example,

□ **QUICK REFERENCE STOP 33-7: PSYCHOLOGICAL CONSIDERATIONS**
Value of Heat and Cold Applications

People do not as a rule appreciate the value of heat and cold applications. They think of them as "home remedies," not as a sophisticated form of medicine such as drugs. Explain the principle of the effects of heat and cold. Many people will be discharged from health care agencies with instructions to continue heat and cold applications at home. Only if they understand their importance will they continue to do them at home.

because they are constantly exposed to environmental effects, tolerate greater heat or cold than areas of the body such as the neck or inner arm or abdomen.

2. *Circulating adaptation capacity.* People with impaired circulation (e.g., those with arteriosclerosis, or narrowed blood vessels) have decreased blood supply to a part. Heat applied to a distal extremity in such a patient may call for more blood in the area than the circulatory system can supply; if cold is applied, the area may already have such a decreased blood supply that cell damage may occur. A large heat application (such as warm soaks to an entire leg) could draw a great deal of fluid into the extremity; in a person with heart disease, this may not leave enough blood in the central system for adequate circulation. If a cold application to a whole extremity is anticipated, a great deal of blood may be shifted back into the central circulation. Again, the person with heart disease or lung disease may not be able to handle this unusual heavy load. Always be aware of the overall circulatory state of a person before applying external heat or cold (see QRS 33-7).

3. *Neurological response capability.* A person with decreased neurological sensations cannot detect heat or cold at normal levels and may therefore readily be burned without even realizing it. To safeguard against burning, never apply any heat that is warmer than is comfortable for you, and never apply ice directly to the skin but always with a protective covering such as a towel between the ice and the skin.

4. *Decreased pain sensation due to medication.* You must be very careful when applying heat or cold to any person who is receiving any medication (a sedative, sleep medicine, an analgesic) that reduces sensation or awareness because the overall nerve conduction capability may be so reduced that the person cannot discern heat and cold at the usual levels. Such a person could easily be burned or frostbitten.

5. *Age of person.* An infant's skin is more tender than adult skin and burns more readily; in addition, infants are unable to describe feelings of heat or cold. Because older adults may have lost some of their ability to perceive pain from heat or cold, this age group also needs extreme caution with heat and cold applications.

6. *New tissue.* New tissue (such as a freshly healed surgical incision or injury) may have decreased sensory capability because nerve tissue at an injured site does not regenerate well. Sections of new tissue may be more tender than older tissue and can stand heat or cold less well than the surrounding tissue. Use caution when working with such tissue.

7. *Presence of malignancy.* Heat is not used as a rule when a malignancy (a cancer) is present in a body part; because heat encourages growth of tissue, it will promote growth of abnormal as well as normal cells.

8. *Kidney adequacy.* Kidneys perform their filtering function in proportion to the blood passing through them. If a large heat application is used on an extremity, so much blood may be drawn away from the central system that kidney perfusion in kidneys already compromised by illness may become inadequate. This could result in kidney failure.

9. *Presence of edema.* Cold applied immediately after an injury reduces the formation of edema by decreasing blood flow and therefore the amount of plasma accumulating in the area. Once edema is present, cold is destructive to edematous tissue because it prevents clearing of the edema. Therefore, cold is applied for the first 24 hours following an injury; after that, heat is applied to promote movement and dissolution of edema by increasing circulation to the area.

10. *Abdominal or oral pain.* As a rule of thumb, never apply heat to the abdomen in the presence of undiagnosed abdominal pain or to the oral cavity in the presence of oral pain. If the abdominal pain is caused by an inflamed appendix or the oral pain by an abscessed tooth, heat may cause such increased blood flow into the area that the appendix or the abscess may rupture. This will spread infectious microorganisms into the bloodstream with possibly fatal consequences.

Types of Heat Application

MOIST HEAT

Heat application may be done by using either a wet or a dry technique. Wet heat has the advantages of penetrating more deeply than dry heat, causing less fluid loss because less sweating occurs during the treatment, and conforming better to body parts, making it easier to apply. However, wet heat applications become cool more readily due to evaporation of water from the surface and therefore need to be changed more frequently during therapy to maintain a warm temperature. Skin exposed to wet heat may become macerated, and burns may occur more frequently because evaporation does not take place at the skin surface to create a local cooling effect.

Moist heat is applied by moist compresses (soaks) or baths. Such a source of heat should be no hotter than would be comfortable against your inner wrist or forearm (an area sensitive to heat). If you have a thermometer to measure the temperature of water put into a container or used with dressings, it should be no hotter than 110°F (43.3°C). To people with low thresholds for sensation, even this temperature may be uncomfortably warm.

Hot Moist Compresses. Hot compresses may be either sterile (both sterile dressings and a sterile solution are used) or nonsterile (clean dressings and a clean solution are used). Sterile technique is necessary when the skin is broken (or when the compress is applied to the eye) because the natural defense mechanisms are limited with these conditions.

The dressings can be wet by submerging them in a basin of warm solution (the temperature should feel warm but not hot to your wrist) and wringing them out so that they are moist but not wet. Excessive wetness will not add to the warmth of the compresses but instead will invite more evaporation and actually cool more. The compresses are then applied to the designated body area. An alternate method is to lay dry compresses on the designated area and then moisten them by squirting the warmed solution onto the compress. In both instances, to prevent evaporation and initiate cooling, the compress must be covered with a waterproof pad. Added heat from a hot water bottle may be used to keep the area warm. Do not keep wet compresses warm by means of a heating pad (wet compresses should not be mixed with electrical appliances to avoid shock or electrocution).

Protect the bedding underneath the wet compresses to prevent it from becoming wet and cool and uncomfortable. If the person's skin becomes macerated easily (and if no open wound is present), the area can be coated with Vaseline (petroleum jelly) prior to the compress application to protect it against the moisture.

If a compress is to be applied with sterile technique, you must be certain to use a sterile solution, a sterile basin, and sterile gloves to handle the compresses. If you are placing the compress first and then wetting it, you must use a sterile syringe for this. (See Chap. 28 for a discussion of sterile technique.)

Baths. Baths are a convenient method of applying moist heat. Frequent types of baths used are soaks of a body part, sitz baths, and whirlpool baths. Paraffin baths are used less frequently.

SOAKS. Soaking an extremity or part of an extremity in a warm basin of water is frequently used to aid in wound healing by drawing leukocytes into the area (causing suppuration). To perform a soak, position the patient comfortably in bed or in a bedside chair, and protect the bedding as necessary with a waterproof pad or rubber sheet covered by a cloth sheet. If the person's skin is broken in the affected area, a sterile basin and solution should be used; if not, a clean basin and clean solution are used. To warm a sterile bottle of solution, set it in a basin of hot water. After about 15 minutes, shake the solution bottle well and pour a few drops onto your wrist without touching the rim of the bottle to your wrist. To test a nonsterile solution for temperature, use the same method or pour some into the basin and submerge your wrist into it.

For the soak, fill the basin about half full with solution. Submerge the affected body part in the basin of solution. Water in a basin stays warm only about 10 minutes, so for a 20-minute soak, you will need to change the water in the middle of the procedure. Have the patient remove the body part from the basin while you change the water so that you do not add solution so warm that it burns. Wrap the wet body part in a towel while you change the solution so that it will not feel cold from evaporation, resulting in vasoconstriction, which is the opposite effect from what you are trying to achieve by a warm soak.

Check the person's body position for good alignment; support an extremity with pillows or other supports as necessary to make the person comfortable. Twenty minutes is a very long time in an uncomfortable position without anything to do, and the patient may resist further therapy if the experience is unpleasant. Provide for stimulation by use of a radio or conversation during the time interval.

At the end of the time period dry the body part gently to reduce the possibility of skin maceration from continued moisture and to prevent excessive cooling due to evaporation.

SITZ BATHS. A sitz bath is a warm water bath that is intended to increase circulation to the anal or perineal region. It is very soothing for patients following perineal or rectal surgery. Most health care agencies today use disposable sitz baths (a plastic shallow basin that fits onto the toilet seat) for this purpose. The advantage of these individual sitz baths is the prevention of bacterial contamination that might otherwise be spread from patient to patient. Almost all hospital units have large sitz baths (shallow, low-lying bathtubs) that can be used instead. If for some reason either of these methods is not acceptable to the patient, a regular bathtub may be used. When using central health care agency equipment such as sitz baths or bathtubs, wash the tub well with a cleansing powder prior to use. Repeat the process after use to discourage the spread of microorganisms.

For a sitz bath, fill the basin about two-thirds full with water that is warm but not hot to your wrist (for a sitz tub or regular tub, fill with enough water to cover the person's rectum and perineum as he sits). Assist the person to a comfortable sitting position; provide privacy as necessary with a towel or bath blanket. Most people for whom sitz baths are prescribed have perineal or rectal pain; the warm water is very relaxing and pain-relieving. The sense of relief from pain plus the change in the circulatory level of blood (vasodilatation in the perineal area draws a supply of blood away from more elevated body parts) has a sedative effect. After 20 minutes of sitting in a warm bath, the patient is often weaker than he thought he would be; he often needs help in replacing clothing and returning to bed. Few people realize how pain-relieving such a warm water application can be; because they have pain, they may be reluctant to walk with you to a bathroom the first time for this procedure. It may be necessary to administer an analgesic (pain-relieving medication) first and then suggest the sitz bath after about 20 minutes when the effect of the analgesic is at its peak. If the person was given an analgesic prior to a sitz bath, the feeling of fatigue and perhaps lightheadedness (particularly if the analgesic was a narcotic) will be even more pronounced at the end of the procedure. Most people quickly realize that warm water is the best pain reliever of the two methods and will begin to use sitz baths for pain relief as a rule.

Many sitz baths (such as the disposable toilet seat type) have a water reservoir (a plastic bag) that hangs from a pole and drains by a plastic tube into the basin, keeping the basin water always circulating (circulating water creates more circulatory stimulation and is even more effective) (Fig. 33-7). Some people may worry that the flowing water will cause them pain because of the motion and will need support to allow the water to circulate until they are convinced that the flowing water adds to their comfort. In a regular bathtub, this same effect can theoretically be created by letting the faucet run slowly with the bottom drain partially open. This can be dangerous if the warmth of the faucet water is affected when anyone else on the nursing unit turns on a source of water because the running water suddenly turns cold or warmer.

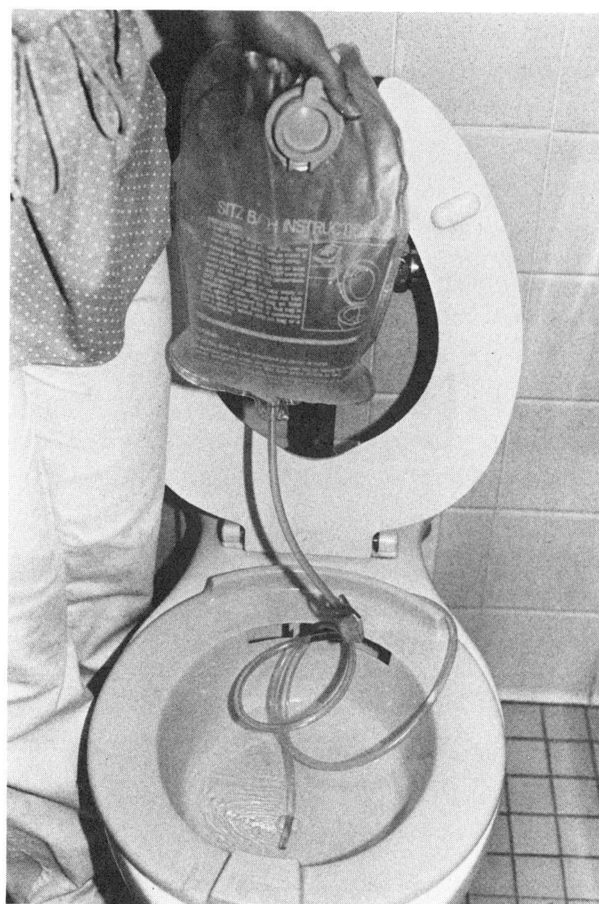

FIGURE 33-7. Sitz baths use warm moving water to increase circulation and promote healing for the perineal or rectal area. Here, a nurse prepares one on a patient toilet.

WHIRLPOOL BATHS. Whirlpool bath units may be small enough to accommodate only one leg or arm but usually are full immersion baths. The term *whirlpool* is derived from the fact that air is bubbled into the water in the tub, creating a bubbling and swirling motion in the water. Such water agitation greatly increases circulatory stimulation; it helps to debride or clean wounds. When a person is submerged in water, his arms and legs become weightless, allowing a passive or active range of motion to be performed easily (Fig. 33-8).

Water in a whirlpool bath is, like all moist heat applications, pleasantly warm (90°—100°F, 32°—38°C); it is controlled by thermostatic adjustments on the whirlpool intake.

Whirlpool baths are generally located in the physical therapy department of health care agencies. Following a 20- to 30-minute soak in such a bath, a person may feel very lightheaded and exhausted. He may need assistance to return to bed and to rest afterward. (Encourage the patient to take a wheelchair to the department; he may be able to walk there very well and feel he does not need it, but he will need it to return.)

Although people tend to be apprehensive about whirlpool baths at first, they are usually able to feel immediately the benefits of the swirling water. For personal privacy while in the bath, the person wears a bathing suit or a patient gown. Ask before transporting the patient to the physical therapy department if you need to supply a gown or not.

If whirlpool baths are used for burn or wound debridement, the bathing itself is enjoyable, but necrotic tissue that is loosened by the effect of the warm water will then be cut away by the physical therapist or the person's physician. This involves a degree of pain.

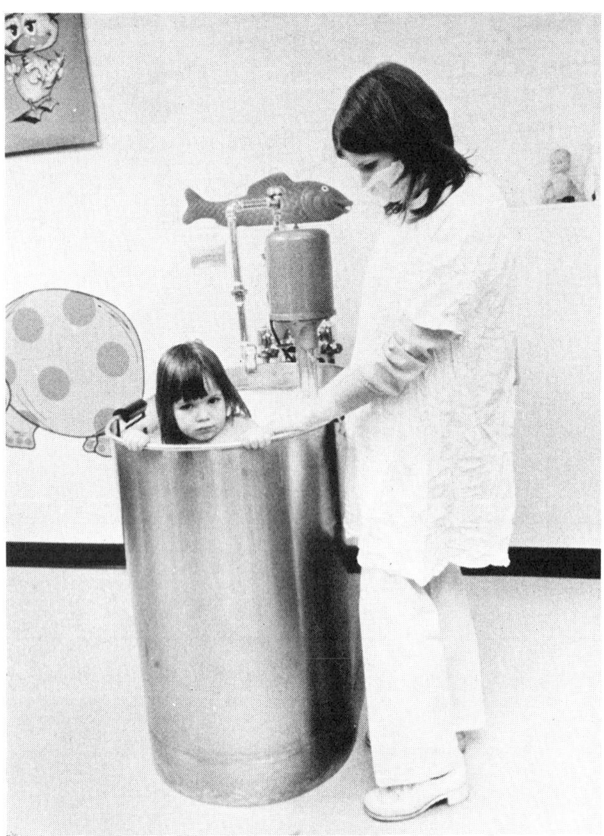

FIGURE 33-8. Whirlpool baths use warm moving water to increase healing or promote body motion. Here a preschooler shows her apprehension at this different from normal bath tub.

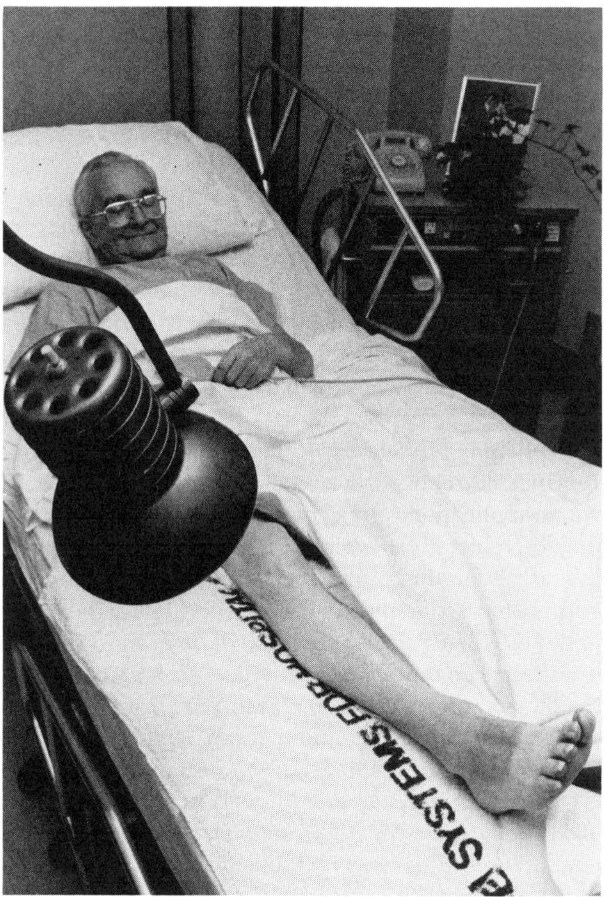

FIGURE 33-9. A heat lamp applied as a source of dry heat. Be certain that heat lamps are kept 18 to 24 inches from the patient. Note the call bell in the patient's hand, available to him should he feel discomfort from the treatment.

The person may appreciate having an analgesic administered before the bath. He needs your support to undergo a procedure of this kind.

PARAFFIN BATHS. Paraffin is the wax used in home canning to seal jar lids. When it is combined with mineral oil (1/2 ounce oil to 1 pint of paraffin) and heated, it melts into a thick waxy liquid. The patient dips the affected body part in the melted solution; as it is slowly removed, paraffin clings to the skin, coating it tightly. Holding it for a few minutes in the room air allows the paraffin to set to a hard wax cover. The body part is dipped five or six times this way until a thick paraffin coating over the skin has been created. Paraffin used this way will keep heat concentrated against an extremity until, at the end of 20 or 30 minutes, it is peeled away.

Paraffin baths are administered in physical therapy departments; they are effective in relieving pain and increasing mobility in people with arthritis. The danger is that the paraffin may reach a temperature that could burn (adding mineral oil lowers the melting point and protects against this possibility).

DRY HEAT

Application of dry heat is a better method than moist heat in many instances because an apparatus such as a heat lamp can be applied to an open wound without fear of contaminating the wound with microorganisms, the bed will not grow damp and cold, and maceration of the skin does not occur. Dry heat may cause more fluid loss due to the evaporation of perspiration at the site, and there is an equal chance of burning the patient. Dry heat does not penetrate as deeply as moist heat, so it is less effective in relieving deep muscle pain. If electricity is used as the heat source, the danger of electrical shock is present.

Heat Lamps. A gooseneck lamp is frequently used to provide dry heat because the flexible frame of the lamp (Fig. 33-9) can be positioned at the bedside to provide heat to a designated body part. The important rules to remember with heat lamps is that they must be kept far enough away from the part so that the heat does not cause a burn, and the part should be exposed to the light for only 20 minutes. The correct distance is 18 inches away for a 40-watt light bulb and 24 inches for a 60-watt bulb. Be certain to position the person comfortably so that he does not move during the 20-minute time interval and by so doing move closer to the lamp. One disadvantage of a heat lamp is that the skin surface of the affected part must be exposed. If the area is an extremity, this is not a problem, but if the perineal area, for example, is the area that needs warmth, the problem of modesty arises. Draw the curtain around the bed or close the room door to provide privacy rather than drawing the bedclothes up over the lamp to form a tent. Forming a tent brings the bedclothing close to the lamp, creating a fire hazard, and because the heat is then concentrated in a small closed space, the temperature is increased. Be sure the rest of the body is covered well so that the person will not feel cool in contrast to the added warmth at one body point.

When using heat lamps with small infants, position the lamp so that if the infant voids (urinates), the urine stream will not strike the light bulb. This could shatter the bulb and send glass fragments into the child's bed.

Radiant Heat Warmers. A radiant heat warmer is another form of dry heat. It is a portable row of lights placed over a person to provide a heat source. Frequently seen in delivery rooms and newborn nurseries, it supplies needed warmth while allowing the infant's body to remain uncovered (Fig. 33-10A). In adults it would be directed toward a specific body part.

Heat Cradles. A heat cradle is a half circle of metal that rests on the bed like a protective shelter over a body part. Inside the frame is a low-wattage (25-watt) light bulb that provides heat (Fig. 33-10B). The cradle is placed over a body part, the light is turned on, and the bedclothing is brought up over the frame to maintain heat. A heat cradle may be used for intermittent heat therapy, or, because its wattage is so low, thus causing no serious rebound vasoconstrictive effect, it may be used continuously. In contrast to a heat lamp, the bedclothing may be pulled over the frame because the wattage of the bulb and the degree of heat are so low. Just be certain that the bedclothes do not rest directly on the light bulb. You should be able to measure 12 to 18 inches between the light bulb and the person's body part. In an extremely obese person with large thighs, for example, a regular size heat cradle applied to the lower extremity would bring the light bulb much closer to the skin surface than this distance. You would need to position the sides of the cradle on folded bath blankets or some sort of solid object (blocks of wood) to lift the cradle away from the bed. Be sure that the rest of the person's body is kept warm enough so that he does not feel cool in contrast to the part being warmed by the heat cradle. Heat cradles are typically used to dry large leg casts or to provide continuous heat to an extremity where there is a thrombophlebitis (inflammation and blood clot formation in a blood vessel).

Electric Heating Pads. Electric heating pads are convenient forms of dry heat for a small body area. Heating pads generally have three heat settings—high, medium, and low. Never use more than a low setting in a health care agency unless you have a prescription to do otherwise. This level of warmth is very mild, and a patient may tell you that he could stand it much hotter. Resist the temptation to increase the heat because analgesics or other factors may have depressed the person's perception of heat to such an extent that he could receive a burn at a higher setting. If there is any doubt that the patient may be tempted to increase the temperature setting himself, place adhesive tape on both sides of the temperature gauge so that it cannot be moved. Do this routinely with children under 12 years of age because such dials and gauges are fun for young children to play with and they do not realize the potential harm in it.

Electric heating pads have a waterproof plastic cover. Never place plastic directly on the skin because it tends to feel very hot after a few minutes. It can also cause skin maceration because perspiration at the site is not absorbed but remains on the skin. Wrap the heating pad in a thin towel or flannel cloth. Never use an electric heating pad to keep wet compresses from cooling or with an infant who might have a wet diaper (electricity and water sources should never be mixed). Do not press the pad tightly against the patient or a coil may be pressed so closely against the skin that a burn results. For the same reason, the patient should not be allowed to lie on a heating pad (turn him on to his side or abdomen and place the pad on top of him). Do not use safety pins with an electric heating pad to secure it in place. The metal of the pin could touch an electric coil and produce a shock for you or the patient.

K Pads. K pads are a miniature form of hyperthermic blanket. They are rubber pads designed in a particular shape to fit a specific body part; hollow channels inside the pad carry warm water that is kept warm and circulated by narrow hoses, which are connected to a bedside portable pump (Fig. 33-11). They can supply heat to both wet and dry dressings.

The temperature of the circulating water is determined by the setting on the pump. After this temperature is set, the key used to set the temperature is removed; the temperature setting cannot be elevated or lowered without the key. In most health care agencies, K pad pumps are filled with distilled water and have the temperature preset in the central supply department so that there is no danger that a patient could change the setting and accidentally burn himself.

Never place a pad directly on the patient's skin (rubber against skin can cause maceration from the perspiration that is not absorbed from the skin); provide a towel or gauze squares between the pad and the skin. Do not use safety pins to secure a K pad in place (you may puncture the water channels). Secure the pad with roller gauze if necessary to achieve a good position. To allow maximum circulation of the water through the pad, place the pad on top of the patient, not the patient on top of the pad.

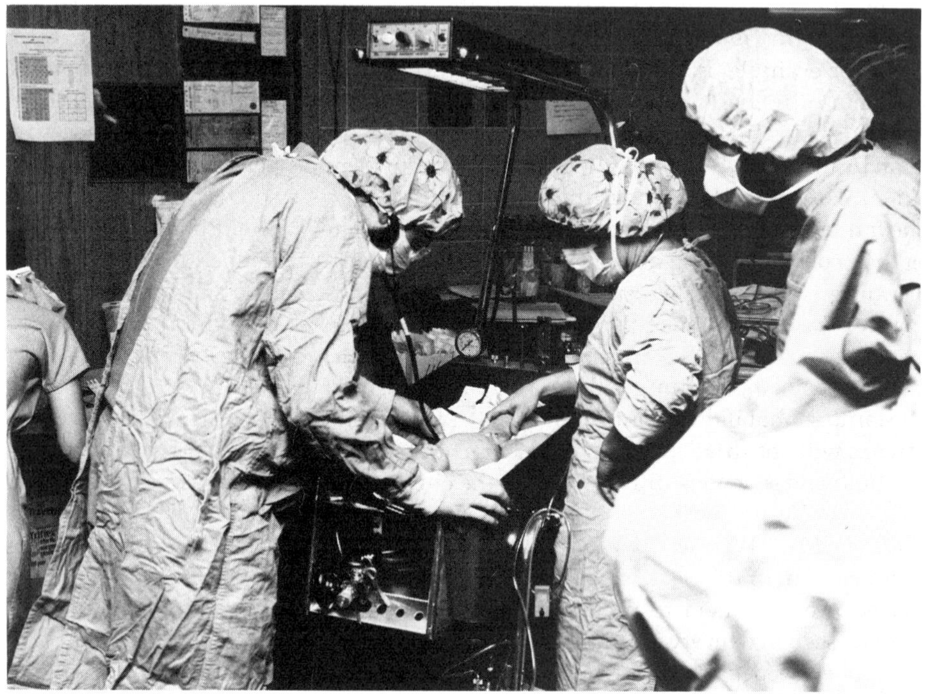

A

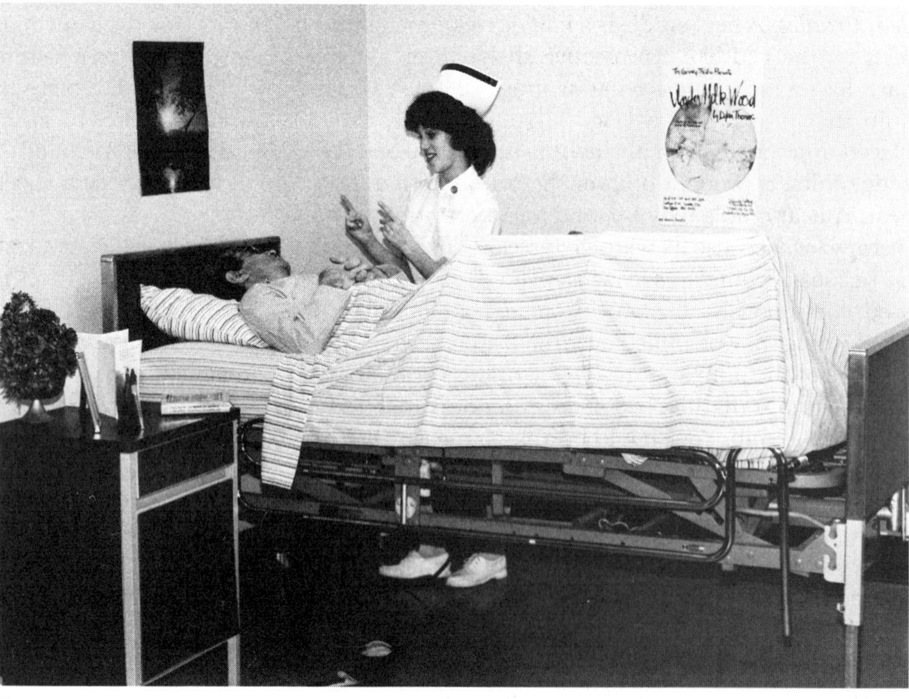

B

FIGURE 33-10. A. Radiant heat warmers are banks of light directed at a surface to produce heat. Here a newborn in a delivery room is kept warm by radiant heat. B. Heat cradles are metal frames with low voltage light bulbs attached to give constant even heat.

Hot Water Bottles. Hot water bottles are a dangerous source of heat if not used properly because they do not have a temperature-setting gauge that allows controlled heat as does a heating pad, for example. To prepare a hot water bottle for use, run water at a sink until it is pleasantly warm to your inner wrist (100°—110°F, 38°—43°C). Fill the hot water bottle and let it remain full for a few minutes, then empty it again. This step warms the rubber. Next, fill the water bottle again with the same pleasantly warm water to no more than two-thirds full. Squeeze the bottle to bring the level of the water up to the opening before you screw the top tight. This removes excess air from the bottle and

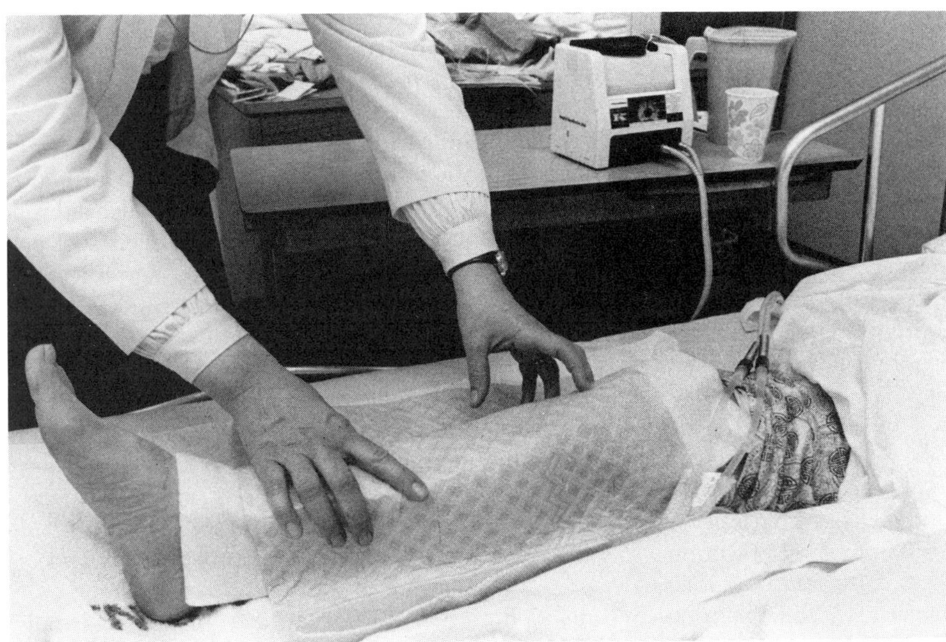

FIGURE 33-11. K pad applied as a source of dry heat. Temperature of the pad is regulated by the control box on the bedside stand. Never apply a plastic or rubber pad directly to the skin. Note the cotton covering underneath.

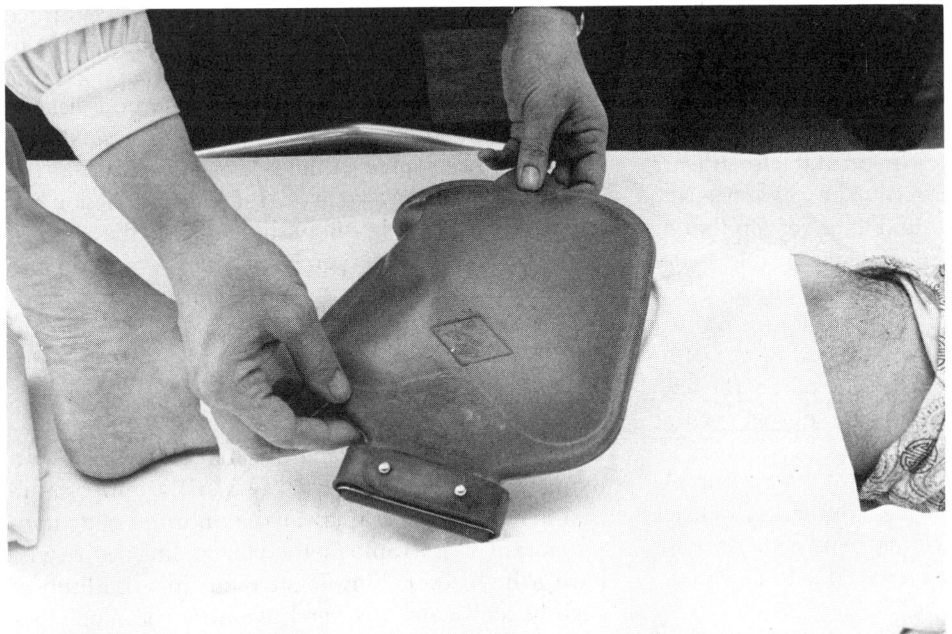

FIGURE 33-12. A hot water bottle used as a source of dry heat. Note that the bottle is pliable since it is not completely filled. Always place a cotton or gauze protection between the bottle and the patient's skin.

makes it more flexible and better able to mold to a body part. *Never use hotter water in a hot water bottle than you would apply directly to your own skin.* The rubber readily becomes the temperature of the inside water and will cause a burn if the water inside is really hot. (For practical purposes, there is no such thing as a hot water bottle; they are always warm water bottles.)

Always cover a hot water bottle with a towel to protect the skin from direct contact with the rubber. Check that the bottle does not leak before placing it on the patient to be certain that the bed will not grow damp and cold.

Chemical Heat Packs. Chemical heat packs are strong plastic bags with two separate compartments filled with chemicals. To heat the pack, knead it or strike it sharply against a counter top according to the manufacturer's instructions. This action breaks the seal between the two chemical compartments; as the chemicals combine, heat is produced. Such a pack reaches a temperature of between 105° and 115°F (40.5° and 46°C), a temperature that should feel pleasantly warm but not hot to your inner arm.

Cover such a pack with a towel before applying it to the patient to keep the plastic covering away from direct contact with the skin. Safety pins should not be used to secure a chemical pack in place. Accidental puncture of the chemical compartments could cause leakage and a severe chemical burn.

Infrared or Ultraviolet Lights. Infrared or ultraviolet light therapy is the use of light rays from the extreme ends of the light spectrum to produce heat. Ultraviolet rays help the liver convert indirect bilirubin released from destroyed red blood cells into direct bilirubin. Indirect bilirubin is a fat-based product and cannot be excreted from the body in that form; it must be transformed into direct bilirubin to keep excessive amounts from accumulating in the body, causing jaundice (yellowing) and, in newborns, brain cell destruction (termed *kernicterus*). Exposing a newborn or immature infant to "bili-lights," or rows of ultraviolet lights, over the Isolette has developed into a common use for this type of light today. Ultraviolet light is so intense that the infant must have his eyes covered during therapy or retinal damage could occur. The heat inside an Isolette with ultraviolet lights above it can increase greatly; for this reason, the portholes of the Isolette are generally left open during therapy. The infant needs to drink an adequate supply of fluid to be certain that he does not become dehydrated from insensible water loss. Therapy may be maintained continually for 2 or 3 days except when the infant is removed for his mother to feed him. Infants with sensory deprivation of this kind (the eyes are covered for the major part of the day) need sensory stimulation from other sources such as touching or sound.

Infrared light is used mainly to relieve muscle spasm. It is administered in physical therapy departments to specific body parts as indicated. As with ultraviolet light, the person's eyes need to be shielded.

Diathermy. Diathermy is the conversion of electrical energy into thermal (heat) energy. It is penetrating heat that is directed by means of a special diathermy machine and pads into deep body layers. Such treatments as a rule are performed in the physical therapy department or in a private physician's office. Be certain that a person undergoing a diathermy treatment does not have any metal (safety pins, hearing aids, religious articles) on his body. So much heat is conducted by diathermy that a metal object in contact with the person could become so hot that it could cause a serious burn.

Diathermy interferes with the functioning of a cardiac pacemaker. *Patients with cardiac pacemakers should not be scheduled for diathermy therapy.*

Types of Cold Application

Cold applications are used to prevent edema formation following trauma or intrusive procedures such as bronchoscopy; they may be used following surgery such as a tonsillectomy because the edema that occurs after such a procedure close to the airway could result in a serious airway obstruction.

Cold, like heat, may be applied in dry or moist forms. The danger sign that cold is too intense is a blue and purple mottling on the skin surface or redness; blisters denote that damage to the cells has occurred.

MOIST COLD

Moist cold can be applied by baths or cold compresses.

Cold Compresses. The usual form of applying moist cold is to wet a washcloth or towel with cool tap water, wring out the excess water, and mold it to the designated body part. Cover it with a plastic or waterproof pad to keep it cool longer. Replace the towel as necessary to keep it cool. You can keep a cold source of water at the patient's bedside by filling one basin with ice cubes and positioning a second basin of cool water in this bottom basin. Be as careful with cold applications as with hot applications; cold *burns* the same as heat. If applying cool compresses to a large body area, always apply a *colder* source to the person's forehead at the same time. Causing a great deal of vasoconstriction in a large area of the body will push blood into the cerebral arteries. The person perceives this as an intense headache, and, in a susceptible individual, the increased intracranial pressure could actually rupture a cerebral artery. Be certain that the head cloth is colder than the other cloth to prevent this.

Tepid Baths. The word *tepid* means "lukewarm," or a temperature of 80° to 98°F (27°—37°C), a temperature that is not a great deal lower than normal body temperature. This is a rapid method for cooling people who have a high fever (simply sit them in a bathtub of slightly cool water). Never leave a person alone in a bathtub because if he is feeling weak and ill from the source of the fever, he may not be able to support himself in the water. Never use water that feels cold. The shock to the person's nervous system from such a great temperature change could cause a reaction as extreme as a convulsion.

An alternate method of applying cool moist bathwater is to place a plastic or rubber sheet on the person's bed, then dip two towels in slightly cool water, wring them out, and place one under the patient and one on top of him, tucking the towels in snugly against the groin and axilla where major arteries pass just under the surface. Although this technique is usually referred to as a "bath," it is really the use of total body compresses.

Make sure that the bathwater or the towel water is not cool enough to cause shivering (shivering will cause heat production and reverse the effect desired). Be sure that a colder cloth is placed on the forehead to prevent vasoconstriction of peripheral vessels from pushing a large supply of blood into the cerebral vessels.

As noted earlier, never use alcohol baths or soaks with children. Not only is the shock of the temperature difference between the evaporating alcohol and the child's temperature so extreme that it could lead to convulsions, but also some children have inhaled so many fumes from this procedure that they died from liver failure. The use of alcohol added to bathwater or applied as a sponge bath has some benefit with adults who are developing extremely high body temperatures.

DRY COLD

The most frequently used methods of applying dry cold are ice bags and chemical packs.

Ice Bags. Ice bags are rubber bags similar in appearance to hot water bottles (in fact, a hot water bottle can be used as an ice bag). Fill such a bag two-thirds full with crushed ice. Do not fill it all the way or it will become too inflexible to mold to a body part; expell all excess air before screwing the top in place for the same reason.

Cover an ice bag with a towel or other cover to protect the skin from moisture (condensation), which will accumulate on the rubber and could cause skin maceration. Test the bag against your forearm for temperature. Provide enough padding so that the bag feels cool, not cold. Do not secure ice bags in place with safety pins to avoid puncturing the bag and causing a leak. Check ice bags frequently for leaks so that the person and his bedding do not become wet and chilled; check the skin underneath to be certain that it is not becoming numb (this is an indication that you have not provided enough padding and the bag is too cold). Never apply ice directly to the skin; it is far too cold and can cause frostbite or destruction of skin cells.

An ice bag can be constructed from a plastic bag (the type used for sandwiches at home or bagging pharmacy supplies in health care agencies) or from a rubber glove. Fill these with ice and tie or secure the top with a rubber band to prevent water leakage. A glove used in this way is a clever ice bag for children because if you paint a face on it with a Magic Marker it looks a lot like a chicken's head, providing not only ice therapy but an amusing chuckle as well (Fig. 33-13).

Chemical Packs. Chemical packs are commercial plastic bags filled with two chemicals in separate compartments that combine to become cold once they are kneaded together (Fig. 33-14). Cover such a pack with a towel or other protective cover to keep the plastic away from direct contact with the skin.

Hypothermia or Hyperthermia Blankets. Hypothermia or hyperthermia blankets are large, body-sized rubber or vinyl blankets with central core coils that are filled with a designated solution (distilled water for warming, or alcohol and distilled water for cooling). The solution circulates through the coils in the blanket back to a large motorized unit at the foot of the patient's bed that cools or warms the fluid passing through it to a set temperature. Such units are used as hypothermia units to reduce high fever; they can also be used to lower a

FIGURE 33-13. An ice pack made from a rubber glove. Drawing a face on it changes its connotation from a form of therapy to a friend.

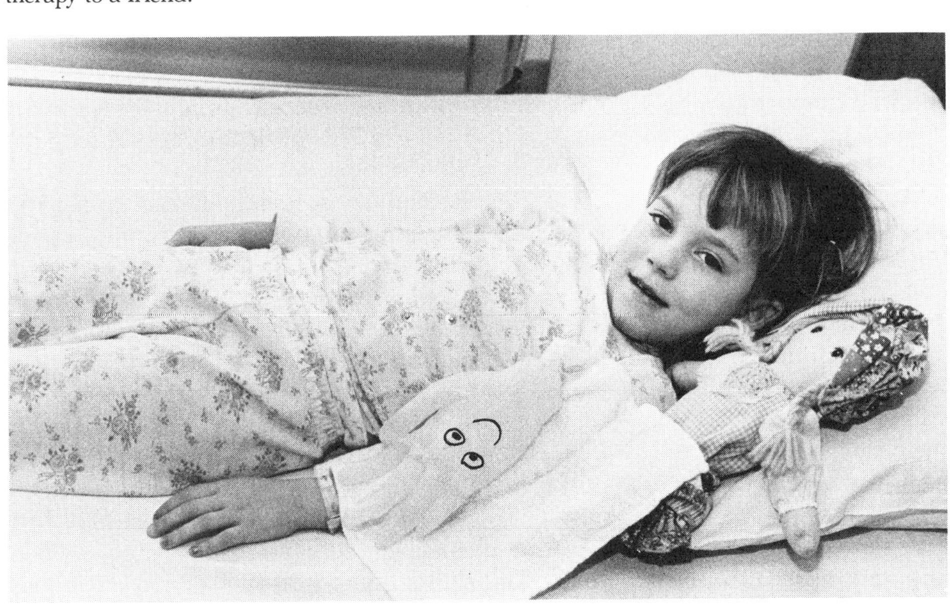

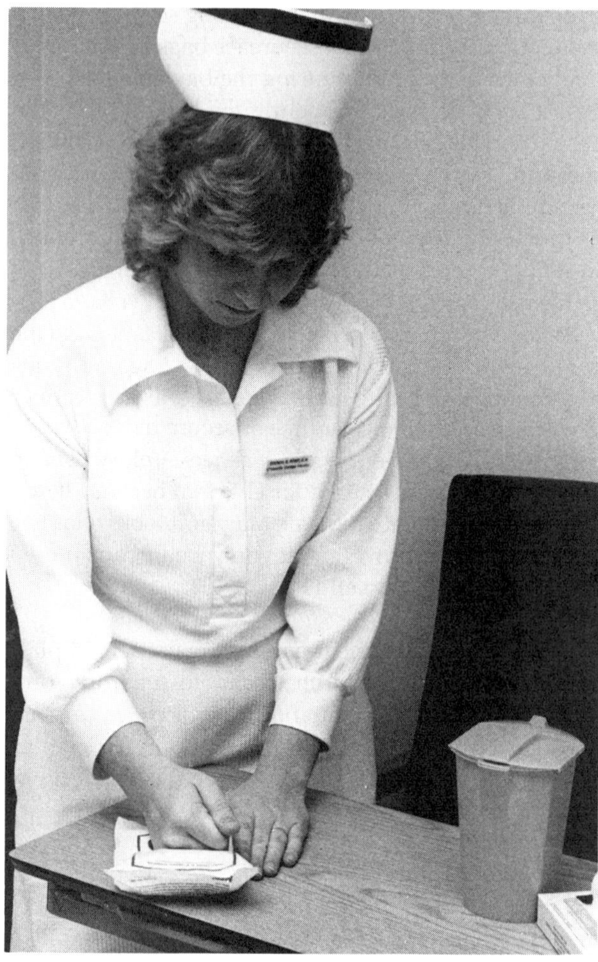

A

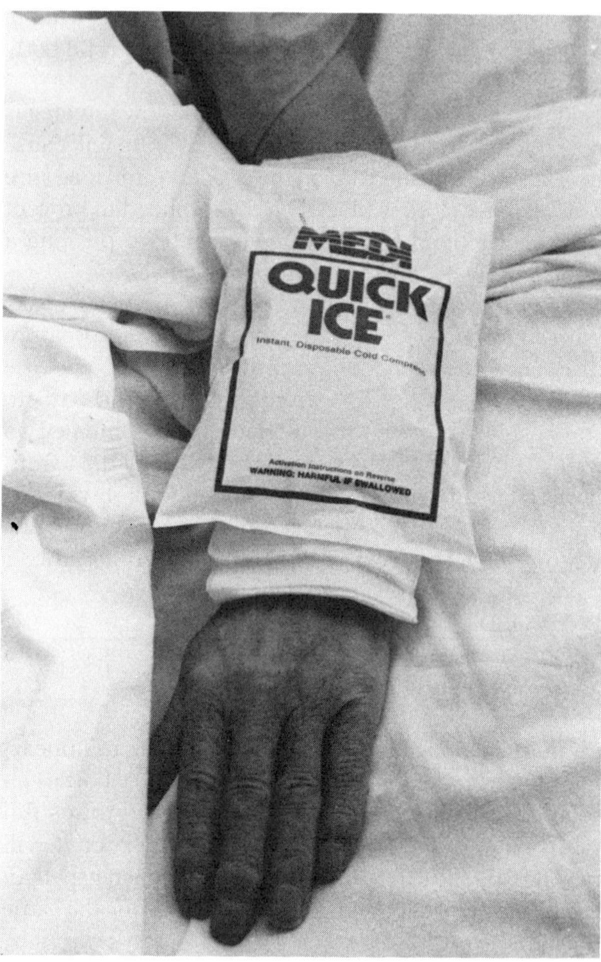

B

FIGURE 33-14. Chemical cold pack. A. Kneading it to mix its contents. B. Cold pack in place. Note gauze underneath to protect skin.

patient's temperature and therefore the metabolic rate prior to surgery such as cardiac surgery. They are used as hyperthermia units to warm a person who has a subnormal temperature following hypothermia from surgery or who has been exposed to cold (a skier lost on a mountaintop, for example).

A continuous rectal temperature probe can be used whenever a hypothermia or hyperthermia blanket is in place to be certain that the patient's temperature can always be immediately assessed. To prevent rectal irritation you can take intermittent temperature readings. The temperature of the blanket and the temperature that the physician desires the patient to reach must be specifically ordered before the blanket is applied. It is good practice to set the dial of the heating or cooling unit at the temperature desired and then place strips of adhesive tape at the maximum and minimum limits so that no one can increase or decrease the temperature of the blanket beyond these limits.

Even for urgent heating and cooling, a sheet should be placed between the rubber or vinyl blanket and the patient to protect the patient's skin from becoming macerated; perspiration or condensation is not absorbed if there is continuous contact of the rubber or vinyl with the skin. Never use a bath blanket for this purpose because it will interfere with the transfer of heat or cold. For urgent cooling, both a bottom and a top blanket may be used; for maintenance, usually just a bottom blanket is necessary. The top blanket is heavy and many people feel fatigued just from the weight of it (and the nurse loses a great deal of opportunity for observation with it in place).

For cooling, the blanket temperature is set slightly lower than the normal body temperature (about 94°—96°F, 34.4°—35.5°C); for warming, it is set one or two degrees above normal body temperature (99°—100°F, 37.2°—37.2°C). For either heating or cooling, the blanket temperature is usually turned off when the patient's temperature reaches to within two degrees of the desired temperature to allow for heating or cooling that will continue for a period of time while the heat or cold in the coils fades.

When cooling is initiated, unless otherwise indicated a coating of lanolin or other cream is usually applied to the person's skin to limit maceration of skin and reduce the possibility of frostbite because lanolin serves as a possible insulator. As with any patient on bed rest, the person must be turned at least every 2 hours. Use supine and prone positions because more body surface tends to be in contact with the blanket in these positions than when the patient is lying on his side. Reapply a coating of ointment as necessary at these times.

Total body warming or cooling in this way places an overall stress on the person's circulatory system. One important measure of compensation for this great an increase or decrease in metabolic rate is maintenance of a normal urine output. Always be extremely aware that urinary output remains normal for the person with a hypothermia or hyperthermia blanket in place. Safety pins should not be used with this type of blanket to avoid puncture of an internal coil and a leak in fluid. To prevent shivering, the person who will receive hypothermia by this method is generally administered a medication before the blanket is first put in place and periodically as needed. A sheet placed between the blanket and the patient's skin may help. Be conscientious in the timing of such medication; if shivering should occur it can very quickly defeat the purpose of the blanket.

LIFE SPAN CONCEPTS AND THERMAL REGULATION

Both heat and cold applications and the technique of temperature-taking differ according to age group.

The Infant

In infants be certain that a rectal thermometer is inserted only for the length of the bulb to prevent rectal mucosal tears. Position an infant either prone or supine (Fig. 33-15). Restrain the infant well during temperature-taking to prevent squirming that may allow the thermometer tip to break or scrape the delicate rectal mucosa.

Never leave an infant alone with any source of electrical heat. Infants may squirm near the heat source and burn themselves.

The Toddler and Preschooler

Preschool-age children fear intrusive procedures so much that even though you believe that a rectal temperature is not a hurting procedure, it is a fearful procedure for a child of this age. Electronic thermometers are ideal to use with this age group because they register so quickly that the child has to be restrained only a few seconds.

When using electrical sources of heat with toddlers and preschoolers, never make a point of the fact that plugging in the apparatus is what makes the light come on or a dial to glow. If plugging something in looks like a game, the child may "play" it after you leave. Electrical outlets in children's rooms should have coverings over the wall plugs to discourage children from playing with electrical equipment.

The Schoolager and Adolescent Child

Schoolagers and adolescents are old enough for oral temperature-taking but grow impatient waiting for thermometers to register and try to fill in the time with conversation or questions. Caution them not to do this so that the thermometer will register accurately. Occasionally a school-age child thinks it will be amusing to hold a thermometer against a radiator or an air conditioner to make the temperature "exciting." Use common sense about evaluating a thermometer reading if you weren't watching the child every second the thermometer was in place (it is unlikely that a 12-year-old sitting up in bed and telling you he is "starved" has the 106°F temperature the thermometer has registered). To avoid this, stay near the child for the entire time the thermometer is in place.

Children of this age have begun to adopt adult values of considering heat and cold applications as an unimportant form of therapy. They need support to accept such procedures. It may be helpful to allow the child to participate in a special activity while the hot or cold application is in place (watching television, playing a board game with him, and so on) so that the procedure is not a chore but an anticipated interval because of the accompanying enjoyable activity.

The Adult

Because adults often think of rectal temperature-taking as a "babyish" technique they need an explanation of why it is necessary to accept it when it is necessary. Many middle-aged adults begin to develop hemorrhoids (distended rectal veins). They occur particularly in women because of the pressure of a fetus resting against the perineal veins during pregnancy. Be extremely careful and gentle when inserting rectal thermometers not to injure hemorrhoidal tissue in this age group.

Adults often need support to accept and value heat and cold applications. They appreciate having something to occupy their time during the treatment such as their telephone or the availability of a magazine or the morning newspaper.

The Older Adult

The older adult often has a decreased peripheral temperature due to some degree of arteriosclerosis. For an axillary temperature to register accurately, it must stay in place for the full 10 minutes.

Older adults may have a decreased sensation of heat and cold so extreme care must be taken when using heat and cold applications in this age group to test the temperature accurately. If the person has little subcutaneous fat, a temperature that feels confortable to you may be uncomfortably warm for him.

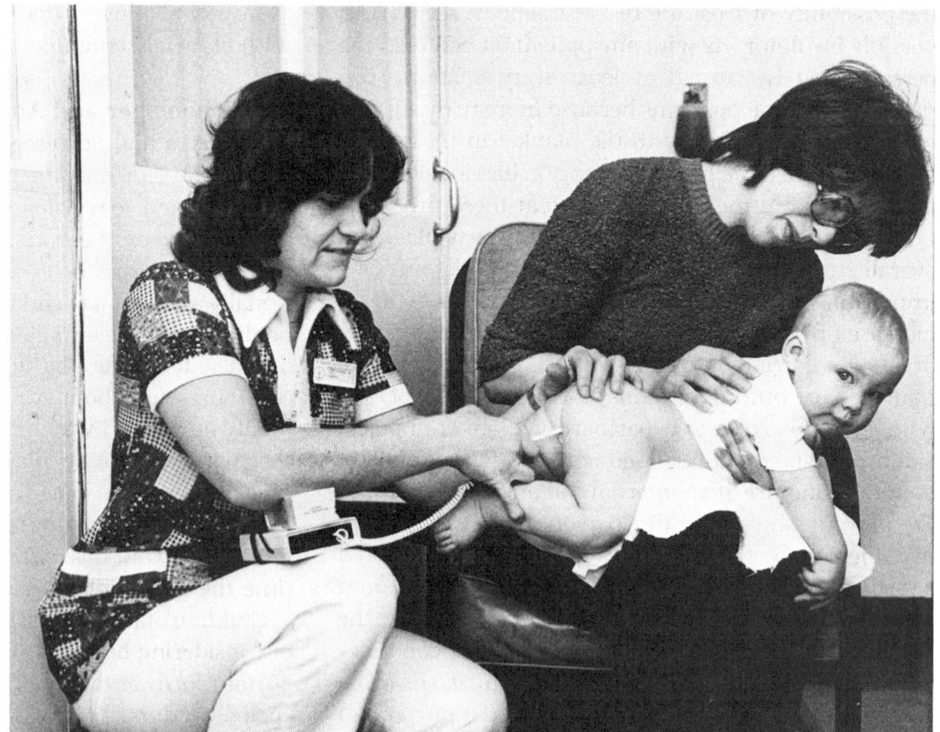

A

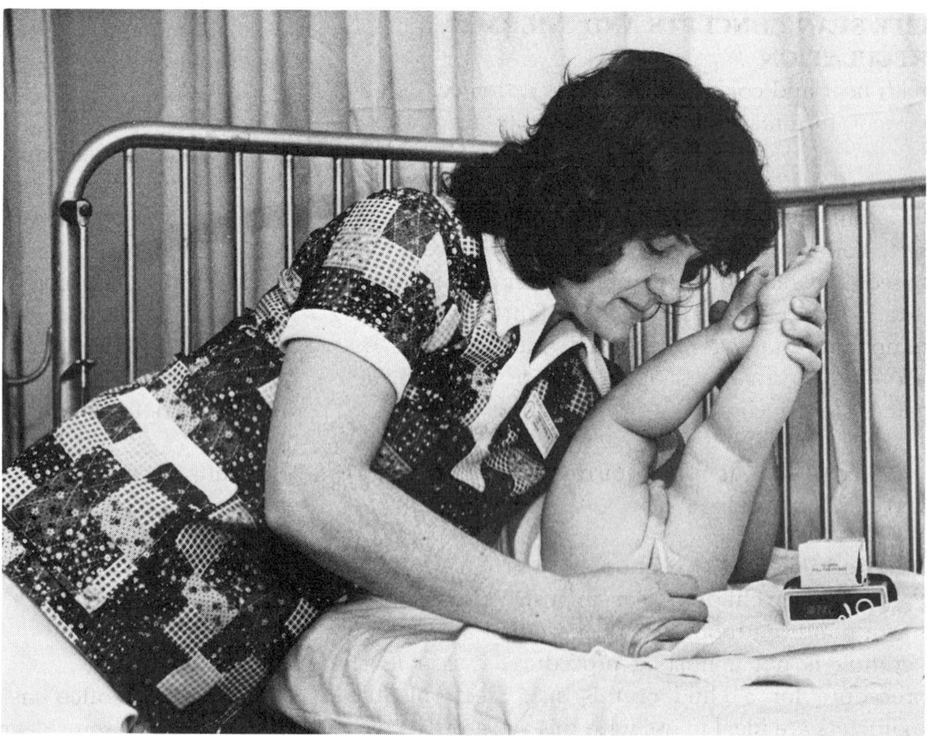

B

FIGURE 33-15. Rectal temperatures in infants can be taken either with the infant prone (A) or supine (B). Note how the infant's legs are grasped to restrain him in the supine position.

UTILIZING NURSING PROCESS

Heat and cold applications are one of the most hazardous areas of nursing practice because the possibility of causing a burn is always present. Temperature-taking is never a truly simple procedure because so many factors can interfere with a correct reading. Both heat and cold applications and temperature-taking need careful planning to be safe.

ASSESSMENT

Always be certain to assess a person's overall condition before taking a body temperature to be sure that you have chosen the best method. In many health care agencies, temperature-taking is done by nursing aides. Because such a person has a shallow knowledge base, be certain that her assessment of a patient's condition is accurate so that her temperature-taking technique is correct for that patient.

Always assess skin appearance halfway through a heat or cold application (about 10 minutes after it is applied) to be sure that the patient does not have an unusual sensitivity to heat or cold and is not developing a circulatory complication from it.

ANALYSIS

The Fourth National Conference of Nursing Diagnosis did not accept any diagnosis specific to thermal regulation. Following the usual format, however, such a diagnosis could be worded "Thermal regulation, impairment of: hyperthermia" or "Thermal regulation, impairment of: hypothermia." A critical defining characteristic would be the presence of an altered body temperature. Additional signs and symptoms would be skin appearance, presence of diaphoresis, and the feel of body warmth to palpation.

PLANNING

Most heat and cold applications are ordered three to four times daily. Plan the times for these treatments so that they do not coincide with such activities as eating if the application will be to an arm, or around visiting times if the procedure will leave the person exposed in any way. Many heat applications involve the use of electricity. Plan the procedure so that it is not scheduled when water will be used with the patient (bath time or shaving).

IMPLEMENTATION

Do not let yourself be caught in the patient's trap of thinking that heat and cold applications are "home remedies" and therefore of low priority or you will discover that you do not have time to do them in a busy day (they are always scheduled as the last thing and last things rarely get accomplished). Resist the thought that if a little heat or cold is good for someone, a lot of it or a longer time interval of it will be even better. Remember the vasoconstriction-vasodilatation rebound effects of heat and cold that affect their time limit. Safety considerations limit the temperature at which heat can be applied (see QRS 33-8).

☐ QUICK REFERENCE STOP 33-8: SAFETY
Safety Measures with Heat and Cold Applications

1. Do not use safety pins to anchor electric heating pads. Metal pins can cause a short circuit leading to a shock to the patient or you. Use roller gauze for the purpose.
2. Do not leave people alone with a heat lamp in place. They may turn toward the light, fall asleep, and become burned.
3. Tape a setting on an electric appliance to the point where you want it left if you have any doubt that the patient will be tempted to change it.
4. Never apply more heat to a person than feels comfortable on your own inner wrist.
5. Never apply ice packs or ice directly to the skin. Ice should always be covered with a towel or other cover to prevent cell damage from cold.
6. Leave heat and cold applications in place for 20 minutes unless otherwise prescribed to avoid rebound vasoconstriction or vasodilatation.
7. Be very cautious about heat or cold applications with a person who is receiving an analgesic, a sedative, or a hypnotic because his perception of heat or cold may be reduced and he could easily be burned.
8. Do not use electric equipment near water; check that all electric cords are intact and have three pronged plugs for proper grounding.

EVALUATION

If heat and cold applications are effective, healing is promoted, edema is reduced, and mobility is improved. Point out to people the improvement that you can detect to help them appreciate that that is the effect of the treatment. Many people return home with instructions to continue such treatments, but they will not do so unless they appreciate the importance of them.

Nursing Care Plan

Bob is a 16-year-old boy who has been admitted to the hospital with a diagnosis of diabetes mellitus. Diabetes not only causes a disturbance in the glucose-insulin balance but also with time creates interference with circulation due to vessel constriction and poor wound healing. Bob has an inflammation of his forearm from a cat scratch suffered just before admission. Warm soaks for his arm have been ordered three times a day.

The following is a nursing care plan you might write in reference to the warm soaks.

Subjective Assessment: Patient states that right forearm is continually painful (dull and nagging pain). States he wants "something better" than warm soaks for arm. Refuses to keep soaks in place longer than 5 minutes at a time. Parent angry with him for lack of cooperation; threatening to discontinue visiting.

Objective Assessment: Erythematous, warm to touch, linear laceration 6 cm long on right forearm. Drainage at site is mucopurulent; laceration surrounded by 2-cm edematous zone. Body temperature 101.6°F. Warm wet dressings applied for 20 minutes at 10 A.M.

Analysis: Knowledge, lack of, related to benefit of heat applications.

Goal: Patient to accept therapy by 24 hours.

Criteria: Patient will allow warm wet dressings to right forearm three times a day for full 20-minute time intervals.

NURSING ORDERS

1. Review with patient the effect of heat on inflammation and infection to increase circulation and white cell count at site and promote healing.
2. Ask him to agree to a cooperative three-day trial period for heat applications.
3. For soaks, use four sterile 4 × 4 gauze and warm sterile normal saline. Cover with plastic gauze and K pad to keep dressing warm for 20 minutes.
4. Test temperature carefully. People with diabetes tend to develop circulatory disturbances and decreased sensations of pain. Assess circulation (by fingerbed check, assessment for warmth midway through procedure to ensure that distal hand is receiving enough blood).
5. Schedule procedure after mealtime. Because of intravenous therapy in other arm, wet dressing limits manual dexterity greatly. Likes backgammon. Use a special activity during time dressing is in place.
6. Evaluate appearance of wound with patient in 3 days to fulfill trial period contract. Establish new 3-day period contract based on positive results.

SUGGESTED READINGS

Barman, M. R. Hypothermia, in summer? *RN* 45(6):42, 1982.

Bauman, B. Update your technique for changing dressings: Dry to dry. *Nursing* (Horsham) 12(1):64, 1982.

Capobianco, J. A. Keeping the newborn warm: How to safeguard the infant against life-threatening heat loss. *Nursing 80* 10:64, 1980.

Castle, M., and Watkins, J. Fever: Understanding a sinister sign. *Nursing 79* 9:27, 1979.

Cunha, B. A. Fever of unknown origin in the elderly. *Geriatrics* 37:30, 1982.

Davis, V. The structure and function of brown adipose tissue in the neonate. *J.O.G.N. Nurs.* 9:368, 1980.

Davis-Sharts, J. Mechanisms and manifestations of fever. *Am. J. Nurs.* 79:1874, 1978.

DeLapp, T. D. Taking the bite out of frostbite and other cold weather injuries. *Am. J. Nurs.* 80:56, 1980.

DeLapp, T. D. Accidental hypothermia. *Am. J. Nurs.* 83(1):67, 1983.

Eoff, M. J., et al. Temperature measurement in children. *Am. J. Nurs.* 81:1010, 1981.

Erickson, R. Oral temperature differences in relation to thermometer and technique. *Nurs. Res.* 29:175, 1980.

Galub, J. Weathering the winter. *Health* 14(11):24, 1982.

Gedrose, J. Prevention and treatment of hypothermia and frostbite. *Nursing 80* 10:34, 1980.

Glen, S. Hypothermia in the neonate: Cold can kill. *Nurs. Mirror* 154(4):36, 1982.

Heineman, H. S. What to do for the patient with fever. *Consultant* 18:21, 1978.

Jarvis, C. M. Vital signs, how to take them more accurately and understand them more fully. *Nursing 76* 6:31, 1976.

Hoyter, J. Hypothermia-hyperthermia in older persons. *J. Gerontol. Nurs.* 6:65, 1980.

Kolanowski, A. M., et al. Thermal stress and the aged. *J. Gerontol. Nurs.* 9(1):13, 1983.

Lorin, M. Elevated body temperature: Symptomatic treatment. *Consultant* 20:130, 1980.

McElroy, C. R. Update on heat illness. *Top. Emerg. Med.* 2:1, 1980.

O'Dell, A. Hot packs for morning stiffness. *Am. J. Nurs.* 75:986, 1975.

Rich, J. Hypothermia. *J.E.N.* 9(1):8, 1983.

Rolnick, M., et al. Hypothermia: Cold weather is only one cause. *Consultant* 20:132, 1980.

Rosenberg, H. Malignant hyperpyrexia. *Am. J. Nurs.* 81:1484, 1981.

Shaver, J. F. The basic mechanisms of fever: Considerations for therapy. *Nurse Pract.* 7(9):15, 1982.

Simpson, C. F. Adult arthritis: Heat, cold or both? *Am. J. Nurs.* 83(2):270, 1983.

Sturzenberger, A. Differentiating among heat syndromes. *J. Emerg. Nurs.* 7:25, 1978.

Takacs, K. M., et al. Temperature measurement in a clinical setting. *Nurs. Res.* 31(6):368, 1982.

Taylor, G. Cold comfort. *Nurs. Times* 78(5):181, 1982.

Thatcher, R. M. 98.6 degrees F: What is normal? *J. Gerontol. Nurs.* 9(1):22, 1983.

Waterson, M. Hot and cold therapy. *Nursing 78* 8:44, 1978.

QUESTIONS FOR REVIEW

Mrs. Jones is a patient in your care. She has a fever of 102°F (38.9°C) caused by an infection. In planning care for her you base your plan on physiological principles.

1. Temperature is the balance between heat production and heat loss. When heat is lost from direct transference to another object, this is heat lost by:
   a. Convection.
   b. Conduction.
   c. Radiation.
   d. Evaporation.

2. Mrs. Jones' fever alternates between periods of elevation and periods of normal temperature. The type of fever this represents is:
   a. Intermittent fever.
   b. Stadium fever.
   c. Remittent fever.
   d. Inconsistent fever.

3. Which of the following would be the best nursing implementation for Mrs. Jones?
   a. Encourage protein-rich foods.
   b. Keep her warmly covered.
   c. Encourage activity.
   d. Encourage fluid.

4. A tepid bath is ordered for Mrs. Jones. The term that best describes tepid is:
   a. Ice cold.
   b. Slightly cool.
   c. Room temperature.
   d. Slightly warm.

5. If Mrs. Jones is very short of breath and breathing heavily, which method of temperature-taking would reflect the best assessment technique?
   a. Rectal temperature.
   b. Oral temperature with an electronic thermometer.
   c. Oral temperature with a glass thermometer.
   d. Axillary temperature with an oral thermometer.

6. Which of the following is considered a normal rectal body temperature?
   a. 97.6°F
   b. 98.6°F
   c. 99.6°F
   d. 100.6°F

7. In an adult, which of the following reflects the best rectal temperature-taking assessment technique?
   a. Slant the thermometer toward the umbilicus.
   b. Slant the thermometer toward the spinal column.
   c. Insert the thermometer only the length of the bulb.
   d. Use a dry, nonlubricated bulb for best accuracy.

8. As an implementation of care, Mrs. Jones has been offered warm wet dressings. The usual length of time that heat applications are left in place is:
   a. 10 minutes.
   b. 20 to 30 minutes.
   c. 40 to 60 minutes.
   d. 60 to 90 minutes.

9. The best place on your body to test the temperature of a warm compress would be:
   a. The palm of your hand.
   b. Your inner wrist.
   c. Your neck.
   d. The lateral surface of your hand.

10. The immediate effect of heat on circulation is:
    a. Vasodilatation.
    b. Vessel spasm.
    c. Decreased viscosity of blood.
    d. Vasoconstriction.

34. NUTRITION IN HEALTH

OBJECTIVES

Upon mastery of the material in this chapter, you should be able to:

1. Define nutrition, malnutrition, overnutrition, and undernutrition.
2. Describe the roles of carbohydrate, protein, fat, vitamins, and minerals in nutrition.
3. Describe the effects of different life span changes on nutrition requirements or preferences.
4. Describe the meaning of food for people.
5. Describe the regulations concerning food labeling and the importance of food labeling in consumer awareness.
6. Describe the Dietary Guidelines for the United States and the implication these guidelines will have on diets.

TERMS

The terms important for an understanding of this chapter are shown below and defined in the glossary:

appetite
basal metabolic rate
hunger
kilocalorie
nutrition
obesity
satiety

Nutrition is the process by which a person receives and utilizes the materials necessary for the maintenance and growth of body cells, synthesis of enzymes and hormones, production of energy, resistance to infection, and capacity for reproduction, activity, and a sense of well-being.

Nutrition is deficient when a person is taking in inadequate amounts of nutrients that are essential for normal body function or when his body cannot utilize the ingested nutrients. The deficiency is *primary* if the diet is at fault. It is *secondary* if some body process interferes with ingestion (taking in of food), digestion (breakdown of food), absorption (transfer of nutrients from the gastrointestinal tract into the bloodstream), transport (movement of nutrients to cells), or utilization (use of nutrients by a cell). Rickets, for example, which is a malformation of bone in children, can occur if there is a deficiency of vitamin D or calcium in the diet. This would be a primary deficiency. Vitamin D is a fat-soluble vitamin. It can be absorbed across the intestine only with fat. Rickets, therefore, may also occur as a secondary deficiency in diseases in which fat cannot be absorbed, such as celiac disease.

NUTRITIONAL STATES

Although sometimes used interchangeably, poor nutritional states can be categorized as malnutrition, undernutrition, or overnutrition.

Undernutrition

Undernutrition occurs when a diet is inadequate in *quantity* (the person does not eat enough because either food is not available or he chooses not to eat). Large numbers of people in developing countries throughout the world are undernourished because not enough food is produced in those countries to supply everyone adequately. Dieters may become undernourished if their food intake is too low. Minimal undernutrition is dangerous because it leads to susceptibility to infection due to lack of body resistance and to lethargy or tiredness. Gross undernutrition is manifest as protein deficiency disease with poor weight gain; when extreme, this is fatal.

Malnutrition

Malnutrition occurs when a diet is inadequate in *quality* (although a person may eat an adequate amount of food, essential nutrients are missing from the diet due to poor food selection).

If a person is minimally malnourished, he will develop signs of illness such as poor weight gain and lethargy or tiredness. Specific nutrient lacks will result in specific diseases such as rickets (malformation of bone structure due to lack of vitamin D), scurvy (malformation of cartilage due to lack of vitamin C), and pellagra (a skin and neurological syndrome caused by lack of niacin). A person with gross malnutrition may develop diseases such as kwashiorkor (imbalance of body fluids) or marasmus (wasted body tissue), both of which are protein-deficiency diseases.

A person is said to be marginally malnourished when he has no overt signs or symptoms of nutrient lack but laboratory analysis of his blood shows deficiencies. Such people are more prone to acquire infectious diseases than those who are well nourished. It is not uncommon for a person who is hospitalized for an extended period of time to become marginally malnourished:

Overnutrition

Overnutrition implies that the person's diet has excessive amounts of calories and fat; at the same time, he may be very deficient in other body needs such as protein and minerals. Such a diet pattern tends to occur only in countries such as the United States where food supplies are plentiful. Overnutrition leads to obesity (a body weight greater than 20 percent of normal weight for height). Obesity is potentially dangerous because it leads to increased stress on cardiac and vascular functions.

METABOLISM OF FOOD

Energy is produced by many actions—electrical, mechanical, and chemical, for example. Electrical energy is measured in kilowatts, mechanical energy in kilogram weight. The energy found in food is chemical energy and is measured in kilocalories (kcal). A kcal is the amount of energy necessary to increase 1 kilogram of water 1 degree Celcius in temperature.

Kilocalorie Measurements

The amount of kilocalories that foods produce has been carefully analyzed, and tables of kilocalories in food are commonly available. Foods differ greatly in the amount of energy they produce depending on the composition of the food. For example, 1 gm of a carbohydrate food releases 4 kcal of energy when metabolized; 1 gm of a protein food also releases 4 kcal. One gram of fat, however, releases 9 kcal; 1 gm of alcohol releases 7 kcal. Depending on which foods are eaten during the day, therefore, the kcal total can increase or decrease by large amounts. The average man needs to consume a diet that supplies about 2700 kcal per day; an average woman needs about 2000 kcal per day. Different kcal needs for different age groups are shown in Table 34-1.

TABLE 34-1. KILOCALORIE REQUIREMENTS FOR DIFFERENT AGE GROUPS

Age group	Kilocalorie requirement (kcal/kg body weight)
Newborn	120
Infant	
0—6 months	115
7—11 months	105
Toddler	
1—3 years	1300
Preschooler	
4—6 years	1700
Schoolager	
7—10 years	2400
Adolescent	
11—14 years	
boys	2700
girls	2200
15—18 years	
boys	2800
girls	2100
Young adult	
19—22 years	
men	2900
women	2100
Middle-aged adult	
23—50 years	
men	2700
women	2000
Older adult	
51—75 years	
men	2400
women	1800
76 years and older	
men	2050
women	1600
Pregnant woman	+300
Lactating woman	+500

Process of Metabolism of Food

The metabolism of food is the process whereby food is broken down and energy is released from it for cell use. The combined processes of chewing, stomach and intestinal mechanical action, intestinal absorption, and transport through the bloodstream are integrated to supply cells with the necessary substances for function—amino acids, glucose, fatty acids, vitamins, minerals, and water.

At any point when not enough nutrients are being supplied by the digestive system (between meals, for example) the body has a failsafe system that it can use to break down glycogen (a storage form of glucose), fat, and protein into their basic components for use in cell maintenance. This breakdown process is termed *catabolism*. Catabolism of food or body substances *releases* energy for cell use.

When a cell is utilizing basic nutrients to make glycogen, fat, or protein, the process is called *anabolism*. The process of anabolism *requires* energy. Following major trauma or surgery, a person needs a good nutrient supply to allow sufficient anabolic healing to take place.

Basal Metabolic Rate

The basal metabolic rate (BMR) is the minimum amount of energy needed by the body at rest or the minimal rate at which kilocalories are spent for such maintenance activities as respiration, circulation, metabolism, gland function, and regulation of temperature. When a person's basal metabolic rate increases for any reason, his need for kilocalories increases. Basal metabolic rates vary greatly from person to person and from periods of resting to strenuous activity. As a rule, the younger the person, the higher the BMR, because BMR decreases by about 2 percent for every 10 years of life. Sex also affects BMR (females have a BMR that is lower than that of males by 5 to 10 percent, probably because they have less muscle mass and require less kilocalories).

A great deal of heat produced by metabolism is spent on maintaining body temperature. People need more calories in winter than in summer because more body heat must be produced in cold weather than in warm. Fever increases the BMR dramatically, calling for a great increase in required kilocalories. The greater the amount of surface area (skin area) a person has, the greater the amount of heat loss, and consequently, the greater the rate of metabolism needed to maintain temperature. The taller a person is, the greater is his surface area. A tall person, therefore, generally has a higher BMR than a shorter person. Adipose (fat) tissue requires little oxygen for maintenance; a person with a high percentage of adipose tissue (an obese person) therefore tends to have a lower BMR than one with a high percentage of muscle tissue. Epinephrine released in response to a stress situation increases the BMR; both the amount of thyroxine released by the thyroid gland and the amount of growth hormone released by the pituitary gland influence the BMR.

BMR increases during pregnancy to supply the energy required for new cell building. The amount of energy needed per day for people of different ages is based not only on the basal metabolic rate but also on physical needs, growth needs, and the energy required for metabolism (specific dynamic action of food).

Recommended Dietary Allowances (RDA)

The Food and Nutrition Board of the National Academy of Sciences has established recommendations not only for kilocalories but for protein and certain vitamins and minerals as well (Table 34-2). Such requirements reflect the needs of healthy people and do not take into consideration special needs arising from infection, metabolic disorders, chronic diseases, or other problems that would require additional dietary considerations. When a single RDA recommendation is quoted, it is usually quoted at the highest level needed for any age group of that nutrient. Adults need, for example, 10 mg of iron daily; adolescent girls need 18 mg. The RDA for iron is often, therefore, listed as 18 mg (the highest level). The exception to this is the recommendation for energy (kcal) requirements. Here, the recommendation is usually quoted at the mean (the average) need.

RDA recommendations are so adequate that many dietitians feel that if a person consumes two-thirds of the RDA they will receive adequate nutrients.

Basic Food Groups and Nutrition

Because no food (with the exception of breast milk for a newborn) contains all nutrients necessary for good nutrition, a person must vary the foods he eats or he will not get enough of the nutrients found principally in the food group he avoids.

To help people choose foods that will provide a balanced diet, the National Dairy Council formerly divided foods into four basic groups. Recently a fifth group including fats has been added. If a person eats foods from all five groups during a week's time, he can feel confident that he is receiving good nutrition.

Table 34-3 shows foods included in the basic five food groups and the recommended number of servings of each group for different age groups. Note that legumes (beans and peas) are included in the meat group because they contain high quantities of protein or are more like meat in protein value than they are like the vegetable group. No recommended amounts are given for the fats group because the recommendations for this group are still controversial.

In addition to the foods recommended by Table 34-3, other foods and beverages may be eaten according to individual preferences.

NUTRIENTS IN HEALTH

There are six classes of nutrients necessary for cell function and growth: carbohydrates, protein, fat, minerals, vitamins, and water. The functions of these are summarized in Table 34-4.

Carbohydrates as Nutrients

Carbohydrates are the chief source of energy for body cells. They are compounds containing carbon, hydrogen, and water (the name *carbohydrate* means "hydrogenated carbon"). They can be divided into three categories: monosaccharides, disaccharides, and polysaccharides.

Monosaccharides. Monosaccharides are termed *simple* sugars because they cannot be broken down into less complex compounds. Glucose is the most abundant of this type of carbohydrate in the human body; it is the only form of carbohydrate that can enter cells to supply energy. Fructose (found in fruit) and galactose (not found free in nature but as a breakdown product of lactose in milk) are other examples of monosaccharides.

Disaccharides. Disaccharides are *compound* sugars formed by the synthesis of two monosaccharides. Common disaccharides found in food are sucrose (table sugar, composed of fructose and glucose), lactose

TABLE 34-2. RECOMMENDED DIETARY ALLOWANCES (RDA), 1980[a]

Age (yr)	Weight (kg)	Weight (lbs)	Height (cm)	Height (in)	Protein (g)	Vitamin A (RE)	Vitamin D (μg)	Vitamin E (mg)	Vitamin C (mg)	Thiamine (mg)	Riboflavin (mg)	Niacin (mg equiv.)	Vitamin B_6 (mg)	Folacin (μg)	Vitamin B_{12} (μg)	Calcium (mg)	Phosphorus (mg)	Magnesium (mg)	Iron (mg)	Zinc (mg)	Iodine (μg)
Infants																					
0.0—0.5	6	13	60	24	kg × 2.2	420	10	3	35	0.3	0.4	6	0.3	30	0.5	360	240	50	10	3	40
0.5—1.0	9	20	71	28	kg × 2.0	400	10	4	35	0.5	0.6	8	0.6	45	1.5	540	360	70	15	5	50
Children																					
1—3	13	29	90	35	23	400	10	5	45	0.7	0.8	9	0.9	100	2.0	800	800	150	15	10	70
4—6	20	44	112	44	30	500	10	6	45	0.9	1.0	11	1.3	200	2.5	800	800	200	10	10	90
7—10	28	62	132	52	34	700	10	7	45	1.2	1.4	16	1.6	300	3.0	800	800	250	10	10	120
Males																					
11—14	45	99	157	62	45	1,000	10	8	50	1.4	1.6	18	1.8	400	3.0	1,200	1,200	350	18	15	150
15—18	66	145	176	69	56	1,000	10	10	60	1.4	1.7	18	2.0	400	3.0	1,200	1,200	400	18	15	150
19—22	70	154	177	70	56	1,000	7.5	10	60	1.5	1.7	19	2.2	400	3.0	800	800	350	10	15	150
23—50	70	154	178	70	56	1,000	5	10	60	1.4	1.6	18	2.2	400	3.0	800	800	350	10	15	150
51+	70	154	178	70	56	1,000	5	10	60	1.2	1.4	16	2.2	400	3.0	800	800	350	10	15	150
Females																					
11—14	46	101	157	62	46	800	10	8	50	1.1	1.3	15	1.8	400	3.0	1,200	1,200	300	18	15	150
15—18	55	120	163	64	46	800	10	8	60	1.1	1.3	14	2.0	400	3.0	1,200	1,200	300	18	15	150
19—22	55	120	163	64	44	800	7.5	8	60	1.1	1.3	14	2.0	400	3.0	800	800	300	18	15	150
23—50	55	120	163	64	44	800	5	8	60	1.0	1.2	13	2.0	400	3.0	800	800	300	18	15	150
51+	55	120	163	64	44	800	5	8	60	1.0	1.2	13	2.0	400	3.0	800	800	300	10	15	150
Pregant					+30	+200	+5	+2	+20	+0.4	+0.3	+2	+0.6	+400	+1.0	+400	+400	+150	[b]	+5	+25
Lactating					+20	+400	+5	+3	+40	+0.5	+0.5	+5	+0.5	+100	+1.0	+400	+400	+150	[b]	+10	+50

[a]The allowances are intended to provide for individual variations among most normal, healthy people in the United States under usual environmental stresses. They were designed for the maintenance of good nutrition. Diets should be based on a variety of common foods in order to provide other nutrients for which human requirements have been less well defined.
[b]Supplemental iron is recommended.
Source: From *Recommended Dietary Alowances*, 9th ed. (1980), with the permission of the National Academy of Sciences, Washington, D.C.

TABLE 34-3. BASIC FIVE FOOD GROUPS

Group	Recommended Servings per Day	Examples of Comparable Servings
Meat	2	2—3 oz cooked lean meat, fish, or poultry 2—3 eggs 1—1-1/2 cup cooked dry beans or dry peas
Milk—dairy	2—3 (children under 9 years)	8 oz milk (whole, skim, or buttermilk; reconstituted, evaporated, or dry)
	3—4 (children 9—12 years)	1-1/3 oz cheddar cheese
	4 (adolescents)	1-1/3 cup cottage cheese
	2 (adults)	1-2/3 cup ice cream
	3—4 (pregnant women)	1 cup yogurt
	4—5 (lactating women)	1 cup pudding (made with milk)
Vegetable—fruit	4 or more servings, including 1-1/2 servings of good sources of vitamin C daily; 1 source of vitamin A 3—4 times per week	3/4 cup fruit juice 1 medium fruit 3/4 cup raw vegetable 1/2 cup cooked vegetable
Bread—cereal	4 or more	1 slice bread 1 oz (1 cup) dry cereal 1/2 to 3/4 cup cooked cereal 1/2 to 3/4 cup cooked spaghetti or macaroni
Fats*		

*Some fat such as butter, margarine, salad dressing, or oil should be included daily. The recommended amount and type of fat has not yet been determined.
Source: National Dairy Council, Rosemont, Ill.

(the sugar of milk, composed of galactose and glucose), and maltose (composed of two glucose units and found in germinating seeds).

Polysaccharides. Polysaccharides consist of many monosaccharide units. Starches, celluloses, and pectin substances are examples. Cellulose is the main component of the cell wall of plants; pectin is a plant cell cement. Human beings have difficulty digesting cellulose and pectin, which are plant fibers. Many of these carbohydrate sources therefore pass unused through the body. They should be included in the diet, however, because they provide bulk that is important for peristaltic movements of the intestine and because they help maintain bowel tone (which apparently prevents diverticulitis or an outpouching of the intestinal walls due to loss of tone); they also lower blood cholesterol levels by absorbing bile salts and removing bile and cholesterol from the body. By absorbing toxic contaminants from food, fiber may reduce the possibility of colon cancer. Interestingly, bran, the fiber of wheat and the fiber most frequently recommended to be included in diets, does not lower blood cholesterol levels, although it is important in all other factors mentioned.

Starches are a plant's stored supply of carbohydrate. Digestive enzymes can effectively change starch into glucose and prepare it for cell use.

METABOLISM OF CARBOHYDRATES

Amylase, a salivary enzyme excreted by the parotid glands, begins the breakdown of carbohydrate. Amylase touches more food and works more efficiently when food is chewed well. Although hydrochloric acid in the stomach acts on strands of carbohydrates to cause further breakdown, the stomach does not play a major role in carbohydrate metabolism. When carbohydrate reaches the intestine, pancreatic amylase acts on starches first to reduce them to maltose, sucrose, and lactose, and then to reduce them ultimately to glucose. Glucose is absorbed across the intestinal walls into the portal bloodstream. It passes through the liver before being released into the systemic bloodstream. Some glucose is used by cells for instant energy; the compound that traps glucose in cells for use is adenosine triphosphate (ATP). Once ATP has caused a cell to store adequate energy, any extra glucose that is taken in (overnourishment) is converted into glycogen (a polysaccharide) and stored in the liver and muscle against future energy requirements. If even more additional glucose is present, it is stored in cells as fat. The body keeps about a half day's supply of glycogen in the liver and muscle. The body's ability to store fat appears to be limitless (the heaviest man known weighed 1,000 pounds).

Glycogen can be readily reconstituted to glucose by the action of epinephrine when it is needed for energy. Although stored fat can be utilized for energy also, it is no longer accessible as a source of glucose. (It is utilized as fatty acids; this provides energy but unfortunately releases an abundance of acid substances that lower the body pH level, making the breakdown of fat for energy a less than preferable source.)

Both insulin and oxygen must be available for utilization of glucose by cells. A person who is without glucose, oxygen, or insulin (secreted by the pancreas), therefore, will suffer cell death (without oxygen or

TABLE 34-4. ESSENTIAL NUTRIENTS FOR NUTRITION

Nutrient	Function in Body	Food Sources	Results of Deficiency
Carbohydrates	Major energy source after it is broken down to glucose	Fruits, table sugar, vegetables (starches in vegetables are reduced to glucose)	Cells cannot function without glucose as energy source
Proteins	Formation of cells, enzymes, antibodies; fluid balance; reserve energy supply	Meats and milk products are complete sources; vegetables are incomplete sources	Stunted growth, susceptibility to infection; edema
Lipids	Structure of cell walls; transport of fat-soluble vitamins; reserve energy supply	Animal sources yield saturated fat; vegetable sources yield polyunsaturated fats	Deficiency of fat-soluble vitamins; poor skin formation
Water	Necessary for metabolism or use of all other nutrients	Drinking water; some water in all foods but dried forms	Dehydration; increased temperature; ineffective body function
Minerals	Necessary for varied functions of cell growth and enzyme production	Found in varied amounts in almost all foods	Reduced body function depending on specific mineral action
Vitamins	Necessary for cell growth and maintenance	Fat-soluble vitamins in fish and plant oils; C vitamin in fruit; B complex vitamins in meat and vegetables	Reduced cell function specific to individual vitamin action

insulin, cells will starve even in the presence of adequate glucose). There is still one more reason why the presence of carbohydrate is important in the diet. Carbohydrate must be present for immediate use by vital brain cells and also has an important "protein-sparing" action. Because the energy needs of the body take precedence over other needs, if inadequate carbohydrate is available in the diet, the body will utilize protein for energy. If this happens over a long period of time, growth will halt because not enough protein is left for normal cell growth.

Foods high in carbohydrates are always plant sources. Foods high in glucose are those that are either naturally high in glucose or are artificially sweetened to improve taste. Table 34-5 summarizes the differences in kcal of a number of common foods.

TABLE 34-5. KILOCALORIE CONTENT OF COMMON FOODS

Food	Portion	Kilocalories
Meat group		
Hamburger	3 oz	245
Tuna (in oil)	3 oz	170
Peanut butter	1 tbs	95
Sirloin steak	3 oz	330
Dairy group		
Whole milk	1 cup	160
Ice cream	1 cup	255
American cheese	1 oz	105
Egg	1	80
Fruit—vegetable group		
Apple	1	70
Orange	1	65
Potato chips	10	115
Raisins	1.5 tbs	40
Bread—cereal group		
White bread	1 slice	75
Yellow cake	1 slice	200
Corn flakes	1 cup	100
Macaroni	1 cup	155
Rice	1 cup	225

DIFFICULTIES OF CARBOHYDRATE METABOLISM

Difficulty with carbohydrate metabolism can lead to either local or systemic body effects.

Dental Caries. Bacteria in the mouth act on sugar to convert sugar into *dextran* or plaque, a thick polymer on which bacteria thrive. Acid (mainly lactic acid) produced by these bacteria lowers the pH of the mouth. When the pH reaches 5.5, saliva is acid enough to begin to etch and erode tooth enamel. As a rule, the more concentrated the sugar load a person ingests, the more cavities will be produced. The longer the time the pH remains lowered, the deeper will be the enamel erosion. Sweet liquids such as soda are particularly cariogenic because their bubbling action carries sugar to hard-to-clean tooth surfaces.

The best rules for keeping teeth cavity-free are to drink fluorinated water and use a fluoride-based toothpaste to strengthen tooth enamel; brush and floss teeth at least once a day to remove food substances and plaque; avoid gummy, sticky sweets that stay in contact with teeth for a long time (eat an easily dissolved chocolate bar, not a chewy taffy one); and eat sweets with meals, not between meals to shorten the number of minutes each day that teeth are surrounded by a low pH level.

Night Bottle Syndrome. When a baby is put to bed at night with a propped bottle of formula or orange juice, the liquid will pool around his teeth and remain in contact with them throughout the night. Because the child's tongue tends to cover his anterior lower teeth, these are protected, but decay of the upper teeth and lower posterior teeth occurs. To prevent this, a mother should hold and feed an infant until he falls asleep and then put him to bed without a bottle. If an infant refuses to fall asleep without a propped bottle, the mother can avoid night bottle syndrome by filling a bottle with only clear water.

Lactose Intolerance. Some people (mainly blacks, Orientals, and persons from South and Central America) lack lactase, the enzyme necessary for the digestion of lactose, the sugar in milk. When lactose is not processed by this enzyme, it passes into the intestine unchanged where, fermented by bacteria, it causes diarrhea and intestinal cramping. The manifestation of lactase deficiency is not necessarily seen in infancy; by school age, children with the deficiency begin to complain of "not liking" milk or "not feeling well" after drinking milk. They may fail to thrive because of chronic nutrient loss due to persistent diarrhea.

Persons who are unable to drink milk need to include other sources that are high in calcium and vitamin D in their diets such as green leafy vegetables (calcium) and fish oils (vitamin D). Such people can usually eat cheese because during cheese processing, lactose is converted to lactic acid. During pregnancy, when calcium needs are very high so that a firm fetal skeleton can be built, people who cannot drink milk may have to take a daily calcium supplement.

Obesity. Obesity is defined as a body weight greater than 20 percent of normal weight for height. It occurs because a person takes in more calories than his body can utilize. These excess calories are converted to fat and stored. People who become obese as infants apparently build *excess* fat cells. People who become obese as adults do not build new cells but merely *expand* existing ones. This may be one reason why people who are obese as infants have such difficulty in losing weight later in life even when strongly motivated (they have more adipose cells than other people).

People from low socioeconomic areas tend to have more obesity than those from upper socioeconomic levels. One reason is that high calorie foods (noodles, spaghetti) are inexpensive; lower calorie foods such as lean meat are more expensive.

Helping an overweight person to take in fewer calories every day is important in helping him to reduce weight. Also important is encouraging the person to increase his activity level. Some people are able to maintain weight reduction programs by themselves; others enjoy and need the companionship of weight-reduction groups to do this successfully. Behavioral modification techniques such as using a small plate so that small portions of food look bigger, eating slowly, putting down the fork between each bite so that a small meal takes longer to consume, and never eating except at a table (to prevent snacking in front of the television set or before falling asleep at night) are effective aids in weight-reduction programs.

Because obesity is strongly associated with heart disease, cerebrovascular accidents (stroke), hypertension (high blood pressure), and adult-onset diabetes weight should be maintained at as near normal a level as possible. Sweet foods are comforting, however. Some people eat (particularly sweets) when they need comfort. Sugar is devoid of vitamins or minerals. A person who uses carbohydrates as his major food source may be nutritionally deficient in body-building nutrients and, although large in weight, not as well nourished as a person of normal weight. If he should become ill, an obese person may feel the effects of his illness acutely because he lacks healthful body nutritional stores. To improve the nutritional habits of such a person, other rewards or positive reinforcement other than eating may need to be provided.

Protein as a Nutrient

Protein is a Greek word that means "of prime importance," thus implying how essential protein is to body health. Proteins are substances composed of carbon, hydrogen, and oxygen (the same components found in carbohydrates, which is why they can be converted into energy if carbohydrates are not present) and, in addition, about 16 percent nitrogen. Protein is the basic constituent of the nucleus and protoplasm of all cells and is important for the manufacture of enzymes, hormones, and antibodies, the regulation of fluid balance (by regulating osmotic pressure), and the pH of blood (by acting as a buffer). In addition, as mentioned earlier, it also serves as an emergency source of energy.

Protein is built from and can be broken down into complex chains composed of 22 amino acids. It is as amino acids that protein functions in the body. If the body is given the component parts, it can construct most amino acids needed for cell growth. Eight amino acids cannot be constructed in the body, however. These are termed *essential* amino acids and must be ingested daily. They are listed below:

Arginine*
Histidine*
Isoleucine
Leucine
Lysine
Methionine
Phenylalanine
Threonine
Tryptophan
Valine

*Whether arginine for all ages and histidine for adults are truly essential has not been fully established.

If a cell begins to synthesize new protein from the amino acids supplied to it by the bloodstream and then discovers it does not have all the amino acids it needs, it does not stop and conserve those amino acids it does have, waiting for the missing one; it rejects everything and allows the amino acids to pass by and be excreted from the body. The lack of the essential amino acids, therefore, does not mean that merely *some* new protein is not formed; it means that *no* new protein is formed. As a rule, protein foods are best metabolized if they are spaced throughout the day to provide cell building material more constantly.

If a protein contains all essential amino acids it is said to be *complete*. Protein from animal sources (meat, milk, eggs) tends to be complete. Protein with less than all the essential amino acids is termed *incomplete*. Vegetable and plant sources of protein are incomplete; this does not mean that these sources are ineffective, however, because by careful balancing and mixing of incomplete proteins, a meal can be constructed that includes all the essential amino acids. Legumes (kidney beans, soybeans, garden peas, black-eyed peas, lentils, and lima beans) are good vegetable sources of incomplete protein. Legumes and grains (beans and rice) generally combine to form sources of complete protein. A rule of thumb that can be used to increase the quality of incomplete protein sources is to combine an incomplete protein with a complete one at the same meal (baked beans and wieners, ham and green pea soup). Two incomplete proteins that when combined include all essential amino acids are termed *complementary* proteins.

Nitrogen Balance. Amino acids and nitrogen are constantly being used by cells. As cells outlive their lifetime and are broken down in the body, nitrogen is released from them and then excreted by the kidneys. A person who retains more nitrogen than he loses, incorporating more of it into cell building than he excretes, is said to be in a *positive* nitrogen balance (a healthy state). When cell breakdown exceeds tissue buildup (or when catabolism exceeds anabolism), a *negative* nitrogen balance exists. This can also occur when protein intake is inadequate. Following a major injury a person may break down so many damaged cells that he is in a negative nitrogen balance.

Sufficient carbohydrate and fat intake along with protein allows protein to be spared for cell building because carbohydrate will be used for energy rather than protein. If carbohydrate particularly is not available for energy, protein will be utilized (protein-sparing action is lost), and no body maintenance or growth will take place. This is one reason why high-protein diets for weight loss are not recommended. As fat is broken down for energy (to spare protein) for the person on such a diet, the person can become quickly acidotic from the buildup of fatty acids.

CONSEQUENCES OF PROTEIN MALNUTRITION

Kwashiorkor. Kwashiorkor is a Ghanian word that means "the evil spirit that infects the first child after the second child is born"; it is a protein-deficiency disease. When a child is breast-fed, he receives adequate protein. When he is weaned at the time a second child is born, he is forced to eat a diet consisting mainly of incomplete plant protein if food supplies are scarce. Protein cannot be formed in the body on such a diet and so levels of blood protein fall. Osmotic pressure causes fluid to leave the blood and invade interstitial tissue (edema) because osmotic pressure always moves fluid from areas of lower concentration to areas of higher concentration. When fluid invades the peritoneal space in the abdomen, the abdomen swells (ascites). These symptoms (failure to gain weight, edema, and ascites) are the symptoms of kwashiorkor or of a person with marked inadequate protein intake.

Marasmus. Marasmus, in contrast to kwashiorkor, is a disease caused by almost no calorie or protein intake (starvation). It tends to occur in children in developing countries where there is no food available, but it can occur in infants who are not fed by their mothers (child neglect) even in very affluent communities. The child fails to gain weight and looks emaciated; skin turgor is poor. Because the infant does not have enough carbohydrate or protein intake for energy, he becomes extremely acidotic from the breakdown of stored fat. There is a grave danger that a child with such severe deprivation of protein has not received adequate nutrients for brain growth, and therefore, even after the deficiency has been corrected, he will be left with long-term mental retardation or neurological deficits.

Lipids as Nutrients

Lipids (fats and oils) are a group of substances that are insoluble in water. About 90 percent of the fat in food and stored in the body is in the form of *triglycerides* (formed by three fatty acids attached to glycerol). *Phospholipids* such as lecithin and *sterols* such as cholesterol comprise the other 10 percent. Lipids form the walls of cells, transport fat-soluble vitamins, serve as a reserve supply of energy, and offer body protection by insulating body organs against blows and heat loss.

One gram of fat supplies 9 kcal of energy in contrast to carbohydrate and protein, each of which supplies only 4 kcal per gram. Hunters and hikers are advised to carry fat with them rather than carbohydrate food (crumbled bacon bits rather than a chocolate bar) because for half the weight bulk, they can thereby carry twice the calories. People who must restrict the number of calories they ingest must be careful of their fat intake because with fats they can easily take in excessive calories.

METABOLISM OF FAT

It takes longer for fat to leave the stomach than protein or sugar; eating a meal heavy in fat often produces a feeling of satiety (and perhaps discomfort) for a long time afterward.

Once the fat reaches the small intestine, bile salts begin to emulsify it, and large globules are broken down into small droplets. Once it is in the form of small droplets, enzymes from the pancreas begin to convert it into fine fatty acids. Because lipids are not soluble in water, they must be covered by a layer of protein to form a lipoprotein that can be transported through the bloodstream to cells. Because fatty acids are surrounded by protein for transport, low protein levels in the blood interfere with fat transport and utilization. An overload in the blood of *low*-density lipoproteins (LDL), which are heavy in cholesterol, may be associated with the occurrence of heart attack; an increase of *high*-density lipoproteins (HDL) does not appear to have this effect.

When lipoproteins reach body cells, the fat is removed by the cell for use. Extra fat that the cells do not need is stored in adipose cells for future use.

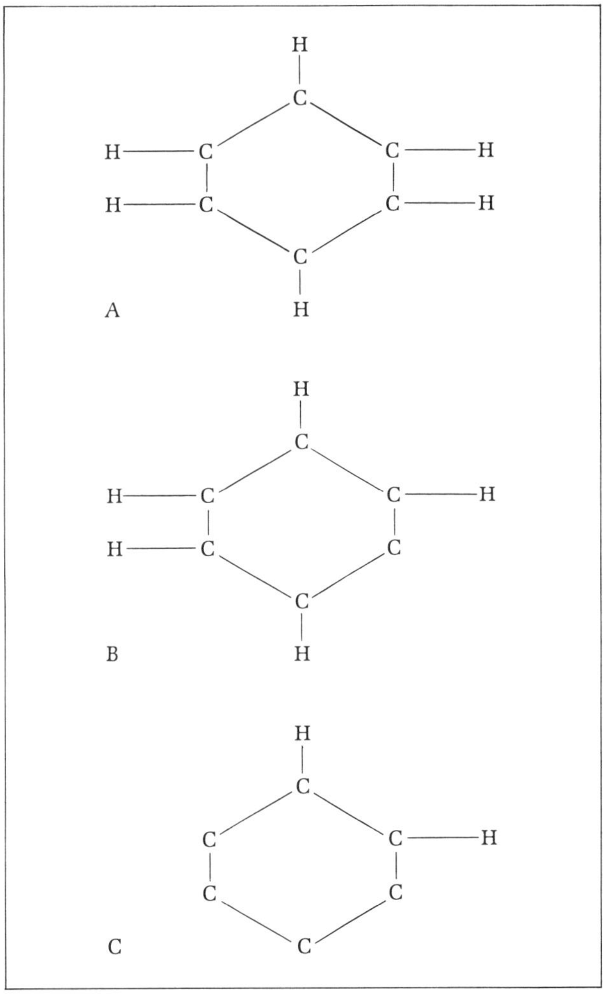

Saturated and Unsaturated Fats. The chemical structure of a fat molecule is shown diagrammatically in Fig. 34-1. If a fat molecule is binding all the hydrogen that it can, it is said to be *saturated* fat. If one hydrogen molecule is missing, the fat is said to be *unsaturated.* If more than one hydrogen molecule is absent, the fat is said to be *polyunsaturated.*

FIGURE 34-1. Chemical structure of fat. A. Saturated fat. B. Unsaturated fat. C. Polyunsaturated fat.

Saturated fats are found in animal sources; they have the effect of increasing cholesterol levels in the bloodstream. Polyunsaturated fats are found in vegetable sources; they tend to lower blood cholesterol levels. Coconut oil, interestingly, although it comes from a plant source, is a saturated oil. Oils can be readily identified as to type because polyunsaturated oils remain liquid at room temperature, whereas hydrogenated or saturated oils are solid at room temperature. Many cooking oils are marked *partially* hydrogenated, which means that they have a higher saturated fat content than those marked low in saturated fats or polyunsaturated.

Essential Fatty Acids. The body can synthesize all essential fatty acids but one—*linoleic acid.* This must be provided in the diet. Linoleic acid is a polyunsaturated fatty acid found widely in plant oils; there is a high content of it in breast milk.

DIFFICULTIES WITH LIPID METABOLISM

Hypercholesterolemia. Cholesterol forms the basic precursor of sex hormones and adrenocortical hormones; it is necessary for the formation of bile salts which aid in the digestion of fat, and it initiates the action that allows sunlight to be converted into vitamin D in the skin. Although cholesterol serves these useful body functions, it has a bad reputation because it can cause plaques to form in the lumina of arteries, narrowing them and blocking blood flow (atherosclerosis) in susceptible individuals. If plaques form in the coronary arteries, the blood supply to the heart may be decreased. If the plugging occurs in the cerebral arteries, a stroke (cerebrovascular accident) may occur.

The cause of plaque formation is controversial, but apparently the smooth muscle that normally lies behind the arterial lining begins to invade the inner wall and spread across its surface. This may happen because of abnormal cell growth similar to malignant growth; perhaps the arterial wall is injured by lack of oxygen, or perhaps cholesterol initiates the change. In any event, once plaque formation begins, the presence of cholesterol contributes to it.

Although a person may have a high blood cholesterol level, only small amounts of cholesterol are ingested. Most of it is manufactured by the body. The liver controls the level of circulating cholesterol and in most people seems to be able to increase excretion of it if the level rises too high. To reduce blood cholesterol levels a person should eat limited amounts of saturated fats (animal sources) and foods with a high cholesterol content (egg yolk and liver), and he should eat more polyunsaturated fats (which seem to lower the circulating level of cholesterol) and a high fiber diet (which removes cholesterol with bile salts from the gastrointestinal tract.) Certain individuals tend to have a high blood cholesterol level despite modified cholesterol intake, probably because of inherited factors.

Linoleic Acid Deficiency. Infants who do not receive enough fat can develop a very severe eczema (dry, flaking, pruritic skin) from a deficiency of linoleic acid. This occurs when an infant is fed skimmed milk (milk from which most of the fat has been removed) as the main dietary staple during the first six months of life.

Minerals as Nutrients

There are 21 minerals that are necessary for body health. Minerals are classified according to the amounts needed daily. If more than 100 mg is needed daily, a mineral is termed a *macronutrient*, or major mineral. If the amount needed is less than 100 mg, it is termed a *micronutrient*, or minor mineral. Major minerals are calcium, phosphorus, chloride, potassium, sulfur, sodium, and magnesium. Minor minerals are fluorine, silicon, vanadium, chromium, manganese, iron, cobalt, nickel, copper, zinc, selenium, molybdenum, tin, and iodine. The classification of a mineral as major or minor does not indicate its importance to the body, only the amount necessary each day. A deficiency of the small amount of iodine needed, for example, would be as serious as a deficiency of calcium or phosphorus, minerals found in large amounts in the body. Sources and functions of minerals are summarized in Table 34-6.

TABLE 34-6. MINERALS ESSENTIAL FOR HEALTH

Mineral	Function in Body	Food Sources	Results of Deficiency
Macronutrients			
Calcium	Formation of bone and teeth; muscle contractility	Milk and milk products, green leafy vegetables	Improper bone growth and maintenance shown by diseases such as rickets in children, osteomalacia and osteoporosis in adults, tetany or muscle spasm
Phosphorus	Formation of bone and teeth; used in cell structure; aids use of glucose	Cheese, milk, whole-grain cereals	Deficiency unlikely as long as calcium and protein needs are met
Sodium	Regulation of fluid volume and pH	Table salt; abundant in most foods except fruit	Deficiency rare but excess leads to hypertension in genetically determined individuals
Chloride	Formation of hydrochloric acid; regulation of body fluid with sodium	Table salt, seafoods, meat, eggs	Deficiency rare except with vomiting, which causes loss of hydrochloric acid
Potassium	Major cation of cells; essential for electrical conduction in muscle and therefore in heart action	Fruits, milk, meat, cereals, legumes, vegetables	Deficiency leading to muscle weakness and heart irritability occurs in people taking diuretics because potassium is excreted with urine
Sulfur	Essential for protein formation and cell growth	Meat, fish, eggs, milk, legumes	Deficiency rare as long as protein intake is adequate
Magnesium	Relaxation of muscles following contraction	Whole-grain cereals, meat, milk, green vegetables	Deficiency leading to muscle contraction may occur with high alcohol consumption because alcohol inhibits metabolism
Micronutrients			
Iodine	Formation of thyroxine and regulation of metabolic rate	Iodized table salt, seafood	Reduced BMR and goiter (enlarged thyroid gland)
Iron	Formation of hemoglobin; transport of oxygen to body cells	Meat, legumes, whole grains, green vegetables	Deficiency leads to microcytic (small) and hypochromic (pale) red blood cells (iron-deficiency anemia); excess leads to infiltration of tissue (hemosiderosis)

TABLE 34-6. (CONTINUED)

Mineral	Function in Body	Food Sources	Results of Deficiency
Copper	Formation of collagen and nerve fiber	Liver, whole grains	No deficiencies known
Fluoride	Reduction of dental caries and demineralization from bone	Drinking water (added by many communities)	Dental caries
Zinc	Formation of eye, male reproductive organs, insulin, and taste sensation	Liver, milk, shellfish	Diabeteslike symptoms due to decreased insulin production; poor taste sensation leading to poor food intake
Manganese	Formation of enzymes	Whole grains, beet greens, legumes	Deficiencies unlikely
Molybdenum	Important for mobilization of iron in body	Legumes, green vegetables, cereals	Deficiencies apparently unknown
Cobalt	Formation of red blood cells in bone marrow	Organ meats, milk (sources of vitamin B_{12})	Deficiencies rare as long as animal food sources are ingested
Selenium	Necessary for immunoglobin formation and prevention of oxidation of cells	Grains, meat, milk	Deficiencies unknown
Chromium	Necessary for glucose metabolism	Whole-grain cereals, meat	Deficiencies seen only in severe malnutrition
Silicon	Necessary for connective tissue and bone growth	Unrefined grains, beer	Retarded growth and bone deformity
Nickel	Necessary for duplication or growth of cells	Grains, vegetables	Deficiencies rare
Vanadium	Necessary for lipid metabolism	Content in foods is little known	Deficiency rare on a well-balanced diet
Tin	Necessary for blood formation	Fat-containing foods	Deficiency rare

MAJOR MINERALS (MACRONUTRIENTS)

Calcium. About 99 percent of the calcium in the body is contained in the bones and teeth. As bone first forms in utero, it is formed as cartilage. Calcium phosphate and calcium bicarbonate crystals gradually invade the cartilage structure and replace it. This makes bones strong enough to support weight by the time the child is born. Bones are never in a static state, however; they consist of cells that are constantly being broken down and reformed, so calcium is constantly necessary for both bone and teeth maintenance.

Although only a small amount of calcium (1 percent) is contained in cells and in blood, its presence in these sites is necessary for muscle contractility and the action of prothrombin in the clotting of blood; it also plays a role in nerve transmission and the function of cells. If the blood level of calcium begins to fall, calcium in bone can be dissolved to maintain the necessary blood level.

Growing children need ample supplies of calcium so that more calcium is deposited in bones than is withdrawn to maintain growth. Calcium absorption from the intestinal tract is influenced by the presence of vitamin D and the presence of hydrochloric acid in the stomach (the more acid there is, the better the absorption) and by the fat content in the stomach (fat and calcium form an insoluble compound preventing absorption); the calcium-phosphorus ratio in the body (calcium and phosphorus are balanced in a 1 : 1 ratio) also influences calcium absorption. Lactose, the sugar in milk, is helpful in making calcium more soluble. Although human breast milk is lower in calcium than cow's milk, it has much more lactose than cow's milk, so actually more calcium is absorbed from breast milk than from cow's milk. Normally, calcium absorption is about 20 percent of that ingested; during pregnancy, a woman absorbs up to 60 percent of calcium ingested, showing the increased need for calcium during this time.

DEFICIENCY OF CALCIUM. If growing children do not receive enough calcium, they may develop rickets, a bone malformation manifested by bowed legs (Fig. 34-2). In adults, osteomalacia (reduced calcium content in bones) is a serious disorder. In both instances, the deficiency may not be lack of calcium in the diet but lack of vitamin D, which prevents absorption of calcium.

Osteoporosis is a disease of older adults in which calcium is withdrawn from the bones and not replaced. This probably is the result of a long-term calcium deficiency. Osteoporosis is most prevalent in women with low estrogen levels. Many nutritionists are now recommending that postmenopausal women take a daily estrogen supplement to prevent osteoporosis. If

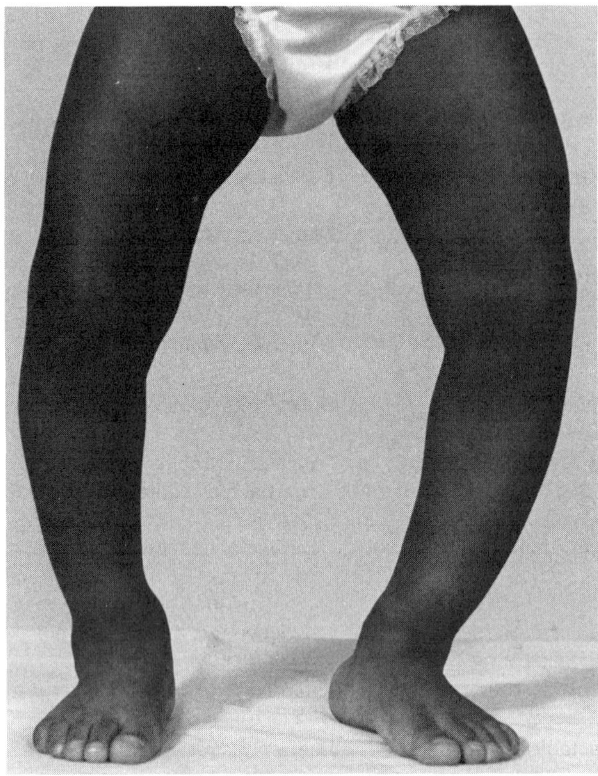

FIGURE 34-2. Bowed legs from rickets, a vitamin D deficiency. Vitamin D is necessary for utilization of calcium.

blood calcium levels fall excessively low, tetany or spasm of muscle occurs. This extreme decrease in calcium is generally the result of metabolic hormone influences, however, rather than a deficiency in food intake.

Milk is the main source of calcium for most people. Yogurt, cheese, and ice cream are also good sources. Butter is not a good source because calcium is not particularly soluble when combined with fat. Dark green vegetables and fish such as salmon with edible bones are fairly good sources. People who cannot drink milk (because they are lactose-intolerant or allergic to milk) are most apt to be calcium deficient.

Phosphorus. About 85 percent of phosphorus is bound in bones as calcium phosphate. It is also a part of all body cells and is therefore important in all cell functions and growth. Because phosphorus is contained in so many foods, a deficiency of phosphorus is almost unknown. Most foods that are high in calcium or protein are also high in phosphorus content. If a person has an adequate calcium and protein intake, he probably will receive enough phosphorus.

Sodium. Sodium is instrumental in regulating the amount of water retained by the body. Kidneys filter sodium out of the body in the proximal tubules and then return as much as is needed in the distal tubules. There is rarely a shortage of sodium in the body because it is found in so many foods and because the kidneys can conserve it if needed. The use of highly salted foods may lead to high blood pressure (hypertension) because a high level of sodium holds excess fluid in the circulatory system. "Soul food" which contains a great deal of salt pork, may tend to cause hypertension in those who eat it. Preserved foods such as cold cuts, pickles, and potato chips are also sources of high sodium content. Sodium has been removed recently from many baby foods so that infants are not exposed to elevated levels that could lead to hypertension at this early stage in life.

Chloride. Chloride is found in salt as sodium chloride. It is found in the body in large amounts in extracellular fluid and as hydrochloric acid in the stomach. It is important for fluid regulation and the pH balance of the body.

Potassium. Potassium is necessary for electrical conduction in muscle and is essential for heart action. An early sign of potassium deficiency is muscle weakness due to lack of proper nervous conduction. Potassium deficiency is rare because potassium occurs in so many foods. People who take diuretics (to promote urine flow) may lose excessive amounts of potassium because it tends to be swept out of the body with large quantities of urine; potassium-sparing diuretics prevent this problem. If a person perspires a great deal, potassium may be lost in large amounts. Foods rich in potassium are fruits, meats, cereals, vegetables, and legumes.

Sulfur. Sulfur is instrumental in helping to form the structure of protein molecules; it is necessary for insulin formation and therefore indirectly for glucose metabolism. There is no RDA for sulfur. Deficiencies are rare.

Magnesium. Magnesium is found in very small amounts in the body; most of it is contained in bones. It works to relax muscles after contraction and promotes resistance to tooth decay by holding calcium in tooth enamel. Deficiencies may occur in people taking diuretics or in those with limited food intake such as post-operative patients.

A serious deficiency can lead to prolonged muscle contraction simulating calcium deficiency. It may be responsible for the hallucinations experienced by alcoholics during alcohol withdrawal (alcohol interferes with magnesium absorption and so increases the need for magnesium). Good sources of magnesium are nuts, cereals, dark green vegetables, seafood, chocolate, and legumes.

MINOR MINERALS (MICRONUTRIENTS)

Iodine. Iodine occurs in the body in extremely small proportions but is vitally important for health and well being. Iodine is necessary for the production of thyroxine, the hormone of the thyroid gland. Thyroxine regulates cell metabolism.

Because sea water is high in iodine, seafood is the chief source of iodine for most people. In areas where the soil is poor in iodine (the Great Lakes and plains states) causing foods grown there to contain small amounts of this mineral, people are advised to use iodized salt to ensure a good iodine intake. Inadequate iodine in the diet causes the thyroid gland to enlarge (hypertrophy) trying to make enough thyroxine. The enlarged gland forms a large bulge in the anterior throat (goiter). The person will be lethargic and may gain excessive weight because of lack of thyroxine and therefore improper metabolism.

Iron. Most iron is found in the body as hemoglobin, the protein substance in red blood cells that carries oxygen to body cells, and as transferrin, iron that is free in the bloodstream. Without iron, hemoglobin formation is inadequate and the person has iron deficiency anemia. With iron deficiency anemia the red blood cells are smaller (microcytic) and paler (hypochromic) than normal; the body is constantly tired due to poor cell oxygenation. It is easy to become deficient in iron because a person absorbs only about 10 to 20 percent of the iron consumed. People need additional iron during periods of rapid growth—infancy, adolescence, and pregnancy; iron is absorbed more efficiently during these times. Iron absorption at all times is most efficient in the presence of vitamin C, an acid medium, and calcium.

Because iron is so important to the body, it is carefully conserved. As red blood cells are broken down, iron is separated and reserved by the bone marrow to be included in the formation of new red blood cells. Even with this conservation of iron, a woman with a heavy menstrual flow may lose considerable amounts of iron each month and become iron deficient. Elderly people tend to have low stomach acidity, which decreases the absorption of iron.

Iron deficiency anemia is a major nutritional problem in the United States. It is most common in areas of low socioeconomic levels (iron-rich foods such as meat are expensive). Infants who drink milk to the exclusion of iron-rich foods are especially at risk. Babies are born with iron stores that will last for three to six months. After this time iron deficiency anemia will occur if foods rich in iron are not ingested. Foods rich in iron are meat, green leafy vegetables, and dried fruits. Eating large quantities of vitamin C increases iron absorption.

Zinc. High concentrations of zinc are present in the eye and in the male reproductive organs. It is important in general protein synthesis and in wound healing; it is associated with insulin production and therefore is necessary for glucose metabolism. People with zinc deficiency experience lack of taste sensation and poor growth; males have poor sexual development or function. Good sources of zinc are meat, oysters, milk, egg yolks, and whole grains.

Copper. Copper is necessary for the formation of hemoglobin; it appears to aid in the formation of collagen and nerve fibers. Good food sources are grains, shellfish, organ meats, and vegetables. Because it occurs in so many foods, copper deficiency is rare.

Fluoride. Fluoride protects children's teeth from tooth decay; it helps to make bone in elderly people more resistant to osteoporosis (loss of calcium). Fluoride is found naturally in drinking water. Many communities add fluoride to the water supply to supplement the natural level and bring the concentration of fluoride up to one part per million. Overfluoridation (over one part per million) can lead to mottled or discolored teeth. People need to be aware that because a little of something is good for them, a lot is not always better.

Selenium. Selenium apparently prevents oxidation of cells in a way that is similar to the action of vitamin E. It is apparently necessary for the formation of immunoglobulins and is therefore helpful in preventing infections. It occurs in so many foods that deficiencies are rare.

Chromium. Chromium works with insulin, facilitating the uptake of glucose by cells. Without it, insulin release is inadequate, and diabetes-like symptoms develop. Brewers yeast is an excellent source, as are whole-grain cereals and meats.

Cobalt. Cobalt is different from other minerals because it is supplied to the body as a component of vitamin B_{12}. It is necessary for the maturation of blood cells.

Silicon. Silicon is necessary for growth of bone and connective tissue. It is found in the body in very minute amounts.

Vanadium. Vanadium is necessary for lipid metabolism. Without it, levels of both cholesterol and triglycerides rise. Little is known about the vanadium content of food, but in a well-balanced diet, a deficiency is unlikely.

Tin. Tin is necessary for blood formation. It is found in fat-containing foods. A deficiency is rare except in severely fat restricted diets.

Manganese. Manganese is necessary for the production of various body enzymes and for reproduction and skeletal integrity. Wheat bran and legumes and instant coffee are rich sources.

Molybdenum. Molybdenum is present in the body in only minute amounts. It appears to be necessary for the mobilization of iron from liver reserves and therefore indirectly for the formation of hemoglobin and cell oxygenation. It is found in leafy vegetables, legumes, and whole-grain cereals. Like so many other minerals, a deficiency is rare because it occurs in so many food sources.

Nickel. Nickel is necessary for enzyme formation and ribonucleic acid (RNA) synthesis. It is found in grains and vegetables; a deficiency is rare except in someone who eats almost no vegetables.

Trace Minerals. A number of other minerals are always present in the body, but whether they are essential or not is unknown. These minerals are aluminum, bromine, arsenic, boron, and cadnium. Cadnium may be important in regulating blood pressure. The actions of the others are undetermined.

Vitamins as Nutrients

Vitamins are a group of unrelated organic compounds that are essential for specific metabolic actions in cells. Unlike protein, carbohydrates, and fat, they do not produce energy.

Although for centuries it was known that the lack of certain foods led to illness, the discovery of vitamins as the essential component in those foods was not isolated until 1912. The word *vitamin* is derived from *vita* (meaning "life") and *amine* (the structure of the first vitamin isolated).

At first vitamins were given letters—A, B, C, and so forth. Further investigation revealed that what was thought to be one B substance was actually several substances, so the B vitamins were then given subnumerals (B_2, B_6, B_{12}). Today, vitamins are more correctly called by the name that refers to their chemical structure (vitamin B_{12} is riboflavin; vitamin B_2 is niacin, and so on).

There are two main types of vitamins: water-soluble and fat-soluble. These are summarized in Table 34-7. Some foods do not contain vitamins but do contain precursors or provitamins, substances that, once taken into the body, are formed into the needed vitamins.

FAT-SOLUBLE VITAMINS

The sources of fat-soluble vitamins are mainly plant oils and fish oils. Such vitamins can leave the gastrointestinal tract only by being absorbed with fat molecules. Once absorbed, they are used by the cells for growth or are stored in the liver and fat cells for later use. Because fat-soluble vitamins can be stored by the body, it is possible for a person to ingest too many of these vitamins (again, people need to be cautioned that because a little of something is good for them, a lot will not necessarily be better). When the body contains too many fat-soluble vitamins, vitamin toxicity occurs in the same way that drug toxicity results when too much of a drug is ingested. If a person is taking mineral oil as a laxative, there is a possibility that fat-soluble vitamins will not be absorbed but will be retained in the mineral oil and removed from the body with feces. Fat-soluble vitamins must be coated by protein carriers to be transported through the bloodstream. A person who is protein-deficient, therefore, may also become deficient in fat-soluble vitamins. A person who has difficulty in absorbing fat may easily become deficient in fat-soluble vitamins.

Vitamin A (Retinol). Vitamin A is necessary for growth of the cornea and the ability to see in dim light, so it is essential for good eyesight. It also plays a major role in the production of mucus, a function of the skin and mucous membranes that helps in resisting infection, and it is important for the growth of bones and teeth. An important provitamin form is carotene, the substance that gives yellow vegetables such as carrots, pumpkin, sweet potatoes, and squash their color. Vitamin A is also found in animal sources. It can be produced synthetically as vitamin tablets. Foods high in vitamin A are fish oil, egg yolk, whole milk, and yellow vegetables.

People who take multivitamin tablets may acquire vitamin A toxicity. Signs of vitamin A toxicity are joint pain, stunted growth, enlargement of the liver and spleen, and gastrointestinal distress. Large amounts of the precursor carotene may color the skin cells so much that the person appears jaundiced (yellowed). A comparison of vitamin A content in common foods is given in Table 34-8.

Vitamin D. About 50 percent of the vitamin D used by the body is ingested. The other 50 percent is formed in the body by the action of ultraviolet rays of the sun reacting with a cholesterollike substance in the skin.

Vitamin D is important in the body's regulation of both calcium and phosphorus. It directs the intestinal absorption of both of these minerals and their integration into bone tissue. Lack of vitamin D in children leads to rickets or abnormal bone growth such as bowed legs (the bones are so soft that they bend under the child's weight; see Fig. 34-2). In adults, deficiency of vitamin D leads to osteomalacia or insufficient deposition of calcium in bones that leaves them brittle and liable to break.

Good food sources of vitamin D are fish oils, butter, egg yolks, liver, and fortified milk. Milk in its natural state is not a rich source of vitamin D, but in the United States it is fortified with vitamin D; many children's cereals are fortified with vitamin D also.

In industrial cities the ultraviolet rays of the sun may be so filtered by smog and smoke that they cannot be counted on as a good source of vitamin D. Elderly people and others who spend little time outdoors cannot depend on this source of the vitamin.

TABLE 34-7. VITAMINS ESSENTIAL FOR HEALTH

Vitamin	Function in Body	Food Sources	Results of Deficiency
*Fat-soluble**			
Vitamin A (retinol)	Important for night vision and corneal integrity and growth	Found as carotene (precursor to vitamin A) in yellow vegetables	Keratinization of the eye (xerophthalmia) and blindness
Vitamin D	Regulates absorption of calcium and phosphorus for bone growth	Fortified milk, fish oils; exposure to sunshine	Rickets (bone deformity) in growing children; osteomalacia (loss of calcium from bones) in adults
Vitamin E	An antioxidant that protects red blood cells from destruction by oxygen	Cereal grains, green vegetables	In immature infants, severe anemia from destruction of red blood cells
Vitamin K	Important in blood clotting (synthesis of prothrombin)	Produced in intestine by bacterial action; green leafy vegetables	Bleeding from lack of sufficient clotting action
Water-soluble			
B complex			
Thiamine	Important for utilization of glucose in cells	Pork, legumes, green vegetables	Beriberi, a disease involving nerve paralysis
Riboflavin	Important for breakdown of fatty acids and amino acids for energy	Milk and milk products	Red swollen tongue, inflamed eyes, fissures of lips
Niacin	Important for conversion of glucose to energy	Enriched breads and cereals	Pellagra-diarrhea, mental confusion, dermatitis, and death
Vitamin B_6 (pyridoxine)	Important for amino acid and glucose metabolism	Meat, whole-grain cereals, vegetables	Neuritis, depression, nausea and vomiting
Vitamin B_{12} (cobalamin)	Important for blood formation	Animal sources only—meat, eggs, milk	Pernicious anemia (large, unfunctional RBCs)
Folic acid (folacin)	Important for red and white blood cell structure	Vegetables, fruit	Excess masks the symptoms of pernicious anemia
Vitamin C (ascorbic acid)	Important for collagen structure	Citrus fruit	Scurvy (weakness, easy bleeding, joint pain)

*All fat-soluble vitamins can be absorbed only in the presence of lipids and can be transported only in the presence of protein.

Vitamin D toxicity is possible. Toxic symptoms are nausea, diarrhea, and headache; excessive calcium deposits in soft tissue may occur as well. If calcium is deposited in the arteries, the blood supply to distal body parts will be greatly compromised.

Children and women during pregnancy and lactation (breast-feeding) need a high intake of vitamin D because of the large amount of bone tissue being formed during these times.

Vitamin E (Tocopherol). Vitamin E is necessary for reproductive function in experimental rats (its name is derived from the word *tokos*, meaning "offspring"). In humans vitamin E appears to act as an antioxidant, protecting the polyunsaturated fats in the body from destruction by oxygen; its role in reproductive function is unproven.

Vitamin E occurs in such a wide variety of foods that it is rare to see a deficiency. The exception occurs in low-birth-weight (premature) babies. Little transfer of vitamin E from mother to fetus occurs until late in pregnancy. Because the low-birth-weight infant is born before this transfer has taken place, his red blood cells are extremely fragile and break easily. This apparently occurs because large amounts of polyunsaturated fatty acids in the red blood cells do not receive adequate protection against oxidation when they are exposed to oxygen in the lungs.

Foods that are good sources of vitamin E are egg yolks, cereal grains, green plants, and butter.

Vitamin K. Vitamin K is necessary for the formation of prothrombin and fibrin, two important components in blood coagulation. It is found in varying amounts in green leafy vegetables.

About half of the vitamin K utilized in the human body is not taken from the ingested substance, however, but is formed by the body in the intestine by the action of intestinal bacteria. Newborn infants are born with a sterile gastrointestinal tract and therefore may

TABLE 34-8. COMMON FOODS COMPARED TO VITAMIN CONTENT

Food (amount)	Vitamin A (IU)	Thiamine (mg)	Riboflavin (mg)	Niacin (mg)	Ascorbic acid (mg)	Folacin (μg)
Beef liver (2 oz)	30,280	0.15	2.37	9.4	15	123
Canned salmon (3 oz)	60	0.03	0.16	6.8	0	17
Chicken (3 oz)	80	0.05	0.16	7.4	0	3
Pork chop (1)	0	0.63	0.18	3.8	0	4
Peanut butter (1 tbsp)	0	0.02	0.02	2.4	0	13
Carrot (1)	5,500	0.03	0.3	0.03	4	19
Collard greens (1 cup)	10,260	0.27	0.37	2.4	87	56
Green peas (1 cup)	860	0.44	0.17	3.7	33	77
Corn (1 ear)	310	0.09	0.08	1.0	7	54
Celery (1 stalk)	100	0.01	0.01	0.1	4	12
Orange (1)	260	0.13	0.05	0.5	66	65
Banana (1)	230	0.06	0.07	0.8	12	33
Tomato juice (1 cup)	1,940	0.12	0.07	1.9	39	63
Peach (1)	1,320	0.02	0.05	1.0	7	8
White bread, enriched (1 slice)	trace	0.07	0.06	0.7	trace	10
Pancake (1)	30	0.05	0.06	0.4	trace	16
Corn muffin (1)	120	0.08	0.09	0.6	trace	10
Spaghetti (1 cup)	0	0.20	0.11	1.5	0	6
Whole milk (1 cup)	350	0.07	0.41	0.2	2	12
Margarine (1 tsp)	170	—	—	—	0	0.5
Egg (1 boiled)	590	0.05	0.15	trace	0	22

have vitamin K deficiency. People who have received an antibiotic to kill intestinal bacteria (a routine practice before extensive bowel surgery) may develop vitamin K deficiency.

As part of routine delivery room care, all newborns in the United States are given one injection of vitamin K (Aquamephyton) to give them a usable amount of vitamin K until bacteria grow in the intestine (about 24—48 hours after birth). One of the important drugs used in heart disease to keep blood from clotting (dicumarol) works by interfering with the vitamin K synthesis of prothrombin.

WATER-SOLUBLE VITAMINS

Unlike fat-soluble vitamins, water-soluble vitamins are not stored well in the body. A person needs a daily intake of these vitamins to maintain effective blood levels. Because they dissolve in water they can be bleached out of foods by excessive boiling during cooking. Toxicity rarely occurs with water-soluble vitamins because they are not readily stored.

B Complex Vitamins. B complex vitamins are nutrients that are similar in nature, are found in similar foods, and are necessary for cell metabolism.

THIAMINE. Thiamine is necessary for use by adenosine triphosphate (ATP) in cells to trap energy and store it for cell use. Thiamine deficiency causes symptoms in those body parts that are dependent on energy, most noticeably nervous tissue and muscle. Extreme thiamine deficiency will cause symptoms of muscle tenderness and nerve paralysis (beriberi).

The richest sources of thiamine are pork, legumes, and green vegetables. Refined flours and polished rice have had their thiamine content removed and so are very poor sources.

RIBOFLAVIN. Riboflavin is necessary for the breakdown of fatty acids and amino acids into energy. Riboflavin deficiency causes a red swollen tongue, cracks at the corners of the mouth, and inflamed eyes. Riboflavin is found in milk and milk products, lean meat, and eggs. It can be destroyed by ultraviolet light (this is one reason why milk is now delivered in cardboard box containers rather than in clear glass bottles).

NIACIN. Niacin is necessary for the conversion of glucose to energy. Niacin deficiency results in pellagra, a condition marked by the "four Ds"—diarrhea, dementia (disturbed mental ability), dermatitis (skin rash), and death. Pellagra occurs most often in people who use corn as a dietary staple because corn is low in niacin in contrast to rice or wheat.

VITAMIN B_6 (PYRIDOXINE). Vitamin B_6 is instrumental in converting one amino acid present in a cell to another that a cell lacks (synthesis of nonessential amino acids); it aids in releasing glucose from glycogen, in the breakdown of linoleic acid, and in the synthesis of hemoglobin and adrenal gland secretions.

A deficiency of vitamin B_6 causes generalized symptoms of neuritis, depression, and nausea and vomiting. Women taking oral contraceptives tend to have low levels of vitamin B_6. A patient with tuberculosis may become deficient in this vitamin because isoniazid (INH), a drug for treatment of tuberculosis, is an antagonist to it.

Rich food sources are muscle meat, vegetables, and whole-grain cereals.

VITAMIN B_{12} (COBALAMIN). Long before vitamin B_{12} was isolated, it was known that to prevent pernicious anemia (large, unfunctional red blood cells) both an extrinsic factor (now known as vitamin B_{12}) and an intrinsic factor found in gastric secretions had to be present. How much vitamin B_{12} is absorbed from the gastrointestinal tract is influenced by the presence of vitamin B_6 and iron as well as by the intrinsic factor. Because absorption tends to decrease with age, lack of vitamin B_{12} may be found in older adults.

In addition to its importance for proper blood formation, vitamin B_{12} is necessary for the formation of the sheath that surrounds and protects nerve fibers (myelin sheath). The vitamin is present only in animal sources, not in plants. People who are strict vegetarians may become deficient in vitamin B_{12} unless they include butter or other sources (such as vitamin tablets) in their diet.

FOLIC ACID (FOLACIN). Folic acid is necessary for the formation of both red and white blood cells. The name is derived from the source of the vitamin—*foliage*, or vegetables or fruits. Folic acid may mask the signs of pernicious anemia (even in the presence of vitamin B_{12} deficiency the red blood cells are normal in shape). This means that in spite of the development of pernicious anemia and permanent nerve damage the blood picture looks normal, so the problem will not be detected until permanent neurologic damage has occurred.

To prevent high levels of folic acid from being taken indiscriminantly, the amount of it in over-the-counter vitamin pills is limited by law. Folic acid is incorporated into vitamins prescribed during pregnancy because of the high number of blood cells that need to be formed during that time. Good sources of the vitamin are liver, kidney, spinach, and broccoli.

ADDITIONAL B VITAMINS. Pantothenic acid and biotin are additional B vitamins necessary for cell maintenance and growth. They are widespread in foods, and there is rarely a problem of deficiency. Little is known about human requirements because people are so rarely deficient in these vitamins. Inositol, choline, and pangamic acid are similar compounds that are probably not essential in humans, although deficiencies can be induced in laboratory animals. All three compounds are found abundantly in foods.

Vitamin C (Ascorbic Acid). As early as the 1700s, it was noticed that when ships carried sufficient citrus fruits on ocean voyages sailors did not develop scurvy (a disease of the cartilage). To ensure that all British sailors remained healthy, the British navy required all of its ships to carry an adequate supply of limes (British sailors are still called "limeys" today).

Vitamin C is important for the formation of collagen, the main supportive protein of connective tissue. Collagen formation is important in the healing of bones and incisions and provides support for blood vessel walls. Vitamin C apparently also aids in fighting infection and in the production of thyroxine from the thyroid gland and the release of the adrenal hormones epinephrine and norepinephrine. It may be associated with the prevention of laryngeal cancer. Iron is absorbed best in the presence of an acid medium, and ascorbic acid is included in some iron compounds to supply this medium.

Levels of vitamin C may be lowered during periods of stress because of its involvement in the formation of epinephrine, which is released during stress. The low levels of this vitamin during stress may account for the fact that people tend to develop upper respiratory infections during periods of stress.

Symptoms of scurvy are related to the breakdown of collagen: tenderness, weakness, bleeding gums, easy bruising, swollen ankles and wrists. Older people who cannot shop frequently and therefore lack fresh fruit and infants who are not receiving vitamin-fortified formula are in danger of being deficient in vitamin C.

The best source of vitamin C are citrus fruits; the fruit may be canned, fresh, or frozen. Cabbage, green leafy vegetables, and broccoli are good vegetable sources. Long cooking tends to destroy vitamin C, however, so cooked vegetables are never as good a source as raw vegetables.

In recent years megavitamin doses of vitamin C (over 2 gm daily) have been proposed as a preventive measure for upper respiratory infections. The worth of this large a dose has not yet been proved; although ordinarily not a problem, toxicity at this high level can occur (see QRS 34-1).

LIFE SPAN CONCEPTS AND NUTRITION

Nutritional requirements differ at different life stages and ages owing to increased or decreased basal metabolic rates and developmental considerations.

Pregnancy

During 9 months, a fetus grows from a two-celled structure to one containing millions of cells and weighing about 7 pounds—a greater than 500-fold weight increase. Because the most rapid growth of the fetus occurs in the first 6 weeks, before the woman may realize that she is pregnant, it is important that she enter pregnancy in a good nutritional state. There is increasing

☐ **QUICK REFERENCE STOP 34-1: PHARMACOLOGY**
Vitamins and Minerals in Nutrition

1. Teach people to meet the requirements for vitamins and minerals through diet whenever possible, not supplements.
2. Advise people not to take mineral oil as a laxative because it interferes with absorption of fat-soluble vitamins.
3. Vitamin K administration may interfere with the action of dicoumarin, a drug used to delay blood clotting.
4. Food or antacids in the stomach change the pH of the stomach. Because iron, for example, is absorbed best from an acid medium, an iron supplement should be taken on an empty stomach if possible. Read drug descriptions carefully to determine when food will interfere with drug interaction or absorption.
5. Women taking oral contraceptives or isonicotinic acid (INH), a drug used in the treatment of tuberculosis, may become vitamin-B_6 deficient.
6. People who ingest a great deal of alcohol may become vitamin-B_6 and protein deficient.
7. Amphetamines (prescribed for hyperactive children) depress the appetite and may lower the total food consumption.
8. Most long-term diuretic therapies may cause potassium deficiency because of increased potassium excretion in urine.
9. People taking monoamine oxidase inhibitors (drugs used to treat depression) may develop acute hypertension if cheese or wine is ingested.

evidence that the good health of the father at the time of conception is equally important to ensure optimal sperm formation.

Early in pregnancy (the first 8 weeks, or the embryonic period) a fetus gains weight mainly by increasing the number of cells present (hyperplastic growth). Later in pregnancy the fetus grows by increasing the size of cells (hypertrophic growth). If a mother does not ingest sufficient nutrients (particularly protein) during the first 8 weeks the fetus may not be able to form enough cells and will therefore always have a lower number of cells in body organs than the average person. If the woman does not ingest adequate nutrients late in pregnancy, cell growth in the fetus may be stunted. Either of these situations will result in an infant who is small-for-gestational age (SGA) at birth. Such a baby will probably always be small for his age. If growth of brain cells was impaired during pregnancy, the child may have severe neurological damage.

The nutrients that are most important during pregnancy are protein, calcium, phosphorus, and magnesium because these are so important for bone and cell growth. A woman doubles her blood volume during pregnancy to supply the placenta (afterbirth) with blood. The rapid increase in blood formation calls for a high intake of folacin, vitamin B_{12}, and iron.

At one time a woman was advised to gain as little weight as possible during pregnancy so that she could regain her figure again as quickly as possible afterward and to prevent the occurrence of hypertension of pregnancy, a disease specific for pregnancy that not only elevates the blood pressure of pregnant women but interferes with the circulation to the fetus and fetal health. Now it is accepted that gaining weight is a normal part of pregnancy and that normal weight gain has no influence on the development of hypertension of pregnancy. There is in fact a correlation between a poor nutritional intake (particularly of protein) and the development of hypertension of pregnancy. A pregnant woman, therefore, should plan on gaining 25 to 30 pounds. If she was obese at the time of conception, she should not attempt to lose weight during pregnancy; dieting often leads to acidosis because of fat breakdown and release of fatty acids. A condition that is as destructive to fetal growth as acidosis may be fatal to the fetus because it interferes with the exchange of oxygen across the placenta.

Women should space children if possible at least 2 years apart to allow their bodies to regain nutrient stores lost during pregnancy. They should try to avoid all alcohol during pregnancy; at least they should limit their alcohol consumption to less than 1 oz per day. This means an intake of at most 1 oz of liquor *or* 4 oz of wine *or* 8 oz of beer per day. A woman cannot "save up" for a party night but must limit her intake every day to this amount. Amounts in excess of this may lead to Fetal Alcohol Syndrome, a cluster of symptoms including distorted facial features and severe mental retardation. Excessive caffeine ingestion (remember that caffeine is found not only in coffee but also in tea, chocolate, and cola beverages as well) may also have teratogenic (harmful to the fetus) effects.

Eating nutritious foods may be difficult early in pregnancy because the woman has "morning sickness" or nausea when she wakes up in the morning, and food does not appeal to her for most of the day during the first three months. A time-honored approach to managing morning sickness is for the woman to eat a few dry crackers or other carbohydrate food in the morning before she arises. Later in the day, after nausea has passed, she often feels extremely hungry. She should be advised to make up for the food intake she neglected earlier (but she must be certain to do this by eating nutritious food, not food chosen quickly and thoughtlessly just because she is hungry).

Later in pregnancy, as the fetus increases in size and presses against the stomach, the woman may develop "heartburn" or discomfort after meals. She may develop constipation from pressure on the bowel. A diet high in fiber, adequate water, and adequate exercise will contribute toward eliminating constipation. Foods that are high in fiber content include the stems of plants (broccoli, celery), large leafy plants (cabbage, spinach), and coarse grains such as bran (see box, p. 914). A woman should be advised *not* to take any over-the-counter medication at anytime during pregnancy. She should consult her physician for a specific prescription to relieve any discomfort rather than choosing her own medication.

An adolescent who is pregnant needs to ingest enough nutrients not only for the growing fetus but for her own growth as well. She may have a difficult time ingesting the high number of calories and protein needed daily to meet this double need.

Recommended daily allowances for women during pregnancy are shown in Table 34-2. A woman must be certain to increase her needs for calcium, iron, and vitamins during pregnancy from nutritiously rich foods, not "empty" calorie foods. A vitamin tablet with iron and folic acid is usually prescribed to help meet recommendations. Early in pregnancy, before a woman is aware of fetal movements (that is, before she makes a psychological change from being pregnant to having a baby), she may need to post a medication chart on her refrigerator door to remind herself to take her daily capsule supplement. WIC (Women, Infants, and Children) programs are federally funded programs that supply food for pregnant women and women who are breast-feeding to help them maintain good nutrition. Nutritionally sound food is also provided for infants and young children of women enrolled in this program.

PICA

Pica (derived from the Latin word for "magpie," a bird that picks up things indiscriminantly) is the eating of inedible substances. Some women during pregnancy develop a strong craving for substances such as laundry starch, clay, or flour. These are probably not harmful in themselves, but they replace foods that would be more nutritious. Pica is often associated with iron deficiency anemia. Women with pica should be examined with this in mind to determine whether iron therapy is necessary, not only to correct the pica but to help the fetus build iron stores in utero.

The Newborn

A newborn infant has rooting, sucking, swallowing, and gag reflexes that prepare him for eating within minutes after birth. A newborn infant needs more calories per pound of body weight than a person at any other age (50—55 kcal per pound compared with 20 kcal per pound in adults) because his basal metabolic rate is so high in the first year of life. A newborn can receive adequate calories and nourishment from breast milk alone or a balanced, iron-fortified commercial formula for the first six months of life.

BREAST-FEEDING

The RDA for a woman who is breast-feeding is even higher than RDA recommendations for a woman during pregnancy (see Table 34-2). If the woman eats a well-balanced diet when she is breast-feeding (being certain to include adequate fluid, at least eight glasses of fluid a day), she needs to take no special supplements during this time. Her infant will need no supplement either.

Breast-fed infants need to nurse as soon after birth as possible (preferably while the mother is still in the delivery or birthing room). Breast-feeding stimulates secretion of oxytocin, a pituitary hormone that aids in uterine contractions, so early breast-feeding is good not only for the baby in that it provides early calories (to prevent hypoglycemia or low blood-sugar level), but also for the mother.

For the first 3 days following birth, colostrum (a thin, watery-appearing fluid high in protein and glucose) is the only breast fluid produced. On about the third day after delivery, breast milk forms, largely from the stimulus of the baby sucking. Although it contains 20 calories per ounce, breast milk appears bluish in color (like skim milk).

Breast-fed infants may not gain weight quite as quickly as formula-fed babies. Because breast milk is so easily digested, babies may need to be fed as frequently as every 2 hours for the first week or two of life. If the baby is sucking adequately, he should complete each feeding in 10 to 20 minutes (Fig. 34-3A).

Breast milk has several advantages over commercially prepared formulas; it contains antibodies to protect against viral and bacterial invasion, it lowers the bacterial content of the gastrointestinal tract to ward off infection further, and it has an ideal electrolyte and mineral composition for human infants. Mothers who are breast-feeding need to be as cautious about taking drugs during this time as they were during pregnancy because almost all drugs are excreted to some degree in breast milk.

FORMULA-FEEDING

When a mother chooses not to (or cannot) breast-feed her infant, the baby may be adequately fed by an iron-fortified commercial formula. Infant formulas are based on cow's milk; the milk is modified, and water and minerals are added to make it as similar to breast milk as possible. After birth, formula-fed infants are given an ounce or two of sterile water for their first feeding (to simulate colostrum) and then started on formula (Fig. 34-3B). A formula-fed infant eats every 3 or 4 hours. If the mother changes from formula to milk before the first year is up, or uses an infant formula she makes herself from evaporated milk, Karo

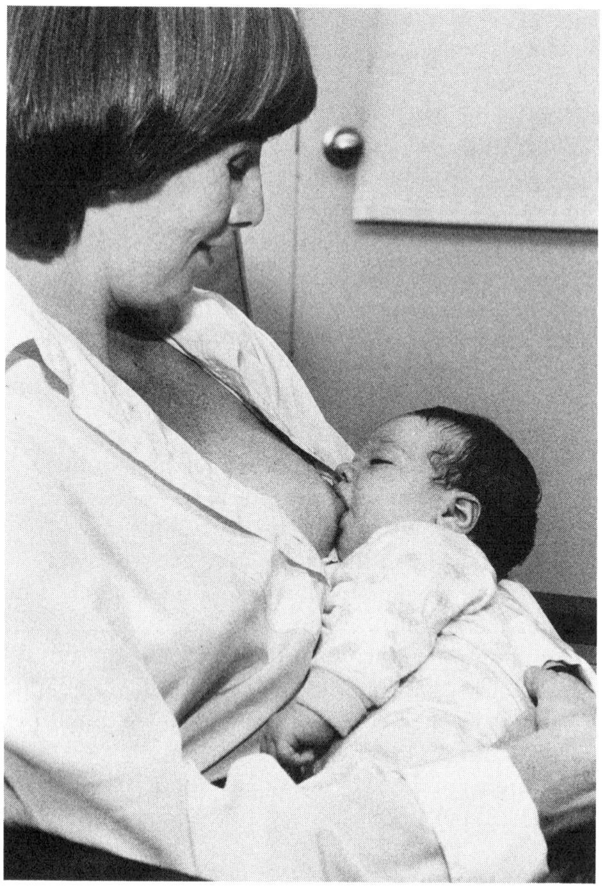

A

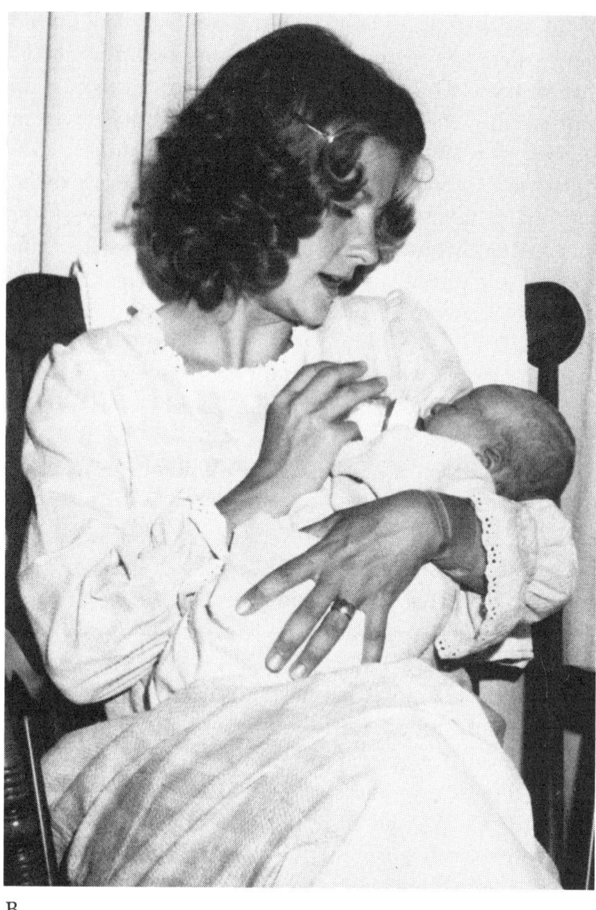

B

FIGURE 34-3. A. Breast-feeding is the preferred form of providing milk for infants. B. Bottle-feeding may be a better choice, however, under certain circumstances. Remember that feeding means more than supplying a substance to alleviate hunger.

syrup, and water, she will need to give a vitamin supplement for the first year. Commercial formulas contain all the vitamins that infants need, so no extra supplement is necessary with these.

The Infant

Infants do not need additional food other than breast milk or an iron-fortified commercial formula until they are 4 to 6 months of age.

Introduction of Solid Food. At about 4 to 6 months of age infants need some solid foods so that their RDA recommendations can be met. These first feedings may consist of commercial strained food, or a mother may prepare her own food by blending or straining it. The first food introduced is generally enriched cereal, followed by vegetables and fruits and then by egg yolk and meat. Foods should be introduced one at a time so that if the infant has an allergy to any food, it can be identified and then omitted from the diet. The first teeth erupt at about six months, and the infant is then ready to bite. He needs soft food for about the first full year (until he has enough teeth to make chewing as well as biting effective).

NUTRITIONAL CONCERNS OF THE FIRST YEAR

Self-Feeding. At about 6 months of age, infants begin to be very interested in feeding themselves. They should be given a spoon and allowed to try this; they should join the family or parents in a high chair at the table for meals. Mothers have to expect some mess when infants begin feeding themselves. It is a developmental step in independence, though a trying one.

Weaning. Many mothers ask questions about how long their baby should continue to be breast-fed or to take a bottle. The decision should be based on both the mother's and the infant's preferences. Some mothers breast-feed for 3 months and then change to bottle-feeding. Many others continue to breast-feed until about 9 months (and some, considerably longer), when most infants are ready to change to taking the major portion of their fluid intake from a cup (the sucking reflex diminishes between 6 and 9 months). A baby who is changed to milk from formula or breast milk before 1 year of age should receive a vitamin supplement until the end of the first year.

Obesity. At one time, a healthy baby was always pictured as a fat baby. Actually, an overweight infant is no different from an overweight schoolage child or adult—he is not a picture of optimal health. Infants who are overweight at this age often form extra fat cells; later in life they may have difficulty losing this weight because of the extra cells. Taking in more milk than necessary (more than a quart daily) is a frequent cause of excess weight gain in infants. This amount of milk not only adds extra calories but also may deprive the infant of other foods, especially iron and protein.

The Toddler

The toddler period is a period of slower growth than the infant stage. The child's appetite, therefore, markedly decreases during these years. Some mothers interpret this decline in desire to eat as illness. They can be shown a growth curve (App. D) to demonstrate that the toddler is undergoing a slow time of growth and his weight is appropriate for his age.

Children should be eating table food by the end of the first year. Using commercial "junior" foods or strained baby foods after this time is an unnecessary expense and prevents the child from feeling like a member of the family (eating the same foods as everyone else).

FINGER FOODS

Toddlers are so independent that they insist on feeding themselves (Fig. 34-4). They need to be supplied with foods from all food groups as "finger foods" so that they can feed themselves completely. Examples of good finger foods for toddlers from the different food groups are (meat) meat balls, shredded chicken, hard-boiled eggs; (fruit and vegetable) chick-peas, cooked carrot slices, peas, pieces of peach or pear; (milk) pieces of cheese; (bread and cereal) dry cereal or bite-size pieces of bread, toast, or crackers; (fat) a touch of margarine on a cracker.

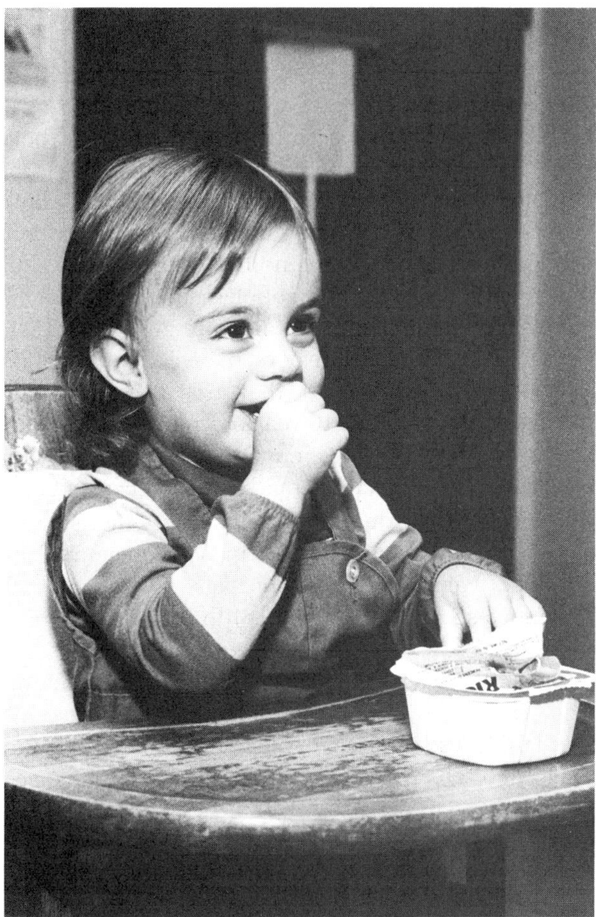

FIGURE 34-4. Finger foods are the best foods for toddlers.

The Preschooler

The preschool period is also a time of relatively slow growth, and the child's appetite does not increase greatly during this time. As preschoolers learn colors, they can be interested in foods for their colors. Because they enjoy imitating adult roles, they can be interested in foods they have helped cook (stirring Jello, washing vegetables, mashing potatoes).

Some mothers report that their child is a "picky eater" during this period. Compare the child's height and weight with a growth curve (App. D) for the period. Some children at this age eat so many snack foods that if the mother makes nutritious snacks, the entire day's food intake is surprisingly adequate when both regular meals and snacks are added together.

The Schoolager

Children are so strongly influenced by their peers during their school years that their friends' diets are strongly reflected in their own food choices. Most schoolage children eat at least one meal away from home each day, so they begin to take increased responsibility for their dietary intake during this time. They may need to be encouraged to eat the lunch packed for them (not exchange a sandwich for a piece of cake, for instance) or to select protein-rich foods in a school cafeteria. They may need to be reminded to take time out of a busy day of activities for sit-down meals.

Learning how to do things well is the developmental task of the schoolage child. A child of this age enjoys cooking foods that are easy to prepare so he can complete the task by himself and feel satisfied with himself. Scrambling eggs, making salad, and frosting a cake are examples.

OBESITY

Many children, particularly boys, become overweight during preadolescence as part of the body's tendency to store excess nutrients for the rapid growth period ahead. If the child is not active and continues to consume a diet high in calories, the temporary obesity may become permanent and will in fact increase in severity. It is important that preadolescents have a balanced program of activity and a nutritious diet to prevent obesity. Children who are overweight may have difficulty in establishing a sense of identity as adolescents because they do not look or feel like the person they want to be.

The Adolescent

Girls begin a growth spurt at 10 or 11 years of age; boys begin such a growth spurt at 12 to 13 years. Greater supplies of nutrients are needed during these rapid growth periods. Girls, as they begin menstruation, especially need increased amounts of iron. Some adolescent girls need an iron supplement to replace the iron lost in menstrual blood. Because girls reach their peak growth period before boys, there is great variation in the number of calories that girls and boys need during adolescence. A 16-year-old boy, for example, may need 2,800 calories a day; a 16-year-old girl with such a high caloric intake would quickly become obese.

Some teenagers do not eat well because they seldom eat a sit-down meal; they eat most of their food by snacking. Parents of such youngsters need to provide nutritious snacks (fruits, cheese) to provide adequate nutrients.

Diets of teenagers tend to be deficient in calcium, iron, vitamin A, and folic acid because adolescents avoid milk (a source rich in calcium but "babyish") and meat and green leafy vegetables (not good snack foods).

ALCOHOL CONSUMPTION AND ADOLESCENTS

As many of 9 out of 10 high school seniors may consume alcohol. In college, alcohol abuse (heavy drinking at least once a month) has become a common occurrence. Alcohol use can interfere with vitamin B_6 utilization; it also can interfere with overall nutrition because it is an empty calorie beverage or replaces needed nutrients in the diet.

ATHLETICS

Athletes need more carbohydrates or energy than do people who do not engage in strenuous activity. The source of carbohydrate that best sustains athletes comes from the breakdown of glycogen. *Glycogen-loading* is a procedure now used to sustain energy. Several days before an athletic event, the athlete lowers his carbohydrate intake and exercises heavily to deplete muscle glycogen stores. Then he switches to a diet high in carbohydrates. Muscle glycogen is stored at about twice the usual level using this system. With high glycogen stores, energy will be readily available at all times during a sports event. Because the effects of frequent glycogen-loading are unknown it is not particularly recommended for adolescents who need nutrients for growth.

To qualify for some sports such as football, an athlete may want to gain weight quickly. This is best done by eating a high fat diet because fat is the most efficient source of calories. The quick weight gain accomplished by this method will be fat, not muscle, however, so weight will increase, not strength. To lose weight rapidly, athletes may starve themselves and, in particular, may decrease fluid intake. This will cause the athlete to lose weight, but it is hazardous because it causes dehydration.

As a rule, the goals of nutrition that are best for everyone, such as eating a well-balanced diet, are also the best rules for athletes rather than diets that interfere with carbohydrate, fluid, or fat intake.

PRESCRIPTION DRUGS

Some drugs such as antacids interfere with iron absorption (iron is absorbed best from an acid medium), thus reducing iron stores. Antacids are prescribed for gastrointestinal tract ulcers and may first be prescribed during adolescence with its natural stresses. Birth control pills alter the use of vitamin B_6 in the body and may also be first prescribed during this time of life.

NONPRESCRIPTION DRUGS

Marijuana increases the desire for sweets. A heavy user of marijuana may eat foods with empty calories ("munchies") to the exclusion of nutritious foods just to satisfy this desire. Mind-altering drugs such as hallucinogens may make mealtime seem unimportant. Amphetamines ("speed") drastically suppress the appetite; some sedatives ("downers") also cause this effect as well as a feeling that food is not important.

FAD DIETS

Many adolescents fall prey to fad diets (high-protein liquids, macrobiotic diets, Mayo diets). At this time of rapid body growth adolescents should be taking in optimal amounts of nutrients, not limiting their diet in some way. High-protein diets are particularly dangerous because when depleted of carbohydrate, the body begins to break down fat to supply energy. This releases fatty acids and leads to acidosis. A macrobiotic diet is a pseudo-oriental diet composed mainly of brown rice (which contains scarce amounts of many nutrients); a diet such as the Mayo diet (grapefruit, eggs, and water) will not meet adolescent growth needs for any length of time.

ANOREXIA NERVOSA

Anorexia nervosa is a condition characterized by extreme weight loss and aversion to food. It is seen particularly often in girls who believe that they are not attractive because they are overweight; they start to diet and continue to lose weight beyond the weight that is ideal for them. Some girls grow nauseated at the sight of food; some eat but then vomit immediately afterward, losing not only the value of the newly ingested food but also chloride from the secretions in the stomach. Anorexia nervosa is not a simple disorder. Some girls report an incident of being threatened by a man (a sexual advance on a bus or in a movie theater) before the illness begins. In these instances girls may starve themselves as a way of psychologically "starving" away an imagined pregnancy. These girls need extensive psychological help before they can return to a normal eating pattern and gain adequate weight again.

BULIMIA

Bulimia is bingelike overeating or episodes of uncontrolled rapid ingestion of large quantities of food during a short period of time. Foods eaten are usually high in calories. Physical discomfort from gastric distention may cause the person to stop eating, or the person may deliberately induce vomiting to relieve the discomfort.

Bulimia, like anorexia nervosa, tends to occur in adolescents and young adults, particularly girls. Following a binge of eating, the person feels guilty, depressed, and filled with self-disgust. He may diet very strictly for a period of time to compensate for the overeating, only to return to the same behavior during a period of stress.

Weight fluctuates widely in a person with bulimia, but weight loss is seldom as severe as it is in anorexia nervosa. Although considered a poor method of responding to stress, bulimia is still poorly understood.

The Young Adult

People in the young adult age group are fully responsible for their own daily nutrition and often for that of a roommate, spouse, or young children as well.

The appetite of a young adult is good. Low incomes from beginning jobs and lack of knowledge about good nutrition are the main reasons why they may fail to consume nutritious diets.

The Middle-Aged Adult

The problems of nutrition and the middle-aged adult are generally job-related (stress-related) or related to health problems such as gallbladder disease that are commonly noticed during this period (with gallbladder disease fatty foods cause indigestion).

Many men and women spend a great deal of time at work because they occupy managerial positions that require extra hours and concern. This may lead to "fast-food" eating. If the person's lifestyle includes luncheons at which alcohol is served as an introduction to business, more alcohol may be ingested than is sensible for health. A busy homemaker may spend too much time feeding other family members when she should eat better herself.

CHOLELITHIASIS

A disease seen frequently at this time of life is cholelithiasis (gallstones) or cholecystitis (inflammation of the gallbladder). It has been said to occur most often in people who are fair (the "fair sex," or women), fat (obese), and forty. Pain tends to occur after fat-rich meals (because bile needed for fat metabolism is not available). It also occurs with increased frequency during pregnancy. Treatment is either avoidance of fatty foods or surgery.

HYPERCHOLESTEROLEMIA

Hypercholesterolemia is an increased cholesterol level in the blood. All adults, particularly males, should have this level analyzed at periodic health assessments. If the blood cholesterol level is elevated (normal, 120—300 mg/100 ml) it is generally recommended that the person make an effort through dietary changes to reduce it to try to avoid atherosclerosis. Development of atherosclerosis is also influenced by hereditary factors, however, so reduction of cholesterol levels in susceptible individuals still may not be successful.

The Older Adult

As people age there is a decrease in the activity and function of body cells. If the sensations of smell and taste are diminished, a great amount of the appeal of food may be lost, and this almost automatically limits food intake. The acid level in the stomach or secretions from the pancreas may decrease with age. This loss of activity may lead to difficulty with digestion, particularly of fatty foods. Fat may infiltrate the liver, generally reducing its function of glucose or protein synthesis. Arteries harden or become lined with plaque, making it more difficult for the body to provide nutrients to body cells. A decrease in blood flow to the kidneys makes them less effective in regulating the sodium nitrogen balance in the body.

As mentioned earlier, a noted change that occurs with aging is the loss of calcium from bones (osteoporosis). This results both because the joints lack mobility and because many older people do not realize that they still need a high calcium intake (they think that milk, a prime source of calcium, is necessary only for young growing people). Missing or loose teeth as well as ill-fitting dentures can make chewing foods such as meat difficult and therefore avoided.

Because of the decreased activity and gradually slowing metabolism of people in this age group, fewer calories are needed (2000 rather than 2600), but minerals such as iron are still needed at high levels; vitamins C and A may be in short supply because these are found in perishable fruits and vegetables. If the older person shops infrequently there may be long periods when these foods are unavailable. The B vitamins found in meats may be deficient if the person's buying power is decreased (meat is expensive). A high level of roughage (fiber) should be retained in the diet to prevent constipation from slowing intestinal peristalsis. If the older adult goes outside infrequently, vitamin D from sunshine may be deficient.

Loneliness. People who are lonely (because they have outlived their family, their friends, even their family doctor) may become so depressed that they lose interest in food; the effort of preparing a meal seems more than they are able to accomplish owing to the lack of self-esteem brought about by loneliness.

Locating new support people to replace those no longer present and locating diversions such as senior citizen groups for otherwise inactive days are measures that may increase the daily dietary intake of many older adults.

Lack of Buying Power. Many older people support themselves on fixed incomes (Social Security payments, pension funds), which remain the same even if food grows more costly. For this reason more expensive foods such as meat and fresh fruit and vegetables may be omitted from the diet.

Two federal programs are available to help increase food buying power in all age groups. Many people in the older age group qualify for the *Food Stamp program* because of their low income; with this program they can receive coupons that reduce the cost of food. *Supplemental Security Income* (SSI) benefits are often another source of income for supplementing buying power. A federally funded nutrition program for the elderly was instituted in 1972. This program provides for low-cost yet nutritious meals served in community settings (often church or school facilities). Transportation to the sites is provided. Meals must supply at least one-third of the RDA for the day; the social interaction of eating with friends is as important for many people as the meal itself. For people who cannot leave their homes, *Meals on Wheels* programs provide meals delivered to the home. When caring for an older adult, investigate the daily diet pattern carefully. This is an area that often needs improvement if good nutrition is to be maintained.

PLANNING DIETARY INTAKE

To ensure that people do receive all the nutrients required for cell growth and maintenance, meal planning must include all five food groups. Table 34-3 shows the recommended number of servings per day for each food group by age group. Although this is only a guide, following it should ensure that people in each age group receive adequate amounts of nutrients daily. Check your own diet today against the guide for your age group. Figure 34-5 shows a scorecard that may be used to rate a diet numerically in relation to the food groups. Make a habit of checking the diet of patients you care for against it (making allowances for restrictions due to a disease process). You will find that in the midst of the best health care available, some people may be receiving less than adequate nutrition (because day after day these people do not eat a single vegetable or piece of meat served to them). Healing will be poor in such people; in children healing needs may be met, but growth needs will halt during this period.

FACTORS THAT INFLUENCE FOOD CHOICES

People eat certain kinds and amounts of foods based on a variety of factors.

THE MEANING OF FOOD

Food means more to people than merely a substance to alleviate hunger. Early in life an infant comes to associate receiving food with comfort. Feeding is a time when he is held and loved. When children are too old to be rocked, giving food is a way of giving them love. On a less intimate level, food is used to show people that they are welcome in your home (offering coffee). Restricting a person's diet, therefore, may be subconsciously interpreted as more than a restriction on food—it may be seen as a restriction on friendship as well. A lonely person often does not eat well because he associates food with friendship.

STRESS

When people are tense or anxious, they tend to react in one of two ways: Either they feel a loss of appetite and so decrease their food intake, or they eat more than the normal amount by constantly snacking. On a particularly bad day, a person may use food as a reward for himself for getting through the day.

CUSTOM

Many people like to brush their teeth before breakfast or wash their hands before eating, and do not enjoy the taste of food until they have done so. Others say grace before a meal and feel guilty eating unless they are allowed a private moment to do this before a meal. Some people expect certain foods to be served as breakfast foods and do not eat eggs, for example, at any meal but breakfast. When caring for people in a hospitalized setting, respect for their customs is extremely important in urging them to eat better.

CULTURE

Adults tend to prefer the types of food that they ate as children (because these are the foods that signify love and comfort for them). Because women tend to cook as they were taught by their mothers, food traditions continue generation after generation in a family (asking a woman to cook other foods may be unreasonable; she does not know *how* to cook any other way). Com-

Food Group and Recommended Intake	Your Score	Your Intake from Group (specify food and amount)
Fruits and vegetables—4 or more servings (1/2 cup cooked edible portion or 3—4 oz, 100 gm, raw); at least one raw daily		
One serving vitamin A-rich dark green or deep orange fruit or vegetable (any food with more than your RDA) = 10 points (no more than 10 points allowed)		
One serving vitamin C-rich fruit or vegetable (any food with more than your RDA) = 10 points (no more than 10 points allowed)		
Other fruits and vegetables, including potatoes = 2.5 each		
Subtotal (no more than 25 points allowed)		
Breads and cereals—4 or more servings of whole-grain or "enriched" (1 oz dry-weight cereal or 1-oz slice bread or equivalent grain product)		
One serving cereal or 2 bread equivalents = 10 points (no more than 10 points allowed)		
Other bread equivalents = 5 points each		
Subtotal (no more than 25 points allowed)		
Milk and milk products—2 or more servings (8 oz fluid milk; calcium equivalents are 1-1/3 oz hard cheese, 1-1/3 cup cottage cheese, 1 pint ice milk or ice cream)		
One serving = 12.5 points		
Subtotal (no more than 25 points allowed)		
Meat and meat substitutes—2 or more servings (2—3 oz cooked lean meat, fish, poultry; protein equivalents are 2 eggs, 2 oz hard cheese, 1/2 cup hard cheese, 1/2 cup cottage cheese, 1 cup cooked legumes, 4 tbsp peanut butter, 1 oz nuts or sunflower seeds); count cheese either in milk group or in meat group, not both		
One serving = 12.5 points		
Subtotal (no more than 25 points allowed)		
Grand total (no more than 100 points)		
The above are FOUNDATION FOODS. ADDITIONAL FOODS are those that do not fit into the above groupings but add flavor, interest, variety and (often) kcalories. List those eaten:		

FIGURE 34-5. Food Selection Scorecard. (Reprinted by permission from E. N. Whitney and E. M. Nunnelley Hamilton, *Understanding Nutrition* [2nd ed.]. Copyright © 1981 by West Publishing Co., St. Paul, Minn. All rights reserved.)

mon cultural differences in people's diets are shown in Table 34-9.

RELIGION

Almost all religions have some associated dietary restrictions. An example, orthodox Jewish people eat only kosher meat (meat that has had all the blood removed); they cannot combine milk products and meat at a meal. On Yom Kippur, the Day of Atonement, they fast. Hindus and Seventh Day Adventists are often vegetarians. Many Roman Catholics still prefer not to eat meat on Fridays, especially during the time of Lent before Easter. People of the Muslim faith typically do not eat pork or drink coffee or alcohol. Mormons also avoid coffee.

GEOGRAPHIC AREA

People living near the seashore tend to eat seafood because it is so plentiful. The diet of people in the southern United States includes much more fruit than the diet of people in the northern United States because of the easy availability of fruit in this region. People in the midwest tend to eat a diet of meat and potatoes. A person living in a new area may not find the foods there appetizing.

SOCIOECONOMIC CONSIDERATIONS

Meat is the most expensive food group. Vegetables and fruit are expensive out of season. Staples such as macaroni, noodles, and rice are the least expensive items. For this reason, people with limited financial resources may be overweight because their diet consists almost

TABLE 34-9. CULTURAL INFLUENCES ON NUTRITION

Culture	Influences on nutrition
Chinese	Diet is rich in vegetables (bean sprouts, broccoli, bamboo shoots, mushrooms) that are stir-fried (fried quickly) so that their vitamins are retained. Meat is served with vegetables; portions may be small. Rice is the dietary staple. Milk is not consumed much because many people tend to have lactase deficiency and cannot digest the lactose in milk. *Nutritional problems:* Lack of protein due to small meat servings. Because bean curd, soybeans, and green leafy vegetables supply calcium, calcium deficiency is not a problem despite the lack of milk. The rice used should be enriched or thiamine deficiency can occur.
Japanese	A Japanese dietary pattern is much like the Chinese pattern. *Nutritional problems:* Lack of protein related to the small portions of meat.
Puerto Rican	Meat is often cooked in stews, so meat portions may be small. Beans and rice are cooked together for complementary protein sources. Little milk is consumed due to lactase deficiency. *Nutritional problems:* Lack of protein due to small meat servings; lack of folic acid in diet.
Mexican-American	Corn is used as the basic grain. Meat is generally mixed with beans and sauce, so individual meat portions may be small. Milk use is limited. *Nutritional problems:* Lack of vitamin A and folic acid; small meat portions may lead to protein deficiency.
Black	The meat consumed is often pork; vegetables are cooked with salt pork for long periods. Little milk is consumed (owing to lactose intolerance). Broad-leaf vegetables (collards, beet greens) are popular and are good sources of calcium. *Nutritional problems:* Iron and protein deficiency may occur; the high level of dietary salt may contribute to chronic hypertension in adults.
Jewish	Level of dietary practices varies according to whether the family is orthodox (follows restrictions firmly), reformed, or conservative (follows rules at individual level). For an orthodox family, food must be *kosher* ("clean"). This means that meat is soaked in salt water to remove the blood; only four-footed animals who are cloven-hoofed and chew a cud are allowed (beef and lamb). Pork and fish without scales (shellfish) are prohibited. Milk and meat cannot be combined. *Nutritional problems:* People may develop increased cholesterol levels owing to the high level of saturated fat used in cooking.
European	Wide range of dietary patterns. The English culture tends to overcook vegetables, thus losing water-soluble vitamins; in the Italian culture a large percentage of pasta is served (leading to obesity). Fresh fruit is not used extensively. *Nutritional problems:* Deficiency of vitamin C.
Vegetarian	A person who is a pure vegetarian by religion or culture eats only vegetables and fruit (all animal foods, dairy products, and eggs are prohibited). A lacto-vegetarian eats vegetables, fruits, milk, and cheese. A lacto-ovovegetarian eats vegetables, fruits, milk, cheese, and eggs. These diets are nutritious and can be well balanced with careful meal planning. *Nutritional problems:* It is easy to develop deficiencies on such a diet unless the person is knowledgeable about complementary protein. Vitamin B_{12} (found only in animal sources) and vitamin D (supplied in normal diets by fortified milk) are apt to be deficient.

wholly of the cheaper but less nutritious and higher calorie foods.

KNOWLEDGE OF GOOD NUTRITION

Teaching people what foods are best for them helps them to select a better diet. Many other factors such as the availability of food and the financial ability to buy food also influence selection, however. Even if a person knows he should eat iron-rich foods, for example, if he cannot afford them or does not like them, he will not eat them.

ENVIRONMENTAL STIMULATION

Hunger at mealtime is influenced by the smells and other stimulation of the environment as well as by the smells and sights of the food itself. Sometimes you are not hungry until you walk into a kitchen and smell food cooking. The hospitalized person lacks the luxury of this sensation for appetite stimulation.

If a person's illness has caused some interference with his ability to smell, food may not appeal to him. If an odor from the hospital unit (urine, cleaning compounds) is strong, it may overpower the food odor and decrease the appetite.

HEALTH

Preparing food, even making a simple snack, involves work. The person who is ill may be so fatigued that he cannot summon enough energy to cook something nutritious for himself and will therefore settle for eating either nothing or something that needs no preparation. If the person has a symptom such as nausea, no food looks good to him, and he will eat nothing. People with inflamed oral mucosa will have difficulty eating because chewing is painful. People with extremely dry mucous membranes may find food tasteless and difficult to swallow. People without dentures (or poorly fitting dentures) must eat a diet of soft foods; if this type of food is not what they prefer, they may not eat as much as they need to maintain a good nutritional status.

EFFECT OF HUNGER

Hunger is the physical sensation that alerts a person to eat food. *Appetite* is the desire or anticipation of food; it is strongly influenced by the sight and smell of food. *Satiety* is the feeling that follows the intake of adequate food.

The amount of food that people eat is apparently regulated by the hypothalamus. Receptors in the hypothalamus are apparently able to analyze the level of nutrients in the bloodstream; when deficiencies are detected, a hunger response is initiated. The stomach contracts; the person feels incomplete or tense until he eats.

Hunger is also caused by a conditioned response. If you are used to eating lunch at noon you become hungry at noon; if during one semester of school you have to delay lunch until 1:00 P.M. each day, you will find that you no longer become hungry until 1:00.

Stretch receptors in the stomach play a part in determining eating patterns. As the stomach is filled to the point of distention, visceral sensations create a feedback reaction in the hypothalamus. Over a period of about 4 hours, as the stomach becomes empty and develops a high level of hydrochloric acid, it registers this as "hunger" or the need to dilute hydrochloric acid by eating again.

NUTRITION TO PREVENT HEALTH PROBLEMS

Good health habits are built in childhood. Because obesity is the major nutrition-based health problem in the United States, parents and health care providers need to examine the habits that lead to obesity. It seems a good practice to most parents to encourage children to eat everything on their plates because this avoids waste. Such a philosophy, however, may encourage overnutrition, not optimal nutrition. To avoid waste it is better to serve smaller portions of food and allow children to ask for second portions as needed.

Encouraging self-esteem in children helps them to avoid eating as a means of comfort. Parents need to evaluate the measures they use for praise to see if they use support measures that are more reassuring and worthwhile (a hug, a "well done") than food. Parents should also evaluate the foods they serve to decide if a well-balanced diet is being provided, not one with a preponderance of starch and glucose.

Iron deficiency anemia is the second most common nutritionally related health problem in the United States. This rarely occurs in infants who are breast-fed or who take iron-fortified commercial formula. It becomes a major problem when children begin to drink cow's milk during the second half of the first year or the second year. It becomes manifest again in adolescence, especially in girls who have a heavy menstrual flow. In pregnant women who do not take their prescribed iron supplement, it is very prevalent. Education should be aimed at helping people to identify iron-rich foods so they can be certain that iron is included in the daily diet.

Dental health is a third problem that can be greatly improved by teaching children not to consume slow-dissolving sugars that remain on the teeth surfaces for a long time; good dental care and fluoride applications or inclusion of fluoride in drinking water are also important aspects of this problem.

The long-term effects of a high sodium diet in causing hypertension and cardiovascular illness are becoming apparent. Common practices such as adding salt to food for infants and toddlers should be modified so that children never become accustomed to a high sodium intake.

In 1977 the Senate Select Committee on Nutrition and Human Needs published a list of Dietary Goals for the United States. In 1979 these were updated as Dietary Guidelines for Americans (see the following box). Figure 34-6 compares current and recommended diets based on these guidelines.

Dietary Guidelines for Americans and Suggestions for Food Choices

1. *Eat a variety of foods daily.* Include these foods everyday: fruits and vegetables; whole grain and enriched breads and cereals; milk and milk products; meats, fish, poultry and eggs; dried peas and beans.
2. *Maintain ideal weight.* Increase physical activity; reduce kcalories by eating fewer fatty foods and sweets and less sugar, and by avoiding too much alcohol; lose weight gradually.
3. *Avoid too much fat, saturated fat, and cholesterol.* Choose low-fat protein sources such as lean meats, fish, poultry, dry peas and beans; use eggs and organ meats in moderation; limit intake of fats on and in foods; trim fats from meats; broil, bake or boil—don't fry; read food labels for fat contents.
4. *Eat foods with adequate starch and fiber.* Substitute starches for fats and sugars; select whole grain breads and cereal, fruits and vegetables, dried beans and peas, and nuts to increase fiber and starch intake.
5. *Avoid too much sugar.* Use less sugar, syrup, and honey; reduce concentrated sweets like candy, soft drinks, cookies, etc.; select fresh fruits or fruits canned in light syrup or their own juices; read food labels—sucrose, glucose, dextrose, maltose, lactose, fructose, syrups, and honey are all sugars; eat sugar less often to reduce dental caries.
6. *Avoid too much sodium.* Reduce salt in cooking; add little or no salt at the table; limit salty foods like potato chips, pretzels, salted nuts; popcorn, condiments, cheese, pickled foods, and cured meats; read food labels for sodium or salt contents especially in processed and snack foods.
7. *If you drink alcohol, do so in moderation.* For individuals who drink—limit all alcoholic beverages (including wine, beer, liquors, etc.) to one or two drinks per day. NOTE: use of alcoholic beverages during pregnancy can result in the development of birth defects and mental retardation called Fetal Alcohol Syndrome.

Source: U.S. Department of Agriculture, 1979.

Some form of diet is used as the method or complement to the therapy of almost all diseases. A knowledge of the basis of good nutrition helps in planning these diets. It helps you in evaluating the nutritional status of the person prior to his illness. Because it is a basic component of health education, it is important in implementing the nursing process in almost all patients in your care.

NUTRITION LABELING

The Federal Food and Drug Administration (FDA) states that a food label must contain the common name of the product, the name and address of the manufacturer, the packer or distributor, the net contents in terms of weight or count, and the ingredients listed in order of descending amount according to weight.

If any nutrient claim is made for a food (such as claiming that a breakfast cereal is good for you), the label must also state the serving size, the number of servings per container, the number of calories per serving, and the amount of protein, carbohydrate, and fat per serving. In addition, the amount of protein, vitamins, and minerals must be stated as a percentage of United States RDA recommendations per day.

If additives are listed, the function of these must be stated. A food said to be *low in calories* (diet breakfast cereal) must be at least one-third lower in calories than the food it most closely resembles; if a food is said to be *nutritionally superior*, it must contain 10 percent more of the RDA nutrients per serving than the food it is compared with.

A food *additive* is any substance added to a food either in preparation or in packaging. Many additives are necessary for keeping foods preserved during their shelf life in stores until they are purchased. When the first law regulating additives was passed in 1958, additives that were presumed to be safe were listed on a GRAS (Generally Recognized As Safe) list. There are over 950 additives on this list; a product does not have to list an additive if it is on this list. To be safe an additive must not have been found to cause cancer in mice or men (this stipulation is called the *Delaney Clause*).

Knowing the meaning of these terms is helpful in educating people about food-buying habits.

FOOD LABELING

Most people today lead such active lives that up to 40 percent of all meals eaten are prepared outside their homes; it is estimated that by 1985, as many as 70 percent of meals may be prepared outside the home. *Fast* foods refer to foods prepared in quick-order restaurants such as hamburger or fried chicken restaurants. *Convenience* foods are those bought from supermarkets

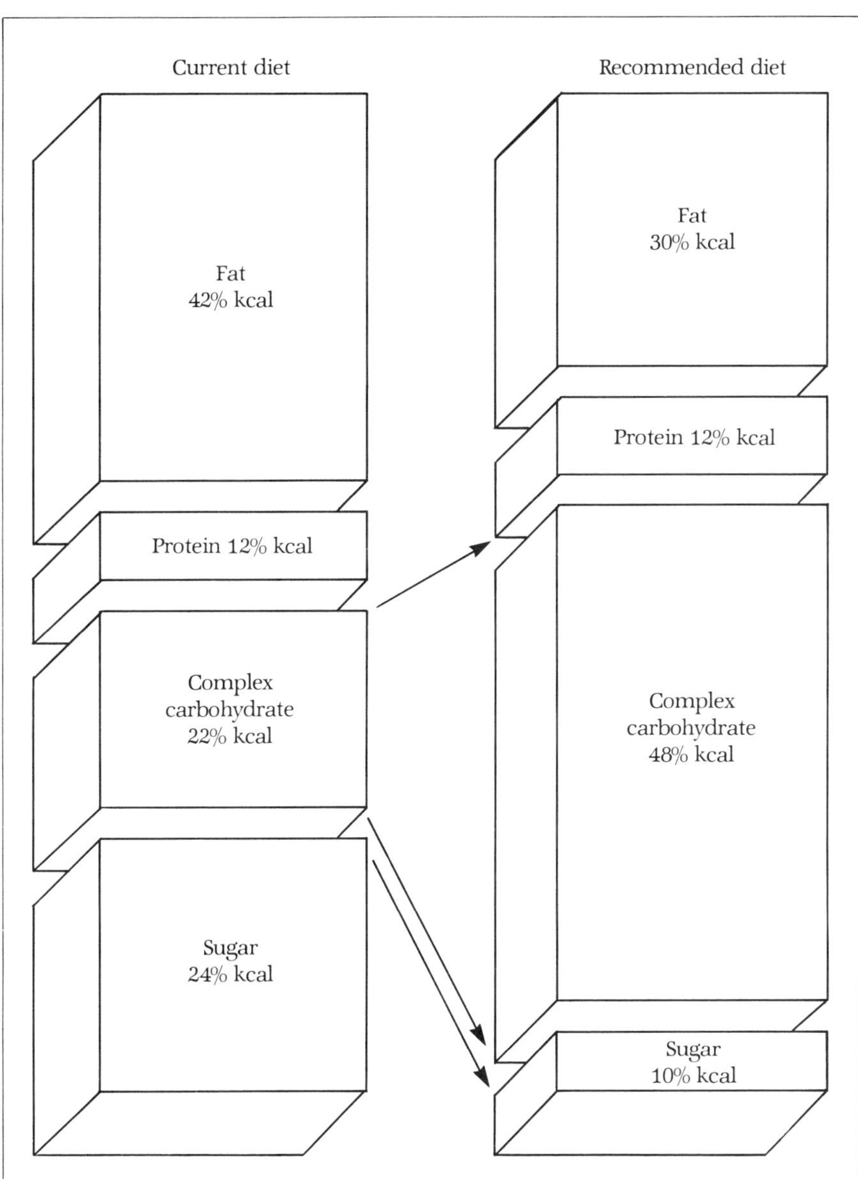

FIGURE 34-6. Proposed U.S. dietary goals. (Reprinted by permission from E. N. Whitney and E. M. Nunnelly Hamilton, *Understanding Nutrition* [2nd ed.]. Copyright © 1981 by West Publishing Co., St. Paul, Minn. All rights reserved.)

already processed such as cold breakfast cereal, canned foods, frozen vegetables, and TV dinners. A food is a *junk* food if it has little or no nutritional value.

An *enriched* food is one to which iron, thiamine, riboflavin, and niacin have been added. In processing grains, these vitamins are removed; in the enrichment process they have been restored to their previous level. *Fortified* means that a nutrient has been added that was not there originally. A fortified breakfast cereal, for example, may have so many nutrients added to it that one serving provides all RDA recommendations for one day. Milk, for another example, is generally fortified with vitamin D, which normally exists in very small amounts in milk. An *imitation* food is one that is produced artificially and is inferior to the food it imitates. If an artificial food contains the same nutrients as the original food, it need not say it is imitation. Imitation vanilla, for example, provides a vanilla taste but is not equal in nutrients to natural vanilla and must be labeled *imitation*.

PROGRAMS THAT PROVIDE FINANCIAL HELP WITH NUTRITION

A number of federally funded programs are available to help people meet the high cost of providing nutritious meals.

FOOD STAMP PROGRAM

Under the Food Stamp program, a family with a low income can buy stamps that can be redeemed at grocery stores for any food item except alcohol or pet food.

The cost of stamps varies but can increase a family's buying power by about 150 dollars a month.

The advantage of this type of program is that it helps to supplement the cost of food yet places almost no restrictions on what foods can be selected and purchased. Rules concerning eligibility for these programs vary from time to time. They can make the difference for a low-income family between being able to eat meat or living on a starch-rich diet.

WIC (SUPPLEMENTAL FOOD PROGRAM FOR WOMEN, INFANTS, AND CHILDREN)

Pregnant and lactating women and infants and children of up to 5 years of age who live in selected project areas and are at nutritional risk qualify for this program. The family is given a voucher that can be exchanged for milk, orange juice, eggs, iron-fortified cereal, iron-fortified formula, or cheese.

An important part of this program is periodic scheduled health care visits that must be kept to continue to qualify for the program. This condition further protects the health of people in these susceptible population groups.

SCHOOL LUNCH PROGRAMS

Millions of school children qualify for free or reduced-price school lunches. Some children qualify for a free school breakfast program as well. A school lunch (type A) provides one-third of a child's RDA. For many children these school lunches may be the only nutritious meals they receive.

NUTRITION PROGRAM FOR THE ELDERLY

As was noted earlier, in 1972 a federally funded program to provide nutritious meals and an opportunity for social interaction, nutrition education, and transportation to the meal site was signed into law (see p. 910).

UTILIZING NURSING PROCESS

Helping people plan a nutritious diet to allow them to remain well is a good example of how the nursing process can be used to promote health as well as to help restore health.

ASSESSMENT

Before people will accept any change in their diet, they need to be aware that their diet is deficient in some way. Assess a person's diet by asking him to describe all the food he ate within the past 24 hours, assuming that the time span was a typical one (this is termed a 24-hour recall). Be certain that the person includes all the snack foods he ate as well as sit-down meals. Compare the types and quantities of the foods listed with those recommended in Table 34-3 and determine whether all five food groups are included. Make a graph of the results on a wheel like the one shown in Fig. 34-7.

Also ask if the person thinks he has any problems with his diet. He may already know his problem (he never eats vegetables) but is unsure how to correct it because he knows no other vegetables he likes except peas and corn (see QRS 34-2).

In addition to these history findings, assess the person's height and weight according to an ideal weight chart or growth chart. Height and weight are such common assessments that it is easy to discount them in terms of importance. In the evaluation of nutritional adequacy, height and weight are the most important assessments. Techniques for measuring height and weight are described in Chap. 19. Growth charts and tables of ideal weight are shown in Appendix D.

People with poor nutrition begin to show physical signs when their bodies can no longer function adequately with missing nutrients. Table 34-10 lists important assessments in the physical examination that suggest a poor nutritional intake.

If a person has had a recent routine health examination, he probably has had a blood sample drawn for hemoglobin or hematocrit evaluation and a urinalysis. These two tests are important in determining the presence of a low iron intake because lack of iron prevents adequate hemoglobin formation; lack of protein causes a disturbed fluid balance, which alters the specific gravity of urine.

NURSING DIAGNOSIS

The Fourth National Conference on Classification of Nursing Diagnosis accepted three diagnoses related to nutrition. These are listed as nutrition, alterations in: less than body requirements; nutrition, alterations in: more than body requirements; and nutrition, alterations in: potential for more than body requirements. These diagnoses and other defining characteristics are listed in Appendix C.

The average person considers his diet adequate, or, if he is aware of deficiencies in it, considers them not too important because, after all, he has been following this diet pattern for a long time and continues to function. Women in particular, who have large iron losses with menstrual periods, may have simply accepted a feeling of chronic fatigue as the way they always feel and are not aware that others do not always feel exhausted.

Plotting the information from the 24-hour recall onto a wheel graph such as that shown in Fig. 34-7 is a helpful way of showing people that what they thought was a "perfect" intake is not perfect or what they thought was a "little" problem involves the loss of an entire food group (the graph shows that the man who knew he didn't eat many vegetables also eats no fruit and therefore lacks an entire food group; the woman who says she knows she is chronically tired eats almost nothing from the meat group). The fact that a picture is

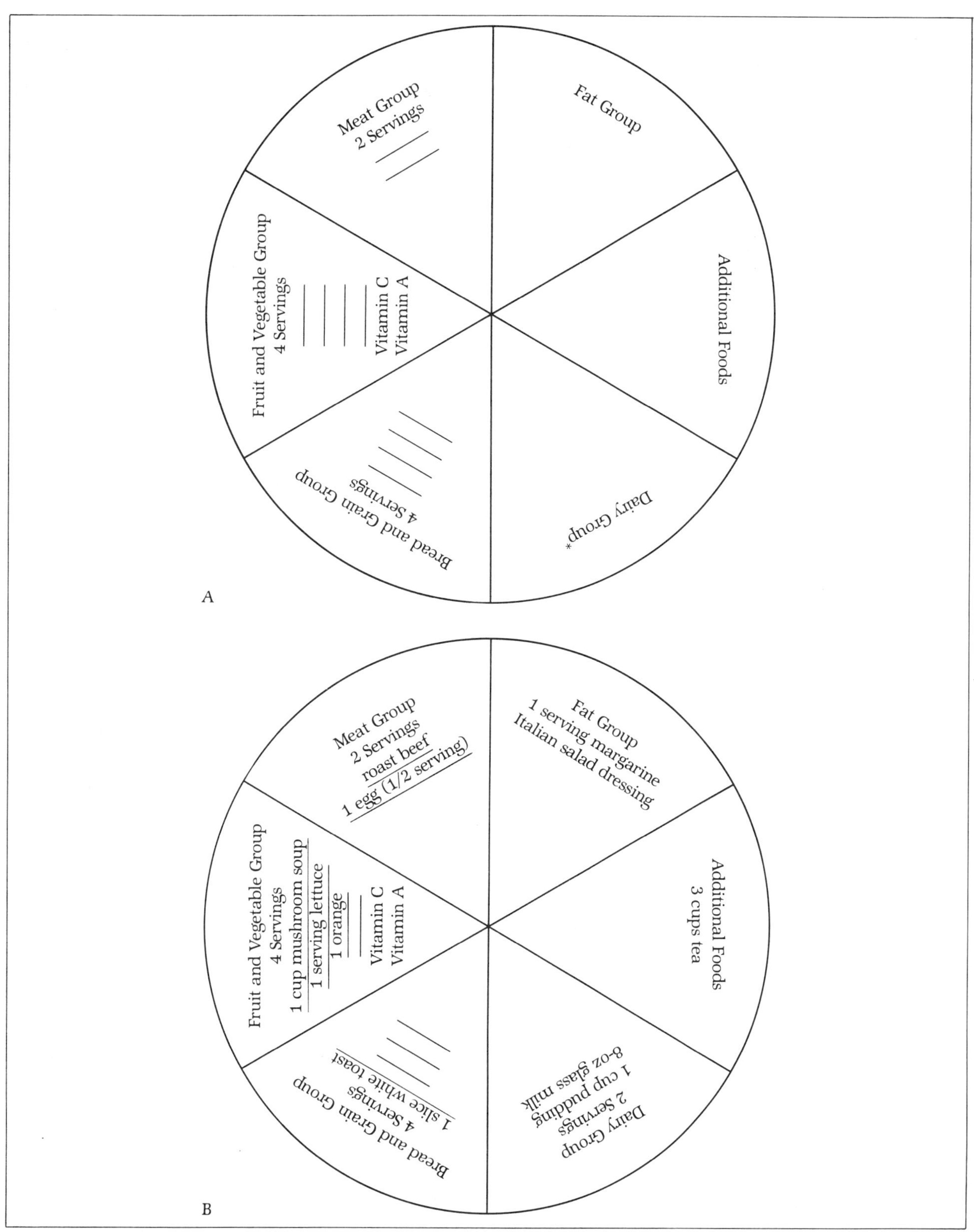

FIGURE 34-7. A. Graph for analysis of food intake. *Dairy group recommendations vary with age: children under 9 years, 2 to 3 servings; children 9 to 12 years, 3 to 4 servings; adolescents, 4 servings; adults, 2 servings; pregnant women, 3 to 4 servings; lactating women, 4 to 5 servings. B. This example of a graph for food group analysis shows a 24-hour recall deficit in 1/2 serving meat group, 1 serving fruit and vegetable group (no strong source of vitamin A), and 3 servings bread and grain group.

☐ **QUICK REFERENCE STOP 34-2: COMMUNITY CONSIDERATIONS**
Meal Preparation and Nutrition

Cooking for one's self can be a lonely and unrewarding endeavor. People who live by themselves may need to be urged to invite others in for occasional meals and to accept all invitations to eat out. A meal prepared for "company" is invariably more balanced than one prepared merely as "something to eat" for oneself.

Remember that with at least 50 percent of mothers of child-bearing age employed outside their homes, many fathers prepare at least one meal a day for their children. Many men have almost no knowledge about balanced diets because high school nutrition courses and meal planning did not seem relevant to them at the time. To prepare such men to be responsible for one-third of their family's dietary pattern, you may need to begin with some very elemental nutrition counseling.

TABLE 34-10. PHYSICAL SIGNS AND SYMPTOMS OF ADEQUATE NUTRITION

Assessment area	Findings
Hair	Shiny, strong, with good body
Eyes	Good eyesight, particularly at night; conjunctiva moist and pink
Mouth	No cavities in teeth; no swollen or inflamed gingiva; no cracks or fissures at corners of mouth; mucous membrane moist and pink; tongue smooth and nontender
Neck	Normal contour of thyroid gland
Skin	Smooth, with normal color and turgor; no ecchymotic or petechial areas present
Extremities	Normal muscle mass and circumference; normal strength and mobility; no edema present; normal reflexes
Finger and toenails	Smooth, pink
Height and weight	Within normal limits of a growth chart or ideal weight chart
Blood pressure	Normal for age

worth a thousand words is important in nutrition counseling; once a person sees that an actual defect exists, he is ready to move on to setting goals to improve his nutrition.

When helping a person set goals to improve his dietary patterns, be certain that you consider all the different things that food means to people other than providing kilocalories and that often a person does not prepare his own meals and must stay within the limits of his finances. Also, rebuilding iron stores or muscle mass is a long-term procedure. Eating an improved diet for a week will probably not make a radical change, but continuing to eat the diet for six months will.

PLANNING

Plans for improving nutritional patterns must be made with the person's life-style, financial resources, customs, habits, and personal desires in mind. Otherwise the person will not maintain the changed eating pattern for longer than a week.

Despite taking a health course in high school that describes the necessity for individual nutrition, most people know very little about what foods are best to supply a particular nutrient. Planning in nutrition counseling, then, invariably begins with education about the components of a good diet and, in consultation with the person, how to improve it (Fig. 34-8).

The man who ate no vegetables, for example, because he likes only peas and corn (and does not want to eat these every day because he is worried that too much of them will be bad for him) could solve his problem in one of two ways—either by agreeing to try some new vegetables to see if he might discover something he likes after all or by eating nothing but peas and corn but eating one or the other every day (they are good basic green and yellow vegetables). The woman who eats almost no meat needs to discover ways to include meat in her diet (slices of ham for lunch, not yogurt, and eggs for breakfast, not a slice of toast; be careful about recommending bacon as meat—it is so fatty it is generally classed in the fat group rather than the meat group). Remember that legumes are meat group foods; incorporating these in the diet also increases the number of meat group choices.

IMPLEMENTATION

Implementation of a changed dietary pattern can be a lonely and seemingly unrewarding endeavor. People often need support by a telephone call or by person-to-person contact to eat a lunch that is different from that eaten by others around them; to get up 15 minutes earlier to prepare breakfast rather than just dashing to work without eating anything more than coffee; to resist a milkshake with a fast food dinner and drink orange juice instead. Asking people to list the foods they eat daily and to bring in the chart to show you at a health maintenance visit is an effective motivating technique for many people (this is the same motivating force as the desire to do well on tests because success is shown on a report card). With this system, the average person will eat better than he normally would so that his list will look better.

EVALUATION

When evaluating whether an improved dietary pattern has been successful or not, rely on your most important

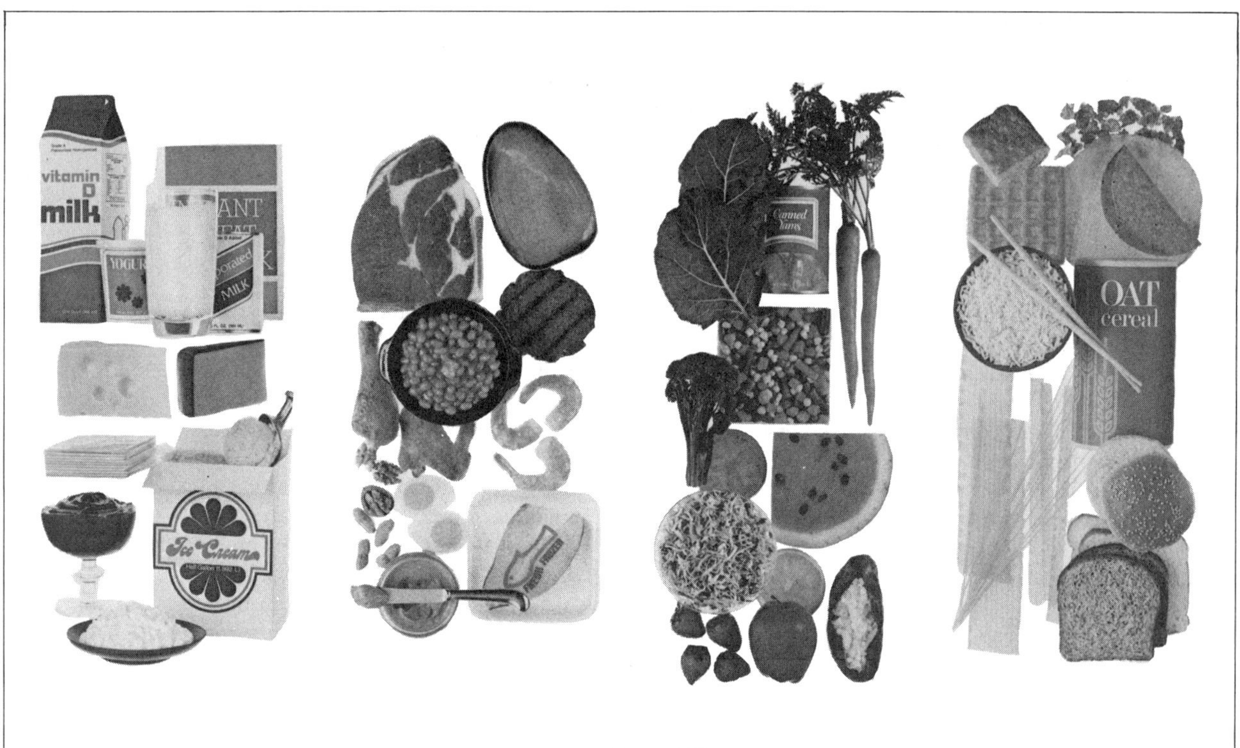

FIGURE 34-8. Education about good nutrition must be included as part of nursing care planning.

assessments—height and weight. Proper bowel function, energy level, general appearance, and, if you have previously assessed them, hemoglobin and urinalysis findings are also useful.

Urge people to be honest about whether they are actually following the new nutritional pattern or not. If they are not, it is not a crime; it simply means that the plan must somehow not have fitted their life-style or degree of motivation, but you cannot know this unless they are honest with you about their success.

Remember that changing a nutritional pattern is difficult. People always have some degree of backsliding during holidays and special events. Respect this as a fact of human nature. If it is of crucial importance that this does not occur on the next holiday, you will need to help the person make definite plans to avoid it or it will happen again.

NURSING CARE PLAN

Mrs. Swanson is an 80-year-old woman whom you visit as a community health nurse in her home.

Subjective Assessment: Patient states, "My daughter only comes every other week to bring food for me." Patient has difficulty chewing food because of poor-fitting dentures; usually "not hungry enough to fix anything by myself." Has tried a meal service to her home but found the food "too dry," "not the way I would have cooked it." Had the service discontinued after a month. Rarely goes outside; has few visitors. Twenty-four-hour food recall graphed.

Objective Assessment: Thin-appearing woman; 5 feet 6 inches in height, 92 pounds (20 percent below ideal weight). Some difficulty in maneuvering right hand; stiffness in right knee due to arthritis. Vision adequate. Mucous membranes in mouth moist but pale. Cupboard and refrigerator are almost bare of food.

Nursing Diagnosis: Nutrition, alteration in: less than body requirements.

Locus of Decision-Making: Shared—Mrs. Swanson and nurse.

GOALS

Short-term: Mrs. Swanson will eat one well-balanced meal daily from now until my next visit in one week's time.

Criteria: Adequate intake to be apparent from a daily list of food she will keep.

Long-Term: Patient will initiate ways to involve herself in community to decrease loneliness and inactivity and increase self-reliance and socialization.

Criteria: Food patterns remain at adequate levels after practice of listing foods eaten is stopped. Patient's weight increases by 10 pounds.

NURSING ORDERS

1. Review with patient the basic food group graph and the importance of nutrients to the older age group.
2. Ask patient to maintain a list for a week of everything she eats.
3. Phone daughter and ask her if patient can accompany her on shopping trips rather than just having food brought to her so patient can choose foods she most prefers to eat.
4. Phone patient daily to ask if she is having difficulty preparing one well-balanced meal daily.
5. Contact local senior citizen's group for a list of activities and transport possibilities so patient can see if there are opportunities there for activities that appeal to her.
6. Continue visits and health education until food intake is adequate without outside support from nursing staff.

SUGGESTED READINGS

Aydelotte, C. Tuning into nutritional education. *Imprint* 29(5):28, 1982.

Bailly, F. E. Socio-economic factors and their effects on the nutrition and dietary habits of the black aged. *J. Gerontol. Nurs.* 8:203, 1982.

Behrends, E. A., et al. Nutrition in neuro science. *J. Neurosurg. Nurs.* 14(1):44, 1982.

Brown, J. G. How to eat right in spite of yourself. *Health* 14(1):25, 1982.

Chilton, T. L., et al. Computerized nutritional assessment: How we do it. *Health Educ.* 13(5):29, 1982.

Crummette, B. D., et al. Mothers' decisions about infant nutrition. *Pediatr. Nurs.* 6:16, 1980.

Deskins, B. B., et al. The community health nurse's nutrition guidelines: A trimester approach for expectant mothers. *M.C.N.* 7(3):202, 1982.

Dickman, S. R. Breast-feeding and infant nutrition. *Fam. Community Health* 1:19, 1979.

Egan, M. C. Nutrition and school health. *J. Sch. Health* 49:516, 1979.

Frankle, R. T. It's never too early for nutrition education. *J. Sch. Health* 50:387, 1980.

Hegsted, M. Priorities in nutrition in the United States. *J. Am. Diet. Assoc.* 71:9, 1977.

Henley, E. C., et al. Nutrition across the woman's life cycle. Special emphasis on pregnancy. *Nurs. Clin. North Am.* 17(1):99, 1982.

Hinkle, M. M. A mixed message: The school vending machine. *J. Sch. Health* 52:20, 1982.

Karvetti, R. L. Effects of nutrition education. *J. Am. Diet. Assoç.* 79(12):660, 1981.

Kuhn, J. G., et al. Vitamins in pediatrics. *Pediatr. Nurs.* 5:25, 1979.

Labson, L. H. Assuring good nutrition prenatally. *Patient Care* 15:20, 1981.

Langford, R. W. Teenagers and obesity. *Am. J. Nurs.* 81:556, 1981.

Lansky, D., et al. Comparison of school-based treatments for adolescent obesity. *J. Sch. Health* 52(8):384, 1982.

Lichtenstein, V. Care of the acutely ill older adult. Part two. Nutritional management. *Geriatr. Nurs.* 3(6):386, 1982.

Mallick, M. J. Health hazards of obesity and weight control in children: A review of the literature. *Am. J. Public Health* 73(1):78, 1983.

Mangham, D. B., et al. Introducing nutrition education. *J. Sch. Health* 51:110, 1981.

Markesberry, B. A., et al. Watching baby's diet: A professional and parental guide. *M.C.N.* 4:177, 1979.

Mowery, B. D. Family-oriented approach to childhood obesity. *Pediatr. Nurs.* 6:40, 1980.

Munro, H. N. Nutritional requirements in the elderly. *Hosp. Pract.* 17(8):143, 1982.

Pittam, M. A symposium on nutrition. Nutritional assessment. *Nursing* (Oxford) 2:94, 1982.

Price, J. H., et al. "Guaranteed in just six weeks": Weight loss fads and fantasies. *Health Educ.* 11:4, 1980.

Rice, B. L. Nutritional problems of developmentally disabled children. *Pediatr. Nurs.* 7(5):15, 1981.

Riordan, J., et al. Preparation for breast-feeding and early optimal functioning. *J.O.G.N. Nurs.* 9:277, 1980.

Schlechter, F. An experiment in group adolescent weight loss guidance. *J. Sch. Health* 51:123, 1981.

Scialabba, M. A. Overview: Nutritional needs of young children. *Child Contemp. Soc.* 12:3, 1978.

Skaien, P. Inadequate nutrition in the elderly: A stumbling block to good health. *Fam. Community Health* 3:61, 1981.

Termini, R. Good food habits for life: Developing a comprehensive nutrition education program. *Health Educ.* 13:26, 1982.

Tredger, J. A symposium on nutrition. Feeding the patient—A team effort. *Nursing* (Oxford) 2:92, 1982.

Veninga, K. S. An easy recipe for assessing your patient's nutrition. *Nursing* (Horsham) 12(11):57, 1982.

Westland, M. A symposium on nutrition. The human diet. *Nursing* (Oxford) 2:89, 1982.

Williams, E. J. Food for thought: Meeting the nutritional needs of the elderly. *Nursing 80* 10:60, 1980.

Wineman, N. M. Obesity: Locus of control, body image, weight loss and age-at-onset. *Nurs. Res.* 29:231, 1980.

Yen, P. What is an adequate diet for the older adult? *Geriatr. Nurs.* 1:64, 1980.

Yen, P. What can you learn from labels? *Geriatr. Nurs.* 1:138, 1980.

Yen, P. K. Nurse-dietitian teamwork . . . keeping elderly people healthy. *Geriatr. Nurs.* 4(1):49, 1983.

QUESTIONS FOR REVIEW

Mrs. Palumbo is a 22-year-old mother with three small children; she works part time, so she does not have much time for meal preparation. Your assessment of her daily dietary pattern reveals a low protein and iron intake according to RDA recommendations.

1. Recommended dietary allowances (RDA) are:
   a. The lowest amount of essential nutrients necessary to maintain health.
   b. Levels of essential nutrients adequate to meet needs of healthy individuals.
   c. Levels of nutrients found in inexpensive foods.
   d. Applicable to children only.

2. To analyze Mrs. Palumbo's diet you plot it on a food graph for her. Which of the following would you plot as *not* a source of complete protein?
   a. Meat.
   b. Fish.
   c. Whole grain.
   d. Milk.

3. Which of the following foods is *not* included in the meat group?
   a. Cottage cheese.
   b. Chicken.
   c. Dried peas.
   d. Peanut butter.

4. One of the first steps of planning is teaching Mrs. Palumbo more about good nutrition. You would teach her that iron functions in the body to:
   a. Form hemoglobin.
   b. Aid in digestion of lactose.
   c. Form thyroxine.
   d. Metabolize protein.

5. A food *not* rich in iron is:
   a. Milk.
   b. Legumes.
   c. Grains.
   d. Beef.

6. Mrs. Palumbo likes to use enriched foods. An enriched food means:
   a. It has more additives than it had before processing.
   b. It is rich in iron and calcium.
   c. It supplies more calories than a nonenriched food.
   d. Substances removed by processing have been replaced.

7. On evaluation, you learn that Mrs. Palumbo does not always prepare the foods you would like her to because she is concerned that she might take in too many calories and that her husband might develop hypercholesterolemia. Which of the following foods contains the greatest number of calories?
   a. A teaspoon of bacon bits.
   b. A teaspoon of sugar.
   c. A teaspoon of hamburger.
   d. A teaspoon of honey.

8. A way to decrease blood cholesterol levels is to:
   a. Decrease the fiber in the diet.
   b. Increase the saturated fat in the diet.
   c. Increase the unsaturated fat in the diet.
   d. Increase the cholesterol in the diet.

9. Which of the following foods does *not* contain saturated fat?
   a. Lean roast beef.
   b. An egg.
   c. Corn oil.
   d. A milk shake.

10. Mrs. Palumbo may be eligible for WIC program funding. With this assistance program, she could receive:
    a. A community-prepared lunch.
    b. Reduced prices at the supermarket.
    c. Free meat and designated poultry.
    d. Free cheese and cereal.

35. MODIFICATIONS IN NUTRITION

OBJECTIVES

Upon mastery of the material in this chapter you should be able to:

1. Describe common interferences with nutrition that occur as a result of illness.
2. Describe methods of assessing nutritional intake during illness.
3. List factors important to consider before asking people to change to a new food pattern.
4. Describe common methods useful in effective diet counseling.
5. Describe common diets used in illness and methods of stimulating optimal intake.
6. Describe the insertion, removal, and feeding technique used with a nasogastric tube.
7. Describe the concept of total parenteral nutrition and important observations of the patient receiving it.
8. List ways to help the handicapped person achieve better nutrition.

TERMS

The terms important for an understanding of this chapter are shown below and defined in the glossary:

anorexia
aspirate
bland diet
clear liquid diet
extubation
full liquid diet
gastric intubation
gastrostomy tube
gavage
lavage
nausea
nasojejunal tube
soft diet
vomiting

Nutrition plays a role in the therapy of almost all illnesses that is equally important as the other components of care. Although a pharmacist prepares the medication and a dietitian directs the nutrition of the patient, a nurse administers the therapy and records observations about its effectiveness. It is a nursing responsibility to educate the patient about both medication and diet so that he can participate more fully in his own care.

ASSESSMENT OF NUTRITIONAL STATUS

Health History

The best method of obtaining factual information about a person's dietary intake is to ask what he has eaten during the last 24 hours (there is termed a 24-hour recall). Ask the person if the preceding day was a typical one (if he is acutely ill you should choose a day before the illness began that is typical of his well state; if the person has a long-term or chronic illness, you are probably interested in an "ill" day because this is his usual state). Ask the person to describe everything he ate on the selected day, both the quantity and the type of food. When discussing an infant, ask how the formula was prepared. In older children and adults, ask how food is prepared to detect the amount of fat or condiments that are normally ingested. Prepare a graph of a 24-hour recall to determine nutritional deficiencies or excesses (see Fig. 34-7).

If you have questions about whether the person omitted or added foods to his usual intake to make it sound better, you can use a second method of eliciting a nutritional history—a food frequency questionnaire (see box, page 924). By asking such questions as "How many times a week do you eat meat? Bread? Milk?" you may find discrepancies in the day history. If the original 24-hour recall is done in a nonthreatening manner, the patient has little reason to prefabricate a nutrition history, so the food frequency inventory is rarely necessary.

A third method is to ask the person to keep a daily log of all food he ingests in the coming week's time. This will give you not only day history information but food frequency information as well. Again, if you present this request in a helpful, nonthreatening way you can expect the person to be honest in listing the foods he actually eats. If at the end of the week the listing is "too good to be true," ask him to continue it for a longer period. When people are asked to record what they eat, it reminds them of what they should eat, and food consumption improves; over a period of time most people will gradually revert to their normal pattern of eating, and omissions or overindulgences of foods will begin to show on the lists.

The box on page 925 lists other areas of information (e.g., alcohol consumption, family setting) that are

Guide for Food Frequency*

Major Food Categories	*No. Times/Day*	*Serving Size*	**or** *No. Times/Week*	*Serving Size*
Milk group				
Milk (what type is it, vitamin D or vitamin A and D fortified?)				
Cheese (what type?)				
Yogurt				
Ice Cream				
Pudding (made from milk)				
Meat group				
Meat				
Fish				
Poultry				
Nuts, peanut butter				
Cooked dried beans (dried peas)				
Fruit and vegetable group				
Vitamin C source				
Vitamin A source				
Fruit juices				
Raw fresh fruits				
Raw fresh vegetables				
Bread and cereal				
Bread, rolls, bagels				
Tacos, burritos				
Crackers				
Cake, pie crust				
Doughnuts				
Cereal				
Fats				
Mayonnaise				
Margarine				
Salad dressing				
Cooking oil				
Butter				

*To be used as a cross-check with the 24-hour recall.

needed to understand fully not only what a person eats but also the total meaning of eating for him.

Physical Examination

A number of physical examination findings are important for determining whether dietary intake has been adequate for an individual and whether related interventions will be necessary to promote good nutrition. Physical examination findings that suggest an adequate dietary intake are summarized in Table 34-10.

In addition, assess the oral cavity to be certain that the patient is capable of chewing and swallowing. This is particularly important in infants (when teeth may still be unformed), in schoolage children who may have multiple cavities (chewing may cause pain), and in older adults (who may have lost teeth). Assess bowel sounds to be sure that intestinal peristalsis is present.

Additional Areas to Be Assessed For a Total Nutrition History

Area of Assessment	*Pertinent Questions*
Food preparation	Who does the cooking? How are foods usually prepared? What spices or condiments are commonly used? What type oil is used for frying?
Food pattern	How many meals does patient eat per day? Which is his big meal? How many snacks does he eat a day? What are they? How many meals are eaten outside the home? Where are outside meals eaten? cafeteria? fast food store? restaurant?
Financial concerns	Is there enough money for food? Has he changed diet lately to economize? Would he eat differently if more money were available?
Family dietary pattern	Does anyone in the family eat a special diet? Is anyone obviously over- or underweight? Has the person had a loss or gain of weight lately? Does the family eat meals together? Is mealtime a social time?
Personal food preference	Are there any foods he particularly enjoys or dislikes? Are there any foods he feels are harmful or particularly beneficial to him? Does he take supplemental vitamins (frequency and type)? Does he drink alcohol? What type? How much?
Health	Does he have any allergies to food that he knows of? Does he have any trouble with chewing or digestion? What is bowel movement frequency? Does he develop intestinal gas? Does he take any medication? Over-the-counter antacids or laxatives?

Evaluate motor coordination of the upper extremities to determine if the person will be able to use a spoon or hold a glass effectively. This is particularly important in young patients (sufficient coordination has not yet developed) and in patients with muscular or neurological disease. Assess whether there are any sensory or mechanical factors that would interfere with optimal nutrition (difficulty with vision, an intravenous fluid line that prevents hand movement, mental confusion).

Assess general mood (a person who is depressed or has low self-esteem may have anorexia or loss of appetite) and activity level (a person who is exhausted may be too tired to expend effort on eating).

Anthropometric Measurements

HEIGHT AND WEIGHT

Height and weight are the prime measurements used in assessing the nutritional status of both well and ill persons. The ideal weight for height for adults is shown in Appendix D as well as growth curves used to determine these measurements in infants and children. Remember that overweight is as serious as underweight, excessive growth as serious as undergrowth when evaluating these measurements.

HEAD CIRCUMFERENCE

Head circumference measurements are routinely taken in children under 2 years of age at health care visits because the size of the growing head reflects the growing brain beneath it (see Chap. 19). A small head circumference may not reflect the present nutritional status of the child as much as it does his nutritional status while in utero. A large head circumference reflects a probable neurological abnormality rather than a nutritional one.

CHEST CIRCUMFERENCE

The chest circumference (measured at the nipple line) may indicate muscle wasting. This measurement is less than the head circumference at birth, equal to head circumference at 2 years of age, and greater than head circumference thereafter.

ABDOMINAL CIRCUMFERENCE

Abdominal circumference is measured at the level of the umbilicus. Such a measurement may reveal an increase in the size of the abdominal organs such as might occur with hepatic or splenic disease or abdominal distention such as occurs with intestinal blockage or obstruction.

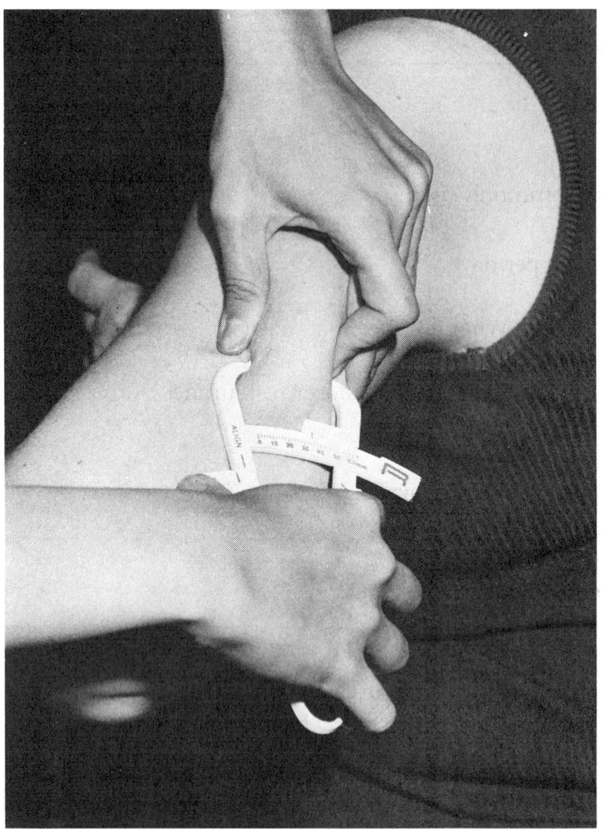

FIGURE 35-1. Measurement of skin-fold thickness using a caliper.

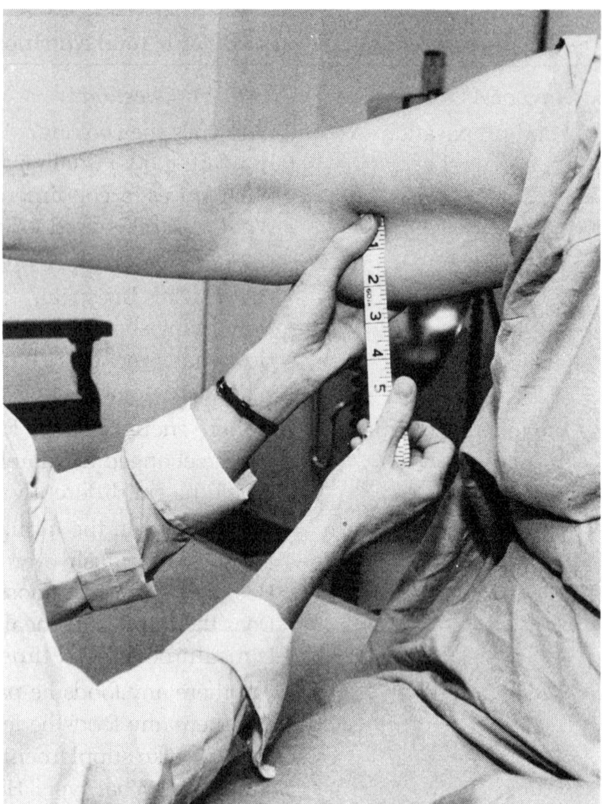

FIGURE 35-2. Measurement of skin-fold thickness using a measuring tape.

SKIN-FOLD THICKNESS

Skin-fold thickness is a determinant of the amount of fat present in subcutaneous tissue over the triceps muscle. To obtain a skin-fold thickness measurement, determine the midpoint of the upper arm (a point halfway between the elbow and the acromion process). Pinch a fold of skin at the midpoint between your finger and thumb and measure its thickness with a skin-fold caliper (Fig. 35-1). This is a painless process, and although it is not routinely used in assessment it can be useful to demonstrate a gain or loss of subcutaneous fat in people on special restricted or additive diets. Because women have a greater amount of subcutaneous fat per square inch than men (24 percent compared with 17 percent), they generally have greater skin-fold measurements than men (Fig. 35-2).

UPPER ARM CIRCUMFERENCE

The upper arm circumference measures arm *muscle.* This measurement reflects calorie and protein intake (which are instrumental in muscle growth) as well as subcutaneous fat. The measurement is made at the upper arm midpoint with a measuring tape; standard measurements are shown in Table 35-1.

Laboratory Tests

A number of standard laboratory tests are helpful in establishing the status of carbohydrates, proteins, fats, minerals, vitamins, and water in the body. Some common tests are blood sugar level, to determine carbohydrate metabolism; blood urea nitrogen (BUN) or total protein, to determine protein level; cholesterol level, to determine saturated fat metabolism; and mineral and vitamin levels. The specific gravity of urine is a helpful determinant of hydration. Appendix G lists the normal values of these tests.

Analysis

After collection of the three prongs of nutritional assessment data it is not unusual to discover that a person who has a primary illness such as pneumonia has developed a secondary nutritional illness due to nausea caused by stress or inability to prepare food because of exhaustion. A secondary problem may also arise from lack of food buying power, preparation of unadvised food (heavy in saturated fat), or omission of certain types of food (no vegetables). The problem might be related to psychological aspects of illness (too depressed to eat), or it can be a direct result of a disease process leading to poor digestion, absorption, transport, or utilization of nutrients.

Establish a locus of decision-making on who will help set patient care goals—the nurse, the patient, or both. Patient participation is particularly important in planning nutritional aspects of care because the best diet is worthless unless it is eaten. If a person is to

TABLE 35-1. MIDARM MUSCLE CIRCUMFERENCE STANDARDS

Age	Male (cm)	Female (cm)
6 months	11.4	11.2
1 year	12.7	12.4
2 years	13.1	12.8
4 years	14.0	13.7
6 years	14.7	14.2
8 years	16.0	15.3
10 years	17.1	16.6
12 years	18.5	18.3
14 years	20.8	19.6
Adult	25.3	23.2

Source: From D. B. Jellife, *The Assessment of the Nutritional Status of the Community.* WHO Monograph 53. Geneva: World Health Organization, 1966.

continue to eat a diet for any length of time, it must be a diet that he enjoys (or at least can tolerate), can afford, and can prepare. Otherwise, within a week or two the patient will be making so many exceptions that the original diet is almost indiscernible.

MOTIVATION FOR DIET CHANGE

A person rarely changes his diet pattern spontaneously for little reason. He needs to see clearly that the new diet will benefit him in some way before he can agree to it. Bad news about his diet, such as being told by a physician that the blood cholesterol level is very high and if he does not make an attempt to eat less saturated fat he could develop a heart attack, has a different effect on different people. Some accept this as a motivation to change, but others tell themselves that the physician said *could* have an attack, not *will.* These people probably are not yet ready for dietary counseling.

When such a person does have a heart attack, he still may not be ready to change, but most people are very susceptible to change when they are told that they have an illness or can recognize that they have an illness and will have to modify their diets to prevent it from becoming worse. Before making plans for dietary changes, consider the factors that are important in food choices.

CULTURAL OR RELIGIOUS IMPORTANCE OF FOOD

People change their dietary patterns most readily if they are allowed to change to other foods familiar to them rather than foods that seem "foreign" to them. A person who is used to eating Italian pasta, for example, who must diet to lose weight might do better if he is encouraged to eat meat sauce without spaghetti rather than cottage cheese and peaches as a low-calorie lunch. Remember that people cook as they learned to cook. A woman from a certain culture does not know *how* to prepare foods other than those she is familiar with.

SYMBOLISM OF FOOD

It is difficult for a person to omit a food from his diet that has a strong symbolic meaning. Milk, for example, is considered by many people to be a perfect food (not true, however—it has a low iron content). They believe that if they do not insist that their child drink milk they are not good parents. It is difficult, therefore, to ask a mother to prepare a milk-free diet for her child.

AVAILABILITY OF ALTERNATE FOODS

People will have difficulty accepting a new or different food in a diet if it is difficult to obtain in their local food stores. Advising a person who has difficulty getting to a store frequently to eat fresh fruit daily will be ineffective. Suggesting frozen orange juice that is made fresh daily will improve his vitamin C intake more effectively because it is a practical and convenient alternate method.

COOPERATION OF PERSON WHO PREPARES FOOD

When discussing changes in dietary patterns, be sure to identify who will be preparing and cooking the food. A low-sodium diet will be unsuccessful if the patient's wife does not understand the diet and continues to add salt in cooking or packs bologna sandwiches in his lunch.

LENGTH OF TIME DIET PATTERN HAS BEEN FOLLOWED

Food habits learned in childhood are difficult to break because they have been with the person for such a long time. Adults who have been obese since they were children, for example, typically have more difficulty changing the built-in habit of overeating than people who only recently have become obese.

COST OF NEW DIET PLAN

Many people eat certain foods because their income is limited and they can afford only the less expensive foods. Investigate whether financial assistance is available that could help increase food buying power (see Chap. 34). Make common suggestions for more economical shopping such as buying day-old bread.

PHYSICAL LIMITATIONS

Dietary planning sometimes fails because the person's physical limitations are not considered. A person with ill-fitting dentures (or no dentures) will have difficulty eating more meat because he cannot chew it well and therefore avoids it. A person who tires quickly may want to prepare three full meals a day but is so tired by dinnertime that a sandwich is all she can accomplish. She may need a second person to prepare and freeze a week's supply of dinners for her, or she might need someone (perhaps a service such as Meals on Wheels) to prepare one meal a day for her.

Hand coordination, motor coordination, and food allergies are other physical limitations that need to be considered. Consider the limitations of the person who cooks as well as the patient if they are different.

SUPPORT PEOPLE AVAILABLE

When people are planning a change in a dietary pattern, they may not be able to use their usual support people as reinforcers. For example, a woman may have difficulty preparing low-calorie meals for herself and normal meals for her family.

FOOD PREFERENCES

Be certain in planning dietary changes that you do not plan a diet that *you* would enjoy; plan one that will be enjoyed by the person who will eat it. If a person who needs to increase his calcium intake chooses to simply drink more milk rather than eating yogurt, cheese, and ice cream, that is his choice.

REINFORCEMENT FOR MAINTAINING A CHANGE IN DIET

People respond better to a reward for good behavior than they do to punishment for bad behavior. In some instances, such as a diet that alleviates the pain of peptic (stomach) ulcers, people *do* receive an immediate reward for following the diet. In most cases, however, people notice no change from following a particular diet (they cannot see more calcium in their bones or more iron in their red blood cells). This lack of visible reward may cause people to become lax in their diet plan after a short period of time.

Discuss with the person how he can measure progress. Showing a person the laboratory study results or height and weight graphs at health care visits is a method of offering encouragement. People on weight-reduction diets are very responsive to this type of reward and often enjoy plotting their own graphs to mark their accomplishment.

Setting both short-term and long-term goals often helps people to stay with a diet longer (a long-term goal is to lose 100 pounds; a short-term goal is to lose 7 pounds a month). Rewards can be given at periodic intervals as a goal is met, and there is a better sense of accomplishment along the way.

Planning and Implementation

Planning care for better nutrition involves a number of actions. It may include education about a special diet or better nutrition in general, supervision of dietary intake, or providing food or fluid through gastric intubation or total parenteral nutrition (a method of intravenous feeding).

EDUCATION FOR GOOD NUTRITION

Education about nutrition can be done either in groups or individually. Most people have learned something about nutrition from a high school class. When counseling people about nutrition, do not tell them to eat "protein-rich foods" or "something with fewer calories" and expect them to know what you mean. Foods are sold as meat, produce, and canned goods, for example, not "high protein" or "low calories." Be specific so that the person knows exactly what you mean. The American Dairy Council has printed forms called Food Comparison Cards that they will supply for nutrition education (Fig. 35-3).

The Dairy Council will also provide colorful pictures of many different foods that can be used to show or to plan a balanced meal. This type of activity is helpful in formal classes in ambulatory or inpatient units and is interesting for a person confined to bed.

Children respond well to board games. A game similar to Monopoly can be constructed in which, to earn money or to stay on a certain space, the player must answer a nutrition or diet question (this interests schoolagers and adolescents). "Flash cards" with nutrition information on them are another form of game that can be devised. Parents can play these games with their children (educating parents, *the food preparers*, about this information is necessary also).

If a person knows almost nothing about what foods are good for him or what foods he will need to change in his diet, do not attempt to teach him too much at one time. Allow time to absorb some elemental information first. Too much diet information makes a diet seem like an overwhelming chore, and the person may not give it a fair trial. For some people, the very word *diet* implies restrictions, or lack of interesting foods, or unappetizing foods. They respond better if you never mention the word diet but refer instead to "foods that would be better for you" or "foods that would be healthier for you not to eat."

COMMON DIET PRESCRIPTIONS

A diet is ordered by a physician with the same care and concern that medications or other therapies are ordered. Many people do not think that their diet prescription is as important as their prescription for medication, however, and often need more reminders to follow a diet than to take a new medication. Making an error in a patient's diet can be as detrimental to them as if you had made an error in medication.

As a person's condition changes, his diet prescription needs changes also, and you may have to remind the physician of this. In most instances you can change the consistency of a diet as an independent nursing action, and often management of diet is given to you as an independent nursing action by an order such as "diet as tolerated" or "proceed to full diet as tolerated."

House or Regular Diets

A "house" diet is a standard diet for a person who does not require a therapeutic diet. It has a total calorie count of about 2000 to 2500 kilocalories and 60 to 90

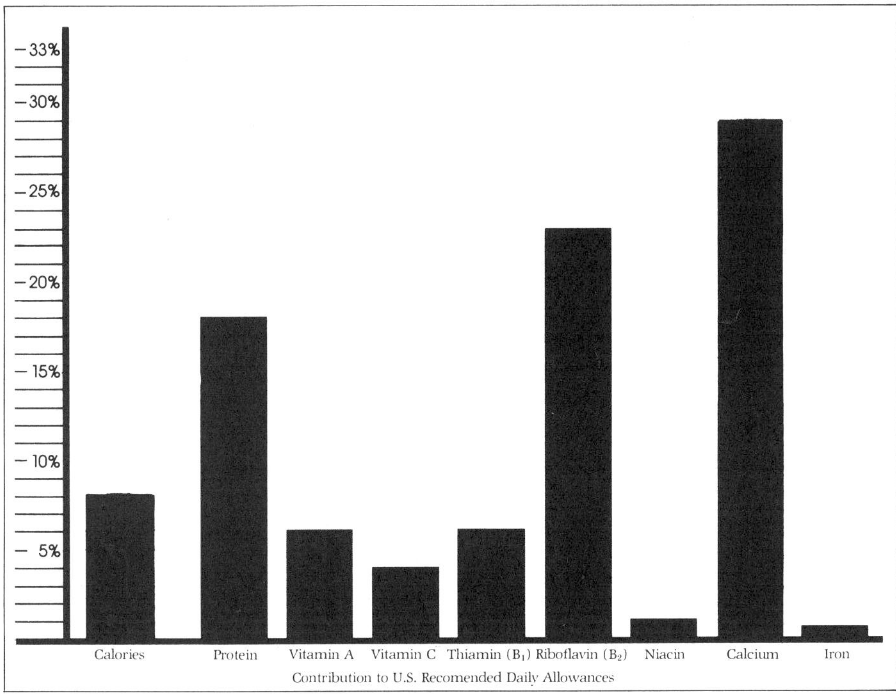

A

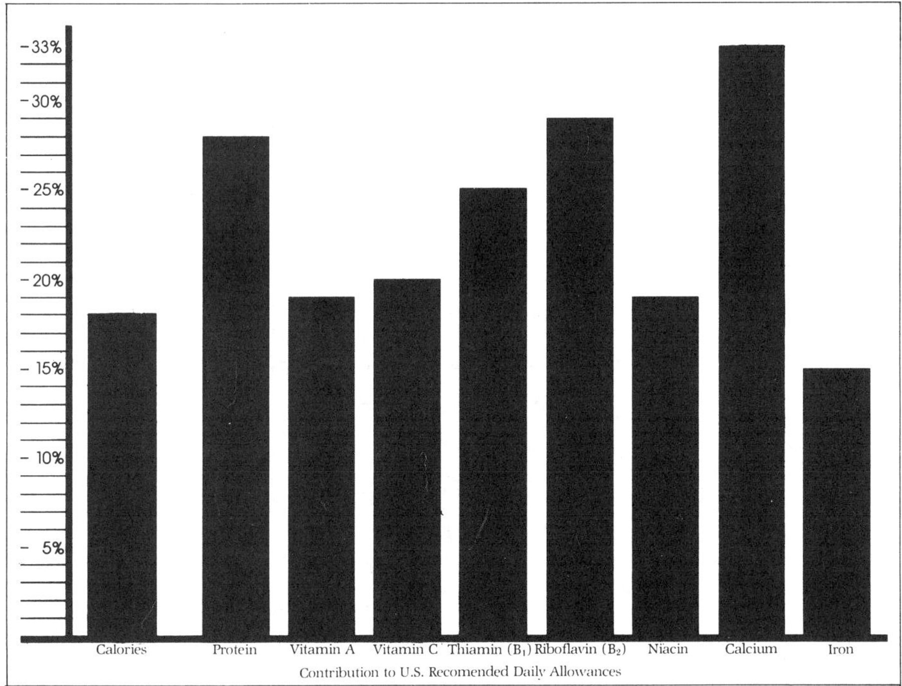

B

FIGURE 35-3. Food Comparison Cards. Notice the difference in the amount of nutrients furnished by (A) milk (1 cup = 8 oz or 244 gm, fortified with vitamin D: 145 calories) and (B) pizza (1/4 of 14-inch pie = 5 oz or 150 gm, with enriched crust: 354 calories). (From National Dairy Council, Rosemont, Ill.)

gm of protein a day. It is adequate for a sedentary person with routine food likes and dislikes. In many health care facilities, the person is allowed to select the foods he would like from a menu. Menu lists for the following day generally arrive on the patient's breakfast or lunch tray. Check that such a list is returned to the dietary department, not disposed of with the tray. A sample house meal plan is shown on page 930.

Children's Diets

House diets for children are usually divided by age group—infant, preschool, child, and adolescent. All these diets are well balanced and contain adequate

House Diet

Description: A house diet is designed for patients who require no special dietary modifications or restrictions. Individual intolerances may necessitate the exclusion of certain food items. Salt, pepper, and sugar are routinely added to the tray.

APPROXIMATE COMPOSITION OF SAMPLE MENU

Calories	2464
Protein (gm)	91
Fat (gm)	115
Carbohydrate (gm)	268

FOODS ALLOWED

Amounts to use daily are based on the Basic Four Food Plan.

Food Group	*Foods Allowed*	*Amount*
Beverages	Milk (any kind), coffee, tea, other beverages	2 or more cups, as desired
Breads	All kinds	3 or more servings, enriched or whole grain
Cereals	All kinds	1 serving
Desserts	All kinds	1—2 servings
Eggs	Any preparation	3—5 per week
Fats	Table spreads, cream, salad dressings	4—6 tsp
Fruits, fruit juices	All	2 or more servings (1 should be citrus)
Meat, fish, poultry, cheese	All kinds	2 servings (5 oz total)
Soups	All kinds	As desired
Sugar, sweets	All kinds	4—6 tsp daily
Vegetables, vegetable juices	All kinds	2 or more servings (1 should be orange or dark green leafy for a source of vitamin A)
Miscellaneous	Salt (iodized), condiments, herbs, spices	As desired

SAMPLE MENU FOR HOUSE DIET

Breakfast	*Luncheon*	*Dinner*
1/2 cup frozen orange juice	3/4 cup creamed chicken on	3 oz roast beef sirloin
1/2 cup farina	1 biscuit	1/2 cup mashed potatoes
1 egg, soft cooked	1/2 cup green beans	1/4 cup beef broth gravy
1 slice toast, white enriched	1/2 sliced tomato on lettuce	1/2 cup cooked carrots
1 tsp butter	2 tsp mayonnaise	3/4 cup tossed lettuce salad
1 tbsp grape jelly	1 slice bread, white enriched	1 tbsp French dressing
1 cup milk	1 tsp butter	1 slice bread, white enriched
2 tsp sugar	1/2 cup canned peaches	1 tsp butter
Coffee or tea	1 slice angel food cake	1/2 cup sherbet
	1 cup milk	3 vanilla wafers
	1 tsp sugar	1 cup milk
	Coffee or tea	1 tsp sugar
		Coffee or tea

Source: Reprinted by permission from University of Iowa Hospitals and Clinics, *Recent Advances in Therapeutic Diets* (3rd ed.).

amounts of calories and nutrients for each age group. An infant diet is composed of soft foods that are easily chewed; a toddler or preschoolage child receives a diet that contains a high proportion of finger foods; a child's diet contains foods that particularly appeal to children (hot dogs instead of roast beef, corn on the cob instead of creamed corn); adolescent diets have high calorie counts and foods that adolescents enjoy (pizza instead of a sandwich). Some adolescent boys have such big appetites that they need extra servings or snacks ordered between meals.

Because children's eating patterns vary greatly, many physicians order a child's diet as a house diet for age and allow you to make a selection of which diet would be most appropriate following your nutrition history. A sample menu for a toddler diet is shown below (Children's Hospital of Buffalo, *Diet Manual*, Buffalo, New York, 1978)*:

BREAKFAST
1 orange (sectioned)
1 serving corn flakes
1 poached egg
1/2 slice toast with butter
1 carton milk

LUNCH
1 cup vegetable soup
2 oz hamburger on bun (quartered)
1 serving tomato wedges
1 skippy cup ice cream
1 carton milk

DINNER
2 oz chicken (cut up)
4 tbsp mashed potatoes
1/2 cup green beans
1/2 slice bread with butter
1/2 slice applesauce cake (sectioned)
1 carton milk

Maternity Diets

A maternity house diet is a diet formulated for a woman following the birth of a baby. She needs a high fluid intake during this time; she feels well and often has a voracious appetite, so portions are large.

Newborn Diets

The diet prescription for a newborn is "breast-feeding" or a specific commercial formula. Breast-feeding is begun shortly after birth. Some physicians prefer to let the infant begin nursing for a limited amount of time (5 minutes on each breast at each feeding the first day, 6 minutes the second day, and up to 10 minutes thereafter). Others specify no particular pattern, and a pattern is then determined by the preferences of the infant and the mother under your guidance.

*A toddler diet is used for children 2 to 5 years of age who can eat table foods. Food items are easily picked up or require little cutting. The diet contains approximately 1600 calories. It meets the RDA for this age group.

TABLE 35-2. COMMON INFANT FORMULAS

Type	Use or Features
Human breast milk	Readily digested protein; contains antibodies to common illnesses; adequate in vitamins and minerals
Similac Enfamil SMA	Similar to human breast milk; vitamins and minerals added
Advance	Designed for infant 9—12 months of age; higher in minerals but lower in calories to promote early growth and prevent early weight gain
ProSobee Neo-Mull-Soy Isomil	Soybean-based formulas for infants allergic to cow's milk; vitamins and minerals added
Portagen	Lactose-free; used for infants with malabsorption problem; vitamins added
Nutramigen	Lactose-free for infants with lactase deficiency
Cho-Free	For infants with carbohydrate intolerance
Lofenalac	Low in phenylalanine; used with children with phenylketonuria
Lonalac	Low in sodium; vitamins added
Meat-base	For infants allergic to soy protein; vitamins and minerals added
Progestimil	Easily digested fat. Used for infants with malabsorption disorders
Skim milk	Inappropriate for infants due to low calorie and fat content
Whole cow's milk	Inappropriate for infants under 6 months of age
Evaporated milk	Inadequate in vitamin C, iron, and possibly fluoride

Commercial formulas are supplied in at least three different strengths (13 calories, 20 calories, and 24 calories per ounce). Feeding the wrong strength could make a big difference in the number of calories the newborn receives. Common brands of infant formula are shown in Table 35-2.

Soft Diets

Soft diets may be prescribed for people who have difficulty with chewing (due to irritated oral mucosa or lack of dentures, for example) or with digestion. A soft diet is composed of low-residue foods (low in cellulose or fiber) and no fried foods for easy digestion. It contains about 1800 to 2500 kcal a day.

Soft diets are not as appetizing as house diets. For most patients they are used for a short period of time. A sample soft diet plan is shown on page 932.

A bland diet is a similar diet designed specifically for the person with gastrointestinal ulcers. It is designed to be as nonirritating to the stomach and duodenal lining as possible. A *pureed* diet is prepared by processing food in a blender. It is used for people who cannot chew to begin breakdown of food.

Soft Diet

Description: The soft diet consists of foods that are tender but not ground or pureed. Whole meats, cooked vegetables, and fruits of moderate fiber content are allowed.

This diet is suitable for patients who cannot tolerate highly seasoned, fried, or raw foods. It is sometimes used as a transition between the full liquid and general diets. The soft diet is *not* designed for the edentulous patient (use a ground or pureed diet).

APPROXIMATE COMPOSITION OF SAMPLE MENU

Calories	2509
Protein (gm)	93
Fat (gm)	117
Carbohydrate (gm)	274

FOODS ALLOWED AND FOODS TO AVOID

Food Group	*Foods Allowed*	*Foods to Avoid*
Beverages	Milk and milk drinks, carbonated beverages, coffee, tea, decaffeinated coffee, cereal beverages	None
Breads	Enriched white, refined whole wheat, and rye breads; saltine and graham crackers	Coarse whole grain breads with seeds, nuts, or raisins; seasoned crackers with seeds or spices
Cereals	Refined cooked and prepared cereals (corn, oats, rice, wheat)	Whole grain cooked and prepared cereals
Desserts	Plain cakes and cookies (thinly iced if desired), plain puddings, smooth ice cream and sherbet, gelatin desserts, fruit whips	Pastries; pies; any desserts containing nuts, coconut, dried fruit, fruits with small seeds
Eggs	Baked, creamed, poached, soft or hard cooked, scrambled, made into soufflé or fondue	Fried eggs
Fats	Butter, margarine, cream, vegetable shortening and oils, lard, crisp bacon, mildly seasoned salad dressings	Fried foods, high fat gravy, spicy salad dressings
Fruits, fruit juices	All fruit juices; raw ripe banana; orange and grapefruit sections without membrane; peeled ripe peach or pear; cooked or canned cherries, applesauce, fruit cocktail, peaches, pears; peeled or pureed plums, apricots, dates	All other raw fruits, all fruits with small seeds, all fruits with tough skins
Meat, fish, poultry, cheese	Baked, broiled, roasted, creamed, or stewed tender beef, lamb, veal, liver, chicken, turkey; crisp bacon; all canned, fresh, or frozen fish and seafood; cottage cheese, cream cheese, mild cheddar or processed cheese	Fried, highly seasoned, or pickled meat, fish, poultry; strongly flavored cheese

Potatoes or substitutes	White and sweet potatoes, spaghetti, macaroni, noodles, rice, hominy	Highly seasoned potatoes or potato substitute, fried potatoes and potato chips, brown or wild rice
Soups	Broth-base and cream soups made from foods allowed	Fatty or highly spiced soups
Sugar, sweets	Sugar, syrup, honey, clear jelly, fruit butters, plain sugar or chocolate candy in moderation	Jams, marmalade, candies containing nuts, seeds, coconut, or tough skins
Vegetables, vegetable juices	All vegetable juices; raw lettuce only; cooked or canned tender vegetables including asparagus tips, beets, carrots, green and wax beans, eggplant, mushrooms, peas, pumpkin, spinach, squash, tomatoes, pureed lima beans and corn	All other raw or cooked vegetables, whole lima beans or corn, frozen peas
Miscellaneous	Salt (iodized), cinnamon, allspice, mild flavorings, dilute vinegar, cocoa powder, smooth peanut butter, cream sauce, nongreasy gravy, lemon juice	Horseradish, mustard, pepper, nuts, coconut, relish, olives, catsup, popcorn, excessive amounts of spices or herbs

SAMPLE MENU FOR SOFT DIET

Breakfast	*Luncheon*	*Dinner*
1/2 cup frozen orange juice	3/4 cup creamed chicken on 1 biscuit	3 oz roast beef sirloin
1/2 cup farina	1/2 cup green beans	1/2 cup mashed potatoes
1 egg, soft cooked	1/2 cup tomato juice	1/4 cup beef broth gravy
1 slice toast, white enriched	1 slice bread, white enriched	1/2 cup cooked carrots
1 tsp butter	1 tsp butter	3/4 cup shredded lettuce salad
1 tbsp grape jelly	1/2 cup canned peaches	2 tsp mayonnaise
1 cup milk	1 slice angel food cake	1 slice bread, white enriched
2 tsp sugar	1 cup milk	1 tsp butter
Coffee or tea	1 tsp sugar	1/2 cup sherbet
	Coffee or tea	3 vanilla wafers
		1 cup milk
		1 tsp sugar
		Coffee or tea

Source: Reprinted by permission from University of Iowa Hospitals and Clinics, *Recent Advances in Therapeutic Diets* (3rd ed.).

Liquid Diets

A liquid diet may be ordered for people who cannot chew or who have had abdominal surgery. These diets can be taken by mouth or administered by nasogastric tube.

FULL LIQUID DIET

A full liquid diet contains about 1300 to 1500 kcal a day. It includes any food that is liquid at room temperature such as ice cream, custard, or Popsicles. It is adequate in all nutrients except fiber. Vitamin or mineral supplements may be added to ensure a good intake of these. Because the diet generally is prepared with a milk base, any problem that leads to an inability to drink milk (lactase deficiency or allergy) will interfere with the success of the diet. The health care agency may prepare its own liquid diet or use a commercial liquid diet. A full liquid diet is described on page 934. Some common types of commercially prepared liquid formulas are shown in Table 35-3.

Full Liquid Diet

Description: The full liquid diet, recommended for temporary use only, includes a variety of foods that are liquid or will become liquid at body temperature. The diet provides nourishment that is easy to consume and is recommended for use when a patient cannot tolerate solid food. Nourishments served between meals and at bedtime increase the caloric and nutrient intake.

Adequacy: This diet will meet the Recommended Daily Dietary Allowances for all nutrients, except iron for women of childbearing age, only if the diet includes the recommended number of servings from the Basic Four Food Plan. The most difficult foods to include are those from the meat, fish, poultry, and cheese group (3-1/2-oz jar pureed meat = 2 oz meat).

APPROXIMATE COMPOSITION

Calories	2249
Protein (gm)	78
Fat (gm)	80
Carbohydrate (gm)	314

FOODS ALLOWED AND FOODS TO AVOID

Food Group	*Foods Allowed*	*Foods to Avoid*
Beverages	Coffee, tea, decaffeinated coffee, cereal beverages, milk drinks, carbonated beverages, fruit drinks	All others
Breads	None	All
Cereals	Cooked refined cereal, cereal gruel	All others
Desserts	Custard, gelatin desserts, rennet dessert, ice cream, sherbet, cornstarch pudding, Popsicles	All products containing seeds, nuts, coconut, fruit, and other foods not allowed
Eggs	Soft custard, eggnog	All other preparations
Fats	Butter, margarine, cream, vegetable oils	All others
Fruits, fruit juices	All fruit juices (include at least 1 serving of citrus juice daily), pureed fruit	All others
Meat, fish, poultry, cheese	Mild cheese sauce, pureed meat added to broth or cream soup	All others
Potatoes or substitutes	Mashed white potato used in cream soup	All others
Soups	Consommé, broth, bouillon, strained cream soup made from foods allowed	All others
Sugar, sweets	Honey, sugar, syrup, hard candy	Jam; marmalade; candy containing coconut, fruit, nuts
Vegetables, vegetable juices	All vegetable juices, pureed vegetables in cream soup	All others
Miscellaneous	Salt (iodized), flavorings, chocolate syrup, cocoa powder, cinnamon, nutmeg	All others

SAMPLE MENU FOR FULL LIQUID DIET

Breakfast	*Luncheon*	*Dinner*
1/2 cup strained orange juice 1 cup farina 1 cup milk 2 tsp sugar 1 cup eggnog Coffee or tea with 1/2 oz half-and-half	3/4 cup cream of potato soup 1/2 cup grape juice 1/2 cup pureed peaches 1/2 cup vanilla ice cream 1 cup milk 1 tsp sugar Coffee or tea with 1/2 oz half-and-half	1 cup pineapple juice 3/4 cup strained cream of chicken soup (1/2 cup soup with 1/4 cup pureed chicken) 3/4 cup chocolate milkshake 1/2 cup flavored gelatin 1/2 cup pureed pears 1 cup milk 1 tsp sugar Coffee or tea with 1/2 oz half-and-half
Midmorning Nourishment	*Midafternoon Nourishment*	*Evening Nourishment*
1/2 cup pureed banana	1/2 cup vanilla flavored yogurt	1 cup chocolate milk

Source: Reprinted by permission from University of Iowa Hospitals and Clinics, *Recent Advances in Therapeutic Diets* (3rd ed.). Copyright © 1979 by Iowa State University Press, Ames, Iowa.

TABLE 35-3. COMMON TOTAL LIQUID FORMULAS FOR TUBE OR ORAL FEEDINGS

Type	Composition	Special Features
Compleat B (Doyle)	Protein: beef; skim milk. Fat: corn oil, beef fat.. Carbohydrate: maltodextrin, lactose, sucrose.	Approximates a normal mixed diet; sterilized, ready to use. Four cans (1600 ml) = 1600 kcal. Fulfills 100% of RDA.
Formula 2 (Cutter)	Protein: milk protein, animal protein, wheat protein. Fat: beef fat, corn oil, egg yolk. Carbohydrate: lactose, sucrose.	Orange-flavored. 2 liters = 2000 kcal. Fulfills 100% of RDA.
Meat-base (Gerber)	Protein: beef hearts. Fat: sesame oil. Carbohydrate: cane sugar.	Low osmolarity, lactose-free. 2.5 liters = 100% RDA except for magnesium and folic acid. Often used with infants because of low osmolarity.
Isocal (Mead-Johnson)	Protein: calcium caseinate, sodium caseinate, soy, protein isolate. Fat: soy oil, MCT oil. Carbohydrate: corn syrup solids.	Lactose-free, nearly isotonic. 2000 kcal = 100% RDA.
Ensure (Ross)	Protein: sodium and calcium caseinate, soy protein isolate. Fat: corn oil. Carbohydrate: corn syrup solids, sucrose.	Lactose-free; polyunsaturated; flavoring may be added. 2000 ml = 100% RDA.
Sustacal (Mead-Johnson)	Protein: skim milk, sodium and calcium caseinates, soy protein isolate. Fat: partially hydrogenated soy oil. Carbohydrate: sucrose, lactose, corn syrup solids.	3 cans (12 oz) = 100% RDA. Flavoring available.
Nutri-1000 (Cutter)	Protein: skim milk. Fat: corn oil. Carbohydrate: sucrose, lactose, dextrin-maltose, dextrose.	2000 ml = 2000 kcal and 100% RDA. Certified Kosher. Flavoring available.
Vivonex (Eaton)	Protein: amino acids. Fat: safflower oil. Carbohydrate: glucose oligosaccharides.	2000 ml = 2000 kcal and 100% RDA.

RDA = Recommended Daily Allowance.

CLEAR LIQUID DIET

A clear liquid diet includes only liquids that are clear when held to the light (apple juice, tea, consommé, ginger ale), not milk or milk products. It includes about 400 to 500 kcal a day. It is used for a transitional period (two or three days) when a person's gastrointestinal tract is unable to accept any foods more difficult to digest than these. *It is not adequate for long-term therapy.* Popsicles are often a pleasant way to take clear fluid; Jello may be included as an acceptable clear liquid. The box on page 936 shows a clear liquid diet.

Restricted Diets

Due to a disease process a diet may have to be restricted in some way.

Clear Liquid Diet

Description: This diet provides clear fluids that will leave little residue and be easily absorbed with a minimum of digestive activity. No milk products are included. The foods are liquid or will become liquid at body temperature. A clear liquid diet is used only for short periods during acute conditions or postoperatively.

Adequacy: This diet does not meet the Recommended Daily Dietary Allowances for any nutrient except ascorbic acid and should not be used more than 3 days without supplementation.

APPROXIMATE COMPOSITION OF SAMPLE MENU

Calories	1154
Protein (gm)	17
Fat (gm)	2
Carbohydrate (gm)	267

FOODS ALLOWED AND FOODS TO AVOID

Food Group	*Foods Allowed*	*Foods to Avoid*
Beverages	Carbonated beverages, coffee, tea, decaffeinated coffee, clear beverages, fruit flavored drinks	Milk, milk drinks
Breads	None	All
Cereals	None	All
Desserts	Clear, flavored gelatin; Popsicles	All others
Eggs	None	All
Fats	None	All
Fruit, fruit juices	Strained fruit juices (apple, cherry, cranapple, cranberry, grape, orange)	Fruit juices with pulp, all fruit
Soups	Clear broth, consommé	All others
Sugar, sweets	Sugar, honey, syrup, stick candy, clear sugar candy	All others

SAMPLE MENU FOR CLEAR LIQUID DIET

Breakfast	*Luncheon*	*Dinner*
1 cup strained orange juice	3/4 cup broth	3/4 cup consommé
1/2 cup broth	1 cup grape juice	1 cup apple juice
1/2 cup flavored gelatin	1/2 cup flavored gelatin	1/2 cup flavored gelatin
1 tsp sugar	2 sticks hard candy	2 sticks hard candy
Coffee or tea	1 tsp sugar	1 tsp sugar
	Coffee or tea	Coffee or tea
Midmorning Nourishment	*Midafternoon Nourishment*	*Evening Nourishment*
1/2 cup flavored gelatin	Popsicle	1 cup cranberry juice

Source: Reprinted by permission from University of Iowa Hospitals and Clinics, *Recent Advances in Therapeutic Diets* (3rd ed.).

MINERAL RESTRICTED DIETS

To correct some disease conditions a person needs a diet that is restricted in a certain mineral. Examples are sodium-restricted diets for people with heart disease (less sodium decreases fluid retention and therefore lessens the work of the heart), potassium-restricted diets for people with kidney disease (high potassium blood levels lead to cardiac arrhythmias; if a person cannot excrete potassium owing to poor kidney function he must ingest a diet low in potassium to prevent potassium buildup), and calcium-restricted diets for people with altered calcium metabolism (high calcium levels can lead to the formation of kidney or bladder stones). A calcium-restricted diet may be deficient in riboflavin and vitamin D because these vitamins are contained in fortified milk, and milk (a high calcium source) is almost totally omitted from a low-calcium diet. The following box gives an example of a sodium-restricted diet.

PROTEIN-RESTRICTED DIETS

Gluten, the protein component of wheat, rye, oats, and barley, cannot be absorbed by people sensitive to this grain protein. A diet devoid of gluten (gluten-free diet) must be constructed for such people. People with kidney disease who cannot excrete the breakdown product of protein (urea) may have to follow a total protein-restricted diet to decrease urea (BUN) in their blood. Phenylketonuria is an inherited disorder in which the affected person is unable to process the essential amino acid phenylalanine. Phenylalanine builds up in the body and exerts a toxic reaction leading to mental retardation as it affects brain tissue. These people need a low-phenylalanine diet to prevent this toxic buildup.

All protein-restricted diets must be planned with care, and evaluation of the actual amounts of food eaten must be made continuously to ensure that enough protein is being consumed for basic cell maintenance.

Sodium-Restricted Diets

Description: The purpose of sodium-restricted diets is to reduce the sodium content of the tissues and to promote loss of body water. Therefore sodium-restricted diets may be useful in the treatment of certain disease entities: cardiovascular diseases such as congestive heart failure and hypertension; diseases associated with fluid retention or electrolyte imbalance such as renal disease or cirrhosis; and diseases requiring treatment with sodium-retaining hormones or drugs such as corticosteroid therapy.

The general hospital diet contains approximately 5—8 gm (217—348 mEq) sodium (Na) daily. Commonly used dietary modifications of sodium content are as follows:

1. Mild sodium restriction—2,000—3,000 mg (87—130 mEq)
2. Mild sodium restriction—1,000 mg (43 mEq)
3. Moderate sodium restriction—800 mg (35 mEq)
4. Strict sodium restriction—500 mg (22 mEq)
5. Extremely strict sodium restriction—200 mg (8.5 mEq)

Notes to the physician: The level of sodium restriction will determine the nutritional adequacy of the diet. Sodium-restricted diets should be ordered in terms of milligrams or milliequivalents of sodium.

The salt substitute used at University of Iowa Hospitals and Clinic contains potassium ions (9.3 mEq K^+ per packet) and will not be given unless ordered by a physician. Because iodized salt is eliminated from the diet, an iodized salt substitute is used to aid in the prevention of endemic goiter.

Many of the special low sodium dietetic foods are processed by a simple ion exchange procedure in which sodium ions are replaced with potassium ions. Therefore some precaution must be taken when using low sodium products for hyperkalemic patients on sodium-restricted diets. A low sodium, low potassium diet may be ordered in such cases.

Sodium and sodium compounds are commonly used in food preparation or processing. It is extremely important that labels on all processed or convenience foods be read carefully by the patient to determine if salt or other sodium compounds have been added. Diets restricted below 2,000—3,000 mg Na will not usually include food products processed with salt or sodium compounds.

The patient should be cautioned to check for "hidden" sodium from sources other than food. Alkalizers for indigestion (e.g., Alka Seltzer or bicarbonate of soda) contain large amounts of sodium and should not be used on any sodium-restricted diet. Drinking water, in particular softened water, can contain rather large amounts of sodium, and the patient should check with the local dietitian or municipal water company to determine the amount. It is usually not necessary to alter water supplies, except for softened water, unless the diet is restricted below 800 mg Na. Chewing tobacco should not be used by patients who must restrict their sodium intake.

MILD SODIUM-RESTRICTED DIET (2,000—3,000 mg OR 87—130 mEq)

Description: The general hospital diet is served without a salt packet and highly salted foods are omitted or replaced with lightly salted substitutes. Milk intake is restricted to 3—4 cups per day.

APPROXIMATE COMPOSITION OF SAMPLE MENU

Calories	2475
Protein (gm)	91
Fat (gm)	117
Carbohydrate (gm)	269

FOODS TO AVOID

Food Group	*Foods High in Sodium*
Beverages	Commercial buttermilk
Breads	Salted crackers
Fats	Gravy, regular peanut butter
Meat, fish, poultry, cheese, substitutes	Cured meats such as ham, bacon, corned beef; chipped beef; wieners; luncheon meats; bologna; regular canned salmon and tuna; all cheeses except cottage cheese
Soups	All regular commercial soups, broth, canned bouillon or bouillon cubes, consommé
Vegetables, vegetable juices	Sauerkraut, regular canned tomato or vegetable juice
Miscellaneous	Free salt packet or salt shaker; seasoned salts such as celery salt, garlic salt; monosodium glutamate (Accent); Kitchen Bouquet; soy sauce; Worcestershire sauce; steak sauce; meat sauces; catsup; chili sauce; prepared mustard; horseradish; pickles; olives; salted snack foods such as pretzels, potato chips, nuts, popcorn; chewing tobacco

SAMPLE MENU FOR MILD SODIUM-RESTRICTED DIET

Breakfast	*Luncheon*	*Dinner*
1/2 cup frozen orange juice	3/4 cup creamed chicken on 1 biscuit	3 oz roast beef sirloin
1/2 cup farina	1/2 cup green beans	1/2 cup mashed potato
1 egg, soft cooked	1/2 sliced tomato on lettuce	1/2 cup cooked carrots
1 slice toast, white enriched	2 tsp mayonnaise	3/4 cup tossed lettuce salad
1 tsp butter	1 slice bread, white enriched	1 tbsp low sodium French dressing
1 tbsp grape jelly	1 tsp butter	1 slice bread, white enriched
1 cup milk	1/2 cup canned peaches	1 tsp butter
2 tsp sugar	1 slice angel food cake	1/2 cup sherbet
Coffee or tea	1 cup milk	3 vanilla wafers
Pepper	1 tsp sugar	1 cup milk
	Coffee or tea	1 tsp sugar
	Pepper	Coffee or tea
		Pepper

Source: Reprinted by permission from University of Iowa Hospitals and Clinics, *Recent Advances in Therapeutic Diets* (3rd ed.).

CARBOHYDRATE-RESTRICTED DIETS

Carbohydrate may be restricted to reduce total caloric intake (weight-reduction diet) or to provide a diet suitable for the person with a metabolic disease such as diabetes that interferes with carbohydrate metabolism.

DIABETIC DIETS

People with diabetes mellitus (decreased or absent production of insulin) tend to have abnormally elevated blood glucose levels because without insulin, glucose cannot enter the cells and builds up in the blood. A paradox exists here: At the same time there is a high glucose level in the blood, the cells are starving from lack of glucose.

To correct this glucose disturbance, diabetics administer insulin to themselves by injection daily and regulate the amount of carbohydrate (glucose) and other nutrients they ingest daily. A diet is designed according to how much carbohydrate, protein, and calories the person is allowed daily. (Daily carbohydrate is generally calculated as one-fifth for breakfast and two-fifths each for lunch and dinner). For the most simple planning of a diet, the American Dietetic Association has devised exchange lists of comparable foods (see the following box) in all food groups.

A person is given a sample day's menu that would constitute a good diet for him; he may substitute foods from exchange lists to plan any day's diet. To fully understand the problems involved in planning diabetic diets, it is necessary to understand the total metabolic activity that occurs in diabetes. The diet is mentioned here because it is frequently encountered and because everyone who assists with serving meals to patients must be aware that although a person with diabetes can have alternate foods if he desires them, foods cannot be substituted or added indiscriminately; if a person does not eat everything supplied on a meal tray he must be observed carefully for signs of hypoglycemia (reduced blood glucose) resulting from the action of the injected insulin and the reduced food intake. Signs of hypoglycemia are lethargy, mental confusion, and trembling.

FAT-RESTRICTED DIETS

Some disease conditions interfere with fat absorption and metabolism, making a low-fat diet necessary. One example is a diet for patients with cystic fibrosis (cystic fibrosis is a condition in which fat-digesting enzymes cannot leave the pancreas to enter the intestine, so fat digestion cannot occur). A fat-free diet may be rather tasteless because fat adds flavor to many common foods.

Additive Diets

Some people need more carbohydrate in their diet than most people (to gain weight) or additional protein or minerals (some people with kidney disease lose so

Fruit Exchange List

Apple—1 small
Apple juice—1/3 cup
Applesauce—1/2 cup
Apricots, fresh—2 medium
Apricots, dried—4 halves
Banana—1/2 small
Berries
  Blackberries—1/2 cup
  Blueberries—1/2 cup
  Raspberries—1/2 cup
  Strawberries—3/4 cup
Cherries—10 large or 15 small
Cider—1/3 cup
Cranberry juice—3/4 cup
Dates—2
Fig, fresh or dried—1 large
Fruit cocktail—1/2 cup
Grapefruit—1/2 small
Grapefruit juice—1/2 cup
Grapes—12
Grape juice—1/4 cup
Mango—1/2 small
Melon
  Cantaloupe—1/4 small
  Honeydew—1/8 medium
  Watermelon—1 cup
Nectarine—1 small
Orange—1 small
Orange juice—1/2 cup
Papaya—3/4 cup
Peach—1 medium
Pear—1 small or 2 halves
Persimmon, native—1 medium
Pineapple—1/2 cup or 2 rings
Pineapple juice—1/3 cup
Plums—2 medium
Prunes, dried—2 medium
Prune juice—1/4 cup
Raisins—2 tbsp
Tangerine—1 medium

Each exchange contains approximately 10 gm carbohydrate and 40 calories.

One exchange of drained sweetened fruit may be substituted for 2 exchanges of unsweetened fruit. Regular fruit nectars may be used (1/3 cup = 1 fruit exchange). If regular cranberry juice cocktail is used, 1/4 cup = 1 exchange. Cranberries may be used as desired if no sugar is added.

Source: American Dietetic Association, Chicago, Ill.

much protein owing to damaged glomeruli that they need protein supplements for cell maintenance. Additive diets often depend on snacks to supply the extra carbohydrate or protein content.

Diagnostic Testing Diets

Sometimes a diet is prescribed not for therapy, but as preparation for a diagnostic procedure. People scheduled for radiographs for gallbladder disease, for example, may be prescribed a low-fat supper the evening before (bile from the gallbladder normally is excreted to digest fat; if there is little fat in the intestine at the time of the test, the gallbladder will remain full and show up better on x-ray film). Following the first film, the person may be given a high-fat meal, and a second film will then be taken (if the bile duct is unobstructed, contraction and emptying of the gallbladder will be visible on this film).

Other examples of this type of diet are urine concentration diets (dry diets to demonstrate that the kidney cannot concentrate urine in spite of a restricted fluid intake) and allergy elimination diets (a food suspected of causing an allergy is removed from the diet and the person's response noted, or almost all foods are eliminated from the diet and then added back gradually).

INTERFERENCES WITH NUTRITION

Anorexia

Anorexia is loss of appetite. This can be caused by a physical illness, medication, or mental stress or anxiety. A person with anorexia may state that he knows he should eat, but when he sees food he is unable to eat anything. Measures to reduce stress, to make mealtime as pleasant as possible, and to prevent the patient from tiring before mealtime may alleviate anorexia in some people. Anorexia is an important problem because it can drastically reduce a person's daily food consumption.

Nausea

Nausea is a feeling of revulsion to food. It may be caused by a disease process (infection, increased intracranial pressure), motion, pain, medication, pregnancy, or psychological stress. As a rule, do not encourage people with nausea to eat except for a limited amount (not over 30 mls every 20 minutes) of clear fluids. Eating anything that requires more digestive activity than simple fluid often turns nausea into vomiting. Offer a person with nausea frequent mouth care because the mucous membrane tends to become dry and the patient develops an unpleasant taste sensation. Assess blood values and skin turgor for evidence that the dietary intake may be becoming too restricted.

Vomiting

Vomiting is the forceful regurgitation of food from the stomach and may be caused by either physical or psychological factors. Vomiting depletes the body of electrolytes (most noticeably chloride, which is lost in hydrochloric acid from the stomach) and fluid. Do not encourage people who are vomiting to eat or drink. Usually this only increases the vomiting and the consequent electrolyte and fluid loss. Resting the gastrointestinal tract for about 4 hours and then introducing fluid gradually again in small amounts (not more than 30 ml every 20 minutes) is a more therapeutic approach. Vomiting should be described according to its duration, amount, frequency, appearance, associated symptoms such as nausea, and abdominal cramping) and the patient's actions. Descriptions of emesis (vomitus) are given in Table 35-4. Types of vomiting are described in Table 35-5. Following vomiting, offer the person clear water or mouthwash to rinse his mouth. Position him with his head elevated (semi-Fowler's position) or on his side or prone so that if vomiting occurs again, the danger of aspiration (vomitus entering the trachea) will be minimized.

Lack of Bowel Tone

Whenever the bowel is handled, as during abdominal or pelvic surgery, bowel functions halt. This may also occur in response to psychological stress or major trauma such as burns or hemorrhage. Without bowel function, nothing eaten can pass through the intestine, a buildup of partially indigested food occurs, accompanied by gaseous distention, pain, vomiting, and possibly aspiration. It is always important, therefore, to be certain that a person has bowel tone before he is fed orally.

Bowel tone can be determined by the presence of the sound of peristaltic action (bowel sounds). On auscul-

TABLE 35-4. APPEARANCE OF EMESIS (VOMITUS)

Type	Possible Importance
Black	Hematemesis (blood in emesis) from old bleeding episode.
Brown, odorous	Fecal stained; has come from the intestine.
Coffee-ground appearance	Dark brown granular appearance of old blood mixed with vomitus.
Green-colored	Bile stained; emesis has come from below the point in the duodenum where the bile duct empties into the duodenum (ampulla of Vater).
Red appearance	Hematemesis (blood in emesis); color suggests current bleeding or very recent bleeding.
Undigested food	Acute irritation of stomach is present—so acute that food is ejected immediately.

TABLE 35-5. TYPES OF VOMITING

Type	Description	Possible Cause
"Spitting-up"	A term used with infants; describes the dribbling of milk from an infant's mouth when he is burped. Usually not over a mouthful (1 tsp) in amount. It is not sour because it does not reach the stomach.	Normal finding in infants under 6 months of age.
Regurgitation	Ejection of fluid from the stomach immediately after being swallowed; small in amount. May smell sour from quick contact with hydrochloric acid in stomach.	Seen mainly in infants whose cardiac sphincter (between stomach and esophagus) is immature; not serious unless fluid loss is great. An upright position after feeding helps to reduce this.
Rumination	Ejection of vomitus from the stomach by physical manipulation such as a finger or the tongue.	Associated with poor mother-child bonding in infants. Psychologically, a pathological condition.
Vomiting	Ejection of undigested food or poorly digested food from the stomach with force.	Associated with disease states or medication effects.
Cyclic vomiting	Vomiting that occurs repeatedly; difficult to establish a physical basis as cause.	May be associated with psychological stress. Could be interpreted as a type of convulsive disorder.
Pernicious vomiting	Severe or long-term vomiting.	A term used to describe vomiting in pregnancy when normal "morning sickness" lasts beyond three months into the pregnancy; could be used to denote any long-term vomiting pattern.
Projectile vomiting	Vomiting so forceful that it is projected some distance from the mouth.	Associated with increased cranial pressure or pyloric stenosis (tight valve between stomach and duodenum) in infants.
Retching	Stomach is contracting to eject food; no vomitus is present because stomach is empty.	Associated with acute gastrointestinal disorders that have made the stomach extremely irritated.

tation of a person's abdomen you should normally be able to hear 5 to 10 bowel sounds (high, tinkling, or pinging sounds) per minute. If no bowel tone is present, there is no sound; if a bowel obstruction is present (the intestine is blocked by a tumor, fecal impaction, or pressure of another organ against it), the area just distal to the block may have very active peristalsis (the intestine trying to move material through the blocked portion) and hyperactive bowel sounds.

Many people are aware that following intestinal surgery they will not be able to eat immediately, but they assume that because other abdominal or pelvic surgery does not involve the intestines, they will not be restricted from eating following this type of surgery. It is true that such surgery is not on the intestine; it is not true that it does not involve the intestine, because intestine is often moved to the side while the abdomen is "explored."

Swallowing and Gag Reflex

A swallowing reflex occurs when any substance is placed on the posterior portion of the tongue (the substance is propelled into the esophagus). A gag reflex is a fail-safe guard to keep foreign substances from entering the trachea because when a foreign substance does enter the trachea, violent coughing to expel it occurs. A person cannot take oral food or fluid safely unless both swallowing and gag reflexes are present.

These reflexes are lost under general anesthesia or unconsciousness; they may be lost with specific neurological disorders. Do not offer oral fluids to people following general anesthesia; if they have been unconscious, wait until full consciousness is regained. If in doubt about a person's ability to swallow safely with neurological impairment, ask for a second person's opinion before offering fluid. Aspiration of oral fluid due to an incomplete swallowing or gag reflex can lead to pneumonia from the irritation of the trachea or death due to edema and inflammation of the trachea that occludes the airway.

Adequate Oral Structure

For food to be properly digested it must be chewed well so that oral enzymes mix with it and begin the breakdown process. People who have no teeth or loose-fitting dentures or painful teeth or gingiva are unable to chew effectively. People with swollen and painful submaxillary or parotid glands (mumps) do not chew well because it hurts too much to move the jaw. People with very sore throats may also experience pain with jaw motion and swallowing. People with jaw injuries find chewing painful. Children with newly applied wire braces often have so much gingival pain that chewing is uncomfortable.

A person with this condition often does not need to omit food intake entirely, but he needs a soft or liquid diet for at least one day's time. Administering an analgesic about 15 minutes before a meal may help him feel comfortable enough to eat.

Respiratory Distress

It is physiologically impossible to swallow food or fluid and breathe at the same time because during swallowing the epiglottis closes over the trachea to keep food out of it. A person who must maintain a very rapid respiratory rate (tachypnea), therefore, has difficulty maintaining an adequate oral intake. Because he also is systemically exhausted from the effort of breathing, he finds that the effort of eating requires more energy than he wants to expend.

Always evaluate carefully the oral intake of a person with respiratory distress. Oral intake may be so low that intravenous supplementation of fluid is needed; he may need his diet modified to high-calorie liquids that are quickly and effortlessly ingested.

Motor Dysfunction

Eating is such a common activity that it is easy to think of it as a simple process. Actually, it requires a complex integration of motor skills. The person must grasp a spoon, direct it toward the food, rotate his wrist to pick up food, redirect the spoon to his mouth, close his lips to remove the food from the spoon, and use his tongue to direct the food to the back of his throat. The throat muscles must be strong enough to effect swallowing. A person with muscle incoordination may be unable to complete all these steps. Because he knows that he is not a neat eater because of muscle incoordination, he may be unwilling to eat in a public setting such as a semi-private hospital room.

Evaluate the food and fluid intake of people with neuromuscular illnesses. Eating calls for *fine* motor skills; lack of such skills may not be noticeable with activities such as ambulating (a gross motor skill) and can be missed if not assessed specifically.

People with poor muscle coordination may need additional time provided for meals or food cut into bite-size portions; if they tire easily, they may need to be fed for the last half of a meal.

Sensory Disturbances

People with sensory disturbances may have loss of taste, so no food is appetizing to them. If they have loss of temperature sensation, they may be unable to detect the temperature of foods and may burn their tongue on hot liquids. Soups, coffee, and tea should be cooled to a drinkable temperature before serving it to such people. Foods that are attractive in color may help a person with a loss of taste to see foods as appetizing; social interaction at mealtime may help to restore appetite.

Decreased Cognitive Ability

Children and adults with impaired mental functioning may not appreciate the importance of eating or the importance of eating one food rather than another. Evaluate both quantity and the quality of food intake in such persons to be sure that they do consume an adequate daily intake.

PROMOTING ADEQUATE NUTRITION IN HOSPITALIZED PATIENTS

Although dietitians supervise what foods are placed on a hospitalized patient's meal tray, the nurse is the person who actually serves it or supervises another person who helps at mealtime. A number of rules are helpful in aiding hospitalized persons to enjoy meals more and thereby increase their dietary intake.

Protect the Temperature and Taste of Food

Food trays are usually delivered to hospital units by the dietary or transport department. The service cart for trays may consist only of metal racks, or it may be a cart that, when plugged into an electrical outlet, furnishes a warmer section for keeping soup or entrees hot. Even with a "hot" cart, food trays should be served to patients as soon as possible to prevent foods from becoming cold or dried out and tasteless.

Arrange procedures or therapy for your patient at other times than meal times so that a meal tray is not left waiting and growing cold.

Promote Patient Comfort at Mealtime

A drug that reduces nausea is an *antiemetic*. If such a drug is ordered, offer it far enough in advance of mealtime (about 20 or 30 minutes) so that it will be working effectively by the time the meal arrives. Try to plan medication for pain relief in the same way (see QRSs 35-1 and 35-2).

Provide a Pleasant Environment

Provide help with washing hands or brushing teeth as necessary to create a pleasant mealtime atmosphere. Many people would rather sit in the chair beside the bed to eat; some patient care units have a dining room where all ambulatory patients can congregate for meals, creating a more homelike setting. Assess patient rooms for odors or any other factor that would decrease meal enjoyment.

Many people think of mealtime as a social time (Fig. 35-4). They often enjoy having someone to talk with while they eat. Others feel self-conscious (eating while you have nothing to eat).

Prevent the Patient from Tiring

People who are ill may tire more easily than they think they will. They may begin to eat eagerly, realize after a few bites that they are too tired to continue, and stop eating. Assess a patient's level of energy as you serve his

☐ QUICK REFERENCE STOP 35-1: PHARMACOLOGY
Antiemetics and Antacids

ANTIEMETICS

Antiemetics are drugs that halt vomiting. All these drugs cause drowsiness to some degree; raise side rails after administration to hospitalized patients. If ambulatory, caution about driving or using machinery.

Name of Drug	*Action*	*Cautions*
Benadryl (diphenhydramine hydrochloride)	Depressant action on labyrinth excitability; depresses vomiting center	Drowsiness or confusion is very common
Compazine (prochlorperazine)	Depresses vomiting center	Toxic effect of extreme spasticity (including laryngeal spasm) must be assessed
Dramamine (dimenhydrinate)	Antihistamine; drug of choice for motion sickness	May cause drowsiness
Tigan (trimethobenzanide hydrochloride)	Depresses vomiting center	May be administered rectally by suppository

ANTACIDS

Antacids act to prevent the formation of, buffer, or neutralize stomach acid. Products with calcium or aluminum may be constipating; those with magnesium may have a laxative effect. Magnesium-containing products should be used cautiously with patients with impaired kidney function because toxic levels of magnesium can occur; sodium-based products must be used cautiously in patients with heart disease because sodium may cause retention of fluid and circulatory overload.

Name of Drug	*Action*	*Cautions*
Amphojel (aluminum hydroxide gel)	Neutralizes acid	May be constipating
Gelusil (aluminum hydroxide and magnesium hydroxide)	Neutralizes acid	
Maalox (aluminum hydroxide and magnesium hydroxide)	Neutralizes acid	
Riopan (magaldrate, aluminum hydroxide and magnesium hydroxide)	Buffers acid	Has a low sodium content; often used in people with a cardiac condition
Tagamet (cimetidine hydrochloride)	Histamine-receptor antagonist (prevents secretions of gastric acid)	Contraindicated during pregnancy and breast-feeding (lactation)

meal tray; decide if any help will be needed such as cutting meat or adding cream to coffee. Check on progress as needed to be sure that mealtime is a therapeutic time, not a stressful one.

Encourage Adequate Exercise
People who exercise little often have little appetite at mealtime. Encourage people to be active within their medical restrictions to promote appetite.

Arrange Medication Schedules to Avoid or Coincide with Mealtime as Appropriate
Some medications cannot be taken with food (some forms of penicillin, for example) because food will neutralize them; some medications are irritating to the stomach unless taken with food (oral potassium, for example). Check a patient's medication schedule to be sure that it is timed appropriately in relation to mealtimes and snacks.

ALTERNATIVE METHODS OF SUPPLYING NUTRITION
People who cannot swallow (or who lack a gag reflex) cannot be fed orally or they may aspirate the food. Intravenous therapy can supply water, glucose, and electrolytes, but because it supplies no fat or protein it is always only a temporary maintenance solution.

☐ **QUICK REFERENCE STOP 35-2: SAFETY**
Precautions When Serving Food

1. One of the greatest dangers of food intake is aspiration (food drawn into the trachea). *Never offer food or fluid to anyone who does not have an intact gag or swallowing reflex.*
2. If a person should begin to choke on food, use a sharp stroke to the upper back or a Heimlich maneuver to dislodge the offending food object (see Fig. 32-27).
3. Think of food as medication in terms of legal responsibility (check identification bands, read labels three times, and so on). A wrong diet prescription could be as hazardous to patient health as a medication error.
4. Be careful that the person does not burn himself drinking hot beverages such as coffee or soup; take care not to burn your fingers from hot liquids splashed while serving trays.
5. Always check placement of a nasogastric tube before tube feeding to prevent aspiration from the tube.

Complete nutrition can be provided by total parenteral nutrition (special intravenous therapy that does include protein and fat) or by nasogastric intubation or gastrostomy feedings.

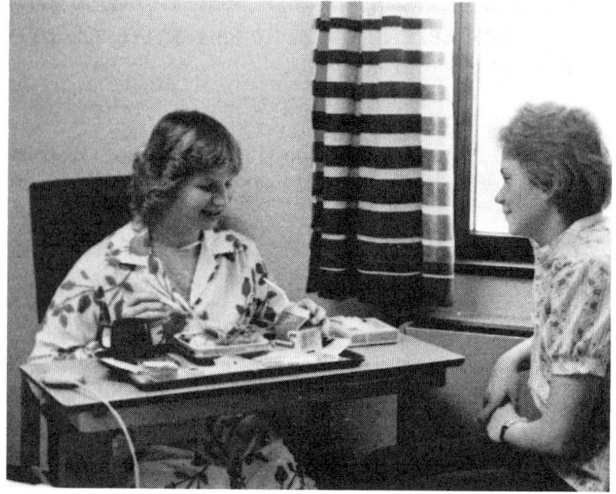

FIGURE 35-4. Mealtime should be a rewarding, not a tiring, experience. Social interaction is generally important to improve appetite.

Nasogastric Intubation

A nasogastric tube is a pliable plastic or rubber tube that is measured and then threaded through the nose (or mouth) into the esophagus and into the stomach (Procedure 35-1, Figs. 1 and 2). Such a tube can be inserted and left in place between feedings or removed after each feeding and replaced just prior to the next feeding. In addition to its use as a feeding (gavage) tube, a tube inserted by this route may also be used to

PROCEDURE 35-1
Passing a Nasogastric Tube

Purpose: To provide a method for introducing liquid feedings for the person who cannot swallow; to provide a route for obtaining laboratory specimens for analysis; to provide a route for irrigation of the stomach (lavage); to provide a means of decompressing the stomach to relieve pressure and prevent vomiting.

Plan	*Principle*
1. Wash hands, identify patient, explain procedure.	1. Prevent spread of microorganisms; ensure patient safety. Remember that even if a patient is comatose, he may be able to hear and needs an explanation.
2. Assess patient condition; analyze appropriateness of procedure; plan modifications as necessary.	2. It is a rare person who likes the thought of a nasogastric tube being passed. Be prepared to offer reassurance throughout procedure.
3. Implement care by assembling supplies: nasogastric tube of correct size, cup of water for lubrication; basin of ice if tube is rubber, towel, tape and tube clamp, glass of tap water and straw (optional).	3. Tube sizes vary depending on age.
4. If tube is rubber, place in ice for approximately 15 minutes.	4. Chilling in ice stiffens the tube; plastic tubes do not need this.
5. Provide for privacy by drawn curtains or closed room door. Raise bed to semi-Fowler's position; place towel across patient's chest.	5. Privacy is a valued right of most people. An elevated head aids gravity and protects against aspiration should vomiting occur. Towel protects bed should vomiting occur.

6. Measure length of tube to be inserted; mark at this point with a clamp or piece of tape.

Measurement is from bridge of nose to ear lobe to xyphoid process of sternum in people over 1 year of age (Fig. 1).

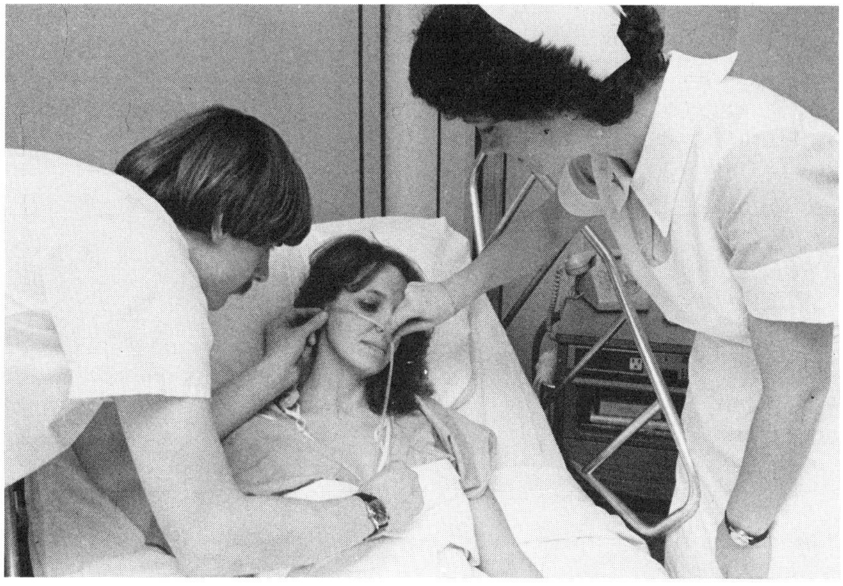

A

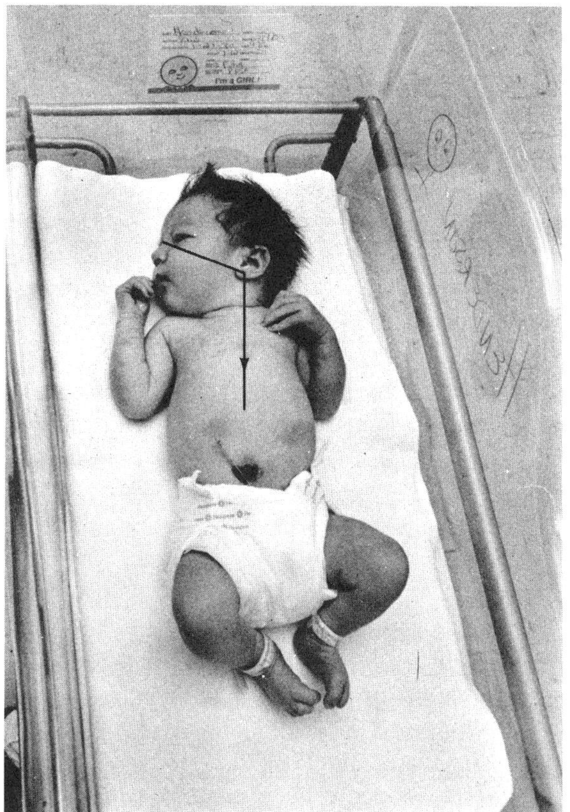

B

FIGURE 1. Measuring the length of a nasogastric tube in an adult (A)—earlobe to tip of nose to xyphoid process—and an infant (B)—earlobe to tip of nose to point halfway between xyphoid process and umbilicus.

7. Lubricate tip of tube by dipping it in water.

7. Do not use an oil-based medium; if the tube should accidentally pass into lungs, oil will cause pneumonia. A water-based lubricant could be used.

8. If patient is alert, give him some distracting activity ("take shallow breaths").

8. Relaxed, a tube passes easily; tense, the procedure is uncomfortable.

9. Steady patient's head with one hand; hold catheter near end; introduce tip of catheter into one nostril; advance the tube forward and downward about 3 inches.

9. This is the distance (in adults) from nostril to pharynx (Fig. 2).

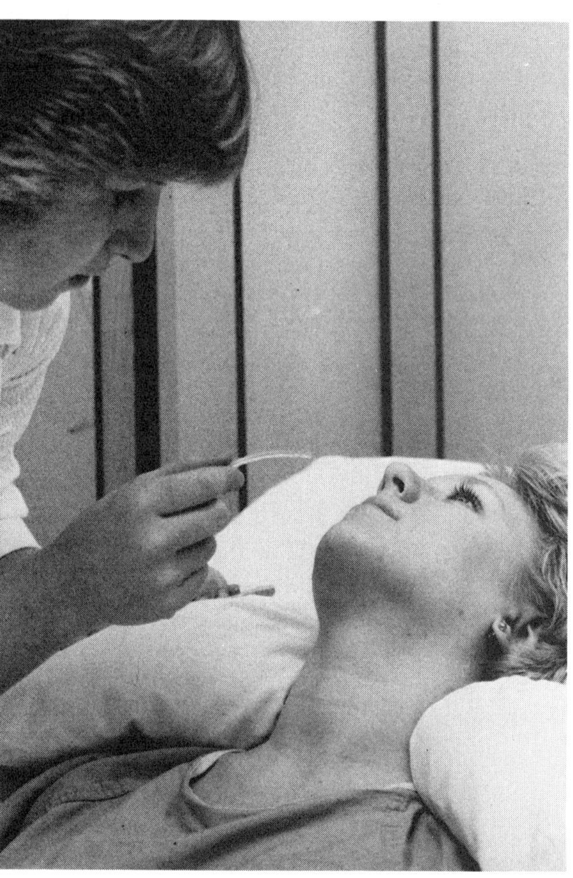

FIGURE 2. Introducing a nasogastric tube into the nostril. As soon as the tube reaches the nasopharynx, ask the patient to flex her neck forward in order to guide it better into the esophagus. Be certain that the head of the bed is elevated at least 30 degrees to decrease possibility of aspiration, should vomiting occur.

10. When tube is in the pharynx, ask patient to flex his neck forward so his chin rests on his chest.

10. A flexed head position helps tube to enter esophagus.

11. Ask the patient to swallow "as if he is swallowing spaghetti" until the tube is inserted the marked distance or the clamp or tape rests next to his nostril. Swallowing water from the glass and straw may be helpful.

11. Swallowing will increase movement into the esophagus.

12. Assess whether tube is in stomach by one of three ways as shown in QRS 35-3.

13. Secure tube to nose or cheek with tape. Do not fold tube toward forehead because this causes pressure on nose and may cause necrosis of tissue.	13. To ensure that tube remains in proper place (Fig. 3).

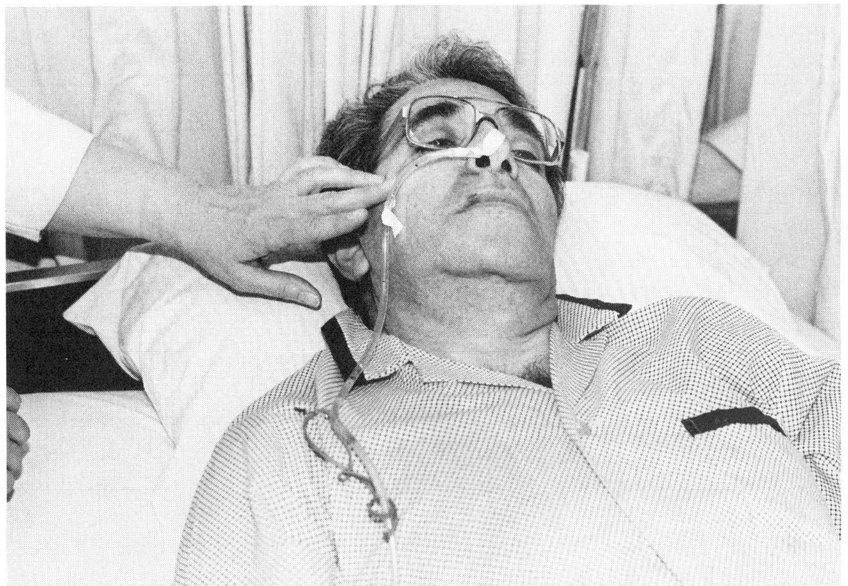

FIGURE 3. Nasogastric tube taped in place. Notice that it is taped across the cheek rather than to the forehead to prevent tension on nares.

14. Follow instructions for tube maintenance—clamp, connect to suction, or prepare for feeding as appropriate.	14. Suction should always be on low pressure to prevent damage to stomach mucosa.
15. Praise patient for cooperation. Evaluate effectiveness, efficiency, cost, safety, and comfort aspects of procedure. Remove equipment and leave room in order; open curtains.	15. Having a tube passed is intrusive and frightening. Any behavior short of hysterical screaming is good behavior. Assure patient he can be observed well.
16. Plan any health teaching measures necessary such as need for nutrition by this route.	16. Health teaching is an independent nursing action always included as part of care.
17. Record procedure and patient status.	17. Documentation of patient status and nursing care.

MODIFICATIONS FOR CARE OF CHILD

1. In an infant (under 1 year old) measure the tube from the bridge of the nose to the earlobe to a space *halfway* between the umbilicus and the xyphoid process instead of just to the xyphoid process for proper placement (see Fig. 1).
2. Infants need to be restrained generally by a mummy restraint before a tube is inserted to keep small hands from pulling at the tube (Fig. 27-10).
3. Following insertion, use restraints as necessary for safety, perhaps clove-hitch restraints to upper extremities to keep hands away from tube.
4. For schoolage children it is important to compare the tube to "swallowing spaghetti." Comparing an unknown to a known is always a good technique with children.

MODIFICATIONS FOR CARE OF OLDER ADULT

Many older adults have one nares that is more patent than the other—a tube will pass through it more easily than through the other. Do not attempt to force a tube to pass. Mucous membranes of the nose are irritated and broken easily; bleeding and infection could result.

TABLE 35-6. COMMONLY USED SIZES OF NASOGASTRIC TUBES

Age	Size
Low birth weight	6, 8
Newborn	8, 10
Infant to adolescent	10, 12, 14
Adult	16, 18

obtain specimens of the stomach contents (gastric analysis) or to decompress the stomach (keep it empty) or to cleanse or irrigate it (lavage).

Nasogastric tubes in some health care agencies are inserted only by physicians. In others, either physicians or nurses insert them. The needed steps to pass a nasogastric tube are shown in Procedure 35-1. The size of the tube used must be evaluated carefully. A tube that is too small will have such a small lumen that it will be difficult to administer liquid feedings through it; a tube that is too large will irritate the walls of the nares and the esophagus. The usual sizes of nasogastric tubes are shown in Table 35-6.Tubes have either an opening at the end or several openings along the sides (French tubes). French tubes have advantages in that they do not plug easily (there are several openings) and they do not tend to become blocked by being pressed against the stomach mucosa.

Almost everyone has a more patent naris on one side than the other; if a tube does not pass easily through the first nostril, do not force it. Remove the tube and try the other nostril. Tubes should be rotated from one nares to another when they are changed if possible to prevent nasal irritation.

When taping a tube in place, tape it to the person's cheek; so that it will not rub against the nasal mucosa (Procedure 35-1, Fig. 3). Do not tape the tube to the person's forehead because this causes upward pressure against the nose. Use allergy-free tape on infants or any person with sensitive skin. Placing a strip of nonallergenic tape under the nose and taping the tube to that strip of tape allows tubes to be changed without tearing tape off the skin each time.

Having a nasogastric tube passed is uncomfortable. It initiates sneezing or may cause a person's eyes to water. Occasionally a person may be so sensitive to irritation at the back of the throat that he gags and vomits. After the tube is in place, these sensations do not persist, and the tube is no longer uncomfortable (see QRS 35-3). The person may be embarrassed that he could not cooperate more or that he vomited. Assure him that you understand that the procedure is stressful. If the tube will be connected to suction for stomach decompression, circle a rubber band on the distal end and pin this to the person's gown so that any pull on the tubing will be registered on the gown rather than at the patient's nose (Procedure 35-1, Fig. 3).

REMOVAL OF A NASOGASTRIC TUBE

Nasogastric tubes are removed by nurses on a physician's order. The tube should be replaced about every other day to keep the bacteria count in its lumen to a low level. If the patient has had esophageal surgery, tubes are *not* changed until the esophageal sutures are healed to prevent irritation or dislodgment of the sutures.

Prior to removing a tube, clamp it securely. This will prevent any fluid remaining in the tube from flowing backward as the tube is withdrawn and being aspirated. Clamping is best done with a clamp rather than just pinching the tube with your fingers to be sure that pressure is maintained during the entire withdrawal process.

Removal of a tube causes the same feelings of distress (coughing, choking, sneezing) as insertion. They are not as intense, however, and disappear quickly because a tube is removed steadily and quickly. The steps used in removing a nasogastric tube are shown in Procedure 35-2. Some people experience a feeling of irritation in the throat following tube removal. A swallow of cold fluid (if medically permitted) generally relieves this feeling.

Tube Feeding (Gavage)

Gavage means to supply food to the stomach through a tube. The type, amount, and frequency of feedings are individually prescribed like any other diet. Use clean technique for gavage feedings. Sterile technique is not needed because of the bactericidal action of hydrochloric acid in the stomach. Many gavage preparations contain milk and therefore sour and spoil if not kept refrigerated (or, if a commercial preparation, sealed) prior to use. Warm refrigerated formula before administration by allowing it to sit in a pan of warm water for about 15 minutes or on a counter for about half an hour to bring it to room temperature. Cold feedings can cause cramping and discomfort. The method of tube feeding is shown in Procedure 35-3.

Feedings must be given slowly in order to guard against reflux. An intermittent adult feeding of 200 to 300 ml requires 30 to 45 minutes. If it is given continuously, a rate of 80 to 150 ml per hour is an average rate. Rapid feedings of a high-calorie solution may cause, in addition to esophageal reflux, rapid emptying into the duodenum, a shift of fluid into the intestine due to increased osmotic pressure, and diarrhea (termed the *dumping syndrome*). To reduce the concentration of gavage feedings and decrease osmotic fluid shifts, feedings may be diluted before administration or followed by a sizable amount of rinse water (100 to 200 ml). Be aware that this amount of water, although called a rinse, is actually part of the diet prescription and is necessary for the person's total fluid intake. Otherwise, it is easy to omit it (realistically, it takes only 30 ml to rinse a tube).

□ **QUICK REFERENCE STOP 35-3: SAFETY**
Methods for Checking Placement of Nasogastric Tube

If a tube accidentally passes into the trachea, patient will cough or facial color will become impaired (cyanotic). In addition to checking patient's general color and comfort:

1. Inject 5 ml of air into tube by syringe; listen over stomach area with stethoscope for sound of rushing air. The sound of air is "popping" or "swooshing" (Fig. 1A).
2. Aspirate stomach contents by using a syringe attached to a tube. No contents can be aspirated unless the tube rests in stomach contents (Fig. 1B).
3. Place end of tube in glass of water and observe for escape of bubbles. If tube is in trachea, air will be exhaled through the tube with this technique. If patient is on a ventilator (respirator), negative respirator pressure may cause the water to be drawn into the lungs (Fig. 1C).

FIGURE 1. Three methods to test that a nasogastric tube is in place. A. Auscultate as air is injected into tube. B. Aspirate stomach content by syringe. C. Submerge distal end in cup of water and observe for bubbles. (To prevent aspiration of water, do not use this method with people with ventilators.)

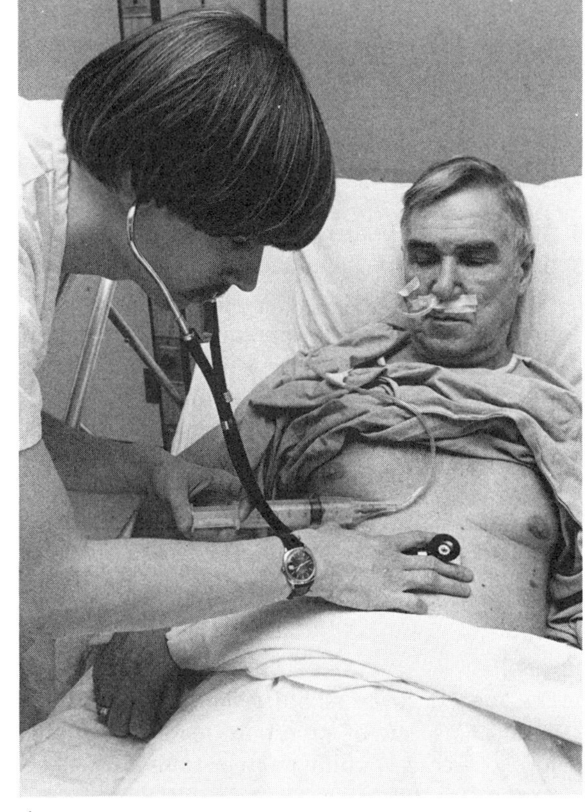

A

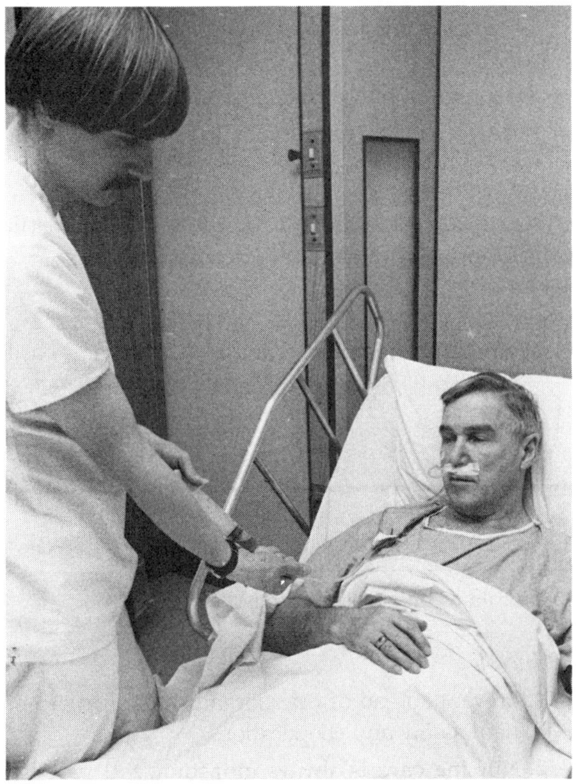

B

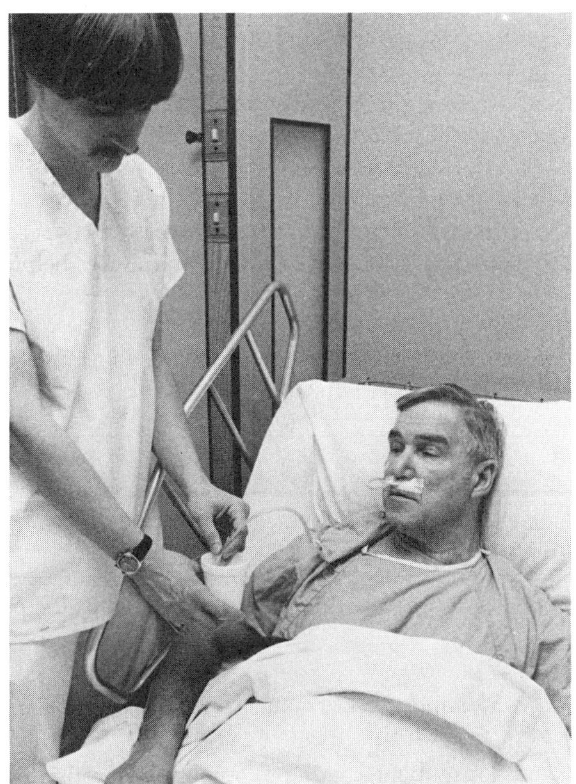

C

PROCEDURE 35-2
Removal of a Nasogastric Tube

Purpose: To remove a nasogastric tube safely without causing aspiration or strong discomfort.

Plan	*Principle*
1. Wash your hands; identify the patient; explain the procedure.	1. Prevent spread of microorganisms; promote patient safety and cooperation.
2. Assess patient condition.	2. Most patients are pleased at having a tube removed; they may not be if another is to be passed.
3. Analyze appropriateness of procedure based on patient condition; plan modifications as necessary.	3. Nursing care is always individualized based on professional judgment of patient needs.
4. Implement care by assembling supplies: clamp and towel. Provide privacy by drawing curtains or room door. Elevate head to semi-Fowler's position.	4. Privacy is a respected right of most people. An elevated head protects against aspiration should vomiting occur.
5. Remove any tape holding tube in place; clamp tube using a hemostat or commercial clamp; place towel across patient's chest.	5. Clamping a tube prevents back-flow of fluid in tube, which could lead to aspiration; towel protects patient should vomiting occur and covers tube after extubation.
6. Pull tube out quickly but gently.	6. Speed in removal decreases sensation of gagging or choking. Gentleness is necessary to protect mucous membrane.
7. Evaluate effectiveness, efficiency, cost, safety, and comfort aspects of procedure; cover tube with towel; discard in utility room or rinse if it will be reused for sterilization.	7. Plastic tubes are disposable; rubber tubes are resterilized. Tubes often smell sour from being in the stomach; do not discard in a patient's room.
8. Plan any health teaching measures; for example, inform the patient that any throat irritation is momentary.	8. Health teaching is an independent nursing action always included as part of nursing care.
9. Record removal of tube and patient condition following extubation.	9. Documentation of nursing care and patient status.

MODIFICATIONS FOR CARE OF CHILD

Preschool-age children and older are often cooperative if a nasogastric tube is referred to as "spaghetti." Associating an unknown to a known is always helpful when working with children.

MODIFICATIONS FOR CARE OF OLDER ADULT

Assess condition of nares carefully following tube removal since mucous membrane is delicate and easily injured in the older adult.

PROCEDURE 35-3
Tube Feeding (Gavage)

Purpose: To provide a method of nutrition for the person unable to take oral feedings.

Plan	*Principle*
1. Wash hands; identify patient; explain procedure.	1. Prevent spread of microorganisms; promote patient safety and cooperation.
2. Assess patient condition. Analyze appropriateness of procedure based on patient condition; plan modifications as necessary.	2. Nursing care is always individualized based on professional judgment of patient needs.

3. Implement care by assembling supplies; asepto syringe or regular syringe; measured amount of feeding at room temperature; measured amount of container of water for rinse.

3. Organization of care. Remember that administration of food or formula has the same legal responsibilities that follow medication administration. Read formula label three times for safety.

4. Provide for privacy by drawn curtains or closed door. Position patient with head of bed elevated at least 30 degrees.

4. Privacy is a respected right of most persons. This position will make fluid flow into the stomach, preventing aspiration.

5. Test that tube is positioned in stomach by one of three methods shown in QRS 35-3.

5. Patient safety.

6. To test if previous feeding has been absorbed, aspirate stomach contents and measure. Return to stomach by tube.

6. Return stomach contents to maintain electrolyte balance.

7. Remove rubber bulb from asepto syringe, barrel from regular syringe; attach syringe to end of feeding tube.

7. Nasogastric feedings should infuse by gravity, not pressure. You do not need the bulb or barrel because using these creates pressure.

8. Pour feeding solution into syringe barrel. Elevate about 12 inches above level of patient's stomach. Let fluid flow by gravity.

8. Elevation higher than 12 inches makes fluid flow too rapidly, leading to possible reflux or aspiration (Fig. 1).

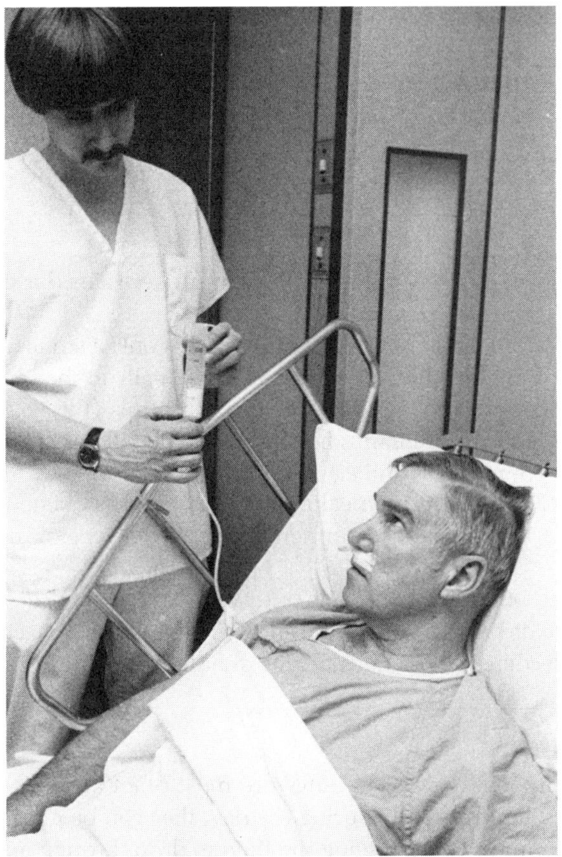

FIGURE 1. Administering a nasogastric feeding. The height of the feeding reservoir should be about 12 inches above the level of the stomach.

9. Continue to add amounts of fluid to syringe until specified amount of feeding is completed. Regulate rate flow by clamp or distance above patient's stomach level.

9. Do not allow syringe to empty so that air enters. Air will fill stomach and lead to reflux and possible aspiration.

10. Following completion of feeding, add the designated milliliters of water to flush feeding from tubing.

10. Maintain patent tubing; milk-base feedings sour if they stand in the tube; also, the person does not receive the full amount of the feeding.

11. If the formula is a commercial one that comes with accompanying tubing, it may be hung like intravenous fluid and allowed to drip slowly but steadily into the patient's stomach after the tubing is attached to the nasogastric tube.

11. This type of commercial feeding system is convenient but does not allow you to leave the room. You must monitor the rate of the infusion to prevent reflux and possible aspiration.

12. Assess patient status during all tube feedings. Stop feeding if person states he has nausea or pain.

12. Pain probably denotes overdistention; nausea may be the forerunner of vomiting.

13. Disconnect the syringe from the nasogastric tube; clamp the tube and cover the end with sterile gauze or remove tube.

13. Clamping the tube prevents the feeding from returning through the tube. Covering the end prevents microorganisms from entering.

14. Leave the patient in a head-elevated position for at least 20 minutes; open curtains or room door.

14. Prevent backflow of feeding into esophagus and aspiration until feeding is absorbed from stomach.

15. Return equipment used to utility room for disposal or resterilization.

15. Asepto syringes are usually made of glass and therefore need resterilization before use with a second patient.

16. Evaluate effectiveness, efficiency, cost, comfort, and safety aspects of procedure; plan health teaching needed such as ability to obtain total nutrition by nasogastric route.

16. Health teaching is an independent nursing action always included as part of care.

17. Chart type, amount of fluid given, and patient reaction to procedure.

17. Documentation of patient status and nursing care.

MODIFICATIONS FOR CARE OF CHILD

1. Infants generally need a mummy restraint during the procedure to prevent their hands from interfering with the procedure.
2. Infants' stomachs are so small that only a small amount of fluid can be used to rinse tube (5—10 ml). This amount should be ordered individually in the same way as the amount of feeding.
3. Many cribs do not have gatch controls (the head of the crib does not elevate). Use sufficient pillows to elevate an infant's head; if adequate pillows are not available, place a box or other solid object under head of mattress and elevate mattress.
4. Children miss mealtime because they associate sitting at a table with people as a time for conversation. Provide periods during the day for this type of mealtime interaction.

MODIFICATIONS FOR CARE OF OLDER ADULT

Older adults, like children, enjoy mealtime conversation. Provide this as part of procedure to make tube feeding a more normal type of nutrition.

Although gavage feedings are most often administered intermittently during the day, they can be given continuously by allowing the fluid to drop through an intravenous tube into a nasogastric tube. Continuous feedings decrease the possibility of esophageal reflux and maintain blood electrolytes at an even level due to the constant infusion.

Esophageal reflux may occur for a third reason. If the stomach contained undigested fluid from the previous feeding, adding the full amount of the present feeding will overdistend it. To prevent this complication stomach secretions can be aspirated through the tube just prior to feeding (this also assures you that the end of the tube is well within the stomach). Measure the amount aspirated and *then return it to the stomach as the first part of the feeding.* Reduce the amount of the feeding by the amount of the aspirated contents. In patients who are on long-term gavage feeding programs and who have no signs or symptoms (abdominal distention, abdominal pain) of feeding intolerance, such aspiration is probably not necessary before every feeding. It is good practice to assess for this at least once every 24 hours as an independent nursing action.

Returning the aspirated stomach contents seems almost contradictory to sensible practice because such aspirated contents contain sour milk. However, such a solution also contains electrolytes (a great deal of chloride), so if aspirated and not returned at every feeding, a severe alkalosis from chloride depletion could result very quickly. Use *clean* technique for aspiration as well as for feeding because the aspirated material will be included in the feeding (do not use a patient's emesis basin to collect this fluid, thinking it is "dirty"; it is sour-smelling but not bacterially contaminated.

Gastrostomy Feedings

Another alternate method of providing liquid feedings is through a gastrostomy tube (a tube inserted through a small surgical opening into the stomach). Gastrostomy tubes have large mushroom-shaped extensions on the tip to hold them in the stomach (Fig. 35-5); a Foley catheter with an inflated balloon tip can be used instead. Gastrostomy tubes are inserted when oral feedings are not possible and nasogastric intubation is contraindicated. They may be either a temporary measure or a long-term one.

Gastrostomy feedings require the same technique as nasogastric feedings. Position the patient with his head elevated to discourage esophageal reflux. If the person has esophageal sutures, the tube is usually left unclamped and elevated following a feeding to allow any air introduced to leave the stomach by way of the tube rather than through the esophagus to decrease the possibility of distention and pressure on the suture line. Apply a protective ointment to the site to prevent excoriation from leakage of hydrochloric acid. Following removal of the tube the insertion site will heal with only a minimal dimple.

FIGURE 35-5. A gastrostomy tube in place.

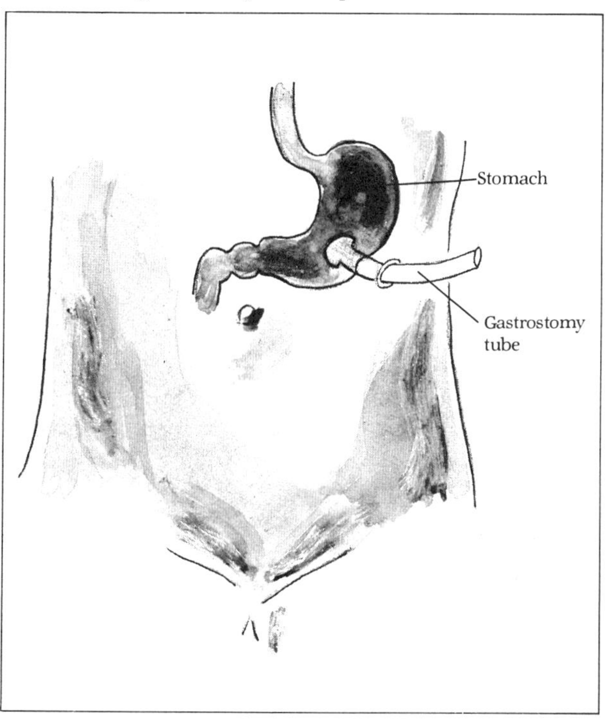

Nasojejunal Feeding

In some instances it is necessary to pass a feeding tube further than the stomach and into the jejunum of the intestine. The tube chosen for this long passage is often a *Levine* or *Miller-Abbott* tube, although other brand names are used as well. Such tubes have a weight on the tip, which is passed through the pyloric valve into the intestine. Tubes are passed in this manner for aspiration and analysis of intestinal contents, although rarely they may be used for feeding. Insertion is basically the same as that used with nasogastric tubes except that the tube will take up to an hour to pass farther into the intestine from the stomach. Positioning the person on his right side in a semi-Fowler's position is thought to help passage during the waiting time.

You can determine whether a tube has passed into the intestine by assessing the pH level of fluid aspirated from it. If it is still in the stomach, the pH of the fluid will be below 7.0 (acid); if in the intestine, the pH will be above 7.0 (alkaline).

Jujunal feedings are not used frequently because introducing food to the intestines bypasses the stomach, an important part of the digestive process, and can lead to a dumping syndrome.

Total Parenteral Nutrition (Hyperalimentation)

Some patients are unable to take food by way of the gastrointestinal tract even by gastric intubation (usually because they have difficulty absorbing nutrients across the gastrointestinal membrane into the bloodstream). These people can be given total nutrition intravenously. Normally, intravenous fluid contains only sugar, water, minerals, and vitamins. It is used for short-term maintenance to supply energy and fluid requirements or to correct electrolyte disturbances. It cannot sustain a person for a long time because it lacks protein and fat.

Total parenteral nutrition (TPN) solutions do contain protein (as amino acids) and lipids and can be used for total nutrition for long periods of time. TPN solutions are ordered by prescription (which specifies what percentage or proportion of nutrients will be given). In most health care agencies the solutions are prepared in a pharmacy under sterile conditions. Solutions are rich in glucose (to initiate protein sparing so that the amino acids given will be used for cell building, not energy). This load of glucose causes such solutions to be hypertonic (have a heavier osmotic pressure) than blood. They must be administered at carefully controlled rates to prevent circulatory overload or hyperglycemia from the heavy sugar load. Although TPN solutions can be administered by way of a peripheral vein, a large vein such as the subclavian or internal jugular vein is more often used. If the fluid empties into a large vein, it is more readily distributed, causes less irritation, and therefore decreases the tendency toward thrombophlebitis formation.

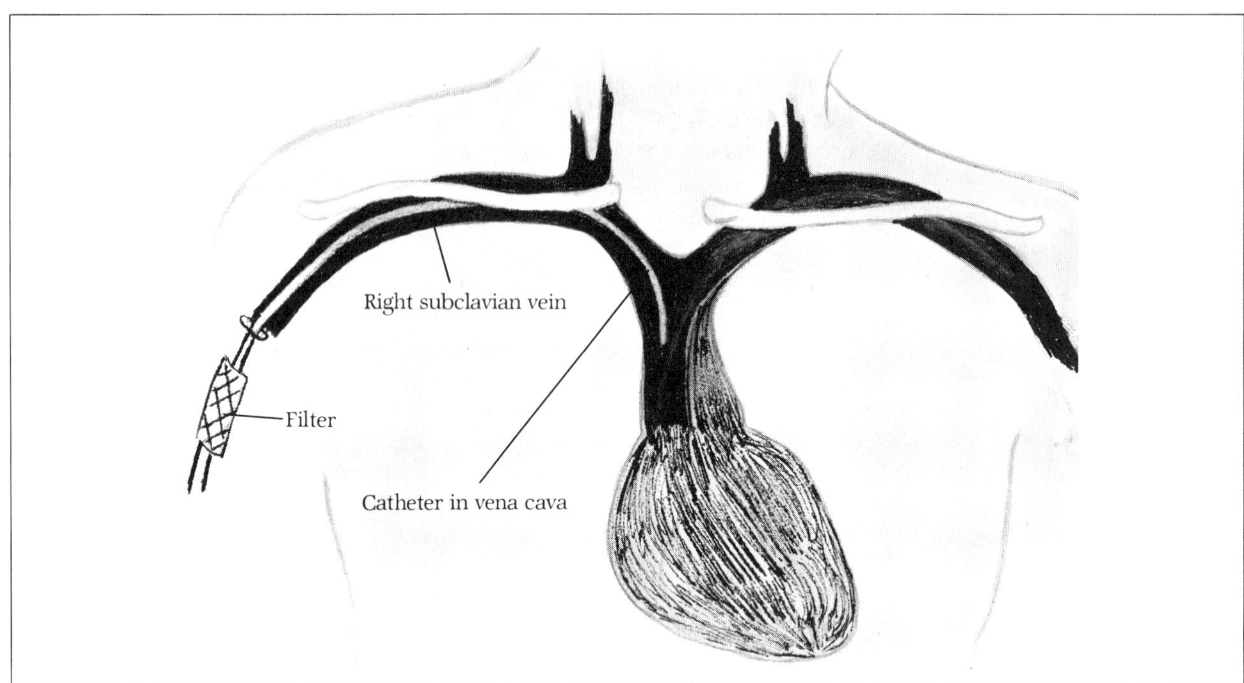

FIGURE 35-6. A total parenteral nutrition catheter in place in the vena cava through the subclavian vein.

Insertion of a TPN line may be done in a patient's room or a treatment room but is usually done in the operating room (or a small emergency surgery room) under strict sterile conditions. A radiograph may be taken following insertion to determine the exact placement of the catheter in the vena cava (Fig. 35-6). The catheter may be sutured to the skin at the insertion site to hold it in place. Antibiotic ointment and a sterile dressing are applied to the insertion site to limit the possibility of infection.

TPN fluid is infused through intravenous tubing with a special micropore filter (Fig. 35-7). The filter removes any undissolved particles from the solution (there is always a possibility that some particles exist because of the number of minerals added). All connections should be covered with tape to ensure that they will not come apart while the infusion is running, allowing air to enter a main vein and cause a pulmonary embolus.

The tubing, solutions of fluid, and the dressing are changed daily or every other day under strict sterile conditions because if infection is introduced, septicemia in a major vessel could occur. The greatest dangers to a person receiving a TPN solution are infection, hyperglycemia, fluid overload, and psychological depression. Measures to prevent these are summarized in Table 35-7.

To compute the caloric content or protein content of a TPN solution or regular intravenous fluid, determine the number of milliliters of glucose or protein in the solution (1 ml is equal to 1 gm). Each gram of glucose or protein produces 4 kcal when metabolized.

FIGURE 35-7. Total parenteral nutrition. The catheter enters the right subclavian vein. Flow is controlled by an IVAC Infusion Pump.

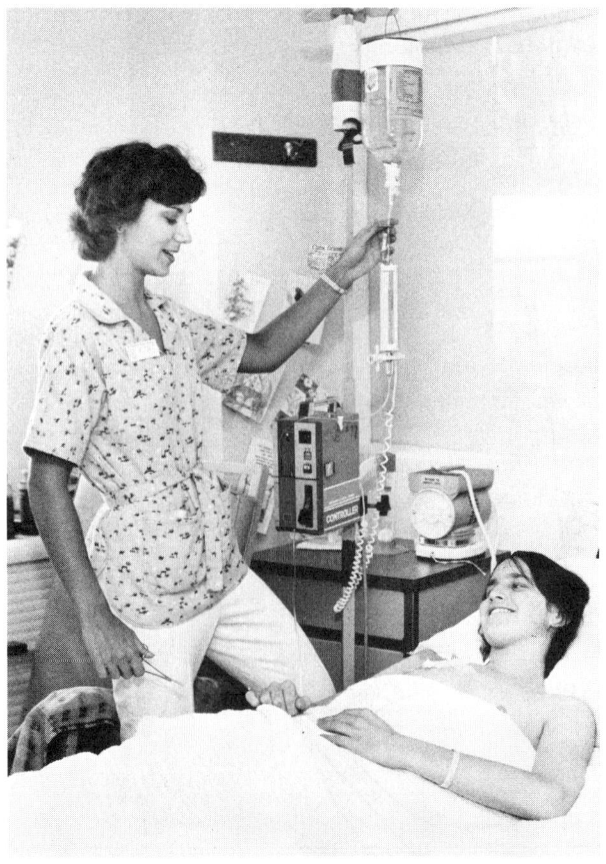

TABLE 35-7. POSSIBLE DIFFICULTIES ARISING FROM TOTAL PARENTERAL NUTRITION (HYPERALIMENTATION)

Problem	Cause	Preventive Intervention
Infection	Rich glucose solution invites bacterial or fungal growth.	Original infusion line is placed under strict sterile conditions. Use sterile technique to change solution bottles, lines, and dressings. Take TPR at least q 8 hours; observe insertion site at dressing change for inflammation, tenderness.
Hyperglycemia (increased blood sugar level)	Solution is high in proportion of glucose to bring about protein-sparing and free protein for cell growth and repair.	Test urine at least once q 8 hours for glucose and acetone. Scant glucose should be present in urine, and no acetone (a breakdown product of fat metabolism). Observe for lightheadedness, mental confusion (signs of hyperglycemia). If a solution falls behind in rate, do not speed up infusion beyond designated speed to "catch up" fluid amount.
Hypoglycemia (decreased blood sugar level)	TPN solution may initiate an insulin rebound effect (the pancreas creates so much insulin in response to the rich glucose level that it overcompensates.	Test urine at least q 8 hours for glucose and acetone. A negative glucose level and positive acetone reading suggests hypoglycemia. Observe for symptoms of dizziness, mental confusion, convulsion; hypoglycemia must be corrected to protect brain cell function (brain cells need constant glucose to function). Blood glucose level will be obtained to document glucose level and serve as basis for correction. Never halt TPN solutions abruptly (amount is gradually tapered day by day to prevent a pancreatic rebound effect).
Fluid overload	A hypertonic solution puts stress on the circulatory system. Subcutaneous fluid is drawn into the bloodstream to equalize osmotic pressure.	Take pulse, respirations, and blood pressure q 8 hours at least. If rate of infusion falls behind, do not speed up rate to catch up volume. Observe for dizziness, mental confusion (symptoms of water intoxication).
Depression	Ingesting food is associated with love and a feeling of normalcy.	Mealtime should include socialization; provide this at what would be mealtimes. Oral care remains important even though no food is being ingested; some patients may be allowed clear candy such as sourballs or gum for oral satisfaction.

If a TPN solution contains 20 gm of protein, at the completion of the infusion the person will have received 20 gm of protein. Glucose is measured by its percentage in solutions. A 5% glucose and water solution means that there are 5 gm of glucose per 100 ml of water. In a 1000-ml bottle, therefore, there are 50 gm (ml) of glucose. Each gram metabolizes to produce 4 kcal. Fifty milliliters of glucose, therefore, supplies 200 kcal.

Assisting the Patient with a Handicap with Nutrition

THE BLIND PATIENT

People who have their eyes temporarily covered following an eye injury or eye surgery generally need to be fed because they cannot accustom themselves to eating without vision in the few days they are unable to see. When feeding a person who cannot see, tell him what foods are on his tray and ask him what he would like to eat first. Do not hurry people when you feed them; tell them what you are doing step by step.

For the person with a permanent vision problem, describe what foods are on the plate and where they are compared to a clock face (roast beef is at 12 o'clock, potatoes are at 3 o'clock). Cut up meat and add butter or other preparation items as needed. Allow the person to feed himself, and check back on progress. When entering the room of a blind person even for a quick check, always announce your presence.

THE PATIENT WITH IMPAIRED MENTAL STATUS

A person with impaired mental status needs help to ingest an adequate intake that is specifically related to the primary source of his difficulty. A person with mental retardation often has a short attention span and may forget that eating is the activity you wanted him to do at a particular time.

People with hallucinogenic distortion may view food as harmful or strange and refuse to eat until their mental status is improved. A person with an extreme fear or suspicion of food may need intravenous supplementation to obtain an adequate fluid intake until he is again able to eat.

THE PATIENT WITH MOTOR DYSFUNCTION

People with unsteady use of their arms may be able to feed themselves after their food is cut and prepared for them. A number of devices are available to help people who cannot hold a spoon well such as the specially adapted spoon shown in Fig. 35-8.

When feeding a person with partial paralysis of the face, always introduce food into the *nonparalyzed* side of the mouth, so they have better control of the tongue and can possibly achieve better swallowing. *Do not offer food or fluid to people who lack a gag reflex* (unconscious or totally paralyzed people) because this invites aspiration.

INTAKE AND OUTPUT

For many hospitalized patients detailed records are kept of the amount of fluid taken in daily (fluid supplied by ingestion or by intravenous or nasogastric routes) and fluid lost daily (through urine, emesis, liquid stools, nasogastric decompression, or suction through a nasogastric tube). For other patients a careful calculation of the number of calories ingested is completed.

FIGURE 35-8. A man using a curved spoon with an easily grasped handle. Using a bowl instead of a plate enables him to feed himself better with one hand.

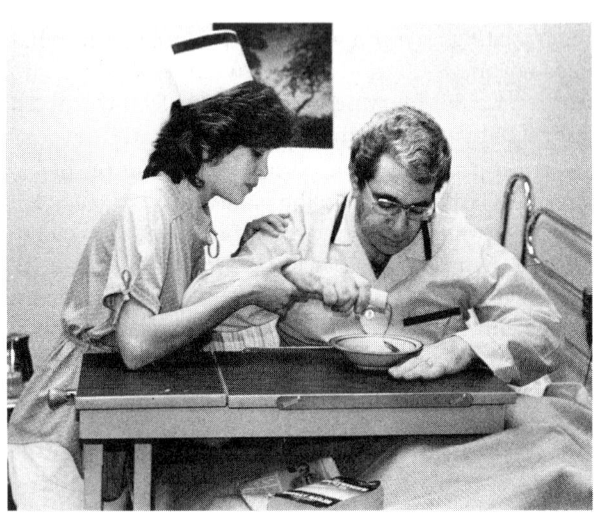

Check whether a person needs documentation of the foods or fluid eaten before you remove a tray from a bedside. Make a habit of observing the amount of fluid and food taken before you remove any tray. Recording intake and output can be done by a patient or his family as a means of participation in self-care; be sure that he understands exactly what is expected of him and that he has a pen or pencil and paper available.

UTILIZING NURSING PROCESS

Nursing Care Plan

The following is a problem-oriented recording of a patient with a nutritional problem demonstrating how well a problem-oriented system can be used to document assessment, analysis, planning, and implementation. John is a 22-year-old man who had esophageal surgery 3 days ago and has a nasogastric tube in place for tube feedings of 250 ml of Ensure and 50 ml of water rinse three times daily. In addition, he will receive intravenous fluid.

NURSING DIAGNOSIS

Nutrition, alteration of: tube feeding related to surgery.

ASSESSMENT

Subjective: States, "How much longer do I have to have this tube in? It hurts my nose every time I turn."

Objective: Tube patency checked by aspiration of gastric secretions (10 ml, clear yellow in appearance); replaced prior to feeding. Head elevated to semi-Fowler's position; 240 ml of Ensure given by slow infusion during 45 minutes. No discomfort from infusion, no regurgitation noted. Tube flushed with 50 ml water and clamped following infusion. Tape on nose changed; slight erythema noted on mucous membrane of right nostril from tube irritation. K-Y jelly applied for comfort.

Analysis: Patient is tolerating nasogastric feedings well nutritionally but is beginning to be impatient and find discomfort related to method.

Locus of Decision-Making: Shared.

Goal: Feeding method will be nutritionally and psychologically acceptable after 1 week.

Short-term Criteria: Patient indicates that method is not that of choice but understands importance of method and is tolerant of it. Weight remains stable.

Long-term Criteria: Patient is able to return to former nutritional pattern in 2 weeks. Takes food orally and weight remains stable.

NURSING ORDERS

1. Assess skin turgor, moist mucous membranes, blood pressure and pulse, and specific gravity of urine q8h as determinants of adequate hydration.
2. Give oral care every 4 hours to prevent mucous membranes drying due to no oral intake.
3. Change tape on nose q8h to prevent excessive nasal irritation.
4. Apply only water-soluble lubricant (K-Y jelly) so that lipid aspiration does not occur.
5. *Do not remove tube and replace in other nostril; patient has sutures in esophagus that could be injured. If it is accidentally dislodged, do not replace.*
6. Becomes dizzy in Fowler's position; raise to semi-Fowler's position before feeding and one-half hour afterward.

7. Give feedings three times daily at 8 A.M., 12 noon, and 5 P.M. to simulate normal mealtime.
8. Review necessity for nasogastric feedings as necessary to help patient accept method; stress this is a temporary alteration for him.
9. Patient to record tube feeding intake and urine output as part of self-care. Nursing staff to record intravenous intake. Patient provided with pencil, chart form, and metric conversion sheet.
10. Support patient by providing a mealtime atmosphere with conversation, information about overall signs of improvement (no increased temperature, skin turgor good, and so on).
11. Weigh daily before morning feeding in patient gown and robe.

SUGGESTED READINGS

Arnold, C. Why that liquid formula diet may not work (and what to do about it). *RN* 44(11):35, 1981.

Borgen, L. Total parenteral nutrition in adults. *Am. J. Nurs.* 77:1605, 1977.

Buergal, N. Monitoring nutritional status in the clinical setting. *Nurs. Clin. North Am.* 14:215, 1979.

Colley, R., and Wilson, J. Meeting patients' nutritional needs with hyperalimentation. *Nursing 79* 9:76, 1979.

Croup, E. H. Feeding the special needs child. *Child Contemp. Soc.* 12:7, 1978.

Ensin, J. Nutritional assessment of a severely head-injured, multi-trauma patient. *J. Neurosurg. Nurs.* 14(5):262, 1982.

Gillis, D. Spotlight on aging. Seniors: A target for nutritional education. *Can. Nurse* 76:28, 1980.

Griggs, B. A., et al. Update: Nasogastric tube feeding. *Am. J. Nurs.* 79:481, 1979.

Hanson, R. L. New approach to measuring adult nasogastric tubes for insertion. *Am. J. Nurs.* 80:1344, 1980.

Hill, M. Helping the hypertensive control sodium intake. *Am. J. Nurs.* 79:906, 1979.

Hinkle, M. M. A mixed message: The school vending machine. *J. Sch. Health* 52(1):20, 1982.

Keithley, J. Proper nutritional assessment can prevent hospital malnutrition. *Nursing 79* 9:68, 1979.

Korczowski, M. M., et al. Strengthen the nurse's role in nutritional counseling . . . guidelines for charting. *Nurs. Health Care* 2:210, 1981.

Kubo, W. G., et al. Fluid and electrolyte problems of tube-fed patients. *Am. J. Nurs.* 76:912, 1976.

Malcom, R., et al. Psychosocial aspects of total parenteral nutrition. *Psychosomatics* 21:115, 1980.

Mandelbaum, J. K. The food square: Helping people of different cultures understand balanced diets. *Pediatr. Nurs.* 9(1):13, 1983.

Mangham, D. B., et al. Introducing nutrition education. *J. Sch. Health* 51:110, 1981.

McConnell, E. Ten problems with nasogastric tubes . . . and how to solve them. *Nursing 79* 9:78, 1979.

McDaniel, J. M. Utilizing the nursing process model to teach nutrition and diet therapy. *J. Am. Diet. Assoc.* 74:568, 1979.

Munro, H. N. Nutritional requirements in the elderly. *Hosp. Pract.* 17(8):143, 1982.

Owen, A. L., et al. Counseling patients about diet and nutrition supplements. *Nurs. Clin. North Am.* 14:247, 1979.

Price, M. R. How nursing diagnosis helps focus your care. The patient is starving . . . but why? *RN* 42:45, 1979.

Rains, B. L. The non-hospitalized tube-fed patient. *Oncol. Nurs. Forum* 8:85, 1981.

Ross, T. The vegetarian diet: Animal, vegetable, mineral. *Nurs. Mirror* 151:22, 1980.

Rowe, N. R. Childhood obesity: Growth charts vs. calipers. *Pediatr. Nurs.* 6:24, 1980.

Salmond, S. W. How to assess the nutritional status of acutely ill patients. *Am. J. Nurs.* 80:922, 1980.

Salmond, S. W. Recognizing protein-calorie malnutrition. *Crit. Care Update* 9(1):5, 1982.

Sheridan, J. F. Current trends in nutritional care of inpatients. *Hosp. Top.* 58:16, 1980.

Stotts, N. Nutritional assessment before surgery. *A.O.R.N. J.* 35(2):207, 1982.

The impact of drugs on nutrition . . . drug-nutrient interactions. *Am. J. Public Health* 72(7):643, 1982.

Tobias, A., and Van Italie, T. Nutritional problems of the hospitalized patient. *J. Am. Diet. Assoc.* 71:253, 1977.

Troupe, C. F. Don't give up on the hopelessly obese. *RN* 44:71, 1981.

White, J. H., et al. When your patient has a weight problem. *Am. J. Nurs.* 81:549, 1981.

Wills, B. B. Food becomes fun for children. *Am. J. Nurs.* 78:2082, 1978.

Yen, P. K. Nutrition. Diet and digestive problems. *Geriatr. Nurs.* 3(6):411, 1982.

Yen, P. K. Nutrition: fast food . . . is it junk? *Geriatr. Nurs.* (New York) 3(3):184, 1982.

QUESTIONS FOR REVIEW

Sally Jackson is a patient of yours. She has emesis.

Match the definition in the left column with the correct term in the right column.

1. Loss of appetite.	a. Pernicious vomiting.
2. Vomiting by tongue manipulation.	b. Anorexia.
3. Long-term vomiting.	c. Rumination.
4. Food ejected from stomach immediately.	d. Regurgitation.
	e. Projectile vomiting.

Match the definition in the left column with the correct term in the right column.

5. Fresh bleeding in stomach.	a. Red-stained emesis.
6. Vomitus from the lower intestine.	b. Green-stained emesis.
7. Vomitus from the upper intestine.	c. Brown-stained emesis.
8. Old bleeding in stomach.	d. Yellow-stained emesis.
	e. Coffee-ground emesis.

9. Mrs. Jackson is placed on a clear liquid diet. When you assess foods on her trays, which of the following would you question?
   a. Apple juice.
   b. Tea.
   c. Orange juice.
   d. Popsicle.

10. Terry is a 4-year-old boy who is unconscious. In planning care for him, the safest statement about his nutrition is:
    a. He should have no oral foods.
    b. He should be fed in an upright position.
    c. He should be given only clear fluid.
    d. He should be fed by gastric intubation.

11. Bill Smith, an adult, has a nasogastric tube inserted for feeding. To measure the length of a nasogastric tube to be inserted, you would measure from:
    a. Nose to earlobe to xyphoid process.
    b. Earlobe to xyphoid process.
    c. Nose to earlobe to umbilicus.
    d. Earlobe to umbilicus.

12. If Bill Smith were an infant, you would measure the tube from:
    a. Nose to xyphoid process.
    b. Nose to earlobe to xyphoid process.
    c. Nose to earlobe to point between umbilicus and xyphoid.
    d. Nose to earlobe to umbilicus.

13. Giving food into the stomach by a tube is termed:
    a. Lavage.
    b. Extubation.
    c. Gavage.
    d. Fluidation.

14. An acceptable method for determining whether a nasogastric tube is positioned in the stomach before a feeding is:
    a. Listen over the stomach while air is infused into the tube.
    b. Listen over the esophagus during exhalation for rushing air.
    c. Lower the tube and observe for stomach contents.
    d. Listen over the stomach while water is infused into the tube.

15. When giving a tube feeding, the height the container of fluid should be elevated is:
    a. 12 inches above stomach level.
    b. 12 inches above heart level.
    c. 24 inches above stomach level.
    d. 18 inches above pubis.

16. Which statement demonstrates good technique for removing a nasogastric tube?
    a. Clamp the tube before removal.
    b. Remove tube slowly.
    c. Remove tube to the pharynx and offer a glass of water.
    d. Remove tube only as far as the cardiac sphincter.

17. Mr. Smith is changed to a soft diet. Which of the following statements is true about a soft diet?
    a. Foods are high in residue.
    b. Soft diets do not appeal to everyone.
    c. Fried foods are allowed.
    d. Protein is very limited.

18. Mr. Smith has paralysis of his left side, including his facial muscles. To introduce food to his mouth, you should:
    a. Introduce it to the right side of his mouth.
    b. Place food far back on his tongue.
    c. Introduce food to the left side of his mouth.
    d. Introduce food to the middle of his mouth.

19. Miss Henry is a patient receiving total parenteral nutrition. How many grams of glucose will she receive from a 1000-ml solution of 5 percent dextrose and water?
    a. 5 gm.
    b. 50 gm.
    c. 100 gm.
    d. 150 gm.

20. TPN solutions are high in glucose to supply calories and to:
    a. Cause hypoglycemia.
    b. Better distribute fat content.
    c. Create an artificial high blood pressure.
    d. Effect protein sparing.

36. REST AND SLEEP

OBJECTIVES

Upon mastery of the material in this chapter, you should be able to:

1. Describe the concept of biorhythms and their relation to sleep and rest.
2. Describe the necessity and benefits of rest.
3. Describe patients who are apt to need periods of rest and nursing implementations to provide for rest.
4. Describe the stages of sleep and conditions necessary for sound sleep.
5. Describe the behaviors that may result from sleep deprivation.
6. Describe nursing implementations to encourage sleep.
7. Discuss the role of sleep medications in inducing sleep.
8. Discuss common sleep problems and approaches to care.

TERMS

The terms important for an understanding of this chapter are shown below and defined in the glossary:

biorhythm
circadian rhythm
hypnotic
insomnia
narcolepsy
obligatory sleep
paradoxical sleep
rest
sedative
sleep
somnambulism

Rest can be defined as a period of quiet activity that promotes a sense of feeling refreshed and able to perform well. *Sleep* is a time of reduced consciousness that restores physical and mental well-being and occurs at periodic intervals. Although everyone needs both rest and sleep (they are first-level needs according to Maslow's hierarchy of needs), the need varies greatly from person to person depending on age and individual differences.

BIORHYTHMS AND REST AND SLEEP

Everyone has an internal rhythm system that guides many body functions—sleep-wake patterns, hormone release, temperature regulation, urinary output, cell synthesis, blood pressure, cardiac output, food intake, muscular activity, and thought processes. Such rhythms are called *biorhythms* because of their influence on these biologic actions.

A rhythm that has a cycle that extends over a long period of time (months or monthly) is called an *infradian* rhythm. Menstrual periods are an example of this type of rhythm. If the rhythm repeats every 24 hours, it is termed a *circadian* rhythm (*circa* means "about"; *die* means "day"). Sleep-wake cycles and most other body rhythms are circadian rhythms. If the rhythm is shorter than a day it is termed an *ultradian* rhythm. Some types of hormone release, such as insulin release, are governed by these shorter rhythms to keep blood levels adequate.

In terms of sleep and rest, some people have a circadian rhythm that sets their most wide-awake time early in the morning; for others this time falls in the midafternoon or late in the evening. Circadian rhythms are established in life at about 3 months of age (Fig. 36-1). The pattern of a particular person may have been influenced by the mother's biorhythm while still in utero.

REST

Rest is an activity that the average well person incorporates into his day without even being aware of it. It is important that you help people returning to wellness to establish suitable rest periods during the day.

Rest is needed for two reasons—physical and mental rejuvenation. Table 36-1 shows the differences between a person with a need for physical rest and one with a need for mental rest.

Physical Benefits of Rest

Resting—sitting or lying down in the middle of the day—reduces the work load on the heart because the heart does not have to pump as forcefully to deliver blood to the lower extremities in a semireclining position. Blood pressure is reduced, freeing the arterial vessels from constant pressure. Venous return from the lower extremities is easier because gravity is not as

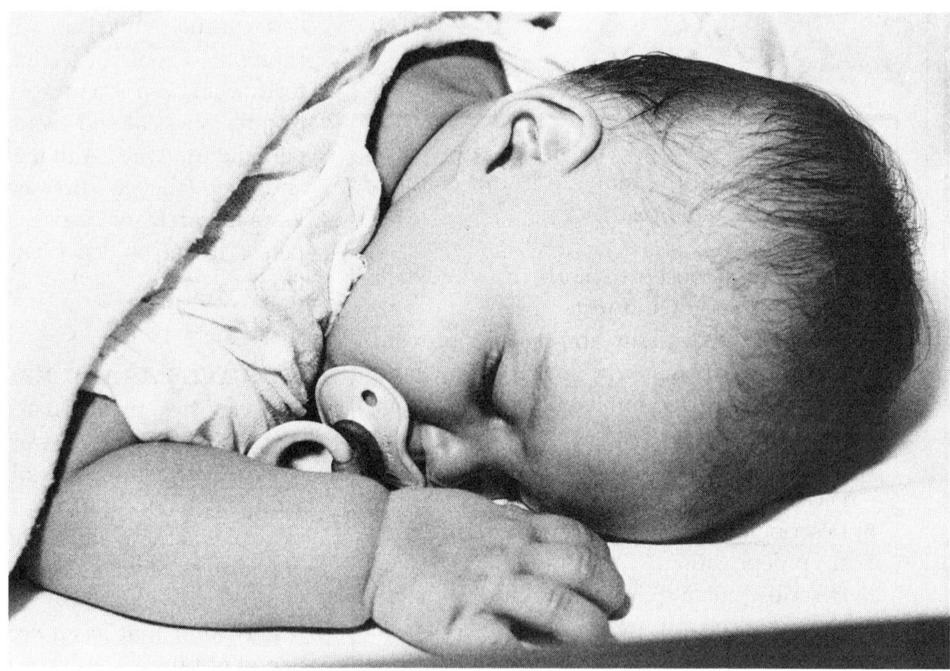

FIGURE 36-1. Infants fall asleep easily when guided by naturally occurring circadian rhythms.

TABLE 36-1. DIFFERENTIATING THE NEED FOR PHYSICAL OR MENTAL REST

Assessment Area	Physical Rest	Mental Rest
Cause of fatigue	Needed following period of active energy expenditure	Needed following emotional or intellectual energy expenditure
Tension level	Relaxed	Tense
Appearance	Lax muscle groups, difficulty keeping eyes open	Headache, stiff neck, eye strain, muscle cramping
Mood	Lethargic	Irritable, easy to anger, difficulty in concentrating
Reaction to attempt to rest	Relaxes easily, sleeps easily	Unable to relax, "fights" sleep

strong a force, and venous pressure in the lower extremities is therefore less. Blood circulation to the cerebral vessels may increase, ensuring good oxygenation of brain cells. The kidneys receive more blood in a semirecumbent position than in a standing position, so kidney output is increased, reducing the possibility of stasis of urine and possibly infection in the kidney pelvis. Muscle groups concerned with maintaining an erect posture have a reduced workload and therefore can restore their metabolic balance. Because less glucose and oxygen are needed for energy, all cells can be well supplied with these nutrients.

Mental Benefits of Rest

To rest mentally means to be able to think of nothing if that is the person's choice or to think of something pleasurable and non-stress-related. Such an activity both improves problem-solving ability and reduces anxiety level. A person who seems to be "always busy," therefore, because he goes from work to an hour of racquetball to coaching a Little League team and then home to write a report for work, has not taken a physical break but may have taken a mental break by mixing activities between those he must do and those he enjoys doing. It is wise planning for everyone to plan a rest period for himself during the day that is his own private time.

Life Span Concepts and Rest

THE INFANT

During the first half of their first year, infants rarely rest; rather, they either are sleeping or are wide awake and active. By the second half of the first year, infants often enjoy a time of rest or quiet "visiting" in the late afternoon.

THE TODDLER AND PRESCHOOLER

Toddlers and preschoolers are often very reluctant to nap in the afternoon because they are afraid they will miss some activity. Rather than stressing sleep for these periods, encouraging a quiet playtime (couch time rather than bed time or reading a story) may be a better plan.

THE SCHOOLAGER AND ADOLESCENT
Beginning with school age, children need time for mental rest as well as physical rest. Rules such as doing homework immediately after school may be unrealistic if the child feels he needs the time before dinner for rejuvenating his thought processes as well as restoring physical energy. Adolescents are undergoing such a growth spurt that chronic fatigue is often a frequent concern of this age group. Adolescents need to reserve some time of their own each day during which they can be guaranteed of being totally undisturbed. Some adolescents with demanding schedules may need some rest time built into the schedule or they find themselves unable to cope with stress due to poor problem-solving ability.

THE ADULT
Young adult women who are pregnant must reserve some time every day for a rest period during which they put their legs up to increase venous circulation from the lower extremities. The woman at home can often do this during her child's "couch time." The woman at work outside her home needs to plan this period. She may need to plan a rest period after work and delay dinner by a half hour.

Many men at middle age become so career-oriented or concerned with work that they literally forget how to rest. Such a person may not be able to take time out merely to rest during the day, but he may be able to play golf or jog or walk. For a person with a desk job, these exercise activities may be more beneficial than quiet rest.

THE OLDER ADULT
Older adults may find themselves cat-napping off and on during the day, not because their bodies or minds need this much rest but because they lack stimulation or an opportunity to be involved in a more interesting activity. Too frequent rest periods may lead to an inability to sleep at night (insomnia). Helping an older person plan responsible activities that must be carried out and encouraging social interaction and independent self-care may help him to be more active.

Providing an Environment for Rest

Because an activity that is restful for one person may not be for another, methods for providing rest differ from person to person. A number of helpful methods, however, are listed in the box on page 964.

Patients in health care facilities or in their own homes who generally need planned periods of rest are discussed in the following sections.

PERSONS WITH RESPIRATORY OR CARDIAC ILLNESS
If a person's heart must work harder than average to circulate blood or if the person must use extra energy for respiratory effort, he will tire physically more quickly than the average person because of the extra energy expenditure.

PERSONS WITH MAJOR TRAUMA
Major trauma such as burns or an amputation always exhausts a person's resources extensively because so much energy is needed for such massive healing. Trauma is also exhausting psychologically.

PERSONS WHO HAVE HEMORRHAGED
A major blood loss leads almost invariably to a lowered hemoglobin level. This makes it more difficult than usual to transport oxygen and nutrients to cells. Following a major blood loss many people are given an oral iron compound to rebuild the hemoglobin level; they may be given a blood transfusion to replace red blood cells quickly. Remind people that rebuilding blood stores can be a lengthy process. They will need to plan a program of combined rest and drug administration to regain their former energy level.

PERSONS WITH INFECTION
Infection creates an elevated body metabolism level and an increased body temperature (fever). To meet the metabolic requirements of this increased basal metabolic rate, the person must use not only whatever carbohydrate and protein he is able to ingest during the illness but must also *catabolize*, or break down, nutrient stores for extra nutrients. At the end of the illness, the person has depleted body stores. He becomes exhausted easily. Many people think that as soon as their temperature returns to normal they will be themselves again. Instead, they need a program of good nutrition and adequate rest to reach that level.

PERSONS WITH DECREASED NUTRIENT INTAKE
People who have a lowered nutrient intake for any reason may have decreased nutrient stores to such a point that a low hemoglobin level or a negative nitrogen balance exists. Oral surgery, gastrointestinal illness or surgery, head injury, and depression are all conditions that can lead to this problem.

PERSONS WITH DEFECTS OF CARBOHYDRATE METABOLISM
Carbohydrate is the nutrient used by the body for instant energy. If a person has a defect in carbohydrate metabolism that makes him unable to utilize carbohydrate or to change glycogen (a stored carbohydrate source) back into glucose, he will have a decreased energy level. Such people need to develop a life-style that

Methods of Providing for Rest

1. Organize care so that a person has sustained intervals with no interruptions between procedures or activities.
2. Divide procedures into steps as necessary so that no one procedure is long enough to be exhausting.
3. Help a person combine activities such as using a bathroom as a time to walk a short distance, not walking the distance and later also walking to the bathroom.
4. If a person is going to work on a project for mental rest, be certain he has all the supplies he needs or he may expend physical energy getting up time after time to get them.
5. Many patients do not like to "bother you" for small things like handing them a magazine from their dresser and will struggle to reach it themselves or get up to get it. Always ask before you leave a room, "Is there anything I can get you? Anything you need?"
6. Assess the number of visitors a person has. If these are his support people, they are psychologically important to him, so even their continual presence is probably not tiring. If visitors are less than primary support people (fellow workers or social acquaintances), he can become fatigued.
7. Teach people that rest is therapeutic. A person who believes in a strong work ethic (not to be busy is lazy) has difficulty saying, "I'd rather just rest."
8. Children under age 12 (who are not influenced by a work ethic) have a good sense of when they need rest and generally reduce their activity accordingly.
9. Give appropriate reassurance that you are observing a person and are pleased with his health status. A person may rest better if his room door is closed to shut out noise; if he is extremely concerned about the intravenous line, however, or that sutures will tear, he may rest better if he knows that he is directly in your line of vision and you can easily observe him.
10. Diminish any feeling of physical discomfort. A person cannot rest mentally or physically if he has pain or pruritus or is too warm or too cold.
11. Meditation is an activity that can be used as a form of conscious rest. Meditation is "centering" or directing thoughts inward to desensitize the mind against worries or concerns.

    Meditation increases self-awareness; it helps strengthen a person's individual philosophy; it aids problem-solving as a person proposes and examines solutions and "works through" concerns.

    Do not disturb people during meditation. Interrupted and half-solved, a problem seems even bigger than it did originally. Mark nursing care plans for "do not disturb" times to respect meditation times.

combines a program of rest with frequent carbohydrate intake to maintain a functioning blood glucose level.

PERSONS WITH A CHANGE IN BODY IMAGE

Loss of a leg, removal of the uterus (hysterectomy), pregnancy, removal of a breast (mastectomy), or a heart attack (coronary thrombosis) can change the way a person thinks about himself. Dealing with such a major change is psychologically stressful. A person may have a general feeling of fatigue for months afterward.

Hazards of Rest

Because a little of something is good for you, it is not necessarily true that a lot will be better. This principle applies strongly to rest. Excessive use of a totally flat bed position for an extended period of time can lead to an increase in cardiac workload (because no blood is "trapped" in the legs, more venous blood constantly arrives at the heart, eventually tiring it); if bones experience a constantly reduced pressure, they will begin to evacuate calcium and become very porous and weak (osteoporosis). The increased level of excreted calcium in urine plus the decreased ureteral flow due to lack of gravity assist can lead to the formation of calcium stones, plugged ureters, and urinary tract infection. Reduction of blood flow through the vessels due to lack of muscle contraction can lead to thrombophlebitis (clot and inflammation) of blood vessels. These hazards of immobility and measures to prevent them are discussed in Chap. 26. An important nursing responsibility is assessment of a patient's needs for rest and for stimulation or activity and helping him achieve these needs.

SLEEP

Although sleep patterns vary from those of a newborn, who sleeps an average of 16 out of 24 hours, to those of an adult, who can make do with 4 hours out of 24, sleep has universal patterns and components. Like rest, sound sleep is influenced by anxiety level, state of health, habit, medications, and environment at the time of sleep.

The Process of Sleep

During sleep, there is a decrease in the tone of the musculoskeletal system. Heart rate, respiratory rate, systolic blood pressure, and body temperature all decrease. Less urine forms during sleep owing to a falling basal metabolic rate. During sleep a person uses less oxygen than when awake; because of the recumbent position, there is increased cerebral blood flow.

Sleep is composed of repeated cycles of 60 to 120 minutes (average, 90 minutes) in length. These cycles are shortest in the newborn (45 to 60 minutes) and become longer (90 to 120 minutes) as the person matures. The average person who sleeps 7 to 8 hours a night has four to six sleep cycles during a night.

As a sleep cycle begins, the person first enters non-rapid-eye movement (NREM) sleep. This type of sleep occurs in up to 80 percent of total sleep time. As a person falls deeper and deeper asleep, he passes from stage I to stage II, III, and IV of NREM sleep over a period of 20 to 30 minutes.

STAGE I NREM SLEEP

This first stage of sleep is the lightest; it is a feeling of "drifting" or falling and is sometimes called "twilight sleep." An electroencephalogram (EEG) or brain wave recording taken during this stage of sleep shows peaked, frequently occurring waves (alpha waves). Temperature and heart rate decrease slightly although this stage lasts only a few minutes. A person can be roused easily from this early sleep by the slightest noise or even the silent presence of another person in the room.

STAGE II NREM SLEEP

This stage is very short (about 2 minutes), but sleep becomes deeper. An EEG tracing taken at this time reveals "spindle waves" or high spikes intermingled with alpha waves. Temperature and heart rate decrease slightly more. It is more difficult to wake someone from sleep when he reaches this point.

STAGE III NREM SLEEP

Sleep deepens still further. An EEG tracing reveals mixed spindle and delta (slow-moving) waves. It is very difficult to wake a person from stage III sleep. Temperature and heart rate decrease further. The period lasts about 10 minutes.

STAGE IV NREM SLEEP

About 20 to 30 minutes after beginning to fall asleep, a person enters stage IV sleep (termed *essential* sleep). Respirations are slow and deep, temperature and heart rate slow even more, and blood pressure decreases. An EEG shows delta (slow, steady) waves. A person will be confused and unable to orient himself readily if awakened from stage IV sleep.

A person remains at a stage IV sleep level for about 30 minutes, then progresses back through stages III, and II until he passes into a phase of rapid eye movement (REM) sleep (Fig. 36-2).

FIGURE 36-2. Stages of sleep. Note how the periods of REM sleep increase in length during the last half of the night.

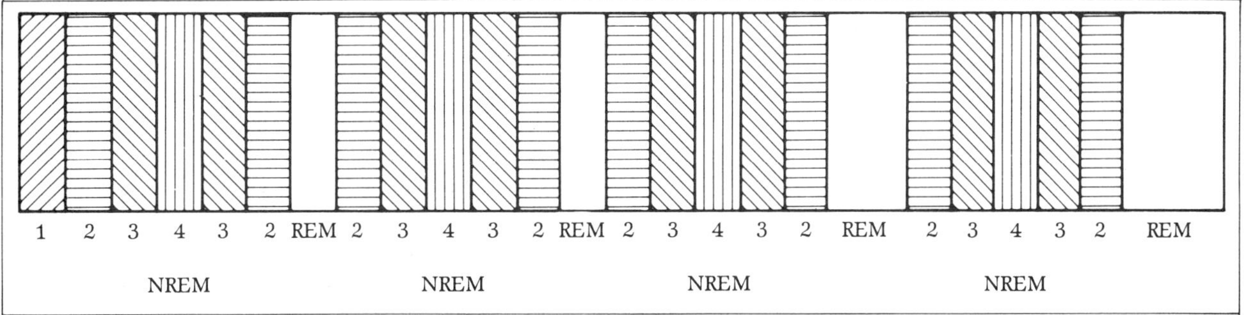

FIGURE 36-3. A night's sleep disturbed by frequent periods of waking. Notice how little REM sleep is allowed.

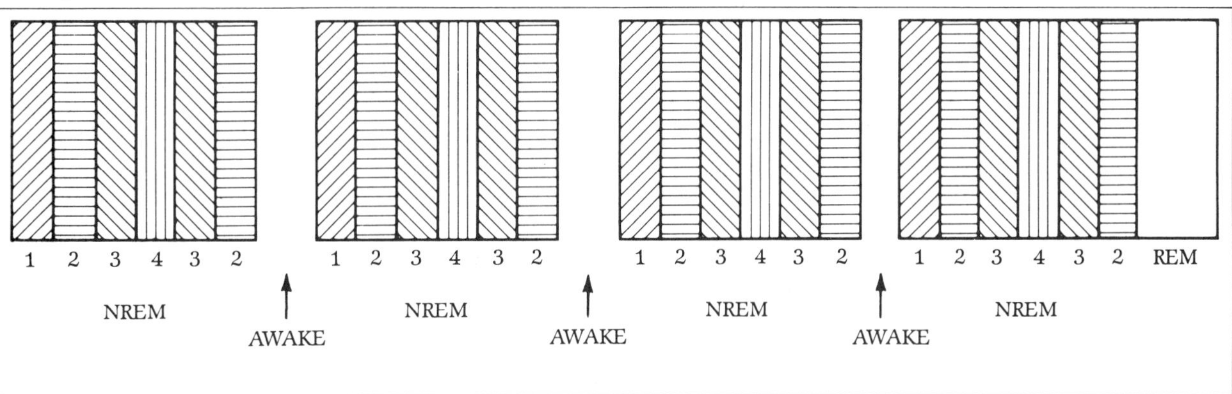

REM SLEEP

During a REM sleep pattern, a person moves his eyes in rapid, involuntary motions. Respirations are irregular; turning, movement, and penile erections may occur. Although dreams occur all through sleep, they are most vivid during REM sleep. REM sleep is termed *paradoxical* sleep because although the person is very sound asleep, he appears to be close to waking because of his active eye movements.

A person remains at a REM sleep level for 10 to 30 minutes and then begins a new sleep cycle with NREM sleep (Fig. 36-2).

Toward morning, the length of REM sleep patterns become longer and periods of NREM sleep become shorter. In infants, a high proportion of sleep time is REM sleep, whereas young adults have the least. If a person is awakened from sleep, he begins again with NREM stage I sleep as he falls asleep again, not at the pattern from which he was awakened. The sleep pattern of someone who was awakened frequently during the night would resemble that shown in Fig. 36-3.

AWAKENING FROM SLEEP

When a person sleeps, the *recticular formation* of the lower brain, composed of nerve fibers that extend from the medulla, pons, and midbrain into the hypothalamus, is not being stimulated. When sensations such as peripheral pain or shaking or touching of the body (by someone else) are transmitted to the central cortex by the reticular chain, a person wakes. Conversely, the initiation of wakefulness may be initiated by the cerebral cortex (a person may wake before his alarm goes off because he is so aware of all the things he must do that day). In this instance, sensation is transmitted from the cortex to the reticular formation to cause wakefulness.

PURPOSES OF SLEEP

The purpose of NREM sleep appears to be rest and restoration of the body. It is termed mandatory or *obligatory* sleep because it keeps the body functioning and healthy. During the periods of stage III and stage IV sleep, the secretion of growth hormone (somatotropic hormone) from the pituitary is at its highest level. Corticosteroids and adrenalin from the adrenal gland are at their lowest levels. Growth hormone is necessary for protein synthesis and growth of new cells and for repair and maintenance of all cells. Corticosteroids and adrenalin are instrumental in the catabolism or breakdown of cells. This balance of hormones is the ideal combination for protein synthesis and cell growth and repair.

The purpose of REM sleep is less clear. The rapid eye movements may serve to coordinate binocular vision; dreams that occur during this time apparently serve as a release of tension or help to integrate new knowledge and experience with old in the brain's memory system. During REM sleep, vital signs rise to near normal levels. These periods of REM sleep interspersed with NREM sleep may be a fail-safe measure to prevent vital signs from falling too low during sleep.

SLEEP DEPRIVATION

The fact that sleep is necessary for well-being can be shown by the altered behavior of people who are deprived of sleep. After about four days of total sleep deprivation, a person has difficulty in concentrating and episodes of disorientation and misperception; he is generally irritable, may manifest feelings of persecution, and of course feels marked fatigue. If a person has less REM sleep than normal, he shows symptoms of increased appetite, irritability, anxiety, and difficulty in concentrating. He has difficulty meeting stressful situations. People who are allowed to sleep for only short periods (for instance, if they are awakened in the hospital to have their temperature taken every hour) suffer REM sleep deprivation because each time they return to sleep they begin with NREM sleep and must progress through its stages before they reach a REM sleep stage. This is shown diagramatically in Fig. 36-3.

In contrast to people who suffer loss of REM sleep, people with lack of stage IV NREM sleep develop apathy and depression. This may occur in hospitalized patients also if they are constantly awakened for procedures or because of pain.

LIFE SPAN CONCEPTS AND SLEEP

The Newborn

A newborn sleeps as much as 16 hours of every 24 and an average of 4 hours at a time. Infants this age wake every 4 hours from thirst because of their high metabolic rate, so a night feeding of solid food, given by some mothers to induce their baby to sleep through the night, actually has no effect.

Newborns should not sleep on their back because they cannot turn readily to avoid aspiration of saliva in this position. They may be placed in either a side-lying or a prone position.

Mattresses for infants should be firm to provide good back support; an infant young enough to be sleeping in a crib should not have a pillow. It is a good rule for a mother to place a newborn on alternate sides each time she puts him to sleep because due to the softness of skull bones, one side of the baby's head could flatten.

The Infant

By 4 months of age, babies sleep an average of 15 hours out of 24. Although this is not much less sleep, it seems less to parents because the baby generally sleeps 8 hours at a time or through the night.

Parents should be cautioned not to induce sleeping by giving the baby a bottle propped in bed. Milk flowing

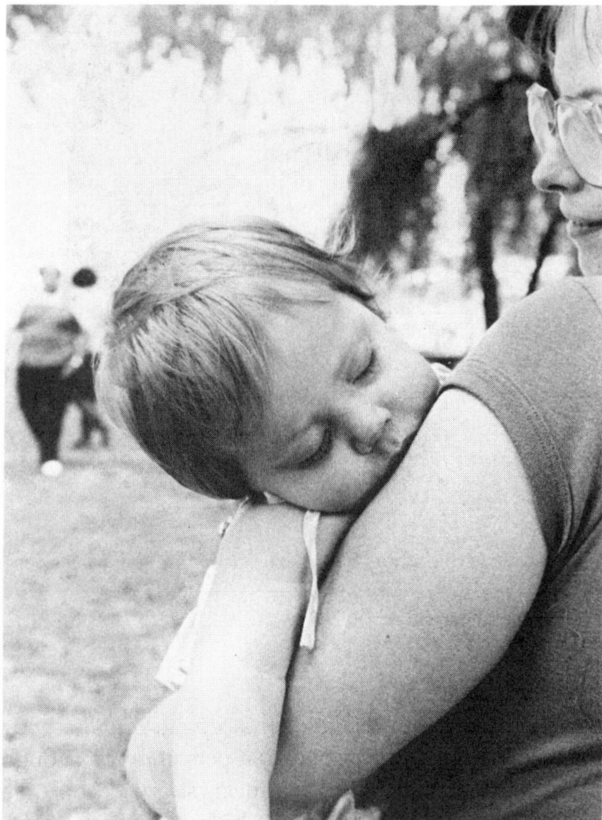

A

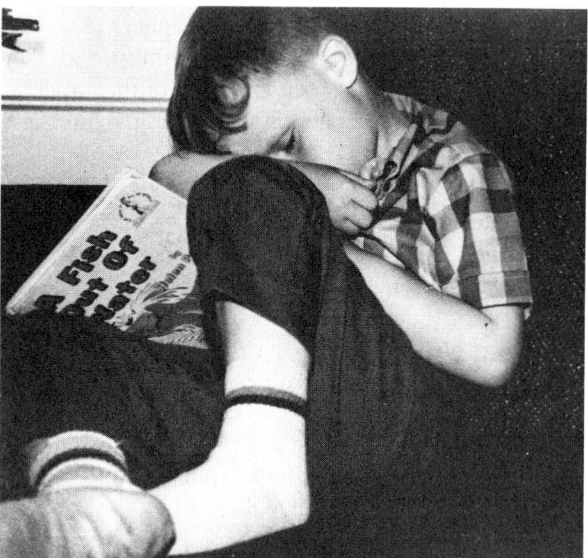

B

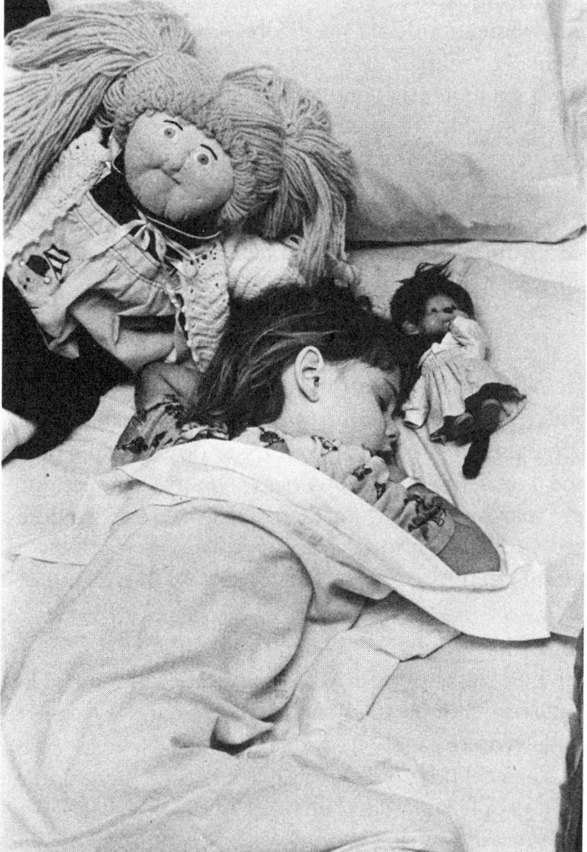

C

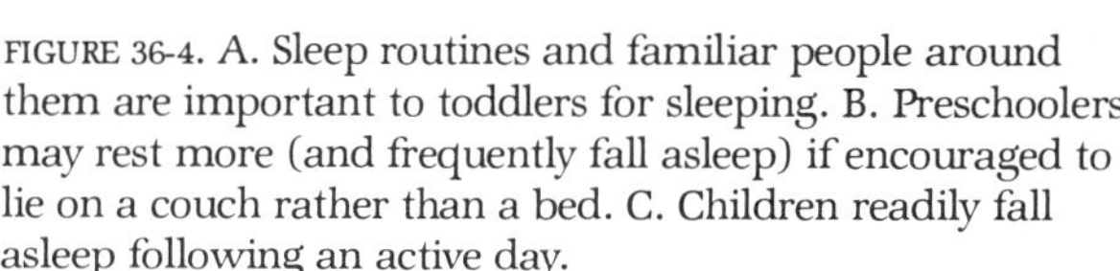

FIGURE 36-4. A. Sleep routines and familiar people around them are important to toddlers for sleeping. B. Preschoolers may rest more (and frequently fall asleep) if encouraged to lie on a couch rather than a bed. C. Children readily fall asleep following an active day.

from the propped bottle into the mouth during the night can cause extensive cavities of the lower teeth (milk-bottle syndrome).

The Toddler

Sleep requirements at this age decrease to 10 to 14 hours per day. Most toddlers are so active that they still need an afternoon nap or at least a quiet "shoes off" time.

Toddlers develop many bedtime rituals. They depend on these rituals to bring order to their lives but have great difficulty falling asleep in strange surroundings unless these routines are followed (Fig. 36-4A). These rituals should be identified when a toddler is admitted to a hospital.

The Preschooler

Many preschoolers refuse to go to bed for an afternoon nap; they may, however, fall asleep on a couch or chair each afternoon (Fig. 36-4B). At night they may have difficulty falling asleep because their imaginations are so stimulated. Fear of the dark is such a universal fear of preschoolers that you should plan to leave on a light in the child's room so that he can sleep.

The Schoolager

School-age children are active and generally sleep soundly (Fig. 36-4C). Toward the end of this period, they may begin to worry about school marks or their appearance and thus lie awake at night worrying about these things.

The Adolescent

Adolescents need proportionately more sleep than school-age children, probably because the growth spurt during this time demands the formation of so many new cells and protein synthesis occurs most rapidly during sleep. Adolescents, not aware of this increased need, often are trying to sleep less than ever before (staying up late is a recognized mark of adulthood) and so always feel tired. Adolescents admitted to a hospital for even a minor illness may sleep as if exhausted for the first few days to make up for lost sleep.

The Young Adult

Many young adults are under pressure to achieve either in school or in their first important work position. Pressure leads to anxiety, and anxiety interferes with sleep.

Parents with infants in the house may lose considerable sleep every night as they wake to respond to an infant's wakefulness. When a young child is admitted to the hospital, his young adult parent may exhibit a very low level of coping ability owing to prolonged sleep deprivation over the last week when the child was ill at home.

The Middle-Aged Adult

Some middle-aged adults may begin to feel that life is slipping away from them and try to do more in a day's time than actually fits. Tenseness and anxiety at bedtime may make it difficult for them to sleep. Many middle-aged adults begin to take sleep medication routinely to initiate sleep.

The Older Adult

Activity increases the need for sleep. Because an older adult is often more sedentary than active and because he has decreased metabolic and activity needs, he requires less sleep than he did formerly (only 6 hours a night). Older people may doze in front of a television set or while reading during the day, discovering at night that they are not tired enough to sleep (Fig. 36-5). Providing interesting activity during the day does a lot toward promoting sleep in the older adult.

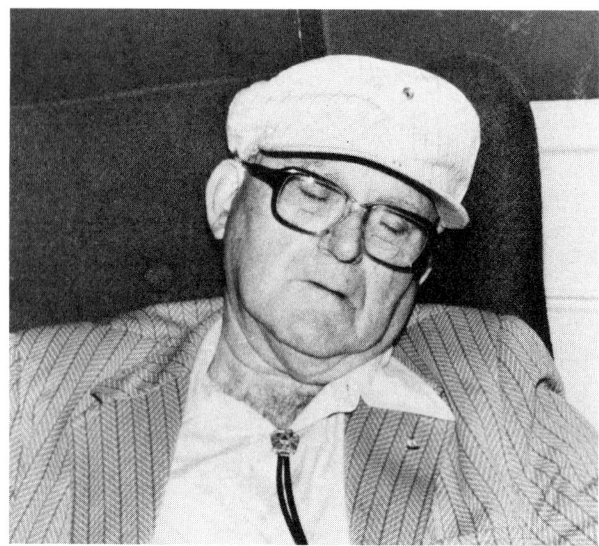

FIGURE 36-5. Older adults who doze during the day may sleep little at night.

FACTORS THAT PROMOTE SLEEP

Sleep is such a common daily occurrence that it is easy to overlook its importance. For the person who is suffering sleep deprivation, however, methods of promoting sleep are important.

Environment

A bed must be comfortable for sleeping. Because body temperature falls during sleep, a person needs enough covers or blankets to be warm during sleep. Most people are unable to sleep if there is a high noise level or if a bright light is on. Hospitals are often poor places for sleeping because mattresses may not be comfortable; the corridors can be noisy at night, and it may be necessary for a bright light to be left on to ensure good observation and safe care.

Timing

Most people have a "usual" bedtime and begin to feel drowsy at that time of day. They are unable to fall asleep before this time. Most people wake at much the same time every morning and are uncomfortable and confused if awakened earlier. People in a hospital are often asked to sleep well before their regular bedtime and are often awakened extremely early in the morning.

Ritual

Almost everyone establishes some type of bedtime ritual and are unable to fall asleep without it. It is important to identify these things on admission to a hospital and to combine as many of them as possible with HS (bedtime) care.

Activity

Exercise performed early in the day promotes sleep. Activity performed close to bedtime, however, may be overstimulating, and thus reduce the chance of sleep. Many hospitalized patients are not very active during the day and so sleep poorly at night. Even if a person cannot be physically active during the day (he is on bed rest), he can be mentally active. Activities such as solving crossword puzzles or playing checkers are sedentary but promote sleep better than watching television because they involve active participation rather than passive watching.

Reduction of Anxiety

Anxiety interferes with falling asleep and may cause a person to wake during the night or early in the morning (3 or 4 A.M.) and then not be able to return to sleep. Some hospitalized patients may need a tranquilizer to reduce their anxiety so that they can sleep. Often a quiet talk near bedtime, a time to review events of the day and to express anxieties, is enough to reduce anxiety to a level that allows sound sleep. Talking about a problem almost always reduces the size of it (see QRS 36-1).

Medication

Sleep medication should never be a prime method of inducing sleep because many such medications reduce REM sleep and are addictive. If other sleep-inducing measures are used, the average person can sleep without medication. Drugs such as amphetamines (used in diet medications) directly interfere with sleep; caffeine (found in coffee, tea, and cola drinks) also interferes with sleep and should not be ingested close to bedtime (see QRS 36-2).

Comfort

Pain will override a feeling of sleepiness. It is important that people be positioned comfortably and pain be relieved prior to bedtime. Medications to induce sleep (hypnotics) do not relieve pain and should not be used if the person has pain. Give an analgesic (medication to reduce pain), and, because he is relaxed, the person will probably sleep.

☐ QUICK REFERENCE STOP 36-1: PSYCHOLOGICAL CONSIDERATIONS
Anxiety

A common reason for not being able to rest or sleep is anxiety. Be certain that a person has a clear understanding of what has happened or will be happening to him. Provide time to talk prior to asking a person to rest or helping him prepare for bed.

Making a definite division between waking activities and bedtime activities establishes a mood for sleep. Encouraging hospitalized people to wear street clothes or their own pajamas during the day and changing to a hospital gown at bedtime can mark this transition. Resting in a comfortable chair during the day and returning to bed for the night can also mark this difference.

☐ QUICK REFERENCE STOP 36-2: NUTRITION
Bedtime Drinks

Foods with caffeine in them are best avoided at bedtime. Common foods with caffeine are coffee, tea, chocolate, and soda beverages other than 7-Up. Drinking a warm fluid such as warm milk is often helpful in promoting sleep.

COMMON SLEEP PROBLEMS

Insomnia

Insomnia is the inability to fall asleep or to stay asleep. Many people use the term to mean restless or unrefreshing sleep. Active exercise during the day increases the need for sleep, particularly stage IV NREM sleep. Because many ill people get little active exercise they may not be able to fall asleep readily and so develop insomnia. Anxiety reduces the ability to fall asleep and remain asleep. Many ill people, anxious about their illness, are likewise unable to sleep.

People who habitually take barbiturates or alcohol to fall asleep develop tolerance to these drugs and after a period of time require greater and greater amounts to induce sleep. Barbiturates and alcohol both depress REM sleep; once tolerance is reached, the person tends to spend a large proportion of time in REM sleep making up for the lack of REM sleep in the past. This is experienced by the person as restless, unfulfilling sleep.

Chloral hydrate is an example of a nonbarbiturate hypnotic that does not suppress REM sleep and so does not cause this rebound effect.

Myoclonic Manifestations

As a person begins to fall asleep he may suddenly feel a part of his body jerk violently (myoclonic spasm). This wakes him and may be strong enough to be frightening. Apparently this occurs as the upper cortical centers begin to relax. It is normal and harmless.

Bedwetting (Nocturnal Enuresis)

Involuntary urination is *enuresis;* when this occurs at night it is called *nocturnal enuresis.* The cause of bedwetting is not definitely known. There is a higher incidence in boys than in girls and in some families rather than others. Children eventually outgrow it with age. It may be associated with small bladder capacity, allergy, extremely deep stage IV sleep, or with the shift into an REM sleep pattern.

Sleepwalking (Somnambulism)

Sleepwalking tends to occur in children, although it may continue into adulthood. Sleepwalking apparently occurs during NREM sleep, probably during the deepest stage IV time. It is frightening for a person to wake and realize that he has been sleepwalking; he is confused

☐ QUICK REFERENCE STOP 36-3: SAFETY Precautions During Sleep

1. Be certain that side rails are raised on the beds of children and any adult who may be confused during sleep.
2. Be certain that the path to the bathroom is clutter-free so that a person will not stumble in a dimly lighted room at night.

because he is waking from such a deep stage of sleep (see QRS 36-3). In a hospital setting sleepwalking may be exceptionally dangerous because, while getting out of bed the person may dislodge intravenous tubing or fall and hurt himself. It is not true that a sleepwalker should not be wakened. He should be wakened gently, helped to orient himself, and then returned to bed after being reassured that he is safe and being looked after so he can sleep again.

Sleeptalking

Sleeptalking occurs apparently during REM sleep. Dreaming of some frightening or puzzling situation, the person calls out a name or instructions such as "Stop!" or cries for help. It is not necessary to wake a person talking in his sleep unless his instructions are upsetting to other patients or unless movements accompanying the talking may dislodge equipment such as intravenous tubing. People can be assured that sleeptalking is normal and harmless.

Narcolepsy

Narcolepsy is a poorly understood neurological disorder that results in an uncontrollable need to sleep at periods during the day. Symptoms usually begin in late adolescence and continue through life. The person may have difficulty holding a full-time job or attending school because of the extra hours he needs to sleep every day.

Such people can be given drugs that cause wakefulness (agrypnotic drugs) such as dextroamphetamine sulfate (Dexedrine), caffeine, and methylphenidate hydrochloride (Ritalin). They must understand the importance of taking their medication conscientiously. They must be cautioned not to drive a car or work with machinery that might harm them if they should fall asleep while operating it.

Sleep Apnea

Apnea means lack of respirations. Some people have such extreme laryngeal relaxation as they sleep that little air is able to enter the trachea. They begin to become oxygen deprived. Adults respond to this oxygen deprivation by stirring and waking, involuntarily "blowing out" air against the larynx and opening it. This makes a loud, brackish, snoring sound. They pull in several deep breaths and then fall asleep again. Within a half hour the problem may develop again and the pattern repeats itself. Although people with sleep apnea appear to sleep for a long time, they may not feel rested in the morning because their sleep has been so constantly disturbed.

In infants, sleep apnea may be the cause of sudden infant death syndrome (SIDS). Sudden infant death syndrome occurs most often in premature infants; it is rarely seen in infants over 6 months of age. Such immature infants may not have sufficient maturation of the larynx to prevent extreme sleep apnea (lack of oxygen for so long a period of time that death results).

UTILIZING NURSING PROCESS

Because sleep is important for tissue healing, mental health, and reducing fatigue, providing adequate sleep time must be considered an important nursing function.

Assessment

Because most people do not sleep soundly in a strange environment they tend not to sleep well their first few nights in a hospital. Not only is the bed different but there is also more sound at night; there may be more light than they are used to, and they are often anxious about their illness. This is particularly true of people in intensive care units. Knowledge of a person's customary nightly routine is a helpful means of promoting sleep.

Analysis

The Fourth National Conference on Nursing Diagnosis accepted only one diagnosis in regard to sleep: sleep pattern disturbance. Its defining characteristics are shown in Appendix C.

Planning

Comfort is of utmost importance for sleep. Give care at bedtime to provide a smooth bed surface and other measures that encourage rest and sleep such as voiding, brushing teeth, washing hands and face, and a backrub.

Planning naps in the morning often helps a patient to feel more rested than if he naps in the afternoon because morning naps tend to have a large REM component; afternoon sleeping tends to include more deep stage IV sleep. Waking from a short period of stage IV sleep makes a person feel groggy and not fully rested.

Planning activity to the limit of the person's ability is helpful. People who are bored tend to nap: by bedtime they have no need to sleep because they have slept so much during the day (but because they may not have experienced much REM sleep they never feel really rested) (see QRS 36-4).

Implementation

Procedures such as establishing comfort and conforming to a previous sleep routine are always preferable to administering medication for sleep. Some common sleep medications are shown in Quick Reference Stop

☐ **QUICK REFERENCE STOP 36-4: PSYCHOLOGICAL CONSIDERATIONS**
Boredom

Although chronic fatigue is a symptom of many illnesses, boredom can also lead to chronic fatigue; the person states that he always needs to rest. Assess whether boredom is not a factor if the person is spending so much time resting that it interferes with his normal functioning.

Some people use sleep as a psychological method of dealing with stress. Although this escapist method has some benefit in temporarily reducing the level of stress, people who use it as a primary or long-term coping mechanism need counseling to learn a better problem-solving technique.

36-5. A drug is a *sedative* if it causes mild depression of incoming stimuli; it is a *hypnotic* if it actively induces sleep. Schedule procedures so that people can sleep for long uninterrupted periods if possible.

Evaluation

A person may sleep a long number of hours yet not feel rested because he experiences little REM sleep. Evaluation must therefore include not only the number of hours a person has slept but also whether he feels rested at the end of the period (see QRSs 36-6 and 36-7).

NURSING CARE PLAN

A nursing note, written in a problem-oriented format, on Ms. White, a 30-year-old woman who is hospitalized

☐ **QUICK REFERENCE STOP 36-5: PHARMACOLOGY**
Common Sedatives and Hypnotics

Generic Name	*Trade Name*	*Use*	*Nursing Considerations*
Barbiturates			
Phenobarbital	Luminal	Sedative, anticonvulsant; long-acting	Barbiturates act by causing central nervous system depression. They are addictive and may cause an excitatory response, especially in elderly people. They should not be used with alcohol because together these drugs have a synergistic effect. Rapid withdrawal may lead to convulsions; always see that the dose is tapered. Because barbiturates decrease respirations they are not generally used with patients with respiratory disease. They cause a decrease in REM sleep patterns.
Secobarbital	Seconal	Sedative, hypnotic, short-acting	
Pentobarbital	Nembutal	Sedative, hypnotic, short-acting	
Nonbarbiturates			
Chloral hydrate	Notec	Sedative, hypnotic	Synergistic with alcohol. Habituation and physical dependence may occur.
Methaqualone	Quaalude	Sedative, hypnotic	May cause physical and psychological dependence.
Glutethimide	Doriden	Sedative, hypnotic	Physical and psychological dependence may occur.

SAFETY RULES OF ADMINISTRATION FOR ALL SLEEPING MEDICATIONS

1. Do not awaken a patient to give a sleeping medication.
2. Use side rails after administration (patient is sleepy).
3. Use caution with heat therapy if a person has received a sedative or hypnotic (he may not perceive heat well).
4. Never just give a sleep medication; enhance effect by backrub, quiet atmosphere, and so on.
5. Sedatives and hypnotics do not relieve pain. (Give an analgesic; free from pain, the person will sleep.)
6. Follow drug control restrictions with barbiturates because they are scheduled drugs (see Chap. 29).

☐ QUICK REFERENCE STOP 36-6: HEALTH TEACHING
Sleep Medications

Teach people not to rely on hypnotics for sleep. If they feel they must use such a medication, encourage them to use a nonbarbiturate. If they do use a barbiturate, caution them not to drink alcohol. Alcohol and barbiturates combine to greatly reduce and even halt respiratory rate.

☐ QUICK REFERENCE STOP 36-7: COMMUNITY CONSIDERATIONS
Rest Following Hospital Discharge

When many people are discharged from the hospital following surgery or an illness they are able to accomplish some aspects of self-care but are unable to accomplish all of it independently, especially without adequate rest during the day. If a parent has been hospitalized for any length of time and his partner has been filling in for him at home, this means that some activities have been curtailed (the kitchen floor was not scrubbed, no blown light bulbs were changed, bedtime stories were greatly shortened). Family members may expect the person returning home to catch up immediately on these activities, and the person himself may feel that he should immediately begin to do this type of work.

You may need to review with him that discharge from a health care facility does not mean that he is well, only that he is no longer so ill that he cannot regain health at home. He may need to make plans for a family member or a neighbor to visit daily to assume some home responsibilities he cannot yet accomplish or to watch small children so he can rest. Many people work too hard during their first few days home from a health care agency and ultimately prolong their recovery. Help them safeguard against this by concrete planning for adequate rest periods until they are completely well again.

for a series of radiographs that will help in the diagnosis of a stomach ulcer, might be as follows:

Subjective Assessment: Patient cries because she says she is exhausted; has not slept at all since being admitted 3 days ago. Although sleep medication (Seconal) has been ordered, she states that she will not take it because it is a barbiturate. Ordinarily knits before she falls asleep but brought no project to hospital with her. Ordinary bedtime is 12 midnight. Patient asks how anyone can sleep when they do not know how a test will turn out.

Objective Assessment: Eyes are darkly lined; night nursing notes confirm that she has slept only sporadically during the last two nights.

Analysis: Sleep pattern disturbance related to anxiety about diagnostic tests.

Locus of Decision-Making: Patient.

GOALS

Short-term Goal: Patient will sleep without difficulty in 2 more nights.

Criteria: Patient will express satisfaction with sleep; appear rested.

Long-term Goal: Patient will express constructive ways to deal with anxiety by time of discharge.

Criteria: Patient will display better coping mechanisms such as ability to help with making plans for home care.

NURSING ORDERS

1. Discuss possibility of increasing exercise during day to correspond more closely with life-style prior to hospitalization (walk to end of hallway six times every morning).
2. Encourage usual bedtime at midnight.
3. Provide time for discussion about concerns prior to bedtime.
4. Remind physician of anxiety about test results so that he can inform her about them as soon as possible.
5. Consult with physician to determine if sleep medication can be changed to a nonbarbiturate but support patient's desire not to depend on it for sleep.
6. Discuss possibility of asking a family member to bring in a knitting project for her to work on prior to bedtime.

SUGGESTED READINGS

Adams, K. Sleep: A time for rest and a time for play. *Nurs. Mirror* 150:17, 1980.

Anders, T. F. Night-waking in infants during the first year of life. *Pediatrics* 63:860, 1979.

Anders, T. F. Sleep and sleepiness in children and adolescents. *Pediatr. Clin. North Am.* 27:29, 1980.

Cohen, D., et al. Sleep disturbances in the institutionalized aged. *J. Am. Geriatr. Soc.* 31(2):79, 1983.

DeLoughery, M. N. Chronic insomnia. *Nurs. Pract.* 7(2):8, 1982.

Deters, G. E. Circadian rhythm phenomenon. *M.C.N.* 5:249, 1980.

Felton, G. Body rhythm effects on rotating work shifts. *Nurs. Digest* 4:29, 1976.

Fosnot, H. Insomnia: When the patterns of sleep go askew. *Patient Care* 14:122, 1980.

Hayter, J. The rhythm of sleep. *Am. J. Nursing* 80:457, 1980.

Hearne, K. Sleep paralysis: Trapped in sleep. *Nurs. Mirror* 154(2):34, 1982.

Kupfer, D. J., et al. Sleep disorders. *Hosp. Pract.* 18(2):101, 1983.

Maslow, A. H. *Motivation and Personality* (2nd ed.). New York: Harper & Row, 1970.

Milne, B. Sleep-wake disorders and what we can do about them. *Can. Nurse* 78(4):24, 1982.

Milner, J. Management of infant sleeping problems. *Midwife Health Visit. Comm. Nurse* 18(3):94, 1982.

Oswald, I. No peace for the worried . . . sleep disorders and their management. *Nurs. Mirror* 150:34, 1980.

Palmer, J. D. *An Introduction to Biological Rhythm.* New York: Academic, 1976.

Prescott-Day, S. Sleep variations in the pre-school child. *Health Visit.* 52:465, 1979.

Rader, J., et al. Circadian rhythms: How the patient's biological timetable affects your care. *RN* 41:100, 1978.

Schirmer, M. S. When sleep won't come. *J. Gerontol. Nurs.* 9(1):16, 1983.

Sebilia, A. J. Sleep deprivation and biological rhythms in the critical care unit. *Crit. Care Nurs.* 1(4):19, 1981.

Tom, C. K., and Lanuza, D. M. Symposium on biological rhythms. *Nurs. Clin. North Am.* 11:569, 1976.

Williams, R. L., et al. Grand rounds in critical care: Problems with sleep. *Heart Lung* 11(3):262, 1982.

Younger, J. B. The management of night waking in older infants. *Pediatr. Nurs.* 8(3):155, 1982.

Zelechowski, G. P. Helping your patient sleep: Planning instead of pills. *Nursing 77* 7:65, 1977.

QUESTIONS FOR REVIEW

1. Mr. Smith is a patient of yours. When planning care for him, one measure you might suggest to encourage sleep might be:
   a. To ask him to do at least 10 sit-ups before bedtime.
   b. To get him a warm drink such as coffee.
   c. To dim the lights in the room.
   d. To encourage him to go to sleep earlier than he does at home.

2. Terry is a 4-year-old girl. One measure you might suggest to encourage her to sleep might be:
   a. To leave the lights in the room on.
   b. To get her a drink such as coca-cola.
   c. To encourage her to go to sleep earlier than she does at home.
   d. To play a game of tag just before bedtime for exercise.

3. In planning further care, you recognize that Terry needs both REM and NREM sleep. Which of the following is true of REM sleep?
   a. Growth hormone is released during this period.
   b. Somnambulism occurs during this time.
   c. Dreams occur.
   d. Protein synthesis is at its highest peak.

4. Which of the following is true of stage IV NREM sleep?
   a. The largest proportion of it occurs during the first half of the night.
   b. Infants do not experience stage IV sleep.
   c. It is not controlled by circadian rhythms.
   d. It is marked by vivid dreams.

5. Implementing care might consist of administering medications for sleep. A barbiturate hypnotic may interfere in what way with restful sleep?
   a. It increases appetite.
   b. It decreases REM sleep.
   c. It decreases stage IV sleep.
   d. It increases stage III sleep.

6. A person can expect to have how many cycles of sleep during one night?
   a. One to two.
   b. Two to four.
   c. Four to six.
   d. Eight to ten.

7. Sleep produces physiological changes. In assessing Terry during the night, which of the following would you *not* expect to notice?
   a. Temperature decrease.
   b. Cerebral blood flow decrease.
   c. Heart rate decrease.
   d. Blood pressure decrease.

8. You wake Mr. Smith every hour during the night to take his pulse. The danger of this practice is:
   a. It may cause REM sleep deprivation.
   b. Pulse rates increase during sleep, so the pulse rate will be inaccurate.
   c. Frequent waking may lead to increased blood pressure.
   d. It may cause lack of stage I sleep.

9. A symptom you would expect Mr. Smith to show if he is deprived of stage IV sleep is:
   a. Anxiety.
   b. Restlessness.
   c. Hallucinations.
   d. Depression.

10. To check your knowledge of the following definitions concerning sleep, find the scrambled word that represents each of them in the box below.
    a. A 24-hour rhythm cycle.
    b. A monthly biorhythm.
    c. A drug that induces sleep.
    d. A drug that initiates rest.
    e. Sleepwalking.
    f. Bedwetting.
    g. A periodic state of rest during which there is lack of conscious thought.
    h. Paradoxical sleep.
    i. Type of drug that causes wakefulness.
    j. A state of refreshing and relaxing inactivity.

potnhicy tnyagroicp bimlnosmmasu plese ters
seirunes lanturnoc tivseeda mre darcician frinianda

37. INTESTINAL ELIMINATION

OBJECTIVES

Upon mastery of the material in this chapter, you should be able to:

1. Describe the normal process of intestinal elimination.
2. Describe factors that promote or impair intestinal elimination.
3. Describe patterns of intestinal elimination and common intestinal elimination problems in reference to different age groups.
4. Describe the technique for obtaining a stool specimen.
5. Describe nursing implementations designed to promote or maintain intestinal elimination.
6. Apply nursing process to give safe and personal care to a patient whose care involves principles of intestinal elimination.

TERMS

The terms important for an understanding of this chapter are shown below and defined in the glossary:

chyme
colostomy
constipation
defecation
diarrhea
enema
feces
flatulence
flatus
guaiac test
Hematest
hemorrhoids
incontinence of stool
meconium
melena
steatorrhea
stool

The body eliminates waste products by four main systems—the urinary tract, gastrointestinal tract, respiratory tract, and integument (skin). Elimination from the gastrointestinal tract is a major route for elimination.

Defecation is the expulsion of feces from the intestine and is a process that most people spend little time thinking about and almost no time worrying about. It is a subject that is often considered "not nice" to discuss with others, but whether or not feces elimination or bowel tone and function remain normal and methods of effecting or maintaining normal bowel movements during health and illness are nursing concerns. Assessing changes in bowel function (the presence of some gallbladder disease is diagnosed by color of feces, for example) is a major nursing responsibility.

NORMAL BOWEL ELIMINATION

Ingested food is broken down into its useful parts (amino acids, glucose, fatty acids, vitamins, minerals, and water) in the stomach and small intestine and then absorbed across the villi into the bloodstream. Left to pass on into the large intestine (colon) to be expelled from the body are the waste products of ingestion and digestion—food residue, bacteria, epithelial cells, bile pigment, inorganic salts, and water (stool or feces).

The large intestine in an adult is about 50 to 60 inches long (125 to 150 cm). It has six divisions—cecum, ascending colon, transverse colon, descending colon, sigmoid, and rectum. It begins with the valve connecting it to the small intestine (the ileocecal valve) and ends at the external opening, the anus.

Stool is very liquid as it enters the large intestine (in this state it is termed *chyme*). As chyme passes through the length of the structure, water is absorbed from it so that when it arrives at the anus it has a semi-solid form. Waste products of food take about 48 hours to reach the anus. If a person eats contaminated food, it will take this long to clear his system; if he has not eaten for days because of surgery, it may be 2 additional days after he begins to eat before he can be expected to have a bowel movement.

Waste products are propelled through the intestine by peristaltic movements or waves of contraction and relaxation. These waves are most prominent following ingestion of food (termed the *gastrocolic* and *duodenal reflexes*); normally they are painless. If an obstruction or inflammation occurs, distending the colon, these waves of contraction and relaxation become painful (intestinal cramps). Intestinal movements are stimulated by the parasympathetic nervous system and inhibited by the sympathetic nervous system. An unusual sensory property of the colon is that it does not register pain when its wall is cut or burnt, only if it is distended or stretched. This property is useful because it means that if a segment of colon is brought out on the abdominal wall during surgery (termed a *colostomy*), the exposed loop of bowel can be cut or cauterized (burned) as a bedside or treatment room procedure without causing pain (loops of bowel are commonly opened this way to drain following surgery).

The anal opening actually consists of two separate sphincters, one just at the skin surface (the external sphincter) and one set about a half inch inside (the internal sphincter). The internal sphincter is controlled by the autonomic nervous system and opens involuntarily to pressure against it. The external sphincter is under voluntary control of motor nerves. When medicine is inserted into the colon (in a suppository form from which it will be absorbed into the bloodstream from the mucous membrane), it is important to place the suppository past the internal sphincter; otherwise, it will be immediately expelled by involuntary muscle action.

Defecation

Defecation is the term used to describe the expulsion of the feces. Stool accumulates in the sigmoid portion of the colon until it reaches considerable bulk and a semiformed consistency. At that point, the internal sphincter opens involuntarily in response to the pressure on it and propels the feces into the rectum. Sensory nerves in the rectal walls begin to register the accompanying distention, and as these sensations are interpreted by brain feedback, the person becomes aware of the need to defecate. Stool is actually expelled when the person voluntarily relaxes his external sphincter and allows feces to pass.

Defecation is aided by a sitting position (which aids the pressure of gravity), the voluntary tension of the abdominal muscles, the downward pressure of the diaphragm (actions that increase intra-abdominal pressure), and contraction of the perineal levator ani muscle.

Defecation is difficult if the abdominal or perineal muscles are tender or injured, diaphragm movement is painful, stool is hard and unmalleable, the anus is unfunctional in some way, or the person cannot assume an upright sitting position.

The sensation of having to defecate is a transitory one; if defecation is not effected within a few minutes, the sensation fades. It returns again in a few hours, and if ignored again, it fades again and so forth until it becomes so forceful that it can no longer be ignored.

Most people have consistent patterns of defecation (every day following breakfast, for example), but there is a wide variation in patterns from person to person. It is important to determine the normal pattern for each individual because this pattern is necessary as an assessment guide for that individual. It is a myth that a daily bowel movement is necessary for health.

TABLE 37-1. COMMON COLORS OF STOOL

Color	Event Suggested by Color
Brown	Normal adult stool.
White (clay-colored acholic)	No bile is entering duodenum or person has had a barium x-ray film and barium is being excreted in stool.
Black	Bleeding into stool has occurred high in gastrointestinal tract and blood has aged, turning black (melena) by time of defecation or ingestion of iron medication.
Red	Bleeding has occurred close to anus or red dye is being excreted in feces.
Blackish-green (tarry)	Meconium of newborn; normal first stool.
Yellow, seedy	Normal stool of infant who is ingesting only breast milk or formula.
Green	Stool has passed very rapidly through the intestinal tract, allowing no time for bile to discolor to brown (diarrhea).

Normal Stool Appearance

COLOR

Stool derives its color from specific foods ingested, the action of intestinal bacteria, and the addition of bile. Bile is manufactured by the liver and stored in the gallbladder; it enters the duodenum very near the stomach at the ampula of Vater. If no bile is added to stool, stool appears white (often termed *clay-colored* or acholic). If stool passes very rapidly through the intestine (diarrhea), bile does not have time to turn the characteristic brown color of normal stool but remains bright green. Food dye can color the stool; barium, a contrast medium ingested for x-ray studies of the gastrointestinal tract, appears white as it is excreted in stool.

If bleeding is occurring in the intestinal tract close to the anus, the stool will appear bright red. If bleeding occurs higher in the tract, the blood is digested and turns black by the time of defecation. To determine if a black or red stool contains blood and not a food dye (a diet rich in red beets or a liquid diet consisting mainly of red Hawaiian Punch will turn stools red; iron compounds ingested as supplemental sources of nutrition will turn stool black), test a stool sample for occult blood as an independent nursing action. Stool color and the possible event it suggests are summarized in Table 37-1.

ODOR

The normal odor of stool is caused by the action of intestinal bacteria. Stools of newborns typically have no odor because the intestine is free of bacteria at birth. If a person is unable to digest or absorb fat the stool will have a high proportion of fat (steatorrhea) and often smells putrid and offensive (often compared to the odor of a cat's feces). If stool has passed through the intestine so rapidly that not even glucose could be absorbed, it may smell sweet from the high carbohydrate content.

CONSISTENCY AND FORM

Normally, stool is semi-formed and assumes the shape of the rectum. Its bulk is formed by the presence of indigestible food substances (largely cellulose from plant stems). If the shape of the rectum or anus is altered in any way, stool may assume this abnormal shape. If the anus or rectum is unusually narrow, for example, the stool may be ribbon-shaped or string-shaped, or the person may be unable to pass any stool that is not liquid or soft in consistency.

If so little water has been removed from stool that it has a liquid consistency, the stool has passed through the intestine very quickly due to irritation and rapid peristaltic action (diarrhea), or else the person is ingesting only liquids so that no cellulose is present to form bulk (sometimes termed a starvation pattern or starvation stool). If stool remains longer than normal in the intestine, more fluid is absorbed than normal, and the stool becomes hard and even pelletlike in consistency (constipation).

CONSTITUENTS

Stool content may be tested to determine if abnormalities are present. Such testing may be done by a laboratory analysis or by a number of quick tests on the patient care unit.

Normally, there is always some fat in stool (about 10 to 20 percent) because fat is the nutrient that is hardest to digest. Stool contains about 75 percent water. It is normally negative for glucose because glucose is the easiest nutrient to absorb; it has an alkaline pH (a pH over 7). It is negative for blood. If diarrhea is present, glucose will be present in the stool, and acid-producing bacteria feasting on the glucose content will test positive for glucose and have an acid pH. If infection is present the specific infective organism can be detected in the stool; blood also may be present with infection due to irritation and inflammation of the bowel wall.

LIFE SPAN CONCEPTS AND INTESTINAL ELIMINATION

THE NEWBORN

Meconium (the first stool of a newborn) begins to form at about the 16th week of intrauterine life; it is a combination of intestinal mucus and shed cells. Meconium is odorless, black in color, and tarlike in consistency. If newborns do not pass a first stool by 24 hours of life some blockage or obstruction in the gastrointestinal tract is suggested.

About the third day of life, newborn stools change to a green color and become loose in consistency. This is a transitional stool; it does not represent diarrhea. Following about 24 hours of transitional stool, the stools become light yellow in color if the infant is breast-fed, a dark or bright yellow in color if the child is formula-fed. Stools may contain small seedlike particles. They remain fairly loose until solid food is added to the diet at 5 to 6 months of age. Newborns may have from one to six stools a day.

THE INFANT

Infants often grow red-faced and make small grunting noises as they defecate. This is normal for infants, and as long as the stool passed is soft, this pattern does not represent unusual difficulty with defecation or constipation. Infants establish a defecation pattern that is unique for them and varies considerably from one infant to another.

Infants may develop diaper rashes if diapers are not changed promptly following defecation; if diarrhea is present and the stool is acid, diaper rash occurs very quickly from the acid irritation.

THE TODDLER AND PRESCHOOLER

Toddlers become interested in stool as a part of normal development. Toilet training of toddlers and preschoolers is discussed in Chap. 9. Because a child of this age has just been recently toilet-trained, it is often difficult to convince him that it is all right to use a bedpan in his room or bed. Ask his mother to explain that it is all right. Ask at a hospital admission what word the child uses to indicate that he has to defecate. It is not unprofessional to use words such as “poopy” or “number 2” when asking a child to defecate if such words will ensure effective communication with the child.

THE SCHOOLAGER AND ADOLESCENT

Schoolagers and adolescents become self-conscious about body functions. A lack of embarrassment on your part aids greatly in making the child feel comfortable about this portion of his care. Providing privacy for defecation is important in reducing his self-consciousness.

THE YOUNG AND MIDDLE-AGED ADULT

People in this age group are active and have little difficulty with defecation. Many women during pregnancy develop constipation (because pressure of the growing fetus against the colon slows peristalsis and causes increased water absorption). Fetal pressure may also cause blockage and congestion of venous return from the lower extremities and rectum (hemorrhoids). Pregnant women need a diet high in water and fiber. Resting in a Sims’ position (see Chap. 26) helps to remove the weight of the fetus from the rectal veins, reducing venous congestion and thereby reducing the possibility of hemorrhoid formation.

THE OLDER ADULT

Older adults were raised at a time when it was believed that a daily bowel movement was necessary to remain healthy. It was thought that if a bowel movement was not achieved daily, toxins from the bacteria in feces would be absorbed back into the person's circulation. Having a daily bowel movement, therefore, is not just a way of monitoring the function of the gastrointestinal system for many older adults but a means of illness prevention as well. Following surgery, when people have not eaten solid food for several days or are on a liquid diet, they may need to be reminded that it is normal not to have a daily bowel movement.

If an older adult has a limited income or limited mobility so that he cannot grocery shop frequently, he may not eat many foods with a cellulose content (fresh vegetables). Unless he understands the importance of a good fluid intake, he may drink very little water. This combination, along with decreased intestinal peristalsis, may lead to constipation. Although not recommended, a great many older adults take a daily laxative or stool softener when at home. Always ask them on hospital admission if they are taking any medicine of this type so that it can be continued.

FACTORS THAT INTERFERE WITH NORMAL ELIMINATION

DIET

As mentioned, fiber in a diet adds bulk to stool and helps the colon move it forward more effectively. Sufficient fiber also improves overall intestinal wall integrity; all fibers but bran (the fiber of wheat) also act to reduce blood cholesterol levels because cholesterol (a component of bile) is incorporated in stool and excreted when such fibers are present. Foods high in fiber are shown in Table 37-2. Lack of sufficient fiber in a diet may lead to constipation.

LACK OF FLUID

Stool is composed of about 75 percent water; when fluid intake is reduced for some reason, stool may become so dried that it is hard and difficult to pass. Passing a hard stool may cause a small anal fissure (tear), which then is painful. The person avoids defecating to avoid pain, and stool remaining in the rectum dries still more, continuing the cycle of constipation.

LACK OF EXERCISE

Activity stimulates intestinal peristalsis. People who can take little exercise, therefore, such as postoperative or bedridden patients, are more prone to constipation than those who are normally active. Effective defecation requires the use of abdominal muscles. People who have little exercise may have poor abdominal tone and are unable to use the abdominal muscles effectively for defecation.

TABLE 37-2. FOODS WITH A HIGH FIBER CONTENT

Type of Food	Example
Vegetables with long fibers	Celery, cabbage, collard greens, broccoli
Fruit with skins	Apples, peaches
Dried fruits	Dates, figs, prunes
Raw fruits and vegetables	Spinach salad, green salad, carrot sticks
Bread with whole grain fibers	Whole wheat bread, bran muffins, brown bread
Cereal with whole grain fibers	Bran flakes, shredded wheat

PARALYTIC ILEUS

Whenever the intestine is handled, such as during abdominal surgery, peristalsis halts for about 24 hours. This occurs not only with intestinal surgery but also with any abdominal surgery because the intestine is handled as it is moved out of the way of the surgical field. The presence of bowel sounds must be assessed following any surgery to be certain that peristalsis has returned before a person can be offered oral fluid.

LACK OF A CONSISTENT PATTERN

People who establish a set pattern of defecation (every morning after breakfast, for example) discover that their body is so used to this pattern that no matter where they are at that time of day, they experience a need to defecate. When a set pattern is broken (when a person is on vacation or hospitalized) and the usual time of day passes without defecation, the person may experience no further need to defecate until the following day. If this occurs day after day, the person can become constipated. People who do not have a set pattern for defecation may allow three or four days to pass before they have a bowel movement; during this time, drying of stool can occur.

MEDICATION

Some medications, particularly narcotics such as morphine and codeine, tend to be constipating due to their effect of slowing gastrointestinal movement. It is important to recognize the possibility of this side effect so it can be counteracted.

EMOTIONS

In some people, stress or anxiety leads to such increased peristalsis that they develop diarrhea. People who are severely depressed may have little body movement, generally eat poorly, and thus may become constipated (general adaptation to stress shifts blood from organs that are not necessary for emergency action to those that are, such as the heart and brain). Because blood is drawn away from the gastrointestinal tract drying and hardening of stool may occur.

> ☐ **QUICK REFERENCE STOP 37-1: PSYCHOLOGICAL CONSIDERATIONS**
>
> Defecation is a private act for most people. Learning to offer bedpans or assisting people to use bathrooms with respect for their feeling of discomfort due to this sudden invasion of privacy is the mark of a professional nurse.

LACK OF PRIVACY

Most people think of defecation as a private act. They are unable to defecate in a setting where the sounds or odors of defecation will be detected by others. This is a particular problem with people in shared hospital units who must use a bedpan (see QRS 37-1).

LACK OF ADEQUATE ABDOMINAL OR PERINEAL MUSCULATURE

Use of the abdominal and perineal muscles is necessary for normal defecation. People with wasted muscle from starvation or muscle disease or neurological impairment may have difficulty with normal elimination. Following abdominal surgery, people have too much pain to use their abdominal muscles for effective defecation.

CULTURAL INFLUENCES

Cultural patterns and values affect elimination. In the United States, defecation is considered a private act, and people may have difficulty defecating without privacy; they may be unwilling to discuss this in a health history. Diapers for infants are used because they absorb feces and completely hide this body process. In contrast, in the Far East, infants typically do not wear diapers. Body elimination is considered a natural process and people speak freely about it at history-taking.

FACTORS THAT PROMOTE EVACUATION

DIET

A diet high in roughage (fiber) stimulates peristalsis; adequate water intake (about 2,000 ml a day in an adult) helps to keep feces soft. Also helpful are regularly spaced meals (because this encourages the bowel to have regularly spaced times of active peristaltic motion). Observe the dietary intake of toddlers carefully; when they choose their own food for the first time they may not choose to eat vegetables (fiber foods).

Observe the diets of schoolagers and adolescents because they may omit eating vegetables if their friends omit them. People with poorly fitting dentures or no dentures may not eat as many vegetables, particularly raw ones, as they otherwise might.

Observe carefully the elimination pattern of people who are dehydrated. In such people, so much water is reabsorbed from stool in the rectum that constipation is almost certain to occur. Encourage fluid intake, unless otherwise contraindicated, in people on bed rest to avoid constipation.

People who normally eat a culturally based diet, such as Japanese or Mexican food, may not enjoy an American diet while in a health care facility; observe the roughage intake of such people carefully to be sure that they are eating enough. (It may be possible to arrange for foods that are more to their liking unless this is medically contraindicated.)

MAINTAINING A PATTERN OF EVACUATION

Ask people who are being admitted to a health care facility about their bowel evacuation pattern as part of a nursing history. Many people might not want to discuss this. Preface such a request with a statement such as "One way we can tell after surgery that your body is returning to normal again is by comparing how it functions then with the way it functions now. Let me ask you some questions about your ordinary habits so I will have a basis for comparison. Then ask about the usual frequency of bowel movements, any problems with elimination, any routine medication taken to help with bowel movements, and the time of the last bowel movement.

In a health care facility, offer to assist people to the bathroom or offer a bedpan periodically. Provide privacy. Be sure to inform people that their usual pattern or stool color probably will change owing to surgery or a special diet or diagnostic study.

MEDICATIONS

A number of medications are effective in aiding bowel evacuation or in slowing rapid peristalsis to halt diarrhea. These types of medications and examples of each are shown in Quick Reference Stop 37-2. Such medications are given orally except for suppository forms, which are administered by rectal insertion. The technique for insertion of suppositories is discussed in Chap. 29 with other types of medication administration. Two important considerations in administration are that they be well lubricated and inserted past the second anal sphincter to avoid being expelled before they can initiate an effect (Fig. 37-1).

ENEMA

An enema is the introduction of a solution into the rectum and sigmoid colon to effect bowel evacuation or instill a medication. An enema may be given to aid bowel evacuation when a person is constipated and cannot effect bowel evacuation by his own initiative, when someone has lost neurological control of his external rectal sphincter and cannot independently effect evacuation, or when the bowel must be thoroughly cleansed in preparation for a diagnostic procedure or surgery.

☐ **QUICK REFERENCE STOP 37-2: PHARMACOLOGY**
Medication to Aid Bowel Evacuation*

Type	*Action*	*Example*
Laxatives		
Bulk-forming	Increase fluid or bulk of intestinal contents, promoting bowel peristalsis. Urge person to drink excess fluid to aid drug's action.	Metamucil (psyllium hydrophilic muciloid)
Wetting agent or emollient (stool softener)	Lower surface tension of fecal material, attracting water to material and increasing bulk.	Colace (diocytl sodium sulfosuccinate)
Lubricant	Soften fecal material and prevent drying even with retention. The oil base may interfere with absorption of fat-soluble vitamins (A, D, E, K) and should not be used for long-term therapy.	Mineral oil
Chemical irritant or stimulant	Increase peristaltic movements by irritating intestine. This type of laxative is contraindicated in young children because so much fluid is lost with bowel movements that the child will become dehydrated. Bowel evacuation is often so complete the person may not have another bowel movement for one to two days.	Cascara sagrada
Saline	Saline salts are not absorbed in the intestine; this increases fecal bulk and draws fluid into the intestine. Termed a *purgative*, such a medicine completely and forcefully empties bowel.	Magnesium hydroxide (Milk of Magnesia)
Local reflex action	Promotes defecation reflex by local space-filling action.	Glycerin
Stimulant action	Promotes defecation by increasing peristaltic movements by a direct effect on intestinal mucosa.	Dulcolax (bisacodyl)

*Caution: Do not administer a laxative to people with undiagnosed abdominal pain. If this pain is a symptom of appendicitis, increased peristaltic action could rupture the appendix, a potentially lethal condition.

Cleansing Enemas. A cleansing enema is designed to wash out feces from the lower colon. It causes defecation by bowel distention. Common solutions used are tap water, soap suds, and normal saline. Any solution used should be room temperature or only slightly warm to your wrist (100° to 105°F; 37.7° to 40.5°C). Cold water could lower body temperature considerably as it touches fold after fold of bowel tissue, cooling a very large surface area; hot water could burn (the bowel has no heat sensation, so a burn could occur without your knowledge).

Tap water cannot be used with children because it is hypotonic to body fluids; if administered into the rectum, therefore, it would very rapidly leave the bowel to enter the capillaries by osmotic pressure. This could lead to fluid overload in the circulatory system, and the effect can be so dramatic in infants that it can actually cause cardiac failure and death. Early symptoms of fluid overload are dizziness, sweating, and vomiting. Although primarily a problem in children, fluid overload can occur in adults.

Normal saline (0.9% sodium chloride and water) must be used with caution in people with heart disease because some sodium chloride is absorbed across bowel membrane and therefore causes retention of water and circulatory overload. A saline solution can be made by adding 2 teaspoons of uniodized table salt to a liter of tap water.

Soap suds enemas are less frequently used today than formerly. Such an enema, made by adding about 5 ml of liquid soap solution to 1,000 ml of tap water, aids bowel evacuation not only by distending the bowel but also by mild irritation of the intestinal lining as well. Castile soap is most frequently used for soap suds enemas because it is mild yet effective. The usual amounts of water used for a cleansing enema are shown in Table 37-3.

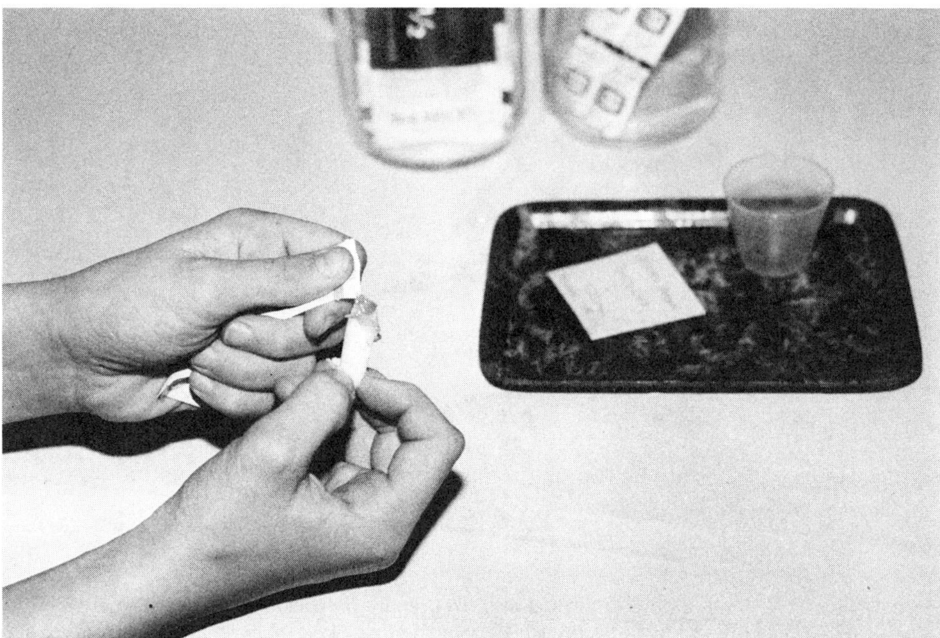

FIGURE 37-1. Suppositories are effective for initiating bowel evacuation. Be certain that they are well lubricated for insertion.

TABLE 37-3. AMOUNT OF SOLUTION USED FOR ENEMA ADMINISTRATION

Age Group	Amount of Fluid
Adult	500—1,000 ml
Schoolager and adolescent	500 ml
Toddler and preschooler*	250—500 ml
Infant*	Under 250 ml

*Exact amount should be stipulated in physician's order.

Oil Retention Enemas. Oil enemas soften feces, thereby aiding evacuation. It is important that oil administered in this way be retained for at least an hour, so small amounts are used with exceptionally gentle technique to minimize the urge to defecate. For an adult, 100 to 200 ml of a mild oil such as mineral oil is administered. Oil enemas are rarely used with children, but the amount would be scaled according to the size of the child and the amount specifically ordered. Oil retention enemas may cause fat-soluble vitamins (A, D, E, K) to be removed in feces with the oil rather than absorbed across the intestinal mucosa as usual. When only one enema is administered, this is not a problem, but if a person needed frequent oil enemas he would probably develop an insufficiency of fat-soluble vitamins and require a vitamin supplement in a water-base form in the diet.

Hypertonic Enemas. A Fleets enema is a commercially prepared enema solution that is an example of a hypertonic enema. Only a small amount of fluid is administered (120 ml). Because the solution is hypertonic, fluid is drawn into the bowel from the subcutaneous tissue and bloodstream, causing rapid distention of the bowel and creating the urge to defecate. Such enemas are convenient because they are commercially packaged and cause little discomfort to the patient. They are unsafe for use in small children because the hypertonic effect will cause such a shift of fluid from the circulatory system as well as the subcutaneous tissue that the child may become hypovolemic (have lowered blood volume). They have the potential for causing this same effect in adults. The term *Fleets enema* is commonly used to denote a small, prepackaged, rapid-acting enema instillation even if the actual brand of solution does not have this name.

TECHNIQUE OF ENEMA ADMINISTRATION

No one likes intrusive procedures; be certain to explain carefully the purpose of the enema and give an overall description of the procedure. Follow this with step-by-step explanations of what is happening or will happen next.

The amount of solution to be used is determined by the physician's order or health agency policy. Prepare to administer an enema by placing a protective plastic pad under the person's buttocks; have the person turn to a Sims' position with his left side down. This places the rectum and sigmoid colon (on the left side of the body) on a slightly downward slant, allowing gravity to act to aid instillation.

A knee-chest position is also effective for administering an enema but is rarely used because it is difficult to

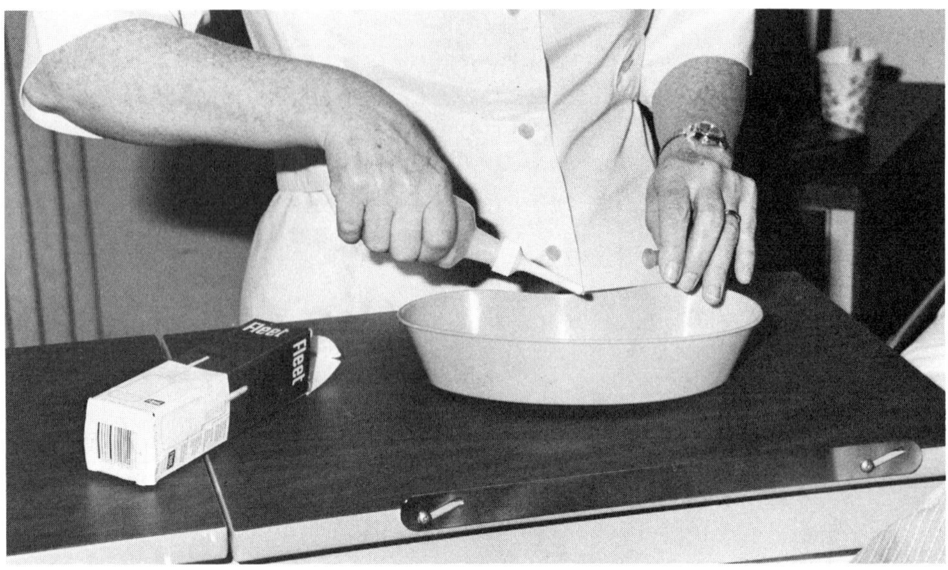

FIGURE 37-2. To prepare prepackaged enemas, expel air from tip. Check that the tip is well lubricated.

maintain. It is important when administering enemas not to add excess air to the bowel because this can cause excessive distention and pain. When using a commercial prepackaged solution, squeeze the bulb (Fig. 37-2) sufficiently to bring the solution to the tip of the tube and eliminate any air present prior to insertion. With water or saline enemas be certain to flush water through the tubing to evacuate all air prior to insertion of the tube into the rectum (Fig. 37-3).

In adults, the tube or applicator tip is inserted about 3 to 4 inches (7.5 to 10 cm), in children 2 to 3 inches (5 to 7 cm), and in infants only 1 inch (2.5 cm). Use gentle pressure for insertion; if the tube meets resistance, never force it. Many middle-aged and older persons have hemorrhoidal tissue (distended rectal veins) externally or internally that make rectal tube insertion painful. Use extreme gentleness and be generous with the use of lubricant to reduce discomfort (Fig. 37-4).

To prevent the solution from flowing too quickly (a condition that will cause severe intestinal cramping), be certain that the height of the solution container is no more than a foot above the level of the sigmoid colon (12 to 18 inches from the bed). Allow the solution to flow at a controlled moderate rate; if the person should experience intestinal cramping, clamp the tubing to halt the flow temporarily and wait until the cramping passes before instilling any more fluid. Taking a deep breath or two usually also helps the cramping sensation to pass. It may take 10 to 15 minutes to instill a large amount of fluid (500 to 1,000 ml).

Following instillation the person should try to retain the solution for at least 5 to 10 minutes; many people are

FIGURE 37-3. To prepare a plain water enema, raise the solution container, allow fluid to flow and expel air from tubing.

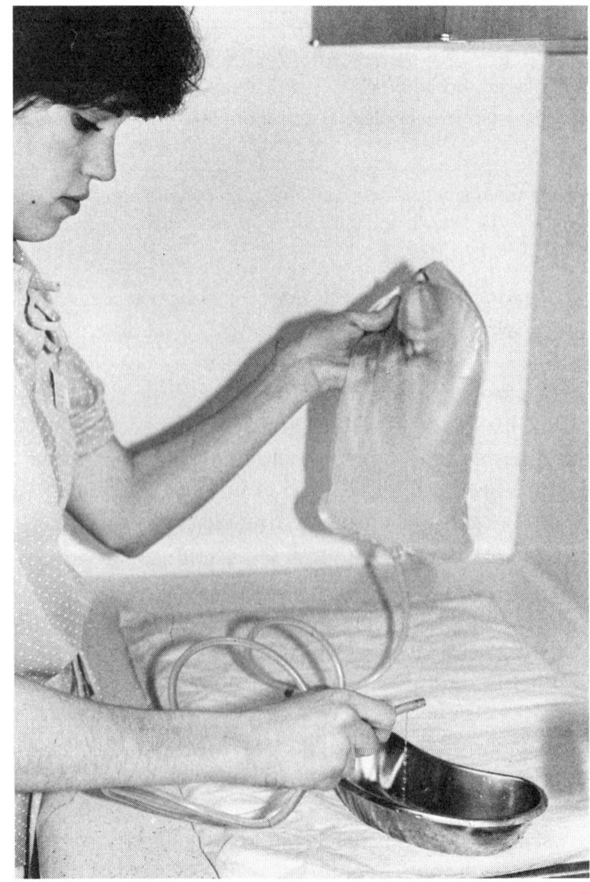

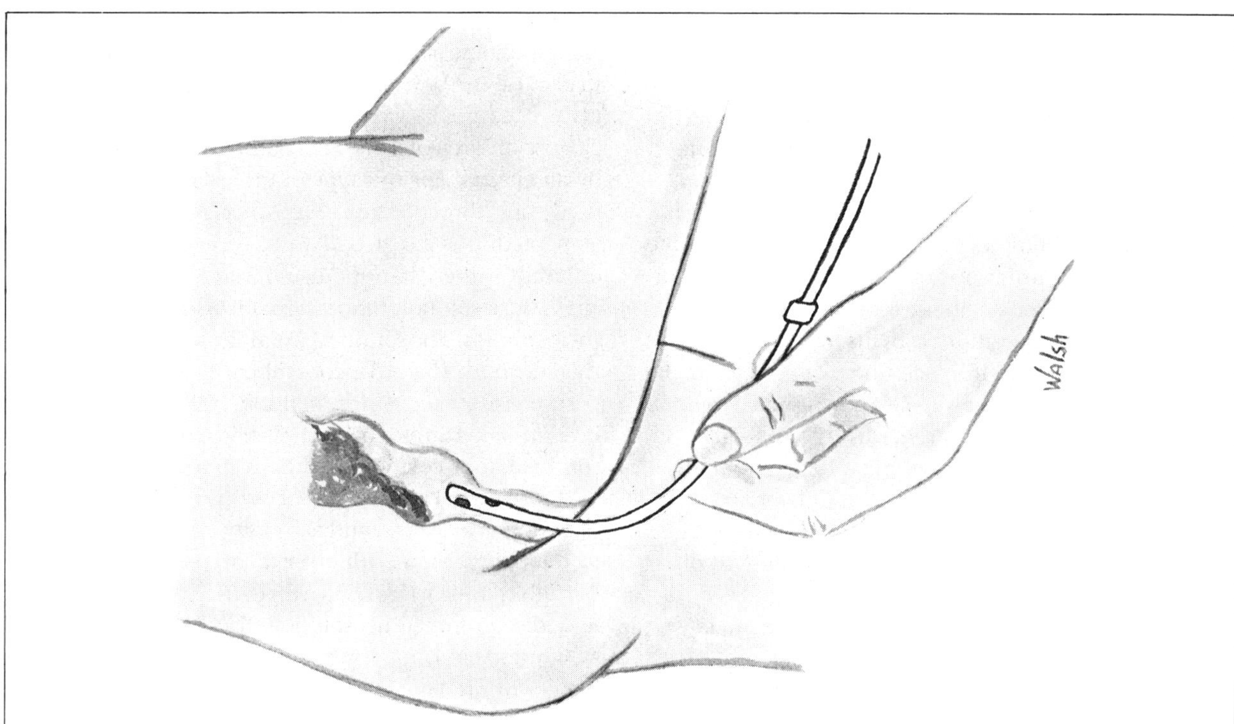

A

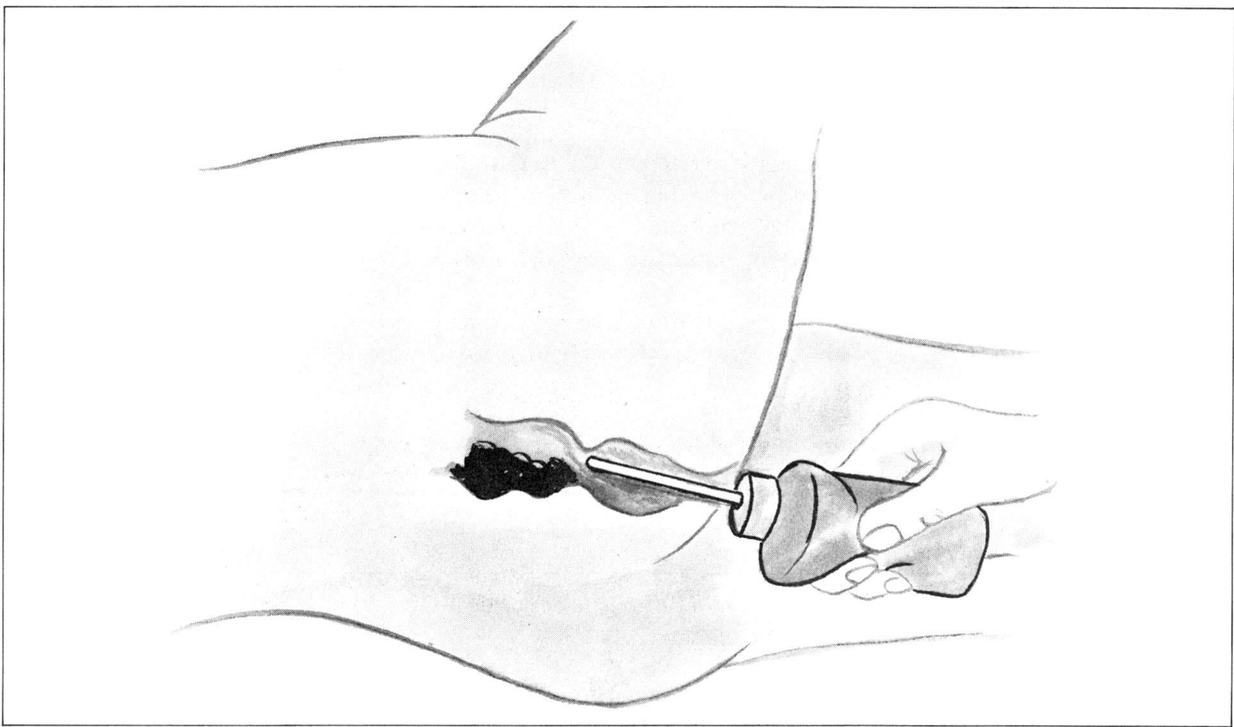

B

FIGURE 37-4. A. Insert an enema tubing 3 to 4 inches. Keep height of solution 12 to 18 inches above bed.
B. Administration of a prepackaged enema.

able to achieve this better if you apply firm pressure to the buttocks as you withdraw the tubing to limit the sensation of having to defecate owing to the tube motion. They can then be helped to a bathroom to expel the solution. Use a commode placed near the bed or offer a bedpan to people who are less mobile.

Some people have such little control of their external rectal sphincter that they are unable to contain the solution during administration. In these instances, administer the solution to the person while he lies in a dorsal recumbent position (on his back with knees raised) with a bedpan in place under his buttocks. Be certain that the edge of the bedpan is not pressing against the person's sacral area; raising the head of the bed about 30 degrees and slipping a folded towel next to the skin over the top of the bedpan helps to ensure comfort. Use a glove to avoid soiling your hand because the solution may be expelled during administration or as you withdraw the tubing. This technique is also useful in children under toilet-training age who still have no sphincter control. To administer a Fleets enema in this position, use a rectal tube and attach it to the short-tipped Fleets enema administration tip.

Although enemas are only a means of facilitating a normal body function, many people find them exhausting. This results possibly from nervous tension and possibly from the physiological effects of minor fluid shifts. Remain nearby while the person expels the solution so that if he does become weak you can help him return to bed. Use the time to be certain that the bed is dry and that you did not accidentally spill solution anywhere but on the extra plastic padding, which can be removed.

If the person shares a bathroom with other patients, check with other patients to be certain that the bathroom will be free when your patient will need to use it. The procedure for a tap water enema administration is shown in Procedure 37-1.

High Colonic Irrigation

A high colonic irrigation is a specially ordered procedure to cleanse the bowel preparatory to diagnostic or surgical procedures. As the name implies, it is designed to cleanse an area of bowel beyond that normally reached by an enema. For this type of procedure, two tubes are used, one threaded into the other so that the tube is elongated. It is inserted 10 to 12 inches (25 to 30 cm) in an adult rather than the usual 3 to 4 inches (7.5 to 10 cm). More solution than normal is used (1,000 to 1,500 ml in adults). The solution container is positioned higher than normal (15 to 18 inches) above the sigmoid colon to ensure greater force of instillation. If the person lies first in a left-sided Sims' position, then in a dorsal recumbent (on his back) position, and then in a right-sided Sims' position, fluid will ideally follow the course of the descending, transverse, and ascending colon, rising higher in the bowel than with an ordinary enema.

High colonic irrigations may cause extreme cramping and discomfort. The solution must be administered slowly and continuously to ensure comfort. The greatest danger of high colonic irrigations is bowel perforation. Using gentle technique and never forcing the tube forward against pressure is the best precaution against this complication. It is a little used procedure due to its inherent risk.

OBTAINING A STOOL SPECIMEN

To give instructions to a patient for obtaining a stool sample, you must know the word that the person uses for such a product. Asking an adult to "move his bowels" is generally well understood. Many people who speak a foreign language as their primary language do not know the English equivalent for "stool" or "urine" even though they appear to understand everything else. Try to obtain

PROCEDURE 37-1
Administering a Plain Water Enema

Purpose: To cleanse the lower bowel prior to a diagnostic or surgical procedure; to soften bowel contents to aid evacuation; and to facilitate bowel evacuation.

Plan	*Principle*
1. Wash your hands, identify patient, explain procedure to patient.	1. Prevent spread of microorganisms; ensure patient safety and cooperation.
2. Assess patient condition; analyze appropriateness of procedure; plan modifications of care. Implement care by organizing equipment: disposable enema tray or separate pieces of equipment such as rectal tube, solution container and tubing, correct solution (type and amount), and lubricant.	2. Some enemas are ordered PRN; do not administer if person has had a normal bowel evacuation. Determine how person will expel enema: into bedpan or commode or in bathroom; check that bathroom will be unused or that commode or bedpan is available. Test water temperature with wrist (room temperature or slightly warm).

3. Prepare bed area by screening for privacy or closing room door; place bath blanket on patient; fanfold cover to foot of bed; place plastic pad under buttocks.	3. It is necessary to expose the person's buttocks for enema administration; protect bed linen from being wet by solution.
4. Ask the person to turn or help him turn to his left side in a Sims' position. If the patient is incontinent (has no control of external rectal sphincter), position him on his back on a bedpan with head of bed elevated about 30 degrees. Use an additional length of rectal tube as necessary if the person is turned on his back.	4. A left side-lying position possibly helps to guide the flow of solution into the rectum.
5. Flush the tubing to clear it of air; lubricate the tip and insert it 3 to 4 inches into the rectum, directing it toward the umbilicus.	5. Reduce possibility of air entering the bowel; prevent mucosal injury by following normal course of bowel.
6. Raise solution container 12 to 18 inches (30 cm) above the bed and allow solution to flow slowly.	6. Slow instillation reduces cramping and prevents irritation to mucosal walls of rectum.
7. If patient experiences any cramping sensation or pain, ask him to take a deep breath and pinch tubing to reduce flow temporarily until sensation passes.	7. Reduce pain to make procedure comfortable for patient.
8. When all solution has been instilled, remove tube gently; press buttocks together firmly until urge to defecate caused by the tube being removed has passed.	8. If a person reports that he has a strong urge to defecate and all fluid is not yet instilled, stop the instillation at this point. People differ slightly, and "usual amount" does not apply to every person.
9. Urge the person to retain the solution for 5 to 10 minutes before using the bathroom or the bedpan or commode.	9. A person's ability to do this varies greatly; allow the person to use common sense in this regard.
10. Remain nearby while the person expels the fluid because this is an exhausting procedure to many people, and he may experience dizziness. Check that bed is dry; assist person to return to bed as necessary.	10. If a person will be using a bedpan in bed, help him to sit up on it; a sitting position is necessary for effective bowel evacuation because it aids use of abdominal muscles.
11. Observe results of enema; evaluate effectiveness, efficiency, cost, comfort, and safety of procedure. Dispose of equipment or rinse and return for sterilizing.	11. If a stool specimen is necessary, place a bedpan on the toilet for the person to use; manually transfer representative specimen to specimen cup by tongue blades.
12. Document procedure, amount, color, and consistency of return. Plan any health teaching necessary such as measures to prevent constipation.	12. Document patient status and nursing care. Health teaching is an independent nursing action always included as part of care.

MODIFICATION FOR CARE OF CHILD

Prior to toilet training, children are incontinent or unable to control external rectal sphincter to retain enema contents. Administer enemas with child in bed with bedpan in place.

Amount of solution to be used should be specifically ordered for children under 2 years of age.

Do not use tap water or Fleets enemas with infants because fatal water intoxication or circulatory depletion could occur.

MODIFICATION FOR CARE OF OLDER ADULT

An older adult who has a neurological disability may have lost control of the external rectal sphincter or may be incontinent. Administer the enema with the person on his back wilth a bedpan in place.

Be extremely careful that the patient is left dry afterward; the skin of older adults becomes denuded readily if it is macerated from continued contact with moisture.

Many older adults have hemorrhoids. Closely observe rectum as you insert the well-lubricated tube to avoid trauma to sensitive hemorrhoidal tissue.

the proper word from the families of these patients as part of an admission history to avoid this problem.

You may be asked to obtain a stool specimen or sample to send for laboratory analysis or for a quick individual test on the patient unit. Most health care agencies have disposable plastic or paper containers to use for stool specimens. Ask the person to use a bedpan for defecation; if it would be more natural, place the bedpan on top of the toilet seat. Most women void (urinate) spontaneously as they defecate because the same perineal muscles are relaxed for both activities. Ask a woman to void first, therefore, wipe her perineum with toilet tissue, and then defecate so that no urine contaminates the stool sample. Ask both men and women not to put the toilet tissue in the bedpan after defecation to avoid contamination by this means also.

To place the specimen in a stool specimen container, first carry the bedpan to a utility room. Always cover the bedpan with a cloth or a disposable waterproof pad for aesthetic reasons and to control odor. Use two clean tongue blades to lift a representative sample into the stool sample cup. If the stool sample is liquid, pour about 30 ml into the specimen cup. Secure the top of the cup tightly, fill out the necessary requisition forms, and see that the specimen is taken to the laboratory promptly because bacteriologic changes in stool may change its composition if it stands at room temperature for a period of time. If there will be a delay in laboratory processing, it is advantageous to refrigerate the specimen in a specimen refrigerator (unless it will be analyzed for ova and parasites; in this case it must be kept at room temperature).

You cannot ask an untoilet-trained child to defecate. Merely wait until he does it spontaneously and then remove a specimen from the diaper with tongue blades.

If a specimen is to be cultured for bacteria, use a sterile culture tube, a sterile applicator, and aseptic culture technique (see Chap. 20). Do not be careless with a specimen, thinking that since fecal material is already filled with bacteria, a few more will make no difference. Isolating a particular microorganism that is causing an illness such as diarrhea is important; if additional bacteria are added to the specimen through careless technique, a wrong diagnosis could be made and the wrong therapy instituted.

Stool specimens can be quickly tested for the presence of blood (do this routinely as an independent activity whenever you see a stool that is red or black in appearance) by a Hematest tablet or guaiac solution; for pH and protein by a dip stick; and for reducing substances (sugars) by a Clinitest tablet. These tests are done routinely with liquid stools to determine if diarrhea is improving (if it is, pH becomes alkaline, and blood, protein, and sugars disappear from the sample, which becomes increasingly solid in consistency). These tests are described in the following box.

COMMON PROBLEMS OF INTESTINAL ELIMINATION

Many people feel more comfortable in discussing a problem with bowel elimination with a nurse than with a physician because although it worries them a great deal, they believe that it is not important enough to interest a physician. When listening to elimination problems be aware that both a change in bowel habits and blood in feces are two of the seven danger signs of bowel cancer. Never take a report of diarrhea lightly, especially in young children. Diarrhea leads to dehydration and can cause death from dehydration within 24 hours in small infants.

Flatulence

Flatulence is the presence of excessive air in the intestine. It creates a feeling of "bloating" or stretching; as the intestine actually becomes stretched, it causes extreme pain. If the intestine is extremely distended, it may press so hard against the diaphragm that the person becomes short of breath. Some flatulence results from the natural bacterial decomposition of food. Flatulence is increased if the mobility of the intestine is slowed; this occurs after the administration of certain drugs such as morphine or codeine, following surgery, from the ingestion of gas-forming foods such as cabbage or beans, or from swallowing air.

Common Techniques of Stool Analysis

Test	*Procedure*
Occult (hidden) blood	To test with a Hematest tablet, use a cotton-tipped applicator to streak a sample of stool onto a piece of filter paper. Place a Hematest tablet on the stool. With a medicine dropper, place one drop of water on the tablet, wait 5—10 seconds and add a second drop, being sure that the second drop runs over the side onto the stool sample and filter paper. In 2 minutes observe the color of the filter paper. If it is blue, there is occult blood in the stool specimen. A guaiac test is another brand of occult blood analysis with similar instructions. Read and follow the instructions for both procedures exactly (Fig. 1).

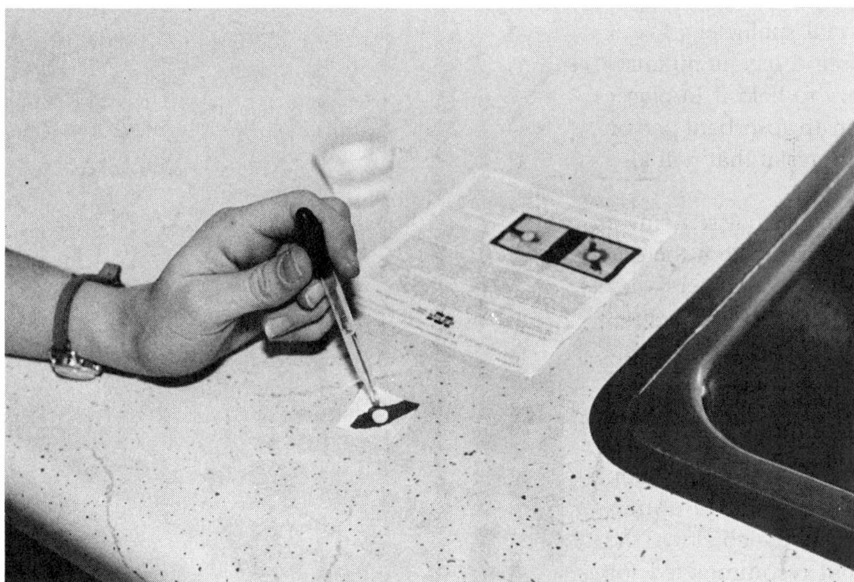

FIGURE 1. Testing of stool for occult (hidden) blood by a Hematest tablet. The color change on the filter paper is compared to the manufacturer's color chart.

Reducing substances (sugars)	Place 10 drops of water in a clean test tube. Liquefy stool if necessary by adding water to specimen. Add five drops of liquid stool to test tube. Drop a Clinitest tablet into mixture in test tube. Observe chemical reaction. At the end of 15 seconds, shake tube and compare color of solution to Clinitest color chart. If solution is blue, sample is negative for sugars. If it is orange to yellow, it is scored as 1^+ to 4^+. Do not hold test tube by bottom while chemical reaction occurs because it becomes boiling hot.
pH	Liquefy stool if necessary by adding water to specimen. Press a dip stick for pH into the liquefied solution. At the end of the designated time period for the brand of test strip, read the strip by comparing it to the color code on bottle.

Flatulence can be relieved by the passage of the air rectally (termed *flatus*) or orally (eructated or belched air). Following surgery, the fact that a person is able to pass flatus is proof that peristalsis has returned and, although perhaps embarrassing, it is a sign of healthful progress.

MEASURES TO RELIEVE EXCESSIVE FLATULENCE

Because air rises, helping a postoperative patient to sit up in bed and ambulate as early as possible helps to relieve the presence of gas in the intestines. Ambulation also aids peristaltic movement, which also contributes to the removal of air. Excessive swallowing of air tends to occur in people who are anxious, so any effort to reduce anxiety helps to relieve this problem. Drinking a carbonated beverage adds to gastrointestinal gases but may also relieve pressure because the carbon dioxide ingested with the drink rises readily, bringing with it additional accumulated air.

INSERTION OF A RECTAL TUBE

A tube inserted into the rectum may offer relief from flatulence through aiding passage of gas rectally. Rectal tubes are made of rubber or pliable plastic. The usual size chosen for adults is 22F to 30F; for preschool and schoolage children, 14F to 16F; for infants, 12F. A small feeding tube (10F or 12F) may be easier to use with infants than a rectal tube because of its greater pliability. The term *French* (abbreviated "F") in reference to catheters or tubes means that the tube has a series of outlet holes on the sides of the tube near the tip, not just one opening at the tip. This type of tube is advantageous for rectal tubes because feces in the rectum will not plug it readily, and the holes help it remain patent.

Lubricate the tube well with a water-based lubricant

and insert it past the internal rectal sphincter (4 to 5 inches in adults; 2 inches in children; 1 inch in infants). Tape it to one buttock if necessary to hold it in place; encase the distal end of the tube in an absorbent pad or towel to collect any liquid fecal material that will also be evacuated by the tube lumen.

Rectal tubes used in this way should not remain in place longer than 30 minutes at a time so that there is not constant pressure against the rectal sphincters; they might be used every 2 to 3 hours for a limited time. Relieving flatulence by this method is only a temporary measure; more important measures are encouraging activity and helping the person assume an upright position. Rectal tube insertion is contraindicated if the person has had rectal or sigmoid surgery as tube insertion might harm a recent suture line. Because rectal stimulation can initiate a vagal response, which slows the heart rate (bradycardia), it is not recommended for people with cardiac disease.

NASOGASTRIC TUBES

A nasogastric tube is a rubber or plastic tube that is inserted into the nose, through the esophagus, and into the stomach. Such a tube can be used for administering feedings (see Procedure 35-1) or, if attached to a suction source, for removing secretions and air from the stomach (decompression). A tube is often placed in this way at the time of abdominal or gastrointestinal surgery, remaining in place to prevent distention of bowel until bowel tone resumes after the surgery (3 to 5 days).

Suction used with nasogastric tubes should always be set at a *low* level to prevent irritation of the gastric lining caused by being drawn into the tube (Fig. 37-5). The technique for measurement and insertion of a nasogastric tube is described in Chap. 35.

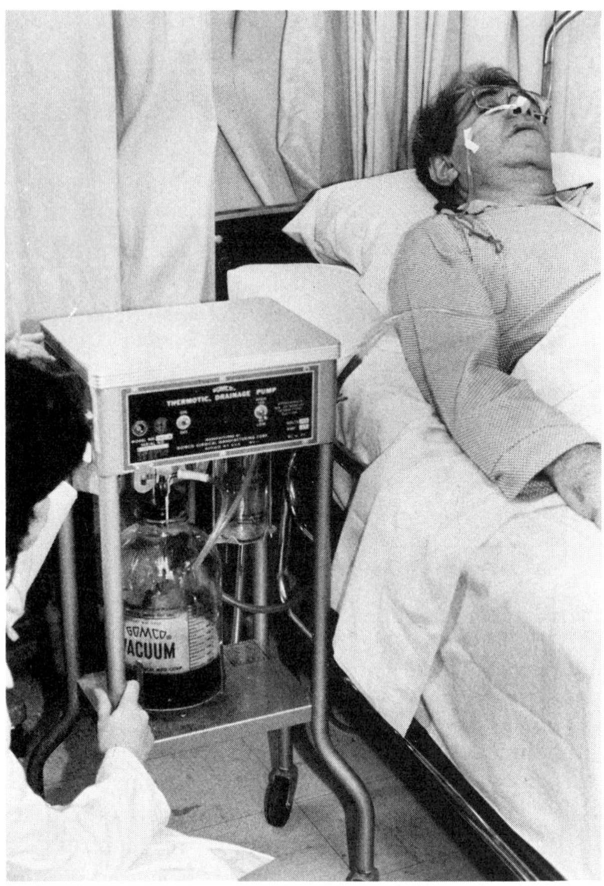

FIGURE 37-5. Set nasogastric suction at a *low* level to prevent irritation to the stomach mucosa.

If a tube with a weight at the tip is used (this is commonly called a Cantor or Miller-Abbott tube), the end of the tube will sink through the pyloric valve by the forces of gravity and peristaltic action; it can then remove secretions and air from the intestine.

Note carefully the amount of drainage obtained from a nasogastric or naso-intestinal tube. Often fluid lost from the body by this route is replaced by an equal amount of intravenous fluid to maintain fluid content and electrolyte balance. Note also the color and consistency of nasogastric drainage. A red or black tinge suggests gastrointestinal bleeding; a green or dark brown color suggests that secretions are not passing through the intestines but are blocked at a point below the ampula of Vater, the point at which bile enters the tract in the duodenum, causing bile-colored secretions to back up into the stomach.

Nasogastric tubes may be irrigated every 3 to 4 hours to keep them clear and ensure that they do not become plugged. In adults the amount of solution used for such a procedure is 10 to 30 ml; in infants the exact amount should be specified by the physician's order. Normal saline is generally used; fill a syringe or a Dakin (bulb type) syringe with the specified amount of fluid. Disconnect the tubing at its suction connection point, and instill the specified amount of solution slowly and gently. Always aspirate as much fluid after irrigation as you instilled (Fig. 37-6). This is important to ensure that the tubing is clear, not only for fluid passing into it but for fluid passing out of it (secretions must pass out of it). Also, if irrigation fluid is constantly instilled and never drawn back, there is a possibility of overdistending or actually rupturing the stomach. Record any fluid obtained over that instilled as output. Record any fluid retained to be subtracted from output.

Constipation

Constipation is the inability to achieve bowel evacuation for a period of time. When stool is passed, it is hard, dry, and painful. Constipation occurs when feces passes through the intestine at such a slow rate that excessive water is absorbed from it.

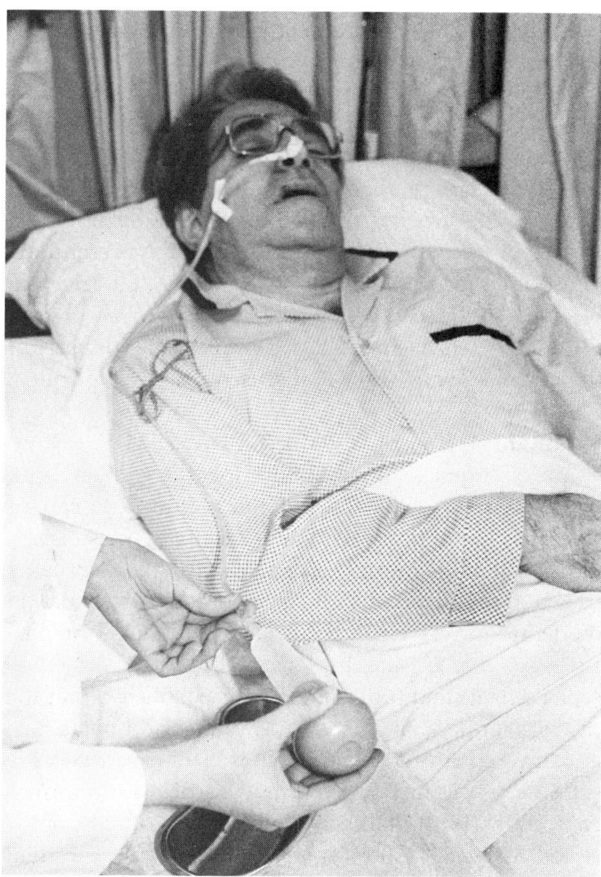

FIGURE 37-6. Irrigating a nasogastric tube. Be certain that as much fluid returns as you instill to prevent stomach distention.

Straining to pass constipated stool is potentially dangerous, especially for people with cardiovascular illness. As a person strains to defecate, he breathes out against a closed glottis (a Valsalva maneuver). This increases intrathoracic pressure, which can interfere with venous return to the heart. As the bowel movement is achieved, the person stops straining, intrathoracic pressure drops greatly, and a great deal of venous blood suddenly returns to the heart; the heart must adjust to this increased amount of blood by increasing stroke volume and rate to avoid being overwhelmed. Exhaling through the mouth during straining helps to reduce or prevent intrathoracic buildup of pressure; it is a technique taught to patients whose hearts are sensitive to changes in chest pressure.

CAUSES OF CONSTIPATION

Constipation occurs for a number of reasons previously discussed—irregular bowel habits, a diet too low in roughage or fiber, insufficient exercise, and use of medications such as codeine or morphine. Additional causes might be overuse of laxatives; (if the person relies on a daily laxative for bowel stimulation, his natural peristaltic movements may not be effective when he does not take it). Disease conditions such as an inability to use the abdominal muscles effectively or painful perineal or rectal disorders such as hemorrhoids will also result in constipation. Long-term stress or depression are other causes.

MEASURES TO RELIEVE CONSTIPATION

Constipation is easier to prevent than to relieve; the most effective nursing measures, therefore, are those aimed at prevention.

Assess Normal Bowel Habits and Patterns. Defecation patterns differ greatly from those who have two bowel movements a day to those who have a bowel movement only once or twice a week. Assessing whether a pattern that you have observed (for instance, no bowel movement during a 3-day hospitalization) is normal or not prevents you from worrying needlessly or missing an important finding. Including assessment for this function in a regular plan of care gives you forewarning of the problem at the earliest possible point when it can best be relieved.

Help People to Follow Their Usual Dietary Patterns. Many middle-aged or older adults consume a naturally laxative food such as prune juice or bran cereal for breakfast everyday. If at all possible, consult with the dietitian about the possibility of continuing these naturally laxative foods while the person is in a health care facility. Be conscious of fluid intake, and urge any person on bed rest or one with only sedentary activity to drink at least one extra glass of water daily above the amount he drinks at meals. Increasing water intake also aids kidney function in people on bed rest, thus serving a twofold purpose.

Monitor and Encourage Ambulation. Some people believe that because they are hospitalized they should be sedentary or rest as quietly as possible. In some instances, this may be true. Most people, however, need to be as active as possible within their limits. Be certain that people who should be out of bed are out of bed and walking; those who must remain in bed must be actively turned every 2 hours during the day to promote not only bowel peristalsis but also circulatory function.

Provide Privacy and Consideration for Bowel Evacuation. It is sometimes necessary to remind a person on bed rest that he has not moved his bowels for 2 days and ask him if he wants to use a bedpan. This is necessary because some people view defecation as such a private function that they are unable to bring up the subject.

Assist people to a high Fowler's position or as near a sitting position as possible while using a bedpan so that they can best use their abdominal muscles in the process.

Administer Medication as Appropriate. Medications that promote normal bowel evacuation are termed *cathartics, cathartic suppositories,* or *laxatives* (see QRS 37-2). People who are confined to bed and are not exercising as much as normal or not eating their regular diet may need a prescription for a cathartic or laxative when normally they would not. Many cathartics are administered at bedtime; they act during the night and the person feels an urge to defecate in the morning. A cathartic suppository is effective in about half an hour. A cathartic is a strong-acting drug, a laxative a mild one. Neither cathartics nor laxatives should be administered to people with undiagnosed abdominal pain. If the pain is a symptom of appendicitis, increased peristaltic action could rupture the appendix, a potentially lethal condition.

Fecal Impaction

A fecal impaction is an extremely hard mass of feces that has formed because of prolonged retention in the rectum; it is so large and hardened that it is impossible to pass rectally. The person will have no bowel movements or only a slight amount of liquid feces that is able to seep around the hard fecal mass. The condition may be mistaken for diarrhea. The patient feels bloated or anorexic (has no appetite); he may have abdominal cramping and an urge to defecate although he is then unable to do so.

Fecal impaction is an extreme form of constipation and occurs for the same reasons. A fecal impaction can be palpated in the rectum by examination with a gloved finger.

Such an impaction can be softened by the administration of an oil retention enema followed in 1 or 2 hours by a cleansing enema. In some instances it is necessary to remove impacted feces manually using one or two fingers of a gloved hand following the softening oil enema (Procedure 37-2). Manipulation in this manner is uncomfortable and should be done only with extremely gentle technique. Many health care agencies require a physician's order for this procedure. If the person has a disease of the bowel, the physician may prefer to do this herself to avoid any risk of injury to the bowel mucosa.

Following removal of a fecal impaction, care must be taken to prevent it from recurring. This involves an active program of adequate fluid, exercise, and roughage in the diet and perhaps laxative, cathartic, or enema administration as necessary.

Diarrhea

Diarrhea is the expulsion of liquid feces, usually more often than normal. Feces remain in a liquid state when they are propelled through the intestine faster than normal or when intestinal peristalsis is more active than normal. The person may have cramping abdominal pain; he may have an uncontrollable urge to defecate that can lead to embarrassing loss of stool if he cannot readily reach a bathroom.

Diarrhea is always serious because, unlike constipation, it is most commonly caused by a disease process, not indiscretion in eating habits or reluctance to defecate. Furthermore, diarrhea can lead to extreme loss of fluid and electrolytes or malnutrition. If an irritating disease process such as a bowel infection is present, the intestinal mucosa may be so irritated that mucosal bleeding with considerable blood loss can result. Chronic diarrhea can be caused by ulcerative diseases of the bowel such as Crohn's disease or ulcerative colitis.

INTERVENTIONS TO COMBAT DIARRHEA

A major nursing intervention for the person with diarrhea is replacing the lost fluid. Oral fluid can be increased, but because drinking stimulates peristalsis, it is usually not the method of choice unless the diarrhea is mild and self-limiting. Fluid is replaced intravenously in moderate to severe diarrhea. Large amounts of potassium are lost in diarrhea; this is generally added to replacement fluid (after it has been established that the person's kidneys are functioning. Never add potassium to intravenous fluid before this is established because extreme potassium overload and cardiac arrhythmias can occur). With diarrhea, the gastrointestinal tract is rested at least 4 hours, and then oral fluid in small amounts (a teaspoon in an infant, an ounce in an adult) may be started. Many people are reluctant to refrain from drinking for this period of time. They need to understand that no food or fluid for a certain period will best slow peristalsis and halt diarrhea.

Be certain that the person with diarrhea has access to a bathroom or place a bedpan or commode where he can reach it easily. If an accident should occur, be sure to give good skin care because diarrhea is invariably acid, not alkaline, and the acid content of the stool will quickly excoriate anal area skin. If the person is having frequent liquid stools, coating the anal area with petroleum jelly (Vaseline) helps to protect the skin from the acid medium. Incontinence from diarrhea is embarrassing, and tact and compassion are needed.

Adults may be given medication to lessen diarrhea. Such medications work by coating the bowel mucosa (demulcents), shrinking swollen and inflamed bowel mucosa (astringents), or absorbing toxic substances from the bowel (absorbents). In addition to these measures to reduce the amount of diarrhea, the cause of the diarrhea must be established and the cause treated.

When caring for people with diarrhea, keep in mind that the diarrhea is not the illness—it is a symptom of illness. Keep accurate intake and output records, be aware of the potassium blood level, and test the specific gravity of urine to help maintain the fluid and electrolyte balance. Respect diarrhea as a symptom that could quickly cause dehydration and electrolyte imbalance.

PROCEDURE 37-2
Removing a Fecal Impaction

Purpose: To restore normal bowel function by nontraumatic removal of an impacted fecal mass.

Plan	*Principle*
1. Wash your hands, identify patient, explain procedure to patient.	1. Prevent spread of microorganisms; ensure patient safety and cooperation.
2. Assess patient status, analyze appropriateness of procedure, plan modifications as appropriate.	2. Fecal impaction is most apt to occur in older adults, people on bed rest, and as a follow-up to a barium enema. The person with painful hemorrhoid formation may need an analgesic 20 minutes before procedure for comfort.
3. Implement care by assembling equipment: clean glove, water, soluble lubricant, bedpan, disposable plastic pad, toilet paper.	3. Organize for efficient use of time.
4. Provide privacy; fanfold top linen to foot of bed, replace with bath blanket. Position patient in Sims' position. Place waterproof pad under buttocks and bedpan.	4. Allow good rectal exposure; protect bed linen. Privacy is a highly regarded value of most people.
5. Lubricate index finger and gently insert it into rectum. Break up mass by digital pressure and remove one piece at a time. Place feces in bedpan.	5. Gentleness is necessary to avoid causing pain and possibly rupturing an internal hemorrhoid.
6. Following removal of impaction, wipe lubricant away from rectum. Position patient comfortably. Clean and replace bedpan in patient stand.	6. Ensure patient safety and comfort.
7. Evaluate effectiveness, efficiency, cost, comfort, and safety of procedure. Plan health teaching such as need for increased fluid intake.	7. Health teaching is an independent nursing action always included in nursing care.
8. Chart results of procedure and patient tolerance. Assess patient after 15 minutes for any evidence of rectal bleeding.	8. Document patient status and nursing care. Ensure safety by checking that an internal hemorrhoid was not ruptured with consequent bleeding.

MODIFICATIONS FOR CARE OF CHILD

Children rarely develop fecal impactions because they have active bowel peristalsis. If procedure is used, it may be necessary to use the little finger to avoid anal trauma.

MODIFICATIONS FOR CARE OF OLDER ADULT

Many older adults have hemorrhoids. Use extreme gentleness to minimize pain.

Incontinence

Anal incontinence is the loss of voluntary control of defecation. Loss of ability to control the voluntary anal sphincter is due to loss of the nerve supply to the sphincter owing to local or central nervous system involvement. Anal incontinence is a serious problem in that it is embarrassing to the person; it leads to skin irritation and loss of self-esteem. Children who have not yet been toilet-trained are not considered incontinent.

ENCOPORESIS

Encoporesis is involuntary defecation in a person who appears to have no physical reason for loss of bowel control. It tends to occur in children 6 to 12 years of age, more often in boys than in girls. It is highly associated with stress (a poor parent-child relationship or a poor teacher-child relationship, for example). After physical reasons for the problem are ruled out, the child is generally given large amounts of mineral oil daily to soften stools and urged to re-establish a consistent bowel routine.

BOWEL RETRAINING

People who have lost the ability to control defecation because they have lost cerebral control but still have an intact spinal reflex are generally begun on bowel retraining programs if possible. The program for each person will vary depending on the cause of the loss of sphincter control, but basically it consists of establishing a regular time each day for defecation and helping the patient to a bathroom or a commode at that time each day. The urge to defecate can be stimulated just prior to this time by inserting a rectal suppository or by using a long-acting laxative that will reach maximum effect at this time.

The person can help evacuate his bowels by leaning forward and pressing on his abdomen or trying to initiate the same action that tensing his abdominal muscles would have achieved. Increasing fluid intake and intake of a stool softener keeps stools soft and nonconstipated. A bowel retraining program may take a considerable amount of time (weeks to months) to be effective; in the meantime the person will have accidents. Treating them lightly and urging continued measures toward retraining will provide the impetus needed to continue with the program. Any improvement in bowel control is generally a great satisfaction to the patient and worth the time involved in improving his self-esteem (see Quick Reference Stop 37-3).

Ostomies

In people who develop a bowel obstruction temporary relief can be achieved by having the bowel above the obstruction brought to the surface of the abdomen by surgery; in patients with bowel cancer or severe inflammation the lower part of the bowel may be removed by surgery and the new lower end of the bowel brought to the abdominal surface. If the portion of the bowel brought to the surface is the colon, this is termed a *colostomy*; if it is the ileum, it is termed an *ileostomy*. The opening itself is termed a *stoma*.

Stool is in a liquid stage as it passes through the ileum, so an ileostomy will drain fairly liquid stool; stool from a colostomy, on the other hand, tends to be well formed (Fig. 37-7). A person with an ileostomy always wears a plastic bag over the stoma opening to contain liquid stool. People with colostomies may feel safer with one in place (Fig. 37-8) if they tend to have only one well-formed stool a day, however, they may use only a small gauze square over the stomal opening. A daily bowel movement through the stoma may occur naturally or may be initiated by colostomy irrigation. A colostomy irrigation is similar to an enema; 500 to 750 ml of tap water is instilled by gravity through a plastic catheter inserted 1 to 3 inches (2 to 8 cm) into the stoma (Fig. 37-9). People who will be performing daily colostomy irrigations are taught this procedure before hospital discharge following the surgical procedure. Colostomy irrigation involves enema administration technique.

☐ QUICK REFERENCE STOP 37-3: ADVOCACY
Bowel Retraining

Bowel retraining can be a lengthy process (weeks to months) requiring cooperation between nursing staff and patient. It is easy for the nursing staff to grow discouraged with the process. You may need to advocate for a patient to continue such a program despite inital unrewarding results.

FIGURE 37-7. A colostomy is a procedure in which sections of the bowel are brought to the abdominal surface. A. Double-barreled colostomy. B. Single-barreled colostomy.

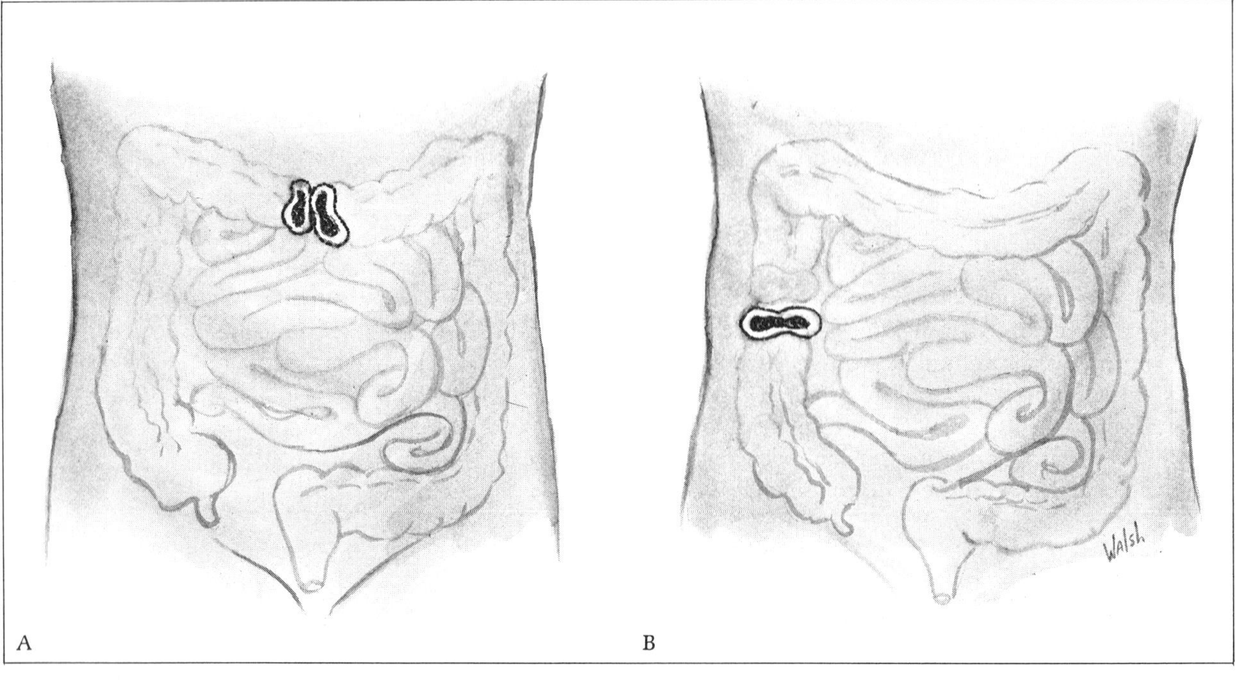

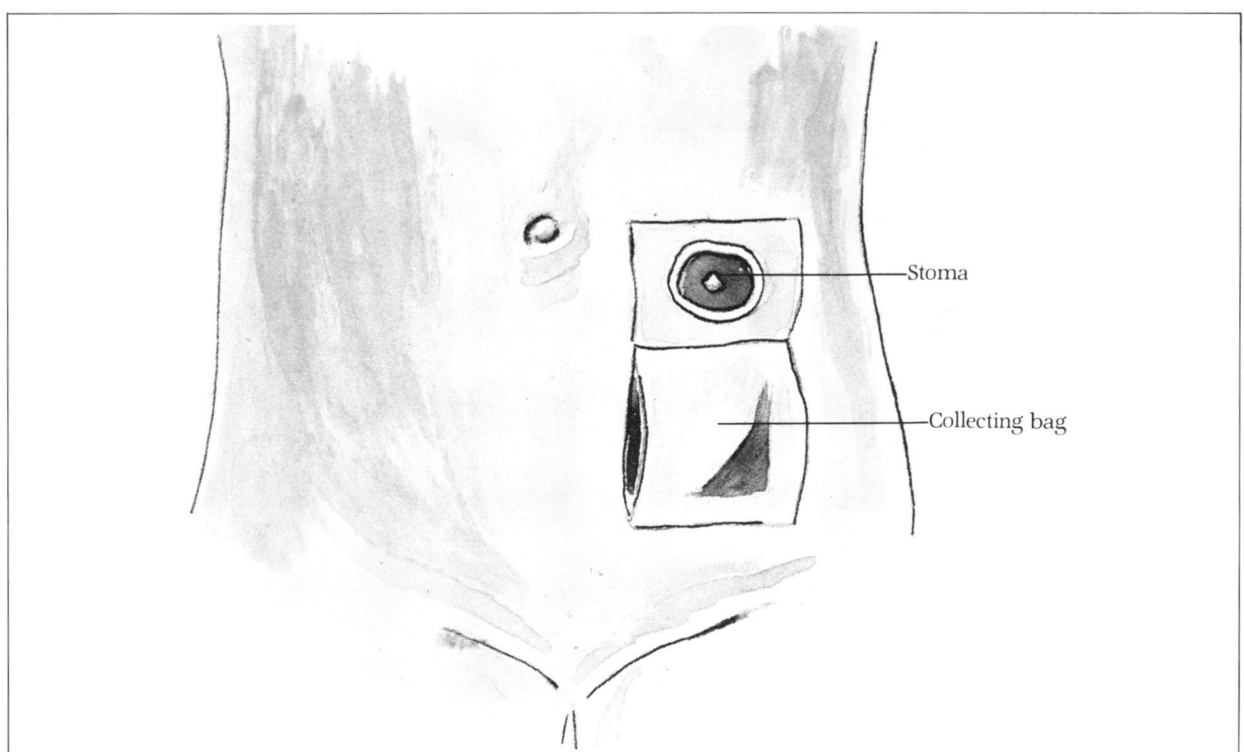

FIGURE 37-8. A disposable colostomy bag in place on a descending cecum stoma.

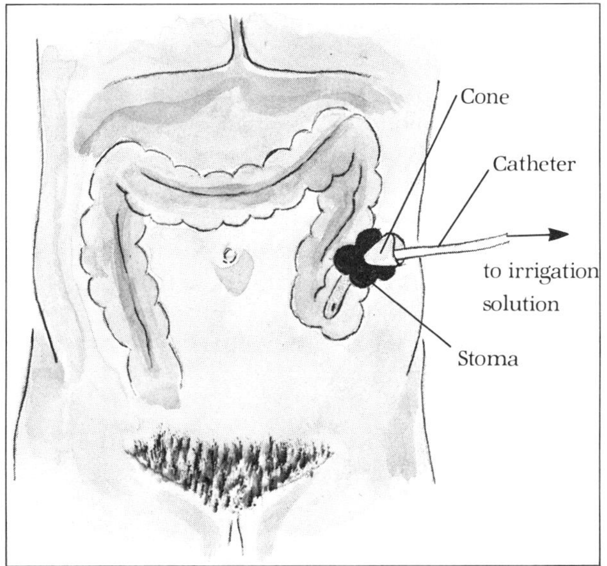

FIGURE 37-9. Irrigation of a colostomy requires enema administration technique.

Important considerations for a colostomy irrigation are shown in the following box.

Care of the skin surrounding a colostomy or ileostomy is necessary to prevent stool from causing excoriation at the site (keep the area clean and dry; for an ileostomy, cover it with a protective coating such as zinc oxide, milk of magnesia, or Karaya powder).

Important Considerations in Colostomy Irrigation

1. Time begun: 5 to 7 days after surgery.
2. Frequency: Same time every day.
3. Solution used: 500—750 ml warm tap water.
4. Equipment: Irrigating solution, container, and tubing.
5. Place: Easiest if the person sits on a toilet so fluid returned is returned to the toilet.
6. Remove appliance from stoma and clean stoma as necessary.
7. Flush air from tubing and insert into stoma 1 to 3 inches.
8. Placing a nipple over the tubing or attaching a commercial irrigating cone helps fluid enter stoma without backflow.
9. Keep height of solution about 18 inches above colon.
10. If cramping occurs, temporarily halt flow of irrigation.
11. At finish of infusion, gently remove tubing. Attach a disposable irrigation bag with open bottom to stoma to allow return solution to flow into toilet.
12. After fluid has returned, dry abdomen well and reapply appliance or dressing.

☐ QUICK REFERENCE STOP 37-4: COMMUNITY CONSIDERATIONS
Ostomies

People with ostomies need empathetic support to adjust to such a drastic change in body image and accept a sense of loss of their former well self. Most large communities have Ostomy Clubs that will supply a member to speak with the patient prior to surgery and act as a support group for him after he returns home. If this type of support group is not available in your community, write to the United Ostomy Association, a self-help group, for teaching materials. The address is 2001 W. Beverly Boulevard, Los Angeles, Calif., 90057.

The *International Association for Enterostomal Therapy* is the professional organization of health care personnel with special preparation in rehabilitation of persons with ostomies. They also can be helpful in supplying information. The address is 505 N. Tustin, Suite 219, Santa Ana, Calif., 92705.

An ostomy is difficult to accept by the average person unless he has support from people who care about him and from health care personnel. This involves a major change in body image and a sense of loss that takes time to adjust to. Most communities have ostomy clubs or organizations of people who have ostomies; such clubs help a person to adjust to the experience and to solve the many accompanying problems (such as how to manage if his job requires him to be away from bathroom facilities for an extended time, the best types of equipment to buy, the proper diet, and social problems) (see QRS 37-4).

An ostomy may be a temporary procedure lasting only a month or two until a second stage of surgery can be accomplished, or it may be a permanent procedure. In most instances, the person has the problem not only of accepting the presence of the ostomy but the initial health problem that necessitated the procedure as well.

UTILIZING NURSING PROCESS

Like other phases of nursing care, care related to intestinal elimination is carried out best if it is guided by a nursing process format.

Assessment

Assessment of intestinal elimination may not be ordered by a person's physician; it will be an independent nursing action. Note not only the frequency of bowel movements but also their consistency and color. Assess whether people under your care in well settings are worried about their elimination patterns.

Analysis

To make an informed judgment about a person's elimination pattern, compare his present pattern with the pattern he described when he was well; this is important because there is such a wide range of normal between different people that it is easy to miss an abnormal pattern.

The Fourth National Conference on Nursing Diagnoses accepted three diagnoses related to intestinal elimination: bowel elimination, alteration in, constipation; bowel elimination, alteration in, diarrhea; and bowel elimination, alteration in, incontinence. These diagnoses with their defining characteristics are described in Appendix C. Although these diagnoses may also be used as medical diagnoses, they are really symptoms that result from medical conditions such as neuromuscular illness or gastrointestinal infection.

Planning

Helping people plan how to maintain good bowel function is health maintenance teaching. Almost everyone has had the experience of being temporarily constipated at a summer camp or on a vacation because they were away from their usual routine and usual foods. Anticipatory planning would have prevented this occurrence.

If a person will be taking a medication such as ferrous sulfate (iron) that you know will color the stool, caution him that this change will occur. If he will be having a barium x-ray series (a diagnostic procedure to discover gastrointestinal pathology), help him plan a diet high in roughage and fluid for the next few days (unless this is contraindicated by the original pathology) in order to help the barium pass through the gastrointestinal tract most rapidly and prevent constipation. If barium has not been passed by three days after the procedure, the physician needs to be notified because the person may need a laxative or enema. Many physicians routinely order these following the procedure.

Implementation

Securing a high fiber cereal for someone in place of a low fiber one and offering a bedpan throughout the day are simple nursing care measures. On the other hand, offering a bedpan so the person feels comfortable in accepting it is a skill that is not comfortable for some people. You may need to practice how to make supportive statements to a person who is concerned about bowel function until you can do it as casually as suggesting a measure to relieve a headache.

Evaluation

Be certain to include this final step of evaluation to be sure that any interventions completed to encourage intestinal elimination have been effective. Administration of a laxative or an enema is not complete until you have evaluated whether the action was successful and bowel elimination has been accomplished.

NURSING CARE PLAN

Mr. Whalen is a 74-year-old man who, following a cerebral vascular accident, has unpredictable fecal incontinence. The following is a nursing care plan you might write for him to initiate bowel retraining.

Assessment: Patient has unpredictable fecal incontinence (two times a day to once every three days). Stools are formed and soft. His mobility is limited on the right side. He is up in a wheelchair twice a day; can use walker but resists it. Fluid intake was less than 1,000 ml for each day last week.

Analysis: Bowel elimination, alteration in, incontinence.

Locus of Decision-Making: Shared.

Goal: Patient to have successful bowel retraining by 2 months' time.

Criteria: Patient will have one bowel evacuation daily following suppository insertion using bedside commode.

NURSING ORDERS

1. Consult with physician for approval of bowel retraining program.
2. Outline program with patient and describe the new responsibilities it will entail for him.
3. Attempt to increase fluid intake daily to 3,000 ml (likes juices, milk, coffee). Divide as 2,000 ml, day shift; 1,500 ml, evening shift; 500 ml, night shift.
4. Consult with physical therapist for ways to increase mobility using walker and how to transfer himself with transfer board to bedside commode.
5. Dulcolax suppository daily at 9:00 A.M. Help as necessary to transfer to commode by 9:15 daily.
6. Provide footstool for use with commode; teach him to breathe out during abdominal straining to avoid Valsalva maneuver.
7. Praise for cooperation with increased mobility and transfer.

EVALUATION

1. Evaluate level of success at 1 week for possible modifications.
2. Re-evaluate at 1 month and restructure plan as necessary for the second month.

SUGGESTED READINGS

Aman, R. A. Treating the patient, not the constipation. *Am. J. Nurs.* 80:1634, 1980.

Amato, E. J. A nursing reference: Gastrointestinal tubes and drains: Intra-abdominal tubes and drains . . . inserted during the intra-operative period. *Crit. Care Nurse* 2(6):50, 1982.

Bass, L. More fiber, less constipation. *Am. J. Nurs.* 77:254, 1977.

Battle, E. H., et al. Evaluation of a dietary regimen for chronic constipation: Report of a pilot study. *J. Gerontol. Nurs.* 6:527, 1980.

Beck, M. L. Guiding your patient a step at a time through a colonoscopy. *Nursing* (Horsham) 11:28, 1981.

Dudas, S. Care of the ostomy patient. *Nurs. Clin. North Am.* 2:389, 1976.

Foroozan, P. Two decades of diarrhea in an elderly woman. *Hosp. Pract.* 17(11):135, 1982.

Habeeb, M., and Kallstrom, M. Bowel program for institutionalized adults. *Am. J. Nurs.* 76:60, 1976.

Hogstel, M. How to give a safe and successful cleansing enema. *Am. J. Nurs.* 77:816, 1977.

Literte, J. Nursing care of patients with intestinal obstruction. *Am. J. Nurs.* 77:1003, 1977.

Rodman, M. J. Diarrhea: Think twice before giving meds. *RN* 43:73, 1980.

Romney, M. L. Nursing research in obstetrics and gynaecology. *Int. J. Nurs. Stud.* 19(4):193, 1982.

Smith, I., et al. Constipation . . . in children . . . in pregnancy . . . in the elderly . . . in the terminally ill. *Nursing* (Oxford) 1:751, 1980.

Stiklorius, C. When patient preparation is the key to success . . . in barium enemas and small bowel studies. *RN* 45:64, 1982.

Taitz, L. Managing toddler diarrhoea. *Health Visit* 56(1):9, 1983.

Thompson, M., et al. Normal and abnormal bowel function. *Nursing* (Oxford) 1:721, 1980.

Watt, R. C. Colostomy irrigation, yes or no? *Am. J. Nurs.* 77:442, 1977.

Welsby, P. D. Present day management of diarrhoea and vomiting. *Midwife Health Visit Comm. Nurse* 18(8):336, 1982.

Whitley, N., and Mack, E. Are enemas justified for women in labor? *Am. J. Nurs.* 80:1339, 1980.

QUESTIONS FOR REVIEW

Mrs. Taylor is one of your patients.

1. She has excessive intestinal gas that causes severe abdominal pain. Excessive intestinal gas that causes distention this way is termed:
   a. Aerobia.
   b. Constipation.
   c. Flatulence.
   d. Gasitis.

2. Mrs. Taylor's physician orders a rectal tube to be inserted every 2 hours as necessary. In planning care, how many minutes at a time would you plan to leave it in place?
   a. 5 minutes.
   b. 20 to 30 minutes.
   c. 40 to 60 minutes.
   d. 60 to 90 minutes.

3. Mrs. Taylor states that she often has constipation. You would assess her diet to be sure that it has:
   a. A low roughage content.
   b. A high protein content.
   c. A low carbohydrate content.
   d. A high fluid content.

4. Besides diet, what other helpful measures can you teach to prevent constipation?
   a. Using deep breaths (moving the diaphragm) three times a day.
   b. Maintaining a standing position for most of the day.
   c. Maintaining a consistent defecation pattern.
   d. Decreasing exercise during the heat of the day.

5. The electrolyte disturbance that is most apt to occur with diarrhea is:
   a. Hypocalcemia.
   b. Hypokalemia.
   c. Hypernatremia.
   d. Hyperkalemia.

6. You collect a stool sample for analysis. For which of the following tests would you not refrigerate the sample?
   a. Ova and parasites.
   b. Occult blood.
   c. Reducing substances.
   d. pH.

7. You begin to administer an enema to Mrs. Taylor and she states that she has abdominal pain. Your best action would be:
   a. Temporarily halt the flow of solution.
   b. Help her to move to a sitting position.
   c. Ask her to turn on her right side.
   d. Stimulate her rectal sphincter to cause expulsion of the solution.

8. The height of an enema solution for a retention enema should be:
   a. 6 to 8 inches.
   b. 8 to 12 inches.
   c. 12 to 18 inches.
   d. 30 to 36 inches.

9. If you administer an oil enema, the instructions you would give Mrs. Taylor following this instillation would be:
   a. Attempt to expel it immediately.
   b. Try to retain it for at least 1 hour.
   c. It will be ineffective if it is not retained for 4 hours.
   d. It will not be expelled but absorbed across the membrane.

10. Oil enemas should not be used routinely because there is a danger that absorption of what substance will be inadequate?
   a. Glucose.
   b. Potassium.
   c. Vitamin A.
   d. Vitamin C.

38. URINARY ELIMINATION

OBJECTIVES

Upon mastery of the material in this chapter, you should be able to:

1. Describe the physiological function of urinary elimination.
2. Describe normal patterns of voiding for each age group.
3. Describe the properties of normal urine and common tests performed on urine.
4. Describe factors that impede or promote urinary elimination.
5. Describe nursing implementations that are helpful in encouraging urinary elimination.
6. Describe the technique of obtaining routine, 24-hour, clean-catch, and catheterized urine specimens from both sexes.
7. Apply nursing process to give safe and planned care to a patient whose care involves principles of urinary elimination.

TERMS

The terms important for an understanding of this chapter are shown below and defined in the glossary:

anuria
calculi
cystitis
diuresis
dysuria
enuresis
frequency
glycosuria
hematuria
incontinence of urine
micturition
nocturia
oliguria
polyuria
pyuria

Urinary elimination, like intestinal elimination, is considered a private act in western civilization: one rarely discussed and certainly taken for granted. Because even grade-school children understand the importance of kidneys to body function, however, and the news media carry stories about kidney transplants, any disturbance of urinary elimination generally carries an underlying fear of serious disease. In fact, because all urinary problems in some way reflect kidney health or could lead to kidney disease, they *are* always potentially serious. In males, because urinary elimination is so closely coupled with sexual performance, urinary disturbances also carry a threat of sexual dysfunction.

When caring for people with urinary elimination problems, remember that although the problem may be an uncomplicated and simple one, the person may be very concerned. He needs good education about what is happening and what he must do to return to wellness again.

NORMAL URINARY ELIMINATION

The two kidneys are located on each side of the spinal column, behind the peritoneal cavity. The upper edge of the kidney is located at the twelfth thoracic vertebra, the bottom at the third lumbar vertebra. The right kidney tends to be a little lower than the left because of the space occupied by the liver. Kidneys tend to be a little more susceptible to trauma in children than in adults because they are located slightly lower than this and thus do not have quite as much protection from the ribs. They also do not have as much perinephritic fat to pad them against sharp blows.

Kidneys are composed of a fatty capsule, an outer portion called the *cortex* and an inner portion called the *medulla*. Urine formed by the cortical and medullar areas is drained into the pelvis of the kidney, from which it empties into the ureter. The portion of the kidney at the junction of the ureter, together with the renal blood vessels and nerves, is called the renal hilus. Because of the number of blood vessels and nerves in this portion, it is important to determine whether the kidney hilus has been injured in cases of trauma.

The cortex and medulla comprise the bulk of the kidney substance; they are composed of minute tubules, connective blood vessels, and nerve fibers. A complex set of tubules, with its accompanying blood supply and glomerulus (filtrating unit) is termed a nephron (Fig. 38-1). The glomerulus is a capillary tuft supplied by a large afferent (ingoing) and a small efferent (outgoing) glomerular artery. It is invaginated into a tubule with proximal and distal portions. In the glomerulus, water and solutes are filtered from the blood. Passage of water and solutes from the blood into the kidney glomeruli will be effective as long as the blood pressure in the glomerular arteries exceeds that in the tubule. Because the smaller efferent (outgoing) artery causes back pressure

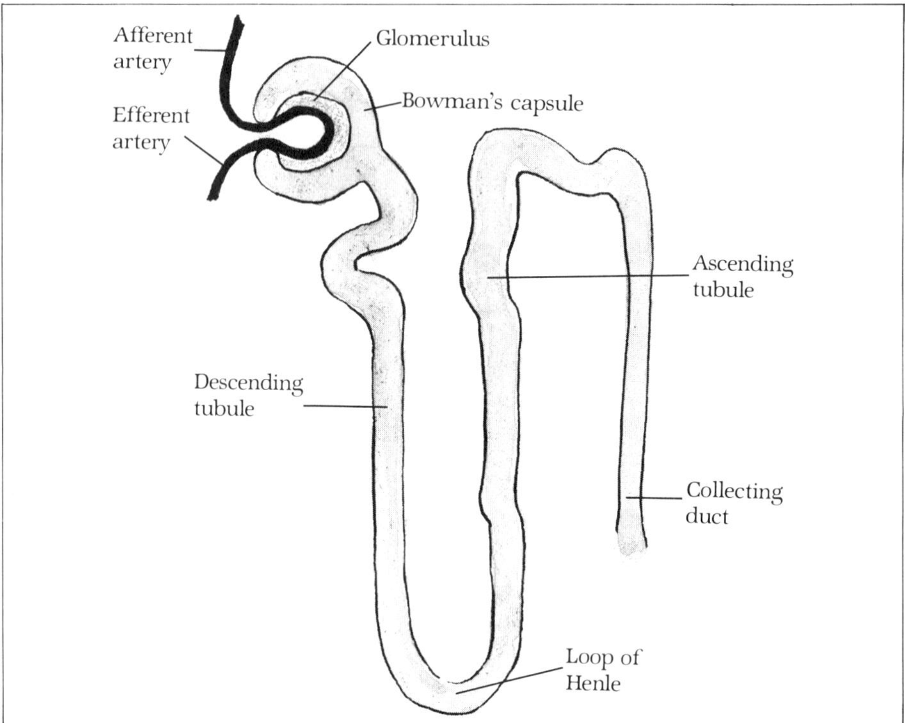

FIGURE 38-1. Anatomy of a glomerulus. Filtration occurs when blood pressure in the arterial circulation exceeds that in the glomeruli.

on the glomerulus, usually filtration occurs readily. If blood pressure in the glomerulus should decrease so that it is below the tubular pressure, little or no filtration can occur. This is why renal function must be observed carefully in persons who are hemorrhaging or who have lowered blood pressure for any reason.

This filtered solution passes through the proximal tubule, the loop of Henle, and the distal tubule. Here, water and electrolytes diffuse back into blood capillaries to such an extent that the volume of the filtrate is reduced by about 90 percent.

The glomerular filtrate enters the proximal tubule at a rate of about 120 ml/min. So much of it is reabsorbed that the final end product (urine) is excreted at a rate of only about 1 ml/min. The proximal tubules cause reabsorbtion of most of the water, glucose, sodium, chloride, phosphate, sulfate, and some bicarbonate ions. This is a passive process, not particularly affected by body needs. The distal tubules have a selective function that responds to body needs; if necessary, sodium and bicarbonate ions and additional water are reabsorbed there. If osmotic pressure increases (due to back pressure in the ureters or pelvis) so that it is greater than glomerular pressure, little reabsorption can be accomplished. The functions of the various kidney structures are summarized in Table 38-1.

TABLE 38-1. SITES OF DIFFERING KIDNEY FUNCTIONS

Site	Activity
Glomerulus	Secretion from blood of water and all solutes but protein.
Proximal convoluted tubule	Reabsorption of 80 percent of glomerular filtrated water, all of glucose, most of sodium, chloride, and ascorbic acid. Secretion of creatinine occurs here.
Descending loop of Henle	Reabsorption of additional water.
Ascending loop	Fluid is neutral in reaction; specific gravity is 1.010.
Distal convoluted tubule	Reabsorption of water, sodium, chloride, phosphate, and sulfate as needed. Secretion of potassium, hydrogen ions, and ammonia. (Secretion of ammonia and hydrogen ions conserves base because hydrogen ions are substituted for sodium ions. Sodium is reabsorbed as sodium bicarbonate.)

Kidney Functions

Excretion of Metabolic Wastes. The kidney excretes breakdown products of protein metabolism (urea, uric acid, creatinine, and ammonia). When these products accumulate in the bloodstream, poor kidney function is suspected.

Regulation of Acid-Base Balance. By regulating the acidity of urine and selecting which electrolytes are excreted, the kidneys help to maintain blood pH within normal limits. When the pH of blood plasma becomes too acid, the kidneys increase the excretion of hydrogen ions. This leaves extra hydroxyl ions in the plasma to bind with hydrogen ions and decrease the acidity of blood plasma.

Regulation of Extracellular Fluid Volume. The kidneys regulate the volume of extracellular fluid by the elimination or retention of water. The specific gravity of the urine indicates the amount of water excreted in proportion to the amount of solute eliminated.

Regulation of Osmotic Pressure of Extracellular Fluid. By regulating the amount of sodium chloride and water excreted, the kidneys regulate the osmotic pressure of the extracellular fluid. If there is a high concentration of sodium in blood plasma, for example, little water will be eliminated by the kidney because it tries to keep the concentration of sodium in the plasma from rising too high.

Regulation of Extracellular Electrolytes. The kidneys regulate electrolyte concentration in the body by selective reabsorption or excretion.

Regulation of Blood Pressure. The kidney produces an enzymelike substance (renin) that can raise blood pressure. Renin is produced in response to decreased blood volume or blood pressure or by stimulation by catecholamines (epinephrine). Renin acts to produce vascular constriction, thereby increasing blood pressure. It also stimulates production of aldosterone by the adrenal gland. This increases the sodium concentration in blood, retaining fluid and increasing blood volume.

Regulation of Red Blood Cell Production. Under stress, the kidney produces erythropoietin, which stimulates the production of red blood cells in bone marrow. Erythropoietin is produced in response to hypoxia (low oxygen level in cells). This is why people with heart diseases, which do not allow good oxygenation of red blood cells, develop an increased number of red blood cells. With many kidney disorders, there is an accompanying anemia due to the halt in erythropoietin production.

Control of Water Excretion. The reabsorption of water in the tubules is controlled by pituitary and hypothalamic action. The posterior pituitary produces an antidiuretic hormone (ADH), which increases the amount of water reabsorbed. The adrenal cortex produces the hormone aldosterone, which influences the reabsorption of sodium and chloride. If there is decreased aldosterone production, the kidney is not stimulated to retain sodium, and large amounts of sodium are excreted. When this occurs, the pituitary limits production of ADH, causing excretion of large amounts of water to balance the hydrostatic pressure of blood plasma. A person could quickly become dehydrated if this condition were allowed to continue.

Ureters, Bladder, and Urethra

Urine collects in the pelvis of the kidney and flows into the ureters. Because of the high position of the kidneys, the ureters are 10 to 12 inches (25 to 30 cm) long in adults, but small in diameter (about 1/2 inch) so that urine moves swiftly through them. This small diameter can be a problem if renal calculi (urine stones) form owing to excess calcium in urine because even a small stone can easily plug such a narrow lumen and cause obstruction. The ureters enter the bladder on the posterior surface under a fold of mucous membrane that acts as a valve to keep large quantities of urine from flowing backward from the bladder. This fold of membrane is not always effective in preventing backflow because the bladder contracts to empty, so almost everyone has some bladder reflux or backflow of urine into the ureters. If reflux is extensive, the ureters may become distended, a quantity of urine is recycled over and over, and, as with any body fluid, when there is stasis, infection tends to occur.

Urine is stored in the bladder until a sufficient amount is present (200 to 500 ml in adults); sensory nerve endings in the bladder register distention, and the person recognizes a need to urinate. An internal sphincter at the junction of the bladder and urethra is under the involuntary control of a spiral reflex. An external sphincter (located distal to the prostate gland in the male, midpoint in the urethra in the female) is under voluntary control, allowing a person to control the release or elimination of urine from the bladder.

The urethra in males is about 8 inches (20 cm) in length; in females it is only 1.5 inches (3.7 cm). This short distance in females accounts for the high incidence of bladder infection in females (bacteria enter easily and can travel the short distance from the perineum). In female infants, this distance is as short as 1/2 inch; in preschoolers it may be 3/4 of an inch (preschool girls have an extremely high incidence of bladder infection).

The actual expulsion of urine is termed *voiding* or *micturition.*

Analysis of Urine

Tests of urine are ordered as an urinalysis. Many of these tests can be done individually as independent nursing actions on the nursing unit. To evaluate the results of such tests it is important to recognize the characteristics of normal urine.

Color. The color of urine is influenced by its concentration and ingredients. Normally it is light yellow. Concentrated urine is more yellow than dilute urine. If fresh blood is present, urine may be red; if old blood is present, it may be brown.

Appearance. Urine is normally clear. It becomes cloudy in the presence of bacteria, excessive crystals, or cells. If urine has a high protein content, it foams like beer when it is poured from a collecting container into the laboratory collector.

pH. Urine normally is slightly acid (pH under 7). It tends to be alkaline (pH over 7) when infection is present or if the person has extreme metabolic alkalosis. Urine left at room temperature for a long period becomes alkaline. Either a fresh specimen must be used or it must be kept refrigerated for accurate testing. pH is tested on a nursing unit by means of a test strip dipped into the urine specimen and read against the color code on the side of the test strip dispenser.

Specific Gravity. Specific gravity is a determination of the concentration of urine. It is important because it shows the ability of the kidneys to concentrate and dilute urine. Specific gravity is elevated in dehydrated persons as the kidneys try to conserve fluid; it is decreased in persons who are overhydrated as the kidneys try to rid the body of as much fluid as possible. Specific gravity is a relative measurement. A concentrated urine specimen gives a higher protein concentration, for example, than a dilute specimen (a fixed amount of protein has been excreted); it is more concentrated in a smaller fluid volume. Normal specific gravity is 1.003 to 1.030. Specific gravity is tested on a nursing unit by use of a urinometer or refractometer.

Protein. If the kidneys are functioning well, few large molecules of protein will pass into the urine. In kidney disease, protein molecules are allowed to pass. Some people have orthostatic (postural) proteinuria, slight to mild proteinuria occurring only when the person is standing upright. The cause of this condition is poorly understood, but it probably results from renal congestion in an upright position. It can be detected by comparing an early morning specimen taken just after the person arises with one taken late in the day. Protein is tested by a test strip.

Ketones. Ketonuria is the result of the breakdown of body fat, generally because of starvation. Diabetes mellitus, if not properly controlled, will also cause ketonuria. Ketonuria is always a symptom demanding careful investigation; it is never normal. Ketones are tested by a test strip.

Glucose. Glucose is found in the urine of people with uncontrolled diabetes mellitus. It may also occur in pregnancy when special problems are present. As with ketonuria, glucosuria is a symptom requiring careful investigation to determine its cause. It is always abnormal. It is tested by a test strip or test tube reaction technique.

Occult Blood. Blood may be present in urine from such diseases as glomerulonephritis, urinary tract infection, cystitis, or trauma. Renal calculi occasionally cause blood in the urine from irritation of ureter walls. Blood in urine may also suggest systemic diseases such as leukemia or blood dyscrasias. As with ketones and glucose, it is never normal; it is tested by a test strip.

Cells. Microscopic examination of urine reveals any cells that may be present. Red blood cells in urine generally suggest trauma or infection. White blood cells suggest infection. Casts are protein configurations that outline the shape of the distal collecting tubules in which they form. Casts are found most often in concentrated urine specimens; when there is cast formation there is generally proteinuria, and vice versa. Casts may be composed of white blood cells, red blood cells, or desquamated renal epithelium. As epithelial casts grow older, they disintegrate into coarse "granular" casts and then finally into "waxy" casts that die translucent and reflect light under the microscope.

The age of casts indicates the amount of urine flow through the kidneys. A cast that has reached the waxy stage by the time it reaches the bladder indicates fairly severe stasis of urine in the tubules. Crystals may be present. Phosphate crystals tend to be present in alkaline urine; uric acid and calcium oxalate crystals may be present in acid urine. Cells or casts are not tested for on a nursing unit but are reported in a laboratory analysis. Normal findings in a routine laboratory urinalysis are summarized in Appendix G.

URINE TESTING

Tests of urine are commonly done using a single urine specimen collected at random during the day, a first-voided specimen in the morning, or collections of urine specimens taken during a 4- to 24-hour period. In most instances urine is collected in clean dry containers except when it is to be cultured. Certain chemical analyses require that a preservative such as acetic acid be added to the urine container. Before obtaining a urine specimen for testing, always be certain you know the type of specimen needed (random, catheterized, 24-hour collection), the proper technique for obtaining the specimen, and the proper laboratory collector.

Many urine tests can be done as independent nursing actions or are ordered as nursing rather than as laboratory actions. The advantage of a nurse performing the test is that the result is known immediately, so that if implementation based on the test result is necessary, it can be begun at once. When doing this type of test be sure that you use clean equipment; leave it clean for the person who uses it after you.

Test (Reagent) Strip Analysis

Test strip or test-tape analysis is the easiest type of analysis to do. Obtain a urine specimen in a clean dry

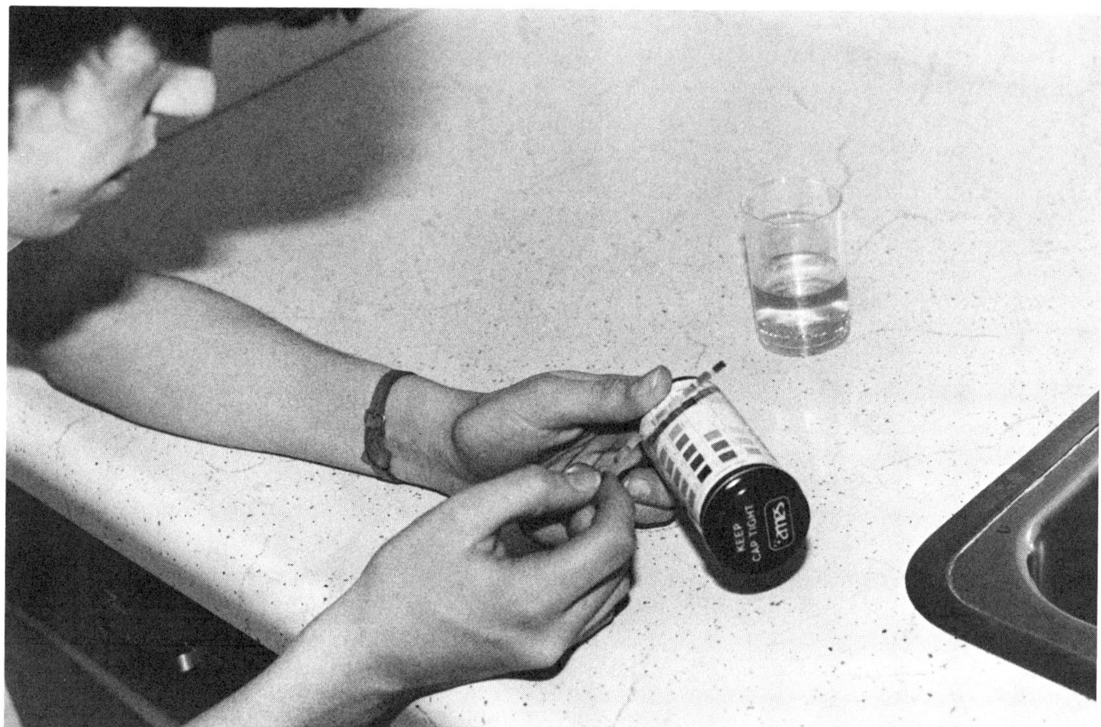

FIGURE 38-2. Testing urine by a dipstick method. Following a predetermined time interval, the color on the strip is read against a manufacturer's color code.

container. Remove a test strip from its commercial bottle. Dip it into the urine sample, observe it for color change according to the manufacturer's stated time period, and compare it to the color code on the bottle to determine the reading. Reading the color at the correct time interval is important because colors often continue to darken from exposure to air and will be very inaccurate if read at a point past the correct time period. Reagent strips are available for glucose, protein, pH, ketones, and occult blood (Fig. 38-2).

Specific Gravity

The specific gravity of urine can be measured by means of a urinometer or a refractometer. To use a urinometer you need 20 to 30 ml of urine. A refractometer needs only one drop. To use a urinometer, set it on a flat counter and fill the glass cylinder three-quarters full of urine. Place the urinometer float in the cylinder and give it a gentle spin to prevent it from resting against the side of the cylinder and distorting the reading. Read the number on the float where the bottom of the miniscus of urine crosses it. Stoop if necessary to read at eye level. The specific gravity (proportion of solute to solvent) of water is 1.000; the specific gravity of urine is only slightly higher, 1.003 to 1.030. Discard the urine and rinse the urinometer cylinder and float to leave it clean for the next person's use (Fig. 38-3A).

To use a refractometer, place one drop of urine on the barrel of the analysis cylinder; cover it with a clean dry slide. Turn on the light at the base of the refractometer, look through the eye piece of the analysis cylinder, and read the number at the point where the screen changes from black to white. Use a tissue to wipe dry the barrel and glass slide to leave the equipment available for the next person's use.

Refractometers require only one drop of urine, so frequent specific gravity determinations do not interfere with output recordings. They are particularly advantageous for use with people who have a reduced urine output when a single specimen may not be enough to use a urinometer (Fig. 38-3B).

Testing for Glucose in Urine

Glucose in urine can be tested in one of two ways: by a test strip method (Clinistix, Diastix, and Tes-Tape), which utilizes the enzyme glucose oxidase, or by a copper sulfate reducing method (Clinitest tablets). Copper sulfate reduction demonstrates all sugars present in the urine; glucose oxidase demonstrates only glucose. Women during pregnancy normally spill some lactose in urine and therefore have abnormally increased results if copper sulfate determination is used.

To use a Clinitest tablet for testing, use a clean medicine dropper and five drops of urine in a clean test tube. Rinse the medicine dropper and add 10 drops of water to the test tube. Being certain not to touch the tablet with your hand (spill it from the bottle cap), drop a Clinitest tablet into the test tube. The chemical reaction that will occur produces instant heat, so hold the test tube by the top to prevent burning your hand. Observe the reaction in the test tube continually. Do not

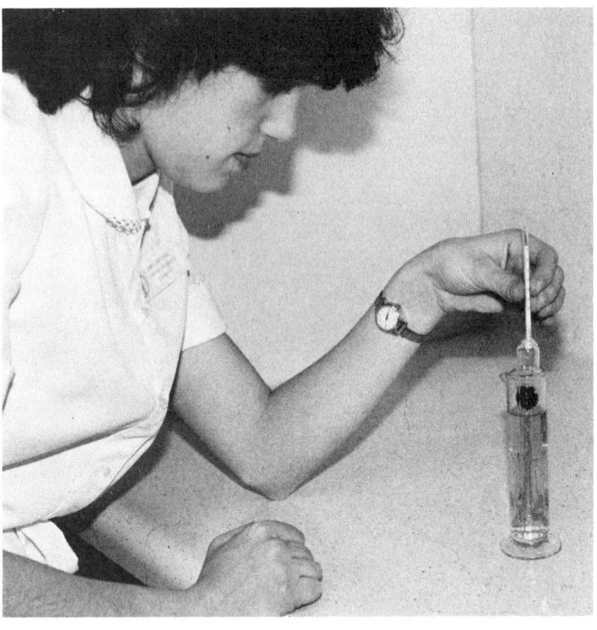

A

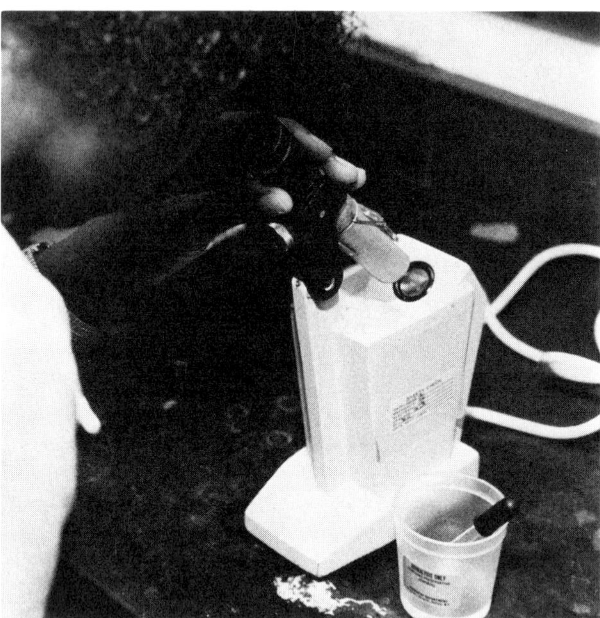

B

FIGURE 38-3. Measurement of specific gravity of urine can be done by a urinometer (A) or a refractometer (B). The advantage of a refractrometer is the small amount of urine needed for analysis.

shake it during this time. At the end of 15 seconds, shake the tube gently and compare the color of the solution to the manufacturer's color chart (Fig. 38-4).

If the color of the liquid is blue, the urine is negative for glucose. Deep yellow to orange shades of color reveal the amount of glucose present. The color change is recorded either on a 1+ to 4+ scale or by the percentage (1/2 to 2 percent) of glucose present, depending on agency policy.

The reason you must constantly observe the chemical reaction in the tube is because if there is more than 2 percent glucose in the specimen, a "pass through" phenomenon will occur—during the 15-second waiting period the specimen will pass through color changes ranging from brown to blue again. If you observed this only at the end of the 15-second period, you would read it as a negative report when instead, it is an indication that a high proportion of glucose is present. A pass through reaction is recorded as 5+ or 2 percent or pass-through, depending on specific agency policy.

Testing for Ketone Bodies

Ketone bodies may be tested for by use of a reagent strip. With people who have diabetes mellitus, a tablet test (Acetest) is generally considered the preferred method. To use the method, place the tablet on a clean paper towel, being careful not to touch it with your fingers as you remove it from the bottle to prevent contamination from any sweat or soap film from your fingers. Following the product directions, place one drop of urine on top of the tablet, using a clean medicine dropper. Thirty seconds after application of urine, compare the color of the tablet with the manufacturer's color chart. Results are recorded as negative (no color change), small, moderate, or large (the tablet turns various deepening shades of purple; see Fig. 38-5).

URINARY ELIMINATION PATTERNS BY AGE GROUP

Differing age groups have typically different patterns of urinary elimination. Table 38-2 summarizes average daily urine output by age.

The Newborn

If a newborn does not void within 24 hours after birth, the presence of an intact urinary tract is in question. The first voiding of urine may be pink-tinged due to an accumulation of uric acid crystals while in utero. The fetus voids in utero from about the fifth month of intrauterine life; voided urine accounts for part of the amniotic fluid (the fluid surrounding the fetus in the uterus). An infant born with less than a normal amount of amniotic fluid needs to be observed critically for urinary function.

The Infant

Infants have no voluntary control of urinary elimination because cephalocaudal (head to tail) development has not yet progressed to the level of the spinal sacral area (where the sensation of bladder fullness is first registered).

Assessment of urinary tract competency in infants involves observation of discomfort during urination,

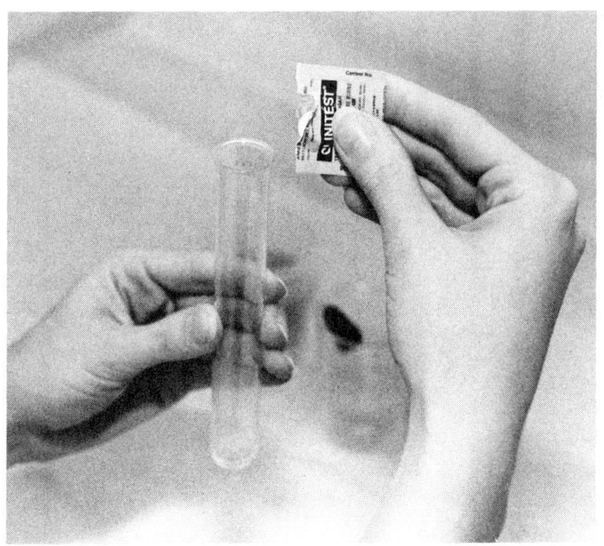

A

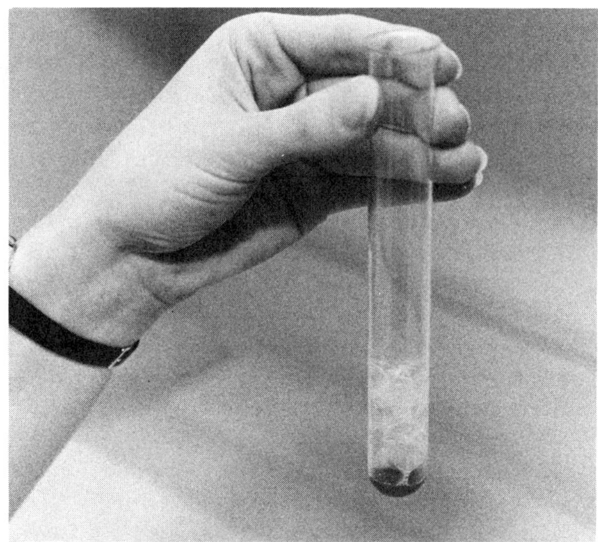

B

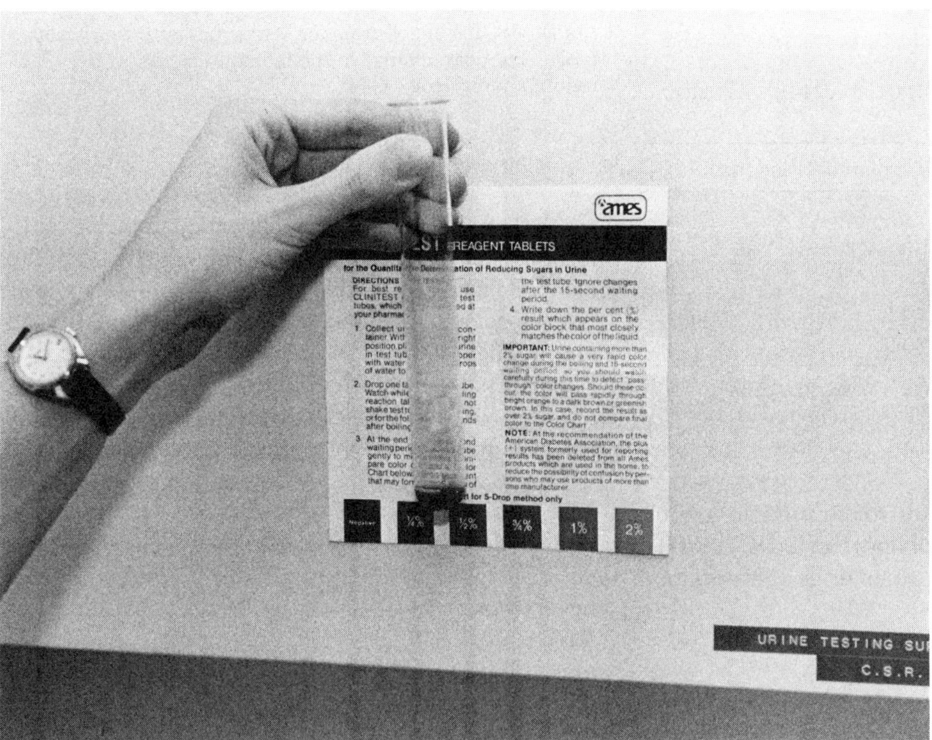

C

FIGURE 38-4. A. Drop Clinitest tablet into test tube containing 5 drops of urine and 10 drops of water. B. Watch boiling reaction; since the test tube becomes extremely hot, hold it at the top. C. Gently shake test tube 15 seconds after the boiling stops, and compare the color of its contents against the manufacturer's color chart.

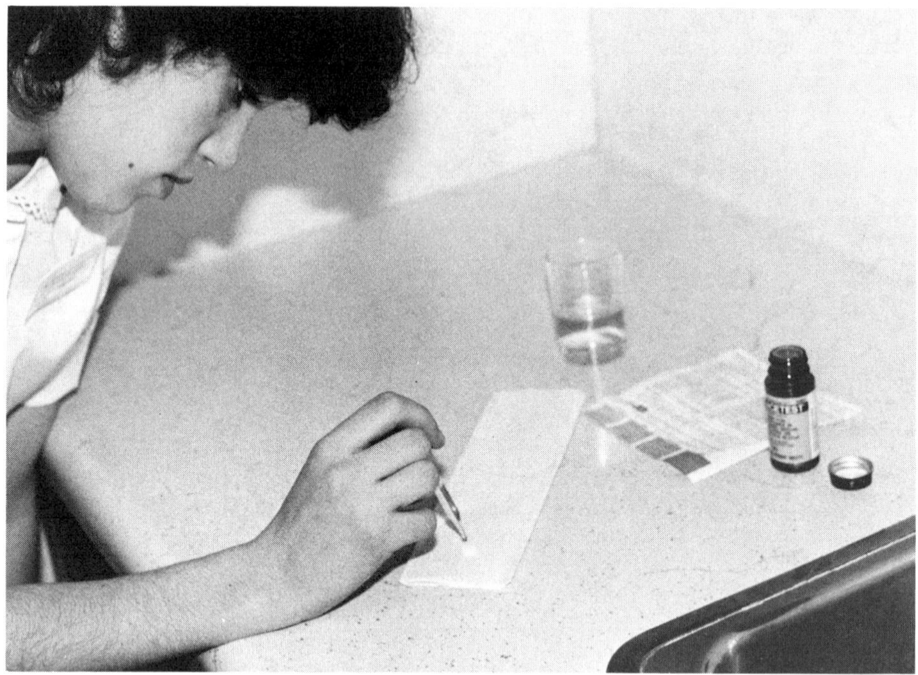

FIGURE 38-5. Testing of urine for ketone bodies by an Acetest tablet. The color change in the tablet is compared to the manufacturer's color chart.

TABLE 38-2. AVERAGE URINE OUTPUT IN A 24-HOUR PERIOD BY AGE

Age	Amount of Urine (ml)
Under 2 years	540—600
2—5 years	500—780
5—8 years	600—1,200
8—14 years	1,000—1,500
Over 14 years to adult	1,500

Source: From V. C. Vaughan III and R. J. McKay, Jr. *Nelson Textbook of Pediatrics* (10th ed.). Philadelphia: Saunders, 1975.

blood in urine, and spacing of voidings (2- to 4-hour intervals, not continual dribbling). In boys, a urine stream should be evident (an arc of urine at least a foot in length).

The Toddler and Preschooler

Toddlers and preschoolers are learning voluntary control of urination. Most children achieve daytime dryness before night-time control. Nocturnal enuresis or bed-wetting persists, especially in boys, often until 6 to 7 years of age. Aspects of toilet training are discussed in Chap. 9.

Because many girls are not taught to clean the perineum with strokes from front to back there is a high incidence of urinary tract infection in these girls. Use of bubble bath may cause perineal irritation and perhaps urinary tract infection.

The Schoolager

Schoolage children are prone to glomerulonephritis, a major kidney disease. This is an inflammation of the renal glomeruli that occurs following streptococcal infections such as tonsillitis or scarlet fever. Symptoms are blood in the urine (often old blood that turns urine "smoke-colored" or dark brown rather than red), pain, and frequency of urination.

Nocturnal enuresis that continues past 8 or 9 years of age needs to be further investigated because by this time it begins to interfere with the child's social contacts.

The Adolescent and Young Adult

The incidence of urinary tract infection rises sharply in girls following the beginning of sexual relations. This is termed *honeymoon cystitis;* it arises from bacteria being forced into the urethra from penal pressure. Adolescents are extremely body conscious and are often unwilling to discuss symptoms of elimination with health care personnel. Because the symptoms of urinary tract infection, however, are acute (burning and frequency of voiding), the person has little choice but to seek help. Many adolescents are afraid that their symptoms are not urinary tract symptoms but those of sexually transmitted disease; they need information about the cause of the problem (gonorrhea, a common sexually transmitted disease, presents with the same symptoms).

Following childbirth, many women have difficulty voiding owing to perineal edema. If the birth of the child was uncomplicated, the edema subsides quickly (within 24 hours). If the anterior wall of the vagina has been stretched by the birth (a condition aggravated by forceps or instrument deliveries), the bladder may herniate into the vagina (a cystocele). This may lead to recurring urinary tract infections due to incomplete emptying and stasis of urine. It can also lead to stress incontinence or involuntary voiding on exercise.

The Middle-Aged Adult

Middle-aged males may begin to have difficulty with normal bladder emptying due to benign (innocent) hypertrophy of the prostate gland. Because the urethra penetrates the prostate gland, the enlarged gland presses on the urethra; the man reports difficulty with beginning urination and interruptions in the stream of urine. Although the cause is usually benign, cancer of the prostate gland is also associated with the same symptoms.

As the perineal muscles begin to relax in women of middle age, many women develop stress incontinence or are incontinent when laughing, coughing or sneezing, or running (whenever intra-abdominal pressure increases). This condition may also be associated with cystocele due to childbirth. With improved obstetric procedures in the last 10 years, stress incontinence now occurs less frequently.

The Older Adult

Older adults may not drink as much fluid as they did formerly, particularly if they have some difficulty in walking. This reduced fluid intake can lead to concentrated urine and a resulting increase in urinary tract infection due to the longer time urine remains in the bladder.

If the older adult has impaired neurological function such as may accompany a cerebral vascular accident, awareness of the need to void may be lost, and the person may become incontinent. This can often be corrected by bladder retraining. Bladder retraining is difficult, however, and in some people, dryness may only be achieved by using an indwelling catheter. This is never the method of choice, however, because it limits the person's activities and feeling of independence.

Many older adults develop nocturia or must void once or twice during the night when previously they slept through the night.

FACTORS THAT INTERFERE WITH URINARY ELIMINATION

DECREASED BLOOD PRESSURE

If blood pressure drops so low that it is lower than glomerular pressure, fluid will not cross from the bloodstream into the glomeruli, and the production of urine stops. This phenomenon is apt to occur in people who have hemorrhaged, have had extreme blood loss during surgery, or have reached such a stage of exhaustion following stress that the peripheral blood vessels are dilated and blood pressure in the internal body core is lowered.

Observation of voiding is most important in a post-surgery patient. Intact circulatory function is shown, not by what the complicated monitors show, but by voiding.

DECREASED FLUID INTAKE

People who are dieting may decrease their fluid intake as sharply as their food intake. This is a potentially dangerous practice because when the body begins to break down cells, high levels of nitrogen and fatty acids are released and must be excreted to prevent acidosis. In addition, with a small fluid intake, urine remains in the bladder for an extended period until enough accumulates to be excreted; such stasis may lead to urinary tract infection.

Adequate fluid intake can be determined by testing the specific gravity of a urine specimen.

EMOTIONS

Under stress, when a general adaptation syndrome occurs, blood is routed from the peripheral circulation and nonessential organs to the core circulation to oxygenate the brain, heart, and skeletal muscles. Therefore, with both physical and emotional stress, the amount of blood circulating through the kidneys is reduced; this decreases the amount of filtrate or the amount of urine produced. When stress is relieved, there is a sensation of having to void because the kidney again begins urine production. Part of this sensation arises also from the effect of mild anxiety, which makes a person more aware than normal of body sensations, including the sensation of a full bladder.

In contrast, people who are severely depressed or acutely anxious may not be aware at all of the need to void. You must be aware of the time interval between voidings in people under stress because their bladder may become severely distended and damaged by the continual pressure.

DIET

Diet influences voiding patterns because certain foods promote diuresis or increase urine volume. Coffee and beer are common examples of such foods. The alkalinity and acid content of urine are also influenced by diet. A high-protein diet, for example, will strongly acidify urine; a total vegetarian diet can cause an alkaline urine. A diet high in sodium can cause fluid retention and decrease urine output. Cranberry juice has a strong acidifying effect and is usually recommended for people on bed rest (who have a high incidence of urinary tract infection due to urine stasis; bacteria grow poorly in a strongly acid medium).

ACTIVITY

The more active a person is, the greater the cardiac output. Consequently, the more blood circulates through the kidneys, the greater the amount of filtrate and urine produced. A sedentary person may, therefore, experience a sharp decrease in the amount of urine produced.

When a small amount of urine is produced, it remains in the bladder longer than normal, so the person becomes more prone to bladder infection than normal (stasis of any fluid invites infection). Lying flat in bed allows good kidney perfusion and output; however, the lack of ability to sit upright or stand for urination may influence the person's ability to void so much that urine may remain in the bladder longer than normal, inviting infection.

HABIT AND SUGGESTION

To a certain extent, people condition themselves to void at various times during the day (when they first rise in the morning, for instance). The person senses bladder fullness very strongly at these times. Passing a public rest-room or hearing running water may stimulate the sensation of having to void. Men void most readily in a standing position and may be almost unable to void in a hospital setting if circumstances such as a cast or traction prohibit this position.

HORMONAL INFLUENCES

Antidiuretic hormone, secreted by the pituitary gland, influences the amount of urine produced. People who have had head injury with resulting edema or inflammation may have such pressure on the pituitary gland that secretion of this hormone decreases (increasing urine flow) or increases (decreasing urine flow). Be aware of the amount of urine volume and the specific gravity of urine in persons with head trauma. Aldosterone, produced by the adrenal gland, controls the amount of sodium retained by the body; the more sodium that is retained, the more fluid is retained and the less urine produced. Any illness affecting the adrenal gland, therefore, may greatly influence urinary elimination. Production of these hormones is also influenced by circadian rhythms or the sleep-wake cycle and basal metabolic rate.

INFECTION

Infection of the bladder or kidneys may result either from an ascending spread of microorganisms from the urethral meatus or from microorganisms already present in the blood entering the kidneys from that route. Women are especially prone to urinary tract infections because of their shorter urethra, which allows microorganisms to gain access more readily to the bladder.

OBSTRUCTION

Obstruction will cause stasis of urine, and stasis of any body fluid invites infection. If the obstruction is complete it may cause such back pressure that the kidney nephrons can be permanently damaged. Obstruction may occur as a congenital defect or as the result of calculi (stones that form in urine) or as an abnormal growth such as a bladder or kidney tumor. Tumors outside the urinary tract often compress the ureters or urethra or cause similar obstructive difficulties.

MEASURES TO PROMOTE PROPER URINARY ELIMINATION

Providing Adequate Fluid Intake

Always be aware of the fluid intake of all of your patients during the previous 24 hours. Make a point of not making suggestions for adequate fluid as vague statements but as direct questions or statements ("I'm concerned with how little you've had to drink today, Mrs. Jones. Can I get you a drink of water right now?").

One method of helping to clear a urinary tract infection is to ask the person to increase his total fluid intake well above average so that more urine is formed and excreted, carrying with it microorganisms present in the bladder. The amount of fluid given to an adult is 2000 to 3000 ml daily. With children the exact amount should be prescribed. Suggestions for encouraging fluids are described further in Chap. 30.

Providing Privacy, Position, and Comfort

The average person is almost unable to void unless he has privacy. Provide this by proper use of curtains or closed doors. A person who needs assistance to walk to the bathroom may grow dizzy if he sits on a toilet for any length of time. Remain close by even though you remove yourself from his immediate range of vision.

Many men have difficulty voiding unless they can stand. Sometimes this helps to provide motivation for men to ambulate following surgery. Women have difficulty voiding unless they are sitting up. When assisting a person to use a bedpan, raise the head of the bed at least to a semi-Fowler's position. Using a commode at the side of the bed is preferable to a bedpan by most people because it simulates a more normal voiding position.

A person who has pain, particularly abdominal pain, may be unable to void because he must tighten his abdominal muscles to do so. Offer analgesic medication as necessary; suggest voiding when the medication reaches its therapeutic peak (about 20 minutes after administration).

Suggestions that may aid voiding are running water within hearing distance or pouring warm water over a woman's genitals to relax the perineal muscle and assist voiding. Do not do this if the urine is to be saved for analysis in any way because the water will change the composition of the urine, particularly the specific gravity, glucose, and protein composition. If the urine is to be assessed only for volume, you can do this and then subtract the known amount of water that was used.

Be certain that bedpans and urinals are warm, not cold. Warm them by running them under warm water for a minute.

Some people are so worried that if they do not void

spontaneously they will have to be catheterized and they are then too tense to void. Clarify concerns about catheterization by giving a true description of it.

Following removal of a catheter, a person may notice a momentary burning sensation the first time he voids (because the urethral lining is slightly irritated). This should happen only once, however.

Offering a Bedpan or Urinal

Women patients who are unable to get out of bed may use a bedpan for urine elimination, male patients a urinal. These are made of either metal or plastic. Thin bedpans for use with people who have little ability to raise themselves off a bed are termed fracture bedpans. Techniques for offering bedpans and urinals are given in Procedure 38-1. Never set bedpans or urinals on a patient's overbed table. Keep such implements off bedside stands also; if a person wants a bedpan or urinal readily available, place it under the top covers of the bed by the person's side.

When handling bedpans or urinals do not touch the inner surface because it is apt to have a bacterial count, especially bedpans. Bedpans and urinals may be emptied into a patient's toilet or taken to a central utility room. When carrying such articles through the hallway, cover them with a cotton cover or a disposable plastic square (Fig. 38-6). After emptying the container, rinse it with water to control odor. Most health care facilities have bedpan flushers (called bedpan sterilizers) that can be used to rinse. Bedpan flushers follow the rinsing process with a minute or two of live steam directed at the bedpan. This makes a metal bedpan extremely hot. Do not be misled by the word *sterilizer;* this limited amount of steam cannot sterilize, only clean more thoroughly.

Using a Bedside Commode

A bedside commode is a portable toilet that can be moved beside the bed of a person with poor mobility to allow him to be independent in elimination functions. A removable container under the seat can be carried to a utility room or bathroom to be emptied. Many women are able to use a bedside commode when they cannot use a bedpan owing to the normal position for voiding this offers. It may be less strain on the heart to use a bedside commode than to lift the entire body weight to use a bedpan by pressing on a mattress.

Medications

Medications that promote urinary flow are termed *diuretics.* Cholinergic drugs may be used to stimulate bladder emptying. Quick Reference Stops 38-1 and 38-2 summarize the properties of a number of common diuretics and cholinergics.

When caring for patients taking diuretics you must provide time in your plan of care for use of a bathroom or a bedpan at fairly frequent intervals to avoid overdistention of the bladder. Diuretics carry the danger that as increased fluid is lost from the body, excessive potassium will be removed. Low potassium levels lead to a general feeling of malaise and lethargy and, at an extreme level, cardiac arrhythmia. As a rule, people taking a diuretic, unless it is a potassium-sparing type, should eat foods high in potassium to avoid becoming potassium defi-

PROCEDURE 38-1
Offering a Bedpan or Urinal

Purpose: To provide a means of elimination for the patient unable to use a bathroom, respecting privacy and sense of self-control.

Plan	*Principle*
1. Wash your hands; identify patient; explain procedure.	1. Prevent spread of microorganisms. Promote patient's safety and well-being.
2. Assess patient status; analyze appropriateness of plan; adjust plan to individual patient need.	2. Nursing care is always individualized based on professional judgment of patient's needs.
3. Implement plan by assembling equipment: urinal or bedpan with cover (use chux or paper towel if no cover is provided), toilet tissue, warm wet washcloth, towel, soap, paper bag for discarding toilet tissue if it is not to be discarded with specimen.	3. Conserve energy by organization and preparation.
4. Raise bed to high position. Provide privacy by curtain or door. Elevate head of bed slightly (30°) if patient condition permits.	4. It is physiologically easier to void or defecate in a sitting position. People appreciate privacy during elimination.

5. Fold back covers but do not expose patient unnecessarily. Position bedpan on side of bed. If person is able to assist, ask him to bend his knees, press down with heels and both hands to raise buttocks off the bed. Slide bedpan under him.

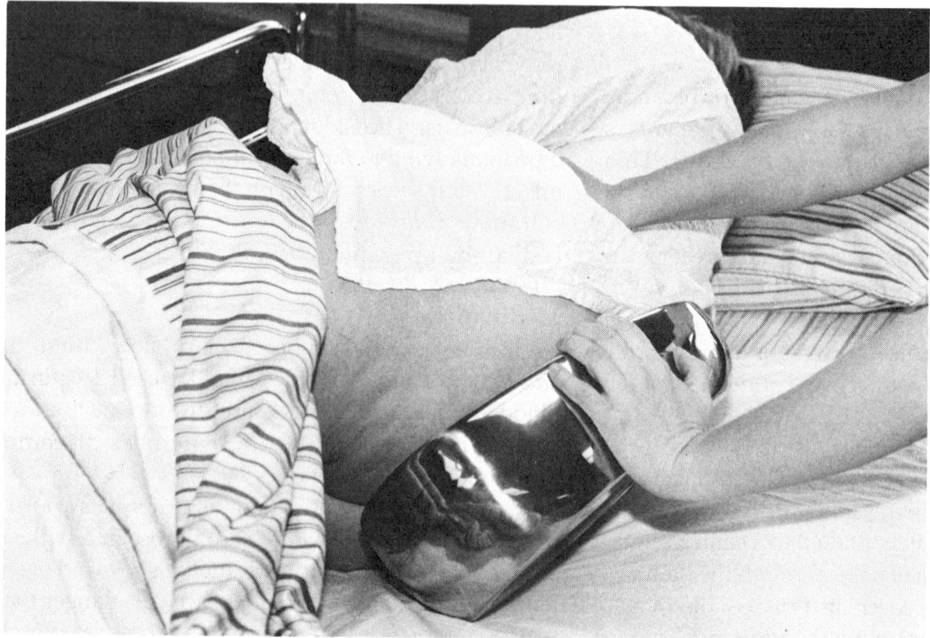

FIGURE 1. Offering a bedpan to a person who cannot assist.

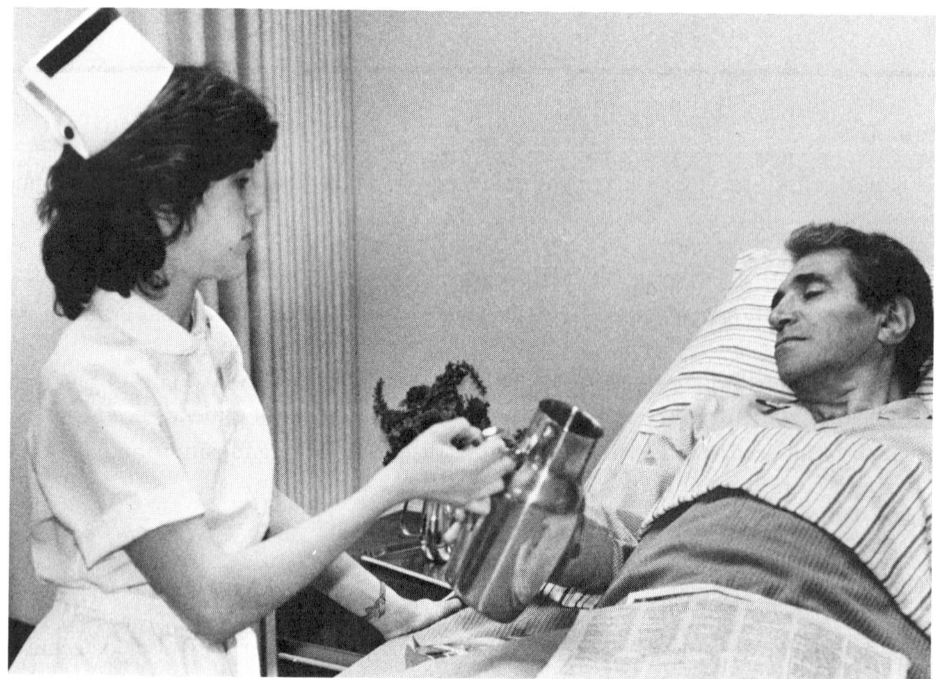

FIGURE 2. Offering a urinal to a man who is able to place it himself.

Action	Rationale
6. If unable to assist, roll patient to side away from you. Place bedpan against buttocks, roll patient onto back with bedpan in place (Fig. 1). Raise head of bed slightly.	6. Ask for help from a second person as necessary.
7. Check that patient's buttocks rest on top edge of bedpan.	7. Avoid injury to skin from sharp edge of bedpan against spine.
8. Allow man to place urinal by himself if he is able (Fig. 2); if not, gently place urinal between legs, being certain that penis is positioned in urinal.	8. Encourage self-care.
9. Place signal device and toilet tissue within easy reach; leave patient by himself if safe to do so.	9. Encourage sense of control.
10. Return in a reasonable time or if patient signals. Remove bedpan using reverse technique in which it was offered. If necessary, wrap toilet tissue around your hand and wipe perineal and anal area clean. With women, always stroke from the pubis to the anus and discard tissue after one stroke. Turn patient on side to clean anal area.	10. Using a front to back stroke reduces the possibility of fecal contamination into vagina or urinary meatus.
11. Place toilet tissue in bedpan to be discarded with specimen. If specimen is going to be saved, discard tissue into paper bag.	
12. Offer washcloth, towel, and soap for hands.	12. Prevent spread of microorganisms.
13. Carry bedpan (covered) to bathroom or utility room for disposal. Wash and rinse bedpan before returning it to unit.	13. Promote aesthetic measures.
14. Position patient comfortably in bed. Evaluate effectiveness, efficiency, cost, comfort, and safety aspects of procedure. Plan appropriate health teaching such as the importance of good fluid intake in promoting good urinary output.	14. Health teaching is an independent nursing action always included as a part of care.
15. Chart the time and amount voided and defecated. Describe any abnormal findings. Test urine and stool as indicated on nursing orders. Document if a specimen was sent for lab analysis.	15. Document nursing care and patient status.

MODIFICATION FOR CARE OF CHILD

Following toilet training, a young child will be reluctant to use a bedpan since he has been taught not to eliminate in bed. Whenever possible, use of a potty seat at the bedside is preferable.

MODIFICATIONS FOR CARE OF OLDER ADULT

Most older adults pride themselves on their ability to provide for themselves. Evaluate each person independently as to his level of self-care and ability to answer his own elimination needs. Use special care to respect modesty; provide privacy. Answer the call light promptly to minimize discomfort and promote self-esteem.

Many older adults have some limitation of body movement, such as occurs with arthritis, which can make it difficult and painful to use a bedpan. A smaller bedpan, commonly called a *fracture bedpan*, is often used with older adults as well as immobilized persons.

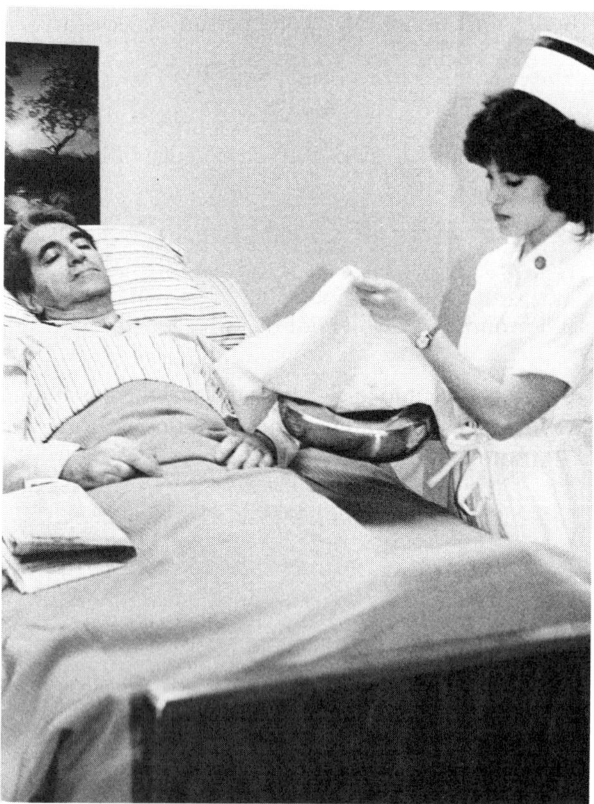

FIGURE 38-6. Cover bedpans or urinals to carry them through hallways for aesthetic reasons and to control odor.

cient due to loss of potassium in the excess urine excreted (Table 38-3). A potassium supplement may be provided as well as the diuretic to maintain an adequate potassium level (see QRS 38-3).

Urinary Catheterization

Urinary catheterization consists of inserting a thin hollow tube through the urethra into the bladder to remove urine from the bladder or to establish a patent urine drainage method.

URINARY CATHETERS

Urinary catheters are of two types—(1) straight and (2) indwelling or retention (Foley). A straight catheter is a narrow rubber or pliable plastic tube in a variety of sizes ranging from 8F to 18F. A French catheter is important for urinary catheterization because a firm insertion tip is needed to follow the length of the urethra. Straight catheters are used only for removal of urine and cannot be left in place. A retention catheter has a double lumen, one lumen similar to that of a straight catheter, the other leading to a rubber balloon near the tip of the catheter. After the catheter has been inserted with the balloon deflated, the balloon is inflated with sterile water or sterile saline. When the balloon is inflated, the catheter will remain in place in the bladder. The usual sizes for both straight and retention catheters are 8 to 10 for children; 12 to 16 for adult females; and 16 to 18 for adult males (Fig. 38-7).

☐ QUICK REFERENCE STOP 38-1: PHARMACOLOGY
Commonly Used Diuretics

Class of Diuretic	*Example*	*Site of Action*	*Precautions or Implications*
Mercurials	Mercaptomerin sodium (thiomerin)	Ascending loop of Henle	Have prompt action; used in severe edematous states. Must be administered intravenously for optimal effect. The addition of theophylline to drug compound increases the absorption and excretion of mercury to avoid mercury intoxication. May cause hypokalemia and hyponatremia.
Carbonic anhydrase inhibitors	Acetazolamide (Diamox)	Proximal and distal tubules	Affect aqueous humor content, so may be used in glaucoma (excessive aqueous humor in eye globe). Hypokalemia and hyponatremia may occur.
Loop diuretics	Furosemide (Lasix)	Ascending loop of Henle and proximal tubule	Hypokalemia and hyponatremia may occur.
	Ethacrynic acid (Edecrin)	Ascending loop of Henle and proximal tubule	Observe for dehydration from excess fluid loss.

Osmotic	Mannitol (Osmitrol)	Increases osmotic pressure in distal tubule	Used to relieve presence of edema in intracranial spaces as fluid is drawn into bloodstream from subcutaneous tissue. May lead to cardiac overload.
Potassium-sparing diuretics	Triamterene (Dyrenium)	Distal tubules and collecting duct	Hyperkalemia may occur. Used in combination with other diuretics to minimize potassium loss.
Thiazide sulfonamides	Hydrochlorothiazide (Hydrodiuril) Chlorothiazide (Diuril)	Ascending loop of Henle and proximal tubule	Hypokalemia and hyponatremia may occur.

GUIDELINES FOR PATIENT CARE

1. Intake and output and weight (at least once a week) should be recorded on all persons taking diuretics.
2. Diuretics should be administered early in the day to avoid nocturnal diuresis.
3. Patients should be encouraged to ingest foods high in potassium unless the diuretic is potassium-sparing to prevent hypokalemia.
4. Assess daily the condition of skin turgor and mucous membrane for signs of dehydration.
5. Laboratory reports should be assessed daily for electrolyte levels.
6. Specific gravity should be measured daily as an independent nursing action.

☐ QUICK REFERENCE STOP 38-2: PHARMACOLOGY
Cholinergic and Antienuretic Agents

Drug	*Precautions or Effects*
Cholinergic agents	Act to cause bladder emptying.
Bethanechol chloride (Urecholine)	These drugs also affect the gastrointestinal tract to cause increased salivation and, in some persons, abdominal cramps and nausea.
Neostigmine methylsulfate (Prostigmin)	Never administer if mechanical obstruction is present.
Antienuretic agents	Act to reduce bladder emptying.
Imipramine hydrochloride (Tofranil)	May cause mild constipation due to slowed gastrointestinal effects.

TABLE 38-3. POTASSIUM-RICH FOODS

	Potassium Level		
Types of Food*	High Quantity	Moderate Quantity	Low Quantity
Grains	Bran, wheat germ	Whole grains	Refined grains
Vegetables	Raw, baked, fried, dried	Steamed	Canned or cooked in water
Fruit	Raw, frozen whole, dried, juices	Canned	Fruit drinks
Liquids	Coffee (brewed, strong)		Instant coffee
Carbohydrates	Chocolate, coconut, raisins, nuts		Hard candy

*Specific examples of foods high in potassium are bananas, oranges and orange juice, fish, fowl, dates, prunes, raisins, cereals, soybeans, and potatoes.

PURPOSE OF URINARY CATHETERIZATION

Urinary catheterization may be performed for a number of reasons. The most frequent reason is removal of urine from the bladder in the presence of urine retention. A catheter can be used to determine how much residual urine remains after the person voids. Bladder catheterization may also be done to reduce the size of the bladder before surgery or another abdominal procedure or to provide a route for voiding if urethral or perineal surgery is performed. It may be done to obtain a sterile urine specimen for analysis or to facilitate strict intake and output measurements. It may be done to place a retention catheter to relieve incontinence when all other measures fail or to provide a route for bladder irrigation.

> ☐ **QUICK REFERENCE STOP 38-3: NUTRITION**
> **Potassium Supplements**
>
> People taking a diuretic (providing it is not a potassium-sparing diuretic) may lose a considerable amount of potassium and should, as a rule, eat foods high in potassium (see Table 38-3) to counteract this loss. In addition, an oral potassium supplement may be prescribed. The person must understand that the potassium is not a "nicety" but a necessity during the time he is taking the diuretic to avoid potassium deficiency.
>
> Be equally certain that the person understands that when the diuretic is no longer prescribed, the potassium supplement should also be discontinued. Excess potassium can lead to cardiac arrhythmias and, in extreme cases, cardiac arrest.

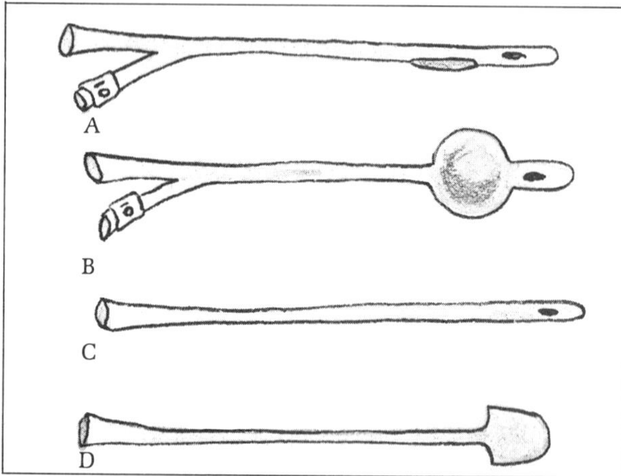

FIGURE 38-7. Types of urinary catheters. A. Deflated retention catheter. B. Inflated retention catheter. C. Straight catheter. D. Mushroom-tipped catheter.

Before performing a catheterization, always ask yourself if the catheter will be left in place following the procedure. If not, you will need a straight catheter; if so, you will use a retention type. Do not use retention catheters when they are not necessary because they increase patient expense and because, since the lumen for urinary drainage is narrower than that in a straight catheter with the same number, it must remain in place longer to drain the same amount of urine, increasing the possibility of urethral trauma.

HAZARDS OF CATHETERIZATION

Catheterization always has certain inherent hazards. Catheterization must always be a strictly sterile procedure to avoid introducing microorganisms into the bladder with catheter insertion. Even with strict technique, microorganisms may be introduced because the urinary meatus can be disinfected but not sterilized. The incidence of urinary tract infections increases greatly when a retention catheter is in place because microorganisms may enter through or beside the catheter. For these reasons, catheterization is kept to a minimum and is used only after other measures have proved unsuccessful.

A second danger of catheterization is trauma to the urethra. Always use extremely gentle technique and the smallest gauge catheter practical. In adults, for example, a 12F catheter is often adequate for obtaining a urine sample and much less traumatic than an 18F. In infants a sterile feeding tube (No. 8 or No. 10) is narrower than a urinary catheter and less traumatic. To prevent urine from leaking around a retention catheter, it is often necessary to use a larger size than would be necessary if the catheter were not going to be left in place.

Loss of bladder tone may occur if a retention catheter is used and the bladder is always kept decompressed.

Another hazard of catheterization is danger to self-esteem. Most people are embarrassed during such a personal, private procedure and have heard stories of how terrible it is. Provide a good explanation of the procedure and use a nonembarrassed, competent attitude to reduce the patient's embarrassment and encourage relaxation. This will also aid catheter insertion.

Be sure of your knowledge of basic anatomy before inserting a urinary catheter. There is a great deal of variation in the location of a female urethra. The slant of the urinary urethra in females is slightly posterior when the woman is lying supine. In males, the curve of the urethra must be visualized when a catheter is inserted to avoid striking the side of the urethra at the angle where it enters the bladder.

FEMALE AND MALE CATHETERIZATION

Female catheterization is outlined in Procedure 38-2. Although female catheterization is usually performed in a dorsal recumbent position, it can be done in a Sims' position; you would then stand behind the woman and spread the labia from your posterior position. This position does not offer good visualization of the urethra, however, so it is useful only if the woman is unable to assume a dorsal recumbent position.

Male catheterization is outlined in Procedure 38-3. Instead of tucking a sterile drape under the buttocks as in a woman, a sterile fenistrated drape (a towel with a circular opening in it), placed over the penis, is used instead. If this is not available, arrange a top and bottom sterile towel snugly around the penis to provide a sterile field.

Clean the urinary meatus, grasp the penis with your left hand, extend the shaft, and, if the man is uncircumcised, gently retract the foreskin to fully reveal the urinary meatus. Hold the penis at a 90-degree angle and pull it slightly upward with gentle pressure to straighten the urethra and allow easy insertion of the catheter (Fig.

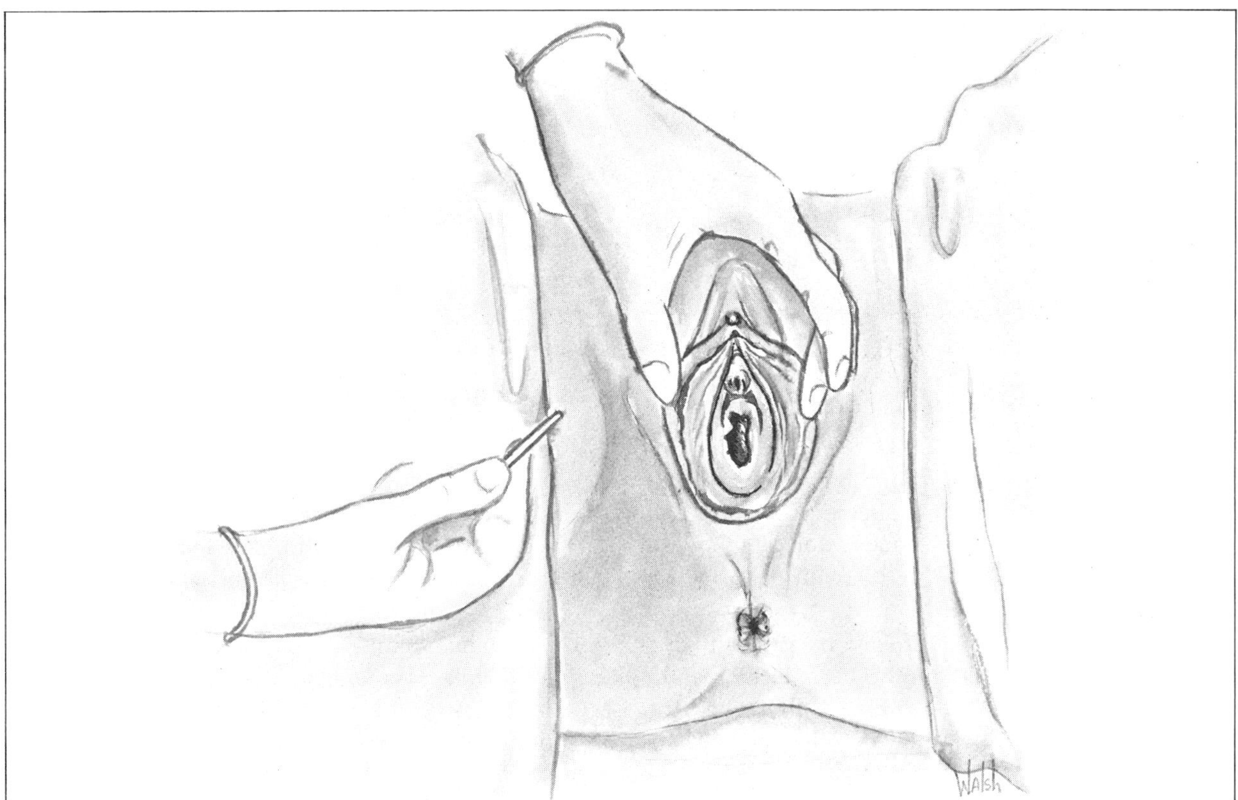

FIGURE 38-8. Female urinary catheterization. Be certain to visualize the urinary meatus well before attempting catheter insertion.

PROCEDURE 38-2
Female Urinary Catheterization

Purpose: To remove urine from the bladder by means of a catheter using sterile technique.

Plan	*Principle*
1. Wash your hands, identify patient; explain procedure.	1. Prevent spread of microorganisms; ensure patient safety and cooperation.
2. Assess patient condition; analyze appropriateness of procedure; plan modifications as necessary.	2. Use the smallest size catheter practical to prevent trauma to the urethra.
3. Implement procedure by assembling equipment: a good light source and a sterile catheterization tray, or separate component parts: sterile cotton balls, sterile basin, specimen container, gloves, drape, lubricant.	3. Strict sterile procedure must be used to reduce the possibility of introducing urinary tract infection. A good light source is crucial to locate urinary meatus.
4. Provide privacy by bed curtains or closed room door. Cover patient with bath blanket or draw sheet to use as a drape to protect modesty. Position her in a dorsal recumbant position; place tray of equipment on bed between her legs.	4. Catheterization requires exposure of the perineum. Proper draping not only protects against undue exposure but prevents chilling. For many women, the loss of modesty involved in catheterization is more uncomfortable than physical pain. Relaxation of the sphincter is important for catheter insertion and privacy aids relaxation.

5. Open the catheterization tray or set up a sterile field. Put on sterile gloves. Open sterile lubricant and drop a spot of it on a section of the tray so the catheter can be dipped into it using only one hand later.

5. Sequence of gloving varies depending on whether the tray is commercially prepared or you are organizing your own tray.

6. Slide a sterile towel or drape under the woman's buttocks by asking her to lift her buttocks.

6. If the woman is unable to cooperate, you may need an assistant not only to help you place the drape but to support her legs in a knee-raised position.

7. Place left hand at anterior surface of labia and gently spread them with your fingers so urinary meatus is evident. Do not allow labia to close over meatus again until catheter is inserted.

7. The left hand is now contaminated and must not be returned to the sterile tray or catheter.

8. With sterile right hand, dip a cotton ball in antiseptic solution, wipe front to back down right side of urinary meatus; discard the cotton ball on rim of tray. Use a second cotton ball to wash left side of meatus, a third cotton ball to wash the center of meatus.

8. Always stroke front to back to avoid carrying microorganisms from the vagina or rectum forward to the meatus. The outer inch of a sterile field is considered contaminated so may be used for disposal of contaminated articles.

9. Use two cotton balls to dry meatus, stroking gently and carefully front to back. Pick up catheter about 3 inches from tip and lubricate it by touching tip to lubricant; place distal end in sterile basin.

9. If an iodine solution was used for disinfection, it is difficult to visualize meatus unless the solution is wiped away. Wiping away also prevents introduction of disinfectant to urethra. Addition of lubricant reduces trauma to urethra and facilitates insertion of catheter.

10. Identify urinary meatus. Ask the woman to take a deep breath while you gently insert catheter into meatus about 2 inches. Do not force the catheter if you meet resistance. Do not allow tip of catheter to touch any surface but the meatus or you must discard it and use a new sterile one.

10. A distraction technique of this kind aids sphincter relaxation and reduces resistance to catheter insertion. The secret of successful catheterization is to be certain that you have identified urinary meatus and not a dimpling under the clitoris or the vaginal opening. In actual practice, perineal anatomy is not as obvious as it is in an anatomical drawing.

11. If the catheter is in the bladder, urine will immediately flow into the sterile basin. If urine does not return, advance catheter another inch.

11. Urine return depends on the length of the individual urethra and the amount of urine in the bladder.

12. If a urine specimen is desired, allow at least 5 ml of urine to flow into sterile specimen container from catheter. Allow remainder to flow into collecting basin. Once catheter is in place, secure it in place by left hand to free right hand to arrange basin and specimen container.

12. As a rule, do not initially remove more than 750 ml of urine from the bladder except under special circumstances; if a bladder is completely distended, removing all urine might cause such a loss of bladder tone that it will not respond to filling afterward. Such a shift in intra-abdominal pressure could also shift blood from the central circulation to the abdominal vessels so that the person grows dizzy from lack of cerebral perfusion.

13. Following removal of the desired amount of urine, remove catheter gently but quickly; dry the perineum well with the towel used as a buttocks pad.

13. Continued perineal moisture can lead to excoriation.

14. Position patient comfortably if in bed or help to return to bed if procedure was done in a treatment room. Evaluate effectiveness, cost, comfort, and safety of procedure. Plan health teaching as needed, such as the fact that the next time she voids she may feel slight pain.

14. Health teaching is an independent nursing action always included as a part of care.

Plan	Principle
15. Record on chart that catheterization was accomplished, amount of urine obtained, whether a specimen was sent for analysis, and any abnormalities observed in procedure or urine.	15. Document nursing care and patient status.

MODIFICATION OF PROCEDURE

Commercial catheterization kits are supplied with tweezers. These may be used to grasp the cotton balls for cleansing and drying the urinary meatus. The advantage of tweezers is that your glove is absolutely sterile when you pick up the catheter; a disadvantage is that they decrease your ability to determine how much pressure against the perineum you are using and may cause pain. You can keep the catheter tip sterile by grasping it 3 inches from the tip, or the length of the urinary urethra, making use of the tweezers optional.

MODIFICATIONS FOR CARE OF CHILD

Because catheterization involves minimal pain, it should be done in a treatment room rather than as a bedside procedure to keep the child's bed area a safe area. For children under 5 years of age, an assistant is needed to help the child remain still and to keep her hands from touching her perineum or the catheter. Young girls' vaginal openings may be much more anterior than you expect from anatomical drawings; take adequate time to locate the meatus. Remember that preschoolers fear intrusive procedures. Catheterization for this age child is, therefore, kept to an absolute minimum. Give praise afterward for cooperation (anything short of hysterical screaming is good cooperation for such a frightening procedure in this age group).

MODIFICATIONS FOR CARE OF OLDER ADULT

Following menopause, the labia of women atrophy, changing the contour of the perineum. Take adequate time to identify the urinary meatus carefully prior to catheter insertion. Some women in this age group have difficulty bending their knees adequately to give you an adequate perineal view without an assistant to help them maintain a correct position.

PROCEDURE 38-3
Male Urinary Catheterization

Purpose: To remove urine from the bladder by means of a catheter using sterile technique.

Plan	*Principle*
1. Wash your hands; identify patient; explain the procedure.	1. Prevent spread of microorganisms; ensure patient safety and cooperation.
2. Assess patient status; analyze appropriateness of procedure; plan modifications as necessary.	2. Use the smallest size catheter practical to prevent trauma to the urethra.
3. Implement procedure by assembling equipment: good light source and sterile catheterization tray, or separate component parts: sterile cotton balls, sterile basin, specimen container, gloves, drape, lubricant.	3. Strict sterile procedure must be used to reduce the possibility of introducing urinary tract infection. A good light source is crucial to locate urinary meatus.
4. Provide privacy by bed curtains or closed room door. Position patient supine with legs slightly spread. Cover legs to midthigh with bath blanket for warmth and modesty. Place tray of equipment on bed at side of patient or between legs.	4. Privacy is a highly valued right of most people.
5. Open the catheterization tray or set up a sterile field. Put on sterile gloves. Open sterile lubricant and drop a spot of it on a section of the tray so the catheter can be dipped into it using only one hand.	5. Sequence of gloving varies depending on whether the tray is commercially prepared or you are organizing your own tray.

6. Place sterile drape over penis by lifting penis with left hand and placing drape with right. If uncircumcised, retract foreskin to reveal urethra and meatus.	6. Left hand is now contaminated and cannot be returned to sterile field or touch catheter.
7. While grasping penis in left hand, use sterile right hand to dip a cotton ball in antiseptic solution, wipe meatal opening with a circular motion; discard soiled cotton ball to rim of tray. Repeat with second and third cotton balls.	7. A circular motion moves bacteria away from meatus. The outer inch of a sterile field is considered contaminated and may be used for disposal of contaminated articles.
8. Use two cotton balls to dry meatus. Pick up catheter 2 or 3 inches from tip and lubricate it by touching tip to lubricant; place distal end in sterile basin.	8. If an iodine solution was used for disinfection, it is difficult to visualize meatus unless solution is wiped away. Wiping away also prevents introduction of disinfectant to urethra. Addition of lubricant reduces trauma to urethra and facilitates insertion of catheter.
9. To insert catheter, extend penis at a 90°-angle using gentle upward traction. Use a distraction technique such as asking the man to take a deep breath. Insert the catheter about a distance of 8 inches (20 cm) until urine begins to flow. Do not allow tip of catheter to touch any surface but the meatus or you must discard it and use a new sterile one.	9. It is important that the penis is held at a 90°-angle to straighten the urethra and allow for easy catheter insertion. Never force the catheter against resistance. If resistance is met, pause a second with insertion because resistance may be only urethral spasm. A distraction technique aids sphincter relaxation and reduces resistance to catheter insertion.
10. If the catheter is in the bladder, urine will immediately flow into the sterile basin. If urine does not return, advance catheter another inch. Once urine begins to flow, the penis need not be held in the extended position any longer.	10. Urine return depends on the length of the individual urethra and the amount of urine in the bladder.
11. If a urine specimen is desired, allow at least 5 ml of urine to flow into sterile specimen container from catheter. Allow remainder to flow into collecting basin. Hold catheter in place with left hand; arrange basin and specimen container with right.	11. As a rule, remove initially no more than 750 ml of urine from the bladder except under special circumstances to prevent rapid filling of abdominal vessels and possibly shock.
12. Following removal of the desired amount of urine, remove catheter gently but quickly; dry the penis well using the drape. In uncircumcised males, replace the foreskin over the glans.	12. If the foreskin is left retracted, it can form a constricting band that will cause edema and impair circulation to penis.
13. Position patient comfortably if in bed or help to return to bed if procedure was done in a treatment room. Evaluate the effectiveness, efficiency, cost, comfort, and safety or procedure. Plan health teaching as needed such as the importance of a good fluid intake for urinary function.	13. Health teaching is an independent nursing action always included as a part of care.
14. Record on chart that catheterization was accomplished, amount of urine obtained, whether a specimen was sent for analysis, and any abnormalities observed in procedure or urine.	14. Document nursing care and patient status.

MODIFICATIONS FOR CARE OF CHILD

Because catheterization involves minimal pain, it should be done in a treatment room rather than as a bedside procedure to keep the child's bed area a safe one.

MODIFICATIONS FOR CARE OF OLDER ADULT

Hypertrophy of the prostate gland may occur with aging. As the prostate presses on the urethra, at the junction of the bladder, catheterization may be very difficult. Do not force a catheter. If resistance is met, discontinue the procedure and alert the patient's physician to the problem. Catheterization may have to be done under anesthesia or suprapubically.

38-9). Never force the catheter against resistance. If resistance is met, pause a second in the event that it is caused by urethral spasm. If resistance continues after a few seconds, discontinue the procedure and notify the person's physician; resistance suggests that a urethral obstruction is present. This is most apt to occur in elderly men who have hypertrophy of the prostate gland causing pressure on the urethra.

Once urine begins to flow, the penis need not be held in the extended position any longer. In uncircumcised men, after catheter removal, be certain that you slide the foreskin forward again to cover the glans. If this is left retracted for an extended period of time, it forms a constricting band that will cause edema at the glans and could actually impair circulation to the anterior portion of the penis.

Penile erection is a normal physiological result of handling and may occur during catheterization. At one time, male catheterization was done only by physicians or male orderlies to reduce this possibility or because female nurses were assumed to be too naive or too embarrassed to deal with this circumstance. Today, the procedure, like female catheterization, is done by both male and female nurses. Erection leads to difficult catheter insertion. Working with a fair degree of speed (but never to the point of neglecting a gentle touch) and using a firm touch, not a light fleeing one, helps to eliminate the problem. Minimal handling prior to catheter insertion is also important. If erection should occur prior to catheter insertion, distracting actions such as conversation or asking the man to take a deep breath may be helpful. The man may be embarrassed, but your sure knowledge that it is caused not by a sexual response but by handling should allow you to keep it in perspective.

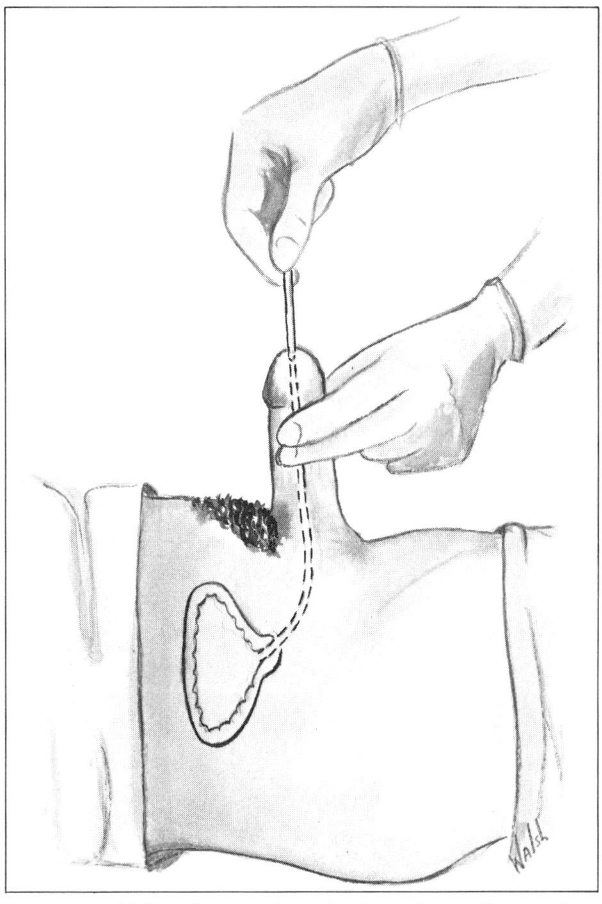

FIGURE 38-9. Male urinary catheterization. The penis must be held at a 90-degree angle to avoid trauma to the urethra.

RETENTION CATHETERS

A retention catheter is inserted with the same catheterization technique as a straight catheter except that extra equipment for inflating the balloon after the catheter is in place must be provided. Figures 38-10A and B show a retention catheter in place.

The size of the balloon on a retention catheter is indicated on the catheter; balloons are either 5 or 30 ml in size; a 5-ml size is the standard size used because it is large enough to allow the catheter to be retained but will not injure the bladder mucosa by constant full pressure. Either sterile distilled water or sterile normal saline can be used for inflating the balloon depending on health care agency policy. The solution used should be sterile so if the balloon should rupture inside the bladder, no microorganisms will be introduced. Additional equipment, therefore, includes a sterile 10-ml syringe filled with the designated amount of the correct solution for insertion of the fluid. For some brands of catheters you need slightly more fluid than the balloon holds or an additional 3 to 5 ml to fill the lumen. Many catheter brands do not require a needle for fluid insertion (Fig. 38-10).

With some brands of catheters it is possible to inflate the balloon and then deflate it prior to insertion to test the efficiency of the balloon. With other brands, the balloon is deflated by cutting off the distal end of the balloon tubing; with this type of catheter, obviously you cannot test the balloon prior to insertion.

As soon as the catheter is in place, hold it in place with your left hand after advancing it another 2 inches to be

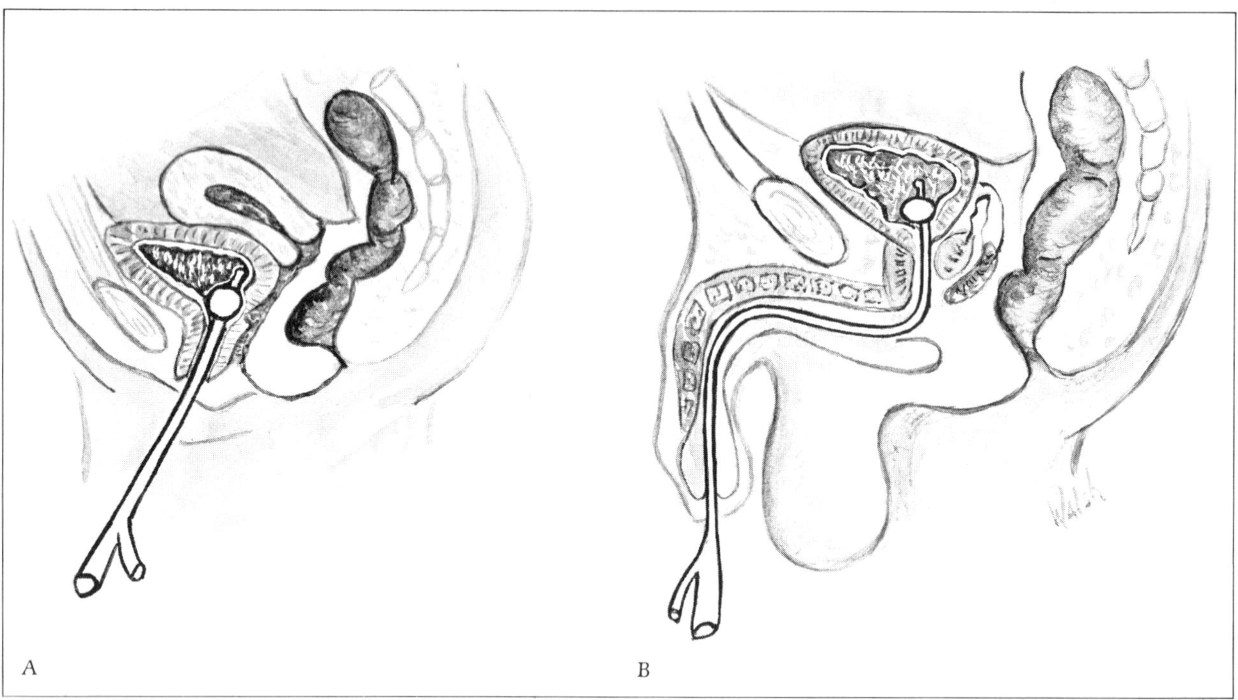

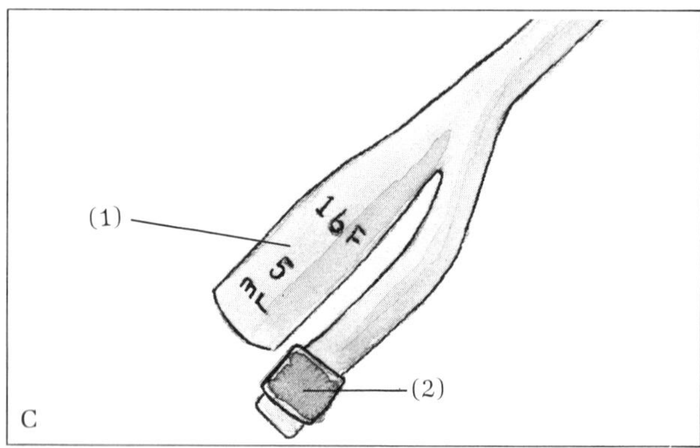

FIGURE 38-10. A retention catheter in place. A. Female catheter. B. Male catheter. C. Inflating the balloon.

certain that the balloon will inflate inside the bladder and not in the urethra (the balloon is not at the tip of the catheter but about a half inch from the tip). Inflate the balloon gently and check that it is inflated by pulling gently on the catheter. If pulling dislodges it because the balloon did not inflate, you will need to insert a second catheter. In males there is a greater chance that the balloon will inflate in the urethra than in females. After the balloon is inflated, move the catheter back and forth to affirm that the balloon is not lodged in the urethra.

Following inflation of the balloon, the catheter will need to be attached to a drainage bag and tubing. Do not touch the end of the catheter or tubing so that the inside of the tubing will remain sterile. You could connect the drainage tubing before insertion.

Establishing a Drainage System. Urine will flow by gravity from the retained catheter through the sterile tube to a drainage container. The drainage container must always be kept lower than the bladder so that urine does not drain from the collecting bag back into the bladder. Although urine is sterile in the bladder, like any fluid, if it stands for any length of time as it does in a collecting bag, it will grow a high proportion of microorganisms. Allowing urine to flow from the collecting bag back to the bladder is a sure way to introduce microorganisms or infection to the bladder. When a person is lying in bed, the collecting bag is generally attached to the lower bedframe; in a wheelchair, the best technique is to bring the tubing under the seat of the chair and hang the bag from the back of the seat (well away from the chair wheels and lower than the bladder) (Fig. 38-11). Be extremely careful when helping people from a bed to a sitting position that you always keep the collecting bag lower than the bladder during the move.

To prevent an accidental tug on the tubing with consequent trauma at the urinary meatus or actual dislodging of the catheter (which could cause severe urethral damage), the catheter is usually taped to a person's leg; if lying in bed, a rubber band may be secured to the tubing and the rubber band pinned to the bed. In a man, the penis should be brought up at an angle onto the abdomen, not taped to the leg to avoid putting pressure on the internal mucosa. If a safety pin cannot be used because of a water or air mattress, secure the tubing by means of adhesive tape to the mattress (Fig. 38-2).

Before helping people to move in bed or turn or sit up, always check that the catheter is not secured so tightly

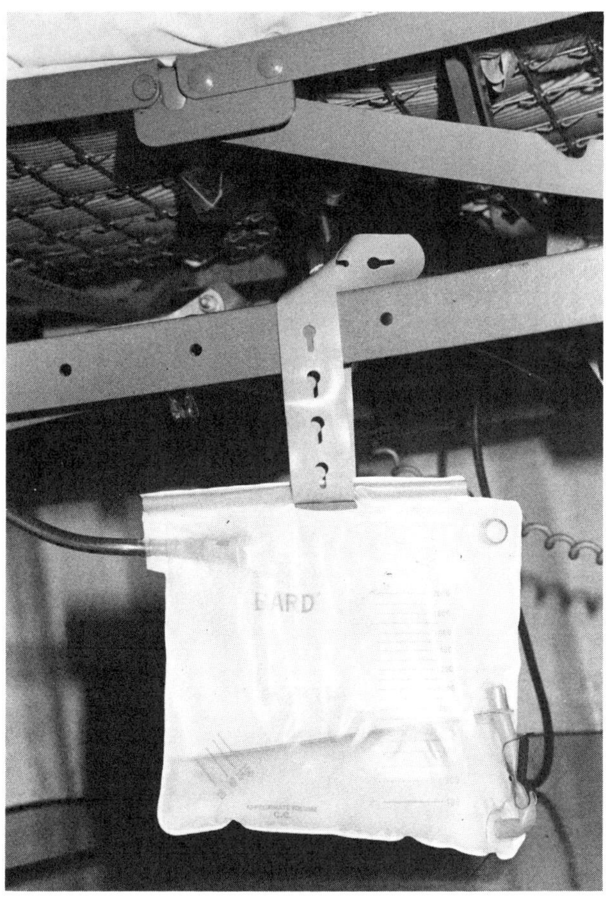

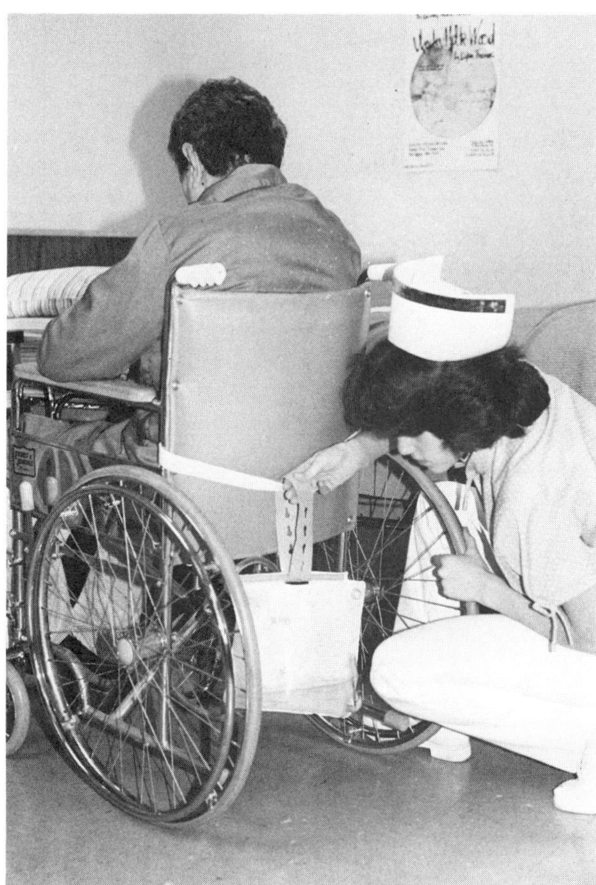

A B

FIGURE 38-11. A. For drainage to occur, the bag must be attached to the bed frame at a point lower than the patient's bladder to allow gravity's effect. B. If the patient is in a wheelchair, bring the tubing underneath and suspend the bag from the back frame of the wheelchair.

that it will pull with movement. After turning or repositioning a patient, always check that the catheter is not kinked or sharply bent so urine can drain freely. When turning a person from side to side, the drainage bag must be moved to the other side of the bed so the tubing is not positioned over the top of the thigh or compressed between legs but lies freely on the bed surface. For ambulatory patients, the physician may choose to have the catheter clamped for short periods (usually not over 2 hours), or it may be attached to a leg bag or a drainage container that attaches to the thigh or lower leg by expandable straps (Fig. 38-3). With this form of drainage bag, the person can be fully ambulatory without any reminder that the bag is in place because it can be fully covered by clothing. When the person returns to bed, the catheter should be reconnected to a regular drainage bag to prevent backflow from the leg bag into the bladder. Rinse the leg bag with clear water and hang it upside down to dry. People who are using leg bags at home may notice that they retain the odor of urine after about two weeks. Allowing them to soak for an hour in a white vinegar solution overnight about once a week will generally prevent the occurrence of this or remedy the problem if it has already occurred.

Perineal-Penile Care. Thorough washing of the urinary meatus and cleansing of any crustations from the catheter with warm soap and water followed by a clear water rinse should be done at least twice a day. Of all the protective measures used, this is probably the most effective. In the uncircumcised male, be certain to retract the foreskin and wash the entire glans well or secretions will form under the foreskin. Following thorough cleansing, an antibiotic ointment or an iodine-povidone ointment is generally applied around the catheter at the insertion point. Use of an individual foil packet of ointment is helpful for this because it can be applied to the catheter directly from the packet. A sterile cotton swab or a sterile disposable glove may be used to be certain the ointment approximates the meatus closely. If using a multidose ointment tube, always place the first drop of ointment on a tissue or other place before using it in case it is contaminated; do not apply it directly to the meatus from the tube because this would contaminate the remainder of the ointment in the tube. Your bare finger should not be used to spread antibiotic

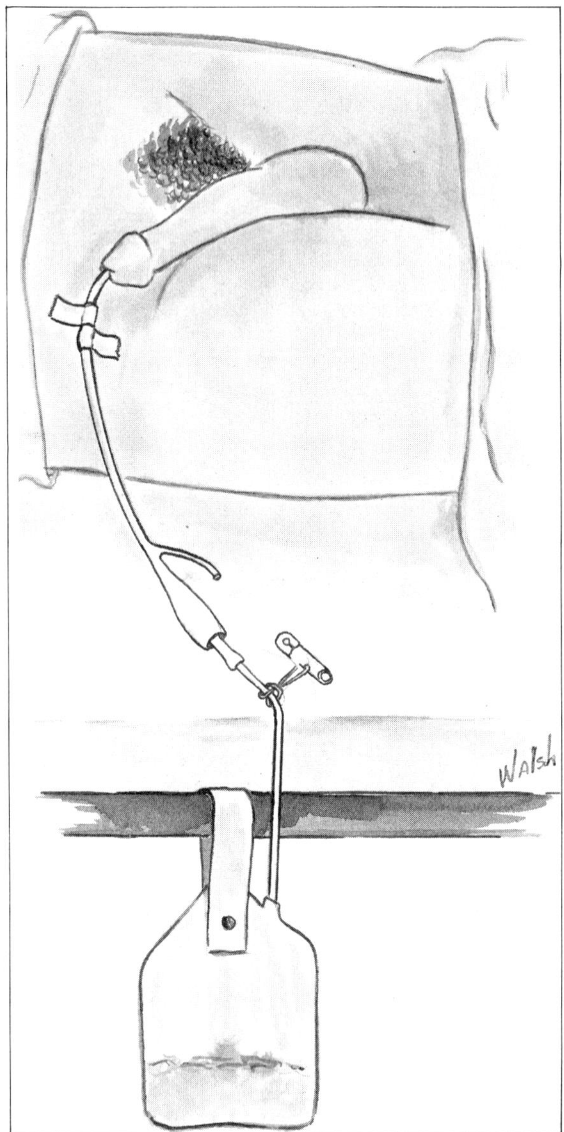

FIGURE 38-12. Taping the catheter to the patient avoids pulling on the tubing. Tape a male catheter on the lower abdomen to decrease compression at the penis-bladder juncture. Tape a female catheter to the leg.

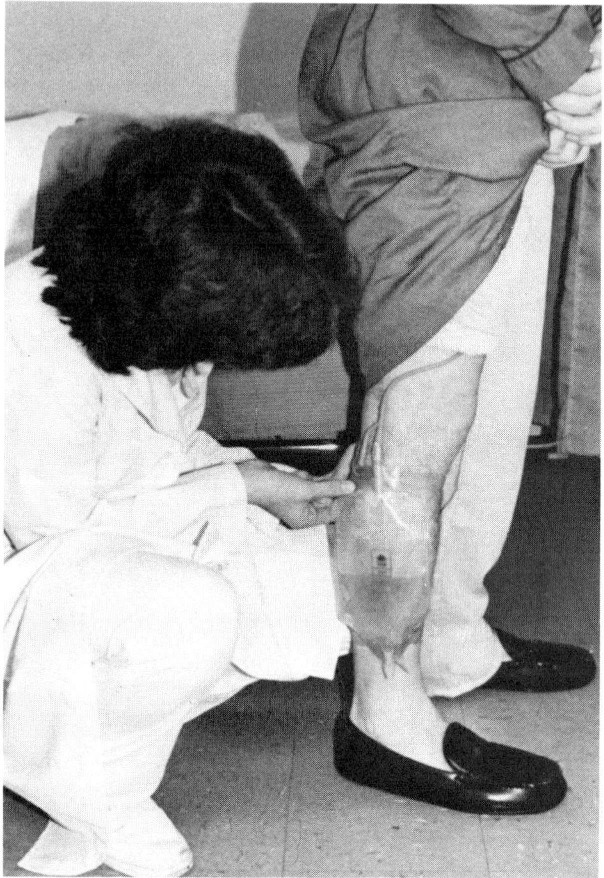

FIGURE 38-13. To encourage ambulation, a catheter may be attached to a leg bag (drainage bag that attaches to the thigh or lower leg by adjustable straps).

ointments (you add microorganisms that you are trying to prevent).

Some men may prefer to perform their own meatal care. Most men can do this independently following good instruction. However, you should still observe the area of catheter insertion at least twice daily to determine that there is no crusting or sign of inflammation at the site. Do not allow a urinary tract infection to develop because of modesty on his or your part.

Women have more difficulty performing their own catheter care because they are unable to view the point of catheter insertion. A woman who wishes to, however, may do this if you supply her with a mirror so she can view the urinary meatus for proper ointment application. Follow the same rule as with men: check at least twice daily for crustations or inflammation with independent patient catheter care. See Quick Reference Stops 38-4, 38-5, and 38-6 for important considerations related to catheterization.

Irrigating Retention Catheters. There is controversy about whether irrigation of retention catheters reduces the tendency toward urinary tract infection or not. In some instances, so much urinary sediment or blood may be present that irrigation is necessary to prevent sediment or a blood clot from clogging the catheter; in such a case the catheter actually becomes an obstruction to urine flow rather than an assisting device. Unfortunately, irrigation may aid the introduction of bacteria and actually cause a urinary tract infection. Follow individual health care agency policy about this process.

Catheter irrigation must be a sterile procedure using a sterile solution such as normal saline or a specially prescribed antiseptic solution. It is done once or twice a day depending on the reason for the irrigation and special circumstances.

Materials needed include the specified irrigation fluid, an asepto syringe, and a collecting basin such as a kidney basin (often furnished as a prepackaged set). For

☐ **QUICK REFERENCE STOP 38-4: SAFETY**
Urinary Output

To protect against urinary tract infection always be certain that a collecting bag for a retention catheter is lower than the bladder so that urine flows from the bladder to the collecting bag and not vice versa.

Use sterile technique with bladder catheterization.

To avoid trauma to the urethral bladder junction in males with retention catheters, tape the catheter to the lower abdomen, not the thigh, to avoid a sharp bend at the junction of the urethra and the bladder.

A Valsalva maneuver occurs when a person takes a deep breath and holds it while contracting the abdominal muscles and straining to void. This maneuver is effective because it increases the intra-abdominal pressure and forces urine out of the bladder. It also increases intrathoracic pressure because of the filled lungs. A Valsalva maneuver is not recommended for people with cardiac conditions because the increased pressure may slow the return of blood to the heart by the inferior vena cava; when the person releases his breath, a great deal of blood returns to the heart all at once, causing tachycardia and possibly a strain on a diseased heart. To counteract this effect, a person who is straining to void should breathe out, not hold his breath.

adults the amount of solution used is 30 to 50 ml; for children, the exact amount should be prescribed (it may be as little as 5 ml in infants). Fill the asepto syringe with the desired fluid (in children you might want to use a 10- to 20-ml syringe with an adaptor tip because of the small amount of fluid involved). At the bedside, wash the connecting portion of the catheter and tubing with an alcohol swab and then separate it at that point. Alcohol is used because when you fit the connection together again, it may not slide back to the same point, and the alcohol wash ensures no microorganisms will be inserted when you do reattach these tubes. Because the end of the collecting tube will be reinserted into the catheter at the end of the irrigation, you must not allow it to be exposed unnecessarily to microorganisms while you irrigate the catheter. You can achieve this by holding it in the same hand in which you hold the end of the catheter as you work, or you can wrap it with a sterile gauze square and tuck it under the edge of the mattress out of your way (Fig. 38-14). The foil wrapper of the alcohol sponge is another effective wrapper; sterile caps are also available. Do not be careless with this connecting tubing; microorganisms can easily travel the 12 to 14 inches of the catheter length from it to the bladder.

☐ **QUICK REFERENCE STOP 38-5: SAFETY**
Trouble Shooting with a Retention Catheter

Before leaving the bedside of a person with a retention catheter, always check the following points.

1. Connections between the catheter and tubing are tight and not leaking.
2. The tubing is not kinked but arranged in well-rounded loops.
3. The drainage bag is lower than the bladder to allow drainage by gravity.
4. There are two security points (tape is attached to the lower abdomen or thigh and a rubber band and pin or tape is attached to the bedsheet so that any pull on the tubing will register at the security point, not at the urinary meatus).
5. There is no tension at the urinary meatus; constant tension will dislodge the catheter or impair circulation at the meatus.
6. The person's body weight is not resting on the tubing to cause obstruction.
7. Observe the level of the urinary drainage in the collection bag. An increase in the amount of urine present in the collecting bag is your assurance that the catheter is functioning properly and the person's urinary output is adequate (an average adult voids about 50 ml per hour).

☐ **QUICK REFERENCE STOP 38-6: PSYCHOLOGICAL CONSIDERATIONS**
Privacy

Urinary elimination is an embarrassing topic for many people, particularly older adults who were raised when modesty was more valued than it is today. Respect this by always providing for proper draping and privacy with procedures that reveal the genitals such as catheterization. If it is necessary to post signs in a patient's room to remind other health care providers to measure or test urine, do not use the word *urine* ("measure I + O," not "measure all urine") because the person may be embarrassed to have his visitors know that he is having some problem with this area of body control.

After the tubing is disconnected, attach the sterile asepto syringe to the distal end of the catheter and, using gentle pressure, inject the specified amount of solution (Fig. 38-15). Remove the syringe and allow the solution to flow back into an emesis basin or other container. This double flow—injecting solution and draining it back—assures you that the catheter is truly patent. Always be certain that as much solution is removed as was

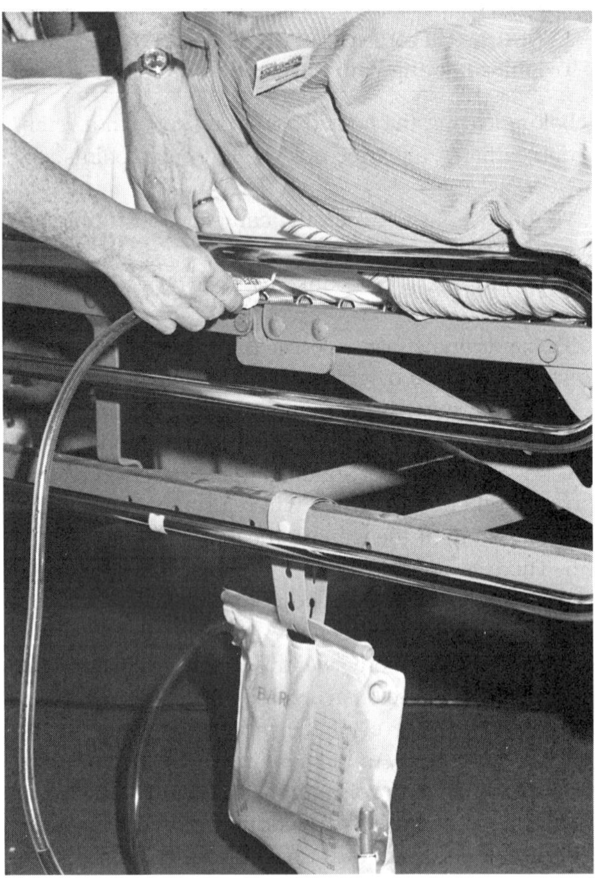

FIGURE 38-14. To keep the distal collecting tube clean, cover it with a sterile cap or foil top wiped with alcohol, and tuck it under the mattress.

FIGURE 38-15. When irrigating a retention catheter, be certain to inject fluid gently to avoid bladder spasm. Shown here is a 3-lumen catheter.

injected. If solution does not return, it may mean that a ball-valve effect is present or that the catheter is patent in only one direction (fluid can flow in but not out).

As the irrigating solution is returned, some urine returns with it. Inspect the return for abnormalities (mucus shreds, heavy sediment, color, odor, blood). Infected urine will be cloudy, pus-filled, and perhaps blood-tinged from mucosal irritation. If the urine is thick with sediment or very concentrated, it suggests that the person needs more fluid than he is currently receiving. Following return of the irrigating solution, reconnect the tubing and catheter and check that the tubing is not kinked and in a good drainage position. Some brands of catheters have resealable ports to use for catheter irrigation; after the tubing is clamped below the port, fluid is introduced into these with a syringe and needle after careful cleansing of the port. This type is preferable because there is less danger of introducing microorganisms.

Record any fluid obtained over the amount of your irrigation solution on the patient's intake and output sheet as urine output. If you did not remove all the solution you injected, record this as a retained amount; it will have to be subtracted from the urine total.

Internal Catheter Irrigation. Another method of irrigating retention catheters is termed *internal* irrigation. In this method one ensures that the person's fluid intake is high, and therefore urine is produced in large amounts, which flush the catheter daily by the large volume of flow. An intake of 2,000 to 3,000 ml a day will be adequate to achieve this flushing effect for an adult and, unless otherwise contraindicated, should always be tried when a person has an indwelling catheter.

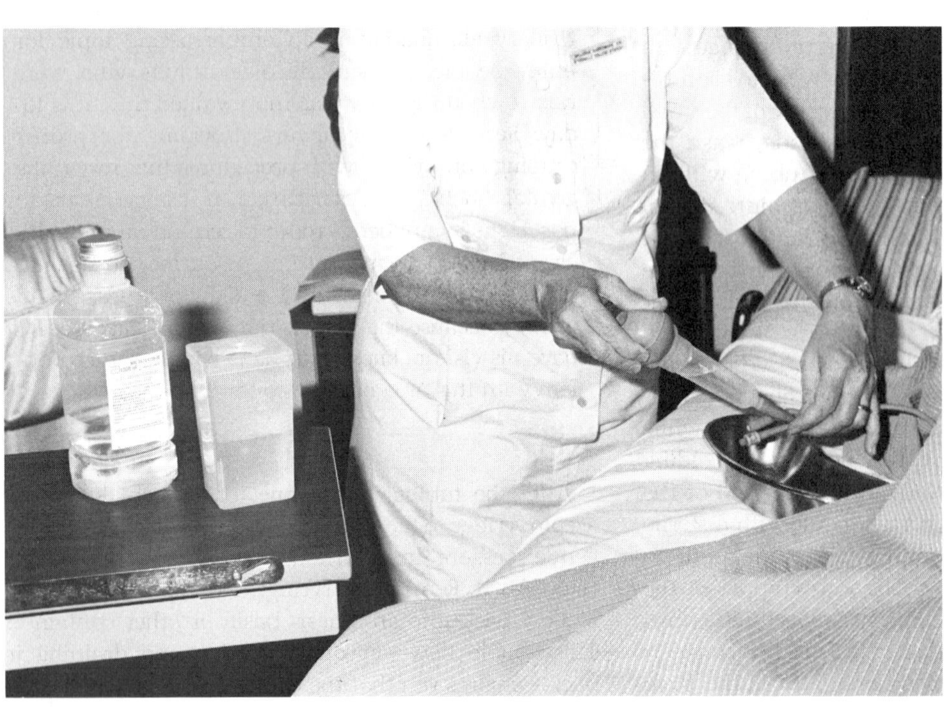

Continuous Bladder Irrigation. Following bladder or prostate surgery to reduce clot formations and to reduce the possibility of urinary tract infection in people with retention catheters, continuous bladder irrigation may be provided. To reduce high bladder bacterial counts by inflation and deflation of the bladder and to help maintain bladder tone, intermittent bladder irrigation may be prescribed. For this type of irrigation, a special type of catheter with three lumens is used. One lumen is used to inflate the balloon, one allows fluid to flow into the bladder, and one allows fluid to flow out of the bladder (Fig. 38-16).

If continuous irrigation is desired, a specified solution is allowed to drip from a bottle attached to the catheter by a tube similar to infusion of intravenous fluid. Fluid mixed with collecting urine will also continuously flow out of the catheter into the collection bag.

If intermittent irrigation is desired, a clamp on the tube to the solution bottle is released and a specified amount of fluid is allowed to enter the bladder; the drainage tubing is clamped during infusion to cause the solution to remain in the bladder for a specified amount of time. Following this designated time interval, the clamp on the drainage tubing is released, and urine and solution drain from the bladder.

FIGURE 38-16. Continuous bladder irrigation.

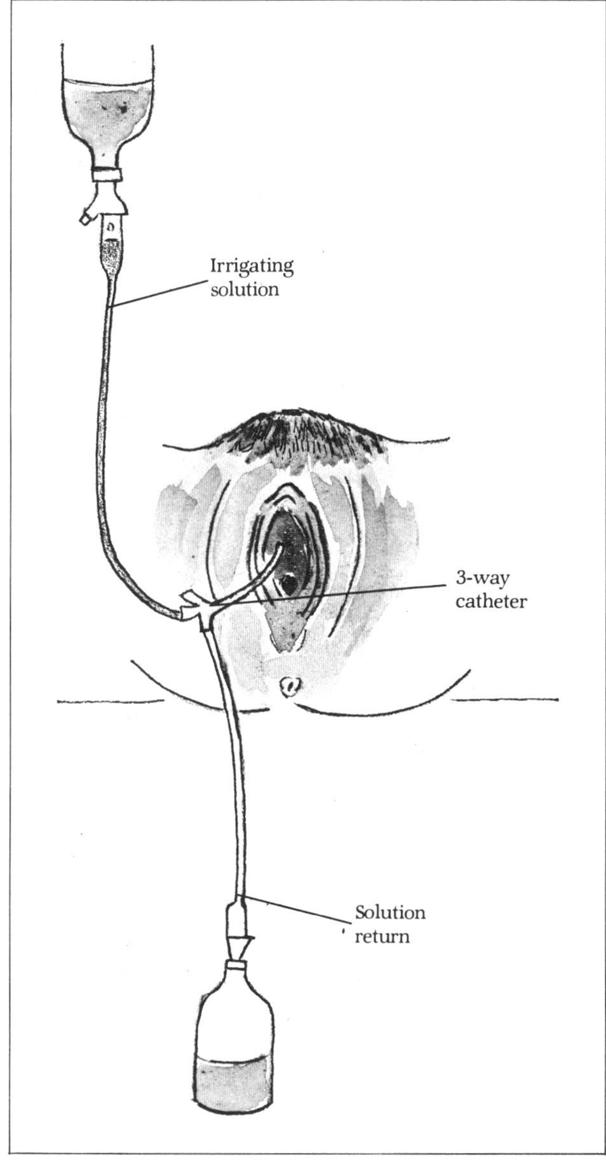

To measure urine output with these systems remember to subtract the amount of fluid infused; otherwise, the amount of urine cannot be accurately determined. You must be aware of how much fluid is collecting in the drainage bag to prevent it from overflowing and forcing solution and urine back into the bladder.

Changing Catheters and Tubing. Microorganisms grow very quickly on the tubing and collecting bags of retention catheters because urine is a good growth medium for organisms, particularly if the person is spilling any protein or glucose in urine. In most health care agencies, tubing and collecting bags are changed every 24 to 48 hours to reduce bacterial counts in these reservoirs. The length of time the catheter is left in place varies with the reason for its insertion. If it was inserted because there was a urethral obstruction, it will be left in place until the obstruction can be relieved because inserting another one past the obstruction would be very difficult; if it was inserted to relieve incontinence, it might be changed every week. Newer systems of collecting apparatus are closed systems. The catheter, tubing, and drainage bag are all connected and cannot be disconnected, so the tubing and drainage bag cannot be changed unless the catheter is changed also. With this apparatus, the entire system is left in place until the catheter is changed.

To change the tubing and collecting bag, clamp the catheter and disconnect the tubing. Because you are going to discard the tubing, you do not need to be concerned with keeping the end of it free of organisms. Tuck it under the mattress of the bed to keep it out of your way. Remove the new drainage tubing from its protective cover and remove the protective cap from the end, being careful not to touch the end of the tubing against your hand or the bedclothes. Insert the new tubing into the catheter and remove the clamp from the catheter. Attach a rubber band or adhesive tape to the new tubing and tape it to a woman's thigh or to a man's lower abdomen; if there should be a tug on the tubing, the force will stop at the attachment point and the catheter will not be dislodged. Be sure that the collecting bag is attached to the bedframe lower than the level of the bladder so that drainage will occur by gravity and urine will not flow from the collecting bag back to the bladder. Never attach the collecting bag to the side railing or raised portion of the bed.

Emptying Collecting Bags. Collecting bags are usually emptied at the end of each 8-hour nursing shift; the amount emptied is recorded so the amount of drainage can be calculated at the end of the 24-hour period.

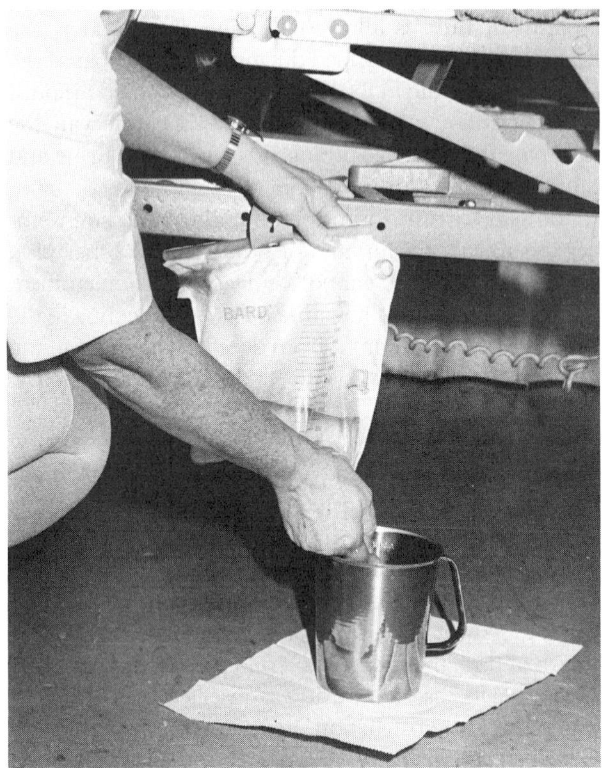

FIGURE 38-17. Emptying urine from a collecting bag.

Collecting bags empty by a bottom outlet attachment. Bring a container for measuring to the bedside, open the bottom valve, and allow the urine to drain into the measuring container (Fig. 38-17). Be certain to include in the total any amount of urine that was removed for a laboratory specimen or with irrigation of the catheter.

Urine Specimens and Retention Catheters. To be sure that a urinary tract infection is not developing, periodic urine cultures are generally ordered. Specimens for protein or glucose analysis are obtained by the same method. To obtain a sterile urine specimen with a retention catheter in place, clamp the tubing for 10 to 15 minutes before attempting to obtain a specimen. Secure a sterile 5-ml syringe, a small-gauge needle (No. 25 to No. 22), and an alcohol swab. After swabbing off the catheter distal to the bifurcation of the balloon tubing, insert the needle into the catheter and withdraw urine with the syringe (Fig. 38-18). Be certain that your insertion site is distal to the bifurcation of the balloon injection tubing or you may accidentally puncture the lumen of the balloon tubing and withdraw the fluid that is inflating the balloon. Many brands of catheters now have special ports for use in withdrawing specimens. Withdraw the needle when 5 ml is obtained and transfer it to a specimen tube or container. This method of obtaining a urine specimen ensures that bladder urine is obtained, and the culture will demonstrate accurately whether an infection is present or not. If you take urine from the tubing or collection bag, the bacterial count may be higher because microorganisms multiply in the collection bag, and the culture report will undoubtedly be falsely positive. Be sure to use a very small needle when puncturing retention catheters for specimens.

Removal of Retention Catheters. People are often worried that a catheter will hurt when it is removed. Provide a good explanation and stress that the actual removal process takes only 1 or 2 seconds.

To remove a retention catheter you need a cover to contain the catheter (a disposable waterproof pad works well), a syringe to remove the fluid from the inflated balloon, and a container such as a medicine cup or emesis basin to contain the balloon solution. Depending on the brand of catheter and health agency policy, you

FIGURE 38-18. Obtaining a urine specimen from a retention catheter. Notice that the puncture is made distal to the bifurcation of the balloon tubing to prevent puncturing of the tubing.

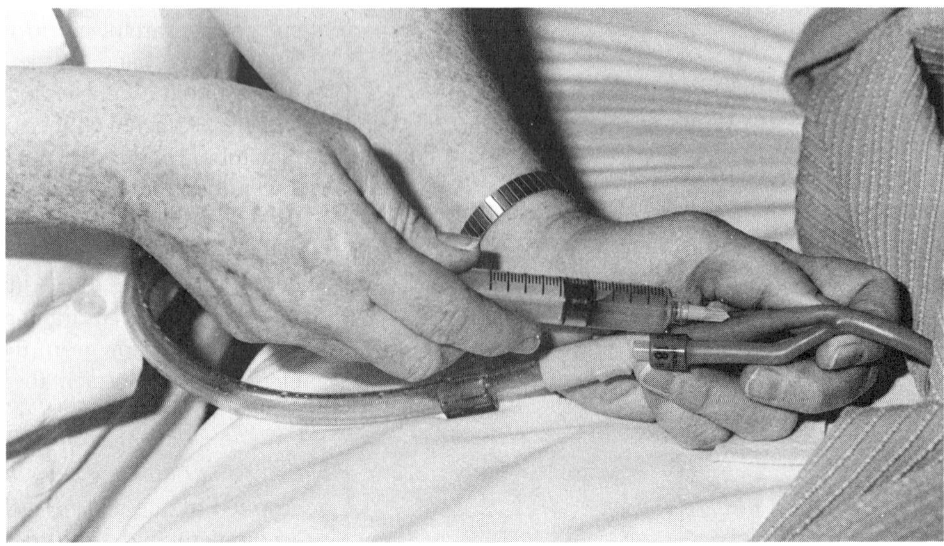

may be able to deflate the balloon by cutting the tube to the balloon with scissors and simply allowing the contained fluid to flow out. A plastic medicine cup can be used to hold the draining balloon solution; measuring the amount obtained assures you that the balloon is fully deflated prior to removal. If you are removing the fluid from the balloon by inserting a syringe and needle into the tubing and withdrawing the fluid, note the size of the balloon (5 to 30 ml) and remove that amount of fluid. If you remove less, the balloon will not be fully deflated and will cause trauma and pressure to the urethra as it is removed. When the correct amount of fluid has been withdrawn into a syringe or has run out of the cut tubing, you know that the balloon is fully collapsed. Use a momentary distraction technique such as asking the person to take a deep breath, inspect the meatal area to be certain that no crusting is present that would cause pain due to an adherent catheter, and gently pull the catheter to remove it. Use a gentle but rapid motion to remove the catheter in 1 or 2 seconds, reducing the possibility of muscle spasm and pain.

Wrap the catheter in the protective pad and dispose of it and the tubing and collection bag in a utility room container. Do not drop it into a wastepaper basket in the patient's room. Measure the amount of urine, and complete the patient's output record. If the person has not voided by 8 hours after removal, assess his bladder for overdistention.

A person may notice some burning when he voids for the first time after removal of a retention catheter. This is caused by irritation of the urethra from the catheter. Urge him to drink fluid readily to keep urine dilute; this will reduce the concentration of urine and minimize burning. Measure urinary output for the first 24 hours after removal of a retention catheter as an independent nursing action. A bladder loses tone with a catheter in place and may not respond to filling as well as previously for the first 24 hours after catheter removal. This can lead to retention of urine.

Monitoring Bladder Tone. Because a urinary bladder never fills entirely when a retention catheter is in place, it may lose its ability to sense filling during this time. One method utilized to encourage bladder tone is to clamp the catheter for about a 2-hour period, open it for a half hour, clamp it again for 2 hours, and so forth to mimic a normal voiding pattern. If such a schedule is prescribed, make out a chart for the person's nursing care plan that specifies the times of opening and closing so that all caregivers can consistently carry out the pattern.

SUPRAPUBIC CATHETERS

A suprapubic catheter is, as the name implies, a catheter inserted, not through the urinary urethra, but through a stab wound in the lower abdomen into the bladder just over the pubis. A retention catheter can be used as a suprapubic tube (the balloon is inflated just as if it were inserted urethrally to keep it in place), or a mushroom-tipped catheter (see Fig. 38-7D) may be inserted. A mushroom tip has a hard rubber base and cannot be inflated or deflated; it will hold the catheter securely in place until time for removal by means of a second small surgical procedure under local anesthesia.

Suprapubic catheters are used following bladder or urethral surgery when the irritation of a urethral catheter might interfere with healing of sutures; they are also used to alleviate incontinence. Women past the age of menopause have a high incidence of monilial (fungal) vaginal infections due to the change in vaginal secretions. A woman who tends to have frequent vaginal infections is more prone to develop urinary tract contamination with a urethral catheter than with a suprapubic catheter because the infection may spread from the vagina to the urethra.

Once a suprapubic catheter has been placed (under local anesthesia a sharp scalpel is inserted into the bladder; the tube is inserted, and two to four stitches are placed in the skin to halt bleeding and secure the tube in place), it is managed as a urethral retention catheter. Drainage is by gravity flow; care and aseptic technique with irrigations are given as if it were a urethral catheter. Many people find the thought of a suprapubic catheter distasteful (mutilating or intrusive) and need support to accept such a procedure. Most suprapubic catheters are used, however, for short time periods such as immediately following surgery; the person can see that it is only a temporary measure and will be removed once the internal suture line has healed. If the catheter is being used to alleviate incontinence, check the bedding when the patient is turned (every 2 hours) to be certain that it is achieving this purpose. If the person has extremely lax urethral sphincter control, he may still have difficulty with incontinence, and the perineal skin will become extremely excoriated from even minor urine flow from the urethra.

Suprapubic catheters typically drain blood-tinged urine for the first 4 hours following insertion because of bleeding caused by the puncture wound used to insert the catheter. If this condition persists or is more than merely blood-tinged, the person's physician should be notified because a "bleeder" or a capillary at the point of insertion might not be fully obliterated.

URETERAL CATHETERS

Following bladder, kidney, pelvic, or ureteral surgery, a person may have extremely thin catheters (called stints) inserted for the length of the ureters. These thread into the bladder and exit usually at a suprapubic point. The drainage from such catheters is usually kept separate from drainage from a urethral catheter or a suprapubic bladder catheter so that urine can be seen flowing through both ureters.

If kidney surgery was performed, drainage will be blood-tinged for the first 24 hours after surgery. Be extremely careful when moving or turning a person with many catheters to trace the length of each catheter and be certain that none will pull out. Be extremely strict with measures to prevent contamination of collecting tubing attached to stint catheters. The opposite end of the catheter is placed very close to or in the kidney pelvis. If microorganisms are introduced due to carelessness, they will be delivered directly to the kidney, and a potentially lethal infection may result. Never clamp ureteral catheters because a kidney pelvis is very small (it holds only 10 to 20 ml) and needs to drain continually to prevent distention with consequent kidney nephron destruction.

SELF-CATHETERIZATION

Self-catheterization is a technique that allows people to be independent in urinary elimination by performing bladder catheterization on themselves. Self-catheterization appears to break all the rules because it is done with clean, not sterile, technique, and is done frequently (every 4 to 6 hours), not as rarely as possible. To perform this, the person washes his hands and the urinary meatus with a washcloth and soap and water (a paper towel if using a public washroom) and then rinses the urinary meatus with the washcloth and clear water. He uses a clean catheter for catheterization, allowing urine to flow into the bathroom toilet. When the bladder is empty, the catheter is removed, washed well with clear water, and stored in a container such as a plastic bag until it is reused.

This procedure leads to a very low incidence of urinary tract infection because the microorganisms in a home setting are generally not pathogenic (disease-causing), unlike the organisms in a health care agency, and because it is done so frequently that urine does not remain in the bladder long enough to become a culture medium for bacterial growth. Also, the filling pressure on the bladder walls never becomes extensive; the pressure that normally occurs in this way may decrease circulation to the bladder mucosa, inviting infection.

Children as young as 6 years of age can be taught self-catheterization and can perform it themselves at school. It allows people to maintain full-time jobs or sports activities without use of collecting tubes. Girls and women need a mirror the first several times they do this so that they can view the urinary meatus, but with practice, they have no difficulty inserting the catheter without it. During menstruation women need to be particularly careful to wash the urinary meatus well to cleanse any accumulated menstrual blood from the meatal opening.

The important criteria for self-catheterization are that it is done with clean, not careless technique (washing hands and the urinary meatus is necessary) and that it is done frequently (no skipping).

An advantage of self-catheterization for males is that it allows a normal sex life, which would not be as

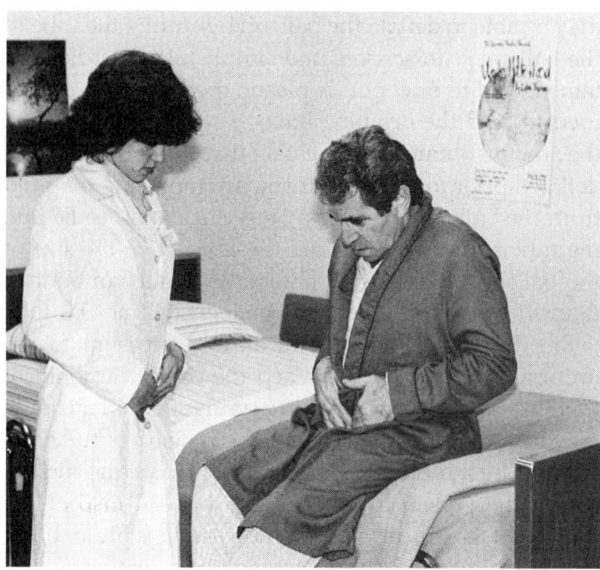

FIGURE 38-19. Teaching a Credé maneuver to a patient.

possible with a retention catheter in place. Both men and women need to be aware of the symptoms of urinary tract infection (pain, frequency, and burning on urination) so that they can contact their physician if these symptoms should occur.

Credé Maneuver

A Credé maneuver is the manual expression of urine by pressing with one or both hands inward and downward over the suprapubic area of the abdomen to evacuate the bladder or urine. People with neurological illnesses such as spinal cord injury who have no sensation of bladder filling use this technique to empty the bladder about every 4 hours during the day (Fig. 38-19).

Bladder Retraining

Bladder retraining is a process of retraining a bladder to empty periodically following some injury or disruption in normal function. This is a long-term process (requiring several months to a year) and requires self-motivation from the patient and cooperation between the patient and caregivers.

For a bladder retraining program, the person is urged to use a bedpan or the bathroom to void every 2 hours whether he feels any need to void or not. Use of a Credé maneuver or listening to the sound of running water are helpful to initiate voiding. Over a period of time, the bladder becomes accustomed to emptying only at these times. Because most people in need of bladder retraining also have some degree of immobility due to a primary neurological or muscular impairment, bladder retraining programs require a great deal of effort, time, and coordination of a nursing staff (being available every 2 hours to offer a bedpan or assist a person to a bathroom). To help the person have a desire to void, fluid may be offered every 2 hours (one half hour before

☐ **QUICK REFERENCE STOP 38-7: COMMUNITY CONSIDERATIONS**
Home Care on Bladder Retraining Program

People may be discharged from a health care facility with retention catheters still in place; they may return home to continue bladder retraining and to learn self-catheterization. Home care and additional supervision and teaching are often provided to such people by a community health nurse.

Be certain before discharge from a health care agency that appropriate referral has been made so that there is no time gap before home care begins; urinary incontinence and urinary tract infection can develop quickly if the person is unable to adjust to a routine without professional support. People who are going to be performing self-catheterization must think through their daily schedule so that they can be sure that a bathroom or restroom will be available to them every 4 hours throughout the day. Remind them that this applies to vacations or Saturdays and Sundays as well as week days. Help the person who has had bladder retraining (or his primary caregiver) to establish a set schedule for voiding. This often involves effort because the person must be helped to transfer to a wheelchair, then to a toilet, back to a wheelchair, and so forth. It may be tempting at the end of a busy day to let a person who has fallen asleep on the living room couch watching television sleep rather than wake him for the regular last voiding of the day. Such neglect, however, might lead to urinary incontinence or defeat a carefully controlled regimen. Support from a community health nurse can offer the motivation a support person needs to continue this type of care day after day.

A person with a retention catheter may choose either to have a community health nurse change the catheter periodically or to learn from her how to change the catheter themselves using sterile technique. Men can do this for themselves; women need a support person to do it for them to maintain sterile technique. A community health nurse is also important for teaching many of the fine points in catheter care and in giving assurance that people are doing well with their own care. School nurses or nurses in industrial settings are instrumental in ensuring that adults or children are able to comply with a self-catheterization schedule and have access to a high fluid intake during the day to ensure good bladder filling.

Adults with retention catheters are often concerned about how to manage sexual relationships with catheters in place. With women, the presence of a catheter should not interfere with penile-vaginal intercourse because the catheter is pliable and compresses easily. Men should be taught to remove the catheter and replace it with a second sterile one following sexual relations. Such men are probably candidates for a self-catheterization program, making this no longer a problem.

the time of voiding). Fluid is kept to a minimum following the evening meal to limit the need to void during sleep.

When setting up a timed program, coordinate voiding times with diuretic administration as well (the voiding time should not fall at 10 o'clock just before the diuretic is administered but closer to 11:00, when the bladder is beginning to fill from the effect of the diuretic administered an hour before). Quick Reference Stop 38-7 discusses further considerations for the person who will return home on a bladder retraining program.

External Urinary Collectors

To avoid the possibility of introducing infection from a urethral or suprapubic catheter, various external urinary collecting devices may be used.

INFANT COLLECTORS

To collect a single urine specimen in infants, a clear pliable plastic bag is attached to the girl's perineum or surrounds the boy's penis with a self-adhesive band. Be certain that the child's skin is clean and dry (no powder or diaper ointment) prior to adhering these devices. Because most infants void when they drink, a bottle or a glass of fluid should be offered as soon as the collector is in place (Fig. 38-20).

For a 24-hour urine collection in an infant, collection devices such as that shown in Fig. 38-20 are available that have an additional tube that is attached to a collecting bag and allow drainage by gravity.

MALE EXTERNAL COLLECTORS

In males an external appliance can be applied to replace an indwelling catheter. Such an external catheter is frequently termed a *condom, Fergusen,* or *Texas catheter.* It can be hand-made from a condom, adhesive tape, and a tube and collection bag such as that used with retention catheters, or a commercially manufactured one may be used.

Use of such a catheter tends to prevent urinary tract infection and trauma to the urethra; it has the disadvantage that urine is constantly in contact with the penis skin surface, and extreme excoriation of the skin can therefore occur. Also, these catheters tend to be difficult

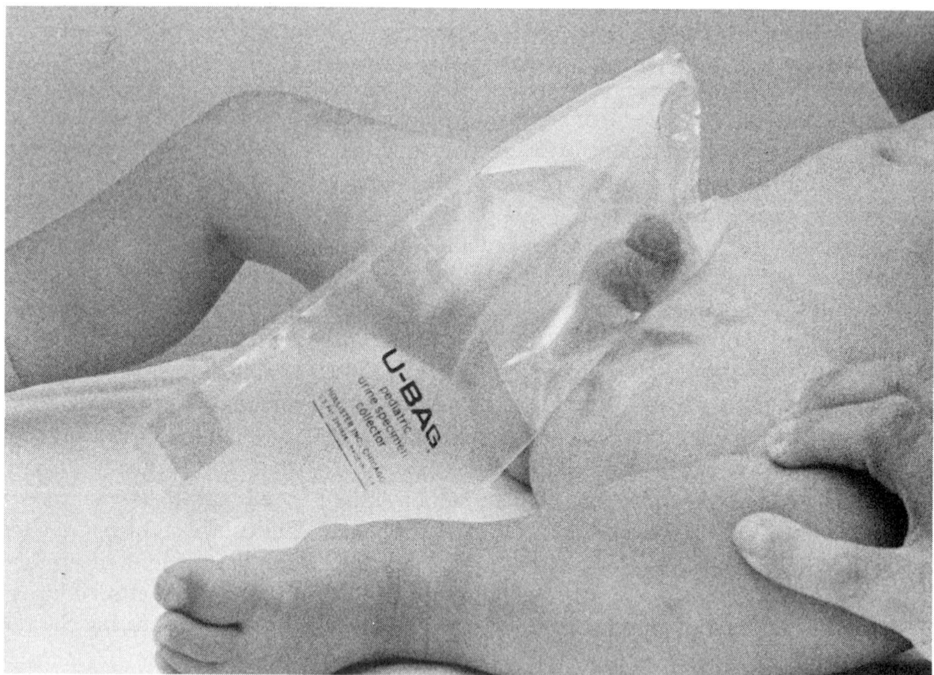

FIGURE 38-20. An external urine collection for an infant.

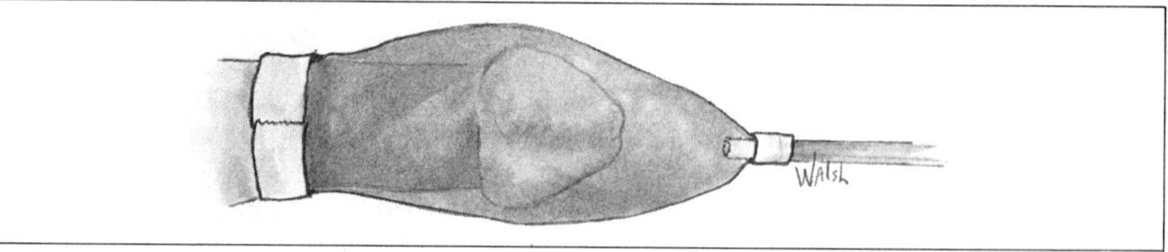

FIGURE 38-21. A male external urine collection.

to keep on and can cause damage to the penis from constricting pressure.

Before application of an external catheter, wash the penis well with soap and water, rinse it, and dry well. In some males pubic hair extends well down over the base of the penis. If an external catheter is going to be in place for longer than 24 hours, it is best to shave this pubic hair to avoid pain each time the apparatus is changed. To make the condom adhere closely, many health care agencies suggest painting the skin of the shaft of the penis with a layer of tincture of benzoin and covering it with surgical adhesive (very thick tacky paste). The condom is rolled into a ring and slipped over the penis against the ring of paste like a rolled stocking being pulled into place (Fig. 38-21).

When placing an external catheter on an uncircumcised male, be sure not to retract the foreskin. If the foreskin is left retracted, it can cause sharp interference with circulation to the distal penis, creating extreme pain and discomfort and actually causing cell anoxia over the gland.

When applying such a catheter, you must handle the penis, which may cause physiological erection. Erection will enlarge the penis, making the condom more difficult to fit, but will also stiffen it, making the procedure faster. Work with speed and handle the penis as little as possible to reduce the erection, which may be embarrassing for the man.

External catheters should be replaced daily and the penile skin washed well and dried between applications. It is helpful if the penis is exposed to air for about a half hour before reapplication to protect the skin from continuous moisture. Removing it before a bath and reapplying it at the end of the bath allows such a time interval.

Check skin condition and drainage about every 2 hours. If the tubing kinks, the kink is usually at the point where it joins the condom. Always check this site to be certain that the tubing is straight.

FEMALE EXTERNAL COLLECTORS

For a woman, unfortunately, no device as convenient as an external appliance has been devised. Women with stress incontinence can achieve dryness by using a sanitary napkin because this form of incontinence usually does not involve a larger amount of urine than a pad can absorb. Commercial waterproof panties with insert lin-

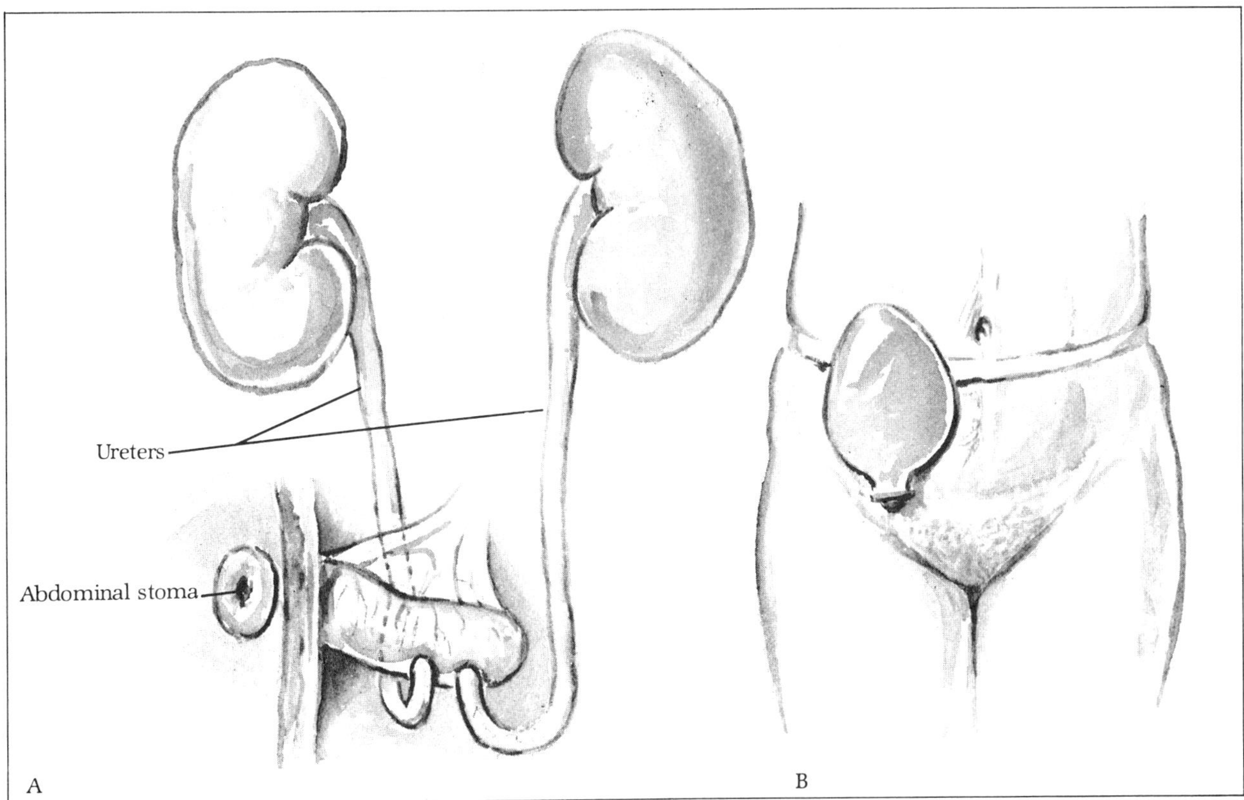

FIGURE 38-22. An ileal conduit. A. Internal view. B. External view with bag in place. (Courtesy Dept. of Medical Illustration, State University of New York at Buffalo, Buffalo, New York.)

ers are available, but these tend to be expensive and appear bulky under clothing.

In a health care setting the use of diapers to keep bed linen dry is never recommended, although in some instances they may be necessary temporarily to keep urine from wetting the suture line of a recent surgical procedure or to keep a recently applied cast dry. Never refer to diapers used this way as diapers in the presence of patients. Refer to them instead as padding or pads. They are never a long-term solution but should be replaced, if at all possible, with alternative techniques such as bladder retraining or self-catheterization programs.

Urinary Diversion

In people who have had extensive disease of the bladder or in children who were born without a functioning bladder, the bladder may be removed and the ureters diverted into an ileal conduit or into the colon. For an ileal conduit, a small segment of the ileum is removed from the intestinal tract and attached to the internal abdominal wall, simulating an ostomy stoma. The ureters are implanted in this section of ileum, and urine drains continually from the ureters into the collecting ileal section and then into a collecting apparatus attached to the abdominal surface (Fig. 38-22). The greatest difficulties with a urinary diversion technique are that the bag must be worn continuously, urine irritates the abdominal skin, and body image problems may occur owing to the abdominal appearance of the stoma and bag.

Ureters may be reimplanted directly into the colon, and urine drains with stool from the rectum. Feces in these individuals will always be more liquid than normal and tend to cause rectal irritation because of the urine acidity contained in them. The procedure is done less often today, although practice varies from one section of the country to another.

COMMON URINARY ELIMINATION PROBLEMS

Urinary Incontinence

Urinary incontinence is involuntary loss of urine. It occurs from inability to control the external sphincter of the bladder. Such loss of control can occur with musculoskeletal illness, spinal cord injury, bladder infection, overdistention of the bladder, or neurological trauma. Incontinence is not only embarrassing but also very frustrating because it involves a loss of self-esteem.

People with musculoskeletal or spinal cord injuries can be taught to empty the bladder periodically (by the Credé method or by self-catheterization, which allows them to remain continent. Bladder retraining, although a long process, is successful in some people.

Assess urinary incontinence to determine whether it is

a constant incontinence (continual dribbling of small amounts of urine) or occasional uncontrolled voiding. This information aids the person's physician in diagnosis and in determining therapy. Differentiation of these types of impairment requires observation over a period of time, so it is best determined by the person giving continuous care.

PERINEAL HYGIENE

Because urine is acid it is excoriating and damaging to the skin. A major problem of the person with incontinence is skin irritation and breakdown from the constant moisture. Check the beds of people who are incontinent frequently (every hour at least) to be certain that linen is dry. Always wash any skin that urine has touched with clear water and dry well. Turn the person so that the area of wet skin is no longer pressed against the bed surface and does dry fully. It is not enough just to add a dry pad to the bottom linen rather than fully changing the bed. In the person who is frequently incontinent, decubitus ulcers will form quickly (in as little as three days) if skin care is neglected.

ACCESS TO BATHROOMS

Many health care facilities have rooms that are small for the amount of equipment used in them; if a person is apt to have poor bladder control, place him in a bed close to the bathroom he will be using; check before you leave the room each time that his bed is in a low position and that no equipment such as a footstool or wheelchair is between his bed and the bathroom so that he can reach it easily and safely. If the person will be using a bedpan or urinal, allow him to keep it within easy reach. Tuck the bedpan or urinal under the edge of the top sheet where it is easily reached but still out of view.

Answer call bells of people who are incontinent promptly. It is second nature to answer the call light of a person with a respiratory or cardiac difficulty promptly. Make it a point to mark the nursing care plan of people who are apt to be incontinent with the same high priority rating. Incontinence is not lethal today, but if it leads to decubitus ulcers and infection, it could be lethal in another month. It is also destructive to self-esteem and therefore damaging to mental health.

PERINEAL AND ABDOMINAL EXERCISES

Strengthening the abdominal muscles by abdominal breathing (using the abdominal muscles rather than the chest muscles to aid inhalation) and perineal exercises (tightening and relaxing the perineal muscles 10 times 3 times a day by starting to void and then deliberately stopping and beginning again) assists in aiding continence. Many people who are incontinent, however, have neuromuscular difficulties, and these techniques may not be applicable. They may be of help with people with stress incontinence.

☐ QUICK REFERENCE STOP 38-8: ADVOCACY
Bladder Retraining

Bladder retraining is a procedure that calls for cooperation between the patient and the nursing staff. It is easy on a busy nursing unit to think of other methods of establishing dryness such as insertion of a retention catheter. It may be the most efficient method, but if it leads to urinary tract infection or loss of self-esteem, it is not the best method. You may need to advocate for a patient to continue a bladder retraining program rather than agree to catheter insertion.

BLADDER RETRAINING PROGRAMS

People who are incontinent are prime candidates for bladder retraining programs. Unfortunately, if the primary illness causing the incontinence has also caused generalized neurological impairment, this technique may not be applicable either. There are few instances, however, when it is not worth at least a trial period (see QRS 38-8).

Enuresis

Enuresis is involuntary loss of urine at night (bedwetting). It is expected in children up until 4 or 5 years of age and persists in many children as late as 9 or 10 years of age. If the child has any symptoms of urinary dysfunction (burning or frequency of urination), he should be referred to a physician because such symptoms suggest urinary tract infection rather than simple bedwetting. Secondary enuresis (the child suddenly begins bedwetting when he had not previously done this) also needs to be referred because it usually reflects a disease condition. The child who is disturbed (or whose parents are disturbed) by enuresis needs a referral when the problem is interfering with the child's perception of himself or with his parents' relationship with him.

In many instances enuresis occurs because of a smaller than usual bladder capacity. In such a case the child is begun on a program of "bladder stretching" exercises daily (he drinks a large quantity of water and then resists voiding for as long as possible to allow his bladder to fill to capacity). Enuresis may occur as a facet of psychological stress (a marital conflict in parents, for example). Measures such as not drinking any fluid after the evening meal and voiding just before sleeping are helpful. Alarms that are triggered by moisture as the child begins to void are a questionable solution. Waking the child during the night to void is also of doubtful benefit. A new medication (Tofranil) may be effective in reducing bladder tone and prolonging the time intervals between voidings.

Enuresis is an embarrassing problem for the child because it limits his ability to attend summer camp or sleep at friends' homes; if he doesn't bathe in the morning before school he may have a strong urine odor about him that other children notice. Ask about enuresis in children's health histories; it may not be mentioned by mothers spontaneously because they consider it just part of growing up. It is, but if it limits the child's ability to relate to friends or parents, it needs to be investigated and some action or care undertaken.

Stress Incontinence

Stress incontinence is the involuntary loss of urine during actions such as laughing, sneezing, or jogging. It occurs because during these times the intra-abdominal pressure increases as the diaphragm descends. It often occurs in women who have weakened perineal muscles from childbirth. Stress incontinence, like enuresis, is an embarrassing situation. Surgery to improve the function of the urethral sphincter is possible. Perineal exercises such as contracting and relaxing the perineal muscles (Kegel exercises) or beginning to void and then stopping the stream of urine may be helpful.

Overflow Incontinence

Overflow incontinence (retention with overflow) occurs when a bladder is filled to capacity and at periodic intervals contracts spasmodically involuntarily to empty partially. The person voids small amounts of urine (under 100 ml) at frequent intervals (every 15 to 60 minutes). This is a potentially dangerous condition because a bladder stretched to capacity can be damaged by the constant pressure; think of this as a possibility whenever a person is frequently incontinent. Assess whether the bladder is full by palpation (the area over the pubis is unusually firm) or by percussion (with an empty bladder the space over the pubis will sound dull; with a taut full bladder it sounds resonant). Retention with overflow is relieved by catheterization to empty the bladder; the disorder that has led to the phenomenon must then be relieved or the situation will undoubtedly recur. For this reason a catheter is usually left in place while the disorder is diagnosed and treated. Although there is little documentation that the practice is warranted, in many health care agencies a bladder that has been stretched to capacity this way is never fully emptied at the time of catheterization to prevent a drastic change in bladder tone from overdistention to completely empty or to cause rapid dilatation of abdominal arteries, which can lead to shock. When this policy is in effect, never initially remove more than 500 to 750 ml of urine when catheterizing to remove urine from an overdistended bladder; allow the remainder to drain gradually through the catheter left in place.

Urgency

Urgency is the sensation that one must void or within minutes the bladder will involuntarily empty. Urgency can be caused by a rapidly filling bladder, such as in the person who has taken a diuretic and is receiving optimal effects from it, or it can accompany urinary tract infection.

Urinary Retention

Urinary retention is the inability to void. This may occur when a bladder becomes overdistended and loses its ability to recognize normal filling; it may occur when the bladder has been traumatized or handled during surgery; or it may be due to obstruction at the neck of the bladder or urethra or to spinal cord trauma. During abdominal surgery, the bladder is often palpated or touched or moved out of the way of the surgical field. In childbirth there is pressure against it as the fetal head descends into the birth canal.

When a person is retaining urine, the bladder may become palpable over the pubis (the suprapubic area feels hard or firm) and, if you percuss at that point, the note will be more ringing than usual because of the tightness of the organ underneath. Urinary retention is relieved by the administration of a cholinergic to relax the urinary sphincter or by catheterization. The catheter may be left in place until the disorder that led to the retention can be identified or the effect of the handling during surgery, for example, has passed.

Urinary retention is a dangerous situation because a bladder can suffer permanent damage if it remains overdistended for too long a time (no longer able to respond to the sensation to void), and back pressure to the kidney pelvis can lead to damage of kidney nephrons.

Residual Urine

When a bladder empties normally, it retains little or no urine. This is important because if a residual amount remains after voiding, its bacterial count tends to increase greatly. Common conditions leading to increased amounts of residual urine are urethral stricture, prostatic hypertrophy, and lack of bladder tone due to neurological illness.

To determine how much residual urine is present, ask a person to void and then immediately catheterize him for urine. A residual urine volume of 50 ml or less indicates normal bladder emptying. In a untoilet-trained child, wait until the child voids spontaneously. Check for a wet diaper every 15 minutes so that you will not miss this.

Before catheterizing, be certain that you understand whether you should leave the catheter in place or not. If a large residual volume is suspected, the physician may wish to leave the catheter in place. Make sure that you and the physician agree on what is a "large amount." If there is a possibility that the catheter will be left in place, you will need to use a retention catheter for the procedure.

Recording Intake and Output

Maintaining an accurate intake and output record is a procedure that many people are able to do as a part of self-care. Be sure that the person understands the importance of the procedure and has adequate measuring equipment, a form to record on, and a pen or pencil.

If an adult voids in the bathroom and does not measure the urine, record the amount as "quantity sufficient" (abbreviated "q.s.") if the person states that it was a large or average amount. If a person is incontinent, this amount of urine is also lost to measurement and is recorded as "incontinent ×1." Urine output in infants who are not toilet trained can be measured by weighing their urine-filled diaper and comparing the weight to that of a dry diaper. Because 1 gm equals 1 ml, the number of extra grams in the wet diaper represents the number of milliliters of urine in the diaper.

UTILIZING NURSING PROCESS

Some problems of urinary elimination arise as a primary illness. Because any illness can affect a person's diet, fluid intake, activity, and usual habits, however, any person with any degree of illness may develop a complication of urinary elimination secondary to his initial problem. Every patient, therefore, needs careful assessment of urinary elimination as a basic component of care.

Health History

Because most people know that kidney function is important to life, they are aware of changes in urinary patterns and report them in giving health histories. Many symptoms of primary urinary tract illness are startling—blood in urine (hematuria), pain and frequency of urination, back pain—and these symptoms are reported quickly. Because many people are not aware that their kidneys are located high in the back, they do not associate back pain in this area as having a kidney origin; they are unaware that excessive fluid accumulating in the body (edema in the lower extremities) is a possible indication of kidney malfunction.

Another aspect of a history that is not often reported is stress incontinence.

Similarly, difficulty with voiding (benign prostatic hypertrophy) in men is also often accepted as a sign of aging. Ask about this in all males over 18 to identify the problem; otherwise, it may not be reported (prostatic cancer begins with the same symptoms, so identifying the problem is important).

Ask about changes in urinary habits (excessive urination is a major symptom of diabetes mellitus; frequent small voidings are a symptom of bladder infection) and whether the person has noticed any abnormality in urine such as the presence of blood or pus.

Note the amount and appearance of urine (concentration, presence of blood, cloudiness, and so on). In people who are ambulatory and are taking care of their own elimination needs, ask if they are voiding without difficulty. You may need to ask them to use a urinal or place a bedpan over a toilet seat so you can measure urine output or test it for specific gravity if you are concerned about output or concentration of urine.

Physical Assessment

Tenderness over the kidneys or bladder area is always suggestive of some pathology. Other signs to look for include the odor of urine (suggests incontinence), inflammation or erythema (redness) at the urinary meatus (suggests infection), and crystals of urine on the skin surface, giving the appearance of a white frost (termed *uremic frost*; this occurs when kidney function fails, so that urine is excreted through perspiration).

A distended bladder can be palpated over the pubis (normally the bladder cannot be felt). It may also be percussed (a full bladder sounds resonant; if it is empty and therefore not present over the pubis, the percussion note is hard or flat). See Fig. 38-23.

Take the time to palpate and percuss the lower abdomen of people who have no difficulty with urination while you are caring for them so that you can recognize the feel and sound of an empty bladder (or rather the absence of a palpable or percussible bladder). When you are caring for a person with a distended bladder you will then be able to recognize the feel and sound of a distended bladder.

Laboratory Testing

Laboratory testing aids greatly in the assessment of a patient with a suspected urinary tract illness. The values of common laboratory tests (urine pH, protein, glucose, and specific gravity) are shown in Appendix G. Common diagnostic procedures such as an intravenous pyelogram (radiograph of the kidney and ureter) and sonogram are discussed in Chap. 20.

COLLECTING URINE FOR ROUTINE URINALYSIS

The technique for urine collection varies according to the age and condition of the patient. In all instances, specimens must be collected in clean containers to prevent contamination by additives.

For adults, you need only give the patient a clean specimen container (many agencies or ambulatory facilities use clean paper cups) and tell him that you need a urine specimen. Most adults can void "on command" and unless the person has very recently voided, he can do this for you almost immediately. Asking him to drink a glass of fluid will enable him to void sooner. Do not encourage him to drink more than a glass of fluid or urine production may be so diluted that the specific gravity and protein and glucose levels may be inaccurate. Adolescents are also able to void on command and can obtain urine specimens by themselves. Remember that adolescents are concerned and self-conscious about

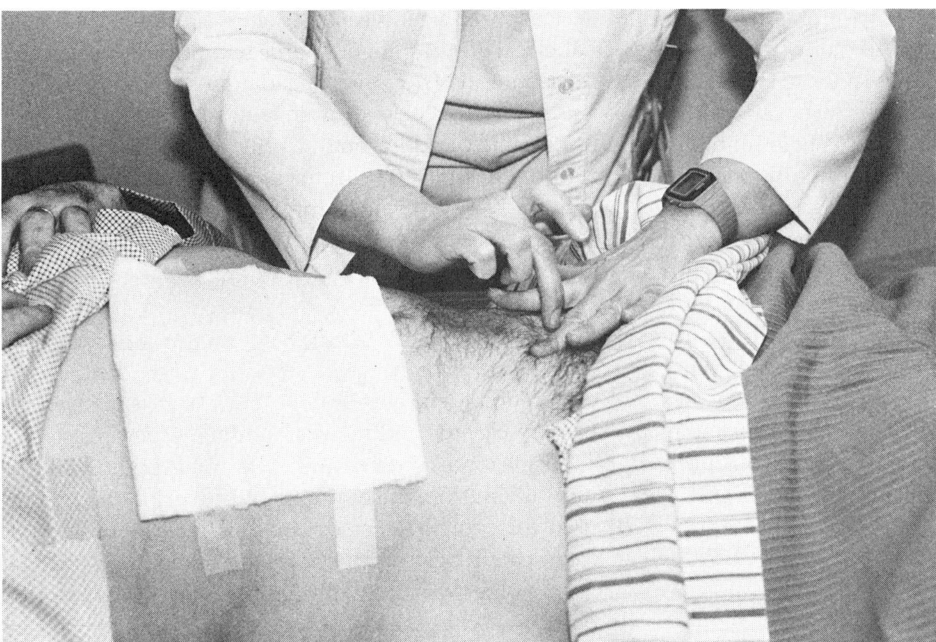

FIGURE 38-23. Percussing for a filled bladder.

body functions. They are often reluctant to carry a urine specimen through a crowded waiting room. Adolescent girls are often embarrassed to point out that they are menstruating; ask them about this so that the presence of red blood cells in the urine can be explained.

Schoolage children find it more difficult than adults to void at a certain time but usually can following a drink of water. It is often difficult to obtain routine urine specimens from preschoolers and toddlers because they cannot void on command but only when they feel a definite urge to do so. Another problem is language. It is not unprofessional to use words such as "pee-pee" if the child will understand them. Provide a potty chair if one is available; if not, put a bedpan on the toilet to simulate one. Offer the child a glass of water or other fluid, and ask the mother to reinforce your request so that the child knows mother approves. Act as if you expect him to be able to void, as if voiding is not a difficult procedure. This approach is generally successful.

Obtaining a urine specimen from an infant who has not been toilet trained presents another problem. You must attach a urine collecting device to a girl's perineum or a boy's penis, then wait for the infant to void. Be certain to wash and dry the place of attachment well. If ointment or powder is on the skin, the sticky adhesive surface of the urine collector will not adhere. Press the collector firmly around the genitalia. If the infant attempts to loosen it, replace the diaper to keep the collector out of sight. Otherwise, it is best to leave it visible so that you or the child's parent can tell when he has voided. Offer the child something to drink. Most infants void shortly after a feeding, so if you put the collector in place just before a regular feeding, voiding will probably result. Remove the collector as soon as the infant voids and transfer the specimen to a specimen cup by clipping a bottom corner of the bag.

Urine may be squeezed from diapers for tests such as dipstick protein, pH, or glucose. Specific gravity of urine may be changed if diaper lint is squeezed into the specimen. With disposable diapers, urine tends to be pulled into the diaper and is best available for testing if the diaper is torn apart and the urine collecting portion used.

COLLECTIONS FOR 24-HOUR URINE SPECIMENS

Although urinalysis of a single urine specimen will reveal the presence of substances such as protein or glucose, a 24-hour urine specimen is necessary to determine the quantitative amount of many substances or how much of the substance is excreted during a day's time. To begin a 24-hour urine collection, ask the patient to void (with an infant, wait for him to void). This specimen (the discard specimen) is then thrown away so that a specific time for the ensuing collection is known. If the urine collection is started early in the morning and this first specimen is counted as part of the collection, the urine collected during the next 24 hours will include the urine that had been forming all night, about a 32-hour collection. This will distort the analysis.

Record the start of the collection period as the time of the discard urine. Save all urine voided for the next 24 hours and place it in one collection bottle. Have the person void at the end of the 24-hour period and add the final specimen to the collection bottle.

For an infant, use a 24-hour urine collector. These are collecting bags similar to single-use collectors except for the presence of a tube attached to them. A collector will adhere only for this length of time if the child's perineum is dry at the time of application. Use no powder because this decreases the ability of the collector to stick. Applying tincture of benzoin to toughen the perineal skin to make removal of the collector easier is helpful; tincture of benzoin also makes the perineum slightly sticky and aids in firm contact. Commercial sprays that encourage adhesiveness are also available. Make certain that the tubing from the collector is pinned out of the child's reach or he will pull the collector free. Place the infant in a semi-Fowler's position, if possible, to encourage urine to flow freely into the collector. You may need to place a diaper on the infant to keep the apparatus out of sight. Provide activities; make sure the mother understands that she can pick up the infant and hold him during this time as long as she takes care not to kink or pull the tubing.

To keep bacterial count to a minimum, 24-hour collections are generally kept refrigerated.

OBTAINING A URINE SPECIMEN FROM THE MENSTRUATING WOMAN

To avoid having a urine specimen contaminated by menstrual blood (which changes the specific gravity, protein, and red blood cell analysis), ask a woman who is menstruating to wash her perineum well with soap and water and rinse and dry it to remove menstrual blood. Next, supply a sterile cotton ball for her to insert gently into her vagina just prior to voiding (it is removed following voiding). Mark the specimen "possibly contaminated by menstrual blood" even though it does not appear discolored because red blood cells may be present microscopically.

SECOND-VOIDED (DOUBLE-VOIDED) SPECIMENS

A second-voided specimen is used to determine the amount of glucose or protein that kidneys are currently spilling rather than the amount they have been spilling during a number of hours. To obtain a second-voided specimen, ask the person to void and discard the specimen; then ask him to void again 20 to 30 minutes later. Test this specimen.

Children under 8 or 9 years old have difficulty voiding when told to do so. Test the first specimen obtained as a backup in case the child is not able to void a second time. Mark it "not double-voided."

FIRST MORNING VOIDINGS

The first morning voiding of urine is most apt to be a concentrated one and is therefore useful for studies such as pregnancy testing in which the presence of a small amount of hormone is tested. Be certain that people receive instructions the evening before.

SERIAL URINE SPECIMENS

Serial urines are collected to demonstrate that there is an increasing or decreasing amount of blood in urine. Collect each voiding in a separate clean specimen container. Label it with the patient's name and time of voiding and refrigerate it. By comparing the gross color of several specimens collected in such a series, it can be determined whether bleeding in urine is decreasing or not. Serial urines can be collected as an independent nursing action. Testing urine samples for occult blood even though they appear clear may reveal that minimal bleeding is still present.

CLEAN-CATCH SPECIMENS

A clean-catch urine specimen is ordered when a urine culture for bacteria is desired. The object is to clean the urinary meatus and the surrounding structures so that the urine is not contaminated by external organisms that increase the organism count of the urine. Specimens used for protein or blood analysis may be ordered as clean-catch specimens because this careful cleaning also reduces the possibility of vaginal or foreskin secretions being added to the specimen.

The technique for this is shown in Procedure 38-4. If clean-catch specimens are obtained with care, they practically eliminate the need for catheterization specimens. Clean-catch urine specimens have many advantages over catheterized specimens—they are not intrusive and they carry no risk of introducing a bladder infection. A clean-catch specimen with a bacterial colony count of over 100,000 per milliliter is considered a positive specimen or evidence that urinary tract infection exists.

SUPRAPUBIC ASPIRATION

Suprapubic aspiration involves the insertion of a sterile needle into the bladder through the anterior wall of the abdomen and withdrawal of urine. It is used to obtain urine for culture. The anterior abdominal wall is cleaned with an antiseptic, and the urinary meatus is blocked by finger pressure. A needle is inserted just above the pubis into the bladder; urine is drawn back into a sterile syringe. Although suprapubic aspiration for urine appears complicated, it is not because the bladder is the most anterior of abdominal organs and, when distended with urine, is readily accessible just under the abdominal wall (Fig. 38-24). Parents may not have heard of this procedure and may wonder why their child had urine drawn by needle and syringe instead of by catheter. The method is used because theoretically the risk of bladder infection from needle insertion is less than that from catheter insertion.

Analysis

Before you make judgments on output, be sure that you are familiar with fluid intake because a person who has been without fluid for a period of time will have a diminished output for the next 24 hours. On the other hand, diminished output may be an important sign that the person's overall intake has been inadequate or his

PROCEDURE 38-4
Obtaining a Clean-Catch Urine Specimen

Purpose: To obtain a midstream urine specimen for culture.

Plan	*Principle*
1. Wash your hands; identify the patient; explain the procedure.	1. Prevent spread of microorganisms; promote patient safety and well-being.
2. Assess patient status; analyze appropriateness of procedure; plan modifications of procedure as appropriate.	2. Adults can obtain clean-catch urine specimens following careful instructions. Assess to determine level of understanding and physical ability to perform procedure.
3. Implement care by assembling supplies: commercial clean-catch urine specimen kit, or five sterile cotton balls, sterile specimen container, appropriate antiseptic solution. Provide privacy.	3. Solution for cleaning differs in various health care agencies. *Thorough* cleansing appears to be more important than solution used.
4. Assist patient to moisten three cotton balls in antiseptic solution and give instructions. Patient will cleanse urinary meatus with three cotton balls (washing front to back, right side of meatus, left side of meatus, directly over meatus in female; three times in circular motion for males) using each cotton ball for only one stroke and then discarding it.	4. Cleansing front to back prevents bringing rectal contamination forward in female. Discarding cotton balls also prevents this.
5. Next, the patient will wipe away the antiseptic solution using the same techniques.	5. Wiping away antiseptic prevents it from entering specimen and, by germicidal action, decreasing bacterial growth and accurate analysis.
6. Next, the patient should begin to void and dip the sterile specimen container into the urine stream to obtain a midstream urine specimen.	6. The flow of urine washes away bacteria from urinary meatus.
7. After 10 to 20 ml is obtained in specimen cup, patient may finish voiding in toilet.	7. If intake and output is being recorded, place a bedpan on top of toilet to collect remainder of urine.
8. Cap specimen container; label with patient's identification; mark "midstream" on label.	8. Most laboratory report slips accompanying specimens being sent for culture also require a list of any antibiotics the person is receiving.
9. Evaluate effectiveness, efficiency, cost, safety, and comfort of procedure. Plan health teaching as needed such as importance of recognizing symptoms of urinary tract infection.	9. Health teaching is an independent nursing action always included as part of care.
10. Document that specimen was obtained, amount of urine obtained, and any abnormalities with voiding or urine.	10. Documentation of patient status and nursing care.

MODIFICATIONS FOR CARE OF CHILD

Schoolage children and younger cannot be depended on to do an adequate job of cleansing themselves for clean-catch specimens. For a girl, have her lie in a dorsal recumbent position on a bed or table so you have a good visualization of her perineum. To obtain the urine specimen, it is often easier to ask the child to kneel over a sterile emesis basin on a bed while he or she begins to void and then dip a sterile container into the urine stream to obtain the specimen. It is not always possible to obtain a midstream urine with young children because if they void only a small amount, there is not time to obtain it. This is the advantage of using a sterile emesis basin for the child to void into. The specimen is still salvageable; simply mark it "not midstream" for the laboratory.

With infants, wash the genitalia and apply a sterile urine collector. This specimen obtained this way is never a "midstream"; mark it as such for the laboratory. If an infant does not void within 2 hours, remove the collecting bag, cleanse the perineum or penis, and reapply a new sterile bag; some microorganisms will have recollected after this amount of time.

MODIFICATIONS FOR CARE OF OLDER ADULT

Older adults who are unstable may appreciate knowing that they can cleanse themselves lying in bed and then walk to a bathroom to void rather than having to accomplish cleansing in the bathroom.

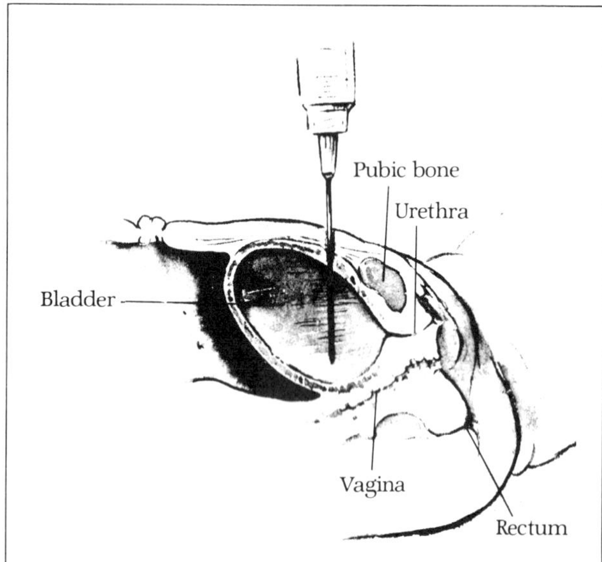

FIGURE 38-24. Suprapubic aspiration for urine. (Courtesy Dept. of Medical Illustration, State University of New York at Buffalo, Buffalo, New York.)

blood pressure has fallen too low for effective kidney perfusion.

The Fourth National Conference on Nursing Diagnoses accepted the diagnosis of urinary elimination, alteration in pattern. Defining characteristics of this are shown in Appendix C.

Planning

Some planning for improving urinary elimination involves temporary measures to relieve urinary retention (insertion of a retention catheter). This type of short-term plan should always be followed with a long-term plan such as maintenance of the catheter and avoidance of urinary tract infection while it is in place. As a rule, before a catheter is inserted, plans for its removal as well as its placement should be established because the longer it remains the greater becomes the risk of urinary tract infection.

Implementation

Implementation of actions to help encourage urinary elimination are often very personal in nature and require

☐ QUICK REFERENCE STOP 38-9: HEALTH TEACHING
Urinary Tract Infections

Some people are embarrassed to go to a physician with urinary system problems and therefore disregard symptoms such as pain and burning or blood in urine as long as possible. Women tend to have a higher incidence of urinary tract infections than men due to the presence of a shorter urethra and the location of the rectum near the urethra. Urinary tract infections are most likely to occur in preschool girls, in adolescents following the first sexual experience, in any patient on bed rest (urinary stasis invites infection), and in any patient with a retention catheter (bacteria enter through or beside the catheter).

Symptoms of burning and pain on urination in sexually active young males are more apt to indicate gonorrheal infection rather than urinary tract infection; such infection needs referral as well, however, to prevent spread from the urethra to the epididimus and testes.

Teach patients the symptoms of urinary tract infection and emphasize that such symptoms are always serious and can lead to a kidney infection if ignored. Teach women good perineal hygiene, to void frequently during the day, to ensure a high fluid intake, and to wear cotton, not rayon or silk underpants to prevent perineal excoriation; these measures help to prevent urinary tract infection.

Teach people with retention catheters the importance of encouraging gravity drainage from the bladder to the collecting bag so that they will be careful not to lie on the tubing and, when getting out of bed to a chair, will never allow the collecting bag to be higher than the bladder, reversing the flow of urine and encouraging urinary tract infection.

☐ **QUICK REFERENCE STOP 38-10: RESEARCH**
Urine Specimens, Urinary Catheterization, and Bladder Reconditioning

Nurses are constantly searching for ways to improve the efficiency of their own delivery of health care to patients. The research presented below questions some of the techniques used in relation to urinary elimination.

Second-voided specimens for sugar and acetone—Necessary?
Most nurses have been taught to obtain a second-voided specimen of urine in order to ensure accurate sugar and acetone readings. This involves asking the patient to void, allowing a short period of time to elapse, and then asking the patient to void again. Readings are obtained from the second specimen of urine; which is believed to reflect glucose levels in the patient most accurately at that point. Congdon (1982) questioned whether or not differences were actually present between first- and second-voided specimens. A large sample of 396 pairs of urine samples were tested, and no significant differences were found between the sugar and acetone readings. The results of this study certainly challenge the current practice of obtaining and testing second specimens, but the authors caution that further duplication of the study is necessary.

How safe is intermittent catheterization?
Intermittent urinary catheterization is often necessary to relieve bladder distention in patients unable to void sufficiently on their own. It provides an alternative to an indwelling catheter as well, especially with chronically ill patients. Concern has often been expressed that periodic invasion into the body with a catheter predisposes a patient to urinary tract infection, even when performed under sterile conditions. Wahlquist et al. (1982) studied a total of 32 patients who had received 662 intermittent catheterizations. A very low infection rate of 0.05 percent was found. Current literature cites the rate of infection among patients with indwelling catheters as much higher. The researchers suggest that the benefits of intermittent catheterization outweigh the risks.

Bladder reconditioning—Effective?
A small experimental study by Williamson (1982) investigated the effectiveness of reconditioning in reducing postcatheter bladder dysfunction. Many patients experience loss of bladder muscle tone as a result of prolonged indwelling catheterization. This often results in incomplete bladder emptying, bladder distention, and bacteriuria. Bladder reconditioning prior to catheter removal involves periodic clamping of the catheter and intermittent drainage. This has been widely practiced by nurses. This study experimentally tested the effectiveness of the technique. It was found that reconditioned subjects resumed natural voiding patterns with less dysfunction significantly sooner than subjects who were not reconditioned. The researcher suggests that replication of the study is necessary with larger samples.

SUGGESTED READINGS

Congdon, J. Are second-voided urine samples needed? *Am. J. Nurs.* 82(9):1394, 1982.

Wahlquist, G. I., McGuire, E., and Herlihy, E. The safety of intermittent catheterization. As presented in: For the research record. *Am. J. Nurs.* 82(12):1880, 1982.

Williamson, M. L. Reducing postcatheterization bladder dysfunction by reconditioning. *Nurs. Res.* 31(1):28, 1982.

sensitivity to the person's feelings. Prevention of urinary tract infection depends heavily on conscientious care by nurses to prevent contamination of closed drainage systems or equipment through poor hand washing during procedures (see QRS 38-9).

Evaluation

Evaluation is an important step in determining whether urinary elimination has been adequate. Evaluate whether a diuretic is truly increasing urinary output or whether it is effective in reducing body edema. Evaluate carefully whether a person continues to void after removal of a catheter. Quick Reference Stop 38-10 presents some of the nursing research related to routine care methods of urinary elimination.

NURSING CARE PLAN

Mrs. O'Connor is a 65-year-old patient who is hospitalized for a persistent urinary tract infection. Her physician is concerned that she maintain an adequate urinary output (1,200 to 1,500 ml of urine a day). The following is a nursing care plan for her.

NURSING DIAGNOSIS

Potential for inadequate urine output due to underlying pathology.

Goal: Patient will maintain an adequate urine output by day 1.

Criteria: Patient will have 24-hour urine total of 1,200 to 1,500 ml.

NURSING ORDERS

1. Encourage fluid intake of 3,000 ml daily. Divide as 2,000 ml, day shift; 750 ml, evening shift; 350 ml, night shift. Favorite fluids are soups, Jello, and grape juice.

2. Encourage voiding at intervals no longer than every 4 hours to reduce bacterial level in bladder.
3. Measure intake and output. Ask patient to use bedpan on toilet.
4. Test one specimen on each nursing shift for specific gravity. Urge additional fluid if this value is above 1.020.
5. Discuss perineal hygiene and implication of good fluid intake to prevent further increase in bacterial level in bladder.
6. Adhere to conscientious administration of prescribed antibiotic to reduce bacteria in bladder.

SUGGESTED READINGS

Altshuler, A., et al. Even children can learn clean self-catheterization. *Am. J. Nurs.* 77:97, 1977.

Anderson, E. Women and cystitis. *Nursing 77* 7:50, 1977.

Bates, P. A troubleshooter's guide to indwelling catheters. *RN* 44:62, 1981.

Baum, M. E. "I want to be dry": The (almost) carefree way to conquer urinary incontinence. *Nursing 78* 8:75, 1978.

Baum, M. Urinary incontinence. *Crit. Care Update* 9(11):27, 1982.

Beber, C. R. Freedom for the incontinent. *Am. J. Nurs.* 80:482, 1980.

Bellfy, L. C. You can improve your catheterized patient's care. *RN* 40:33, 1977.

Blannin, J. P. Catheter management. *Nurs. Times* 78(11):438, 1982.

Cannon, J. Urinary incontinence: A disposable flannel and wipe for incontinent patients. *Nurs. Times* 78(4):165, 1982.

Chesmore, G. Nursing management . . . the most common urological emergencies. *Nurs. Mirror* 155(16):37, 1982.

Dipalma, J. Drugs that induce changes in urine color. *RN* 40:34, 1977.

Freed, S. Urinary incontinence in the elderly. *Hosp. Pract.* 17:81, 1982.

Friedman, F. B. Why not use a Foley? *RN* 45(11):71, 1982.

Green, J., et al. Promoting continence . . . a course for nurses. *Nurs. Times* 79(5):30, 1983.

Holloran, S. D. Teaching male catheterization: An application of change theory for an entire nursing staff. *Nurs. Educ.* 7(1):11, 1982.

Hooley, B. C., et al. Help, dignity and independence for patients with catheters. *Nurs. Times* 78(11):440, 1982.

Juliani, L. Assessing renal function. *Nursing 78* 8:34, 1978.

Karrei, I. Hickman catheters: Your guide to troublefree use. *Can. Nurse* 78(11):25, 1982.

Kennedy, A. P., et al. The nursing management of patients with long-term indwelling catheters. *J. Adv. Nurs.* 7(5):411, 1982.

Killian, A. Reducing the risk of infection from indwelling urethral catheters. *Nursing* (Horsham) 12(5):84, 1982.

Lapides, J., et al. Clean intermittent self-catheterization in treatment of urinary tract disease. *J. Urol.* 107:458, 1972.

McConnell, E. A. Urinalysis: A common test, but never routine. *Nursing* (Horsham) 12:108, 1982.

McCoy, J. A. Preliminary diagnosis of urinary tract infection in symptomatic children. *Nurs. Pract.* 7:28, 1982.

McGill, S. Catheter management: It's the size that's important. *Nurs. Mirror* 157(14):48, 1982.

Nortridge, J. A. Ambulatory nursing: Helpful hints for assessing the ostomate. *Nursing* (Horsham) 12(4):72, 1982.

Ozanne, S. Nursing care study—total cystectomy: Going home. *Nurs. Mirror* 154(17):56, 1982.

Pierson, C. A. Urinary incontinence: New methods of diagnosis and treatment. *J.O.G.N. Nurs.* 10:407, 1981.

Sheahan, S. L., et al. Understanding urinary tract infection in women: The first step to controlling it. *Nursing* (Horsham) 12(11):68, 1982.

Shelter, M. G., and Bartos, H. Culture specimens: How to collect and what to expect. *RN* 43:65, 1980.

Thomas, C. K. Childhood urinary tract infection. *Pediatr. Nurs.* 8:114, 1982.

Toner, M. Urinary tract obstruction: The hidden threats in treatment. *RN* 45:58, 1982.

Turtill, A. T. Urinary incontinence: The female cone—a urine transfer device. *Nurs. Times* 78(4):168, 1982.

Wright, B. T., et al. Test for glucose in the urine: Understanding test specificity and interferences. *Pediatr. Nurs.* 8:44, 1982.

QUESTIONS FOR REVIEW

1. Mrs. Jones is one your patients. You notice that she has had diarrhea for three days. Based on this fact, you would expect her urinary output to be:
   a. Increased in amount from normal.
   b. Same in amount as usual but more dilute.
   c. Decreased in amount from normal.
   d. Decreased in amount from normal but more dilute.

2. You would assess the amount of residual urine in Mrs. Jones' bladder by which of the following methods?
   a. Asking her to void at half hour intervals.
   b. Measuring drainage from an indwelling catheter.
   c. Palpating her abdomen for fullness.
   d. Catheterization immediately following voiding.

3. Mrs. Jones' urinalysis shows a specific gravity of 1.010. You would interpret this assessment as:
   a. Concentrated urine.
   b. Abnormally dilute urine.
   c. Normal specific gravity.
   d. Acidic urine.

4. In establishing a nursing diagnosis of Mrs. Jones, you consider hormonal influences. The hormone responsible for the reabsorption of sodium in the distal kidney tubule is:
   a. Aldosterone
   b. Antidiuretic hormone
   c. Pituitary oxytocin
   d. Hypothyroid hormone

5. If Mrs. Jones asks for a bedpan at frequent intervals but voids only 20 to 30 ml at a time, your nursing diagnosis would most likely be:
   a. Retention of urine.
   b. Severe diuresis.
   c. Urine suppression.
   d. Kidney atrophy.

6. In planning care for Mrs. Jones, you could anticipate that when the kidney is unable to concentrate urine adequately, one of the following problems may occur. Which one?
   a. Glycosuria.
   b. Nocturia.
   c. Proteinuria.
   d. Infection.

7. An indwelling catheter might be ordered for Mrs. Jones for which of the following situations?
   a. To obtain a sterile specimen for culture.
   b. To prevent repeated catheterizations.
   c. To prevent infection.
   d. To improve bladder tone.

8. You implement care for Mrs. Jones in several areas. Preventing infection in a patient who has an indwelling catheter is best done by:
   a. Keeping the urine alkaline.
   b. Irrigating the catheter frequently.
   c. Keeping the meatal area clean.
   d. Replacing the catheter frequently.

9. If Mrs. Jones were on a bladder retraining program, it would be important to schedule voidings at what time interval?
   a. Every half hour.
   b. Every 2 hours.
   c. Every 4 hours.
   d. Immediately following meals.

10. In evaluating care for Mrs. Jones, you must decide whether the diuretic prescribed for her is effective. A diuretic should:
    a. Increase urine output.
    b. Decrease proteinuria.
    c. Increase body fluid.
    d. Decrease kidney circulation.

X. HEALTH CARE IN ACTION

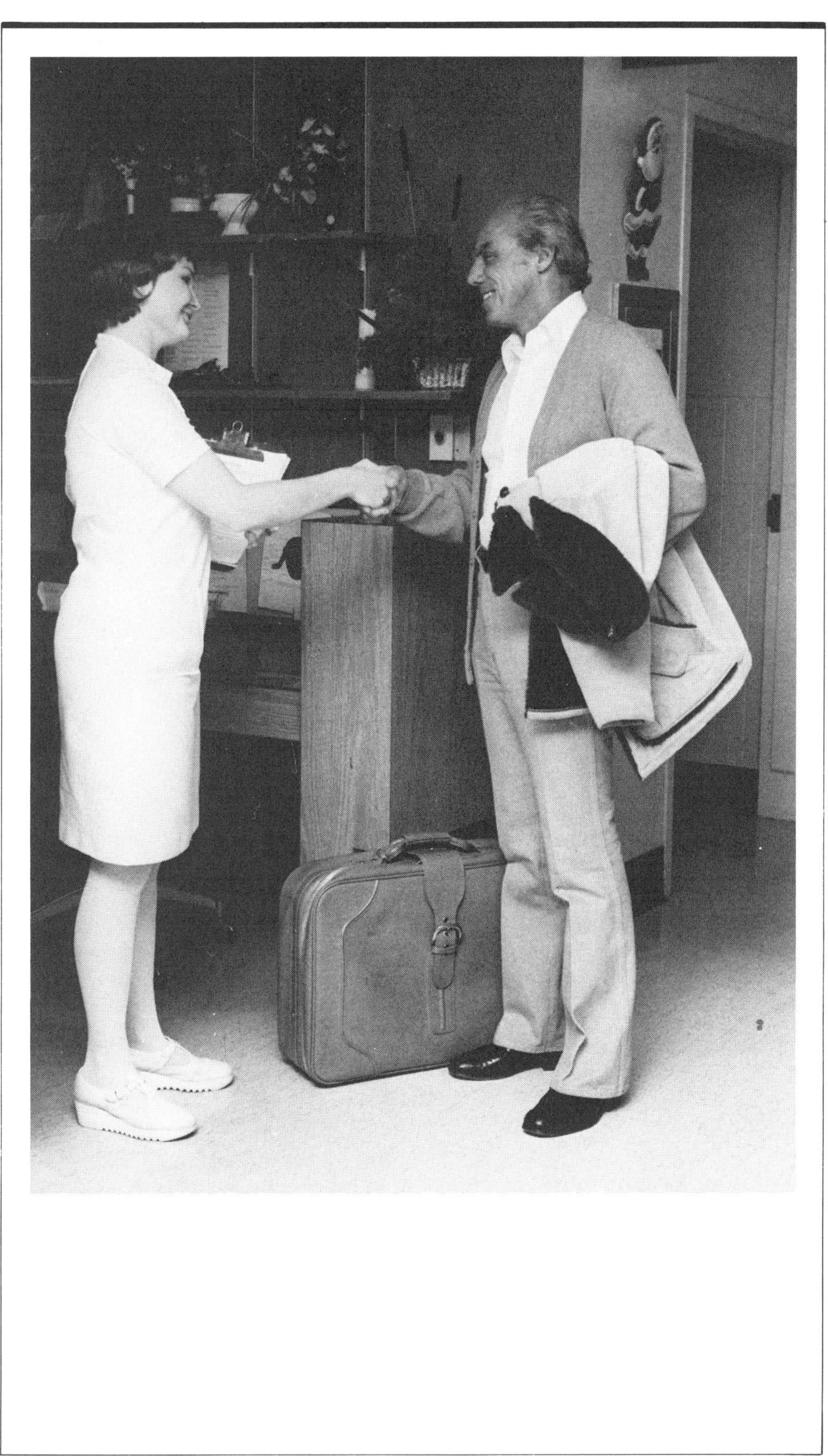

39. ADMISSION AND DISCHARGE

OBJECTIVES

Upon mastery of the material of this chapter, you should be able to:

1. Describe the nurse's role in ambulatory and inpatient settings on admission of a patient.
2. Describe assessments necessary on admission to a health care facility.
3. Describe the documentation responsibilities of the nurse on admission to a health care facility.
4. Describe the stress that patients experience during admission and discharge.
5. Describe the nurse's role in ambulatory and inpatient settings on discharge.
6. Describe the documentation responsibilities of the nurse at patient discharge.
7. Apply nursing process to give safe and planned care to the patient whose care involves a time of admission or discharge.

TERMS

The terms important for an understanding of this chapter are shown below and defined in the glossary:

ambulatory setting
discharge planning
inpatient setting
maternal deprivation
triage

A person is admitted to the health care delivery system the first time he contacts any health caregiver or when a caregiver supervises his birth. He is not discharged from the system until he dies. Even after death, health care concerns continue to be extended to his support people to ensure that they can cope effectively with the death. If the deceased person wished any body organ such as a cornea or a kidney donated to another person or institution, caregivers at death conserve these organs and see that the person's wishes are honored.

Admission and discharge to different facilities or care points in the health care delivery system may occur frequently. Whenever change occurs—whether it is a good change (an ill person has recovered and is ready to return home) or an unwelcome change (a person has been told he should be hospitalized)—it is a time of stress due to the number of unknowns present (the ill person may not get better, and the well person may become ill again). Both admission and discharge, therefore, are times when people need special care and consideration. Not only must physical care needs (oxygen, nutrition, rest) be met but psychological needs (security and comfort) must be dealt with as well.

ADMISSION TO AN AMBULATORY SETTING

The term *ambulatory* denotes a setting in which a patient is seen for health care but does not remain overnight (a clinic, for example). Such facilities were formerly termed *outpatient departments* of hospitals, in contrast to the inpatient section, where people remained overnight for care. Today, many ambulatory settings are not part of hospitals or at a physical distance from the main hospital, so the term *ambulatory* is now more descriptive of the intent of such facilities (to keep people ambulatory or able to care for themselves at home with guidance as necessary from health care providers).

People may be seen in ambulatory care settings for health maintenance care (well people learning better ways to remain well or receiving assurance at scheduled health assessment visits that they are well) or for illness care. In either case, they usually have some concern about the visit (the well person worries that a routine physical examination will reveal that he is ill; the ill person worries that he will be told he is seriously ill). No visit, therefore, even in these settings, is without stress for the person being seen.

Ambulatory settings are structured to provide a reception area where the person gives his name, type of health care payment, age, address, and reason for the visit to a health care provider assigned that function (secretary or receptionist). In illness settings, this initial contact person may be a nurse because the reason for the visit needs evaluation of its seriousness. A person who is very short of breath, for example, cannot wait to be seen;

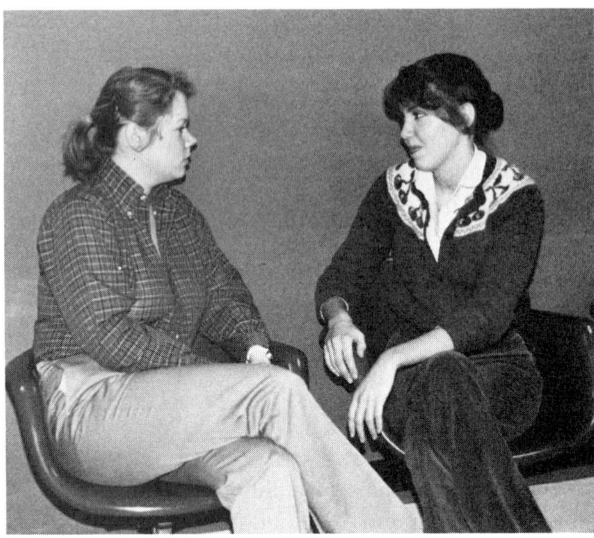

FIGURE 39-1. A waiting room in an ambulatory care setting. Triage, the determination of which patients need to be seen first, is often a nursing responsibility.

a person with a skin rash probably can. Making this type of decision (seriousness of illness and priority of visit) is termed *triage.*

In an ambulatory setting, the reception area should be sufficiently separate from the waiting area to afford privacy. Some people are reluctant to tell a receptionist the reason for the visit if they know that people in the waiting room can overhear them. Receptionists may not be as aware of maintaining patient privacy as they could be unless they are well oriented to the concept that people have a right to keep their health confidential; in some settings, architectural design may be at fault.

Waiting rooms should be supplied with an ample number of chairs. Waiting room chairs are typically made not for comfort but for their ability to be washed and moved to accommodate people in wheelchairs or stretchers. If the wait will be lengthy, reading material or children's toys should be furnished (Fig. 39-1). At their best, waiting rooms serve as space for educational programs (posters or pamphlets) on such subjects as good dental hygiene or the advantages of not smoking. In some settings, individually played videotape machines are provided so that people can watch a tape on such topics as normal growth and development of children or, in a specialty setting, breathing exercises for adults or the best sports programs for children with respiratory illness.

When a health care provider is available, a person is asked to come into an examining room, where his height and weight and perhaps temperature are recorded. Additional history is taken. The person will then be seen by his primary caregiver (a physician or nurse practitioner). Following an examination, he may need medicine administered by injection, instructions for additional medicine or improved diet, or procedures such as having blood drawn or obtaining a urine specimen. This followup care is an important role of a nurse in an ambulatory care setting.

Be certain before a person leaves an ambulatory setting after a first visit that he fully understands any instructions given him and knows the name and number of the person he should call if disease symptoms should grow worse or if he has any questions after he returns home.

Complaints from consumers about ambulatory care often center around a long waiting period and inadequate time provided by the primary caregiver. Nurses can be instrumental in ensuring that appointments for ambulatory services are made at staggered intervals to prevent many people arriving at one time and that each person is addressed by name and made to feel welcome. Only when people feel relaxed can they concentrate on explaining an illness fully and listening to instructions of procedures or care they should continue at home.

Be aware that for many people having blood drawn or receiving an injection is the worst part of any health care visit. These procedures are so feared by some people that they reject health care rather than submit to them. Give support while these procedures are done (because many people are seen in ambulatory settings for diagnosis of illness, a great many visits do involve drawing of blood; although they are routine procedures for you, they are never routine for the patient.

Also, be aware of the importance of telling a person he is well. For many people there is no material gift as wonderful as a primary care provider telling them that all test results have returned with negative results and they are being given a clean bill of health. There is ceremony attached to ambulatory visits such as a diagnosis of pregnancy. This type of visit is not routine for such patients and they enjoy having health care providers share good news with them.

Some ambulatory settings are staffed with a rotating group of physicians; every time a patient visits he sees a different physician. A nurse in such a setting is often the person who can best interpret new disease symptoms or whether a person's illness is becoming better or worse because she may be the only one who has seen the person before.

The use of ambulatory care settings is growing. Because an ambulatory care setting is often a person's first contact with the system (from the physician's office he will be admitted to the hospital for further care), it is important that his admission be carried out with skill and nursing expertise.

ADMISSION TO AN INPATIENT SETTING

An inpatient setting is one in which the person will remain at least overnight for care. Such settings as hospitals, extended care facilities, and nursing homes are examples.

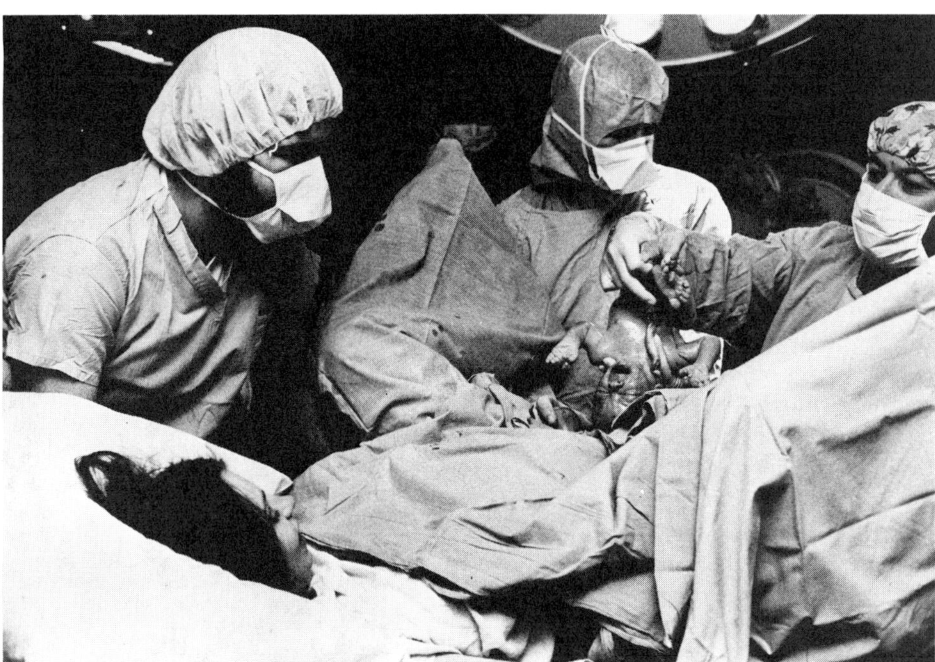

FIGURE 39-2. A newborn enters the hospital through the delivery room. His father observes from a place by his mother's head.

Delivery Rooms

In the United States, the majority of infants are born in hospitals. Traditionally, the room provided for birth was a surgerylike room (a delivery room, Fig. 39-2). Today, to make birth a more family-centered experience, hospitals are providing more relaxed settings for birth (birthing rooms). Fathers are allowed to watch their child being born in both birthing rooms and delivery rooms; mothers are encouraged to use childbirth preparation techniques to enable them to be awake and to cooperate with the birth.

Parents bond with their child by spending time with the child immediately after birth, holding him and just "getting acquainted" for the first time. A nurse in a birthing or delivery room helps to provide this time for parents and child to be together. Before the child leaves the room he should be properly identified with arm bands or necklace designating his hospital number and his name.

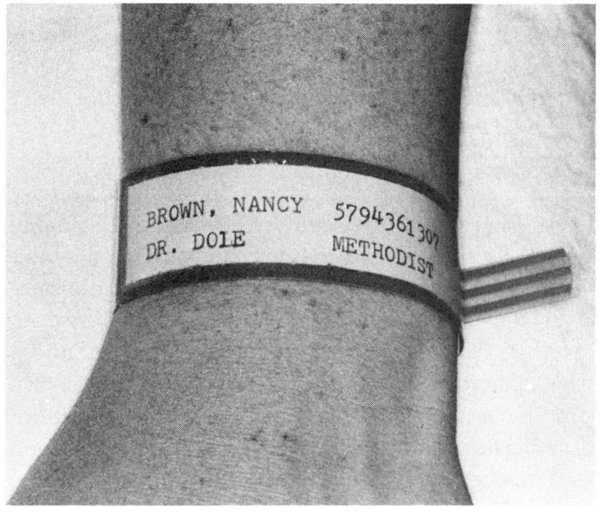

FIGURE 39-3. Upon admission, every patient receives an identification bracelet noting his name and hospital number; usually his religious affiliation and physician's name are also included.

Hospital Admission

People are admitted to a hospital for either diagnostic studies or therapy. In either event, a hospital admission is interpreted by most people as a stressful, serious event.

Provided it is not an emergency, in most cases the person has been seen in an ambulatory setting recently, and his physician has phoned the hospital and arranged for an admission date. When the person arrives at this time, he reports to the Admissions Department. There he is asked to fill out forms that include his name, age, physician, type of health payment, and reason for admission; he signs a permission form for therapy or care.

Depending on the reason he is being admitted and his age, he may have blood drawn for preliminary testing in the Admissions Department; he may have an electrocardiogram (a tracing of heart conduction patterns), or a radiograph and be asked to provide a urine specimen. He will be given an identification bracelet with his name and assigned hospital number (Fig. 39-3).

Because of the number of people who are admitted at one time and the availability of hospital beds, a person may have to wait a considerable time in an Admissions Department. It is usually an unpleasant wait because once a person has agreed to be hospitalized he wants to get on with it; a delay at this point is frustrating because it appears to be delaying his treatment.

As soon as these admission procedures are completed, the Admissions Department phones the nursing unit that the patient will be arriving shortly and provides his name, diagnosis, physician, and bed placement. This notification is invariably given only 10 to 15 minutes before the person actually arrives on the unit. It is enough time for initial planning among the nursing staff about who will admit the patient and checking the preparation of a room. Evaluate this information from an Admissions Department carefully to find your first clues for patient care (will you need a crib or a bed depending on the age?) and to decide whether the information is consistent with your knowledge of other patients in the room (if the other patient in that room has an infection, is it sound to put this patient who will be going to surgery in the same room?). Although Admissions Department personnel have some assessment skill, they are unable to individualize care or assess patient condition and need at your level. Question room placement or reason for admission if it is not clear.

Room preparation should consist of opening the bed and, if the person is ambulatory, lowering it for easy access. Check that towels and a washcloth are available as well as patient care equipment such as a water basin, emesis basin, and bedpan. Secure equipment that you will need for admission: a blood pressure cuff, a stethoscope, a thermometer, a patient gown, and a urine specimen container for a routine urinalysis. In some instances a urine sample has already been obtained in the Admissions Department. Determine if you need to assemble other equipment such as an intravenous pole or nasogastric suction. Often you cannot anticipate this type of equipment because no orders for therapy have yet been written.

A patient usually arrives on a nursing unit accompanied by a person from the Admissions Department. It is important to remember that when people arrive at a nursing unit they have probably already been through a waiting period. It may seem unreasonable to them if they are told at this point that no one is really ready for them or that they have to wait still longer. Take a minute to stand by the elevator that opens onto a nursing unit and consider how it must appear to someone looking at it for the first time. If it is a busy time of day, the number of people you see may be confusing, and the language they are using is confusing. The atmosphere may be tense (everyone concerned over a patient who has just had a sudden complication). To someone already under stress, the confusion and tension may be overwhelming (Fig. 39-4). Always make an effort to greet a newly arrived patient warmly to attempt to relieve these feelings.

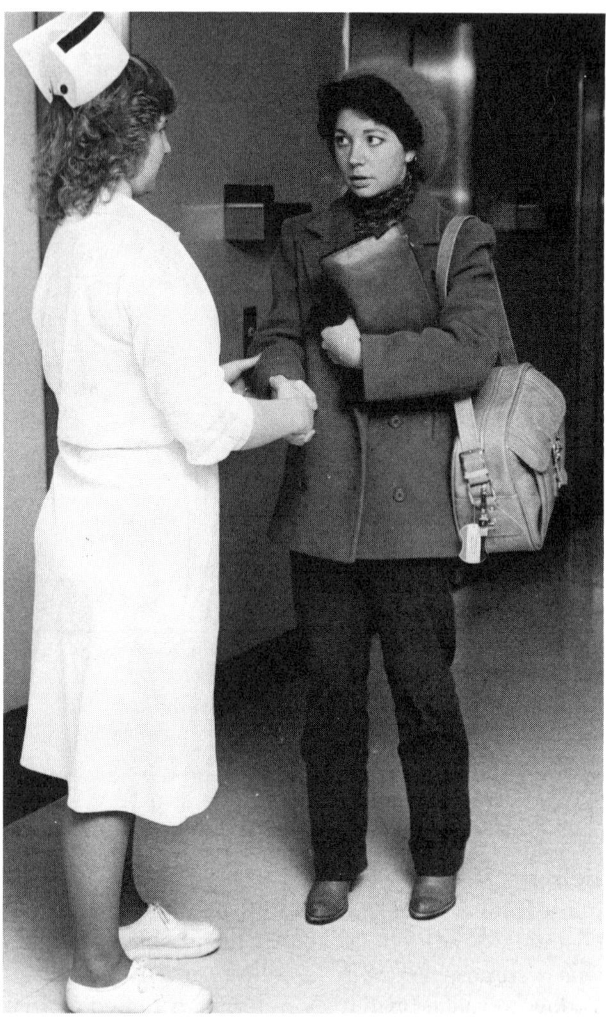

FIGURE 39-4. A nurse welcomes a new patient to the hospital unit. Note the clenched purse and look of apprehension. You need to serve as a primary support person at the time of admission.

Check the person's identification band. Introduce yourself and your status; learn the patient's name correctly (ask how he pronounces it if you are not certain). A frightening situation almost automatically becomes less frightening when you know the name of someone who can be depended on to help you. Most people remember the nurse who admitted them to the hospital long after they have forgotten other caregivers' names.

Admitted patients are generally shown immediately to their assigned room. Procedures 39-1 and 39-2 describe preparation of a hospital room for an adult and child. If there should be a delay because a room is not yet ready, show the person to a waiting area and explain the unfortunate delay. If the delay will be lengthy, admission procedures can be done in a treatment room or a private conference room. Preparing a treatment room is shown in Procedure 39-3. If the person will

PROCEDURE 39-1
Preparing a Hospital Unit for an Adult

Plan	*Principle*
1. Make bed or convert bed from a closed to an open bed.	1. Offers an expected, welcoming appearance.
2. Check room for good ventilation, temperature, and light.	2. Ill persons are very aware of odors, "stuffiness," and so on.
3. Lower the bed if the patient is ambulatory; raise it if the patient will be admitted by stretcher.	3. To ensure easy and safe access.
4. Provide routine bedside equipment (washbasin, emesis basin, bedpan or urinal, water pitcher and glass).	4. Ensure that items necessary for comfort are present.
5. Place gown on bedside stand.	5. Item will be necessary for initial physical assessment.
6. Position call light so that it is easily available.	6. To ensure patient safety.
7. Add additional supplies according to patient condition (if intravenous fluid will be needed, provide an IV pole; if oxygen will be needed, check functioning oxygen outlet).	7. Ensure that necessary procedures can be initiated quickly.
8. Arrange the bedside stand near the bed if the patient is ambulatory; away from it so the stretcher can fit next to the bed if admitted by stretcher.	8. Ensure easy transfer of patient to bed.
9. Secure a stethoscope, blood pressure cuff, thermometer, and urine specimen container for admission procedure.	9. Ensure a welcoming prepared atmosphere for the patient.

PROCEDURE 39-2
Preparing a Hosptial Unit for a Child

Plan	*Principle*
1. Choose proper bed: (a) Isolette for baby under 10 pounds if warmth is needed; cover mattress with pillow case. (b) Crib (most children up to 3 years of age sleep in cribs); cover mattress with full sheet, no draw sheet. Provide blanket if needed for warmth. *No pillows are used in cribs.* (c) Bed (if child sleeps in a bed at home). Make it the same as an adult bed.	1. Children sleep best in the type of bed they sleep in at home. Children who are used to side rails need them for safety and comfort in a hospital setting. A child young enough to be in a crib might suffocate with a pillow.
2. Check room for good ventilation, temperature, and light. Close windows unless equipped with safety screens.	2. Ill persons are very aware of odors, "stuffiness," and so on. Young children might crawl out windows not properly secured.
3. Lower the bed if the patient is ambulatory; raise it to a high position if the child is admitted by stretcher. Lower one side rail of a crib. Do not open an Isolette until the baby arrives to ensure that warmth is maintained.	3. To ensure easy, safe access.
4. Check routine equipment (washbasin, emesis basin, bedpan or urinal, water pitcher, and glass) Do not provide bedpan, urinal, emesis basin, or water pitcher and glass for infant.	4. To ensure that items necessary for comfort are present.
5. Position call light so it is easily available for older child.	5. To ensure patient safety.

6. Choose and provide a suitable toy.	6. Play is a primary method by which children relate to their environment.
7. Add additional supplies according to patient condition (if intravenous fluid will be needed, provide an IV pole; if oxygen will be needed, check for functioning oxygen outlet; if child is not toilet trained, provide diapers).	7. To ensure that necessary procedures can be initiated quickly.
8. Position bedside stand near bed if the older child is ambulatory; away from the bed so the stretcher can fit next to the bed if he is to be admitted by stretcher. Position the bedside stand away from a crib so a young child cannot use it to stand on to climb out of bed or reach for equipment he should not touch.	8. Ensure easy transfer of patient to bed.
9. No need to provide examining equipment at bedside. Children are admitted first to a treatment room to keep their bed area a safe area free from procedures that cause pain.	9. To minimize the effects of hospitalization on young children.

PROCEDURE 39-3
Preparing an Examining Room

Plan	*Principle*
1. Cover the examining table with clean paper.	1. To discourage cross infection between patients.
2. Provide two chairs and a writing surface.	2. To facilitate a meaningful interview.
3. Check room for proper ventilation, temperature, and light.	3. Ill persons are very aware of odors, "stuffiness," and so on.
4. Provide privacy by curtains or door that closes.	4. The right to privacy is a highly valued right by most people.
5. Provide equipment for examination: otoscope, ophthalmoscope, blood pressure cuff, stethoscope, tongue blade.	5. To facilitate the physical examination.
6. Provide a gown if the patient is an adult or older child.	6. To ensure protection of privacy.

have a roommate, make introductions. Show the person what closet space and what bedside stand are his, where the bathroom is, and how to operate an automatic bed control or call bell system (Fig. 39-5). Help him as necessary with unpacking personal articles.

Be certain when handling personal articles to do so with respect and care. Many people bring articles to the hospital with them that have little material value but great sentimental or personal value. Although there is little financial loss to the person if these are accidentally discarded, the sentimental loss is great, and rapport or confidence between health care providers and the patient may never fully develop because of it. A person who is admitting himself to a hospital is putting his life in your hands. He must develop confidence in the people who will be performing his surgery or giving him medication or he may not be able to withstand the emotional stress of this experience. Treat all articles as if they were priceless because that is the price of trust.

Ask the person if he has money or valuables with him that he would like to place in the hospital safe. Many health care agencies have policies that restrict the amount of cash a person may keep with him. If he has more than this, particularly if it is a large amount, investigate the reason. Some people are so worried that someone will break into their apartment while they are hospitalized that they bring their life savings with them. Some older people think of a hospital as a place to die and bring money with them for their spouse to use for funeral expenses. Other people always carry a great deal of money with them and may have hundreds of dollars in their wallet or purse as usual. It helps you to know the reason for bringing such a large amount of money because you may need to initiate some interventions de-

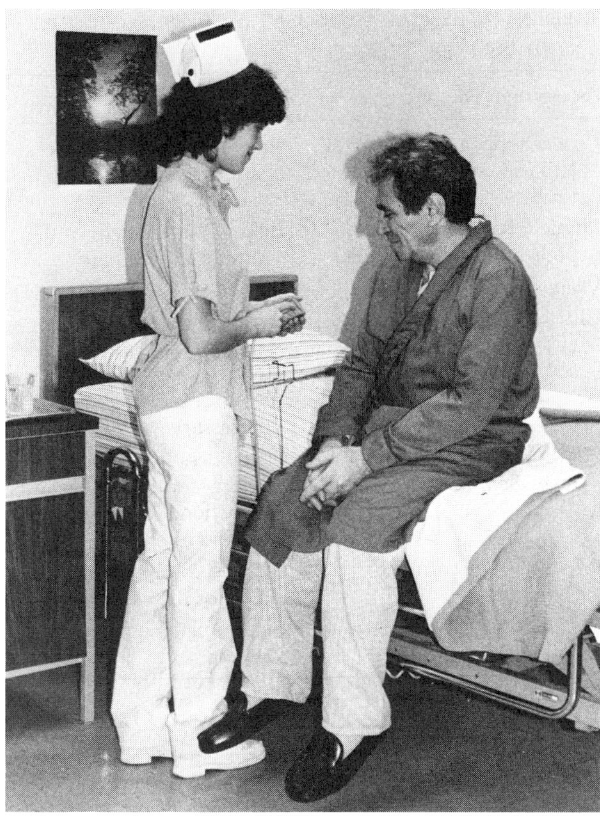

FIGURE 39-5. Orienting a patient to a hospital unit. Here a nurse explains the electric bed controls.

pending on the reason. If the person is convinced that he is going to die, for example, he probably needs better presurgery or pretherapy information than the average person about the outcome or he will not participate well in such postsurgical therapies as coughing and deep breathing exercises. Similarly, if he is worried about his apartment being robbed, he cannot concentrate on procedures in the hospital (and may insist on leaving before he is completely well). You might plan some interventions aimed at locating a neighbor or friend who will check frequently that his home is safe (the police department will do this in small communities). In most health care agencies, money to be deposited in the cashier's office is counted in the presence of the patient and then both the patient and a representative from the cashier's office sign an envelope stating the amount of money inside and seal it before it is taken to the hospital safe. Record on the nursing care plan or nursing kardex file that the person does have valuables in the hospital safe so that these are not overlooked at discharge.

Ask if the person has any medication with him and if he has ever had an allergic reaction to any prescribed or over-the-counter medicine that he has taken; remember, many commonly used medicines such as aspirin can cause drug allergies (see QRS 39-1). Explain that his physician will prescribe any medication that will be necessary for him during his stay in the hospital. Ask him to have his family take home the medicine he has

QUICK REFERENCE STOP 39-1: PHARMACOLOGY
Allergies and Medication Instructions

1. Be certain to ask for known allergies to medication on admission to a health care facility. Document these in a conspicuous place on the patient's chart, nursing care plan, and physician order sheet. If the person cannot name the medicine he knows he is allergic to, ask him what he took it for and to describe what it looked like (small white tablet). Ask the pharmacist to identify such a medicine for you. If the allergic reaction occurred during a previous hospitalization, the old patient chart should include this information.
2. On health care agency discharge, take time to give careful medication instructions. If people arrive home and cannot remember the type, frequency, or dosage of medicine they are to take, they usually handle the problem by not taking the medication at all. Write out instructions as well as giving them orally to increase compliance.

with him or bring it out to the unit medication area to be stored for him until discharge. Record in your admission note the type of medicine he had been taking (medication effects or side effects may have been causing or aggravating some of his recent symptoms). Write a memo for the physician listing the patient's current medications. If the patient has a chronic illness such as recurrent convulsions or asthma, he will probably need to continue this medication during his hospital stay, but if he is being admitted for a reason unrelated to his chronic illness, it is easy for a physician to be concentrating so much on the immediate concerns that she neglects to write orders for the chronic medication. Reminders of types and dosages of medicine help to better coordinate care.

A great many first admission procedures seem to be basically host or hostess measures. But some people are better hosts or hostesses than others because they are more aware of individual concerns and the measures needed to make people feel comfortable and relaxed. Helping patients to feel relaxed and confident in the people who will be their caregivers is not a small accomplishment.

Baseline Measurements

On admission, vital signs are taken (pulse, blood pressure, temperature, and respiratory rate), height and weight are measured, and a urine specimen is obtained. A person will have blood drawn for preliminary base values if this was not done in the Admissions Department. A physical examination is performed by a physician, nurse practitioner, or physician's assistant. This information establishes baseline data; all other measurements taken during the hospital stay will be compared to these. If a person is extremely apprehensive on admission, the first vital signs you measure may be falsely elevated (stress increases pulse, respiratory rate, and blood pressure). In some instances, therefore, you need to repeat these measurements about an hour after admission and mark these determinations as the baseline levels rather than the initial ones.

A urine specimen is obtained to detect metabolic diseases such as diabetes, which might interfere with medication or anesthesia administration. Kidney function that must be assessed before surgery or administration of medication is also revealed by analysis of such a specimen.

Height and weight are taken as an overall guide to good health status and because the doses of medication and anesthesia to be prescribed are influenced by body surface area derived from height and weight. Blood is obtained for determination of a hemoglobin and hematocrit level (estimation of the number of red blood cells present). These measures reflect overall hydration and nutritional status. Additional blood and urine samples are obtained depending on the specific reason for hospital admission.

A person can remain in his street clothing while you assess his vital signs (if his shirt sleeve will roll up far enough for you to fit a blood pressure cuff in place). He will usually need to change to a hospital gown for a physical examination. Patients are urged to wear their own clothing if possible while hospitalized because this generally gives them a feeling of independence.

Nursing Assessment

Even though a complete physical examination will be done by a member of the hospital medical staff, there are some physical factors that you need to assess independently to plan your care (Table 39-1).

TABLE 39-1. PHYSICAL ASSESSMENT FACTORS TO CONSIDER ON ADMISSION

Assessment Factor	Rationale
General appearance (alert, lethargic, thin, obese, tired)	Help to plan activity level, assess level of illness
Physical handicaps (limp, poor manipulative skills)	Help to plan activity and ability for self-care
Vision and hearing	Help to plan for safety
Difficulty in breathing or circulation (cyanosis, coughing, dyspnea)	Establish necessity for immediate care measures; cough suggests infection control measures are necessary
Condition of skin (bruises, rash, cleanliness)	Cleanliness is estimation of energy level; rash suggests infection. Control measures are necessary
Presence of discomfort (pain, pruritus)	Establish necessity for immediate care measures
Prosthesis (contact lenses, artifical leg)	Help to plan activity and safety

Admission History

The person who performs the physical examination will also take a comprehensive health history. In addition, you need to obtain a nursing history of factors that will be important in establishing problems and goals of nursing care. Such a history is discussed in Chap. 18.

Admission Orientation

Review with the patient hospital routines as appropriate (meal hours, visiting regulations, and roles of such people as the dietitian who will be helping to plan care) (QRS 39-2). Be sure that the person knows what specific things will be required of him (for example, he must not eat anything but the food furnished him by the dietitian because he will be on a special diet). Review the projected outline of events that are scheduled for him (he will be going to surgery in the morning; he will be in the hospital a certain number of days, and so on; see QRS 39-3). If you do not know his expected course (and you may not know until the laboratory reports are returned or his physician makes such a determination), do not guess at answers. State simply, "I can't predict anything yet until I get more information." Nothing is as worrisome to people who are already worried as conflicting information. In addition, you may overpredict (making the illness seem more severe than it is) or underpredict. Remember that patients and their support people are under stress at the time of a hospital admission. You may need to repeat instructions concerning procedures at a later date.

QUICK REFERENCE STOP 39-2: NUTRITION
Food Habits

1. Include questions of food habits and likes and dislikes on admission to a health care facility. People have very definite habits related to food consumption. When healthy, they are unwilling to change these habits; if they are ill, it is even more difficult.
2. On discharge, if you anticipate that a person will feel fatigued for a period of time, ask in particular about the plan for home food preparation. If people are too exhausted to cook nutritious food their intake can fall drastically and their full recovery may be very prolonged.

ESTABLISHING SAFETY AND COMFORT

Before you leave a newly admitted patient, be sure to check his immediate environment to be certain it is safe for him. This should be based on data from your history

QUICK REFERENCE STOP 39-3: HEALTH TEACHING
Patient's Knowledge Level

On admission to or discharge from a health care facility, a person cannot know too much about what he can expect to happen to him. No fear is as great for most people as fear of the unknown. People's imaginations are at a high peak at times of stress; often the information you offer (you are going to have intravenous therapy for three days) is good news compared to what a person imagines (he will never be able to eat regularly again).

Many people have only a little factual information about their illness even if they have been ill for a considerable period of time. They may have learned some of what they do know from a neighbor or friend. A little information or wrong information is dangerous because it distorts the person's interpretation of his illness or his therapy. Make a habit of thorough teaching on admission and discharge to prepare the person better for the stress associated with these times.

QUICK REFERENCE STOP 39-4: SAFETY
Self-Care and Support People

1. Ask enough questions and make enough observations on admission so that you can make a sound analysis of a person's ability to perform self-care and to report circumstances accurately. Over- or underestimating a person's potential based on inadequate assessment data can lead to severe injury and increased stress.
2. Ask specifically about the presence of support people on health care facility discharge. No problem ever seems too big or unsolvable if a person has adequate support people around him; the smallest problem can seem overwhelming if no support people are present. Your best assurance of successful posthospital care is the presence of adequate support people.

and physical assessment. Be certain that the bed is in a low position if the person will be ambulatory and that the bedside stand is nearby and easily accessible. The call bell should be pinned to the bottom sheet or within easy reach, and there should be no obstructions between the bed and the bathroom, especially if the patient has any difficulty with vision (see QRS 39-4) or mobility.

If the person is uncomfortable due to pain or nausea, alert his primary care provider. Try to get an order if possible to alleviate such symptoms, and meanwhile, establish independent comfort measures—a quiet environment, shaded lights, comfortable body position. Nausea and pain always seem worse when other factors such as uncertainty are present. Making the person feel welcome and assured that he is going to be cared for by people who are sincerely concerned about him go a long way toward making such symptoms less troublesome.

DOCUMENTATION OF ADMISSION

An initial nurse's note documenting patient status and nursing care must be made on admission. Such a note should contain the date and time and method of admission (ambulatory, by wheelchair, through the emergency room, and so on), physical and interview assessment findings, vital signs, height, weight, and specimens for laboratory analysis that were secured. Communicate findings that need immediate implementation such as dyspnea (difficulty with breathing) or pain so that therapy can be coordinated and begun.

NURSING CARE PLAN

Based on the information obtained from the initial interview, physical assessment, laboratory data, and physician's orders, patient problems can be established and patient care goals and individualized implementations of care can be planned. The use of nursing process to do this is discussed later in this chapter.

ADMISSION THROUGH THE EMERGENCY ROOM

Because some people are already very ill at the time they see a physician or come to a hospital emergency room, they are admitted immediately to the hospital not through the Admissions Department but through the emergency room. In such cases the Admissions Department is contacted by emergency room personnel, and the person is brought to the nursing unit not by an Admissions officer but by emergency room personnel (Fig. 39-6).

A person admitted by this route is under severe stress because of the speed with which events have occurred and the obvious severity of his symptoms. He is usually in severe pain, which is characteristic of most acute illnesses. Because events move quickly in the emergency room, there may have been less time for explanations than in ordinary circumstances; one important first aspect of care on the nursing unit is to provide the patient with explanations to catch up with the circumstances.

A person who has been cared for in the emergency room is grateful for his care there; he feels insecure when his care must be transferred to the nursing unit. Awareness of this feeling helps you to make an extra effort to give the necessary reassurance.

People who are ill enough to come to an emergency room are often in so much pain or so uncomfortable in some other way that they have had little time for planning before admission about practical or family matters. Do they need to notify their family where they are? Did

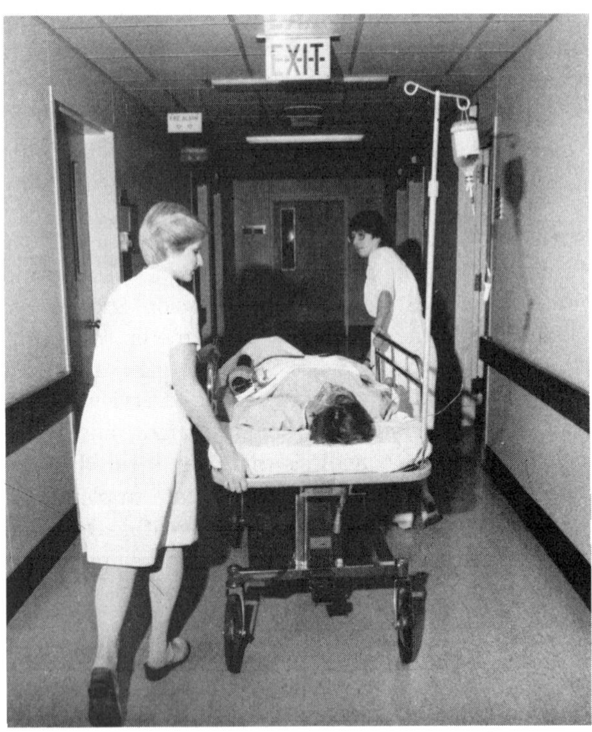

FIGURE 39-6. Transferring a patient from the emergency room to the nursing unit with a stretcher. Because this is an emergency admission, the stress level of patient and family is increased.

they leave small children alone unsupervised? Ask these questions as part of your initial assessment.

Secure a thorough report of the care initiated in the emergency room such as administration of intravenous fluid or any medication. This is important because drug errors can be made if medicine is administered twice, and care measures can be duplicated if they are unknown.

LIFE SPAN CONCEPTS

The Young Child

The admission of a child to a hospital is always a stressful occurrence because it involves separation from parents. In admitting a child, always introduce yourself to both the mother and the child (Fig. 39-7). Think of mother and child as a linked pair.

Rene Spitz, a psychoanalyst, was one of the first modern researchers to document the effects of hospitalization on children (Spitz, 1945). He observed young children in a penal nursery and a foundling home, children separated from their mothers for both short and long periods of time. When a child had been separated from his mother, he noted that the child's first response was crying, a loud demanding sound, suggesting that the child was reaching out and demanding help or comfort. This was the main response of the child for the first month of separation. During the second month of continuous separation, the child's cry changed to a

FIGURE 39-7. The admission of a child to a hospital unit. The nurse stoops to the level of the child to greet and introduce herself. It is important that the nurse also introduce herself to the mother.

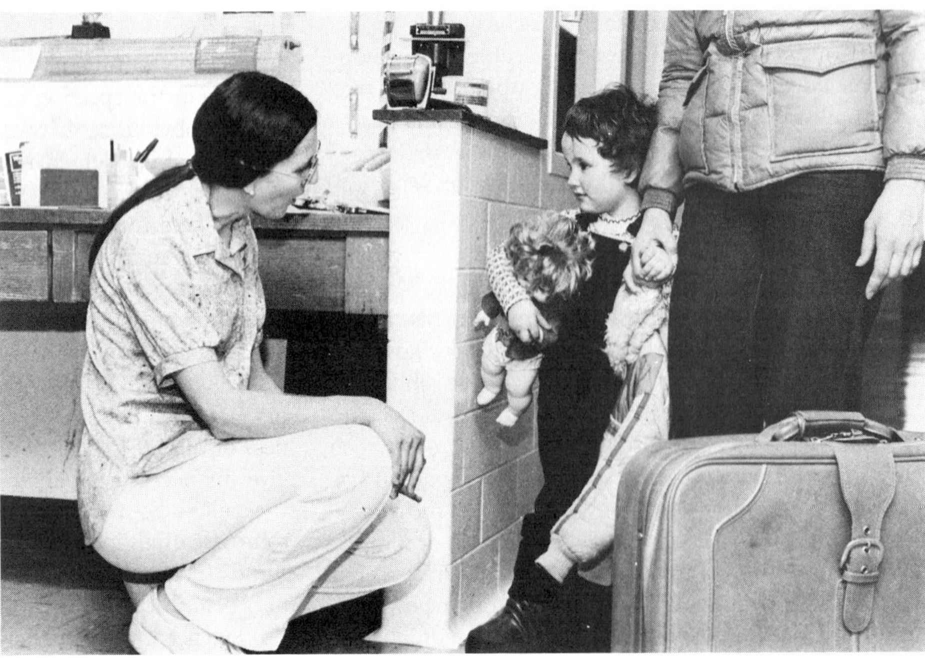

sound more like a scream than a demanding tone. He tended to withdraw when approached; he began to lose weight, and his level of development (such as ability to walk or talk) declined.

During the third month of separation, the child characteristically assumed a position of lying flat on his abdomen. He screamed incessantly if disturbed. He became prone to minor ailments such as upper respiratory tract infections. His IQ level might test as low as 12 points below its preseparation level.

A child who had shown these changes in a separation of less than 3 months and was then returned to his mother usually regained his normal relationship with her in a few days; the changes were only temporary. If separation continued beyond this time, the chances that changes would become permanent increased.

During the fourth month of separation, the child's facial expression became flat; he no longer screamed when approached but had a more pathetic, sad cry. He lost previously acquired skills, and his measured IQ continued to fall. During the fifth month of separation these changes became worse. In some children who were returned to their mothers at this point, the changes were reversible; in others they were not. These 2 months seem to reflect a transition period.

After more than 6 months of separation, irreversible changes occur. The child became silent, his facial expression rigid and fixed. He did not reach out to people around him or expect people to reach out and interact with him. In accordance with Erikson's theory of development, he had failed to develop or lost his sense of trust (Erikson, 1968).

John Bowlby, an English psychoanalyst, documented these earlier findings by studying the reaction of children who were removed from London to the countryside during World War II to keep them safe from the nightly German bombing raids (Bowlby, 1966). Although most of these children were shielded from the terror of the war by this action, they were removed from their parents for more than six months and showed the same inability to interact with people around them as children in the early studies. Bowlby termed loss of maternal attachment in this way *maternal deprivation.* Today, because so many primary caregivers are men, a better term might be *parental deprivation.*

Robertson is another researcher who supplied labels for the effects of separation or maternal deprivation observed by Spitz and Bowlby (Robertson, 1958). He divided such a reaction into three phases: protest, despair, and denial (Table 39-2). The protest and despair stages are comparable to the reversible and transitional stages described by Spitz; the denial stage is the final irreversible stage that will leave a child unable to interact deeply with people again (he does not dare to offer love and risk being so overwhelmingly hurt again). This same phenomenon can occur if a parent dies.

TABLE 39-2. STAGES OF SEPARATION ANXIETY

Stage	Manifestations
Protest	Child cries loudly and demandingly; rejects attempts to comfort him.
Despair	Child wails rather than cries. May turn away at parent's approach. Often lies on abdomen; facial expression is flat. May lose weight and develop insomnia; loses developmental skills. Prone to minor ailments such as upper respiratory infections. IQ will measure lower than formerly.
Denial	Child is silent, face expressionless. Deterioration in developmental milestones. May respond very quickly but very superficially to all caregivers. Will have difficulty forming close relationships during life.

Separation of this kind is most damaging to a child between 6 months and 5 years of age. Special measures to prevent damaging effects during hospitalization must be initiated at hospital admission for children between these ages. These measures include limiting admission to cases that are absolutely necessary, limiting the length of a hospital stay as much as possible, allowing open visiting, providing adequate play space and activities, providing a substitute mother (one nurse should give consistent care, not a multitude—a staffing pattern termed *primary care*), and preparing children adequately for the hospitalization experience and all procedures at their age level. Preschool children especially need good explanations of why they are going to the hospital and what will happen to them. Fear of abandonment is one of their greatest fears; they need assurance not only that they will be well cared for while in the hospital but that they will be going home again. On discharge from the hospital a child in this early age group may demonstrate symptoms of regressive behavior such as thumbsucking or bedwetting for as long as three months past the time of hospitalization.

The Schoolager and Adolescent

Because schoolagers and adolescents are better able to understand explanations and have had some experience with separation before, they adapt better to the hospital experience. Most children do not enjoy missing school more than one or two days because they begin to worry about the large amount of homework they are missing and will have to make up and they miss the companionship of their friends. Help them maintain contact with friends and with school if their physical condition warrants. Help to make arrangements for school work to be brought in or a hospital-based tutor to spend time with them.

The Young and Middle-Aged Adult

Young and middle-aged adults are busy people due to school or work commitments. Some people in these age

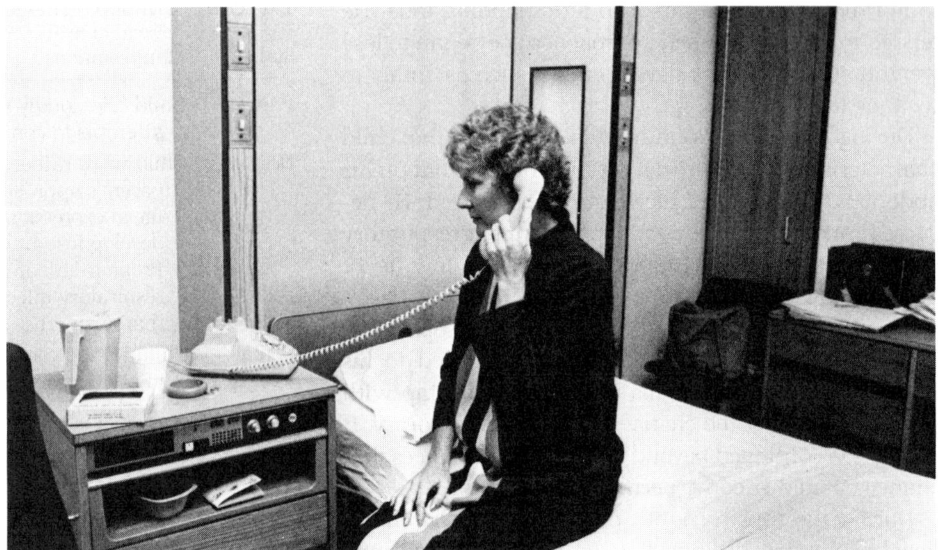

FIGURE 39-8. This patient calls her office daily. Hospitalization interrupts her professional and personal life.

groups are reluctant to take a few days out of their busy life for a hospital admission. They may wait until they are seriously ill before they go for health care, and may be extremely distressed by any delay that prevents them from returning as soon as possible to their outside life (Fig. 39-8).

Discharge planning for this age group needs to concentrate on helping them maintain a schedule that will not exhaust them on discharge and will allow them to return to their regular activity level gradually.

The Older Adult

Fifty years ago, people were admitted to hospitals only when they were extremely ill; hospitals were viewed as places where people were taken to die. Today, hospitals are utilized to promote health as well as restore it, but an older adult may still interpret a hospital admission as a pronouncement of impending death. Many older adults have had little experience with hospitals. They are accustomed to feeling competent in handling their everyday affairs, but in a hospital suddenly they are in a world where they have little information or experience. They may also feel a very distinct age difference from the average health care provider (in a modern hospital the majority of the house medical and nursing staff are under 30 years of age).

On discharge, be sure that the older adult has adequate support people available. Some older adults have outlived their family and neighbors and friends. They need help in locating new support people so they can return to their community again for self-care. Otherwise, they will be readmitted shortly because of their inability to manage alone.

DISCHARGE FROM A HEALTH CARE FACILITY

Discharge planning for a patient begins on the day of admission so that by the day of discharge, all the arrangements for patient care at home will fall smoothly into place. Many people need a referral to a community health nurse to help coordinate or supervise their care at home. Other persons are discharged from the hospital to an extended care setting.

Before a person can be discharged from a health care facility, he must have a discharge order written by his physician. Most people (including you) know well in advance what day they will be discharged, however, so planning can begin well before this. The actual order serves as a confirmation.

The average person is pleased at going home; he is usually weaker than he realizes, however. You need to help him conserve his strength on the day of discharge and during discharge activities so he does not arrive home exhausted. Help him pack his personal articles as necessary. Ask a representative from the cashier's office to bring any valuables the patient placed in the hospital safe up to the patient's unit.

To be released from the facility, a family member as a rule must take the discharge notice from the nursing unit to the business office and return it to the nursing unit showing that payment for the hospitalization has been made or arranged for. No patient can be kept in a hospital, however, if he does not want to stay (unless he presents a health risk to the community such as someone with a communicable disease or self-destructive tendencies) or because he has not paid his bill. Keeping a person under these conditions legally constitutes false imprisonment. People who wish to leave against medical advice are asked to sign a form that states that they are aware they are leaving against medical advice and doing so may be harmful to them. Your responsibility to these people is to help them understand why their actions may be detrimental to their health, but, if they decide that that is their choice, it is truly their choice. Health care is a right, not an obligation. People who insist on leaving without paying their hospital bill are, from your standpoint, free to do so also.

Many health care agencies have a policy stating that people being discharged must be taken to the lobby of the hospital by wheelchair to conserve their strength and to prevent accidental falls on stairways or in the elevator. Many people consider riding in a wheelchair a nuisance and ask to walk. If this is hospital policy, however, explain it as such and ask the patient to comply, stressing that he needs to conserve energy. Wait with him while a family member brings the car to the lobby or discharge entrance; assist him with getting into the car and as necessary with a suitcase and personal articles.

The Patient's Room After Discharge

Following discharge, the patient's bed must be stripped of all linen, and all supplies such as unused intravenous fluid or dressings must be removed from the room. Do not return any supplies from a patient's room to an area for reuse. Depending on hospital policy, these will either be discarded or resterilized. Before another person can be admitted to the room, it will need to be cleaned by the housekeeping department and the bed remade; supplies such as washbasin, towels, and washcloth will be replaced. Because cleaning of rooms must be done between patients to reduce the possibility of spread of microorganisms, there is sometimes a delay in admitting a new patient.

Documentation of Discharge

You need to record in your nursing note the time and means of discharge (by wheelchair, in mother's arms, or ambulatory), general physical and psychological condition of the patient (pleased to go home, walked steadily), where he was discharged to (home or an extended care facility), and who he was discharged to if a child (most health care agencies do not allow a minor child to be discharged to anyone but his parents or foster parents). Comment on whether the original goals that were established for the patient on admission were fully accomplished or not. This information will be important if the person is readmitted because it also documents his condition on discharge.

Discharge Instructions

Most physicians review with patients the care they want them to continue at home (can walk upstairs, must take medicine). Because people under stress do not "hear" well, however, and discharge is a stressful situation, the physician also writes these instructions on an order sheet so that you can review them with the patient. Begin discharge instructions by asking what the person has been told. Fill in details and elaborate as necessary. Sometimes the first time a person is told something he first thinks only that he must do it; then he begins to wonder how to do it. Help people to think through their individual circumstances and solve problems they can anticipate (how can I take a bath with a cast on my leg?). You will learn to answer many of these questions because the solution for most people will be the same (he can't take a bath but he can shower if he covers the cast tightly with a plastic bag). Directions such as "sparingly" may be as difficult for you to understand as for the patient. Recheck with the physician for clarification as necessary. If instructions are not clear, most people handle the problem by simply ignoring the instruction.

If more than one medicine is involved in the instructions, it may be necessary to make out a chart as a medicine reminder. It is easy to confuse two types of medicine or forget to take them when everyday problems of a family or home are superimposed on medication administration (see Chap. 29).

Be certain that the person knows where he should return for a check-up visit and when. In some instances the person will be told to telephone the physician's office or a clinic the next day and make an appointment for a return visit. If this is so, be sure he knows what number (his physician, a clinic) to telephone if he has some questions about his care after he returns home or if his condition changes markedly before it is time for his return follow-up visit (Fig. 39-9).

The Concept of Discharge Planning

In many health care agencies a discharge planner is assigned to help people with planning home care, but even when such people are available, you, as the person who knows the patient best, should review home care plans (well enough in advance of discharge that changes can be made; see QRS 39-5). Factors to consider in planning discharge include activity allowed, supplies the person will need to purchase (including medications), nutrition, support people available, and arrangements for follow-up care (Fig. 39-10).

ACTIVITY

A person who will need to limit his activity following hospitalization (for a heart attack or heart surgery, for example) may have difficulty in doing so unless someone helps him make definite plans. If he lives in a second-floor apartment he cannot even arrive home without climbing a flight of stairs. If he has no refrigeration and therefore has to go out daily to buy milk and other perishable food, he must climb stairs at least once a day. In such cases, the person's physician may delay discharge from the hospital until he is ready to climb stairs.

If the person lives in a two-story home and has his bedroom on the upper floor, his family may have to temporarily convert a downstairs room to a bedroom so

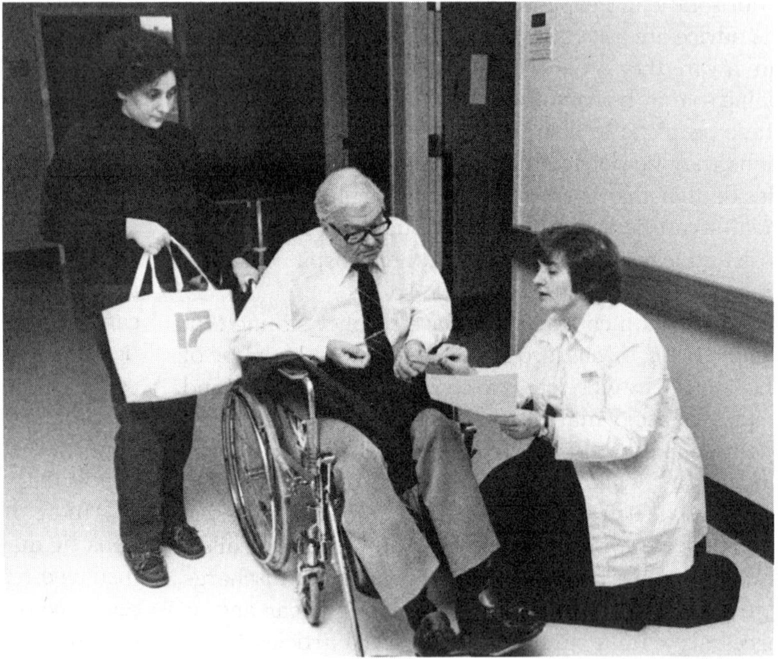

A

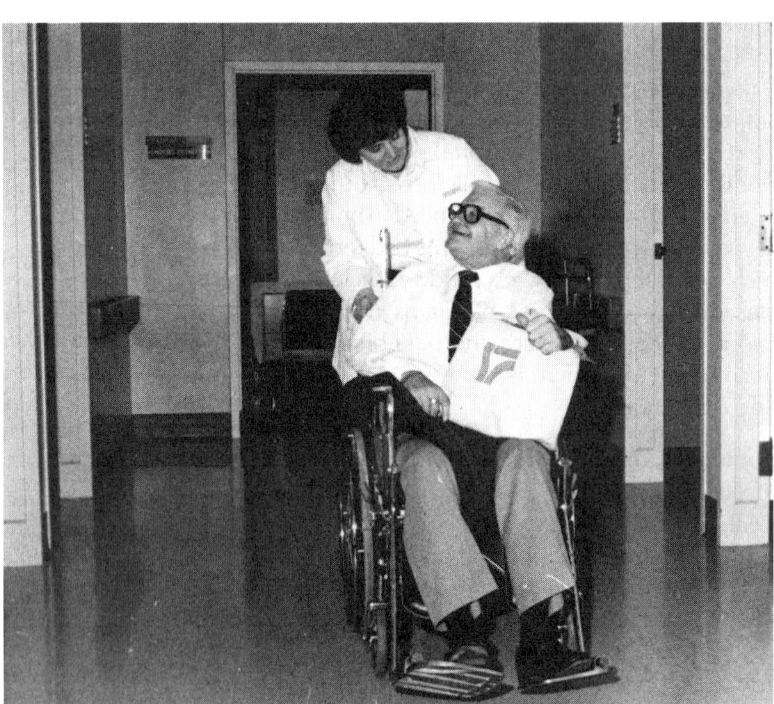

B

FIGURE 39-9. A. Preparation for discharge begins at the time of hospital admission and continues throughout hospitalization. Because people under stress do not "hear" well, the nurse reviews this man's clinic appointment card and written instructions one final time before discharge. Notice the level of concentration. B. This nurse-patient relationship is one of concern and trust. The nurse can function in a supportive role for the patient following discharge as well as she did during his hospitalization.

QUICK REFERENCE STOP 39-5: ADVOCACY
Discharge to Proper Setting

A person can be discharged to many different places following hospitalization in an acute care setting: his home, an extended care facility, a hospice, a nursing home, a relative's home, another acute care setting, or a specialty care setting. Because you are often the person who knows a patient best, you are often the person most aware of the patient's desires or capabilities. You may need to advocate for a patient to see that his wishes are respected and his discharge plans are in his best interests.

that he will not have to climb stairs. In some families this may create a major change and will need time to make plans.

In other instances, encouraging activity may be the problem you need to deal with. Following bone or muscle surgery, for example, the person may have instructions to walk a specified distance or amount of time every day. If it is summer and no stairs are involved, this should be no problem. If the front walk is icy, however, and the patient worries about falling on slippery stairs, he may not be able to walk further than the distance between his living room and the bathroom. A person may need help to realize that exercise is exercise whether it is outside or inside.

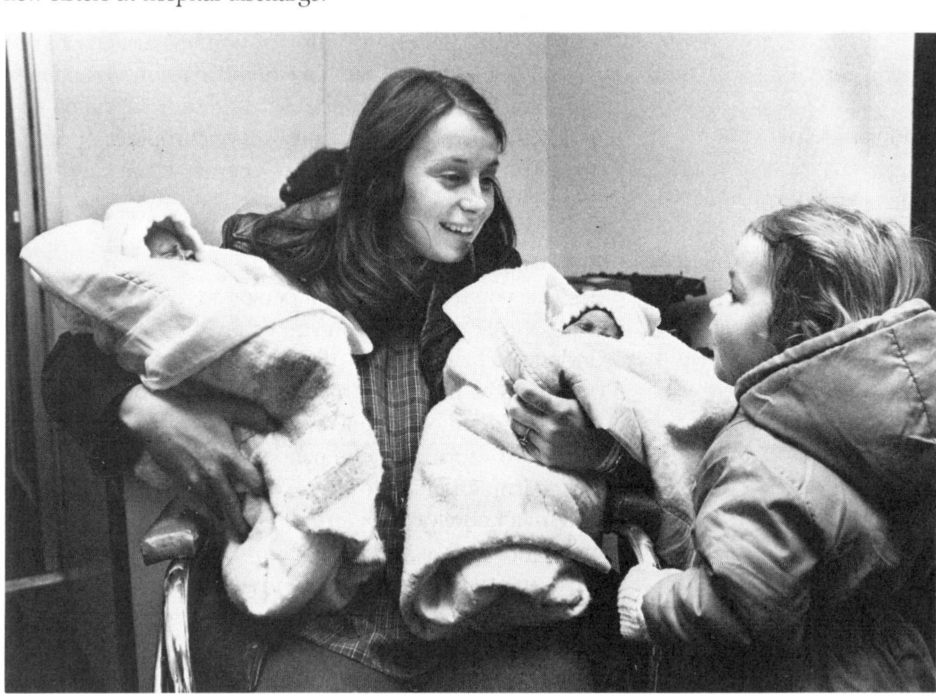

FIGURE 39-10. People assume increased responsibility at the time of discharge. Here a mother introduces a sibling to two new sisters at hospital discharge.

SUPPLIES

If a person will be taking medicine when he returns home or changing a dressing, he will need to secure the medicine or dressings needed. Discuss with him whether this will involve financial difficulty (his hospital insurance may have covered all of his hospital expenses but will not pay for ambulatory expenses, for example). The physician may be able to order medicine by its generic name rather than a brand name, or the social services department of the hospital might be able to suggest other forms of health care financing as alternatives. Ask whether transportation to a pharmacy for medication refills or dressings will be a problem. This is the type of problem that is usually solved easily but appears difficult to a person under stress.

NUTRITION

Management of a nutritious diet requires special investigation. If the person cannot accomplish this, none of the other measures of therapy will be as effective as they could be. Food is an expensive budget item; ask if cost will be a problem. Buying food requires transportation or assistance, and cooking may require assistance. Will either of these aspects be a problem?

SUPPORT PEOPLE AVAILABLE

In some instances the person who is ill does not have ready support people around him because he is his family's chief support person. People who normally are helpful may be as distraught by the illness as the ill person and unexpectedly provide no support. In such cases, you need to help the ill person locate other support people. These may be family members such as aunts, cousins, or uncles rather than immediate family members; they may be secondary support people such as friends and neighbors, or they may be tertiary support people such as members of the family's church or synagogue or an organization such as Parents of Retarded Children. Health care providers who will offer followup care (physician or clinic) may serve this function, as may a community health nurse.

CONTINUED CARE

If a family member or the patient himself will be performing a procedure such as injecting medicine or changing a dressing, he should have ample opportunity to practice and redemonstrate the procedure under your guidance before the patient is discharged from the health care facility; his proficiency requires individual assessment.

If the patient will be giving self-injections, a family member is generally taught the procedure as well so that someone else is available for this task in an emergency. To be eligible for home health service care under a third-party payment program, the patient must be in need of skilled nursing care or need a service such as those listed in the following box. Although a family member can be taught to do many of these things, if the family is eligible for third-party payment for a community health nursing service, this is probably their best option (they not only will receive the technical aspects of care but will have an active teacher and support person available to them). Many people who are not eligible for third-party payment programs want to be referred to a community health nurse because they recognize that they will need continued support while at home. See the box, Situations That Suggest Continuing Care.

COMMUNITY HEALTH NURSE REFERRAL FOR THIRD-PARTY PAYMENTS
Eligibility Factors

To be eligible for a third-party program, a patient must be in need of skilled nursing care:

1. Administration of intravenous therapy
2. Wound care or dressing
3. Rehabilitative nursing care
4. Postcataract care
5. Indwelling bladder catheter irrigation or instillation
6. Chest physiotherapy (percussion or postural drainage)
7. Venipuncture for blood drawing
8. Establish bowel or bladder training
9. Injections of medication
10. Nasogastric tube feedings
11. Tracheostomy care
12. Oxygen or inhalation therapy
13. Health teaching for such subjects as diabetic care, terminal illness, ostomy care
14. Skilled observations such as vital signs

Situations That Suggest Continuing Care

A functional handicap
Emotional or psychological handicap
No known support people
Alcohol or drug dependence
Person has suffered a violent crime (includes child, spouse, or older age abuse)
Terminal illness
Indigency
Elderly person or minor child

UTILIZING NURSING PROCESS

Assessment

A great deal of information must be gathered quickly during admission to a health care facility. Interview and physical assessment information is gathered immediately. In many instances you are aware of the person's status and needs hours before other members of the health care team. Ability to assess on admission with a degree of speed comes with practice. Thoroughness in the beginning is a better quality to strive for. If you think speed first, you may never learn to become thorough, and your initial assessments will always be incomplete and not of high quality.

Assessment findings on the day of admission serve a twofold purpose. They serve both as assessment information and as discharge information because discharge planning begins on the day of admission. Discharge planning information should be kept updated by periodic reassessment to prevent incomplete or inappropriate information by the time of actual discharge due to changing patient status.

Analysis

Because you may be the first person to realize a patient's status on admission, you are often the first person to understand how uncomfortable he is or how many questions he has about his illness. Once you have established a nursing diagnosis based on your findings (analysis) there are many independent nursing actions that can be implemented to relieve discomfort or increase the patient's knowledge before the remainder of the health care team arrives. Because you often know patients better than other caregivers, you are often in the best position to establish nursing diagnosis for problems that are still present and need followup care when the person returns home.

Planning

Any life change involves modifications of actions; planning with a person for changes at both admission and discharge from a health care facility is a major nursing role. It is important to discuss plans with the patient as well as alternative or modifications of these plans.

The following box lists patient situations that will need careful discharge planning. Discharge plans must often be discussed with support persons because it is these people who will actually be carrying out the plan (cooking a low sodium diet, administering a medicine, and so on).

Situations That Suggest Careful Discharge Planning

Dietary restrictions
Infection
Major surgery or illness
Multiple diagnoses
A varying or complicated therapy program
A history of past complications performing self-care
Limitation of body function in any area
Progressive disease process

Implementation

On any nursing unit, the measures carried out when a person is admitted vary greatly depending on patient condition and age, diagnosis, and plan of care. In some instances so many immediate physical care measures are needed that your immediate time is occupied with technical aspects of care such as vital signs recording or beginning intravenous therapy; as soon as the patient's condition is stabilized, return to the measures that are designed to make him feel comfortable and confident in his situation because without this assurance and teaching, a hospital experience can be overwhelming (see QRS 39-6).

DISCHARGE INSTRUCTIONS

ERIE COUNTY HEALTH CENTER
Discharge Instruction Sheet

Name: Robert Colton

DIET

Your diet at home will be: 2500 calorie diabetic diet

Restrictions: Use exchange lists (attached)

MEDICATIONS

Medication	*Time and Frequency*	*Possible Side Effects*
Regular insulin 5 units	Daily 7:00 A.M.	Call physician if nausea, vomiting, dizziness, or disorientation occur.
NPH insulin 10 units	Daily 7:00 A.M.	
	Combine in one syringe and inject subcutanously.	

ACTIVITY

You may: Shower _X_ Tub bath _X_ Sponge bath __ Climb stairs _X_
Drive a car _X_ Resume sexual activity _X_
Other Resume full phys. ed. program in school.

SPECIAL INSTRUCTIONS

Test urine twice daily, before 7:00 A.M. insulin and 12:00 noon. Call nurse practitioner if urine tests reveals glucose 2^+ or over or any acetone. Followup Care: Return to Diabetic Clinic in 1 week with urine test results. Call Diabetic Clinic (695-2124) if any concerns arise within 1 week.

Signature: M. Smith R.N.

QUICK REFERENCE STOP 39-6: PSYCHOLOGICAL CONSIDERATIONS
Importance of Admission and Discharge

Admission to and discharge from a health care agency both involve change, and change is one of the hardest circumstances for a person to accept. Do not allow yourself to begin to think of these procedures as routine.

Evaluation

Evaluation tells you if your initial plan of care was therapeutic or not. Because first plans on a hospital admission are based on information gathered the first time you meet a person, interventions planned at this time may turn out to be less than optimal when you know the person better. Evaluation allows you to discover these discrepancies and make corrections as needed.

One of the dissatisfactions in nursing is that although you care for a person for many days when he is critically ill and are interested in how well he returns to health, you never see or hear from him again after discharge. If you know that people will be returning for a followup visit to a clinic in the hospital, tell them to stop by the nursing unit to let you know how they are doing. If they will be followed in a physician's office outside the hospital, ask them to call the nursing unit in a week or a month and let you know how they are. This is an aspect not only of evaluation but of job satisfaction as well. You impart a great deal of physical and mental effort in helping a person recover from a serious illness. You deserve the satisfaction of seeing a man who was exhausted by taking only six steps the last time you saw him now walk the full length of the hallway and tell you that he is back at work again. That is both an evaluation of your skill as a professional nurse and your reward for hours of concern and care.

Discharge Instructions

Bobby is a 16-year-old patient of yours. He is admitted to the hospital for 10 days for diagnosis of diabetes mellitus, regulation of diet, and insulin injection. The teaching plan for Bobby was shown in Chap. 16. The box on page 1059 shows an example of discharge instructions that would be given to him.

SUGGESTED READINGS

Aish, A. Not all patients need hospitals. *Canad. Nurse* 75:23, 1979.

Armitage, S. K. Negotiating the discharge of medical patients. *J. Adv. Nurs.* 6:385, 1981.

Atkins, D. M. Evaluation of preadmission preparation programs: Goals clarification as the first step. *Child Health Care* 10:48, 1981.

Avery, M. D., et al. An early postpartum hospital discharge program: Implementation and evaluation. *J.O.G.N. Nurs.* 11(4):233, 1982.

Bowlby, J., et al. *Maternal Care and Mental Health.* New York: Schocken Books, 1966.

Bristow, C., et al. *Discharge Planning for Continuity of Care.* New York: National League of Nursing, 1976.

Britton, C., et al. Innovative discharge planning—Try it: the result may surprise you. *Nursing 80* 10:44, 1980.

Broomfield, F. Involving staff in discharge planning. *Supervisor Nurse* 10:35, 1979.

Combined functions ensure patient's continuity of care. *Hosp. Prog.* 64(3):26, 1983.

Conger, S. A., et al. Is there a gap in communication between acute care facilities and nursing homes? *Health Soc. Work* 7(4):274, 1982.

Connolly, M. L. Organize your workday for more effective discharge planning. *Nursing* (Horsham) 11(7):44, 1981.

Coulton, C. J., et al. Discharge planning and decision making. *Health Soc. Work* 7(4):253, 1982.

DeYoung, M. Care of the acutely ill older adult: Planning for discharge. *Geriatr. Nurs.* 3(6):396, 1982.

Erikson, E. H. *Childhood and Society.* New York: Norton, 1968.

Glover, J. C. Reducing discharge planning paperwork with a pocket-size discharge planning record. *Nursing* (Horsham) 11(12):50, 1981.

Harvey, B. Your patient's discharge plan. *Nursing 81* 11:48, 1981.

Johnson, J., et al. Planning patient's discharge. *Supervisor Nurse* 12:44, 1981.

Kucler, M. A. Discharge dilemma for an ED nurse. *Am. J. Nurs.* 81:2010, 1981.

Mandell, S. Post discharge follow-up. *Issues Compr. Pediatr. Nurs.* 4:1, 1980.

Mezzanotte, E. J. A checklist for better discharge planning. *Nursing* (Horsham) 10(11):64, 1980.

Minor, H. E., et al. The nurse as admission evaluator . . . for a 30 bed rehabilitation medicine unit. *Am. J. Nurs.* 81:118, 1981.

Noga, K. M. High-risk infants: The need for nursing follow-up. *J.O.G.N. Nurs.* 11(2):112, 1982.

Reichelt, P. A., et al. Organizational factors in discharge planning—four models. *J. Nurs. Admin.* 10:30, 1980.

Robertson, J. *Young Children in Hospitals.* London: Tavistock, 1958.

Scupholme, A. Postpartum early discharge: An inner city experience. *J. Nurse Midwife* 26(6):19, 1981.

Smith, I., et al. Psychiatry/mental handicap forum. 9. Return to the world of everyday living. *Nurs. Mirror* 155(12):20, 1982.

Spitz, R. A. Hospitalism: An inquiry into the genesis of psychiatric conditions in early childhood. *Psychoanal. Study Child.* 1:53, 1945.

Trofino, J. Reducing workloads for staff nurses. *Nurs. Manage.* 13(3):37, 1982.

Van Putte, A. A student contribution to excellence in the unification model. *Nurs. Adm. Q.* 6(1):41, 1981.

QUESTIONS FOR REVIEW

The following is a Bingo card. Cross out the appropriate answer for each question. When you think you have a Bingo (five across or diagonally) check the Answers to Questions for Review to see if you are correct.

1. The day that discharge planning should begin.
2. Important aspect to ask about in relation to medicine on admission.
3. An important aspect of the reception area in an ambulatory setting.
4. The term that describes determining priority for care.
5. The person who usually offers the most consistency in an ambulatory health care setting.
6. An important aspect of care for someone admitted through a birthing room.
7. Type of measures carried out on admission to a health care facility.
8. Important aspect to check before you leave a newly admitted patient.
9. Hazard of hospitalization in preschool and younger children.
10. Concept of the purpose of hospitals for some older adults.
11. Refusing to allow a person to leave a health care facility is ______ .
12. Persons to whom a minor child can be discharged.

B	I	N	G	O
MEDICINE	DAY DIAGNOSIS IS ESTABLISHED	IDENTIFICATION	PHYSICIAN	DAY OF ADMISSION
SELECTIVE PROCESSING	A PLACE TO DIE	TRIAGE	BASELINE DETERMINATIONS	NUTRITION
SAFETY	ALLERGIES	FREE	FALSE IMPRISONMENT	PRIVACY
DAY OF DISCHARGE	NURSE	FINANCIAL AID	TYPE OF PATIENT	PHYSICAL THERAPIST
MATERNAL DEPRIVATION	RESTRAINT AGAINST COMMON PRACTICE	PARENTS	A PLACE OF HEALTH PROMOTION	THIRD-PARTY PAYMENT

40. PREOPERATIVE, INTRAOPERATIVE, AND POSTOPERATIVE MEASURES OF CARE

Surgery, like all branches of health care, grows in complexity every year. Types of surgery possible increase, as do their safety requirements. As types and extents of surgery expand, so does the responsibility of nursing care.

OBJECTIVES

Upon mastery of the material in this chapter, you should be able to:

1. List the important components of a preoperative nursing interview.
2. Assess a patient in terms of surgical risk in order to plan nursing care.
3. Describe preoperative teaching measures.
4. Describe the experience a person can expect to encounter in surgery.
5. List common preoperative medications and their effects.
6. Describe the criteria for informed surgical consent.
7. Describe how surgery is affected by differing age groups.
8. Describe common postoperative care measures.
9. Describe common complications of surgery and the common measures used to prevent them.
10. Apply nursing process to give safe and planned care to a patient whose care involves principles of preoperative, intraoperative, or postoperative care.

TERMS

The terms important for an understanding of this chapter are shown below and defined in the glossary:

anesthesia
dehiscence
evisceration
general anesthesia
hemostasis
keloid
local anesthesia
paralytic ileus
regional anesthesia
saddle-back anesthesia
spinal anesthesia

TYPES OF SURGERY

Surgery may be done to provide a diagnosis (biopsy) or elective therapy (plastic surgery for cosmetic affect), to prevent or cure infection (incision and drainage of an infected wound), to treat disease (removal of an inflammed gall bladder), to remove symptoms (palliative surgery such as severing a nerve to alleviate pain), or to preserve life (relief of intestinal obstruction).

Surgery may be done on an *emergency* basis if the cause for surgery is life threatening, such as appendicitis or skull fracture. The preoperative phase is shortened in these situations but still must include all necessary preparations.

Other surgery, termed *imperative*, is scheduled to be performed as soon as the operating schedule will accommodate the procedure (6 to 8 hours); an example is a gall bladder removal (cholecystectomy). It is important that a person maintain optimal physical condition during this waiting period in order to enter surgery in the best physical condition possible. Still other surgery is *required* but not immediate, such as tonsillectomy, so it is scheduled weeks or months in advance.

Some surgical procedures are two-stage procedures, and a person may actually be discharged from the hospital between stages. Be certain that the person understands the importance of returning for the second stage of surgery.

Still other surgery is *elective* or optional surgery (a procedure with little immediate cause) and is scheduled at the convenience of the surgeon and patient. Revision of scar tissue is an example of this type of surgery. Some insurance policies do not pay for elective surgery. Be certain that you do not note the term wrongly on a chart. Because a person elected to be hospitalized for surgery on a certain date does not make the surgery elective.

HOLISTIC EFFECTS OF SURGERY

If a body cavity is opened but no organs are cut or repaired, the procedure is described as an *otomy* (a *laparotomy* is an exploration of the abdominal cavity, for example). If an organ is repaired or removed, the procedure is described with the suffix *ectomy* (*tonsillectomy*, for example, is removal of tonsils).

Minor surgery is surgery that involves a simple procedure and is performed in a brief time with minor blood loss and anesthesia. Biopsies (removal of a small tissue sample for laboratory analysis) or simple hernia repairs are examples. In actual practice, however, there is no such thing as truly *minor* surgery, since a person's entire

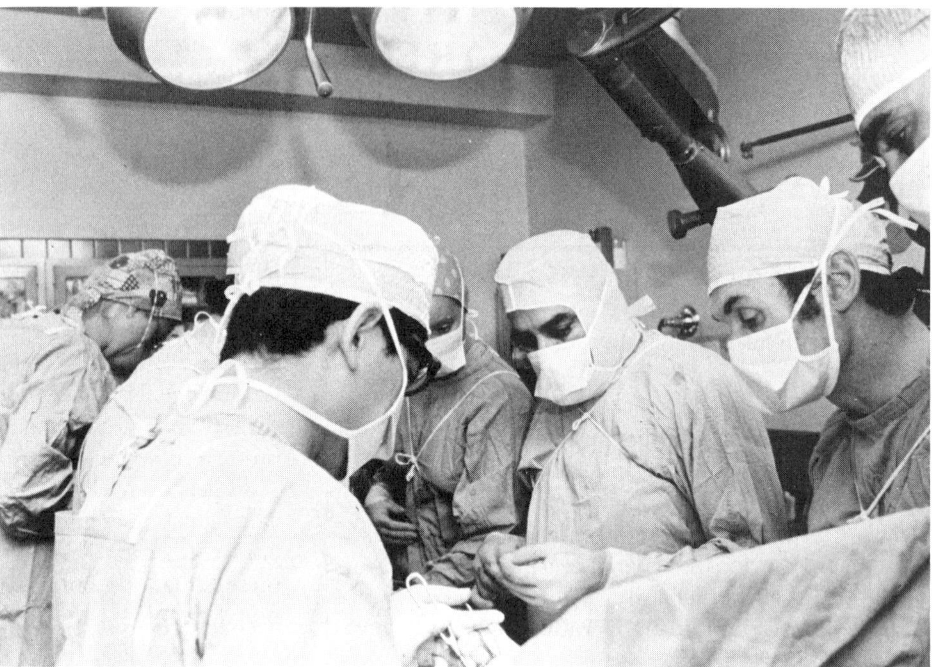

FIGURE 40-1. Surgery is always a risk because of the physical and psychosocial factors involved.

physical and psychosocial self is affected by any surgical procedure, no matter how limited (Fig. 40-1). *Major* surgery is surgery that involves major body structures, takes a long time to complete, and has the potential for extensive blood loss. Cholecystectomy, hysterectomy (removal of the uterus), and heart surgery are examples.

EFFECT OF STRESS RESPONSE ON BODY SYSTEMS

Whenever the body is subjected to stress, either physical or psychosocial, it responds with measures to preserve the function of major body systems. Because a surgical experience involves both physical and psychosocial aspects, it readily activates this "fight or flight" mechanism.

A stress response results in release of epinephrine and norepinephrine from the adrenal gland medulla. Epinephrine causes an increased heart rate, bronchial dilatation, and elevation of blood glucose level. Norepinephrine leads to peripheral vasoconstriction, which forces a good blood supply to the central circulation and an increased blood pressure.

These normally positive responses (the person is tensed or ready for action with good heart and lung function and glucose for energy) may contradict anesthetic action (which is aimed at minimizing body activity) and therefore not be beneficial for the surgical patient. Combined with interferences to major body systems, these effects can add to the risk of surgery.

INTERFERENCE WITH BODY DEFENSES

The skin serves as the primary line of defense against bacterial invasion. When skin is incised (cut) for a surgical procedure the important line of defense is automatically lost. Strict adherence to aseptic technique during surgery and the days following the procedure must be maintained to compensate for the impaired defense.

INTERFERENCE WITH CIRCULATORY FUNCTION

The cutting of blood vessels is required in even the simplest of surgical procedures. Although cut vessels are immediately clamped and ligated (tied off) during surgery, there will always be some blood loss. Extensive blood loss leads to hypovolemia with lowered blood pressure. This could lead to ineffective perfusion of body tissues. Controlling or stopping blood loss is termed *hemostasis*. Close observation of vital signs (pulse, respiratory rate, and blood pressure) during and following the procedure is important to determine that hemostasis is complete and that no "bleeders" are still present.

INTERFERENCE WITH BODY ORGAN FUNCTION

When any body organ is handled, cut, or repaired in surgery, it may respond with a temporary disruption in function. Pressure of edema or inflammation as fluid moves into the injured area will further impair function of the organ involved and that of surrounding organs. If blood vessels are compressed, distant organs may be deprived of blood flow and thus function will be reduced. Following a surgical procedure, therefore, broad

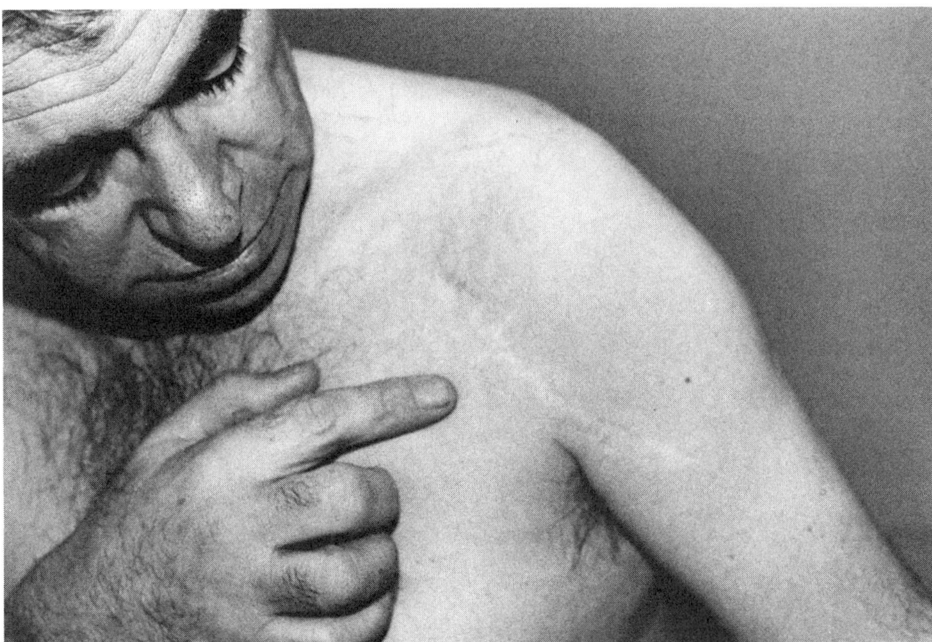

FIGURE 40-2. Surgical scars can interfere with self-esteem. Here a patient describes how a scar from past surgery makes him feel self-conscious.

observation of not only the one organ involved but of total body function is necessary to assess the total disruption present.

INTERFERENCE WITH SELF-IMAGE OR SELF-ESTEEM

Surgery always leaves an incisional scar; if clearly visible, the scar may cause the person later to feel self-conscious (Fig. 40-2). If surgery involves removal of a major organ such as the uterus or intestine, a person may feel less or inferior to others afterward. If the outcome of surgery is not optimal, the person may need to adjust his life style to compensate for a continuing health problem. People who anticipate that the outcome of surgery will not be favorable generally do not participate in its preparation as much as others and so may develop more postoperative complications, such as pneumonia from inability to perform coughing or breathing exercises. Assessing a person's self-esteem is an important preoperative measure.

LIFE SPAN CONCEPTS

People's attitude toward surgery as well as the actual risks they face are influenced by age.

The Newborn

Newborn infants (provided that they were born without respiratory or nutritional defects) are good candidates for surgery. Their parents, however, are generally reluctant to agree to surgery for such a young infant. Birth of a child is a stressful situation; parents under stress are less able to reason or problem solve than those who are not. Parents need very clear explanations of the risks and benefits involved in surgery; you may have to repeat yourself before they feel that they understand. If the mother has no support person with her, she may be unwilling to make a decision for surgery until a person whose judgment she trusts arrives.

Bonding is a tenuous phenomenon. Mothers who feel well cared for during the immediate birth period appear better able to offer warm care to their infants. Remembering this, be certain that the mother learns that surgery has gone well and her infant is in the recovery room as soon as possible; prepare her for any equipment that is being used with her child following surgery, such as nasogastric tubes. Help her to hold and care for the infant as soon as possible. Until she does this, the birth of the infant does not seem real and bonding cannot occur.

The Infant

The hemoglobin level of infants reaches a low point at about 3 months of age as fetal hemoglobin reaches the end of its life span and adult type hemoglobin has not yet reached full production. Within a short time, the hemoglobin level returns to normal and infants do well with surgery. Mothers often have difficulty judging an infant's needs and degree of illness, so the information that the infant is so ill he needs surgery may be totally unexpected. It may also destroy the mother's confidence in herself as a mother. During the postoperative period, a major nursing responsibility is to reinstate a mother's confidence in herself by allowing her to hold

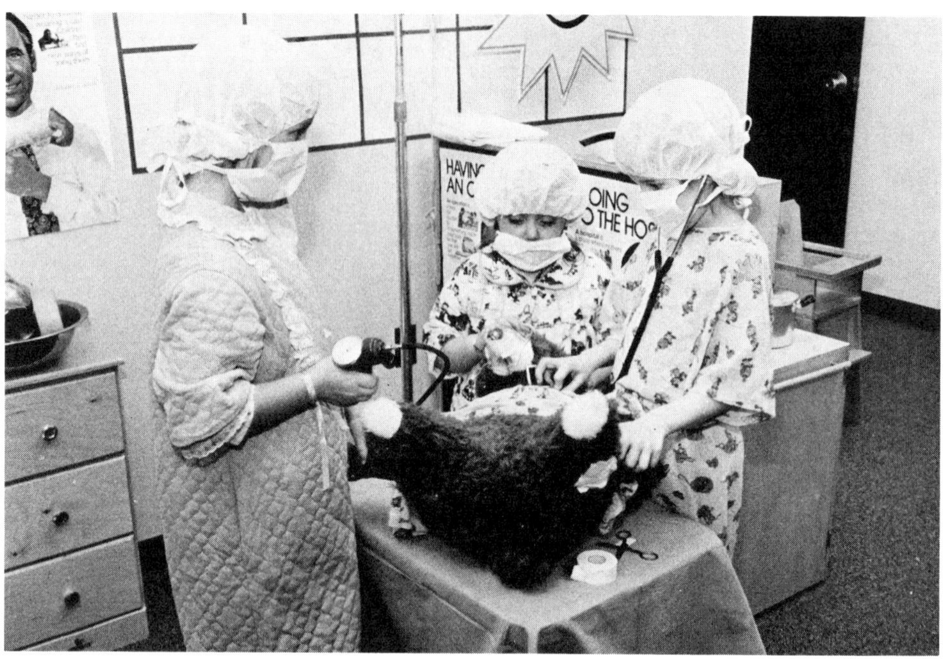

FIGURE 40-3. To reduce their fear of new procedures, toddlers and preschoolers can "act them out." Here three preschoolers give anesthesia to a bear with a face mask.

and give care to the infant and re-prove her capabilities to herself.

The Toddler and Preschooler

Toddlers and preschoolers often have minor surgical procedures such as umbilical hernia repair, testicular repair for undescended testes, and tonsillectomy. Since these procedures do not require emergency surgery, they can be planned for well in advance. Preschoolers have an extreme fear of abandonment, so they may need to have a parent accompany them to surgery and remain with them until they are induced; they may need to have a parent with them in the recovery room before they are able to relax and rest. A second major fear of preschoolers is mutilation. Talk about fixing, not cutting, with preschoolers. Preschoolers need some time to handle hospital equipment or role play surgery in order to reduce their fear of it (Fig. 40-3).

Children this age appear to have minimal pain following surgery, ambulate early, and have extremely rapid postoperative courses.

The Schoolager and Adolescent

Schoolage children are not yet aware of which body organs are necessary for life and which are expendable; they may therefore misinterpret the seriousness of surgery, thinking that a small procedure is a major one unless they are given clear preoperative explanations including body anatomy.

Schoolagers are very aware of family stories concerning surgery (Aunt Helen had an operation and died'). Ask in a preoperative interview if the child has heard of a person having a poor surgical outcome or has listened to a television program recently that portrayed an unsuccessful surgical outcome. Make well-considered preoperative plans to counteract misconceptions.

Adolescents are so aware of body image that any surgery may be difficult for them. They may worry more about the size of the incision and its appearance in the postoperative period than about measures to help them to return to wellness. Provide reassurance and clear explanations in order to reduce these identity fears. You can assure them that scars whiten with time and become much less noticeable.

Many surgical procedures in this age group are the result of traumatic injury (skateboard, bicycle, motor vehicle accidents). The child often has reason to feel guilty about the cause of the accident (was told not to use his skateboard on a hill). In the postoperative period he may need to spend time talking to reestablish self-esteem (yes, he did do an unwise thing; no, one unwise act does not make him a bad person) in order to deal effectively with a surgical experience.

The Young Adult

Young adulthood is generally a surgery-free age except for procedures resulting from traumatic injury (motor vehicle accidents) or cosmetic surgery. Young adults who have always been healthy may expect to feel well immediately after surgery and need help to understand that they will feel tired and have pain afterward. Check the person's plans for self-care carefully after hospital discharge. A young adult may be returning to a college dormitory or apartment where he lives alone following a hospital admission. Be certain that he has adequate support people available to help him until he feels well again.

The Middle-Aged Adult

Surgical procedures in the middle-aged adult are often scheduled after a period of medical illness (gallbladder disease, intestinal bleeding, inadequate circulation to the heart). The person is relieved that the surgery will cure his illness but is also apprehensive that the surgeon will discover an even bigger problem (what was diagnosed a gallbladder stone is really a cancerous tumor). Be certain that people receive good explanations following a surgical procedure regarding the outcome. Assess middle-aged adults carefully before surgery for fluid, electrolyte, and nutritional balance. People who have been ill prior to surgery are at high risk for imbalances in these areas.

Many middle-aged adults are at the peak of their careers and are important and knowledgeable people in their chosen fields. Do not assume, however, that someone well versed in nuclear science or accounting has an appreciation for the importance of postoperative measures such as deep breathing and coughing. Such teaching is just as important with this age group as any other.

The Older Adult

Older adults may postpone seeing a physician because they are worried about dying in surgery. Although this age group is indeed at high risk for surgery due to decreased air exchange in their lungs and possible poor healing caused by decreased circulation, even major surgery is performed successfully in older adults today and delaying a procedure only invites complications. Assess older adults carefully before surgery for nutritional status; it is apt not to be optimal if they have been ill for a period of time. Be certain that they have adequate support people to help them after they return home.

THE PREOPERATIVE PHASE

The preoperative phase begins with the person's awareness that he has an illness and ends when the person is anesthetized for surgery. Many people report that this phase of surgery is the most distressing. The waiting for surgery (an unknown) is often worse than the actual procedure or any discomfort felt afterward. The length of this waiting period depends on the immediacy of the procedure.

No matter what surgery is planned, preoperative preparation always consists of well-defined steps: admission to the hospital unit, the preoperative interview, establishment of surgical risk, scheduling of diagnostic tests, preoperative teaching, assessment that informed consent has been obtained, and immediate preoperative care measures.

Admission to the Hospital Unit

People admitted for elective or required but not immediate surgery generally feel well on admission. Yesterday they were working, taking care of their families, attending school; today they are being asked to change suddenly from that independent "well" role to a dependent "ill" one.

Because he has had more time to worry, a person who has expected surgery for weeks or months is often more worried about the procedure than the person who is admitted for emergency surgery. He needs specific time put aside following routine admission procedures to talk about his fears; he needs encouragement to do as much as possible for himself preoperatively (and thus accept his ill role).

A person who is admitted for an emergency procedure often feels pain that should be alleviated as soon as possible. He cannot begin to think about what surgery represents as long as pain absorbs all his attention. Although steps of preoperative care are done more quickly in emergencies than in planned procedures, people undergoing emergency surgery still need them to ensure a safe outcome.

Admission steps for the surgical patient include orienting him to the hospital unit; taking and recording vital signs (an increased temperature may be reason to cancel or postpone surgery; an irregular heart beat may cause his physician to order an additional heart evaluation before surgery; a rapid respiratory rate may lead to scheduling of additional respiratory assessments); and carefully measuring weight and height (measurements will influence the amount and type of preoperative medication or anesthesia used).

People undergoing surgery cannot begin to relax as long as their support people are nervous and worried. Make a point of including these people in all explanations and admission routines (Fig. 40-4).

The Preoperative Interview

Both the physician and anesthesiologist will interview the patient preoperatively to obtain a medical history and make an assessment and decision for safe anesthetic administration. In addition, a nursing interview must be held. Specific information you need to obtain is the person's knowledge about (1) the procedure he will undergo (does he view this as major, serious but not major, or minor surgery? what will be done in surgery—will something be repaired or removed?), (2) the length of the hospitalization, and (3) any postsurgical equipment that will be used for therapy (oxygen, tubes, a cast).

Remember that because the thought of being cut is very frightening for children under 12, they are told instead that they will be "fixed" (even tonsils are "fixed"). Be certain to use this terminology when discussing surgery with this age group.

Record the information you obtain. When the sur-

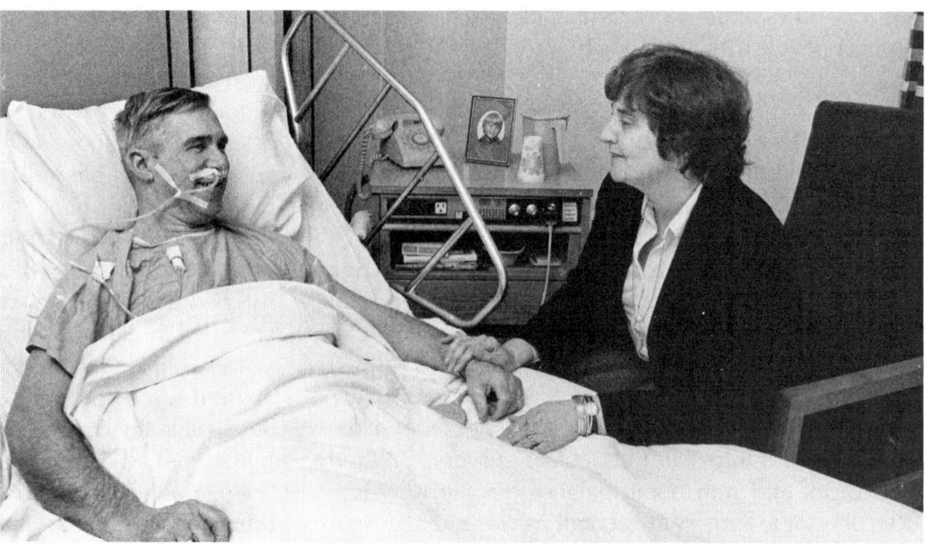

FIGURE 40-4. Waiting is for many people the most difficult part of surgery. Here a patient has had a nasogastric tube inserted prior to surgery. Both he and his support person need to be included in preparations to reduce their anxiety.

geon's plans for the procedure are complete, compare his plans with the patient's perceptions. A person who views a serious procedure as minor will think something terrible has occurred when he is not able to feel well again quickly after surgery. A women who will probably be hospitalized for 7 to 10 days but expects to be hospitalized for only 4 days may need to modify her plans for safe child care. Furthermore, if a person has a wrong perception of surgery, he cannot sign a true "informed" consent.

To help ensure a safe surgical outcome, you also need to obtain health information. Determine whether the patient has had any past surgery, has any illness other than the surgical reason for which he was admitted, is currently taking any medication, or has any allergies to foods or drugs.

Review Chap. 18 for other areas necessary to obtain total information for a nursing history. Use the information gained to prepare a preoperative nursing care plan.

The Establishment of Operative Risk

For surgery to be performed safely, a person must be in the best possible physical and psychological state before surgery. People who have less than optimal physical or psychological health are at risk for a complicated surgical outcome unless the risk factor is identified and special precautions to lessen it are undertaken. Areas that create surgical risk follow.

NUTRITIONAL STATUS

A person who is obese or who has a protein or vitamin deficiency is at risk for surgery because such a condition interferes with wound healing. Tissue that contains an abundance of fatty cells is difficult to suture, so the incision may take longer to heal; an increased healing period invites infection and rupture of the incision (dehiscence). Such a person's heart may also have an increased workload; the physiological shock of surgery may place too much stress on an already overworked organ. In addition, an obese person often has more difficulty moving and turning postoperatively than a person of normal weight and thus has an increased risk for developing respiratory or circulatory complications (pneumonia or blood clots).

Protein and vitamins C and D are necessary for new cell formation at the incision site. Vitamin K is necessary for blood clotting to effect homeostasis following surgery.

Protein and vitamin deficiencies are found most frequently in the elderly person whose income or food preparation ability is limited or in people who have been ill for some time before surgery (too nauseated or too tired to prepare or eat well-balanced meals). Someone who has been attempting to lose weight, a person who depends a great deal on fast-food sources, or an adolescent or homemaker who eats "on the run" may also have serious nutritional deficiencies. Evaluate all people preoperatively by asking for a "typical day history." Assess the adequacy of their diet.

AGE

Age affects surgical risk since it influences size and circulatory and urinary function. An infant, for example, is a much more difficult surgical subject than an average-sized adult purely because of the small size of his body organs in contrast to that of the surgeon's hands. A 300-ml blood loss (normal for an adult) would be extremely serious in the neonate as a far greater percentage of circulatory blood would be depleted. Since an infant also has increased difficulty shifting fluid from one body compartment to another, he has more difficulty compensating for fluid loss.

Children, who are engaged in rapid growth, are at risk because they must postoperatively organize adequate resources not only for wound healing but also for normal growth.

Elderly patients may have decreased circulatory function due to arteriosclerosis (hardening of the arteries) and decreased respiratory function such as emphysema (stretched alveoli). These conditions make it more difficult for them to adjust to the physiological shock of surgery; wound healing may be slower (inviting infection).

GENERAL HEALTH

A person who has a secondary disease (cardiac disease, diabetes mellitus, anemia, kidney disease, any infection) is at surgical risk depending on the extent of the primary disease because the pathology present from the secondary illness may not allow him to make the physiological adjustments demanded by surgery. People with secondary illness may also have accompanying nutritional or electrolyte imbalance related to their other illness.

Be certain to ask in your preoperative nursing history if the person has any illness other than the cause for surgery (Fig. 40-5). Prior to surgery, people are under stress, which may limit their reasoning ability. It is not unusual for a person admitted for an appendectomy not to tell anyone that he also has diabetes.

Also ask if the patient is currently taking any medications (either prescriptive or over-the-counter) since some drugs will increase surgical risk by interfering with either the effect of the anesthetic or the surgical procedure itself. Drugs most likely to cause these effects are summarized in Quick Reference Stop 40-1.

FIGURE 40-5. A preoperative nursing interview helps the nurse establish a nursing care plan by uncovering the amount of knowledge her patient has about upcoming surgery.

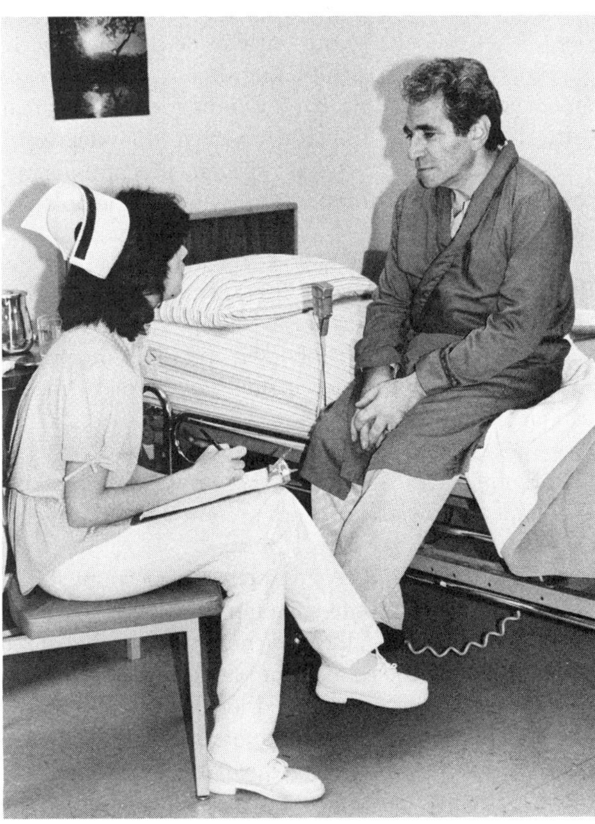

FLUID AND ELECTROLYTE BALANCE

Blood loss will occur during surgery. A person who enters surgery with a lower than normal blood volume (hypovolemia) will feel the effect of normal blood loss more than the person with a normal blood volume. Hypovolemia may result from vomiting, diarrhea, bleeding, or a poor fluid intake prior to surgery. Equally as important as the amount of fluid present is the balance of electrolytes. Imbalances of potassium, mag-

☐ **QUICK REFERENCE STOP 40-1: PHARMACOLOGY**

Drugs that may Result in Complications of Surgery

Type of Drug	*Action*
Anticoagulants	May cause hemorrhage due to lack of hemostasis during surgery.
Tranquilizers	May cause hypotension following anesthesia.
Antibiotics	Specific antibiotics may predispose to renal insufficiency or increase neuromuscular blockage.
Antihypertensives	May result in hypotension following anesthesia.
Anticonvulsants	May increase liver action and metabolism of anesthetic agent.
MAO inhibitors	May lead to hypertensive crisis if sympathomimetic drug is given as anesthetic.
Insulin	May lead to hypoglycemia during NPO period.
Corticosteroids	May block body's response to shock and lead to lack of adrenal function.
Thiazide diuretics	May lead to potassium deficiency due to potassium excretion.
Propranolol (Inderol)	May result in cardiac depression from anesthetic interaction.

nesium, calcium, and acid-base (pH) lead to difficulty in regulating heart function, muscle tone, and oxygen distribution, and thus increase operative risk appreciably.

To prevent fluid and electrolyte imbalances, and to correct those present, many people are begun on intravenous fluid therapy preoperatively. Correction is continued postoperatively.

PSYCHOLOGICAL CONDITION

A person who is frightened when an anesthetic is induced is at greater risk for cardiac arrest than the person who is calm and relaxed. How frightened a person is of surgery depends not as much on the seriousness of the surgery as on his perception of the seriousness. Elicit from people preoperatively their expectations of the procedure and their general attitudes toward it. People who are extremely worried need a more detailed than usual explanation of the procedure before they can enter surgery without intense fear.

A surgical experience can reduce the ability of some people to cope with the stresses around them so much that it actually moves them from a well mental state to mental instability. Aside from the fear of the surgical procedure itself (losing control while under anesthesia, hemorrhage, shock, death, pain), the person may be worried about a poor outcome (since he has cancer, he will never be able to walk or work again) or some other facet of his life (financial inability to pay his hospital bill, unsupervised children). In many instances, just helping the patient acknowledge that fear of surgery is normal is beneficial. The procedure does not become any less awesome but the patient can view himself as "normal" and competent.

EXTENT OR TYPE OF SURGERY

Obviously a major surgical procedure carries more risk than a minor one; one performed under general anesthesia carries more risk than one performed under local anesthesia. Surgery on body organs crucial for life, such as the heart, lungs, kidneys, brain, and liver, carry more risk than surgery on organs not necessary for life, such as the gall bladder or hand (see QRS 40-2).

CARE FACILITIES AND STAFF AVAILABLE

The risk of surgery performed in a well-equipped operating suite with accompanying optimal preoperative and postoperative facilities and personnel available is less than that of surgery performed, for example, in battlefield conditions. If people are going to be transferred to an intensive care unit following surgery, they often are very relieved by seeing this setting preoperatively. The presence of so much equipment and personnel almost certainly assures them that any change in postoperative condition will be quickly noted and corrected. Seeing an intensive care unit preoperatively may be overwhelming for small children. A more effective way to acquaint them with postoperative equipment such as monitors is to show them play models (Fig. 40-6).

Report operative risk factors you identify to the patient's physician. Utilize them too as important points of planning in your care plan.

☐ QUICK REFERENCE STOP 40-2: ADVOCACY

People may ask how they can know for certain that the type or extent of surgery planned for them is really needed. Advise people that they have a right to a second opinion. They can feel free to tell their surgeon that they are seeking a second opinion; a legitimate surgeon is not threatened by such an action but welcomes confirmation of his opinion.

Preoperative Diagnostic Procedures

In order for surgery to be performed safely, not only must a person be in the best physical condition possible but the exact nature of his illness must be pinpointed as accurately as possible. Tests ordered to determine these two areas will vary depending on the patient's age and condition, but common assessments made are the following.

Urinalysis. All surgical patients have a urinalysis done prior to surgery to estimate metabolic and kidney function. It would be dangerous, for example, for a person with undetected diabetes (a metabolic disease in which glucose levels cannot be regulated) to undergo surgery without extra precautions (infusions of intravenous fluid containing glucose could be extremely dangerous). That diabetes is present can be detected by the presence of glucose spilling into the urine. Surgery is a systemic insult to the body. It is dangerous for a person with poor kidney function to face this degree of physiological shock unless special precautions are taken. Poor kidney function is revealed by the presence of protein in urine.

BUN. Blood urea nitrogen (BUN) is a blood test to confirm or rule out poor kidney function. With poor kidney function, urea, the breakdown product of protein metabolism, accumulates in the bloodstream since it cannot be filtered and removed.

FBS. Fasting blood sugar (FBS) is a method of checking that undetected diabetes is not present prior to surgery.

CBC with Differential. A complete blood count (CBC) with differential measures the number and types of red and white blood cells, the oxygen-carrying ability of red blood cells, and the number of platelets. Every surgical procedure involves some blood loss. It is important to know that a person has adequate blood components before surgery so that subsequent blood loss will not reduce his functioning blood components below a safe level. If a person has a low hemoglobin level preopera-

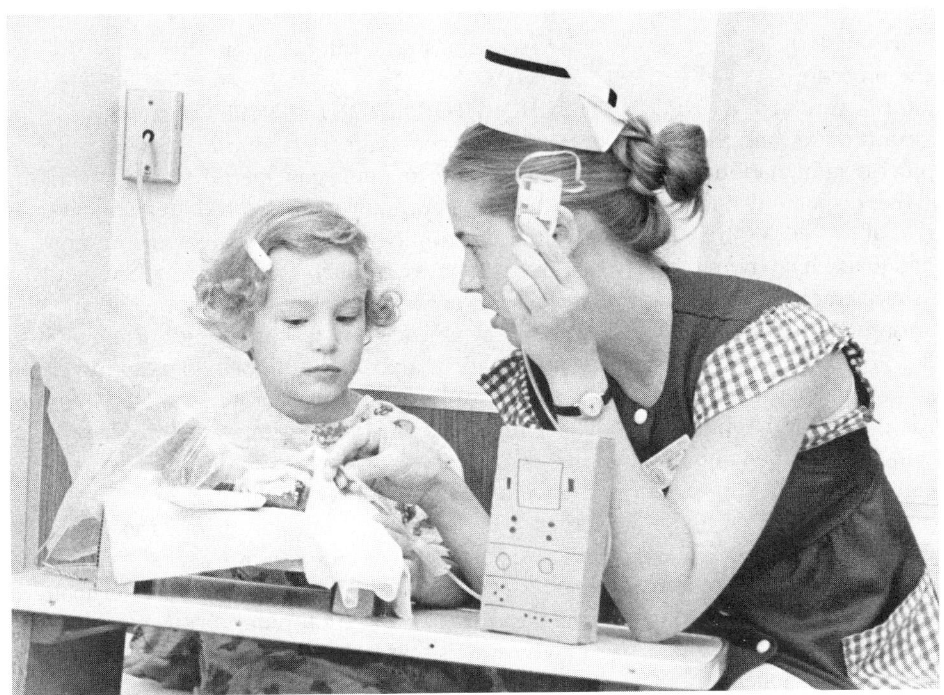

FIGURE 40-6. A nurse prepares a preschool child for heart surgery by explaining equipment that will be used following surgery. Such play equipment is handmade from boxes and medicine bottles.

tively, a blood loss that appears normal could be fatal. A person with inadequate blood platelets will not have normal blood clotting ability and so blood loss will be appreciably more than usual. A person with an inadequate leukocyte count will have a difficult time resisting infection following surgery; elevated leukocyte count suggests that the person already has an infection or inflammation, which will compound his illness.

Serum Electrolytes and pH. If people have been ill prior to surgery, they may experience serious electrolyte imbalance. This happens very quickly with vomiting (alkalosis develops) or diarrhea (acidosis develops). People with an electrolyte imbalance cannot cope with the physiological shock of surgery or the time interval of fasting involved. If electrolyte imbalance is revealed, it should be corrected by intravenous therapy infusion before surgery.

Chest X-ray. During surgery a person's respiratory level is decreased as respirations become slow and shallow due to anesthesia. A person with respiratory disease may suffer from anoxia at this time unless special precautions to institute good oxygen exchange are initiated. Chest x-rays are taken on middle-aged and older adults prior to surgery to determine if lung disease is present since the incidence of lung disease is increased in this age group. X-rays are never taken routinely in children to reduce the amount of exposure to radiation that they will receive in a lifetime.

ECG. An electrocardiogram (ECG) may be ordered for middle-aged and older adults to detect any cardiac abnormalities prior to surgery. The effect of blood loss and physiological shock could cause cardiac arrhythmia in a person with cardiac disease unless special precautions are undertaken.

Specific Diagnostic Tests. To determine the exact point of pathology, the person may have a biopsy, endoscopy, or radio-opaque or radiation study performed. Chapter 25 discusses these specific diagnostic tests.

Preoperative Teaching

Fear of the unknown is one of the hardest fears to conquer. Preoperative teaching is aimed at acquainting the person with the procedure and any special equipment used so that he will be as informed about the surgery as possible. Activities to help maintain respiratory and skeletal function in order to prevent postsurgical complications from stasis of body secretions or circulation are also taught.

PRINCIPLES OF TEACHING

Be certain that you determine how much the patient already knows about surgery before you begin. The patient who had the cartilege in one knee repaired last year and is now having the cartilege in his other knee repaired may have a better idea of his surgery than you do. People admitted for a repeat procedure, however, do appreciate having their memory refreshed and recall confirmed. Be certain to answer all specific questions and fill in gaps in knowledge.

Be certain that all information you offer is accurate. If you are unsure whether the postoperative course will necessitate using oxygen, a cast, or a nasogastric tube, for example, do not guess. Confirm with the surgeon or another nurse familiar with the procedure.

Be certain not to use hospital jargon such as NPO (nothing by mouth) or EUA (exam under anesthesia). People under stress do not process information well. They cannot process at all what they do not understand.

Receiving a lot of information at one sitting may be more stressing than helpful. Plan to teach no more than one activity at a time. Have the patient demonstrate activities such as coughing and deep breathing to show you that he can do them well.

Use visual aids as necessary. Many people do not even know about body organs such as a ureter or diaphragm. They think the stomach is low in the abdomen and are perplexed why everyone is concerned that an upper abdominal surgery incision will limit their depth of respirations after surgery. Draw people pictures or show them illustrations of anatomy if necessary to help them understand exactly what the procedure involves. Do not leave textbooks that detail disease conditions with patients. The patient has to know possible complications of the procedure in order to sign an informed consent, but he may frighten himself by reading about complications that are rare for his type of surgery.

If a person is going to have surgery such as an amputation, colostomy (opening of the intestine onto the abdomen), or open heart surgery, he might appreciate talking to another patient in whom the same procedure was performed successfully. Some communities have support clubs that will gladly supply someone to offer preoperative information of this kind.

Be certain to include the patient's support people in teaching. A mother may be more effective at getting her 3-year-old to cough postoperatively than you, and will do so gladly if she understands the importance of the procedure; a wife or husband can be very reassuring once their fears are calmed by good explanations. Their fears can reinfect the patient and render your preoperative teaching and support ineffective.

PARTICULAR POINTS OF TEACHING

Explain preoperative measures that will be necessary such as use of an enema, surgical skin preparation, the NPO state, premedication, and method of transport to surgery.

Inform the patient where his incision will be and whether or not a dressing will be used (for example, an incision in the groin area of a child is often covered with collodion, a waterproof translucent coating, rather than a dressing to prevent urine from a wet diaper from contaminating the incision). Explain as well equipment such as chest tubes, a nasogastric tube, intravenous therapy, or oxygen that will surround him postoperatively; the fact that he will go to the recovery room before returning to his own room (or the intensive care unit); and frequent determinations such as blood pressure and pulse recordings that will be taken after surgery.

TEACHING TO PREVENT COMPLICATIONS

Patients who cooperate to maintain good respiratory and circulatory function postoperatively will probably have a postoperative course freer of respiratory and circulatory complications than people who do not.

These preventive measures are best taught during the preoperative period, when the person is free of pain and can concentrate on your teaching. Such teaching also gives the patient a positive outlook about his surgery (a sense of control as well as reassurance that, since you are taking time to teach him postoperative measures, you think he is going to recover safely from surgery). His surgeon and anesthesiologist both say to him, "I'll see you in the operating room tomorrow morning." By teaching postoperative care, you are saying, "I'll see you safely back here in your room tomorrow afternoon," a message with a strong subliminal message for the person who knows that there will be a tomorrow morning but has serious doubts that there will be a tomorrow afternoon.

Deep Breathing. Periodic deep breathing exercises fully aerate the lungs and help to prevent stasis of lung mucus (stasis tends to occur because the lungs are relatively quiet during surgery). Since it always has the potential for causing infection, stasis must be prevented as far as possible.

The person will need to take 5 to 10 deep breaths every hour. He does this simply by inhaling as deeply as possible, holding his breath for a second or two and then exhaling as deeply as possible. He must be certain that he inhales and exhales fully or he will feel lightheaded from hypoventilation.

Coughing. Coughing every hour helps move lung mucus and, again, prevent stasis. Teach the person to inhale deeply, exhale deeply, inhale again, and attempt to cough. The irritation of air passing over bronchial mucus often spontaneously initiates the coughing reflex, which is why breathing in and out first is important. If the person has a chest or abdominal incision, coughing will hurt. Teach him to splint his incision area with his interlaced hands or a pillow to reduce this "tugging" or "cutting" feeling (Fig. 40-7).

Be certain that the person not only clears his throat but uses his chest muscles when coughing. This action truly raises bronchial mucus. It is usually necessary to demonstrate the coughing technique to be certain that the patient understands the depth of movement required.

Young children cannot do deep breathing or coughing exercises as such but can imitate your actions. Play a game of "Simon Says" with them before surgery to fami-

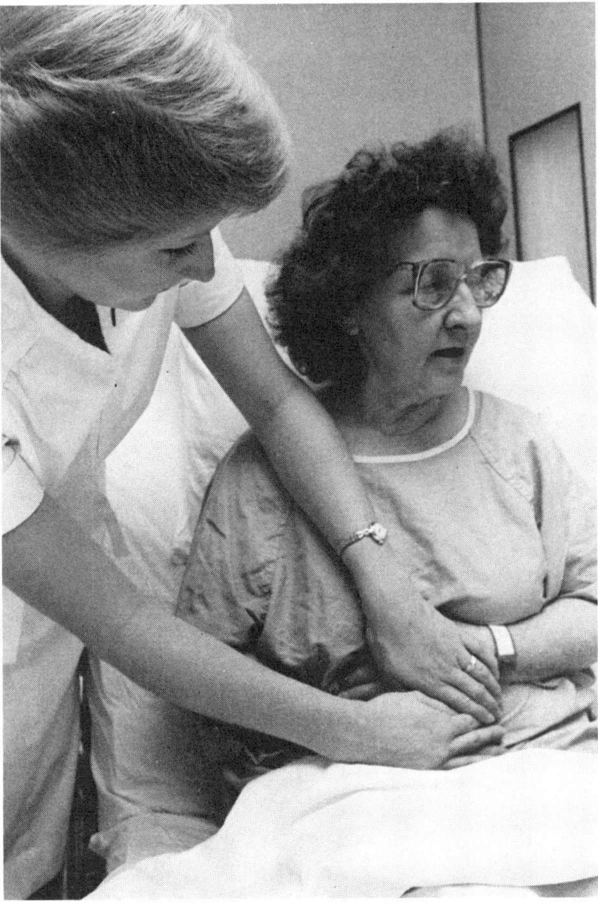

A

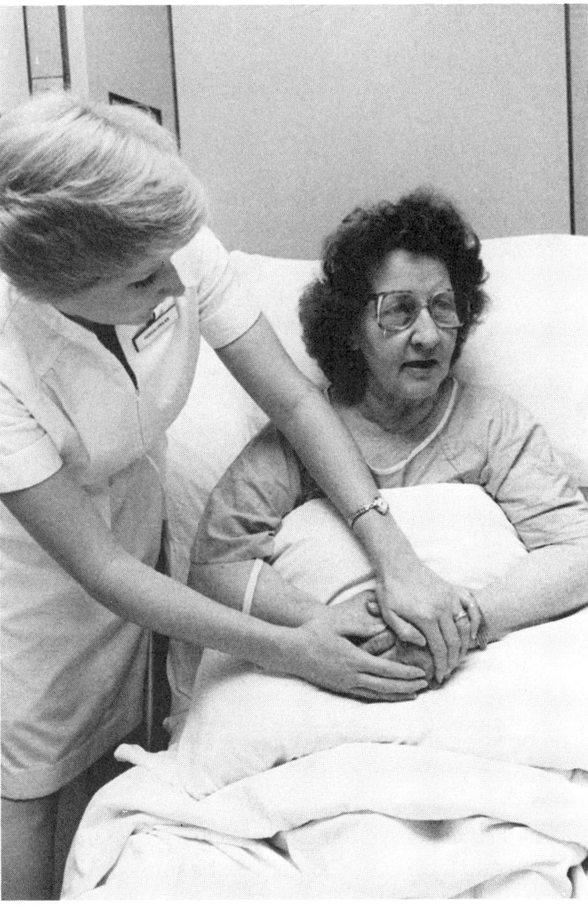

B

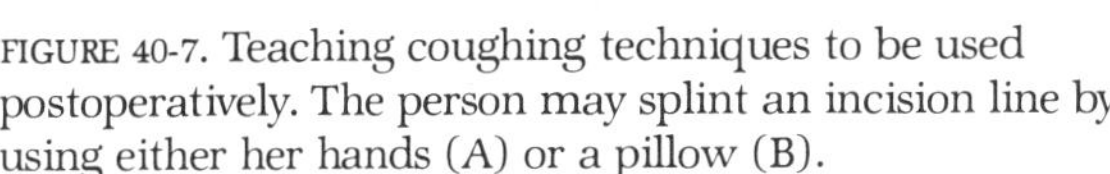

FIGURE 40-7. Teaching coughing techniques to be used postoperatively. The person may splint an incision line by using either her hands (A) or a pillow (B).

liarize them with deep breathing and coughing (Simon says touch your nose; Simon says take a deep breath in and out; Simon says take another deep breath; Simon says cough).

Turning. Patients do not need to practice turning side to side prior to surgery unless they have some additional handicapping condition but do need to understand its importance (to prevent both respiratory and circulatory stasis). If a special turning procedure such as logrolling (keeping the back straight and unbending following spinal surgery) will be used, it should be explained and demonstrated.

Leg Exercises. Another means of preventing circulatory stasis postoperatively is ankle, knee, and hip flexion and extension about five times every hour. Lifting each foot off the mattress and moving it in a circle (circumduction) is also an effective motion to teach (Fig. 40-8). If the person cannot do active exercises, passive exercises should be done by you. Full range-of-motion exercises including leg flexion are shown in Chap. 26.

Obtaining Informed Consent

Every person going to surgery, no matter how minor the procedure, must sign an operative permission consent form prior to the procedure. The patient must have a full explanation of the procedure involved, its possible complications, and the risks to him if the procedure is not performed at this time. If a body organ will be removed, he must be told of this.

Obtaining operative consent is the surgeon's responsibility but seeing that it is obtained is everyone's responsibility. You are often asked to witness the patient's signature on such a form; be certain you agree that it was informed consent (patient was explained the risks and benefits of the procedure in terms that he could understand) before signing as a witness.

Operative permits must be signed before the person is given his preoperative medication. (Since premedication makes the patient sleepy, the permission is not considered valid if signed after administration.) Adults sign their own permits; those of children are signed by their parent or guardian. Emancipated minors (children under legal age of consent who provide for the majority of their own care or are the mother of a child) are given the right in some states to sign their own permission

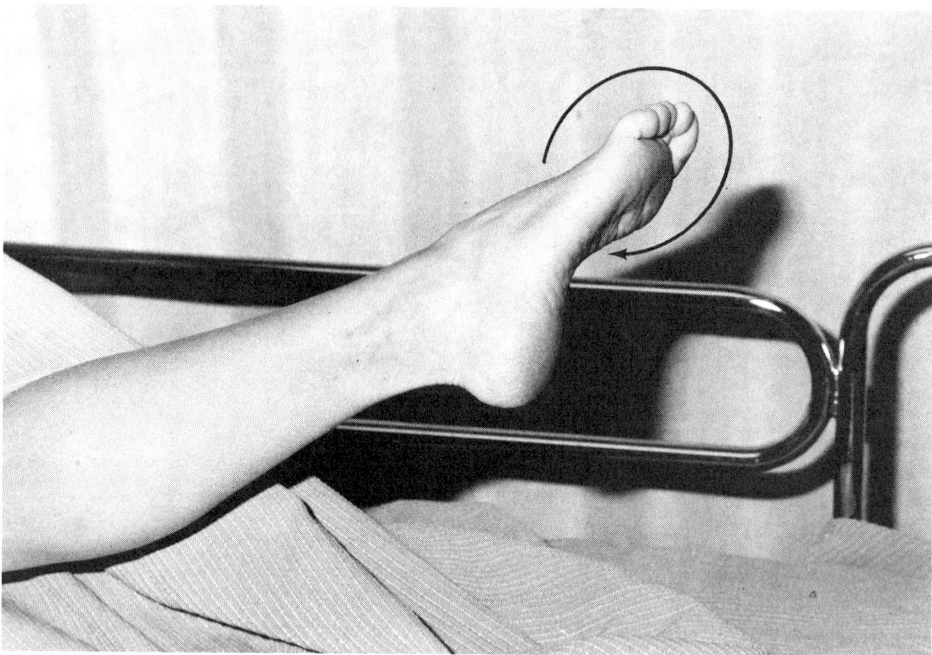

FIGURE 40-8. Leg circumduction (moving the foot in a circle) in addition to knee and hip flexion and extension is a good postoperative exercise to promote venous return.

forms. Be certain you know the legal requirements of consent and legal age of consent in the state in which you practice.

If the surgical procedure involves abortion or sterilization, some health care agencies require a spouse to sign the permission form also. This is agency, not legal, policy, however. Legally, abortion and sterilization procedures are agreements between only the patient and the physician.

Immediate Preoperative Care Measures

The evening before surgery, routine measures toward preparing the patient's skin and gastrointestinal tract, and promoting rest are performed. On the day of surgery, measures to safeguard the patient and his property, premedication, and transport to surgery are undertaken.

PREOPERATIVE SKIN PREPARATION

Reducing the number of bacteria on the skin prior to surgery automatically reduces the possibility of bacteria entering the incision at the time of surgery.

The extent of skin preparation varies according to the surgical procedure. Some patients may have an order for a complete tub bath with an antiseptic soap the evening prior to surgery; other patients may have orders to have the area of the surgical incision "scrubbed" or washed thoroughly with an antiseptic soap several times in the 2 days preceding surgery. All patients have the area of incision shaved and washed either the evening prior to surgery or the morning of surgery. A newer form of preoperative care requires shaving to be done minutes before surgery in a specially prepared surgery "hold" room; theoretically this makes best use of the antiseptic properties of the soap used and achieves a surgical site most free of surface hair (Fig. 40-9). In some hospitals

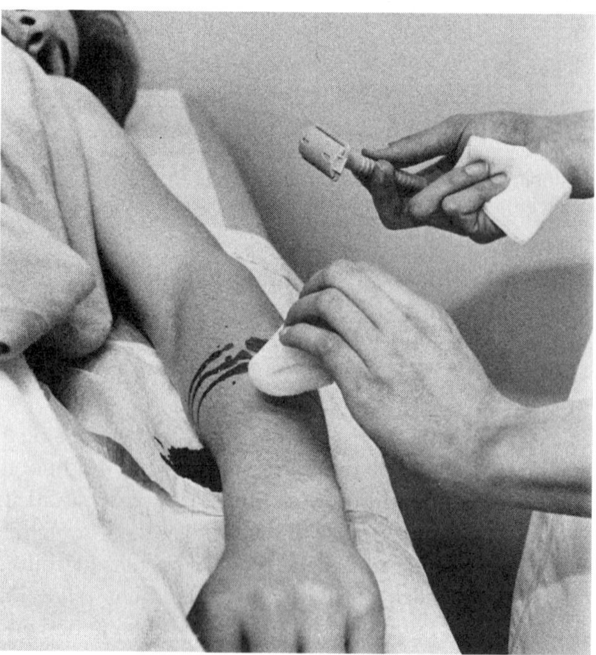

FIGURE 40-9. Preoperative shaving of body parts is done to remove hair from the area of incision and to reduce bacteria count. Here an arm is prepared with an antiseptic soap that will foam when rubbed.

this type of preparation for surgery is done by a "prep team" or personnel hired especially for this duty. In other instances the nurse caring for the patient the day or evening before surgery is responsible.

A much wider skin area than the actual incision site is prepared to ensure a wide safe area as free as possible from bacteria. Steps in preoperative skin preparation are shown in Procedure 40-1. If orthopedic surgery is planned, even more caution to prevent bacteria from entering the wound must be taken (bacteria might invade the bone and cause osteomyelitis, a severe debilitating bone infection). For orthopedic surgery, antiseptic scrubbing of skin area is usually included in preparation. Figure 40-10 shows usual skin preparation areas for various surgical procedures. Be certain to alert people that the skin preparation area is a wide one; otherwise they may be alarmed that the procedure planned is more extensive than they had anticipated.

To ensure that you do not cut or irritate skin, which would invite infection, use a generous supply of shaving lather and a sharp razor. Use small, controlled, smooth strokes; shave with the grain of the hair shaft for comfort; provide a good light for yourself so you can accurately see that all hair has been removed from the area.

In order to be effective, skin preparation before surgery must be thorough. Do not allow the patient's or

PROCEDURE 40-1
Preoperative Skin Preparation

Purpose: To provide a skin area clear of body hair to reduce chance of infection at a surgical incision site.

Plan	*Principle*
1. Wash your hands; identify patient; explain procedure.	1. Prevent spread of microorganisms; ensure patient safety and cooperation.
2. Assess patient status; analyze appropriateness of procedure; plan modifications as necessary.	2. Hair on the head is usually not shaved unless additional permission has been signed.
3. Implement care by assembling supplies: safety razor with new blade, shaving soap or lather according to agency policy, waterproof pad, emesis basin, dry gauge sponges, good light source. Determine extent of skin area to be prepared.	3. A good light source is important to be certain that all hair is removed. Check with the surgeon or surgical suite if you are uncertain as to the extent of the preparation.
4. Provide privacy; fanfold covers as necessary to reveal body area to be prepared. Place waterproof pad under area to protect bed. Fill basin with warm water to use to rinse razor.	4. Protect against chilling; protect bed linen.
5. Lather area well with a moistened sponge, using predetermined soap or lather. Stretch skin taut; shave off all hair using short strokes in direction of hair shafts. Be careful not to nick skin.	5. Lather softens hair and reduces friction to skin. Any open area would be an invitation to infection.
6. Wipe away all removed hair; dry area well. Inspect it carefully for additional hair. Evaluate effectiveness, efficiency, cost, comfort, and safety of procedure. Plan health teaching as necessary, for example, inform the patient of the importance of remaining NPO prior to surgery.	6. Health teaching is an independent nursing action always included as a part of care.
7. Leave patient comfortable. Chart area prepared and time of preparation.	7. Document patient status and nursing care.

MODIFICATIONS FOR CARE OF CHILD

Many children have been told that they will be cut if they play with razors, and consequently are very afraid of them. You may need to demonstrate on your own arm that the razor does not hurt but only removes hair.

MODIFICATIONS FOR CARE OF OLDER ADULT

Many older adults have very fine hair that is not readily observable except in a bright light. Looking across an area at eye level often best reveals any fine hairs that were not removed.

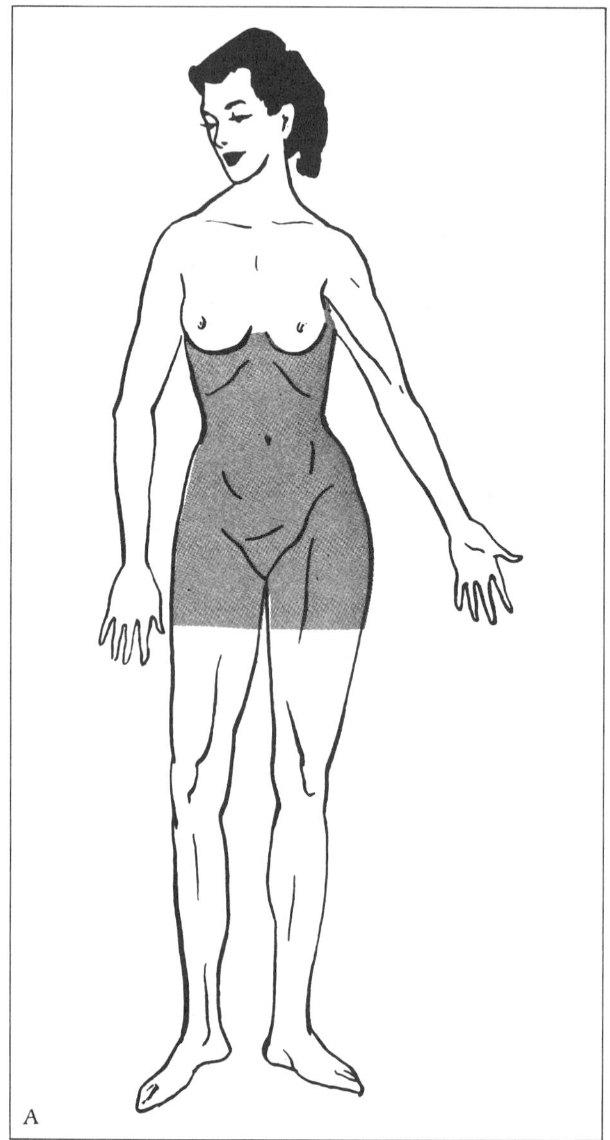

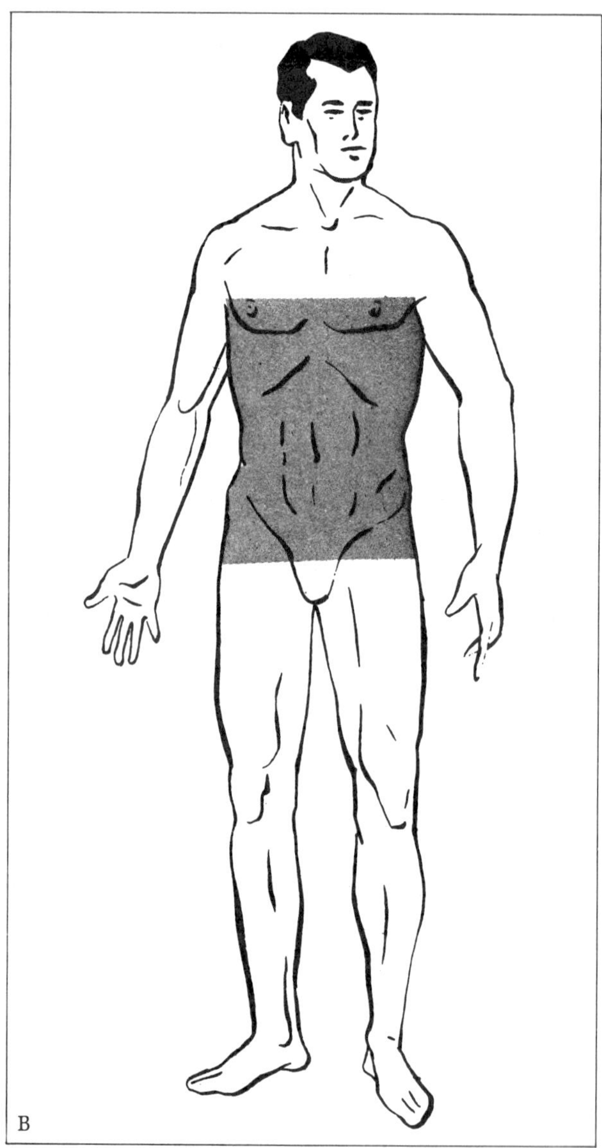

FIGURE 40-10. Common skin preparation areas for surgical procedures. Alert patients that skin preparation areas are wide and do not reflect the actual length of the incision. A. Gynecological operations, laparotomy, abdomen-perineal laparotomy. B. Gastrectomy, splenectomy, cholecystectomy. C. Mastectomy. D. Neck operations. E. Thoracic operations. F. Vein ligation. (Courtesy Johnson & Johnson, New Brunswick, New Jersey.)

your modesty to compromise the thoroughness or extent of a preparation.

GASTROINTESTINAL TRACT PREPARATION

Special preparation of the patient's gastrointestinal tract is carried out to reduce the possibility of vomiting (and therefore aspiration) during anesthesia administration and to prevent bowel obstruction or fecal impaction, which leads to difficulty in moving bowels following surgery due to tender abdominal muscles. If the gastrointestinal tract will be entered during surgery, measures to reduce the bacterial flora of the tract may be undertaken; measures to reduce fecal contamination into the peritoneal cavity from the tract may also be undertaken.

Measures to Reduce Vomiting. An important measure to reduce vomiting in the surgical patient is to restrict food and fluid intake for about 8 hours prior to surgery. In most instances this is achieved by preventing the patient who will have early morning surgery from eating or drinking after midnight. Persons who will have afternoon surgery may be allowed a light breakfast, then nothing more to eat until surgery.

It is dangerous for infants to be kept NPO for this long a period (they could become severely dehydrated) so their food and fluid intake is usually restricted for no longer than 4 hours. If fluid restriction for a period longer than this is necessary, intravenous fluid will be begun.

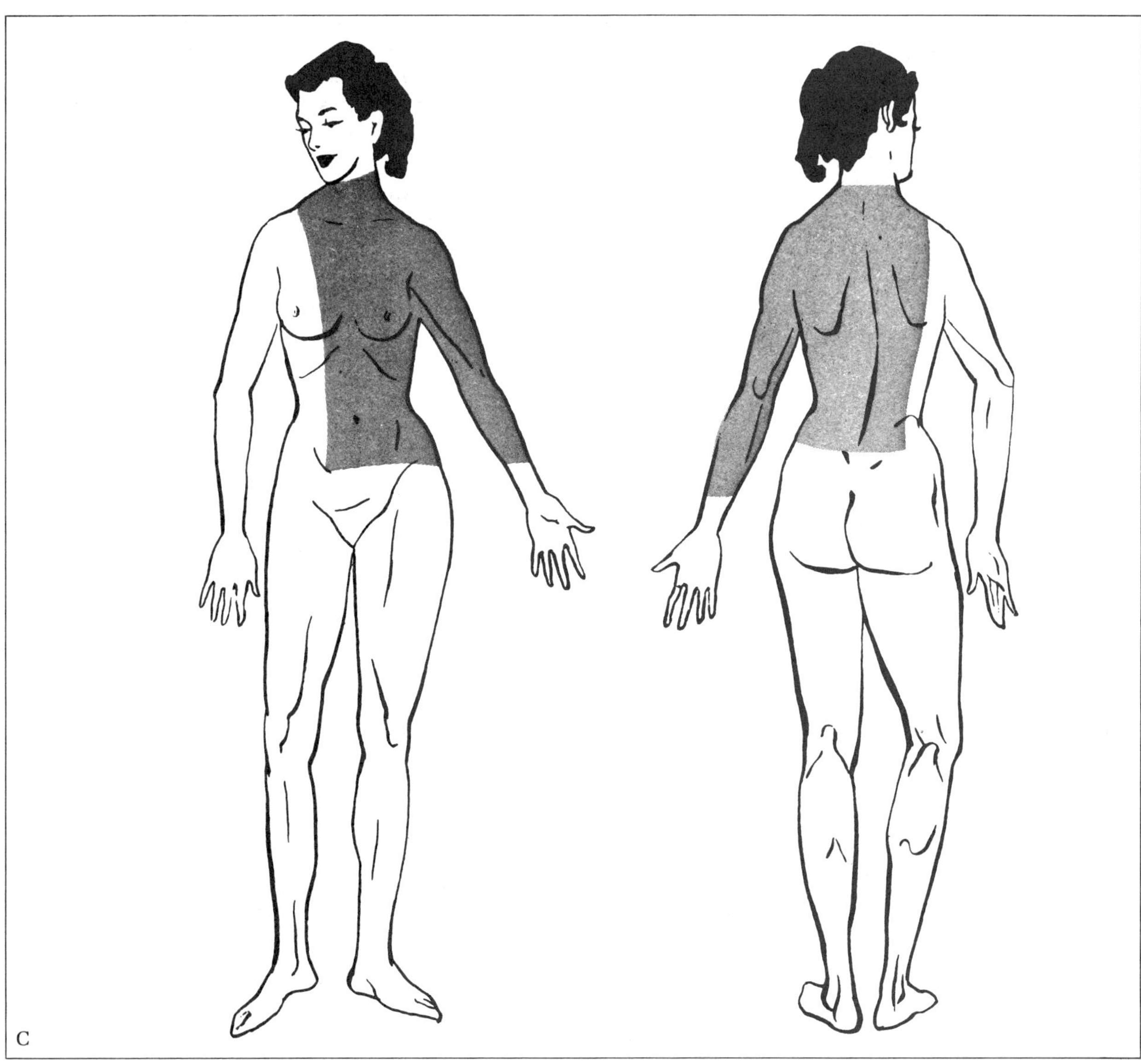

Tell patients and parents the reason for this restriction. Make a point of actually removing all food and fluid from the patient room at the specified time and cancel their diet order with the diet kitchen. Even though a person knew the evening before surgery that he was not to drink anything the following morning, his level of anxiety may cause him to forget. If there is no water present on his bedside stand, he is reminded of the restriction. Mark the door and the bed area with an NPO sign and mark the nursing Kardex or care plan so someone else does not offer him fluid. Do not allow children under 8 or 9 years to have water to rinse their mouth for teethbrushing if they are NPO. Many children this age swallow the water instead of spitting it out.

If a person should accidentally eat or drink on the morning of surgery, the anesthesiologist and surgeon must be informed. In most instances, the surgery will subsequently be canceled.

If gastrointestinal surgery is planned the person may have a nasogastric tube inserted the evening before surgery. As a rule, such a tube is connected to low suction after insertion so that the upper gastrointestinal tract will be kept empty of secretions (decompressed) prior to surgery. Instructions for inserting nasogastric tubes are given in Chap. 35.

Measures to Prevent Fecal Impaction. With gastrointestinal or abdominal surgery, the person's surgeon may order an enema administered the evening before surgery to clean the lower gastrointestinal tract of fecal material. If the person will have a large abdominal or chest incision, it may hurt him to use his abdominal muscles to effect a bowel movement following surgery. Use of an enema to clean the lower colon of fecal material will eliminate the need for the person to initiate a bowel movement for 2 to 4 days after surgery and so save him

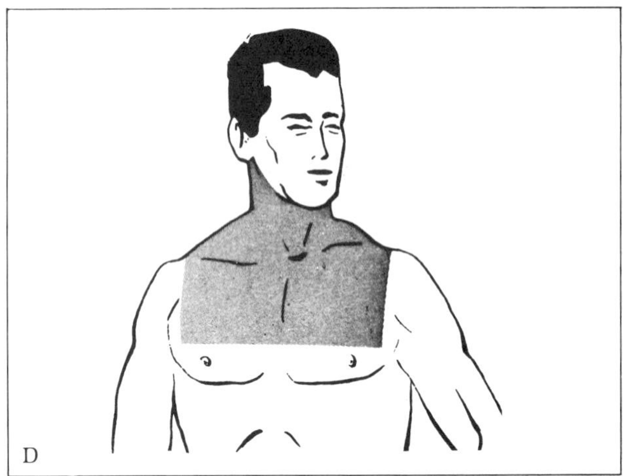

pain. When administering an enema before surgery, inform the patient that he will not have a bowel movement for 2 to 3 days following surgery to prevent him from worrying. Enemas may also be administered prior to cranial or heart surgery since straining during bowel movements tends to increase intracranial pressure and cause a Valsalva maneuver (see Chap. 37).

When gastrointestinal surgery is planned, some patients may also receive oral antibiotics such as neomycin for 2 or 3 days prior to surgery to reduce the number of flora in the gastrointestinal tract. These medications are given orally rather than intramuscularly to make as much use of local action as possible. Check that preoperative orders do not contradict themselves in

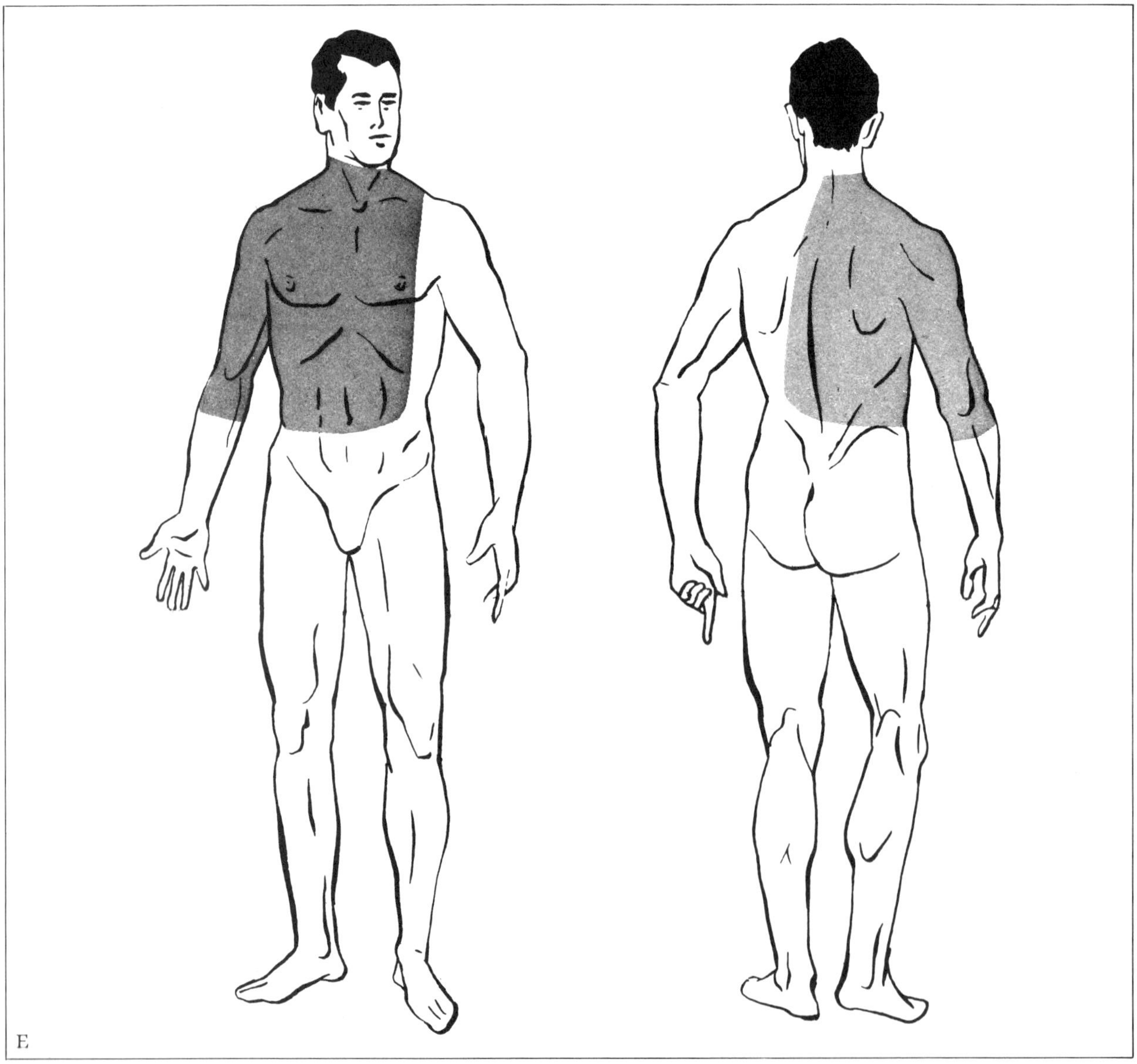

E

FIGURE 40-10 (CONTINUED)

these instances (give an oral medication and keep the patient NPO at the same time).

PROMOTING SLEEP AND RELAXATION
Most surgeons order a sleep medication for a patient on the evening before surgery to ensure that the person has a good night's sleep prior to surgery. Be certain that you complement the administration of this medication by a soothing backrub, a freshly made bed, and a last opportunity to answer any questions about surgery. Talking to relieve anxiety may be more effective in promoting a good night's sleep than the ordered medication.

SAFEGUARDING THE PATIENT AND HIS PROPERTY
On the morning of surgery, various measures to assess the patient's overall condition are carried out.

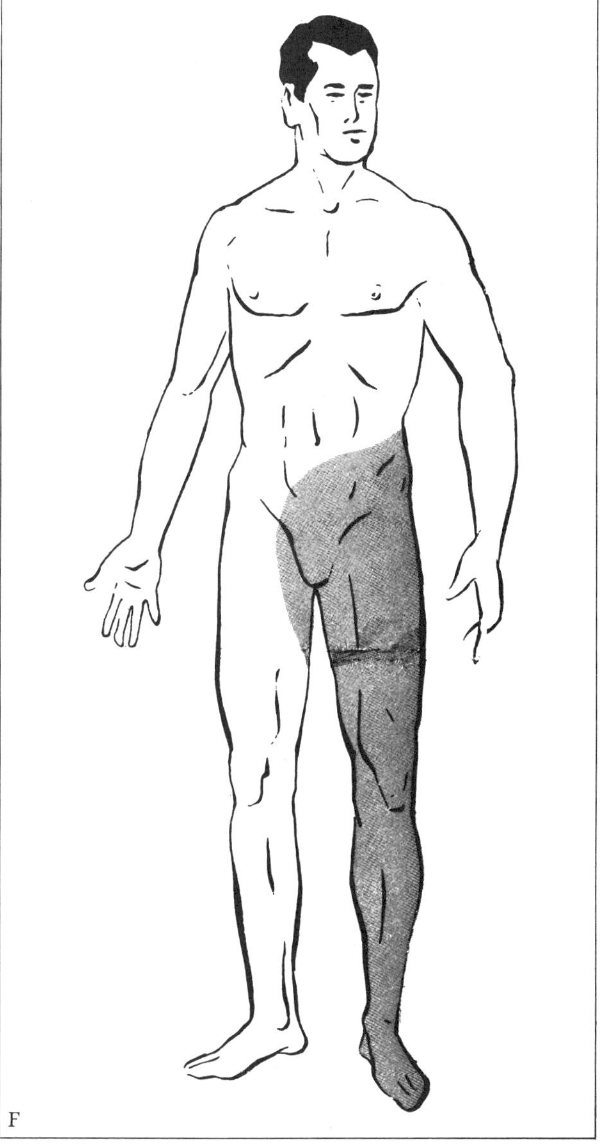

Vital Signs. Assess vital signs; take particular care in temperature recording since an elevated temperature on the morning of surgery may be an indication of an upper respiratory tract infection. If the surgery is not immediately necessary, such an infection may increase the risk of anesthesia enough to postpone the procedure. Make certain that an increase in temperature or any new variation in vital signs is reported promptly to the surgeon so she can make a new patient assessment before scrubbing for surgery.

Morning Care. The patient needs to wash or shower on the morning of surgery to reduce the overall level of skin bacteria. Provide him with a clean hospital gown (his own might be lost in surgery or stained with iodine from the surgical skin preparation). If a woman's hair is long, braid it or put it in a ponytail so that it will more easily fit under the surgical cap worn by a patient in the operating room (hair contained by a cap is less likely to spread microorganisms than hair uncontained). Do not use bobbypins in hair since these can lacerate skin unnoticed when a person is unconscious. Check women's nailbeds for nailpolish; if present, have it removed from at least two fingers on each hand to allow determining whether or not nailbed color is remaining pink during anesthesia administration (a good check that lack of oxygen is not occurring). Some agency policies require removal of all nailpolish. Caution women not to apply cosmetics on the morning of surgery since extreme paleness or cyanosis from lack of oxygen could be hidden by blush or lipstick. Remove all jewelery except a wedding ring so that it will not be lost during the time the person is unconscious. Use adhesive tape to secure the ring in place.

Some patients have elastic stockings ordered to be applied prior to surgery to ensure venous return during surgery. Apply these using gentle technique with the person in a supine position (see Chap. 31).

Give good oral care (brush and rinse teeth or clean dentures well) so that the oral cavity is as clean as possible. An endotracheal tube passed through the mouth to the trachea will consequently carry the least number of organisms with it. Respiratory tract infection is a threat following surgery from stasis of secretions; do not introduce additional bacteria in this way.

Check your hospital policy to determine whether or not dentures should be removed. When intubation tubes were fairly nonpliable, all dentures had to be removed prior to surgery (to many a person's embarrassment); now that newer anesthesia techniques are available, full dentures are sometimes left in place. Partial dentures and children's retainers (plastic appliances fitted to be worn for additional correction following oral braces), which fit more loosely, generally need to be removed. Note on the chart if dentures are in place. Remove contact lenses. It is unsafe to leave these in eyes of an unconscious person as they might cause undetected corneal abrasions. Examine the skin preparation area to be certain that it is cleanly shaven.

Identification Ensurance. Examine the patient's identification band to be certain that it is correct and secure. Infants should have two bands (bands slide off more easily from infants because of the smaller difference in circumference between wrist and hand). If a band is missing, secure one from the admissions department. Once unconscious, a person has no way of identifying himself or guarding his well-being; that responsibility is yours.

Establish Baseline for Intake and Output. Ask the person to void prior to surgery, and note the time and amount as a baseline output calculation. One of the gravest dangers of surgery is that kidneys may fail under the physiological stress of surgery or lack of blood flow to them because of decreased blood pressure. Knowing the exact time of the last voiding helps to establish how long the person has been without urine output. If the person is going to have abdominal surgery, this act also serves to reduce bladder size and remove it more completely from the surgical area.

If a suction machine for nasogastric drainage or a catheter to bladder drainage was in place before surgery, empty these containers to avoid confusing amounts drained following surgery with amounts drained prior to surgery. Measure these amounts if indicated and add them to the person's preoperative total fluid balance.

Perform Specific Procedures. Check the surgeon's orders to be certain that there is no special procedure to be carried out just prior to surgery, such as an enema, bladder catheterization, neurological baseline assessment, or eye drops. Check that results of diagnostic studies such as urinalysis and hematocrit have been returned. If abnormal results were obtained, alert the patient's surgeon.

Complete Patient Chart and Presurgery Checklist. You must finish your recording of nursing care up to the time the patient leaves the nursing care unit. Many hospitals use an additional preoperative checklist, such as that shown in the following box, to remind you of all neces-

Preoperative Check List

Action	*Completed*
Patient concerns	
Skin preparation:	______
Identification in place:	______
Temperature, pulse, respiration ______	______
Blood pressure ______	______
Height ______ Weight ______	______
Voided ______ Time ______ Amount ______	______
NPO after ______	______
Hospital gown	______
Hairpins removed	______
Nailpolish removed	______
Jewelry removed	______
Preoperative medication: ______	______
Dentures removed ______ In place ______	______
Contact lenses removed ______	______
Prosthetic devices removed ______	______
Chart concerns	
Addressograph plate attached	______
Operative permit obtained	______
Urinalysis	______
Hematocrit	______
Electrocardiogram	______
Chest x-ray	______
Blood order of ______	______

Signature ______ R.N.

sary measures to be taken. Checking and signing such a form indicates that you have completed the measures.

Preoperative Medication. Almost all patients receive a premedication injection prior to leaving the patient unit (it may be administered in a presurgery "hold" room in the operating suite itself). Preoperative drugs have four main purposes: (1) to sedate or tranquilize, (2) to act as an analgesic, (3) to decrease respiratory tract secretions, and (4) to decrease the possibility of nausea.

SEDATION AND TRANQUILIZATION. Almost all people admit to nervousness immediately before surgery. A preoperative drug with a sedative or tranquilizing effect, therefore, is often a welcome medication. Preoperative drugs are never given orally since a person is not allowed oral fluid so close to administration of an anesthetic. Before administering the injection, be certain to caution the person that it will make him feel sleepy and relaxed. Some people expect to fall sound asleep after taking premedication and are disappointed to discover that, although they feel less tense, they are still conscious of their surroundings.

ANALGESIA. People who are in pain cannot relax as long as the pain is present. An analgesic given in combination with a sedative as premedication, therefore, aids (potentiates) the action of the sedative.

RESPIRATORY DRYING (VAGOLYTIC) AGENTS. The gag and cough reflexes are obliterated in an anesthetized patient, and it is important that large amounts of secretions do not pool in the pulmonary system, which could lead to aspiration. Administration of a drug with parasympathetic action not only reduces the amount of saliva and respiratory tract mucus present but also prevents bradycardia, a possible effect of vagal-stimulating anesthetics. Caution the person before giving the injection that the medication may make his mouth feel dry so that he is not alarmed by the sensation (and does not take a drink of water to relieve it); the person's face may flush and feel warm.

ANTINAUSEA AGENTS. When ether was a frequently used anesthetic, many people had severe nausea and vomiting following surgery. Today, although newer anesthetic agents do not have the same nausea-inducing effect, it is still dangerous for a person to vomit following anesthesia before his cough and gag reflexes return. For this reason, a drug with an anti-emetic effect may be included as a preoperative medication.

PRECAUTIONS WITH PREMEDICATIONS. Common preoperative medications are summarized in Quick Reference Stop 40-3. General rules for administering premedications are given in Quick Reference Stop 40-4.

TRANSPORT TO SURGERY

To transfer the patient to surgery, help him move to a stretcher. Use optimal safety features for transport (siderails up and cart straps secure). Since the person may be extremely sleepy from the preoperative medication, you generally need help to transfer him to the stretcher safely.

Cover him with a blanket as well as a sheet to prevent him from feeling chilled in the cool surgical suite (Fig. 40-11). His chart with the surgical checklist must accompany him. Check that his identification is secure one final time before he leaves the patient unit.

PREPARATION OF A POST-SURGICAL ROOM

Prepare a surgical bed for the patient's return (see Chap. 27). Be certain that you place an emesis basin and a waterproof pad on the bed, which is in a raised position and easily reached by a stretcher.

☐ QUICK REFERENCE STOP 40-3: PHARMACOLOGY
Common Premedication Drugs

Drug	*Effect and Concern*
Sedative Pentobarbital sodium (Nembutal) Secobarbital sodium (Seconal)	Causes sleepiness; overdose can lead to severe respiratory depression.
Tranquilizer Promethazine (Phenergan) Chlorpromazine (Thorazine) Diazapan (Valium)	Relaxes; reduces anxiety. Can have an extreme hypotensive effect.
Narcotic analgesic Meperidine (Demerol) Morphine sulfate	Can cause severe respiratory depression (especially morphine sulfate); relaxes.
Vagolytic agent Atropine sulfate Scopolamine (Hyoscine)	Causes extreme mouth dryness; increases heart rate dramatically; causes flushing of face. Scopolamine may cause severe hallucinations and confusion.
Anti-nausea agent Hydroxyzine (Atarax)	Reduces sensation of nausea; provides mild relaxation. Used mainly with children.

□ **QUICK REFERENCE STOP 40-4: PHARMACOLOGY**
Safe Preoperative Medication Administration

1. Preoperative medications are ordered to be given at a set time (7:00 A.M., for example) or "on call" (when surgical personnel call to say to administer it) because they must be administered 1 to 2 hours prior to anesthetic administration for maximum effect. Give preoperative medications on time to coordinate their administration with the anesthesia administration.
2. Never give preoperative medications orally. Patients should be on NPO status this soon before anesthesia administration.
3. Complete all surgery preparations, including voiding, prior to medication administration so that the person can rest and the drug has optimum effect.
4. Always raise siderails on bed following preoperative drug administration since person will feel relaxed and sleepy.
5. Be certain that the patient's call bell is nearby so that he will not be tempted to rise should he need anything.
6. Be certain that the surgical permit is signed prior to preoperative drug administration. Permits signed while the person due to drowsiness is not reasoning clearly are not valid.

Secure any equipment that will be necessary for postoperative care, such as oxygen equipment, an IV pole, suction, or clamps for chest tubes.

RESPONSIBILITY FOR SUPPORT PEOPLE
While surgery is performed, the patient's support people generally wait in the patient's room or, depending on hospital policy, a waiting room outside the surgical unit. Assure them that the surgeon will tell them following surgery of the procedure's outcome. Remind them that the patient will go to a recovery room for an hour or two before returning to the patient unit so they will need to wait to see the patient. Answer any questions they have. Their support postoperatively will be instrumental in the patient's recovery, and they need support themselves while they wait for surgery to be completed.

THE INTRAOPERATIVE PHASE

The intraoperative phase takes place from the induction of anesthesia to the awakening of the patient from anesthesia. Although it is usually the shortest of the three surgical phases, it may also be the most hazardous for the patient.

Operating Suite Personnel

The operating suite is a separate section of the hospital and maintains its own separate staff as an infection control measure.

STERILE (SCRUBBED) PERSONNEL
Personnel who will participate in the actual surgery must scrub (wash thoroughly) and put on sterile gloves, caps, and masks. All equipment or items that they touch are sterile (all microorganisms and their spores have been killed). These people are the operating surgeon, her assistant, and the "scrub" nurse.

FIGURE 40-11. A surgical suite "hold room." Nursing unit personnel on the left help familiarize this schoolage girl with operating room personnel on the right.

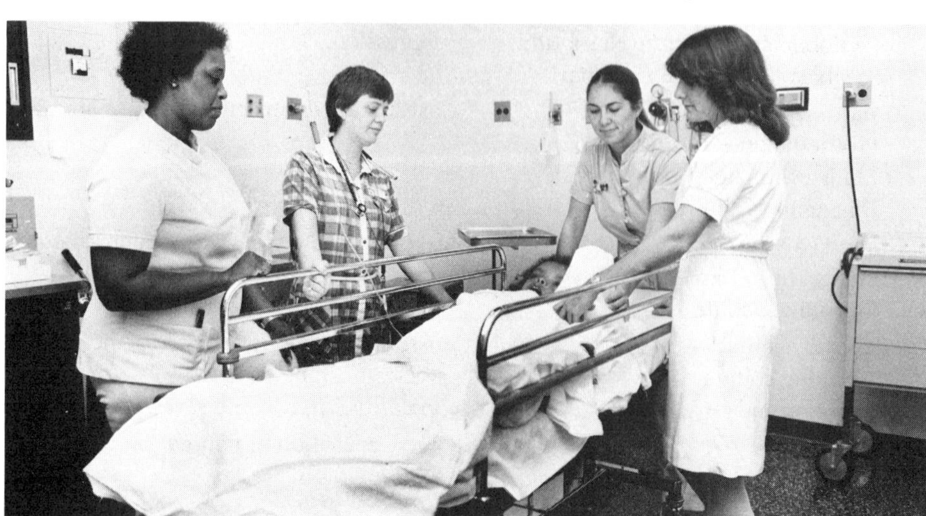

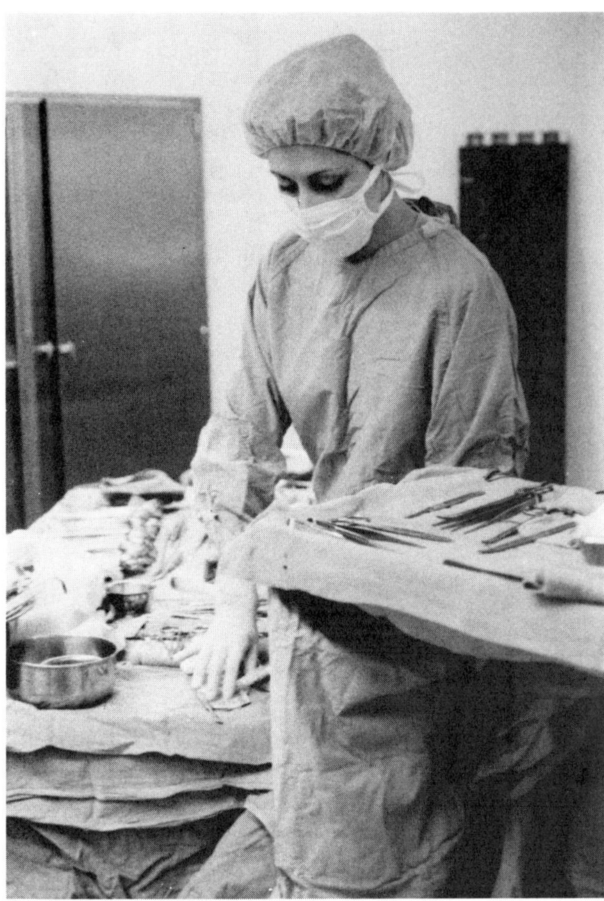

FIGURE 40-12. A scrub nurse is an example of sterile personnel in an operating suite. Here a nurse prepares sutures to finish readying the sterile instrument table.

Scrub Nurse. A scrub nurse (Fig. 40-12) is also referred to as the *sterile* or *suture* nurse. She is responsible for preparing and arranging instruments and supplies for the particular surgery planned; and assisting the surgeon and her assistants during the procedure by providing sterile instruments as needed. By maintaining strict sterile technique, she is the patient's best safeguard against the introduction of infection during surgery. In many hospitals today, this role is filled by a technician rather than a nurse.

UNSTERILE (UNSCRUBBED) PERSONNEL

People other than those participating in the actual surgery serve as support people, regulating the patient's body temperature or fluid administration and anesthesia, and handing additional sterile supplies to the sterile personnel. These people include the anesthesiologist or anesthetist and the circulating nurse.

Circulating Nurse. The circulating nurse is not sterile, so she is free to leave or enter the operating room as necessary. She greets the patient in the surgery corridor to ease any last minute apprehension. She has supervised the preparations for surgery; she acts as coordinator of supplies and equipment during surgery. She will help position the patient on the operating table and, after he is anesthetized, complete the surgical skin preparation. She is the manager of the operating room, assuring a procedure free of unnecessary delay or absent supplies (Fig. 40-13).

Positions for Surgery

A patient is placed on an operating table in the position that will allow the greatest exposure of the incision site. General rules to observe when helping position people on the operating room table are to (1) preserve modesty (even sedated people are aware of being exposed unnecessarily), (2) secure table straps firmly but with good padding to protect pressure on nerves or tissue (the person will lie in this position for a long time and, while unconscious, will have no means of indicating that a strap is accidentally interfering with circulation), and (3) assess that good respiratory function is maintained in this position (anesthetic administration will not be effective without good air exchange).

Anesthesia

The type of anesthesia used for a surgical procedure depends on the extent and type of the procedure, and the patient's preference and past experiences with anesthesia.

PRESURGICAL INTERVIEW

Prior to surgery, the anesthesiologist (a doctor) or anesthetist (possibly a specially prepared nurse) who will administer the anesthetic meets with the patient to discuss the type of anesthesia planned. She interviews the patient about previous experiences with anesthesia. She notes smoking and drinking habits (smoking may make it difficult to reduce the cough reflex; liver function, which is needed to metabolize the anesthetic, may be limited due to heavy alcohol consumption). She asks for any knowledge of renal, liver, pulmonary, or cardiovascular disease.

Medications that the patient is currently taking are noted to be certain that none of these will interfere with the anesthetic selected. Any drugs that cause an allergic reaction are also noted so that the anesthetic chosen is not similar.

A preoperative anesthesiologist interview also serves the psychological purpose of allowing the patient to meet the person who will literally control his life while his body is held under a general anesthetic. Most people place more trust in someone they have actually met than in a faceless stranger.

TYPES OF ANESTHESIA

Types of anesthesia available vary from the simple forms that block the peripheral stimulus for pain at its origin to the type that produces general anesthesia.

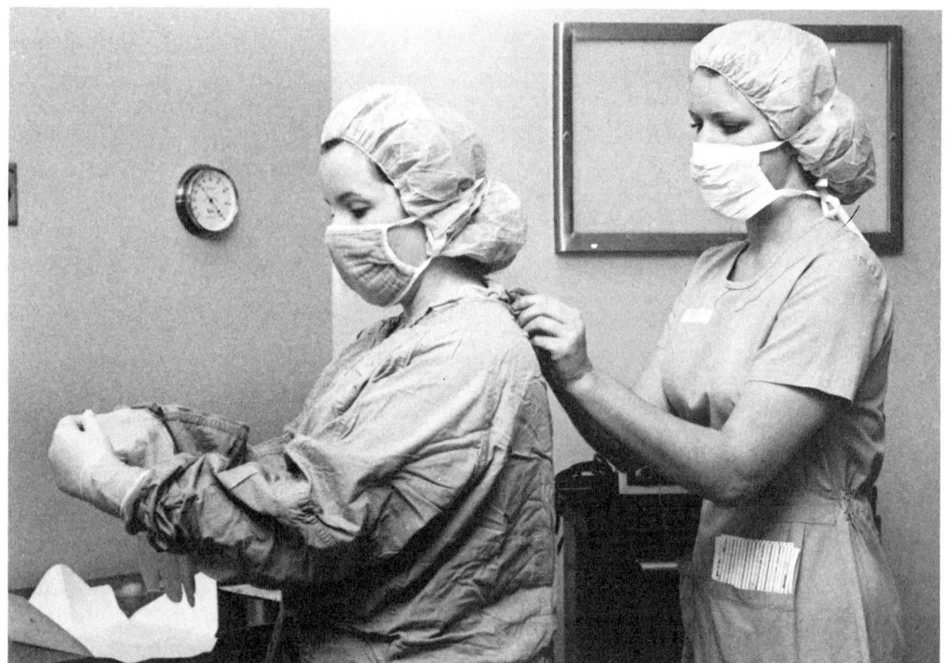

FIGURE 40-13. A scrub nurse (left) puts on sterile gloves while a circulating nurse (right) ties a sterile gown. Circulating nurses serve as operating room managers to ensure patient safety.

Agents that Block Peripheral Nerves at Their Origin. This type of anesthesia is the easiest to administer. Such administration has limitations since it does not relieve anxiety or allow for relaxation of tissue, and only a local area of the body can be anesthetized.

TOPICAL ANESTHESIA APPLICATION. Because mucus membrane absorbs an anesthetic agent such as xylocaine very rapidly, anesthesia for a minor procedure such as a bronchoscope or rectal biopsy may be given by spraying the area with a xylocaine solution. Such application provides anesthesia almost immediately; unfortunately, however, the effect is very short-term. During a procedure, several applications may be necessary to keep the area anesthetized and pain-free.

LOCAL INFILTRATION. For surgery such as placing sutures (stitches) in a small laceration or for a diagnostic procedure such as a biopsy (excision of a small piece of tissue) or removal of a tooth, the peripheral nerve impulses from the site may be blocked by the injection of an anesthetic such as xylocaine intracutaneously or subcutaneously.

The anesthetic is drawn into the syringe from its vial with a small No. 25 needle. This small bore needle is inserted intracutaneously and xylocaine is injected to raise a small wheal in the skin. A larger needle (No. 19 or 20) is then used to inject anesthetic into the deeper area. Anesthesia is obtained in 2 to 5 minutes, and lasts about 20 minutes. The duration of anesthesia can be prolonged if epinephrine, a vasoconstrictor, is added to the anesthetic before injection. Vasoconstriction at the site decreases blood flow and allows the drug to remain at the site longer and therefore exert its effect longer.

In rare instances, anaphylactic shock can occur from the administration of xylocaine if the person is sensitive to the drug. Anaphylactic shock is marked by shortness of breath leading to respiratory and cardiac arrest. Even this simplest type of anesthetic administration, therefore, is never a simple procedure.

Agents that Block Transmission of Nerve Impulses. When anesthesia is placed at a distance from the surgical site to block the transmission of nerve impulses to their point of reception in the central nervous system, a larger area of the body is anesthetized.

REGIONAL BLOCK ANESTHESIA. Regional block anesthesia involves injecting anesthesia (xylocaine) into the large afferent nerve bundles proximal to a given area. An ulnar or radial block, for example, anesthetizes the entire hand; a brachial plexus block the entire arm. Anesthetizing such a large area allows for greater manipulation of soft tissue than that permitted by a local block. Relief of pain from labor contractions may be accomplished with this technique by injection of an anesthetic at the sides of the uterine cervix (Fig. 40-14A).

For a regional nerve block, the anesthetic is injected into the site close by the nerve bundle; it is absorbed into the nerves at that point. Loss of sensation becomes apparent in 10 to 30 minutes; anesthesia will last 30 to 60 minutes. The danger of a regional anesthetic block is that the drug will be injected by error into a blood vessel; injection of xylocaine into the vascular system could lead to sudden cardiac arrythmia and cardiac arrest.

Agents that Block Spinal Cord Conduction. An anesthetic (xylocaine) may be injected into the epidural space (outside the dura mater of the spinal cord) or into the subdural space to obtain anesthesia of the lower body (Fig. 40-14). The advantage of an epidural block is that the anesthetic does not enter the cerebrospinal fluid; only the high number of nerves leaving the cord through this space are anesthetized. Epidural anesthesia is injected at the third or fourth lumbar interspace. It is often used in childbirth.

Intradural anesthesia is placed at the same lumbar-level; the anesthetic, however, is actually injected into the cerebrospinal fluid. When this space is entered, there is a possibility that a small amount of air will also enter the space. The combination of the presence of the air and the stretching of meningeal tissue may cause the person to have a severe "spinal headache" following administration of a "spinal" anesthetic. Lying prone and flat (only a small pillow under his head) for eight hours after the procedure (until air has been reabsorbed) helps best to relieve this type of headache.

Many people are frightened at having a spinal anesthetic because they have heard that the injection will harm nerves in the spinal cord and leave them with lower extremity paralysis. People can be assured that the spinal cord ends at the first or second lumbar vertebrae. The anesthetic is injected below this point at the third or fourth level (Fig. 40-15).

Epidural or intradural anesthesia is used for childbirth, hernia, and gynecological and neurological procedures. The chief danger of such anesthesia is hypotension from sympathetic nerve blockage. The patient is positioned in the same sitting position for epidural administration as for lumbar puncture (see Chap. 20). The procedure is the same as that of lumbar puncture except that injection of an anesthetic agent occurs rather than withdrawal of a sample of cerebrospinal fluid.

Agents that Produce Unconsciousness (General Anesthesia). An agent that produces unconsciousness directly affects the brain. Such anesthesia may be administered by inhalation, intravenously, or, on rare occasions, rectally.

INHALATION ANESTHESIA. Inhalation anesthesia is administered through either a mask held close to the face (Fig. 40-16) or a flexible tube passed from the oral or nasal cavity to the trachea. As the anesthetic is inhaled, it crosses the alveoli into the vascular system and circulates to the brain.

Inhalation agents are gases or volatile liquids. Common ones are nitrous oxide (laughing gas) and halothane. Halothane has a rapid action but must be processed by the liver, so it is not used with people with liver disease.

Inhalation agents have the advantage of being easily administered. They are unsafe if administered by anyone unfamiliar with their properties since an irritating

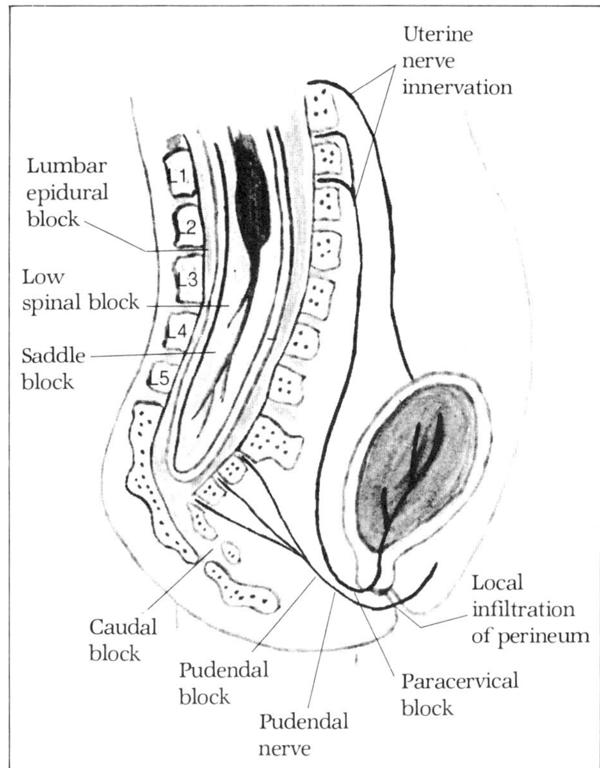

A

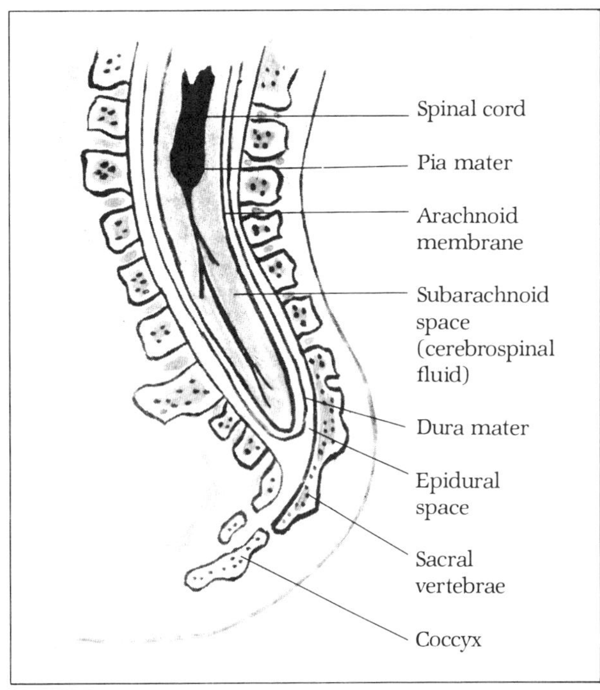

B

FIGURE 40-14. Different sites of anesthesia administration produce differing levels of anesthesia. A. Common injection sites and types. B. Anatomy of the spinal canal.

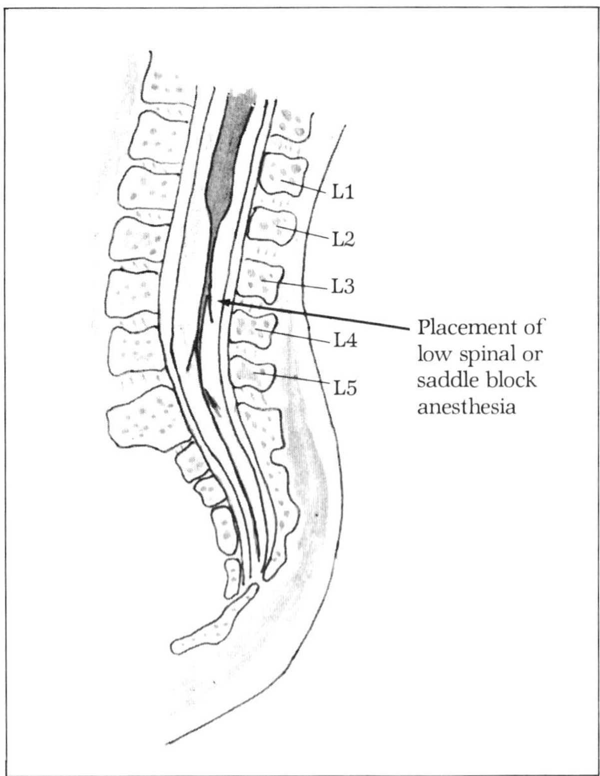

FIGURE 40-15. Spinal anesthesia is injected into the third or fourth lumbar space. Notice how the spinal cord ends at the first lumbar space.

effect on the respiratory mucosa may lead to bronco-spasm or laryngospasm, and thus airway constriction. This complication is most apt to occur in the heavy smoker or person with chronic lung disease or upper respiratory infection (the reason why surgery is usually canceled if the person has cold symptoms on the morning of surgery). Because inhalation agents must be administered with a combination of oxygen, the circulating air in operating suites is a rich mixture of oxygen able to support combustion easily, and special care is taken to reduce the possibility of static sparks.

INTRAVENOUS ANESTHESIA. Intravenous anesthesia is administered through an intravenous fluid line typically placed in a dorsal vessel of the hand or antecubital space. Induction is rapid and pleasant with these agents, but analgesia is not complete unless very large doses are used. Today an agent such as thiopental sodium is first used to induce anesthesia; then an inhalation anesthetic is used to maintain unconsciousness. As with an inhalation anesthetic, laryngospasm may occur with thiopental, so a person must be observed continuously during induction.

STAGES OF ANESTHESIA

As a person becomes anesthetized, he passes through the set stages or levels of anesthesia summarized in Table 40-1. Note that the person becomes agitated in stage II. He may thrash his arms and appear to fight a breathing mask. This stage of induction is dangerous because the person's nervous system is so stressed that should a sudden noise or undue stress occur at this point he could convulse or have a cardiac arrythmia. Surgery is performed at stage III. Stage IV, during which the person is so depressed that vital life functions may no longer be operational is again a danger stage.

FIGURE 40-16. Inhalation anesthesia is given by mask. Here a preschooler gains a feeling of control by being allowed to help hold a mask.

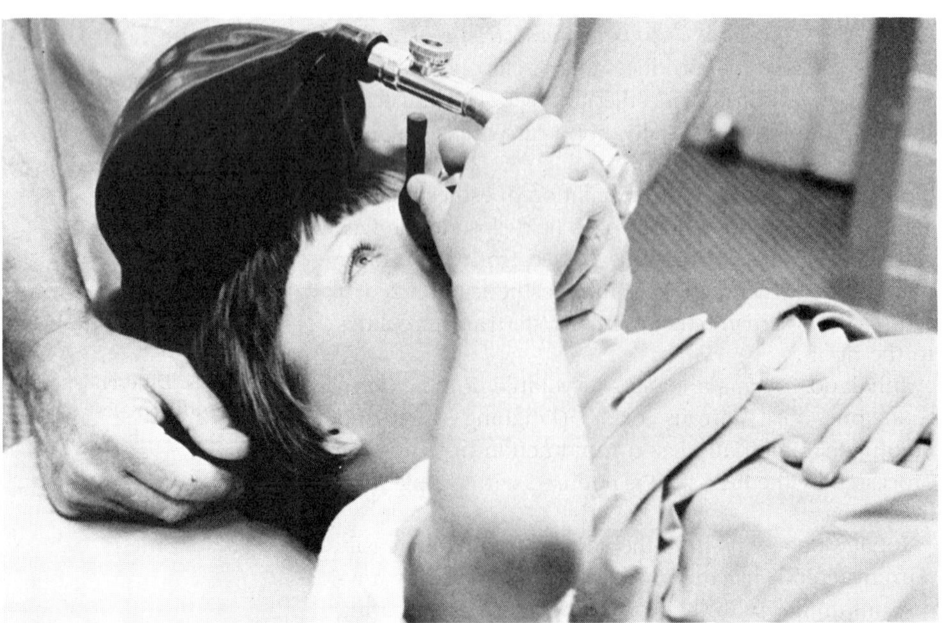

TABLE 40-1. STAGES OF ANESTHESIA

Stage	Time Interval	Importance
I	From beginning of induction to loss of consciousness	Patient feels drowsy and then will remember nothing following this point.
II	From loss of consciousness to relaxation phase	Patient becomes excited; breathing is irregular; thrashing with extremities may occur. Stress at this point, e.g., from a loud noise or a change in position, might cause him to convulse.
III	From relaxation phase to loss of reflexes (surgery stage)	No auditory sensation present; breathing slow and regular; reflexes absent.
IV	Anesthesia stage is too deep and respiratory failure or cardiac arrest occur	No respiratory or cardiac action is present.

COMPLICATIONS OF GENERAL ANESTHESIA

Vomiting and Aspiration. General anesthesia blocks the gag reflex; if pressure on the stomach during the surgical procedure should cause vomiting, vomitus will easily enter the trachea or bronchus, leading to bronchospasm and acute anoxia. This complication is reduced by being certain that the stomach is empty at the time of surgery. Use of a cuffed intubation tube during anesthesia also helps to prevent this complication (the cuff makes a seal around the tube and so prevents fluid from entering the trachea).

Respiratory Obstruction. As the tongue relaxes with general anesthesia, it may fall backward and obstruct the airway; saliva may also obstruct the airway. Such complications are prevented by use of an intubation tube or airway during surgery and use of a parasympathetic agent prior to surgery to dry oral secretions.

Hypotension. The vasodilation effects of some anesthetics combined with the blood loss from surgery may lead to extreme lowered blood pressure. Blood pressure is maintained by intravenous therapy to replace lost fluid. Postsurgical hematocrit counts are important in documenting the amount of blood lost and the need for continued replacement.

ACUPUNCTURE

Although acceptance of acupuncture is growing in the United States, the technique is rarely used to achieve anesthesia. The principle of acupuncture is to distract the patient through needle insertion and thus achieve "gating" of nerve impulses. Gating to reduce pain sensation is discussed in Chap. 27.

HYPNOSIS

Hypnosis is a technique to achieve pain relief that is used only occasionally in the United States for childbirth and dental extraction. Not all people are susceptible enough to hypnotic suggestion for the procedure to be effective.

HYPOTHERMIA

Hypothermia (lowered body temperature) is a select type of anesthesia used in cardiac surgery. When a person's body temperature is lowered to 82 to 86°F (28—30°C), the metabolic rate slows so dramatically that oxygen requirements by body tissue are minimal and anesthesia occurs. Cooling is accomplished by cooling blankets, ice water immersion, or circulation of blood through a cooled heart-lung machine after initial anesthesia induction. Hypothermia is effective anesthesia for cardiac surgery because the heart discontinues beating at this low temperature, allowing the cardiac surgeon to operate without heart action present.

Following surgery, warming is accomplished by warming the blood in the heart-lung machine to body temperature and by using warming blankets.

CONTRAINDICATIONS OF ANESTHESIA

The type of anesthesia chosen depends on the person's preference and physical condition. A person with poor blood coagulation, for example, should not be administered an epidural or spinal anesthetic, which could cause bleeding into the spinal canal. People with cardiac disorders may respond poorly to epidural anesthesia because the hypotension that occurs may place a great strain on an already strained body system. People with liver damage cannot tolerate halothane as it is detoxified by the liver; those with chronic lung disease may not tolerate an irritating inhalation agent. A person who has had an idiosyncratic reaction to an anesthetic should not be administered that type again.

The Operating Room Experience

Observing or participating in an operation offers you information about specific areas to explain to patients before surgery and complications to watch for in patients after surgery. In order to observe or participate, you must be free of infection, particularly cutaneous (skin) or respiratory infection. Before entering the operating room suite (or going any farther than the hallway of the suite) you must change to scrub clothing (cap, mask, gown, and shoe covers) and thoroughly wash your hands and arms. This procedure automatically reduces the level of bacteria in the operating suite.

Scrub clothing generally consists of soft green cotton, pajama-like tops and bottoms or straight house dresses. The color green does not glare under bright light so is

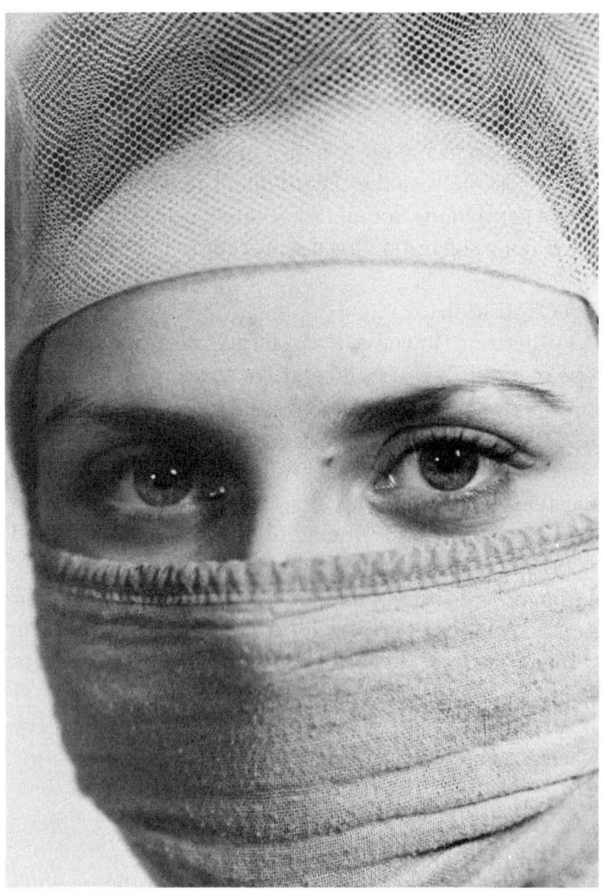

FIGURE 40-17. A properly fitted operating room mask covers both nose and mouth securely.

used a great deal in operating suites for apparel, drapes, and even walls and floor tiles. Scrub clothing is form-fitting to prevent it from brushing carelessly against sterile areas. The cap should completely cover the hair; the mask covers both mouth and nose and should be pulled snugly against the edges of the face by ties at the back (Fig. 40-17). In order that shoes do not conduct sparks, which could cause the explosion of some anesthetic gases, they should be rubber-soled; covering them with a cloth or paper impregnated with conduction strips further reduces their capacity to conduct electricity. Most operating suites have a conductometer or instrument to detect static electricity; you will be shown how to use this device to verify that your shoes are nonconductive. If no flammable gases are being used, such a precaution may not be necessary.

SURGICAL SCRUB

It is impossible to make skin sterile, but it is possible to reduce the number of bacteria present on skin to a bare minimum through careful washing. Be certain that your fingernails are trimmed short and that you are not wearing nailpolish or rings, which could lodge bacteria. If you forget and wear a ring to an operating room, ask for a safety pin and pin it to your underwear. Do not pin it to the front of your scrub dress or top. You may forget its location and toss it into a laundry hamper at the end of the procedure.

To clean your hands, take a sterile hand brush from the container by the scrub sink; allow liquid soap to run onto it (some brands have self-contained soap); turn on the water at the sink by using the foot or knee pedal. Scrub with the brush from your fingertips to 2 inches above your elbow, touching every inch of skin on fingers, hand, and arm as you progress. It should take 10 minutes to complete a thorough scrub of both arms. Rinse each hand and arm by elevating your hand so that water runs from your fingertips to your elbow, effectively removing soapy water from your arm. Dry each hand and arm with a sterile towel from the fingertips to the elbow to prevent moving germs from the unwashed skin surface above the elbow down onto your clean hands (see QRS 40-5).

☐ QUICK REFERENCE STOP 40-5: SAFETY
Basic Aseptic Principles

1. A sterile pack that is found opened or torn is no longer considered sterile.
2. A sterile pack that is found moist is no longer considered sterile.
3. Reaching over a sterile table contaminates the table.
4. Every area below the waist level is unsterile.
5. Any article of doubtful sterility is considered unsterile.
6. Any article past its specified outdate is unsterile.

IMPORTANT OBSERVATIONS TO MAKE

An operating suite has so many new sights that it is easy to miss focusing on the most important ones. Try to remember how strange everything seems to you; the operating room is this strange to patients also and, because of the strangeness, intimidating and frightening.

Operating room suite corridors are cool. Be certain that patients being transported to surgery are covered with a cotton blanket; if not, they may become chilled if they have to wait in the corridor. There is little for a patient resting on a stretcher to see in a corridor except overhead lights and green tile walls, and little to think about except the chance that something may go wrong.

Depending on the surgery planned and the particular surgical suite, the patient may be either wheeled into the operating room for anesthesia induction or taken to a special anesthesia induction room. Being wheeled into an operating room (and seeing tables of instruments, the bright overhead light, the ominous operating table, people wearing gowns and masks), is the epitomy of fright; a special induction room is preferable.

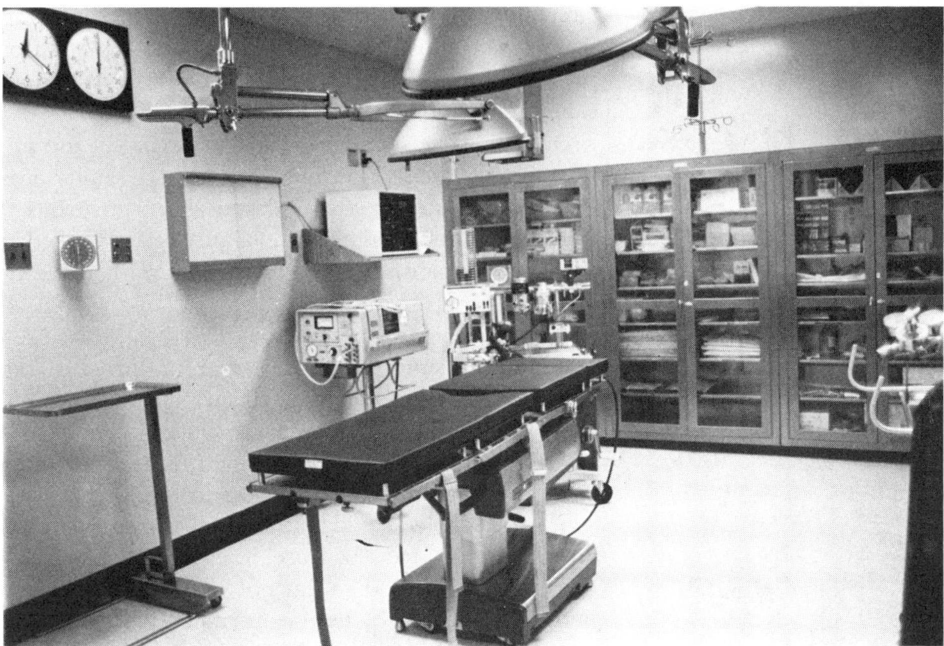

FIGURE 40-18. An empty operating room. Note cupboards for supplies at the back; an x-ray view box and a cardiac monitor hang on the wall. Anesthetic equipment sits by the head of the table.

As you enter the operating room, take a minute to look at it from the patient's view. Think how much you would appreciate a nurse for having stood by your stretcher as you waited in the hallway. Think how good you would feel if a nurse stepped forward from the row of personnel in the room to greet you with reassuring words. These are the responsibilities of a circulating nurse.

In a typical operating room, the operating table is located in the center of the room under a large overhead light (Fig. 40-18). The light is attached to a track so that it can be tilted or focused by means of an overhead handle. The table is built so that it can be tilted in many directions, allowing patients to be positioned with good support for different surgical approaches. Anesthesiology equipment (the portable machine for administering inhalation anesthesia with accompanying oxygen and suction equipment) is placed at the head of the table, and an instrument table at the foot of the table. Additional equipment includes a small Mayo (over-the-table stand) for instruments that will be used first during surgery, a table for surgeon's gloves and gown, and kickbuckets (stainless steel buckets on wheels) for disposal of used sponges. The walls may be lined with cupboards with sterile supplies, additional intravenous equipment, and an x-ray box.

The circulating nurse will assist the patient to move from the transport stretcher to the operating room table and remain with him until anesthesia is administered (if it is not given in an induction room). Once administration of the anesthetic is begun, the anesthesiologist will announce to the room at large that she is beginning. Stand still and do not talk until the anesthesiologist announces that induction is complete as this is the most dangerous time of anesthesia for a patient. A loud noise at this point (bumping against a table, dropping an instrument, talking suddenly) could be so shocking to the person's nervous system that he might convulse or have laryngopasm.

GOWNING

All personnel who are going to participate in the actual surgery must not only scrub but don a sterile cover gown and gloves as well. The scrub nurse puts on her own cover (long-sleeved) gown, taking care to touch only its inner surfaces. Using sterile technique, she puts on her own sterile gloves. She cannot tie her gown in back since the back of a gown is considered contaminated; tying is done by the circulating nurse.

Once she is gowned and gloved, the scrub nurse sets up sterile supplies for the operators. She places sterile pillowcases or drapes over tables and stands, opens sterile instrument trays, and arranges instruments in the order in which they will be used on the back table and the Mayo stand. With the circulating nurse, she counts all the "sponges" (gauze squares used to absorb blood) and "lap" pads (thick heavy pads used to absorb moisture during the operation); the circulating nurse notes this count on a conspicuous "count" sheet somewhere in the room. If more sponge packs are opened and added to the setup during the procedure, this additional number will be added to the list. At the conclusion of surgery, the number of sponges (both used and unused) in the room will again be added to be

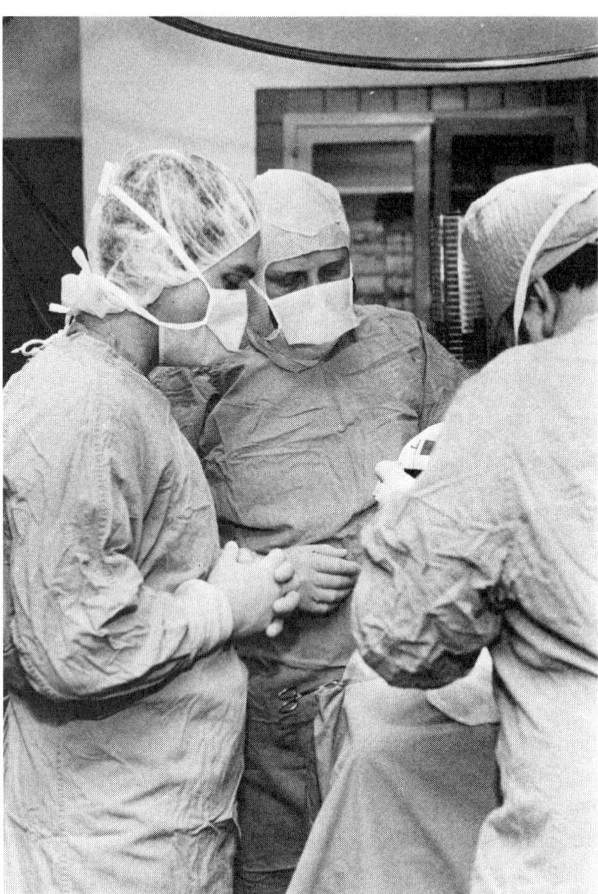

FIGURE 40-19. Sterile operating room personnel checks a sterile piece of equipment to be used with surgery. Note that the hands are kept at waist level to avoid contamination.

certain that no sponge was left inside the incision. Explain this safeguard to patients, who sometimes fear such an accident.

When the setup is complete, the scrub nurse assists the surgeon and her assistants in gowning and gloving as they finish their "scrubs." The circulating nurse ties the rear strings of their gowns to prevent them from contaminating their gloves. As a nonsterile observer in an operating room, you may be asked to help with gown tying. Watch someone do it first to be sure you understand the technique. You are allowed to touch any area of the inside surface of a gown, but only the bottom hem and the ties of the outside surface. To keep gloves sterile, they cannot be lowered below the waist. Notice how people waiting at any point in a procedure are careful not to lower their hands to their sides (Fig. 40-19).

SURGICAL PROCEDURE

Following assurance that the patient is fully anesthetized, the patient is positioned for that particular procedure. A metal screen is placed at the patient's shoulder level and covered with a sterile drape to block the flow of bacteria from the patient's respiratory tract to the incision site. The incision site is cleaned by the circulating nurse or a surgeon's assistant using a predetermined antiseptic such as iodine. Sterile cloth or plastic drapes are then placed around the area of incision to expose only a small area of skin.

Operating incisions are made with careful precautions against excess bleeding. First, just the skin layer is cut. Capillaries at the edge of the cut skin begin to bleed. Hemostats (small metal clamps) are quickly applied to compress these miniature "bleeders" and halt bleeding. Sutures (strings of absorbable gut) are then placed over each hemostat and tied to ligate (tie off) bleeding. The hemostats are then removed and returned to the Mayo stand. The layer of fat is cut and bleeders are clamped and ligated in the same way. The incision is extended deeper and deeper through fascia and muscle using the same cut, clamp, ligate technique.

The scalpel blade used for the initial skin cut is considered contaminated (because it cut through surface bacteria that the iodine did not remove) so is folded under a sterile towel after use and not reused during the procedure. If you have the opportunity to observe surgery by "scrubbing in" next to the scrub nurse, remember that this knife is contaminated and cannot be used again.

Once the surgical incision is complete, retractors (long metal curved instruments) are slipped into the incision. Gentle traction on these handles by an assistant keeps the incision spread apart and allows for good visualization of the operative site. Sterile towels may be placed in the incision to separate body organs or they may be pushed aside with lap pads.

Although the pace of surgery is rapid, an extensive procedure can easily take 2 hours, during which time abdominal contents have remained shifted and people surrounding the table have leaned on the sides of the patient. As a result, many people have an overall aching feeling following surgery.

As the surgeon begins to close the incision, the scrub nurse and circulating nurse begin the sponge count. Before the incision can be fully closed, this count must be correct. As the last suture is placed and the incision is covered with a sterile dressing, the anesthesiologist begins to lighten the level of anesthesia to keep the period of anesthesia as short as possible. The person will then be transferred to a stretcher and taken to the recovery room until he can state his name, what day it is, and where he is (orientation to person, time, and place).

Types of Sutures. Many people envision that their bodies will remain filled with sutures following a surgical procedure. Sutures are designed, however, to prevent this occurrence. They are divided into two types: internal and external. Those used internally are absorbable (will be digested and absorbed by body tissue after a period of time). They consist of catgut (rapidly absorbed), chromic catgut (coated with chromic acid to make it slowly absorbed), or synthetic catgut (also slowly absorbed). Sutures used externally for a final skin incision may consist of absorbable material or of silk, cotton, nylon, or synthetic threads, which must be removed 4 to 7 days following surgery to prevent irritation from longer exposure. A newer technique often used in abdominal surgery is the use of metal staples rather than sutures to close incisions. These are placed rapidly and removed easily. With still other incisions, steristrips (plastic coatings) are used to seal the wound.

Sutures may be either used as "ties" to ligate bleeders or threaded into needles for actual sewing of body tissues. Tissue needles are often curved; the scrub nurse clamps the needle to a hemostat before handing it to the surgeon for easier handling. Notice that needles are counted as cautiously as sponges to prevent the possibility of a needle left in the incision.

Ambulatory Surgery

If a person's health problem is not complex and his general health is good, he may choose not to be admitted to a hospital but to have surgery done on an ambulatory basis through the outpatient department.

Ambulatory surgery has the advantages of being less costly, eliminating the psychological stress of an overnight stay (particularly important with children), and encouraging early ambulation (very important for the most rapid postoperative course). It also frees hospital staff to attend to patients with more serious illnesses.

A person scheduled for ambulatory surgery generally comes to the hospital a week or several days beforehand for blood and urine studies. He then reports to the outpatient department early on the day of surgery. He is given a physical and preoperative interview and receives his preoperative medication.

Following surgery, he remains in the recovery room until awake, then is returned to a special "hold" or "observation" room for an additional 1 to 4 hours. Following this time he returns home, provided that no complications have developed.

Ambulatory surgery places the responsibility on the patient to report to the hospital on the day of surgery without eating or drinking anything, and to monitor his own care and condition following surgery. Good teaching is needed to ensure that the person understands the importance of postoperative measures and knows when to seek help for signs or symptoms that unexpectedly develop.

THE POSTOPERATIVE PHASE

The postoperative phase can be divided into the recovery room period, the intermediate postoperative period, and the extended postoperative period.

Recovery Room Period

Patients are redressed in a hospital gown and transferred from the operating room table to a stretcher for transfer to the recovery room. The recovery room is adjacent to the operating room suite; people remain on stretchers in the room until they are awake enough from anesthesia to tell you their name, their age or the date, and where they are, and until vital signs are stable (a 1- to 2-hour period). Attached to the wall near each stretcher are oxygen and suction outlets, readily available airways, additional intravenous and blood transfusion equipment, emergency drugs, and cardiac and respiratory monitors (Fig. 40-20).

Recovery rooms have the advantage of being situated near the operating room so if a sudden complication such as hemorrhage develops, the person can be returned immediately to the operating room suite for further care. Such a room centralizes care and safeguards in the best way possible the person in the immediate postsurgical period.

People who have had major surgery or who have been identified preoperatively as poor surgical risks may be transferred to an intensive care unit (ICU) rather than a recovery room for this period of care.

When moving people postoperatively, always use gentle motions to avoid disrupting sutures; turn people slowly to avoid hypotension from a quick change of posture. Be certain that the person is kept warm to avoid having to increase metabolism to maintain body temperature, an unnecessary stress at an already stressful time. Always use full safety precautions—siderails and stretcher straps—since a person may be confused and disoriented for a few minutes after waking from anesthesia.

POSITIONING

When people are first moved to a stretcher in the operating room and while they remain in the recovery room, they are placed on their side with their head tipped slightly forward (Sim's position) to prevent their tongue from falling backward or saliva or mucus from obstructing their airway. Place a pillow securely behind the person's back to keep him in this position. In certain instances, such as spinal or cranial surgery, a special postoperative position may be required. Observe any person who is not placed on his side or in a Sim's position very carefully for airway obstruction until he is fully awake. A prone position with the head turned to the side allows saliva to drain from the mouth but may interfere with chest expansion.

HEMORRHAGE

The possibility of hemorrhage following surgery exists until all blood vessels cut and ligated during surgery have thrombosed, sclerosed, and permanently sealed closed. The danger of hemorrhage is most acute in the first hour following surgery; it remains an acute problem for the first 24 hours. That hemorrhage is occurring is revealed by a fall in blood pressure, increased pulse, and rapid respirations. The person may be restless and feel thirsty.

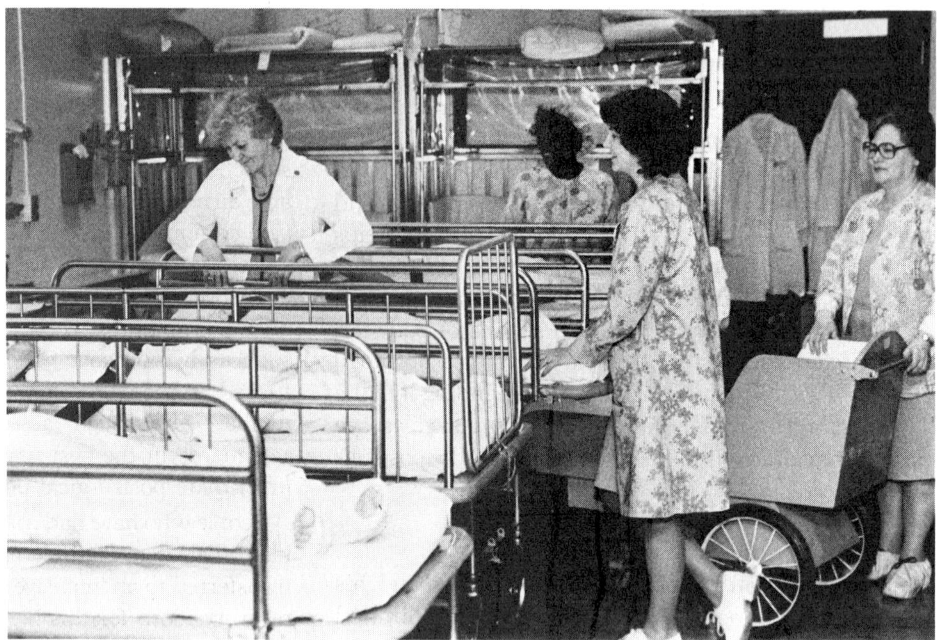

FIGURE 40-20. A recovery room. The child in the third stretcher is awake and ready to return to her hospital unit.

To detect the earliest signs of hemorrhage, blood pressure, pulse, and respiration rates should be taken every 15 minutes for the first hour after surgery, every 30 minutes for the next 2 hours, every hour for the next 4 hours, or as specifically ordered. The dressing over the surgical incision should be checked for blood stains every time the vital signs are taken. Be certain to turn the person to look under their body for bleeding. Blood oozing from a surgical wound can pool to a great amount under a sedated patient before it is visible unless you conscientiously check for it.

The person's physician must be notified of changes in vital signs that might indicate hemorrhage in order that action can be taken to infuse additional fluid to replace loss or to return the patient to surgery. Following some surgical procedures, the physician will leave specific orders such as to notify her if blood pressure falls below 70 or 50 diastolic, or heart rate rises above 100 to 120. In most instances, a continued change in vital signs (pulse steadily increasing, blood pressure steadily declining) will alert you to danger even before these cut-off points are reached.

RESPIRATORY OBSTRUCTION

People who had intubation tubes in place during surgery may have edema of the upper airway, which can compromise air exchange. An anesthetized patient does not have an operational gag reflex and so saliva from his mouth may pool in the back of his throat and flow into his trachea, causing obstruction or aspiration. The best way to prevent these complications is to be certain that the person is positioned on his side or in a Sim's position. These positions also prevent the person's tongue from falling backward to cause obstruction. Signs of obstruction are noisy respirations, restlessness, cyanosis, and increasing respiratory rate.

An airway is a hollow plastic tube that slips inside the person's mouth and presses on top of the base of the tongue to keep it forward and from obstructing the airway. As soon as a person regains consciousness, he feels uncomfortable and pushes the airway forward and out of his mouth with his tongue.

BASELINE OBSERVATIONS

As soon as a patient is received in the recovery room, baseline assessments are taken of blood pressure, pulse, respirations, temperature, skin color, condition of dressing, and any equipment present such as an intravenous infusion, airway, or catheter. These observations are recorded together with a statement regarding the patient's overall condition, presence or absence of pharyngeal reflex (swallowing or gag reflex), and level of responsiveness (responds to voice? deep pressure? pain?).

Whether or not a dressing is dry and intact is an important baseline determination for predicting the amount of blood lost from the incision. Any drains present in the incision are recorded. Drains are flat (penrose) or round rubber catheters used to allow infected material or blood to drain from a wound. A dressing over an incision with a drain will invariably become soiled with drainage more quickly than a dressing over an incision without a drain.

This first nursing note serves as the baseline document of respiratory and circulatory status and incision condition; consequently, it is important not only to nurses working in the recovery room but to every nurse who gives care during the postoperative period.

Intermediate Postoperative Period

As soon as the patient's immediate condition has stabilized and he is able to respond to his name, he is transferred to a patient unit accompanied by a nurse from the recovery room.

The person is transferred to his patient unit bed and positioned appropriately (on his side unless wide awake). Check the patient's dressing immediately after transfer to be certain that it is intact; review the patient's postoperative course to that point with the nurse accompanying him and check that all equipment being used by the patient (intravenous fluid, urinary catheters, nasogastric tubes) is functioning. Check the person's level of consciousness and vital signs (pulse, respirations, and blood pressure).

PHYSICIAN'S ORDERS

All previous physician's orders are automatically halted while a person is in surgery. New physician's orders are written while the patient is in the recovery room. Those that require immediate interventions are begun by the recovery room nurse (attach nasogastric tube to suction, administer intravenous fluid). Review the orders with her to establish which have been begun and which have not. This is particularly important for orders concerning intravenous fluid, blood transfusion, and postoperative medications. Typical postoperative orders are shown in the following box. If, in this example, the nurse in the recovery room already administered 1,000 ml of fluid, you would only administer 2,000 ml, not the full 3,000 ml. If the nurse in the recovery room already administered the analgesic (Demerol), you could not administer it for 4 hours from that time. Good communication between recovery room and patient unit personnel is the best safeguard against errors in intravenous or medication administration following the transfer of a patient from one unit to another.

COMMON POSTOPERATIVE ORDERS

1. Vital signs q15min for 1 hour; then q30min for 2 hours; then q1h × 4 hours.
2. Infuse 3,000 ml 5% D/W over 24 hours.
3. Demerol 50 mg IM q4h PRN for pain.
4. NPO until wide awake; ice chips as tolerated when alert.
5. Record intake and output.
6. Turn, cough, and deep breathe q2h.
7. Hematocrit determination in A.M.
8. Catheterize × 1 if patient does not void in 8 hours.

Notice how the physician's orders are a list of specific functions. Your observations and plan of nursing orders must be added to this list or the patient's care will be very incomplete. Positioning, for example, is not mentioned. The rate of intravenous fluid is not specified (you would have to calculate how rapidly to infuse the solution to administer it in 24 hours); it will be your evaluation that will determine when the analgesic is needed. The physician's orders do not mention checking the dressing; they do not delineate any action concerning voiding until 8 hours time. Postoperative care is a good example of how nursing and physician's orders complement each other to provide optimal care.

PATIENT'S FAMILY

The first time that the patient's support people are able to see him following surgery is after his return to the patient unit. To prevent people from over-reading the seriousness of the patient's condition, prepare them outside the patient's room for any equipment being used such as intravenous fluid or nasogastric tube; explain the purpose of the equipment and, particularly if it is temporary, how soon it will be removed. You may also need to explain that the patient is still sleepy from the anesthetic.

Extended Postoperative Period

Although the time following surgery that a person will be hospitalized depends on the patient and the type of surgery, it averages 4 to 10 days or until healing has progressed enough so that the person may safely return home to monitor his own care. During this period there are a number of interventions necessary to promote healing and prevent postoperative complications.

PROMOTION OF ADEQUATE RESPIRATORY EXCHANGE

While the patient is anesthetized, he breathes very shallowly. Following a return to consciousness, he may not breathe as deeply as normally in order to limit chest movement and prevent pain at his surgical site. This limited motion, along with increased respiratory secretions due to the irritation of the anesthetic gas or oral-tracheal tube, may lead to a great deal of fluid pooling in the respiratory tract. Pooling of fluid invites infection or atelectasis (collapse of lung alveoli that occurs when oxygen is unable to reach alveoli through the concentration of mucus).

A person who is having signs of poor respiratory exchange will have rapid shallow respirations and may be restless and apprehensive; his pulse will become rapid and he may insist on remaining in an upright position. To prevent poor air exchange, begin encouraging deep breaths and coughing every 2 hours. Splint an abdominal incision for the patient with your hands or help him press a small pillow against his abdomen while he coughs. This relieves pain and helps assure the person that coughing will not harm his incision. Be certain that he is turned to a different position every 2 hours. Both these measures help to prevent pooling of respiratory secretions and increase the depth of respirations. Young children can be encouraged to deep breathe by playing "Simon Says" or by imitating your movements.

Some patients have intermittent positive pressure breathing (IPPB) treatments ordered for them to encourage deep breathing. An IPPB machine is a machine that blows oxygen and air through a mouthpiece into the patient's lungs at a set rate and strength. The patient seals his lips around the mouthpiece; as he starts to breathe in, the machine "assists" him by pushing air into his lungs. The patient may experience a smothering feeling at first. At the instant that the person starts to breathe out, however, the machine clicks off. The person, therefore, controls the machine; the machine does not control him. The patient needs to be reassured of this before beginning IPPB treatments.

Another device used postoperatively to encourage deep breathing is the incentive spirometer, a system of plastic tubes with colored Ping-Pong balls suspended in each tube or a similar tube system that flashes lights. With most incentive spirometers, the person places his lips around the mouthpiece and inhales. The harder he inhales, the farther the Ping-Pong ball rises in the hollow tube (or the more the light flashes). Such an exerciser is fun to operate and gives a patient a sense of reward for his effort. Patients need a good explanation before using an incentive spirometer since their initial impression is usually that the balls rise or lights flash as a result of blowing into the instrument. Its purpose is to cause the person to take deep breaths and fully aerate lung spaces, however, so most models are triggered by inhalations, not exhalations. Both IPPB machines and incentive breathing devices are shown in Chap. 32.

PROMOTION OF ADEQUATE NUTRITION AND FLUID BALANCE

The length of time before a person can eat postoperatively depends on the type and extent of surgery performed. To prevent aspiration, *no patient should be given anything by mouth until he is wide awake from the anesthesia.* Anesthesia and handling during surgery causes the intestine to halt or slow its function; it takes about 24 to 48 hours before full function is restored (if full function does not return, the condition is termed *paralytic ileus*). Patients with abdominal surgery, therefore, often have a nasogastric tube in place after surgery to prevent stomach distention from gas and stomach secretions from being unable to pass through this temporary blockage. They will be NPO until this tube is removed in 24 to 48 hours.

Introduce fluid slowly (ice chips for the first hour, then sips of clear fluid such as ginger ale, Jello, tea, Popsicles); gradually return the person to a soft and then regular diet as ordered. Many people assume that they will not be allowed to eat for a long time following surgery and are surprised to learn that they can have something to drink only hours after surgery. Other people try to drink and eat too soon (their mouth is dry from the preoperative medication) and become nauseated. Help the person to find the level that is right for him by introducing ice chips first. Ice chips dissolve slowly so the person receives very little fluid from them; they feel cool, however, so quickly take away the "cottony" feeling caused by preoperative medication. You may need to assure people who are too nauseated after surgery to drink that they can receive enough fluid intravenously to sustain them until they are able to drink freely (see QRS 40-6).

> ☐ **QUICK REFERENCE STOP 40-6: NUTRITION**
>
> People tend either to assume that they will not be allowed anything to eat after surgery, and consequently are surprised to be offered ice chips shortly afterward, or to grow impatient with the length of time that elapses before they are allowed to eat more than fluid. Teach the importance of restoring intestinal function before beginning to eat again.

Ask people if they are passing gas rectally; assess for bowel sounds to establish that bowel function is returning. Note carefully the time and number of bowel movements that the person is having after surgery. If he has no bowel movement by the third or fourth day after surgery (and is eating well), the physician may order a stool softener or a suppository or enema to assist with stool evacuation. Assure people who are not receiving much food yet that it is normal not to have bowel movements for 3 or 4 days postoperatively (providing that bowel sounds are returning), especially if they had an enema administered prior to surgery.

Adequate fluid intake is important following surgery in order to replace blood loss from surgery and to maintain blood pressure and renal function. It must be monitored carefully to prevent giving it at too rapid a rate (which could lead to cardiac overload) or too slow a rate (which could lead to inadequate circulatory compensation). Keeping an accurate intake and output record on all postsurgical patients for at least the first 48 hours helps to ascertain an adequate fluid balance.

PROMOTION OF ADEQUATE RENAL FUNCTION

If the bladder was displaced or handled during surgery, its tone may be inadequate to initiate voiding following surgery. If the person does not receive or take in adequate fluid to promote kidney function, he does not produce adequate urine. Inadequate kidney function will result in the body being unable to rid itself sufficiently of waste products. Inadequate bladder emptying may also result in bladder infection (stasis of any body fluid leads to infection).

Normally a person voids within 8 hours following surgery. You can determine whether or not a bladder is filling by pressing lightly over the symphysis pubis to assess fullness and by percussion (an empty bladder sounds dull, a full bladder resonant, an extended bladder hyperresonant). If a bladder has filled to capacity but cannot empty properly, the person may have "retention with overflow," or void 30 to 60 ml of urine every 15 to 20 minutes. This voiding pattern is potentially dangerous because it means that the person's bladder is held continuously under tension, which may result in permanent bladder damage if the condition is not detected and the bladder emptied by catheterization.

Measures to help people void are to administer an analgesic (helps to relax abdominal musculature), provide privacy for voiding, help the man to stand to void if possible, pour warm water over a woman's vulva (measure the amount of water used so that it can be differentiated from urine), and run water from a tap within hearing distance.

Keeping an accurate intake and output record on all patients for at least 48 hours following surgery helps to remind you to check for voiding. This type of monitoring does a great deal toward ensuring the safe return of renal function after surgery. Do not underestimate the importance of a first voiding within 6 to 8 hours following surgery; it proves not only renal competency but also circulatory competency since the kidneys must have adequate blood flow through them to function.

PROMOTION OF ADEQUATE CIRCULATION

Adequate cardiovascular circulation is necessary for perfusion of body tissue and nutrient and oxygen supply to body cells. Because of blood loss during surgery and the vasodilation of blood vessels due to the action of some anesthetics, it may be difficult for a person to maintain adequate blood pressure following surgery. If he is required to rest in bed for an extended period of time following surgery, it is difficult for him to maintain venous return especially from lower extremities. A physician may order a cut-off point on blood pressure that she wants reported to her. If no specific numbers are indicated by her, use the following guide (helpful for all, not just postoperative, patients):

Fall in systolic blood pressure > 20 mm Hg
Systolic blood pressure < 80 mm Hg
Blood pressure dropping 5 to 10 mm Hg over several readings
Pulse > 110 beats per minute, < 60 beats per minute

Turning the patient every 2 hours postoperatively helps to increase circulation. Allowing the patient to assist in his care as much as possible also helps. Some patients will have thromboembolitic stockings, which promote venous return, ordered for them after surgery (see Chap. 31).

Sitting on the side of the bed the evening of surgery, getting out of bed to a bedside chair the next morning, and walking to the hallway the second morning are typical physician orders concerning early ambulation. Make a habit of taking a person's pulse before you help him sit up following surgery so that you have a baseline measurement. Always let a patient sit up and stand up slowly. If blood volume is slightly decreased, rapid shifts of position will cause him to become extremely dizzy and lightheaded.

Observe closely the amount of blood loss from the surgical incision; monitor carefully replacement intravenous fluid or oral fluid. Elicit a Homan's sign (pain in the calf of the leg on dorsiflexion of the foot) or Luke's sign (pain in the calf on standing) to detect if a blood clot (thrombus) is present in the calf before ambulation. It would be dangerous to ambulate anyone with this sign since a thrombus could shift and become an embolus, a potentially lethal situation. Unless contraindicated, ask people to flex and extend their legs every 2 hours at the same time that you ask them to cough and deep breathe to prevent thrombus formation (see Chap. 31). Any person on bed rest is prone to thrombus formation due to stasis in venous circulation.

It is difficult for people to appreciate how important it is for them to turn and ambulate as soon as their condition allows following surgery. Still in pain, they would like to spend the first few days following surgery just resting quietly in bed. Give analgesia as necessary in the first postoperative few days so that movement and ambulation are possible.

PROMOTION OF PSYCHOLOGICAL WELL-BEING

Some surgery is scheduled so quickly that the person does not have much time preoperatively to think about how he will feel after surgery; others are too ill prior to surgery to think about how they will feel afterward. Most people, therefore, are surprised at how well they feel afterward but also at how quickly they become fatigued and how painful a simple surgical incision can be. Being assured that they are recovering well and that surgery is a physiological shock to their system helps them to accept temporary discomforts.

Some people do not receive good news following surgery. They are told that their condition could not be completely repaired or that the tumor that was removed was cancerous. A postoperative course for these people is very difficult as they experience a sense of loss (their former well self is gone) and may even anticipate death. Knowing that the course ahead of them does not lead to wellness, no matter how great their effort, makes it very difficult for these patients to bear pain or to be interested in early ambulation.

PROMOTION OF ACTIVITY AND REST

Early ambulation promotes both increased depth of respirations (helping to prevent respiratory complications) and circulatory function (helping to prevent venous stasis and promote wound healing). Encourage the patient to do as much for himself as he can as soon as possible following surgery in order to achieve these benefits of early movement. Many people are afraid to move following surgery, particularly from bed, because they are worried that their sutures will tear. This event is extremely unlikely, except in obese individuals. Show people how to press a pillow against the incision line while they cough or move to splint the incision if they are worried; support the incision line for them with your hand while you help them out of bed to assure them that, although not worried yourself, you appreciate their concern. Supporting the incision line in this way reduces pain and so serves a secondary function of facilitating early ambulation.

While a person needs active movement after surgery, he also needs adequate rest. Be certain at bedtime that he has adequate analgesic administered to allow him a pain-free night. Provide a time in the middle of the morning and again in the afternoon for a noninterrupted rest. Help the patient plan a routine after discharge that will continue to counterbalance these two opposites: activity and rest.

PROMOTION OF COMFORT

Because surgery involves incising the skin and muscle layers, a degree of pain will be present following surgery until the incised tissue heals again. Physicians generally order narcotic analgesics to be given for the first 24 to 48 hours after surgery, and then weaker analgesics such as Tylenol. A person who is worried about the outcome of his surgery may feel more pain than the person who believes that his cure is complete since tenseness causes pressure on sutures.

Be certain when administering analgesics following surgery that you supplement them with other comfort measures such as change of position or straightening of bed linen. Check for an uncomfortable distended abdomen, which suggests intestinal gas pain rather than incision pain.

Pain in an area of the body other than the incision suggests a complication of surgery or a secondary illness rather than the usual postoperative discomfort. A person who still requires a narcotic analgesic for pain relief after the third day following surgery either is experiencing more than ordinary pain or has an inordinate level of pain perception. He needs careful assessment of the reason for the continued pain that entertains the possibility of dependency on the narcotic analgesic. Implementations for pain are further discussed in Chap. 27.

PROMOTION OF WOUND HEALING

Wounds heal by the gradual removal and replacement of dead or damaged cells at the wound site with new cells produced by the surrounding tissue. Within minutes after injury, circulation to the area increases, bringing additional nutrients and leukocytes (white blood cells) to the area. This results in a clear plasma-like exudate coating the edges of the wound. The exudate is composed of macrophages (to clear away damaged cells) and fibrin (which quickly knits together an incision, thus sealing it off from contaminants).

New identical cells are produced by regeneration at the edges of the wound; scar (fibrous) tissue or tough, thick collagenous tissue is manufactured to bridge any gap that regenerating cells cannot fill. The closer wound edges are approximated, therefore, and the less strain that is put on a suture line, the smaller will be the gap and the less the amount of scar tissue.

Wounds may heal in one of three different ways: primary, secondary, or tertiary intention.

Primary Intention. In primary intention, the sides of the wounds are brought together and the wound heals side to side. This form of healing is the fastest and leaves the least scar formation. It is the usual intention following surgery.

Secondary Intention. In some instances, such as burns or wounds that involve removal of a large amount of skin or subcutaneous tissue, the sides of the wound cannot be approximated since they are too far apart to touch. In these cases, the wound will not be sutured but will be left open to heal from the bottom up (secondary intention). This process is longer than primary intention, making it more difficult to keep a wound free of infection. The final healing, moreover, always results in more scar tissue than closure by primary intention.

Tertiary Intention. Tertiary intention is primary intention that is delayed because a wound is too contaminated at first to close. The wound is cleaned by soaks and antibiotic administration; delayed closure is completed 4 to 5 days after the wound occurrence. Although the final healing will be side to side, scar formation due to the presence of some secondary intention regeneration will probably be present with the final healing.

TECHNIQUES OF WOUND MANAGEMENT

The best assurance that rapid noncomplicated wound healing will take place is use of strict aseptic technique in surgery, wound dressing, and irrigation. Changing dressings using sterile technique is discussed in Chap. 28.

In addition, be certain to maintain good circulation to the wound area. Check that body alignment favors good venous return, and that pressure on an arm or leg will not interfere with blood supply to that part. In some instances an arm or leg will be ordered to be kept elevated to ensure good venous return from that part.

Antibiotics are ordered for many people following surgery to prevent wound infection. If an antibiotic is given intravenously, check that the intravenous fluid is infusing well before adding the antibiotic to ensure that the drug enters the vascular circulation, not the subcutaneous tissue. Some intravenous antibiotics cause subcutaneous skin damage, and infiltration of this nature prevents their rapid absorption and preventive function. If you are giving antibiotics intramuscularly, ensure that they are always well absorbed by rotating body sites. If giving antibiotics orally, check to be certain that food does not interfere with absorption. You want to make the drug as effective as possible.

Monitor and encourage good fluid and nutritional intake so that protein for new cell growth and fluid for adequate blood circulation are available. Protect the incision from excessive movement or strain that could disturb newly forming tissue by showing the person how to support it as he moves (or support it yourself). To reduce strain on an abdominal suture line, people may have binders ordered postoperatively. There are two types of binders: (1) a Scultetus' binder, which is made of many tails and is applied by overlapping first one left-sided, then one right-sided tail (Fig. 40-21A), and (2) a firm cotton type with a velcro fastener (Fig. 40-21B).

Binders slide out of position and loosen readily as the person moves. Be certain that a binder is not so high on a person's abdomen that it interferes with full rib expansion when lungs are fully aerated. Remove and reapply them as necessary to assess the suture line or dressing. Remove them to give back care as they cover the sacral area or the portion of the back most apt to suffer pressure and damage from bed rest.

SCAR FORMATION

A wound takes about 6 months to reach its final appearance following surgery. Caution people as you are changing their dressings in the immediate postoperative period that the way the incision looks at the moment (reddened and raised) will not be its eventual appearance.

In a few people, scar tissue does not form simply to fill in the gap between skin edges, but overgrows into a raised, irregular structure on the skin surface. Such overgrowths are termed *keloids.* They tend to occur in people with dark pigmentation and are most prevalent in blacks. Although keloids can be removed for a better cosmetic appearance at a later date, this surgery is not usually done because the new surgical incision made to remove the keloid may itself overgrow into a keloid.

If the wound is over a body joint, there is a danger that scar formation (because it is thick and fibrotic) will leave a degree of immobility in the joint. In order to prevent this problem, the wound may be closed utilizing a skin graft or the person may have to return for physical therapy or learn exercises to maintain mobility of the joint. The surgeon may ask you to position the joint continually in an overextended position so that, as the scar tissue contracts, the joint will contract to normal position from the overextended one you have maintained.

WOUND DEHISCENCE AND EVISCERATION

Wound dehiscence is the opening of an incision line; evisceration is the protrusion of body contents (generally bowel) through the dehiscence. Dehiscence and evisceration result from faulty wound healing; they are most apt to occur between the third and seventh day following surgery in the presence of wound infection, obesity (tissue is difficult to suture), or excess strain on the suture line. A dehiscence is generally revealed by the sudden escape of serosanguinous fluid from the incision. If you notice this phenomenon, immediately put pressure on the suture line with your hand and assist the patient to lie back in bed or, if sitting, to remain quiet. Stay with him and maintain firm pressure on the suture line; lift the dressing carefully to inspect the suture line. If sutures have torn away, maintain pressure until a surgeon can arrive to inspect the incision. These actions will prevent a wound dehiscence from becoming an evisceration.

If evisceration occurs, again, maintain firm and steady pressure on the suture line to prevent further evisceration. Ask another nurse to obtain vital signs on the patient (he will become pale with irregular respirations due to shock) and to cover any protruding intestine with sterile towels wetted with normal saline. Do not attempt to replace eviscerated intestine, which could result in volvulus (twisting) of the intestine and introduction of bacteria into the peritoneal cavity.

Wound evisceration is a frightening event. Remain calm and remember that the patient is even more upset by the occurrence than you. He needs your support during this devastating surgical complication.

DRAINS

If a collection of blood, lymph, or other fluid is anticipated inside the incision, a drain will be placed in the incision to allow the fluid to drain freely and not well up behind and put pressure on the incision line.

A penrose drain is a flat rubber drain that allows accumulated fluid to drain by capillary action. It is placed either near the incision by means of a "stab wound" or in the incision and is secured to the skin with stitches. In case the drain should accidentally slip back inside the wound, it usually has a sterile safety pin passed through one end in order that it can be located by x-ray. The surgeon notes in the surgery summary whether or not drains were placed. Read this report for the presence of drains before changing dressings; always remove dressings around drains carefully so you do not inadvertently remove the drain. If a drain is present, a dressing may become soaked with serosanguinous fluid quickly following surgery, proof that the drain is functioning.

In other instances, a drain (a Foley catheter or t-tube)

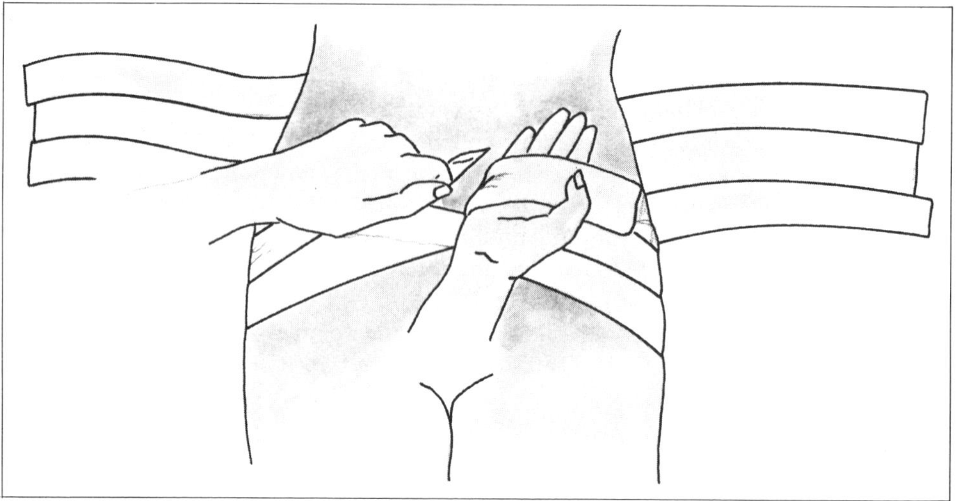

A

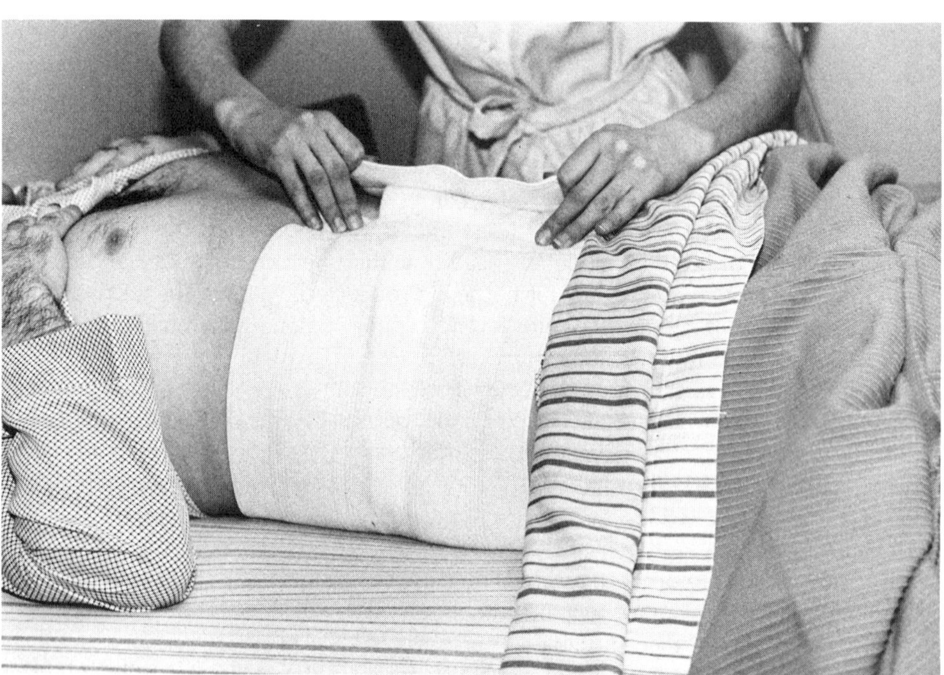

B

FIGURE 40-21. Two types of abdominal binders. A. A Scultetis'. B. A velcro-fastened type.

may be inserted near the incision and attached to low suction to continue draining the body cavity. Assessment of this type and amount of drainage will assure you that the drain is functioning properly.

Hemovac Drains. Hemovac drains are plastic drains the size of intravenous tubing that are inserted near an incision at the time of surgery and drain back to a circular, low suction device. When the circular device is compressed, it gradually begins to rise and expand. This expansion creates constant low suction to remove collecting pus, blood, or serum from the wound. Hemovac drains are generally emptied and measured every 8 hours; not only the amount of drainage obtained but a description of it are important assessments of wound healing.

SUTURE REMOVAL

Skin sutures are removed 4 to 7 days following surgery. The surgeon needs a sterile instrument set (hemostat, scissors, and small forceps) to remove sutures. If a suture is surrounded by blood or lymph, the patient feels a slight stinging sensation when it is cut and removed. Stay with a patient while sutures are removed and, if he cannot see the area, describe the procedure to him.

Many people are afraid to move or turn following suture removal for fear that their incision will now come apart. You can assure them that the sutures were removed because the incision line had healed well.

In some instances, a surgeon will remove every other suture on one day and then write an order for you to

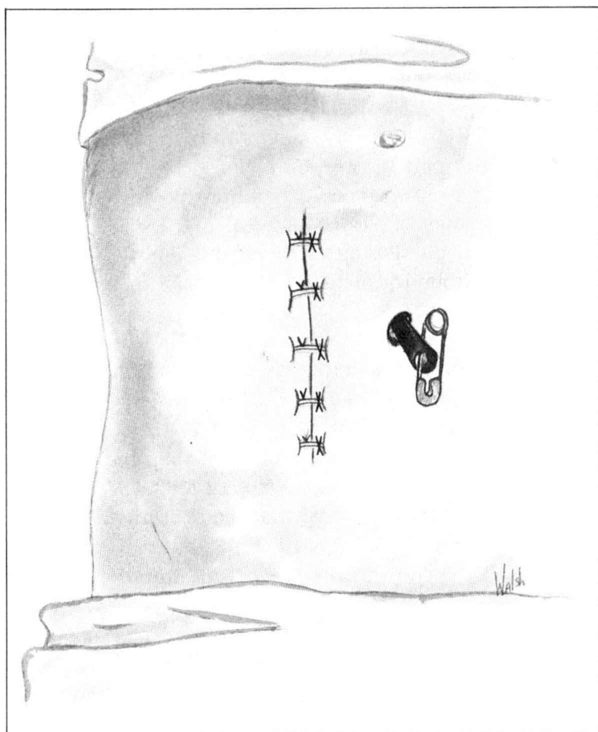

FIGURE 40-22. Suture removal. A suture is cut as close as possible to the skin (at x marks) to minimize pulling underneath the skin surface. These sutures would then be pulled toward the left.

> ☐ **QUICK REFERENCE STOP 40-7: COMMUNITY CONSIDERATIONS**
>
> Although people are discharged early from health care agencies following surgery, they may not be able to return to work or school for an additional few weeks or many months. During checkups or visits, assess if patients are taking in an adequate nutrient level and getting enough (or too much) exercise. If they become discouraged with their progress or exhausted, their nutrient intake will invariably fall and decrease their healing potential.

remove the remaining sutures on the following day; in ambulatory settings, you may be asked to remove sutures when people return for follow-up care. To remove silk sutures, lift the suture with the forceps, cut the suture as close to the skin as possible, and then, with gentle effort, pull the cut end under the skin and clear. It is important that the suture be cut as close to the skin surface as possible to reduce the exposure of the suture, which has been in room air and thus has bacteria to underlying areas of tissue (Fig. 40-22). Inspect the suture line as you work to be certain that healing has taken place. If healing has not occurred, do not remove any remaining sutures but refer to the person's physician for further evaluation and care.

UTILIZING NURSING PROCESS

Assessment

Always ask a surgical patient during the admission interview what the scheduled surgery means to him and what he expects it to be like. Be certain that people know they will have pain afterward; otherwise the degree of pain may frighten them. Assure them that they will be given medicine for pain relief. "Walk through" the stages of a typical day of surgery. Try to elicit fears such as fear of saying something that they would rather a spouse did not know while under anesthesia (assure patients that what they say as they wake from anesthesia is not repeated as part of patient confidentiality), fear of failing to be a "good" patient following surgery (assure patients that surgery is not a test, and they should only try to be themselves), or fear of the outcome. You cannot always alleviate this latter worry; alerting the surgeon and anesthesiologist to the concern is important, however, as a high level of anxiety may affect safe anesthesia administration.

Analysis

Nursing diagnoses are derived from those concerns that the patient voices (fear of surgery, fear of poor outcome) or physical problems that may interfere with a safe surgery outcome (fluid and electrolyte balance, alteration in; or nutritional balance, alteration in). The higher the risk of surgery, the more nursing diagnoses are generally established.

Planning and Implementation

Be certain that preoperative planning includes measures that will be introduced postoperatively such as deep breathing and coughing. Allowing the patient to participate in planning permits him a sense of control over events. Many people secretly fear that they will be confused with someone else in surgery and the wrong surgical procedure will be performed. Being asked to help make decisions regarding their care helps patients to see that your approach is organized and cautious.

Following surgery, help the person to find the level of activity most conducive for healing; otherwise, some people overdo and some underdo. People need to talk about their experience in the operating room (the sensation of falling asleep before they could count to 10, the strange disorientation of waking in what seemed to be only a second later). Allow time for this tension relief as a planned part of care. Talking about events invariably reduces their frightening aspects (see QRS 40-7).

Evaluation

Preparation of discharge from a hospital must begin on the day of surgery because people remain in the hospital only a short time following surgery. Help the person plan how he will manage at home based on your evaluation of his postoperative condition. Ascertain that he has adequate support people at home until he feels well enough to be able to perform self-care again (4 to 6 weeks following major surgery).

NURSING CARE PLAN

Mr. Burrows is a 40-year-old construction worker admitted for a right inguinal hernia repair. He was hospitalized 5 years ago for a thrombophlebitis in his right leg following a tibial fracture. Below is a preoperative nursing care plan that you might write for him in regard to circulatory function.

Assessment: Patient states he is more worried about a thrombophlebitis returning than he is about the hernia surgery. Toes on right foot are warm to touch; nails blanch and refill in less than 5 seconds. Negative Homan's and Luke's signs. Observed sitting with knees crossed in chair.
Nursing Diagnosis: Circulation, potential alteration in, related to thrombophlebitis formation.
Locus of Decision-Making: Patient.
Goal: Patient's venous circulation will be free of complication until discharge.
Criteria: Homan's and Luke's signs remain negative.
NURSING ORDERS

1. Caution patient not to sit or lie with knees crossed.
2. Encourage him to be ambulatory until administration of preoperative medication; maintain good fluid intake until midnight.
3. Teach hip and knee flexion and extension and leg circumduction exercises, importance of early ambulation, adequate fluid intake, and turning q2h while in bed following surgery.
4. Alert surgeon and anesthesiologist of primary concern.
5. Mark chart "previous thrombophlebitis" for attention of surgical and recovery room personnel.

New nursing orders written for him postoperatively might be:

1. IV of 2,000 lactated ringers to infuse over 12 hours. Monitor infusion rate carefully to ensure adequate intake; if it should infiltrate, do *not* restart in legs.
2. Begin ice chips (per M.D. order) when patient is alert.
3. Help to turn q2h when patient is alert; when patient is on side, do not allow top leg to rest on bottom leg.
4. Begin leg exercises (flexion, extension, circumduction) q1h when patient is awake.
5. Test for Homan's or Luke's sign q8h.
6. Assess warmth of toes, ability to blanch, and ability to sense touch q8h.
7. Review importance of good fluid intake, positioning with pressure on leg, early ambulation to prevent thrombophlebitis.

THE SURGICAL EXPERIENCE

A surgical experience is a major undertaking for an individual because it involves both physical and psychological stress. It is a time of fear, pain and loss of independence; a nurse who can meet the needs of people during the preoperative, intraoperative, and postoperative phases is a nurse who is a very valued member of a health care team.

SUGGESTED READINGS

Abbott, N. K., et al. The impact of preoperative assessment on intraoperative nurse performance. *A.O.R.N. J.* 37(1):43, 1983.

Aish, A., et al. How to use risk factors and assessment skills to individualize patient care. *Can. Nurse* 78(11):46, 1982.

AORN . . . recommended practices for preoperative skin preparation of patients. *A.O.R.N. J.* 37(2):244, 1983.

Cooper, D. M., et al. Postoperative nursing intervention as an adjunct to wound healing. *Nurs. Clin. North Am.* 14:713, 1979.

Croushore, T. M. Postoperative assessment: The key to avoiding the most common nursing mistakes. *Nursing 79* 9:46, 1979.

Dunphy, J. E., et al. *Current Surgical Diagnosis and Treatment* (3rd ed.). Los Altos, Calif.: Lange, 1977.

Dzierbejke, M. M., and Larkin, J. C. Including the family in preoperative teaching. *Am. J. Nurs.* 78:1892, 1978.

Ennis, C. E., et al. Nutritional management of the surgical patient. *A.O.R.N. J.* 31:1217, 1980.

Finn, K. L. Postoperative ambulation. *Crit. Care Update* 7:22, 1980.

Fordham, M. The recovery of physical fitness. *Int. J. Nurs. Stud.* 19(4):205, 1982.

Gault, P. L. Plan for a patchwork of problems when your patient is elderly. *Nursing* (Horsham) 12(1):50, 1982.

Greenwood, B. S. The before and after of good postop pulmonary care. *Nursing* (Horsham) 12(12):68, 1982.

Hinshaw, A. S., et al. The use of predictive modeling to test nursing practice outcomes. *Nurs. Res.* 32(1):35, 1983.

Hosking, K. J. Postoperative pain: Preoperative preparation. Part 1. *Nurs. Mirror* 155(14):25, 1982.

Jackson, B. S., et al. How post-op complications can burgeon into crisis. *RN* 44:26, 1981.

Keithley, J. K., et al. A unified approach to assessment of the surgical patient. *Am. J. Nurs.* 82(4):612, 1982.

King, I. The effect of structured and unstructured preoperative teaching: A replication. *Nurs. Res.* 31(6):324, 1982.

Leonard, C. Preoperative teaching. *Nurs. Times* (suppl.)77:19, 1981.

Marshall, C. Operative count down: How a patient might feel as she waits for surgery. *Nurs. Mirror* 153:31, 1981.

McClintic, J. Preoperative care of the pediatric patient. *Today's OR Nurse* 2:7, 1980.

McClurg, E. Developing an effective teaching program. *A.O.R.N. J.* 34:474, 1981.

McConnell, E. Toward complication-free recoveries for your surgical patients. *RN* 43:30, 1980.

McConnell, E. A. After surgery: How you can avoid the obvious . . . and the not so obvious . . . hazards. *Nursing* (Horsham) 13(2):74, 1983.

Meng, A. L. Parents' and children's reactions toward impending hospitalization for surgery. *Mat. Child Nurs. J.* 9:83, 1980.

Methany, N. Preoperative fluid balance assessment. *A.O.R.N. J.* 33:51, 1981.

Nyberg, K. G. When diabetes complicates your pre- and post-op care. *RN* 46(1):42, 1983.

Paritzky, J. F., et al. Preoperative teaching on a gynecology unit. *J.O.G.N. Nurs.* 11(6):384, 1982.

Phippen, M. L. Nursing assessment of preoperative anxiety. *A.O.R.N. J.* 31:1019, 1980.

Schumann, D. Preoperative measures to promote wound healing. *Nurs. Clin. North Am.* 14:683, 1979.

Smith, B.J. Safeguarding your patient after anesthesia. *Nursing 78* 8:53, 1978.

Steele, B. G. Test your knowledge of postoperative pain management. *Nursing 80* 10:76, 1980.

Test your knowledge of surgical nursing problems. *Nursing* (Horsham) 11(11):177, 1981.

Voshall, B. The effects of preoperative teaching on postoperative pain. *Top. Clin. Nurs.* 2:39, 1980.

Wainwright, P. Information and the surgical patient . . . the relation of postoperative pain. *Nurs. Times* 78(35):1480, 1982.

Watson, P. G. The effects of short-term postoperative counseling on cancer/ostomy patients. *Cancer Nurs.* 6(1):21, 1983.

Wong, J., et al. Surgical care of the aged. *Can. Nurse* 77:30, 1981.

QUESTIONS FOR REVIEW

Mrs. Brinder is a 28-year-old woman admitted to the hospital to have a cholecystectomy (surgical operation to remove gall bladder).

1. In making a nursing care plan, which measure for Mrs. Brinder would you want to include in preoperative teaching?
   a. She should turn every 4 hours.
   b. She should exercise both legs every 2 hours.
   c. She should deep breathe twice a day.
   d. She should cough every 8 hours.

2. In making preoperative assessments, which of the following facts would cause you to categorize Mrs. Brinder as at possibly high risk for surgery?
   a. She does not eat regular meals due to care of three small children.
   b. She had jaundice as a newborn.
   c. She takes aspirin for occasional headache.
   d. She is in the young adult age group.

3. You implement preoperative care. Which of the following is a true statement about usual preoperative medications?
   a. They cause loss of consciousness.
   b. They cause excessive salivation.
   c. They are given at least 4 hours prior to surgery.
   d. They generally include an analgesic.

4. You remove Mrs. Brinder's nail polish prior to surgery to:
   a. Avoid contaminating intravenous lines.
   b. Stimulate circulation.
   c. Prevent contamination of the surgical incision.
   d. Assist in circulatory assessment.

5. If you are nonsterile when observing her surgery, which of the following would you *not* do?
   a. Touch the overhead light to straighten it as requested.
   b. Touch the scrub nurse's gown above her waist.
   c. Talk just prior to anesthesia administration.
   d. Ask the scrub nurse to name instruments for you prior to surgery.

6. Following surgery, a question you would ask Mrs. Brinder to assess whether she is awakening from general anesthesia would be:
   a. What type of surgery did she have?
   b. What is her name?
   c. What is her home address?
   d. What is her age?

7. The main purpose of assessing an incision dressing following surgery is to check for:
   a. Wound dehiscence.
   b. Inflammation.
   c. Infection.
   d. Bleeding.

8. The best position in which to place Mrs. Brinder until she fully regains consciousness is:
   a. Prone, head turned to her side.
   b. Supine, arms at her side.
   c. Sim's position.
   d. Side-lying, neck sharply flexed.

9. People may not void immediately after surgery. As a general rule, you should note in a patient's nursing care plan that he has not voided if voiding has not occurred within:
   a. 2 hours
   b. 4 hours
   c. 8 hours
   d. 16 hours

10. A prime implementation for stimulating circulation after surgery is to:
   a. Massage lower extremities.
   b. Administer blood for replacement.
   c. Encourage early ambulation.
   d. Encourage deep breathing.

APPENDIXES

A. ADDRESSES OF NURSING ORGANIZATIONS

1. American Association of Colleges of Nursing (AACN)
   11 Dupont Circle, Suite 430
   Washington, D.C. 20036

2. American Association of Critical Care Nurses (AACCN)
   P.O. Box C-19528
   Irvine, California 92713

3. American Association of Nephrology Nurses and Technicians (AANNT)
   2 Talcott Road, Suite 8
   Park Ridge, Illinois 60068

4. American Association of Neurosurgical Nurses (AANN)
   304 East 45th Street
   New York City, New York 10017

5. American Association of Nurse Anesthetists (AANA)
   216 West Higgins
   Park Ridge, Illinois 60068

6. American Association of Occupational Health Nurses (AAOHN)
   575 Lexington Avenue
   New York, New York 10022

7. American College of Nurse-Midwives (ACNM)
   1012 14th Street, Suite 801 N.W.
   Washington, D.C. 20005

8. American Indian/Alaskan Native Nurses' Association (AIANNA)
   P.O. Box 1588
   Norman, Oklahoma 73070

9. American Nurses' Association (ANA)
   2420 Pershing Road
   Kansas City, Missouri 64108

10. American Urological Association, Allied (AUAA)
    21510 South Main Street
    Carson, California 90745

11. Association for Practitioners in Infection Control (APIC)
    1557 North Pinecrest
    Wichita, Kansas 67208

12. Association of Operating Room Nurses (AORN)
    10170 East Mississippi Avenue
    Denver, Colorado 80231

13. Association of Rehabilitation Nurses (ARN)
    1701 Lake Avenue, Suite 470
    Glenview, Illinois 60025

14. Department of School Nurses/National Education Association (DSN/NEA)
    1201 16th Street N.W.
    Washington, D.C. 20036

15. Emergency Department Nurses' Association (EDNA)
    666 North Lake Shore Drive, Suite 1729
    Chicago, Illinois 60611

16. International Council of Nurses (ICN)
    P.O. Box 42
    1211 Geneva 20, Switzerland

17. International Association for Enterostomal Therapy, Inc. (IAET)
    1701 Lake Avenue
    Glenview, Illinois 60025

18. National Association of Hispanic Nurses (NAHN)
    12044 7th Avenue N.W.
    Seattle, Washington 98177

19. National Association of Pediatric Nurse Associates and Practitioners (NAP-NAP)
    North Woodbury Road, Box 56
    Pitman, New Jersey 08071

20. National Black Nurses' Association (NBNA)
    318 The Ohio Building
    175 South Main Street
    Akron, Ohio 44308

21. Nurses' Coalition for Action in Politics (NCAP)
    1030 15th Street, Suite 108 N.W.
    Washington, D.C. 20005

22. National Intravenous Therapy Association, Inc. (NITA)
    850 Third Avenue,
    New York, New York 10022

23. National League for Nursing (NLN)
    10 Columbus Circle
    New York, New York 10019

24. National Male Nurse Association (NMNA)
    2309 State Street
    Saginaw, Michigan 48602

25. National Nurses' Society on Alcoholism (NNSA)
    733 Third Avenue
    New York, New York 10017

26. National Student Nurses' Association (NSNA)
    10 Columbus Circle
    New York, New York 10019

27. Nurses' Association of the American College of Obstetricians and Gynecologists (NAACOG)
    1 East Wacker Drive, Suite 2700
    Chicago, Illinois 60601

28. Nurses' Christian Fellowship (NCF)
    233 Langdon Street
    Madison, Wisconsin 53703

29. Oncology Nursing Society (ONS)
    P.O. Box 33
    Oakmont, Pennsylvania 15139

30. Sigma Theta Tau
    1100 West Michigan Street
    Indianapolis, Indiana 46223

31. World Health Organization
    1211 Geneva 27, Switzerland

B. RIGHTS OF SPECIAL GROUPS

RIGHTS OF PEOPLE IN NURSING HOMES*

1. The right to be fully informed, as evidenced by the patient's written acknowledgement of rules and regulations.
2. The right to be fully informed of services available and related charges.
3. The right to be fully informed, by a physician, of his medical condition and afforded the opportunity to participate in planning care and treatment; he has a right to refuse to participate in experimental research.
4. The right to be transferred or discharged only for medical reasons or for his welfare or that of other patients; he should be given reasonable notice of such action.
5. The right to be encouraged and assisted to exercise his rights as a patient and as a citizen; he may voice grievances and recommend changes in policies and services to facility staff.
6. The right to manage his personal financial affairs or be given at least a quarterly statement of financial transactions.
7. The right to be free from mental and physical abuse and free from chemical and physical restraints except as authorized in writing by a physician.
8. The right to be assured confidential treatment of his personal and medical records.
9. The right to be treated with consideration, respect, and full recognition of his dignity and individuality, including privacy in treatment and in care for his personal needs.
10. The right not to be required to perform services for the facility that are not included for therapeutic purposes in his plan of care.
11. The right to associate and communicate privately with persons of his choice and send and receive his personal mail unopened, unless medically contraindicated.
12. The right to meet with and participate in activities of social, religious, and community groups at his discretion, unless medically contraindicated.
13. The right to retain and use his personal clothing and possessions as space permits.
14. The right, if married, to be assured privacy for visits by his/her spouse; if both are inpatients in the facility, they are permitted to share a room.

THE DYING PERSON'S BILL OF RIGHTS†

1. I have the right to be treated as a living human being until I die.

*Modified from U.S. Department of Health and Human Resources, Skilled nursing facilities. *Federal Register* 39(193):35775, Oct. 3, 1974.
†From Dying person's bill of rights. *Am. J. Nurs.* 75:99, 1975.

2. I have the right to maintain a sense of hopefulness, however changing its focus may be.
3. I have the right to be cared for by those who can maintain a sense of hopefulness, however changing this might be.
4. I have the right to express my feelings and emotions about my approaching death in my own way.
5. I have the right to participate in decisions concerning my care.
6. I have the right to expect continuing medical and nursing attention, even though cure goals must be changed to comfort goals.
7. I have the right to not die alone.
8. I have the right to be free from pain.
9. I have the right to have my questions answered honestly.
10. I have the right not to be deceived.
11. I have the right to die in peace and dignity.
12. I have the right to retain my individuality and not be judged for my decisions which may be contrary to beliefs of others.
13. I have the right to discuss and enlarge my religious and/or spiritual experiences, whatever these may mean to others.
14. I have the right to expect that the sanctity of the human body will be respected after death.
15. I have the right to be cared for by caring, sensitive, knowledgeable people who will attempt to understand my needs and will be able to gain some satisfaction in helping me face my death.

DECLARATION OF THE RIGHTS OF DISABLED PERSONS*

1. The term *disabled person* means any person unable to ensure by himself or herself wholly or partly the necessities of a normal individual and/or social life, as a result of a deficiency, either congenital or not, in his or her physical or mental capabilities.
2. Disabled persons shall enjoy all the rights set forth in this Declaration. These rights shall be granted to all disabled persons without any exception whatsoever and without distinction or discrimination on the basis of race, color, sex, language, religion, political or other opinions, national or social origin, state of wealth, birth, or any other situation applying either to the disabled person himself or herself or to his or her family.
3. Disabled persons have the inherent right to respect for their human dignity. Disabled persons, whatever the origin, nature, and seriousness of their handicaps and disabilities, have the same fundamental rights as their fellow-citizens of the same age, which implies first and foremost the right to enjoy a decent life, as normal and full as possible.
4. Disabled persons have the same civil and political rights as other human beings; article 7 of the Declaration of the Rights of Mentally Retarded Persons applies to any possible limitation or suppression of those rights for mentally disabled persons.
5. Disabled persons are entitled to the measures designed to enable them to become as self-reliant as possible.
6. Disabled persons have the right to medical, psychological, and functional treatment, including prosthetic and orthetic appliances, to medical and social rehabilitation, education, vocational education, training and rehabilitation, aid, counselling, placement services, and other services which will enable them to develop their capabilities and skills to the maximum and will hasten the process of their social integration or reintegration.
7. Disabled persons have the right to economic and social security and to a decent level of living. They have the right, according to their capabilities, to secure and retain employment or to engage in a useful, productive, and remunerative occupation and to join trade unions.
8. Disabled persons are entitled to have their special needs taken into consideration at all stages of economic and social planning.
9. Disabled persons have the right to live with their families or with foster parents and to participate in all social, creative, or recreational activities. No disabled persons shall be subjected, as far as his or her residence is concerned, to differential treatment other than that required by his or her condition or by the improvement which he or she may derive therefrom. If the stay of a disabled person in a specialized establishment is indispensable, the environment and living conditions therein shall be as close as possible to those of the normal life of a person of his or her age.
10. Disabled persons shall be protected against all exploitation, all regulations, and all treatment of a discriminatory, abusive, and degrading nature.
11. Disabled persons shall be able to avail themselves of qualified legal aid when such aid proves indispensable for the protection of their persons or property. If judicial proceedings are instituted against them, the legal procedures applied shall take their physical and mental condition fully into account.
12. Organizations of disabled persons may be usefully consulted in all matters regarding the rights of disabled persons.
13. Disabled persons, their families, and communities shall be fully informed, by all appropriate means, of the rights contained in this Declaration.

*From United Nations, *Declaration of the Rights of Disabled Persons*. New York: United Nations Publications, 1975.

DECLARATION OF THE RIGHTS OF MENTALLY RETARDED PERSONS*

1. The mentally retarded person has, to the maximum degree of feasibility, the same rights as other human beings.
2. The mentally retarded person has a right to proper medical care and physical therapy and to such education, training, rehabilitation, and guidance as will enable him to develop his ability and maximum potential.
3. The mentally retarded person has a right to economic security and to a decent standard of living. He has a right to perform productive work or to engage in any meaningful occupation to the fullest possible extent of his capabilities.
4. Whenever possible, the mentally retarded person should live with his own family or with foster parents and participate in different forms of community life. The family with which he lives should receive assistance. If care in an institution becomes necessary, it should be provided in surroundings and other circumstances as close as possible to those of normal life.
5. The mentally retarded person has a right to a qualified guardian when this is required to protect his personal well-being and interests.
6. The mentally retarded person has a right to protection from exploitation, abuse, and degrading treatment. If prosecuted for any offence, he shall have a right to due process of law with full recognition being given to his degree of mental responsibility.
7. Whenever mentally retarded persons are unable, because of the severity of their handicap, to exercise all their rights in a meaningful way or it should become necessary to restrict or deny some or all of these rights, the procedure used for that restriction or denial of rights must contain proper legal safeguards against every form of abuse. This procedure must be based on an evaluation of the social capability of the mentally retarded person by qualified experts and must be subject to periodic review and to the right of appeal to higher authorities.

THE MENTAL PATIENT'S BILL OF RIGHTS†

1. The right to be treated with as much decency and respect as is accorded any other human being.
2. Every right established by the Declaration of Independence and guaranteed by the Constitution of the United States of America as an American citizen.
3. The right to the integrity of your own mind and the integrity of your own body.
4. The right to have treatment and medication administered to you only with your consent and to be given all relevant information regarding said treatment and/or medication.
5. The right to access to your own legal and medical counsel.
6. The right to refuse to work in a mental hospital, to choose what work you shall do, and to receive for such work the minimum wage set by the state labor laws.
7. The right to decent medical attention.
8. The right to uncensored communication by telephone, letter, and in person with whomever and at any time you wish.
9. The right not to be locked up against your will, not to be committed involuntarily, and not to be fingerprinted or photographed.
10. The right to decent living conditions.
11. The right to retain your own personal property.
12. The right to bring grievance against those who have mistreated you and to counsel and a court hearing.
13. The right to refuse experimental drugs and treatments and to be used as learning material for students.
14. The right not to have your character questioned or defamed.
15. The right to request an alternative to legal commitment or incarceration in a mental hospital.

THE PREGNANT PATIENT'S BILL OF RIGHTS‡

1. The pregnant patient has the right, prior to the administration of any drug or procedure, to be informed by the health professional caring for her of any potential direct or indirect effects, risks, or hazards to herself or her newborn infant that may result from the use of a drug or procedure prescribed for or administered to her during pregnancy, labor, birth, or lactation (breast-feeding).
2. The pregnant patient has the right, prior to the proposed therapy, to be informed, not only of the benefits, risks, and hazards of the proposed therapy, but also of known alternative therapy, such as available childbirth education classes which could help to prepare the pregnant patient physically and mentally to cope with the discomfort or stress of pregnancy and the experience of childbirth, thereby reducing or eliminating her need for drugs and obstetric intervention. She should be offered such in-

*From United Nations, *Declaration of the Rights of Mentally Retarded Persons.* New York: United Nations Publications, 1971.

†Modified from *Mental Patient's Bill of Rights,* Mental Patients' Liberation Project.

‡Courtesy Doris Haire, President, American Foundation for Maternal and Child Health, and Consultant, International Childbirth Education Association.

formation early in her pregnancy in order that she may make a reasoned decision.

3. The pregnant patient has the right, prior to the administration of any drug, to be informed by the health professional who is prescribing or administering the drug to her that any drug that she receives during pregnancy, labor, and birth, no matter how or when the drug is taken or administered, may adversely affect her unborn baby, directly or indirectly, and that there is no drug or chemical that has been proven safe for the unborn child.
4. The pregnant patient has the right, if cesarean section is anticipated, to be informed prior to the administration of any drug, and preferably prior to her hospitalization, that minimizing her and, in turn, her baby's intake of nonessential preoperative medicine will benefit her baby.
5. The pregnant patient has the right, prior to the administration of a drug or procedure, to be informed if there is no properly controlled follow-up research that has established the safety of the drug or procedure with regard to its direct and/or indirect effects on the physiological, mental, and neurological development of the child exposed, via the mother, to the drug or procedure during pregnancy, labor, birth, or lactation.
6. The pregnant patient has the right, prior to the administration of any drug, to be informed of the brand name and generic name of the drug in order that she may advise the health professional of any past adverse reaction to the drug.
7. The pregnant patient has the right to determine for herself, without pressure from her attendant, whether she will accept the risks inherent in the proposed therapy or refuse a drug or procedure.
8. The pregnant patient has the right to know the name and qualifications of the individual administering a medication or procedure to her during labor and birth.
9. The pregnant patient has the right to be informed, prior to the administration of any procedure, whether that procedure is being administered to her for her or her baby's benefit (medically indicated) or as an elective procedure (for convenience or teaching purposes).
10. The pregnant patient has the right to be accompanied during the stress of labor and birth by someone she cares for and to whom she looks for emotional comfort and encouragement.
11. The pregnant patient has the right after appropriate medical consultation to choose a position for labor and for birth which is least stressful to her baby and to herself.
12. The obstetric patient has the right to have her baby cared for at her bedside if her baby is normal, and to feed her baby according to her baby's needs rather than according to the hospital regimen.
13. The obstetric patient has the right to be informed in writing of the name of the person who actually delivered her baby and the professional qualifications of that person. This information should also be on the birth certificate.
14. The obstetric patient has the right to be informed if there is any known or indicated aspect of her or her baby's care or condition that may cause her or her baby later difficulty or problems.
15. The obstetric patient has the right to have her and her baby's hospital medical records complete, accurate, and legible and to have their records, including nurses' notes, retained by the hospital until the child reaches at least the age of majority, or, alternatively, to have the records offered to her before they are destroyed.
16. The obstetric patient, both during and after her hospital stay, has the right to have access to her complete hospital records, including nurses' notes, and to receive a copy upon payment of a reasonable fee and without incurring the expense of retaining an attorney.

SUPPORT PEOPLE'S BILL OF RIGHTS

1. Support people have the right to the same degree of consideration and respectful care as the patient they support.
2. Following the patient's permission to release such information to them, support people have a right to explanations of health progress or therapy from the appropriate people consistent with their level of understanding.
3. Support people have the right to be asked if they wish to be present for procedures, depending on whether they feel they can be supportive during that time (if acceptable to the patient).
4. Support people have the right to opportunities to visit with a patient at times that will be most helpful to the patient (preoperatively, postoperatively, during special treatments, for example) and not be restricted during these times to agency visiting policies.
5. Support people have a right to a degree of comfort such as a chair to sit in and "respite time" for meals.

C. CLASSIFICATION OF NURSING DIAGNOSES

Nursing Diagnosis	Defining Characteristics
Airway clearance, ineffective	Abnormal breath sounds (rales [crackles], rhonchi [wheezes]) Changes in rate or depth of respiration Tachypnea Cough, effective or ineffective (with or without sputum) Cyanosis Dyspnea
Bowel elimination, alteration in	
Constipation	Decreased activity level Lower than usual frequency Hard formed stool Palpable mass Reported feeling of pressure in rectum Reported feeling of rectal fullness Straining at stool *Other possible defining characteristics* Abdominal pain Appetite impairment Back pain Headache Interference with daily living Use of laxatives
Diarrhea	Abdominal pain Cramping Increased frequency Increased frequency of bowel sounds Loose, liquid stools Urgency *Other possible defining characteristics* Changes in color
Incontinence	Involuntary passage of stool
Breathing pattern, ineffective	Dyspnea Shortness of breath Tachypnea Fremitus Abnormal arterial blood gas Cyanosis Cough Nasal flaring Respiratory depth changes Assumption of 3-point position Pursed-lip breathing/prolonged expiratory phase Increased anteroposterior diameter Use of accessory muscles Altered chest excursion
Cardiac output, alteration in: decreased	Variations in blood pressure readings Arrhythmias Fatigue Jugular vein distention Color changes, skin and mucous membranes Oliguria Decreased peripheral pulses Cold, clammy skin

Nursing Diagnosis	Defining Characteristics
	Rales Dyspnea Orthopnea Restlessness *Other possible defining characteristics* Changes in mental status Shortness of breath Syncope Vertigo Edema Cough Frothy sputum Gallop rhythm Weakness
Comfort, alteration in: pain	*Subjective* Communication (verbal or coded) of pain descriptors *Objective* Guarding behavior, protective Self-focusing Narrowed focus (altered time perception, withdrawal from social contact, impaired thought process) Distraction behavior (moaning, crying, pacing, seeking out other people and/or activities, restlessness) Facial mask of pain (lackluster eyes, "beaten look," fixed or scattered movement, grimace) Alteration in muscle tone (may span from listless to rigid) Autonomic responses not seen in chronic stable pain (diaphoresis, blood pressure and pulse rate change, pupillary dilatation, increased or decreased respiratory rate)
Communication, impaired verbal	[a]Unable to speak dominant language [a]Speaks or verbalizes with difficulty [a]Does not or cannot speak Stuttering Slurring Difficulty forming words or sentences Difficulty expressing thought verbally Inappropriate verbalization Dyspnea Disorientation
Coping, ineffective individual	[a]Verbalization of inability to cope or to ask for help [a]Inability to problem-solve Inability to meet role expectations Inability to meet basic needs Alteration in societal participation Destructive behavior toward self or others Inappropriate use of defense mechanisms Change in usual communication patterns Verbal manipulation High illness rate High accident rate
Coping, ineffective family Compromised	*Subjective* Client expresses or confirms a concern or complaint about significant other's response to his or her health problem Significant person describes preoccupation with personal reactions (e.g., fear, anticipatory grief, guilt, anxiety) to client's illness, disability, or to other situational or developmental crises Significant person describes or confirms an inadequate understanding or knowledge base that interferes with effective assistive or supportive behaviors

[a]Critical defining characteristic.

Nursing Diagnosis	Defining Characteristics
	Objective Significant person attempts assistive or supportive behaviors with less than satisfactory results Significant person withdraws or enters into limited or temporary personal communication with the client at time of need Significant person displays protective behavior disproportionate (too little or too much) to the client's abilities or need for autonomy
Disabling *Definition:* The behavior of a significant person (family member or other primary person) disables his or her own capacities and the client's capacities to address effectively tasks essential to either person's adaptation to the health challenge.	Neglectful care of the client in regard to basic human needs and/or illness treatment Distortion of reality regarding the client's health problem, including extreme denial about its existence or severity Intolerance Rejection Abandonment Desertion Carrying on usual routines, disregarding client's needs Psychosomaticism Taking on illness signs of client Decisions and actions by family that are detrimental to economic or social well-being Agitation, depression, aggression, hostility Impaired restructuring of a meaningful life for self, impaired individualization, prolonged overconcern for client Neglectful relationships with other family members Client's development of helpless, inactive dependence
Coping, family: potential for growth *Definition:* The family member has effectively managed adaptive tasks involved with the client's health challenge and is exhibiting desire and readiness for enhanced health and growth in regard to self and in relation to the client.	Family member attempts to describe growth impact of crisis on his or her own values, priorities, goals, or relationships Family member is moving in direction of health-promoting and enriching life style, which supports and monitors maturational processes; audits and negotiates treatment programs; and generally chooses experiences that optimize wellness Individual expresses interest in making contact on a one-to-one basis or on a mutual-aid group basis with another person who has experienced a similar situation.
Diversional activity, deficit	Patients statements regarding boredom; his wish for something to do, to read, and so on; his usual hobbies cannot be undertaken in hospital
Fear *Definition:* Fear is a feeling of dread related to an identifiable source validated by the person.	Ability to identify object of fear
Fluid volume deficit Actual (1) *Comments:* Consider further development as subcategories of alterations in nutrition.	Dilute urine Increased urine output Sudden weight loss *Other possible defining characteristics* Possible weight gain Hypotension Decreased venous filling Increased pulse rate Decreased skin turgor Decreased pulse volume/pressure Increased body temperature Dry skin Dry mucous membranes Hemoconcentration Weakness Edema Thirst

Nursing Diagnosis	Defining Characteristics
Actual (2) *Comments:* Consider further development as subcategories of alterations in nutrition.	Decreased urine output Concentrated urine Output greater than intake Sudden weight loss Decreased venous filling Hemoconcentration Increased serum sodium *Other possible defining characteristics* Hypotension Thirst Increased pulse rate Decreased skin turgor Decreased pulse volume/pressure Change in mental state Increased body temperature Dry skin Dry mucous membranes Weakness
Potential	Increased output Urinary frequency Thirst Altered intake
Gas exhange, impaired	Confusion Somnolence Restlessness Irritability Inability to move secretions Hypercapnea Hypoxia
Grieving	
Anticipatory	Potential loss of significant object Expression of distress at potential loss Denial of potential loss Guilt Anger Sorrow Choked feelings Changes in eating habits Alterations in sleep patterns Alterations in activity level Altered libido Altered communication patterns
Dysfunctional	Verbal expression of distress at loss Denial of loss Expression of guilt Expression of unresolved issues Anger Sadness Crying Difficulty in expressing loss Alterations in eating habits, sleep patterns, dream patterns, activity level, libido Idealization of lost object Reliving of past experiences Interference with life functioning Developmental regression Labile effect Alterations in concentration on and/or pursuits of tasks
Home maintenance management, impaired *Definition:* The client is unable to maintain independently a safe, growth-promoting, immediate environment.	*Subjective* [a]Household members express difficulty in maintaining their home in a comfortable fashion [a]Household requests assistance with home maintenance [a]Household members describe outstanding debts or financial crises

[a]Critical defining characteristic.

Nursing Diagnosis	Defining Characteristics
	Objective [a]Unwashed or unavailable cooking equipment, clothes, or linen [a]Accumulation of dirt, food wastes, or hygienic wastes [a]Overtaxed family members, e.g., exhausted, anxious family members [a]Repeated hygienic disorders, infestations, or infections Disorderly surroundings Offensive odors Inappropriate household temperature Lack of necessary equipment or aids Presence of vermin or rodents
Injury, potential for *Etiology:* Interactive conditions between individual and environment that impose a risk to the defensive and adaptive resources of the individual *Internal factors, host* Biological Chemical Physiological Psychological perception Developmental *External environment* Biological Chemical Physiological Psychological People/provider	*Internal* Biochemical Regulatory function Sensory dysfunction Integrative dysfunction Effector dysfunction Tissue hypoxia Malnutrition Immune-autoimmune Abnormal blood profile Leukocytosis/leukopenia Altered clotting factors Thrombocytopenia Sickle cell Thalassemia Decreased hemoglobin Physical Broken skin Altered mobility Developmental Age Physiological Psychosocial Psychological Affective Orientation *External* Biological Immunization level of community Microorganism Chemical Pollutants Poisons Drugs Pharmaceutical agents Alcohol Caffeine Nicotine Preservatives Cosmetics and dyes Nutrients (vitamins, food types) Physical Design, structure, and arrangement of community, building, and/or equipment Mode of transport, transportation Nosocomial agents People/provider Nosocomial agent Staffing patterns Cognitive, affective, and psychomotor factors

[a]Critical defining characteristic.

Nursing Diagnosis	Defining Characteristics
Poisoning, potential for *Definition:* The client has accentuated risk of accidental exposure to or ingestion of drugs or dangerous products in doses sufficient to cause poisoning.	*Internal* Reduced vision Verbalization of occupational setting without adequate safeguards Lack of safety or drug education Lack of proper precaution Cognitive or emotional difficulties Insufficient finances *External* Large supplies of drugs in house Medicines stored in unlocked cabinets accessible to children or confused persons Dangerous products placed or stored within the reach of children or confused persons Availability of illicit drugs potentially contaminated by poisonous additives Flaking, peeling paint or plaster in presence of young children Chemical contamination of food and water Unprotected contact with heavy metals or chemicals Paint, lacquer, and so on, in poorly ventilated areas or without effective protection Presence of poisonous vegetation Presence of atmospheric pollutants
Suffocation, potential for *Definition:* The client has accentuated risk of accidental suffocation (air available for inhalation is inadequate).	*Internal* Reduced olfactory sensation Reduced motor abilities Lack of safety education Lack of safety precautions Cognitive or emotional difficulties Disease or injury process *External* Pillow placed in an infant's crib Propped bottle placed in an infant's crib Vehicle warming in closed garage Children playing with plastic bags or inserting small objects into their mouths or noses Discarded or unused refrigerators or freezers without removed doors Children left unattended in bathtubs or pools Household gas leaks Smoking in bed Use of fuel-burning heaters not vented to outside Low strung clothesline Pacifier hung around infant's head Person who eats large mouthfuls of food
Trauma, potential for *Definition:* The client has accentuated risk of accidental tissue injury, e.g., wound, burn, fracture.	*Internal* Weakness Poor vision Balancing difficulties Reduced temperature and/or tactile sensation Reduced large or small muscle coordination Reduced hand-eye coordination Lack of safety education Lack of safety precautions Insufficient finances to purchase safety equipment or effect repairs Cognitive or emotional difficulties History of previous trauma

Nursing Diagnosis	Defining Characteristics
	External Slippery (e.g., wet or highly waxed) floors Snow or ice collected on stairs, walkways Highly flammable children's toys or clothing Overloaded fuse boxes Contact with rapidly moving machinery, industrial belts, or pulleys Wearing plastic aprons or flowing clothing around open flame Children playing with matches, candles, cigarettes Inadequately stored combustible or corrosive material, e.g., matches, oily rags, lye Smoking in bed or near oxygen Overloaded electrical outlets Grease waste collected on stoves Use of thin or worn pot holders or mitts Unrestrained babies riding in car Nonuse or misuse of seat restraints Nonuse or misuse of necessary headgear for motorized cyclists or young children carried on adult bicycles Unsafe road or road-crossing conditions Play or work near vehicle pathways, e.g., driveways, laneways, railroad tracks Unanchored rugs Bathtub without hand grip or antislip equipment Use of unsteady ladders or chairs Entering unlighted rooms Unsturdy or absent stair rails Unanchored electrical wires Litter or liquid spills on floors or stairways High beds Children playing without gates at the top of stairs Obstructed passageways Unsafe window protection in homes with young children Inappropriate call-for-aid mechanisms for bed-resting client Pot handles facing toward front of stove Bathing in very hot water, e.g., unsupervised bathing of young children Potentially igniting gas leaks Delayed lighting of gas burner or oven Experimenting with chemicals or gasoline Unscreened fires or heaters Sliding on coarse bed linen or struggling within bed restraints Faulty electrical plugs, frayed wires, or defective appliances Contact with acids or alkalis Playing with fireworks or gunpowder Contact with intense cold Overexposure to sun, sun lamps, radiotherapy Use of cracked dishware or glasses Knives stored uncovered Guns or ammunition stored unlocked Large icicles hanging from roof Exposure to dangerous machinery Children playing with sharp-edged toys High-crime neighborhood and vulnerable client Driving a mechanically unsafe vehicle Driving after partaking of alcoholic beverages or drugs Driving at excessive speeds Driving without necessary visual aids Children riding in the front seat of a car

Nursing Diagnosis	Defining Characteristics
Knowledge deficit	Verbalization of the problem Inaccurate follow-through of instruction Inadequate performance of test Inappropriate or exaggerated (e.g., hysterical, hostile, agitated, apathetic) behaviors
Mobility, impaired physical	Inability to move purposefully within the physical environment, including bed mobility, transfer, and ambulation Reluctance to attempt movement Limited range of motion Decreased muscle strength, control, and/or mass Imposed restrictions of movement, including mechanical, medical protocol Impaired coordination
Noncompliance (specify) *Definition:* Noncompliance is a person's informed decision not to adhere to a therapeutic recommendation.	[a]Behavior indicative of failure to adhere by direct observation, statements by patient or significant others Objective tests (physiological measures, detection of markers) Evidence of development of complications Evidence of exacerbation of symptoms Failure to keep appointments Failure to progress
Nutrition, alterations in	
Less than body requirements	Loss of weight with adequate food intake 20% or more below ideal body weight Reported inadequate food intake less than RDA Weakness of muscles required for swallowing or mastication Reported or evidence of lack of food Lack of interest in food Perceived inability to ingest food Aversion to eating Reported altered taste sensation Satiety immediately after ingesting food Abdominal pain with or without pathology Sore, inflamed buccal cavity Capillary fragility Abdominal cramping Diarrhea and/or steatorrhea Hyperactive bowel sounds Pale conjunctiva and mucous membranes Poor muscle tone Excessive loss of hair Lack of information, misinformation Misconceptions
More than body requirements	Weight 10% over ideal for height and frame [a]Weight 20% over ideal for height and frame [a]Triceps skin fold greater than 15 mm in men and 25 mm in women Sedentary activity level Reported or observed dysfunctional eating patterns Pairing food with other activities Concentrating food intake at end of day Eating in response to external cues, e.g., time of day, social situation Eating in response to internal cues other than hunger, e.g., anxiety

[a]Critical defining characteristic.

Nursing Diagnosis	Defining Characteristics
Potential for more than body requirements	[a]Reported or observed obesity in one or both parents [a]Rapid transition across growth percentiles in infants or children Reported use of solid food as major food source before 5 months of age Observed use of food as reward or comfort measure Reported or observed higher baseline weight at beginning of each pregnancy Dysfunctional eating patterns Pairing food with other activities Concentrating food intake at end of day Eating in response to external cues, e.g., time of day, social situation Eating in response to internal cues, other than hunger, e.g., anxiety
Parenting, alterations in: actual or potential *Definition:* Parenting is the ability of a nurturing figure(s) to create an environment that promotes the optimum growth and development of another human being. It is important to state as a preface to this diagnosis that adjustment to parenting in general is a normal maturational process that elicits nursing behaviors of prevention of potential problems and health promotion.	Actual and potential [b]Lack of parental attachment behaviors Inappropriate visual, tactile, auditory stimulation Negative identification of infant/child's characteristics Negative attachment of meanings to infant/child's characteristics Constant verbalization of disappointment in infant/child's gender or physical characteristics Verbalization of resentment toward infant/child Verbalization of role inadequacy [a]Inattention to infant/child's needs Verbal disgust at infant/child's body functions Noncompliance with health appointments for self and/or infant/child [a]Inappropriate caretaking behaviors (toilet training, sleep/rest, feeding) Inappropriate or inconsistent discipline practices Frequent accidents Frequent illness Growth and development lag in the child [a]History of child abuse or abandonment by primary caretaker Verbalization of desire to have child call himself or herself by first name versus traditional cultural tendencies Infant/child receives care from multiple caretakers without consideration for his needs Compulsive seeking of role approval from others Actual [b]Abandonment Runaway [b]Verbalization of inability to control child [b]Evidence of physical and psychological trauma
Rape-trauma syndrome *Definition:* Rape is forced, violent sexual penetration against the victim's will and without the victim's consent. The trauma syndrome that develops from this attack or attempted attack includes an acute phase of disorganization of the victim's life style and a long-term process of reorganization of life style. This syndrome includes the following three components: (1) rape trauma, (2) compound reaction, and (3) silent reaction.	

[a]Critical defining characteristic.
[b]Highly critical defining characteristic.

Nursing Diagnosis	Defining Characteristics
Rape trauma	*Acute phase* Emotional reactions Anger Embarrassment Fear of physical violence and death Humiliation Revenge Self-blame Multiple physical symptoms Gastrointestinal irritability Genitourinary discomfort Muscle tension Sleep pattern disturbance *Long-term phase* Changes in life style (changing residence, dealing with repetitive nightmares and phobias, seeking family support, seeking social network support)
Compound reaction	All defining characteristics listed under Rape trauma Reactivated symptoms of such previous conditions, i.e., physical illness, psychiatric illness Reliance on alcohol and/or drugs
Silent reaction	Abrupt changes in relationships with men Increase in nightmares Increasing anxiety during interview, i.e., blocking of associations, long periods of silence, minor stuttering, physical distress Marked changes in sexual behavior No verbalization of the occurrence of rape Sudden onset of phobic reactions
Self-care deficit	
Self-feeding deficit (level 0 to 4)[b]	Inability to bring food from a receptacle to the mouth
Self-bathing/hygiene deficit (level 0 to 4)[b]	[a]Inability to wash body or body parts Inability to obtain or get to water source Inability to regulate temperature or flow
Self-dressing/grooming deficit (level 0 to 4)[b]	[a]Impaired ability to put on or take off necessary items of clothing Impaired ability to obtain or replace articles of clothing Impaired ability to fasten clothing Inability to maintain appearance at a satisfactory level
Self-toileting deficit (level 0 to 4)[b]	[a]Inability to get to toilet or commode [a]Inability to sit on or rise from toilet or commode [a]Inability to manipulate clothing for toileting [a]Inability to carry out proper toilet hygiene [a]Inability to flush toilet or empty commode
Self-concepts, disturbance in *Definition:* A disturbance in self-concept is a disruption in the way one perceives one's body image, self-esteem, role performance, and/or personal identity. These four components, in turn, have their own etiologies and defining characteristics.	
Body image, disturbance in	Either A or B must be present to justify the diagnosis of Body image, disturbance in: [a]A. Verbal response to actual or perceived change in structure and/or function [a]B. Nonverbal response to actual or perceived change in structure and/or function

[a]Critical defining characteristic.
[b]0 = completely independent; 1 = requires use of equipment or device; 2 = requires help from another person; 3 = requires both help from another person and equipment or device; 4 = dependent; does not participate in activity.

Nursing Diagnosis	Defining Characteristics
	Objective Missing body part Actual change in structure and/or function Not looking at body parts Not touching body part Hiding or overexposing body part (intentionally or unintentionally) Trauma to nonfunctioning part Change in social involvement Change in ability to estimate spatial relationship of body to environment *Subjective* Verbalization of: Change in life style Fear of rejection or of reaction by others Focus on past strength, function, or appearance Negative feelings about body Feelings of helplessness, hopelessness, or powerlessness Preoccupation with change or loss Emphasis on remaining strengths, heightened achievement Extension of body boundary to incorporate environmental objects Personalization of part or loss by name Depersonalization of part or loss by impersonal pronouns Refusal to verify actual change
Self-esteem, disturbance in	Inability to accept positive reinforcement Lack of follow-through Nonparticipation in therapy Not taking responsibility for self care (self-neglect) Self-destructive behavior Lack of eye contact
Role performance, disturbance in	Change in self-perception of role Denial of role Change in others' perception of role Conflict in roles Change in physical capacity to resume role Lack of knowledge of role Change in usual patterns of responsibility
Personal identity, disturbance in *Definition:* Inability to distinguish between self and nonself.	Defining characteristics not yet developed
Sensory-perceptual alterations: visual, auditory, kinesthetic, gustatory, tactile, and olfactory perception	Disoriented in time, in place, or with persons Altered abstraction Altered conceptualization Change in problem-solving abilities Reported or measured change in sensory acuity Change in behavioral pattern Anxiety Apathy Change in usual response to stimuli Indication of body image alteration Restlessness Irritability Altered communication patterns *Other possible defining characteristics* Complaints of fatigue Alteration in posture Change in muscular tension Inappropriate responses Hallucinations

Nursing Diagnosis	Defining Characteristics
Sexual dysfunction	Verbalization of problem Alteration in achieving perceived sex role Actual or perceived limitation imposed by disease and/or therapy Conflicts involving values Alteration in achieving sexual satisfaction Inability to achieve desired satisfaction Seeking confirmation of desirability Alteration in relationship with significant other Change of interest in self and others
Skin integrity, impairment of	
Actual	Disruption of skin surface Destruction of skin layers Invasion of body structures
Potential	*External* Hypothermia, hyperthermia Chemical substance Mechanical factors: shearing forces, pressure, restraint Radiation Physical immobilization Excretions, secretions Humidity *Internal* Medication Alteration in nutritional state (obesity, emaciation) Altered metabolic state Altered circulation Altered sensation Altered pigmentation Skeletal prominence Developmental factors Alteration in skin turgor (change in elasticity) Psychogenic Immunologic
Sleep pattern disturbance *Definition:* Disruption of sleep time that causes discomfort to a patient or interferes with the patient's desired life style.	[a]Verbal complaints of difficulty falling asleep [a]Awakening earlier or later than desired [a]Interrupted sleep [a]Verbal complaints of not feeling well-rested Changes in behavior and performance Increased irritability Restlessness Disorientation Lethargy Listlessness Physical signs Mild, fleeting nystagmus Slight hand tremor Ptosis of eyelid Expressionless face Thick speech with mispronunciation and incorrect words Dark circles under eyes Frequent yawning Changes in posture

[a]Critical defining characteristic.

Nursing Diagnosis	Defining Characteristics
Spiritual distress (distress of the human spirit) *Definition:* Distress of the human spirit is a disruption in the life principle that pervades a person's entire being and integrates and transcends his biological and psychosocial nature.	[a]Expresses concern with meaning of life, death, and/or belief systems Anger toward God Questions meaning of suffering Verbalizes inner conflict about beliefs Verbalizes concern about relationship with deity Questions meaning for own existence Unable to participate in usual religious practices Seeks spiritual assistance Questions moral and ethical implications of therapeutic regime Gallows humor Displacement of anger toward religious representatives Description of nightmares or sleep disturbances Alteration in behavior or mood evidenced by anger, crying, withdrawal, preoccupation, anxiety, hostility, apathy, and so on
Thought processes, alteration in	Inaccurate interpretation of environment Cognitive dissonance Distractibility Memory deficit, problems Egocentricity Hypervigilance, hypovigilance *Other possible defining characteristic* Inappropriate or nonreality-based thinking
Tissue perfusion, alteration in: cerebral, cardiopulmonary, renal, gastrointestinal, peripheral	[bg]Skin temperature: cold extremities [cg]Skin color: dependent, blue or purple [abe]Pale on elevation, and color does not return on lowering leg [abe]Diminished arterial pulsations [bg]Skin quality: shining [bf]Lack of lanugo Round scars covered with atrophied skin [de]Gangrene [bf]Slow-growing, dry, thick, brittle nails [ce]Claudication Blood pressure changes in extremities [cf]Bruits [bg]Slow healing of lesions
Urinary elimination, alteration in pattern	Dysuria Frequency Hesitancy Incontinence Nocturia Retention Urgency

[a]Critical defining characteristic.
[b]High chance that defining characteristic will be present, given diagnosis.
[c]Moderate chance that defining characteristic will be present, given diagnosis.
[d]Low chance that defining characteristic will be present, given diagnosis.
[e]High chance that defining characteristic is not explained by any other diagnosis.
[f]Moderate chance that defining characteristic is not explained by any other diagnosis.
[g]Low chance that defining characteristic is not explained by any other diagnosis.

Nursing Diagnosis	Defining Characteristics
Violence, potential for (self-directed or directed at others)	Body language: clenched fists, angry facial expressions, rigid posture, tautness indicating intense effort to control Hostile threatening verbalizations; boasting of prior abuse to others Increased motor activity, pacing, excitement, irritability, agitation Overt and aggressive acts; goal-directed destruction of objects in environment Possession of destructive means, e.g., gun, knife, other weapon Rage Self-destructive behavior; active, aggressive suicidal acts Substance abuse or withdrawal Suspicion of others, paranoid ideas, delusions, hallucinations *Other possible defining characteristics* Increased anxiety levels Fear of self or others Inability to verbalize feelings Repetition of verbalizations: continued complaints, requests, and demands Anger Provocative behavior: argumentative, dissatisfied, overreactive, hypersensative Vulnerable self-esteem Depression (specifically, active, aggressive, suicidal acts)

Source: North American Nursing Diagnosis Association. Clearinghouse for Nursing Diagnosis, Saint Louis University, Department of Nursing.; and M. Kim and D. Moritz (Eds.), *Classification of Nursing Diagnoses: Proceedings of the Third and Fourth Conferences.* New York: McGraw-Hill, 1982.

D. GROWTH CHARTS

1983 METROPOLITAN HEIGHT AND WEIGHT TABLES

TABLE 1. MEN*

Height				
Feet	Inches	Small Frame (lb)	Medium Frame (lb)	Large Frame (lb)
5	2	128—134	131—141	138—150
5	3	130—136	133—143	140—153
5	4	132—138	135—145	142—156
5	5	134—140	137—148	144—160
5	6	136—142	139—151	146—164
5	7	138—145	142—154	149—168
5	8	140—148	145—157	152—172
5	9	142—151	148—160	155—176
5	10	144—154	151—163	158—180
5	11	146—157	154—166	161—184
6	0	149—160	157—170	164—188
6	1	152—164	160—174	168—192
6	2	155—168	164—178	172—197
6	3	158—172	167—182	176—202
6	4	162—176	171—187	181—207

*Weights at ages 25—59 based on lowest mortality. Weight in pounds according to frame (in indoor clothing weighing 5 lb, shoes with 1-in. heels).

TABLE 2. WOMEN*

Height				
Feet	Inches	Small Frame (lb)	Medium Frame (lb)	Large Frame (lb)
4	10	102—111	109—121	118—131
4	11	103—113	111—123	120—134
5	0	104—115	113—126	122—137
5	1	106—118	115—129	125—140
5	2	108—121	118—132	128—143
5	3	111—124	121—135	131—147
5	4	114—127	124—138	134—151
5	5	117—130	127—141	137—155
5	6	120—133	130—144	140—159
5	7	123—136	133—147	143—163
5	8	126—139	136—150	146—167
5	9	129—142	139—153	149—170
5	10	132—145	142—156	152—173
5	11	135—148	145—159	155—176
6	0	138—151	148—162	158—179

*Weights at ages 25—59 based on lowest mortality. Weight in pounds according to frame (in indoor clothing weighing 3 lb, shoes with 1-in. heels).

Source of basic data: *1979 Build Study*, Society of Actuaries and Association of Life Insurance Medical Directors of America, 1980.

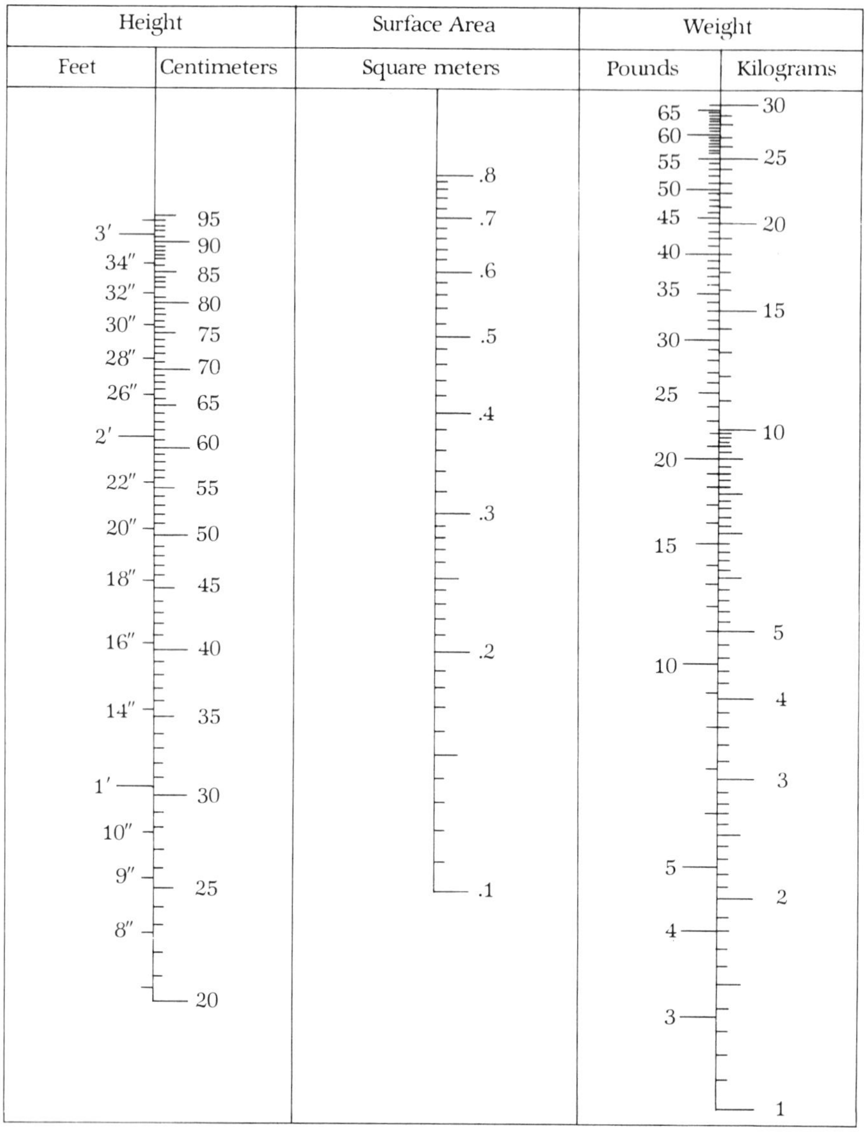

Height		Surface Area	Weight	
Feet	Centimeters	Square meters	Pounds	Kilograms

Height — Feet: 3′, 34″, 32″, 30″, 28″, 26″, 2′, 22″, 20″, 18″, 16″, 14″, 1′, 10″, 9″, 8″

Height — Centimeters: 95, 90, 85, 80, 75, 70, 65, 60, 55, 50, 45, 40, 35, 30, 25, 20

Surface Area — Square meters: .8, .7, .6, .5, .4, .3, .2, .1

Weight — Pounds: 65, 60, 55, 50, 45, 40, 35, 30, 25, 20, 15, 10, 5, 4, 3

Weight — Kilograms: 30, 25, 20, 15, 10, 5, 4, 3, 2, 1

FIGURE 1. Nomogram for estimating surface area of infants and young children. To determine the surface area of the patient, draw a straight line between the point representing his or her height on the left vertical scale to the point representing his or her weight on the right vertical scale. The point at which this line intersects the middle vertical scale represents the patient's surface area in square meters. (Courtesy Abbott Laboratories, Chicago, Illinois.)

E. COMMON MEDICAL ABBREVIATIONS

ā before (*ante*)
abd abdomen
ac before meals (*ante cibum*)
ADL activities of daily living
ad lib as desired
Amb ambulatory (able to move about)
BID twice a day (*bis in die*)
BM bowel movement
BP blood pressure
Br bathroom or bedrest
BRP bathroom privileges
C Celsius (centigrade)
c̄ with (c̄um)
CBC complete blood count
CBR complete bedrest
cc cubic centimeter
CC chief concern
CCU cardiac care unit
CO_2 carbon dioxide
CSR central supply room
C+S culture and sensitivity
DAT diet as tolerated
DC discontinue
DD differential diagnosis
Dx diagnosis
eg for example
ENT ear, nose, and throat
EENT eye, ear, nose, and throat
ER emergency room
EUA examination under anesthesia
F Fahrenheit
FMH family medical history
GI gastrointestinal
gm gram
gr grain
gtt drop (*guttae*)
GU genitourinary
Hct hematocrit
Hgb hemoglobin
H/O history of
HPI history of present illness
HR heart rate
hr hour
HS hour of sleep (*hora somni*); bedtime
Hx history
I&D incision and drainage
I&O intake and output
ICN intensive care nursery
ICU intensive care unit
IM intramuscular
IV intravenous
L left or liter
m minim
mg milligram
mEq milliequivalent
ml milliliter
NB note well (*nota bene*)

Neg negative
N/G nasogastric
NKA no known allergies
NPO nothing by mouth (nothing *per os*)
N/S normal saline
NYD not yet diagnosed
Ø none, no
O_2 oxygen
OOB out of bed
OD right eye (*oculus dextra*)
OPD outpatient department
OR operating room
OS left eye (*oculus sinister*)
os mouth
OT occupational therapy
OU both eyes (*oculus uterque*)
oz ounce
$\bar{p}$ after (*post*)
P pulse
pc after meals (*post cibum*)
PE physical examination
per by
PI present illness
PO by mouth (*per os*)
post-op postoperative
pre-op preoperative
prep preparation
prn as necessary (*pro renata*)
PT physical therapy
pt patient
q every (*quaque*)
qd everyday
qh every hour
QID four times a day (*quater in die*)
QOD every other day
qs sufficient quantity (*quantum satis*)
R right or respiration
RBC red blood cells
ROM range of motion
RR respiratory rate
Rx treatment or take
$\bar{s}$ without (*sine*)
sc subcutaneous
SG specific gravity
$\overline{ss}$ a half
SOB shortness of breath
S/P after a happening (*status post*)
STAT immediately (*statim*)
Sx symptoms
T temperature
TID three times a day (*ter in die*)
TLC tender loving care
TPR temperature, pulse, respiration
U/A urinalysis
$\underline{ug}$ microgram
$\underline{uug}$ picogram
UO unknown origin
VS vital signs
wc wheelchair
w/d well developed
WNL within normal limits
$>$ greater than
$<$ less than
↓ decreasing
↑ increasing
2° secondary to
= equals
♀ female
♂ male
number

F. TEMPERATURE CONVERSION

TABLE 1. FAHRENHEIT TO CELSIUS

°C	°F	°C	°F
34.0	93.2	38.6	101.5
34.2	93.6	38.8	101.8
34.4	93.9	39.0	102.2
34.6	94.3	39.2	102.6
34.8	94.6	39.4	102.9
35.0	95.0	39.6	103.3
35.2	95.4	39.8	103.6
35.4	95.7	40.0	104.0
35.6	96.1	40.2	104.4
35.8	96.4	40.4	104.7
36.0	96.8	40.6	105.2
36.2	97.2	40.8	105.4
36.4	97.5	41.0	105.9
36.6	97.9	41.2	106.1
36.8	98.2	41.4	106.5
37.0	98.6	41.6	106.8
37.2	99.0	41.8	107.2
37.4	99.3	42.0	107.6
37.6	99.7	42.2	108.0
37.8	100.0	42.4	108.3
38.0	100.4	42.6	108.7
38.2	100.8	42.8	109.0
38.4	101.1	43.0	109.4

Note: (°C) × (9/5) + 32 = °F; (°F − 32) × (5/9) = °C. °C = temperature in Celsius (centigrade) degrees; °F = temperature in Fahrenheit degrees.

G. CLINICAL APPLICATION AND NORMAL VALUES OF COMMON LABORATORY STUDIES

TABLE 1. COMMON HEMATOLOGY STUDIES

Study	Clinical Application	Normal Value
Complete blood count (CBC)	Basic screening for normal structure of blood components. Consists of all of the following tests.	
White blood count (WBC)	Total number of leukocytes present.	4,000—11,000 mm^3
Differential count	Analysis of types and amounts of white cells present.	
	Granular form	
	Neutrophils (active in acute bacterial infections).	1,800—7,000 mm^3 40—60%
	Eosinophils (increased in allergies and parasitic infections).	0—500 mm^3 0—5%
	Basophils (increased with inflammation).	0—100 mm^3 0—1%
	Nongranular form	
	Lymphocytes (T-cells react with antigens directly to combat infection. B-cells produce antibodies against infection). Tend to increase in viral infections.	2,000—4,500 mm^3 20—45%
	Monocytes (act as back up for neutrophils in acute infections).	0—600 mm^3 2—6%
Red blood count (RBC)	Total number of erythrocytes present.	Men: 4.6—6.2 million/mm^3 Women: 4.2—5.4 million/mm^3
Hematocrit (HCT)	Analysis of the concentration of RBCs in reference to plasma volume.	Men: 40—52% Women: 38—48%
Hemoglobin (HGB)	Analysis of the amount of hemoglobin in RBCs.	Men: 13.5—18.0 gm/100 ml Women: 12—16 gm/100 ml

TABLE 1. (CONTINUED)

Study	Clinical Application	Normal Value
Red blood cell indices	Determination of the size of a single red blood cell.	
Mean corpuscular volume (MCV)	Determination of the size of a single red blood cell.	82—98 mm^3
Mean corpuscular-hemoglobin (MCH)	Measurement of the amount of hemoglobin in a single red blood cell.	27—32 pg
Mean corpuscular hemoglobin concentration (MCHC)	Measurement of the average concentration of hemoglobin in average red blood cell.	32—36%
Stained erythrocyte examination	Microscopic inspection of cells for size, color, and shape after blood is smeared on slide.	No report of or few abnormal cells.
Platelet count	Total number of platelets present.	140,000—450,000 mm^3
Erythrocyte sedimentation rate (ESR)	Determination of the rate at which red blood cells settle in a tube of blood on standing.	Men: 0—5 mm/hr (Wintrobe); 0—15 mm/hr (Westergren) Women: 0—15 mm/hr (Wintrobe); 0—20 mm/hr (Westergren)
Reticulocyte count	Total number of immature red blood cells present.	0.5—2.0%
Sickle cell (hemoglobin S)	Determination if inherited hemoglobin S is present.	0

Source: Normal values adapted from J. Stein (Ed.), *Internal Medicine*. Boston: Little, Brown, 1983.

TABLE 2. COMMON BLOOD COAGULATION STUDIES

Study	Purpose	Normal Value
Bleeding time	Determination of time required for bleeding at site of earlobe incision to cease. Reveals deficiencies in platelet formation and vasoconstrictive ability.	Duke: 1—4 min Ivy: 1—9 min
Clot retraction	Determination of the interval from placement of blood in a tube until the clot shrinks and expels serum. Measures platelet function.	Retraction is apparent in 30—60 min; complete in 24 hr.
Partial thromboplastin time (PTT)	Determination of activity of thromboplastin after incomplete thromboplastin is added to sample. Reveals deficiencies in thromboplastin and Factors VIII—XII.	Standard: 68—82 sec Activated: 24—38 sec
Plasma fibrinogen	Determination of the level of fibrinogen in blood. Measures stage 4 of the clotting process.	200—400 mg/ml
Prothrombin time (PT)	Determination of action of prothrombin after complete thromboplastin is added to the sample. Reveals deficiencies in prothrombin, Factors V, VII, and X.	11—14 sec
Tourniquet	Determination of response of tissue to the application of a tourniquet to forearm for 5—10 minutes. Measures capillary fragility and platelet function.	<10 petechiae at site.
Venous clotting time (Lee-White)	Determination of time it takes venous blood to clot in a test tube. Measures factor defects in stages 2 and 4.	5—15 min

Source: Normal values adapted from J. Stein (Ed.), *Internal Medicine*. Boston: Little, Brown, 1983.

TABLE 3. COMMON BLOOD CHEMISTRY STUDIES

Study	Clinical Application	Normal Value
Acid phosphatase	An enzyme that rises when the prostate gland is injured or diseased.	0—0.8 μ/ml
Alkaline phosphatase	An enzyme that rises in liver or bone disease.	15—20 years: 40—200 IU/L >20 years: 35—125 IU/L
Bilirubin	Bilirubin is a breakdown product of red blood cells. The level of the first form (indirect) denotes the rate of red cell breakdown. Indirect bilirubin is processed by the liver and converted to direct bilirubin. Levels of direct bilirubin reflect liver function.	Total: 0.2—1.2 mg/100 ml Direct: 0—0.4 mg/100 ml Indirect: determined by subtracting direct from total.
Blood urea nitrogen (BUN)	Urea is the breakdown product of protein metabolism. It is measured in patients with kidney disease who are unable to excrete urea so it accumulates in the blood.	5—22 mg/100 ml
Calcium (Ca)	Calcium level reflects parathyroid function and mineralization of skeleton. Influenced by vitamin D.	8.7—10.6 mg/100 ml
Chloride (Cl)	Chloride in combination with sodium maintains osmotic pressure in the intravascular system. It is decreased in people with vomiting because of loss of hydrochloric acid.	95—105 mEq/L
Cholesterol	Cholesterol levels may be associated with the development of coronary artery disease. Increased levels arise from dietary and hereditary factors.	150—250 mg/100 ml
Creatinine	Creatinine is a breakdown product of muscle metabolism. It is increased in people with kidney disease since it cannot be excreted; decreased in people with lessened muscle mass.	Female: 0.5—1.3 mg/100 ml Male: 0.7—1.5 mg/100 ml
Folic acid (folate)	Folic acid is necessary for red blood cell formation.	1.9—14.0 ng/ml
Glucose (fasting blood sugar-FBS)	Normal glucose metabolism is necessary for function of all body cells. It is assessed in patients with diabetes or liver disease.	Serum: 70—110 mg/100 ml Whole blood: 60—110 mg/100 ml Postprandial blood sugar (2 hr following a meal): <140 mg/100 ml
Magnesium (Mg)	Magnesium is necessary for enzyme systems function.	1.5—2.5 mEq/L
Phosphorus (P)	Phosphate contributes to skeletal growth. There is a strong inverse factor between phosphorus and calcium (if Ca decreases, P increases).	2.0—4.3 mg/100 ml
Potassium (K)	Potassium is necessary for electrical conduction of impulses in body tissues. Heart muscle is particularly sensitive to potassium level.	3.5—5.0 mEq/L
Serum glutamic oxaloacetic transaminase (SGOT)	This enzyme is released if liver, heart, or muscle cells are damaged. The amount of enzyme present suggests extent of drainage.	5—40 IU/L
Serum glutamic pyruvic transaminase (SGPT)	This enzyme is released if there is liver cell damage.	0—48 IU/L

TABLE 3. (CONTINUED)

Study	Clinical Application	Normal Value
SMA-12/60 (sequential multiple analyzer)	This is a battery of chemistry analyses done by computer. Included in this scan is: total protein, albumin, calcium, phosphorous, cholesterol, glucose, blood urea nitrogen, uric acid, creatinine, total bilirubin, alkaline phosphatase, and serum glutamine oxalocetic transaminase (SGOT).	
Sodium (Na)	Sodium controls fluid metabolism. It is measured in patients with cardiac or kidney disease who have fluid retention.	135—145 mEq/L
Total blood proteins: albumin-globulin (A/G) ratio	Proteins are necessary for all cell metabolism and enzyme production. It is measured largely in patients with kidney disease, when proteins are easily excreted in urine.	Total: 6—8 gm/dl Albumin: 4—4.5 gm/100 ml Globulin: 1.5—3 gm/100 ml A/G ratio: 1.5—2.5:1

Source: Normal values adapted from J. Stein (Ed.), *Internal Medicine.* Boston: Little, Brown, 1983; and F. Fischbach, *A Manual of Laboratory Diagnostic Tests.* Philadelphia: Lippincott, 1980.

TABLE 4. COMMON ARTERIAL BLOOD GAS STUDIES

Assessment Factor	Clinical Application	Normal Value
Oxygen		
Partial pressure (PO_2)	Measurement of oxygen tension; decrease indicates inadequate oxygenation of body cells.	80—150 mm Hg
Saturation (SO_2)	Measurement of proportion of hemoglobin saturated with oxygen in red blood cells.	95—97%
Carbon dioxide (PCO_2)	Measurement of partial pressure of carbon dioxide; increase indicates poor respiratory function.	38—44 mm Hg
pH	Measurement of acid-base balance; blood is always slightly alkaline. Decrease indicates acidosis; with acidosis, hemoglobin is less well saturated with oxygen, resulting in inadequate oxygenation of body cells. A pH of 7.0 is incompatible with life.	7.35—7.45

Source: Normal values from J. Stein (Ed.), *Internal Medicine.* Boston: Little, Brown, 1983.

TABLE 5. COMMON CEREBROSPINAL FLUID STUDIES

Assessment Factor	Clinical Application	Normal Value
Albumin-globulin (A/G) ratio	Abnormal value suggests infection or neurological disorder.	8 : 1
Chloride	Decrease suggests bacterial infection.	110—129
Color	Cloudiness suggests infection; red tinge suggests bleeding.	Colorless
Glucose	Decrease suggests that bacteria are present and utilizing glucose.	45—85 mg/100 ml or 20 mg $<$ blood glucose level
Pressure	Increase suggests obstruction to the flow of fluid.	75—150 mm H_2O
Protein	Increase suggests infection or neurological disorder.	15—45 mg/100 ml
Total cell count	Increase suggests infection.	0—8 mm^3

Source: Normal values adapted from J. Stein (Ed.), *Internal Medicine.* Boston: Little, Brown, 1983; and F. Fischbach, *A Manual of Laboratory Diagnostic Tests.* Philadelphia: Lippincott, 1980.

TABLE 6. COMMON URINE STUDIES

Assessment Factor	Clinical Application	Normal Value
Color	Gross determination of concentration; the yellower the color, the greater the concentration.	Straw-colored
Appearance	Cloudy appearance suggests the presence of bacteria or excessive crystals or cells.	Clear
pH	Urine becomes alkaline (pH > 7.0) in the presence of bacteria or when exposed to room temperature.	4.6—8.0
Specific gravity	Specific determination of concentration; elevated value indicates dehydration.	1.003—1.030
Protein	Protein molecules pass into urine in the presence of kidney disease.	Qualitative: 0 Quantitative: 0—2.4 mg/24 hr
Ketones	Presence of ketones is abnormal and results from breakdown of body fat. Ketonuria is found in starvation and in poorly controlled diabetes mellitus.	0
Glucose	Presence of glucose is abnormal. Glucosuria is present in uncontrolled diabetes mellitus.	Qualitative: 0 Quantitative: 16—300 mg/24 hr
Occult blood	Bleeding suggests urinary tract infection or trauma; present also in kidney disorders.	0
Red blood cells	Presence suggests bleeding caused by trauma or infection.	< 1/high-power field
White blood cells	Increase suggests infection.	< 5/high-power field
Casts	Casts are composed of epithelial cells, pus cells, red blood cells, granules, and fat globulins. Present in concentrated urine specimens. Increase suggests kidney disorder.	Occasionally, 1/high-power field
Bacteria	Presence indicated infection.	100,000/ml bacterial colony count in clean-catch specimen; 0 bacterial colony count in suprapubic or catheterized specimen.

Source: Normal values adapted from J. Stein (Ed.), *Internal Medicine.* Boston: Little, Brown, 1983.

H. FRACTIONAL DRUG CALCULATIONS

QUESTIONS

1. You have an order for aspirin gr xx. The bottle you have supplies tablets of 300 mg. How many tablets would you administer?
2. You have an order for 1,050 mg of medicine. The tablets you have are 350 mg each. How many tablets would you administer?
3. You have an order for penicillin 800,000 units. The bottle of penicillin you have provides 250,000 units in each 0.5 ml. How many milliliters would you administer?
4. How many minims of the above solution would you administer?
5. You have an order for erythromycin 400 mg. If the vial you have supplies 1 gm in 5 ml, how many milliliters would you administer?
6. You have an order for gr 1/300 of atropine sulfate. It comes supplied as 0.4 mg/ml. How many milliliters will you administer?
7. You have an order for 250 mg of an antibiotic. When reconstituted from its dry powder, the vial will supply 100 mg/0.8 ml. How many milliliters will you administer?
8. You have an order for 1 tsp of liquid oral erythromycin. The bottle label tells you there is 250 mg in each 7 ml of solution. How many milligrams are you administering in each teaspoon?
9. You have an order for 2 gm of oral medicine. It is supplied 400 mg in 3 ml. How many milliliters will you administer?
10. You have an order for gr v of cough syrup. It is supplied as 120 mg in 10 ml. How many milliliters will you administer?
11. You have an order for nitroglycerine gr 1/150. You have on hand tablets of 0.2 mg nitroglycerine per tablet. How many tablets will you give?
12. You have an order for liquid tylenol of gr v. The bottle states there is 120 mg in each 5 ml. How many teaspoons should a mother administer?

ANSWERS

1. Using the short formula (conversion factor gr i = 60 mg):

   amount ordered × conversion factor × dose on hand = answer

$$\frac{\overset{i}{\cancel{\text{gr xx}}}}{1} \times \frac{60\text{ mg}}{\text{gr i}} \times \frac{1\text{ tablet}}{\underset{15}{\cancel{300}\text{ mg}}} = \frac{60}{15} = 4\text{ tablets}$$

2. No conversion factor needed.

amount ordered × dose on hand = answer

$$\frac{\overset{21}{\cancel{1050}}\text{ mg}}{1} \times \frac{1\text{ tablet}}{\underset{7}{\cancel{350}}\text{ mg}} = \frac{21}{7} = 3\text{ tablets}$$

3. No conversion factor needed.

amount ordered × dose on hand = answer

$$\frac{\overset{16}{\cancel{800,000}}\text{ units}}{1} \times \frac{0.5\text{ ml}}{\underset{5}{\cancel{250,000}}\text{ units}} = \frac{8}{5} = 1.6\text{ ml}$$

4. Conversion factor necessary (15 minims = 1 ml):

amount ordered × conversion factor = answer

$$\frac{1.6\text{ ml}}{1} \times \frac{15\text{ minims}}{1\text{ ml}} = 24\text{ minims}$$

5. Conversion factor necessary (1,000 mg = 1 gm):

amount ordered × conversion factor × dose on hand = answer

$$\frac{\overset{4}{\cancel{400}}\text{ mg}}{1} \times \frac{1\text{ gm}}{\underset{10}{\cancel{1000}}\text{ mg}} \times \frac{5\text{ ml}}{1\text{ gm}} = \frac{20}{10} = 2\text{ ml}$$

6. Conversion factor necessary (gr i = 60 mg):

amount ordered × conversion factor × dose on hand = answer

$$\frac{\text{gr i}}{\underset{5}{\cancel{300}}} \times \frac{\overset{1}{\cancel{60}}\text{ mg}}{\text{gr i}} \times \frac{1\text{ ml}}{0.4\text{ mg}} = 0.5\text{ ml}$$

7. No conversion factor needed.

amount ordered × dose on hand = answer

$$\frac{\overset{5}{\cancel{250}}\text{ mg}}{1} \times \frac{\overset{0.4}{\cancel{0.8}}\text{ ml}}{\underset{2}{\cancel{100}}\text{ mg}} = 2.0\text{ ml}$$

8. Conversion factor necessary (1 tsp = 5 ml):

amount ordered × dose on hand = answer

$$\frac{5\text{ ml}}{1\text{ tsp}} \times \frac{250\text{ mg}}{7\text{ ml}} = \frac{1{,}250}{7} = 178\text{ mg}$$

9. Conversion factor necessary (1,000 mg = 1 gm):

amount ordered × conversion factor × dose on hand = answer

$$\frac{2\text{ gm}}{1} \times \frac{\overset{20}{\cancel{1000}}\text{ mg}}{1\text{ gm}} \times \frac{3\text{ ml}}{\underset{8}{\cancel{400}}\text{ mg}} = \frac{120}{8} = 15\text{ ml}$$

10. Conversion factor necessary (gr i = 60 mg):

amount ordered × conversion factor × dose on hand = answer

$$\frac{\text{gr v}}{1} \times \frac{\overset{1}{\cancel{60}}\text{ mg}}{\text{gr i}} \times \frac{\overset{5}{\cancel{10}}\text{ ml}}{\underset{\underset{1}{\cancel{2}}}{\cancel{120}}\text{ mg}} = 25\text{ ml}$$

11. Conversion factor necessary (gr i = 60 mg):

amount ordered × conversion factor × dose on hand = answer

$$\frac{\text{gr i}}{\underset{15}{\cancel{150}}} \times \frac{\overset{6}{\cancel{60}}\text{ mg}}{\text{gr i}} \times \frac{1\text{ tablet}}{0.2\text{ mg}} = \frac{6}{3} = 2\text{ tablets}$$

12. This is a difficult problem because you have three different systems of measurement (grains, milligrams and milliliters, and teaspoons) involved. Solve the problem first in milliliters and then convert into teaspoons for the mother. You could do this by adding the extra conversion factor (5 ml = 1 tsp) to the short formula or:

amount ordered × conversion factor (gr i = 60 mg) × dose on hand × conversion factor (5 ml = 1 tsp) = answer

$$\frac{\text{gr v}}{1} \times \frac{\overset{1}{\cancel{60}}\text{ mg}}{\text{gr i}} \times \frac{\overset{1}{\cancel{5}}\text{ ml}}{\underset{2}{\cancel{120}}\text{ mg}} = \frac{1\text{ tsp}}{\underset{1}{\cancel{5}}\text{ ml}} = 2.5\text{ tsp}$$

General Guidelines

1. When fitting numbers into the formula be certain always to arrange measurements from *top* to *bottom*. For example, in the following formula grains is the top unit of the first fraction, and therefore will be the bottom unit of the conversion factor fraction. The measurement (mg) at the top of the conversion factor will be the bottom measurement of the dose on hand factor:

amount ordered × conversion factor × dose on hand = answer

$$\frac{\text{gr } \overset{\text{i}}{\cancel{\text{ii}}}}{1} \times \frac{\overset{1}{\cancel{60}}\text{ mg}}{\text{gr i}} \times \frac{1\text{ tablet}}{\underset{\underset{1}{\cancel{2}}}{\cancel{120}}\text{ mg}} = 1\text{ tablet}$$

2. The measurement unit that is the *top* of the last fraction will be the unit of measurement of the answer (tablets plus tablets in the above example).

I. ANSWERS TO REVIEW QUESTIONS

CHAPTER 1

1. d 2. c 3. b 4. d 5. d 6. a 7. b 8. b

9. 1. Associate degree
   2. Diploma program
   3. Hospitals
   4. State level
   5. Environmental control
   6. *American Journal of Nursing*
   7. Baccalaureate degree
   8. Nurse practitioner
   9. Men
   10. Sets own standards

CHAPTER 2

1. b 2. d 3. b 4. d 5. a 6. d 7. b 8. b

CHAPTER 3

1. c 2. c 3. a 4. d 5. b 6. d 7. d 8. c 9. a 10. c

CHAPTER 4

1. c 2. a 3. c 4. c 5. a 6. b 7. b 8. a 9. d

10. a. 10
    b. 4
    c. 8
    d. 2
    e. 3
    f. 9
    g. 1
    h. 5
    i. 7
    j. 6

CHAPTER 5

1. Deductive 2. Mode 3. Sample 4. Variable
5. Inductive 6. Assumption 7. Mean 8. Correlation
9. Rights 10. Median 11. Range 12. Data
13. Hypothesis 14. Population 15. T test
A role of a professional nurse: researcher.

CHAPTER 6

1. c 2. b 3. b 4. a 5. d 6. b 7. a 8. c 9. d
10. c

CHAPTER 7

1. a. 4
   b. 8
   c. 1
   d. 7
   e. 6
   f. 2
   g. 3
   h. 5

2. a. 4
   b. 1
   c. 2
   d. 3
   e. 5

CHAPTER 8

1. T 2. T 3. F 4. T 5. T 6. F 7. F 8. F 9. T 10. T 11. F 12. F 13. F 14. F 15. T

CHAPTER 9

1. a. 8
   b. 5
   c. 2
   d. 6
   e. 3
   f. 7
   g. 4
   h. 1
2. a. 6
   b. 5
   c. 1
   d. 4
   e. 3
   f. 2
3. a. 2
   b. 4
   c. 5
   d. 6
   e. 1
   f. 3
4. a. 7
   b. 1
   c. 6
   d. 9
   e. 2
   f. 4
   g. 8
   h. 5
   i. 3
5. a. 7
   b. 8
   c. 1
   d. 2
   e. 4
   f. 3
   g. 6
   h. 5

CHAPTER 10

1. b 2. c 3. a 4. d 5. a 6. c

CHAPTER 11

1. b 2. a 3. c 4. b 5. b 6. d 7. b 8. b

CHAPTER 12

1. b 2. b 3. b 4. a 5. d 6. a 7. b 8. d

CHAPTER 13

1. a 2. a 3. a 4. d 5. a 6. b 7. d 8. c 9. b 10. b 11. a 12. d

B	M	X	P	B	A	N	O	R	T	V	E	F	T	B	X	W	M
K	E	P	R	I	O	R	I	T	Y	S	E	T	T	I	N	G	P
M	V	T	M	V	R	S	B	Q	C	D	W	X	M	A	D	C	Y
W	I	M	V	R	B	E	V	A	L	U	A	T	I	O	N	L	T
N	T	O	O	V	K	T	T	Q	P	D	N	A	K	C	A	D	K
L	C	N	U	R	S	I	N	G	D	I	A	G	N	O	S	I	S
Y	E	E	U	S	C	O	E	Y	F	J	L	K	G	Y	I	R	M
P	J	E	Q	Y	A	L	M	P	M	R	Y	Z	G	B	C	S	K
Z	B	D	N	V	L	O	S	T	E	K	S	M	F	J	X	I	N
D	O	V	Y	W	Q	G	S	Z	W	M	I	B	N	O	L	Y	S
W	X	U	P	M	M	Y	E	R	H	N	S	T	N	P	Q	Z	U
L	A	C	T	E	Z	P	S	H	D	N	L	L	K	O	D	X	N
M	A	R	T	E	P	W	S	W	R	U	T	V	G	U	R	S	A
T	P	W	S	G	H	T	A	P	B	C	X	R	U	H	F	W	B

13. a. Nursing Diagnosis
    b. Assessment
    c. Need
    d. Etiology
    e. Objective
    f. Priority setting
    g. Goal
    h. Evaluation
    i. Analysis

CHAPTER 14

1. a 2. d 3. c 4. c 5. d 6. d 7. d 8. a 9. b 10. d

CHAPTER 15

1. c 2. a 3. d 4. d 5. b 6. a 7. c 8. d 9. c 10. c

CHAPTER 16

1. b 2. a 3. d 4. a 5. a 6. b 7. d 8. b 9. a

CHAPTER 17

1. September 18, 1983 (7:00—3:30)

7:00 A.M. Patient (1) complaining of pain in right foot. States pain is sharp and penetrating. Foot feels cold to (2) percussion.

7:30 Demerol 50 mg. (3)

8:00 Breakfast taken (4) poor. States "I hate this place. I'm glad I'm going home tomorrow."

8:30 Bath given. Two (5) red areas evident on back. Massaged. Lotion applied. I (6) made bed and talked to her.

9:00 (7) Up to wheelchair; daughter visited for 15 minutes.

10:00 (8) Complaining of pain in foot. I (9) think real problem, however, is loneliness.

(12) 2:00 Returned to bed. States (10) toes feel numb and cold.

3:00 In bed. States toes feel numb and cold.

(11) *Mary Smith*

1. The word *complaining* is unprofessional. Say that patient reports sharp and penetrating pain.
2. Percussion is used wrongly; assessing by feel is palpation.
3. Route of administration of a medication should be recorded. Draw line to end of page.
4. *Breakfast taken poor* is both poor grammar and a poor description. *Drank 1/2 glass orange juice*, etc., would be better.
5. *Erythematous* is a more professional word than *red*; size of area would be important to add.
6. "I made bed and talked to her" is nurse, not patient action. Describing content of exhange would be better.
7. Incomplete description of activity. Does patient move without pain? Does she grow dizzy in upright position? Was there any change with daughter's visit?
8. The word *complaining* again.
9. This is a conclusion unwarranted by information given. Either just describe appearance (sad, crying, and so on) or document reason for conclusion.
10. Incomplete assessment. How did they feel to you? Can she move them?
11. Signature incomplete. Usually the first initial only is used; title should be added.
12. Space should not be left between the columns, permitting the recording to be changed or distorted.

2. Tracey Burns (1)
   Problem: Pain in left knee

   S: (2) Temperature: 100°F. States "My knee is no better and I'm bored." Limps when walks. (3)

O: (4) Mother states, "I think the swelling is less than yesterday." Left knee feels warm to touch; appears erytematus; (5) aspirin (6) given once during morning; child refused (7) it at noon.

A: (11) 6-year-old with no improvement in pain.

Goal: Patient to have pain in right knee reduced to acceptable level. (8)

P: Therapeutic: Ask M.D. if she could be out of bed more to go to playroom. (9)

Education: Educate about pill taking. (10)

S. Ashley, J.U.S.N.

1. Additional identifying information about the patient needed: Hospital number? Address?
2. Temperature is an objective finding.
3. Observing her limping is an objective finding.
4. Mother's statement is a subjective finding.
5. *Erythematous* misspelled.
6. Medication time, dose, and route of administration all need to be recorded.
7. Reason for refusing medicine should be given.
8. Criteria to measure goal should be included.
9. Asking for more information is diagnostic, not therapeutic, information.
10. Vague order; educate about *what*?
11. Space should not be left between the columns, permitting the recording to be changed or distorted.

CHAPTER 18

1. i 2. e 3. n 4. t 5. b 6. m 7. h 8. r 9. a 10. g 11. u 12. d 13. l 14. v 15. o 16. c 17. q 18. w 19. f 20. j 21. s 22. p 23. k

CHAPTER 19

1. a 2. d 3. a 4. d 5. a 6. d 7. c 8. b 9. a 10. a

CHAPTER 20

1. T 2. F 3. T 4. F 5. F 6. F 7. F 8. T 9. T 10. T 11. T 12. F 13. T 14. F 15. F

CHAPTER 21

1. b 2. b 3. b 4. d 5. d 6. d 7. c 8. b 9. c 10. b 11. c 12. a

CHAPTER 22

1. Overload 2. Cognitive 3. Premature 4. Explain 5. Bed rest 6. Calendar 7. Television 8. Confused 9. Homework 10. Older

CHAPTER 23

1. a 2. c 3. d 4. d 5. b 6. a 7. a 8. b

CHAPTER 24

1. b 2. c 3. d 4. b 5. c 6. d 7. c 8. a 9. d 10. c

CHAPTER 25

1. c 2. b 3. a 4. a 5. b 6. c 7. b 8. c 9. b 10. a 11. d 12. d 13. d

CHAPTER 26

1. a 2. d 3. a 4. b 5. a 6. a 7. b

CHAPTER 27

1. b 2. e 3. a 4. c 5. b 6. a 7. d 8. b 9. c 10. d 11. a

CHAPTER 28

1. c 2. d 3. c 4. d 5. b 6. d 7. c 8. b

CHAPTER 29

A1. 4 B1. 3 C1. 1 D1. 3 E1. 4 F1. 2 G1. 4 H1. 1 I1. 1

CHAPTER 30

1. a 2. a 3. b 4. c 5. c 6. b 7. d 8. b

CHAPTER 31

1. c 2. c 3. b 4. a 5. a 6. b 7. b 8. d 9. d 10. a

CHAPTER 32

1. b 2. c 3. c 4. d 5. b 6. c 7. d 8. a 9. b 10. d 11. a

CHAPTER 33

1. b 2. a 3. d 4. b 5. d 6. c 7. a 8. b 9. b 10. a

CHAPTER 34

1. b 2. c 3. a 4. a 5. a 6. d 7. a 8. d 9. c 10. d

CHAPTER 35

1. b 2. c 3. a 4. d 5. a 6. c 7. b 8. e 9. c 10. a 11. a 12. c 13. c 14. a 15. a 16. a 17. b 18. a 19. b 20. d

CHAPTER 36

1. c 2. a 3. c 4. a 5. b 6. c 7. b 8. a 9. d
10. a. Circadian (darcician)
 b. Infradian (friniand)
 c. Hypnotic (potnhicy)
 d. Sedative (tivseeda)
 e. Somnambulism (bimlnosmmasu)
 f. Nocturnal enuresis (seirunes lanturnoc)
 g. Sleep (plese)
 h. REM (mre)
 i. Agrypnotic (tnyagroicp)
 j. Rest (ters)

CHAPTER 37

1. c 2. b 3. d 4. c 5. b 6. a 7. a 8. c 9. b 10. c

CHAPTER 38

1. c 2. d 3. c 4. a 5. a 6. b 7. b 8. c 9. b 10. a

CHAPTER 39

You should have a diagonal pattern when you answer question 9.

1. Day of admission 2. Allergies 3. Privacy 4. Triage 5. Nurse 6. Identification 7. Baseline determinations 8. Safety 9. Maternal deprivation 10. A place to die 11. False imprisonment 12. Parents

CHAPTER 40

1. b 2. a 3. d 4. d 5. b 6. b 7. d 8. c 9. c 10. c

GLOSSARY

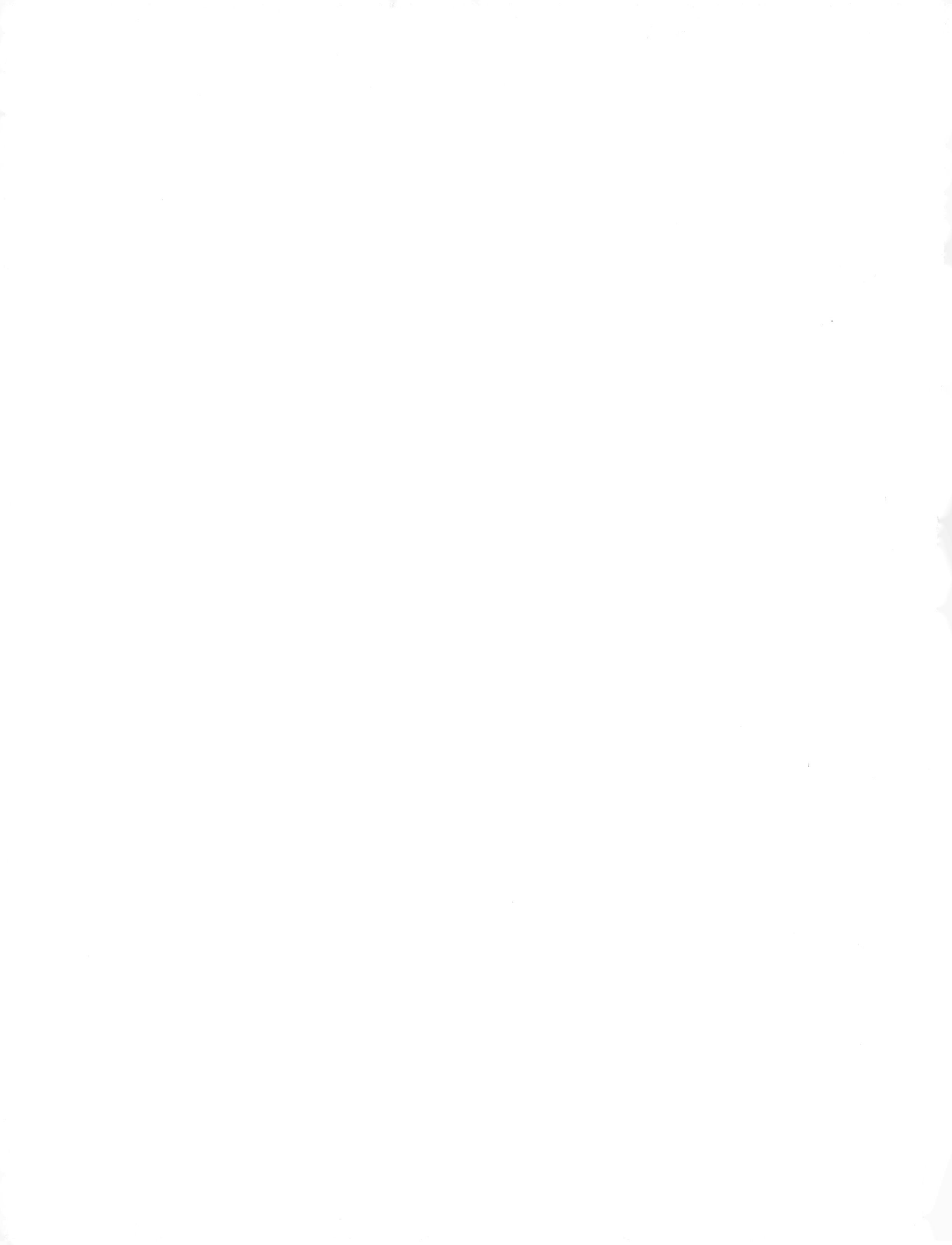

GLOSSARY

accommodation a cognitive realization that other people's views may be different from yours
adaptation the final resolution to a problem
adverse effect a detrimental effect of medicine
advocacy the act of speaking for another for the benefit of the other
advocate one who pleads another's cause
ambulatory setting a place where a person is seen for health care and returns home
anal sex insertion of the penis into the anus
analingus anal stimulation with the tongue
analysis the study of assessment data to identify the patient's health care needs and to select goals of nursing care
anesthesia loss of feeling or sensation
anorexia loss of appetite
antagonistic effect A lessened effect that occurs when two drugs are administered simultaneously
anuria absence of urine
antipyretic a medication used to reduce body temperature
antiseptic a substance used to achieve asepsis of a skin surface
anxiety a state of feeling threatened or uneasy in response to threat
Apgar score a rating given infants at birth as to body function
aphasia lack of speech or inability to speak
apical heart rate a count of the heart rate over the apex of the heart; the place where the mitral valve sound is heard best
apnea cessation of respirations
appetite desire for or anticipation of food
asepsis state of being free of pathogenic microorganisms
aspirate to allow a foreign substance to enter the trachea
aspiration studies procedures requiring the removal of fluid or gases from a body cavity
assault the threat of harm to someone
assertiveness the ability to express your feelings in a socially acceptable manner, respecting others' rights and feelings
assessment the systematic collection of data in order to establish a data base for a patient
assumptions statements whose correctness can be taken for granted
atarxy apathetic; not anxious. Drugs used to reduce anxiety are ataractics
atrophy to stop growing or recede in growth
audit methodical examination of patient records to evaluate quality of care given. In a nursing audit, nursing care is evaluated
auscultation listening with your ears; listen for four qualities of sound: duration, frequency, intensity (loudness), and pitch (high or low)

autoclave the instrument used to achieve sterilization

autopsy medical examination after death to further medical science or to document the cause of death

bacteriocidal a substance that kills bacteria

bacteriostatic a substance that halts bacterial growth

basal metabolic rate minimum amount of energy needed by the body at rest

battery the intentional touching of another's body without his consent

behavior modification a learning mode based on erasing undesirable behavior by rewarding acceptable behavior

Bill of Rights a statement of fundamental expectations or rights

biorhythm an internal rhythm system that regulates biological functions

bland diet a diet that is nonirritating to the stomach and duodenal lining

blood pressure measurement of the force exerted by arterial blood against vessel walls

bone marrow aspiration the removal of a specimen of bone marrow

bradycardia slow heart rate; under 60 beats per minute in the adult

bradypnea slow respiratory rate; under 16 breaths per minute in an adult

Brazelton Neonatal Behavioral Assessment Scale a standardized scale for rating the responsiveness of newborns

calculi "stone" in urine

caries decay of the teeth

celibacy a conscious choice to abstain from sexual activity

cephalocaudal growth proceeding from head to tail

change to alter a pattern of behavior

chaplain a spiritual advisor assigned to a health care agency

charting in common usage, refers to the act of writing nurse's notes

chemistry studies analysis of blood samples concerning the plasma portion or the chemical component of blood

Cheyne-Stokes respirations a cycle of increased depth, then decreased depth, then apnea in respirations

chyme liquid waste products entering the large intestine

circadian rhythm a 24-hour body rhythm

civil law law controlling most offenses against individuals

clean state of being free of pathogenic microorganisms (medically aseptic)

clear liquid diet a diet containing only liquids that are clear when held to the light such as tea or broth

climacteric male menopause or a lessening of sexual function in males

cognitive development intellectual growth

cognitive stimulation the interest or excitement of thought processes, as in thinking through a problem

coitus motivated insertion of the penis into the vagina

colostomy a surgical procedure that brings a portion of the large intestine to the abdominal surface for elimination

comedones plugged sebaceous glands associated with acne

comfort possessing a sense of well-being over and above freedom from pain and aggravating factors

common law law of precedent or judicial law

communicable disease an illness that can be transmitted from one person to another

community a limited geographic area in which the residents relate to and interact among themselves

community assessment examination of the various systems present in most communities to see if they are functioning adequately

community health nurse a nurse who practices in community settings such as schools, industry, ambulatory clinics, and homes

complete health history patient information elicited and recorded in the areas of present illness, family profile, past illnesses, family health history, and body systems (review of systems—ROS)

comprehensive data base patient information gained from three sources: the complete health history, the physical examination, and laboratory data

conduction loss of heat to an adjacent colder object

conservation a cognitive realization that although substances change shape they do not necessarily change mass

constipation the passage of hardened stool; inability to defecate or difficult defecation

consumer one who uses a product

contraception voluntary prevention of pregnancy

control group a group of subjects who are like the test group except for the research variable

convection loss of heat to a moving air or liquid current

coping a mechanism used to counteract or control threat

correlation the degree of relationship between two or more factors

criminal law law designed to protect the physical safety and property of people at large

crisis prolonged stress; severe stress

culture beliefs and practices shared by a specific social group, passed from generation to generation

cunnilingus stimulation of the female genitalia by the mouth and tongue

cyanosis blue tinge to skin or mucous membrane from lack of oxygen in red blood cells
cystitis bladder inflammation

data pieces of information gained by a study
death cessation of life functions
decoder the person who receives and interprets a message
decubitus ulcer an erosion of skin caused by compromised blood circulation to the area
deductive reasoning reasoning that proceeds from the general to the specific
defecation elimination of feces from the intestine
defendant a person accused in court
dehiscence separation of the layers of an incision or wound
Denver Developmental Screening Test (DDST) a standardized test to determine development in children up to 6 years of age
dependent variable an effect or response being measured
development an increase in the ability to perform tasks
developmental crisis a task that an individual normally seeks to complete at a specific point in time
diagnostic-laboratory studies tests or procedures done to establish or confirm a medical diagnosis or to provide information on the effect of therapy
dialect the intonation and pronunciation of words
diarrhea loose, watery bowel movements due to the rapid passage of stool through the intestines
diastole the second heart sound heard; the sound of the pulmonary and aortic valves closing (the *dub* of "lub-dub")
diastolic blood pressure the last sound heard when taking a blood pressure; the point where the sound muffles and is described as blowing
discharge planning instructions and arrangements for care following hospital discharge
diuresis excessive amount of urination
documentation the keeping of original, official, or legal records
drug any substance that is capable of affecting a person's state of health or ability to function
dysarthria difficulty with articulation or pronunciation of words
dyspnea difficulty breathing for any reason
dysuria pain on urination

edema excessive amount of fluid in interstitial tissues
electrocardiogram (ECG or EKG) a graph of the electrical conduction of the heart
electroencephalogram (EEG) a graph of the electrical activity of the brain
electrolytes substances that dissociate into particles termed *ions* when dissolved in water; positively charged ions are *cations*, negatively charged ions are *anions*
electromyogram (EMG) a recording of the electrical potential created by contraction of muscle
embryo growth in utero during the first 5 to 8 weeks of life
empathy ability to experience an emotion as the person is experiencing it
encoder the person who originates and sends a message
endemic an illness that is always present in a population
endoscopic studies procedures for direct visualization of a body area; the procedure is named for the body part involved, e.g., colonoscopy
enema the instillation of fluid into the rectum to effect defecation
enuresis bedwetting or involuntary loss of urine at night
epidemic an illness that is occurring at above average incidence in a population
erythematous reddened
ethnic pertaining to traits and customs shared by a race or large group of people, passed from generation to generation
ethnicity the racial or cultural heritage of a person, the ethnic group into which he is born
euthanasia the taking of someone's life to prevent suffering (mercy-killing)
evaluation a systematic method of determining the extent to which goals have been met
evaporation loss of heat due to the energy released as a liquid is changed to a gas
eviseration escape of abdominal organs through a wound dehiscence
extracellular fluid compartment fluid in spaces outside the cells; composed of two compartments—intravascular (fluid within blood vessels) and interstitial (fluid surrounding cells)
extubation removal of a tube

family a group of people who depend on each other for interaction and support
feces waste products in or excreted from the large intestine (stool)
fellatio stimulation of the male genitalia by the mouth and tongue
fetishism sexual arousal by the use of objects
fetus growth in utero after the 5th to 8th week
fever elevation in body temperature over normal limits
flatulence accumulation of excess gas in the intestine
flatus air expelled from the rectum
frequency sensation of having to urinate at short time intervals

frequency distribution a systematic arrangement of values from the lowest to highest value
full liquid diet a diet that includes any food that is liquid at room temperature (soup, milk, ice cream, custard)

gastrostomy tube a tube inserted into the stomach through the abdominal wall
gastric intubation insertion of a tube through the nose into the stomach
gavage introduction of fluid into the stomach by a tube
general adaptation syndrome (GAS) the physiologic responses to a threat
general anesthesia state of unconsciousness produced by the administration of an anesthetic agent
geriatrics science of health care and treatment of older persons
gerontology science of aging and its problems and process
glycosuria sugar in urine
growth an increase in size
guaiac test a test for occult blood in stool

halitosis an odor to the breath
Hawthorne effect the effect of increased productivity that occurs in observed workers
health a state of physical, psychological, and sociological well-being
health care delivery system the network of health care providers, agencies, and services that supplies health care to a designated area
heart rate the number of times the heart beats in 1 minute
hematest a test for occult blood in stool
hematology studies analysis of blood samples concerning the function or structure of blood cells
hematuria blood in urine
hemorrhoids congested, tender blood vessels just inside or outside the anus
hemostasis stoppage of blood flow
high-level wellness state of optimum physical and psychosocial health
homeodynamics a state of physiological balance; implies that even at rest the body is not static but constantly working to maintain balance
hospice a health care facility specifically designed for the care of dying persons to aid them to a peaceful death
hunger physical sensation that alerts a person to eat food
hydrostatic pressure, also **oncotic pressure** the pressure exerted on blood cells and plasma by volume
hygienics science of health and cleanliness
hypercapnea increased level of carbon dioxide in arterial blood
hyperpnea increased depth of respirations
hypertension elevated blood pressure
hyperthermia abnormally elevated body temperature (107°F, 41°C)
hypertonic solution with more molecular weight than blood plasma (high concentration of solute to solvent)
hyperventilation increased rate and depth of respirations
hypervolemia increased blood volume, which can result in pulmonary edema
hypnotic a medication to induce sleep
hypotension decreased blood pressure
hypothermia abnormally decreased body temperature (80.6°F, 27°C)
hypothesis statement of the expected relationship between phenomena under study
hypotonic solution with less molecular weight than blood plasma (low concentration of solute to solvent)
hypoventilation shallow breathing
hypovolemia reduction of blood volume causing cell perfusion to be inadequate
hypoxemia decreased level of oxygen in bloodstream

idiosyncratic effect abnormal effect caused by an individual response to a medicine
illness a state in which there is psychological, physical, or social malfunction of a body part
implementation the initiation and completion of predetermined actions to accomplish established goals
incontinence of stool involuntary loss of stool
incontinence of urine involuntary loss of urine
independent variable a characteristic that can be manipulated
individuality the uniqueness of a person; those characteristics that make him different from any other person
inductive reasoning reasoning that proceeds from the specific to the general
infection an illness caused by the invasion and action of a microorganism
infiltration intravenous fluid enters the local subcutaneous tissue from the needle that has pierced the vein wall
infusion pump machine that automatically pushes intravenous fluid into a vein at a predetermined rate
inpatient setting a place where a person is admitted for health care and remains overnight
insomnia inability to fall asleep or to stay asleep
inspection examination based on sight; smelling is a less often used but also important phase of inspection
intracellular fluid compartment fluid within body cells

intravenous fluid sterile fluid introduced into the circulatory system by means of venipuncture

intravenous medication medicine added to an intravenous solution bottle or volume control chamber or directly into the venipuncture site; immediately enters the circulatory system

isolation a medical aseptic technique for protecting a patient or health care provider from the spread of microorganisms (barrier technique)

isometric exercises increasing tension in muscles without joint movement

isotonic solution with molecular weight equal to that of blood plasma

karyotype arrangement of chromosomes so that they can be studied

keloid an overgrowth of scar tissue

kilocalorie amount of energy necessary to increase 1 kilogram of water 1 degree Celcius in temperature

Korotkoff's sounds four distinct sounds (or lack of sounds) heard when taking a blood pressure

Kussmaul respirations rapid and deep respirations

lavage irrigation or washing of the stomach by introducing fluid through a tube

leadership the art of guiding others to accomplish goals

learning a two-step process of acquiring new information and changing behavior accordingly

learning style the individual manner in which a person grasps and processes new information

libel a written derogatory statement about someone

libido sexual motivation; the desire or urge for sexual activity

local anesthesia loss of pain sensation in a limited body area due to the injection or application of an anesthetic agent into the direct operative site

local public health department a public agency administered and operated within a political jurisdiction such as a county

lumbar puncture (LP) insertion of a sterile needle into the spinal canal to remove cerebral spinal fluid (CSF); commonly called a "spinal tap"

masochism sexual arousal by receiving pain

masturbation stimulation of genitals for sexual arousal; may be self-stimulation or mutual with partner

maternal deprivation psychological changes that occur in young children when they are separated from their primary caregiver

maturity state of full development of a person's judgment and reasoning ability

mean the sum of values divided by the number of values; also the arithmetical average

meconium black, tarry first stool of a newborn

median the middle value when values are arranged in order of magnitude

medication Any substance that improves a person's state of health or ability to function

melena blood in stool

menarche the first menstrual period

menopause A period of decreasing hormone function and cessation of menstruation

micturition urination

mode the most common value in a distribution of measurements

murmur a blowing sound heard on auscultation due to interference of blood flow through the heart

narcolepsy uncontrollable need for sleep during the day

nasojejunal tube a tube introduced into the jejunum of the intestine

nausea a feeling of revulsion to food

neonate individual during the first 28 days of life

nocturia unable to sleep through night without urination

nosocomial infection a hospital-acquired infection

nuclear medicine studies procedures that require the use of a radioactive substance

nurse a professionally educated person who cares for and about individuals, families, and communities, in health and illness

nurses' notes the recording of patients' actions or responses, not the nurse's actions. Traditional recording: information recorded in chronological order in narrative form in a separate section of the patient record. Problem-oriented recording (POR): information recorded based on patient problems; all health care professionals use the same pages in the patient record

nursing a professional discipline based on theory, practice, and research

nursing history health interview performed by the nurse; depending on the nurse's role and agency policy, this may or may not be the complete health history

nursing Kardex a series of index cards in a flip-type file kept on the nursing unit desk; a temporary reference system for coordinating nursing care

nutrition process by which a person receives and utilizes materials necessary for the maintenance and growth of body cells

obesity a body weight greater than 20 percent of normal weight for height

obligatory sleep nonrapid eye movement sleep

oliguria decreased quantity of urine

ophthalmoscope-otoscope instrument used to examine the ear canal, tympanic membrane and eye

orthopnea subjective difficulty in breathing unless the head and chest are elevated

osmolarity the proportion of dissolved particles (solute) present in a solution in contrast to fluid (solvent) present

osmotic pressure flow of fluid between compartments from an area of greater concentration to one of lesser concentration

pain a subjective feeling of discomfort

palpation examining by touch, using the tips of your fingers

pandemic an illness that is occurring over a large area of the world

panic disintegration of personality organization due to extreme threat

paracentesis aspiration of fluid from the peritoneal cavity

paradoxical sleep rapid eye movement sleep

paralytic ileus loss of function of the intestine due to surgical handling

pathogenic a microorganism capable of causing illness in humans

patient record confidential documentation of a person's state of wellness or illness; commonly called a "patient chart"

percussion assessment of the consistency of a body structure by evaluating the sound that you hear in response to striking the part with an examining finger

pharmacodynamics study of biochemical and physiological effects of drugs

pharmacokinetics study of drug absorption, distribution, biotransformation, and excretion

pharmacology the study of drugs and their effects on cells and cell products

pharmacotherapeutics use of chemicals with living organisms for the treatment of illness

pharmacy the science of preparing and dispensing of drugs

phlegm respiratory secretions in mouth

physical stimulation that which leads to physical activity, increasing heart rate and body metabolism; movement toward or away from a stimulus

placenta the organ that furnishes oxygen and nutrients to the fetus in utero; also called "afterbirth"

plaintiff a person bringing a law suit to court

planning the designing of necessary actions and strategies to reach established goals

plaque bacteria-laden film on teeth

polyuria increased amount of urine

population all the subjects to be studied

premature beat a variation in heart rate where an extra beat is interspaced in a normal rhythm

preventive focus a concern with keeping people well and, if ill, helping to restore health again

profession a discipline that requires an extensive educational practice period, has a well-defined body of knowledge, provides necessary human services, is autonomous in practice, and whose members practice under a code of ethics

pruritus itchiness

puberty time of life when secondary sex characteristics appear

pulse ventricular contraction (systole) that can be felt at points where an artery passes close to the skin surface

pulse deficit difference between radial and apical pulse rates

pulse pressure difference between systolic and diastolic blood pressure readings

pyrexia fever

pyrogen agent that increases body temperature

pyuria pus in urine

radiation loss of heat to a distant colder object

radiograph (x-ray) the direction of radiation with short wave lengths toward body tissue to determine density of tissue

range-of-motion exercises exercises that move joints through their full capabilities

regional anesthesia loss of pain sensation in a body part due to interruption of sensory nerve conduction from that body part

religion an organized form of worship

resident flora microorganisms that are difficult to remove from skin or objects

response reaction initiated by a stimulus

rest a period of quiet activity that promotes a sense of refreshment and ability to perform well

rigor mortis stiffening of the body following death

saddle-block anesthesia loss of pain sensation in a body region corresponding to the area of the buttocks, perineum, and inner thighs due to injection of an anesthetic agent into the dural sac; used for childbirth

sadism sexual arousal by inflicting pain

sample a representative number of subjects to be studied, randomly chosen

satiety feeling that follows the intake of adequate food

sebum secretions from sebaceous glands

sedative a medication to induce relaxation by limiting incoming stimuli

sensory deprivation lack of adequate sensory, cognitive, social, or physical stimulation

sensory overload greater stimulation than a person can tolerate or process

sensory stimulation receiving stimulation through one of the five basic senses—sight (visual), hearing (auditory), touch (tactile), taste (gustatory), and smell (olfactory)—or from muscle (kinetic) or body organs (visceral)

sexual dysfunction a perceived problem in achieving desired sexual gratification

sexual identity an inner feeling or sense of being male or female

sexuality maleness or femaleness, including attitudes and activities

sexually transmitted disease (STD) a disease transmitted through intercourse, commonly called "veneral disease" (VD)

sick role the expected pattern of behavior of someone who is ill

side effect effect of a medication other than its intended therapeutic effect

sign an observable condition of malfunction or illness (an objective finding)

sinus arrhythmia variation in heart rate due to pressure changes in the chest during respiration

slander a spoken derogatory statement about someone

sleep a time, occurring periodically, of reduced consciousness; it is restorative to physical and mental well-being

social stimulation stimulation that results from interaction with other people; combines sensory and cognitive stimulation

soft diet a diet low in cellulose, easy to chew and digest

somnambulism sleepwalking

sordes crust on teeth or gum

sphygmomanometer instrument used to measure blood pressure (a blood pressure cuff)

spinal anesthesia loss of pain sensation in the lower extremities and the perineum produced by injection of anesthesia into the lower spinal canal

spiritual belief a trust that a higher power than oneself guides life

sputum expectorated respiratory secretions

standard a rule or statement that can be used as a basis of measuring

statistical significance a statement that determinations are truly different and not a matter of chance

steatorrhea fat in stool

sterile state of being free of all microorganisms and their spore form

sterilization the act of making an object free of all microorganisms and their spore form

stethoscope instrument used to auscultate (listen to) sounds produced by the body

stimulation inciting a person to mental or physical action through sensory reception and central nervous system interpretation of stimuli; Response to the stimulus may be emotional (pleasure or fright), cognitive (thoughtful), or motor (physical movement)

stimulus a factor that initiates a response

stool waste products in or excreted from the large intestine (feces)

stress the rate of wear and tear in the body (Selye); the body reaction to threat

stressor a threatening experience that can elicit a general adaptation response

symptom an awareness of disease or malfunction experienced by the patient (a subjective finding)

synergistic effect a complementary effect that occurs when two drugs are administered together

system a set of interrelated parts that joined together produce a meaningful whole

systole the first heart sound heard; the sound of the mitral and tricuspid valves closing (the *lub* of "lub-dub")

tachycardia increased heart rate; over 100 beats per minute in the adult

tachypnea rapid respiratory rate; over 20 breaths per minute in an adult

Tanner scale a scale to rate secondary sex characteristic development

teaching the act of providing knowledge or insight

temperament the characteristic manner in which a person responds to situations

terminal illness an illness for which there is no reasonable expectation of recovery

thanatology the study of death

theory a set of interrelated concepts that can be tested and used to explain a phenomenon systematically

therapeutic effect the helpful, intended effect of a medication

therapeutic environment surroundings conducive to comfort and well-being and maintaining wellness

thorocentesis aspiration of fluid from the pleural cavity

tolerance ability to take greater amounts of a drug without experiencing increased effects

tort a violation of civil law

toxic effect effect caused by an overdose or excessive accumulation of a normal dose of a drug

transient flora easily removed microorganisms

triage determination of seriousness of illness and priority of care

trial period a short-term period during which new behavior is practiced

turgor the degree of elasticity of skin; indicates body hydration

Valsalva's maneuver breath holding during exercise that increases intrathoracic pressure and results in tachycardia

value something believed in or prized over other things

value clarification a process for evaluating and determining the things you believe in or desire most

variable an isolated characteristic to be studied

venipuncture the removal of a blood sample from a vein

volume control set calibrated chamber of 100 to 250 ml in size that can be added to intravenous tubing as a safety control and port of medication administration

vomiting forceful regurgitation of food from the stomach

voyeurism sexual arousal by viewing sexual activity of others

CREDITS

CREDITS

Chapter 1

Figure 1-1 courtesy Millard Fillmore Hospital, Buffalo, New York

Figure 1-3 courtesy Department of Medical Photography, Children's Hospital, Buffalo, New York

Chapter 2

Figure 2-2 courtesy Donald Abbott

Figure 2-4 courtesy Millard Fillmore Hospital, Buffalo, New York

Chapter 3

Figure 3-2 courtesy Donald Abbott

Chapter 4

Figure 4-1 courtesy Department of Medical Photography, Children's Hospital, Buffalo, New York

Figures 4-2, 4-5, 4-6 courtesy Millard Fillmore Hospital, Buffalo, New York

Chapter 5

Figures 5-1, 5-2 courtesy Millard Fillmore Hospital, Buffalo, New York

Chapter 6

Figure 6-6 courtesy Millard Fillmore Hospital, Buffalo, New York

Figure 6-7 courtesy Department of Medical Photography, Children's Hospital, Buffalo, New York

Chapter 8

Figure 8-1 courtesy Millard Fillmore Hospital, Buffalo, New York

Figure 8-2 courtesy Department of Medical Photography, Children's Hospital, Buffalo, New York

Chapter 9

Figure 9-1 from R. E. Scammon, The Measurement of the Body in Childhood. In J. A. Harris et al. (Eds.), *The Measurement of Man.* Minneapolis: University of Minnesota Press, 1930.

Figure 9-2 reprinted by permission of Dr. W. Frankenburg, University of Colorado Medical Center, Denver, Colorado

Figure 9-4 courtesy Department of Embryology, Davis Division, Carnegie Institution of Washington

Figures 9-5, 9-6, 9-8, 9-9, 9-11, 9-12, 9-16 courtesy Department of Medical Photography, Children's Hospital, Buffalo, New York

Figure 9-7 courtesy Millard Fillmore Hospital, Buffalo, New York

Figure 9-13 from E. Fuller, A physician's guide to sexual maturity. *Patient Care* 13:122, 1979. Copyright © 1979, Patient Care Publications, Inc., Darien, Conn. All rights reserved.

Figure 9-19 from M. W. Blackwell, *Care of the Mentally Retarded.* Boston: Little, Brown, 1979

Chapter 13

QRS 13-1 from D. Little and D. Carneveli, *Nursing Care Planning.* Philadelphia: Lippincott, 1976.

Figures 13-3, 13-6, 13-10 courtesy Millard Fillmore Hospital, Buffalo, New York

Figure 13-8 courtesy Department of Medical Photography, Children's Hospital, Buffalo, New York

Chapter 14

Figures 14-1, 14-3, 14-4 courtesy Millard Fillmore Hospital, Buffalo, New York

Chapter 15

Figures 15-2, 15-5 courtesy Department of Medical Photography, Children's Hospital, Buffalo, New York

Figures 15-3, 15-6 courtesy Donald Abbott

Chapter 16

Figures 16-1, 16-3 courtesy Department of Medical Photography, Children's Hospital, Buffalo, New York

Figures 16-4, 16-7 courtesy Millard Fillmore Hospital, Buffalo, New York

Chapter 17

Figures 17-1, 17-2, 17-6 courtesy Department of Medical Photography, Children's Hospital, Buffalo, New York

Figures 17-5, 17-9 courtesy Millard Fillmore Hospital, Buffalo, New York

Chapter 18

Figure 18-1 courtesy Millard Fillmore Hospital, Buffalo, New York

Chapter 19

Figures 19-2, 19-3, 19-4, 19-5, 19-6, 19-8, 19-9, 19-11, 19-15A, B, 19-16, 19-18, 19-24, 19-28A—F courtesy Department of Medical Photography, Children's Hospital, Buffalo, New York

Figure 19-17 courtesy Department of Medical Illustrations, State University of New York at Buffalo, Buffalo, New York

Chapter 20

Figures 20-1A, B, 20-3, 20-4, 20-5A, B, 20-7, 20-8, 20-9, 20-11, 20-14A, B, 20-15, 20-17, 20-19 courtesy Department of Medical Photography, Children's Hospital, Buffalo, New York

Figure 20-12 courtesy Jerald P. Kuhn, M.D., Children's Hospital, Buffalo, New York

Figure 20-16A courtesy Millard Fillmore Hospital, Buffalo, New York

Figure 20-18 courtesy Richard W. Munchauer, M.D., Children's Hospital, Buffalo, New York

Chapter 22

Figure 22-2B courtesy Millard Fillmore Hospital, Buffalo, New York

Figures 22-3, 22-4, 22-5, 22-6 courtesy Department of Medical Photography, Children's Hospital, Buffalo, New York

Chapter 24

Figure 24-1A, B courtesy Millard Fillmore Hospital, Buffalo, New York

Figure 24-2 courtesy Department of Medical Photography, Children's Hospital, Buffalo, New York

Chapter 25

Figures 1 (Procedure 25-12), 25-3 courtesy Donald Abbott

Figure 1 (Procedure 25-9) courtesy Department of Medical Photography, Children's Hospital, Buffalo, New York

Chapter 26

Figures 1 (Procedure 26-1), 1 (Procedure 26-2), 1 (Procedure 26-3), 1 (Procedure 26-5), 26-1, 26-2, 26-3, 26-5, 26-30, 26-39 courtesy Department of Medical Photography, Children's Hospital, Buffalo, New York

Figures 26-6, 26-8A, B, 26-9, 26-10, 26-12, 26-13, 26-14, 26-18, 26-19A—D, 26-20A—D, 26-21, 26-22A—F, 26-23A, B, 26-24A—F, 26-25A—D, 26-26A—D, 26-27A, B, 26-28A—E, 26-29A, B, 26-30C, 26-32, 26-33, 26-34A—C, 26-35, 26-36 courtesy Millard Fillmore Hospital, Buffalo, New York

Figure 26-28F courtesy Mead Johnson & Company, Evansville, Indiana

Figure 26-40 courtesy Hoyer & Company, Inc., Oshkosh, Wisconsin

Chapter 27

Figures 27-1, 27-2, 27-3, 27-8, 27-10A—C courtesy Department of Medical Photography, Children's Hospital, Buffalo, New York

Figures 6, 7 (Procedure 27-1), 27-6, 27-7 courtesy Millard Fillmore Hospital, Buffalo, New York

Chapter 28

Figures 28-1, 28-2 courtesy Department of Medical Photography, Children's Hospital, Buffalo, New York

Figures 28-3, 28-4, 28-5, 28-6, 28-7, 28-8, 28-14 courtesy Millard Fillmore Hospital, Buffalo, New York

Figures 28-10, 28-11 courtesy Donald Abbott

Chapter 29

Figures 29-1, 29-6, 29-9A, 29-40A, B courtesy Millard Fillmore Hospital, Buffalo, New York

Figures 29-2, 29-4, 29-7B, 29-8, 29-9B, 29-11, 29-12, 29-15, 29-16B, 29-21, 29-22, 29-23, 29-24, 29-31B, 29-33 courtesy Department of Medical Photography, Children's Hospital, Buffalo, New York

Figure 29-3 courtesy Beth Israel Hospital, Boston (photo by Michael Lutch)

Figures 29-10, 29-17, 29-25, 29-26A, 29-32 courtesy Donald Abbott

Chapter 30

Figures 1, 2 (Procedure 30-1), 2, 3 (Procedure 30-2), 30-4, 30-5A, B, 30-6A, B, 30-8, 30-9, 30-12, 30-13, 30-14A, B, 30-15, 30-16, 30-17, 30-18A, B courtesy Department of Medical Photography, Children's Hospital, Buffalo, New York

Figure 30-7 courtesy Millard Fillmore Hospital, Buffalo, New York

Chapter 31

Figure 31-1 courtesy Ross Laboratories, Columbus, Ohio, 1970 (Clinical Education Aid No. 7)

Figure 31-3 courtesy Millard Fillmore Hospital, Buffalo, New York

Figures 31-5, 31-6 courtesy Department of Medical Photography, Children's Hospital, Buffalo, New York

Chapter 32

Figures 32-2, 32-3, 32-4, 32-7, 32-13, 32-14, 32-22, 32-23, 32-30, 32-31, 32-32A, B, 32-34 courtesy Department of Medical Photography, Children's Hospital, Buffalo, New York

Figures 2 (Procedure 32-4), 32-6, 32-8, 32-9, 32-10, 32-15, 32-16, 32-17, 32-18, 32-19, 32-21, 32-26 courtesy Millard Fillmore Hospital, Buffalo, New York

Figure 32-28 courtesy Donald Abbott

Chapter 33

Figures 1 (Procedure 33-3), 33-2, 33-3 courtesy Donald Abbott

Figures 2 (Procedure 33-3), 33-5, 33-6, 33-8, 33-10A, 33-13, 33-15A, B courtesy Department of Medical Photography, Children's Hospital, Buffalo, New York

Figures 33-9, 33-11, 33-12, 33-14A, B courtesy Millard Fillmore Hospital, Buffalo, New York

Chapter 34

Figures 34-2, 34-3A, 34-4 courtesy Department of Medical Photography, Children's Hospital, Buffalo, New York

Figure 34-3B courtesy Millard Fillmore Hospital, Buffalo, New York

Chapter 35

Figure 35-1 courtesy Donald Abbott

Figures 1A, 2 (Procedure 35-1), 1 (Procedure 35-3), 1A—C (QRS 35-3), 35-4 courtesy Millard Fillmore Hospital, Buffalo, New York

Figures 1B (Procedure 35-1), 35-2, 35-7 courtesy Department of Medical Photography, Children's Hospital, Buffalo, New York

Chapter 36

Figures 36-1, 36-4C courtesy Department of Medical Photography, Children's Hospital, Buffalo, New York

Chapter 37

Figures 37-1, 37-2 courtesy Donald Abbott

Chapter 38

Figures 38-3B, 38-20 courtesy Department of Medical Photography, Childen's Hospital, Buffalo, New York

Figures 38-14, 38-15, 38-17, 38-18 courtesy Donald Abbott

Chapter 39

Figures 39-2, 39-3, 39-4, 39-7, 39-10 courtesy Department of Medical Photography, Children's Hospital, Buffalo, New York

Figures 39-6, 39-8, 39-9A, B, 39-10 courtesy Millard Fillmore Hospital, Buffalo, New York

Chapter 40

Figures 40-1, 40-2, 40-4, 40-7A, B, 40-12, 40-13, 40-17, 40-18 courtesy Millard Fillmore Hospital, Buffalo, New York

Figures 40-3, 40-6, 40-9, 40-11, 40-16, 40-19, 40-20 courtesy Department of Medical Photography, Children's Hospital, Buffalo, New York

Figure 40-8 courtesy Donald Abbott

Part Frontispieces

Parts I, X courtesy Millard Fillmore Hospital, Buffalo, New York

Part II courtesy Harvard Community Health Plan, Boston

Parts III, VII courtesy Jeffrey Grosscup

Parts IV, V, VIII courtesy Michael Lutch

Parts VI, IX courtesy Department of Medical Photography, Children's Hospital, Buffalo, New York

INDEX

INDEX